NINTH EDITION

HISTOLOGY

A TEXT AND ATLAS

With Correlated Cell and Molecular Biology

T0290918

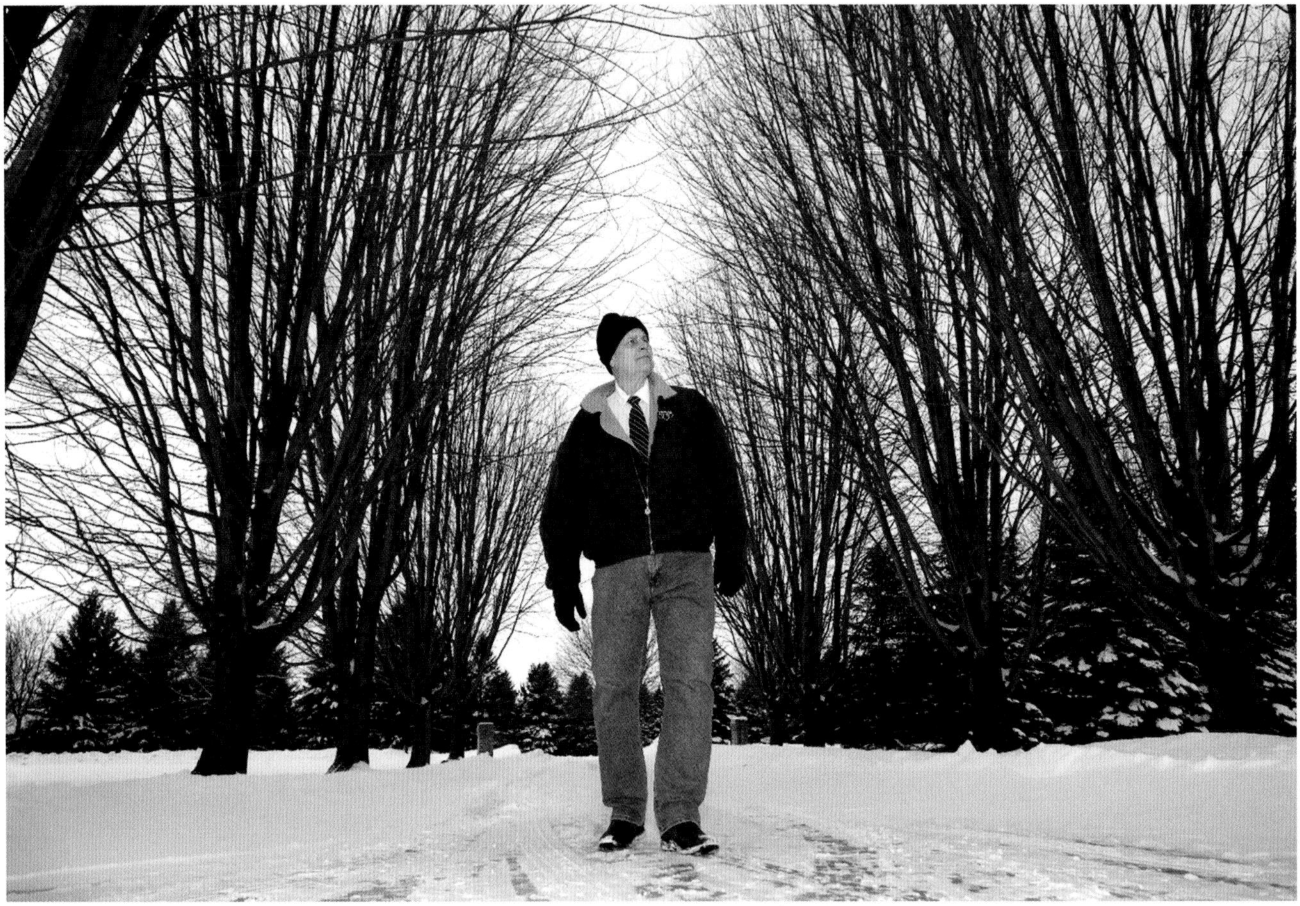

Wojciech Pawlina

Walking in freezing winter cold weather (−22°C) on his driveway in Rochester, Minnesota contemplating on snow-white histologic structures: white blood cells, white adipocytes, white pulp of the spleen, white matter of the brain and spinal cord, white muscle fibers, and perhaps corpus albicans, and tunica albuginea. (Photograph by Kevin J. Ness.)

NINTH EDITION

HISTOLOGY

A TEXT AND ATLAS

With Correlated Cell and Molecular Biology

WOJCIECH PAWLINA, MD, FAAA

Professor of Anatomy and Medical Education
Consultant and Past Chair, Department of Clinical Anatomy
Joint Consultant, Department of Obstetrics and Gynecology
Past Medical Director of Procedural Skills Laboratory
Mayo Clinic College of Medicine and Science
Rochester, Minnesota
Fellow of the American Association of Anatomists

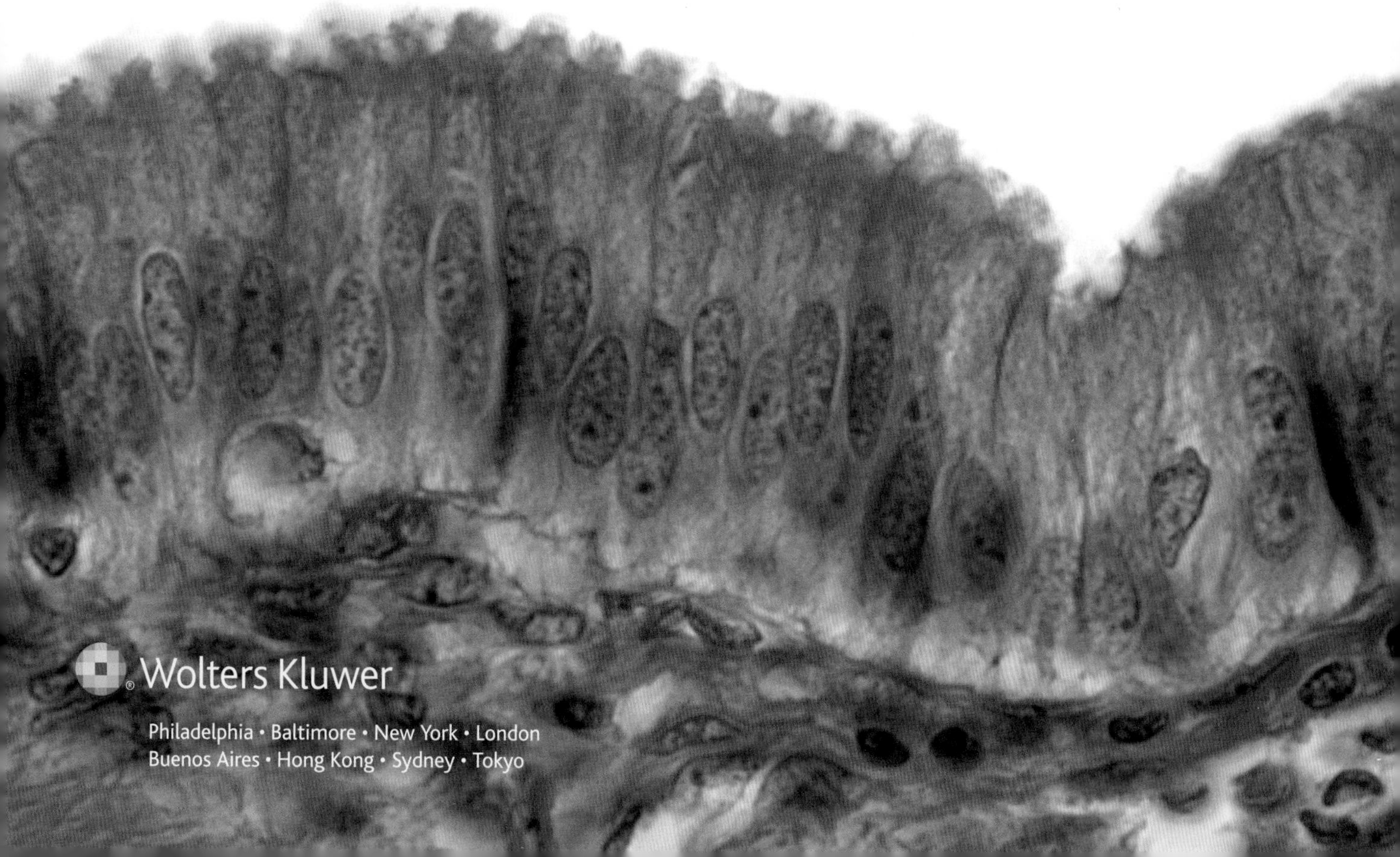

Wolters Kluwer

Philadelphia • Baltimore • New York • London
Buenos Aires • Hong Kong • Sydney • Tokyo

Acquisitions Editor: Crystal Taylor
Development Editor: Andrea Vosburgh/Deborah Bordeaux
Freelance Editor: Kathleen H. Scogna
Production Project Manager: Kirstin Johnson
Marketing Manager: Danielle Klahr
Manager, Graphic Arts & Design: Steve Druding
Art Director: Jennifer Clements
Manufacturing Coordinator: Margie Orzech-Zarenko
Prepress Vendor: S4Carlisle Publishing Services

Top cover image: Courtesy of Drs. Daniel Berger and Jeff W. Lichtman, Harvard University, Cambridge, MA

Ninth Edition

Copyright © 2024 Wolters Kluwer.

Copyright © 2020, 2016 Wolters Kluwer Health. Copyright © 2011, 2006, 2003 Lippincott Williams & Wilkins. Copyright © 1995, 1989 Williams & Wilkins. Copyright © 1985 Harper & Row, Publisher, J. B. Lippincott Company. All rights reserved. This book is protected by copyright. No part of this book may be reproduced or transmitted in any form or by any means, including as photocopies or scanned-in or other electronic copies, or utilized by any information storage and retrieval system without written permission from the copyright owner, except for brief quotations embodied in critical articles and reviews. Materials appearing in this book prepared by individuals as part of their official duties as U.S. government employees are not covered by the above-mentioned copyright. To request permission, please contact Wolters Kluwer at Two Commerce Square, 2001 Market Street, Philadelphia, PA 19103, via email at permissions@lww.com, or via our website at shop.lww.com (products and services).

9 8 7 6 5 4 3 2 1

Printed in Mexico

Library of Congress Cataloging-in-Publication Data

ISBN-13: 978-1-975181-51-2
ISBN-10: 1-975181-51-4

Library of Congress Control Number: 2023907331

This work is provided "as is," and the publisher disclaims any and all warranties, express or implied, including any warranties as to accuracy, comprehensiveness, or currency of the content of this work.

This work is no substitute for individual patient assessment based upon healthcare professionals' examination of each patient and consideration of, among other things, age, weight, gender, current or prior medical conditions, medication history, laboratory data, and other factors unique to the patient. The publisher does not provide medical advice or guidance, and this work is merely a reference tool. Healthcare professionals, and not the publisher, are solely responsible for the use of this work including all medical judgments and for any resulting diagnosis and treatments.

Given continuous, rapid advances in medical science and health information, independent professional verification of medical diagnoses, indications, appropriate pharmaceutical selections and dosages, and treatment options should be made and healthcare professionals should consult a variety of sources. When prescribing medication, healthcare professionals are advised to consult the product information sheet (the manufacturer's package insert) accompanying each drug to verify, among other things, conditions of use, warnings, and side effects and identify any changes in dosage schedule or contraindications, particularly if the medication to be administered is new, infrequently used, or has a narrow therapeutic range. To the maximum extent permitted under applicable law, no responsibility is assumed by the publisher for any injury and/or damage to persons or property, as a matter of products liability, negligence law or otherwise, or from any reference to or use by any person of this work.

shop.lww.com

QUADM0823

This edition is dedicated to **Teresa Pawlina,** *my wife, colleague, and best friend, whose love, patience, and endurance created a safe haven for working on this textbook*

and

to my children **Conrad Pawlina** *and* **Stephanie Pawlina Fixell,** *whose stimulation and excitement are always contagious*

and

to my grandchildren **Alexander Conrad Fixell** *and* **Zofia Marie Pawlina,** *whose capability to learn new life skills is simply breathtaking.*

PREFACE

This ninth edition of *Histology: A Text and Atlas With Correlated Cell and Molecular Biology* continues its tradition of introducing Health Professions students to the foremost world of histology with cell and molecular biology combined. In addition, to better understand the nature of cells and tissues, the presented material is immersed in basic anatomy, embryology, and physiology and is accompanied by relevant clinical commentaries. As in previous editions, this book is a combination "text-atlas" in that the standard textbook descriptions of histologic concepts are supplemented by an array of schematics, tissue and cell images, and clinical photographs. The separate atlas sections conclude each chapter to provide large-format, labeled atlas plates with detailed legends that highlight and summarize the elements of microscopic anatomy. *Histology: A Text and Atlas* is, therefore, "two books in one."

This edition of *Histology: A Text and Atlas With Correlated Cell and Molecular Biology* is intended to serve as a reliable resource and clinical viewpoint for those who seek to understand histology from medical, dental, graduate, undergraduate, and other health professions perspective. Inclusion of current and up-to-date information provides a solid framework on which to build further scientific exploration and clinical application. As a student resource, it should not be approached with the goal of memorizing detailed facts but rather as a guide for learning by extracting from all explanations key concepts that will serve future academic pursuits.

The following improvements have been made to this edition:

All figures in this book have been carefully reviewed, revised, and updated. Several new figures have been added to show the latest interpretation of important concepts based on recent discoveries in molecular and cellular research. All drawings maintain a uniform style throughout the chapters with a palette of eye-pleasing colors. Several new conceptual drawings have been aligned with photomicrographs or electron micrographs, a feature carried over from previous editions that has received wide acclaim from reviewers, students, and faculty members. In addition, all atlas plates have been renumbered to be consistent with chapter numbers.

Cellular and molecular biology content has been updated. Text material from the eighth edition has been carefully revised and updated to include the latest advancements in cellular and molecular biology, stem cell biology, cellular markers, and cell signaling. The ninth edition focuses on key concepts to help students comprehend these rapidly increasing fields. To accommodate reviewers' suggestions, the ninth edition integrates new information in cell biology with clinical correlates, which readers will see as new clinical information items highlighted in blue text and in clinical correlations and functional considerations folders. For example, the last few years of the COVID-19 pandemic has sparked interest about the changes in normal tissue when infected by the severe acute respiratory syndrome coronavirus 2 (SARS-CoV-2) virus. Several chapters contain descriptions of these changes with underlying explanations of cellular and molecular mechanisms and clinical features presented by patients. Additional changes include the following:

- A new discussion on the mononuclear phagocyte system and the cell biology of resident tissue macrophages has been added.
- The latest research findings in immune cell activation have been incorporated.
- Updated cellular biology topics include beige adipose tissue, the epithelial–mesenchymal transition, conjunctiva-associated lymphatic tissue, biogenesis and function of peroxisomes, and exosomes as the newest discovered form of cell-to-cell communication.
- New, more detailed information about the histology of the female and male external genitalia has been included.
- The skin chapter has been supplemented and updated with many new images and discussion on skin color and skin aging.
- With the constant improvement in microscopic methods, a new basic discussion on three-dimensional (3D) microscopy methods was incorporated in the methods chapter.

"Histology 101" sections have been revised and updated. These sections contain clear and concise summaries for a quick review of the material listed in a "sticky notes" format posted on the notebook pages at the end of each chapter. The bullet-point format is designed specifically for students needing a quick review and is especially useful for quiz and examination preparation. These reader-friendly sections allow fast information retrieval with concepts and facts grouped on separate sticky notes. The colored sticky notes have been designed with ample free space to allow readers to write their own notes to complement the bulleted points.

Reader-friendly innovations have been implemented. Similar to the previous editions of this book, the aim is to provide ready access to important concepts and essential information. Changes introduced in previous editions, such as bolded key terms, clinical information in blue text, pages with color-coded edges, and a fresh design for clinical correlation folders, were all enthusiastically approved by the new generation of textbook users and have been maintained in this edition. Essential terms within each specific section are introduced within the text in eye-catching, oversized, bold, red font. Text containing clinical information and the latest research findings is presented in blue, with terminology pertaining to diseases, conditions, symptoms, or causative mechanisms highlighted in oversized bold blue font. Each clinical folder contains updated clinical text with even more illustrations and drawings and is easily found within each chapter. As in previous editions, all changes have been made with students in mind. The author–editor team strived for clarity and concision to aid student comprehension of the subject matter, familiarity with the latest information, and application of newfound knowledge.

Wojciech Pawlina

ACKNOWLEDGMENTS

I remain grateful to the creator of this book, **Dr. Michael H. Ross**, my mentor, colleague, and dear friend, for the ability to carry on his vision for teaching histology. Many changes in histology education have occurred in the last two decades. In today's medical curricula, histology courses continue to lose their identity as they become integrated into larger didactic blocks. In the digital world of virtual histology, often driven by self-directed instructions, there is a need for a comprehensive textbook from which students can pick small chunks of knowledge for their specific learning assignments across many disciplines. The classical descriptive histology of the past is no longer sufficient for understanding the structure and function of cells and tissues. Modern histology is increasingly becoming the study of cell and molecular biology, a trend we had foreseen in the early 2000s. From the fifth edition of this textbook (2006), we increased emphases on topics of cell and molecular biology that are aligned with histology; as acknowledged by adding the subtitle "*With Correlated Cell and Molecular Biology*" to the fifth and subsequent editions of this textbook. Dr. Ross vision to provide the best quality modern histology text with superior imaging integrated with the most recent advances in cell and molecular biology and supporting clinical facts remained unchanged.

Changes to the ninth edition arise largely from comments and suggestions of students from around the world who have taken the time and effort to send me messages about what they like about the book and, more importantly, how the book might be improved to help them better learn histology. I have also received thoughtful comments from my first-year histology students who often direct me to explore new discoveries and achievements in the many fields related to histology. I am grateful to them for their keen sense of sharpening this work.

Also, many of my colleagues who teach histology, cell biology, immunology, and physiology courses have helped improve this new edition. Many have suggested a stronger emphasis on clinical relevance and new discoveries, especially in cell and molecular biology, which I strive to include as new research emerges. Others have provided new photomicrographs, electron micrographs, access to their virtual slide collections, proposals for new tables, and have suggested which existing diagrams and figures need to be redrawn.

Specifically, I owe my thanks to the following reviewers, who have spent time to provide me with constructive feedback that had an impact on this current edition.

Jan Aten, PhD
Amsterdam University Medical Center
Amsterdam, The Netherlands

Stefanie Attardi, PhD
Oakland University William Beaumont School of Medicine
Rochester, Michigan

Barış Baykal, MD
Gülhane Faculty of Medicine
University of Health Sciences
Ankara, Türkiye

Paul B. Bell, Jr., PhD
University of Oklahoma
Norman, Oklahoma

Jalaluddin Bin Mohamed, MBBS, PhD
National Defence University of Malaysia
Kuala Lumpur, Malaysia

David E. Birk, PhD
University of South Florida, College of Medicine
Tampa, Florida

Christy Bridges, PhD
Mercer University School of Medicine
Macon, Georgia

Craig A. Canby, PhD
Des Moines University
Des Moines, Iowa

Stephen W. Carmichael, PhD
Mayo Clinic College of Medicine and Science
Rochester, Minnesota

Yasmin Carter, PhD
University of Massachusetts Chan Medical School
Worcester, Massachusetts

Pike See Cheah, PhD
Universiti Putra Malaysia
Serdang, Selangor, Malaysia

Kevin N. Christensen, MD
Winona Health
Winona, Minnesota

Sookja K. Chung, PhD
Macau University of Science and Technology
Taipa, Macau

John Clancy, Jr., PhD
Loyola University Medical Center
Maywood, Illinois

Rita Colella, PhD
University of Louisville School of Medicine
Louisville, Kentucky

Iris M. Cook, PhD
State University of New York Westchester Community College
Valhalla, New York

Robert D. Cottrell, MHS, PA (ASCP)^{CM}
Quinnipiac University School of Health Sciences
Hamden, Connecticut

Dongmei Cui, MD, PhD
University of Mississippi Medical Center
Jackson, Mississippi

Eduard I. Dedkov, MD, PhD
Cooper Medical School of Rowan University
Camden, New Jersey

Andrea Deyrup, MD, PhD
University of South Carolina School of Medicine Greenville
Greenville, South Carolina

Lori B. Dribin, PhD
Nova Southeastern University
Fort Lauderdale, Florida

Jennifer Eastwood, PhD
Burrell College of Osteopathic Medicine
Las Cruces, New Mexico

Rodrigo Enrique Elizondo-Omaña, MD, PhD
Autonomous University of Nuevo León, School of Medicine
Monterrey, Nuevo León, Mexico

Tamira Elul, PhD
Touro University College of Osteopathic Medicine
Vallejo, California

Francis A. Fakoya, MBChB, MSc, PhD
St. George's University School of Medicine
True Blue, Grenada, West Indies

Bruce E. Felgenhauer, PhD
University of Louisiana at Lafayette
Lafayette, Louisiana

G. Ian Gallicano, PhD
Georgetown University School of Medicine
Washington, District of Columbia

Joaquin J. Garcia, MD
Mayo Clinic College of Medicine and Science
Rochester, Minnesota

Mathangi Gilkes, MBBS, MSc
St. George's University School of Medicine
True Blue, Grenada, West Indies

Ferdinand Gomez, MS
Herbert Wertheim College of Medicine
Florida International University
Miami, Florida

Amos Gona, PhD
University of Medicine & Dentistry of New Jersey
New Brunswick, New Jersey

Ervin M. Gore, PhD
Middle Tennessee State University
Murfreesboro, Tennessee

Joseph P. Grande, MD, PhD
Mayo Clinic College of Medicine and Science
Rochester, Minnesota

Joseph A. Grasso, PhD
University of Connecticut Health Center
Farmington, Connecticut

Shannon Haley, MD, PhD
Thomas Jefferson University
Philadelphia, Pennsylvania

Brian H. Hallas, PhD
New York Institute of Technology
Old Westbury, New York

Arthur R. Hand, DDS
University of Connecticut School of Dental Medicine
Farmington, Connecticut

Robert J. Hillwig, MD
Kentucky College of Osteopathic Medicine
University of Pikeville
Pikeville, Kentucky

Charlene Hoegler, PhD
Pace University—Pleasantville Campus
Pleasantville, New York

Christopher Horst Lillig, PhD
University of Greifswald
Greifswald, Germany

Michael Hortsch, PhD
University of Michigan Medical School
Ann Arbor, Michigan

Jim Hutson, PhD
Texas Tech University
Lubbock, Texas

John-Olov Jansson, MD, PhD
University of Gothenburg
Gothenburg, Sweden

Malsawmzuali (JC) Joute Chawngvawr, MS
Cardiovascular Research, Mayo Clinic
Rochester, Minnesota

Cynthia J. M. Kane, PhD
University of Arkansas for Medical Sciences
Little Rock, Arkansas

Punnose K. Kattil, MBBS, MD
Mayo Clinic College of Medicine and Science
Rochester, Minnesota

Nazanin Yeganeh Kazemi, MD, PhD
Mayo Clinic College of Medicine and Science
Rochester, Minnesota

Michael J. Kern, PhD
Medical University of South Carolina
Charleston, South Carolina

G. M. Kibria, MD
National Defence University of Malaysia
Kuala Lumpur, Malaysia

Thomas S. King, PhD
University of Texas Health Science Center at San Antonio
San Antonio, Texas

Bruce M. Koeppen, MD, PhD
Quinnipiac University
Frank H. Netter MD School of Medicine
North Haven, Connecticut

Andrew Koob, PhD
University of Wisconsin—River Falls
River Falls, Wisconsin

Craig Kuehn, PhD
Western University of Health Sciences
Pomona, California

Ton La, MD, JD, LLM
Baylor College of Medicine
Houston, Texas

Nirusha Lachman, PhD
Mayo Clinic College of Medicine and Science
Rochester, Minnesota

Gavin R. Lawson, PhD
Western University of Health Sciences
Pomona, California

Susan LeDoux, PhD
University of South Alabama
Mobile, Alabama

Karen Leong, MD
Drexel University College of Medicine
Philadelphia, Pennsylvania

Kenneth M. Lerea, PhD
New York Medical College
Valhalla, New York

Frank Liuzzi, PhD
Lake Erie College of Osteopathic Medicine
Bradenton, Florida

Donald J. Lowrie, Jr., PhD
University of Cincinnati College of Medicine
Cincinnati, Ohio

Kuo-Shyan Lu, PhD
National Taiwan University College of Medicine
Taipei, Taiwan

Andrew T. Mariassy, PhD
Nova Southeastern University College of Medical Sciences
Fort Lauderdale, Florida

Geoffrey W. McAuliffe, PhD
Rutgers Robert Wood Johnson Medical School
Piscataway, New Jersey

Kevin J. McCarthy, PhD
Louisiana State University Health Sciences Center Shreveport
Shreveport, Louisiana

David L. McWhorter, PhD
Georgia Campus—Philadelphia College of Osteopathic Medicine
Suwanee, Georgia

Fabiola Medeiros, MD
Cedars-Sinai Medical Center
Los Angeles, California

William D. Meek, PhD
College of Osteopathic Medicine
Oklahoma State University
Tulsa, Oklahoma

Björn Meister, MD, PhD
Karolinska Institutet
Stockholm, Sweden

Amir A. Mhawi, DVM, PhD
Saba University School of Medicine
Saba, Dutch Caribbean

Siobhan Moyes, PhD
University of Plymouth
Plymouth, United Kingdom

Frank E. Nelson, PhD
Temple University
Philadelphia, Pennsylvania

Christine E. Niekrash, DMD
Frank H. Netter MD School of Medicine
Quinnipiac University
North Haven, Connecticut

Diego F. Nino, PhD
Louisiana State University Health Sciences Center
Delgado Community College
New Orleans, Louisiana

Sasha N. Noe, DO, PhD
Saint Leo University
Saint Leo, Florida

Mohammad (Reza) Nourbakhsh, PhD
University of North Georgia
Dahlonega, Georgia

Ivón T. C. Novak, PhD
National University of Córdoba
Córdoba, Argentina

Joanne Orth, PhD
Temple University School of Medicine
Downingtown, Pennsylvania

Fauziah Othman, DVM, PhD
Universiti Putra Malaysia
Serdang, Selangor, Malaysia

Claus Oxvig, PhD
Aarhus University
Aarhus C, Denmark

Scott Paterson, PhD
University of Bristol
Bristol, United Kingdom

Malin Petersson, MD
Karolinska Institutet
Stockholm, Sweden

Thomas E. Phillips, PhD
University of Missouri
Columbia, Missouri

Stephen R. Planck, PhD
Oregon Health & Science University
Portland, Oregon

Harry H. Plymale, PhD
San Diego State University
San Diego, California

Rebecca L. Pratt, PhD
Oakland University William Beaumont School of Medicine
Rochester, Michigan

Margaret Pratten, PhD
Medical School, University of Nottingham
Nottingham, United Kingdom

Rongsun Pu, PhD
Kean University
East Brunswick, New Jersey

Edwin S. Purcell, PhD
University of Medicine and Health Sciences
Basseterre, St. Kitts & Nevis

Romano Regazzi, PhD
Faculty of Biology and Medicine
University of Lausanne
Lausanne, Switzerland

Herman Reid, DVM, MD
Saba University School of Medicine
Saba, Dutch Caribbean

Mary Rheuben, PhD
Michigan State University
East Lansing, Michigan

Michael S. Risley, PhD
Albert Einstein College of Medicine—Jack and Pearl Resnick Campus
Bronx, New York

Melvin G. Rosenfeld, PhD
New York University School of Medicine
New York, New York

Jeffrey L. Salisbury, PhD
Mayo Clinic College of Medicine and Science
Rochester, Minnesota

David K. Saunders, PhD
University of Northern Iowa
Cedar Falls, Iowa

Roger C. Searle, PhD
School of Medical Sciences, Newcastle University
Newcastle, United Kingdom

Lorenzo R. Sewanan, MD, PhD
Yale School of Medicine
New Haven, Connecticut

Allen A. Smith, PhD
Barry University
Miami Shores, Florida

Carles Solsona, PhD
Faculty of Medicine, University of Barcelona
Barcelona, Spain

Jamil Talukder, DVM, PhD
University of Wisconsin—Stout
Menomonie, Wisconsin

Sehime G. Temel, MD, PhD
Uludağ University
Bursa, Türkiye

Barry Timms, PhD
Sanford School of Medicine, University of South Dakota
Vermillion, South Dakota

James J. Tomasek, PhD
University of Oklahoma Health Science Center
Oklahoma City, Oklahoma

John Matthew Velkey, PhD
University of Michigan
Ann Arbor, Michigan

Suvi Kristiina Viranta-Kovanen, PhD
University of Helsinki
Helsinki, Finland

Robert Waltzer, PhD
Belhaven University
Jackson, Mississippi

Scott A. Weed, PhD
West Virginia University School of Medicine
Morgantown, West Virginia

Taylor M. Weiskittel, MD, PhD
Mayo Clinic College of Medicine and Science
Rochester, Minnesota

Brandon A. Wilbanks, PhD
Mayo Clinic College of Medicine and Science
Rochester, Minnesota

Anne-Marie Williams, PhD
School of Medical Sciences, University of Tasmania
Hobart, Australia

Joan W. Witkin, PhD
College of Physicians and Surgeons, Columbia University
New York, New York

Robert W. Zajdel, PhD
State University of New York Upstate Medical University
Syracuse, New York

As in every new edition, several colleagues have made especially notable contributions to this textbook. I am extremely grateful to Dr. **Ivón T. C. Novak** from the National University of Córdoba in Argentina for providing a detailed review of the immune system with many helpful suggestions for improvements; to Dr. **Nazanin Yeganeh Kazemi** for editing and adding helpful comments to the chapter on lymphatic system; to Dr. **Michael Hortsch** from the University of Michigan Medical School for providing guidance in obtaining permission to use their outstanding virtual microscopy slide collection; to Dr. **Kevin N. Christensen** from Winona Health for providing original histologic images of skin specimens and for interesting discussions on dermatopathology; to Dr. **Nirusha Lachman** from the Mayo Clinic College of Medicine and Science who provided me with many ideas and feedback for improvements; to Dr. **Barış Baykal**, a Turkish translation editor from the University of Health Sciences, Gülhane Faculty of Medicine in Ankara, Türkiye, for providing a list of improvements he compiled while translating the eighth edition; and to the many other clinicians, researchers, and educators who gave me permission to use their original, unique digital images; electron micrographs; photomicrographs; and 3D reconstruction images in this edition. They are all acknowledged in the appropriate figure legends.

When Wolters Kluwer initiated this ninth edition in early 2020, we had no idea that this revision would take longer than expected. The unforeseen factor, the COVID-19 pandemic, impacted our schedule as new demands on developing emergency online virtual resources took precedence over the scheduled activities of many histology educators. With pandemic restrictions, the limited access to our medical school laboratories, specimens and specimen processing facilities, and imaging equipment delayed many scheduled material developments for this edition.

Despite these challenges, there have been many bright spots in the development of this edition. **Crystal Taylor**, senior acquisitions editor, is acknowledged for her long-lasting (more than 20 years) support and encouragement throughout the development and improvement of this book. **Kathleen H. Scogna**, freelance editor, as in all previous editions since the fourth edition (2003), edited the manuscript and provided comments and suggestions with honest feedback and constructive advice. For any author, a relationship built on mutual respect with a trusted editor is essential for a successful textbook. I am fortunate to experience such a relationship while working with Kathleen.

I was once again privileged that **Rob Duckwall** from the Dragonfly Media Group (Baltimore, Maryland), one of the most talented medical illustrators working today, whom I have referred to in previous edition as the "Michelangelo of Histology's Sistine Chapel," agreed to work on this ninth edition. Rob added several new illustrations and improved many old illustrations in this edition. His commitment and willingness to work as an artist–author team provided an unprecedented creative dynamic that has made all the difference. Rob has made each and every drawing an unparalleled work of fine art.

I also wish to extend my appreciation to **Jennifer Clements**, the art director, for relabeling and replacing images in the text and atlas sections of this book. Finally, special thanks go to **Deborah Bordeaux**, development editor, who joined the team for this ninth edition, for managing all revised chapters and figures.

CONTENTS

20 Urinary System 768

21 Endocrine Organs 814

22 Male Reproductive System 862

23 Female Reproductive System 908

1 METHODS

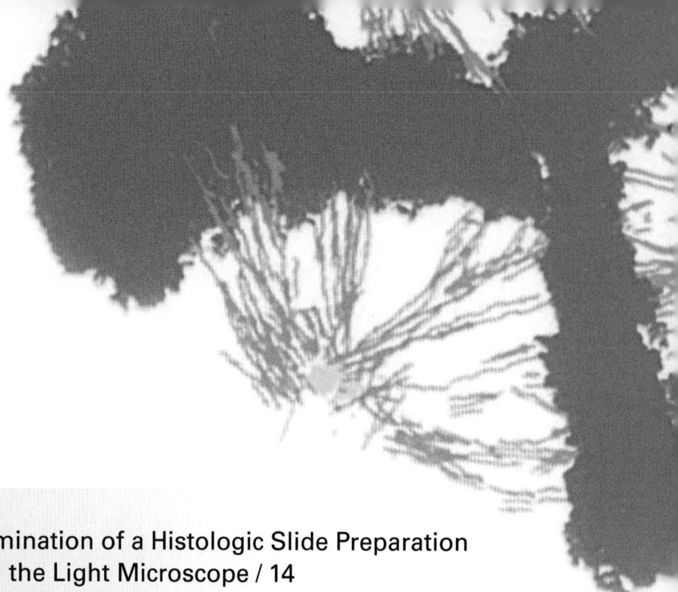

■ OVERVIEW OF METHODS USED IN HISTOLOGY

The objective of a histology course is to lead the student to understand the microanatomy of cells, tissues, and organs and to correlate structure with function.

Histology *[Gr., histos, tissue; Gr., logia, science]*, also called **microscopic anatomy**, is the scientific study of microscopic structures of tissues and organs of the body. Modern histology is not only a descriptive science but also includes many aspects of molecular and cell biology, which help describe cell organization and function. The methods used by histologists are extremely diverse. Much of the histology course content can be framed in terms of light microscopy. Today, students in histology laboratories use either **light microscopes** or, with increasing frequency, **virtual microscopes**, where digitized microscopic specimens are viewed on a computer screen or mobile devices. In the past, more detailed interpretation of microscopic structures was done with the **electron microscope (EM)**—both the **transmission electron microscope (TEM)** and the **scanning electron microscope (SEM)**. Now, the **atomic force microscope (AFM)** and a variety of **super-resolution microscopic techniques** can provide images that are comparable or higher (e.g., AFM) in resolution to those obtained with the TEM. Both EM and AFM, because of their greater resolution and useful magnification, are often the last step in data acquisition from many auxiliary techniques of cell and molecular biology. However, usage of super-resolution techniques is increasing in cell and molecular biology research, mainly because high-resolution images can be captured directly from living cells using fluorescence microscopy. These **auxiliary techniques** include the following:

- Variety of staining methods to enhance contrast of microscopic images
- Histochemistry and cytochemistry techniques
- Immunocytochemistry and hybridization techniques
- Autoradiography
- Organ and tissue culture
- Cell and organelle separation by differential centrifugation

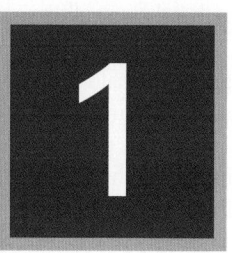

- Specialized tissue preparation (e.g., in expansion microscopy)
- Specialized microscopic techniques (e.g., super-resolution microscopy)
- Specialized optical systems (e.g., polarizing microscope, confocal scanning microscope, or light sheet fluorescence microscope)
- Image analysis software that allow for three-dimensional reconstruction of cells and organelles

The student may feel removed from such techniques and experimental procedures because direct experience with them is usually not available in current curricula. Nevertheless, it is important to know about these specialized procedures and the types of data they yield. *This chapter provides a survey of methods and offers an explanation of how the data provided by these methods can help the student acquire a better understanding of cells, tissues, and organ function.*

One problem that students of histology face is understanding the nature of the two-dimensional (2D) image of a histologic slide or an electron micrograph and how the image relates to the three-dimensional (3D) structure from which it came. To bridge this conceptual gap, we first briefly describe how glass slides and electron microscopic specimens are produced and examined. In addition, we discuss several new methods of light and electron microscopy that have been developed to reconstruct 3D cellular objects from imaged structures.

■ TISSUE PREPARATION

Hematoxylin and Eosin Staining With Formalin Fixation

The routinely prepared hematoxylin and eosin–stained section is the specimen most commonly studied.

The slide set given to each student to study with the light microscope consists mostly of **formalin-fixed, paraffin-embedded, hematoxylin and eosin (H&E)-stained** specimens. Nearly all of the light micrographs in the Atlas section of this book are of slides from actual student sets. Also, most photomicrographs used to illustrate tissues and organs in histology lectures and conferences are taken from such slides. Other staining techniques are sometimes used to demonstrate specific cell and tissue components; several of these methods are discussed later.

The first step in preparation of a tissue or organ sample is fixation to preserve structure.

Fixation, usually by a chemical or mixture of chemicals, permanently preserves the tissue structure for subsequent treatments. Specimens should be immersed in fixative immediately after they are removed from the body. Fixation is used to

- terminate cell metabolism;
- prevent enzymatic degradation of cells and tissues by autolysis (self-digestion);
- kill pathogenic microorganisms such as bacteria, fungi, and viruses; and
- harden the tissue as a result of either cross-linking or denaturing protein molecules.

Formalin, a 37% aqueous solution of formaldehyde, at various dilutions and in combination with other chemicals and buffers, is the most commonly used fixative. Formaldehyde preserves the general structure of the cell and extracellular components by reacting with the amino groups of proteins (most often cross-linked lysine residues). Because formaldehyde does not significantly alter their 3D structure, proteins maintain their ability to react with specific antibodies. This property is important in immunocytochemical staining methods (see pages 8-10). The standard commercial solution of formaldehyde buffered with phosphates (pH 7) acts relatively slowly but penetrates the tissue well. However, because it does not react with lipids, it is a poor fixative of cell membranes.

In the second step, the specimen is prepared for embedding in paraffin to permit sectioning.

Preparing a specimen for examination requires its infiltration with an **embedding medium** that allows it to be thinly sliced, typically in the range of 5–15 μm (1 μm = 1/1,000 mm; Table 1.1). The specimen is **washed** after fixation and **dehydrated** in a series of alcohol solutions of ascending concentration as high as 100% alcohol to remove water. In the next step, **clearing**, organic solvents such as xylol or toluol, which are miscible in both alcohol and **paraffin**, are used to remove the alcohol before infiltration of the specimen with melted paraffin.

When the melted paraffin is cool and hardened, it is trimmed into an appropriately sized block. The block is then attached to a specially designed slicing machine—a **microtome**—and cut with a steel knife. The resulting sections are then mounted on glass slides using a **mounting medium** as an adhesive. Mounting medium is a solution that hardens into a permanent mount that keeps the specimen attached to the glass and prevents deterioration of the specimen over time (i.e., darken, fade, leach, crystalize, etc.). The most commonly used nonaqueous permanent mounting media include toluene-based synthetic resins (Permount), Canada balsam (a turpentine made from the resin of the balsam fir tree), and many others. Aqueous-based media are often used in immunocytochemistry and include glycerol-based products and gelatin.

In the third step, the specimen is stained to permit examination.

Because paraffin sections are colorless, the specimen is not yet suitable for light microscopic examination. To color or stain the tissue sections, the paraffin must be dissolved out, again with xylol or toluol, and the slide must then be rehydrated through a series of solutions of descending alcohol concentration. The tissue on the slides is then stained with **hematoxylin** in water. Because the counterstain, **eosin**, is more soluble in alcohol than in water, the specimen is again dehydrated through a series of alcohol solutions of

TABLE 1.1 Commonly Used Linear Equivalents

1 picometer	=	0.01 angstrom (Å)
1 angstrom	=	0.1 nanometer (nm)
10 angstroms	=	1.0 nanometer
1 nanometer	=	1,000 picometers (pm)
1,000 nanometers	=	1.0 micrometer (μm)
1,000 micrometers	=	1.0 millimeter (mm)

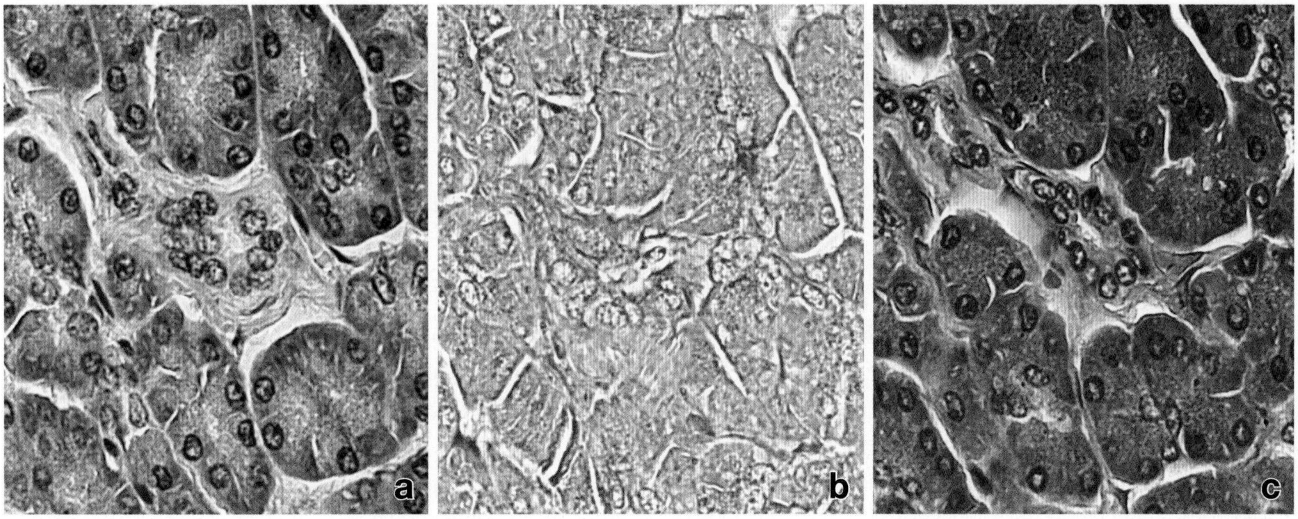

FIGURE 1.1. Hematoxylin and eosin (H&E) staining. This series of specimens from the pancreas are serial (adjacent) sections that demonstrate the effect of H&E used alone and H&E used in combination. **a.** This photomicrograph reveals the staining with hematoxylin only. Although there is a general overall staining of the specimen, those components and structures that have a high affinity for the dye are most heavily stained—for example, the nuclear DNA and areas of the cell containing cytoplasmic RNA. **b.** In this photomicrograph, eosin, the counterstain, likewise has an overall staining effect when used alone. Note, however, that the nuclei are less conspicuous than in the specimen stained with hematoxylin alone. After the specimen is stained with hematoxylin and then prepared for staining with eosin in alcohol solution, the hematoxylin that is not tightly bound is lost, and the eosin then stains those components to which it has a high affinity. **c.** This photomicrograph reveals the combined staining effect of H&E. ×480.

ascending concentration and stained with eosin in alcohol. Figure 1.1 shows the results of staining with hematoxylin alone, eosin alone, and hematoxylin with counterstain eosin. After staining, the specimen is then passed through xylol or toluol to a nonaqueous mounting medium and covered with a coverslip to obtain a permanent preparation.

Other Fixatives

Formalin does not preserve all cell and tissue components.

Although H&E-stained sections of formalin-fixed specimens are convenient to use because they adequately display general structural features, they cannot elucidate the specific chemical composition of cell components. Also, many components are lost in the preparation of the specimen. To retain these components and structures, other fixation methods must be used. These methods are generally based on a clear understanding of the chemistry involved. For instance, the use of alcohols and organic solvents in routine preparations removes neutral lipids.

To retain neutral lipids, such as those in adipose cells, frozen sections of formalin-fixed tissue and dyes that dissolve in fats must be used; to retain membrane structures, special fixatives containing heavy metals that bind to the phospholipids, such as permanganate and osmium, are used (Folder 1.1). The routine use of **osmium tetroxide** as a fixative for electron microscopy is the primary reason for the excellent preservation of membranes in electron micrographs.

Other Staining Procedures

Hematoxylin and eosin are used in histology primarily to display structural features.

Despite the advantages of H&E staining, the procedure does not adequately reveal certain structural components of histologic sections such as elastic material, reticular fibers, basement membranes, and lipids. When it is desirable to display these components, other staining procedures, most of them selective, can be used. These procedures include the use of orcein and resorcin-fuchsin for elastic material and silver impregnation for reticular fibers and basement membrane material. The chemical bases of many staining methods are not completely understood. Understanding the basic concepts of a staining procedure is often more important than knowing precisely all the steps that are involved in that process.

■ HISTOCHEMISTRY AND CYTOCHEMISTRY

Specific chemical procedures can provide information about the function of cells and the extracellular components of tissues.

Histochemical and cytochemical procedures may be based on **specific binding** of a dye, use of a **fluorescent dye–labeled antibody** with a particular cell component, or the **inherent enzymatic activity** of a cell component. In addition, many large molecules present in cells can be localized by the process of **autoradiography**, in which radioactively tagged precursors of the molecule are incorporated by cells and tissues before fixation. Many of these procedures can be used with both light microscopic and electron microscopic preparations.

Before discussing the chemistry of routine staining and histochemical and cytochemical methods, it is useful to examine briefly the nature of a routinely fixed and embedded section of a specimen.

Chemical Composition of Histologic Samples

The chemical composition of a tissue ready for routine staining differs from living tissue.

The components that remain after fixation consist mostly of large molecules that do not readily dissolve, especially after treatment with the fixative. These large molecules, particularly those that react with other large molecules to form

FOLDER 1.1

CLINICAL CORRELATION: FROZEN SECTIONS

Sometimes, a pathologist may be asked to immediately evaluate tissue obtained during surgery, especially when instant pathologic diagnosis may determine how the surgery will proceed. There are several indications to perform such an evaluation, routinely known as a **frozen section**. Most commonly, a surgeon in the operating room requests a frozen section when no preoperative diagnosis was available or when unexpected intraoperative findings must be identified. In addition, the surgeon may want to know whether all of a pathologic mass within the healthy tissue limit has been removed and whether the margin of the surgical resection is free of diseased tissue. Frozen sections are also done in combination with other procedures such as endoscopy or thin-needle biopsy to confirm whether the obtained biopsy material will be usable in further pathologic examinations.

Three main steps are involved in frozen-section preparation:

- **Freezing the tissue sample**. Small tissue samples are frozen either by using compressed carbon dioxide or by immersion in a cold fluid (isopentane) at a temperature of −50°C. Freezing can be achieved in a special high-efficiency refrigerator. Freezing makes the tissue solid and allows sectioning with a microtome.
- **Sectioning the frozen tissue**. Sectioning is usually performed inside a cryostat, a refrigerated compartment containing a microtome. Because the tissue is frozen solid, it can be cut into extremely thin (5–10 μm) sections. The sections are then mounted on glass slides.
- **Staining the cut sections**. Staining is done to differentiate cell nuclei from the rest of the tissue. The most common stains used for frozen sections are hematoxylin and eosin (H&E), methylene blue (Fig. F1.1.1), and periodic acid–Schiff (PAS) stains.

The entire process of preparation and evaluation of frozen sections may take as little as 10 minutes to complete. The total time to obtain results largely depends on the transport time of the tissue from the operating room to the pathology laboratory, the pathologic technique used, and the experience of the pathologist. The findings are then directly communicated to the surgeon waiting in the operating room.

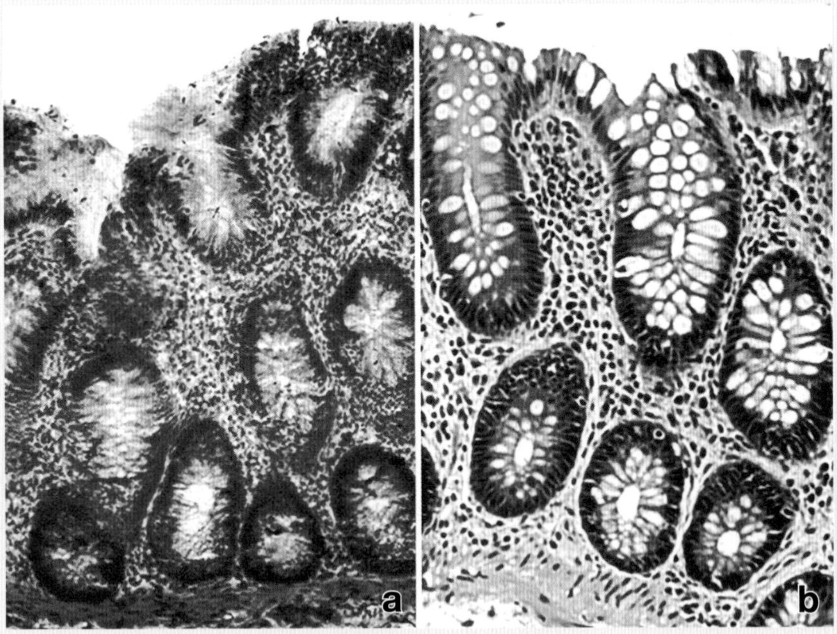

FIGURE F1.1.1. Evaluation of a specimen obtained during surgery by the frozen-section technique. a. This photomicrograph shows a specimen obtained from the large intestine that was prepared by the frozen-section technique and stained with methylene blue. ×160. **b.** Part of the specimen was fixed in formalin and processed as a routine hematoxylin and eosin (H&E) preparation. Examination of the frozen section revealed it to be normal. This diagnosis was later confirmed by examining the routinely prepared H&E specimen. ×180. (Courtesy of Dr. Daniel W. Visscher.)

macromolecular complexes, are usually preserved in a tissue section. Examples of such large macromolecular complexes include the following:

- **Nucleoproteins** formed from nucleic acids bound to protein
- **Intracellular cytoskeletal proteins** complexed with associated proteins
- **Extracellular proteins** in large insoluble aggregates, bound to similar molecules by cross-linking of neighboring molecules, as in collagen fiber formation
- **Membrane phospholipid–protein (or carbohydrate) complexes**

These molecules constitute the structure of cells and tissues—that is, they make up the formed elements of the tissue. They are the basis for the organization that is seen in tissue with the microscope.

In many cases, a structural element is also a functional unit. For example, in the case of proteins that make up the contractile filaments of muscle cells, the filaments are the visible structural components and the actual participants in the contractile process. The RNA of the cytoplasm is visualized as part of a structural component (e.g., ergastoplasm of secretory cells, Nissl bodies of nerve cells) and is also the actual participant in the synthesis of protein.

Many tissue components are lost during the routine preparation of H&E-stained sections.

Although nucleic acids, proteins, and phospholipids are mostly retained in tissue sections, many tissue components are also lost. Small proteins and small nucleic acids, such as transfer RNA, are generally lost during the preparation of the tissue. As previously described, neutral lipids are usually dissolved by the organic solvents used in tissue preparation. Other large molecules also may be lost, for example, by being hydrolyzed because of the unfavorable pH of the fixative solutions. Examples of large molecules lost during routine fixation in aqueous fixatives are

- **glycogen** (an intracellular storage carbohydrate common in liver and muscle cells) and
- **proteoglycans** and **glycosaminoglycans** (extracellular complex carbohydrates found in connective tissue).

These molecules can be preserved, however, by using a nonaqueous fixative for glycogen or by adding specific binding agents to the fixative solution that preserve extracellular carbohydrate-containing molecules.

Soluble components, ions, and small molecules are also lost during the preparation of paraffin sections.

Intermediary metabolites, glucose, sodium, chloride, and similar substances are lost during preparation of routine H&E paraffin sections. Many of these substances can be studied in special preparations, sometimes with considerable loss of structural integrity. These small soluble ions and molecules do not make up the formed elements of a tissue; they participate in synthetic processes or cellular reactions. When they can be preserved and demonstrated by specific methods, they provide invaluable information about cell metabolism, active transport, and other vital cellular processes. Water, a highly versatile molecule, participates in these reactions and processes and contributes to the stabilization of macromolecular structure through hydrogen bonding.

Chemical Basis of Staining

Acidic and Basic Dyes

Hematoxylin and eosin are the most commonly used dyes in histology.

An **acidic dye**, such as **eosin**, carries a *net negative charge* on its colored portion and is described by the general formula $[Na^+dye^-]$.

A **basic dye** carries a *net positive charge* on its colored portion and is described by the general formula $[dye^+Cl^-]$.

Hematoxylin does not meet the definition of a strict basic dye but has properties that closely resemble those of a basic dye. The color of a dye is not related to whether it is basic or acidic, as can be noted by the examples of basic and acidic dyes listed in Table 1.2.

TABLE 1.2 Some Basic and Acidic Dyes

Dye	Color
Basic Dyes	
Methyl green	Green
Methylene blue	Blue
Pyronin G	Red
Toluidine blue	Blue
Acidic Dyes	
Acid fuchsin	Red
Aniline blue	Blue
Eosin	Red
Orange G	Orange

Basic dyes react with anionic components of cells and tissue (components that carry a net negative charge).

Anionic components include the phosphate groups of nucleic acids, the sulfate groups of glycosaminoglycans, and the carboxyl groups of proteins. The ability of such anionic groups to react with a basic dye is called **basophilia** *[Gr., base-loving]*. Tissue components that stain with hematoxylin also exhibit basophilia.

The reaction of the anionic groups varies with pH:

- At a *high pH* (about 10), all three groups are ionized and available for reaction by electrostatic linkages with the basic dye.
- At a *slightly acidic to neutral pH* (5–7), sulfate and phosphate groups are ionized and available for reaction with the basic dye by electrostatic linkages.
- At a *low pH* (below 4), only sulfate groups remain ionized and react with basic dyes.

Therefore, staining with basic dyes at a specific pH can be used to focus on specific anionic groups; because the specific anionic groups are found predominantly on certain macromolecules, the staining serves as an indicator of these macromolecules.

As mentioned, **hematoxylin** is not, strictly speaking, a basic dye. It is used with a **mordant** (i.e., an intermediate link between the tissue component and the dye). The mordant causes the stain to resemble a basic dye. The linkage in the **tissue–mordant–hematoxylin complex** is not a simple electrostatic linkage; when sections are placed in water, hematoxylin does not dissociate from the tissue. Hematoxylin is best suited to staining sequences in which it is followed by aqueous solutions of acidic dyes. True basic dyes, as distinguished from hematoxylin, are not generally used in sequences in which the basic dye is followed by an acidic dye. True basic dye would dissociate from the tissue during the aqueous washes between the basic and acidic dye solutions.

Acidic dyes react with cationic groups in cells and tissues, particularly with the ionized amino groups of proteins.

The reaction of **cationic groups** with an acidic dye is called **acidophilia** *[Gr., acid-loving]*. Reactions of cell and tissue components with acidic dyes are neither as specific nor as precise as reactions with basic dyes.

Although electrostatic linkage is the major factor in the primary binding of an acidic dye to the tissue, it is not the only one; because of this, acidic dyes are sometimes used in combinations to color different tissue constituents selectively. For example, three acidic dyes are used in the **Mallory staining technique**: aniline blue, acid fuchsin, and orange G. These dyes selectively stain collagen, ordinary cytoplasm, and red blood cells, respectively. Acid fuchsin also stains nuclei.

In other multiple acidic dye techniques, hematoxylin is used to stain nuclei first, and then acidic dyes are used to stain cytoplasm and extracellular fibers selectively. The selective staining of tissue components by acidic dyes is attributable to relative factors such as the size and degree of aggregation of the dye molecules and the permeability and "compactness" of the tissue.

Basic dyes can also be used in combination or sequentially (e.g., methyl green and pyronin to study protein synthesis and secretion), but these combinations are not as widely used as acidic dye combinations.

A limited number of substances within cells and the extracellular matrix display basophilia.

Substances that display basophilia include the following:

- **Heterochromatin** and **nucleoli** of the nucleus (chiefly because of ionized phosphate groups in nucleic acids of both)
- **Cytoplasmic components** such as the ergastoplasm (also because of ionized phosphate groups in ribosomal RNA)
- **Extracellular materials** such as the complex carbohydrates of the matrix of cartilage (because of ionized sulfate groups)

Staining with acidic dyes is less specific, but more substances within cells and the extracellular matrix exhibit acidophilia.

Substances that exhibit acidophilia include the following:

- Most **cytoplasmic filaments**, especially those of muscle cells
- Most **intracellular membranous components** and much of the otherwise unspecialized cytoplasm
- Most **extracellular fibers** (primarily because of ionized amino groups)

Metachromasia

Certain basic dyes react with tissue components that shift their normal color from blue to red or purple; this absorbance change is called *metachromasia*.

The underlying mechanism for **metachromasia** is the presence of **polyanions** within the tissue. When these tissues are stained with a concentrated basic dye solution, such as **toluidine blue**, the dye molecules are close enough to form dimeric and polymeric aggregates. The absorption properties of these aggregations differ from those of the individual nonaggregated dye molecules.

Cell and tissue structures that have high concentrations of ionized sulfate and phosphate groups—such as the ground substance of cartilage, heparin-containing granules of mast cells, and rough endoplasmic reticulum of plasma cells—exhibit metachromasia. Therefore, toluidine blue will appear purple to red when it stains these components.

Aldehyde Groups and the Schiff Reagent

The ability of bleached basic fuchsin (Schiff reagent) to react with aldehyde groups results in a distinctive red color and is the basis of the periodic acid–Schiff and Feulgen reactions.

The **periodic acid–Schiff (PAS) reaction** stains carbohydrates and carbohydrate-rich macromolecules. It is used to demonstrate glycogen in cells, mucus in various cells and tissues, the basement membrane that underlies epithelia, and reticular fibers in connective tissue. The Schiff reagent is also used in **Feulgen stain**, which relies on a mild hydrochloric acid hydrolysis to stain DNA.

The PAS reaction is based on the following facts:

- Hexose rings of carbohydrates contain adjacent carbons, each of which bears a hydroxyl (−OH) group.

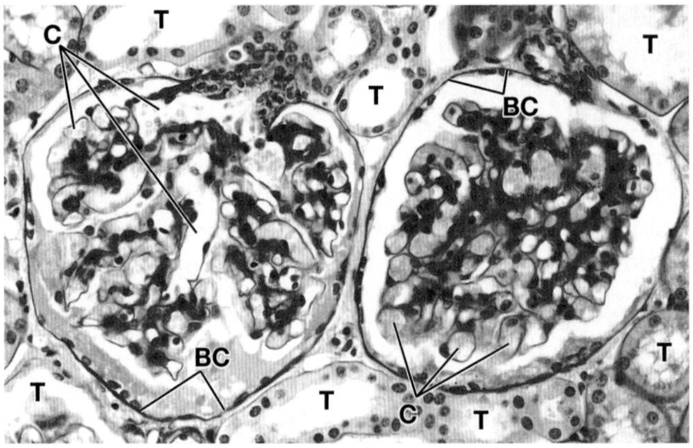

FIGURE 1.2. Photomicrograph of kidney tissue stained by the periodic acid–Schiff (PAS) method. This histochemical method demonstrates and localizes carbohydrates and carbohydrate-rich macromolecules. The basement membranes are PAS-positive as evidenced by the magenta staining of these sites. The kidney tubules (*T*) are sharply delineated by the stained basement membrane surrounding the tubules. The glomerular capillaries (*C*) and the epithelium of Bowman capsule (*BC*) also show PAS-positive basement membranes. The specimen was counterstained with hematoxylin to visualize cell nuclei. ×320.

- Hexosamines of glycosaminoglycans contain adjacent carbons, one of which bears an −OH group, whereas the other bears an amino (−NH_2) group.
- Periodic acid cleaves the bond between these adjacent carbon atoms and forms aldehyde groups.
- These aldehyde groups react with the Schiff reagent to give a distinctive magenta color.

The PAS staining of basement membrane (Fig. 1.2) and reticular fibers is based on the content or association of proteoglycans (complex carbohydrates associated with a protein core). PAS staining is an alternative to silver impregnation methods, which are also based on reaction with the sugar molecules in the proteoglycans.

The **Feulgen reaction** is based on the cleavage of purines from the deoxyribose of DNA by mild acid hydrolysis; the sugar ring then opens with the formation of aldehyde groups. Again, the newly formed aldehyde groups react with the Schiff reagent to impart its distinctive magenta color. The reaction of the Schiff reagent with DNA is **stoichiometric**, meaning that the product of this reaction is measurable and proportional to the amount of DNA. This property makes it ideal for use in spectrophotometric methods to quantify the amount of DNA in the nucleus of a cell. RNA does not stain with the Schiff reagent because it lacks deoxyribose.

Enzyme Digestion

Enzyme digestion of a section adjacent to one stained for a specific component—such as glycogen, DNA, or RNA—can be used to confirm the identity of the stained material.

Intracellular material that stains with the PAS reaction may be identified as glycogen by pretreatment of sections with diastase or amylase. Elimination of the staining after these treatments positively identifies the stained material as glycogen.

Similarly, pretreatment of tissue sections with deoxyribonuclease (DNAse) will abolish the Feulgen staining in those sections, and treatment of sections of protein secretory epithelia with ribonuclease (RNAse) will abolish the staining of the ergastoplasm with basic dyes.

FOLDER 1.2

FUNCTIONAL CONSIDERATIONS: FEULGEN MICROSPECTROPHOTOMETRY

Feulgen microspectrophotometry is a technique developed to study DNA increases in developing cells and to analyze *ploidy*—that is, the number of times the normal DNA content of a cell is multiplied (a normal, nondividing cell is said to be *diploid*; a sperm or egg cell is *haploid*). Two techniques, **static cytometry** for tissue sections and **flow cytometry** for isolated cells, are used to quantify the amount of nuclear DNA.

Static cytometry of Feulgen-stained sections of tumors uses microspectrophotometry coupled with a digitizing imaging system to measure the absorption of light emitted by cells and cell clusters at 560-nm wavelength. In contrast, flow cytometry uses instrumentation able to scan only single cells flowing past a sensor in a liquid medium. This technique provides rapid, quantitative analysis of a single cell based on the measurement of fluorescent light emission.

Currently, Feulgen microspectrophotometry is used to study changes in the DNA content in dividing cells undergoing differentiation. It is also used clinically to analyze abnormal chromosomal number (i.e., ploidy patterns) in malignant cells. Some malignant cells that have a largely diploid pattern are said to be well differentiated; tumors with these types of cells have a better prognosis than tumors with *aneuploid* (nonintegral multiples of the haploid amount of DNA) and tetraploid cells. Feulgen microspectrophotometry has been particularly useful in studies of specific adenocarcinomas (epithelial cancers), breast cancer, kidney cancer, colon and other gastrointestinal cancers, endometrial (uterine epithelium) cancer, and ovarian cancer. It is one of the most valuable tools for pathologists in evaluating the metastatic potential of these tumors and in making prognostic and treatment decisions.

Enzyme Histochemistry

Histochemical methods are also used to identify and localize enzymes in cells and tissues.

To localize enzymes in tissue sections, special care must be taken in fixation to preserve the enzyme activity. Usually, mild aldehyde fixation is the preferred method. In these procedures, the reaction product of the enzyme activity, rather than the enzyme itself, is visualized. In general, a **capture reagent**, either a dye or a heavy metal, is used to trap or bind the reaction product of the enzyme by precipitation at the site of reaction. In a typical reaction to display a hydrolytic enzyme, the tissue section is placed in a solution containing a substrate (AB) and a trapping agent (T) that precipitates one of the products as follows:

$$AB + T \xrightarrow{\text{enzyme}} AT + B$$

where AT is the trapped end product and B is the hydrolyzed substrate.

By using such methods, the lysosome, first identified in differential centrifugation studies of cells, was equated with a vacuolar component seen in electron micrographs. In lightly fixed tissues, the acid hydrolases and esterases contained in lysosomes react with an appropriate substrate. The reaction mixture also contains lead ions to precipitate (e.g., lead phosphate derived from the action of acid phosphatase). The precipitated reaction product can then be observed with both light and electron microscopy. Similar histochemical procedures have been developed to demonstrate alkaline phosphatase, adenosine triphosphatases (ATPases) of many varieties (including the Na^+/K^+ ATPase that is the enzymatic basis of the sodium pump in cells and tissues), various esterases, and many respiratory enzymes (Fig. 1.3a).

One of the most common histochemical methods (often used in conjunction with immunocytochemistry) employs horseradish peroxidase for enzyme-mediated antigen detection. A widely used substrate for horseradish peroxidase is

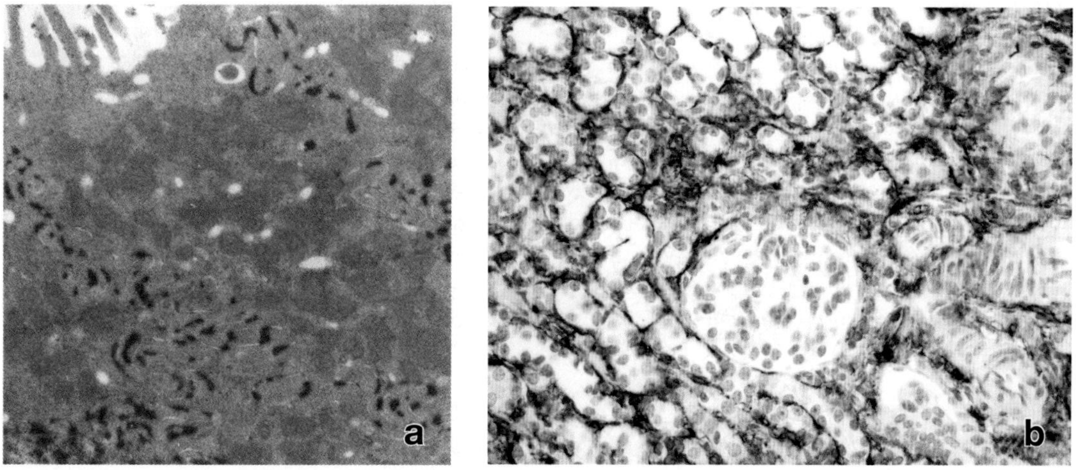

FIGURE 1.3. Electron and light microscopic histochemical procedures. a. This electron micrograph shows localization of membrane ATPase in epithelial cells of rabbit gallbladder. *Dark areas* visible on the electron micrograph show the location of the enzyme ATPase. This enzyme is detected in the plasma membrane at the lateral domains of epithelial cells, which correspond to the location of sodium pumps. These epithelial cells are involved in active transport of molecules across the plasma membrane. ×26,000. **b.** This photomicrograph shows macrophages stained with a histochemical method using peroxidase-labeled antibodies and 3,3′-diaminobenzidine (DAB) reagent. A paraffin-embedded section of mouse kidney with renal vascular hypertension disease was stained for the presence of F4/80+ specific marker protein expressed only on the surface of macrophages. Initially, sections were exposed to primary rat anti-mouse F4/80+ antibodies followed by incubation with secondary goat anti-rat immunoglobulin G (IgG) antibodies labeled with horseradish peroxidase. The specimen was washed and treated with a buffer containing DAB. A brown precipitate (product of DAB oxidation by horseradish peroxidase) is localized in the areas where macrophages are present. The specimen was counterstained with hematoxylin to visualize cell nuclei. ×400. (Courtesy of Dr. Joseph P. Grande.)

3,3′-diaminobenzidine (DAB), a colorless organic compound that produces a brown insoluble product at the site of enzymatic reaction (Fig. 1.3b). The product of this enzymatic reaction can be easily localized in cells, yielding high-resolution images in both light and electron microscopy.

Immunocytochemistry

The specificity of a reaction between an antigen and an antibody is the underlying basis of immunocytochemistry.

Antibodies, also known as **immunoglobulins**, are glycoproteins that are produced by specific cells of the immune system in response to a foreign protein or **antigen**. In the laboratory, antibodies can be purified from blood and conjugated (attached) to a fluorescent dye. In general, **fluorescent dyes (fluorochromes)** are chemicals that absorb light of different wavelengths (e.g., ultraviolet light) and then emit visible light of a specific wavelength (e.g., green, yellow, red). **Fluorescein**, the most commonly used dye, absorbs ultraviolet light and emits green light. Antibodies conjugated with fluorescein can be applied to sections of lightly fixed or frozen tissues on glass slides to localize an antigen in cells and tissues. The reaction of antibody with antigen can then be examined and photographed with a fluorescence microscope or confocal microscope that produces a 3D reconstruction of the examined tissue (Fig. 1.4).

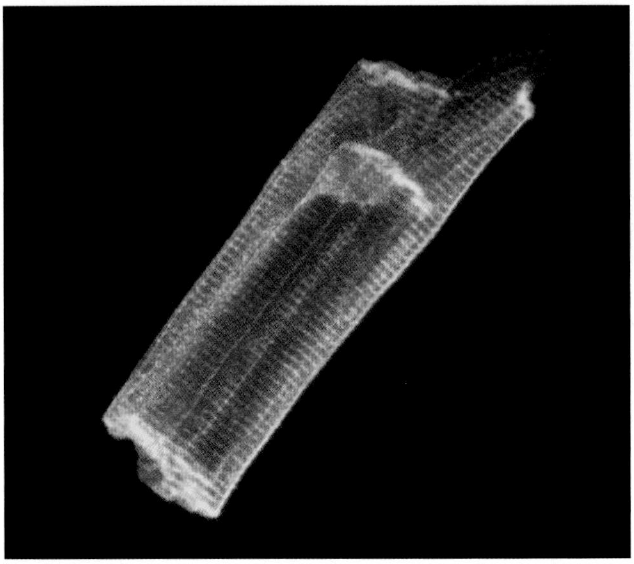

FIGURE 1.4. Confocal microscopy image of a rat cardiac muscle cell. This image was obtained with the confocal microscope using the indirect immunofluorescence method. Two primary antibodies were used. The first primary antibody recognizes a specific lactate transporter (MCT1) and is detected with a secondary antibody conjugated with rhodamine (*red*). The second primary antibody is directed against the transmembrane protein CD147, which is tightly associated with MCT1. This antibody was detected by a secondary antibody labeled with fluorescein (*green*). The *yellow* color is visible at the point at which the two labeled secondary antibodies exactly colocalize within the cardiac muscle cell. This three-dimensional image shows that both proteins are distributed on the surface of the muscle cell, whereas the lactate transporter alone is visible deep to the plasma membrane. (Courtesy of Drs. Andrew P. Halestrap and Catherine Heddle.)

Two types of antibodies are used in immunocytochemistry: polyclonal antibodies that are produced by immunized animals and monoclonal antibodies that are produced by immortalized (continuously replicating) antibody-producing cell lines.

In a typical procedure, a specific protein, such as actin, is isolated from a muscle cell of one species, such as a rat, and injected into the circulation of another species, such as a rabbit. In the immunized rabbit, the rat's actin molecules are recognized by the rabbit immune system as a foreign antigen. This recognition triggers a cascade of immunologic reactions involving multiple groups (clones) of immune cells called **B lymphocytes**. The cloning of B lymphocytes eventually leads to the production of anti-actin antibodies. Collectively, these **polyclonal antibodies** represent mixtures of different antibodies produced by many clones of B lymphocytes that each recognize different regions of the actin molecule. The antibodies are then removed from the blood, purified, and conjugated with a fluorescent dye. They can now be used to locate actin molecules in rat tissues or cells. If actin is present in a cell or tissue, such as a fibroblast in connective tissue, then the fluorescein-labeled antibody binds to it, and the reaction is visualized by fluorescence microscopy.

Monoclonal antibodies (Folder 1.3) are those produced by an **antibody-producing cell line** consisting of a single group (clone) of identical B lymphocytes. The single clone that becomes a cell line is obtained from an individual with **multiple myeloma**, a tumor derived from a single antibody-producing plasma cell. Individuals with multiple myeloma produce a large population of identical, homogeneous antibodies with an identical specificity against an antigen. To produce monoclonal antibodies against a specific antigen, a mouse or rat is immunized with that antigen. The activated B lymphocytes are then isolated from the lymphatic tissue (spleen or lymph nodes) of the animal and fused with the myeloma cell line. This fusion produces a **hybridoma**, an immortalized individual antibody-secreting cell line. To obtain monoclonal antibodies against rat actin molecules, for example, the B lymphocytes from the lymphatic organs of immunized rabbits must be fused with myeloma cells.

FOLDER 1.3
CLINICAL CORRELATION: MONOCLONAL ANTIBODIES IN MEDICINE

Monoclonal antibodies are now widely used in immunocytochemical techniques and also have many clinical applications. Monoclonal antibodies conjugated with radioactive compounds are used to detect and diagnose tumor metastasis in pathology, differentiate subtypes of tumors and stages of their differentiation, and in infectious disease diagnosis to identify microorganisms in blood and tissue fluids. Monoclonal antibodies conjugated with immunotoxins, chemotherapy agents, or radioisotopes are now being used to deliver therapeutic agents to specific tumor cells in the body.

Both direct and indirect immunocytochemical methods are used to locate a target antigen in cells and tissues.

The oldest immunocytochemistry technique used for identifying the distribution of an antigen within cells and tissues is known as **direct immunofluorescence**. This technique uses a fluorochrome-labeled **primary antibody** (either polyclonal or monoclonal) that reacts with the antigen within the sample (Fig. 1.5a). As a one-step procedure, this method involves only a single labeled antibody. Visualization of structures is not ideal because of the low intensity of the signal emission. Direct immunofluorescence methods are now being replaced by the indirect method because of suboptimal sensitivity.

Indirect immunofluorescence provides much greater sensitivity than direct methods and is often referred to as the "sandwich" or "double-layer technique." Instead of conjugating a fluorochrome with a specific (primary) antibody directed against the antigen of interest (e.g., a rat actin molecule), the fluorochrome is conjugated with a **secondary antibody** directed against a rat primary antibody (i.e., goat anti-rat antibody; Fig. 1.5b). When the fluorescein is conjugated directly with the specific primary antibody, the method is direct; when fluorescein is conjugated with a secondary antibody, the method is indirect. The indirect method considerably enhances the fluorescence signal emission from the tissue. An additional advantage of the indirect labeling method is that a single secondary antibody can be used to localize the tissue-specific binding of several different primary antibodies (Fig. 1.6). For microscopic studies, the secondary antibody can be conjugated with different fluorescent dyes so that multiple labels can be shown in the same tissue section (see Fig. 1.4). Drawbacks of indirect immunofluorescence are that it is expensive, labor-intensive, and not easily adapted to automated procedures.

It is also possible to conjugate polyclonal or monoclonal antibodies with other substances, such as enzymes (e.g., horseradish peroxidase), that convert colorless substrates (e.g., DAB) into an insoluble product of a specific color that precipitates at the site of the enzymatic reaction. The staining that results from this **immunoperoxidase method** can be observed in the light microscope (see Fig. 1.3b) with either direct or indirect immunocytochemical methods. In another variation, colloidal gold or ferritin (an iron-containing molecule) can be attached to the antibody molecule. These electron-dense markers can be visualized directly with the EM.

Hybridization Techniques

Hybridization is a method of localizing messenger RNA (mRNA) or DNA by hybridizing the sequence of interest to a complementary strand of a nucleotide probe.

In general, the term **hybridization** describes the ability of single-stranded RNA or DNA molecules to interact (hybridize) with complementary sequences. In the laboratory, hybridization requires the isolation of DNA or RNA, which is then mixed with a complementary nucleotide sequence (called a **nucleotide probe**). Hybrids are detected most often using a radioactive label attached to one component of the hybrid.

Binding of the probe and sequence can take place in a solution or on a nitrocellulose membrane. In **in situ hybridization**, the binding of the nucleotide probe to the DNA or RNA sequence of interest is performed within cells or tissues, such as cultured cells or whole embryos. This technique allows the localization of specific nucleotide sequences as small as 10–20 copies of mRNA or DNA per cell.

Several nucleotide probes are used in in situ hybridization. **Oligonucleotide probes** can be as small as 20–40 base pairs. Single- or double-stranded DNA probes are much longer and can contain as many as 1,000 base pairs. For specific

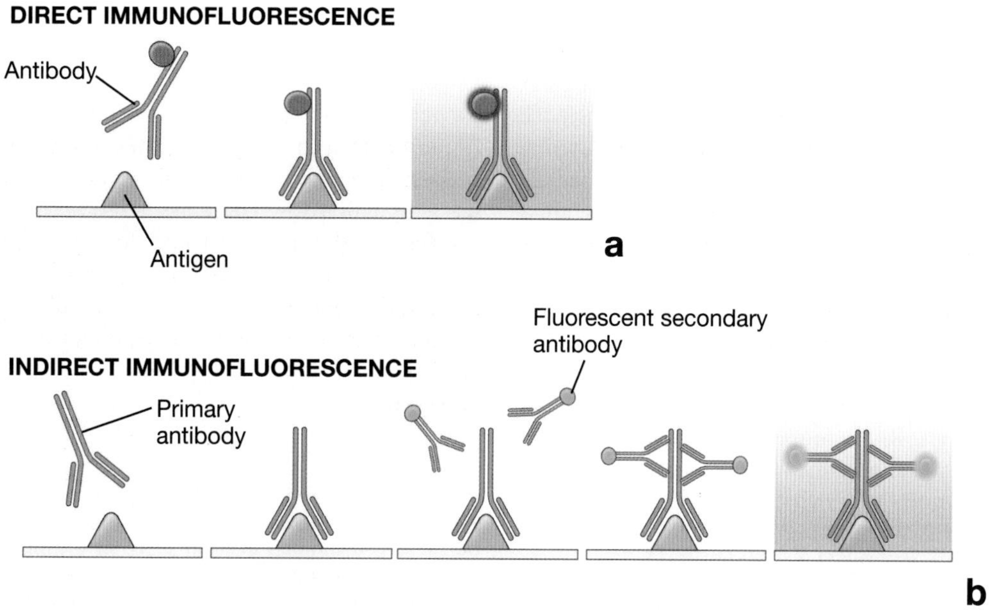

FIGURE 1.5. Direct and indirect immunofluorescence. a. In direct immunofluorescence, a fluorochrome-labeled primary antibody reacts with a specific antigen within the tissue sample. Labeled structures are then observed in the fluorescence microscope in which an excitation wavelength (usually ultraviolet light) triggers the emission of another wavelength. The length of this wavelength depends on the nature of the fluorochrome used for antibody labeling. **b.** The indirect method involves two processes. First, specific primary antibodies react with the antigen of interest. Second, the secondary antibodies, which are fluorochrome labeled, react with the primary antibodies. The visualization of labeled structures within the tissue is the same in both methods and requires the fluorescence microscope.

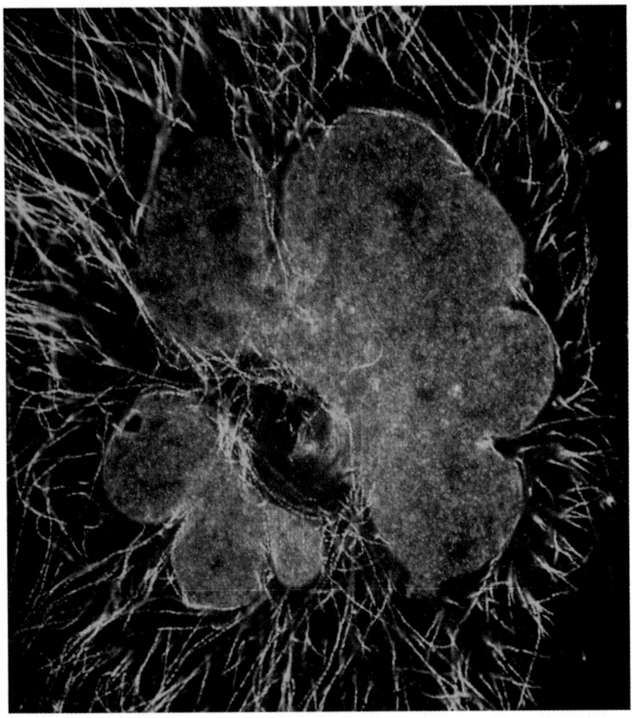

FIGURE 1.6. Microtubules and nuclear-specific histone proteins visualized by immunocytochemical methods using expansion microscopy. Distribution of microtubules (elements of the cell cytoskeleton labeled in green) and nuclear-specific phospho-histone H3 (Ser10) proteins (labeled in magenta) obtained from the HeLa human cervical cancer cell line can be studied in vitro using the fluorescence microscope. By use of indirect immunofluorescence techniques, microtubules were labeled with primary rabbit anti–α-tubulin polyclonal antibodies and visualized by secondary goat anti-rabbit antibodies conjugated with green fluorescent dye (Alexa Fluor 488). The histone proteins were labeled with monoclonal mouse anti–phospho-histone H3 (Ser10) primary antibodies and visualized by secondary goat anti-mouse antibodies conjugated with fluorescent dye (CF633). DNA in the nucleus has been counterstained with a nonspecific blue stain (DAPI stain). The microtubule network is well visualized because of the high resolution afforded by the expansion microscopy procedure (expansion factor: 4.2). (Photomicrograph courtesy of Drs. Yongxin Zhao and Edward S. Boyden, Massachusetts Institute of Technology, Cambridge, MA.)

localization of mRNA, complementary RNA probes are used. These probes are labeled with radioactive isotopes (e.g., ^{32}P, ^{35}S, ^{3}H), a specifically modified nucleotide (digoxigenin), or biotin (a commonly used covalent multipurpose label). Radioactive probes can be detected and visualized by autoradiography. Digoxigenin and biotin are detected by immunocytochemical and cytochemical methods, respectively.

The strength of the bonds between the probe and the complementary sequence depends on the type of nucleic acid in the two strands. The strongest bond is formed between a DNA probe and a complementary DNA strand and the weakest between an RNA probe and a complementary RNA strand. If a tissue specimen is expected to contain a minute amount of mRNA or a viral transcript, **polymerase chain reaction (PCR)** amplification for DNA or **reverse transcription-PCR (RT-PCR)** for RNA can be used. The amplified transcripts obtained during these procedures are usually detected using labeled complementary nucleotide probes using standard in situ hybridization techniques.

Recently, fluorescent dyes have been combined with nucleotide probes, making it possible to visualize multiple probes at the same time (Fig. 1.7). This technique, called **fluorescence in situ hybridization (FISH)**, is extensively used in the clinical setting for genetic testing. For example, a probe hybridized to metaphase chromosomes can be used to identify the chromosomal position of a gene. **FISH** is used to simultaneously examine chromosomes, gene expression, and the distribution of gene products such as pathologic or abnormal proteins. Many specific **fluorescent probes** are now commercially available and are used clinically in **screening procedures** for cervical cancer or for the detection of human immunodeficiency virus (HIV)-infected cells. FISH is also used in **prenatal diagnostic testing** to visualize chromosomes in fetal cells obtained from amniocentesis or chorionic villus sampling to detect chromosomal abnormalities. In addition, FISH is used to examine the chromosomes in the lymphocytes of astronauts to estimate their absorbed radiation dose after their return from space. The frequency of chromosome translocations in lymphocytes is proportional to the absorbed radiation dose.

Autoradiography

Autoradiography makes use of a photographic emulsion placed over a tissue section to localize radioactive material within tissues.

Many small molecular precursors of larger molecules, such as the amino acids that make up proteins and the nucleotides that make up nucleic acids, may be tagged by incorporating a radioactive atom or atoms into their molecular structure. The radioactivity is then traced to localize the larger molecules in cells and tissues. Labeled precursor molecules can be injected into animals or introduced into cell or organ cultures. For instance, **radioactive precursors** of **DNA (^{3}H-thymidine)** or **RNA (^{3}H-uridine)** can be introduced to living cells to study synthesis of DNA and subsequent cell division, synthesis of mRNA, and localization of protein synthesis in the cell. Other radioactive precursors can trace protein secretion by cells and localization of synthetic products within cells and in the extracellular matrix.

Sections of specimens that have incorporated radioactive material are mounted on slides. In the dark, the slide is usually

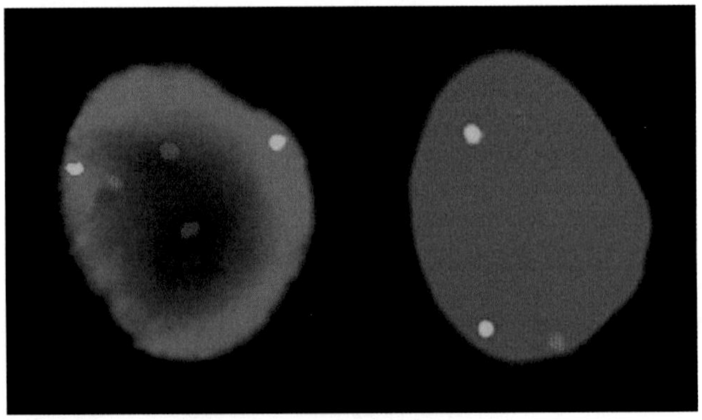

FIGURE 1.7. Example of the fluorescence in situ hybridization (FISH) technique used in prenatal diagnostic testing. Interphase nuclei of cells obtained from amniotic fluid specimens were hybridized with two specific DNA probes. The *orange* probe (LSI 21) is locus-specific for chromosome 21, and the *green* probe (LSI 13) is locus-specific for chromosome 13. The *right* nucleus is from a normal amniotic fluid specimen and exhibits two *green* and two *orange* signals, which indicates two copies of chromosomes 13 and 21, respectively. The nucleus on the *left* has three *orange* signals, which indicate trisomy 21 (Down syndrome). DNA has been counterstained with a nonspecific blue stain (DAPI stain) to make the nucleus visible. ×1,250. (Courtesy of Dr. Robert B. Jenkins.)

dipped in a melted photographic emulsion, thus producing a thin photographic film on the surface of the slide. After appropriate exposure in a light-tight box, usually for days to weeks, the exposed emulsion on the slide is developed by standard photographic techniques and permanently mounted with a coverslip. The slides may be stained either before or after exposure and development. The silver grains in the emulsion over the radioactively labeled molecules are exposed and developed by this procedure and appear as dark grains overlying the site of the radioactive emission when examined with the light microscope (Fig. 1.8a).

These grains may be used simply to indicate the location of a substance, or they may be counted to provide semiquantitative information about the amount of a given substance in a specific location. For instance, after injection of an animal with tritiated thymidine, cells that have incorporated this nucleotide into their DNA before they divide will have approximately twice as many silver grains overlying their nuclei as will cells that have divided after incorporating the labeled nucleotide.

Autoradiography can also be performed using thin plastic sections for examination with the EM. Essentially, the same procedures are used, but as with all TEM preparation techniques, the processes are much more delicate and difficult; however, they also yield much greater resolution and more precise localization (Fig. 1.8b).

Expansion Microscopy

Expansion microscopy is a method for improving the resolution of light microscopy by implementing a specific preparation that physically expands the specimen.

Expansion microscopy (ExM) refers to a process in which specimens are infiltrated with **swellable polymers** (hydrogels—very absorbent materials commonly found in baby diapers), which form hydrophilic polymer networks that are able to absorb large amounts of water and increase their volumes. The structure and physical integrity of these networks are due to the presence of strong and stable cross-links that allow the hydrogel to withstand expansion forces generated by the addition of water, thus stabilizing the gel. As a result of the **isotropic expansion** of the specimen, the molecules within the cells, plasma membrane, and extracellular matrix are separated from each other equally in all directions. Preparation of the specimen for ExM involves the following steps (Fig. 1.9):

- **Fixation**. The fixation process for ExM is the same as for light microscopy immunostaining protocols.
- **Anchoring**. The cellular structure of interest is labeled with a molecular probe (e.g., antibodies conjugated with fluorescein dye, fluorescent proteins, and others) and incubated with an anchoring reagent expressing specific

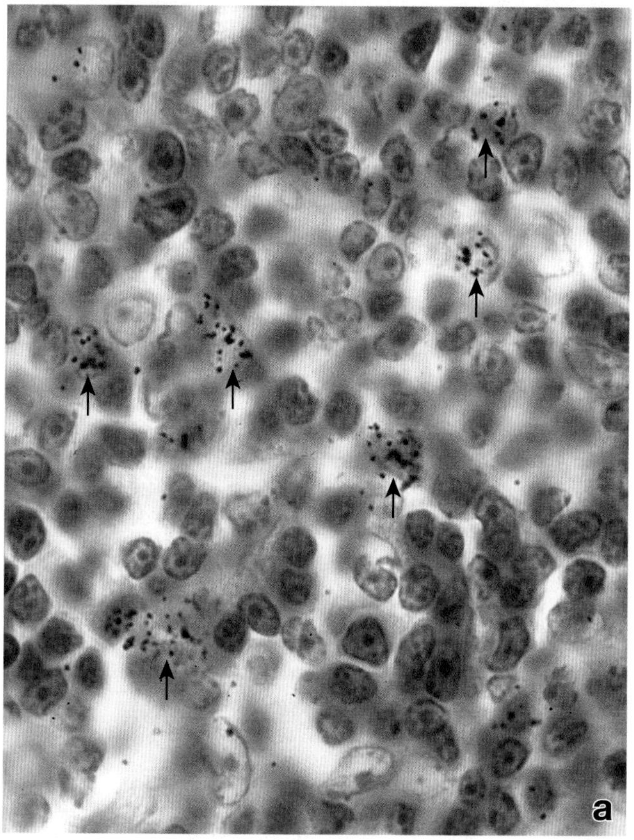

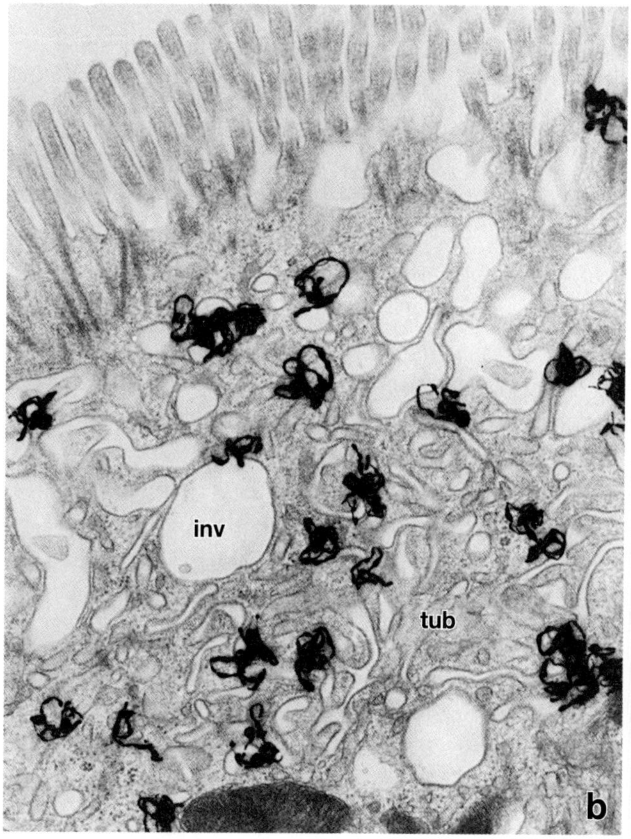

FIGURE 1.8. Examples of autoradiography used in light and electron microscopy. a. Photomicrograph of a lymph node section from an animal injected with tritiated [^{3}H]thymidine. Some of the cells exhibit aggregates of metallic silver grains, which appear as small black particles (*arrows*). These cells synthesized DNA in preparation for cell division and have incorporated the [^{3}H]thymidine into newly formed DNA. Over time, the low-energy radioactive particles emitted from the [^{3}H]thymidine strike silver halide crystals in a photographic emulsion covering the specimen (exposure) and create a latent image (much like light striking photographic film in a camera). During photographic development of the slide with its covering emulsion, the latent image—actually the activated silver halide in the emulsion—is reduced to the metallic silver, which then appears as black grains in the microscope. ×1,200. (Original slide specimen courtesy of Dr. Ernst Kallenbach.) **b.** Electron microscopic autoradiograph of the apical region of an intestinal absorptive cell. In this specimen, ^{125}I bound to nerve growth factor (NGF) was injected into the animal, and the tissue was removed 1 hour later. The specimen was prepared in a manner similar to that for light microscopy. The relatively small size of the silver grains aids precise localization of the ^{125}I–NGF complexes. Note that the silver grains are concentrated over apical invaginations (*inv*) and early endosomal tubular profiles (*tub*). ×32,000. (Electron micrograph courtesy of Dr. Marian R. Neutra.)

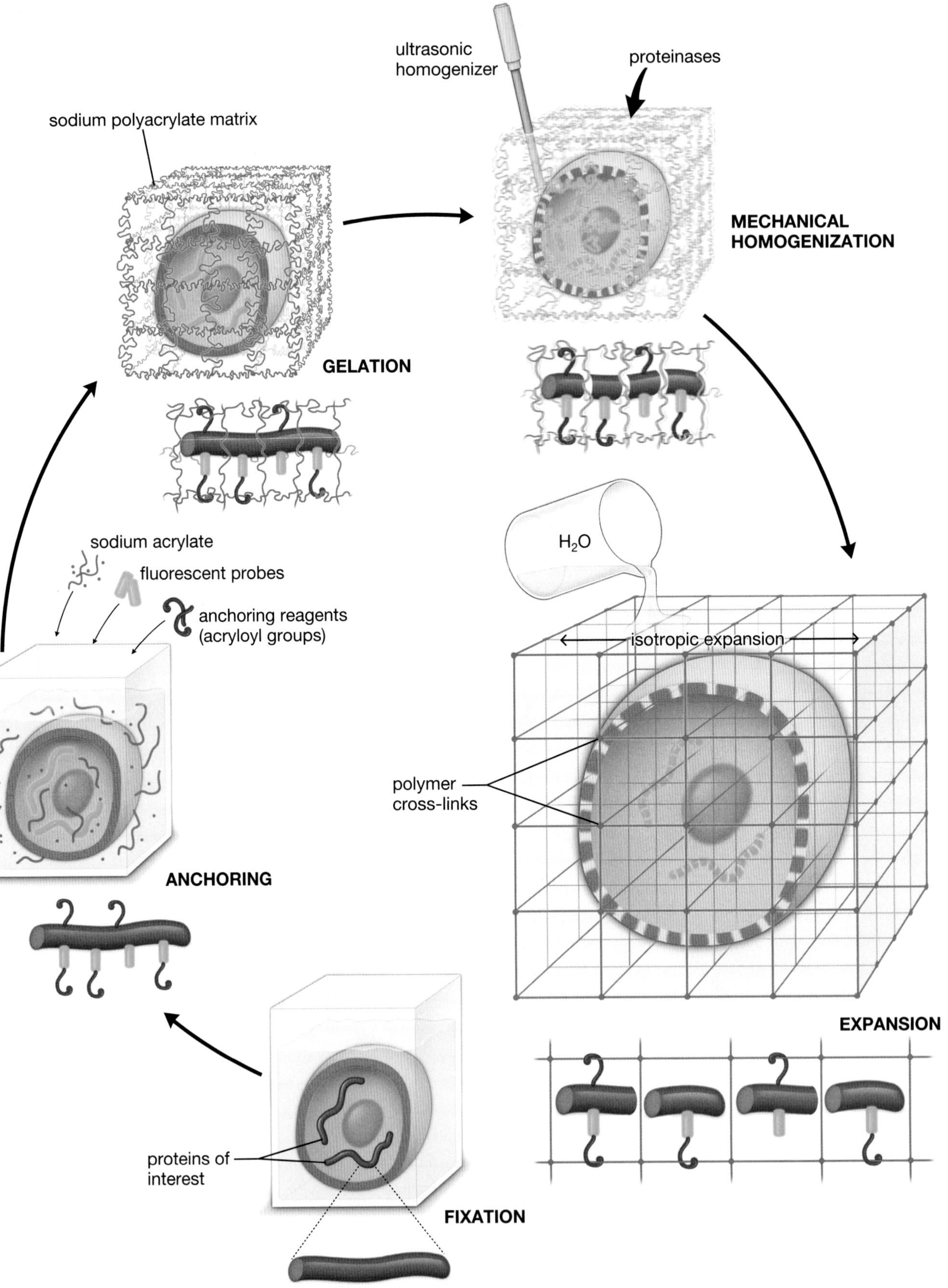

FIGURE 1.9. Steps in tissue processing for expansion microscopy. This diagram shows the consecutive steps in preparation of a specimen for expansion microscopy. After conventional fixation (in formaldehyde), the specimen is treated with anchoring reagents that bind to proteins or other molecules of interest and molecular probes conjugated with fluorescent labels. The addition of sodium acrylate monomers triggers development of a dense three-dimensional hydrogel polymer matrix. After mechanical homogenization that allows the cells to break open, the specimen, now embedded in a hydrogel matrix, is ready for physical expansion by the addition of water. Proteins of interest remain connected to the expanded polymer network, which pulls them apart. The integrity of the expanded gel is maintained by strong and stable cross-links that resist expansion forces generated by the addition of the water. After the expansion (approximately 4.5 times), the specimen is ready for examination with the fluorescence microscope.

binding sites for molecular probes and with gel monomers. In addition, some molecules (e.g., proteins or RNA) can also be anchored directly to the gel.

- **Gelation.** The specimen is infiltrated with gel monomers (i.e., sodium acrylate) that polymerize within the cells and tissues. The resulting polymers (sodium polyacrylate) form a dense 3D matrix that is firmly anchored to the cell molecules via binding sites on the anchoring reagent.
- **Mechanical homogenization.** The polymer-embedded specimen undergoes mechanical homogenization. This process, which breaks open the cells, involves denaturation and/or digestion of structural molecules by specific proteases.
- **Expansion.** A solvent is added to the specimen (water in the case of sodium polyacrylate polymers), causing expansion of specimen in all three dimensions (more than 100-fold in volume).

Following this preparation, the expanded specimen is ready for examination using standard fluorescence microscopy.

Expansion microscopy, which utilizes inexpensive chemicals and commonly used optical microscopes, provides super-resolution imaging by increasing the size of the observed specimen.

The main advantage of ExM lies in its ability to separate tightly spaced molecules that were not initially detectable as separate structures because of the light microscope's innate resolution and diffraction limitations. In expanded specimens, these molecules are pulled far enough apart to be easily resolved without changing the resolution limits of the optical instrument. Linear expansion to 4.5 times is possible, which correlates to an increase in resolution in the range of 60–70 nm. Interestingly, after an initial expansion, the specimen can be subject to repeated expansions with a second swellable polymer network. This process, called **iterative expansion microscopy (iExM)**, may be used to expand biologic specimens up to 20 times and obtain images of cells and tissues with a resolution of approximately 25 nm when viewed with conventional fluorescence microscopy (Fig. 1.10).

Recently, ExM protocols have been applied to routine H&E slide preparations of pathologic specimens to convert glass slides into ExM-compatible preparations. This method, known as **expansion pathology (ExPath)**, allows for the optical microscopic examination and diagnosis of diseases that previously required electron microscopy.

■ MICROSCOPY

Light Microscopy

A microscope, whether simple (one lens) or compound (multiple lenses), is an instrument that magnifies an image and allows visualization of greater detail than is possible with the unaided eye. The simplest microscope is a magnifying glass or a pair of reading glasses.

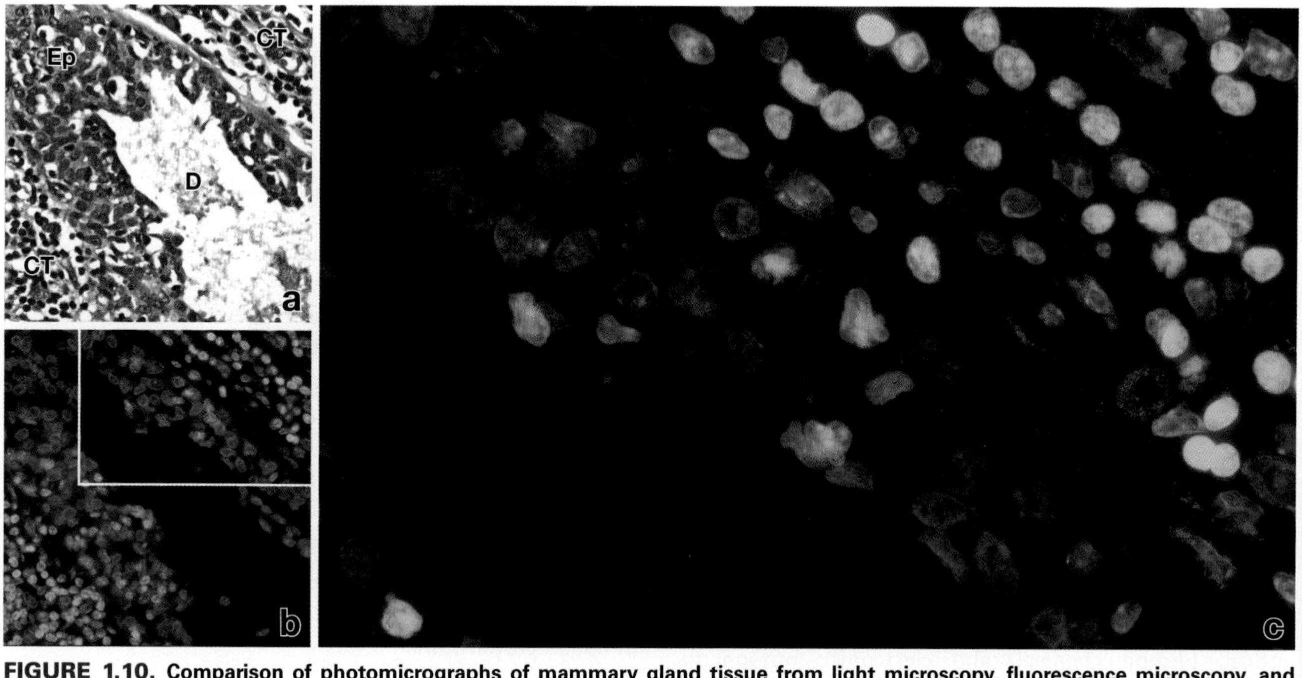

FIGURE 1.10. Comparison of photomicrographs of mammary gland tissue from light microscopy, fluorescence microscopy, and expansion microscopy. All images were obtained from serial sections of the same tissue and processed according to specific microscopy techniques. All images were obtained with the same 40× objective lens. **a.** This photomicrograph of a routine hematoxylin and eosin (H&E)-stained section shows the mammary duct (*D*) and surrounding connective tissue (*CT*). There is noticeable increase of cell layers within the ductal epithelium (*Ep*) that is indicative of usual ductal hyperplasia (UDH). Nuclei are stained blue with hematoxylin, and the pink elongated line beneath the epithelium represents connective tissue fibers stained with eosin. Note that the small and more intensely stained nuclei within the *CT* belong to infiltrating lymphocytes. ×460. **b.** This immunofluorescent image was obtained from the section stained for vimentin intermediate filaments. The vimentin proteins stained in magenta were labeled with polyclonal chicken antivimentin primary antibodies and visualized by secondary goat antichicken antibodies conjugated with fluorescent dye (Alexa Fluor 488). DNA has been counterstained with a nonspecific blue stain (DAPI stain) to make the nuclei visible. At this magnification, many nuclei are difficult to discern because of borderline resolution. ×460. **c.** Adjacent section of the same tissue shown in image b was processed for expansion microscopy. The specimen was embedded in the polyacrylate polymer and expanded 4.25 times. The image shows part of the section included within the rectangle in image **b** that was photographed at the same magnification ×460. Because of expansion of the tissue, resolution of this image is markedly improved compared with the routine immunofluorescent image taken at the same magnification. (Photomicrographs courtesy of Drs. Yongxin Zhao and Edward S. Boyden, Massachusetts Institute of Technology, Cambridge, MA.)

TABLE 1.3 Eye Versus Instrument Resolution

Distance Between Resolvable Points	
Human eye	0.2 mm
Bright-field microscope	0.2 μm
Super-resolution optical microscope	10–100 nm
Scanning electron microscope	2.5 nm
Transmission electron microscope	
Theoretical	0.05 nm
Tissue section	1.0 nm
Atomic force microscopy	50.0 pm

The **resolving power of the human eye**—that is, the distance by which two objects must be separated to be seen as two objects **(0.2 mm)**—is determined by the spacing of the photoreceptor cells in the retina. The role of a microscope is to magnify an image to a level at which the retina can resolve the information that would otherwise be below its limit of resolution. Table 1.3 compares the resolution of the eye with that of various instruments.

Resolving power is the ability of a microscope lens or optical system to produce separate images of closely positioned objects.

Resolution depends not only on the optical system but also on the wavelength of the light source and other factors such as specimen thickness, quality of fixation, and staining intensity. With light of wavelength 540 nm (see Table 1.1), a green-filtered light to which the eye is extremely sensitive, and appropriate objective and condenser lenses, the greatest attainable **resolving power of a bright-field microscope** is approximately **0.2 μm** (see Folder 1.4, page 15, for method of calculation). This theoretical resolution depends on all conditions being optimal. *The ocular or eyepiece lens magnifies the image produced by the objective lens, but it cannot increase resolution.*

Various **light microscopes** are available for general and specialized use in modern biologic research. Their differences are based largely on such factors as the wavelength of specimen illumination, physical alteration of the light coming into or leaving the specimen, and specific analytic processes that can be applied to the final image. Modern light microscopes are expensive and immensely complex, combining a growing number of optical, photomechanical, and electronic components. However, **low-cost, 3D-printed, open-source light microscopes** (i.e., UC2, μCube, etc.) are being designed that may be more widely available. Many of the light-, electron-, and nonoptical instruments used in education and research and their applications are described briefly in the following sections.

The microscope used by most students and researchers is the bright-field microscope.

The **bright-field microscope** is the direct descendant of the microscopes that became widely available in the 1800s and inaugurated the first major era of histologic research. The bright-field (light) microscope (Fig. F1.4.1 in Folder 1.4) essentially consists of

- a **light source** for illumination of the specimen (e.g., a substage lamp),
- a **condenser lens** to focus the beam of light at the level of the specimen,
- a **stage** on which the slide or other specimen is placed,
- an **objective lens** to gather the light that has passed through the specimen, and
- an **ocular lens** (or a pair of ocular lenses in the more commonly used binocular microscopes) through which the image formed by the objective lens may be examined directly.

A specimen to be examined with the bright-field microscope must be sufficiently thin for light to pass through it. Although some light is absorbed while passing through the specimen, the optical system of the bright-field microscope does not produce a useful level of contrast in unstained specimens. For this reason, various staining methods as discussed earlier are used.

Examination of a Histologic Slide Preparation in the Light Microscope

Organs are three-dimensional, whereas histologic sections are only two-dimensional.

As discussed in the earlier "Tissue Preparation" section, every tissue sample prepared for light microscopic examination must be sliced into thin sections. Thus, 2D sections are obtained from an original 3D sample of tissue. One of the most challenging aspects for students using the microscope to study histology is the ability to mentally reconstruct the "missing" third dimension.

For example, slices in different planes through an orange are shown in Figure 1.11. Note that each cut surface (indicated by the dotted line) of the whole orange reveals different sizes and surface patterns, depending on the orientation of the cut. Thus, it is important when observing a given section cut through the orange to be able to mentally reconstruct the organization of the structure and its component parts. An example of a histologic structure—in this case, a kidney renal corpuscle—is shown as it would appear in different sectional planes (see Fig. 1.11). Note the marked differences in size, orientation, and organization of surrounding tissue in each section of the renal corpuscle. By examining a number of such 2D sections, it is possible to perceive the 3D configuration of the examined structure.

Artifacts in histologic slides can be generated in all stages of tissue preparation.

The preparation of a histologic slide requires a series of steps beginning with the collection of the specimen and ending with the placement of the coverslip. During each step, an **artifact** (a defect caused by an error in the preparation process) may be introduced. In general, artifacts that appear on the finished glass slide are linked to methodology, equipment, or reagents used during preparation. The inferior purity of chemicals and reagents used in the process (fixatives, reagents, and stains), imperfections in the execution of the methodology (too short or too long intervals of fixation, dehydration, embedding, or staining, or careless mounting and placement of the coverslip), or improper equipment (e.g., a microtome with a

FOLDER 1.4

FUNCTIONAL CONSIDERATIONS: PROPER USE OF THE LIGHT MICROSCOPE

This brief introduction to the proper use of the light microscope is directed to those students who will use the microscope for the routine examination of tissues. If the following comments appear elementary, it is only because most users of the microscope fail to use it to its fullest advantage. Despite the availability of today's fine equipment, relatively little formal instruction is given on the correct use of the light microscope.

Expensive and highly corrected optics perform optimally only when the illumination and observation beam paths are centered and properly adjusted. The use of proper settings and proper alignment of the optic pathway will contribute substantially to the recognition of minute details in the specimen and to the faithful display of color for the visual image and for photomicrography.

Köhler illumination is one key to good microscopy and is incorporated in the design of practically all modern laboratory and research microscopes. Figure F1.4.1 shows a typical light path and the controls for alignment on a modern laboratory microscope; it should be referred to in following the instructions given here to provide appropriate illumination in your microscope.

The **alignment steps** necessary to achieve good Köhler illumination are few and simple:

- Focus the specimen.
- Close the field diaphragm.
- Focus the condenser by moving it up or down until the outline of its field diaphragm appears in sharp focus.
- Center the field diaphragm with the centering controls on the (condenser) substage. Then, open the field diaphragm until the light beam covers the full field observed.
- Remove the eyepiece (or use a centering telescope or a phase telescope accessory if available) and observe the exit pupil of the objective. You will see an illuminated circular field that has a radius directly proportional to the numeric aperture of the objective. As you close the condenser diaphragm, its outline will appear in this circular field. For most stained materials, set the condenser diaphragm to cover approximately two-thirds of the objective aperture. This setting results in the best compromise between resolution and contrast (contrast simply being the intensity difference between dark and light areas in the specimen).

Using only these five simple steps, the image obtained will be as good as the optics allow. Now, let us find out why.

First, why do we adjust the field diaphragm to cover only the field observed? Illuminating a larger field than the optics can "see" only leads to internal reflections or stray light, resulting in more "noise" or a decrease in image contrast.

Second, why do we emphasize the setting of the condenser diaphragm—that is, the illuminating aperture? This diaphragm greatly influences the resolution and the contrast with which specimen detail can be observed.

For most practical applications, the **resolution** is determined by the following equation:

$$d = \frac{\lambda}{NA_{objective} + NA_{condenser}}$$

where

d = point-to-point distance of resolved detail (in nm),
λ = wavelength of light used (green = 540 nm),
NA = numeric aperture or sine of half angle picked up by the objective or condenser of a central specimen point multiplied by the refractive index of the medium between objective or condenser and specimen.

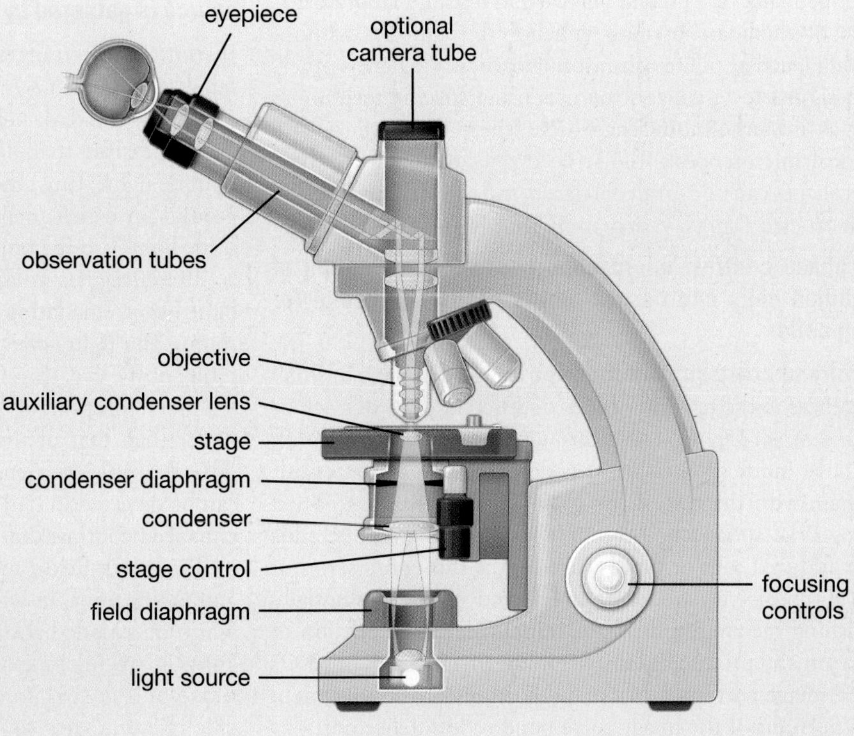

FIGURE F1.4.1. Diagram of a typical light microscope. This drawing shows a cross-sectional view of the microscope, its operating components, and light path.

(*continued*)

FOLDER 1.4

FUNCTIONAL CONSIDERATIONS: PROPER USE OF THE LIGHT MICROSCOPE (*continued*)

How do wavelength and numeric aperture directly influence resolution? Specimen structures diffract light. The diffraction angle is directly proportional to the wavelength and inversely proportional to the spacing of the structures. According to physicist Ernst Abbé, a given structural spacing can be resolved only when the observing optical system (objective) can see some of the diffracted light produced by the spacing. The larger the objective's aperture, the more diffracted the light that participates in the image formation, resulting in resolution of smaller detail and sharper images.

Our simple formula, however, shows that the condenser aperture is just as important as the objective aperture. This point is only logical when you consider the diffraction angle for an oblique beam or one of higher aperture. This angle remains essentially constant but is presented to the objective in such a fashion that it can be picked up easily.

How does the aperture setting affect the contrast? Theoretically, the best contrast transfer from object to image would be obtained by the interaction (interference) between nondiffracted and all the diffracted wave fronts.

For the transfer of contrast between full transmission and complete absorption in a specimen, the intensity relationship between diffracted and nondiffracted light would have to be 1:1 to achieve full destructive interference (black) or full constructive interference (bright). When the condenser aperture matches the objective aperture, the nondiffracted light enters the objective with full intensity, but only part of the diffracted light can enter, resulting in decreased contrast. In other words, closing the aperture of the condenser to two-thirds of the objective aperture brings the intensity relationship between diffracted and nondiffracted light close to 1:1 and thereby optimizes the contrast. Closing the condenser aperture (or lowering the condenser) beyond this equilibrium will produce interference phenomena or image artifacts such as diffraction rings or artificial lines around specimen structures. Most microscope techniques used for the enhancement of contrast—such as dark field, oblique illumination, phase contrast, or modulation contrast—are based on the same principle (i.e., they suppress or reduce the intensity of the nondiffracted light to improve an inherently low contrast of the specimen).

By observing the steps outlined earlier and maintaining clean lenses, the quality and fidelity of visual images will vary only with the performance capability of the optical system.

defective blade) can produce artifacts in the final preparation. It is important for students to recognize that not every slide in their slide collection is perfect and to be familiar with the most common artifacts found on their slides.

Other Optical Systems

Besides bright-field microscopy, which is commonly used for routine examination of histologic slides, other optical systems (described later) are used in clinical and research laboratories. Some of them are used to enhance the contrast without staining (such as phase contrast microscopes), whereas others are designed to visualize structures using specific techniques such as immunofluorescence (light sheet fluorescence and confocal microscopes). The serial images obtained by these microscopes can be captured in layers and three-dimensionally reconstructed using a variety of 3D image analysis software.

The phase contrast microscope enables examination of unstained cells and tissues and is especially useful for living cells.

The **phase contrast microscope** takes advantage of small differences in the refractive index of different parts of a cell or tissue sample. Light passing through areas of relatively high refractive index (denser areas) is deflected and becomes out of phase with the rest of the beam of light that has passed through the specimen. The phase contrast microscope adds other induced, out-of-phase wavelengths through a series of optical rings in the condenser and objective lenses, essentially abolishing the amplitude of the initially deflected portion of the beam and producing contrast in the image. Dark portions of the image correspond to dense portions of the specimen; light portions of the image correspond to less dense portions of the specimen. The phase contrast microscope is used to examine living cells and tissues (such as cells in tissue culture) and extensively to examine unstained semithin (approximately 0.5 μm) sections of plastic-embedded tissue.

Two modifications of the phase contrast microscope are the **interference microscope**, which also allows quantification of tissue mass, and the **differential interference microscope** (using Nomarski optics), which is especially useful for assessing surface properties of cells and other biologic objects.

In dark-field microscopy, no direct light from the light source is gathered by the objective lens.

In **dark-field microscopy**, only light that has been scattered or diffracted by structures in the specimen reaches the objective. The dark-field microscope is equipped with a special condenser that illuminates the specimen with strong, oblique light. Thus, the field of view appears as a dark background on which small particles in the specimen that reflect some light into the objective appear bright.

The effect is similar to that of dust particles seen in the light beam emanating from a slide projector in a darkened room. The light reflected off the dust particles reaches the retina of the eye, thus making the particles visible.

The resolution of the dark-field microscope cannot be better than that of the bright-field microscope, using, as it does, the same wavelength source. Smaller individual particles can be detected in dark-field images, however, because of the enhanced contrast that is created.

The dark-field microscope is useful in examining autoradiographs, in which the developed silver grains appear white in a dark background. Clinically, **dark-field microscopy** is useful in examining urine for crystals, such as those of uric acid and oxalate, and in demonstrating specific bacteria such as **spirochetes**, particularly *Treponema pallidum*, the microorganism that causes **syphilis**, a sexually transmitted disease.

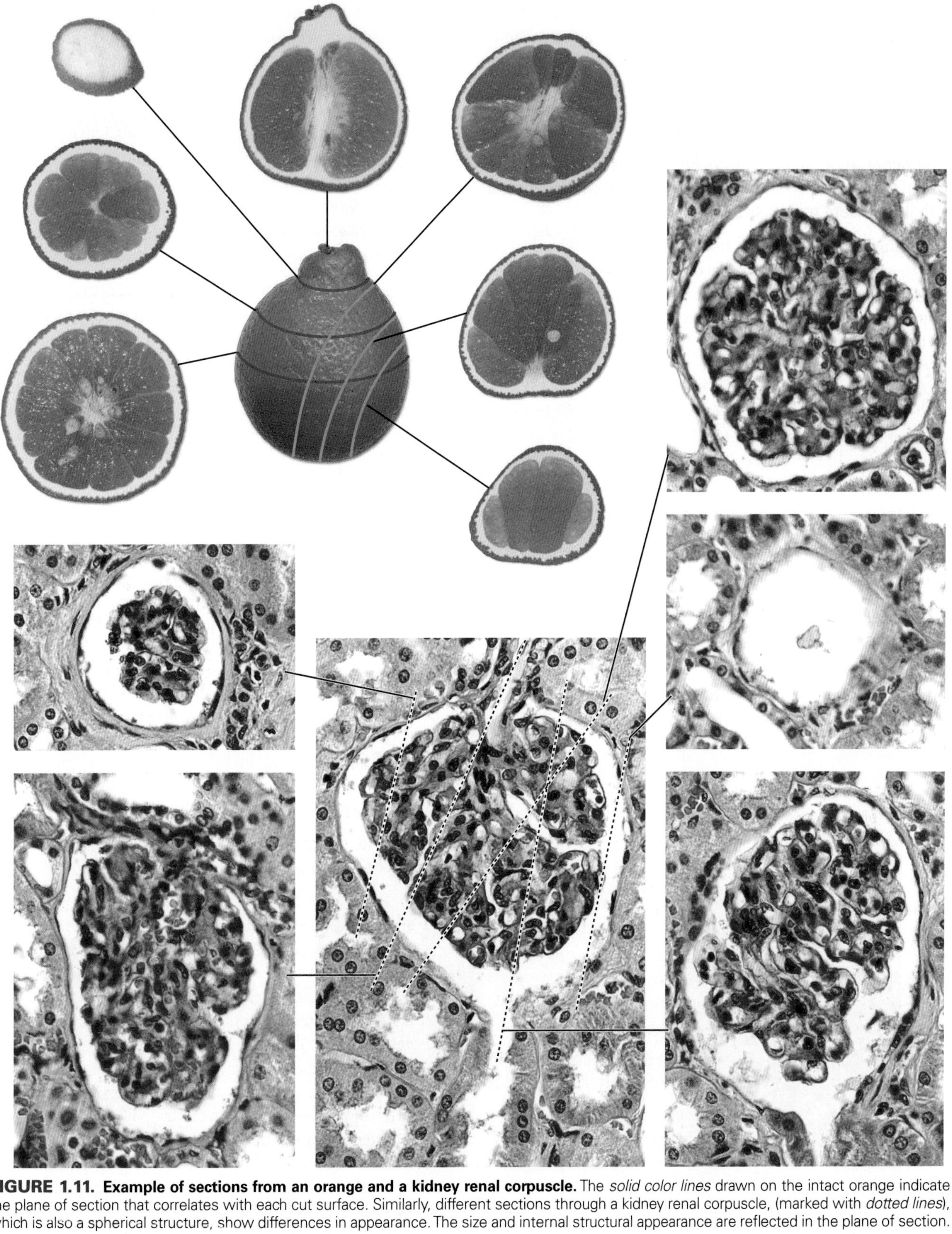

FIGURE 1.11. Example of sections from an orange and a kidney renal corpuscle. The *solid color lines* drawn on the intact orange indicate the plane of section that correlates with each cut surface. Similarly, different sections through a kidney renal corpuscle, (marked with *dotted lines*), which is also a spherical structure, show differences in appearance. The size and internal structural appearance are reflected in the plane of section.

The fluorescence microscope makes use of the ability of certain molecules to fluoresce under ultraviolet light.

Fluorescent molecules are those that emit light of wavelengths in the visible range when exposed to an ultraviolet (UV) source. The **fluorescence microscope** is used to display naturally occurring fluorescent (autofluorescent) molecules such as vitamin A and some neurotransmitters. Because autofluorescent molecules are not numerous, the microscope's most common application is the display of introduced fluorescence, as in the detection of antigens or antibodies in immunocytochemical staining procedures (see Fig. 1.6). Specific **fluorescent molecules (fluorophores)** can also be injected into an animal or directly into cells and used as tracers. Such methods have been useful in studying intercellular (gap) junctions, tracing the pathway of nerve fibers in neurobiology, and detecting fluorescent growth markers of mineralized tissues. Various filters are inserted between the

UV light source and the specimen to produce monochromatic or near-monochromatic (single-wavelength or narrow-band-wavelength) light. A second set of filters inserted between the specimen and the objective allows only the narrow band of wavelength of the fluorescence to reach the eye or to reach an image sensor in the digital recording device.

Light sheet fluorescence microscopy utilizes a thin plane of light to optically section a transparent specimen labeled with fluorescent molecules.

Light sheet fluorescence microscopy (LSFM) utilizes a light sheet that is formed by a flat laser beam. This **thin sheet of light** is formed in the focal plane and optically sections transparent specimen labeled with fluorescent dyes. The fluorescent light emitted from the specimen is then collected perpendicularly to the light path by the objective of the microscope and recorded by an imaging sensor (e.g., a charge-coupled device or CCD). The specimen is illuminated only in a **single focal plane** at a time, avoiding excitation from out-of-focus areas of the specimen. The light sheet itself can be static or dynamically formed by a moving (scanning) laser beam approximating a light sheet over a short period of time. By moving the sample through the light sheet, images can be recorded in layers and three-dimensionally reconstructed (Fig. 1.12).

Fluorescence microscopy is currently one of the more powerful and versatile techniques available for studies of biologic specimens.

Most modern research laboratories utilize fluorescence microscopy as a primary tool in biologic research. Fluorescent molecules (fluorophores) have been engineered to absorb light at a specific wavelength and to emit light at a longer wavelength. These molecules appear very bright and are readily distinguishable in tissue sections from other background signals. In addition, with the development of genetically encoded **fluorescent proteins (FPs)**, it has become possible to visualize and create images of protein expression, localization, and activity in living cells. The combination of fluorescence and confocal microscopic techniques with fast data processing hardware allows investigators to render the images in three dimensions.

The ultraviolet microscope uses quartz lenses with an ultraviolet light source.

The image in the **ultraviolet (UV) microscope** depends on the absorption of UV light by molecules in the specimen. The UV source has a wavelength of approximately 200 nm. Thus, the UV microscope may achieve a resolution of 0.1 μm. The general principle behind UV microscopy resembles that of a spectrophotometer; the results are usually recorded photographically. The specimen cannot be inspected directly through an ocular lens because the UV light is not visible and is injurious to the eye.

UV microscopy is useful in detecting nucleic acids, specifically the purine and pyrimidine bases of the nucleotides. It is also useful for detecting proteins that contain certain amino acids. Using specific illuminating wavelengths, UV spectrophotometric measurements are commonly made through the UV microscope to determine quantitatively the amount of DNA and RNA in individual cells. As described in Folder 1.2 on page 7, **Feulgen microspectrophotometry** is used clinically to evaluate the degree of ploidy (multiples of normal DNA quantity) in sections of tumors.

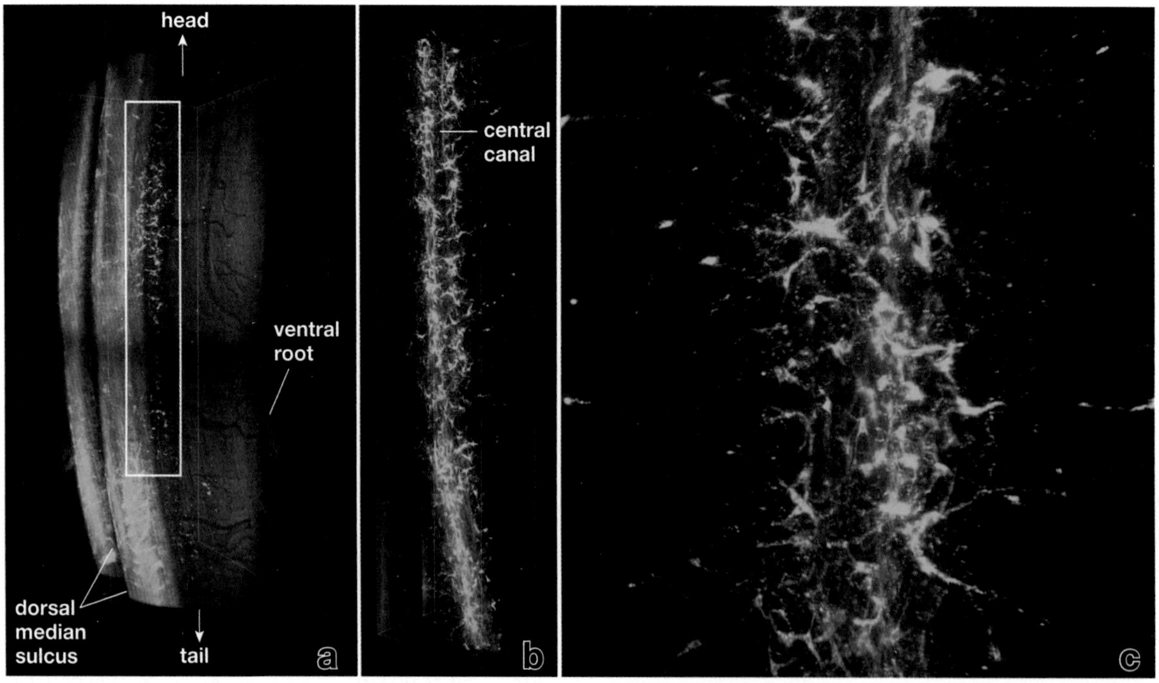

FIGURE 1.12. Light sheet fluorescence microscopy (LSFM) image of cells expressing galanin neuropeptide in the spinal cord of an adult male rat. a. This photomicrograph shows a three-dimensional (3D) rendering of an LSFM image of the rat spinal cord at the L3 and L4 vertebral levels. Within the *rectangle*, note the immunofluorescent labeling of galanin neuropeptide expressed in the spinothalamic cells. This neuropeptide was detected by the indirect immunofluorescence method using polyclonal rabbit anti-galanin primary antibodies and then visualized by using goat anti-rabbit secondary antibodies conjugated with fluorescein dye (Alexa Fluor 647). After immunostaining, the specimen was cleared in dibenzyl ether (DBE) and the transparent tissue was imaged in the horizontal plane using bidirectional LSFM. Stacks of TIFF images were collected at 4 μm optical intervals and linked together using specialized imaging software. The reconstructed image was then artificially colored in *green*. The 3D rendering allows the image to be rotated and examined from all possible directions. ×10. **b.** This image represents a higher magnification of galanin-positive spinothalamic cells with the spinal cord background shown in the *rectangle* subtracted. Note that galanin-positive cells are in close proximity to the central canal. ×22. **c.** High-magnification view of galanin-expressing spinothalamic cells showing their interconnecting pattern. ×110. (Courtesy of Drs. Aleisha M. Moore, Michael N. Lehman, and Lique M. Coolen.)

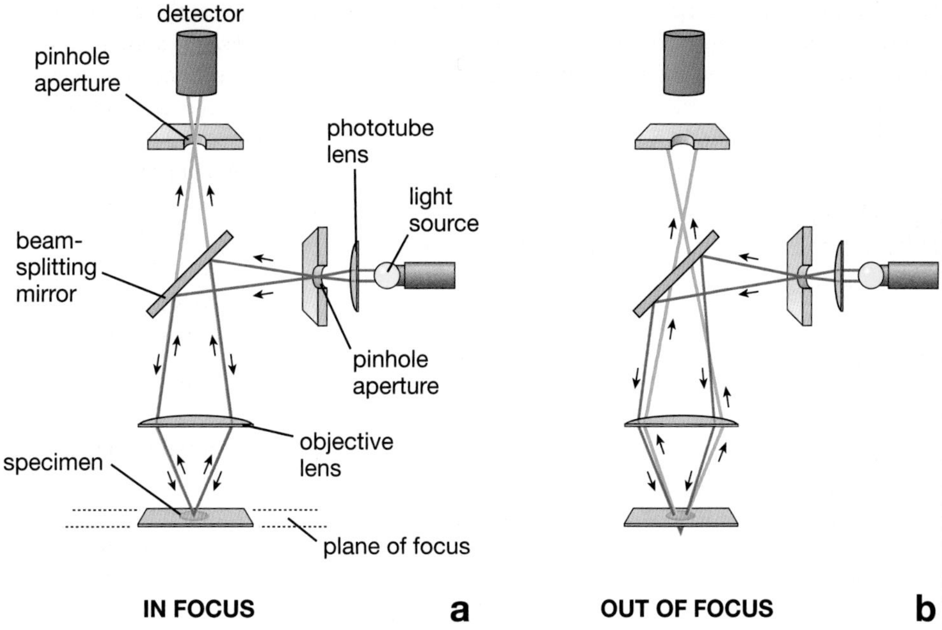

FIGURE 1.13. Diagram of the in-focus and out-of-focus emitted light in the confocal microscope. **a.** This diagram shows the path of the laser beam and emitted light when the imaging structure is directly at the focus of the lens. The screen with a pinhole at the other side of the optical system of the confocal microscope allows the light from the structure in focus to pass through the pinhole. The light is then translated into an image by computer software. Because the focal point of the objective lens of the microscope forms a sharp image at the level at which the pinhole is located, these two points are referred to as *confocal points.* **b.** This diagram shows the path of the laser beam and the emitted light, which is out of focus in relation to the pinhole. Thus, the light from the specimen that gets blocked by the pinhole is never detected.

The confocal scanning microscope combines components of a light optical microscope with a scanning system to dissect a specimen optically.

The **confocal scanning microscope** allows visualization of a biologic specimen in three dimensions. The two lenses in the confocal microscope (objective and phototube lens) are perfectly aligned to focus light from the focal point of one lens to the focal point of the other lens. The major difference between a conventional and a confocal microscope is the addition of a **detector aperture** (pinhole) that is *con*jugate with the *focal* point of the lens; therefore, it is **confocal**. This precisely positioned pinhole allows only "in-focus" light to pass into a photomultiplier (detector) device, whereas the "out-of-focus" light is blocked from entering the detector (Fig. 1.13). This system has the capability to obtain exceptional resolution (0.2–0.5 μm) and clarity from a thin section of a biologic sample simply by rejecting out-of-focus light.

The light source in a confocal microscope comes from an illuminating laser light system that is strongly convergent and therefore produces a high-intensity excitation light in the form of a shallow scanning spot. A mirror system is used to move the laser beam across the specimen, illuminating a single spot at a time (Fig. 1.14). Many single spots in the same focal plane are scanned, and a computer software program reconstructs the image from the data recorded during scanning. In this aspect, confocal microscopy resembles the imaging process in a computerized axial tomography (CAT) scan.

Furthermore, by using only the narrow depth of the in-focus image, it is possible to create multiple images at varying depths within the specimen. Thus, one can literally dissect layer by layer through the thickness of the specimen. It is also possible to use the computer to make 3D reconstructions of a series of these images. Because each individual image located at a specific depth within the specimen is extremely sharp, the resulting assembled 3D image is equally sharp. Moreover, once the computer has assembled each sectioned image, the reconstructed 3D image can be animated for viewing on the computer from any orientation desired (see Fig. 1.4).

The polarizing microscope exploits the fact that highly ordered molecules or arrays of molecules can rotate the angle of the plane of polarized light.

The **polarizing microscope** is a simple modification of the light microscope in which a polarizing filter (the **polarizer**) is located between the light source and the specimen, and a second polarizer (the **analyzer**) is located between the objective lens and the viewer.

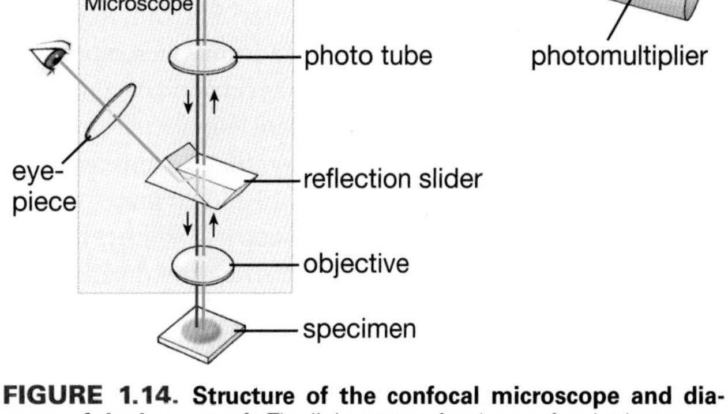

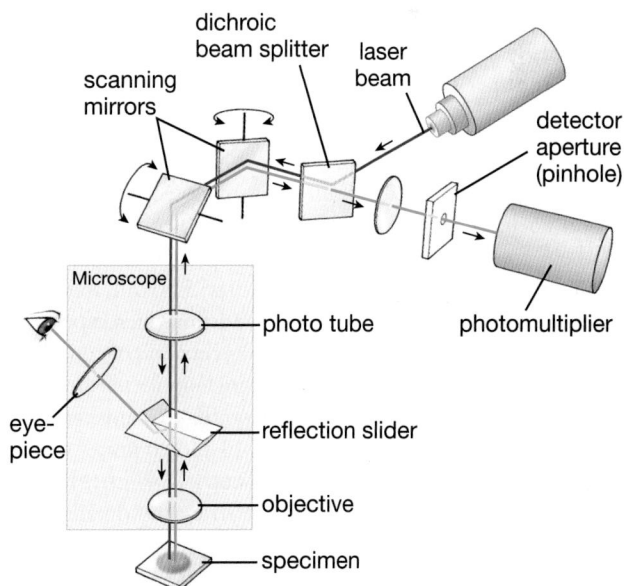

FIGURE 1.14. Structure of the confocal microscope and diagram of the beam path. The light source for the confocal microscope comes from a laser. The laser beam (*red line*) travels to the tissue sample via a dichroic beam splitter and then to two movable scanning mirrors; these mirrors scan the laser beam across the sample in both *x* and *y* directions. Finally, the laser beam enters the fluorescence microscope and travels through its optical system to illuminate an examined tissue sample. The emitted light by the illuminated tissue sample (*blue line*) travels back through the optical system of the microscope, through both scanning mirrors, passes through the beam splitter, and is focused onto the pinhole. The light that passes through the pinhole is received and registered by the detector attached to a computer that builds the image one pixel at a time.

Both the polarizer and the analyzer can be rotated; the difference between their angles of rotation is used to determine the degree by which a structure affects the beam of polarized light. The ability of a crystal or paracrystalline array to rotate the plane of polarized light is called **birefringence** (double refraction). Striated muscle and the crystalloid inclusions in testicular interstitial cells (Leydig cells), among other common structures, exhibit birefringence.

Super-Resolution Microscopy

Conventional optical microscopes have an inherent limitation in resolving power because of the wavelength of light. The resolution, which is defined by the minimum point-to-point distance between two distinguishable details, is restricted by the diffraction limit of the light. Diffraction causes the light signal from the specimen to spread as it travels to the eye of the observer or other light detector devices. As discussed earlier, the resolution of an optical microscope with an optimal alignment of the objective and condenser lenses is limited to 0.2 μm; therefore, it is unable to resolve many detailed cellular structures.

Newer super-resolution microscopy techniques are able to overcome the resolution limit of conventional light microscopy.

For decades, researchers have been searching for techniques that could exceed the resolution limit of the optical microscope. Recent conceptual advances and technical innovation resulted in increases in optical resolution from 0.2 μm to ~10 nm. Any microscopy technique that increases the resolution of a conventional light microscope dictated by the diffraction barrier by at least a factor of 2 is called **super-resolution microscopy**.

Several super-resolution microscopy techniques have been developed to study living cells under fluorescence light microscopy. In general, there are three methods that are utilized in super-resolution microscopy:

- **Single-molecule localization methods**, which include photoactivated localization microscopy (PALM), fluorescence photoactivated localization microscopy (FPALM), and stochastic optical reconstruction microscopy (STORM). These methods involve the use of photoactivatable and photoswitchable fluorescent molecules that can transition between the state of dark and bright emission when exposed to specific wavelengths of light. Computer analysis of combined data obtained from thousands of single-molecule intensity profiles and microscope diffraction profile are converted into an image with a resolution between 10 and 20 nm.
- **Structured illumination microscopy (SIM) methods**, which are based on extracting fine structural details from the interference of a structure with predetermined illumination patterns. Because this method utilizes spatial frequencies, which are also limited by diffraction, SIM microscopy can only improve the resolution by a factor of 2 (resolution ~100 nm).
- **Point-scanning methods**, which include stimulated emission depletion (STED) microscopy and isotropic stimulated emission depletion (isoSTED) microscopy. These methods are based on laser scanning confocal microscopy with the addition of a depletion laser, which stimulates excited molecules to revert back to the ground state. Using STED microscopy, image resolution of 30–80 nm can be achieved.

Super-resolution microscopy methods offer new opportunities for revealing details of cellular structures in living cells at a higher resolution that was not previously achievable with conventional fluorescence microscopy.

Electron Microscopy

In general, two kinds of EMs can provide morphologic and analytic data about cells and tissues: the **transmission electron microscope (TEM)** and the **scanning electron microscope (SEM)**. The primary improvement in the EM versus the light microscope is that the wavelength of the EM beam is approximately 1/2,000th that of the light microscope beam, thereby increasing resolution by a factor of 10^3.

The TEM uses the interaction of a beam of electrons with a specimen to produce an image.

The optics of the TEM are, in principle, similar to those of the light microscope (Fig. 1.15), except that the TEM uses a beam of electrons rather than a beam of light. The principle of the microscope is as follows:

- An electron source (**cathode, electron emitter, electron gun**), such as a heated tungsten filament, emits electrons.
- The negatively charged **electrons** are attracted toward an **anode**, which is the positively charged electron collector.
- An electrical difference between the cathode cover and the anode imparts an accelerating voltage of between 20,000 and 200,000 volts to the electrons, creating the **electron beam**.
- The beam then passes through a series of **electromagnetic lenses** that serve the same function as the glass lenses of a light microscope.

The **condenser lens** shapes and changes the diameter of the **electron beam** that reaches the specimen plane. The beam that has passed through the specimen is then focused and magnified by an **objective lens** and then further magnified by one or more **projector lenses**. The final image is viewed on a phosphor-coated **fluorescent screen** or captured on a **photographic plate**. Portions of the specimen through which electrons have passed appear bright; dark portions of the specimen have absorbed or scattered electrons because of their inherent density or because of heavy metals added during specimen preparation. Often, an electron detector with a light-sensitive sensor such as a **charge-coupled device (CCD)** is placed above or below the viewing screen to observe the image in real time on a monitor. This allows images or videos to be archived in digital format for storage on computers.

Specimen preparation for transmission electron microscopy is similar to that for light microscopy except that it requires finer methods.

The principles used in the preparation of sections for viewing with the TEM are essentially the same as those used in light microscopy, with the added constraint that at every step one must work with specimens three to four orders of magnitude smaller or thinner than those used for light microscopy. The TEM, which has an electron beam wavelength of approximately 0.1 nm, has a theoretical resolution of 0.05 nm.

Because of the exceptional resolution of the TEM, the quality of fixation—that is, the degree of preservation of subcellular structure—must be the best achievable.

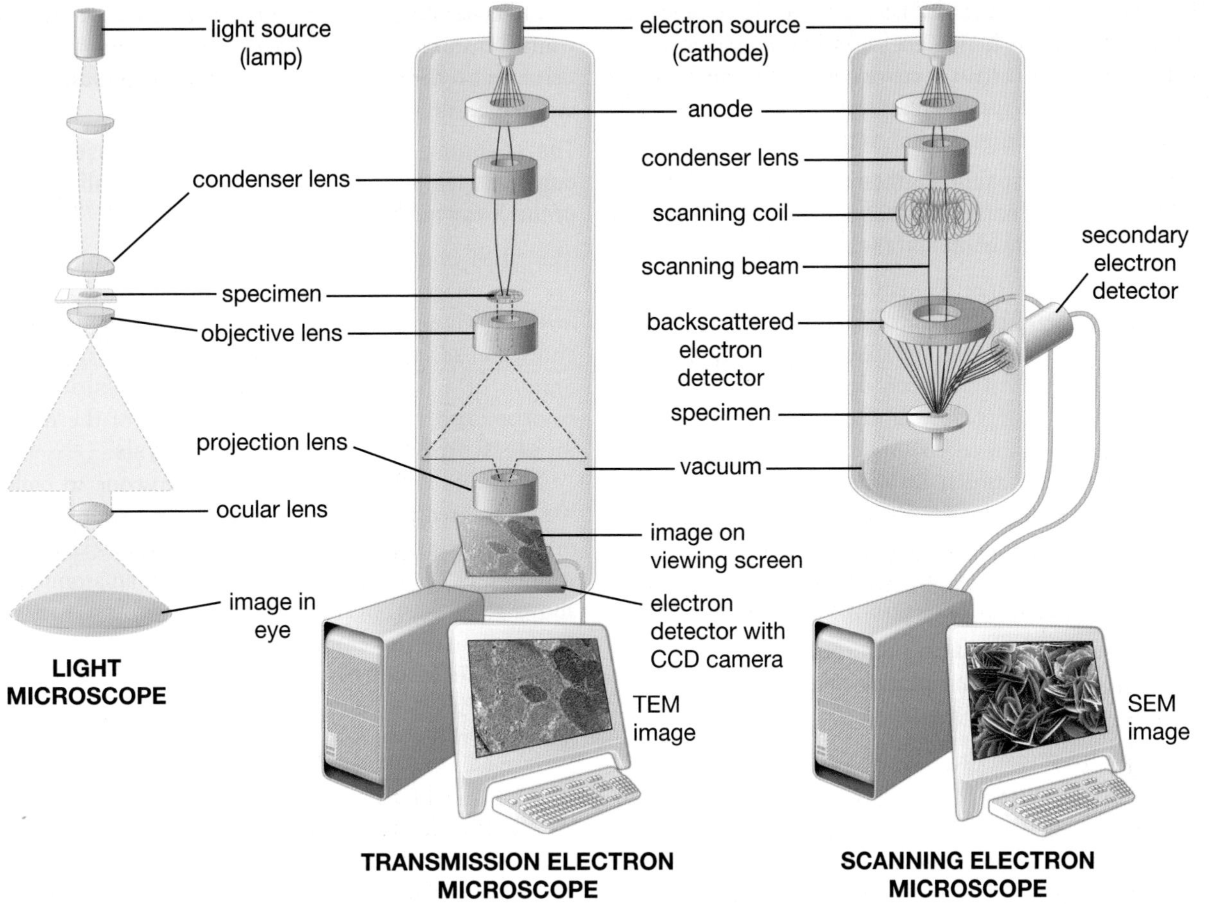

FIGURE 1.15. Diagram comparing the optical paths in different types of microscopes. For better comparison among all three types of microscopes, the light microscope (*left*) is shown as if it were turned upside down. Note that in both the transmission electron microscope (*TEM*) and the scanning electron microscope (*SEM*), specimens need to be inserted into a high-vacuum (10^{-4} to 10^{-7} Pa) environment.

Routine preparation of specimens for transmission electron microscopy begins with glutaraldehyde fixation followed by a buffer rinse and fixation with osmium tetroxide.

Glutaraldehyde, a dialdehyde, preserves protein constituents by cross-linking them; **osmium tetroxide** reacts with lipids, particularly phospholipids. The osmium also imparts electron density to cell and tissue structures because it is a heavy metal, thus enhancing subsequent image formation in the TEM.

Ideally, tissues should be perfused with buffered glutaraldehyde before excision. More commonly, tissue pieces no more than 1 mm^3 are fixed for the TEM (compared with light microscope specimens, which may be measured in centimeters). The dehydration process is identical to that used in light microscopy, and the tissue is infiltrated with a monomeric resin, usually an **epoxy resin**, that is subsequently polymerized.

The plastic-embedded tissue is sectioned on specially designed microtomes using diamond knives.

Because of the limited penetrating power of electrons, sections for routine TEM range from 50 nm to no more than 150 nm. Also, for the reason that abrasives used to sharpen steel knives leave unacceptable scratches on sections viewed in the TEM, **diamond knives** with a nearly perfect cutting edge are used. Sections cut by the diamond knife are much too thin to handle; they are floated away from the knife edge on the surface of a fluid-filled trough and picked up from the surface onto plastic-coated copper mesh grids. The grids have 50–400 holes per inch or special slots for viewing serial sections. The beam passes through the specimen and then through the holes in the copper grid, and the image is then focused on the viewing screen, CCD, or photographic film.

Routine staining of transmission electron microscopy sections is necessary to increase the inherent contrast of cell structures so that details are readily visible and photographable.

In general, TEM sections are stained by adding materials of great density, such as ions of heavy metals, to the specimen. **Heavy metal ions** may be bound to the tissues during fixation or dehydration or by soaking the sections in solutions of ions after sectioning. **Osmium tetroxide**, routinely used in the fixative, binds to the phospholipid components of membranes, imparting additional density to the membranes.

Uranyl nitrate is often added to the alcohol solutions used in dehydration to increase the density of components of cell junctions and other sites. Sequential soaking in solutions of **uranyl acetate** and **lead citrate** is routinely used to stain sections before viewing with the TEM to provide high-resolution, high-contrast electron micrographs.

Sometimes, special staining is required to visualize results of histocytochemical or immunocytochemical reactions with the TEM. Phosphatase and esterase procedures are used for this purpose (see Fig. 1.3). Substitution of a **heavy metal–containing compound** for the fluorescent dye that has been conjugated with an antibody allows the adaptation of immunocytochemical methods to TEM. Similarly, routine **EM autoradiography techniques** have been refined for use with TEM (see Fig. 1.8b). These methods have been particularly useful in elucidating the cellular sources and intracellular pathways of certain secretory products, the location on the cell surface of specific receptors, and the intracellular location of ingested drugs and substrates.

Freeze fracture is a special method of sample preparation for transmission electron microscopy; it is especially important in the study of membranes.

Freeze fracture is a special method of sample preparation that physically breaks apart (fractures) a frozen specimen to reveal its internal structures. The tissue to be examined may be fixed or unfixed; if it has been fixed, then the fixative is washed out of the tissue before proceeding. A cryoprotectant such as glycerol is allowed to infiltrate the tissue, and the tissue is then rapidly frozen to about −160°C. Ice crystal formation is prevented by the use of cryoprotectants, rapid freezing, and extremely small tissue samples. The frozen tissue is then placed in a vacuum in the freeze fracture apparatus and struck with a knife edge or razor blade.

The fracture plane passes preferentially through the hydrophobic portion of the plasma membrane, exposing the interior of the plasma membrane.

The resulting fracture of the plasma membrane produces two new surfaces. The surface of the membrane that is backed by the extracellular space is called the **E-face**; the face backed by the protoplasm (cytoplasm) is called the **P-face**. The specimen is then coated, typically with evaporated platinum and carbon, to create a replica of the fracture surface. The tissue is dissolved, and the surface replica, not the tissue itself, is picked up on grids to be examined with the TEM. Such a replica displays planar views of the internal organization of membranes with details at the macromolecular level (see Fig. 2.5, page 34). One of the most common uses of the freeze fracture technique is to examine zonula occludens junctions, where integral membrane proteins bind cells together (see Fig. 5.15c, page 141).

In scanning electron microscopy, the electron beam does not pass through the specimen but is scanned across its surface.

In many ways, the images obtained from the SEM more closely resemble those seen on a television screen than on the TEM monitor. They are 3D in appearance and portray the surface structure of an examined sample. For the examination of most tissues, the sample is fixed, dehydrated by critical point drying, coated with an evaporated gold–carbon film, mounted on an aluminum stub, and placed in the vacuum chamber of the SEM. For mineralized tissues, it is possible to remove all the soft tissues with bleach and then examine the structural features of the mineral.

Scanning is accomplished by the same type of raster that scans the electron beam across the face of a television tube. Electrons reflected from the surface (**backscattered electrons**) and electrons forced out of the surface (**secondary electrons**) are collected by one or more detectors and reprocessed to form a high-resolution 3D image of a sample surface (see Fig. 1.15). In earlier models of microscopes, images were captured on a high-resolution cathode ray tube (CRT) or photographic plate; modern instruments, however, capture digital images using sensitive detectors and CCD for display on a high-resolution computer monitor.

Other detectors can be used to measure X-rays emitted from the surface, cathodoluminescence of molecules in the tissue below the surface, and very-low-energy Auger electrons emitted at the surface.

The scanning-transmission electron microscope (STEM) combines features of the TEM and SEM to allow electron-probe X-ray microanalysis.

The SEM configuration can be used to produce a transmission image by inserting a grid holder at the specimen level, collecting the transmitted electrons with a detector, and reconstructing the image on a CRT. This latter configuration of a SEM or **scanning-transmission electron microscope (STEM)** facilitates the use of the instrument for **electron-probe X-ray microanalysis.**

Detectors can be fitted to the microscope to collect the X-rays emitted as the beam bombards the section; with appropriate analyzers, a map can be constructed that shows the distribution in the sections of elements with an atomic number above 12 and a concentration sufficient to produce enough X-rays to analyze. Semiquantitative data can also be derived for elements in sufficient concentration. Thus, both the TEM and the SEM can be converted into sophisticated analytical tools in addition to being used as "optical" instruments.

Three-dimensional electron microscopy is used for reconstructing entire cells, their connections, and their organelles.

Single 2D images obtained from TEM impose several limitations in interpreting different cellular structures, such as their size, shape, number, and relationship to neighboring structures. However, single 2D images (in serial sections) can be used to recreate 3D models of a structure of interest. Reconstructed 3D models of imaged structures allow researchers to obtain new information on volume, surface area, spatial distribution, and contact area between different structures.

In the last decade, the **three-dimensional electron microscopy (3DEM)** has rapidly developed to include several powerful imaging modalities. In general, 3D reconstruction is possible with both TEM and SEM that allows multiple views of specimens to be collected and analyzed using 3D reconstruction software. Several methods, such as serial section TEM, focused ion beam SEM, serial block-face SEM, image segmentation, and 3D reconstructions of cells and tissues, are currently utilized for obtaining 3D images at the ultrastructural level. 3D reconstruction is especially helpful in **connectomics**, a field that specializes in studying the brain's structural and functional connections between nerve cells. With the recent imaging of the entire network of synaptic connections within the brain of *Drosophila melanogaster* (fruit fly), mapping of all neural connections in the human brain using 3DEM techniques may be possible in the distant future. The following approaches to 3D visualization at the EM level are frequently used:

- **Serial section TEM (SSTEM).** This technique involves sectioning epoxy resin–embedded tissues using an ultramicrotome and collecting the arrays of consecutive aligned sections throughout the specimen. Each section from the collected ribbons is placed on a grid and separately imaged using TEM. The advantage of using SSTEM is that all individual sections can be preserved, archived, and reimaged. Using image analysis software, EM images can be aligned, segmented, and modeled to generate 3D images of selected structures.

- **Focused ion beam SEM (FIBSEM).** This technique takes advantage of dual beam instruments with two imaging columns. The first column is a standard electron column found in SEMs, and the second ion column generates positively charged ions (frequently, liquid metal gallium is used as a source of ions). Both columns have scan coils, which allow the beams of electrons and ions to move across the surface of the imaging sample. As the high-momentum ion beam is moved over the specimen, it mills away (removes) a very thin layer of the specimen. The imaging beam of electrons follows, allowing the SEM detector to capture backscattered and emitted secondary electrons to visualize the block surface between rounds of milling. A series of images are generated that are assembled into 3D images.
- **Serial block-face SEM (SBFSEM).** The basic principle of this technique is the presence of an ultramicrotome within the vacuum chamber of a SEM that removes thin slices of the embedded specimen. The top of the block face is imaged before the surface is shaved away by a diamond knife at a specified depth, revealing a new block face, which is again imaged. This cyclical repetition captures an automatically aligned stack of serial images of tissues sequentially removed from the block. Collected images are then reconstructed using 3D image analysis software. Specific organelles of interest can be segmented out and recreated in 3D (Fig. 1.16).

Image segmentation allows for visualization of structures of interest by assigning a label to every pixel associated with the structure

In generating 3D models, **image segmentation** allows for visualizing selected structures of interest. In this process, individual pixels are assigned to objects, giving them a "label." Segmentation can be performed manually by a researcher or automatically using computer algorithms. For example, identifying and assigning all pixels related to the nuclear membrane to a "nuclear membrane" label allows the user to tract the pixel distribution throughout serial sections and reconstruct them into a 3D object (Fig. 1.16).

- **Manual segmentation** is a labor-intensive and time-consuming process. It is often done by tracing selected structures with a computer mouse, pen, or stylus on a drawing tablet or touch-sensitive screen. The user then "paints" labels onto the 3D stack of images.
- **Automatic segmentation** uses image **segmentation algorithms** based on user-defined or preexisting criteria. Most commonly, a **basic thresholding segmentation** algorithm is the most successful in achieving good 3D imaging. During this procedure, the researcher selects a specific threshold value of pixel intensity, and all pixels with an intensity equal to or above the selected intensity value are automatically assigned to an object label. This approach is especially suited to images with highly contrasted and selectively stained structures of interest (i.e., individual neurons with biocytin stain or where osmium tetroxide

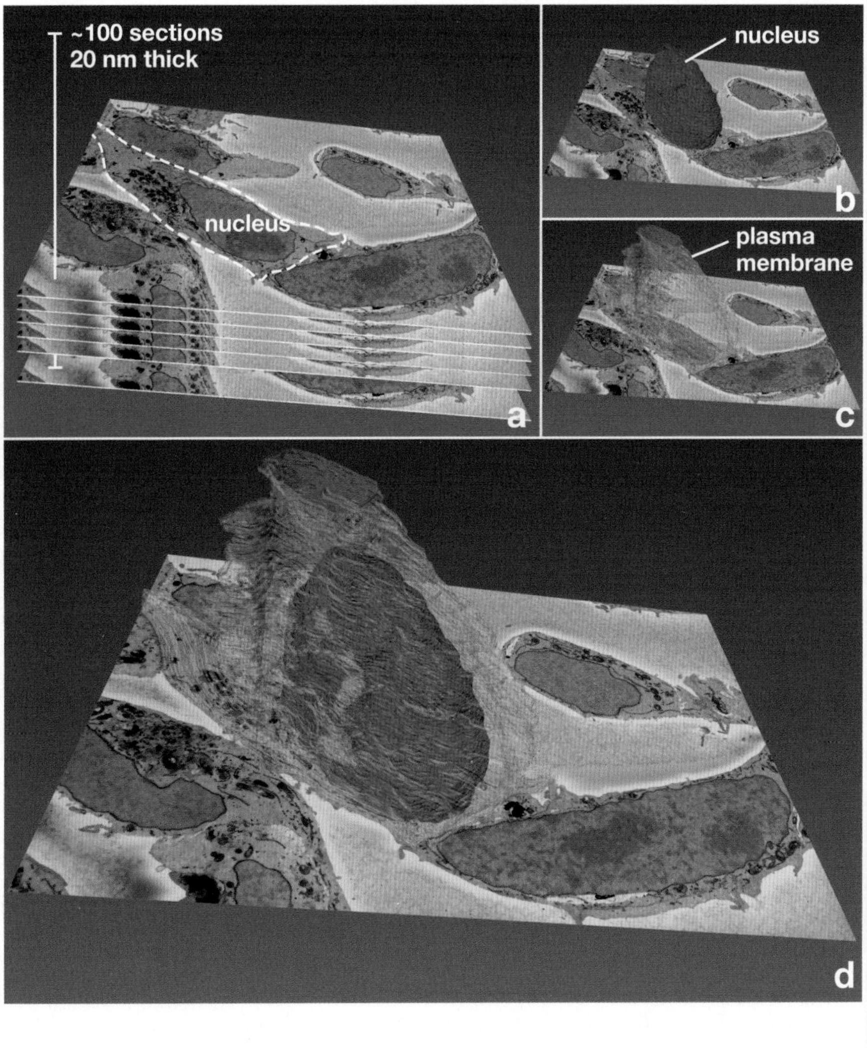

FIGURE 1.16. Serial block-face scanning electron microscopy (SBFSEM) image of the cell membrane and nuclear envelope. This image of human embryonic kidney cells growing in culture (HEK-293 cell line) was obtained using SBFSEM. Cells were routinely prepared for SEM, and an epoxy resin block containing the sample was placed in the vacuum chamber containing an ultramicrotome. **a.** The top of the block face was imaged by an electron beam before the block face was cut off by the microtome at a thickness of ~20 nm, revealing a new block face that was again imaged. This process was repeated until ~100 images of sequential sections were collected. The *dashed line* outlines the cell of interest for three-dimensional (3D) reconstruction. The black inclusions in the cytoplasm represent gold nanoparticles taken up by cells. The block-imaged face and subsequent serial sections that were scanned and removed are shown. The collected 3D data set was manually segmented by tracing the nuclear envelope shown in panel **b** (*blue structure*) and the cell membrane shown in panel **c** (*green structure*). Panel **d** shows a superimposed reconstructed 3D image of the cell membrane and the nucleus within the cell. ×8,000 (panel d). (Courtesy of Dr. Louis J. Maher and Brandon A. Wilbanks, Mayo Clinic, Rochester, MN.)

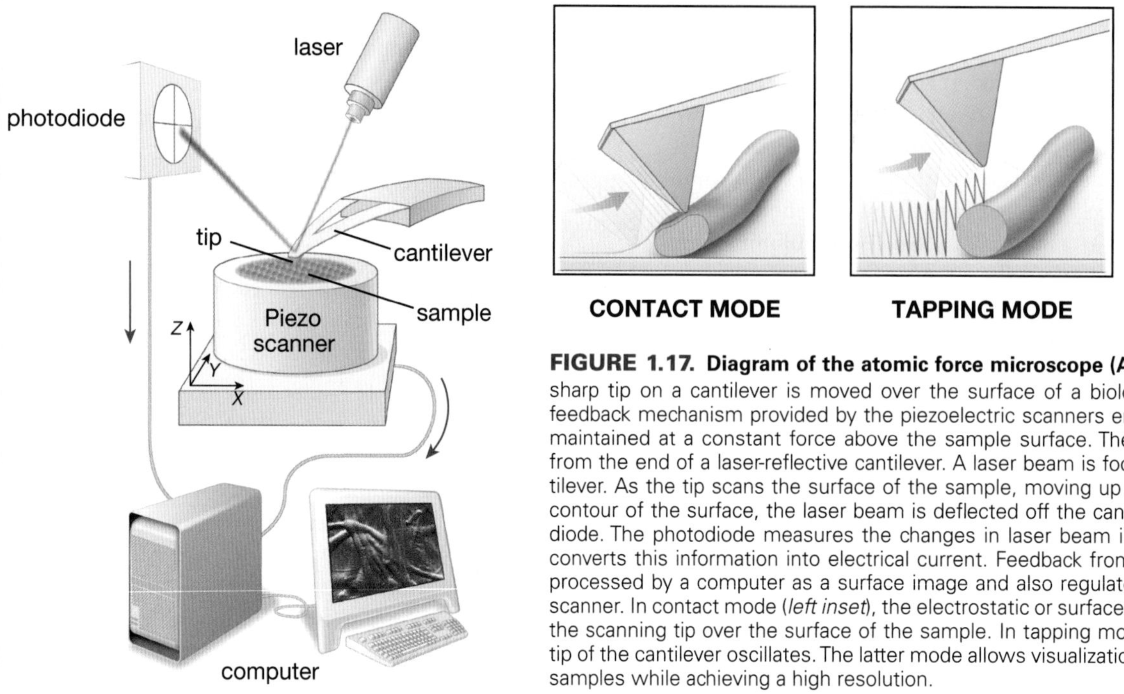

FIGURE 1.17. Diagram of the atomic force microscope (AFM). An extremely sharp tip on a cantilever is moved over the surface of a biologic specimen. The feedback mechanism provided by the piezoelectric scanners enables the tip to be maintained at a constant force above the sample surface. The tip extends down from the end of a laser-reflective cantilever. A laser beam is focused onto the cantilever. As the tip scans the surface of the sample, moving up and down with the contour of the surface, the laser beam is deflected off the cantilever into a photodiode. The photodiode measures the changes in laser beam intensities and then converts this information into electrical current. Feedback from the photodiode is processed by a computer as a surface image and also regulates the piezoelectric scanner. In contact mode (*left inset*), the electrostatic or surface tension forces drag the scanning tip over the surface of the sample. In tapping mode (*right inset*), the tip of the cantilever oscillates. The latter mode allows visualization of soft and fragile samples while achieving a high resolution.

staining is low in the lumen of T tubules compared with the surrounding cytoplasm of skeletal muscle cells). Automatic segmentation is the fastest method of generating 3D models. However, it often does not work in reconstructions of tissue samples because of the heterogeneous distribution of pixel intensities in the sample. Currently, fully automated segmentation protocols are still in development. More powerful algorithms are being developed that, in the future, will fully automate 3DEM image analysis.

Atomic Force Microscopy

The AFM has emerged as one of the most powerful tools for studying surface topography at molecular and atomic resolution.

One newer microscope that has proved most useful for biologic studies is the **atomic force microscope (AFM)**. It is a **nonoptical microscope** that works in the same way as a fingertip, which touches and feels the skin of our face when we cannot see it. The sensation from the fingertip is processed by our brain, which is able to deduce surface topography of the face while touching it.

In the AFM, an ultrasharp, pointed probe, approaching the size of a single atom at the tip, scans the specimen following parallel lines along the *x*-axis, repeating the scan at small intervals along the *y*-axis. The sharp tip is mounted at the end of a highly flexible **cantilever** so that the tip deflects the cantilever as it encounters the "atomic force" on the surface of the specimen (Fig. 1.17). The upper surface of the cantilever is reflective, and a laser beam is directed off the cantilever to a diode. This arrangement acts as an "optical lever" because extremely small deflections of the cantilever are greatly magnified on the diode. The AFM can work with the tip of the cantilever touching the sample (**contact mode**), or the tip can tap across the surface (**tapping mode**) much like the cane used by individuals with visual impairment (see Fig. 1.17, insets).

As the tip moves up and down in the *z*-axis as it traverses the specimen, the movements are recorded on the diode as movements of the reflected laser beam. A piezoelectric device under the specimen is activated in a sensitive feedback loop with the diode to move the specimen up and down so that the laser beam is centered on the diode. As the tip dips down into a depression, the piezoelectric device moves the specimen up to compensate, and when the tip moves up over an elevation, the device compensates by lowering the specimen. The current to the piezoelectric device is interpreted as the *z*-axis, which along with the *x*- and *y*-axes renders the topography of the specimen at a molecular, and sometimes an atomic, resolution (Fig. 1.18).

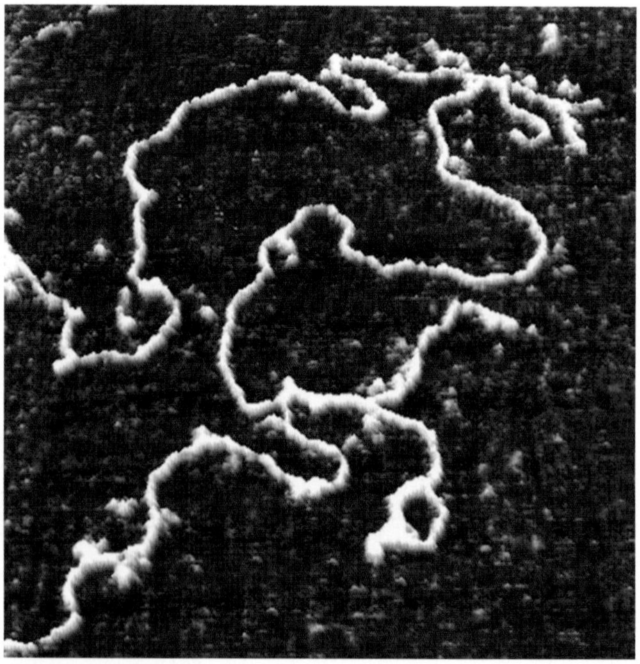

FIGURE 1.18. Atomic force microscopic image of a single DNA molecule. This image was obtained in the contact mode in which the sharp scanning tip "bumps" up and down as it is moved back and forth over the surface of the sample. The sample lies on an ultrasmooth mica surface. An individual molecule of DNA easily produces enough of a bump to be detected. Thickenings along the DNA molecule are produced by proteins bound to the molecule, and these thickenings produce an even larger movement of the scanning tip. The scan field measures 540 by 540 nm. The length of the DNA molecule ranges from 0 to 40 nm. ×185,000. (Courtesy of Dr. Gabriela Bagordo, JPK Instruments AG, Berlin, Germany.)

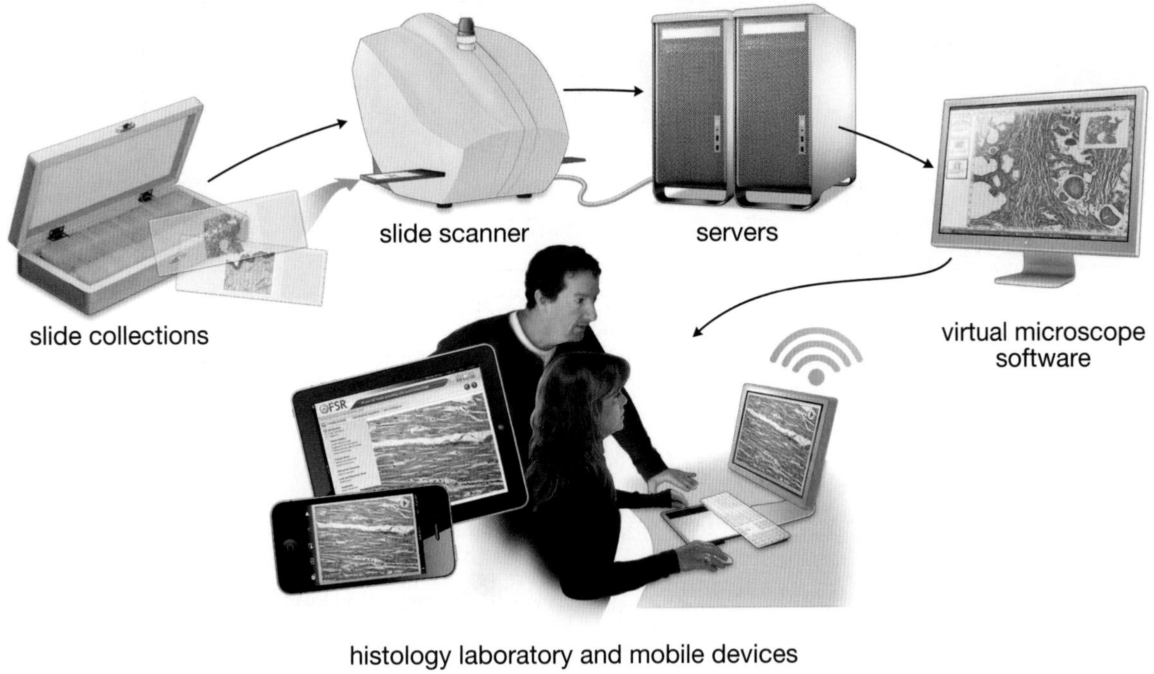

FIGURE 1.19. Virtual microscopy. Glass slides are scanned using a high-resolution automated slide scanner to create digital files that are stored typically in dedicated virtual microscopy servers. The virtual slide is a digital representation of a glass slide and can be displayed by using a specialized software viewer referred to as a virtual microscope. Virtual slides are distributed over a computer network or the Internet for remote viewing. Note that the virtual slides may be viewed individually or in groups on any mobile device, such as tablet computers or smartphones with virtual microscopy applications.

A major advantage of the AFM for examining biologic specimens is that unlike high-resolution optical instruments (i.e., TEM or SEM), the specimen does not have to be in a vacuum; it can even be submerged in water. Thus, it is feasible to image living cells and their surrounding environments.

Virtual Microscopy

Virtual microscopy is a digital procedure that is an alternative to the examination of glass slides using a light microscope.

Virtual microscopy integrates conventional light microscopy with digital technologies. Using optical image acquisition systems with automatic focus, glass slides are scanned to create 2D digital files that typically are stored on dedicated virtual microscopy servers (Fig. 1.18). The process of scanning involves acquiring images from a glass slide. Different systems acquire images either as tiles or as linear strips that are stitched together to create a virtual slide. The **virtual slide** is a digital representation of a glass slide, which can be viewed remotely without a light microscope. Glass slides are commonly digitized in a single focal plane (e.g., 40× objective lens), but they can be captured in multiple focal planes.

Many commercially available software packages called **virtual microscopes** provide Internet access to viewers for exploring digital slides on any network device in a manner similar to light microscopy. Virtual microscopes offer new possibilities for specimen viewing and handling that are not available on a standard light microscope. These include the following:

- Remote viewing of any digitized slide on any network device (e.g., tablet computers, smartphones) containing a virtual microscopy viewer
- Seamless progressive zooming in and out (usually ranging from 0.06 to 40×)
- Switching with ease between very low- and high-power magnifications without altering the field of view or plane of focus
- An orientation (navigation) thumbnail image of the whole slide that shows the location of the main screen image on the slide in real time (This orientation image remains present on the screen even while zooming.)
- A magnified glass thumbnail image that displays a digitally enlarged view of the region correlated to the position of the pointer on the screen
- Additional features such as drag, rotate, and measuring tools; arrays of color adjustment; and a focus feature to choose between different planes in images captured at multifocal planes

From an educational perspective, students using virtual microscopes are able to compare side-by-side images of different tissues and/or the same tissues stained by different stains. An important feature not available on light microscopes is the ability of students or instructors to make personalized annotations on each virtual slide, including freehand drawings as well as typed text. These annotations can be easily saved as overlay files with the virtual microscopy slides. In addition, virtual microscopy facilitates collaborative and team-based learning approaches between multiple students sharing a virtual microscope in a laboratory environment (see Fig. 1.19).

Virtual microscopy is also utilized in pathology education, research, and remote pathology practice (**telepathology**). It can be performed in a virtual environment by sharing virtual slides online among pathology specialists. Telepathology is currently used for many different applications, including histopathology diagnoses that are rendered from a distance. Use of digitalized slides (virtual microscopy) is preferred; however, in some developing countries, an analog imaging is still used in telepathology.

HISTOLOGY 101 NOTEBOOK

METHODS

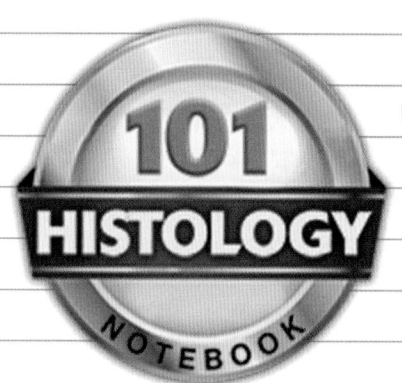

OVERVIEW OF METHODS USED IN HISTOLOGY

- **Histology (microscopic anatomy)** is the scientific study of microscopic structures of tissues and organs of the body.
- **Light microscopy** (for viewing glass slides) and **virtual microscopy** (for viewing digitized microscopic specimens on a computer screen or mobile device) are the most commonly taught methods for examining cells, tissues, and organs in histology courses.

TISSUE PREPARATION

- Routinely prepared **hematoxylin and eosin (H&E)**-stained sections of **formalin**-fixed tissue are the specimens most commonly examined for histologic studies with the **light microscope.**
- The first step in preparation of a tissue sample is **fixation**, which preserves structure and prevents enzymatic degradation.
- In the second step, the **specimen is dehydrated**, cleared, and then **embedded in paraffin** or epoxy resins to permit sectioning.
- In the third step, the **specimen is mounted** on a glass slide and **stained** to permit light microscope examination.
- Specific preparations are required for **expansion microscopy (ExM)** in which specimens are infiltrated with hydrogels that cause physical expansion of specimens.
- Steps in specimen preparation for the **transmission electron microscope (TEM)** are similar to that for light microscopy except that they require different fixatives (glutaraldehyde and osmium tetroxide), embedded media (plastic and epoxy resins), and staining dyes (heavy metals).

STAINING PROCEDURES

- **Eosin** is an **acidic dye** (pink) and carries a **net negative charge.** It reacts with positively charged cationic groups in cells and tissues, particularly amino groups of proteins (eosinophilic structures).
- **Hematoxylin** acts as a **basic dye** (blue) and carries a **net positive charge.** It reacts with negatively charged ionized phosphate groups in nucleic acids (basophilic structures).
- The **periodic acid–Schiff (PAS) reaction** stains carbohydrates and carbohydrate-rich molecules a distinctive magenta color. It is used to demonstrate glycogen in cells, mucus in cells and tissues, the basement membrane, and reticular fibers in connective tissue.
- **Immunocytochemistry** is based on the specificity of the reaction between an antigen and an antibody that is conjugated either to a fluorescent dye (for light microscopy) or gold particles (for electron microscopy). Both **direct** and **indirect immunocytochemical methods** are used to locate a target antigen in cells and tissues.
- **Histochemical** and **cytochemical** procedures are based on **specific binding** of a dye with a particular cell component exhibiting **inherent enzymatic activity.**
- **Hybridization** is a method of localizing mRNA or DNA by hybridizing the sequence of interest to a complementary strand of a nucleotide probe.
- **Fluorescence in situ hybridization (FISH) procedure** utilizes fluorescent dyes combined with nucleotide probes to visualize multiple probes at the same time. This technique is used extensively in genetic testing.
- **Autoradiography** makes use of a photographic emulsion placed over a tissue section to localize radioactive material within tissues.

MICROSCOPY

- Correct interpretation of microscopic images is important because organs are 3D, whereas histologic sections are only 2D.
- **Resolving power** is the ability of a microscope lens or optical system to produce separate images of closely positioned objects. The resolving power of a **bright-field microscope** (most commonly used by students and researchers) is about 0.2 µm.
- In addition to bright-field microscopy, other optical systems include **phase contrast microscopy, dark-field microscopy, fluorescence microscopy, confocal scanning microscopy, ultraviolet microscopy,** and **super-resolution microscopy.**
- **Transmission electron microscopes** (TEMs; theoretical resolving power of 0.05 nm) use the interaction of a beam of electrons with a specimen to produce an image.
- **Scanning electron microscopes** (SEMs; resolving power of 2.5 nm) use electrons reflected or forced out of the specimen surface that are collected by detectors and reprocessed to form an image of a sample surface.
- **Three-dimensional electron microscopy** (3DEM) is used for the reconstruction of entire structures including cells, their connections, and their organelles. The most frequently used 3DEM methods are **serial section TEM (SSTEM), focused ion beam SEM (FIBSEM),** and **serial block-face SEM (SBFSEM).**
- **Atomic force microscopes** (AFMs; resolving power of 50 pm) are nonoptical microscopes that utilize an ultrasharp, pointed probe (**cantilever**) that is dragged across the surface of a specimen. The up-and-down movements of the cantilever are recorded and transformed into a graphic image.

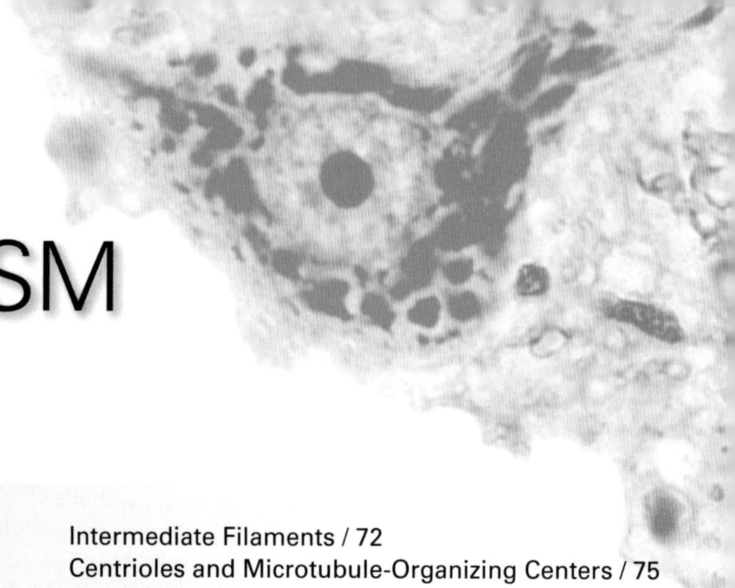

2 CELL CYTOPLASM

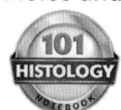

■ OVERVIEW OF THE CELL AND CYTOPLASM

Cells are the basic structural and functional units of all multicellular organisms.

The processes we normally associate with the daily activities of organisms—protection, ingestion, digestion, absorption of metabolites, elimination of wastes, movement, reproduction, and even death—are all reflections of similar processes occurring within each of the billions of cells that constitute the human body. To a large extent, cells of different types use similar mechanisms to synthesize protein, transform energy, and move essential substances into the cell. They use the same kinds of molecules to engage in contraction, and they duplicate their genetic material in the same manner.

Specific functions are identified with specific structural components and domains within the cell.

Some cells develop one or more of these functions to such a degree of specialization that they are identified by the function and the cell structures associated with them. For example, although all cells contain contractile filamentous proteins, some cells, such as **muscle cells**, contain large amounts of these proteins in specific arrays. This allows them to carry out their specialized function of contraction at both the cellular and tissue level. The specialized activity or function of a cell may be reflected not only by the presence of a larger amount of the specific structural component performing the activity but also by the shape of the cell, its organization with respect to other similar cells, and its products (Fig. 2.1).

Cells can be divided into two major compartments: the cytoplasm and the nucleus.

In general, the **cytoplasm** is the part of the cell located outside the **nucleus**. The cytoplasm contains **organelles** ("little organs"), **cytoskeleton** (made of polymerized proteins that form microtubules, intermediate filaments, and actin filaments), and **inclusions** suspended in an aqueous gel called the **cytoplasmic matrix**. The matrix consists of a variety of solutes, including inorganic ions (Na^+, K^+, Ca^{2+}) and organic molecules such as intermediate metabolites, carbohydrates, lipids, proteins, and RNAs. The cell controls the concentration of solutes within the matrix, which influences the rate of metabolic activity within the cytoplasmic compartment.

The nucleus is the largest organelle within the cell and contains the genome along with the enzymes necessary for DNA

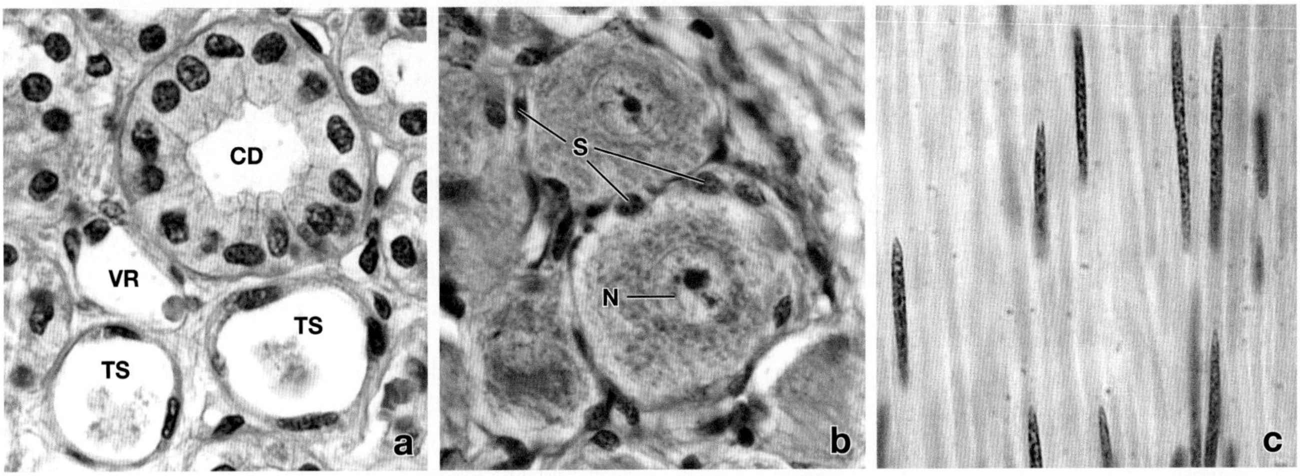

FIGURE 2.1. Histologic features of different cell types. These three photomicrographs show different types of cells in three different organs of the body. The distinguishing features include size, shape, orientation, and cytoplasmic contents that can be related to each cell's specialized activity or function. **a.** Epithelial cells in the kidney. Note several shapes of epithelial cells: columnar cells with well-defined borders in the collecting duct (*CD*), squamous cells in the thin segment (*TS*) of the nephron, and even more flattened cells lining blood vessels, the vasa recta (*VR*) in the kidney. ×380. **b.** Dorsal root ganglion cells. Note the large size of these nerve cell bodies and the large, pale (euchromatic) nuclei (*N*) with distinct nucleoli. Each ganglion cell is surrounded by flattened satellite cells (*S*). The size of the ganglion cell and the presence of a euchromatic nucleus, prominent nucleolus, and Nissl bodies (rough endoplasmic reticulum visible as darker granules within the cytoplasm) reflect the extensive synthetic activity required to maintain the exceedingly long processes (axons) of these cells. ×380. **c.** Smooth muscle cells of the small intestine. Note that these cells are typically elongated, fusiform-shaped, and organized in a parallel array. The nuclei are also elongated to conform to the general shape of the cell. ×380.

replication and RNA transcription. The cytoplasm and nucleus not only play distinct functional roles but also work in concert to maintain the cell's viability. The structure and function of the nucleus is discussed in Chapter 3, The Cell Nucleus, page 87.

Organelles are described as membranous (membrane-limited) or nonmembranous.

Organelles include the membrane systems of the cell and the membrane-limited compartments that perform the metabolic, synthetic, energy-requiring, and energy-generating functions of the cell as well as nonmembranous structural components. All cells have the same basic set of intracellular organelles, which can be classified into two groups: (1) **membranous organelles** with plasma membranes that separate the internal environment of the organelle from the cytoplasm and (2) **nonmembranous organelles** without plasma membranes.

The membranes of membranous organelles form vesicular, tubular, and other structural patterns within the cytoplasm that may be convoluted (as in smooth endoplasmic reticulum) or plicated (as in the inner mitochondrial membrane). These membrane configurations greatly increase the surface area on which essential physiologic and biochemical reactions take place. The spaces enclosed by the organelles' membranes constitute the **intracellular microcompartments** in which substrates, products, and other substances are segregated or concentrated. In addition, each type of organelle contains a set of unique proteins; in membranous organelles, these proteins are either incorporated into their membranes or sequestered within their lumens. For example, the enzymes of lysosomes are separated by a specific enzyme-resistant membrane from the cytoplasmic matrix because their hydrolytic activity would be detrimental to the cell. In nonmembranous organelles, the unique proteins usually self-assemble into polymers that form the structural elements of the **cytoskeleton**.

Besides organelles, the cytoplasm contains **inclusions**, structures that are not usually surrounded by a plasma membrane. They consist of such diverse materials as crystals, pigment granules, lipids, glycogen, and other stored waste products (for details, see pages 81-82).

Membranous organelles include the following:

- **Plasma (cell) membrane**, a lipid bilayer that forms the cell boundary as well as the boundaries of many organelles within the cell
- **Rough endoplasmic reticulum (rER)**, a region of endoplasmic reticulum associated with ribosomes and the site of protein synthesis and modification of newly synthesized proteins
- **Smooth endoplasmic reticulum (sER)**, a region of endoplasmic reticulum involved in detoxifying xenobiotics (foreign drugs or chemicals) and synthesis of lipids and steroids but not associated with ribosomes
- **Golgi apparatus**, a membranous organelle composed of multiple flattened cisternae responsible for modifying, sorting, and packaging proteins and lipids for intracellular or extracellular transport
- **Endosomes**, membrane-bounded compartments interposed within endocytic pathways that have the major function of sorting proteins delivered to them via endocytic vesicles and redirecting them to different cellular compartments for their final destination
- **Exosomes**, small (average 100 nm in diameter), endosome-derived, membrane-bound vesicles that originate within the lumen of **multivesicular bodies**. They are released via exocytosis into the extracellular space. Exosomes carry nucleic acids, proteins, lipids, and metabolites secreted by cells to the extracellular space. They act as mediators for near- and long-distance communication between cells.
- **Lysosomes**, small organelles containing digestive enzymes that are formed from endosomes by targeted delivery of unique lysosomal membrane proteins and lysosomal enzymes
- **Transport vesicles**—including **pinocytic vesicles**, **endocytic vesicles**, and **coated vesicles**—that are involved in both endocytosis and exocytosis and vary in shape and the material that they transport
- **Mitochondria**, organelles that provide most of the energy to the cell by producing adenosine triphosphate (ATP) in the process of oxidative phosphorylation

- **Peroxisomes**, small organelles involved in an oxidative type of metabolism. They are involved in the degradation of fatty acids and production and degradation of reactive oxygen intermediates.

Nonmembranous organelles include the following:

- **Microtubules**, which together with actin and intermediate filaments form elements of the **cytoskeleton** and continuously elongate (by adding tubulin dimers) and shorten (by removing tubulin dimers), a property referred to as **dynamic instability**
- **Filaments**, which are also part of the cytoskeleton and can be classified into two groups—**actin filaments**, which are flexible chains of actin molecules, and **intermediate filaments**, which are rope-like fibers formed from a variety of proteins—provide tensile strength to withstand tension and confer resistance to shearing forces.
- **Centrioles**, or short, paired cylindrical structures found in the center of the **microtubule-organizing center (MTOC)** or **centrosome** and whose derivatives give rise to basal bodies of cilia
- **Ribosomes**, structures essential for protein synthesis and composed of ribosomal RNA (rRNA) and ribosomal proteins (including proteins attached to membranes of the rER and proteins free in the cytoplasm)
- **Proteasomes**, which are protein complexes that enzymatically degrade damaged and unnecessary proteins into small polypeptides and amino acids

An outline of the key features of cellular organelles and inclusions is provided in Table 2.1. The normal function and related pathologies of the organelles are summarized in Table 2.2.

TABLE 2.1 Review of Organelles and Cytoplasmic Inclusions: A Key to Light Microscopic and Electron Microscopic Identification

Organelle or Inclusion	Size (μm)	Light Microscopic Features	Electron Microscopic Features
Nucleus	3–10	Largest organelle within the cell with distinct boundary Often visible nucleoli and chromatin pattern regions	Surrounded by two membranes (nuclear envelope containing nuclear pore complexes and perinuclear cisternal space Regions with condensed and diffused chromatin pattern (heterochromatin and euchromatin)
Nucleolus	1–2	Roughly circular, basophilic region within the nucleus Visible in living cells throughout interphase with interference microscopy	Dense, nonmembranous structure containing fibrillar and granular material
Plasma membrane	0.008–0.01	Not visible	External membrane and membranes surrounding membranous organelles of cell; two inner and outer electron-dense layers separated by intermediate electron-lucent layer
rER	Area ~5–10	Often observed as basophilic region of cytoplasm referred to as *ergastoplasm*	Flattened sheets, sacs, and tubes of membranes with attached ribosomes
sER	Throughout cytoplasm	Not visible Cytoplasm in region of sER may exhibit distinct eosinophilia	Flattened sheets, sacs, and tubes of membranes *without* attached ribosomes
Golgi apparatus	Area ~5–10	Sometimes observed as "negative staining" region Appears as network in heavy metal–stained preparations Visible in living cells with interference microscopy	Stack of flattened membrane sheets, often adjace to one side of nucleus
Secretory vesicles	0.05–1.0	Observed only when vesicles are very large (e.g., zymogen granules in pancreas)	Many relatively small, membrane-bounded vesicles uniform diameter, often polarized on one side of ce
Mitochondria	0.2–7	Sometimes observed in favorable situations (e.g., liver or nerve cells) as miniscule, dark dots; visible in living cells stained with vital dyes (e.g., Janus Green)	Two-membrane system: outer membrane and inner membrane arranged in numerous folds (cristae) In steroid-producing cells, inner membrane arranged in tubular cristae
Endosomes	0.02–0.5	Not visible	Tubulovesicular structures with subdivided lumen containing electron-lucent material or other smaller vesicles
Exosomes	0.03–0.1	Not visible	Intraluminal vesicles inside the multivesicular bodies (MVBs). They are released into extracellular space fusion of MVBs with the cell membrane.
Lysosomes	0.2–0.5	Visible only after special enzyme histochemical staining	Membrane-bounded vesicles, often electron dense
Peroxisomes	0.1–0.5	Visible only after special enzyme histochemical staining	Membrane-bounded vesicles, often with electron-dense crystalloid inclusions
Cytoskeletal elements	0.006–0.025	Only observed when organized into large structures (e.g., muscle fibrils)	Long, linear staining pattern with width and features characteristic of each filament type
Ribosomes	0.025	Not visible	Minute dark dots, often associated with the rER
Proteasomes	0.015	Not visible	Difficult to distinguish from other matrix proteins
Glycogen	0.010–0.040	Observed as a "purple haze" region of cytoplasm metachromasia with toluidine blue–stained specimen	Nonmembranous, extremely dense grape-like inclusions
Lipid droplets	0.2–5, up to 80	Readily visible when extremely large (e.g., in adipocytes) Appear as large empty holes in section (lipid itself is usually removed by embedding solvents)	Nonmembranous inclusions Generally appear as a void in the section

rER, rough endoplasmic reticulum; sER, smooth endoplasmic reticulum.

TABLE 2.2 Organelles and Cytoplasmic Inclusions: Functions and Pathologies

Organelle or Inclusion	Functions	Pathologies
Nucleus	Storage and use of genome	Inherited genetic diseases; environmentally induced mutations
Nucleolus	Synthesis of rRNA and partial assembly of ribosomal subunits Involved in regulation of cell cycle	Werner syndrome (premature aging disease) Malfunctions of cell cycle leading to cancerogenesis
Plasma membrane	Ion and nutrient transport Recognition of environmental signal Cell-to-cell and cell-to-extracellular matrix adhesions	Cystic fibrosis Intestinal malabsorption syndromes Lactose intolerance
rER	Binds ribosomes engaged in translating mRNA for proteins destined for secretion or for membrane insertion Also involved in chemical modifications of proteins and membrane lipid synthesis	Pseudoachondroplasia Calcium pyrophosphate dihydrate crystal deposition disease (CPPD disease; pseudogout)
sER	Involved in lipid and steroid metabolism	Hepatic endoplasmic reticular storage disease
Golgi apparatus	Chemical modification of proteins Sorting and packaging of molecules for secretion or transport to other organelles	I-cell disease Polycystic kidney disease
Secretory vesicles	Transport and storage of secreted proteins to plasma membrane	Lewy bodies of Parkinson disease Proinsulin diabetes
Mitochondria	Aerobic energy supply (oxidative phosphorylation, ATP) Initiation of apoptosis	Mitochondrial myopathies such as MERRF syndrome, MELAS syndrome, Kearns–Sayre syndrome, and Leber hereditary optic atrophy
Endosomes	Transport of endocytosed material Biogenesis of lysosomes	M-6-P receptor deficiency (I-cell disease)
Exosomes	Transport vehicles for intercellular communication and material exchange between cells	Depending on their transported cargo, they can promote neoplasia, tumor growth, metastasis formation, and resistance to therapy.
Lysosomes	Digestion of macromolecules	Lysosomal storage diseases (see Folder 2.1, Clinical Correlation: Lysosomal Storage Diseases)
Peroxisomes	Oxidative digestion (e.g., fatty acids), lipid biosynthesis, metabolism of reactive oxygen intermediates	Zellweger spectrum diseases (peroxisomal biogenesis disorders): Zellweger syndrome, Refsum disease, and X-linked adrenoleukodystrophy
Cytoskeletal elements	Various functions, including cell motility, cell adhesions, and intracellular and extracellular transport Maintenance of cellular skeleton	Immotile cilia syndrome, Alzheimer disease, epidermolysis bullosa
Ribosomes	Synthesis of protein by translating protein-coding sequence from mRNA	Ribosomal dysfunction in Alzheimer disease; Diamond–Blackfan anemia Many antibiotics act selectively on bacterial ribosomes: for example, tetracyclines, aminoglycosides (gentamicin, streptomycin).
Proteasomes	Degradation of unnecessary and damaged proteins that are labeled for destruction with ubiquitin	Diseases characterized by cytoplasmic accumulation of misfolded proteins: Parkinson disease, Alzheimer disease, Angelman syndrome, inclusion body myopathies
Glycogen	Short-term storage of glucose in the form of branched polymer Found in liver, skeletal muscle, and adipose tissue	Several known glycogen-storage diseases, including major groups of hepatic–hypoglycemic and muscle-energy pathophysiologies
Lipid droplets	Storage of esterified forms of fatty acids as high-energy storage molecules	Lipid storage diseases such as Gaucher and Niemann–Pick disease, liver cirrhosis

ATP, adenosine triphosphate; MELAS, mitochondrial encephalopathy, lactic acidosis, and stroke-like episodes; MERRF, myoclonic epilepsy with ragged red fiber; mRNA, messenger RNA; rER, rough endoplasmic reticulum; ROIs, reactive oxygen intermediates; rRNA, ribosomal RNA; sER, smooth endoplasmic reticulum.

■ MEMBRANOUS ORGANELLES

Plasma Membrane

The plasma membrane is a lipid-bilayered structure visible with transmission electron microscopy.

The **plasma membrane (cell membrane, plasmalemma)** is a dynamic structure that actively participates in many physiologic and biochemical activities essential to cell function and survival. When the plasma membrane is properly fixed, sectioned, stained, and viewed in cross section with the transmission electron microscope (TEM), it appears as two electron-dense layers separated by an intermediate, electron-lucent (nonstaining) layer (Fig. 2.2). The total thickness of the plasma membrane is about 8–10 nm.

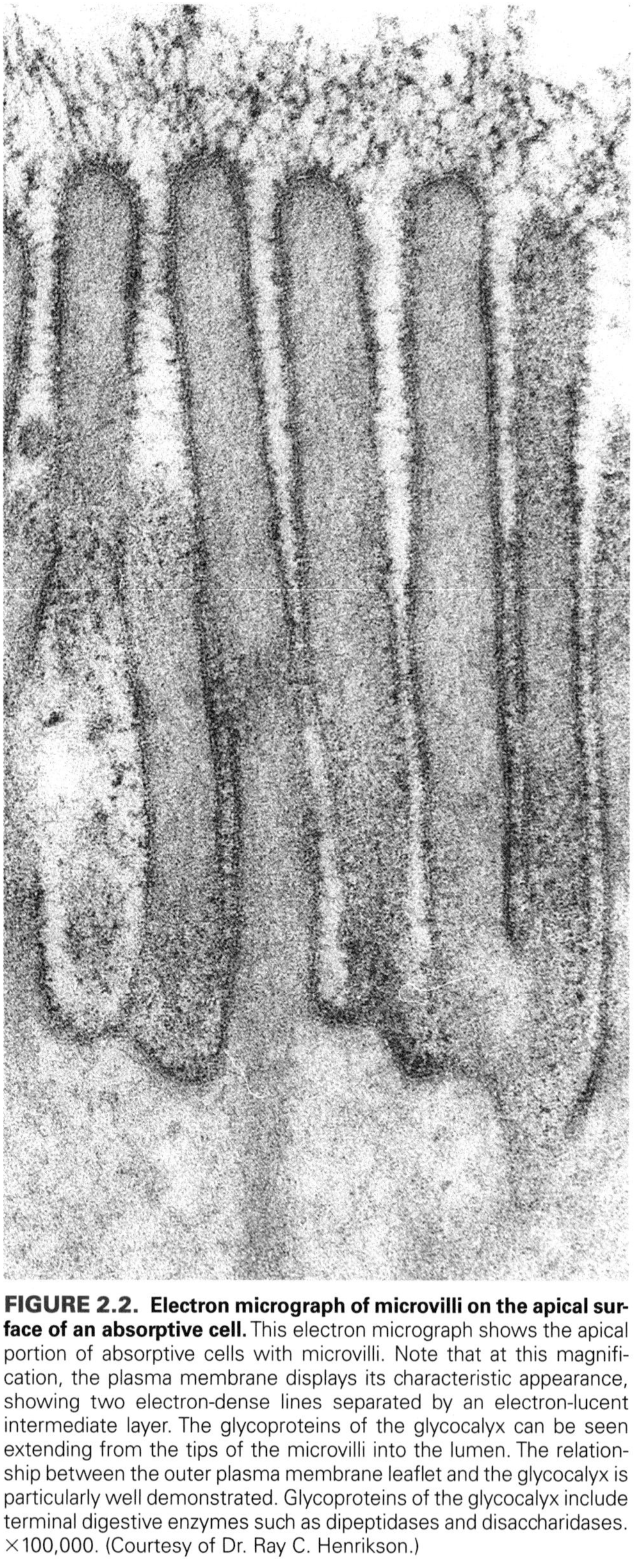

FIGURE 2.2. Electron micrograph of microvilli on the apical surface of an absorptive cell. This electron micrograph shows the apical portion of absorptive cells with microvilli. Note that at this magnification, the plasma membrane displays its characteristic appearance, showing two electron-dense lines separated by an electron-lucent intermediate layer. The glycoproteins of the glycocalyx can be seen extending from the tips of the microvilli into the lumen. The relationship between the outer plasma membrane leaflet and the glycocalyx is particularly well demonstrated. Glycoproteins of the glycocalyx include terminal digestive enzymes such as dipeptidases and disaccharidases. ×100,000. (Courtesy of Dr. Ray C. Henrikson.)

The plasma membrane is composed of an amphipathic lipid layer containing embedded integral membrane proteins with peripheral membrane proteins attached to its surfaces.

The current interpretation of the molecular organization of the plasma membrane is referred to as the **modified fluid–mosaic model** (Fig. 2.3). The membrane consists primarily of **phospholipid**, **cholesterol**, and **protein molecules**. The lipid molecules form a lipid bilayer with an amphipathic character (it is both hydrophobic and hydrophilic). The fatty acid chains of the lipid molecules face each other, making the inner portion of the membrane **hydrophobic** (i.e., having no affinity for water). The surfaces of the membrane are formed by the polar head groups of the lipid molecules, thereby making the surfaces **hydrophilic** (i.e., they have an affinity for water). Lipids are distributed asymmetrically between the inner and outer leaflets of the **lipid bilayer**, and their composition varies considerably among different biologic membranes.

In most plasma membranes, protein molecules constitute approximately half of the total membrane mass. Most of the proteins are embedded within the lipid bilayer or pass through the lipid bilayer completely. These proteins are called **integral membrane proteins**. The other types of protein—**peripheral membrane proteins**—are not embedded within the lipid bilayer. They are associated with the plasma membrane by strong ionic interactions, mainly with integral proteins on both the extracellular and intracellular surfaces of the membrane (see Fig. 2.3). In addition, on the extracellular surface of the plasma membrane, carbohydrates may be attached to proteins, thereby forming **glycoproteins**, or to lipids of the bilayer, thereby forming **glycolipids**. These surface molecules constitute a layer at the surface of the cell, referred to as the **cell coat** or **glycocalyx** (see Fig. 2.2). They help establish extracellular microenvironments at the membrane surface that have specific functions in metabolism, cell recognition, and cell association and serve as receptor sites for hormones.

Microdomains of the plasma membrane, known as lipid rafts, control the movement and distribution of proteins within the lipid bilayer.

The fluidity of the plasma membrane is not revealed in static electron micrographs. Experiments reveal that the membrane behaves as though it were a two-dimensional lipid fluid. For many years, it was thought that integral membrane proteins moved freely within the plane of the membrane; this movement was compared to the movement of icebergs floating in the ocean (see Fig. 2.3). However, the distribution and movement of proteins within the lipid bilayer is not as random as once thought. The plasma membrane appears to be patchy with localized regions that are distinct in structure and function and vary in thickness and composition. These localized regions contain high concentrations of **cholesterol** and **glycosphingolipids** and are called **lipid rafts.** Because of the high concentration of cholesterol and the presence of longer, highly saturated fatty acid chains, the lipid raft area is thicker and exhibits less fluidity than the surrounding plasma membrane (Fig. 2.4). Cholesterol is the dynamic "glue" that holds the raft together; its removal from the raft results in dispersal of raft-associated lipids and proteins.

In general, there are two types of lipid rafts:

- **Planar lipid rafts** contain a family of 47-kDa proteins known as **flotillins** as well as specific lipids and cholesterol. Flotillins are regarded as the molecular markers of lipid rafts and are considered to be scaffolding proteins. They also participate in the recruitment of specific membrane proteins into the rafts and work as active partners in various signaling pathways.
- **Caveolar rafts**, or **caveolae** ("little caves"), represent small (50–100 nm in diameter), flask-shaped invaginations of the plasma membrane containing 18- to 24-kDa integral membrane proteins called **caveolins**. Oligomerization of caveolins produces the caveolin scaffold essential to creating invaginations within the plasma membrane. These proteins also bind to cholesterol and a variety of proteins

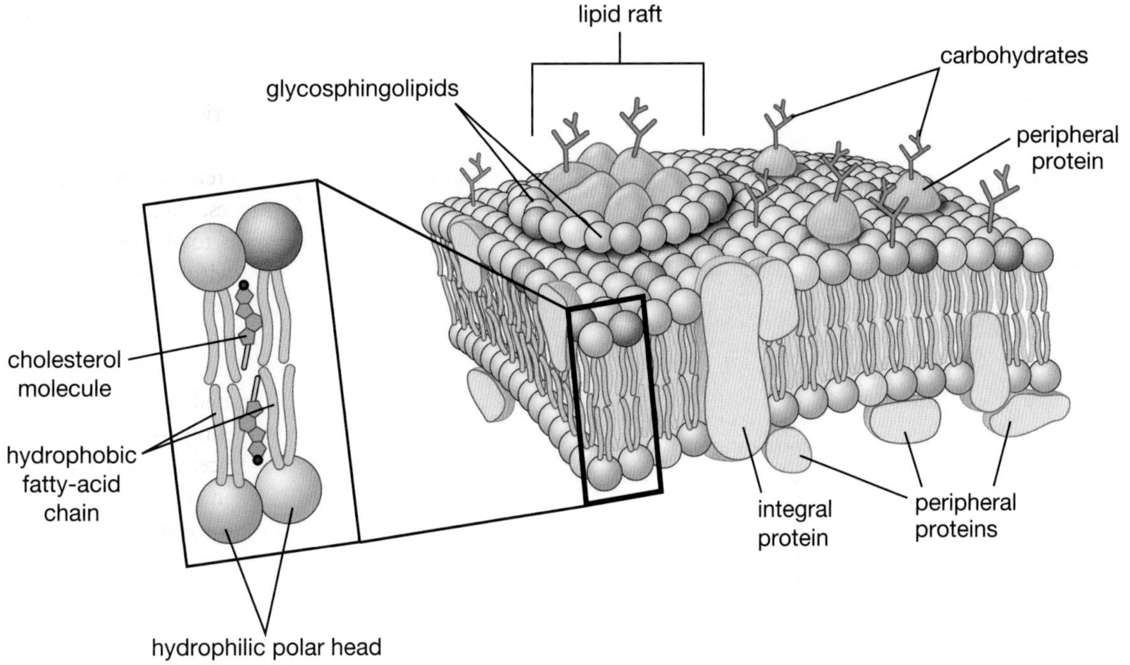

FIGURE 2.3. Diagram of a plasma membrane showing the modified fluid–mosaic model. The plasma membrane is a lipid bilayer consisting primarily of phospholipid molecules, cholesterol, and protein molecules. The hydrophobic fatty acid chains of phospholipids face each other to form the inner portion of the membrane, whereas the hydrophilic polar heads of the phospholipids form the extracellular and intracellular surfaces of the membrane. Cholesterol molecules are incorporated within the gaps between phospholipids equally on both sides of the membrane. Note the elevated area of the lipid raft that is characterized by a high concentration of glycosphingolipids and cholesterol. It contains large numbers of integral and peripheral membrane proteins. The raft protrudes above the level of asymmetrically distributed phospholipids in the membrane bilayer (*indicated by the different colors of the phospholipid heads*). Carbohydrate chains attach to both integral and peripheral membrane proteins to form glycoproteins as well as to polar phospholipid heads to form glycolipids.

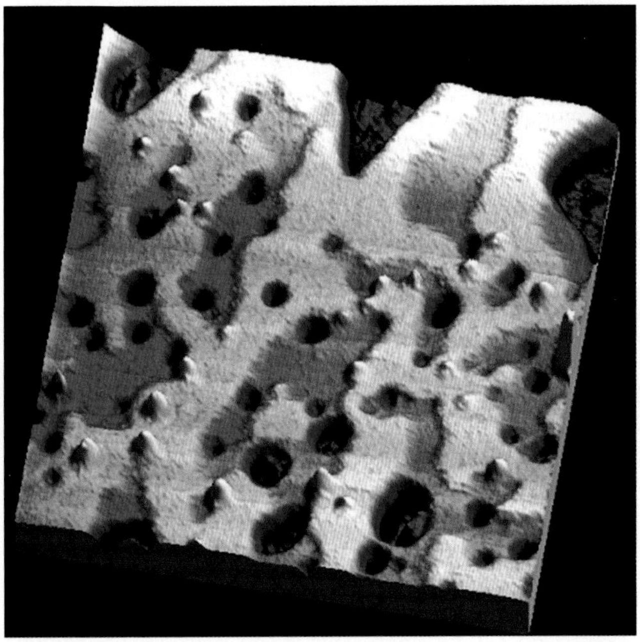

FIGURE 2.4. Image of lipid rafts obtained with tapping-mode atomic force microscopy (AFM). This image shows a 5-nm-thick lipid bilayer spread on a mica support. The bilayer is composed of dioleoyl phosphatidylcholine (dioleoyl-PC), sphingomyelin, and cholesterol. Sphingomyelin and cholesterol together form lipid rafts represented on the image by the *pink areas*; the *blue-purple areas* are the nonraft background of the bilayer. Because the sphingomyelin molecules are longer than the dioleoyl-PC molecules, the rafts protrude from the nonraft background by about 0.8 nm, and the AFM is sensitive enough to detect this protrusion. The black regions represent the mica support. The image also shows molecules of the *Helicobacter pylori* toxin VacA (*white particles*), which preferentially bind to protein receptors on the raft domains. The area depicted in this image is 800 nm^2. (Courtesy of Drs. Nicholas A. Geisse, Timothy L. Cover, Robert M. Henderson, and J. Michael Edwardson.)

involved in signal transduction. Caveolae are prominent in **smooth muscle cells** (see page 370), where they contain various Ca^{2+} channels, Na^+/Ca^{2+} exchangers, and G protein–coupled receptors involved in ligand-mediated regulation of intracellular Ca^{2+} levels.

Lipid rafts contain a variety of integral and peripheral membrane proteins involved in cell signaling. They can be viewed as "**signaling platforms**" floating in the ocean of lipids. Each individual raft is equipped with all of the necessary elements (receptors, coupling factors, effector enzymes, and substrates) to receive and convey specific signals. Signal transduction in lipid rafts occurs more rapidly and efficiently because of the close proximity of interacting proteins. In addition, different signaling rafts allow for the separation of specific signaling molecules from each other.

In bacterial and viral infections, the initial contact of the microorganism with the cell occurs at the lipid raft. For example, some bacteria (e.g., *Shigella flexneri, Salmonella typhimurium*) hijack the rafts with their signaling mechanism and use them to support their own entry into the cell. Many bacteria use rafts to avoid phagocytosis and subsequent destruction in lysosomes. In other cases, invading bacteria use raft-associated receptors to generate vacuoles made of raft components. These vacuoles are then used to transport bacteria into the cell without the risk of being detected by phagocytic compartments.

Integral membrane proteins can be visualized with the freeze fracture tissue preparation technique.

The existence of proteins within the substance of the plasma membrane (i.e., integral proteins) was confirmed by the

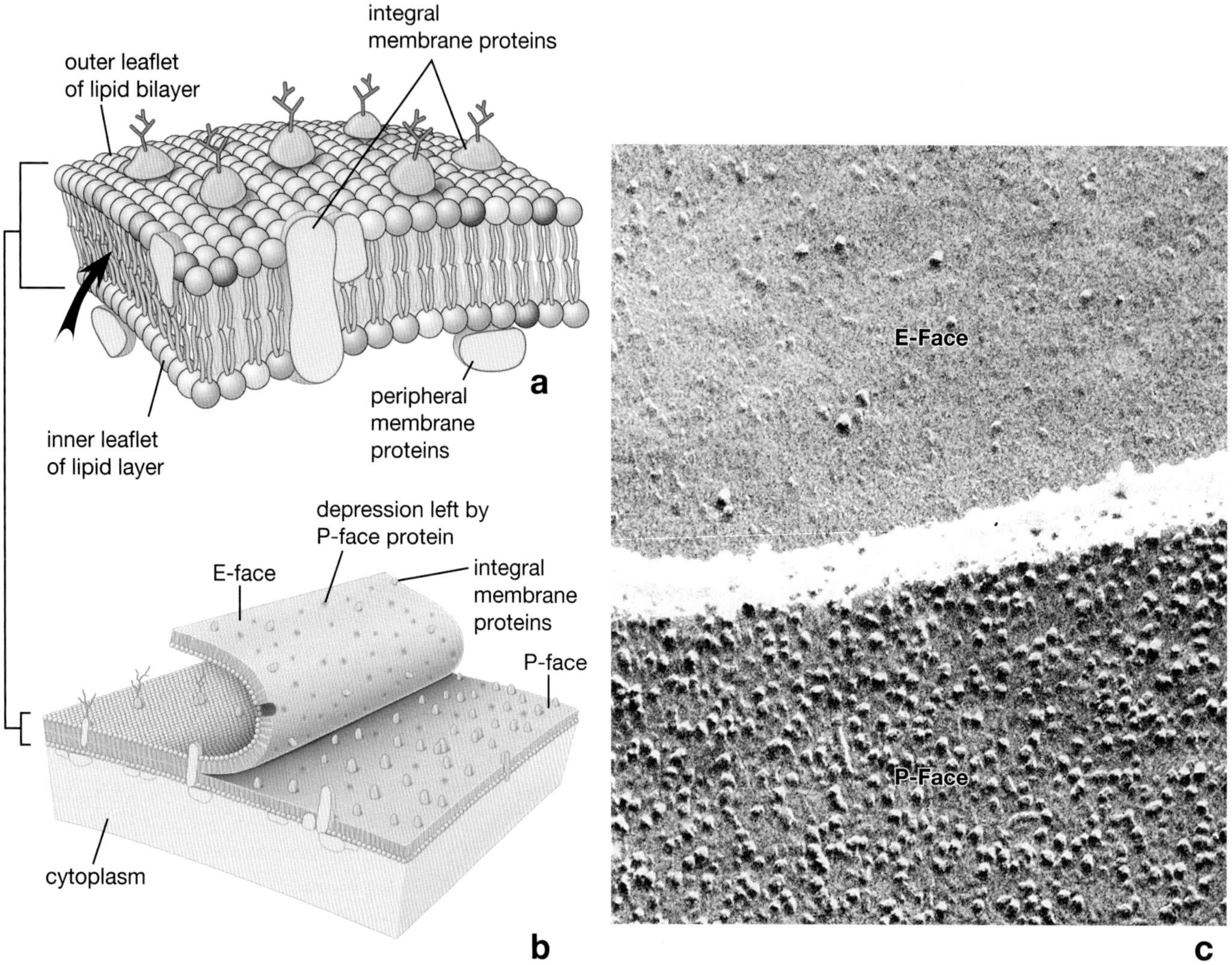

FIGURE 2.5. Freeze fracture examination of the plasma membrane. a. View of the plasma membrane seen on edge, with *arrow* indicating the preferential plane of splitting of the lipid bilayer through the hydrophobic portion of the membrane. When the membrane splits, some proteins are carried with the outer leaflet, although most are retained within the inner leaflet. **b.** View of the plasma membrane with the leaflets separating along the cleavage plane. The surfaces of the cleaved membrane are coated, forming replicas; the replicas are separated from the tissue and examined with the transmission electron microscope (TEM). Proteins appear as bumps. The replica of the inner leaflet is called the *P-face*; it is backed by cytoplasm (*p*rotoplasm). A view of the outer leaflet is called the *E-face*; it is backed by the *e*xtracellular space. **c.** Electron micrograph of a freeze fracture replica shows the E-face of the membrane of one epithelial cell and the P-face of the membrane of the adjoining cell. The cleavage plane has jumped from the membrane of one cell to the membrane of the other cell, as indicated by the clear space (intercellular space) across the middle of the figure. Note the paucity of particles in the E-face compared with the P-face, from which the majority of the integral membrane proteins project. (Courtesy of Dr. Giuseppina d'Elia Raviola.)

preparation technique known as **freeze fracture**. When tissue is prepared for electron microscopy (EM) by the freeze fracture process (Fig. 2.5a), membranes typically split or cleave along the hydrophobic plane (i.e., between the two lipid layers) to expose two interior faces of the membrane, an E-face and a P-face (Fig. 2.5b). For details on tissue preparation using freeze fracture technique, see Chapter 1, Methods, page 22.

The **E-face** is backed by the *e*xtracellular space, whereas the **P-face** is backed by the cytoplasm (*p*rotoplasm). The numerous particles seen on the E- and P-faces with the TEM represent the integral proteins of the membrane. Usually, the P-face displays more particles, thus more protein, than the E-face (Fig. 2.5c).

Integral membrane proteins have important functions in cell metabolism, regulation, integration, and cell signaling.

Six broad categories of membrane proteins have been defined in terms of their function: pumps, channels, receptors, linkers, enzymes, and structural proteins (Fig. 2.6). These categories are not mutually exclusive (e.g., a structural membrane protein may simultaneously serve as a receptor, an enzyme, a pump, or any combination of these functions):

- **Pumps** transport certain ions, such as Na^+, actively across membranes. Pumps also transport metabolic precursors of macromolecules, such as amino acids and sugars, across membranes, either by themselves or linked to the Na^+ pump.
- **Channels** allow the passage of small ions, molecules, and water across the plasma membrane in either direction (i.e., passive diffusion). Gap junctions formed by aligned channels in the membranes of adjacent cells permit passage of ions and small molecules involved in signaling pathways from the cytoplasm of one cell to the cytoplasm of adjacent cells.
- **Receptor proteins** allow recognition and localized binding of ligands (molecules that bind to the extracellular surface of the plasma membrane) in processes such as hormonal stimulation, coated vesicle endocytosis, and antibody reactions. Receptors that bind to signaling molecules transmit the signal through a sequence of

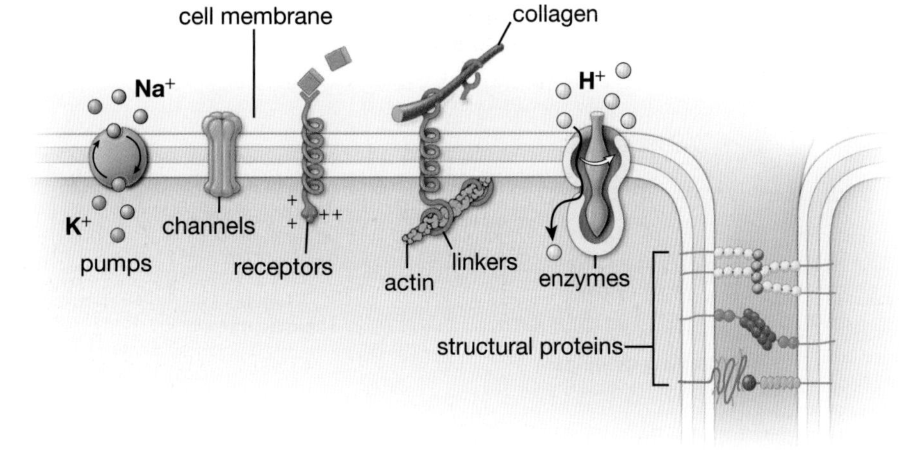

FIGURE 2.6. Different functions of integral membrane proteins. The six major categories of integral membrane proteins are shown in this diagram: pumps, channels, receptors, linkers, enzymes, and structural proteins. These categories are not mutually exclusive. A structural membrane protein involved in cell-to-cell junctions might simultaneously serve as a receptor, enzyme, linker, or a combination of these functions.

molecular switches (i.e., second messengers) to the cell's internal signaling pathways, thereby initiating a physiologic response.

- **Linker proteins** anchor the intracellular cytoskeleton to the extracellular matrix. Examples of linker proteins include the family of integrins that link cytoplasmic actin filaments to an extracellular matrix protein (fibronectin).
- **Enzymes** have a variety of roles. ATPases have specific roles in ion pumping: ATP synthase is the major protein of the inner mitochondrial membrane, and digestive enzymes such as disaccharidases and dipeptidases are integral membrane proteins.
- **Structural proteins** are visualized by the freeze fracture method, especially where they form junctions with neighboring cells. Often, certain proteins and lipids are concentrated in localized regions of the plasma membrane to carry out specific functions. Examples of such regions can be recognized in polarized cells such as epithelial cells.

Integral membrane proteins move within the lipid bilayer of the membrane.

Particles bound to the membrane can move on the surface of a cell; even integral membrane proteins, such as enzymes, may move from one cell surface to another (e.g., from apical to lateral) when barriers to flow, such as cell junctions, are disrupted. The fluidity of the membrane is a function of the types of phospholipids in the membrane and variations in their local concentrations.

As previously mentioned, lipid rafts containing integral membrane proteins may move to a different region of the plasma membrane. The movement of an integral protein anchored on a lipid raft makes signaling more precise and prevents nonspecific interactions. The lateral migration of proteins is often limited by physical connections between membrane proteins and intracellular or extracellular structures. Such connections may exist among

- proteins associated with cytoskeletal elements and portions of the membrane proteins that extend into the adjacent cytoplasm,
- the cytoplasmic domains of membrane proteins, and
- peripheral proteins associated with the extracellular matrix and the integral membrane proteins that extend from the cell surface (i.e., the extracellular domain).

Through these connections, proteins can be localized or restricted to specialized regions of the plasma membrane or can act as transmembrane linkers between intracellular and extracellular filaments (see the next section).

The plasma membrane undergoes continuous remodeling.

The cell membrane and internal plasma membranes of organelles are continually remodeling. Video microscopy reveals that the plasma membrane undergoes bulging, invagination, budding, tubulation, ruffling, fusion, and fission. These processes are essential for virtually all the major functions of the cell, including synthesis and degradation of molecules, endocytosis, exocytosis, signaling, immunologic defense mechanisms, cell division, and migration. In general, there are two types of membrane remodeling:

- Remodeling that **excludes cytoplasm** from the lumen of forming vesicles or tubules, such as during the formation of **endocytic vesicles** (Fig. 2.7). This process involves proteins residing on the inner (cytoplasmic) surface of the membrane (i.e., clathrin, caveolins, COP-I and COP-II, and others) that help change the shape of the plasma membrane into vesicle-like invaginations (see page 41). The **dynamin** family of membrane scission proteins is essential to mediate the liberation of the vesicles from the plasma membrane. Similar invaginations can be found in skeletal muscle cells, where **T tubules** are connected to the external cell environment. In smooth muscle cells, **caveolae** and endocytic vesicles help regulate Ca^{2+} homeostasis.
- Remodeling that **includes cytoplasm** within the newly formed structures. This process occurs when cytoplasmic-embedded **viral particles** bud from the cell membrane (Fig. 2.8). As the cell membrane envelops the viral particles and surrounds them with cytoplasm, the connection of this forming vesicle to the cell membrane narrows. The membrane constricts until the budding vesicles are connected to the cell by only a thin, cytoplasm-filled stalk (membrane neck) that must be severed to liberate the vesicle. Formation of vesicles containing viral particles can also occur inside the cell from intracellular membranes such as rER, Golgi, or membrane-bounded replication complexes for the virus (Fig. 2.8). Remodeling of the membrane and the liberation of vesicles or scission of tubules filled with cytoplasm are controlled by

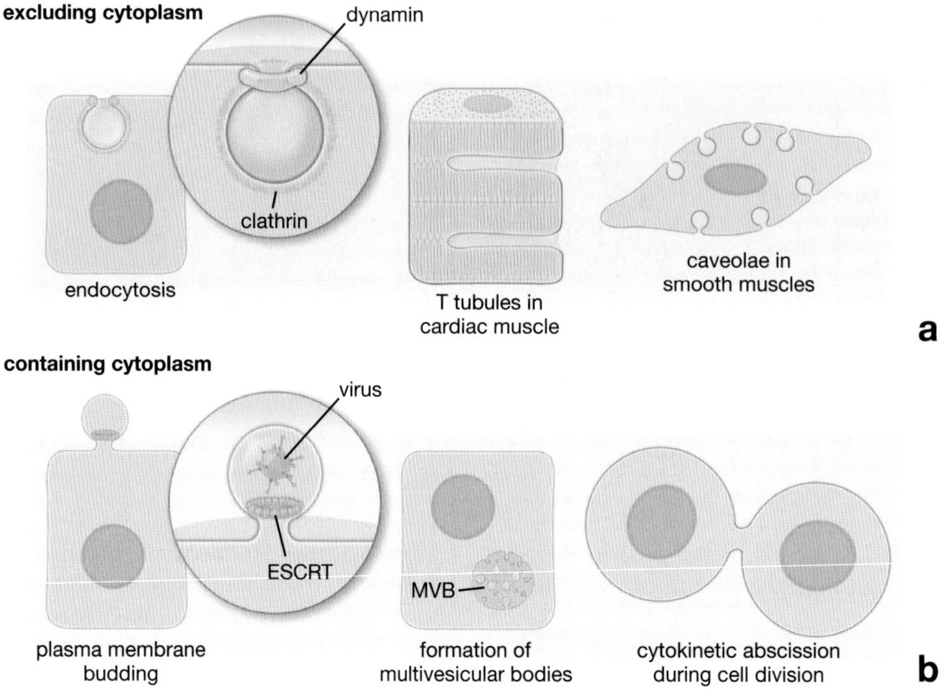

FIGURE 2.7. Remodeling process of the plasma membrane. a. Examples of plasma membrane remodeling that excludes cytoplasm from the lumen of forming vesicles (i.e., endocytic vesicles or caveolae) are shown here. This process involves proteins such as clathrin, caveolins, COP-I, and COP-II that help in the formation of coated vesicles. The dynamin family of membrane scission proteins is essential to liberate the vesicles from the plasma membrane. Tubular invaginations can also be found in skeletal muscle cells, where the lumen of the T-tubule is connected to the external cell environment. **b.** Examples of plasma membrane remodeling that includes cytoplasm within the newly formed structures are shown here. This process occurs in budding vesicles from cell membranes or intracellular structures. The liberation of vesicles or tubular structures filled with cytoplasm is controlled by endosomal sorting complex required for transport (ESCRT) complexes of proteins. Note that the separation of membranes mediated by ESCRT occurs from the inside surface of the membrane contiguous with the cytoplasm, whereas vesicles and tubules that exclude cytoplasm are liberated from the plasma membrane by the dynamin family of membrane scission proteins.

endosomal sorting complex required for transport (ESCRT) complexes of proteins. ESCRT complexes also participate in the formation of **multivesicular bodies (MVBs)**, **exosomes**, **microvesicles**, **apoptotic bodies**, **resealing of the post-mitotic nuclear envelope**, and **closure of autophagosomes**. In addition, cell division requires remodeling of the plasma membrane during cytoplasmic separation (**cytokinetic abscission**) into two daughter cells. The separation of membranes mediated by ESCRT occurs from the surface of the membrane that is contiguous with the inside of the cytoplasm-filled membrane neck (see Fig. 2.7). This mechanism is opposite to that of the dynamin family of membrane scission proteins, which cleaves the membrane neck by constricting it from the outside (see Fig. 2.7).

Cell injury often manifests as morphologic changes in the cell's plasma membrane that result in the formation of **plasma membrane blebs.** These are dynamic cell protrusions of the plasma membrane that are commonly observed in acute cell injury, in dividing and dying cells, and during cell movement. Blebbing is caused by the detachment of the plasma membrane from underlying actin filaments of the cell cytoskeleton. **Cytoskeletal toxins** that act on actin filaments such as phalloidin and cytochalasin B cause extensive membrane blebbing. In addition, in **viral infections** such as human immunodeficiency virus (HIV), Ebola, and human T-lymphotropic virus, the ESCRT complex is "hijacked" during virus budding at the surface of infected host cells, where they catalyze the scission of the membrane stalk that connects the budding virus to the host cell.

Signaling Processes

Cell signaling involves integral membrane proteins such as cell surface receptors, cell surface channels, and molecules released from exosomes.

Cell signaling is the process by which extracellular stimuli are received, processed, and conveyed by the cell to regulate its own physiologic responses. A single cell may receive many different signals at the same time, and it needs to integrate all information into a unified action plan. Signaling processes often are involved in the regulation of gene expression, exocytosis, endocytosis, differentiation, cell growth and death, cytoskeletal reorganization, movement, contraction, and/or cell relaxation. Individual cells also send out signaling molecules to other cells both near (e.g., neurotransmitters in nerve synapses) and far away (e.g., hormones acting on distant cells).

Signal transduction pathways are mechanisms by which cells respond to the external environment. They are hierarchical cascades of molecular events that mediate tissue and cell specificity, allow for amplification and modulation of the signal, and are involved in biochemical and physiologic regulation. They are initiated by external **signaling molecules** (also referred to as **primary messengers** or *ligands*) that can be soluble, act locally (autocrine or paracrine control as discussed in Chapter 21, Endocrine Organs, pages 816-818), or be transmitted to cellular targets via blood vasculature (endocrine signaling). They can also be insoluble, tethered to cell membranes, or localized in the extracellular matrix. Signaling molecules in sensory systems often are of exogenous origin (i.e., odorants, mechanical signals, vibration, light).

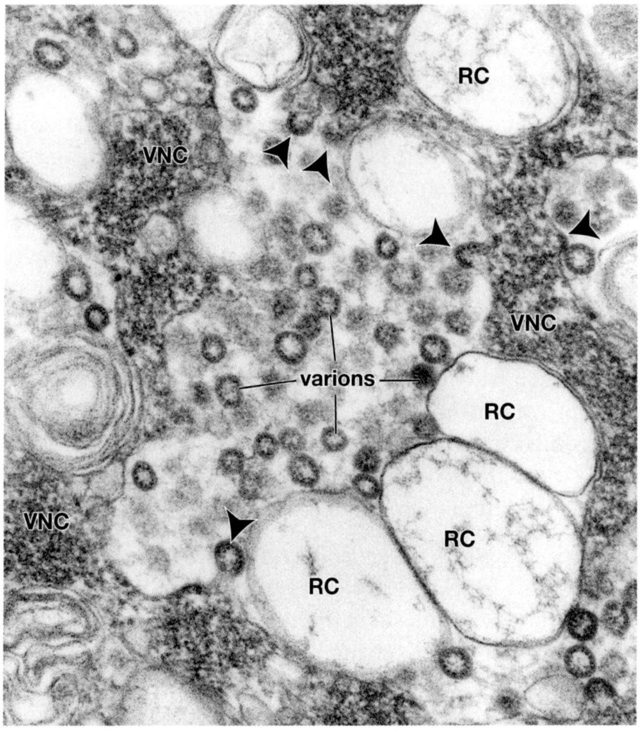

FIGURE 2.8. Budding vesicles containing viral particles. This electron micrograph shows a kidney epithelial cell in culture derived from the African green monkey cell line (Vero E6) infected by a coronavirus (severe acute respiratory syndrome [SARS]-CoV). Vero E6 cells are susceptible to virus infection because they have a deficiency in the interferon gene cluster and cyclin-dependent kinase inhibitor genes; therefore, they do not secrete α or β interferon. Three to five days after inoculation with the SARS-CoV virus, Vero E6 cells were harvested, inactivated by γ-irradiation, and processed for standard EM examination. Arrowheads indicate budding vesicles into the cisternae of rough endoplasmic reticulum or Golgi apparatus that contain viral particles (varions). These cisternae represent cellular compartments in which vesicles containing viral particles are stored within the cytoplasm before the entire compartment migrates to the cell surface to release its contents into the extracellular space. The area labeled *VNC* represents viral intracellular inclusions of the viral nucleocapsid. The large cisternae labeled *RC* represent double-membrane vesicles that serve as replication complexes for this virus. ×55,000. (Courtesy of Dr. Cynthia Goldsmith, Centers for Disease Control and Prevention, Atlanta, Georgia).

The majority of signaling pathways are initiated by the binding of primary messengers to specific receptors, which exist in an inactive state in the absence of ligands. Signals from receptors are conveyed to target molecules inside the cell by the **second messenger system**. Receptors are typically classified into three groups, which are discussed in earlier sections and later chapters: **channel proteins** (page 34), **intracellular receptors**, and **cell surface receptors** (see Chapter 21, Endocrine Organs, pages 817-818). The latter group includes members of the G-protein–linked receptor family (see Chapter 12, Nerve Tissue, page 400), the enzyme-linked (catalytic) receptor family (see Chapter 21, Endocrine Organs, page 816), and the integrin family of cell-to-extracellular matrix receptors (see Chapter 5, Epithelial Tissue, page 146).

Exosomal signaling represents an intercellular communication pathway in which functional proteins, metabolites, and nucleic acids are delivered to recipient cells using exosomes as transfer vehicles. Exosomes represent very small, membrane-bound **cargo vesicles** secreted into extracellular space by virtually every prokaryotic and eukaryotic cell. The detailed structure and function of exosomes are discussed on pages 47-48. Exosomes are present in the blood and all body fluids and transfer messages and cargo molecules from the parent cells to the target destination via autocrine, paracrine, and endocrine mechanisms.

Exosomes with their cargo molecules interact with a target cell, fusing either directly with the plasma membrane of recipient cells (mediated by SNAREs and Rab interactions) or using receptor–ligand-mediated interaction pathways, that is, phagocytosis, macropinocytosis, or micropinocytosis (pages 39-40). Exosomes then release their contents directly into the cytoplasm of the target cell, initiating downstream signaling cascades. After delivering their cargo, exosomes undergo degradation in the cytoplasm of the recipient cell in a typical endosomal pathway.

Activation of cell surface receptors leads to posttranslational modifications, which contribute to the amplification of the signal.

There are several **posttranslational modifications** of intracellular proteins that contribute to the amplification of a signal that the cell receives. These include the following:

- **Phosphorylation** (addition of phosphate groups—PO_4^{3-})
- **Glycosylation** (addition of a diverse selection of sugar moieties)
- **Acetylation** (attaching acetyl functional groups—$COCH_3$)
- **Methylation** (adding methyl groups—CH_3)
- **Nitrosylation** (reaction of nitric oxide [NO] with protein-free cysteine residues)
- **Ubiquitination** (attaching ubiquitin protein)
- **SUMOylation** (addition of small ubiquitin-related modifier [SUMO] protein)

Common to the activation of cell surface receptors is the triggering of kinase-linked cascades of intracellular reactions. **Protein kinases** and **protein phosphatases** are families of enzymes that mediate the phosphorylation and dephosphorylation of cellular proteins, respectively. Phosphorylation of seryl, threonyl, or tyrosyl residues can alter activity, levels, or subcellular location of proteins.

Multiple protein kinases exist in cells and are classified as follows:

- **Second messenger-dependent protein kinases**, such as cyclic adenosine monophosphate (cAMP)-dependent protein kinase (PKA, see Fig. 13.12), cyclic granulocyte/monocyte progenitor (cGMP)-dependent protein kinase (PKG, see Fig. 13.12), and calcium/calmodulin-dependent kinases, including myosin light chain kinase (MLCK, see Fig. 11.28)
- **Second messenger-independent protein kinases**, such as enzymes of the mitogen-activated protein kinase (MAPK, see Fig. 3.21), cyclin-dependent kinase (Cdk, see Fig. 3.11), and protein tyrosine kinase (see Fig. 21.4)

Consequently, the intracellular spatial–temporal patterns of specific phosphorylation events are tightly linked to many of the cellular responses highlighted in subsequent chapters.

Membrane Transport and Vesicular Transport

Substances that enter or leave the cell must traverse the plasma membrane.

Some substances (small, fat-soluble, uncharged molecules and gases) cross the plasma membrane by **simple** or

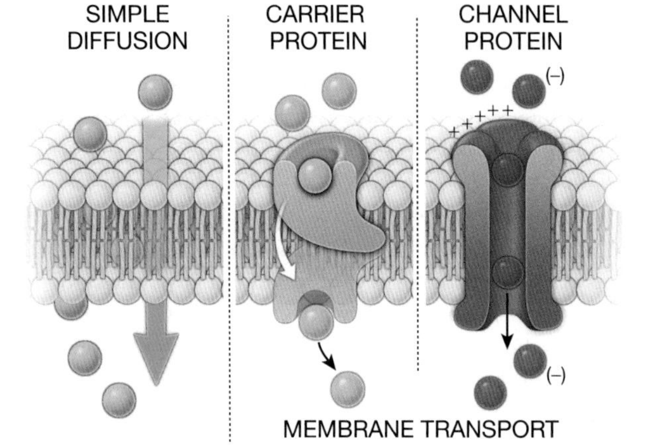

FIGURE 2.9. Movement of molecules across the plasma membrane. Fat-soluble and other small, uncharged molecules (in *green*) cross the plasma membrane by simple diffusion down their concentration gradient. Other molecules require membrane transport proteins to provide them with individual passage across the plasma membrane. Small water-soluble molecules (in *blue*) require highly selective carrier proteins to transfer them across the plasma membrane. After binding with a molecule, the carrier protein undergoes a series of conformational changes and releases the molecule on the other side of the membrane. If the process requires energy, it is called *active transport* (e.g., transport of H^+ ions against their concentration gradient). If the process does not require energy, it is called *passive transport* (e.g., glucose transport). Ions and other small charged molecules (in *purple*) are transported across the plasma membrane by ion-selective channel proteins. In neurons, for instance, ion transport is regulated by membrane potentials (voltage-gated ion channels); in skeletal muscle cells, neuromuscular junctions possess ligand-gated ion channels.

passive diffusion down their concentration gradient without expenditure of metabolic energy and without help of transport proteins (Fig. 2.9). All other molecules require **membrane transport proteins** to provide them with individual passage across the plasma membrane.

There are generally two classes of transport proteins:

- **Carrier proteins** transfer small, water-soluble molecules. They are highly selective, often transporting only one type of molecule. After binding to a molecule designated for transport, the carrier protein undergoes a series of conformational changes and releases the molecule on the other side of the membrane (see Fig. 2.9). Some carrier proteins, such as the Na^+/K^+ pump or H^+ pump, require energy for **active transport** of molecules against their concentration or electrochemical gradient. Other carrier proteins, such as glucose carriers, do not require energy and participate in **passive transport**.
- **Channel proteins** also transfer small, water-soluble molecules. In general, channels are made of transmembrane proteins with several membrane-spanning domains that create hydrophilic channels through the plasma membrane. Usually, channel proteins contain a **pore domain** that partially penetrates the membrane bilayer and serves as an ion-selectivity filter. The pore domain is responsible for exquisite ion selectivity, which is achieved by regulation of its three-dimensional structure (see Fig. 2.9). Channels are ion-selective and are regulated on the basis of the cell's needs. Channel protein transport can be regulated by membrane potentials (e.g., **voltage-gated ion channels** in neurons), neurotransmitters (e.g., **ligand-gated ion channels** such as acetylcholine receptors in muscle cells), or mechanical stress (e.g., **mechanically gated ion channels** in the internal ear).

Vesicular transport maintains the integrity of the plasma membrane and also provides for the transfer of molecules between different cellular compartments.

Some substances enter and leave cells by **vesicular transport**, a process that involves configurational changes in the plasma membrane at localized sites and subsequent formation of vesicles from the membrane or fusion of vesicles with the membrane (Fig. 2.10).

The major mechanism by which large molecules enter, leave, and move within the cell is called **vesicle budding**. Vesicles formed by budding from the plasma membrane of one compartment fuse with the plasma membrane of another compartment. Within the cell, this process ensures intercompartmental transfer of the vesicle contents.

Vesicular transport involving the cell membrane may also be described in more specific terms:

- **Endocytosis** is the general term for processes of vesicular transport in which substances enter the cell. Endocytosis controls the composition of the plasma membrane and the cellular response to changes in the external environment. It also plays key roles in nutrient uptake, cell signaling, and cell shape changes.
- **Exocytosis** is the general term for processes of vesicular transport in which substances (cargo molecules) leave the cell. Exocytosis is also the process by which all cells deliver the intracellular plasma membrane (that forms cytoplasmic vesicles) to the cell surface. Both processes can be visualized with the EM.

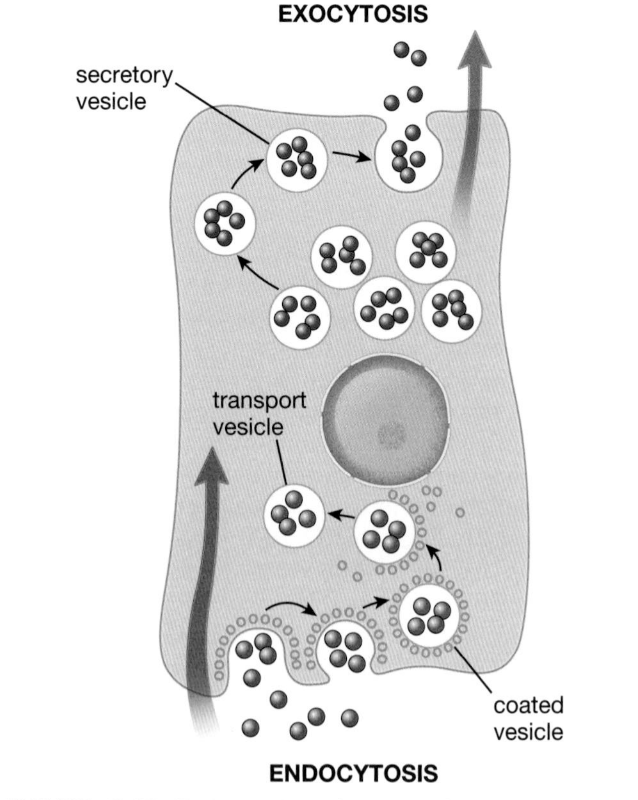

FIGURE 2.10. Endocytosis and exocytosis. These processes are the two major forms of vesicular transport. Endocytosis brings molecules and other substances into the cell. In exocytosis, synthesized molecules and other substances leave the cell. Endocytosis is associated with the formation and budding of vesicles from the plasma membrane; exocytosis is associated with the fusion of vesicles originating from intracellular organelles with the plasma membrane, and it is a primary secretory modality.

Exocytosis and endocytosis are coupled together: When exocytosis is abolished, no endocytosis takes place.

Fusion of a vesicle with the plasma membrane releases cargo proteins into the extracellular space. Following exocytosis, the vesicular membrane and its associated proteins are retrieved from the plasma membrane through endocytosis, which recycles vesicles and prevents secretory cells from swelling or shrinking. Recent experimental studies revealed that tetanus or botulinum neurotoxins that **block exocytosis** also **block endocytosis** in nerve terminals. These studies indicate that exocytosis and endocytosis are coupled together and that the proteins mediating exocytosis and vesicular membrane fusion (i.e., **SNARE proteins**; see pages 42-44) have a role in **initiating endocytosis**.

Endocytosis

Endocytosis is the cellular process that facilitates the uptake of membrane proteins, fluids, nutrients, lipids, and signaling molecules from the extracellular environment into the cell by endocytic vesicles. Following endocytosis, the contents of endocytic vesicles and their membrane components are either recycled to the cell surface or are transported to late endosomes for future degradation.

Uptake of fluid and macromolecules during endocytosis depends in general on three different mechanisms.

Some **endocytic mechanisms** require special proteins during vesicle formation. The best-known protein that interacts with the plasma membrane in vesicle formation is **clathrin**. Although the presence of clathrin is certainly important for endocytic vesicle formation, many vesicles are formed in a clathrin-independent manner utilizing different proteins (i.e., caveolins or flotillins). Therefore, endocytosis can be classified as either **clathrin dependent** or **clathrin independent**. In general, three major mechanisms of endocytosis are recognized in the cell. They include **pinocytosis** *[Gr., cell drinking]*, **phagocytosis** *[Gr., cell eating]*, and **receptor-mediated endocytosis**. Pinocytosis can occur via two different pathways, micropinocytosis and macropinocytosis, which are discussed separately:

- **Micropinocytosis** is the nonspecific ingestion of fluid and small protein molecules via small vesicles, usually smaller than 150 nm in diameter. Micropinocytosis is performed by virtually every cell in the organism, and it is **constitutive** (i.e., it involves a continuous dynamic formation of small vesicles at the cell surface) (Fig. 2.11a). The vesicle formation in micropinocytosis is usually associated with the presence of **caveolin** and **flotillin** proteins that are found in lipid rafts. Caveolin-1 and caveolin-2 are found in all nonmuscle cells, except neurons and white blood cells, whereas caveolin-3 is muscle cell specific. Flotillin-1 and flotillin-2 are found in vesicles distinct from caveolae. Also, mechanoenzymes such as **dynamin**, a GTPase family of membrane scission proteins, are involved in pinocytic vesicle scission (the process of pinching off from the plasma membrane). Pinocytic vesicles are visible with the TEM, and they have a smooth surface. They are especially numerous in the endothelium of blood vessels (Fig. 2.11b) and in smooth muscle cells. Because caveolin-1 forms complexes (of 14–16 monomers) that effect changes in membrane curvature leading to vesicle formation, micropinocytosis does not require clathrin. Micropinocytosis also does not require remodeling of the actin cytoskeleton and therefore may be referred to as **clathrin-independent** and **actin-independent endocytosis.**
- **Macropinocytosis** represents a nonspecific uptake mechanism for extracellular fluids, solutes, nutrients, and antigens. In this actin-dependent process, the actin cytoskeleton is rearranged at the plasma membrane, leading to formation of **surface membrane ruffles.** The membrane

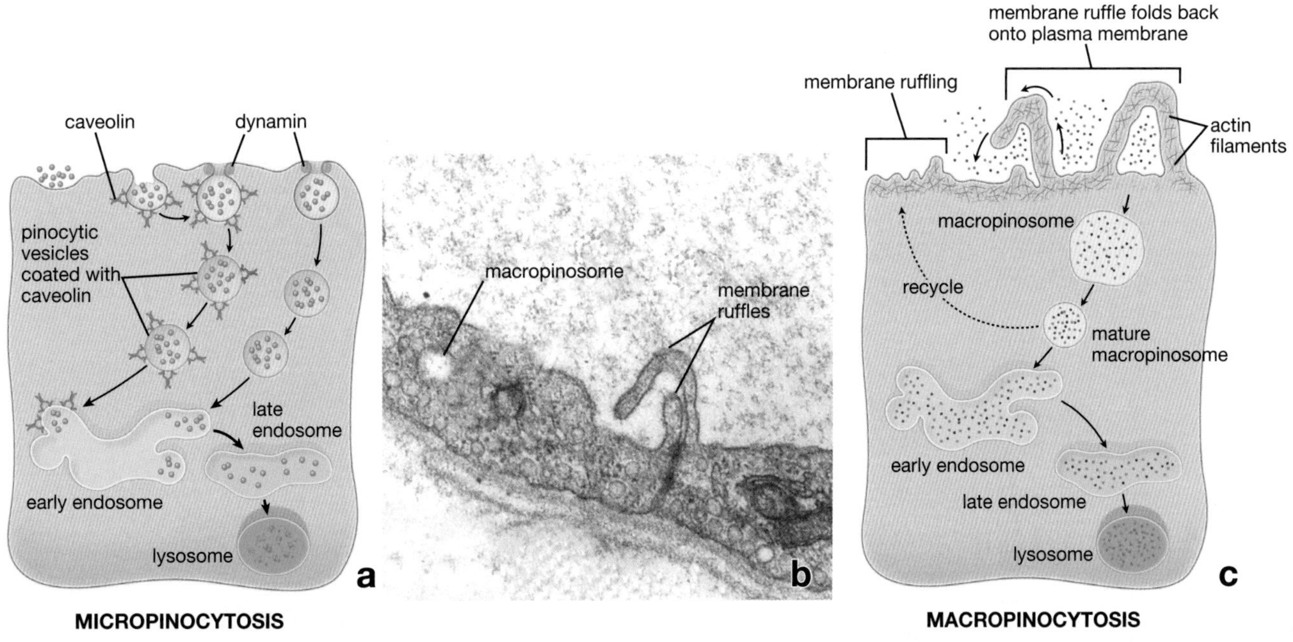

FIGURE 2.11. Pinocytosis. a. Micropinocytosis involves the dynamic formation of small vesicles at the cell surface. First, substances to be pinocytosed (e.g., small soluble proteins, colloidal tracers) make contact with the extracellular surface of the plasma membrane. Next, the surface becomes invaginated, and dynamin (a GTPase) pinches off the vesicle from the membrane to become a pinocytic vesicle within the cell. Pinocytosis of certain substances may be associated with caveolin. **b.** This electron micrograph shows numerous smooth-surfaced pinocytic vesicles within the cytoplasm of endothelial cells of a blood vessel. Also membrane ruffles are visible on this image. They are essential in the formation of large macropinosomes. ×55,000. **c.** Macropinocytosis involves the rearrangement of the plasma membrane and underlying actin cytoskeleton to form surface membrane ruffles that entrap large volumes of extracellular fluid. The large vesicles (macropinosomes) enter the cell cytoplasm, undergo maturation, and either fuse with early lysosomes or return to the plasma membrane for recycling.

ruffles become elongated and then fold back onto the plasma membrane to entrap extracellular fluid. They give rise to large (>0.2 μm in diameter) endocytic vacuoles called **macropinosomes** (see Fig. 2.11c). The large fluid-carrying capacity of macropinosomes is utilized by cells of the immune system (e.g., macrophages and dendritic cells) in order to sample as much of their extracellular environment as possible. The amount of solutes and membranes internalized during macropinocytosis exceeds that of any other endocytic pathways. Macropinocytosis is a regulated process and occurs in response to various growth factors, such as macrophage colony-stimulating factor-1 (CSF-1), epidermal growth factor (EGF), or platelet-derived growth factor (PDGF). The macropinosomes undergo a defined sequence of maturation steps in which their contents are either degraded in the late endosome or lysosome or recycled back to the plasma membrane. Because of the initial increase in actin cytoskeleton remodeling in distinct regions of the cell surface leading to formation of plasma membrane ruffles, macropinocytosis is referred to as **clathrin-independent** but **actin-dependent endocytosis**.

- **Phagocytosis** is the ingestion of large particles such as cell debris, bacteria, and other foreign materials. In this nonselective process, the plasma membrane sends out pseudopodia to engulf phagocytosed particles into large vesicles (larger than approximately 250 nm in diameter) called **phagosomes**. Phagocytosis is performed mainly by a specialized group of cells belonging to the mononuclear phagocyte system (MPS). Phagocytosis is generally a receptor-mediated process in which receptors on the cell surface recognize non–antigen-binding domains (F_c fragments) of antibodies coating the surface of an invading microorganism or cell (Fig. 2.12a). Phagocytosis is also triggered by recognition of **pathogen-associated molecular patterns (PAMPs)** that are commonly expressed on pathogen surfaces by toll-like receptors (page 309). PAMP recognition leads to activation of nuclear factor kappa B (NF-κB) transcription factor, which regulates genes that control cell responses in phagocytosis. Nonbiologic materials, such as inhaled carbon particles, inorganic dusts, and asbestos fibers, as well as biologic debris from inflammation, wound healing, and dead cells are sequestered by cells of the mononuclear phagocyte system (MPS) without involvement of F_c receptors (Fig. 2.12b). This process does not require clathrin for phagosome formation. Because of the initial extension of pseudopods by the plasma membrane that contributes to the formation of phagosome, the actin cytoskeleton must be rearranged in a process that requires depolymerization and repolymerization of the actin filaments. Thus, phagocytosis is referred to as **clathrin-independent** but **actin-dependent endocytosis**.
- **Receptor-mediated endocytosis** allows entry of specific molecules into the cell. In this mechanism, receptors for specific molecules, called **cargo receptors**, accumulate in well-defined regions of the cell membrane. These regions, which are represented by the lipid rafts in the plasma membrane, eventually become **coated pits** (Fig. 2.13a). The name *coated pit* is derived from these regions' appearance in the EM as an accumulation of electron-dense material that represents aggregation of **clathrin** molecules on

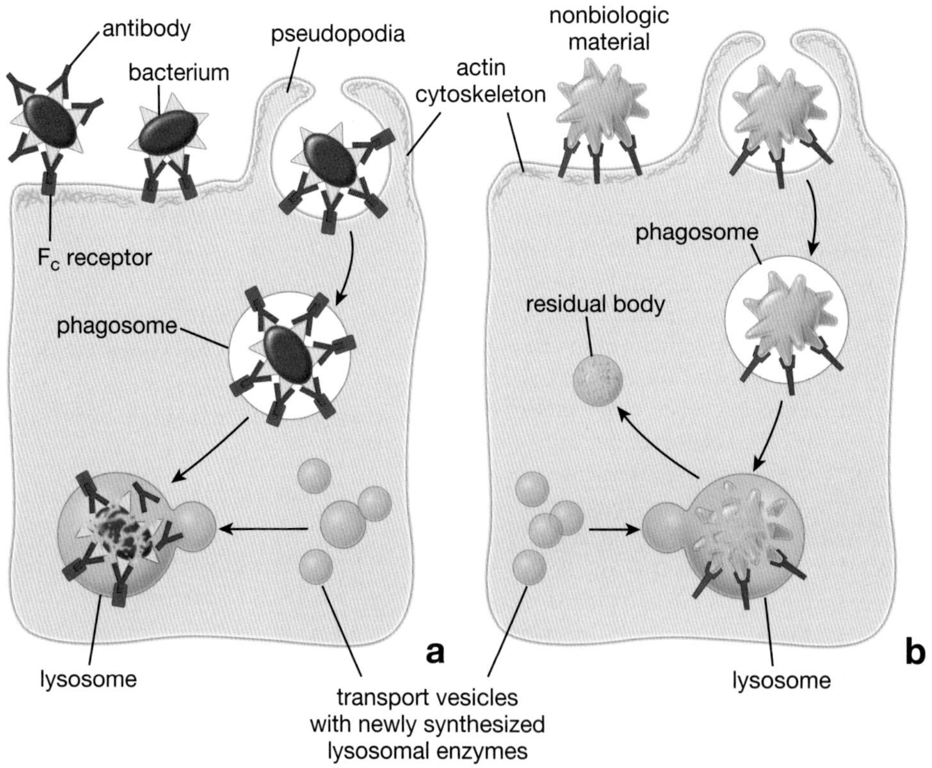

FIGURE 2.12. Phagocytosis. a. This drawing shows the steps in the phagocytosis of a large particle, such as a bacterium, that has been killed as a result of an immune response. The bacterium is surrounded by antibodies attached to the bacterial surface antigens. F_c receptors on the surface of the plasma membrane of phagocytic cells recognize the F_c portion of the antibodies. This interaction triggers rearrangement of the actin cytoskeleton. Depolymerizations and repolymerizations of actin filaments produce temporary projections of the plasma membrane called *pseudopodia*. They surround the phagocytosed particle, forming a phagosome. By targeted delivery of lysosomal enzymes, a phagosome matures into a lysosome that digests its phagocytosed contents. **b.** Nonbiologic materials such as inhaled carbon particles, inorganic dusts, and asbestos fibers, as well as cellular debris resulting from inflammation, are internalized without involvement of antibodies and F_c receptors. These particles are bound to multiple receptors on the plasma membrane.

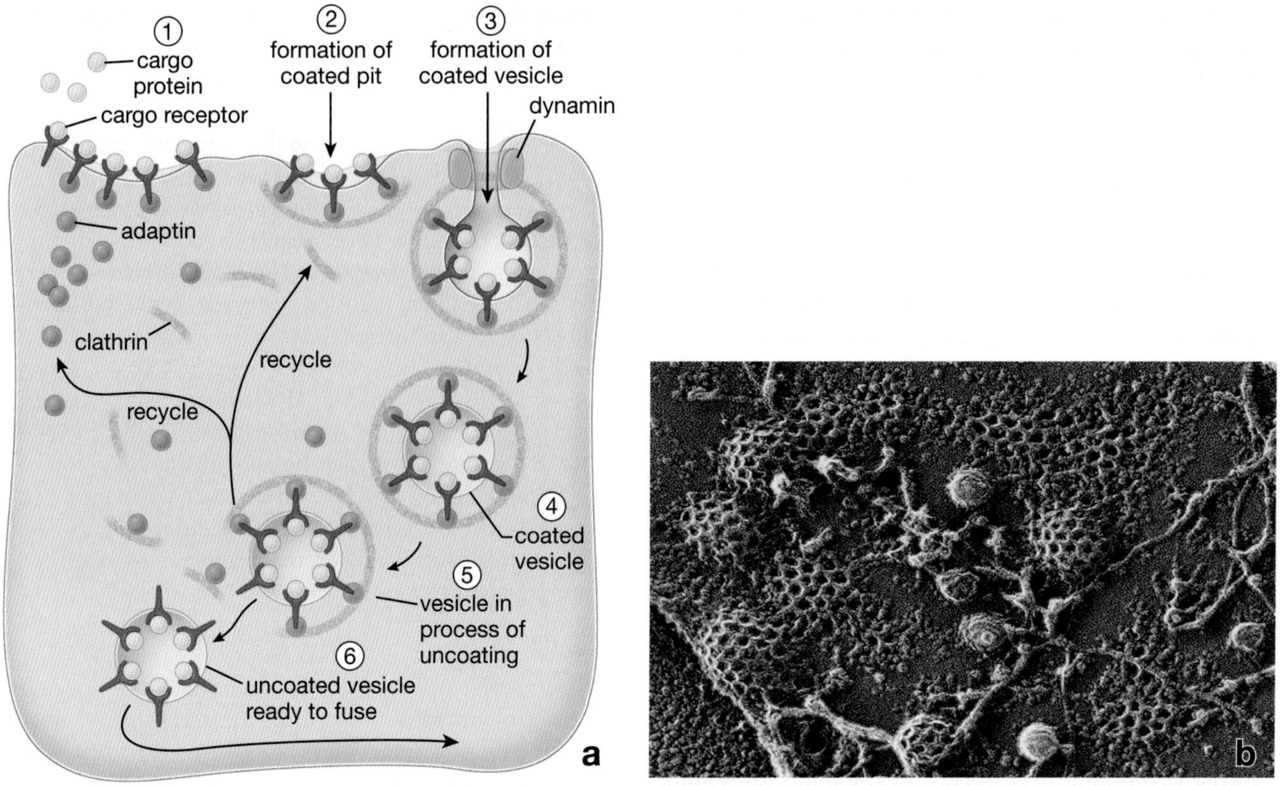

FIGURE 2.13. Receptor-mediated endocytosis. a. This diagram shows the steps in receptor-mediated endocytosis, a transport mechanism that allows selected molecules to enter the cell. Cargo receptors recognize and bind specific molecules that come in contact with the plasma membrane. Cargo receptor–molecule complexes are recognized by adaptin, a protein that helps select and gather appropriate complexes in specific areas of the plasma membrane for transport into cells. Clathrin molecules then bind to the adaptin–cargo receptor–molecule complex to assemble into a shallow basket-like cage and form a coated pit. Clathrin interactions then assist the plasma membrane to change shape to form a deep depression, a fully formed coated pit that becomes pinched off from the plasma membrane by the protein complex dynamin as a coated vesicle (i.e., budding from the membrane). Selected cargo proteins and their receptors are thus pulled from the extracellular space into the lumen of a forming coated vesicle. After budding and internalization of the vesicle, the coat proteins are removed and recycled for further use. The uncoated vesicle travels to its destination to fuse with a cytoplasmic organelle. **b.** Electron micrograph of the cytoplasmic surface of the plasma membrane of A431 cells prepared by the quick-freeze, deep-etch technique. This image shows coated pits and clathrin-coated vesicles in different stages of their formation. Note that the coated pits and clathrin-coated vesicles are formed in areas devoid of actin filaments. The small uniform pinocytic vesicles do not have a clathrin coat and are located in close proximity to actin filaments. ×200,000. (Courtesy of Dr. John E. Heuser, Washington University School of Medicine.)

the cytoplasmic surface of the plasma membrane. Cargo receptors recognize and bind to specific molecules that come in contact with the plasma membrane. Clathrin molecules then assemble into a basket-like cage that helps change the shape of the plasma membrane into a vesicle-like invagination (Fig. 2.13b). Clathrin interacts with the cargo receptor via **clathrin adaptor proteins (adaptin, AP180)**, which are instrumental in selecting appropriate cargo molecules for transport into the cells. Thus, selected cargo proteins and their receptors are pulled from the extracellular space into the lumen of a forming vesicle. The large (100-kDa) mechanoenzyme GTPase from the family of membrane scission proteins, called **dynamin**, mediates the liberation of forming clathrin-coated vesicles from the plasma membrane during receptor-mediated endocytosis. The type of vesicle formed as a result of receptor-mediated endocytosis is referred to as a **coated vesicle**, and the process itself is known as **clathrin-dependent endocytosis**. Clathrin-coated vesicles are also involved in the movement of the cargo material from the plasma membrane to early endosomes and from the Golgi apparatus to the early and late endosomes.

Exocytosis

The movement of secretory vesicles to the plasma membrane is essential for normal cell function. The fusion of secretory vesicles with the plasma membrane is a complex process and involves various types of proteins and lipids. Understanding the underlying molecular mechanisms of exocytosis and membrane fusion provides a solid foundation for pharmacologic treatment of many diseases.

Exocytosis is the process by which a vesicle moves from the cytoplasm to the plasma membrane, where it discharges its contents to the extracellular space.

A variety of molecules produced by the cell for export are initially delivered from the site of their formation to the Golgi apparatus. The next step involves sorting and packaging the secretory product into transport vesicles that are destined to fuse with the plasma membrane in a process known as **exocytosis**. Intracellular traffic of these vesicles is achieved by the presence of specific proteins on their surface (coatomers such as COP-I and COP-II) that mediate their movements (see page 56). The molecules that travel this route are often chemically modified (e.g., glycosylated, sulfated) as they pass through different cellular compartments. The membrane that is added to the plasma membrane by exocytosis is recovered into the cytoplasmic compartment by an endocytic process. There are two general pathways of exocytosis:

- In the **constitutive pathway**, substances designated for export are continuously delivered in transport vesicles to the plasma membrane. Proteins that leave the cell by this process are secreted immediately after their synthesis and exit from the Golgi apparatus, as seen in the secretion of immunoglobulins by plasma cells and of procollagen by fibroblasts. This pathway is present to some degree in all cells. The TEM reveals that these cells lack secretory granules.

- In the **regulated secretory pathway**, specialized cells, such as endocrine and exocrine cells and neurons, concentrate secretory proteins and transiently store them in secretory vesicles within the cytoplasm (Fig. 2.14). In this case, a regulatory event (hormonal or neural stimulus) must be activated for secretion to occur, as in the release of secretory vesicles by chief cells of the gastric mucosa and by acinar cells of the pancreas. The signaling stimulus causes a transient influx of Ca^{2+} into the cytoplasm, which in turn stimulates secretory vesicles to fuse with the plasma membrane and discharge their contents (Fig. 2.15). In the past, secretory vesicles containing inactive precursor (zymogen) were called zymogen granules.

In addition to excretory pathways, proteins can be transported between the Golgi apparatus and other organelles along endosomal pathways. These pathways are used for delivery of organelle-specific proteins, such as lysosomal structural proteins, into the appropriate organelles.

The precise targeting of vesicles to the appropriate cellular compartment is initially controlled by docking proteins, and specificity is ensured by interactions between soluble NSF attachment receptor (SNARE) proteins.

As discussed previously, newly formed vesicles that bud off from the donor membrane (such as cell membrane or Golgi cisternae) can fuse with a number of possible target membranes within the cell. Shortly after budding and shedding its clathrin coat, a vesicle must be targeted to the appropriate cellular

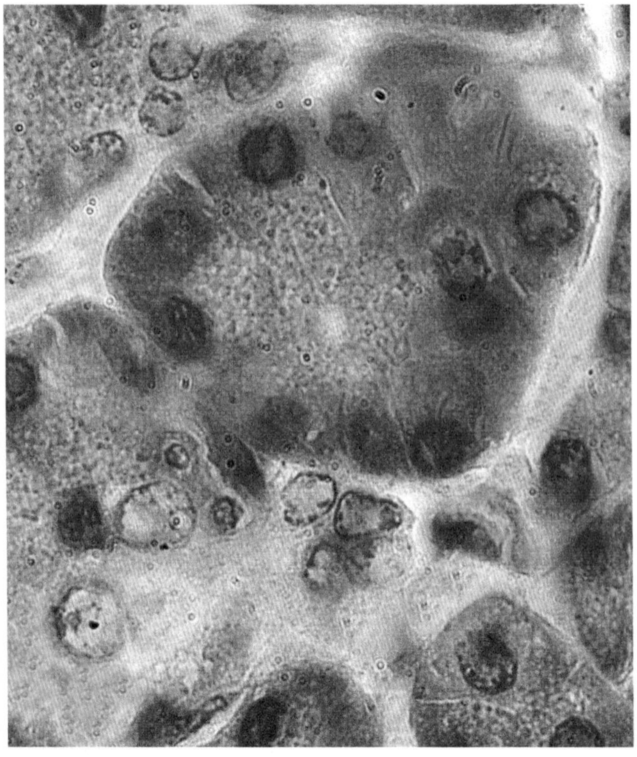

FIGURE 2.14. Photomicrograph of secretory cells of the pancreas. Note that secretory vesicles containing protein ready for secretion fill the apical portion of the cells. This process requires an external signaling mechanism for the cell to discharge the accumulated granules. ×860.

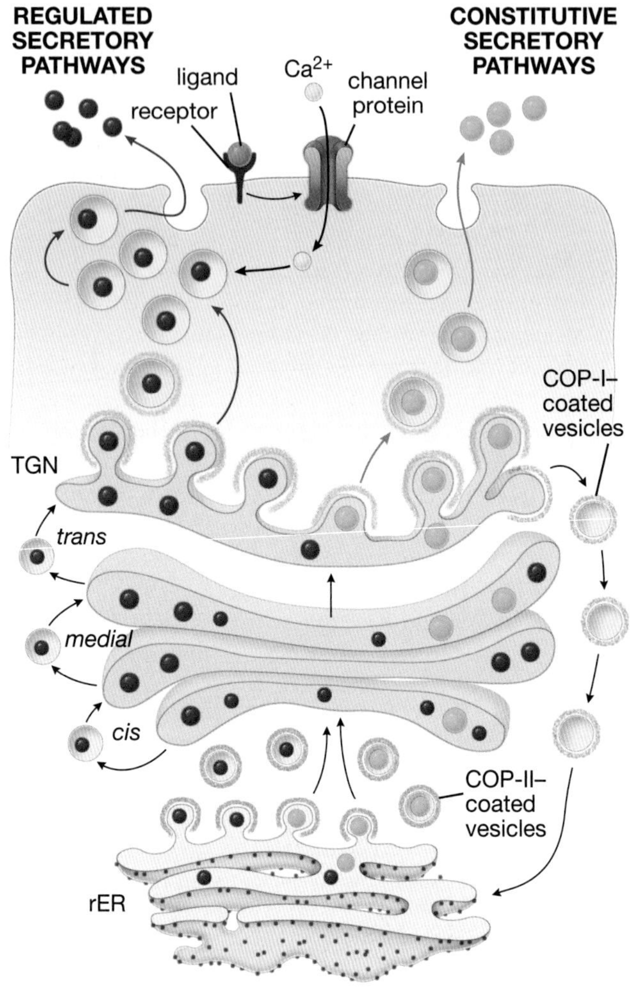

FIGURE 2.15. Diagram showing two pathways for exocytosis. Newly synthesized proteins are synthesized in the rough endoplasmic reticulum (*rER*). After their initial posttranslational modification, they are delivered in COP-II-coated vesicles to the Golgi apparatus. After additional modification in the Golgi apparatus, sorting, and packaging, the final secretory product is transported to the plasma membrane in vesicles that form from the *trans*-Golgi network (*TGN*). Note that retrograde transport is present between Golgi cisternae and is mediated by the COP-I-coated vesicle. Two distinct pathways are recognized. *Blue arrows* indicate the constitutive pathway in which proteins leave the cell immediately after their synthesis. In cells using this pathway, almost no secretory product accumulates, and thus, few secretory vesicles are present in the cytoplasm. *Red arrows* indicate the regulated secretory pathway in which protein secretion is regulated by hormonal or neural stimuli. In cells using this pathway, such as the pancreatic acinar cells in Figure 2.14, secretory proteins are concentrated and transiently stored in secretory vesicles within the cytoplasm. After appropriate stimulation, the secretory vesicles fuse with the plasma membrane and discharge their contents.

compartment. A **targeting mechanism** can be likened to a taxi driver in a large city who successfully delivers a passenger to the proper street address. In the cell, the street address is recognized by **Rab-GTPase** bound to the membrane of the traveling vesicle. Rab-GTPase interacts with **tethering proteins** located on the target membrane. This initial interaction provides recognition of the vesicle and recruits the necessary number of tethering proteins to dock the incoming vesicle. The **docking complex** between Rab-GTPase and its receptor immobilizes the vesicle near the target membrane (Fig. 2.16).

The **SNARE** family of small transmembrane proteins (name derived from "**S**oluble **N**SF **A**ttachment **RE**ceptor") is expressed on both the vesicles and target membranes to mediate accurate vesicle trafficking and subsequent membrane fusion. SNAREs are originally grouped according to their location within the vesicle or target membrane. A **vesicle-specific SNARE** called **v-SNARE** interacts with the target plasma membrane that contains a **target-specific SNARE** called **t-SNARE.** When a vesicle reaches its destination membrane, both groups of SNARE proteins located on separate membranes must recognize each other and assemble into a tight α-helical configuration called the ***trans*-SNARE complex.** Successful assembly of the trans-SNARE complex guarantees the specificity of interaction between a particular vesicle and its target membrane. It also pulls the vesicle and plasma membrane together, initiating a membrane fusion.

After the membrane fuses, proteins of the trans-SNARE complexes are located in this single fused membrane and are now referred as ***cis*-SNARE complexes.** These complexes are dismantled with the help of the **NSF/α-SNAP protein complex** and recycled for use in another round of vesicle fusion.

The SNARE proteins and their interactions have been extensively studied in neuromuscular junctions and other nerve terminals. In nerve terminals, three specific SNARE proteins control trafficking and fusion of synaptic vesicles (containing neurotransmitter) with the presynaptic plasma membrane:

- **Synaptobrevin** is an 18-kDa integral membrane protein found in the synaptic vesicle (v-SNARE).
- **Syntaxin** is a 33-kDa integral membrane protein found in the presynaptic plasma membrane (t-SNARE).
- **SNAP-25** is a 23-kDa peripheral membrane protein covalently attached to the intracellular surface of the presynaptic plasma membrane via modified lipid (palmitic acid) in the process called palmitoylation. SNAP-25 is essential for neurotransmitter release from synaptic terminals and it is considered a t-SNARE protein.

Interactions of these three SNARE proteins are required for the formation of *trans*-SNARE complexes and neurotransmitter release. Their intracellular domains have an ability to form coiled-coil structures. All three SNARE proteins contribute their own coiled-coil regions for the formation of the *trans*-SNARE complex, creating a parallel four-helical bundle. Synaptobrevin and syntaxin each contribute a single helical region, and SNAP-25 contributes two helical regions to form the complex.

Malfunction of any one of these three proteins leads to neurotransmitter release defects in nerve endings. For instance, **botulinum neurotoxin**, produced by the anaerobic bacterium *Clostridium botulinum*, blocks neuromuscular transmission. This toxin binds to the neuronal cell membrane and is subsequently endocytosed. Next, the toxin penetrates the membrane of the endocytic vesicle to enter the cytoplasm of the nerve terminal at the neuromuscular junction. There are seven distinct serotypes (A to G) of botulinum toxins, with each toxin cleaving the SNARE proteins

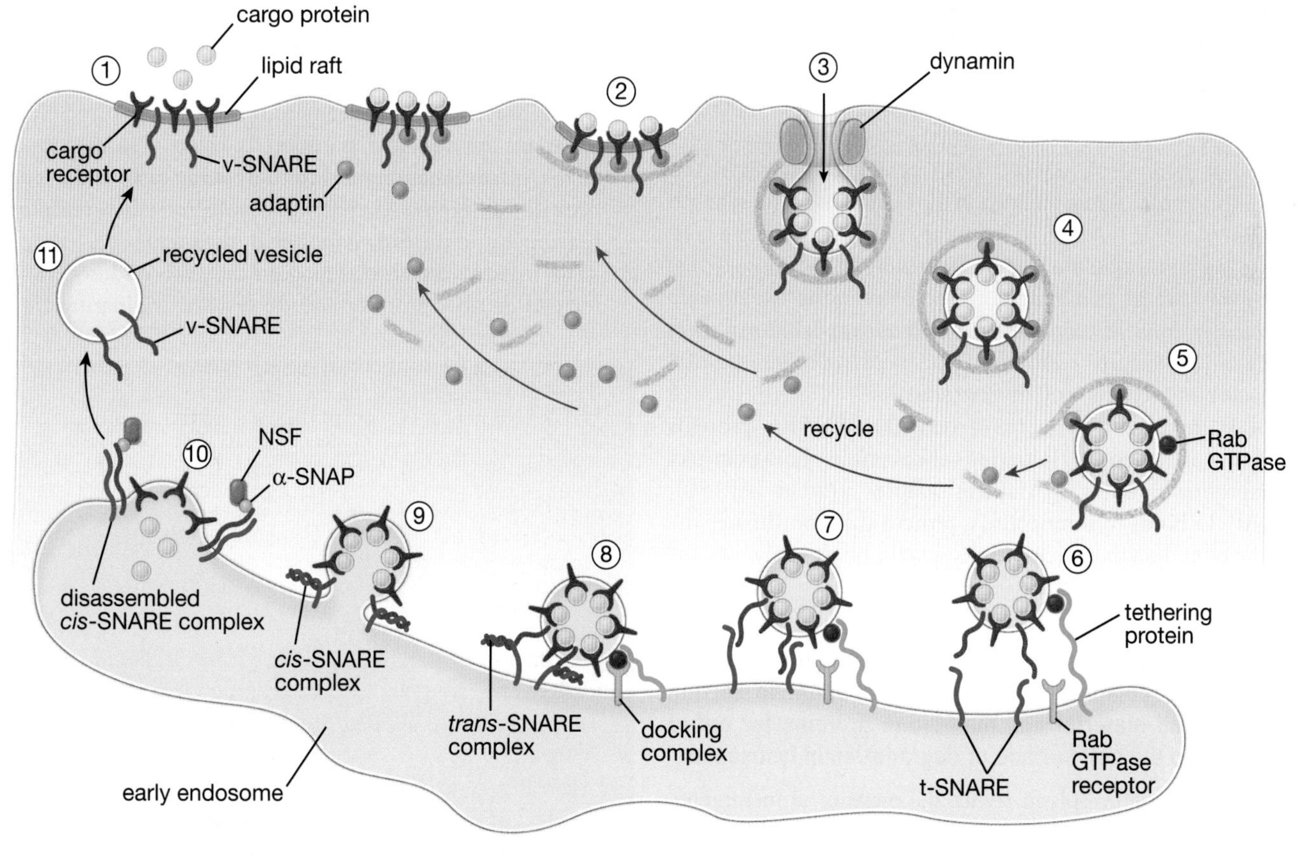

FIGURE 2.16. Steps in formation, targeting, docking, and fusion of transport vesicles with the target membrane. (1) Lipid raft with cargo receptors ready to interact with cargo protein. Note the presence of the specific targeting protein v-SNARE. **(2)** Initial step in vesicle formation: The binding of the adaptin complex and clathrin forms a coated pit. **(3)** Formation (budding) of the fully assembled coated vesicle. **(4)** Transport of the coated vesicle to its destination. **(5)** Disassembly of clathrin coat. Note the expression of Rab-GTPase activity. **(6)** Tethering of the vesicle to the target membrane by the interaction between Rab-GTPase and tethering proteins. **(7)** Beginning of the docking process (recruitment of tethering proteins). **(8)** Formation of the docking complex between Rab-GTPase and its protein in the target membrane: v-SNAREs on the immobilized vesicle interact with t-SNAREs on the target membrane to form the *trans*-SNARE complex. **(9)** Fusion of the vesicle to the target membrane, *trans*-SNARE becomes *cis*-SNARE complex. **(10)** Discharge of the cargo protein into the early endosomal compartment and disassembly of the *cis* complex by the interaction of the NSF/α-SNAP protein complex. **(11)** Recycling of v-SNAREs in the transport vesicles for use in another round of vesicle targeting and fusion.

at different sites. This prevents the release of the neurotransmitter acetylcholine from the neuromuscular terminal and depolarization of muscle cell. Serotypes B, D, F, and G cleave **synaptobrevin**; serotypes A, C, and E cleave **SNAP-25**; and serotype C cleaves **syntaxin**. In humans, the A, B, and E serotypes are responsible for **botulism**, a life-threatening disease characterized by progressive muscle weakness. Symptoms include descending paralysis that begins with the muscles controlling eye movement, facial expression, and swallowing and spreads subsequently to the upper limbs, thorax (respiratory muscles), and lower limbs. Paralysis of respiratory muscles (e.g., diaphragm) hampers breathing and eventually results in respiratory failure.

The botulin toxin serotypes A and B are used therapeutically to treat patients with nerve and muscle disorders. Injection of a small amount of botulin toxin into specific muscles is used in ophthalmology for treating **blepharospasm** (excessive blinking) or **strabismus** (not aligned eyes). In strabismus, the toxin is used to paralyze the muscle on one side of the eye that is pulling the eye into the abnormal position. In **movement disorders** such as **dystonia**, uncontrollable repetitive skeletal muscle contractions as well as **gastrointestinal smooth muscle and sphincter spasms** are also treated by injections of botulin toxin. In addition, injection of extremely small quantities of botulin toxin (**onabotulinumtoxinA** or **botox**) into muscles of facial expression is used for the cosmetic treatment of facial wrinkles.

Another anaerobic bacterium, *Clostridium tetani*, produces **tetanospasmin toxin**, which causes **tetanus**. Tetanospasmin cleaves **synaptobrevin** (v-SNARE protein) and prevents the release of inhibitory neurotransmitters (mainly glycine and γ-aminobutyric acid [GABA]) from synaptic vesicles at the inhibitory motor nerve endings in the central nervous system. The physiologic function of inhibitory neurotransmitters is to decrease and modulate excitatory activity of motor neurons. With the loss of this inhibition, motor neurons excessively stimulate muscle contractions, producing stiffness and rigidity (particularly in the jaw and neck muscles), painful muscle contractions, and muscle spasms.

It is important to mention here that SNARE proteins are also involved in initiating endocytosis. For example, synaptobrevin binds to clathrin adaptor protein (AP180); SNAP-25 binds to intersectin, a protein that coordinates the traffic of endocytic vesicles; and syntaxin binds to dynamin.

Endosomes

Endosomes represent a network of membrane-enclosed cytoplasmic compartments that are essential in sorting endocytosed material and membrane proteins for either transport to the cell surface or degradation in lysosomes.

TEM of the cell cytoplasm reveals the presence of membrane-enclosed compartments associated with all endocytic pathways (Fig. 2.17). These compartments, called **early sorting endosomes** or **early endosomes**, are restricted to a portion of the cytoplasm near the cell membrane. The sorting function of early endosomes enables the return of many vesicles budding from their surface to the plasma membrane. Early endosomes are formed de novo from the invagination of the plasma membrane, forming vesicles containing cell surface proteins and soluble content from the extracellular space. These newly formed endocytic vesicles directly merge with each other or with preexisting early endosomes. In addition, vesicles originating from the trans-Golgi network (TGN) and endoplasmic reticulum can also contribute to the formation and content of the early endosomes.

The contents of vesicles incorporated into early endosomal compartments remain in this compartment. As the early endosome matures, it becomes more acidic and sinks into deeper regions of the cytoplasm to become **late-sorting endosomes** or **late endosomes**. The ESCRT cytoplasmic protein complex controls membrane remodeling (pages 35-36), which is the basis of the sorting and maturation of early endosomes into late endosomes. The sorting function continues in late endosomes. The endosomal membrane of some late endosomes undergoes inward invagination to generate intraluminal vesicles. These structures, called intracellular **multivesicular bodies (MVBs)** or multivesicular endosomes, are also sorted. Some mature into **lysosomes** (where their contents will be degraded), and others fuse with the plasma membrane to release intraluminal vesicles by exocytosis. These extracellular vesicles originating from MVBs are called **exosomes**.

Endosomes can be viewed either as stable cytoplasmic organelles or as temporary structures formed by endocytosis.

Recent experimental observations of endocytic pathways conducted in vitro and in vivo suggest two different models that explain the origin and formation of the endosomal compartments in the cell:

- The **stable compartment model** describes early and late endosomes as stable cellular organelles that maintain their connection to the external environment of the cell and Golgi apparatus by vesicular transport. Coated vesicles formed at the plasma membrane fuse only with early endosomes because they express specific surface receptors; these receptors remain part of the early endosomal membrane.
- The **maturation model** suggests that early endosomes are formed de novo from endocytic vesicles originating from

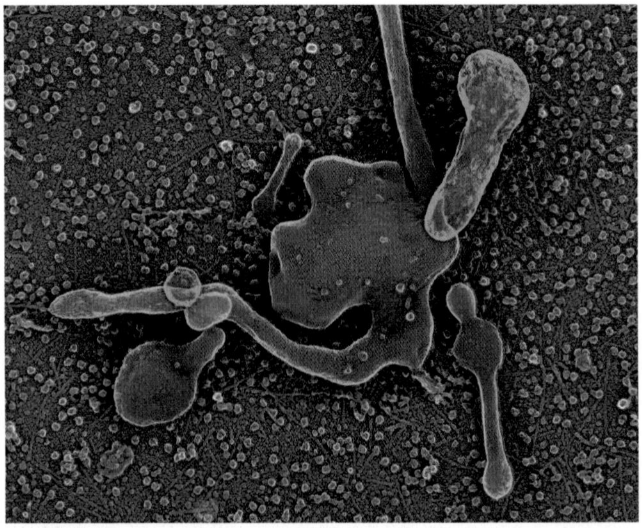

FIGURE 2.17. Electron micrograph of an early endosome. This deep-etch electron micrograph shows the structure of an early endosome in *Dictyostelium*. Early endosomes are located near the plasma membrane and, as in many other sorting compartments, have a typical tubulovesicular structure. The tubular portions contain the majority of integral membrane proteins destined for membrane recycling, whereas the luminal portions collect secretory cargo proteins. The lumen of the endosome is subdivided into multiple compartments, or *cisternae*, by the invagination of its membrane and undergoes frequent changes in shape. ×15,000. (Courtesy of Dr. John E. Heuser, Washington University School of Medicine.)

the plasma membrane. Therefore, the composition of the early endosomal membrane changes progressively as some components are recycled between the cell surface and the Golgi apparatus. This maturation process leads to the formation of late endosomes and, subsequently, lysosomes. As this compartment matures, specific receptors present on early sorting endosomes (e.g., for coated vesicles) are removed by recycling, degradation, or inactivation.

Both models complement rather than contradict each other in describing, identifying, and studying the pathways of internalized molecules.

The major function of early endosomes is to sort and recycle proteins internalized by endocytic pathways.

As their name implies, **early endosomes** sort proteins that have been internalized by endocytic processes. The sorting process is primarily regulated by **ESCRT** (pages 35-36). ESCRT represents an assembly of four separate protein subcomplexes (ESCRT 0 through III) that mediate the scission of membrane necks from the inside. The shape and geometry of the tubules and vesicles emerging from the early endosome create an environment where localized changes in pH constitute the basis of the endosome sorting mechanism. This mechanism includes the dissociation of ligands from their receptor proteins. In addition, the narrow diameter of the tubules and vesicles may also aid in sorting large molecules, which can be mechanically prevented from entering specific sorting compartments. After sorting, most proteins are rapidly recycled or destined for digestion, and the excess membrane is returned to the plasma membrane.

The fate of the internalized ligand–receptor complex depends on the sorting and recycling ability of the early endosome.

The following four pathways for processing internalized ligand–receptor complexes are present in the cell:

- **The receptor is recycled and the ligand is degraded.** Surface receptors allow the cell to bring in substances selectively through the process of endocytosis. This pathway occurs most often in the cell; it is important because it allows surface receptors to be recycled. Most ligand–receptor complexes dissociate in the acidic pH of the early endosome. The receptor, most likely an integral membrane protein (see page 35), is recycled to the surface via vesicles that bud off the ends of narrow-diameter tubules of the early endosome. Ligands are usually sequestered in the spherical vacuolar part of the endosome that will later form MVBs, which will transport the ligand to late endosomes for further degradation in the lysosome (Fig. 2.18a). This pathway is utilized by the **low-density lipoprotein (LDL)–receptor complex**, **insulin–glucose transporter (GLUT) receptor complex**, and a variety of **peptide hormones** and their receptors.
- **Both receptor and ligand are recycled**. Ligand–receptor complex dissociation does not always accompany receptor recycling. For example, the low pH of the endosome dissociates iron from the iron-carrier protein **transferrin**, but transferrin remains associated with its receptor. However, transferrin is released once the

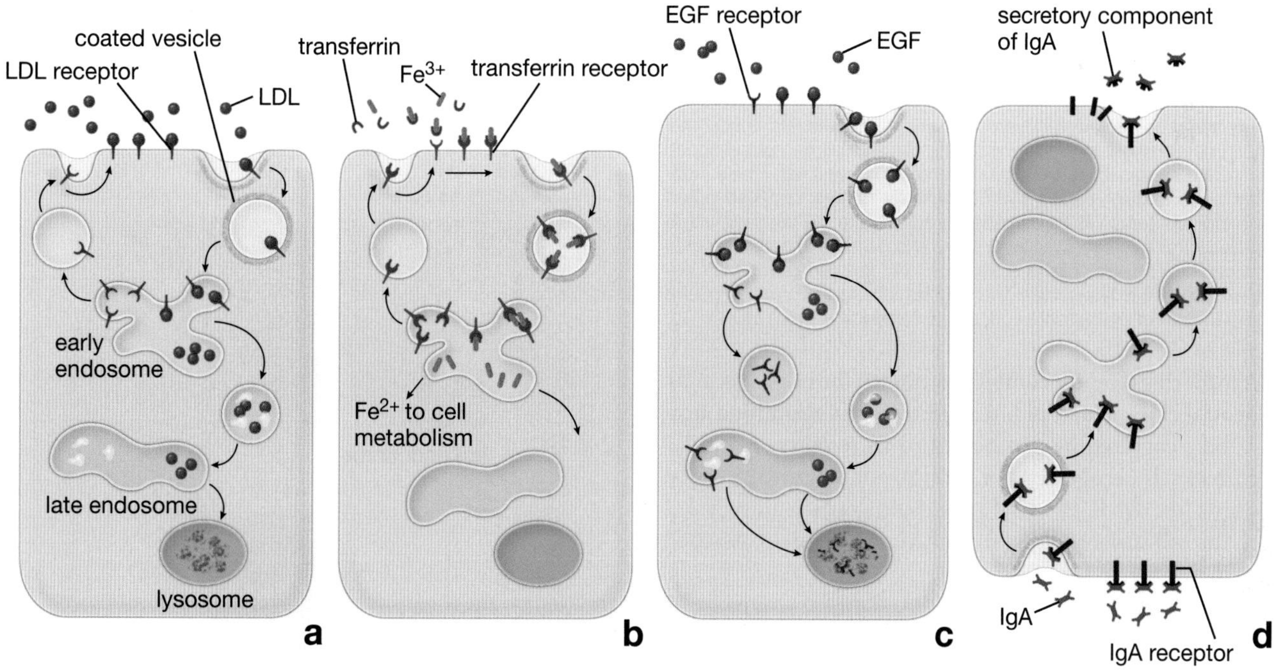

FIGURE 2.18. Fate of receptor and ligand in receptor-mediated endocytosis. This diagram shows four major pathways along which the fate of internalized ligand–receptor complexes is determined. **a.** The internalized ligand–receptor complex dissociates, the receptor is recycled to the cell surface, and the ligand is directed to late endosomes and eventually degraded within lysosomes. This processing pathway is used by the LDL–receptor complex, insulin–GLUT receptor complex, and a variety of peptide hormone–receptor complexes. LDL, low-density lipoprotein; GLUT, glucose transporter. **b.** Both internalized receptor and ligand are recycled. Ligand–receptor complex dissociation does not occur, and the entire complex is recycled to the surface. An example is the iron–transferrin–transferrin receptor complex that uses this processing pathway. Once iron (Fe^{3}+) is released from transferrin in the endosome, the transferrin–transferrin receptor complex returns to the cell surface, where transferrin is released. In early endosomes, the Fe^{3}+ ions are reduced to the ferrous state (Fe^{2}+) by ferrireductase and are released into the cell cytoplasm. **c.** The internalized ligand–receptor complex dissociates in the early endosome. The free ligand and the receptor are directed to the late endosomal compartment for further degradation. This pathway is used by many growth factors (e.g., the EGF–receptor complex). EGF, epidermal growth factor. **d.** The internalized ligand–receptor complex is transported through the cell. Dissociation does not occur, and the entire complex undergoes transcytosis and release at a different site of the cell surface. This pathway is used during secretion of immunoglobulins (secretory IgA) into saliva. The antibody IgA–receptor complex is internalized at the basal surface of the secretory cells in the salivary gland and released at the apical surface. IgA, immunoglobulin A.

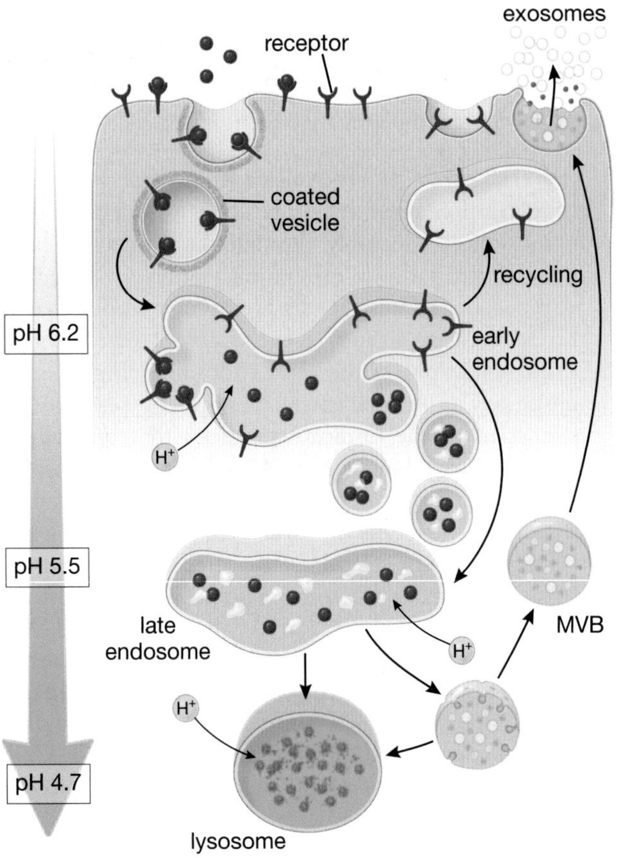

FIGURE 2.19. Schematic diagram of endosomal compartments of the cell. This diagram shows the fate of protein (*red circles*) endocytosed from the cell surface and destined for lysosomal destruction. Proteins are first found in endocytic (coated) vesicles that deliver them to early endosomes, which are located in the peripheral part of the cytoplasm. Because of the sorting capability of early endosomes, receptors are usually recycled to the plasma membrane, and endocytosed proteins are transported via vesicles to late endosomes positioned near the Golgi apparatus and the nucleus. The proteins transported to late endosomes will eventually be degraded in lysosomes. Note that the late endosomal compartment makes vesicles in which the endosomal membrane undergoes inward invaginations to generate intraluminal vesicles. These intracellular multivesicular bodies (*MVBs*) typically mature into lysosomes where their contents will be degraded or fused with the cell membrane to release intraluminal vesicles (now called exosomes) and other contents by exocytosis. The acidification scale (*left*) illustrates changes in pH from early endosomes to lysosomes. The acidification is accomplished by the active transport of protons into endosomal compartments.

transferrin–receptor complex returns to the cell surface. At neutral extracellular pH, transferrin must again bind iron to be recognized by and bound to its receptor. A similar pathway is recognized for **major histocompatibility complex (MHC) I and II molecules**, which are recycled to the cell surface with a foreign antigen protein attached to them (Fig. 2.18b).

- **Both receptor and ligand are degraded.** This pathway has been identified for **epidermal growth factor (EGF)** and its receptor. Like many other proteins, EGF binds to its receptor on the cell surface. The complex is internalized and carried to early endosomes. Here, EGF dissociates from its receptor, and both are sorted, packaged in separate vesicles, and transferred to the late endosome, often detected in the MVBs. From there, both ligand and receptor are destined to be degraded within lysosomes (Fig. 2.18c).
- **Both receptor and ligand are transported through the cell.** This pathway is used for secretion of **immunoglobulins (secretory IgA)** into the saliva and human milk. During this process, commonly referred to as **transcytosis**, substances can be altered as they are transported across the epithelial cell (Fig. 2.18d). Transport of maternal immunoglobulin G (IgG) across the placental barrier into the fetus also follows a similar pathway.

Early and late endosomes differ in their cellular localization, morphology, and state of acidification and function.

Early and late endosomes are localized in different areas of the cell. **Early endosomes** can be found in the more peripheral cytoplasm, whereas late endosomes are often positioned near the Golgi apparatus and the nucleus. An early endosome has a tubulovesicular structure: The lumen is subdivided into cisternae separated by invaginations of its membrane. Within early endosomes, proteins destined to be transported to late endosomes are sorted and separated from proteins destined for recycling and packaged into vesicles. Early endosomes exhibit only a slightly more acidic environment (pH 6.2–6.5) than the cell cytoplasm.

In contrast, **late endosomes** have a more complex structure and often exhibit onion-like internal membranes. Invagination of late endosomal membranes results in the formation of **MVBs** containing **intraluminal vesicles.** The pH of late endosomes is more acidic, averaging 5.5. TEM studies reveal specific vesicles that transport substances between early and

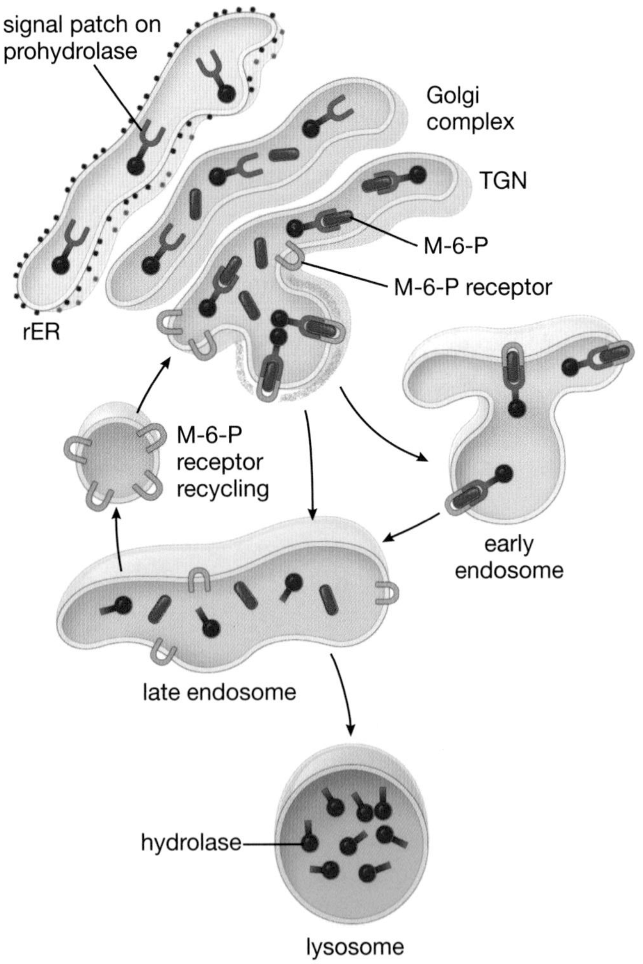

FIGURE 2.20. Pathways for delivery of newly synthesized lysosomal enzymes. Lysosomal enzymes (such as lysosomal hydrolases) are synthesized and glycosylated within the rough endoplasmic reticulum (*rER*). The enzymes then fold in a specific way so that a signal patch is formed to which mannose-6-phosphate (*M-6-P*) is added. This additional modification allows the enzyme to be targeted to specific proteins that possess M-6-P receptor activity. M-6-P receptors are present in the *trans*-Golgi network (*TGN*) of the Golgi apparatus, where the lysosomal enzymes are sorted and packaged into vesicles later transported to the early or late endosomes. The M-6-P receptors are recycled back to the Golgi apparatus.

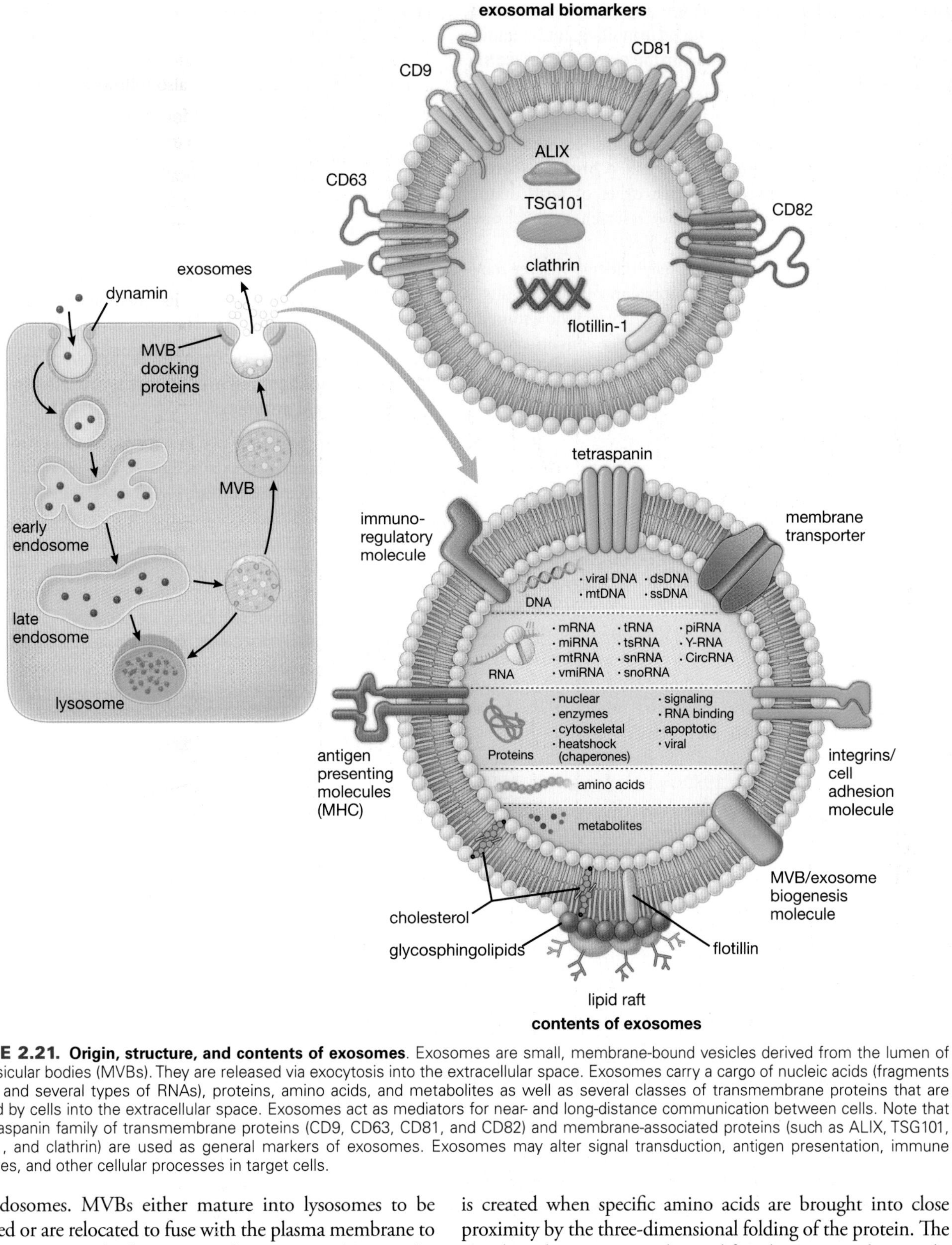

FIGURE 2.21. Origin, structure, and contents of exosomes. Exosomes are small, membrane-bound vesicles derived from the lumen of multivesicular bodies (MVBs). They are released via exocytosis into the extracellular space. Exosomes carry a cargo of nucleic acids (fragments of DNA and several types of RNAs), proteins, amino acids, and metabolites as well as several classes of transmembrane proteins that are released by cells into the extracellular space. Exosomes act as mediators for near- and long-distance communication between cells. Note that the tetraspanin family of transmembrane proteins (CD9, CD63, CD81, and CD82) and membrane-associated proteins (such as ALIX, TSG101, flotillin-1, and clathrin) are used as general markers of exosomes. Exosomes may alter signal transduction, antigen presentation, immune responses, and other cellular processes in target cells.

late endosomes. MVBs either mature into lysosomes to be degraded or are relocated to fuse with the plasma membrane to release exosomes and other contents by exocytosis (Fig. 2.19).

Late endosomes destined to become lysosomes receive newly synthesized lysosomal enzymes that are targeted via the mannose-6-phosphate (M-6-P) receptor.

Some endosomes also communicate with the vesicular transport system of the rER. This pathway provides constant delivery of newly synthesized lysosomal enzymes, or **hydrolases**. A hydrolase is synthesized in the rER as an enzymatically inactive precursor called a **prohydrolase**. This heavily glycosylated protein then folds in a specific way so that a **signal patch** is formed and exposed on its surface. This recognition signal is created when specific amino acids are brought into close proximity by the three-dimensional folding of the protein. The signal patch on a protein destined for a lysosome is then modified by several enzymes that attach **mannose-6-phosphate (M-6-P)** to the prohydrolase surface. M-6-P acts as a target for proteins possessing an **M-6-P receptor**. M-6-P receptors are present in early and late endosomes, lysosomes, and the Golgi apparatus, which is involved in sorting and retrieving secreted prohydrolases destined for transport to endosomes (Fig. 2.20). The acidic environment of late endosomes causes the release of prohydrolases from the M-6-P receptors, which are recycled back (retrograde transport) to the TGN. Prohydrolases are next activated by cleavage and by removing phosphate groups from the mannose residues.

The contents of late endosomes are degraded in lysosomes; however, intraluminal vesicles found in multivesicular bodies are often released as exosomes into the extracellular matrix.

In general, substances transported to late endosomes are eventually degraded in lysosomes in a default process that does not require any additional signals. Because late endosomes mature into lysosomes, they are also called **prelysosomes**. Late endosomes may fuse with each other or with mature lysosomes. Video microscopy allows researchers to observe the complex behavior of these organelles.

A population of late endosomes may undergo further transformation. Invagination of late endosomal membranes results in the formation of **intraluminal vesicles** (they reside within the lumen of the late endosomes). These vesicles contain cytosolic components and certain proteins derived from the invaginated late endosomal membrane. The formation of intraluminal vesicles is aided by ESCRT cytoplasmic protein complex (pages 35-36).

Exosomes

Exosomes originate from multivesicular bodies and represent a novel mode of intercellular communication.

Exosomes represent very small (40–100 nm in diameter) endosome-derived membrane-bound vesicles secreted by cells into the extracellular space. These nano-sized vesicles are released from the cell when MVBs fuse with the plasma membrane (Fig. 2.21). High concentrations of exosomes are present in all body fluids, including blood, lymph, cerebrospinal fluid, vitreous body, interstitial fluids, saliva, breast milk, amniotic fluid, semen, and urine.

The presence of exosomes in the extracellular space was discovered in the late 1980s when they were initially characterized as cellular waste products. Recent studies confirm that exosomes are functional vesicles that act as transport vehicles for near- and long-distance intercellular communication and material exchange between cells. Exosome membranes contain various transmembrane proteins originating from the plasma membrane of the cell of origin (i.e., adhesion molecules, receptors, and signaling molecules). Exosomes also carry a cargo of nucleic acids (fragments of DNA and several types of RNAs), proteins, lipids, cytokines, transcription factor receptors, growth factors, and other bioactive substances that can be delivered to target cells (see Fig. 2.21). Because the tetraspanin family of transmembrane proteins (such as CD9, CD63, CD81, and CD82) and membrane-associated proteins (such as ALIX, TSG101, flotillin-1, and clathrin) are most common, they are often used as general markers of exosomes. However, many more cell markers specific to the cell type from which the exosome originated have been identified. Exosomes released from cancer cells can promote neoplasia, tumor growth, metastasis formation, and resistance to therapy. For instance, exosomes originating from breast and prostate cancer cells induce neoplastic transformation of other cells through the transfer of their miRNA cargo.

The delivery of the exosome contents is achieved by the selective binding of exosomes to cell surface receptors (triggering specific intracellular signaling), by endocytosis, or by the direct transfer of intra-exosomal contents, such as messenger RNA (mRNA), into the recipient cells by fusion of the exosome with the cell membrane. Exosomes, therefore, represent a novel mode of intercellular communication in signal transduction, antigen presentation, immune responses, and many other cellular processes.

Clinical research into exosomes is rapidly evolving. Exosomes offer a novel approach for effective vaccine development. Recently, **exosome-based mRNA vaccines** that drive the expression of the immunogenic COVID-19 viral nucleocapsid and spike proteins have been tested. This vaccine shows long-lasting cellular and humoral responses, demonstrating that exosome-based mRNA formulations represent a new approach to protecting against COVID-19 and other infectious diseases. In addition, exosomes are being tested for delivery of gene-based agents, such as DNA and RNA, to patients with genetic disorders and for targeted delivery of therapeutic agents encapsulated into exosomes.

Lysosomes

Lysosomes are digestive organelles that were recognized only after histochemical procedures were used to demonstrate lysosomal enzymes.

Lysosomes are organelles rich in **hydrolytic enzymes** such as proteases, nucleases, glycosidases, lipases, and phospholipases. A lysosome represents a **major digestive compartment** in the cell that degrades macromolecules derived from endocytic pathways as well as from the cell itself in a process known as autophagy (removal of cytoplasmic components, particularly membrane-bounded organelles, by digesting them within lysosomes). For more information about autophagy, see pages 50-53.

The **original hypothesis for lysosomal biogenesis**, formulated almost a half century ago, postulated that lysosomes arise as complete and functional organelles budding from the Golgi apparatus. These newly formed lysosomes were termed **primary lysosomes** in contrast to **secondary lysosomes**, which had already fused with incoming endosomes. However, the primary and secondary lysosome hypothesis has proved to have little validity as new research data allow a better understanding of the details of protein secretory pathways and the fate of endocytic vesicles. It is now widely accepted that **lysosomes are formed** in a complex series of pathways that converge at the late endosomes, transforming them into lysosomes. These pathways are responsible for **targeted delivery of newly synthesized lysosomal enzymes and structural lysosomal membrane proteins into late endosomes**. As stated earlier, lysosomal enzymes are synthesized in the rER and sorted in the Golgi apparatus based on their binding ability to M-6-P receptors (see pages 46-47).

Lysosomes have a unique membrane that is resistant to the hydrolytic digestion occurring in their lumen.

Lysosomes contain a collection of hydrolytic enzymes and are surrounded by a unique membrane that resists hydrolysis by their own enzymes (Fig. 2.22). The **lysosomal membrane** has an unusual phospholipid structure that contains cholesterol and a unique lipid called **lysobisphosphatidic acid**. Most of the structural lysosomal membrane proteins are classified into **lysosome-associated membrane proteins (LAMPs)**, **lysosomal membrane glycoproteins (LGPs)**, and **lysosomal integral membrane proteins (LIMPs)**. LAMPs, LGPs, and LIMPs represent more than 50% of the total membrane proteins in lysosomes and are highly glycosylated on the luminal surface. Sugar molecules cover almost the entire luminal surface of these proteins, thus protecting them from digestion by hydrolytic enzymes. Lysobisphosphatidic acids within the lysosomal membrane may play an important role in restricting the activity of hydrolytic enzymes directed

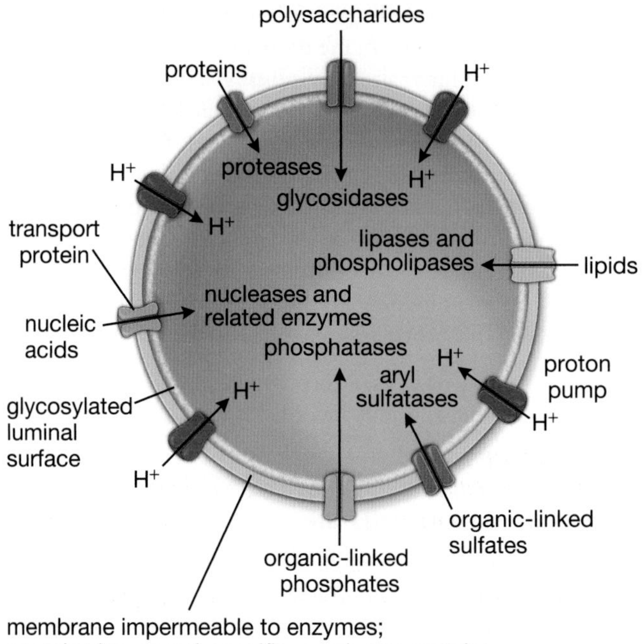

FIGURE 2.22. Schematic diagram of a lysosome. This diagram shows a few selected lysosomal enzymes residing within a lysosome and their respective substrates. The major lysosomal membrane-specific proteins, as well as a few other proteins associated with membrane transport, are also shown. LAMP, lysosome-associated membrane protein; LGP, lysosomal membrane glycoprotein; LIMP, lysosomal integral membrane protein.

against the membrane. The same family of membrane proteins is also detected in late endosomes. In addition, lysosomes and late endosomes contain **proton (H^+) pumps** that transport H^+ ions into the lysosomal lumen, maintaining a low pH (~4.7). The lysosomal membrane also contains **transport proteins** that transport the final products of digestion (amino acids, sugars, nucleotides) to the cytoplasm, where they are used in the synthetic processes of the cell or are exocytosed.

Certain drugs can affect lysosomal function. For example, **chloroquine**, an agent used in the treatment and prevention of malaria, is a **lysosomotropic agent** that accumulates in the lysosomes. It raises the pH of the lysosomal content, thereby inactivating many lysosomal enzymes. The action of chloroquine on lysosomes accounts for its antimalarial activity; the drug concentrates in the acidic food vacuole of the **malaria parasite** (*Plasmodium falciparum*) and interferes with its digestive processes, eventually killing the parasite.

Lysosomal membrane proteins are synthesized in the rER and have a specific lysosomal targeting signal.

As mentioned previously, the intracellular trafficking leading to the delivery of many soluble lysosomal enzymes to late endosomes and lysosomes involves the M-6-P signal and its receptor. All membrane proteins destined for lysosomes (and late endosomes) are synthesized in the rER and transported to and sorted in the Golgi apparatus. However, because they do not contain M-6-P signals, they must be targeted to lysosomes by a different mechanism. The targeting signal for integral membrane proteins is represented by a short cytoplasmic C-terminus domain, which is recognized by adaptin protein complexes and packaged into clathrin-coated vesicles. These proteins reach their destination by one of two pathways:

- In the **constitutive secretory pathway**, LIMPs exit the Golgi apparatus in coated vesicles and are delivered to the cell surface. From there, they are endocytosed and, via the early and late endosomal compartments, finally reach lysosomes (Fig. 2.23).
- In the **Golgi-derived coated vesicle secretory pathway**, LIMPs, after sorting and packaging, exit the Golgi apparatus in clathrin-coated vesicles (see Fig. 2.23). These transport vesicles travel and fuse with late endosomes as a result of interaction between endosome-specific components of v-SNARE and t-SNARE docking proteins (see pages 42-43).

Three different pathways deliver material for intracellular digestion in lysosomes.

Depending on the nature of the digested material, different pathways deliver material for digestion within the lysosomes (Fig. 2.24). In the digestion process, most of the digested material comes from endocytic processes; however, the cell also uses lysosomes to digest its own obsolete parts, nonfunctional organelles, and unnecessary molecules. Three pathways for digestion exist:

- **Extracellular large particles** such as bacteria, cell debris, and other foreign materials are engulfed in the process of phagocytosis. A **phagosome**, formed as the material is internalized within the cytoplasm, subsequently receives hydrolytic enzymes to become a late endosome, which matures into a lysosome.

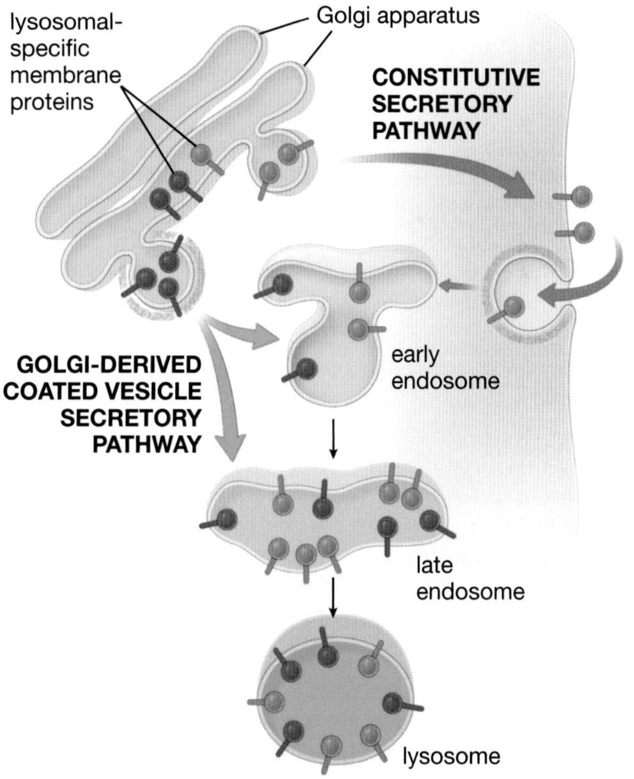

FIGURE 2.23. Lysosome biogenesis. This diagram shows regulated and constitutive pathways for delivery of lysosomal-specific membrane proteins into early and late endosomes. The lysosomal membrane possesses highly glycosylated specific membrane proteins that protect the membrane from digestion by lysosomal enzymes. These lysosome-specific proteins are synthesized in the rough endoplasmic reticulum, transported to the Golgi apparatus, and reach their destination by two pathways. *Blue arrows* indicate the constitutive secretory pathway in which certain lysosomal membrane proteins exit the Golgi apparatus and are delivered to the cell surface. From there, they are endocytosed and, via the early and late endosomal compartments, finally reach lysosomes. *Green arrows* indicate the endosomal Golgi-derived coated vesicle secretory pathway. Here, other lysosomal proteins, after sorting and packaging, exit the Golgi apparatus in clathrin-coated vesicles to fuse with early and late endosomes.

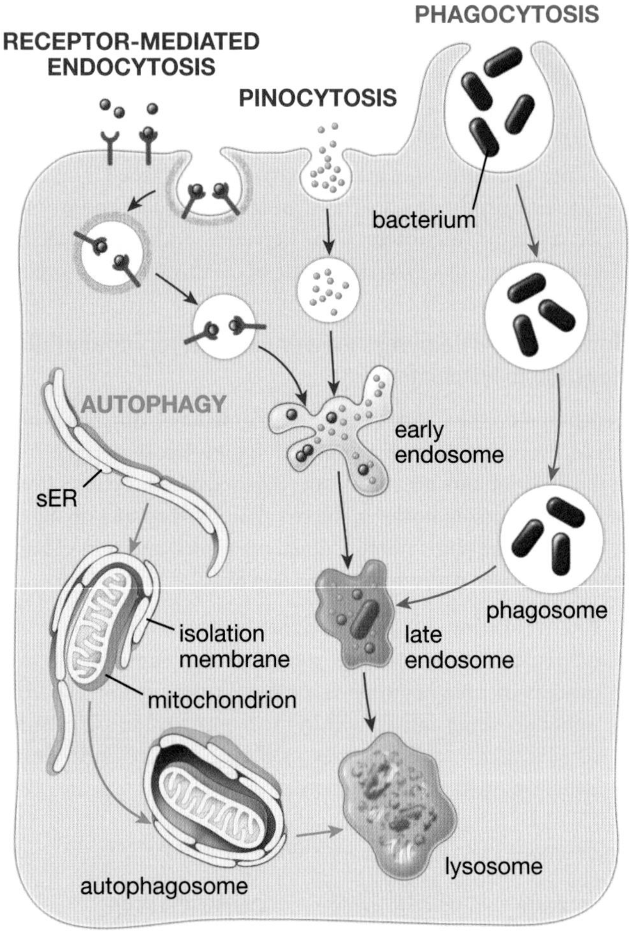

FIGURE 2.24. Pathways of delivery of materials for digestion in lysosomes. Most of the small extracellular particles are internalized by both receptor-mediated endocytosis and pinocytosis. These two endocytic pathways are labeled with *red arrows*. Large extracellular particles such as bacteria and cellular debris are delivered for cellular digestion via the phagocytic pathway (*blue arrows*). The cell also uses lysosomes to digest its own organelles and other intracellular proteins via the autophagic pathway (*green arrows*). Intracellular particles are isolated from the cytoplasmic matrix by the isolation membrane of the smooth endoplasmic reticulum (*sER*), transported to lysosomes, and subsequently degraded.

- **Extracellular small particles** such as extracellular proteins, plasma membrane proteins, and ligand–receptor complexes are internalized by **pinocytosis** and **receptor-mediated endocytosis**. These particles follow the endocytic pathway through early and late endosomal compartments and are finally degraded in lysosomes.
- **Intracellular particles** such as entire organelles, cytoplasmic proteins, and other cellular components are isolated from the cytoplasmic matrix by endoplasmic reticulum membranes, transported to lysosomes, and degraded. This process is called **autophagy**.

In addition, some cells (e.g., osteoclasts involved in bone resorption and neutrophils involved in acute inflammation) may release lysosomal enzymes directly into the extracellular space to digest components of the extracellular matrix.

Lysosomes in some cells are recognizable in the light microscope because of their number, size, or contents.

The numerous azurophilic granules of **neutrophils** (white blood cells) represent lysosomes and are recognized in aggregate by their specific staining. Lysosomes that contain phagocytized bacteria and fragments of damaged cells are often recognized in **macrophages**.

Hydrolytic breakdown of the contents of lysosomes often produces a debris-filled vacuole called a **residual body** that may remain for the entire life of the cell. For example, in neurons, residual bodies are called **age pigment** or **lipofuscin granules**. Residual bodies are a normal feature of cell aging. The absence of certain lysosomal enzymes can cause the pathologic accumulation of undigested substrate in residual bodies. This can lead to several disorders collectively termed **lysosomal storage diseases** (see Folder 2.1).

Autophagy

Autophagy represents the major cellular pathway in which a number of cytoplasmic proteins, organelles, and other cellular structures are degraded in the lysosomal compartment (Fig. 2.25). This important process maintains a well-controlled balance between anabolic and catabolic cell functions and permits the cell to eliminate unwanted or unnecessary organelles. Digested components of organelles are recycled and reused for normal cell growth and development.

FOLDER 2.1

CLINICAL CORRELATION: LYSOSOMAL STORAGE DISEASES

Many genetic disorders have been identified in individuals who have mutations in a gene that encodes lysosomal proteins. These diseases are termed **lysosomal storage diseases (LSDs)** and are characterized by dysfunctional lysosomes. The defective protein in most cases is a hydrolytic enzyme or its cofactor; less commonly, lysosomal membrane proteins or proteins that are involved in sorting, targeting, and transporting lysosomal proteins are defective. The result is an accumulation in cells of the specific products that lysosomal enzymes normally use as substrates in their reactions. These undigested, accumulated products disrupt the normal function of the cell and lead to its death.

Currently, 49 disorders are known LSDs with a collective incidence of about 1 in 7,000 live births. The life expectancy across the entire group of people with these disorders is 15 years. The first LSD was described in 1881 by British ophthalmologist Warren Tay, who reported symptoms of retinal abnormalities in a 12-month-old infant with severe neuromuscular symptoms. In 1896, U.S. neurologist Bernard Sachs described a patient with similar eye symptoms found earlier by Tay. This disease is now known as **Tay–Sachs disease**. It is caused by the absence of one enzyme, a lysosomal galactosidase (β-hexosaminidase) that catalyzes a step in lysosomal breakdown of gangliosides in neurons. The resulting accumulation of the GM_2 ganglioside that is found within concentric lamellated structures in residual bodies of neurons interferes with normal cell function.

Children born with LSDs usually appear normal at birth; however, they soon show clinical signs of the disease. They often experience slower growth, show changes in facial features, and develop bone and joint deformities that lead to significant restrictions of limb movement. They may lose already attained skills such as speech and learning ability. Behavioral problems as well as severe intellectual disability may occur. They are prone to frequent lung infections and heart disease. Some children have enlarged internal organs such as the liver and spleen (hepatosplenomegaly). The most common LSDs in children are Gaucher disease, Hurler syndrome (mucopolysaccharidosis [MPS] I), Hunter syndrome (MPS II), and Pompe disease.

Not long ago, LSDs were seen as neurodegenerative disorders without any potential treatment. In the last two decades, there has been limited success in treating the symptoms of LSDs. Considerable effort has been devoted to genetic research and finding methods to replace the missing enzymes that cause various forms of LSD. **Enzyme replacement therapy**, which requires the cellular delivery of a manufactured recombinant enzyme, is available for some LSDs such as cystinosis and Gaucher disease. Enzymes have also been supplied by transplantation of bone marrow containing normal genes from an unaffected person. Success of the enzyme replacement therapy is often limited by insufficient biodistribution of recombinant enzymes and high costs. Recently, emerging strategies for the treatment of LSDs include **pharmacologic chaperone therapy** in which chaperone molecules are delivered to affected cells. In some cases, synthetic chaperones can assist in the folding of mutated enzymes to improve their stability and advance their lysosomal delivery. In the future, the combination of different therapies such as enzyme replacement, pharmacologic chaperone, and **gene transfer therapies** with the development of newborn screening tests will enable early detection and improve clinical outcome of patients with LSDs.

Summary of Common Lysosomal Storage Diseases

Disease	Protein Deficiency	Accumulating Product (or Defective Process)
Disorders of Sphingolipid Degradation		
Gaucher disease	Glucocerebrosidase	Glucosylceramide
Tay–Sachs disease	β-Hexosaminidase, α-subunit	GM_2 ganglioside
Sandhoff disease	β-Hexosaminidase, β-subunit	GM_2 ganglioside, oligosaccharides
Krabbe disease	Galactosylceramidase	Gal-ceramide, gal-sphingosine
Niemann–Pick disease A, B	Sphingomyelinase	Sphingomyelin
Disorders of Glycoprotein Degradation		
Aspartylglycosaminuria	Aspartylglycosaminidase	*N*-linked oligosaccharides
α-Mannosidosis	α-Mannosidase	α-Mannosides
Disorders of Glycosaminoglycan Degradation		
Hurler syndrome (MPS I)	α-L-iduronidase	Dermatan sulfate, heparan sulfate
Hunter syndrome (MPS II)	L-iduronate sulfatase	Dermatan sulfate, heparan sulfate
Maroteaux–Lamy syndrome (MPS VI)	GalNAc 4-sulfatase/arylsulfatase B	Dermatan sulfate
Other Disorders of Single Enzyme Deficiency		
Pompe disease (glycogenosis II)	α-1,4-Glucosidase	Glycogen
Wolman disease (familial xanthomatosis)	Acid lipase	Cholesterol esters, triglycerides
Canavan disease (aspartoacylase deficiency)	Aspartoacylase	*N*-acetylaspartic acid
Disorders of Lysosomal Biogenesis		
Inclusion-cell (I-cell) disease, mucolipidosis II	GlcNAc-1-phosphotransferase (GlcNAcPTase); leads to defective sorting of most soluble hydrolytic lysosomal enzymes	Lysosomal hydrolases are not present in lysosomes
Disorders of the Lysosomal Membrane		
Danon disease	LAMP2	Presence of autophagic vacuoles
Cystinosis	Cystinosin (cystine transporter)	Cystine

LAMP2, lysosome-associated membrane protein 2; MPS I, II, VI, mucopolysaccharidosis type I, II, VI.

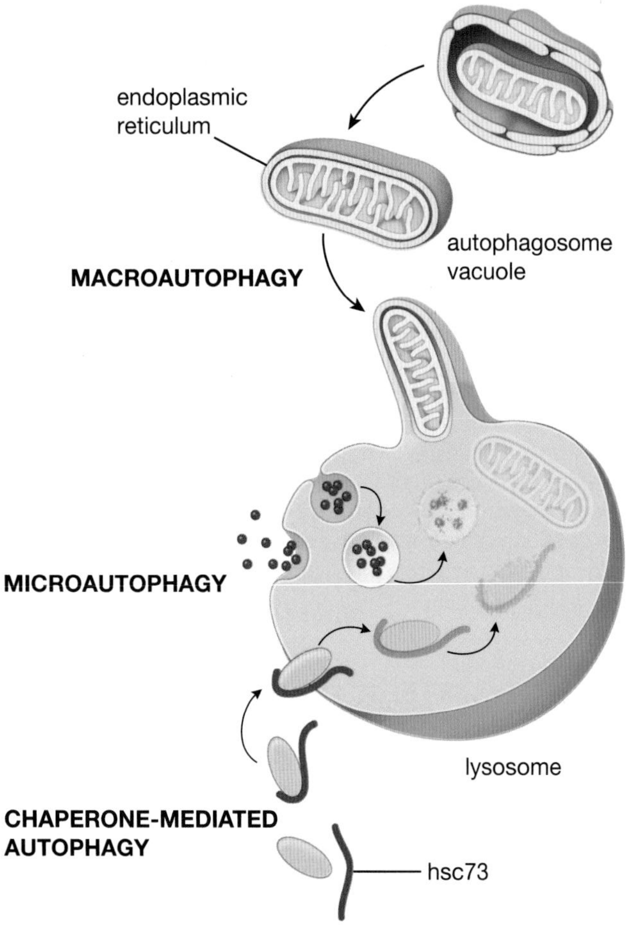

FIGURE 2.25. Three autophagic pathways for degradation of cytoplasmic constituents. In *macroautophagy*, a portion of the cytoplasm or an entire organelle is surrounded by an intracellular membrane of the endoplasmic reticulum to form a double-membraned autophagosome vacuole. After fusion with a lysosome, the inner membrane and the contents of the vacuole are degraded. In *microautophagy*, cytoplasmic proteins are internalized into lysosomes by invagination of the lysosomal membrane. *Chaperone-mediated autophagy* to lysosomes is the most selective process for degradation of specific cytoplasmic proteins. It requires assistance of proteins called *chaperones*. The chaperone protein (hsc73) binds to the protein and helps transport it into the lysosomal lumen, where it is finally degraded.

Cytoplasmic proteins and organelles are substrates for lysosomal degradation in the process of autophagy.

Autophagy plays an essential role during starvation, cellular differentiation, cell death, and cell aging. Applying genetic screening tests originally developed for yeasts, researchers have discovered a number (approximately 33) of **autophagy-related genes (Atg genes)** in the mammalian cell genome and have been able to trace the activation or inhibition of these genes under specific conditions. The presence of adequate nutrients and growth factors stimulates enzymatic activity of a serine/threonine kinase known as **mammalian target of rapamycin (mTOR)**. High mTOR activity exerts an inhibitory effect on autophagy. The opposite occurs in nutrient starvation, hypoxia, and high temperatures, where lack of mTOR activity causes activation of Atg genes. This results in the formation of an **Atg1 protein kinase autophagy–regulatory complex** that initiates the process of autophagy. Generally, autophagy can be divided into three well-characterized pathways:

- **Macroautophagy**, or simply autophagy, is a nonspecific process in which a portion of the cytoplasm or an entire organelle is first surrounded by a double or multilamellar intracellular membrane of endoplasmic reticulum, called the **isolation membrane**, to form a vacuole called an **autophagosome**. This process is aided by proteins encoded by several Atg genes. First, the complex containing **Atg12–Atg5–Atg16L proteins** attaches to a portion of the endoplasmic reticulum and localizes in the isolation membrane. Subsequently, **Atg8** is recruited and bound to the membrane. Together, these proteins change the shape of the isolation membrane, which bends to enclose and seal an organelle destined for digestion within the lumen of the autophagosome. Once the autophagosome is completed, the Atg12–Atg5–Atg16L complex and Atg8 dissociate from this structure. After targeted delivery of lysosomal enzymes, the autophagosome matures into a lysosome. The isolation membrane disintegrates within the hydrolytic compartment of a lysosome. Macroautophagy occurs in the liver during the first stages of starvation (Fig. 2.26).
- **Microautophagy** is also a nonspecific process in which cytoplasmic proteins are degraded in a slow, continuous process under normal physiologic conditions. In microautophagy, small cytoplasmic soluble proteins are internalized into the lysosomes by invagination of the lysosomal membrane.

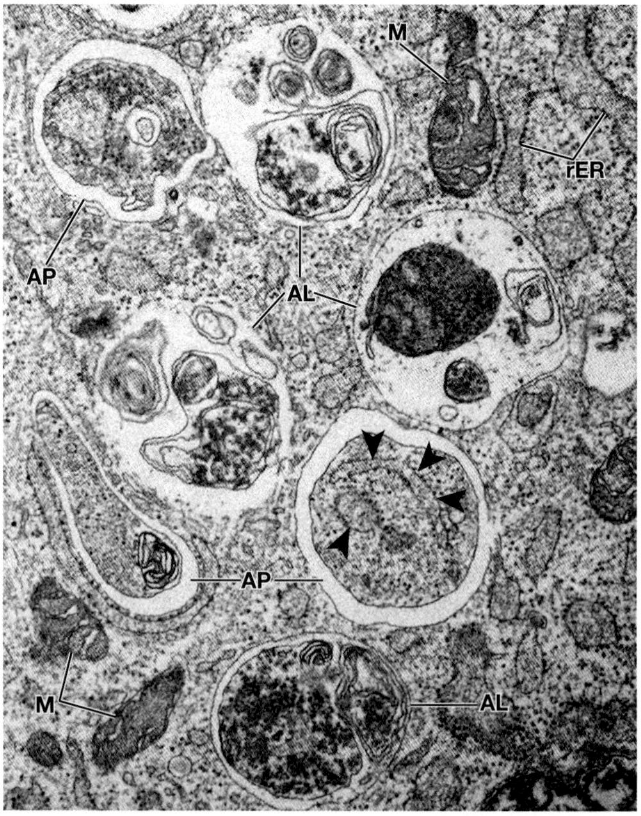

FIGURE 2.26. Electron micrograph of nutrient-starved mouse embryonic fibroblasts. This electron micrograph shows several autophagosomes (*AP*). Note that autophagosomes are double-membraned structures containing undigested intracellular organelles, such as mitochondria or fragments of the endoplasmic reticulum (*arrowheads*). After the autophagosome fuses with a lysosome, it forms an autolysosome (*AL*) that degrades the enclosed materials including the inner autophagosomal membrane. *M*, mitochondria, *rER*, rough endoplasmic reticulum. ×26,300. (Courtesy of Drs. Chieko Kishi-Itakura and Noboru Mizushima.)

- **Chaperone-mediated autophagy** is the only selective process of protein degradation and requires assistance from specific cytosolic chaperones such as a **heat-shock chaperone protein** called **hsc73**. This process is activated during nutrient deprivation and requires the presence of targeting signals on the degraded proteins and a specific receptor on the lysosomal membrane. Chaperone-mediated direct transport resembles the process of protein importation to various other cellular organelles: hsc73 binds to the protein and assists in its transport through the lysosomal membrane into the lumen, where it is finally degraded. Chaperone-mediated autophagy is responsible for the degradation of approximately 30% of cytoplasmic proteins in organs such as the liver and kidney.

Proteasome-Mediated Degradation

In addition to the lysosomal pathway of protein degradation, cells are able to destroy proteins without involvement of lysosomes. Such a process occurs within large cytoplasmic or nuclear protein complexes called **proteasomes.** They represent ATP-dependent protease complexes that destroy proteins that have been specifically tagged for this pathway. **Proteasome-mediated degradation** is used by cells to destroy abnormal proteins that are misfolded, are denatured, or contain abnormal amino acids. This pathway also degrades normal short-lived regulatory proteins that need to be rapidly inactivated and degraded, such as mitotic cyclins that regulate cell cycle progression, transcriptional factors, tumor suppressors, and tumor promoters.

Proteins destined for proteasome-mediated degradation must be recognized and specifically tagged by the polyubiquitin chain.

Degradation of a protein in the proteasome-mediated pathway involves two successive steps:

- **Polyubiquitination**, in which proteins targeted for destruction are repeatedly tagged by covalent attachments of a small (8.5-kDa) protein called **ubiquitin**. The tagging reaction is catalyzed by three ubiquitin ligases called **ubiquitin-activating enzymes E1, E2, and E3**. In a cascade of enzymatic reactions, the targeted protein is first marked by a single ubiquitin molecule. This creates a signal for consecutive attachment of several other ubiquitin molecules, resulting in a linear chain of ubiquitin conjugates. A protein target for destruction within the proteasome must be labeled with at least four ubiquitin molecules in the form of a **polyubiquitin chain** that serves as a degradation signal for proteasome complex.
- **Degradation of the tagged protein by the 26S proteasome complex**. Each proteasome consists of a hollow cylinder, shaped like a barrel, containing a **20S core particle (CP)** that facilitates the multicatalytic protease activity in which polyubiquitinated proteins are degraded into small polypeptides and amino acids. On both ends of the CP cylinder are two **19S regulatory particles (RPs)**. The RP that forms the lid of the barrel recognizes polyubiquitin tags, unfolds the protein, and regulates its entry into the destruction chamber. The RP on the opposite side (on the base) of the barrel releases short peptides and amino acids after degradation of the protein is completed. Free ubiquitin molecules are released by **deubiquitinating (DUB) enzymes** and recycled (Fig. 2.27).

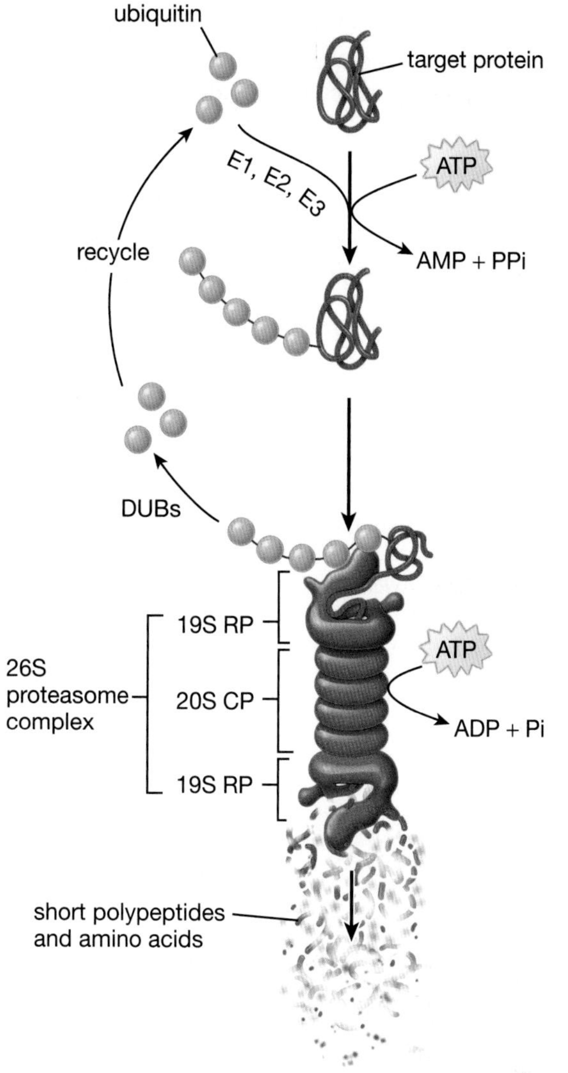

FIGURE 2.27. Proteasome-mediated degradation. This degradation pathway involves tagging proteins destined for destruction by a polyubiquitin chain and its subsequent degradation in a proteasome complex with the release of free reusable ubiquitin molecules. Ubiquitin in the presence of adenosine triphosphate (*ATP*) is activated by a complex of three ubiquitin-activating enzymes (E1, E2, and E3) to form a single polyubiquitin chain that serves as the degradation signal for the 26S proteasome complex. The regulatory particle (19S RP) that forms the lid of the main protein destruction chamber (20S core particle [CP]) recognizes polyubiquitin tags, unfolds the protein, and inserts and regulates its entry into the destruction chamber. The regulatory particle on the opposite side of the chamber releases short peptides and amino acids after degradation of the protein is completed. Free ubiquitin molecules are released by deubiquitinating enzymes (*DUBs*) and recycled. ADP, adenosine diphosphate.

Two groups of pathologic conditions are associated with **malfunction of proteasome-mediated degradation.** The first group results from a loss of proteasome function because of mutations in the genes encoding ubiquitin-activating enzymes. This leads to a decrease in protein degradation and their subsequent accumulation in the cell cytoplasm (e.g., in **Angelman syndrome** and **Alzheimer disease**). The second group is caused by overexpression of proteins involved in the proteasome-mediated degradation pathway that causes accelerated degradation of cellular proteins (e.g., infections with human papillomavirus). Use of a specific proteasome inhibitor has been successful in treating multiple myeloma, and researchers hope to develop additional inhibitors for the treatment of other diseases.

Rough Endoplasmic Reticulum

The protein synthetic system of the cell consists of the rough endoplasmic reticulum and ribosomes.

The cytoplasm of a variety of cells engaged chiefly in protein synthesis stains intensely with basic dyes. The basophilic staining is caused by the presence of RNA. The portion of the cytoplasm that stains with the basic dye is called **ergastoplasm**. The ergastoplasm in secretory cells (e.g., pancreatic acinar cells) is the light microscopic image of the organelle called the **rough endoplasmic reticulum (rER)**.

With the TEM, the rER appears as a series of interconnected, membrane-limited, flattened sacs called **cisternae**, with particles studding the exterior surface of the membrane (Fig. 2.28). These particles, called **ribosomes**, are attached to the membrane of the rER by ribosomal docking proteins. Ribosomes measure 15–20 nm in diameter and consist of a small and large subunit. Each subunit contains **ribosomal RNA (rRNA)** of different lengths as well as numerous types of proteins. In many instances, the rER is continuous with the outer membrane of the nuclear envelope (see the next section). Groups of ribosomes form short spiral arrays called **polyribosomes** or **polysomes** (Fig. 2.29) in which many ribosomes are attached to a thread of **messenger RNA (mRNA)**.

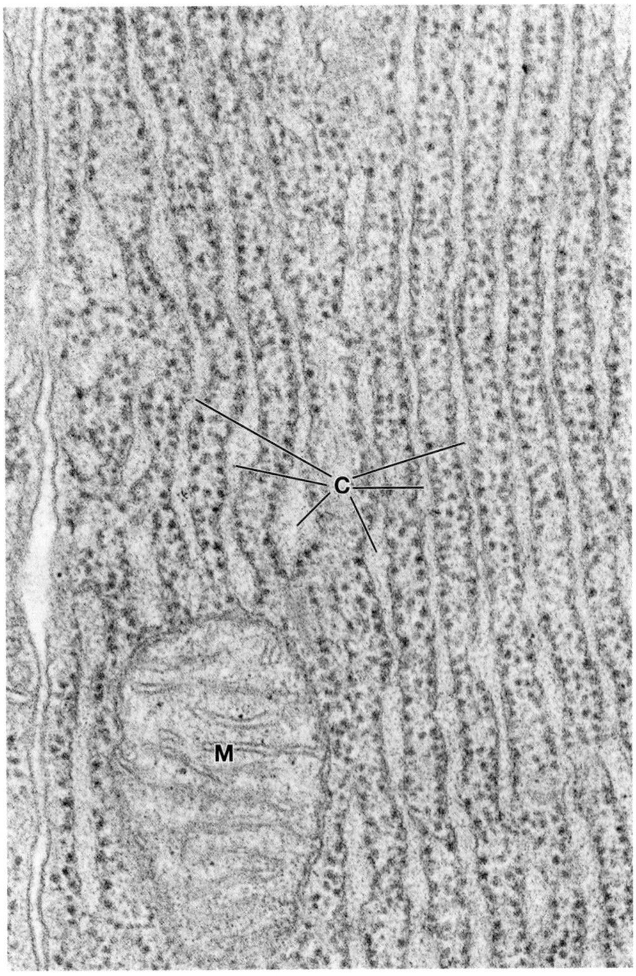

FIGURE 2.28. Electron micrograph of the rough endoplasmic reticulum (rER). This image of the rER in a chief cell of the stomach shows the membranous cisternae (*C*) closely packed in parallel arrays. Polyribosomes are present on the cytoplasmic surface of the membrane surrounding the cisternae. The appearance of a ribosome-studded membrane is the origin of the term *rough endoplasmic reticulum.* A few ribosomes are free in the cytoplasm. *M,* mitochondrion. ×50,000.

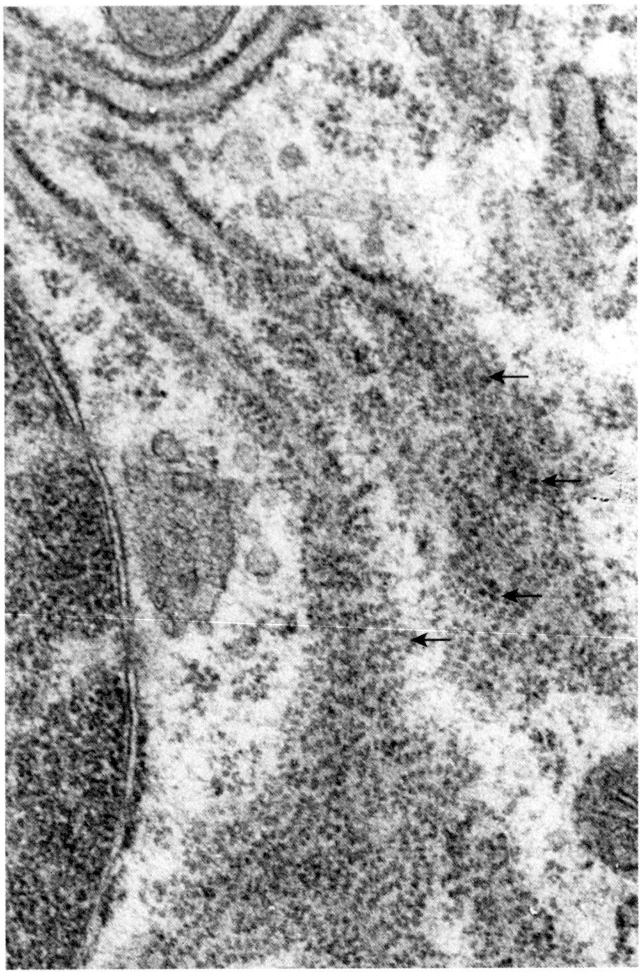

FIGURE 2.29. Electron micrograph of the rough endoplasmic reticulum (rER) and polyribosome complexes. This image shows a small section of the rER adjacent to the nucleus sectioned in two planes. The reticulum has turned within the section. Thus, in the *upper right and left,* the membranes of the reticulum have been cut at a right angle to their surface. In the *center,* the reticulum has twisted and is shown as in an aerial view (from above the membrane). The large spiral cytoplasmic assemblies (*arrows*) are chains of ribosomes that form polyribosomes that are actively engaged in translation of the mRNA molecule. ×38,000.

Protein synthesis involves transcription and translation.

The production of proteins by the cell begins within the nucleus with **transcription**, in which the genetic code for a protein is transcribed from DNA to **pre-mRNA**. After posttranscriptional modifications of the pre-mRNA molecule—which includes RNA cleavage, excision of introns, rejoining of exons, and capping by the addition of poly(A) tracks at the 3′ end and a methylguanosine cap [M(7) GPPP] at the 5′ end—the resulting **mRNA** molecule leaves the nucleus and migrates into the cytoplasm (Fig. 2.30). Transcription is followed by **translation**, in which the coded message contained in the mRNA is read by ribosomal complexes to form a polypeptide. A typical single cytoplasmic mRNA molecule binds to many ribosomes spaced as close as 80 nucleotides apart, thus forming a **polyribosome complex** or **polysome**. A polysome attached to the cytoplasmic surface of the rER can translate a single mRNA molecule and simultaneously produce many copies of a particular protein. In contrast, **free ribosomes** reside within the cytoplasm. They are not associated with any intracellular membranes and are structurally and functionally identical to polysomes of the rER.

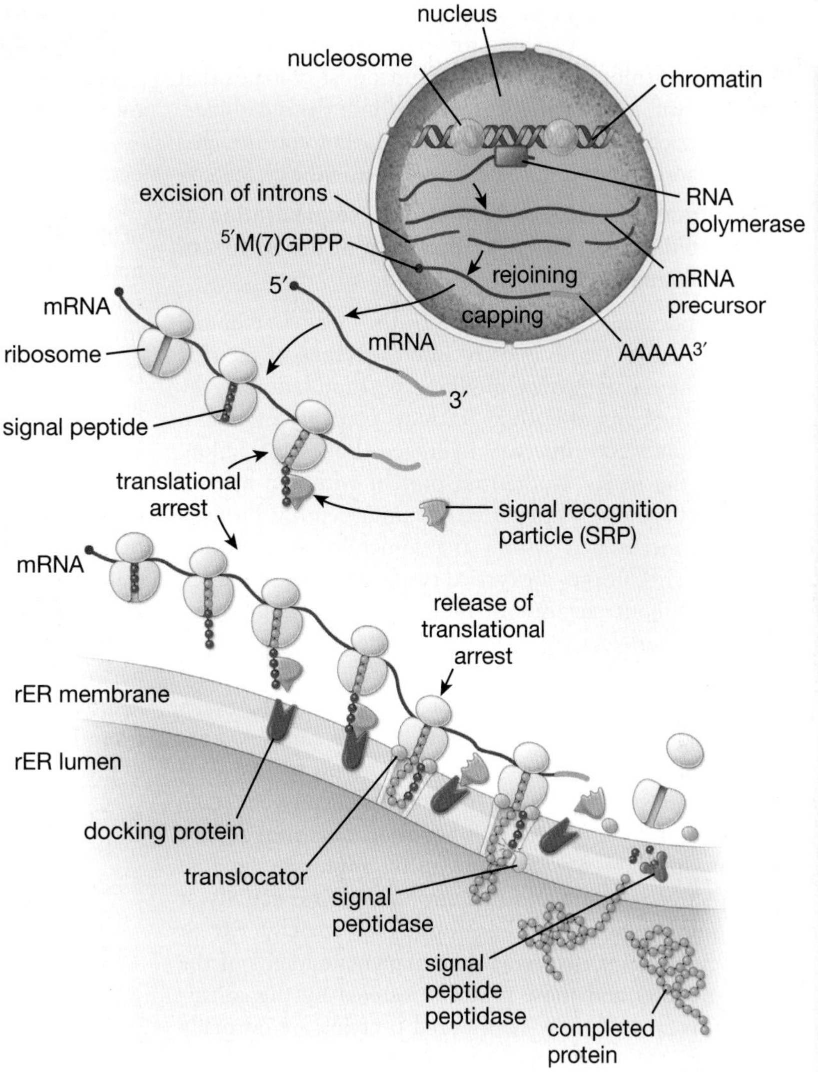

FIGURE 2.30. Summary of events during protein synthesis. Protein synthesis begins within the nucleus with transcription, during which the genetic code for a protein is transcribed from DNA to messenger RNA (mRNA) precursors. After posttranscriptional modifications of the pre-mRNA molecule—which include RNA cleavage, excision of introns, rejoining of exons, and capping by addition of poly(A) tracks at the 3′ end and methylguanosine cap at the 5′ end—the resulting mRNA molecule leaves the nucleus and enters the cytoplasm. In the cytoplasm, the mRNA sequence is read by the ribosomal complex in the process of translation to form a polypeptide chain. The first group of 15–60 amino acids on the amino-terminus of a newly synthesized polypeptide forms a signal sequence (signal peptide) that directs the protein to its destination (i.e., lumen of rough endoplasmic reticulum [*rER*]). The signal peptide interacts with a signal recognition particle (*SRP*), which arrests further growth of the polypeptide chain until its relocation toward the rER membrane. Binding of the SRP to a docking protein on the cytoplasmic surface of the rER aligns the ribosome with the translocator protein. Binding of the ribosome to the translocator causes dissociation of the SRP–docking protein complex away from the ribosome, and protein synthesis is resumed. The translocator protein guides the polypeptide chain into the lumen of the rER cisterna. The signal sequence is cleaved from the polypeptide by signal peptidase and is subsequently digested by signal peptide peptidases. On completion of protein synthesis, the ribosome detaches from the translocator protein.

The differences between the structure of **prokaryotic (bacterial) and eukaryotic ribosomes** were exploited by researchers, who discovered chemical compounds (antibiotics) that bind to bacterial ribosomes. Antibiotics are able to kill bacteria without harming the cells of the infected individual. Several types of antibiotics, such as aminoglycosides (streptomycin), macrolides (erythromycin), lincosamides (clindamycin), tetracyclines, and chloramphenicol, inhibit protein synthesis by binding to different portions of bacterial ribosomes.

Signal peptides direct the posttranslational transport of a protein.

Most proteins that are synthesized for export or that will become a part of specific organelles (such as the plasma membrane, mitochondrial matrix, endoplasmic reticulum, or nucleus) require sorting signals that direct proteins to their correct destinations. These **signal sequences (signal peptides)** are often found in the sequence of the first group of 15–60 amino acids on the amino-terminus of a newly synthesized protein. Signal sequences can be compared to airline tags on luggage. Just as the tags ensure that baggage moves correctly from one aircraft to another at airports, so signal peptides ensure that the newly synthetized protein is properly identified as it passes through the organelles of the cell. During this transit, a series of synthetic events and posttranslational modifications occur before the polypeptides ultimately arrive at their proper destination.

For example, almost all proteins that are transported to the endoplasmic reticulum have a signal sequence consisting of 5–10 hydrophobic amino acids on their amino-termini. The signal sequence of the nascent peptide interacts with a **signal recognition particle (SRP)**, which arrests further growth of the polypeptide chain. The complex containing the SRP–polyribosome complex that arrests polypeptide synthesis is then relocated toward the rER membrane. Binding of the SRP to a **docking protein** on the cytoplasmic surface of rER aligns the ribosome with the **translocator**, an integral membrane protein of the rER. Binding of the ribosome to the protein translocator causes dissociation of the SRP–docking protein complex from the ribosome and rER membrane, releasing the translational block and allowing the ribosome to resume protein synthesis (see Fig. 2.30). The translocator protein inserts the polypeptide chain into its aqueous pore, allowing the newly formed protein to be discharged into the lumen of the rER cisterna.

For simple secretory proteins, the polypeptide continues to be inserted by the translocator into the lumen as it is synthesized. The signal sequence is cleaved from the polypeptide by signal peptidase residing on the cisternal face of the rER membrane, even before the synthesis of the entire chain is completed. For integral membrane proteins, sequences along the polypeptide may instruct the forming protein to pass back and forth through the membrane, creating the functional domains that the protein will exhibit once it is inserted into the membrane. On completion of protein synthesis, the ribosome detaches from the translocator protein and is again free in the cytoplasm.

The posttranslational modification and sequestration of proteins within the rER is the first step in the export of proteins destined to leave the cell.

As polypeptide chains are synthesized by the membrane-bound polysomes, the protein is injected into the lumen of the rER cisterna, where it is further modified posttranslationally by enzymes. These modifications include core glycosylation, disulfide bond and internal hydrogen bond formation, folding of the newly synthesized protein with the help of molecular chaperones, and partial subunit assembly. Proteins are then concentrated within the lumen of neighboring cisternae of rER, or they are carried to another part of the cell in the continuous channels of the rER. Some antibiotics, such as **tunicamycin (A, B, C, and D),** collectively act on rER to inhibit *N*-linked glycosylation in glycoprotein synthesis. By preventing glycoprotein synthesis, these compounds impede the formation of the surface coat (glycocalyx) of virus-infected cells and the protective viral capsid of replicating viruses. The name tunicamycin (*Lat., tunica,* coat) reflects this antibiotic's mechanism of action. Although tunicamycin is a powerful antibiotic against gram-positive bacteria and has strong antiviral activity, it has no therapeutic use because of its high toxicity. Except for the few proteins that remain permanent residents of the rER membranes and those proteins secreted by the constitutive pathway, the newly synthesized proteins are normally delivered to the Golgi apparatus within minutes. A few diseases are characterized by an inability of the rER to export posttranslationally modified proteins to the Golgi apparatus. For example, in **α1-antitrypsin deficiency**, a single amino acid substitution renders the rER unable to export α1-antitrypsin (A1AT). This leads to decreased activity of A1AT in the blood and lungs and abnormal deposition of defective A1AT within the rER of liver hepatocytes, resulting in **emphysema** (chronic obstructive pulmonary disease) and impaired liver function.

In cells in which the constitutive pathway is dominant—namely, plasma cells and activated fibroblasts—newly synthesized proteins may accumulate in the rER cisternae, causing their engorgement and distention.

The rER also serves as a **quality checkpoint** in the process of protein production. If the newly synthesized protein is not properly posttranslationally modified or is misfolded, it is then exported from the rER back to the cytoplasm via the mechanism of retrotranslocation. Here, defective proteins are deglycosylated, polyubiquitinated, and degraded within proteasomes (see page 53).

The rER is most highly developed in active secretory cells.

The rER is particularly well developed in those cells that synthesize proteins destined to leave the cell (secretory cells) as well as in cells with large amounts of plasma membrane, such as neurons. Secretory cells include glandular cells, activated fibroblasts, plasma cells, odontoblasts, ameloblasts, and osteoblasts. The rER is not limited, however, to secretory cells and neurons. Virtually every cell of the body contains profiles of rER. However, they may be few in number, a reflection of the amount of protein the cell secretes, and dispersed so that in the light microscope, they are not evident as areas of basophilia.

The rER is most highly developed in active secretory cells because secretory proteins are synthesized exclusively by the ribosomes of the rER. In all cells, however, the ribosomes of the rER also synthesize proteins that are to become permanent components of lysosomes, Golgi apparatus, rER, or nuclear envelope (these structures are discussed in the next sections) or integral components of the plasma membrane.

Coatomers mediate bidirectional traffic between the rER and Golgi apparatus.

Two classes of coated vesicles are involved in the transport of protein from and to the rER. A protein coat similar to clathrin surrounds vesicles transporting proteins between the rER and the Golgi apparatus (page 41). However, unlike clathrins, which mediate bidirectional transport from and to the plasma membrane, one class of proteins is involved only in **anterograde transport** from the rER to the *cis*-Golgi network (CGN), the Golgi cisternae closest to the rER. Another class of proteins mediates **retrograde transport** from the CGN back to the rER (Fig. 2.31). These two classes of proteins are called **coatomers** or **COPs**.

- **COP-I** mediates transport vesicles originating in the CGN back to the rER (Fig. 2.32a). This **retrograde transport** mediates a salvage operation that returns rER proteins mistakenly transferred to the CGN during normal anterograde transport. In addition, COP-I is also responsible for maintaining retrograde transport between the Golgi cisternae.
- **COP-II** is responsible for **anterograde transport**, forming rER transport vesicles destined for the CGN

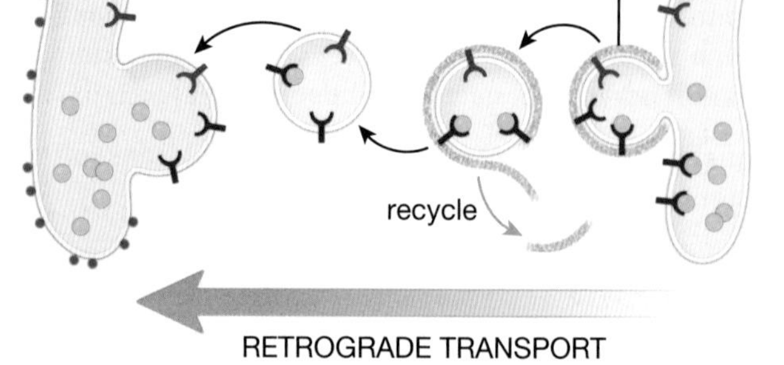

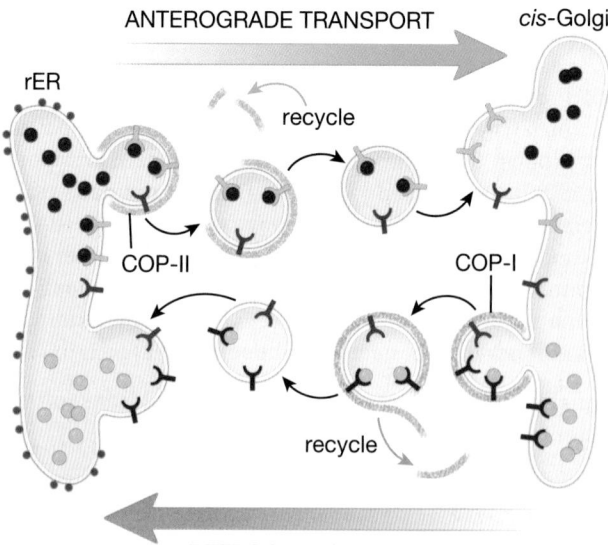

FIGURE 2.31. Anterograde and retrograde transport between the rough endoplasmic reticulum (rER) and *cis*-Golgi network (CGN). Two classes of coated vesicles are involved in protein transport to and from the rER. These vesicles are surrounded by COP-I and COP-II protein coat complexes, respectively. COP-II is involved in anterograde transport from the rER to the CGN, and COP-I is involved in retrograde transport from the CGN back to the rER. After a vesicle is formed, the coat components dissociate from the vesicle and are recycled to their site of origin. The COP-I protein coat is also involved in retrograde transport between cisternae within the Golgi apparatus (see Fig. 2.15).

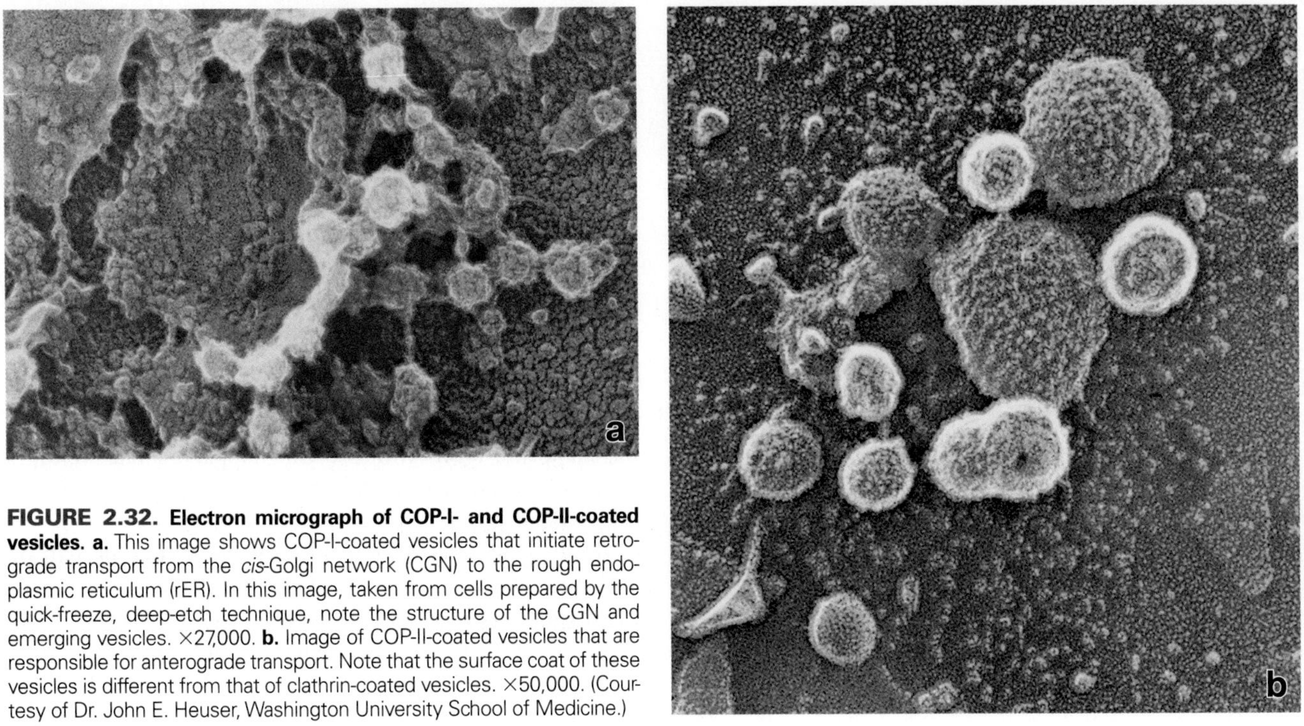

FIGURE 2.32. Electron micrograph of COP-I- and COP-II-coated vesicles. a. This image shows COP-I-coated vesicles that initiate retrograde transport from the *cis*-Golgi network (CGN) to the rough endoplasmic reticulum (rER). In this image, taken from cells prepared by the quick-freeze, deep-etch technique, note the structure of the CGN and emerging vesicles. ×27,000. **b.** Image of COP-II-coated vesicles that are responsible for anterograde transport. Note that the surface coat of these vesicles is different from that of clathrin-coated vesicles. ×50,000. (Courtesy of Dr. John E. Heuser, Washington University School of Medicine.)

(Fig. 2.32b). COP-II assists in the physical deformation of rER membranes into sharply curved buds and the further separation of vesicles from the rER membrane. Most proteins produced in the rER use COP-II-coated vesicles to reach the CGN.

Shortly after formation of COP-I- or COP-II-coated vesicles, the coats dissociate from the newly formed vesicles, allowing the vesicle to fuse with its target. The coat components then are recycled to their site of origin.

"Free" ribosomes synthesize proteins that will remain in the cell as cytoplasmic structural or functional elements.

Proteins targeted to the nucleus, mitochondria, or peroxisomes are synthesized on **free ribosomes** and released into the cytosol. Some have a short targeting signal (e.g., for peroxisomes, the targeting signal consists of three amino acid motif, Ser-Lys-Leu) and may use specialized proteins (soluble chaperones) to guide them to specific organelles (pages 64-66). However, most proteins synthesized on free ribosomes lack a signal sequence and thus remain in the cytosol. Cytoplasmic basophilia is associated with cells that produce large amounts of protein that will remain in the cell. Such cells and their products include developing red blood cells (hemoglobin), developing muscle cells (the contractile proteins actin and myosin), nerve cells (neurofilaments), and keratinocytes of the skin (keratin). In addition, most enzymes of the mitochondrion are synthesized by free polysomes and transported into that organelle.

Basophilia in these cells was formerly called ergastoplasm and is caused by the presence of large amounts of RNA. In this case, the ribosomes and polysomes are free in the cytoplasm (i.e., they are not attached to membranes of the endoplasmic reticulum). The large basophilic bodies of nerve cells, which are called **Nissl bodies**, consist of both rER and large numbers of free ribosomes (Fig. 2.33). All ribosomes contain RNA; it is the phosphate groups of the RNA of the ribosomes, not the membranous component of the endoplasmic reticulum, that account for basophilic staining of the cytoplasm.

Smooth Endoplasmic Reticulum

The sER consists of short anastomosing tubules that are not associated with ribosomes.

Cells with large amounts of **smooth endoplasmic reticulum** may exhibit distinct cytoplasmic eosinophilia (acidophilia) when viewed in the light microscope. The sER is structurally similar to the rER but lacks the ribosome docking proteins. It tends to be tubular rather than sheet-like, and it may be separate from the rER or an extension of it. The sER is abundant in cells that function in **lipid metabolism** (i.e., cells that synthesize fatty acids and phospholipids), and it proliferates in hepatocytes when animals are challenged with lipophilic drugs. The sER is well developed in cells that synthesize and **secrete steroids**, such as in adrenocortical cells and testicular Leydig (interstitial) cells (Fig. 2.34). In skeletal and cardiac muscle, the sER is also called the **sarcoplasmic reticulum**. It sequesters Ca^{2+}, which is essential for the contractile process and is closely apposed to the plasma membrane invaginations that conduct the contractile impulses to the interior of the cell. The sER is also involved in de novo biogenesis of peroxisomes (pages 64-65).

The sER is the principal organelle involved in the detoxification of the xenobiotics.

The sER is particularly well developed in the liver and contains a variety of **detoxifying enzymes** related to **cytochrome P450**. These enzymes are anchored directly into sER plasma membranes (especially in the liver). The cytochrome P450 enzymatic compound represents a group of heme-containing enzymes that participate in the metabolism of many xenobiotics (foreign drugs or chemicals), steroids, and carcinogens. Cytochrome P450 enzymes modify and detoxify hydrophobic compounds such as drugs, pesticides, and carcinogens by chemically converting them into water-soluble conjugated products that can be eliminated from the body. In essence, cytochrome P450 enzymes in the sER of the liver control the speed at which drugs are metabolized and the duration for which the drugs are present in the body. Cytochrome P450 compound is also important in the synthesis of

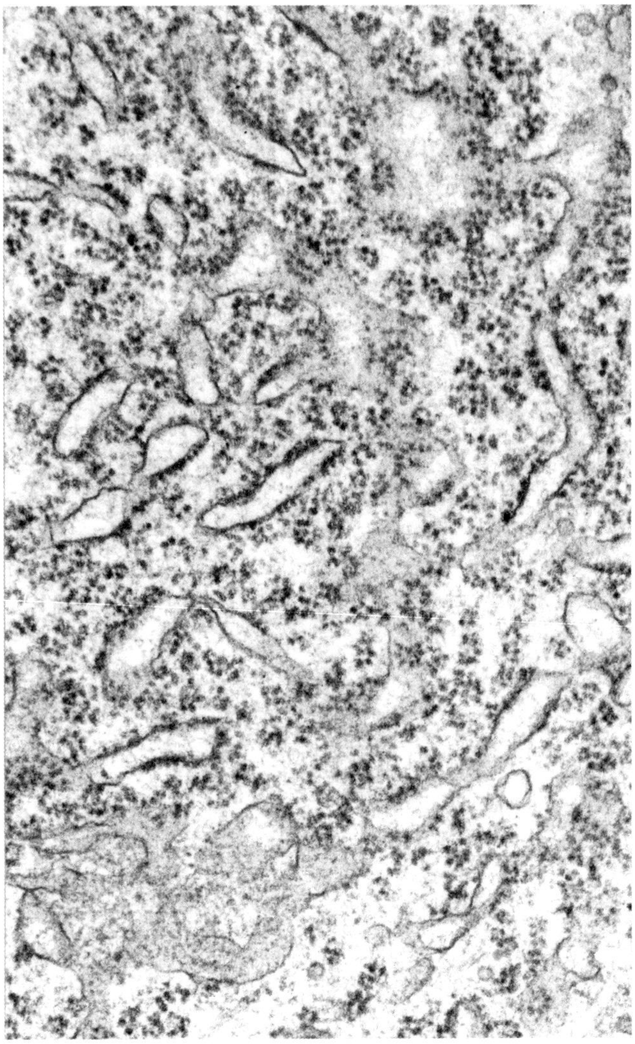

FIGURE 2.33. Electron micrograph of a nerve cell body showing the rough endoplasmic reticulum (rER). This image shows rER profiles as well as numerous free ribosomes located between the membranes of the rER. Collectively, the free ribosomes and membrane-attached ribosomes are responsible for the characteristic cytoplasmic basophilia (Nissl bodies) observed in the light microscope in the perinuclear cytoplasm of neurons. ×45,000.

steroid hormones (i.e., estrogen and testosterone), fatty acids, and sterols (such as cholesterol and bile acids).

Characterizing an individual's **cytochrome P450** enzymes may provide information about optimal therapeutic drug dosage levels, thus preventing complications of overdose or, conversely, ineffective treatment. For example, the **CYP2C9 gene** that encodes a member of the cytochrome P450 enzyme family metabolizes the anticoagulant **warfarin (blood thinner)** and other drugs such as phenytoin, tolbutamide, and ibuprofen. The ability to metabolize drugs is genetically determined, and a person can be classified as an ultrarapid, rapid, extensive, intermediate, or poor metabolizer. By identifying the specific gene variant an individual possesses and thus the type of metabolizer the person is, the warfarin dosage can be tailored to prevent internal bleeding, a common and potentially dangerous complication of this drug. Such personalization of therapeutics has been called **personalized medicine**.

The degree to which the liver is involved in detoxification at any given time may be estimated by the amount of sER present in liver cells. The sER is also involved in

- lipid and steroid metabolism,
- glycogen metabolism, and
- membrane formation and recycling.

Because of these widely disparate functions, numerous other enzymes—including hydrolases, methylases, glucose-6-phosphatase, ATPases, and lipid oxidases—are associated with the sER, depending on its functional role.

Golgi Apparatus

The Golgi apparatus is well developed in secretory cells and does not stain with hematoxylin or eosin.

The **Golgi apparatus** was described more than 100 years ago by the histologist Camillo Golgi. In studies of osmium-impregnated nerve cells, he discovered an organelle that formed networks around the nucleus. It was also described as well developed in secretory cells. Changes in the shape and location of the Golgi apparatus relative to its secretory state were described even before it was viewed with the EM and before its functional relationship to the rER was established. It is active both in cells that secrete protein by exocytosis and in cells that synthesize large amounts of membrane and membrane-associated proteins such as nerve cells.

In the light microscope, secretory cells that have a large Golgi apparatus (e.g., plasma cells, osteoblasts, and cells of the epididymis) typically exhibit a clear area partially surrounded by ergastoplasm (Fig. 2.35). In the EM, the Golgi apparatus appears as a series of stacked, flattened, membrane-limited sacs or cisternae and tubular extensions embedded in a network of microtubules near the microtubule-organizing center or MTOC (see pages 75-77). Small vesicles involved in vesicular transport are seen in association with the cisternae.

The Golgi apparatus is polarized both morphologically and functionally. The flattened cisternae located closest to the rER represent the forming face, or the ***cis*-Golgi network (CGN)**; the cisternae located away from the rER represent the maturing face, or the ***trans*-Golgi network (TGN)** (Figs. 2.36 and 2.37). The cisternae located between the TGN and CGN are commonly referred as **the medial-Golgi network**.

The Golgi apparatus functions in the posttranslational modification, sorting, and packaging of proteins.

Small **COP-II-coated transport vesicles** carry newly synthesized proteins (both secretory and membrane) from the rER to the CGN. From there, they travel within **transport**

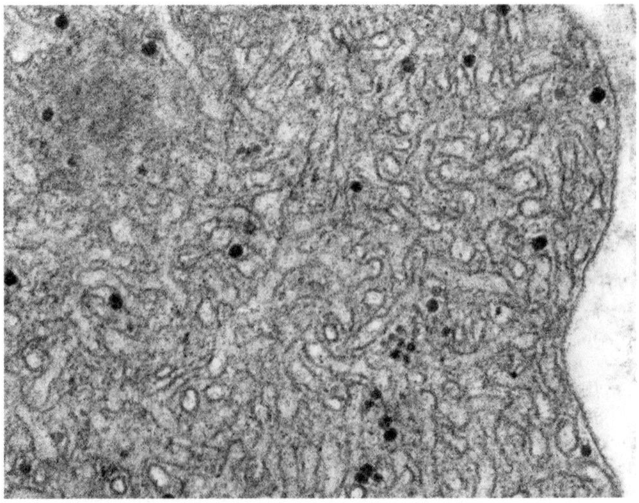

FIGURE 2.34. Electron micrograph of the smooth endoplasmic reticulum (sER). This image shows numerous profiles of sER in an interstitial (Leydig) cell of the testis, a cell that produces steroid hormones. The sER seen here is a complex system of anastomosing tubules. The small, dense objects are glycogen particles. ×60,000.

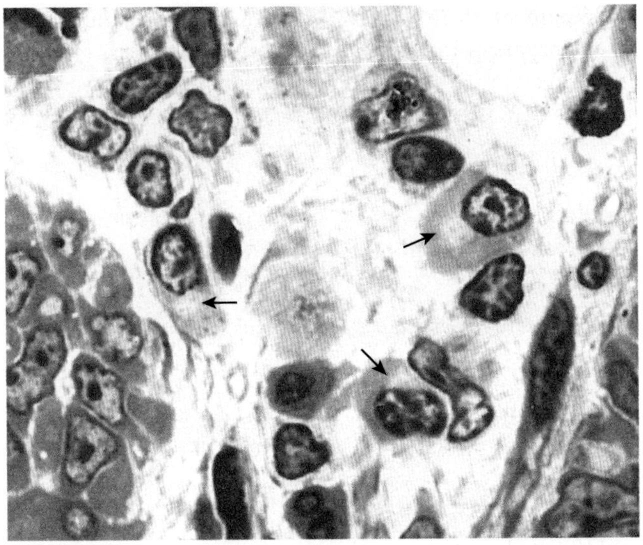

FIGURE 2.35. Photomicrograph of plasma cells. This photomicrograph of a plastic-embedded specimen showing the lamina propria of the small intestine is stained with toluidine blue. The plasma cells, where appropriately oriented, exhibit a clear area in the cytoplasm near the nucleus. These negatively stained regions (*arrows*) represent extensive accumulation of membranous cisternae that belong to the Golgi apparatus. The surrounding cytoplasm is deeply metachromatically stained because of the presence of ribosomes associated with the extensive rough endoplasmic reticulum (rER). ×1,200.

vesicles from one cisterna to the next. The vesicles bud from one cisterna and fuse with the adjacent cisternae (Fig. 2.38).

As proteins and lipids travel through the Golgi stacks, they undergo a series of **posttranslational modifications** that involve remodeling of *N*-linked oligosaccharides previously added in the rER. In general, oligosaccharides present in glycoproteins and glycolipids are trimmed and translocated.

Proteins and lipids undergo glycosylation by several carbohydrate-processing enzymes that add, remove, and modify sugar moieties of oligosaccharide chains. M-6-P is added to those proteins destined to travel to late endosomes and lysosomes (see pages 44-46). In addition, glycoproteins are phosphorylated and sulfated. The proteolytic cleavage of certain proteins is also initiated within the cisternae.

Four major pathways of protein secretion from the Golgi apparatus disperse proteins to various cell destinations.

As noted, proteins exit the Golgi apparatus from the TGN. This network and the associated tubulovesicular array serve as the sorting station for shuttling vesicles that deliver proteins to the following locations (Fig. 2.39):

- **Apical plasma membrane**. Many extracellular and membrane proteins are delivered to this site. This constitutive pathway most likely uses non–clathrin-coated vesicles. In most cells, secretory proteins destined for the apical plasma membrane have specific sorting signals that guide their sorting process in the TGN. Proteins are then delivered to the apical cell surface.
- **Basolateral plasma membrane**. Proteins targeted to the basolateral domain also have a specific sorting signal attached to them by the TGN. This constitutive pathway uses vesicles coated with unique proteins that bind to epithelium-specific adaptor proteins. The transported membrane proteins are continuously incorporated into the basolateral cell surface. This type of targeting is present in most polarized epithelial cells. In liver hepatocytes, however, the process of protein sorting into the basolateral and apical domains is quite different. All integral plasma membrane proteins that are destined for both apical and basolateral domains are first transported from the TGN to the basolateral plasma membrane. From there, both proteins are endocytosed and sorted into early endosomal compartments. Basolateral proteins are recycled back into the basolateral membrane, whereas apical

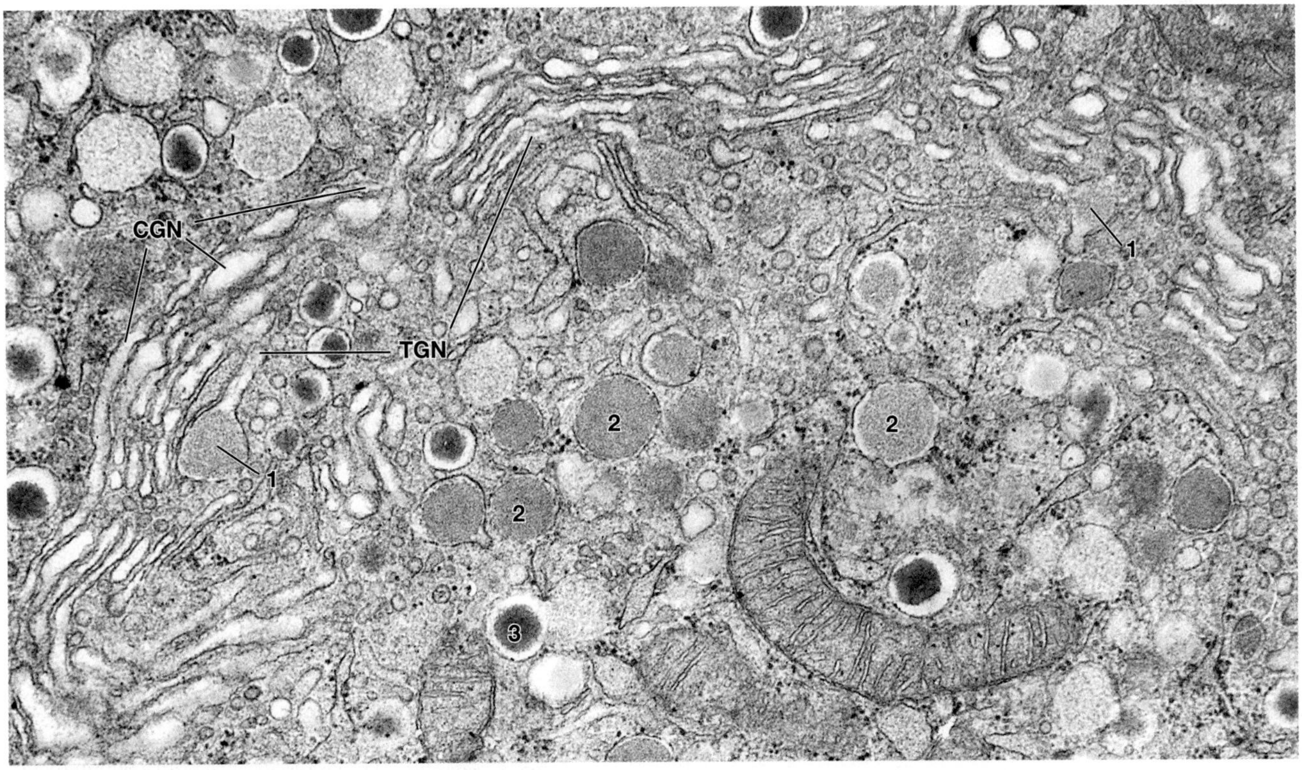

FIGURE 2.36. Electron micrograph of the Golgi apparatus. This electron micrograph shows the extensive Golgi apparatus in an islet cell of the pancreas. The flattened membrane sacs of the Golgi apparatus are arranged in layers. The *cis*-Golgi network (*CGN*) is represented by the flattened vesicles on the outer convex surface, whereas the flattened vesicles of the inner convex region constitute the *trans*-Golgi network (*TGN*). Budding off the TGN are several vesicles **(1)**. These vesicles are released **(2)** and eventually become secretory vesicles **(3)**. ×55,000.

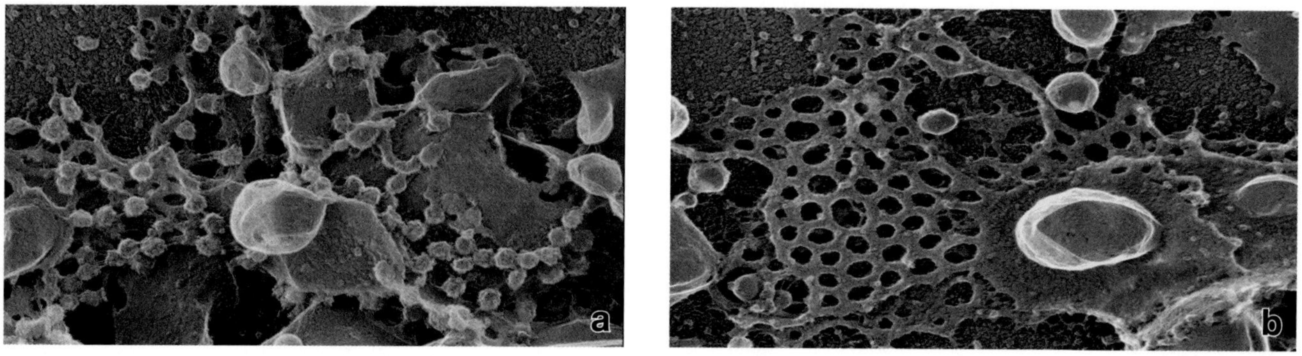

FIGURE 2.37. Electron micrograph of Golgi cisternae. a. This transmission electron micrograph shows a quick-frozen isolated Golgi apparatus replica from a cultured Chinese hamster ovary (CHO) cell line. The *trans*-Golgi cisternae are in the process of coated vesicle formation. **b.** Incubation of the *trans*-Golgi cisternae with the coatomer-depleted cytosol shows a decrease in vesicle formation activity. Note the lack of vesicles and the fenestrated shape of the *trans*-Golgi cisternae. ×85,000. (Courtesy of Dr. John E. Heuser, Washington University School of Medicine.)

proteins are transported across the cytoplasm to the apical cell membrane via transcytosis.

- **Endosomes or lysosomes.** Most proteins destined for organelles bear specific signal sequences. They are sorted in the TGN and delivered to specific organelles. However, TGN sorting mechanisms are never completely accurate. For instance, about 10% of LIMPs instead travel directly into early or late endosomes, traveling an extended route via the apical plasma membrane (see Fig. 2.23), and from there move back into the endosomal pathways. Enzymes destined for lysosomes using M-6-P markers (see pages 46-47) are delivered into early or late endosomes as they develop into mature lysosomes.
- **Apical cytoplasm.** Proteins that were aggregated or crystallized in the TGN as a result of changes in pH and Ca^{2+} concentration are stored in large **secretory vesicles**. These vesicles undergo a maturation process in which secretory proteins are retained within the vesicle. All other nonsecretory proteins are recycled into the endosomal compartment or TGN in clathrin-coated vesicles (see Fig. 2.38). Mature secretory vesicles eventually fuse with the plasma membrane to release the secretory product by

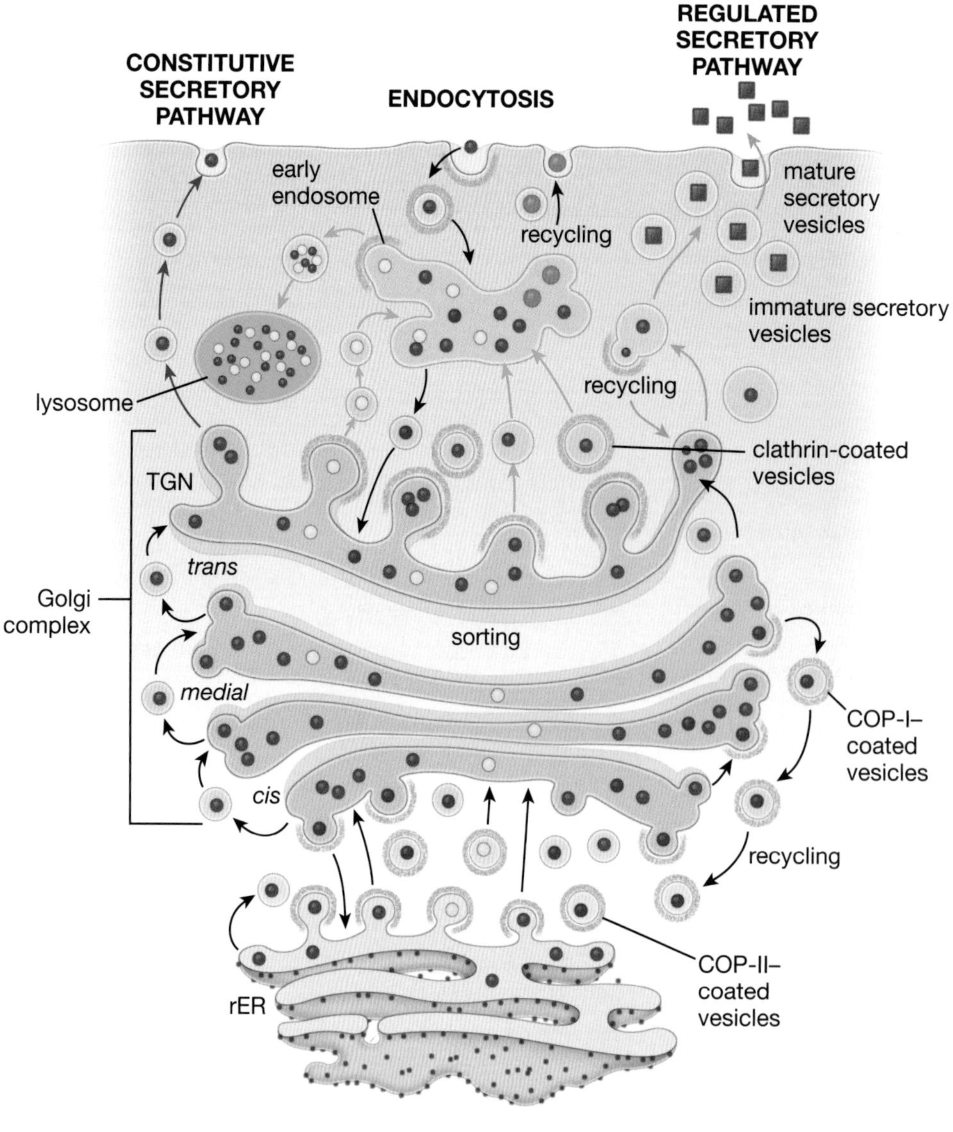

FIGURE 2.38. The Golgi apparatus and vesicular trafficking. The Golgi apparatus contains several stacks of flattened cisternae with dilated edges. The Golgi cisternae form separate functional compartments. The closest compartment to the rough endoplasmic reticulum (*rER*) represents the *cis*-Golgi network (CGN), to which COP-II-coated transport vesicles originating from the rER fuse and deliver newly synthesized proteins. Retrograde transport from the CGN to the rER, as well as retrograde transport between Golgi cisternae, is mediated by COP-I-coated vesicles. Once proteins have been modified within the CGN, the transport vesicles bud off dilated ends of this compartment, and proteins are transferred into *medial*-Golgi cisternae. The process continues; in the same fashion, proteins are translocated into the *trans*-Golgi cisternae and further into the *trans*-Golgi network (*TGN*), where they are sorted into different transport vesicles that deliver them to their final destinations.

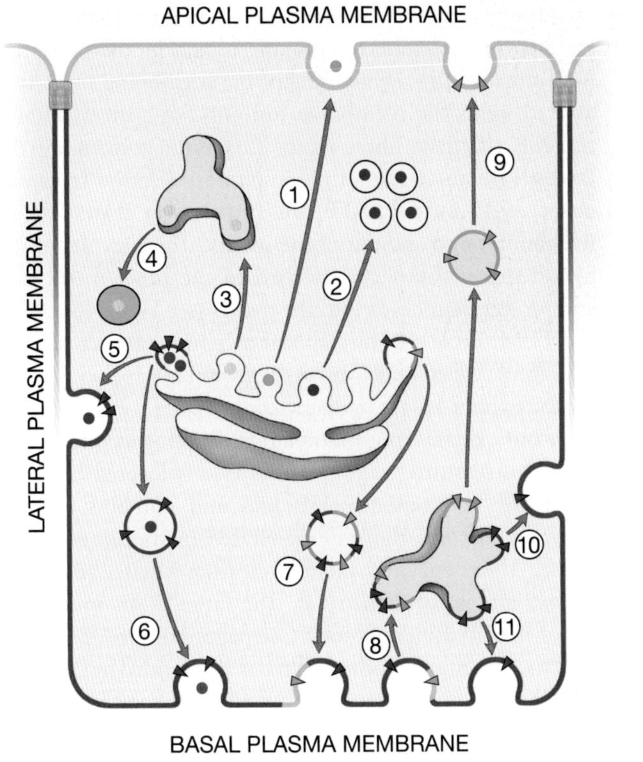

FIGURE 2.39. Summary of events in protein trafficking from the *trans*-Golgi network (TGN). The tubulovesicular array of the TGN serves as the sorting station for transporting vesicles that deliver proteins to the following destinations: **(1)** apical plasma membrane (i.e., epithelial cells); **(2)** apical region of the cell cytoplasm where proteins are stored in secretory vesicles (i.e., secretory cells); **(3)** early or late endosomal compartment; **(4)** selected proteins containing lysosomal signals, which are targeted to lysosomes; **(5)** lateral plasma membrane (i.e., epithelial cells); **(6)** basal plasma membrane (i.e., epithelial cells); **(7)** proteins destined for apical, basal, and lateral surfaces of plasma membrane, which are delivered to the basal plasma membrane (i.e., in hepatocytes); **(8)** all proteins endocytosed and sorted in early endosomes; **(9)** apical plasma membrane from early endosomes; **(10)** lateral plasma membrane; and **(11)** basal plasma membrane. Note the two targeting mechanisms of proteins to different surfaces of plasma membrane. In epithelial cells, proteins are directly targeted from the TGN into the appropriate cell surface as shown in steps **1**, **5**, and **6**. In hepatocytes, all proteins are secreted first to the basal cell surface, after which they are distributed to the appropriate cell surface via the endosomal compartment as shown in steps **7–11**.

exocytosis. This type of secretion is characteristic of highly specialized secretory cells found in exocrine glands.

Sorting and packaging of proteins into transport vesicles occurs in the *trans*-Golgi network.

Proteins that arrive in the TGN are distributed to different intracellular locations within transport vesicles. The intracellular destination of each protein depends on the sorting signals that are incorporated within the polypeptide chain of the protein. The actual sorting and packaging of proteins in TGN is primarily based on sorting signals and physical properties.

- **Sorting signals** are represented by the linear array of amino acid or associated carbohydrate molecules. This type of signal is recognized by the sorting machinery, which directs the protein into the appropriately coated transport vesicle.
- **Physical properties** are important for packaging functionally associated protein complexes. These groups of proteins are first partitioned into separate lipid rafts that are later incorporated into transport vesicles destined for a targeted organelle.

Mitochondria

Mitochondria are abundant in cells that generate and expend large amounts of energy.

Mitochondria were also known to early cytologists who observed them in cells vitally stained with Janus Green B. It is now evident that mitochondria increase in number by division throughout interphase, and their divisions are not synchronized with the cell cycle. Video microscopy confirms that mitochondria can both change their location and undergo transient changes in shape. They may therefore be compared to mobile power generators as they migrate from one area of the cell to another to supply needed energy.

Because mitochondria generate ATP, they are more numerous in cells that use large amounts of energy, such as striated muscle cells and cells engaged in fluid and electrolyte transport. Mitochondria also localize at sites in the cell where energy is needed, as in the middle piece of sperm cells, the intermyofibrillar spaces in striated muscle cells, and adjacent to the basolateral plasma membrane infoldings in the cells of the proximal convoluted tubule of the kidney.

Mitochondria evolved from aerobic bacteria that were engulfed by eukaryotic cells.

Mitochondria are believed to have evolved from an aerobic prokaryote (*Eubacterium*) that lived symbiotically within primitive eukaryotic cells. This hypothesis received support with the demonstration that mitochondria possess their own genome, increase their numbers by division, and synthesize some of their structural (constituent) proteins. **Mitochondrial DNA (mtDNA)** is a small, closed circular molecule that encodes 13 enzymes involved in the oxidative phosphorylation pathway, 2 mitochondrial rRNAs that are essential components of its own translational apparatus, and 22 transfer RNAs (tRNAs) used in the translation of the mitochondrial mRNA. The mitochondrial **DNA is haploid** in nature and is **inherited exclusively from the mother**.

Mitochondria possess a **complete system for protein synthesis**, including the synthesis of their own ribosomes. The remainder of the mitochondrial proteins is encoded by nuclear DNA; new polypeptides are synthesized by free ribosomes in the cytoplasm and then imported into mitochondria with the help of two protein complexes. These include **translocase of the outer mitochondrial membrane (TOM) complexes** and **translocase of the inner mitochondrial membrane (TIM) complexes**. Translocation of proteins through mitochondrial membranes requires energy and assistance from several specialized chaperone proteins.

Mitochondria are present in all cells except red blood cells and terminal keratinocytes.

The number, shape, and internal structure of mitochondria are often characteristic for specific cell types. When present in large numbers, mitochondria contribute to the acidophilia of the cytoplasm because of the large amount of membrane they contain. Mitochondria may be stained specifically by histochemical procedures that demonstrate some of their constituent enzymes, such as those involved in ATP synthesis and electron transport.

Mitochondria possess two membranes that delineate distinct compartments.

Mitochondria display a variety of shapes, including spheres, rods, elongated filaments, and even coiled structures. All mitochondria, unlike other organelles described earlier, possess two membranes (Fig. 2.40). The **inner mitochondrial membrane** surrounds a space called the **matrix**. The **outer mitochondrial membrane** is in close contact with the cytoplasm. The space between the two membranes is called the **intermembrane space**. The following structural components of mitochondria possess specific characteristics related to their functions.

- **Outer mitochondrial membrane.** This 6- to 7-nm-thick smooth membrane contains many **voltage-dependent anion channels** (also called **mitochondrial porins**). These large channels (approximately 3 nm in diameter) are permeable to uncharged molecules as large as 5 kDa. Thus, small molecules, ions, and metabolites can enter the intermembrane space but cannot penetrate the inner membrane. The environment of the intermembrane space is therefore similar to that of cytoplasm with respect to ions and small molecules. The outer membrane possesses receptors for proteins and polypeptides that translocate into the intermembrane space. It also contains several enzymes, including phospholipase A_2, monoamine oxidase, and acetyl coenzyme A (CoA) synthase.
- **Inner mitochondrial membrane.** The TEM reveals that this membrane is thinner than the outer mitochondrial membrane. It is arranged into numerous **cristae** (folds) that significantly increase the inner membrane surface area (see Fig. 2.40). These folds project into the matrix that constitutes the inner compartment of the organelle. In some cells involved in steroid metabolism, the inner membrane may form tubular or vesicular projections into the matrix. The inner membrane is rich in the phospholipid **cardiolipin**, which makes the membrane impermeable to ions. The membrane forming the cristae contains proteins that have three major functions: performing the **oxidation reactions** of the respiratory electron transport chain, **synthesizing ATP**, and **regulating transport** of metabolites into and out of the matrix. The enzymes of the **respiratory chain** are attached to the inner membrane and project their heads into the matrix (see Fig. 2.40). With the TEM, these enzymes appear as tennis racquet–shaped structures called **elementary particles**. Their heads measure about 10 nm in diameter and contain enzymes that carry out oxidative phosphorylation, which generates ATP.
- **Intermembrane space.** This space is located between the inner and outer membranes and contains specific enzymes that use the ATP generated in the inner membrane. These enzymes include creatine kinase, adenylate kinase, and **cytochrome *c*.** The latter is an important factor in initiating apoptosis (see pages 104-107).
- **Matrix.** The mitochondrial matrix is surrounded by the inner mitochondrial membrane and contains the soluble enzymes of the **citric acid cycle (Krebs cycle)** and the enzymes involved in **fatty acid β-oxidation.** The major products of the matrix are CO_2 and reduced NADH, which is the source of electrons for the electron transport chain. Mitochondria contain dense **matrix granules** that store Ca^{2+} and other divalent and trivalent cations. These granules increase in

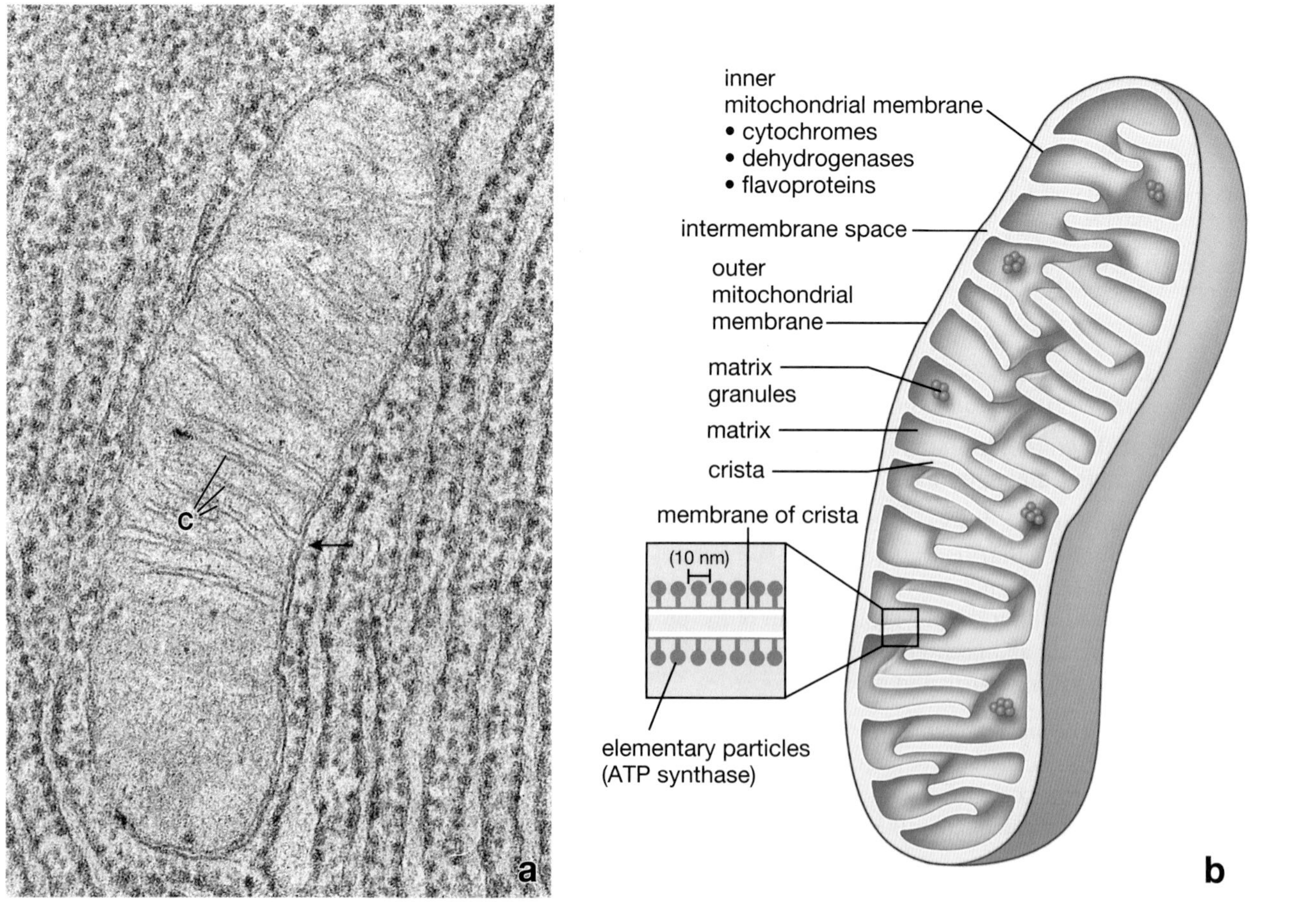

FIGURE 2.40. Structure of the mitochondrion. a. This electron micrograph shows a mitochondrion in a pancreatic acinar cell. Note that the inner mitochondrial membrane forms the cristae (*C*) through a series of infoldings, as is evident in the region of the *arrow*. The outer mitochondrial membrane is a smooth continuous envelope that is separate and distinct from the inner membrane. ×200,000. **b.** Schematic diagram showing the components of a mitochondrion. Note the location of the elementary particles (*inset*), the shape of which reflects the three-dimensional structure of adenosine triphosphate (*ATP*) synthase.

number and size when the concentration of divalent (and trivalent) cations increases in the cytoplasm. Mitochondria can accumulate cations against a concentration gradient. Thus, in addition to ATP production, mitochondria also regulate the concentration of certain ions of the cytoplasmic matrix, a role they share with the sER. The matrix also contains mitochondrial DNA, ribosomes, and tRNAs.

Mitochondria contain the enzyme system that generates ATP by means of the citric acid cycle and oxidative phosphorylation.

Mitochondria generate ATP in a variety of metabolic pathways, including oxidative phosphorylation, the citric acid cycle, and β-oxidation of fatty acids. The energy generated from these reactions, which take place in the mitochondrial matrix, is represented by hydrogen ions (H^+) derived from reduced NADH. These ions drive a series of **proton pumps** located within the inner mitochondrial membrane that transfer H^+ from the matrix to the intermembrane space (Fig. 2.41). These pumps constitute the **electron transport chain** of respiratory enzymes (see Fig. 2.40). The transfer of H^+ across the inner mitochondrial membrane establishes an **electrochemical proton gradient**. This gradient creates a **large proton motive force** that causes the movement of H^+ to occur down its electrochemical gradient through a large, membrane-bound enzyme called **ATP synthase**. ATP synthase provides a pathway across the inner mitochondrial membrane in which H^+ ions are used to drive the energetically unfavorable reactions leading to synthesis of ATP. This movement of protons back to the mitochondrial matrix is referred to as **chemiosmotic coupling**. The newly produced ATP is transported from the matrix to the intermembrane space by the voltage gradient–driven **ATP/ADP exchange protein** located in the inner mitochondrial membrane. From here, ATP leaves the mitochondria via **voltage-dependent anion channels (VDACs)** in the outer membrane to enter the cytoplasm. At the same time, ADP produced in the cytoplasm rapidly enters the mitochondria for recharging.

Several **mitochondrial defects** are related to defects in enzymes that produce ATP. Metabolically active tissues that use large amounts of ATP, such as muscle cells and neurons, are the most commonly affected. For example, **myoclonic epilepsy with ragged red fibers (MERRF)** is characterized by muscle weakness, ataxia, seizures, and cardiac and respiratory failure. Microscopic examination of muscle tissue from affected patients shows aggregates of abnormal mitochondria that provide a ragged appearance of red muscle fibers. MERRF is caused by mutation of the mitochondrial DNA gene encoding tRNA for lysine. This defect produces two abnormal complexes in the electron transport chain of respiratory enzymes affecting ATP production.

Mitochondria decide whether the cell lives or dies.

Experimental studies indicate that mitochondria sense cellular stress and are capable of deciding whether the cell lives or dies by initiating **apoptosis** (programmed cell death). The major cell death event generated by the mitochondria is the release of cytochrome *c* from the mitochondrial intermembranous space into the cell cytoplasm. Changes in the **voltage-dependent anion channels (VDACs)**

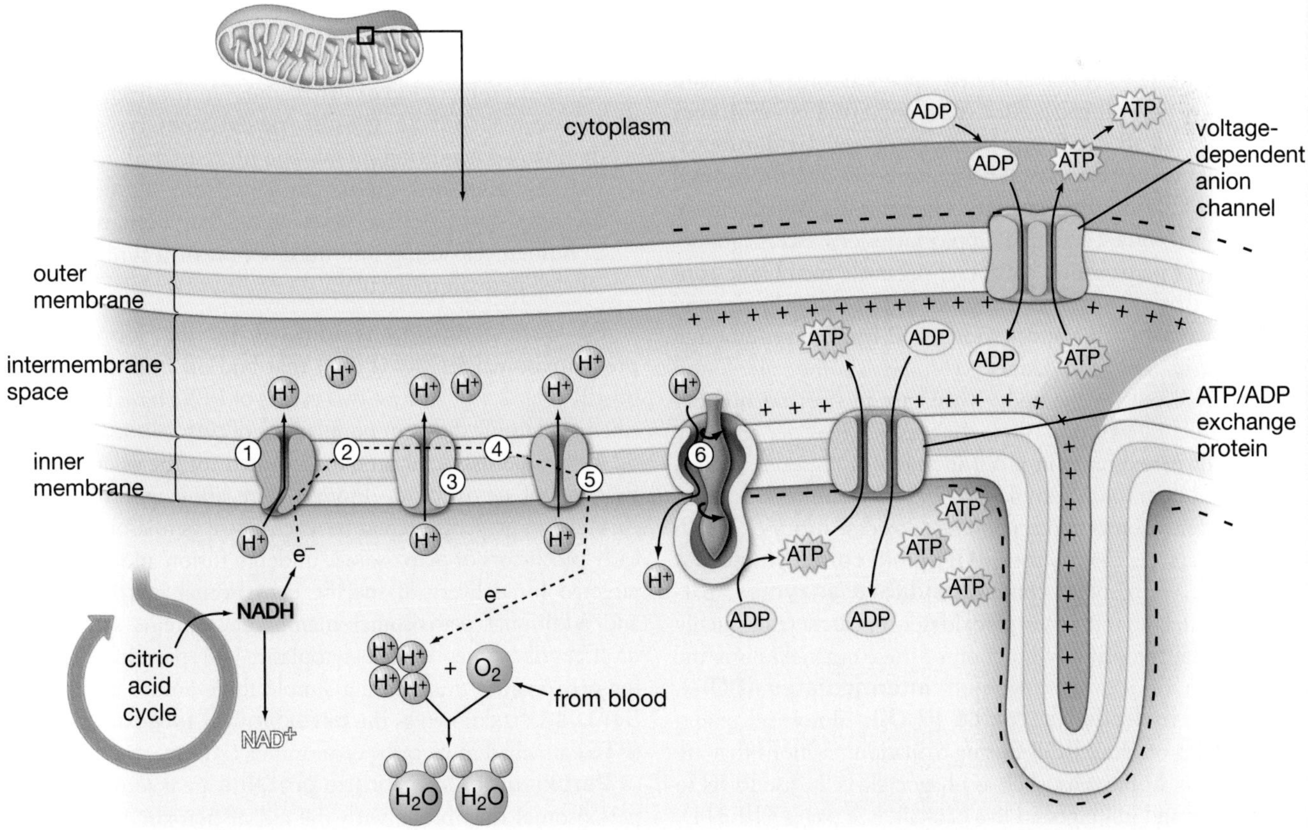

FIGURE 2.41. Schematic diagram illustrating how mitochondria generate energy. The diagram indicates the adenosine triphosphate (*ATP*) synthase complex and the electron transport chain of proteins located in the inner mitochondrial membrane. The electron transport chain generates a proton gradient between the matrix and intermembrane space that is used to produce ATP. *Numbers* represent sequential proteins involved in the electron transport chain and ATP production: *1*, NADH dehydrogenase complex; *2*, ubiquinone; *3*, cytochrome b–c_1 complex; *4*, cytochrome *c*; *5*, cytochrome oxidase complex; and *6*, ATP synthase complex. *ADP*, adenosine diphosphate.

at the outer mitochondrial membrane are responsible for this release. This event, regulated by the proapoptotic **Bcl-2 protein family** (see pages 106-107), initiates the cascade of proteolytic enzymatic reactions that lead to apoptosis. The Bcl-2 family of proteins thus controls cell death primarily by regulating permeability of the outer mitochondrial membrane, which leads to the irreversible release of cytochrome *c*, subsequent caspase activation, and apoptosis. However, in certain conditions (e.g., translational modifications), the Bcl-2 proteins may act as antiapoptotic agents.

Mitochondria undergo morphologic changes related to their functional state.

TEM studies show mitochondria in two distinct configurations. In the **orthodox configuration**, the cristae are prominent, and the matrix compartment occupies a large part of the total mitochondrial volume. This energized mitochondrion configuration is observed in healthy cells. In this configuration, most of the cytochrome *c* is sequestered within the cristae and is resistant to release by agents that disrupt the mitochondrial outer membrane. Matrix remodeling to the **condensed configuration** results in depolarization of mitochondrial membranes. This configuration is characterized by unfolded cristae that are not easily recognized in the TEM. The matrix is reduced in volume and appears more concentrated, whereas the intermembrane space increases to as much as 50% of the total volume of the organelle. These changes expose cytochrome *c* to the intermembrane space, facilitating its release from the mitochondria during apoptosis.

Peroxisomes

Peroxisomes are single-membrane-bound organelles containing a variety of oxidative enzymes.

Peroxisomes (historically called microbodies) are dynamic, multifunctional membrane-limited spherical organelles with an oxidative type of metabolism. When observed in TEM, they resemble small (0.1–0.5 μm in diameter) vesicles distributed throughout the cell cytoplasm. Because peroxisomes are involved in cellular lipid metabolism, they interact with the ER, mitochondria, lysosomes, and lipid droplet inclusions. Recent studies indicate that peroxisomes have inter-organelle membrane contact sites that allow the exchange of metabolites, lipids, and proteins with the ER, mitochondria, and lysosomes. Although abundant in liver and kidney cells, peroxisomes are found in almost all cells in the body. They vary in size and number and typically range from 10^2 to 10^3 peroxisomes per cell. The number of peroxisomes in a cell increases in response to diet, drugs, and hormonal stimulation. In most animals, but not humans, peroxisomes also contain urate oxidase (uricase), which often appears as a characteristic **crystalloid core inclusion**.

Because peroxisomes contain **oxidative enzymes**, particularly catalase and other peroxidases, researchers originally thought that the primary function of these organelles was the metabolism of **reactive oxygen intermediates (ROIs)**, particularly **hydrogen peroxide (H_2O_2)**. Almost all oxidative enzymes produce ROIs during oxidation reactions that are toxic to cells. Some cells, such as phagocytic cells, use ROIs to immobilize and kill ingested live bacteria (see pages 310-311). The catalase in peroxisomes carefully regulates the **removal of ROIs**, thus protecting the cell. For example, hydrogen peroxide is broken down into water (H_2O) and oxygen (O_2). Oxidative enzymes are particularly important in liver cells (hepatocytes), where they perform a variety of detoxification processes. For instance, peroxisomes in hepatocytes are responsible for detoxifying ingested alcohol by converting it to acetaldehyde.

However, recent evidence suggests that peroxisomes play a primary function in lipid metabolism, contributing to the breakdown and detoxification of fatty acids. Although medium and long chain fatty acids are mainly oxidized in mitochondria, peroxisomes almost exclusively metabolize very long chain fatty acids (**β-oxidation of very long chain fatty acids**) and branched chain fatty acids (**α-oxidation of branched chain fatty acids**). In addition, peroxisomes in mammalian cells are involved in lipid biosynthesis of cholesterol, dolichol, and fatty acid–linked phospholipids (e.g., ether phospholipids found in the myelin sheath). In the liver, peroxisomes are also involved in the synthesis of bile acids, which are derived from cholesterol. As mentioned earlier, β-oxidation also occurs in mitochondria. Peroxisomal β-oxidation in some cells may equal that occurring in mitochondria and thus aids in maintaining metabolic fatty acid cell homeostasis. A summary of the functions of peroxisomes is shown in Figure 2.42.

In addition to their metabolic roles, peroxisomes have recently been implicated in cellular signaling in various metabolic pathways. Different levels of peroxisomal reactive oxygen species in peroxisomes may influence intracellular processes promoting autophagy, improving cell survival, and modulating cellular immunity.

Peroxisomal biogenesis is complex; they may arise from preexisting peroxisomes, or they can be synthesized de novo.

The biogenesis of peroxisomes is still incompletely understood. In general, two models of biogenesis are generally accepted:

- In the **classical model**, peroxisomes arise from preexisting peroxisomes through growth and division. This observation is supported by TEM studies of pharmacologically induced proliferation of peroxisomes in the liver.
- In the **alternative model**, peroxisomes are generated de novo by acquiring membrane proteins and lipids from the sER and their matrix proteins from the cytoplasm. De novo formation of peroxisomes has been confirmed in human cells using immunofluorescent techniques with labeled peroxin molecules.

De novo formation is initiated by the formation of pre-peroxisomal vesicles (PPVs) that bud off from the surface of sER (Fig. 2.43). At least two classes of PPVs have been identified containing different populations of **peroxins**, a family of 32 known peroxisomal proteins required for the assembly and function of peroxisomes. Protein segregation within the two PPV classes prevents premature assembly of peroxisomes. These early precursors of peroxisomes undergo fusion and are further targeted for delivery of specific peroxisomal matrix proteins and additional peroxisomal membrane proteins synthesized on free ribosomes in the cytoplasm. All proteins destined for peroxisomes must have a simple three amino acid motif, **Ser-Lys-Leu**, known as the **peroxisomal targeting signal (PTS)** attached to its carboxy-terminus (PTS1).

Peroxisomal membrane proteins are inserted into the peroxisomal membrane with the aid of peroxin 19 (**Pex19**) protein. This soluble chaperone binds to peroxisomal membrane proteins in the cytoplasm and transports them to the place of docking (Pex3 and Pex16) and insertion into the peroxisomal membrane. After insertion, Pex19 is recycled back to the cytoplasm.

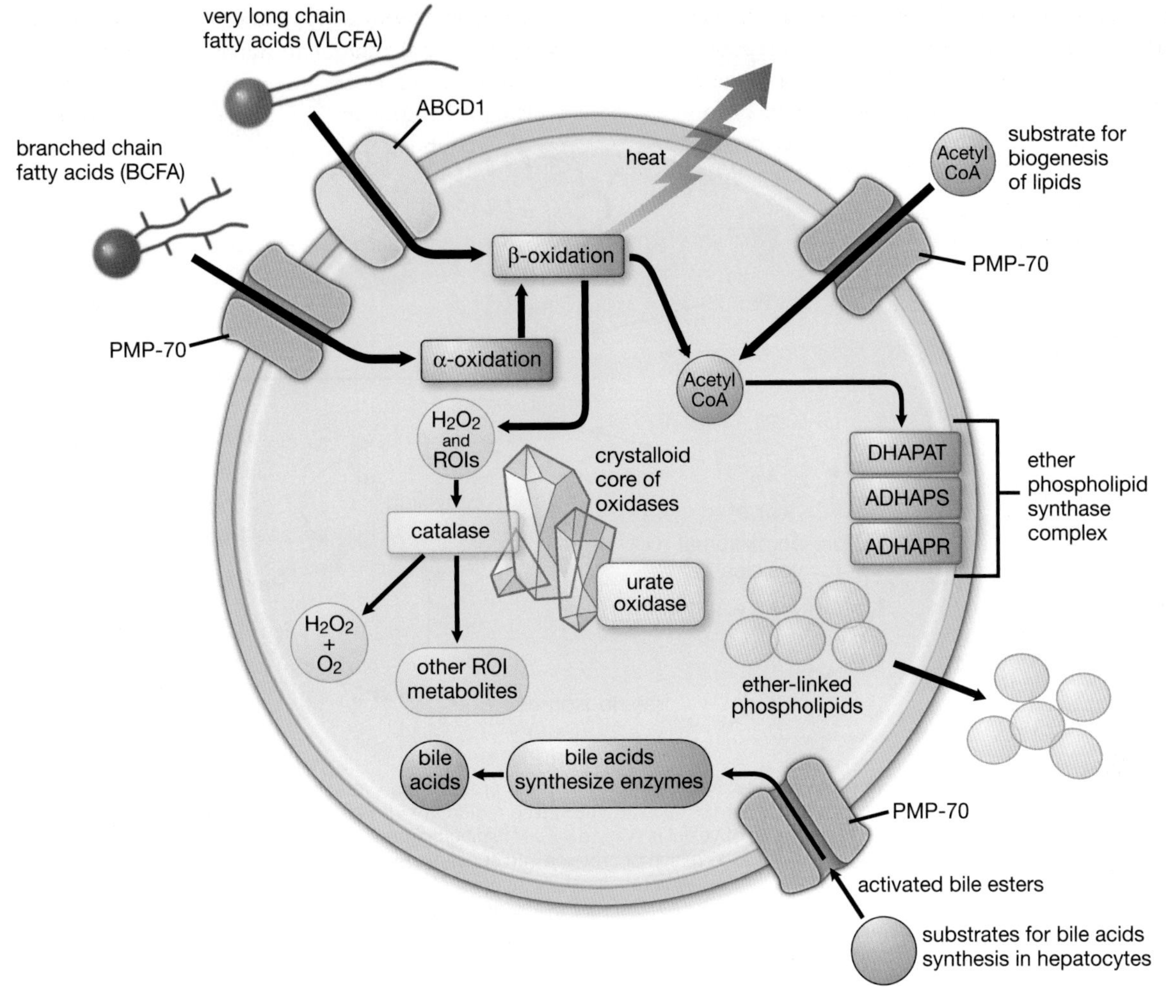

FIGURE 2.42. Schematic diagram of a peroxisome. This diagram shows peroxisomal enzymes residing within the peroxisome matrix and their respective metabolic pathways. Selected peroxisomal membrane proteins are also shown. The crystalloid core of oxidases may not be present in all species. ABCD1, ATP-binding cassette (ABC) transporters in subfamily D; ADHAPR, alkyl dihydroxyacetone phosphate reductase; ADHAPS, alkyl dihydroxyacetone phosphate synthase; DHAPAT; dihydroxyacetone phosphate acyltransferase; PMP-70, peroxisomal membrane protein-70; ROI, reactive oxygen intermediate.

Peroxisomal matrix proteins also utilize peroxins (**Pex5** and **Pex7**) as import receptors. These receptors bind peroxisomal matrix proteins in the cytoplasm and transport them to docking receptors (Pex3 and Pex16) at the peroxisomal membrane, where the proteins are delivered to the peroxisomal lumen. The receptors recycle back to the cytoplasm.

In general, peroxisomal disorders are caused by impaired peroxisomal activity or lack of peroxisomes because of defective peroxisomal biogenesis. Various human metabolic disorders are caused by mutations in the **PEX genes** encoding the **peroxisomal proteins** (peroxins) required for peroxisome biogenesis and function. These mutations result in the inability to import peroxisomal matrix and membrane proteins into the organelle. **Peroxisomal disorders** are associated with impaired peroxisomal lipid metabolism (e.g., resulting in the accumulation of very long chain fatty acids, branched chain fatty acids) and defective synthesis of ether lipids and bile acids. **Peroxisomal biogenesis disorders** include **Zellweger spectrum disorders (ZSDs)** and **rhizomelic chondrodysplasia punctata type 1 (RCDP1).** The most common inherited Zellweger spectrum disorders are **cerebrohepatorenal Zellweger syndrome**, **neonatal adrenoleukodystrophy (NALD)**, and **infantile Refsum disease**. Zellweger syndrome is the most severe of these three disorders. It causes craniofacial malformations, hepatomegaly, neurologic and developmental abnormalities, retinal degeneration, and deafness. Most infants affected by Zellweger syndrome do not survive past 1 year of age. The clinical features of neonatal adrenoleukodystrophy and infantile Refsum disease are similar to those of Zellweger syndrome; however, these disorders progress more slowly. Mutations in Pex3, Pex16, and Pex19 genes cause the most severe phenotypes, which result in the complete absence of peroxisomes. Therapies for peroxisomal disorders have been unsatisfactory to date.

■ NONMEMBRANOUS ORGANELLES

Microtubules

Microtubules are nonbranching and rigid hollow tubes of polymerized protein that can rapidly assemble and equally rapidly disassemble. In general, microtubules are found in the cytoplasm, where they originate from the **microtubule-organizing center (MTOC)**. They grow from the MTOC located near the nucleus and extend toward the cell periphery. Microtubules are also present in cilia and flagella, where they form the axoneme and its anchoring basal body; in centrioles and the mitotic spindle; and in elongating processes of the cell, such as those in growing axons.

Microtubules are involved in numerous essential cellular functions:

- **Intracellular vesicular transport** (i.e., movement of secretory vesicles, endosomes, and lysosomes). Microtubules

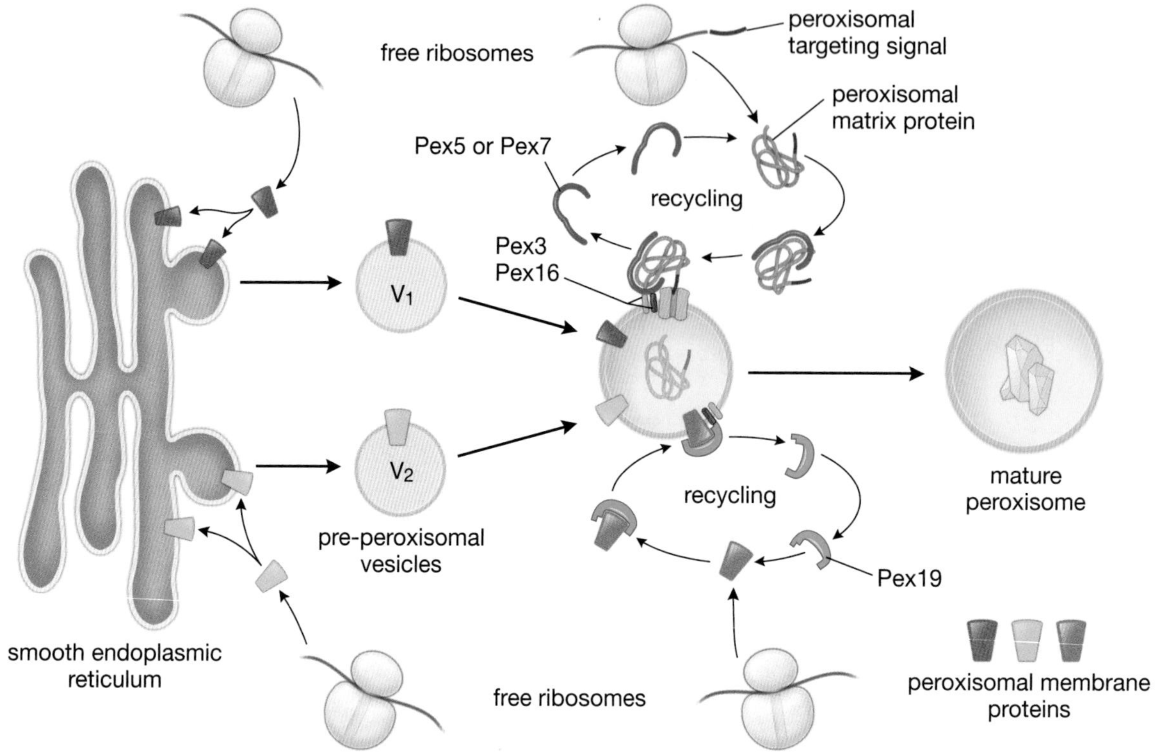

FIGURE 2.43. De novo formation of peroxisomes. Peroxisomal membrane proteins are synthesized on free ribosomes in the cytoplasm. Initially, they are incorporated into the smooth endoplasmic reticulum (sER). The region of sER rich in peroxisomal membrane proteins buds off the sER to form pre-peroxisomal vesicles. Two classes of vesicles (V_1 and V_2) containing different classes of peroxisomal membrane proteins are depicted in the initial stage of peroxisome formation. Segregation of proteins into separate vesicles prevents their interaction and the premature assembly of peroxisomes. Fusion of the two classes of vesicles results in a precursor of the peroxisome. This precursor is further targeted for delivery of specific peroxisomal matrix and membrane proteins. Delivery of these proteins to the peroxisome is aided by soluble cytoplasmic receptor (chaperone) proteins. Chaperones bind to respective peroxisomal proteins in the cytoplasm, transport them to the place of docking (Pex3 and Pex16), and insert them either into the peroxisomal membrane (Pex19) or act as import receptors (Pex5 or Pex7) to guide matrix proteins into the lumen. After the insertion of proteins, chaperones are recycled back into the cytoplasm. Note that proteins destined for the peroxisomes have a peroxisomal targeting signal.

create a system of connections within the cell, frequently compared with railroad tracks originating from a central station, along which vesicular movement occurs.

- **Movement of cilia and flagella**
- **Attachment of chromosomes to the mitotic spindle** and their movement during mitosis and meiosis
- **Maintenance of cell shape**, particularly its asymmetry
- **Regulatory effect on cell elongation and movement** (migration)

Although microtubules may exert a regulatory effect on cell elongation and movement, they are not essential for these functions, which are mediated by actin polymerization (see pages 69-70). Microtubules play an indirect role by regulating actin polymerization, organizing transport of vesicles to the leading edge of migrating cells, and facilitating disassembly of focal adhesions (see pages 160-161). In addition, microtubules may restrain cell locomotion by slowing the retraction of the trailing edge (tail) of the migrating cell, thus influencing the direction of cell migration.

Microtubules are elongated polymeric structures composed of equal parts of α-tubulin and β-tubulin.

Microtubules measure 20–25 nm in diameter. The wall of the microtubule is approximately 5 nm thick and consists of 13 circularly arrayed globular **dimeric tubulin molecules.** The tubulin dimer has a molecular weight of 110 kDa and is formed from an α-tubulin and a β-tubulin molecule, each with a molecular weight of 55 kDa (Fig. 2.44). The dimers polymerize in an end-to-end fashion, head to tail, with the α molecule of one dimer bound to the β molecule of the next dimer in a repeating pattern. Longitudinal contacts between dimers link them into a linear structure called a **protofilament.** Axial periodicity seen along the 5-nm-diameter dimers corresponds to the length of the protein molecules. A small, 1-μm segment of microtubule contains approximately 16,000 tubulin dimers.

Microtubules grow from γ-tubulin rings within the MTOC that serve as nucleation sites for each microtubule.

Microtubule formation can be traced to hundreds of **γ-tubulin rings** that form an integral part of the MTOC and function as templates for the correct assembly of microtubules. Their nucleation pattern initiated in the MTOC can be studied in vitro (Fig. 2.45). The α- and β-tubulin dimers are added to a γ-tubulin ring in an end-to-end fashion. The most simplistic model used in the past described microtubule assembly as a process of adding tubulin dimers one by one onto the growing end of a fully formed microtubule. However, a number of experimental studies using cryoelectron microscopy have shown that the initial assembly occurs from a curved sheet made of tubulin dimers, which in turn closes into a tube at the growing end of the microtubule (see Fig. 2.44).

Polymerization of tubulin dimers requires the presence of **guanosine triphosphate (GTP)** and **Mg^{2+}**. Each tubulin molecule binds GTP before it is incorporated into the

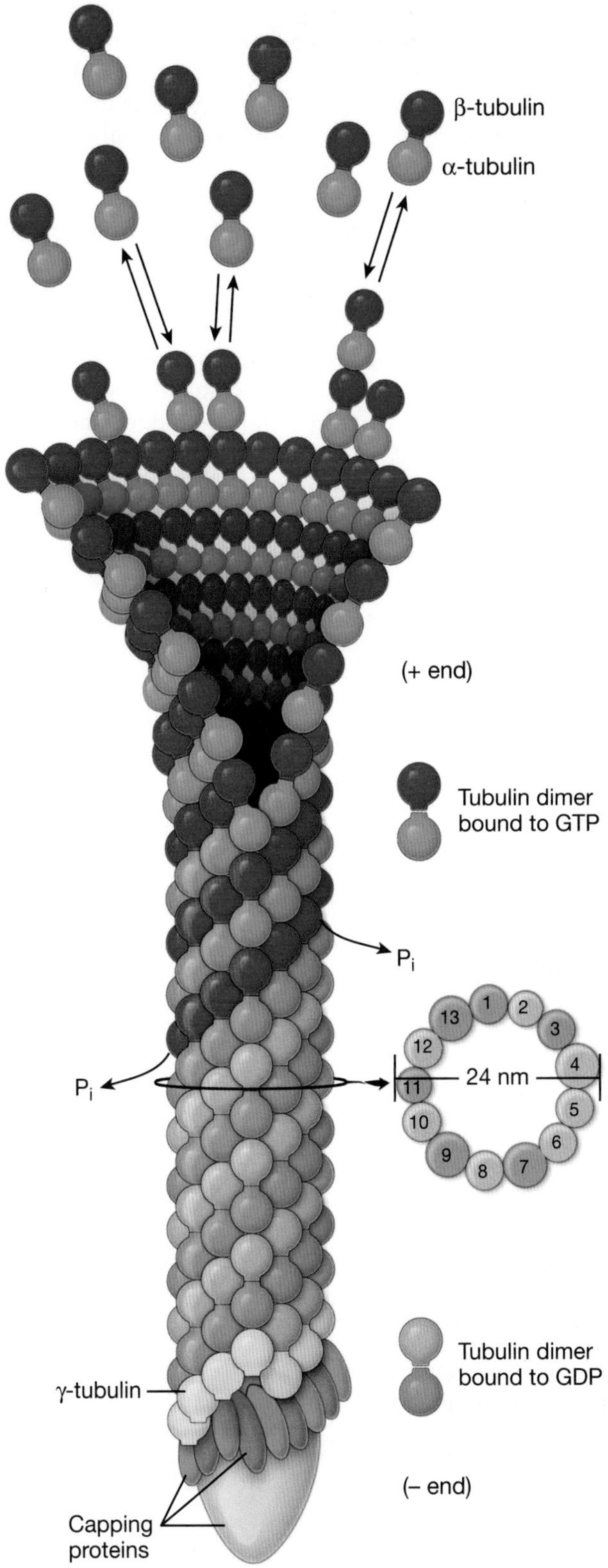

FIGURE 2.44. Polymerization of microtubules. On the *left*, the diagram depicts the process of polymerization of tubulin dimers during microtubule assembly. Each tubulin dimer consists of an α-tubulin and β-tubulin subunit. The plus (+) end of the microtubule is the growing end to which tubulin dimers bound to guanosine triphosphate (*GTP*) molecules are incorporated into a curved sheet, which in turn closes into a tube. Incorporated tubulin dimers hydrolyze GTP, which releases the phosphate groups to form polymers with guanosine diphosphate (*GDP*)-tubulin molecules. The minus (−) end of the microtubule contains a ring of γ-tubulin, which is necessary for microtubule nucleation. This end is usually embedded within the microtubule-organizing center (MTOC) and possesses numerous capping proteins. On the *right* is a diagram showing that each microtubule contains 13 tubulin dimers within its cross section.

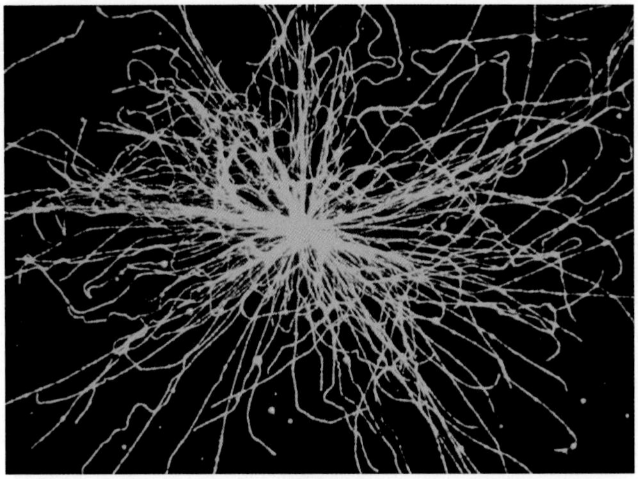

FIGURE 2.45. Nucleation activity of microtubules observed in vitro using immunocytochemical methods. The behavior of microtubules obtained from human breast cancer cells can be studied in vitro by measuring their nucleation activity. Microtubules were labeled with a mixture of anti-α-tubulin and anti-β-tubulin monoclonal antibodies (primary antibodies) and visualized by secondary antibodies conjugated with fluorescein dye (fluorescein isothiocyanate–goat antimouse immunoglobulin G). Polymerization of tubulin dimers is responsible for the formation of more than 120 microtubules visible on this image. They originate from the microtubule-organizing center (MTOC) and extend outward approximately 20–25 μm in a uniform radial array. ×1,400. (Photomicrograph courtesy of Drs. Wilma L. Lingle and Vivian A. Negron.)

forming microtubule. The tubulin dimers containing GTP have a conformation that favors stronger lateral interactions between dimers resulting in polymerization. At some point, GTP is hydrolyzed to guanosine diphosphate (GDP).

As a result of this polymerization pattern, microtubules are polar structures because all of the dimers in each protofilament have the same orientation. Each microtubule possesses a **nongrowing (−) end** that corresponds to α-tubulin; in the cell, it is usually embedded in the MTOC and often stabilized by actin-capping proteins (see Fig. 2.44). The **growing (+) end** of microtubules corresponds to β-tubulin and extends the cell periphery. Tubulin dimers dissociate from microtubules in the steady state, which creates a pool of free tubulin dimers in the cytoplasm. This pool is in equilibrium with the polymerized tubulin in the microtubules; therefore, polymerization and depolymerization are in equilibrium. The equilibrium can be shifted in the direction of depolymerization by exposing the cell or isolated microtubules to low temperatures or high pressure. Repeated exposure to alternating low and high temperatures is the basis of the purification technique for tubulin and microtubules. The speed of polymerization or depolymerization can also be modified by interaction with specific **microtubule-associated proteins (MAPs)**. These proteins, such as MAP-1, MAP-2, MAP-3, and MAP-4; MAP-τ; and TOG-ρ, regulate microtubule assembly and anchor the microtubules to specific organelles. MAPs are also responsible for the existence of stable populations of nondepolymerizing microtubules in the cell, such as those found in cilia and flagella.

The length of microtubules constantly changes as dimers are added or removed in a process of dynamic instability.

Microtubules observed in cultured cells with real-time video microscopy appear to be constantly growing toward the cell periphery by addition (polymerization) of tubulin dimers and then suddenly shrinking in the direction of the MTOC by removal (depolymerization) of tubulin dimers (Fig. 2.46). This

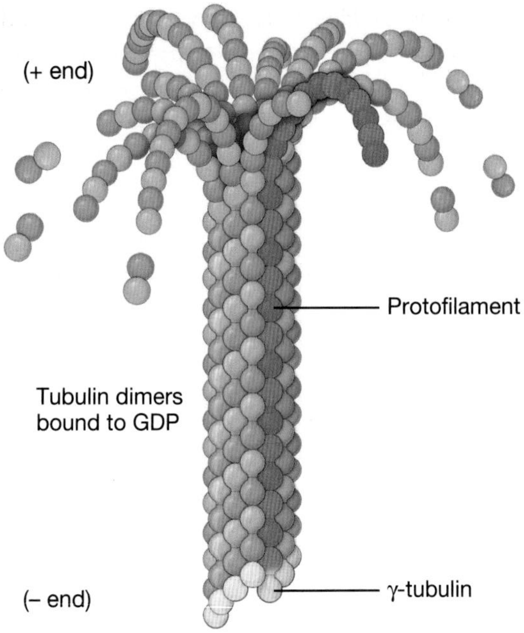

FIGURE 2.46. Depolymerization of microtubules. Microtubules are dynamic structures involved in a constant remodeling process known as dynamic instability. They elongate by addition (polymerization) of tubulin dimers bound to guanosine triphosphate (*GTP*) and then quickly shrink by removal (depolymerization) of tubulin dimers that hydrolyzed GTP. The tubulin dimers bound to guanosine diphosphate (*GDP*) are prone to depolymerization by losing lateral interactions between each other. This allows for protofilaments to curl away from the end of the microtubule. Note the arrangement of tubulin dimers in a single protofilament highlighted in *pink*.

constant remodeling process, known as **dynamic instability**, is linked to a pattern of GTP hydrolysis during the microtubule assembly and disassembly process. The tubulin dimers bound to GTP at the growing (+) end of the microtubule protect it from disassembly. In contrast, tubulin dimers bound to GDP are prone to depolymerization that leads to rapid microtubule disassembly and shrinking. During disassembly, the tubulin dimers bound to GDP lose lateral interaction with each other and protofilaments of the tubulin dimers curl away from the end of the microtubule, producing "split ends" (see Fig. 2.46). The process of switching from a growing to a shrinking microtubule is often called a **microtubule catastrophe**.

The MTOC can be compared to a feeding chameleon, which fires its long, projectile tongue to make contact with potential food. The chameleon then retracts its tongue back into its mouth and repeats this process until it is successful in obtaining food. The same strategy of "firing" dynamic microtubules from the MTOC toward the cell periphery and subsequently retracting them enables microtubules to search the cytoplasm. When the fired microtubule encounters stabilization factors (such as MAPs), it is captured and changes its dynamic behavior. This **selective stabilization process** allows the cell to establish an organized system of microtubules linking peripheral structures and organelles with the MTOC.

As mentioned earlier, the association of a microtubule with MAPs (e.g., within the axoneme of a cilium or flagellum) effectively blocks this dynamic instability and stabilizes the microtubules. In certain cells, such as neurons, some microtubules that nucleated at the MTOC can be released by the action of a **microtubule-severing protein** called **katanin**. Short, detached polymers of microtubules are then transported along existing microtubules by molecular motor proteins such as kinesins.

The structure and function of microtubules in mitosis and in cilia and flagella are discussed later in this chapter and in Chapter 5, Epithelial Tissue, pages 128-134.

Microtubules can be visualized with a variety of imaging methods.

EM of both in vitro isolated microtubules and in vivo microtubules within the cell cytoplasm is an essential tool for examining their structure and function. Microtubules can be readily visualized with the TEM as shown in Figure 2.47.

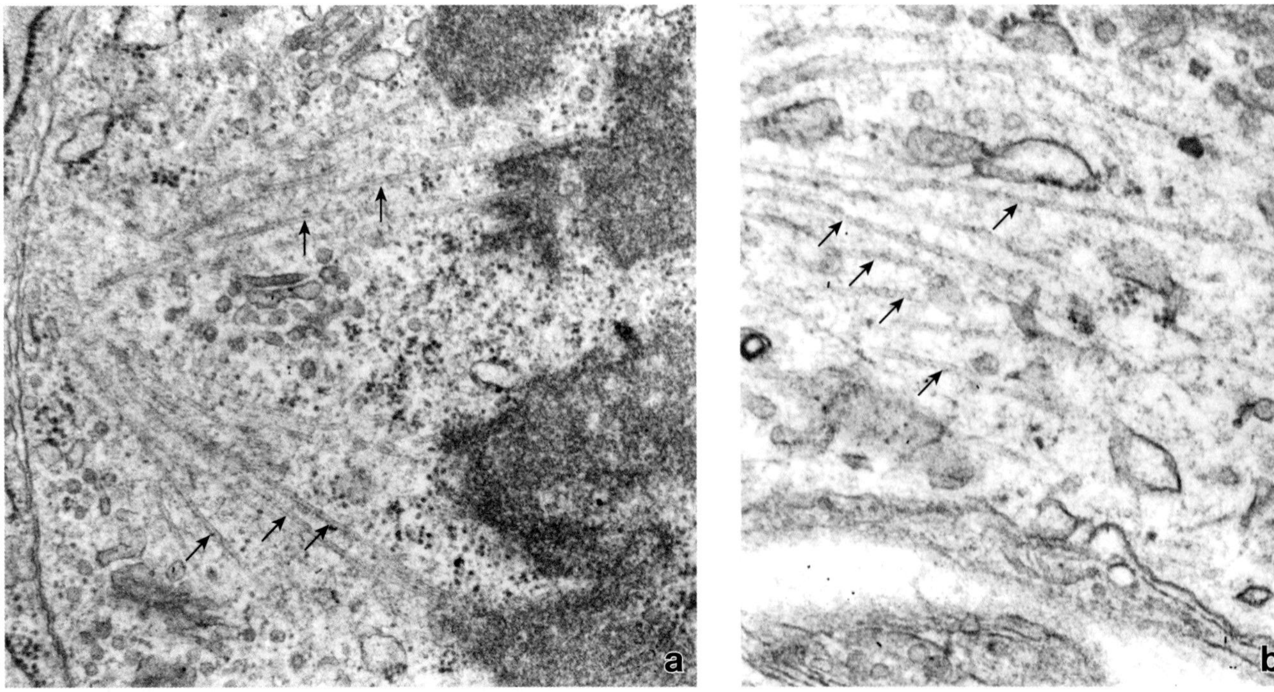

FIGURE 2.47. Electron micrographs of microtubules. a. Micrograph showing microtubules (*arrows*) of the mitotic spindle in a dividing cell. On the *right*, the microtubules are attached to chromosomes. ×30,000. **b.** Micrograph of microtubules (*arrows*) in the axon of a nerve cell. In both cells, the microtubules are seen in longitudinal profile. ×30,000.

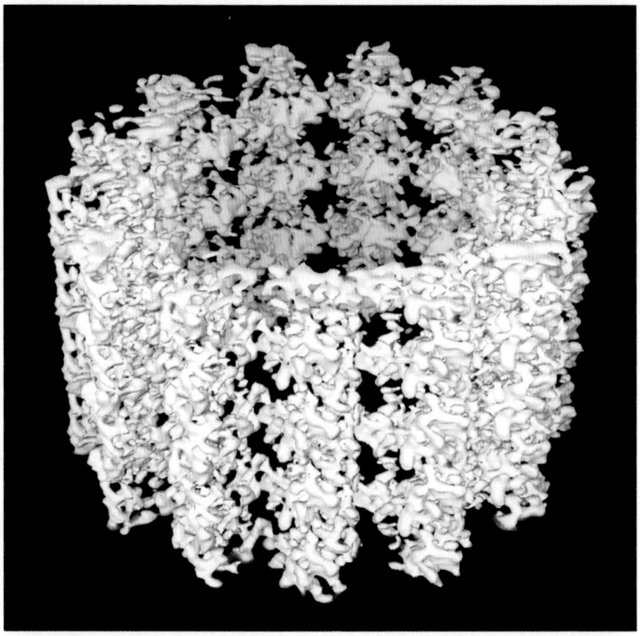

FIGURE 2.48. Three-dimensional reconstruction of an intact microtubule. This image was obtained using cryoelectron microscopy. Tomographic (sectional) images of a frozen hydrated microtubule were collected and digitally reconstructed at a resolution of 8 Å. The helical structure of the α-tubulin molecules is recognizable at this magnification. ×3,250,000. (Courtesy of Dr. Kenneth Downing.)

High-resolution images of microtubules have been obtained with cryoelectron microscopy aided by tomographic reconstruction of their unique molecular structure (Fig. 2.48). In addition, high-resolution images of microtubules can also be obtained using atomic force microscopy. In the past, microtubules were observed in the light microscope by using special stains, polarization, or phase contrast optics. Because of the limited resolution of the light microscope, microtubules may now be easily distinguished from other components of the cell cytoskeleton with immunocytochemical methods using tubulin antibodies conjugated with fluorescent dyes (Fig. 2.49).

Movement of intracellular organelles is generated by molecular motor proteins associated with microtubules.

In cellular activities that involve movement of organelles and other cytoplasmic structures—such as transport vesicles, mitochondria, and lysosomes—microtubules serve as guides to the appropriate destinations. **Molecular motor proteins** attach to these organelles or structures and ratchet along the microtubule track (Fig. 2.50). The energy required for the ratcheting movement is derived from ATP hydrolysis. Two families of molecular motor proteins have been identified that allow for unidirectional movement:

- **Dyneins** constitute one family of molecular motors. They move along the microtubules **toward the minus (−) end** of the tubule. Therefore, **cytoplasmic dyneins** are capable of transporting organelles from the cell periphery toward the MTOC. One member of the dynein family, **axonemal dynein**, is present in cilia and flagella. It is responsible for the sliding of one microtubule against an adjacent microtubule within the axoneme, thus effecting their movement.
- **Kinesins**, members of the other family, move along the microtubules **toward the plus (+) end**; therefore, they are capable of moving organelles from the cell center toward the cell periphery.

Both dyneins and kinesins are involved in mitosis and meiosis. In these activities, dyneins move the chromosomes along the microtubules of the mitotic spindle. Kinesins are simultaneously involved in movement of polar microtubules. These microtubules extend from one spindle pole past the metaphase plate and overlap with microtubules extending from the opposite spindle pole. Kinesins located between these microtubules generate a sliding movement that reduces the overlap, thereby pushing the two spindle poles apart toward each daughter cell (Fig. 2.51).

Actin Filaments

Actin filaments are present in virtually all cell types.

Actin molecules (42 kDa) are abundant and may constitute as much as 20% of the total protein of some nonmuscle cells (Fig. 2.52). Similar to the tubulin in microtubules, actin molecules also assemble spontaneously by polymerization into a linear helical array to form filaments 6–8 nm in diameter. They are thinner, shorter, and more flexible than microtubules. Free actin molecules in the cytoplasm are referred to as **G-actin (globular actin)**, in contrast to the polymerized actin of the filament, which is called **F-actin (filamentous actin)**. An actin filament or microfilament is a polarized structure; its fast-growing end is referred to as the **plus (barbed) end**, and its slow-growing end is referred to as the **minus (pointed) end**.

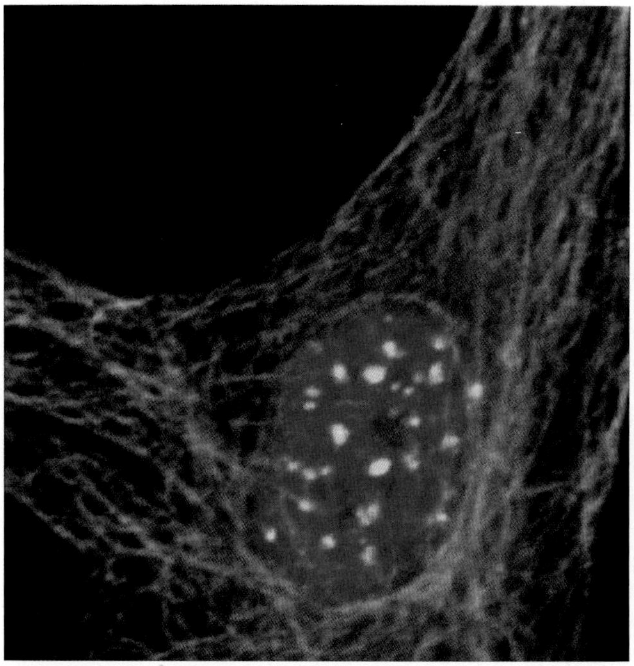

FIGURE 2.49. Staining of microtubules with fluorescent dye. This confocal immunofluorescent image shows the organization of the microtubules within an epithelial cell in tissue culture. In this example, the specimen was immunostained with three primary antibodies against tubulin (*green*), centrin (*red*), and kinetochores (*light blue*) and then incubated in a mixture of three different fluorescently tagged secondary antibodies that recognized the primary antibodies. Nuclei were stained (*dark blue*) with a fluorescent molecule that intercalates into the DNA double helix. Note that the microtubules are focused at the microtubule-organizing center (MTOC) or centrosome (*red*), located adjacent to the nucleus. The cell is in the S phase of the cell cycle, as indicated by the presence of both large unduplicated kinetochores and smaller pairs of duplicated kinetochores. ×3,000. (Courtesy of Drs. Wilma L. Lingle and Vivian A. Negron.)

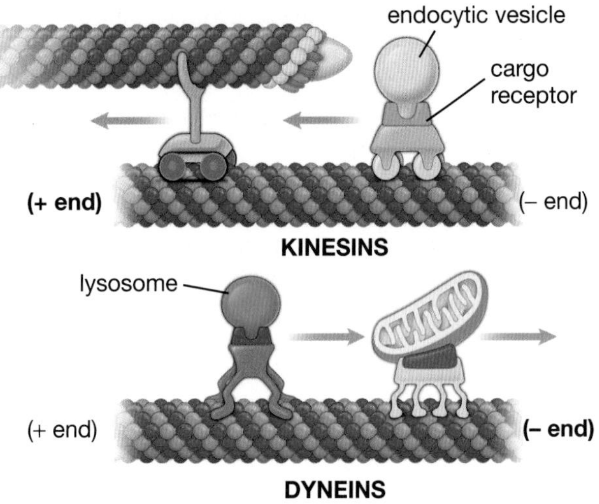

FIGURE 2.50. Molecular motor proteins associated with microtubules. Microtubules serve as guides for molecular motor proteins. These adenosine triphosphate (ATP)-driven microtubule-associated motor proteins are attached to moving structures (such as organelles) that ratchet them along a tubular track. Two types of molecular motors have been identified: dyneins that move along microtubules toward their minus (−) end (i.e., toward the center of the cell) and kinesins that move toward their plus (+) end (i.e., toward the cell periphery).

Actin is preferentially added to the plus end of the actin filament, and it dissociates from the minus end.

The dynamic process of actin polymerization that occurs mainly at the plus end of the actin filament requires the presence of **K^+**, **Mg^{2+}**, and **ATP**. After each G-actin molecule is incorporated into the filament, ATP is hydrolyzed to ADP. However, the phosphate group release from the ATP hydrolysis is not immediate, and the transient form of actin bound to ADP and the free phosphate group persist in filaments (Fig. 2.53).

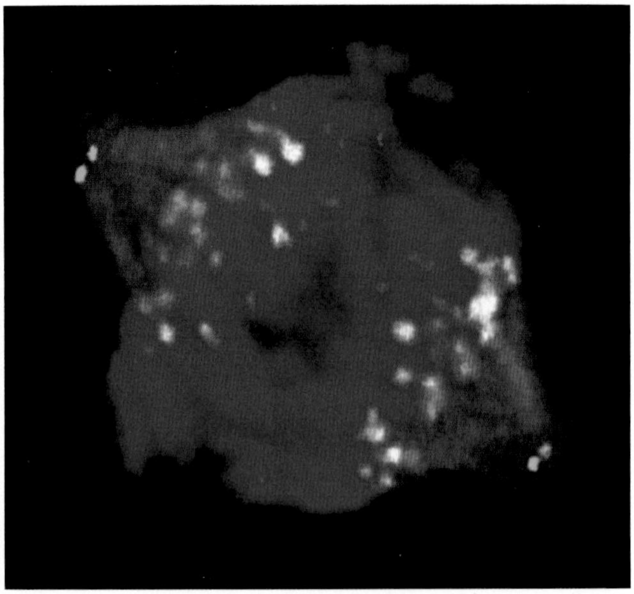

FIGURE 2.51. Distribution of kinesin-like motor protein within the mitotic spindle. This confocal immunofluorescent image shows a mammary gland epithelial cell in anaphase of mitosis. Each mitotic spindle pole contains two centrioles (*green*). A mitosis-specific kinesin-like molecule called Eg5 (*red*) is associated with the subset of the mitotic spindle microtubules that connect the kinetochores (*white*) to the spindle poles. The motor action of Eg5 is required to separate the sister chromatids (*blue*) into the daughter cells. This cell was first immunostained with three primary antibodies against Eg5 (*red*), centrin (*green*), and kinetochores (*white*) and then incubated in three different fluorescently tagged secondary antibodies that recognize the primary antibodies. Chromosomes were stained with a fluorescent molecule that intercalates into the DNA double helix. ×3,500. (Courtesy of Drs. Wilma L. Lingle and Vivian A. Negron.)

Under physiologic conditions, G-actin molecules are preferentially incorporated into the plus end and preferentially dissociated from the minus end of the actin filament. Thus, each new G-actin molecule that is added to the plus end travels the length of the actin filament as additional actin molecules are added behind it and eventually leaves the actin filament from the minus end. This phenomenon is called **treadmilling** (see Fig. 5.5).

When the rate at which free G-actin is added at the plus end is greater than the rate of subunit loss at the minus end, the filament appears to grow. Conversely, when the rate at which free G-actin is added is lower than the rate of subunit loss, the actin filament appears to shrink. When the rate at which G-actin is added is equal to the rate of its dissociation at the minus end, the length of filament is unchanged. This state is referred to as the **steady state of treadmilling**.

The control and regulation of the polymerization process depends on the local concentration of G-actin and the interaction of **actin-binding proteins (ABPs)**, which can prevent or enhance polymerization.

Several natural toxins that have been found and isolated from mushrooms, fungi, and sponges bind to actin filaments and affect their polymerization and disassembly. **Phalloidin**, a seven-amino-acid polypeptide found in the death cap mushroom (*Amanita phalloides*), inhibits actin filament disassembly by stabilizing adjacent actin molecules within the filament. Because of its strong binding to F-actin, phalloidin molecules linked to fluorescent tags are used as staining reagents for microscopic visualization of actin filaments. The **cytochalasins** produced by a variety of fungi bind to the plus end of actin filaments to prevent actin filament assembly and disassembly at that end. **Latrunculin A**, a toxin produced by the Red Sea sponge (*Latrunculia magnifica*), binds to G-actin monomers to inhibit their polymerization into actin filaments. **Jasplakinolide**, a small compound present in the marine sponge (*Jaspis johnstoni*) found in the Fuji and Palau islands, stabilizes actin monomers, thereby enhancing polymerization and assembly of actin filaments.

Actin-binding proteins are responsible for assembly, disassembly, and organization of actin filaments.

In addition to controlling the rate of polymerization of actin filaments, ABPs are responsible for the filaments' organization. For example, a number of proteins can modify or act on actin filaments to give them various specific characteristics:

- **Actin-bundling proteins** cross-link actin filaments into parallel arrays, creating actin filament bundles. An example of this modification occurs inside the microvillus, where actin filaments are cross-linked by the actin-bundling proteins **fascin** and **fimbrin**. This cross-linkage provides support and imparts rigidity to the microvilli.
- **Actin filament–severing proteins** cut long actin filaments into shorter fragments. An example of such a protein is **gelsolin**, a 90-kDa ABP that normally initiates actin polymerization but at high Ca^{2+} concentrations causes severing and capping of the actin filaments, converting an actin gel into a fluid state. **Cofilin**, an 18-kDa protein

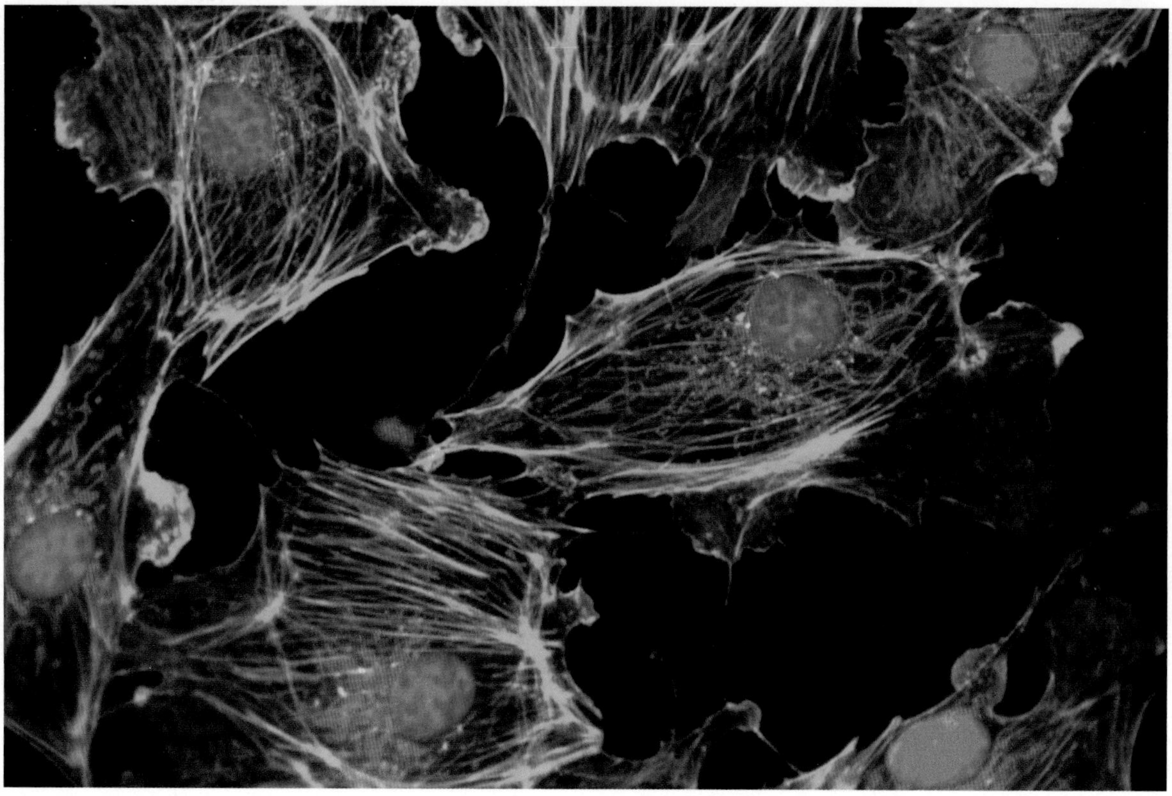

FIGURE 2.52. Distribution of actin filaments in pulmonary artery endothelial cells in culture. Cells were fixed and stained with NDB-phallacidin stain conjugated with fluorescein dye. Phallacidin binds and stabilizes actin filaments, preventing their depolymerization. Note the accumulation of actin filaments at the periphery of the cell just beneath the plasma membrane. These cells were also stained with two additional dyes: a mitochondria-selective dye (MitoTracker Red) that allows the visualization of mitochondria (*red*) in the middle of the cell and DAPI stain that reacts with nuclear DNA and exhibits *blue* fluorescence over the nucleus. ×3,000. (Courtesy of Molecular Probes, Inc., Eugene, OR.)

involved in rapid remodeling of the actin cytoskeleton, severs actin filaments to create free plus and minus ends that are available for polymerization or depolymerization of free actin molecules.

- **Actin-capping proteins** block further addition of actin molecules by binding to the free end of an actin filament. An example is **tropomodulin**, which can be isolated from skeletal and cardiac muscle cells. Tropomodulin binds to the free end of actin myofilaments, regulating the length of the filaments in a sarcomere.
- **Actin cross-linking** proteins are responsible for cross-linking actin filaments with each other. An example of such proteins can be found in the cytoskeleton of erythrocytes. Several proteins—such as **spectrin**, **adducin**, **protein 4.1**, and **protein 4.9**—are involved in cross-linking actin filaments.

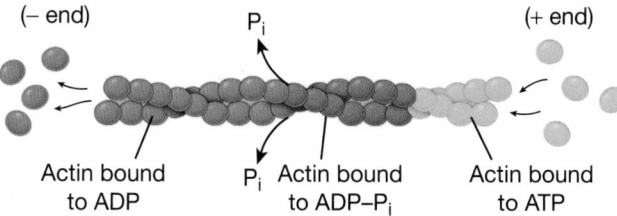

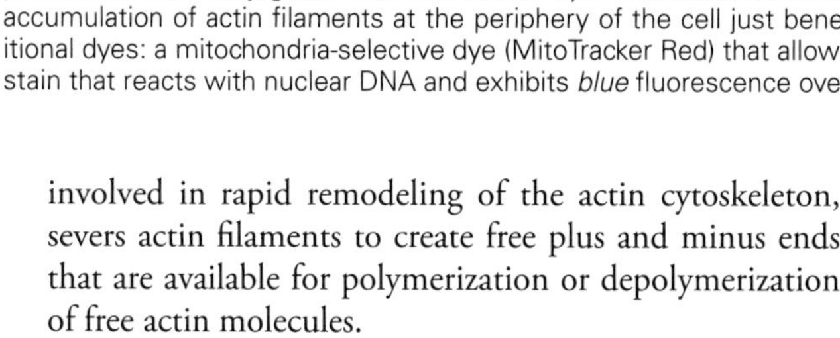

FIGURE 2.53. Polymerization of actin filaments. Actin filaments are polarized structures. Their fast-growing end is referred to as the *plus* (+) or *barbed end*; the slow-growing end is referred to as the *minus* (−) or *pointed end*. The dynamic process of actin polymerization requires energy in the form of an adenosine triphosphate (*ATP*) molecule that is hydrolyzed to adenosine diphosphate (*ADP*) after a G-actin molecule is incorporated into the filament. The phosphate groups are not immediately released; therefore, a transient form of actin bound to ADP–P_i is detectable in the filament.

- **Actin motor proteins** belong to the myosin family, which hydrolyzes ATP to provide the energy for movement along the actin filament from the minus end to the plus end. Some cells, such as muscle cells, are characterized by the size, amount, and nature of the filaments and actin motor proteins they contain. There are two types of filaments (**myofilaments**) present in muscle cells: 6- to 8-nm actin filaments (called **thin filaments**; Fig. 2.54) and 15-nm filaments (called **thick filaments**) of myosin II, which is the predominant protein in muscle cells. **Myosin II** is a double-headed molecule with an elongated rod-like tail. The specific structural and functional relationships among actin, myosin, and other ABPs in muscle contraction are discussed in Chapter 11, Muscle Tissue, pages 349-352.

In addition to myosin II, nonmuscle cells contain **myosin I**, a protein with a single globular domain and short tail that attaches to other molecules or organelles. Extensive studies have revealed the presence of a variety of other nonmuscle myosin isoforms that are responsible for motor functions in many specialized cells, such as melanocytes, kidney and intestinal absorptive cells, nerve growth cones, and inner ear hair cells.

Actin filaments participate in a variety of cell functions.

Actin filaments are often grouped in bundles close to the plasma membrane. Functions of these membrane-associated actin filaments include the following.

- **Anchorage and movement of membrane proteins.** Actin filaments are distributed in three-dimensional networks throughout the cell and are used as anchors within specialized cell junctions such as focal adhesions.

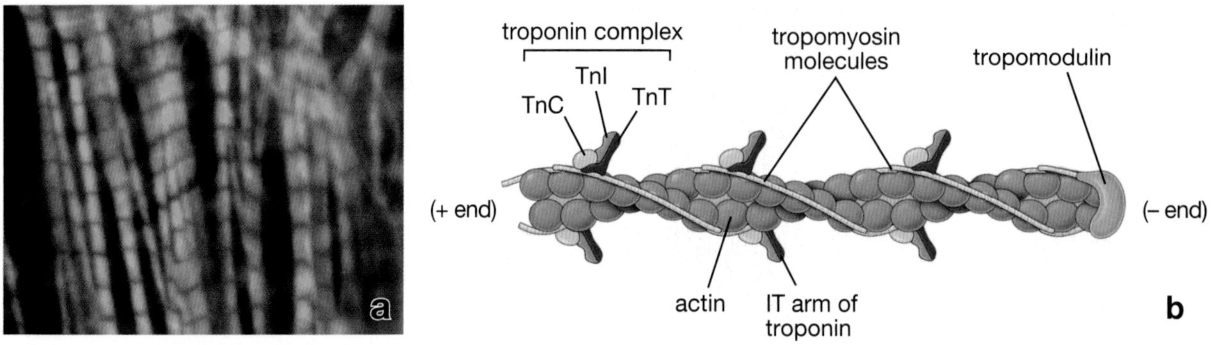

FIGURE 2.54. Thin filament organization and structure in cardiac cells. a. Immunofluorescence micrograph of a chick cardiac myocyte stained for actin (*green*) to show the thin filaments and for tropomodulin (*red*) to show the location of the slow-growing (−) ends of the thin filaments. Tropomodulin appears as regular striations because of the uniform lengths and alignment of the thin filaments in sarcomeres. ×320. **b.** Diagram of a thin filament. The polarity of the thin filament is indicated by the fast-growing (+) end and the slow-growing (−) end. Only a portion of the entire thin filament is shown for clarity. Tropomodulin is bound to actin and tropomyosin at the slow-growing (−) end. The troponin complex binds to each tropomyosin molecule every seven actin monomers along the length of the thin filament. (Courtesy of Drs. Velia F. Fowler and Ryan Littlefield.)

- **Formation of the structural core of microvilli** on absorptive epithelial cells. Actin filaments may also help maintain the shape of the apical cell surface (e.g., the apical **terminal web** of actin filaments serves as a set of tension cables beneath the cell surface).
- **Locomotion of cells**. Locomotion is achieved by the force exerted by actin filaments undergoing polymerization at their growing ends. This mechanism is used in many migrating cells, particularly in transformed cells of invasive tumors. As a result of actin polymerization at their **leading edge**, cells extend processes from their surface by pushing the plasma membrane ahead of the growing actin filaments. Although the leading edge is extending, the actin filaments in the **trailing edge** (tail) of the cell undergo depolymerization, causing its retraction. The leading edge extensions of a crawling cell are called **lamellipodia**; they contain elongating organized bundles of actin filaments with their plus ends directed toward the plasma membrane.
- **Extension of cell processes**. These processes can be observed in many other cells that exhibit small protrusions called **filopodia**, located around their surface. As in lamellipodia, these protrusions contain loose aggregations of 10–20 actin filaments organized in the same direction, again with their plus ends directed toward the plasma membrane. Actin filaments are also essential in cytoplasmic streaming (i.e., the stream-like movement of cytoplasm that can be observed in cultured cells).

In **listeriosis**, an infection caused by *Listeria monocytogenes*, the actin polymerization machinery of the cell is hijacked by the invading pathogen and utilized for its intracellular movement and dissemination throughout the tissue. Following internalization into the host phagosome (see Fig. 2.24), *L. monocytogenes* lyses the membrane of the phagosome and escapes into the cytoplasm. Within the cytoplasm, one end of the bacterium triggers polymerization of the host cell's actin filaments, which propels it through the cell like a space rocket, leaving a characteristic tail of polymerized actin behind. Actin polymerization allows bacteria to pass into a neighboring cell by forming protrusions in the host plasma membrane.

Intermediate Filaments

Intermediate filaments play a supporting or general structural role. These rope-like filaments are called *intermediate* because their diameter of 8–10 nm is between those of actin filaments and microtubules. Nearly all intermediate filaments consist of subunits with a molecular weight of about 50 kDa. Some evidence suggests that many of the stable structural proteins in intermediate filaments evolved from highly conserved enzymes, with only minor genetic modification.

Intermediate filaments are formed from nonpolar and highly variable intermediate filament subunits.

Unlike those of microfilaments and microtubules, the protein subunits of intermediate filaments show considerable diversity and tissue specificity. In addition, they do not possess enzymatic activity and form nonpolar filaments. Intermediate filaments also do not typically disappear and re-form in the continuous manner characteristic of most microtubules and actin filaments. For these reasons, intermediate filaments are believed to play a primarily structural role within the cell and to compose the cytoplasmic link of a tissue-wide continuum of cytoplasmic, nuclear, and extracellular filaments (Fig. 2.55).

Intermediate filament proteins are characterized by a conserved central **rod-shaped domain** with highly variable **globular domains** at either end (Fig. 2.56). Although the various classes of intermediate filaments slightly differ in the amino acid sequence of the rod-shaped domain and show some variation in molecular weight, they all share a homologous region that is important in filament self-assembly. Intermediate filaments are assembled from a pair of **helical monomers** that twist around each other to form **coiled-coil dimers**. Next, two coiled-coil dimers twist around each other in antiparallel fashion (parallel but pointing in opposite directions) to generate a **staggered tetramer** of two coiled-coil dimers, thus forming the nonpolarized unit of the intermediate filaments (see Fig. 2.56). Each tetramer, acting as an individual unit, is aligned along the axis of the filament. The ends of the tetramers are bound together to form the free ends of the filament. This assembly process provides a stable, staggered, helical array in which filaments are packed together and additionally stabilized by lateral binding interactions between adjacent tetramers.

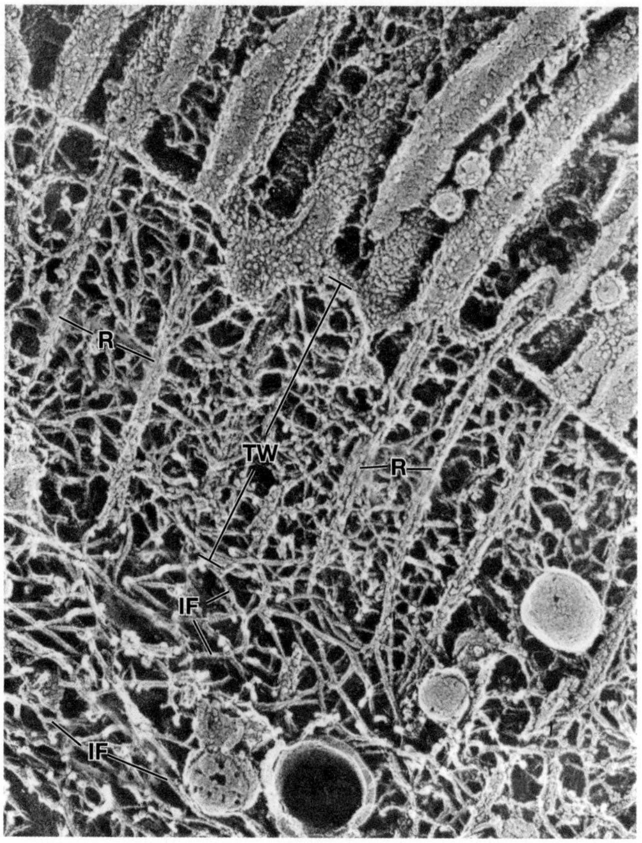

FIGURE 2.55. Electron micrograph of the apical part of an epithelial cell demonstrating intermediate filaments. This electron micrograph, obtained using the quick-freeze, deep-etch technique, shows the terminal web (*TW*) of an epithelial cell and underlying intermediate filaments (*IF*). The long, straight actin filament cores or rootlets (*R*) extending from the microvilli are cross-linked by a dense network of actin filaments containing numerous actin-binding proteins. The network of intermediate filaments can be seen beneath the TW anchoring the actin filaments of the microvilli. ×47,000. (Reprinted with permission from Hirokawa N, Keller TC 3rd, Chasan R, et al. Mechanism of brush border contractility studied by the quick-freeze, deep-etch method. *J Cell Biol.* 1983;96:1325–1336.)

Intermediate filaments are a heterogeneous group of cytoskeletal elements found in various cell types.

Intermediate filaments are organized into six major classes on the basis of gene structure, protein composition, and cellular distribution (Table 2.3).

- **Classes 1 and 2**. These are the most diverse groups of intermediate filaments and are called **keratins (cytokeratins)**. These classes contain more than 50 different isoforms and account for most of the intermediate filaments (about 54 genes of the total 70 human intermediate filament genes are linked to keratin molecules). Keratins only assemble as heteropolymers; an **acid cytokeratin** (class 1) and a **basic cytokeratin** (class 2) molecule form a heterodimer. Each keratin pair is characteristic of a particular type of epithelium; however, some epithelial cells may express more than one pair. Keratin filaments are found in different cells of epithelial origin and are divided into three expression groups: **keratins of simple epithelia**, **keratins of stratified epithelia**, and **structural keratins**, also called **hard keratins**. Hard keratins are found in skin appendages, such as hair and nails. Keratin filaments span the cytoplasm of epithelial cells and, via desmosomes, connect with keratin filaments in neighboring cells. Keratin subunits do not coassemble with other classes of intermediate filaments; therefore, they form a distinct cell-specific and tissue-specific recognition system.

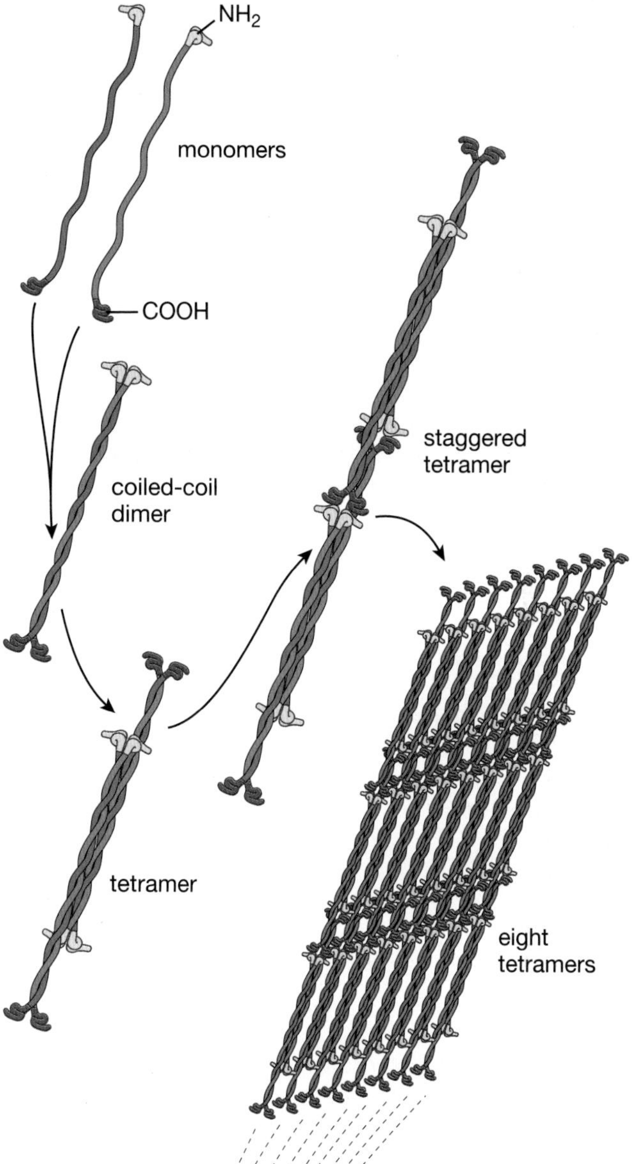

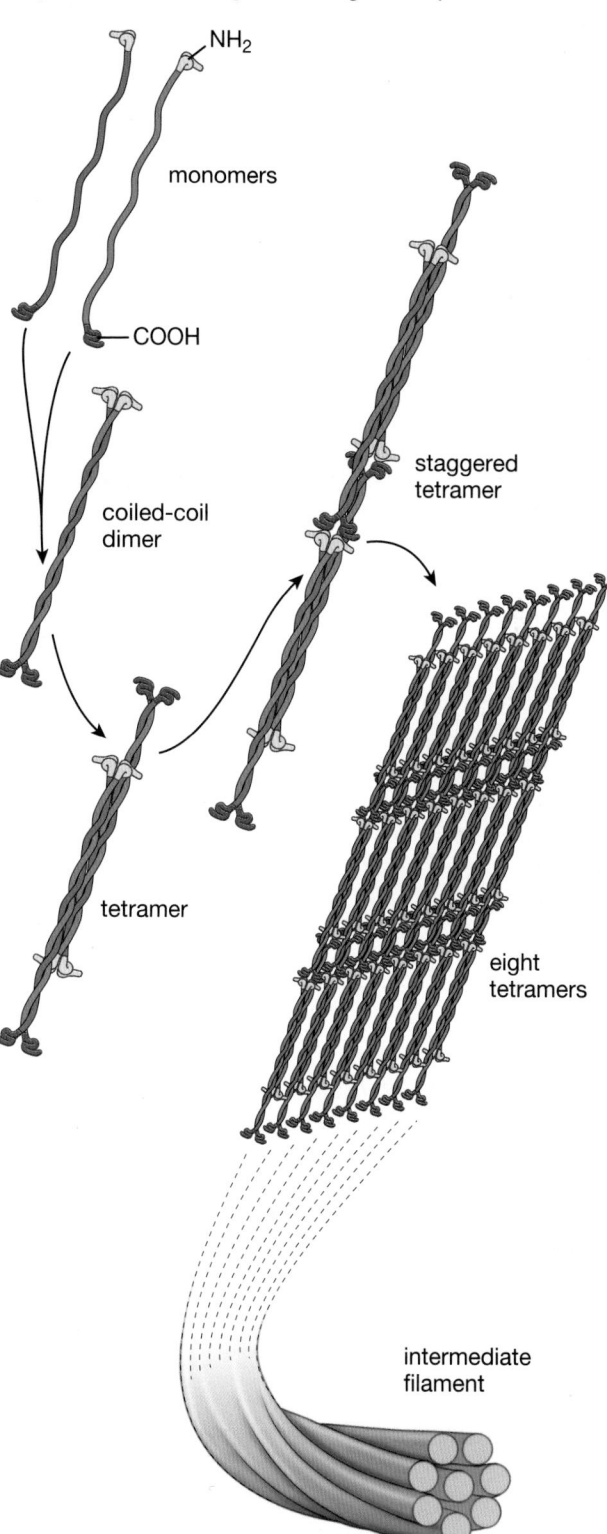

FIGURE 2.56. Polymerization and structure of intermediate filaments. Intermediate filaments are self-assembled from a pair of monomers that twist around each other in parallel fashion to form a stable dimer. Two coiled-coil dimers then twist around each other in antiparallel fashion to generate a staggered tetramer of two coiled-coil dimers. This tetramer forms the nonpolarized unit of the intermediate filaments. Each tetramer, acting as an individual unit, aligns along the axis of the filament and binds to the free end of the elongating structure. This staggered helical array is additionally stabilized by lateral binding interactions between adjacent tetramers.

TABLE 2.3 Classes of Intermediate Filaments, Their Location, and Associated Diseases

Type of Protein	Molecular Weight (kDa)	Where Found	Examples of Associated Diseases
Class 1 and 2: Keratins			
Acid cytokeratins	40–64	All epithelial cells	Epidermolysis bullosa simplex
Basic cytokeratins	52–68	All epithelial cells	Keratoderma disorders caused by keratin mutations Meesmann corneal dystrophy
Class 3: Vimentin and Vimentin-Like			
Vimentin	55	Cells of mesenchymal origin (including endothelial cells, myofibroblasts, some smooth muscle cells) and some cells of neuroectodermal origin	Desmin-related myopathy (DRM) Dilated cardiomyopathy Alexander disease Amyotrophic lateral sclerosis (ALS)
Desmin	53	Muscle cells; coassembles with nestin, synemin, and paranemin	
Glial fibrillary acidic protein (GFAP)	50–52	Neuroglial cells (mainly astrocytes; to lesser degree, ependymal cells), Schwann cells, enteric glial cells, satellite cells of sensory ganglia, and pituicytes	
Peripherin	54	Peripheral neurons	
Class 4: Neurofilaments			
Neurofilament L (NF-L)	68	Neurons Coassembles with NF-M or NF-H	Charcot–Marie–Tooth disease Parkinson disease
Neurofilament M (NF-M)	110	Neurons Coassembles with NF-L	
Neurofilament H (NF-H)	130	Neurons Coassembles with NF-L	
Nestin	240	Neural stem cells, some cells of neuroectodermal origin, muscle cells Coassembles with desmin	
α-Internexin	68	Neurons	
Synemin α/β[a]	182	Muscle cells Coassembles with desmin	
Syncoilin	64	Muscle cells	
Paranemin	178	Muscle cells Coassembles with desmin	
Class 5: Lamins			
Lamin A/C[b]	62–72	Nucleus of all nucleated cells	Emery–Dreifuss muscular dystrophy
Lamin B	65–68	Nucleus of all nucleated cells	Limb girdle muscular dystrophy
Class 6: Beaded Filaments			
Phakinin (CP49)[c]	49	Eye lens fiber cells Coassembles with filensin	Juvenile-onset cataracts Congenital cataracts
Filensin (CP115)	115	Eye lens fiber cells Coassembles with phakinin	

[a]Synemin α and synemin β represent two alternative transcripts of the DMN gene.

[b]Lamin C is a splice product of lamin A.

[c]The molecular weight of filensin/phakinin heterodimer is 131 kDa.

- **Class 3**. This group contains four proteins: **vimentin**, the most widely distributed intermediate filament protein in the body, and vimentin-like proteins such as **desmin**, **glial fibrillary acidic protein (GFAP)**, and **peripherin**. They represent a diverse family of cytoplasmic filaments found in many cell types. In contrast to keratins, class 3 proteins (with the exception of desmin) preferentially form homopolymeric filaments containing only one type of intermediate protein. Vimentin is the most abundant intermediate filament found in all mesoderm-derived cells, including fibroblasts (Fig. 2.57); desmin is characteristic of muscle cells; GFAP is found in glial cells (highly specific for astrocytes), and peripherin is found in many peripheral nerve cells.
- **Class 4**. Historically, this group has been called **neurofilaments**; they contain intermediate filament proteins that are expressed mostly in the axons of nerve cells. The three types of neurofilament proteins are of different molecular weights: **NF-L** (a low-weight protein), **NF-M** (a medium-weight protein), and **NF-H**

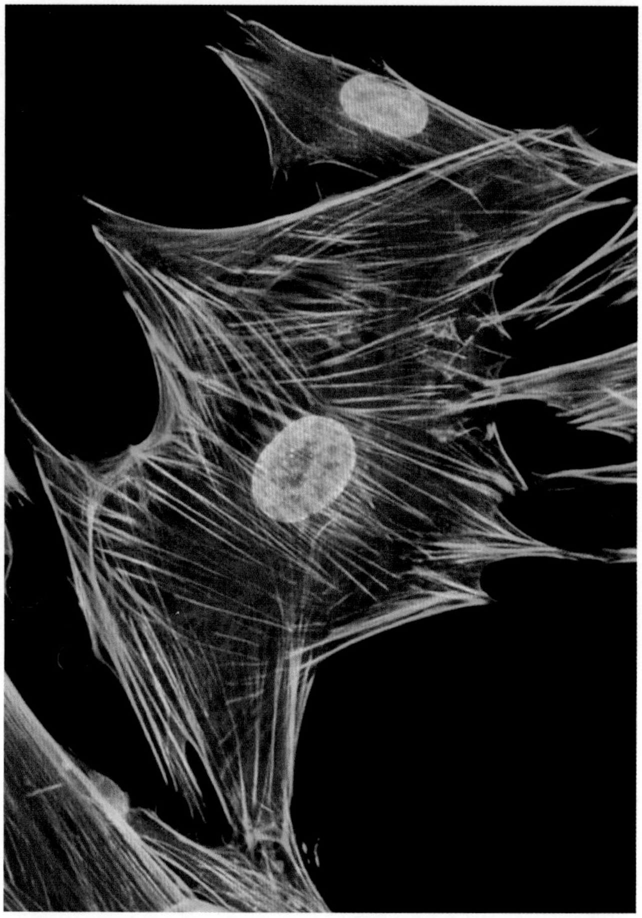

FIGURE 2.57. Distribution of intermediate filaments in human fetal lung fibroblasts. Distribution of vimentin (*red*) and actin filaments (*green*) is shown in cultured fibroblasts from human fetal lung. Vimentin is an intermediate filament protein expressed in all cells of mesenchymal origin. In cultured fibroblasts, vimentin filaments are visible centrally within the cell cytoplasm, whereas the actin filaments are aggregated primary near the cell surface. This immunofluorescent image was obtained using indirect immunofluorescence techniques in which vimentin filaments were treated with mouse antivimentin primary antibodies followed by goat antimouse secondary antibodies conjugated with Texas red fluorescent dye. Actin filaments were counterstained with phalloidin conjugated with a green fluorescent dye. Nuclei were stained blue with Hoechst fluorescent stain. ×3,500. (Reprinted with permission from Michael W. Davidson, Florida State University.)

(a high-weight protein). They coassemble to form a heterodimer that contains one NF-L molecule along with one of the other two proteins. All three proteins form neurofilaments that extend from the cell body into the ends of axons and dendrites, providing structural support. However, genes for class 4 proteins also encode several other intermediate filament proteins. These include **nestin** and **α-internexin** in nerve cells as well as **synemin**, **syncoilin**, and **paranemin** in muscle cells. Members of this group preferentially coassemble in tissues as heteropolymers.

- **Class 5. Lamins**, specifically nuclear lamins, form a network-like structure that is associated with the nuclear envelope. Lamins are represented by two types of proteins, **lamin A** and **lamin B**. In contrast to other types of intermediate filaments found in the cytoplasm, lamins are located within the nucleoplasm of almost all differentiated cells in the body. A description of their structure and function can be found on page 94.
- **Class 6.** This is a lens-specific group of intermediate filament, or "**beaded filaments**," containing two proteins, **phakinin** and **filensin**. The periodic bead-like surface appearance of these filaments is attributed to the globular structure of the carboxy-terminus of the filensin molecule, which projects out from the assembled filament core.

Intermediate filament–associated proteins are essential for the integrity of cell-to-cell and cell-to-extracellular matrix junctions.

A variety of **intermediate filament–associated proteins** function within the cytoskeleton as integral parts of the molecular architecture of cells. Some proteins, such as those of the **plectin family**, possess binding sites for actin filaments, microtubules, and intermediate filaments and are thus important in the proper assembly of the cytoskeleton. **Lamins**, the intermediate filaments in the nucleus, are associated with numerous proteins in the inner nuclear membrane, including **emerin**, **lamin B receptor (LBR)**, **nurim**, and several **lamina-associated polypeptides**. Some of these proteins have multiple binding sites to intermediate filaments, actin, chromatin, and signaling proteins; thus, they function in chromatin organization, gene expression, nuclear architecture, and cell signaling and provide an essential link between the nucleoskeleton and cytoskeleton of the cell. Another important family of intermediate filament–associated proteins consists of **desmoplakins**, **desmoplakin-like proteins**, and **plakoglobins**. These proteins form the attachment plaques for intermediate filaments, an essential part of **desmosomes** and **hemidesmosomes**. The interaction of intermediate filaments with cell-to-cell and cell-to-extracellular matrix junctions provides mechanical strength and resistance to extracellular forces. Table 2.4 summarizes the characteristics of the three types of cytoskeletal filaments.

Centrioles and Microtubule-Organizing Centers

Centrioles represent the focal point around which the MTOC assembles.

Centrioles, visible in the light microscope, are paired, short, rod-like cytoplasmic cylinders built from **nine microtubule triplets**. In resting cells, centrioles have an **orthogonal orientation**: One centriole in the pair is arrayed at a right angle to the other. **Centrioles** are usually found close to the nucleus, often partially surrounded by the Golgi apparatus, and associated with a zone of amorphous, dense **pericentriolar material**. The region of the cell containing the centrioles and pericentriolar material is called the **microtubule-organizing center** or **centrosome** (Fig. 2.58). The MTOC is the region where most microtubules are formed and from which they are then directed to specific destinations within the cell. The MTOC controls the number, polarity, direction, orientation, and organization of microtubules formed during the interphase of the cell cycle. During mitosis, duplicated MTOCs serve as mitotic spindle poles. Development of the MTOC itself depends solely on the presence of centrioles. When

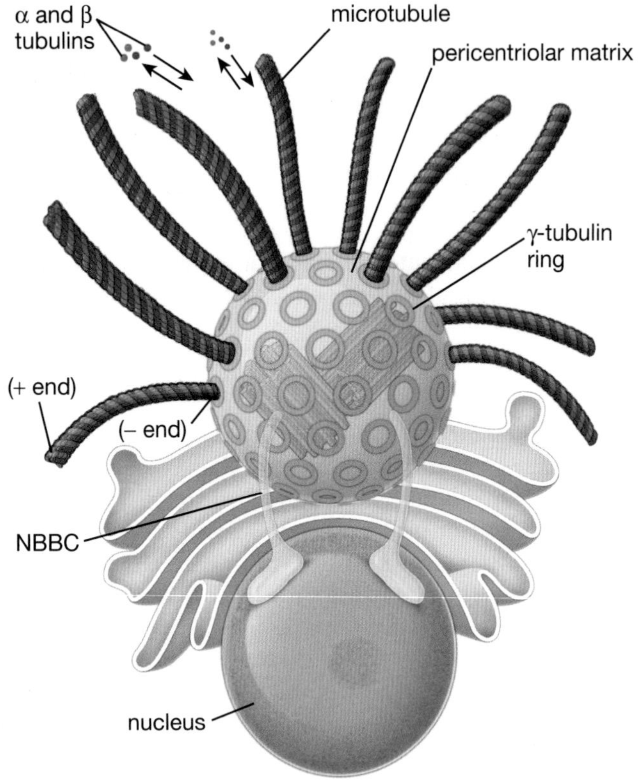

FIGURE 2.58. Structure of the microtubule-organizing center (MTOC). This diagram shows the location of the MTOC in relation to the nucleus and the Golgi apparatus. In some species, the MTOC is tethered to the nuclear envelope by a contractile protein, the nucleus–basal body connector (*NBBC*). The MTOC contains the centrioles and an amorphous protein matrix with an abundance of γ-tubulin rings. Each γ-tubulin ring serves as the nucleation site for the growth of a single microtubule. Note that the minus (−) end of the microtubule remains attached to the MTOC, and the plus (+) end represents the growing end directed toward the plasma membrane.

centrioles are missing, the MTOCs disappear, and formation of microtubules is severely impaired.

The pericentriolar matrix of MTOC contains numerous ring-shaped structures that initiate microtubule formation.

The MTOC contains centrioles and an amorphous pericentriolar matrix of more than 200 proteins, including γ-tubulin that is organized in ring-shaped structures. Each **γ-tubulin ring** serves as the starting point (nucleation site) for the growth of one microtubule that is assembled from tubulin dimers; α- and β-tubulin dimers are added with specific orientation to the γ-tubulin ring. The minus end of the microtubule remains attached to the MTOC, and the plus end represents the growing end directed toward the plasma membrane (see Fig. 2.58).

Centrioles provide basal bodies for cilia and flagella and align the mitotic spindle during cell division.

Although centrioles were discovered more than a century ago, their precise functions, replication, and assembly are still under intense investigation. The known functions of centrioles can be organized into two categories:

- **Basal body formation**. One of the important functions of the centriole is to provide basal bodies, which are necessary for the assembly of cilia and flagella (Fig. 2.59). Basal bodies are formed either de novo without contact with the preexisting centrioles (the **acentriolar pathway**) or by duplication of existing centrioles (the **centriolar pathway**). About 95% of the centrioles are generated through the acentriolar pathway. Both pathways give rise to multiple immediate precursors of centrioles, known as **procentrioles**, which mature as they migrate to the appropriate site near the apical cell membrane, where they become **basal bodies** (Fig. 2.60). The basal body acts as the organizing center for a cilium. Microtubules grow upward from the basal body, pushing the cell membrane outward, and elongate to form the mature cilium. The process of centriole duplication is described on pages 76-79.
- **Mitotic spindle formation**. During mitosis, the position of centrioles determines the location of mitotic spindle poles. Centrioles are also necessary for the formation of a fully functional MTOC, which nucleates mitotic spindle–associated microtubules. For instance, **astral microtubules** are formed around each individual

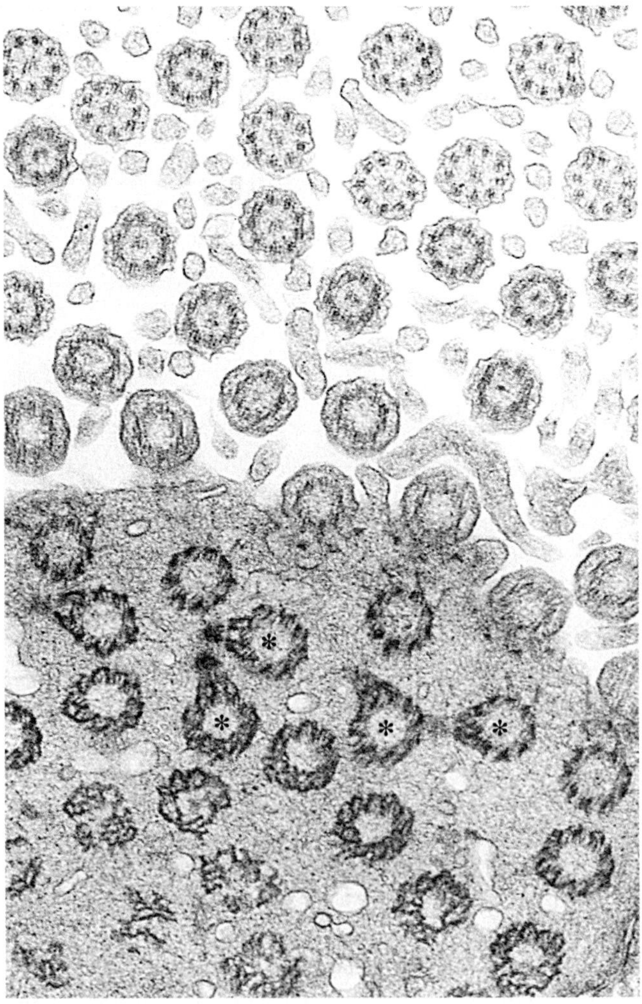

FIGURE 2.59. Basal bodies and cilia. This electron micrograph shows the basal bodies and cilia in cross-sectional profile as seen in an oblique section through the apical part of a ciliated cell in the respiratory tract. Note the 9 + 2 microtubule arrangement of the cilia in which nine microtubules at the periphery of the cilia surround two central microtubules. The basal bodies lack the central tubule pair. On several cross sections, the basal foot is visible as it projects laterally from the basal body (*asterisks*). ×28,000. (Courtesy of Patrice C. Abell-Aleff.)

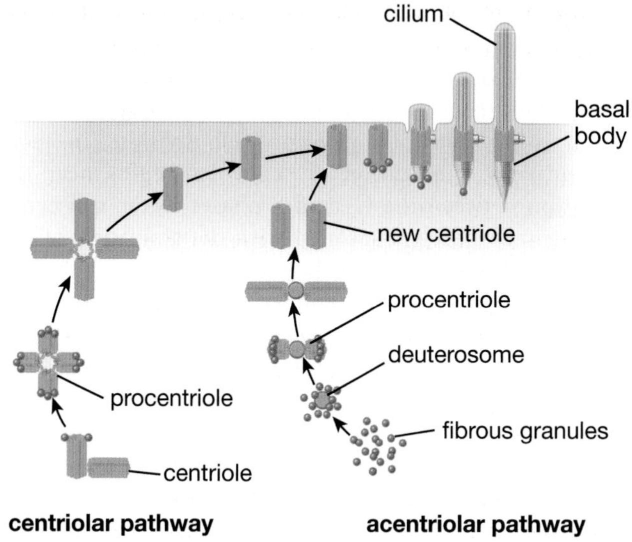

FIGURE 2.60. Two pathways of basal body formation. In the centriolar pathway, a pair of existing centriole serves as an organizing center for the duplication of new centrioles. Utilizing this pathway, ciliated cells have the ability to assemble large number of centrioles in the vicinity of an old mature centriole. In the acentriolar pathway, which plays a major role in the formation of basal bodies in ciliated cells, new centrioles are formed de novo from fibrous granules located in close proximity to nonmicrotubular structures called deuterosomes. Both pathways give rise to procentrioles, which mature as they migrate to the appropriate site near the apical cell membrane, where they become basal bodies. Fibrous granules contribute to the formation of the striated rootlet. (Based on Hagiwara H, Ohwada N, Takata K. Cell biology of normal and abnormal ciliogenesis in the ciliated epithelium. *Int Rev Cytol.* 2004;234:101–139.)

centriole in a star-like fashion. They are crucial in establishing the axis of the developing mitotic spindle. In some animal cells, the mitotic spindle itself (mainly kinetochore microtubules) is formed by MTOC-independent mechanisms and consists of microtubules that originate from the chromosomes. Data from experimental studies indicate that in the absence of centrioles, astral microtubules fail to develop, causing errors in mitotic spindle orientation (Fig. 2.61). Thus, the primary role of centrioles in mitosis is to position the mitotic spindle properly by recruiting the MTOC from which astral microtubules can grow and establish the axis for the developing spindle.

The dominant feature of centrioles is the cylindrical array of triplet microtubules with associated proteins.

The TEM reveals that each rod-shaped centriole is about 0.2 μm long and consists of **nine triplets of microtubules** that are oriented parallel to the long axis of the organelle and run in slightly twisted bundles (Fig. 2.62). The three microtubules of the triplet are fused, with adjacent microtubules sharing a common wall. The innermost or **A microtubule** is a complete ring of 13 protofilaments containing α- and β-tubulin dimers; the middle and outer **B and C microtubules**, respectively, appear C-shaped because they share tubulin dimers with each other and with the A microtubule. The microtubules of the triplets are not equal in length. The C microtubule of the triplet is usually shorter than A and B.

The microtubule triplets of the centriole surround an internal lumen. The distal part of the lumen (away from the nucleus) contains a 20-kDa Ca^{2+}-binding protein, **centrin** (Fig. 2.63). The proximal part of the lumen (close to the nucleus) is lined by **γ-tubulin**, which provides the template for the arrangement of the triplet microtubules. In addition, a family of newly discovered **δ-**, **ε-**, **ζ-**, and **η-tubulin** molecules as well as **pericentrin** protein complexes have been localized with the centrioles. Other proteins, such as **protein p210**, form a ring of molecules that appears to link the distal end of the centriole to the plasma membrane. Filamentous connections between the centriole pair have been identified in human lymphocytes. In other organisms, two protein bridges, the **proximal** and **distal connecting fibers**, connect each centriole in a pair (see Fig. 2.63).

In dividing cells, these connections participate in segregating the centrioles to each daughter cell. In some organisms, the proximal end of each centriole is attached to the nuclear envelope by contractile proteins called **nucleus–basal body connectors (NBBCs)**. Their function is to link the centriole to the mitotic spindle poles during mitosis. In human cells, the centrosome–nucleus connection appears to be maintained by filamentous

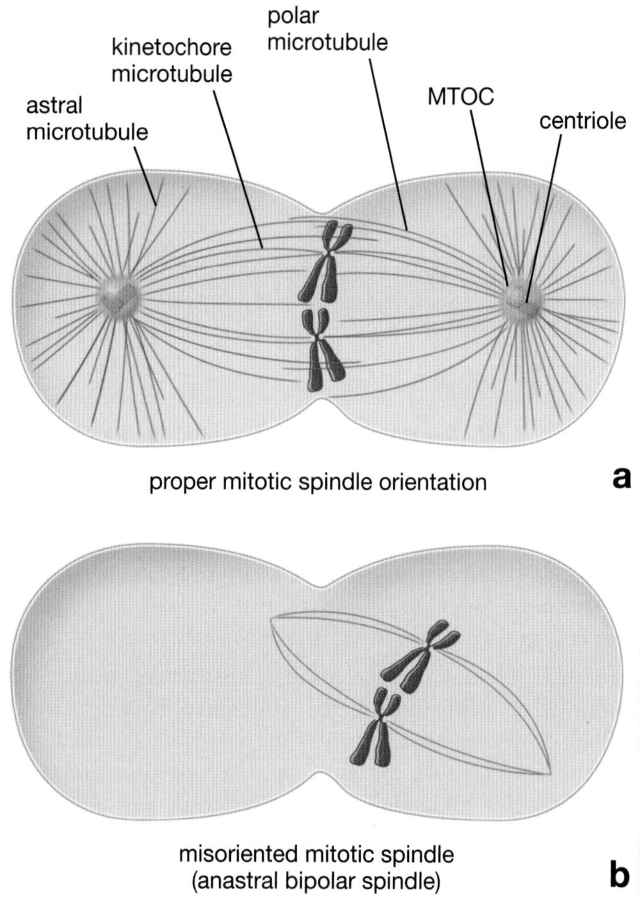

FIGURE 2.61. Mitotic spindle during normal cell division and in cells lacking centrioles. a. This schematic drawing shows the orientation of the mitotic spindle in a normal cell undergoing mitosis. Note the positions of the centrioles and the distribution of the spindle microtubules. *MTOC*, microtubule-organizing center. **b.** In a cell that lacks centrioles, mitosis occurs and a mitotic spindle containing only kinetochore microtubules is formed. However, both poles of the mitotic spindle lack astral microtubules, which position the spindle in the proper plane during mitosis. Such a misoriented spindle is referred to as an *anastral bipolar spindle*. (Based on Marshall WF, Rosenbaum JL. How centrioles work: lessons from green yeast. *Curr Opin Cell Biol.* 2000;12:119–125.)

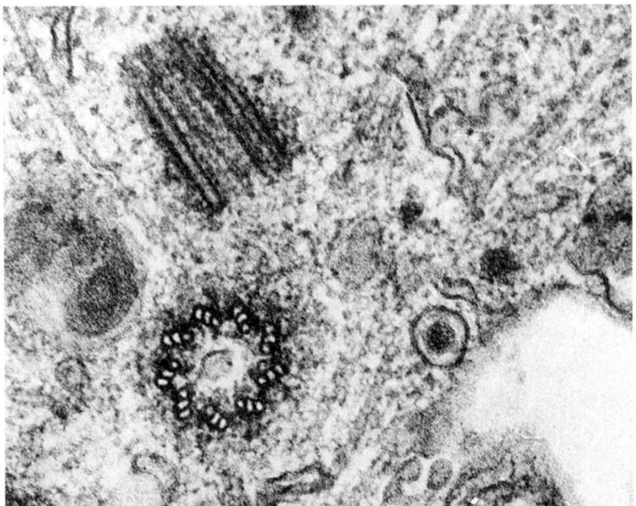

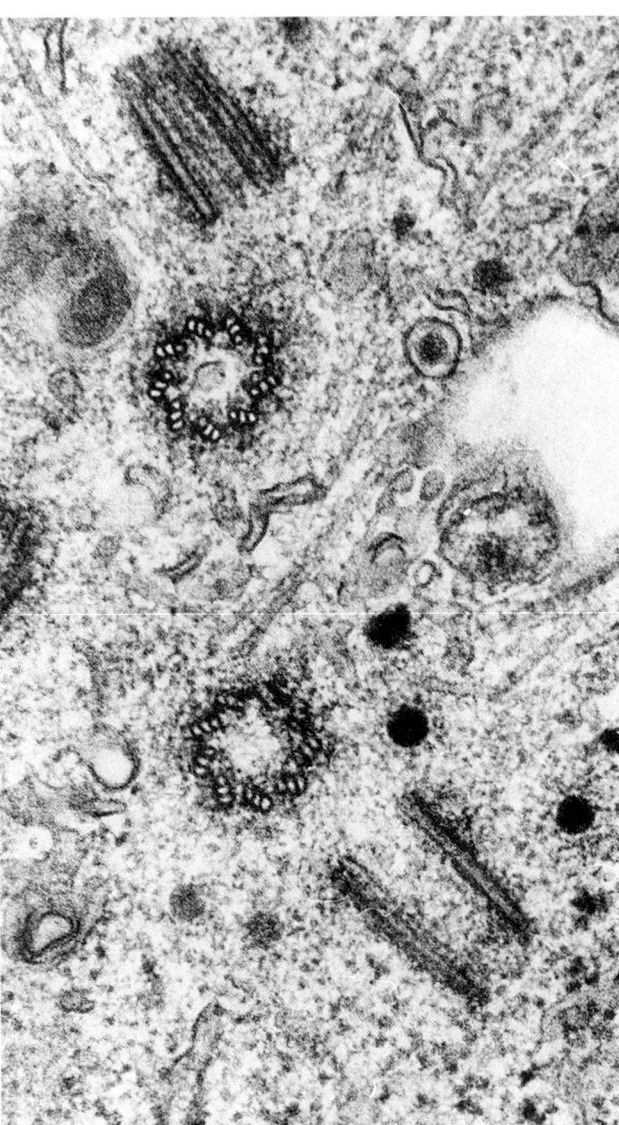

FIGURE 2.62. Electron micrograph showing parent and daughter centrioles in a fibroblast. Note that the transverse-sectioned centriole in each of the pairs reveals the triplet configuration of microtubules. The *lower right* centriole represents a mid-longitudinal section, whereas the *upper left* centriole has also been longitudinally sectioned but along the plane of its wall. ×90,000. (Courtesy of Drs. Manley McGill, D. P. Highfield, T. M. Monahan, and Bill R. Brinkley.)

structures of the cytoskeleton. A distinctive feature of mammalian centrioles is the difference between individual centrioles in the pair. One centriole (termed the **mature centriole**) contains stalk-like satellite processes and sheet-like appendages whose function is not known (see Fig. 2.63). The other centriole (termed the **immature centriole**) does not possess satellites or appendages.

Centrosome duplication is synchronized with cell cycle events and linked to the process of ciliogenesis.

Centrosome dynamics, such as duplication or formation of basal bodies for ciliogenesis, are synchronized with cell cycle progression. Cilia are assembled during the G_1 phase; they are most abundant in G_0 and are disassembled before the cell enters the M phase. These events are depicted in Figure 2.64, which shows the relationships between centrosome duplication, primary cilium formation, and progression through the cell cycle.

Because each daughter cell receives only one pair of centrioles after cell division, the daughter cells must duplicate existing centrioles prior to cell division. In most somatic cells, duplication of centrioles begins near the transition between the G_1 and S phases of the cell cycle. This event is closely associated with the activation of the **cyclin E–Cdk2 complex** during the S phase of the cell cycle (see Fig. 3.11). This complex directly phosphorylates the nucleus-chaperoning protein **nucleophosmin/B23**, which is responsible for initiating the duplication of centrioles.

In most cells, duplication begins with the splitting of a centriole pair, followed by the appearance of a small mass of fibrillar and granular material at the proximal lateral end of each original centriole. Because the existing pair of centrioles serves as a core for new organelle formation, this process of centriole duplication is referred as the **centriolar pathway** (see Fig. 2.60).

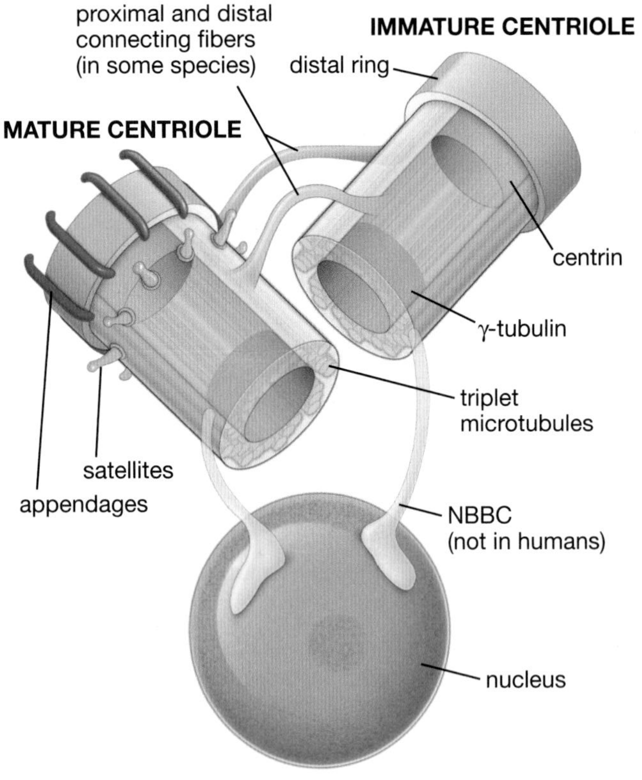

FIGURE 2.63. Schematic structure of centrioles. In nondividing cells, centrioles are arranged in pairs in which one centriole is aligned at a right angle to the other. One centriole is also more mature (generated at least two cell cycles earlier) than the other centriole, which was generated in the previous cell cycle. The mature centriole is characterized by the presence of satellites and appendages. Centrioles are located in close proximity to the nucleus. The basic components of each centriole are microtubule triplets that form the cylindrical structure surrounding an internal lumen. The proximal part of the lumen is lined by γ-tubulin, which provides the template for nucleation and arrangement of the microtubule triplets. The distal part of each lumen contains the protein centrin. In some species, two protein bridges, the proximal and distal connecting fibers, connect each centriole in a pair. In some species, but not in humans, the proximal end of each centriole is attached to the nuclear envelope by a contractile protein known as the nucleus–basal body connector (*NBBC*).

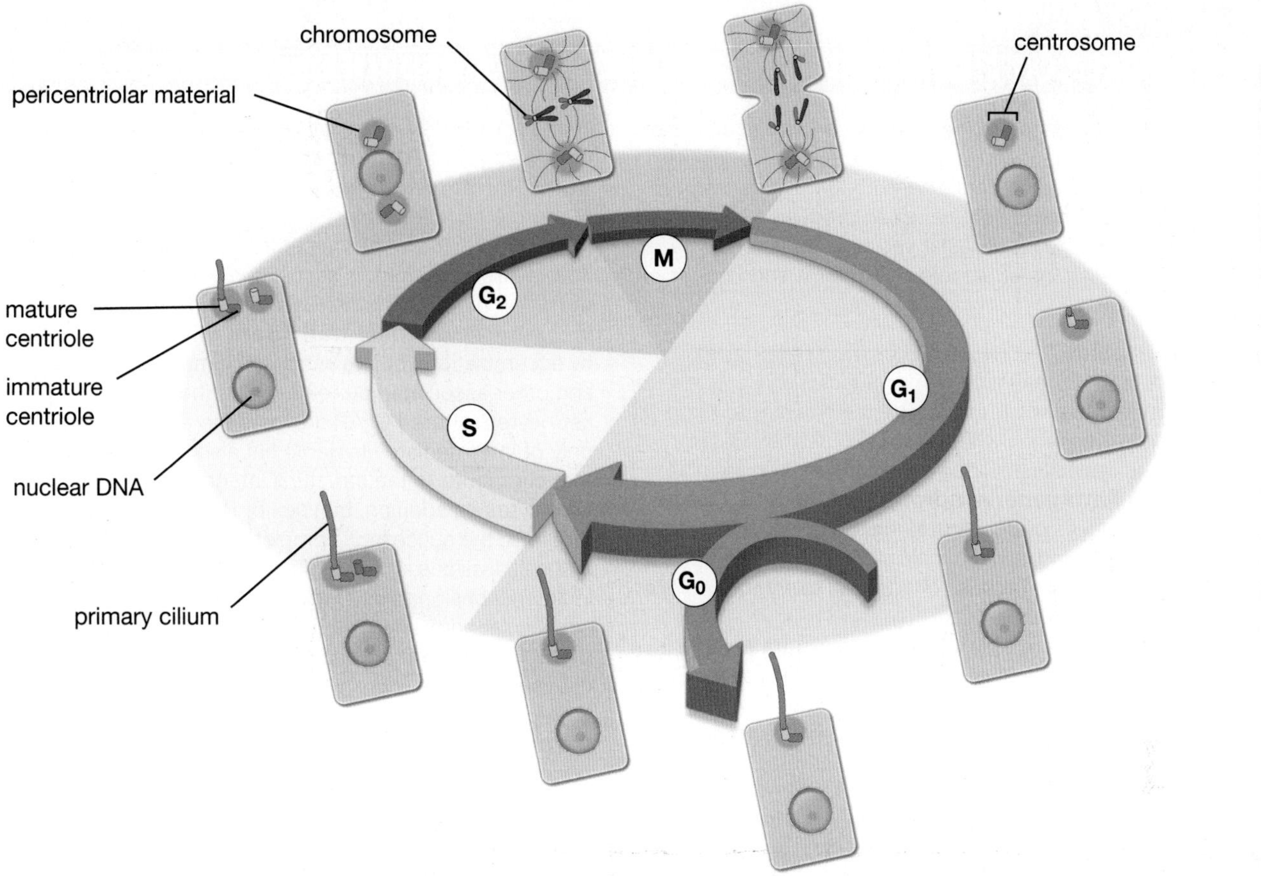

FIGURE 2.64. Association of the centrosome duplication and primary cilium formation with the cell cycle. After a cell emerges from mitosis, it possesses a single centrosome (microtubule-organizing center [MTOC]) surrounded by amorphous pericentriolar material. The primary cilium formation first occurs during the G_1 phase in which the centrosome migrates toward the cell membrane and initiates the process of ciliogenesis. Necessary structural and transport proteins are acquired and activated to build the primary cilium axoneme (9 + 0) directly on top of the mature centriole. During the end of the G_1 phase, as well as in G_0, the primary cilium functions as an external receiver antenna sensing and interpreting signals from the extracellular environment. Duplication of centrioles begins near the transition between the G_1 and S phases of the cell cycle, and the two centrioles are visible in S phase. During the late G_2 phase, centrioles reach their full maturity, whereas the primary cilium is disassembled. This allows centrioles to migrate away from the cell membrane and participate in mitotic spindle formation. Once cell division is complete, the centrioles can proceed to ciliary reassembly in the G_1 phase. (Based on Santos N, Reiter JF. Building it up and taking it down: the regulation of vertebrate ciliogenesis. *Dev Dyn.* 2008;237:1972–1981.)

In this pathway, the **fibrous granules** coalesce into dense spherical structures called **deuterosomes**, and they give rise to the **procentriole** (or bud), which gradually enlarges to form a right angle appendage to the parent (see Fig. 2.60). Microtubules begin to develop in the mass of fibrous granules as it grows (usually during the S to late G_2 phases of the cell cycle), appearing first as a ring of nine single tubules, then as doublets, and finally as triplets. As procentrioles mature during the S and G_2 phases of the cell cycle, each parent–daughter pair migrates around the nucleus. Before the onset of mitosis, centrioles with surrounding amorphous pericentriolar material position themselves on opposite sides of the nucleus and produce astral microtubules. In doing so, they define the poles between which the bipolar mitotic spindle develops.

The important difference between duplication of centrioles during mitosis and during ciliogenesis is the fact that during mitosis, only one daughter centriole buds from the lateral side of parent organelle, whereas during ciliogenesis, as many as 10 centrioles may develop around the parent centriole.

Basal Bodies

Development of cilia on the cell surface requires the presence of basal bodies, structures derived from centrioles.

Each cilium requires a **basal body**. The generation of centrioles, which occurs during the process of **ciliogenesis**, is responsible for the production of basal bodies. The newly formed centrioles migrate to the apical surface of the cell and serve as organizing centers for the assembly of the microtubules of the cilium. The core structure (axoneme) of a motile cilium is composed of a complex set of microtubules consisting of two central microtubules surrounded by nine microtubule doublets (9 + 2 configuration). The organizing role of the basal body differs from that of the MTOC. The axonemal microtubule doublets are continuous with the A and B microtubules of the basal body from which they develop by addition of α- and β-tubulin dimers at the growing plus end. A detailed description of the structure of cilia, basal bodies, and the process of ciliogenesis can be found in Chapter 5, Epithelial Tissue, pages 137-139.

FOLDER 2.2

CLINICAL CORRELATION: ABNORMALITIES IN MICROTUBULES AND FILAMENTS

Abnormalities related to the organization and structure of microtubules, actin, and intermediate filaments underlie many pathologic disorders. These abnormalities lead to defects in the cytoskeleton and can produce a variety of defects related to intracellular vesicular transport, intracellular accumulations of pathologic proteins, and impairment of cell mobility.

Microtubules

Defects in the organization of microtubules and microtubule-associated proteins can immobilize the cilia of respiratory epithelium, interfering with the ability of the respiratory system to clear accumulated secretions. This condition, known as **Kartagener syndrome** (see Folder 5.2, page 139), also causes dysfunction of microtubules, which affects sperm motility and leads to male sterility. It may also cause infertility in women because of impaired ciliary transport of the ovum through the oviduct.

Microtubules are essential for vesicular transport (endocytosis and exocytosis) as well as cell motility. Certain drugs, such as **colchicine**, bind to tubulin molecules and prevent their polymerization. Used in the treatment of acute attacks of gout, this prevents neutrophil migration and decreases their ability to respond to urate crystal deposits in the tissues. **Vinblastine** and **vincristine (Oncovin)** represent another family of drugs that bind to microtubules and inhibit the formation of the mitotic spindle essential for cell division. These drugs are used as antimitotic and antiproliferative agents in cancer therapy. Another drug, **paclitaxel (Taxol)**, is used in chemotherapy for breast cancer. It stabilizes microtubules, preventing them from depolymerizing (an action opposite to that of colchicine), and thus arrests cancer cells in various stages of cell division.

Actin Filaments

Actin filaments play essential roles in various stages of leukocyte migration as well as the phagocytic functions of various cells. Some chemical substances isolated from fungi, such as **cytochalasin B** and **cytochalasin D**, prevent actin polymerization by binding to the plus end of the actin filament, inhibiting lymphocyte migration, phagocytosis, and cell division (cytokinesis). Several toxins of poisonous mushrooms, such as **phalloidin**, also bind to actin filaments, stabilizing them and preventing their depolymerization. Conjugated with fluorescein dyes, derivatives of the phallotoxin family (i.e., NDB-phallacidin) are frequently used in the laboratory to stain actin filaments (see Figs. 2.47 and 2.51). Prolonged exposure of the cell to these substances can disrupt the dynamic equilibrium between F-actin and G-actin, causing cell death.

Intermediate Filaments

As noted, the molecular structure of intermediate filaments is tissue specific and consists of many different types of proteins. Several diseases are caused by defects in the proper assembly of intermediate filaments. These defects have also been induced experimentally by mutations in intermediate filament genes in laboratory animals. Changes in neurofilaments within brain tissue are characteristic of **Alzheimer disease**, which produces **neurofibrillary tangles** containing neurofilaments and other microtubule-associated proteins.

Another disorder of the central nervous system, **Alexander disease**, is associated with mutations of the GFAP gene. The pathologic feature of this disease is the presence of **Rosenthal fibers**, which are formed by accumulations of intermediate filament protein GFAP and other associated proteins within the cytoplasm of astrocytes. Altered GFAP prevents the assembly not only of intermediate filaments but also of other proteins that contribute to the structural integrity and function of astrocytes. In addition, bundles of Rosenthal fibers interfere with the successful completion of astrocyte mitosis and cell divisions. Infants with Alexander disease develop leukoencephalopathy (infection of the brain) with macrocephaly (abnormally large head), seizures, and psychomotor impairment, leading to death usually within the first decade of life.

A prominent feature of **alcoholic liver cirrhosis** is the presence of eosinophilic intracytoplasmic inclusions composed predominantly of keratin intermediate filaments. These inclusions, called **Mallory bodies**, are visible in light microscopy within the hepatocyte cytoplasm (Fig. F2.2.1).

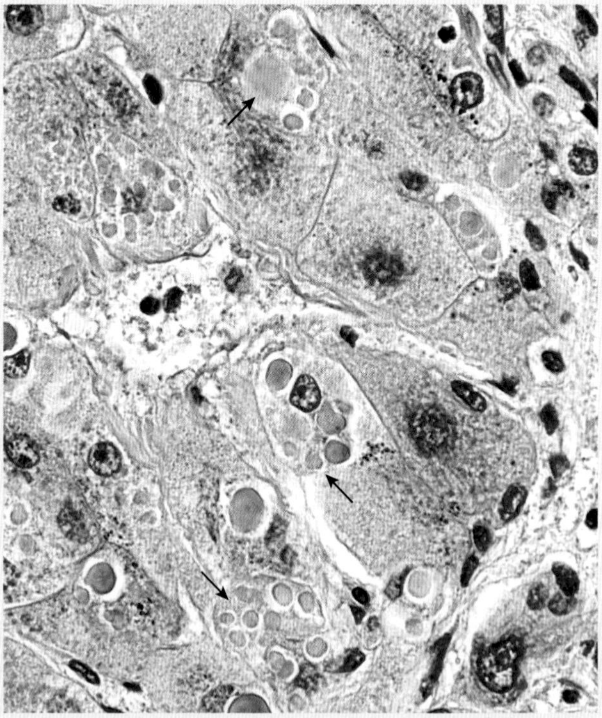

FIGURE F2.2.1. Photomicrograph of Mallory bodies. Accumulation of keratin intermediate filaments forming intracellular inclusions is frequently associated with specific cell injuries. In alcoholic liver cirrhosis, hepatocytes exhibit such inclusions (*arrows*), which are known as Mallory bodies. Lymphocytes and macrophages responsible for an intense inflammatory reaction surround cells containing Mallory bodies. ×900.

TABLE 2.4 Summary Characteristics of Three Types of Cytoskeletal Elements

	Actin Filaments (Microfilaments)	Intermediate Filaments	Microtubules
Shape	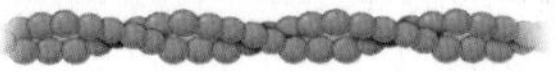 Double-stranded linear helical array	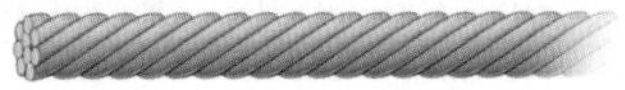 Rope-like fibers	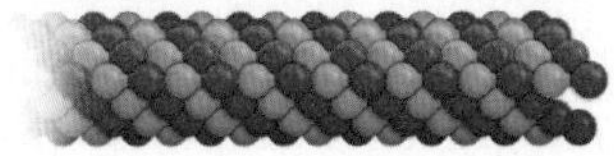 Nonbranching long, hollow cylinders
Diameter (nm)	6–8	8–10	20–25
Basic protein subunit	Monomer of G-actin (MW 42 kDa)	Various intermediate filament proteins (MW ~50 kDa)	Dimers of α- and β-tubulin (MW 54 kDa); γ-tubulin found in MTOC is necessary for nucleation of microtubules; δ-, ε-, ζ-, η-tubulins are associated with MTOC and basal bodies.
Enzymatic activity	ATP hydrolytic activity	None	GTP hydrolytic activity
Polarity	Yes; minus (−) or pointed end is slow-growing end. Plus (+) or barbed end is faster growing end.	Nonpolar structures	Yes; minus (−) end is nongrowing end embedded in MTOC. Plus (+) end is the growing end.
Assembly process	Monomers of G-actin are added to growing filament. Polymerization requires presence of K^+, Mg^{2+}, and ATP, which is hydrolyzed to ADP after each G-actin molecule is incorporated into the filament.	Two pairs of monomers form two coiled-coil dimers, and then two coiled-coil dimers twist around each other to generate a staggered tetramer, which aligns along the axis of the filament and binds to the free end of the elongating structure.	At the nucleation site, α- and β-tubulin dimers are added to γ-tubulin ring. Each tubulin dimer binds to GTP before it becomes incorporated into the microtubule in the presence of Mg^{2+}. After polymerization, GTP is hydrolyzed to GDP.
Source of energy required for assembly	ATP	N/A	GTP
Characteristics	Thin, flexible filaments	Strong, stable structures	Exhibit dynamic instability
Associated proteins	Variety of ABPs with different functions: fascin = bundling; gelsolin = filament severing; CP protein = capping; spectrin = cross-linking; myosin I and II = motor functions	Intermediate filament–associated proteins: plectins bind microtubules, actin, and intermediate filaments; desmoplakins and plakoglobins attach intermediate filaments to desmosomes and hemidesmosomes.	Microtubule-associated proteins: MAP-1, MAP-2, MAP-3, MAP-4, MAP-τ, and TOG-ρ regulate assembly, stabilize, and anchor microtubules to specific organelles; motor proteins—dyneins and kinesins—required for organelle movement
Location in cell	Core of microvilli Terminal web Concentrated beneath plasma membrane Contractile elements of muscles Contractile ring in dividing cells	Extend across cytoplasm connecting desmosomes and hemidesmosomes In nucleus just beneath inner nuclear membrane	Core of cilia Emerge from MTOC and spread into periphery of cell Mitotic spindle Centrosome
Major functions	Provide essential components (sarcomeres for muscle cells)	Provide mechanical strength and resistance to shearing forces	Provide network ("railroad tracks") for movement of organelles within cell Provide movement for cilia and chromosomes during cell division

ABP, actin-binding protein; ADP, adenosine diphosphate; ATP, adenosine triphosphate; GDP, guanosine diphosphate; GTP, guanosine triphosphate; MAP, microtubule-associated protein; MTOC, microtubule-organizing center; MW, molecular weight; N/A, not applicable.

■ INCLUSIONS

Inclusions contain products of metabolic activity of the cell and consist largely of pigment granules, lipid droplets, and glycogen.

Inclusions are cytoplasmic or nuclear structures with characteristic staining properties that are formed from the metabolic products of cell. They are considered nonmoving and nonliving components of the cell. Some of them, such as pigment granules, are surrounded by a plasma membrane; others (e.g., lipid droplets or glycogen) instead reside within the cytoplasmic or nuclear matrix.

- **Lipofuscin** is a brownish-gold pigment visible in routine hematoxylin and eosin (H&E) preparations. It is easily seen in nondividing cells such as neurons and skeletal and cardiac muscle cells. Lipofuscin accumulates over time in most eukaryotic cells as a result of cellular senescence (aging); thus, it is often called the **"wear-and-tear" pigment**. Lipofuscin is a conglomerate of oxidized lipids, phospholipids, metals, and organic molecules that accumulate within the cells as a result of oxidative degradation of mitochondria and lysosomal digestion. Phagocytic cells such as macrophages may also contain lipofuscin, which accumulates from the digestion of bacteria, foreign particles, dead cells, and their own organelles. Experimental studies indicate that lipofuscin accumulation may be an accurate indicator of cellular stress.

- **Hemosiderin** is an **iron-storage complex** found within the cytoplasm of many cells. It is most likely formed by the indigestible residues of hemoglobin, and its presence is related to phagocytosis of red blood cells. Hemosiderin is most easily demonstrated in the spleen, where aged erythrocytes are phagocytosed, but it can also be found in alveolar macrophages in the lung tissue, especially following pulmonary infection accompanied by a small hemorrhage into the alveoli. It is visible in light microscopy as a deep brown granule, more or less indistinguishable from lipofuscin. Hemosiderin granules can be differentially stained using histochemical methods for iron detection.
- **Glycogen** is a highly branched polymer used as a storage material for glucose. It is not stained in routine H&E preparations. However, it may be seen in the light microscope with special fixation and staining procedures (such as toluidine blue or the periodic acid–Schiff [PAS] method). Liver and striated muscle cells, which usually contain large amounts of glycogen, may display unstained regions where glycogen is located. Glycogen appears in the EM as granules 25–30 nm in diameter or as clusters of granules that often occupy significant portions of the cytoplasm (Fig. 2.65).
- **Lipid inclusions (fat droplets)** are usually nutritive inclusions that provide energy for cellular metabolism. The lipid droplets may appear in a cell for a brief time (e.g., in intestinal absorptive cells) or may reside for a long period (e.g., in adipocytes). In adipocytes, lipid inclusions often constitute most of the cytoplasmic volume, compressing the other formed organelles into a thin rim at the margin of the cell. Lipid droplets are usually extracted by the organic solvents used to prepare tissues for both light microscopy and EM. What is seen as a fat droplet in light microscopy is actually a hole in the cytoplasm that represents the site from which the lipid was extracted. In individuals with genetic defects of enzymes involved in lipid metabolism, lipid droplets may accumulate in abnormal locations or in abnormal amounts. Such diseases are classified as **lipid storage diseases**.
- **Crystalline inclusions** contained in certain cells are recognized in the light microscope. In humans, such inclusions are found in the Sertoli (sustentacular) and Leydig (interstitial) cells of the testis. With the TEM, crystalline inclusions have been found in many cell types and in virtually all parts of the cell, including the nucleus and most cytoplasmic organelles. Although some of these inclusions contain viral proteins, storage material, or cellular metabolites, the significance of others is not clear.

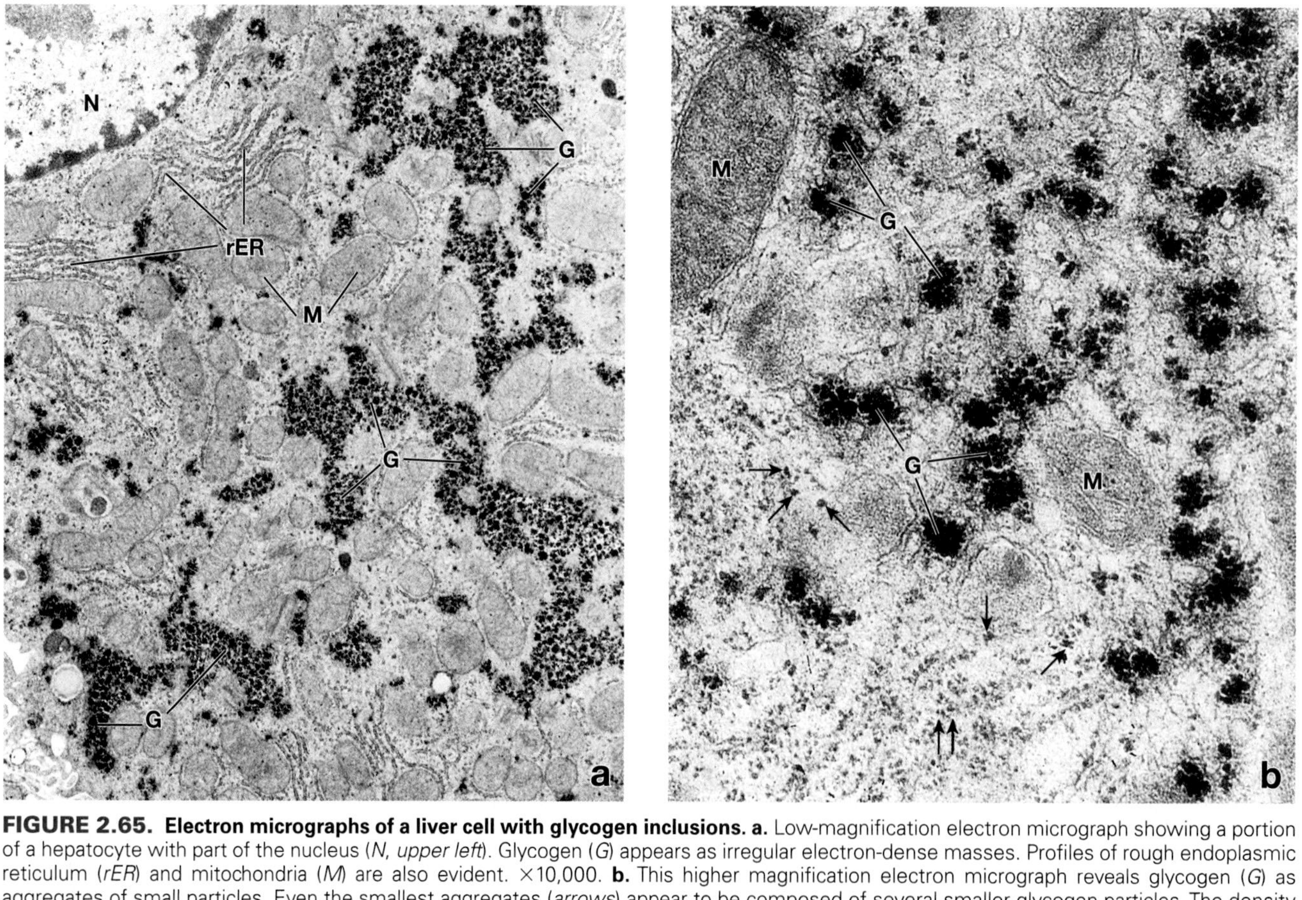

FIGURE 2.65. Electron micrographs of a liver cell with glycogen inclusions. a. Low-magnification electron micrograph showing a portion of a hepatocyte with part of the nucleus (*N, upper left*). Glycogen (*G*) appears as irregular electron-dense masses. Profiles of rough endoplasmic reticulum (*rER*) and mitochondria (*M*) are also evident. ×10,000. **b.** This higher magnification electron micrograph reveals glycogen (*G*) as aggregates of small particles. Even the smallest aggregates (*arrows*) appear to be composed of several smaller glycogen particles. The density of the glycogen is considerably greater than that of the ribosomes (*lower left*). M, mitochondria. ×52,000.

FOLDER 2.3

CLINICAL CORRELATION: ABNORMAL DUPLICATION OF CENTRIOLES AND CANCER

One of the critical components of normal cell division is the precise redistribution of chromosomes and other cell organelles during mitosis. Following replication of chromosomal DNA in the S phase of the cell cycle, centrioles undergo a single round of duplication that is closely coordinated with cell cycle progression. During mitosis, centrioles are responsible for forming the bipolar mitotic spindle, which is essential for equal segregation of chromosomes between daughter cells. Alterations of mechanisms regulating centriole duplication may lead to multiplication and abnormalities of centrioles and surrounding centrosomes (microtubule-organizing center [MTOC]). Cells with multiple centrosomes that overcome tumor-suppressor protein (p53)-mediated cell cycle arrest and spindle assembly checkpoint inhibition can enter cell divisions with distortions of the mitotic spindle (i.e., the presence of multipolar or misoriented spindles) (Fig. F2.3.1), leading to abnormal sorting of chromosomes during cell division. Multipolar cell divisions lead to aneuploidy, resulting in cell death.

However, some cancer cells can cluster their extra centrosomes into two poles and then undergo cell division resulting in viable daughter cells. Centrosome clustering, which depends on interaction of astral microtubules with the cell membrane, can lead to aneuploidy and defective asymmetric cell division. Centrosome clustering is most likely a unique requirement for the survival of certain tumor cells in which increased numbers of centrioles are frequently observed.

Also, additional centrosomes may lose pericentriolar matrix proteins essential for microtubule nucleation (i.e., γ-tubulin). This process silences MTOC activity in extra centrosomes, blocking their participation in spindle formation.

The resulting changes in chromosomal number may increase the activity of oncogenes or decrease protection from tumor suppressor genes. These changes are known to promote malignant cell transformation.

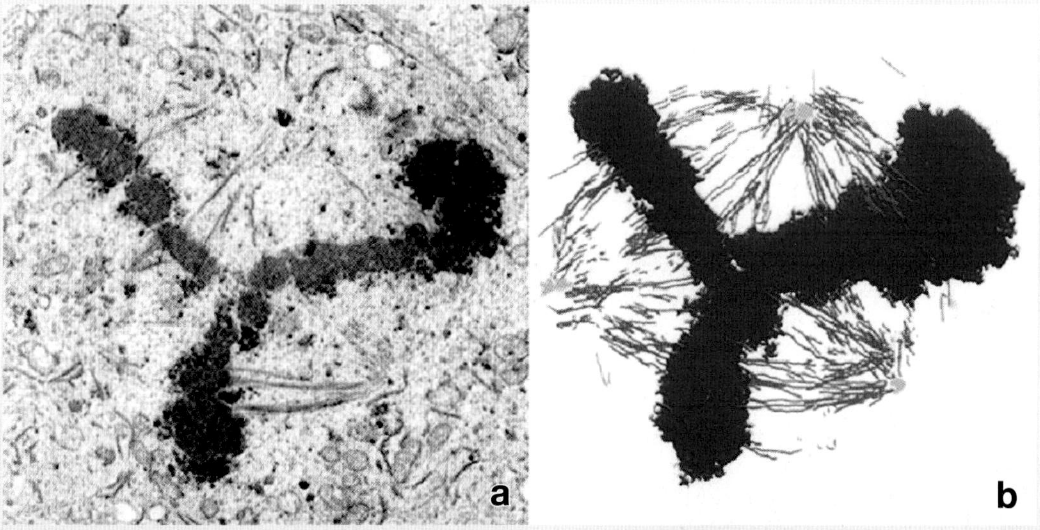

FIGURE F2.3.1. Multipolar mitotic spindle in a tumor cell. a. Electron micrograph of an invasive breast tumor cell showing abnormal symmetrical tripolar mitotic spindle in the metaphase of cell division. ×16,000. **b.** This drawing composed of color tracings of microtubules (*red*), mitotic spindle poles (*green*), and metaphase chromosomes (*blue*) (obtained from six nonadjacent serial sections of dividing tumor cell) shows more clearly the organization of this abnormal mitotic spindle. Detailed analysis and three-dimensional reconstruction of the spindle revealed that each spindle pole had at least two centrioles and that one spindle pole was composed of two distinct but adjacent foci of microtubules. (Reprinted with permission from Lingle WL, Salisbury JL. Altered centrosome structure is associated with abnormal mitoses in human breast tumors. *Am J Path.* 1999;155:1941–1951.)

■ CYTOPLASMIC MATRIX

The cytoplasmic matrix is a concentrated aqueous gel consisting of molecules of different sizes and shapes.

The **cytoplasmic matrix** (ground substance or **cytosol**) shows little specific structure by light microscopy or conventional TEM and has traditionally been described as a concentrated aqueous solution containing molecules of different size and shape (e.g., electrolytes, metabolites, RNA, and synthesized proteins). In most cells, it is the largest single compartment. The cytoplasmic matrix is the site of physiologic processes that are fundamental to the cell's existence (protein synthesis and degradation, breakdown of nutrients). Studies with high-voltage EM (HVEM) of 0.25- to 0.5-μm sections reveal a complex three-dimensional structural network of thin **microtrabecular strands** and **cross-linkers**. This network provides a structural substratum on which cytoplasmic reactions occur, such as those involving free ribosomes, and along which regulated and directed cytoplasmic transport and movement of organelles occur.

CELL CYTOPLASM

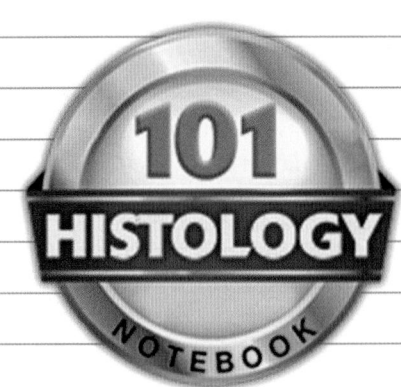

OVERVIEW OF THE CELL AND CYTOPLASM

- **Cells** are the basic structural and functional units of all multicellular organisms.
- Cells have two major compartments: the **cytoplasm** (which contains **organelles** and **inclusions** surrounded by **cytoplasmic matrix**) and the **nucleus** (which contains the genome).
- Organelles are metabolically active complexes or compartments that are classified as **membranous** and **nonmembranous organelles**.

PLASMA MEMBRANE

- The **plasma membrane** is an amphipathic lipid-bilayered structure visible with the transmission electron microscope (TEM). It is composed of phospholipids, cholesterol, embedded integral membrane proteins, and associated peripheral membrane proteins.
- **Integral membrane proteins** have important functions in cell metabolism, regulation, and integration. They include pumps, channels, receptor proteins, linker proteins, enzymes, and structural proteins.
- **Lipid rafts** represent microdomains in the plasma membrane that contain high concentrations of cholesterol and glycosphingolipids. They are movable signaling platforms that carry integral and peripheral membrane proteins.
- The **cell membrane** and **internal plasma membranes** of organelles are **continuously remodeling**. Cytoplasm can be included or excluded in the remodeling process that is mediated by complexes of proteins (i.e., family of **ESCRT** or **dynamin** proteins).
- The plasma membrane invaginates, which allows for **vesicle budding**. Vesicle budding permits molecules to enter the cell (**endocytosis**), leave the cell (**exocytosis**), or travel within the cell cytoplasm in transport vesicles.

MEMBRANE TRANSPORT AND VESICULAR TRANSPORT

- Small molecules (fat-soluble, uncharged) and gases cross the plasma membrane by **simple (passive) diffusion** without energy expenditure. All other molecules require **membrane transport proteins** (carrier proteins or channels) for passage across the plasma membran
- **Active transport** requires energy because molecules are transported across the plasma membrane against their concentratio or electrochemical gradient. **Passive transport** requires carrier proteins but does not consume energy.
- **Endocytosis** is the cellular uptake of fluids and macromolecules. It is dependent on three different mechanisms: **pinocytos** (both micro- and macropinocytotic uptake of fluids and solutes in small or large vesicles, respectively); **phagocytosis** (uptake large particles); and **receptor-mediated endocytosis** (uptake of specific molecules that bind to receptors).
- **Early** and **late endosomes** represent a network of membrane-enclosed cytoplasmic compartments that are essential in sorti endocytosed material and membrane proteins for either transport to the cell surface or degradation in lysosomes.
- **Vesicle formation** during receptor-mediated endocytosis involves interaction with the protein **clathrin**, which assembles basket-like cages visible in the EM as **coated pits** or **coated vesicles**.
- **Exocytosis** is the process of cellular secretion in which transport vesicles, when fused with plasma membrane, discharge their conte into the extracellular space. **SNARE proteins** are necessary for membrane fusion in exocytosis and for endocytosis initiation.
- **Exosomes** are very small endosome-derived membrane-bound vesicles secreted by cells into extracellular space. They act transport vehicles for near- and long-distance intercellular communication and material exchange between cells.
- **Constitutive exocytosis** is an ongoing process in which the contents of transport vesicles are continuously delivered discharged at the plasma membrane. In **regulated secretory exocytosis**, the contents of vesicles are stored within the and released pending hormonal or neural stimulation.

DEGRADATION OF PROTEINS

- **Lysosomes** are digestive organelles containing hydrolytic enzymes that degrade substances derived from endocytosis and from the cell itself (autophagy). They have a unique membrane made of specific structural proteins resistant to hydrolytic digestion.
- **Lysosomes develop from endosomes** by receiving newly synthesized lysosomal proteins (enzymes and structural proteins) that are targeted via the **mannose-6-phosphate (M-6-P)** lysosomal targeting signals.
- The endosomal membrane of some **late endosomes undergoes inward invagination** to generate intraluminal vesicles. These intracellular **multivesicular bodies (MVBs)** are either degraded in lysosomes or fused with the plasma membrane to release intraluminal vesicles into extracellular space as **exosomes**.
- **Proteasomes** are nonmembranous organelles that also function in degradation of proteins. They represent cytoplasmic protein complexes that destroy damaged (misfolded) or unnecessary proteins that have been labeled for destruction with **ubiquitin** without the involvement of lysosomes.

ENDOPLASMIC RETICULUM

- The **rough endoplasmic reticulum (rER)** represents a region of endoplasmic reticulum associated with **ribosomes**. It is the site of protein synthesis and posttranslational modification of newly synthesized proteins. The rER is most highly developed in active secretory cells and is visible in light microscopy as a basophilic region (**ergastoplasm**).
- The **smooth endoplasmic reticulum (sER)** consists of anastomosing tubules that are not associated with ribosomes. It contains **cytochrome P450 detoxifying enzymes** (liver) and enzymes for glycogen and **lipid metabolism**. sER also serves as a Ca^{2+} reservoir in skeletal muscle cells.

GOLGI APPARATUS AND OTHER MEMBRANOUS ORGANELLES

- The **Golgi apparatus** represents a series of stacked, flattened cisternae and functions in the posttranslational modification, sorting, and packaging of proteins directed to four major cellular destinations: **apical and basolateral plasma membrane, endosomes** and **lysosomes**, and **apical cytoplasm** (for storage and/or secretion).
- **Mitochondria** are elongated, mobile organelles containing the **electron transport chain** of respiratory enzymes to generate adenosine triphosphate (ATP). They are abundant in cells that generate and expend large amounts of energy, and they regulate **apoptosis** (programmed cell death).
- **Peroxisomes** are small organelles involved in an oxidative type of metabolism. They degrade **fatty acids**, synthesize ether phospholipids, and produce and degrade **reactive oxygen intermediates** such as H_2O_2.

MICROTUBULES

- **Microtubules** are elongated, rigid hollow tubes (20–25 nm in diameter) composed of **α-tubulin** and **β-tubulin**. They originate from **γ-tubulin rings** within the microtubule-organizing center (MTOC), and their length changes dynamically as tubulin dimers are added or removed in a constant remodeling process known as **dynamic instability**.
- Microtubules form tracts for intracellular **vesicular transport** and **mitotic spindles**; they are also responsible for the movement of **cilia** and **flagella** and for the maintenance of cell shape.
- **Movement of intracellular organelles** along microtubules is generated by molecular motor proteins (**dyneins** and **kinesins**).
- **Centrioles** are paired, short, rod-like cytoplasmic cylinders built from **nine microtubule triplets**. They represent the focal point around which the MTOC assembles, and they provide **basal bodies** for cilia and flagella and align the mitotic spindle during cell division.

ACTIN FILAMENTS

- **Actin filaments** (microfilaments) are thinner (6–8 nm in diameter), shorter, and more flexible than microtubules. They are composed of polymerized **G-actin (globular actin)** molecules that form **F-actin (filamentous actin)**.
- Actin filaments are also responsible for **cell-to-extracellular matrix attachment (focal adhesions)**, movement of membrane proteins, formation of the structural core of microvilli, and cell motility through the creation of cell extensions (**lamellipodia** and **filopodia**).
- **Actin motor proteins** (myosin family), which hydrolyze ATP to provide energy for movement along the actin filament, are responsible for muscle contraction.

INTERMEDIATE FILAMENTS

- **Intermediate filaments** are rope-like filaments (8–10 nm in diameter) that add stability to the cell and interact with cell junctions (desmosomes and hemidesmosomes).
- Intermediate filaments are formed from nonpolar and highly variable intermediate filament subunits that include **keratins** (found in epithelial cells), **vimentin** (mesodermally derived cells), **desmin** (muscle cells), **neurofilament proteins** (nerve cells), **lamins** (nucleus), and **beaded filament proteins** (eye lens).

INCLUSIONS

- **Inclusions** contain products of metabolic activity of the cell and consist largely of pigment granules (**lipofuscin** is the most common **"wear-and-tear" pigment**), **lipid droplets**, and **glycogen**.

3 THE CELL NUCLEUS

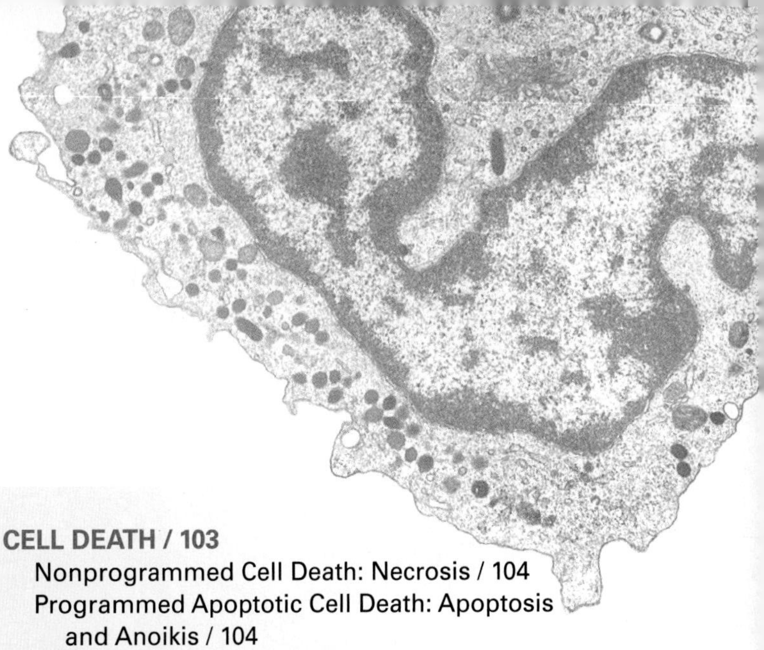

■ OVERVIEW OF THE NUCLEUS

The nucleus is a membrane-limited compartment that contains the genome (genetic information) in eukaryotic cells.

The **nucleus** contains genetic information, together with the machinery for DNA replication and RNA transcription and processing. The nucleus of a nondividing cell, also called an **interphase cell**, consists of the following components:

- **Chromatin** is nuclear material organized as **euchromatin** or **heterochromatin**. It contains DNA associated with roughly an equal mass of various nuclear proteins (e.g., histones) that are necessary for DNA to function.
- The **nucleolus** (pl., **nucleoli**) is a small area within the nucleus that contains DNA in the form of transcriptionally active ribosomal RNA (rRNA) genes, RNA, and proteins. The nucleolus is the site of rRNA synthesis and contains regulatory cell cycle proteins.
- The **nuclear envelope** is a double membrane system that surrounds the nucleus of the cell. It consists of an inner and an outer membrane separated by a perinuclear cisternal space and perforated by **nuclear pores**. The outer membrane of the nuclear envelope is continuous with that of the rough-surfaced endoplasmic reticulum (rER) and is often studded with ribosomes (Fig. 3.1).
- The **nucleoplasm** is nuclear content other than the chromatin and nucleolus.

A simple microscopic evaluation of the nucleus provides a great deal of information about a cell's well-being. Evaluation of nuclear size, shape, and structure plays an important role in cancer. For instance, **dying cells** have visible nuclear alterations. These include the following findings:

- **Karyolysis**, or the disappearance of nuclei due to complete dissolution of DNA by increased activity of DNAse
- **Pyknosis**, or condensation of chromatin leading to shrinkage of the nuclei (they appear as dense basophilic masses)
- **Karyorrhexis**, or fragmentations of nuclei (these changes are usually preceded by pyknosis)

■ NUCLEAR COMPONENTS

Chromatin

Chromatin, a complex of DNA and proteins, is responsible for the characteristic basophilia of the nucleus.

Each eukaryotic cell contains about 6 billion bits of information encoded within a DNA molecule, which measures about 1.8 m in length. The length of the DNA molecule is 100,000 times longer than that of the nuclear diameter. Therefore, DNA must be highly folded and tightly packed in the cell nucleus. This is accomplished by the formation of a unique nucleoprotein complex called **chromatin**.

The chromatin complex consists of DNA and structural proteins. Further folding of chromatin, such as that which occurs

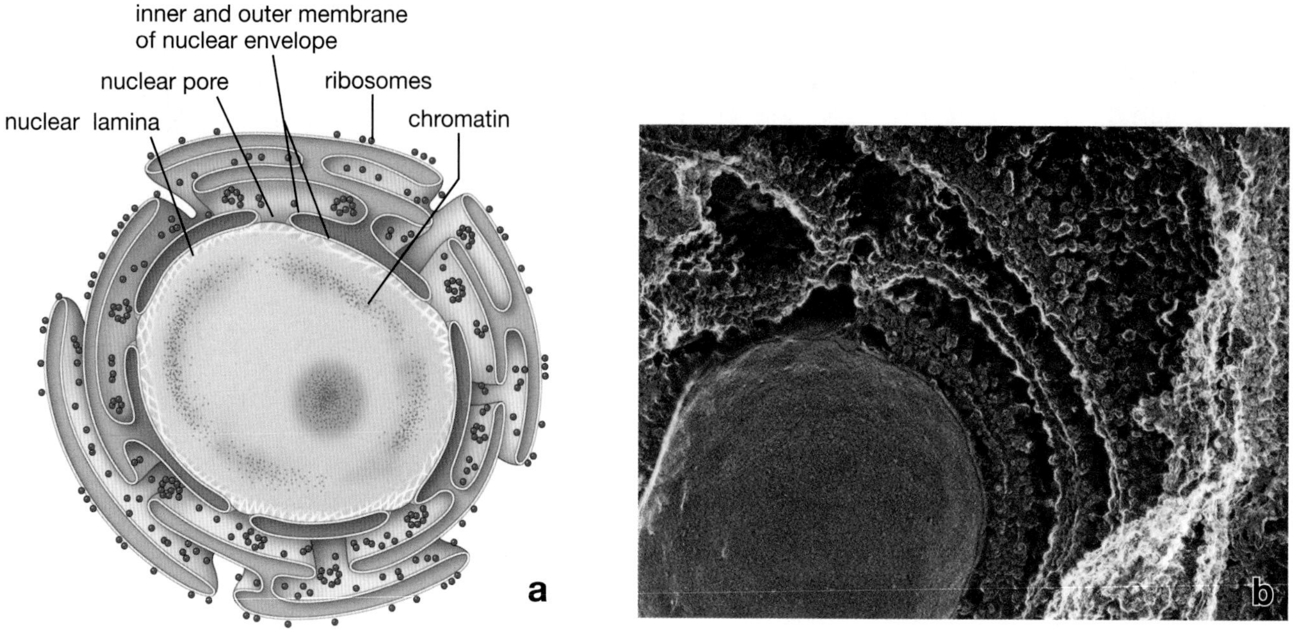

FIGURE 3.1. Nucleus and its relationship to the rough-surfaced endoplasmic reticulum (rER). a. The nuclear wall consists of a double membrane envelope that surrounds the nucleus. The outer membrane is continuous with the membranes of the rER; thus, the perinuclear space communicates with the rER lumen. The inner membrane is adjacent to nuclear intermediate filaments that form the nuclear lamina. **b.** This electron micrograph, prepared by the quick-freeze, deep-etch technique, shows the nucleus, the large spherical object, surrounded by the nuclear envelope. Note that the outer membrane possesses ribosomes and is continuous with the rER. ×12,000. (Courtesy of Dr. John E. Heuser, Washington University School of Medicine.)

during mitosis, produces structures called **chromosomes.** Each human cell contains 46 chromosomes. Chromatin proteins include five basic proteins called **histones** along with other **nonhistone proteins.** A unique feature of chromatin packaging is that it permits the transcriptional machinery to access those regions of the chromosomes required for gene expression.

Sequencing the human genome was successfully completed in 2003.

The **human genome** encompasses the entire length of human DNA that contains the genetic information packaged in all 46 chromosomes. Sequencing of the human genome took approximately 13 years and was successfully completed in 2003 by the Human Genome Project. The human genome contains a 2.85 billion base pair consensus sequence of nucleotides, which are arranged in approximately 23,000 protein-coding genes. For years, it was thought that genes were usually present in two copies in a genome. However, recent discoveries have revealed that large segments of DNA can vary in numbers of copies. For instance, genes that were thought to always occur in two copies per genome have sometimes one, three, or more copies. Such **copy number variations (CNVs)** are widespread in the human genome and most likely lead to genetic imbalances. Previously defined as a segment of DNA involved in producing a polypeptide chain, a **gene** is now defined as a union of genomic sequences encoding a coherent set of potentially overlapping functional products.

In general, two forms of chromatin are found in the nucleus: a condensed form called *heterochromatin* and a dispersed form called *euchromatin*.

In most cells, chromatin does not have a homogeneous appearance; rather, clumps of densely staining chromatin are embedded in a more lightly staining background. The densely staining material is highly condensed chromatin called **heterochromatin**, and the lightly staining material (where most transcribed genes are located) is a dispersed form called **euchromatin.** It is the phosphate groups of the chromatin DNA that are responsible for the characteristic basophilia of chromatin (page 6).

There are two recognizable types of heterochromatin: constitutive and facultative. **Constitutive heterochromatin** contains the same regions of genetically inactive, highly repetitive sequences of DNA that are condensed and consistently packaged in the same regions of the chromosome when compared with other cells. Large amounts of constitutive heterochromatin are found in chromosomes near the centromeres and telomeres. **Facultative heterochromatin** is also condensed and is not involved in the transcription process. In contrast to constitutive heterochromatin, facultative heterochromatin is not repetitive, and its location within the nucleus and chromosomes varies when compared with other cells. Facultative heterochromatin may undergo active transcription in certain cells (see the description of Barr bodies on page 91) owing to specific conditions, such as certain cell cycle stages, nuclear localization changes (i.e., migration from the center to the periphery), or the active transcription of only one allele of a gene (monoallelic gene expression).

Heterochromatin is found in the following three locations (Fig. 3.2):

- **Marginal chromatin** is found at the periphery of the nucleus; the structure that light microscopists formerly referred to as the *nuclear membrane* actually consists largely of marginal chromatin.
- **Karyosomes** are discrete bodies of chromatin irregular in size and shape that are found throughout the nucleus.
- **Nucleolar-associated chromatin** is chromatin found in association with the nucleolus.

Heterochromatin stains with hematoxylin and basic dyes; it is also readily displayed with the Feulgen stain (a specific

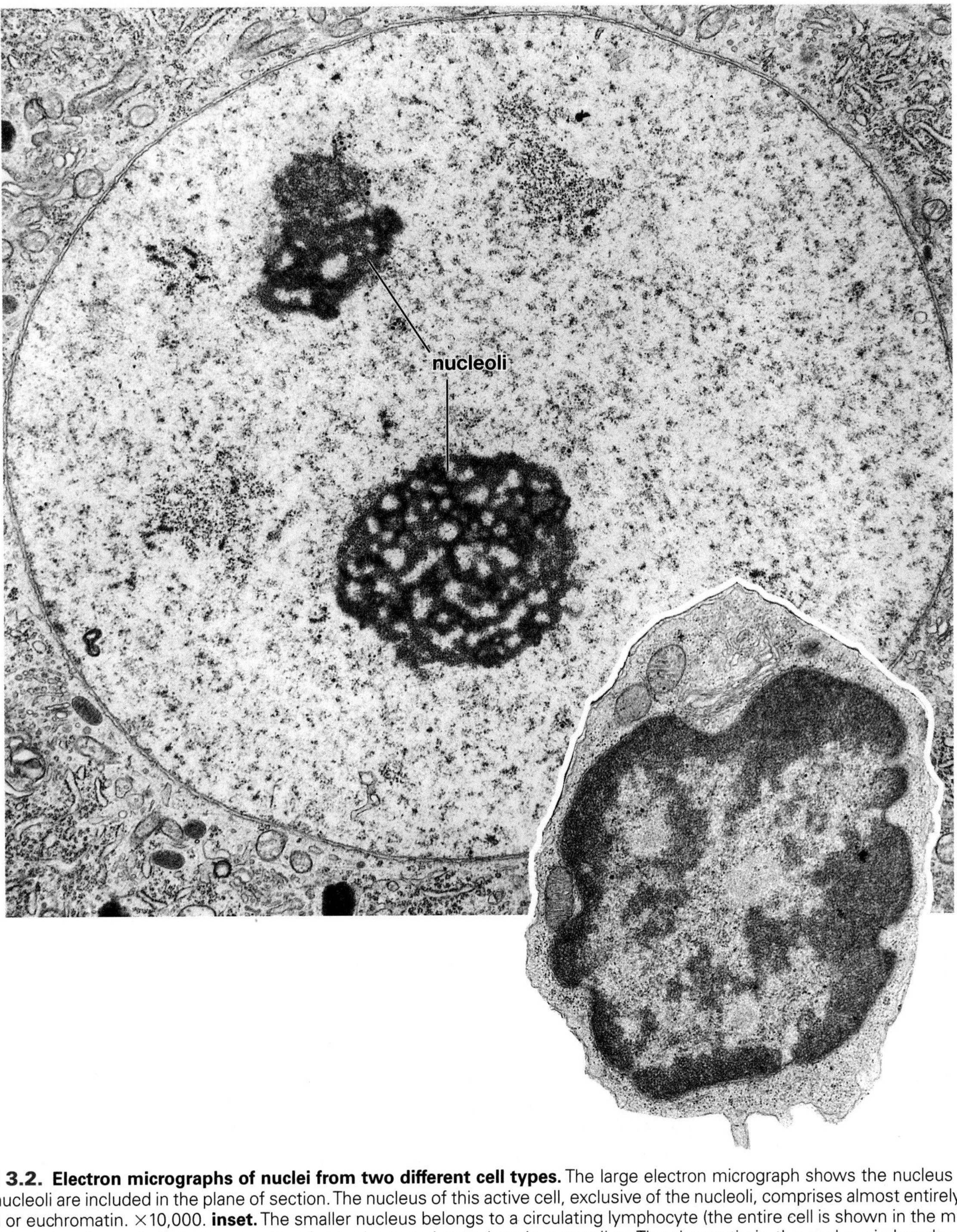

FIGURE 3.2. Electron micrographs of nuclei from two different cell types. The large electron micrograph shows the nucleus of a nerve cell. Two nucleoli are included in the plane of section. The nucleus of this active cell, exclusive of the nucleoli, comprises almost entirely extended chromatin or euchromatin. ×10,000. **inset.** The smaller nucleus belongs to a circulating lymphocyte (the entire cell is shown in the micrograph). It is a relatively inactive cell. Note the paucity of cytoplasm and cytoplasmic organelles. The chromatin in the nucleus is largely condensed (heterochromatin). The lighter areas represent euchromatin. ×13,000.

histochemical reaction for the deoxyribose of DNA, page 6) and fluorescent vital dyes such as Hoechst dyes and propidium iodide. It is the heterochromatin that accounts for the conspicuous staining of the nucleus in hematoxylin and eosin (H&E) preparations.

Euchromatin is not evident in the light microscope. It is present within the nucleoplasm in the "clear" areas between and around the heterochromatin. In routine electron micrographs, there is no sharp delineation between euchromatin and heterochromatin; both have a granular, filamentous appearance, but the euchromatin is less tightly packed.

Euchromatin indicates active chromatin—that is, chromatin that is stretched out so that the genetic information in the DNA can be read and transcribed. It is prominent in metabolically active cells, such as neurons and liver cells. Heterochromatin predominates in metabolically inactive cells, such as small circulating lymphocytes and sperm cells, or in cells that produce one major product, such as plasma cells.

The smallest units of chromatin structure are macromolecular complexes of DNA and histones called nucleosomes.

Nucleosomes are found in both euchromatin and heterochromatin and in chromosomes. These 10-nm-diameter particles represent the first level of chromatin folding and are formed by the coiling of the DNA molecule around a protein core. This step shortens the DNA molecule by approximately sevenfold relative to the unfolded DNA molecule. The core of the nucleosome consists of eight **histone molecules** (called an **octamer**). Two loops of DNA (~146 nucleotide pairs) are wrapped around the core octamer. The DNA extends between each particle as a 2-nm filament that joins adjacent nucleosomes. When chromatin is extracted from the nucleus, the nucleosomal substructure of chromatin is visible in transmission electron microscopy (TEM) and is often described as "**beads on a string**" (Fig. 3.3a).

In the next step of chromatin folding, a long strand of nucleosomes is coiled to produce a **30-nm chromatin fibril**. Six nucleosomes form one turn in the coil of the chromatin fibril, which is approximately 40-fold shorter than unfolded DNA. Long stretches of 30-nm chromatin fibrils are further organized into **loop domains** (containing 15,000–100,000 base pairs), which are anchored into a **chromosome scaffold** or **nuclear matrix** composed of nonhistone proteins. In heterochromatin, the chromatin fibers are tightly packed and folded on each other; in euchromatin, the chromatin fibrils are more loosely arranged.

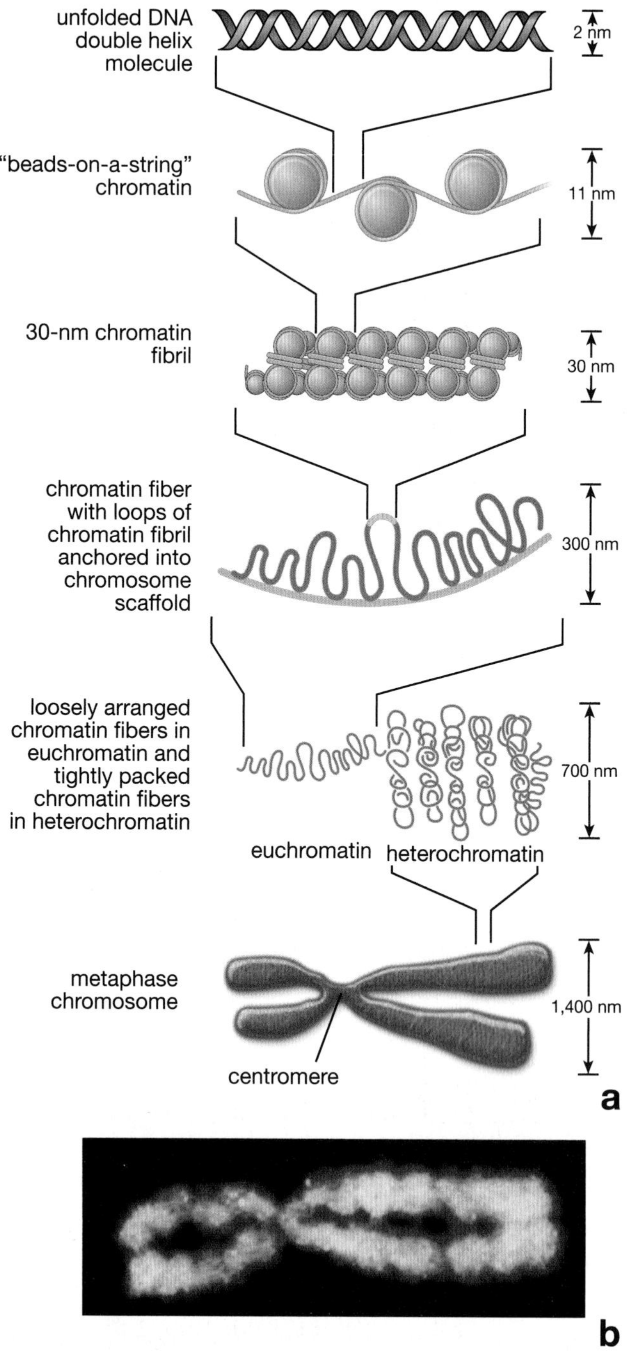

FIGURE 3.3. Packaging of chromatin into the chromosomal structure. a. Sequential steps in the packaging of nuclear chromatin are shown in this diagram, beginning with the DNA double helix and ending with the highly condensed form found in chromosomes. **b.** Structure of human metaphase chromosome 2 as visible in atomic force microscopic image. ×20,000. (Courtesy of Dr. Tatsuo Ushiki.)

In dividing cells, chromatin is condensed and organized into discrete bodies called chromosomes.

During mitotic division, **chromatin fibers** formed from chromatin loop domains attached to a flexible protein scaffold undergo condensation to form **chromosomes** *[Gr., colored bodies]*. Each chromosome is formed by two **chromatids** that are joined together at a point called the **centromere** (Fig. 3.3b). The double nature of the chromosome is produced in the preceding synthetic (S) phase of the cell cycle (see pages 97-99), during which DNA is replicated in preparation for the next mitotic division.

The area located at each end of the chromosome is called the **telomere**. Telomeres shorten with each cell division. Recent studies indicate that telomere length is an important indicator of the life span of the cell. To survive indefinitely (become "immortalized"), cells must activate a mechanism that maintains telomere length. For example, in cells that have been transformed into malignant cells, an enzyme called **telomerase** is present that adds repeated nucleotide sequences to the telomere ends. Expression of this enzyme has been shown to extend the life span of cells, thus promoting cell growth. Telomerase is being studied as a potential target for use as an anticancer treatment.

With the exception of the mature gametes, the egg and sperm, human cells contain **46 chromosomes** organized as **23 homologous pairs** (each chromosome in the pair has the same shape and size). Twenty-two pairs have identical chromosomes (i.e., each chromosome of the pair contains the same portion of the genome) and are called **autosomes**. The 23rd pair of chromosomes are the **sex chromosomes**, designated **X** and **Y**. Females contain two X chromosomes (46,XX); males contain one X and one Y chromosome (46,XY).

The chromosomal number, 46, is found in most of the somatic cells of the body and is called the **diploid (2n)** number. To simplify the description of chromosomal number and DNA changes during mitosis and meiosis, we use the lowercase letter **(n)** for chromosome number and lowercase letter **(d)** for DNA content. Diploid chromosomes have the **(2d)** amount of DNA immediately after cell division. They have twice that amount **(4d)** after the S phase (see pages 99-101).

As a result of **meiosis**, eggs and sperm have only 23 chromosomes, the haploid **(1n)** number, as well as the haploid **(1d)** amount of DNA. The somatic chromosome number **(2n)** and the diploid **(2d)** amount of DNA are restored at **fertilization** by the fusion of the sperm nucleus with the egg nucleus (see pages 102-103).

In a karyotype, chromosome pairs are sorted according to their size, shape, and emitted fluorescent color.

A preparation of chromosomes derived from mechanically ruptured, dividing cells that are then fixed, plated on a microscope slide, and stained is called a **metaphase spread**. In the past, chromosomes were routinely stained with Giemsa stain; however, with the recent development of in situ hybridization techniques, the fluorescent in situ hybridization (FISH) procedure is now more often used to visualize a chromosomal spread. These spreads are observed with fluorescence microscopes, and computer-controlled cameras are then used

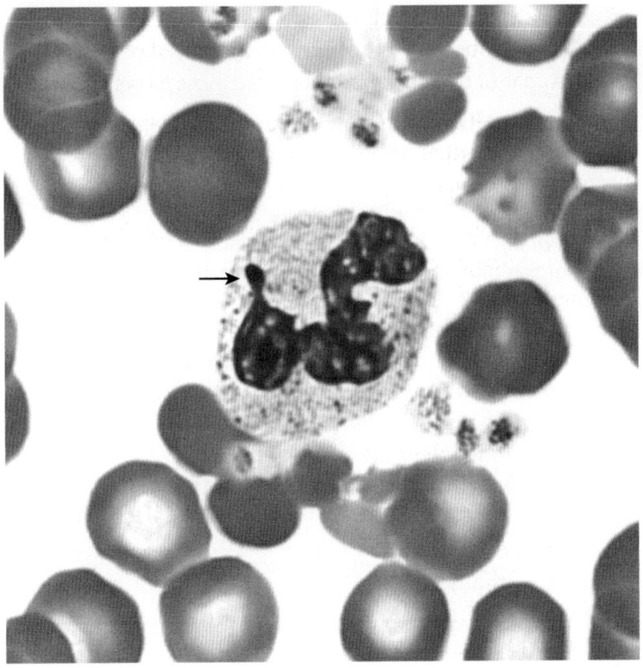

FIGURE 3.4. Photomicrograph of a neutrophil from a female patient's blood smear. The second X chromosome of the female patient is repressed in the interphase nucleus and can be demonstrated in the neutrophil as a drumstick-appearing appendage (*arrow*) on a nuclear lobe. ×250.

to capture images of the chromosome pairs. Image-processing software is used to sort the chromosome pairs according to their morphology to form a **karyotype** (see Fig. F3.1.1a). A variety of molecular probes that are now commercially available are used in **cytogenetic testing** to diagnose disorders caused by chromosomal abnormalities, such as nondisjunctions, transpositions (see Fig. F3.1.1a), deletions (see Fig. F3.1.1b), and duplications of specific gene sites. Karyotypes are also used for prenatal determination of sex in fetuses and for prenatal diagnosis of certain genetic diseases (see Fig. 1.7).

The Barr body represents a region of facultative heterochromatin that can be used to identify the sex of a fetus.

Some chromosomes are repressed in the interphase nucleus and exist only in the tightly packed heterochromatic form. One **X chromosome** of the female is an example of such a chromosome and can be used to identify the sex of a fetus. This chromosome was discovered in 1949 by Barr and Bartram in nerve cells of female cats, where it appears as a well-stained round body, now called the **Barr body**, adjacent to the nucleolus. In females, the Barr body represents a region of **facultative heterochromatin** that is condensed and not involved in the transcription process. During embryonic development, one randomly chosen X chromosome in the female zygote undergoes chromosome-wide chromatin condensation, and this state is maintained throughout the lifetime of the organism.

Although the Barr body was originally found in sectioned tissue, it was subsequently shown that any relatively large number of cells prepared as a smear (e.g., scrapings of the oral mucous membrane from the inside of the cheeks or neutrophils from a blood smear) can be used to search for the Barr body. In cells of the oral mucous membrane, the Barr body is located adjacent to the nuclear envelope. In neutrophils, the Barr body forms a drumstick-shaped appendage on one of the nuclear lobes (Fig. 3.4). In both sections and smears, many cells must be examined to find those whose orientation is suitable for the display of the Barr body.

Nucleolus

The nucleolus is the site of ribosomal RNA (rRNA) synthesis and initial ribosomal assembly.

The **nucleolus** is a nonmembranous region of the nucleus that surrounds transcriptionally active rRNA genes. It is the primary site of ribosomal production and assembly. The nucleolus varies in size but is particularly well developed in cells active in protein synthesis. Some cells contain more than one nucleolus (Fig. 3.5). The nucleolus has three morphologically distinct regions:

- **Fibrillar centers** contain DNA loops of five different chromosomes (13, 14, 15, 21, and 22) that contain rRNA genes, RNA polymerase I, and transcription factors.
- **Fibrillar material (pars fibrosa)** contains ribosomal genes that are actively undergoing transcription and large amounts of rRNA.
- **Granular material (pars granulosa)** represents the site of initial ribosomal assembly and contains densely packed preribosomal particles.

The network formed by the granular and the fibrillar materials is called the **nucleolonema**. rRNA is present in both granular and fibrillar material and is organized, respectively, as both granules and extremely fine filaments packed tightly together. Genes for the ribosomal subunits are localized in the interstices of this network and are transcribed by RNA polymerase I. After further processing and modification of rRNA by small nucleolar RNAs (snoRNAs), the subunits of rRNA are assembled using ribosomal proteins imported from the cytoplasm. The partially assembled ribosomal subunits (preribosomes) are exported from the nucleus via nuclear pores for full assembly into mature ribosomes in the cytoplasm.

The nucleolus is involved in the regulation of the cell cycle.

Nucleostemin is a p53-binding protein found within the nucleolus that regulates the cell cycle and influences cell differentiation. As cellular differentiation progresses, the level of this protein decreases. The presence of nucleostemin in **malignant cells** suggests that it could play a role in their

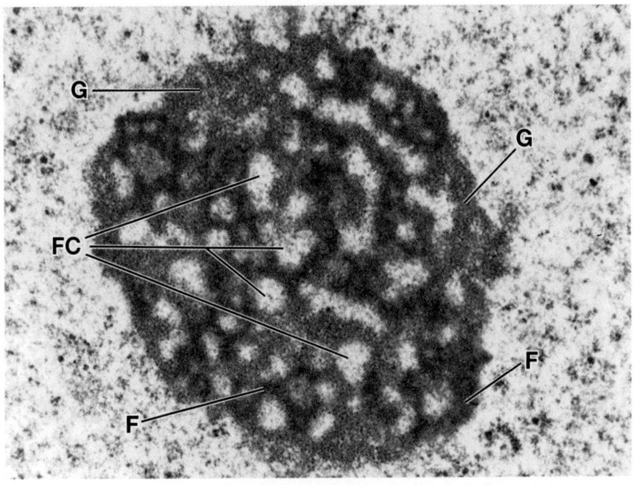

FIGURE 3.5. Electron micrograph of the nucleolus. This nucleolus from a nerve cell shows fibrillar centers (*FC*) surrounded by the fibrillar (*F*) and granular (*G*) materials. Such a network of both materials is referred to as the *nucleolonema*. The ribosomal RNA (rRNA), DNA-containing genes for the rRNA, and specific proteins are localized in the interstices of the nucleolonema. ×15,000.

FOLDER 3.1

CLINICAL CORRELATION: CYTOGENETIC TESTING

Cytogenetic testing is an important component in the diagnosis and evaluation of genetic disorders and refers to the analysis of chromosomes. Chromosomal abnormalities occur in ~0.5% of all live births and are detected in ~50% of first-trimester miscarriages (spontaneous abortions) and 95% of various tumor cells. Chromosome analysis can be performed on peripheral blood, bone marrow, tissues (such as skin or chorionic villi obtained from biopsies), and cells obtained from amniotic fluid during amniocentesis.

Studies of chromosomes begin with the extraction of whole chromosomes from the nuclei of dividing cells. These chromosomes are then placed on glass slides, hybridized with special fluorescence probes (fluorescent in situ hybridization [FISH] technique), and examined under a microscope. A single fluorescent DNA probe produces a bright microscopic signal when the probe is hybridized to a specific part of a particular chromosome. To obtain an image of all of the chromosomes, a mixture of different probes is used to produce different colors in each chromosome. Karyotypes labeled by this method allow cytogeneticists to perform a comprehensive analysis of changes in the number of chromosomes and chromosomal abnormalities, such as additions or deletions. The paired chromosomes are numbered in the karyotype, and the male sex is indicated by the presence of chromosomes X and Y (Fig. F3.1.1a). The *white box* inset in Figure F3.1.1a shows the XX chromosome pair as it appears in the female.

Sometimes, part of a chromosome will break off and attach to another chromosome. When this happens, it is referred to as a **translocation**. Note that the *red box* inset in Figure F3.1.1a shows a translocation between chromosomes 8 and 14 (t8;14). It is clearly visible in this color image that a part of the original chromosome 8 (*aqua blue region*) is now attached to chromosome 14, and a small portion of chromosome 14 (*red region*) is now part of chromosome 8. Such chromosomal translocations are present in lymphomas (cancers of blood cells), such as acute myeloid leukemia (AML), non-Hodgkin lymphoma (NHL), and Burkitt lymphoma.

In Figure F3.1.1b, a metaphase spread obtained from cultured lymphocytes of a patient with suspected **Prader-Willi/Angelman syndrome (PWS/AS)** has been hybridized with several DNA probes reacting with chromosome 15 (an enlarged chromosomal pair from chromosome 15 is shown in the *yellow box* inset). The *green* probe (D15Z1) indicates the centromere of chromosome 15. The adjacent *orange* probe (D15S10) reacts with the PWS/AS region of chromosome 15. Deletion of this region is associated with PWS/AS. Note that one homolog of chromosome 15 has lost that region (no orange signal is visible). The third *red* probe (PML) recognizes the distal long arm of chromosome 15 and is visible in both chromosomes. Severe intellectual disability, muscular hypotonia, short stature, hypogonadism, and insulin-resistant diabetes are characteristics of PWS/AS. When the deletion is inherited from the mother, patients develop AS; when inherited from the father, patients develop PWS. This preparation is counterstained with DAPI that reacts with double-stranded DNA and exhibits *blue* fluorescence.

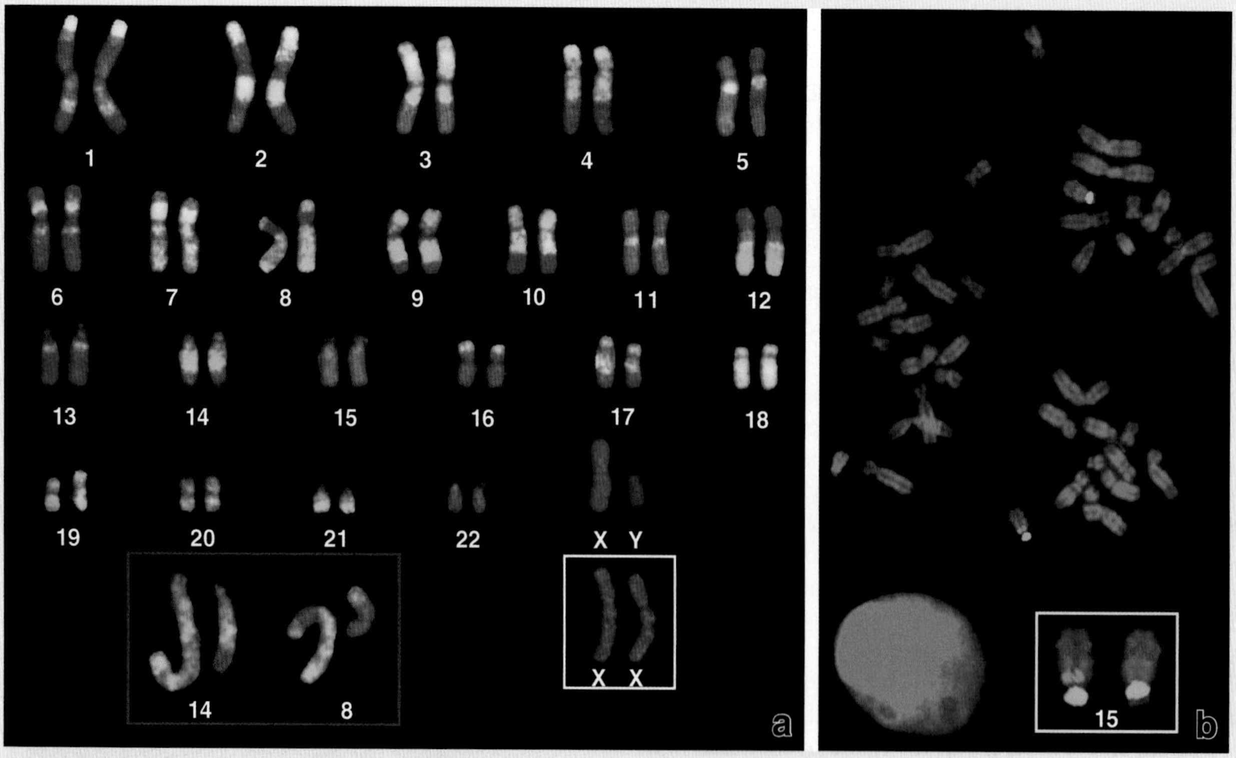

FIGURE F3.1.1. Karyotypes obtained with the fluorescent in situ hybridization technique. a. Karyotype of a normal male. The *white box inset* shows the XX chromosome pair of a normal female. The *red box inset* reveals an abnormality in chromosomes 14 and 8. (Courtesy of the Applied Imaging International Ltd., Newcastle upon Tyne, United Kingdom.) **b.** A metaphase spread from a patient with Prader-Willi/Angelman syndrome. The *yellow box inset* shows the enlarged pair of chromosome 15. (Courtesy of Dr. Robert B. Jenkins.)

uncontrolled proliferation (Folder 3.2). In addition, DNA, RNA, and retroviruses and their viral proteins interact with the nucleolus and cause redistribution of fibrillar and granular materials during the course of viral infection. These viruses may use components of the nucleolus as part of their own replication process. Evidence suggests that viruses may target the nucleolus and its components to favor viral transcription and translation and perhaps alter the cell cycle to promote viral replication.

The nucleolus stains intensely with hematoxylin and basic dyes and metachromatically with thionine dyes.

The relation of basophilia and metachromasia of the nucleolus to the phosphate groups of the nucleolar RNA is confirmed by predigestion of specimens with ribonuclease (RNAse), which abolishes the staining. As mentioned earlier, DNA is present in the nucleolus; however, its concentration is below the detection capability of the Feulgen reaction. Thus, when examined in the light microscope, nucleoli appear Feulgen-negative with Feulgen-positive nucleolus-associated chromatin that often rims the nucleolus.

Nuclear Envelope

The nuclear envelope, formed by two membranes with a perinuclear cisternal space between them, separates the nucleoplasm from the cytoplasm.

The **nuclear envelope** provides a selectively permeable membranous barrier between the nuclear compartment and the cytoplasm, and it encloses the chromatin. The nuclear envelope is assembled from two (outer and inner) nuclear membranes with a **perinuclear cisternal space** between them. The perinuclear clear cisternal space is continuous with the cisternal space of the rER (see Fig. 3.1). The two membranes of the envelope are perforated at intervals by **nuclear pores** that mediate the active transport of proteins, ribonucleoproteins, and RNAs between the nucleus and the cytoplasm. The membranes of the nuclear envelope differ in structure and functions:

- The **outer nuclear membrane** closely resembles the membrane of the ER and in fact is continuous with the rER membrane (Fig. 3.6). Polyribosomes are often attached to ribosomal docking proteins present on the cytoplasmic side of the outer nuclear membrane.
- The **inner nuclear membrane** is supported by a rigid network of intermediate protein filaments attached to its inner surface called the **nuclear (fibrous) lamina** (see Fig. 3.6). In addition, the inner nuclear membrane contains specific lamin receptors and several lamina-associated proteins that bind to chromosomes and secure the attachment of the nuclear lamina.

The nuclear lamina is formed by intermediate filaments and lies adjacent to the inner nuclear membrane.

The **nuclear lamina**, a thin, electron-dense intermediate filament network-like layer, resides underneath the nuclear membrane. In addition to its supporting or "nucleoskeletal" function, nuclear lamina is essential in many nuclear activities, such as DNA replication, transcription, and gene regulation. If the membranous component of the nuclear envelope is disrupted by exposure to detergent, the nuclear lamina remains, and the nucleus retains its shape.

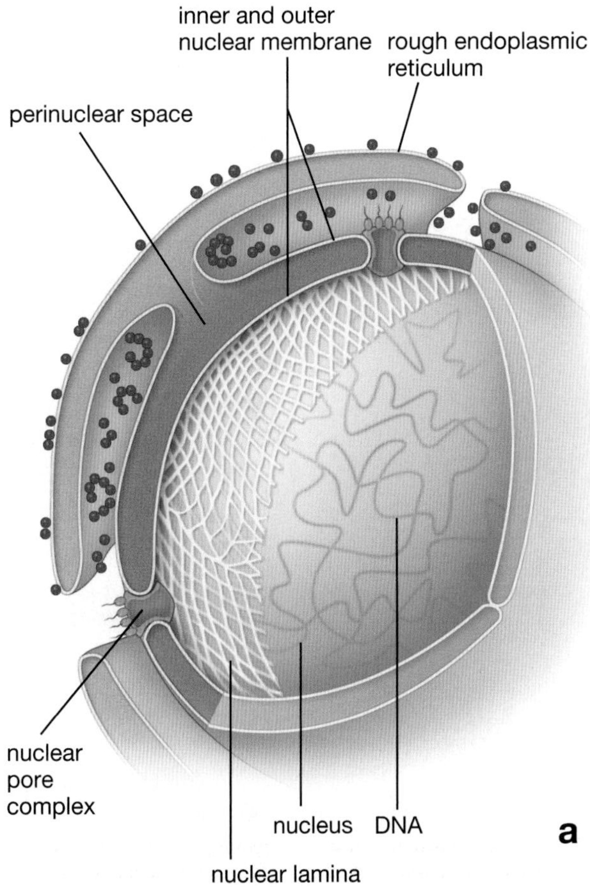

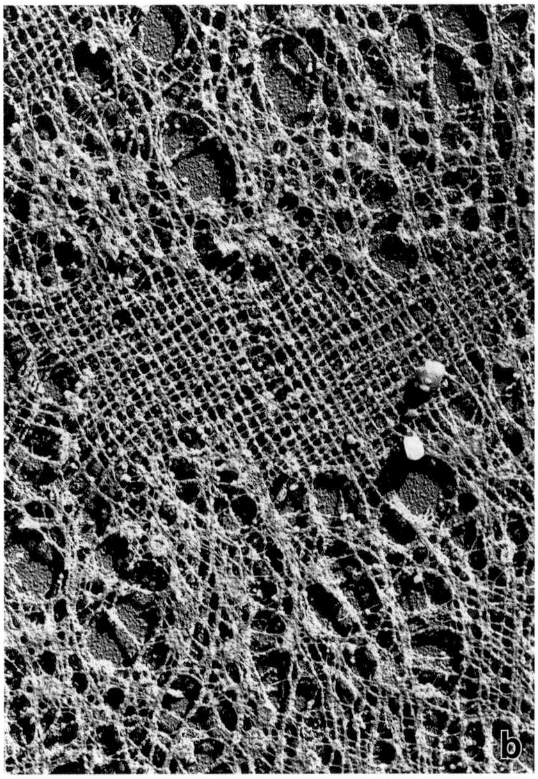

FIGURE 3.6. Structure of the nuclear lamina. a. This schematic drawing shows the structure of the nuclear lamina adjacent to the inner nuclear membrane. The cut window in the nuclear lamina shows the DNA within the nucleus. Note that the nuclear envelope is pierced by nuclear pore complexes, which allow for selective bidirectional transport of molecules between the nucleus and the cytoplasm. **b.** Electron micrograph of a portion of the nuclear lamina from a *Xenopus* oocyte. It is formed by intermediate filaments (lamins) that are arranged in a square lattice. ×43,000. (Adapted from Aebi U, Cohn J, Buhle L, et al. The nuclear lamina is a meshwork of intermediate-type filaments. *Nature*. 1986;323:560–564.)

FOLDER 3.2

CLINICAL CORRELATION: REGULATION OF CELL CYCLE AND CANCER TREATMENT

Understanding the details of **cell cycle regulation** has had an impact on cancer research and has contributed to the development of new treatments. For instance, inactivation of tumor suppressor genes has been shown to play a role in the growth and division of cancer cells. The proteins encoded by these genes are used by the cell throughout several DNA-damage checkpoints. For instance, mutations in the **breast cancer susceptibility gene 1 (BRCA-1)** and **breast cancer susceptibility gene 2 (BRCA-2)** are associated with an increased risk for bilateral breast cancer and ovarian cancer. Both protein products of these tumor suppressor genes—namely, BRCA-1 and BRCA-2 proteins—are directly involved in multiple cellular processes in response to DNA damage, including checkpoint activation, gene transcription, and repair of DNA double-strand breaks. Together with **RAD-51 protein**, which is involved in the homologous recombination and repair of DNA, they maintain the stability of the human genome. The defective BRCA proteins are unable to interact with RAD-51. By screening patients for mutations in these genes, enhanced screening and prophylactic mastectomy and/or oophorectomy can be offered to those who test positive for these mutations.

It is also now known why in some individuals, **p53 mutations** make their tumors resistant to radiotherapy. DNA damage caused by therapeutic radiation procedures is detected by DNA-damage checkpoints, which cause cancer cells to be arrested in the cell cycle. However, these cells will not die because of the absence of functional p53, which triggers apoptosis.

The major components of the lamina, as determined by biochemical isolation, are **nuclear lamins**, a specialized type of nuclear intermediate filament (see pages 73-75), and **lamin-associated proteins.** Nuclear lamina is essentially composed of lamin A and lamin C proteins that form intermediate filaments. These filaments are cross-linked into an orthogonal lattice (see Fig. 3.6), which is attached mainly via lamin B protein to the inner nuclear membrane through its interactions with lamin receptors. The family of lamin receptors includes **emerin** (34 kDa) that binds both lamin A and B; **nurim** (29 kDa) that binds lamin A; and a 58-kDa **lamin B receptor (LBR)** that, as its name suggests, binds lamin B.

Unlike other cytoplasmic intermediate filaments, lamins disassemble during mitosis and reassemble when mitosis ends. The nuclear lamina appears to serve as scaffolding for chromatin, chromatin-associated proteins, nuclear pores, and the membranes of the nuclear envelope. In addition, it is involved in nuclear organization, cell cycle regulation, differentiation, and gene expression.

Impairment in nuclear lamina architecture or function is associated with certain genetic diseases (laminopathies) and apoptosis. Mutations in **lamin A/C** cause tissue-specific diseases that affect striated muscle, adipose tissue, peripheral nerve or skeletal development, and premature aging. Two hereditary forms of **Emery–Dreifuss muscular dystrophy (EDMD)** are associated with mutations in either lamins or lamin receptors. The X-linked recessive form of EDMD is caused by mutations of **emerin**, whereas the autosomal dominant form of EDMD is caused by mutations in lamin A/C. In general, EDMD is characterized by early-onset contractures of major tendons, slowly progressive muscle weakness, muscle wasting in the upper and lower limbs, and cardiomyopathy (weakening of the heart muscle).

The nuclear envelope has an array of openings called nuclear pores.

At numerous sites, the paired membranes of the nuclear envelope are punctuated by 70- to 80-nm "openings" through the envelope. These **nuclear pores** are formed from the merging of the inner and outer membranes of the nuclear envelope. With an ordinary TEM, a diaphragm-like structure appears to cross the pore opening (Fig. 3.7). Often, a small, dense body

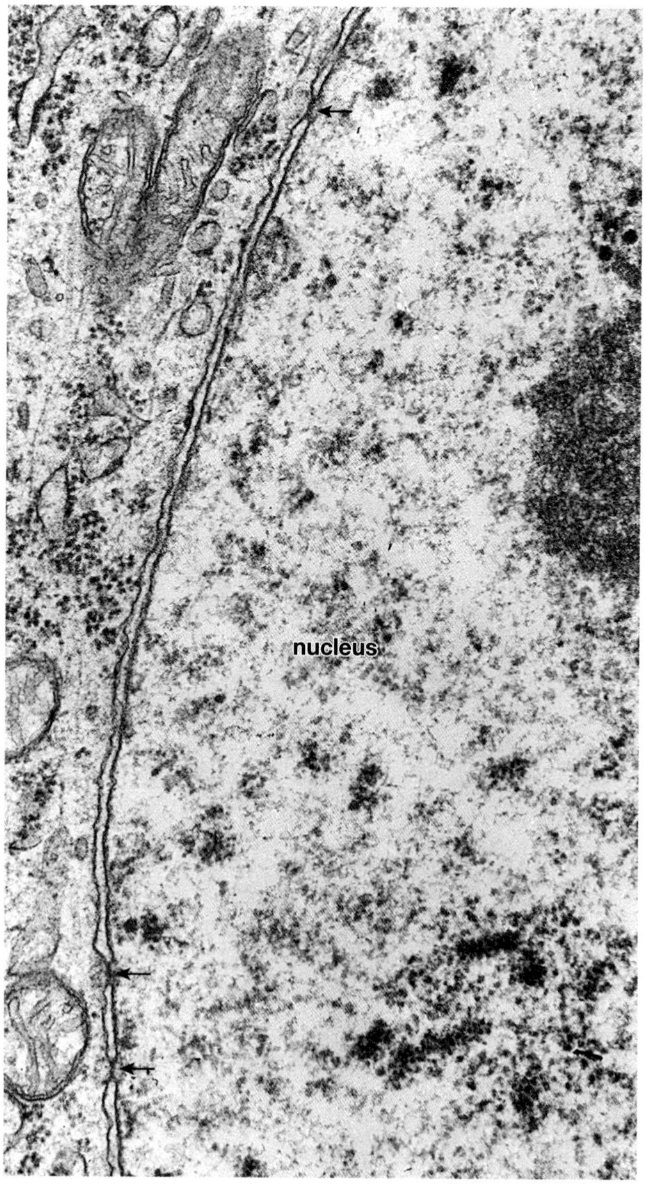

FIGURE 3.7. Electron micrograph of the nuclear envelope. Note the visible nuclear pore complexes (*arrows*) and the two membranes that constitute the nuclear envelope. At the periphery of each pore, the outer and inner membranes of the nuclear envelope appear continuous. ×30,000.

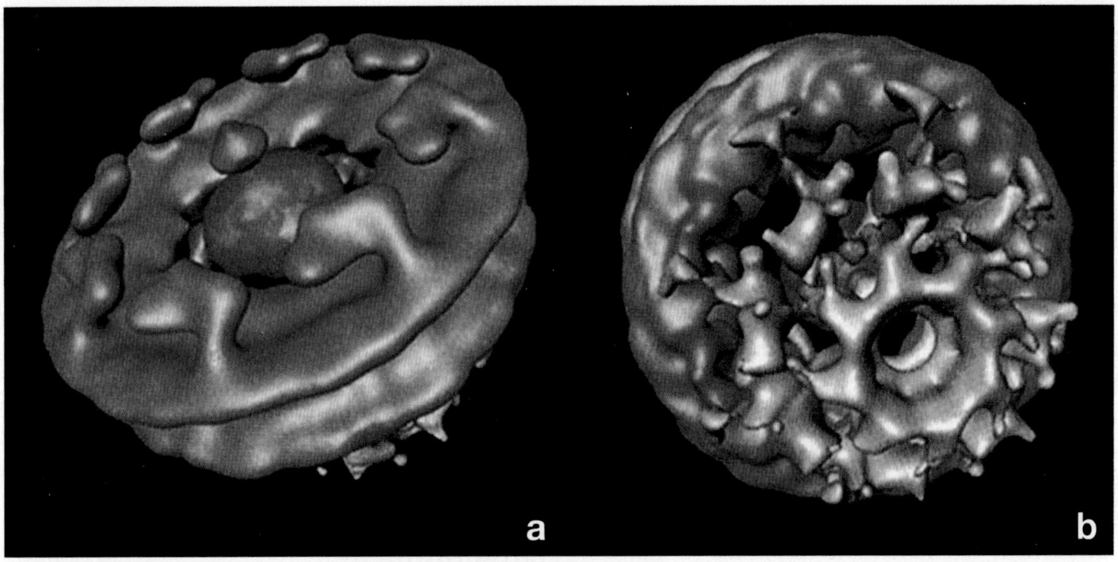

FIGURE 3.8. Cryoelectron tomography of the nuclear pore complex (NPC). These surface renderings of electron tomograms obtained from the frozen-hydrated *Dictyostelium* nuclei show detailed structure of the NPC. ×320,000. **a.** Cytoplasmic face of the NPC shows eight protein fibrils arranged around the central channel. They protrude from the cytoplasmic ring subunits and point toward the center of the structure. Note a presence of the central plug or transporter within the central pore, which represents either ribosomes or other protein transporters captured during their passage through the NPC. **b.** Nuclear face of the NPC shows the nucleoplasmic ring subunits connected by nuclear filaments with the basket indicated in *brown* color. (Adapted from Beck M, Förster F, Ecke M, et al. Nuclear pore complex structure and dynamics revealed by cryoelectron tomography. *Science.* 2004;306:1387–1390.)

is observed in the center of the opening (Fig. 3.8). Because such profiles are thought to represent either ribosomes or other protein complexes (transporters) captured during their passage through the pore at the time of fixation, the term **central plug/transporter** is commonly used to describe this feature.

With special techniques—such as negative staining and high-voltage TEM, or, recently, cryoelectron tomography—the nuclear pore exhibits additional structural detail (see Fig. 3.8). Eight multidomain protein subunits arranged in an octagonal **central framework** at the periphery of each pore form a cylinder-like structure known as the **nuclear pore complex (NPC)**. The NPC, which has an estimated total mass of 125 $\times 10^6$ Da, is composed of approximately 50 different NPC proteins collectively referred to as **nucleoporins (Nup proteins)**. This central framework is inserted between the **cytoplasmic ring** and the **nuclear ring** (Fig. 3.9). From

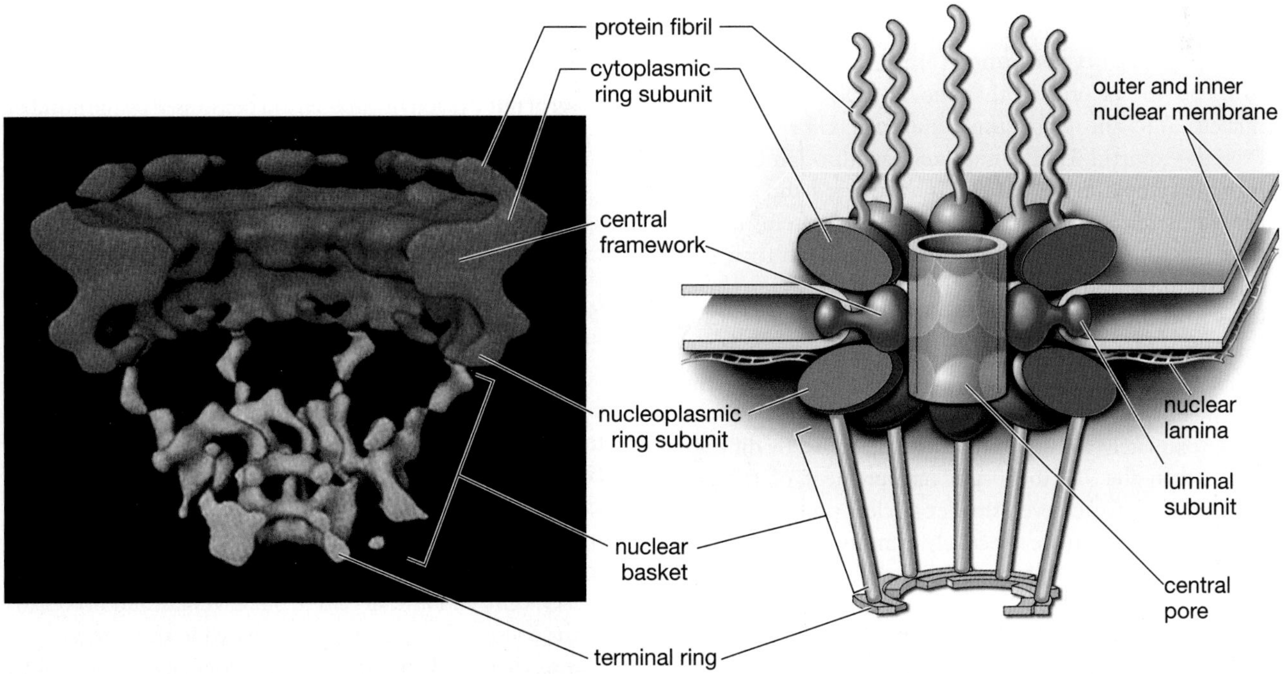

FIGURE 3.9. Sagittal section of the nuclear pore complex. Cryoelectron tomographic view of a sagittal section of the nuclear pore complex—shown in Figure 3.8—is compared with a schematic drawing of the complex. Note that the central plug/transporter has been removed from the central pore. ×320,000. Each pore contains eight protein subunits arranged in an octagonal central framework at the periphery of the pore. These subunits form a nuclear pore complex that is inserted between two cytoplasmic and nucleoplasmic rings. Eight short protein fibrils protrude from the cytoplasmic rings into the cytoplasm. The nuclear ring anchors a basket assembled from eight thin filaments joined distally into the terminal ring. The diameter of the ring can be adjusted to meet nuclear pore transport requirements. The cylindrical central framework encircles the central pore, which acts as a close-fitting diaphragm. (Adapted from Beck M, Förster F, Ecke M, et al. Nuclear pore complex structure and dynamics revealed by cryoelectron tomography. *Science.* 2004;306:1387–1390.)

the cytoplasmic ring, eight short **protein fibrils** protrude into the cytoplasm and point toward the center of the structure. The nucleoplasmic ring complex anchors a **nuclear basket** (or nuclear "cage" that resembles a fish trap) assembled from eight thin 50-nm-long filaments joined distally by an adjustable **terminal ring** 30–50 nm in diameter (see Fig. 3.9). The cylinder-shaped central framework encircles the **central pore** of the NPC, which acts as a close-fitting diaphragm or gated channel. In addition, each NPC contains one or more water-filled channels for the transport of small molecules.

The nuclear pore complex mediates bidirectional nucleocytoplasmic transport.

Various experiments have shown that the NPC regulates the passage of proteins between the nucleus and the cytoplasm. The significance of the NPC can be readily appreciated, as the nucleus does not carry out protein synthesis. Ribosomal proteins are partially assembled into ribosomal subunits in the nucleolus and are transported through nuclear pores to the cytoplasm. Conversely, nuclear proteins, such as histones and lamins, are produced in the cytoplasm and are transported through nuclear pores into the nucleus. Transport through the NPC largely depends on the size of the molecules:

- **Large molecules** (such as large proteins and macromolecular complexes) depend on the presence of an attached signal sequence called the **nuclear localization signal (NLS)** for passage through the pores. Proteins labeled with NLS destined for the nucleus then bind to a soluble cytosolic receptor called a **nuclear import receptor (importin)** that directs them from the cytoplasm to an appropriate NPC. They are then actively transported through the pore by a **GTP energy–dependent mechanism**. Export of proteins and RNA from the nucleus is similar to the import mechanism into the nucleus. Proteins that possess a **nuclear export sequence (NES)** bind in the nucleus to **exportin** (a protein that moves molecules from the nucleus into the cytoplasm) and to a GTP molecule. Protein–exportin–GTP complexes pass through the NPC into the cytoplasm where GTP is hydrolyzed and the NES protein is released. The NPC transports proteins and all forms of RNA as well as ribosomal subunits in their fully folded configurations.
- **Ions and smaller water-soluble molecules** (<9 Da) may cross the **water-filled channels** of the NPC by simple diffusion. This process is nonspecific and does not require nuclear signal proteins. The effective size of the pore is approximately 9 nm for substances that cross by diffusion rather than the 70- to 80-nm measurement of the pore boundary. However, even smaller nuclear proteins that are capable of diffusion are selectively transported, presumably because the rate is faster than with simple diffusion.

During cell division, the nuclear envelope is disassembled to allow chromosome separation and is later reassembled as the daughter cells form.

In late prophase of cell division, enzymes (kinases) are activated that cause phosphorylation of the nuclear lamins and other lamina-associated proteins of the nuclear envelope. After phosphorylation, the proteins become soluble, and the nuclear envelope disassembles. The lipid component of the nuclear membranes then disassociates from the proteins and is retained in small cytoplasmic vesicles. The replicated chromosomes then attach to the microtubules of the mitotic spindle and undergo active movement.

Reassembly of the nuclear envelope begins in late anaphase, when phosphatases are activated to remove the phosphate residues from the nuclear lamins. During telophase, the nuclear lamins begin to repolymerize and form the nuclear lamina material around each set of daughter chromosomes. At the same time, vesicles containing the lipid components of the nuclear membranes and structural membrane protein components fuse, and an envelope is formed on the surface of the already-reassembled nuclear lamina. By the end of telophase, formation of a nuclear envelope in each daughter cell is complete.

Nucleoplasm

Nucleoplasm is the material enclosed by the nuclear envelope exclusive of the chromatin and the nucleolus.

Although crystalline, viral, and other inclusions are sometimes found in the **nucleoplasm**, until recently, morphologic techniques showed it to be amorphous. It must be assumed, however, that many proteins and other metabolites reside in or pass through the nucleus in relation to the synthetic and metabolic activity of the chromatin and nucleolus. Structures that have been identified within the nucleoplasm include intranuclear lamin–based arrays, the protein filaments emanating inward from the NPCs, and the active gene–tethered RNA transcription and processing machinery itself.

■ CELL RENEWAL

Somatic cells in the adult organism may be classified according to their mitotic activity.

The level of mitotic activity in a cell can be assessed by the number of mitotic metaphases visible in a single high-magnification light microscopic field or by autoradiographic studies of the incorporation of tritiated thymidine into the newly synthesized DNA before mitosis. Using these methods, cell populations may be classified as static, stable, or renewing:

- **Static cell populations** consist of cells that no longer divide (postmitotic cells), such as cells of the central nervous system and skeletal or cardiac muscle cells. Under certain circumstances, some of these cells (i.e., cardiac myocytes) may enter mitotic division.
- **Stable cell populations** consist of cells that divide episodically and slowly to maintain normal tissue or organ structure. These cells may be stimulated by injury to become more mitotically active. Periosteal and perichondrial cells, smooth muscle cells, endothelial cells of blood vessels, and fibroblasts of the connective tissue may be included in this category.
- **Renewing cell populations** may be slowly or rapidly renewing but display regular mitotic activity. Division of such cells usually results in two daughter cells that differentiate both morphologically and functionally or two cells that remain as stem cells. Daughter cells may divide 1 or more times before their mature state is reached. The differentiated cell may ultimately be lost from the body.

- **Slowly renewing populations** include smooth muscle cells of most hollow organs, fibroblasts of the uterine wall, and epithelial cells of the lens of the eye. Slowly renewing populations may actually slowly increase in size during life, as do the smooth muscle cells of the gastrointestinal tract and the epithelial cells of the lens.
- **Rapidly renewing populations** include blood cells, epithelial cells and dermal fibroblasts of the skin, and the epithelial cells and subepithelial fibroblasts of the mucosal lining of the alimentary tract.

■ CELL CYCLE

Phases and Checkpoints Within the Cell Cycle

The cell cycle represents a self-regulated sequence of events that controls cell growth and cell division.

For renewing cell populations and growing cell populations, including embryonic cells and cells in tissue culture, the goal of the **cell cycle** is to produce two daughter cells, each containing chromosomes identical to those of the parent cell. The cell cycle incorporates two principal phases: **interphase**, representing continuous growth of the cell, and **M phase (mitosis)**, characterized by the partition of the genome. Three other phases, **G_1 (gap 1) phase, S (synthesis) phase**, and **G_2 (gap 2) phase**, further subdivide interphase (Fig. 3.10).

Rapidly renewing populations of human cells progress through the full cell cycle in about 24 hours. Throughout the cycle, several internal quality control mechanisms or **checkpoints** represented by biochemical pathways control the transition between cell cycle stages. The cell cycle stops at several checkpoints and can only proceed if certain conditions are met—for example, if the cell has reached a certain size. Checkpoints monitor and modulate the progression of cells through the cell cycle in response to intracellular or environmental signals.

The G_1 phase is usually the longest and the most variable phase of the cell cycle, and it begins at the end of the M phase.

During the **G_1 phase**, the cell gathers nutrients and synthesizes RNA and proteins necessary for DNA synthesis and chromosome replication. The cell's progress through this phase is monitored by two checkpoints: (1) the **restriction checkpoint**, which is sensitive to the size of the cell, the state of the cell's physiologic processes, and its interactions with extracellular matrix, and (2) the **G_1 DNA-damage checkpoint**, which monitors the integrity of newly replicated DNA. For instance, if the DNA has irreparable damage, the G_1 DNA-damage checkpoint detects high levels of **tumor suppressor protein p53** and does not allow the cell to enter the S phase. The cell will then most likely undergo programmed cell death (apoptosis).

The **restriction checkpoint (or "point of no return")** is the most important checkpoint in the cell cycle. At this checkpoint, the cell self-evaluates its own replicative potential before deciding to either enter the S phase and the next round of cell division or retire and leave the cell cycle. A cell that leaves the cycle in the G_1 phase usually begins **terminal differentiation (G_{TD})** by entering the **G_O phase** ("O" stands for "outside" the cycle). Thus, the G_1 phase may last for only a few hours (average 9–12 hours) in a rapidly dividing cell, or it may last a lifetime in a nondividing cell. This checkpoint is mediated by interactions between the **retinoblastoma susceptibility protein (pRb)** and a family of **essential transcription factors (E2F)** with target promoters. In normal cells, proper interaction between pRb and E2F turns off many genes and blocks cell cycle progression.

In the S phase, DNA is replicated.

Initiation of DNA synthesis marks the beginning of the **S phase**, which is about 7.5–10 hours in duration. The DNA of the cell is doubled during the S phase, and new chromatids are formed that will become obvious at prophase or metaphase of the mitotic division. Chromosome replication is

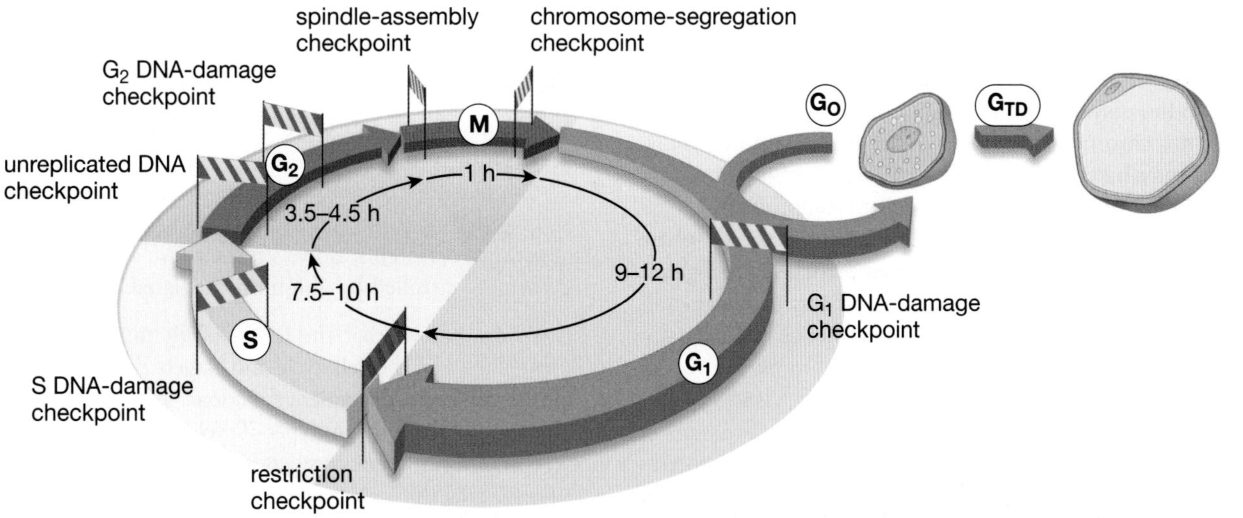

FIGURE 3.10. Cell cycle and checkpoints. This diagram illustrates the cell cycle of rapidly dividing cells in relation to DNA synthesis. After mitosis, the cell is in interphase. G_1 represents the period during which a gap occurs in DNA synthesis. S represents the period during which DNA synthesis occurs. G_2 represents a second gap in DNA synthesis. G_O represents the path of a cell that has stopped dividing; however, such a cell may reenter the cell cycle after an appropriate stimulus. The cell residing in G_O may undergo terminal differentiation (G_{TD}) and produce a population of permanent nondividing cells (e.g., mature fat cells). The average timing of each phase of the cell cycle is indicated on the diagram. Each phase contains several checkpoints that ensure that the system only proceeds to the next stage when the previous stage has been completed and no damage to the DNA is detected.

initiated at many different sites called **replicons** along the chromosomal DNA. Each replicon has a specifically assigned time frame for replication during the S phase. The presence of the **S DNA-damage checkpoint** in this phase monitors the quality of replicating DNA.

In the G_2 phase, the cell prepares for cell division.

During this phase, the cell examines its replicated DNA in preparation for cell division. It is also a period of cell growth and reorganization of cytoplasmic organelles. The **G_2 phase** may be as short as 1 hour in rapidly dividing cells or of nearly indefinite duration in some polyploid cells and in cells that are arrested in G_2 for extended periods, such as primary oocytes. Two checkpoints monitor DNA quality: the **G_2 DNA-damage checkpoint** and the **unreplicated DNA checkpoint**. The latter checkpoint prevents the progression of the cell into the M phase before DNA synthesis is complete.

Mitosis occurs in the M phase.

Mitosis nearly always includes both **karyokinesis** (division of the nucleus) and **cytokinesis** (division of the cell) and lasts about 1 hour. Mitosis takes place in several stages described in more detail later. Separation of two identical daughter cells concludes the **M phase**. The M phase possesses two checkpoints: the **spindle-assembly checkpoint**, which prevents premature entry into anaphase, and the **chromosome-segregation checkpoint**, which prevents the process of cytokinesis until all of the chromosomes have been correctly separated.

A mitotic catastrophe caused by malfunction of cell cycle checkpoints may lead to cell death and tumor cell development.

Malfunction of any of the three DNA-damage checkpoints at the G_1, S, and G_2 phases of the cell cycle and the spindle-assembly checkpoint at the M phase may lead to a **mitotic catastrophe**. Mitotic catastrophe is defined as the failure to arrest the cell cycle before or at mitosis, resulting in aberrant chromosome segregation. Under normal conditions, death in these cells will occur by activation of the apoptotic cycle. Cells that fail to execute the apoptotic cycle in response to DNA or mitotic spindle damage are likely to divide asymmetrically in the next round of cell division. This leads to the generation of **aneuploid cells** (cells containing abnormal chromosome numbers). Thus, a mitotic catastrophe may be regarded as one of the mechanisms contributing to oncogenesis (tumor cell development).

Malfunction of the restriction checkpoint at the G_1 phase may also result in malignant transformation of cells. Malignant cells lose contact inhibition, a normal process in which cells inhibit their division when they contact other cells. Malignant cells in culture continue to divide and may grow on top of one another rather than discontinuing growth when the plate is fully covered in a monolayer of cells. The malfunction of the restriction checkpoint may be facilitated by viral proteins of several cancer-causing viruses, such as the **T antigen of simian virus (SV40)** that binds to pRb. This binding alters the configuration of the pRb–T antigen complex and renders the restriction checkpoint inoperable, thus facilitating the cell's progression from the G_1 to S phase of the cell cycle. This mechanism of carcinogenesis occurs in **mesothelioma** (cancer of the lining epithelium of the pleural cavities in the thorax), **osteosarcoma** (a type of bone cancer), and **ependymoma** (a type of childhood brain tumor).

The reserve stem cell population may become activated and reenter the cell cycle.

Cells identified as **reserve stem cells** are essentially G_0 cells that may be induced to reenter the cell cycle in response to injury. Activation of these cells may occur in normal **wound healing** and in repopulation of the seminiferous epithelium after intense acute exposure of the testis to X-irradiation or during regeneration of an organ, such as the liver, after removal of a major portion. If damage is too extensive, even the reserve stem cells die, and there is no potential for regeneration.

Regulation of the Cell Cycle

Passage through the cell cycle is driven by proteins that are cyclically synthesized and degraded during each cycle.

A number of cytoplasmic protein complexes regulate and control the cell cycle. Some of these proteins function as biochemical oscillators, whose synthesis and degradation are coordinated with specific phases of the cycle. Cellular and molecular events induced during the increase and decrease of different protein levels are the basis of the cell cycle "engine." Other proteins actively monitor the quality of the molecular processes at the different checkpoints distributed throughout the cycle (described earlier). The protein complexes at the checkpoints may drive the cell into and out of the cell cycle, stimulating growth and division when conditions are favorable and, conversely, stopping or reducing the rate of cell division when conditions are not favorable.

A two-protein complex consisting of cyclin and a cyclin-dependent kinase (Cdk) helps power the cells through the checkpoints of cell cycle division.

The first milestone in understanding the regulation of the cell cycle was the discovery in the early 1970s of a protein called **maturation-promoting factor (MPF)**. MPF appeared to control the initiation of mitosis. When injected into the nuclei of immature frog oocytes, which are normally arrested in G_2, the cells immediately proceeded through mitosis. MPF was eventually found to consist of two proteins:

- **Cdc2** (also known as **Cdk-1**), a 32-kDa member of the Cdk family of proteins
- **Cyclin B**, a 45-kDa member of the cyclin family, which are key regulators of the cell cycle. Cyclins are synthesized as constitutive proteins; however, their levels during the cell cycle are controlled by ubiquitin-mediated degradation.

It is now known that the **cyclin–Cdk complex** acts at different phases of the cell cycle and targets different proteins to control cell cycle–dependent functions. Table 3.1 shows the combination of the different types of cyclins with different types of Cdks and how interactions between these two proteins affect cells progressing through the cell cycle. Passage through the cell cycle requires an increase in cyclin–Cdk activity in some phases followed by a decline of activity in other phases (Fig. 3.11). The increased activity of cyclin–Cdk is achieved by the stimulatory action of cyclins and is counterbalanced by the inhibitory action of proteins, such as Inks (inhibitors of kinase), Cips (Cdk inhibitory proteins), and Kips (kinase inhibitory proteins).

TABLE 3.1 **Functional Summary of Cyclin–Cyclin-Dependent Kinase Complexes Used in Regulating the Human Cell Cycle**

Cyclin Type	Associated Cyclin-Dependent Protein Kinase	Targeted Phase of Cell Cycle	Targeted Effector Proteins
Cyclin D	Cdk4/6	G_1 phase progression	Tumor suppressor protein p53, retinoblastoma susceptibility protein (pRb)
Cyclin E	Cdk2	S phase entry	ATM or ATR protein kinases, tumor suppressor protein p53
Cyclin A	Cdk2	S phase progression	Replication protein A, DNA polymerase, minichromosome maintenance (MCM) protein
Cyclin A	Cdk1	S phase through G_2 phase and M phase entry	Cdc25 phosphatase, cyclin B
Cyclin E	Cdk1	M phase progression	Chromatin-associated proteins, histone H1, nuclear lamins, myosin regulatory proteins, centrosomal proteins, transcription factors c-*fos/jun*, c-*myb*, *oct*-1, SWI5; p60src protein kinases, casein kinase II, c-mos protein kinases

ATM, ataxia-telangiectasia–mutated protein kinase; *ATR*, ATM- and Rad3-related kinase; *Cdk*, cyclin-dependent kinase.

Mitosis

Cell division is a crucial process that increases the number of cells, permits renewal of cell populations, and allows wound repair.

Mitosis is a process of chromosome segregation and nuclear division followed by cell division that produces two daughter cells with the same chromosome number and DNA content as the parent cell.

The term **mitosis** is used to describe the **equal partitioning of replicated chromosomes** and their genes into two identical groups. The process of cell division includes division of both the nucleus (**karyokinesis**) and the cytoplasm (**cytokinesis**). The process of cytokinesis results in distribution of nonnuclear organelles into two daughter cells. Before entering mitosis, cells duplicate their DNA. This phase of the cell cycle is called the *S* or *synthesis phase*. At the beginning of this phase, the chromosome number is **(2n)**, and the DNA content is also **(2d)**; at the end, the chromosome number remains the same **(2n)**, and the DNA content doubles to **(4d)**.

Mitosis follows the S phase of the cell cycle and is divided into four phases.

Mitosis consists of four phases (Fig. 3.12):

- **Prophase** begins as the replicated chromosomes condense and become visible. As the chromosomes continue to condense, each of the four chromosomes derived from each homologous pair consists of two **chromatids**. The sister chromatids are held together by a ring of proteins called **cohesins** and the **centromere**. In late prophase or **prometaphase** (sometimes identified as a separate phase of mitosis), the nuclear envelope begins to disintegrate into small transport vesicles and resembles the smooth ER (sER). The nucleolus, which may still be present in some cells, also completely disappears in prometaphase. In addition, a highly specialized protein complex called a **kinetochore** appears on each chromatid opposite to the centromere (Fig. 3.13). The protein complexes that form kinetochores in the centromere region of the chromatids are attached to specific repetitive DNA sequences known as **satellite DNA**, which are similar in each chromosome. Microtubules of the developing mitotic spindle attach to the kinetochores and thus to the chromosomes.
- **Metaphase** (Fig. 3.14) begins as the mitotic spindle becomes organized around the microtubule-organizing centers (MTOCs) located at opposite poles of the cell. The mitotic spindle consists of three types of microtubules:
- **Astral microtubules** that are nucleated from γ-tubulin rings in a star-like manner around each MTOC (see Fig. 2.61, page 77). They are responsible for positioning the spindle within the cell.
  - **Polar microtubules**, also originating from the MTOC. They constitute all microtubules that lie between spindle poles that are not connected to kinetochores. Polar microtubules from opposite poles interact with each other via motor proteins in an antiparallel manner pushing the spindle poles apart to ensure its bipolarity.
  - **Kinetochore microtubules** that emanate from the MTOC to probe the cytoplasm in search of kinetochores. When a kinetochore is finally captured by a kinetochore microtubule, it is pulled toward the MTOC. This allows for attachment of additional microtubules to the kinetochore. The kinetochore is capable of binding between 30 and 40 microtubules to each

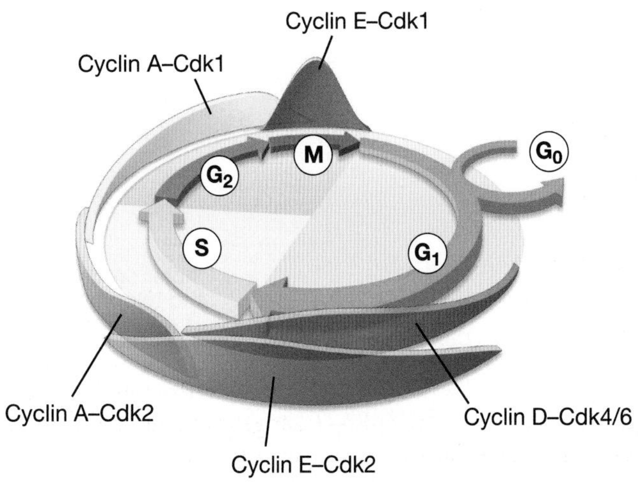

FIGURE 3.11. Regulation of the cell cycle by cyclin–Cdk complexes. This diagram shows the changing pattern of cyclin–Cdk activities during different phases of the cell cycle. *Cdk*, cyclin-dependent kinase.

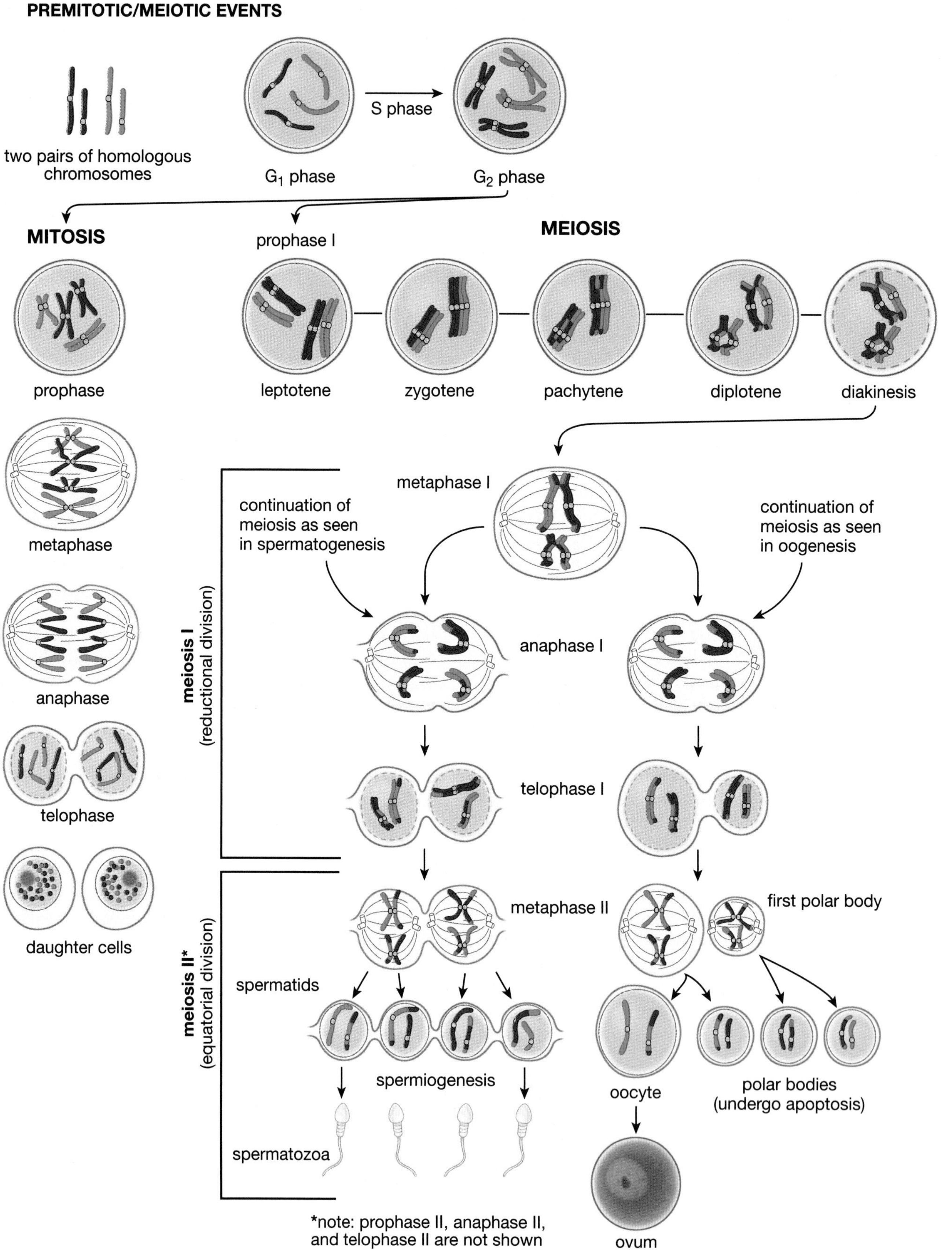

FIGURE 3.12. Comparison of mitosis and meiosis in an idealized cell with two pairs of chromosomes (2n). The chromosomes of maternal and paternal origin are depicted in *red* and *blue*, respectively. The mitotic division produces daughter cells that are genetically identical to the parental cell (2n). The meiotic division, which has two components, a reductional division and an equatorial division, produces a cell that has only two chromosomes (1n). In addition, during the chromosome pairing in prophase I of meiosis, chromosome segments are exchanged, leading to further genetic diversity. It should be noted that in humans, the first polar body does not divide. Division of the first polar body does occur in some species.

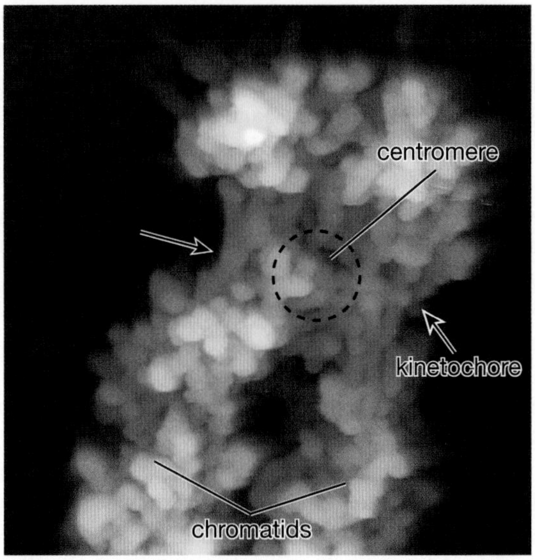

FIGURE 3.13. Atomic force microscopic image of the centromeric region of a human metaphase chromosome. The facing surfaces of two sister chromatids visible in this image form the centromere, a point of junction of both chromatids. On the opposite side of the centromere, each chromatid possesses a specialized protein complex, the kinetochore, which serves as an attachment point for kinetochore microtubules of the mitotic spindle. Note that the surface of the chromosome has several protruding loop domains formed by chromatin fibrils anchored into the chromosome scaffold. ×40,000. (Courtesy of Dr. Tatsuo Ushiki.)

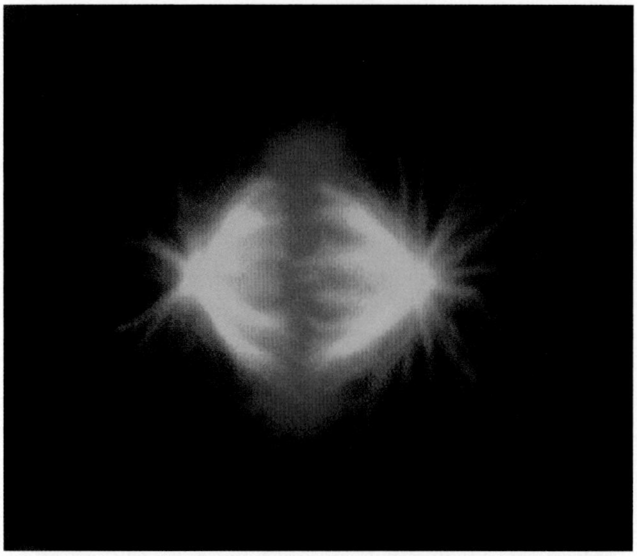

FIGURE 3.14. Mitotic spindle in metaphase. Using indirect immunofluorescence techniques, the mitotic spindle in a *Xenopus* XL-177 cell was labeled with an antibody against α-tubulin conjugated with fluorescein (*green*). DNA was stained *blue* with fluorescent DAPI stain. In metaphase, the nuclear membrane disassembles, DNA is condensed into chromosomes, and microtubules form a mitotic spindle. The action of microtubule-associated motor proteins on the microtubules of the mitotic spindle creates the metaphase plate along which the chromosomes align in the center of the cell. ×1,400. (Courtesy of Dr. Thomas U. Mayer.)

chromatid. In some species, kinetochore microtubules are formed by MTOC-independent mechanisms that involve kinetochores. Kinetochore microtubules and their associated motor proteins direct the movement of the chromosomes to a plane in the middle of the cell, the **equatorial** or **metaphase plate**.

- **Anaphase** (Fig. 3.15) begins at the initial separation of sister chromatids. This separation occurs when the cohesins that have been holding the chromatids together break down. The chromatids then begin to separate and are pulled to opposite poles of the cell by the molecular motors (dyneins) sliding along the kinetochore microtubules toward the MTOC.
- **Telophase** (Fig. 3.16) is marked by reconstitution of the nuclear envelope around the chromosomes at each pole. The chromosomes uncoil and become indistinct, except at regions that will remain condensed in the interphase nucleus. The nucleoli reappear, and the cytoplasm divides (cytokinesis) to form two daughter cells. Cytokinesis begins with the furrowing of the plasma membrane midway between the poles of the mitotic spindle. Separation at the **cleavage furrow** is achieved by a **contractile ring** consisting of a very thin array of actin filaments positioned around the perimeter of the cell. Within the ring, **myosin II** molecules are assembled into small filaments that interact with the actin filaments, causing the ring to contract. As the ring tightens, the cell is pinched into two daughter cells. Because the chromosomes in the daughter cells contain identical copies of the duplicated DNA, the daughter cells are genetically identical and contain the same kind and number of chromosomes. The daughter cells are **(2d)** in DNA content and **(2n)** in chromosome number.

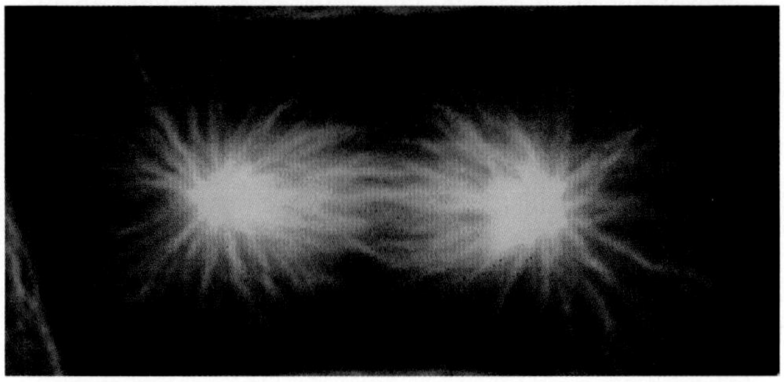

FIGURE 3.15. Mitotic spindle in anaphase. This immunofluorescent image comes from the same cell type and identical preparation as in Figure 3.13. Connections that hold the sister chromatids together break at this stage. The chromatids are then moved to opposite poles of the cell by microtubule-associated molecular motors (dyneins and kinesins) that slide along the kinetochore microtubules toward the centriole and are also pushed by the polar microtubules (visible between the separated chromosomes) away from each other, thus moving opposite poles of the mitotic spindle into the separate cells. ×1,400. (Courtesy of Dr. Thomas U. Mayer.)

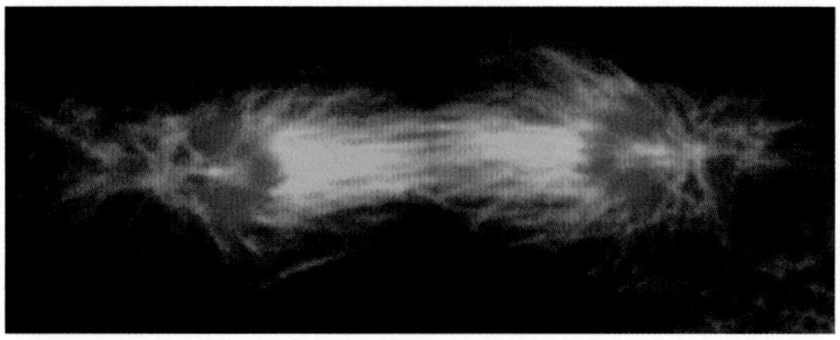

FIGURE 3.16. Mitotic spindle in telophase. In this phase, DNA is segregated, and a nuclear envelope is reconstituted around the chromosomes at each pole of the mitotic spindle. The cell divides into two during cytokinesis. In the middle of the cell, actin, septins, myosins, microtubules, and other proteins gather as the cell establishes a ring of proteins that will constrict, forming a bridge between the two sides of what was once one cell. The chromosomes uncoil and become indistinct, except at regions that remain condensed in interphase. The cell types and preparation are the same as those in Figures 3.13 and 3.14. ×1,400. (Courtesy of Dr. Thomas U. Mayer.)

Meiosis

Meiosis involves two sequential nuclear divisions followed by cell divisions that produce gametes containing half the number of chromosomes and half the DNA found in somatic cells.

The **zygote** (the cell resulting from the fusion of an ovum and a sperm) and all the somatic cells derived from it are **diploid (2n)** in chromosome number; thus, their cells have two copies of every chromosome and every gene encoded on this chromosome. These chromosomes are called **homologous chromosomes** because they are similar, but not identical; one set of chromosomes is of maternal origin, the other is from the male parent. The **gametes**, having only one member of each chromosome pair, are described as **haploid (1n)**. During gametogenesis, reduction in chromosome number to the haploid state (23 chromosomes in humans) occurs through **meiosis**, a process that involves two successive divisions, the second of which is not preceded by an S phase. This reduction is necessary to maintain a constant number of chromosomes in a given species. Reduction in chromosome number to **(1n)** in the first meiotic division is followed by reduction in DNA content to the haploid **(1d)** amount in the second meiotic division.

During meiosis, the chromosome pair may exchange chromosome segments, thus altering the genetic composition of the chromosomes. This genetic exchange, called *crossing-over*, and the random assortment of each member of the chromosome pairs into haploid gametes give rise to infinite genetic diversity.

The cytoplasmic events associated with meiosis differ in the male and female.

The nuclear events of meiosis are the same in males and females, but the cytoplasmic events are markedly different. Figure 3.12 illustrates the key nuclear and cytoplasmic events of meiosis as they occur in spermatogenesis and oogenesis. The events of meiosis through metaphase I are the same in both sexes. Therefore, the figure illustrates the differences in the process as they diverge after metaphase I.

In males, the two meiotic divisions of a **primary spermatocyte** yield four structurally identical, although genetically unique, haploid **spermatids**. Each spermatid has the capacity to differentiate into a **spermatozoon**. In contrast, in females, the two meiotic divisions of a **primary oocyte** yield one haploid **ovum** and three haploid **polar bodies**. The ovum receives most of the cytoplasm and becomes the functional gamete. The polar bodies receive very little cytoplasm and degenerate.

The nuclear events of meiosis are similar in males and females.

Meiosis consists of two successive mitotic divisions without the additional **S phase** between the two divisions. During the S phase that precedes meiosis, DNA is replicated forming sister chromatids (two parallel strands of DNA) joined together by the centromere. The DNA content becomes **(4d)**, but the chromosome number remains the same **(2n)**. The cells then undergo a **reductional division (meiosis I)** and an **equatorial division (meiosis II)**.

During **meiosis I**, as the name **reductional division** implies, the chromosome number is reduced from diploid **(2n)** to haploid **(1n)**, and the amount of DNA is reduced from **(4d)** to **(2d)**. During prophase I, double-stranded chromosomes condense, and homologous chromosomes (normally, one inherited from the mother and one from the father) are paired at centromeres. At this point, recombination of genetic material between the maternal and paternal chromosome pairs may occur. In metaphase I, the homologous chromosomes with their centromeres line up along the equator of the mitotic spindle and, in anaphase I, are separated and distributed to each daughter cell. This results in reduction of both the chromosome number **(1n)** and the DNA to the **(2d)** amount.

No DNA replication precedes **meiosis II**. The division during meiosis II is always **equatorial** because the number of chromosomes does not change. It remains at **(1n)**, although the amount of DNA represented by the number of chromatids is reduced to **(1d)**. During metaphase II, each chromosome aligns along the equator of the mitotic spindle, and at anaphase II, sister chromatids are separated from each other. Thus, each chromosome splits into two single-stranded chromosomes that are then distributed to each haploid daughter cell.

Phases in the process of meiosis are similar to the phases of mitosis.

Prophase I

The prophase of meiosis I is an extended phase in which **pairing** of homologous chromosomes, **synapsis** (close association of homologous chromosomes), and **recombination** of genetic material on homologous chromosomes are observed. Prophase I is subdivided into the following five stages (see Fig. 3.12).

- **Leptotene.** This stage is characterized by the condensation of chromatin and appearance of chromosomes. Sister chromatids also condense and become connected with each other by **meiosis-specific cohesion complexes (Rec8p)**. At this phase, pairing of homologous chromosomes of maternal and paternal origin is initiated. Homologous pairing can be described as a process in which chromosomes actively search for each other. After finding their mates, they align themselves side by side with a slight space separating them.
- **Zygotene.** Synapsis, the close association of homologous chromosomes, begins at this stage and continues throughout pachytene. This process involves the formation of a **synaptonemal complex**, a tripartite structure that binds the chromosomes together. The synaptonemal complex is often compared to railroad tracks with an additional third rail positioned in the middle between two others. The cross ties in this track are represented by the transverse filaments that bind the scaffold material of both homologous chromosomes together.
- **Pachytene.** At this stage, synapsis is complete. **Crossing-over** occurs early in this phase and involves transposition of DNA strands between two different chromosomes.
- **Diplotene.** Early in this stage, the synaptonemal complex dissolves, and the chromosomes condense further. Homologous chromosomes begin to separate from each other and appear to be connected by newly formed junctions between chromosomes called **chiasmata** (sing., *chiasma*). Sister chromatids still remain closely associated with each other. Chiasmata indicate that crossing-over may have occurred.
- **Diakinesis.** The homologous chromosomes condense and shorten to reach their maximum thickness, the nucleolus disappears, and the nuclear envelope disintegrates.

Metaphase I

Metaphase I is similar to the metaphase of mitosis, except that the paired chromosomes are aligned at the **equatorial plate** with one member on either side. The homologous chromosomes are still held together by chiasmata. At late metaphase, chiasmata are cleaved, and the chromosomes separate. Once the nuclear envelope has broken down, the spindle microtubules begin to interact with the chromosomes through the multilayered protein structure, the **kinetochore**, which is usually positioned near the centromere (see Fig. 3.13). The chromosomes undergo movement to ultimately align their centromeres along the equator of the spindle.

Anaphase I and telophase I

Anaphase I and **telophase I** are similar to the same phases in mitosis, except that the centromeres do not split. The sister chromatids, held together by cohesin complexes and by the centromere, remain together. A maternal or paternal member of each homologous pair, now containing exchanged segments, moves to each pole. **Segregation** or **random assortment** occurs because the maternal and paternal chromosomes of each pair are randomly aligned on one side or the other of the metaphase plate, thus contributing to genetic diversity. At the completion of meiosis I, the cytoplasm divides. Each resulting daughter cell (a **secondary spermatocyte** or **oocyte**) is haploid in chromosome number **(1n)** and contains one member of each homologous chromosome pair. The cell is still diploid in DNA content **(2d)**.

Meiosis II

After meiosis I, the cells quickly enter meiosis II without passing through an S phase. **Meiosis II** is an equatorial division and resembles mitosis. During this phase, the proteinase enzyme **separase** cleaves the cohesion complexes between the sister chromatids. Cleavage of the cohesin complexes in the region of the centromere releases the bond between both centromeres. This cleavage allows the sister chromatids to separate at anaphase II and move to opposite poles of the cell. During meiosis II, the cells pass through prophase II, metaphase II, anaphase II, and telophase II. These stages are essentially the same as those in mitosis, except that they involve a haploid set of chromosomes **(1n)** and produce daughter cells that have only haploid DNA content **(1d)**. Unlike the cells produced by mitosis, which are genetically identical to the parent cell, the cells produced by meiosis are genetically unique.

■ CELL DEATH

In humans, as in all other multicellular organisms, cell death, survival, proliferation, and differentiation represent fundamental life processes. The rates of cell proliferation and cell death determine net cell production. An abnormality in any of these rates can cause **disorders of cell accumulation** (e.g., hyperplasia, cancer, autoimmune diseases) or **disorders of cell loss** (atrophy, degenerative diseases, AIDS, ischemic injury). In cancer, the ratio of cell death to cell division is altered, resulting in a net gain of malignant tissue. Therefore, the balance (homeostasis) between cell production and cell death must be carefully maintained (Fig. 3.17).

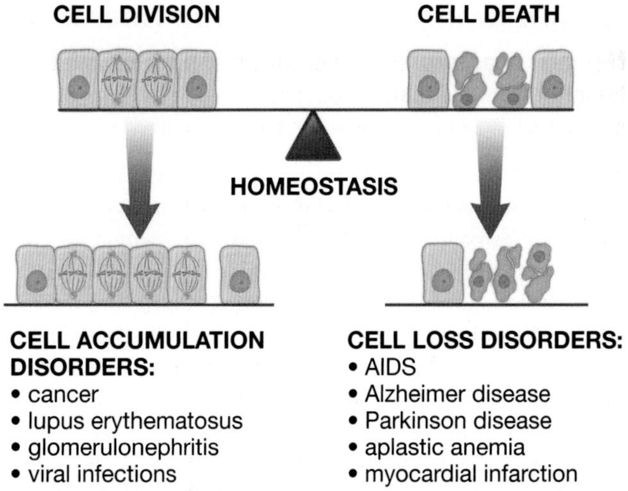

FIGURE 3.17. Schematic diagram showing the relationship between cell death and cell division. Under normal physiologic conditions (homeostasis), the rates of cell division and cell death are similar. If the rate of cell death is higher than that of cell division, then a net loss of cell number will occur. Such conditions are categorized as cell loss disorders. When the situation is reversed and the rate of cell division is higher than the rate of cell death, then the net gain in cell number will be prominent, leading to a variety of disorders of cell accumulation.

Cell death may occur as a result of acute cell injury or an internally encoded suicide program.

Cell death may result from accidental cell injury or mechanisms that cause cells to self-destruct. Recently, several novel cell death modalities have been identified and characterized based on their stimuli, molecular mechanisms, and morphologies. Microscopic studies of dying cells in the tissue reveal that different forms of cell death can occur simultaneously and that dying cells can share features of different types of cell death (some cell death modalities share overlapping but not identical signaling pathways). There are many different classifications of cell death mechanisms that are rather complex. In this section, a simplified classification based on cell morphology, molecular machinery, and types of stimuli is presented.

Two major mechanisms of cell death can be categorized into programmed or nonprogrammed cell death based on their specific signaling mechanisms:

- **Programmed cell death** is a physiologic process driven by highly regulated intracellular signal transduction pathways. The term *programmed cell death* is applied broadly to any cell death mediated by an intracellular death program, irrespective of the trigger mechanism or molecular machinery involved. However, this internally encoded suicide program can be further divided into **apoptotic cell death**, which is controlled by **caspases** and preserves the integrity of cell membranes, and **nonapoptotic cell death**, which is a caspase-independent process that likely compromises cell membrane integrity.
- **Nonprogrammed cell death** or **necrosis** is a pathologic process of accidental cell death. It occurs when cells are exposed to an unfavorable physical or chemical environment (e.g., hypothermia, hypoxia, radiation, low pH, cell trauma) that causes acute cellular injury and damage to the plasma membrane. Rapid **cell swelling** and **lysis** are two characteristic features of this process.

Nonprogrammed Cell Death: Necrosis

Necrosis begins with an impairment of the cell's ability to maintain homeostasis.

Death by **necrosis** occurs when the cell is exposed to extreme environmental conditions or adverse or excessive stimuli that cause acute cellular injury. The injury is accompanied by damage to the plasma membrane, which may also result from infections (e.g., bacterial or viral), toxins, or physical injury, leading to cytoplasmic swelling and the subsequent loss of organelle function. As a result of cell injury, damage to the cell membrane leads to an influx of water and disruption of ion pumps with an influx of extracellular ions (e.g., Ca^{2+}). Intracellular organelles, such as the mitochondria, rER, and nucleus, undergo irreversible changes caused by cell swelling and cell membrane rupture (cell lysis). As a result of the breakdown of the plasma membrane, the cytoplasmic contents, including lysosomal enzymes, are released into the extracellular space. Therefore, necrotic cell death is often associated with extensive surrounding tissue damage and an **intense inflammatory response** (Fig. 3.18). Necrosis is often observed in ischemia and trauma. It is considered a messy, chaotic, and destructive process that leads to the unavoidable demise of the cell otherwise not destined to die.

Programmed Apoptotic Cell Death: Apoptosis and Anoikis

Apoptosis is a mode of caspase-dependent cell death that occurs under normal physiologic conditions.

Apoptosis *[Gr., falling off, as petals from flowers]* is a physiologic process in which cells that are no longer needed are eliminated from the organism. This process involves a series of enzymatic events controlled by specific enzymes known as **caspases**, leading to cell shrinkage, membrane blebbing, DNA fragmentation, and loss of organelle function. Apoptosis may occur during normal embryologic development or other normal physiologic processes, such as follicular atresia in the ovaries. Cells can initiate their own death by activating an internally encoded suicide program (intrinsic mitochondrial pathways), or it can be initiated by extrinsic pathways (death receptors or interaction with cytotoxic T lymphocytes). Apoptosis is characterized by controlled autodigestion, which maintains cell membrane integrity; thus, the cell "dies with dignity" without spilling its contents and damaging its neighbors.

Certain cells or their secretions found in the immune system are toxic to other cells (e.g., **cytotoxic T lymphocytes**, **natural killer [NK] cells**); they initiate processes that destroy designated cells (e.g., cancer-transformed or virus-infected cells). This death modality does not involve one specific mechanism. For example, cell death mediated by cytotoxic T lymphocytes, in which proteins called *perforins* and *granzymes* are inserted into the plasma membrane, combines some aspects of both necrosis (alterations of plasma membrane) and apoptosis (stimulation of **caspase-3 enzyme**). For an overview of apoptosis and necrosis, see Table 3.2.

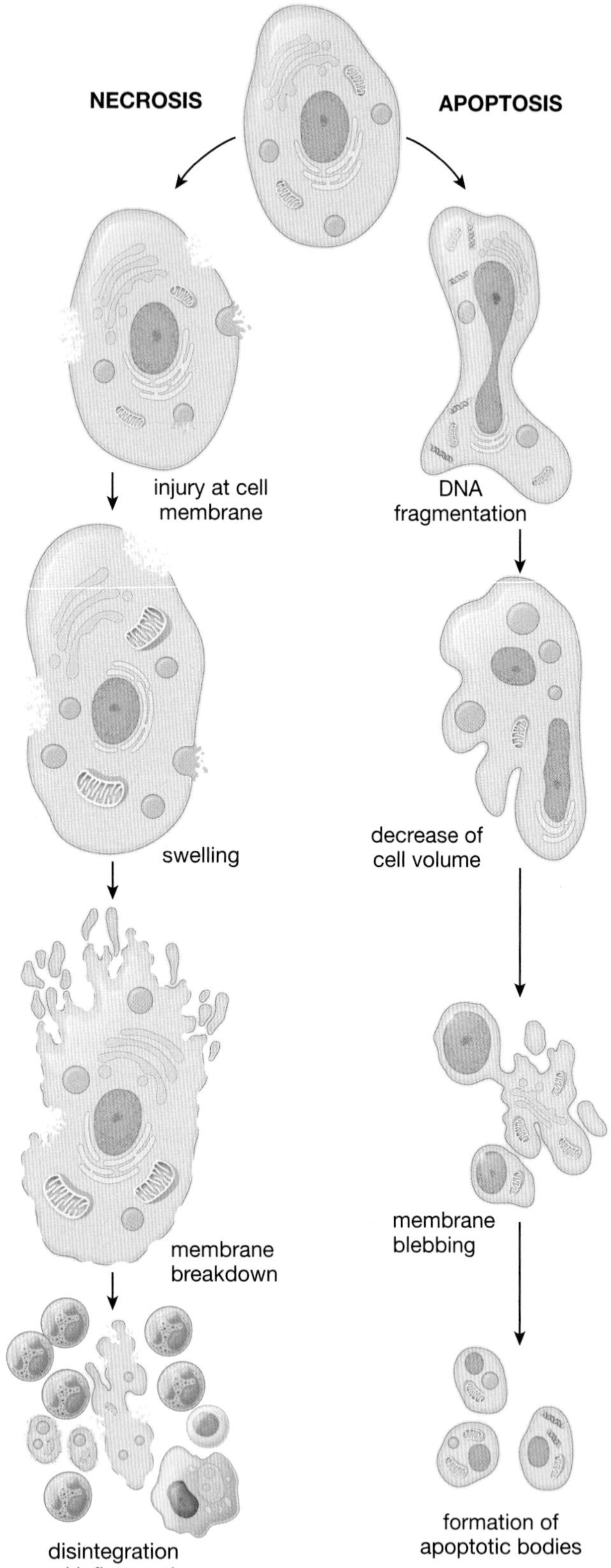

FIGURE 3.18. Schematic diagram of changes occurring in necrosis and apoptosis. This diagram shows the major steps in necrosis and apoptosis. In necrosis (*left side*), breakdown of the cell membrane results in an influx of water and extracellular ions, causing the organelles to undergo irreversible changes. Lysosomal enzymes are released into the extracellular space, causing damage to neighboring tissue and an intense inflammatory response. In apoptosis (*right side*), the cell undergoes characteristic morphologic and biochemical changes such as DNA fragmentation, decrease in cell volume, membrane blebbing without loss of membrane integrity, and formation of apoptotic bodies, causing cell breakage. Apoptotic bodies are later removed by phagocytotic cells without causing an inflammatory reaction.

Apoptosis is characterized by a series of typical morphologic and biochemical features.

In **apoptosis**, the cell is an active participant in its own demise ("cellular suicide"). This process is activated by a variety of extrinsic and intrinsic signals. Cells undergoing apoptosis show the following characteristic morphologic and biochemical features (see Fig. 3.18):

- **DNA fragmentation** occurs in the nucleus and is an irreversible event that commits the cell to die. DNA fragmentation is a result of Ca^{2+}- and Mg^{2+}-dependent activation of nuclear endonucleases. These enzymes selectively cleave DNA, generating small oligonucleosomal fragments. Nuclear chromatin then aggregates, and the nucleus may divide into several discrete fragments bounded by the nuclear envelope.
- **Decrease in cell volume** is achieved by shrinking of the cytoplasm. The cytoskeletal elements become reorganized in bundles parallel to the cell surface. Ribosomes become clumped within the cytoplasm, the rER forms a series of concentric whorls, and most of the endocytotic vesicles fuse with the plasma membrane.
- **Loss of mitochondrial function** is caused by changes in the permeability of the mitochondrial membrane channels. The integrity of the mitochondrion is breached, the mitochondrial transmembrane potential drops, and the electron transport chain is disrupted. Proteins from the mitochondrial intermembrane space, such as **cytochrome *c*** and **SMAC/DIABLO** (second mitochondria-derived activator of caspases/direct inhibitor of apoptosis-binding protein with low isoelectric point [pI]), are released into the cytoplasm to activate a cascade of proteolytic enzymes called **caspases** that are responsible for dismantling the cell. The regulated release of cytochrome *c* and SMAC/DIABLO suggests that mitochondria, under the influence of regulatory **Bcl-2 proteins** (see page 106), are the decision makers for initiating apoptosis. Thus, many researchers view mitochondria as either the "headquarters for the leader of a crack suicide squad" or a "high-security prison for the leaders of a military coup."
- **Membrane blebbing** results from cell membrane alterations. One alteration is related to translocation of certain molecules (e.g., phosphatidylserine) from the cytoplasmic surface to the outer surface of the plasma membrane. These changes cause the plasma membrane to change its physical and chemical properties and lead to blebbing without loss of membrane integrity (see Fig. 3.18).
- **Formation of apoptotic bodies**, the final step of apoptosis, results in cell breakage (Fig. 3.19a–c). These membrane-bounded extracellular vesicles originate from the cytoplasmic bleb containing organelles and nuclear material. They are rapidly removed without a trace by phagocytotic cells. The removal of apoptotic bodies is so efficient that no inflammatory response is elicited. Apoptosis occurs more than 20 times faster than mitosis; therefore, it is challenging to find apoptotic cells in a routine H&E preparation (Fig. 3.19d).

TABLE 3.2 Overview of Characteristic Features Distinguishing Necrosis From Apoptosis

Features of Dying Cells	Necrosis	Apoptosis
Cell swelling	+	–
Cell shrinkage	–	+
Damage to the plasma membrane	+	–
Plasma membrane blebbing	–	+
Aggregation of chromatin	–	+
Fragmentation of the nucleus	–	+
Oligonucleosomal DNA fragmentation	–	+
Random DNA degradation	+/–	–
Release of cytochrome *c* and SMAC/DIABLO from mitochondria	–	+
Caspase cascade activation	–	+

Mitotic catastrophe is a programmed apoptotic cell death that occurs during cell division.

- **Mitotic catastrophe** (discussed earlier in the chapter) is a type of cell death that occurs during mitosis. It results from a combination of cellular damage and malfunction of several **cell cycle checkpoints**, such as the G_1, S, and G_2 DNA-damage checkpoints or the spindle-assembly checkpoint (see pages 97-98). Failure to arrest the cell cycle before mitosis occurs causes problems with chromosome separation. Cell death occurs during the metaphase/anaphase transition and is characterized by the activation of caspase-2 in response to DNA damage, which triggers the apoptotic pathway and cell death.

Apoptosis is regulated by external and internal stimuli.

Apoptotic processes can be activated by a variety of external and internal stimuli. Some factors, such as **tumor necrosis factor (TNF)**, acting on cell membrane receptors, trigger apoptosis by recruiting and activating the caspase cascade. Consequently, the TNF receptor (TNFr) belongs to the so-called **death receptor** family that can induce apoptosis. Other external activators of apoptosis include transforming growth factor β (TGF-β), certain neurotransmitters, free radicals, oxidants, and ultraviolet (UV) ionizing radiation.

Caspases represent a class of cysteine proteases that convey the apoptotic signal in a form of proteolytic cascade, with caspases cleaving and activating other caspases that then degrade other cellular targets that lead to cell death. The upper end of the caspase cascade includes **caspase-8** and **caspase-9**, whereas **caspase-3**, **capsase-6**, and **caspase-7** are downstream effector caspases that cleave cellular targets.

Apoptosis is also activated by the insertion of pore-forming proteins **perforins** and **granzymes** (serine proteases) into the cell membrane of virus-infected and/or virus-transformed cells by cytotoxic T lymphocytes. Granzyme acts directly on caspase-3 enzyme and activates proapoptotic members of the

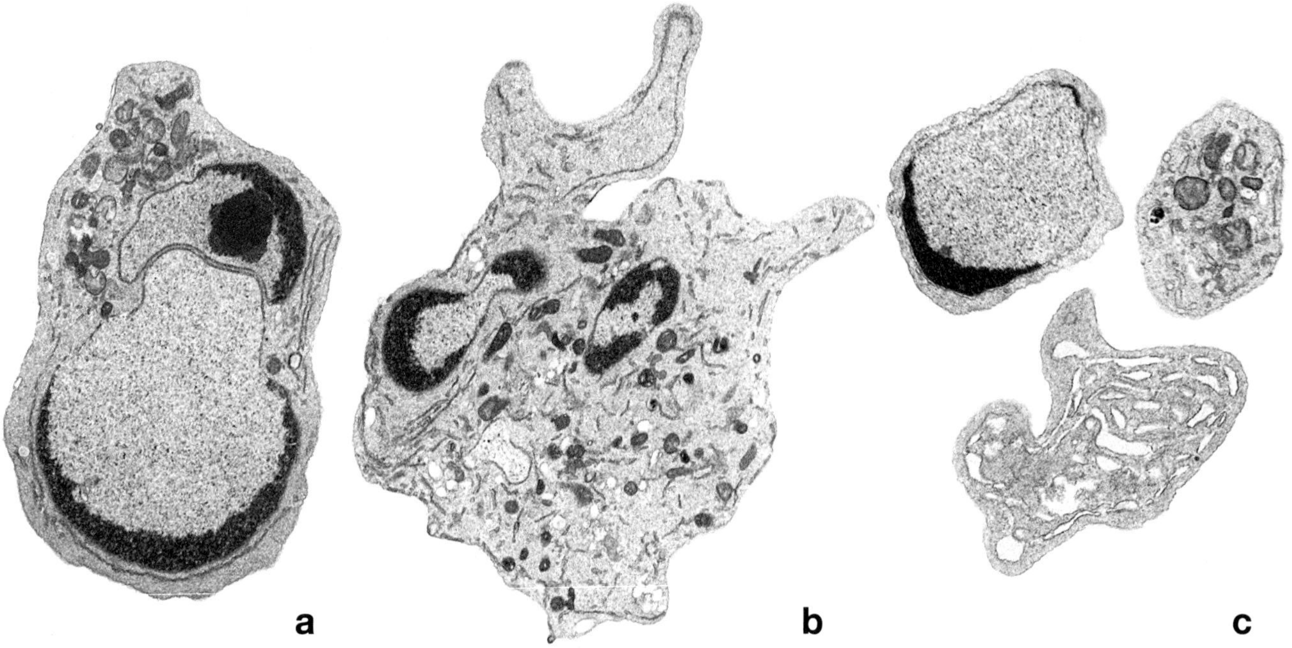

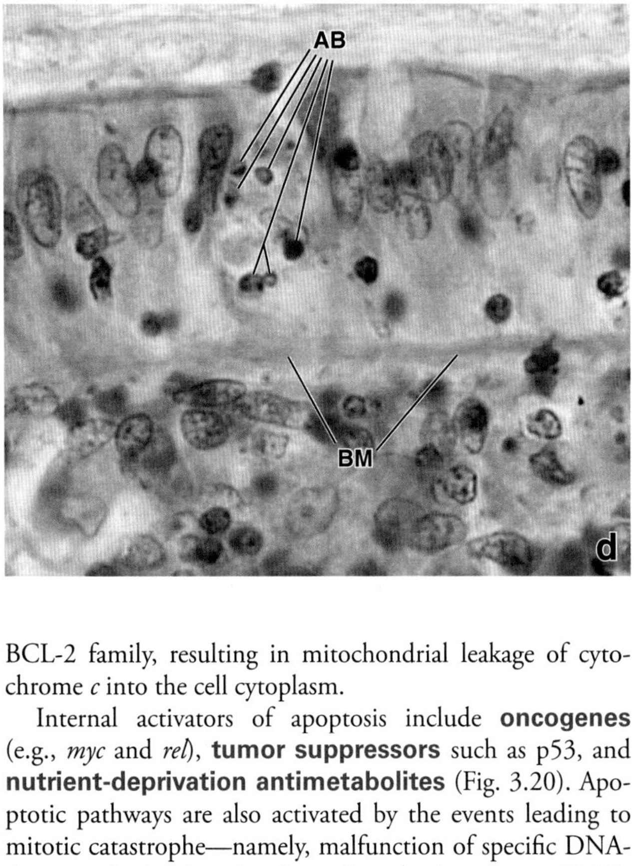

FIGURE 3.19. Electron micrographs of apoptotic cells. a. This electron micrograph shows an early stage of apoptosis in a lymphocyte. The nucleus is already fragmented, and the irreversible process of DNA fragmentation is turned on. Note the regions containing condensed heterochromatin adjacent to the nuclear envelope. ×5,200. **b.** Further fragmentation of DNA. The heterochromatin in one of the nuclear fragments (*left*) begins to bud outward through the envelope, initiating a new round of nuclear fragmentation. Note the reorganization of the cytoplasm and budding of the cytoplasm to produce apoptotic bodies. ×5,200. **c.** Apoptotic bodies containing fragments of the nucleus, organelles, and cytoplasm. These bodies will eventually be phagocytosed by cells from the mononuclear phagocyte system. ×5,200. (Courtesy of Dr. Scott H. Kaufmann.) **d.** This photomicrograph taken with light microscopy of intestinal epithelium from the human colon shows apoptotic bodies (*AB*) within a single layer of absorptive cells. *BM*, basement membrane. ×750.

BCL-2 family, resulting in mitochondrial leakage of cytochrome *c* into the cell cytoplasm.

Internal activators of apoptosis include **oncogenes** (e.g., *myc* and *rel*), **tumor suppressors** such as p53, and **nutrient-deprivation antimetabolites** (Fig. 3.20). Apoptotic pathways are also activated by the events leading to mitotic catastrophe—namely, malfunction of specific DNA-damage checkpoints in the cell cycle (see pages 97-98). Mitotic catastrophe is accompanied by chromatin condensation, mitochondrial release of cytochrome *c*, activation of the caspase cascade, and DNA fragmentation.

Apoptosis can be inhibited by signals from other cells and the surrounding environment via the so-called *survival factors*, including growth factors, hormones such as estrogen and androgens, neutral amino acids, zinc, and interactions with extracellular matrix proteins. The functions of activated caspases are inhibited by the binding of **apoptosis inhibitors (IAPs)**, which are regulated by the proapoptotic SMAC/DIABLO complex. Several cellular and viral proteins act as caspase inhibitors; for instance, nerve cells contain neuronal apoptosis inhibitory protein (NAIP) to protect them from premature apoptosis.

The Bcl-2 family of proteins is a key factor in the regulation of the apoptotic process.

The most important regulatory function in apoptosis is ascribed to internal signals from the **Bcl-2 (B-cell lymphoma 2) family** of proteins. Members of this family consist of proapoptotic and antiapoptotic members that determine the life or death of a cell.

- The **proapoptotic** members of the Bcl-2 family of proteins include **Bad** (Bcl-2–associated death promoter), **Bax** (Bcl-2–associated X protein), **Bak** (Blc-2 antagonist killer), **Bid** (Bcl-2–interacting domain), and **Bim** (Bcl-2–interacting mediator of cell death). Bak or Bax is required to form apoptotic pores in the mitochondrial outer membrane to allow for the release of cytochrome *c*.

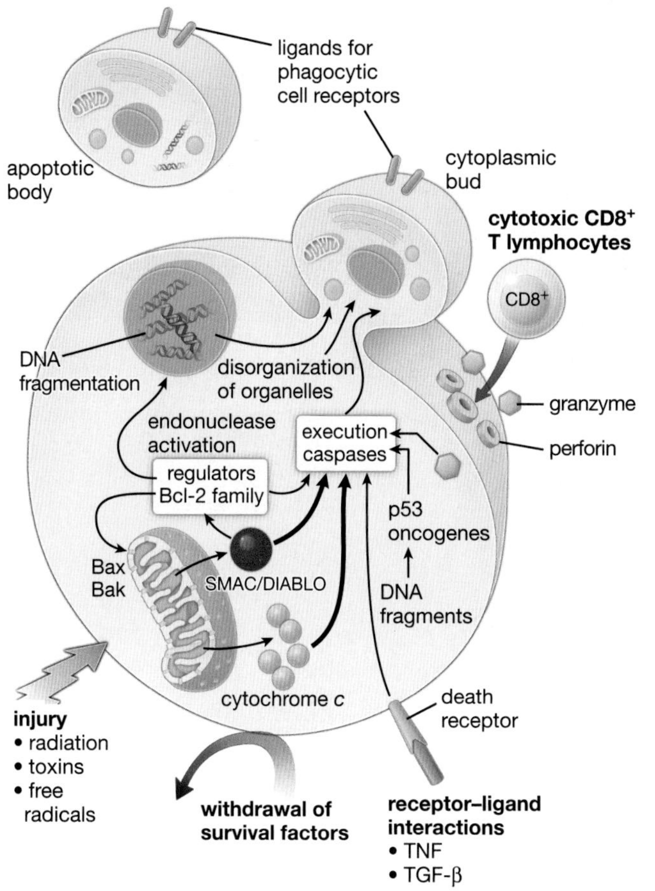

FIGURE 3.20. Schematic drawing of mechanisms leading to apoptosis. Both external and internal stimuli can trigger apoptosis by activating the enzymatic caspase cascade. Many external activators act on the cell to initiate signals leading to apoptosis; note that tumor necrosis factor (TNF) and transforming growth factor β (TGF-β) act through a "death receptor." Another external perforin/granzyme pathway is shown in which apoptosis is triggered by the action of cytotoxic ($CD8^+$) T lymphocytes. Controlled release of cytochrome *c* and SMAC/DIABLO from mitochondria is an important internal step in the activation of the intrinsic (mitochondrial) pathway of apoptosis. Anoikis shares identical signaling pathways with apoptosis; however, it is triggered by inadequate or inappropriate cell-matrix interactions. *SMAC/DIABLO*, second mitochondria-derived activator of caspases/direct inhibitor of apoptosis-binding protein with low isoelectric point.

- The **antiapoptotic** member of the Bcl-2 family of proteins is **Bcl-xL** (B-cell lymphoma-extra large). Bcl-xL blocks the action of Bax and Bak, thus preventing the release of cytochrome *c* and subsequent activation of the caspase cascade.

Proteins from the Bcl-2 family interact to suppress or propagate their own activity by acting on the downstream activation of various execution steps of apoptosis. They also act independently on mitochondria to regulate the release of cytochrome *c* and SMAC/DIABLO, the most potent apoptosis-inducing agents. Tumor cells may acquire resistance to apoptosis by expressing antiapoptotic proteins or by the downregulation or mutation of proapoptotic mediators.

Anoikis is a form of apoptosis induced by a lack of cell-to-extracellular matrix interactions.

Anoikis *[Gr., homeless wanderer]* is a cell detachment–induced apoptosis that prevents detached cells from further growth and reattachment to the extracellular matrix. Anoikis shares identical pathways with apoptosis; however, it is triggered by inadequate or inappropriate cell-to-extracellular matrix interactions. Under these conditions, the cell cycle is arrested, and apoptosis initiated. Signals from the extracellular matrix are sensed by **integrins** that form an integral part of anchoring cell-to-extracellular matrix junctions (see pages 145-150). Because of their connections with the cell cytoskeleton, integrins are involved in the intrinsic pathway signaling mechanisms that control apoptosis, DNA-damage responses, and the function of death receptors. Defects in these signaling pathways lead to anoikis, which is triggered by activating the proapoptotic Bcl-2 family of proteins. Anoikis leads to the release of cytochrome *c* and SMAC/DIABLO into the cytosol, which, in turn, leads to the activation of the caspase enzymatic cascade and initiation of apoptosis. In **metastatic cancer**, cells develop mechanisms to survive the anoikis process, including changes in integrin receptor types, activation of antiapoptotic factors, oncogene activation, and growth factor receptor signaling.

Programmed Nonapoptotic Cell Death

Several forms of programmed nonapoptotic cell death are characterized by ruptured cell membrane, pathologic changes in organelles, and involvement of immune cells with no caspase cascade activation.

Several different forms of programmed cell death do not conform to the classic definitions of programmed apoptotic cell death. By contrast, nonapoptotic cell death is mostly characterized by a lack of plasma membrane integrity and caspase independence. Under microscopic examination, the affected cells exhibit different cytoplasmic and nuclear features, such as large cytoplasmic vacuoles (autophagy, entosis, and paraptosis), mitochondrial deformations (mitoptosis), changes in morphology of immune cells (pyroptosis and NETosis), as well as other changes resembling necrosis (necroptosis) (Fig. 3.21). These programmed nonapoptotic cell death modalities include the following:

- **Autophagy** is a regulated cellular process that enables cells to recycle their contents through lysosomal degradation of their own components. It starts when an intracellular membrane (often part of the sER cistern) wraps around an organelle or portion of the cytoplasm, forming a closed double membrane–bound vacuole. This vacuole, called an **autophagosome**, is initially devoid of any lysosomal enzymes until it fuses with a lysosome and initiates digestion. For a detailed description of three pathways utilized in autophagy, see pages 50-52.
- **Entosis** *[Gr., inside]* is a nonapoptotic cell death process in which one cell can actively internalize a similar cell that became detached from the extracellular matrix. After internalization, the "swallowed" cell remains alive within the vacuole of the host cell until it is either degraded by the **lysosomal mechanism** or released. Entosis is a specific receptor-regulated process that involves **cadherins** and the formation of anchoring cell-to-cell junctions between two similar types of cells (i.e., within the epithelium). This process should be distinguished from **cell cannibalism**, which is a nonspecific process observed in metastatic tumors that involves cancer cells "eating" and killing immune cells that are directed against them.

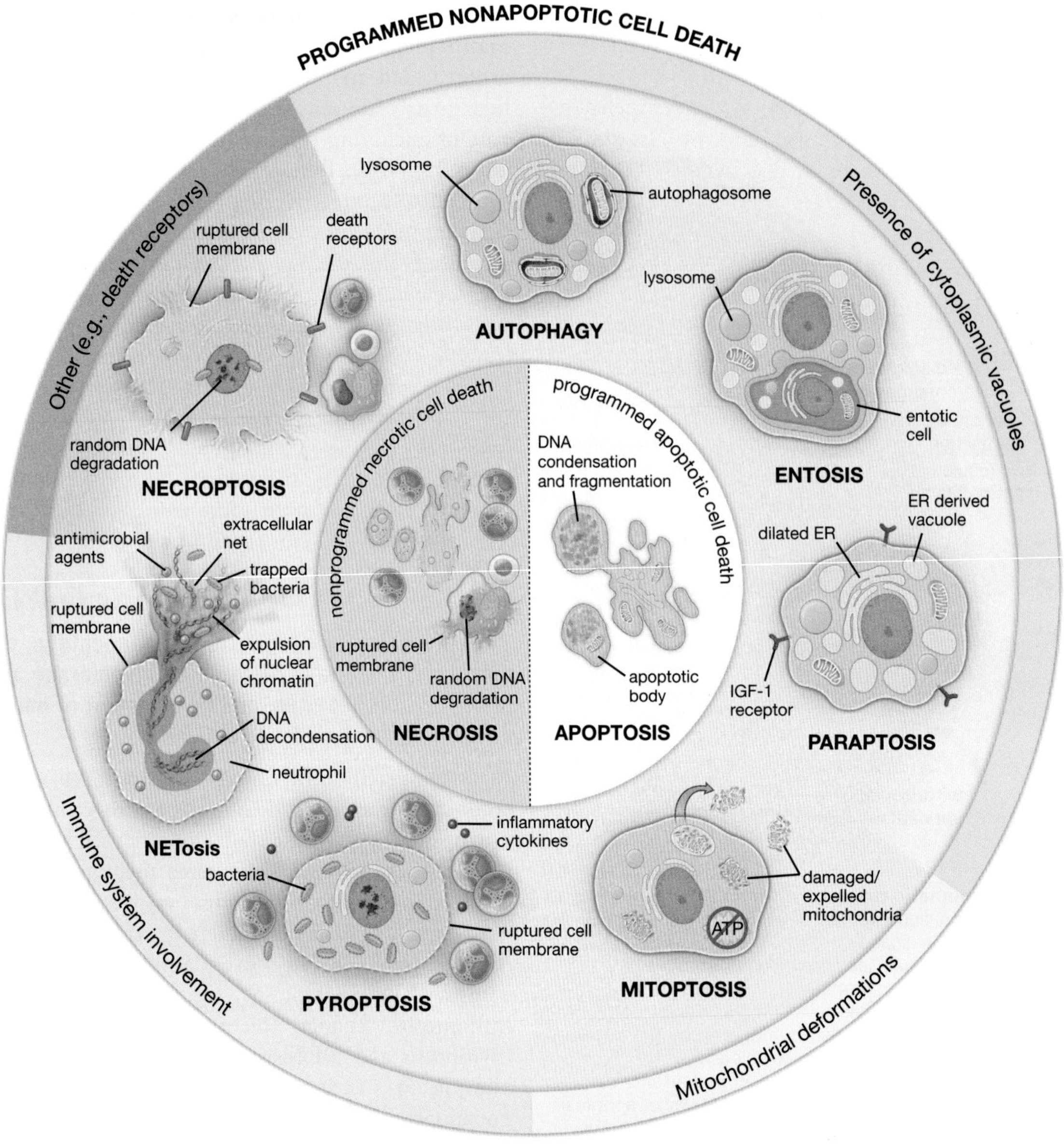

FIGURE 3.21. Classification of programmed nonapoptotic cell deaths. This diagram shows the current classification of programmed nonapoptotic cell death modalities based on their signal dependency, morphologic characteristics, and molecular mechanisms. For comparison, necrosis (nonprogrammed cell death) and apoptosis (programmed cell death) are shown in the *center*. *ER*, endoplasmic reticulum; *IGF*, insulin growth factor 1.

- **Paraptosis** is an alternative, nonapoptotic cell death that is induced by growth factor receptors (i.e., insulin growth factor [IGF-1] receptor). In contrast to apoptosis, cell death is not mediated by caspases but by **mitogen-activated protein kinases (MAPKs)**. On a cellular level, paraptosis is characterized by the formation of multiple large vacuoles within the cell cytoplasm along with mitochondrial swellings.
- **Mitoptosis** represents a programmed process of fragmentation and fusion of the mitochondria with diminished production of adenosine triphosphate (ATP). This process is also known as "**mitochondrial suicide**." Mitochondrial fragments undergo degradation by autophagic vacuole or become mitoptotic bodies expelled by the cell. Extensive mitochondrial fragmentation leads to a lack of ATP production and cell death.
- **Pyroptosis** *[pyro, Gr., fire; ptosis, Gr., to fall]* is a form of cell death induced by infection with certain microorganisms that generates intense inflammatory reactions in immune cells. This pathway is uniquely dependent on the **caspase-1 enzyme**, which is not involved in the caspase cascade in apoptotic cell death. Caspase-1 activates inflammatory cytokines such as interleukin-1 (IL-1) and IL-18 that mediate intense inflammatory reactions in surrounding tissue.
- **Neutrophil extracellular trap–associated cell death (NETosis)** is a unique form of cell death triggered by the presence of pathogens within neutrophils. Upon recognition of phagocytosed pathogens, some neutrophils modify their nuclear histone structures, resulting in chromatin decondensation and disruption of the nuclear membrane. The nuclear chromatin enters the cytoplasm and is subsequently released by the compromised plasma membrane into the extracellular matrix, forming an extracellular net (Fig. 3.21). This process leads to neutrophil death known as "**suicidal NETosis.**" The decondensed chromatin fibers and histones combined with antimicrobial granular contents form a large web of extracellular

strands (**neutrophils extracellular traps**) that capture and kill a wide range of pathogens (bacteria, viruses, fungi, parasites).

- **Necroptosis** is a regulated caspase-independent cell death mechanism that can be induced in different cell types. It is initiated by the activation of **the TNFRs (or death receptors)** and the **Fas signaling pathway**. Although it occurs under regulated conditions, necroptotic cell death is characterized by the same morphologic features as unregulated necrotic death. **Necrostatin-1** is a specific inhibitor of necroptosis that significantly reduces ischemic damage in affected tissues.

Different cell death modalities are not isolated from each other.

The different cell death modalities interact with each other. For instance, the activation of death receptors can stimulate both apoptosis and necroptosis. The destruction of mitochondria during mitoptosis can lead to autophagic cell death or apoptotic cell death. In general, necrosis-like cell death is associated with membrane rupture and may occur in several programmed nonapoptotic cell death modalities. In such conditions, the release of intracellular inflammatory factors can give rise to an inflammatory tissue response, such as that observed in necroptosis, NETosis, or pyroptosis.

HISTOLOGY 101 NOTEBOOK

CELL NUCLEUS

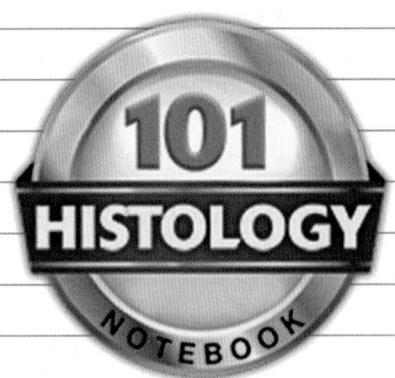

OVERVIEW OF THE NUCLEUS

- The **nucleus** is a membrane-limited compartment that contains the **genome** (genetic information) in eukaryotic cells.
- The nucleus of a nondividing cell consists of **chromatin** (contains DNA) and the **nucleolus** (site of rRNA synthesis), which are suspended in the **nucleoplasm** and surrounded by the **nuclear envelope**.

NUCLEAR CHROMATIN

- **Chromatin**, a complex of DNA and associated proteins, is responsible for basophilic staining of the nucleus in hematoxylin and eosin (h&E) preparation.
- Two forms of chromatin are found in the nucleus: a dispersed form called **euchromatin** and a condensed form called **heterochromatin**.
- **Nucleosomes** are the smallest units of chromatin structure. They represent the initial folding of the DNA molecule.
- In dividing cells, chromatin is condensed and organized into discrete bodies called **chromosomes.**

NUCLEOLUS

- The **nucleolus** is the site of **rRNA synthesis** and initial **ribosomal assembly**, and it is involved in regulation of the cell cycle.
- The nucleolus has three distinct regions: **fibrillar centers** (include DNA loops of chromosomes containing rRNA genes), **fibrillar material** (includes actively transcribed ribosomal genes), and **granular material** (site of initial ribosomal assembly).

NUCLEAR ENVELOPE

- The **nuclear envelope**, formed by two membranes with a **perinuclear cisternal space** between them, separates the nucleoplasm from the cytoplasm. The **outer nuclear membrane** binds ribosomes and is continuous with the rough-surfaced endoplasmic reticulum (rER) membrane. The **inner nuclear membrane** is supported by the **nuclear (fibrous) lamina.**
- The **nuclear lamina** is composed of **nuclear lamins**, a specialized type of intermediate filaments, and **lamin-associated proteins**. Lamins disassemble during mitosis and reassemble when mitosis ends.
- The nuclear envelope has an array of openings called **nuclear pores**. Nuclear pores contain a cylinder-like structure known as the **nuclear pore complex (NPC)**, which mediates bidirectional nucleocytoplasmic transport.

CELL CYCLE

- The **cell cycle** represents a self-regulated sequence of events that controls cell growth and cell division. Progress through the cell cycle is monitored at different **checkpoints**.
- The **G_1 phase** is usually the longest and the most variable phase of the cell cycle; it begins at the end of mitosis (M phase). During the G_1 phase, the cell gathers nutrients and synthesizes RNA and proteins necessary for DNA synthesis and chromosome replication. This phase also contains the most important checkpoint in the cell cycle, the **restriction point**, at which the cell evaluates its own replicative potential.
- In the **S phase**, DNA is replicated, and the quality of DNA synthesis is monitored at the **S DNA-damage checkpoint**.
- In the **G_2 phase**, the cell prepares for division during mitosis (M phase) and continues to assess the quality of the newly synthesized DNA (at the **G_2 DNA-damage checkpoint** and the **unreplicated DNA checkpoint**).
- Mitosis occurs in the M phase and is controlled by the spindle-assembly and chromosome-segregation checkpoints.
- Passage through the cell cycle is driven by a two-protein complex consisting of **cyclin** and **cyclin-dependent kinase (Cdk)**. These proteins are synthesized and degraded at regular intervals during each cycle.

MITOSIS

- **Mitosis** is a process of chromosome segregation, nuclear division, and eventual cell division that produces two daughter cells with the same chromosome number and DNA content as the parent cell.
- Mitosis **follows the S phase** of the cell cycle and contains four phases: **prophase**, during which chromosomes condense and become visible, the nuclear envelope disassembles, and the mitotic spindle develops from microtubules; **metaphase**, which involves the alignment of chromosomes in the equatorial plate; **anaphase**, during which the sister chromatids begin to separate and are pulled to opposite poles of the cell; and **telophase**, which involves the reconstruction of the nuclear envelope and the division of cytoplasm.
- **Mitosis** ends with the formation of two daughter cells that are genetically identical (containing the **same number of chromosomes and amount of DNA**).

MEIOSIS

- **Meiosis** involves two sequential nuclear divisions followed by cell divisions that produce gametes containing half the amount of chromosomes and DNA found in somatic cells.
- During the prophase of **meiosis I** (reductional division), homologous chromosomes are paired, and the recombination of genetic material occurs between maternal and paternal pairs. These pairs (with exchanged segments) form two daughter cells that contain a haploid number of chromosomes and a diploid amount of DNA.
- **Meiosis II** occurs quickly without passing through the S phase. The second meiotic division separates the sister chromatids into two final cells, each containing a **haploid number of chromosomes and a haploid amount of DNA**.

CELL DEATH

- **Cell death** may occur due to acute cell injury **(nonprogrammed necrosis)** or programmed apoptotic **(apoptosis, anoikis)** or programmed nonapoptotic cell death.
- **Apoptosis** occurs under normal physiologic conditions to eliminate defective or senescent cells without an inflammatory response by the tissue. Cells retain cell membrane integrity, and death occurs in a caspase-dependent manner.
- Molecular regulation of apoptotic cell death involves a cascade of events controlled by the proapoptotic members of the **Bcl-2 family** of proteins. They increase the permeability of the mitochondrial membrane, causing the release of **cytochrome *c*** and **SMAC/DIABLO** into the cytoplasm.
- In **programmed apoptotic cell death**, cytochrome c and SMAC/DIABLO activate the cascade of cytoplasmic proteases called **caspases**. They dismantle the cell by digesting cytoplasmic proteins.
- **Anoikis** is a form of apoptosis that is induced by a lack of cell-to-extracellular matrix interactions.
- **Programmed nonapoptotic cell death** involves cell death that is mostly characterized by membrane rupture and caspase independence. Examples include autophagy, entosis, paraptosis, mitoptosis, pyroptosis, NETosis, and necroptosis.

4 TISSUES: CONCEPT AND CLASSIFICATION

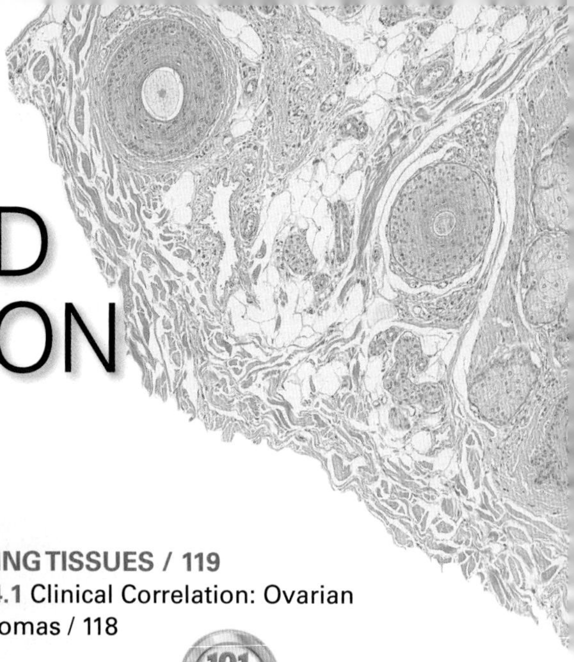

■ OVERVIEW OF TISSUES

Tissues are aggregates or groups of cells organized to perform one or more specific functions.

At the light microscope level, the **cells** and **extracellular components** of the various organs of the body exhibit a recognizable and often distinctive pattern of organization. This organized arrangement reflects the cooperative effort of cells performing a particular function. An organized aggregation of cells that functions in a collective manner is called a **tissue** *[Fr., tissu, woven; L., texo, to weave]*.

Although it is frequently said that the cell is the basic functional unit of the body, it is really the tissues, through the collaborative efforts of their individual cells, that are responsible for maintaining body functions. Cells within tissues are connected to each other by specialized junctions (cell-to-cell adhesions, pages 139-150). Cells also sense their surrounding extracellular environment and communicate with each other by specialized intercellular junctions (gap junctions, pages 150-153); facilitating this collaborative effort allows the cells to operate as a functional unit. Other mechanisms that permit the cells of a given tissue to function in a unified manner include specific membrane receptors that generate responses to various stimuli (i.e., hormonal, neural, or mechanical).

Despite their disparate structure and physiologic properties, all organs are made up of only four basic tissue types.

The tissue concept provides a basis for understanding and recognizing the many cell types within the body and how they interrelate. Despite the variations in general appearance, structural organization, and physiologic properties of the various body organs, the tissues that compose them are classified into four basic types:

- **Epithelium (epithelial tissue)** covers body surfaces, lines body cavities, and forms glands.
- **Connective tissue** underlies or supports the other three basic tissues, both structurally and functionally.
- **Muscle tissue** is made up of contractile cells and is responsible for movement.
- **Nerve tissue** receives, transmits, and integrates information from outside and inside the body to control the activities of the body.

Each basic tissue is defined by a set of general morphologic characteristics or functional properties. Each type may be further subdivided according to the specific characteristics of its various cell populations and any special extracellular substances that may be present.

In classifying the basic tissues, two different definitional parameters are used. The basis for the definition of epithelial and connective tissue is primarily morphologic; for muscle and nerve tissue, it is primarily functional. Moreover, the same parameters exist in designating the tissue subclasses. For example, whereas muscle tissue itself is defined by its function, it is subclassified into smooth and striated categories: a purely morphologic distinction, not a functional one. Another kind of contractile tissue, myoepithelium, functions as muscle tissue but is typically designated epithelium because of its location.

For these reasons, tissue classification cannot be reduced to a simple formula. Rather, students are advised to learn the features or characteristics of the different cell aggregations that define the four basic tissues and their subclasses.

■ EPITHELIUM

Epithelium is characterized by close cell apposition and presence at a free surface.

Epithelial cells, whether arranged in a single layer or in multiple layers, are always contiguous with one another. In addition, they are usually joined by specialized cell-to-cell junctions that create a selective barrier between the external environment and the underlying connective tissue. The **intercellular space** between epithelial cells is minimal and devoid of any structure, except where junctional attachments are present.

Free surfaces are characteristic of the exterior of the body, the outer surface of many internal organs, and the lining of the body cavities and tubes that ultimately communicate with the exterior of the body. The enclosed body cavities and tubes include the pleural, pericardial, and peritoneal cavities as well as the cardiovascular system. All of these structures are lined by epithelium. The epithelium also forms **glands** and their ducts that help secrete their products onto a free surface or into the lumen of a tube.

Classifications of epithelium are usually based on the shape of the cells and the number of cell layers rather than on function. Cell shapes include squamous (flattened), cuboidal, and columnar. Layers are described as **simple** (single layer) or **stratified** (multiple layers). Figure 4.1 shows epithelia from three sites. Two of them (see Fig. 4.1a and b) are simple epithelia (i.e., one cell layer) that line a free surface that is exposed to the lumen of the structure. The major distinction between these two simple epithelia is the shape of the cells: cuboidal (see Fig. 4.1a) versus columnar (see Fig. 4.1b). The third example (see Fig. 4.1c) is a stratified squamous epithelium that contains multiple layers of cells. Only the top layer of squamous cells is in contact with the lumen; the other cells are connected with each other by specialized cell-to-cell occluding and anchoring junctions or to the underlying connective tissue by specialized cell-to-extracellular matrix–anchoring junctions expressed in the lower dark-stained bottom layer of the epithelium.

The free surface of the epithelium exhibits special structural **surface modifications** that perform specific functions. Simple epithelia may possess microvilli, stereocilia, or cilia. Stratified epithelia may be keratinized on the exterior of the body or nonkeratinized within the lumen of internal organs.

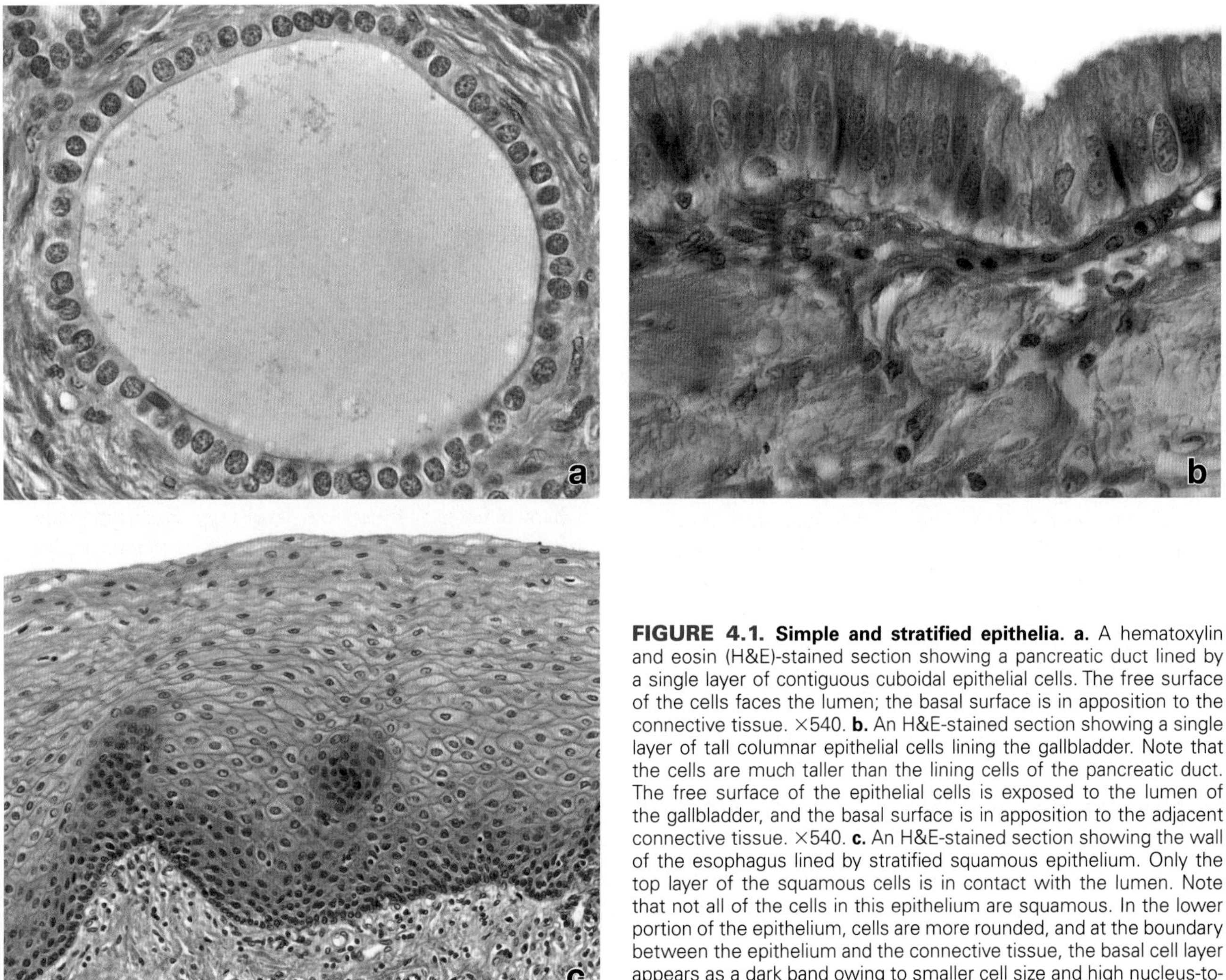

FIGURE 4.1. Simple and stratified epithelia. a. A hematoxylin and eosin (H&E)-stained section showing a pancreatic duct lined by a single layer of contiguous cuboidal epithelial cells. The free surface of the cells faces the lumen; the basal surface is in apposition to the connective tissue. ×540. **b.** An H&E-stained section showing a single layer of tall columnar epithelial cells lining the gallbladder. Note that the cells are much taller than the lining cells of the pancreatic duct. The free surface of the epithelial cells is exposed to the lumen of the gallbladder, and the basal surface is in apposition to the adjacent connective tissue. ×540. **c.** An H&E-stained section showing the wall of the esophagus lined by stratified squamous epithelium. Only the top layer of the squamous cells is in contact with the lumen. Note that not all of the cells in this epithelium are squamous. In the lower portion of the epithelium, cells are more rounded, and at the boundary between the epithelium and the connective tissue, the basal cell layer appears as a dark band owing to smaller cell size and high nucleus-to-cytoplasmic ratio. ×240.

All epithelia rest on the **basal lamina**, the structural attachment site for overlying epithelial cells and underlying connective tissue. Normally, blood vessels from connective tissue are restricted from passing through the basal lamina; epithelium is thus an **avascular** tissue. All nutrients to epithelial cells must pass through either absorption from the free surface or diffusion from underlying tissues.

■ CONNECTIVE TISSUE

Connective tissue is characterized on the basis of its extracellular matrix.

Unlike epithelial cells, connective tissue cells are conspicuously separated from one another. The intervening spaces are occupied by material produced by the cells. This extracellular material is called the **extracellular matrix**. The nature of the cells and matrix varies according to the function of the tissue. Thus, classification of connective tissue takes into account not only the cells but also the composition and organization of the extracellular matrix.

Embryonic connective tissue derives from the mesoderm, the middle embryonic germ layer, and is present in the embryo and within the umbilical fold. It gives rise to various connective tissues in the body.

A type of connective tissue found in close association with most epithelia is **loose connective tissue** (Fig. 4.2a). In fact, most epithelia rest on connective tissue. The extracellular matrix of loose connective tissue contains loosely arranged collagen fibers and numerous cells. Some of these cells, the fibroblasts, form and maintain the extracellular matrix. However, most of the cells are migrants from the vascular system and are associated with the immune system. In contrast, where only strength is required, collagen fibers are more numerous and densely packed. Also, the cells are relatively sparse and limited to the fiber-forming cell, the fibroblast (see Fig. 4.2b). This type of connective tissue is described as **dense connective tissue**.

Examples of **specialized connective tissues** include bone, cartilage, and blood. These connective tissues are characterized by the specialized nature of their extracellular matrix. For instance, **bone** has a matrix that is mineralized by calcium and phosphate molecules that are associated with collagen fibers. **Cartilage** possesses a matrix that contains a large amount of water bound to hyaluronan aggregates. Bone and cartilage provide a supporting framework for organs and tissues. **Blood** consists of cells and an extracellular matrix in the form of a protein-rich fluid called *plasma* that circulates throughout the body transporting oxygen (O_2) and nutrients and removing carbon dioxide CO_2) and metabolites from the tissues. Again, in all of these tissues, it is the extracellular material that characterizes the tissue, not the cells.

Adipose tissue is another example of specialized connective tissue; however, it is different from other connective tissues because the predominant distinguishing features are related to the cells (**adipocytes**) and not to the extracellular matrix. Adipose tissue plays an important role in energy homeostasis. Adipocytes store energy reserves within intracellular lipid droplets and regulate energy metabolism by secreting specific hormones (Chapter 9, Adipose Tissue, page 280).

■ MUSCLE TISSUE

Muscle tissue is categorized on the basis of a functional property, the ability of its cells to contract.

Muscle cells are characterized by large amounts of the contractile proteins actin and myosin in their cytoplasm and by their particular cellular arrangement in the tissue. To function efficiently to effect movement, most muscle cells are aggregated into distinct bundles that are easily distinguished from the surrounding tissue. Muscle cells are typically elongated and oriented with their long axes in the same direction (Fig. 4.3). The arrangement of nuclei is also consistent with the parallel orientation of muscle cells.

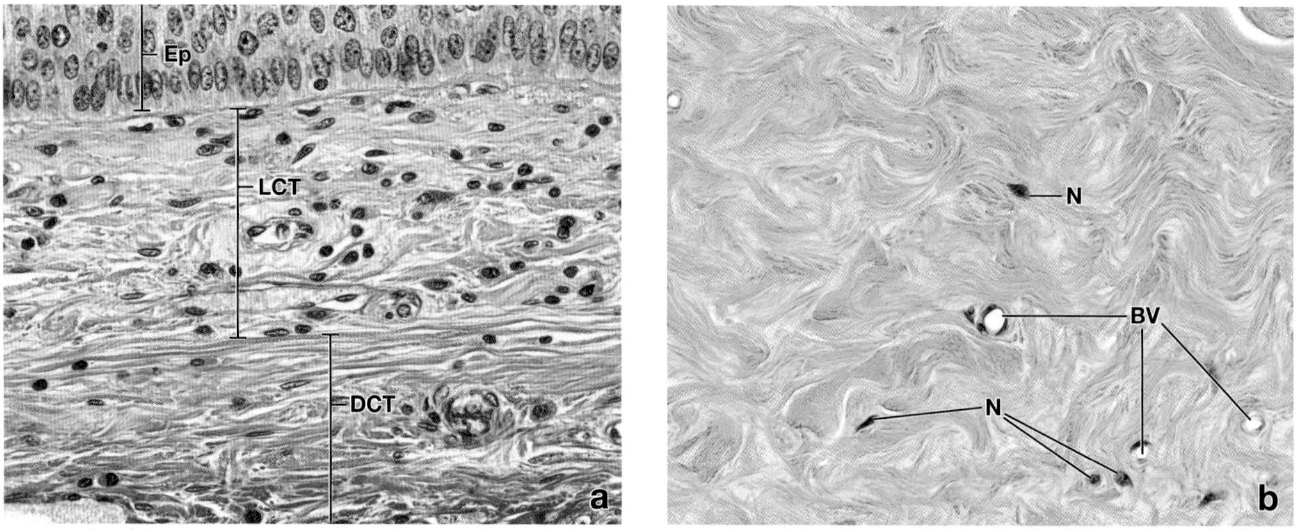

FIGURE 4.2. Loose and dense connective tissue. a. Mallory-Azan–stained specimen of a section through the epiglottis showing the lower part of its stratified epithelium (*Ep*), subjacent loose connective tissue (*LCT*), and dense connective tissue (*DCT*) below. Loose connective tissue typically contains many cells of several types. Their nuclei vary in size and shape. The elongated nuclei most likely belong to fibroblasts. Because dense connective tissue contains thick collagen bundles, it stains more intensely with the blue dye. Also, note the relatively fewer nuclei. ×540. **b.** A Mallory-stained specimen of dense connective tissue showing a region composed of numerous, densely packed collagen fibers. The few nuclei (*N*) that are present belong to fibroblasts. The combination of densely packed fibers and the paucity of cells characterize dense connective tissue. Relatively few small blood vessels (*BV*) are shown in this section. ×540.

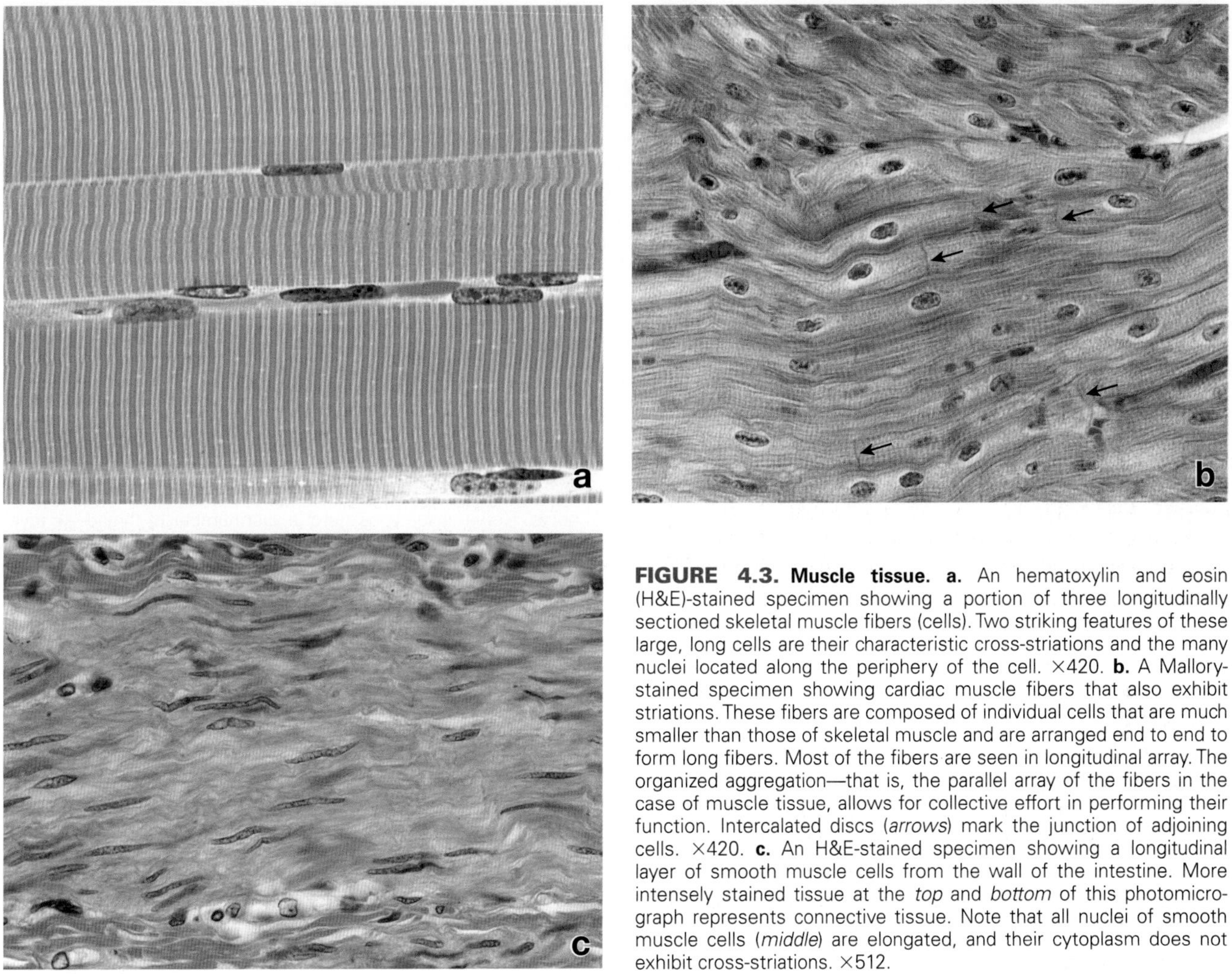

FIGURE 4.3. Muscle tissue. a. An hematoxylin and eosin (H&E)-stained specimen showing a portion of three longitudinally sectioned skeletal muscle fibers (cells). Two striking features of these large, long cells are their characteristic cross-striations and the many nuclei located along the periphery of the cell. ×420. **b.** A Mallory-stained specimen showing cardiac muscle fibers that also exhibit striations. These fibers are composed of individual cells that are much smaller than those of skeletal muscle and are arranged end to end to form long fibers. Most of the fibers are seen in longitudinal array. The organized aggregation—that is, the parallel array of the fibers in the case of muscle tissue, allows for collective effort in performing their function. Intercalated discs (*arrows*) mark the junction of adjoining cells. ×420. **c.** An H&E-stained specimen showing a longitudinal layer of smooth muscle cells from the wall of the intestine. More intensely stained tissue at the *top* and *bottom* of this photomicrograph represents connective tissue. Note that all nuclei of smooth muscle cells (*middle*) are elongated, and their cytoplasm does not exhibit cross-striations. ×512.

Although the shape and arrangement of cells in specific muscle types (e.g., smooth muscle, skeletal muscle, and cardiac muscle) are quite different, all muscle types share a common characteristic. The bulk of the cytoplasm consists of the contractile proteins actin and myosin, which form thin and thick myofilaments, respectively. **Skeletal muscle** (see Fig. 4.3a) and **cardiac muscle** (see Fig. 4.3b) cells exhibit cross-striations that are produced largely by the specific arrangement of myofilaments. **Smooth muscle** cells (see Fig. 4.3c) do not exhibit cross-striations because the myofilaments do not achieve the same degree of order in their arrangement.

The contractile proteins **actin** and **myosin** are ubiquitous in all cells. But only in muscle cells are they present in such large amounts and organized in such highly ordered arrays that their contractile activity can produce movement in an organ or organism.

■ NERVE TISSUE

Nerve tissue consists of nerve cells (neurons) and associated supporting cells of several types.

Although all cells exhibit electrical properties, nerve cells or **neurons** are highly specialized to transmit electrical impulses from one site in the body to another; they are also specialized to integrate those impulses. Nerve cells receive and process information from the external and internal environment and may have specific sensory receptors and sensory organs to accomplish this function.

Neurons are characterized by two different types of processes through which they interact with other nerve cells and with cells of the epithelia and muscle. A single, long **axon** (sometimes longer than a meter) carries impulses away from the **cell body**, which contains the neuron's nucleus. Multiple **dendrites** receive impulses and carry them toward the cell body. (In histologic sections, it is usually impossible to differentiate axons and dendrites because they have the same structural appearance.) The axon terminates at a neuronal junction called a **synapse** at which electrical impulses are transferred from one cell to the next by secretion of **neuromediators**. These chemical substances are released at synapses to generate electrical impulses in the adjacent communicating neuron.

In the **central nervous system (CNS)**, which comprises the brain and spinal cord, the supporting cells are called **neuroglial cells**. In the **peripheral nervous system (PNS)**, which comprises the nerves in all other parts of the body, the supporting cells are called **Schwann (neurilemmal) cells** and **satellite cells**. Supporting cells are responsible for several important functions. They separate

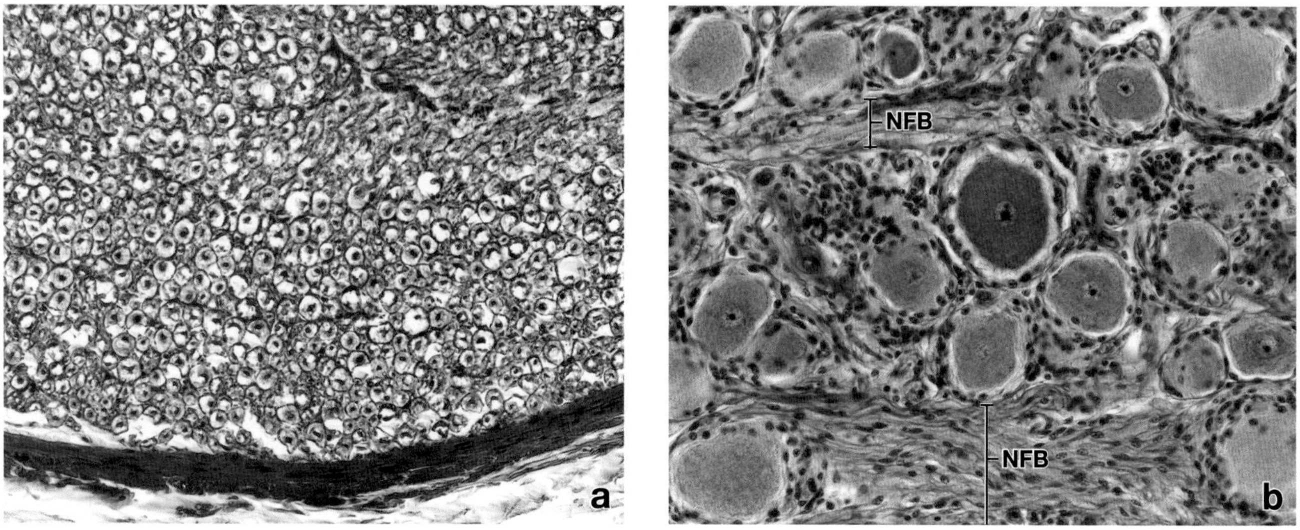

FIGURE 4.4. Nerve tissue. a. A Mallory-stained section of a peripheral nerve. Nerve tissue consists of a vast number of thread-like myelinated axons held together by connective tissue. The axons have been cross-sectioned and appear as small, red, dot-like structures. The clear space surrounding the axons previously contained myelin that was dissolved and lost during preparation of the specimen. The connective tissue is stained blue. It forms a delicate network around the myelinated axons and ensheathes the bundle, thus forming a structural unit, the nerve. ×270. **b.** An Azan-stained section of a nerve ganglion showing the large, spherical nerve cell bodies and the nuclei of the small satellite cells that surround the nerve cell bodies. The axons associated with the nerve cell bodies are unmyelinated. They are seen as nerve fiber bundles (*NFB*) between clusters of the cell bodies. ×270.

neurons from one another, produce the **myelin sheath** that insulates and speeds conduction in certain types of neurons, provide active phagocytosis to remove cellular debris, and contribute to the blood–brain barrier in the CNS.

In an ordinary hematoxylin and eosin (H&E)-stained section, nerve tissue may be observed in the form of a nerve, which consists of varying numbers of neuronal processes along with their supporting cells (Fig. 4.4a). Nerves are most commonly seen in longitudinal or cross sections in loose connective tissue. Nerve cell bodies in the PNS, including the autonomic nervous system (ANS), are seen in aggregations called **ganglia**, where they are surrounded by satellite cells (see Fig. 4.4b).

Neurons and supporting cells are derived from neuroectoderm, which forms the neural tube in the embryo. Neuroectoderm originates by invagination of an epithelial layer, the dorsal ectoderm of the embryo. Some nervous system cells, such as **ependymal cells** and cells of the choroid plexus in the CNS, retain the absorptive and secretory functions characteristic of epithelial cells.

■ HISTOGENESIS OF TISSUES

In the early developing embryo during the gastrulation phase, a **trilaminar embryo** (trilaminar germ disc) is formed. The three germ layers include the **ectoderm**, **mesoderm**, and **endoderm**, which give rise to all the tissues and organs.

Ectodermal Derivatives

The **ectoderm** is the outermost of the three germ layers. The derivatives of the ectoderm may be divided into two major classes: surface ectoderm and neuroectoderm.

Surface ectoderm gives rise to the

- **epidermis** and its derivatives (hair, nails, sweat glands, sebaceous glands, and the parenchyma and ducts of the mammary glands),
- **cornea** and **lens epithelia** of the eye,
- **enamel organ** and **enamel** of the teeth,
- components of the **internal ear**,
- **adenohypophysis** (anterior lobe of the pituitary gland), and
- mucosa of the **oral cavity** and lower part of the **anal canal**.

Neuroectoderm gives rise to

- the **neural tube** and its derivatives, including **components of the CNS**, ependyma (epithelium lining the cavities of the brain and spinal cord), pineal body, posterior lobe of the pituitary gland (neurohypophysis), and the sensory epithelium of the eye, ear, and nose;
- the **neural crest** and its derivatives, including **components of the PNS** (cranial, spinal, and autonomic ganglia; peripheral nerves; and Schwann cells); glial cells (oligodendrocytes and astrocytes); chromaffin (medullary) cells of the adrenal gland; enteroendocrine cells, also called *amine precursor uptake and decarboxylation* (APUD) system cells of the diffuse neuroendocrine system; melanoblasts, the precursors of melanocytes; the mesenchyme of the head and its derivatives (such as pharyngeal arches that contain muscles, connective tissue, nerves, and vessels); odontoblasts; and corneal and vascular endothelium.

Mesodermal Derivatives

Mesoderm is the middle of the three primary germ layers of an embryo. It gives rise to

- **connective tissue**, including embryonic connective tissue (mesenchyme), connective tissue proper (loose and dense connective tissue), and specialized connective tissues (cartilage, bone, adipose tissue, blood and hemopoietic tissue, and lymphatic tissue);
- **striated muscles** and **smooth muscles**;
- **heart**, **blood vessels**, and **lymphatic vessels**, including their endothelial lining;

- **spleen**;
- **kidneys** and the **gonads** (ovaries and testes) with genital ducts and their derivatives (ureters, uterine tubes, uterus, ductus deferens);
- **mesothelium**, the epithelium lining the pericardial, pleural, and peritoneal cavities; and
- the **adrenal cortex**.

Endodermal Derivatives

Endoderm is the innermost layer of the three germ layers. In the early embryo, it forms the wall of the primitive gut and gives rise to epithelial portions or linings of the organs arising from the primitive gut tube. Derivatives of the endoderm include the

- **alimentary canal epithelium** (excluding the epithelium of the oral cavity and lower part of the anal canal, which are of ectodermal origin);
- **extramural digestive gland epithelium** (e.g., the liver, pancreas, and gallbladder);
- lining **epithelium of the urinary bladder** and most of the **urethra**;
- **respiratory system epithelium**;
- **thyroid**, **parathyroid**, and **thymus gland** epithelial components;
- parenchyma of the **tonsils**; and
- lining **epithelium of the tympanic cavity** and **auditory (Eustachian) tubes**.

Thyroid and parathyroid glands develop as epithelial outgrowths from the floor and walls of the pharynx; they then lose their attachments from these sites of original outgrowth. As an epithelial outgrowth of the pharyngeal wall, the thymus grows into the mediastinum and also loses its original connection. Figure 4.5 summarizes the derivatives of the three germ layers.

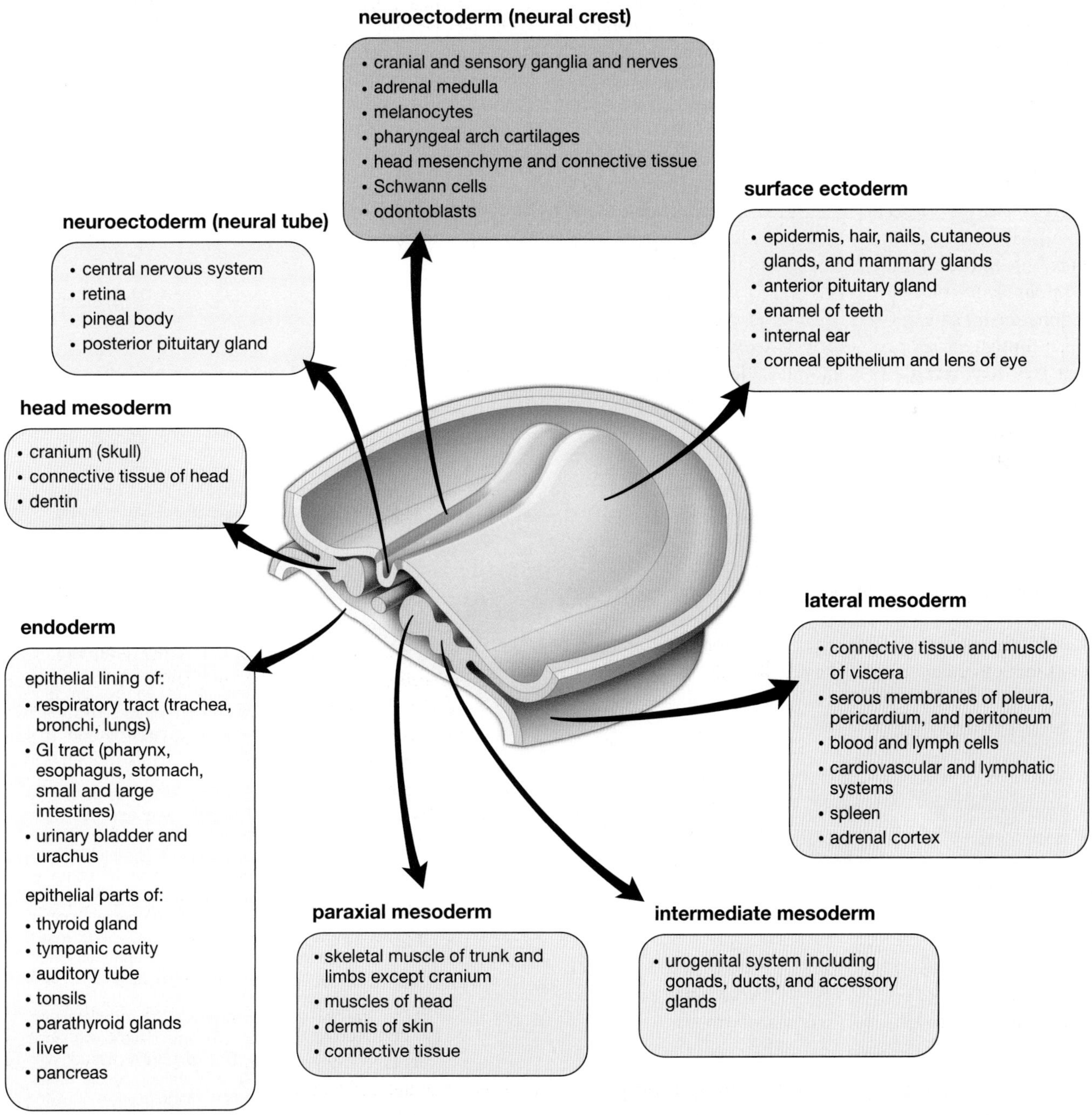

FIGURE 4.5. Derivatives of the three germ layers. Schematic drawing illustrates the derivatives of the three germ layers: ectoderm, endoderm, and mesoderm. *GI*, gastrointestinal. (Based on Moore KL, Persaud TVN. *The Developing Human, Clinically Oriented Embryology*. WB Saunders; 1998.)

FOLDER 4.1

CLINICAL CORRELATION: OVARIAN TERATOMAS

Under certain conditions, abnormal cellular differentiation may occur and lead to tumor formation. Human embryonic stem cells derived from early embryos are considered pluripotent stem cells, capable of differentiating into various somatic cells and tissues. Most tumors are derived from cells that originate from a single germ cell layer. However, if tumor cells arise from pluripotential stem cells, the tumor may contain cells that differentiate and resemble cells originating from all three germ layers. The result is the formation of a tumor that contains a variety of mature tissues arranged in an unorganized manner. Such masses are referred to as **teratomas**.

Because pluripotential stem cells are primarily encountered in gonads, teratomas almost always occur in this location. In the ovary, these tumors usually develop into solid masses that contain characteristics of mature basic tissues. Although the tissues fail to form functional structures, frequently organ-like structures may be seen (i.e., teeth, hair, epidermis, nerves, bowel segments, etc.). Teratomas may also develop in the testis, but they are rare. Moreover, ovarian teratomas are usually benign, whereas teratomas in the testis are composed of less differentiated tissues that usually lead to malignancy. An example of a solid mass ovarian teratoma containing fully differentiated tissue is shown in the *center* micrograph of Figure F4.1.1. The low power reveals the lack of organized structures but does not allow identification of the specific tissues present. However, with higher magnification, as shown in **insets** (a–f), mature differentiated tissues are evident. This tumor represents a **mature teratoma** of the ovary, often called a **dermoid cyst**. This benign tumor has a normal female karyotype 46,XX; based on genetic studies, these tissues are thought to arise through parthenogenetic oocyte development. Mature teratomas are common ovarian tumors in childhood and during the early reproductive years.

The example given in Figure F4.1.1 shows that one can readily identify tissue characteristics, even in an unorganized structure. Again, the important point is the ability to recognize aggregates of cells and to determine the special characteristics that they exhibit.

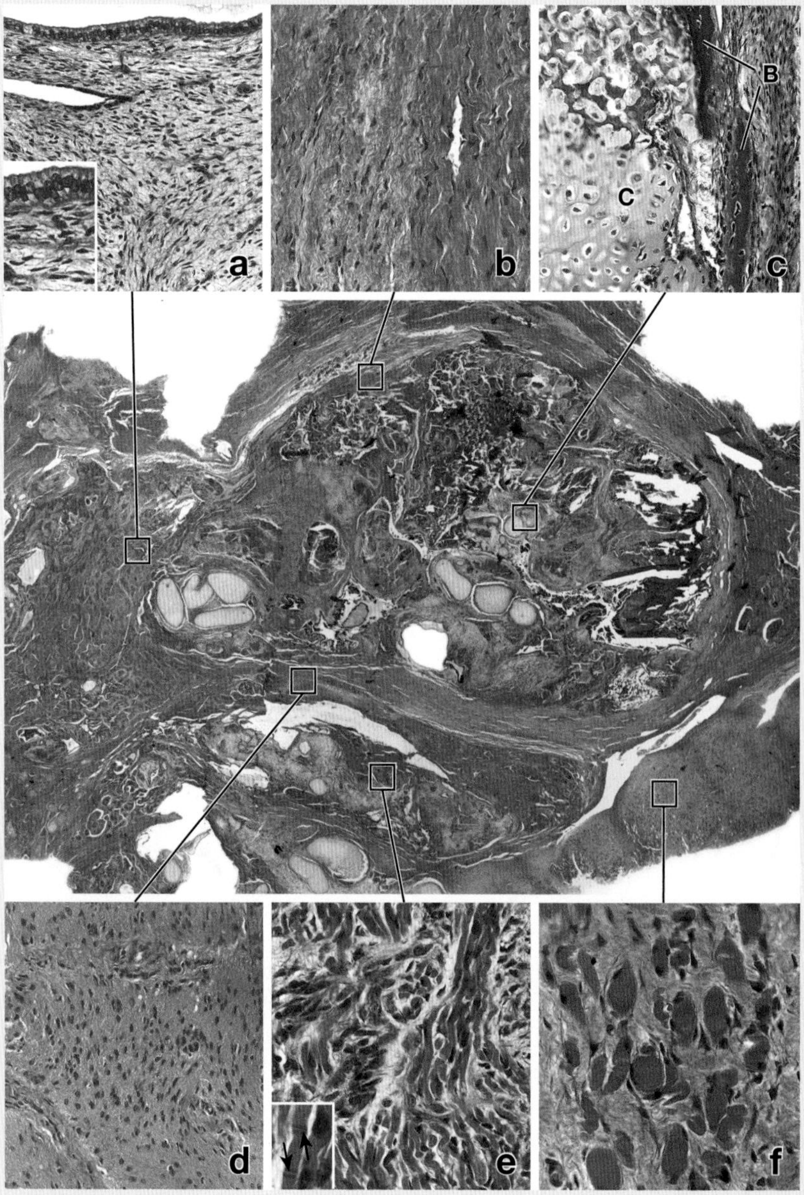

FIGURE F4.1.1. Ovarian teratoma. In the *center* is a hematoxylin and eosin (H&E)-stained section of an ovarian teratoma seen at low magnification. This mass is composed of various basic tissues that are well differentiated and easy to identify at higher magnification. The abnormal feature is the lack of organization of the tissues to form functional organs. The tissues within the *boxed areas* are seen at higher magnification in micrographs **a–f**. The higher magnification allows identification of some of the basic tissues that are present within this tumor. ×10. **a.** Simple columnar epithelium lining a cavity of a small cyst. ×170. **Inset.** Higher magnification of the epithelium and the underlying connective tissue. ×320. **b.** Dense regular connective tissue forming a tendon-like structure. ×170. **c.** Area showing hyaline cartilage (*C*) and developing bone spicules (*B*). ×170. **d.** Brain tissue with glial cells. ×170. **e.** Cardiac muscle fibers. ×220. **Inset.** Higher magnification showing intercalated discs (*arrows*). ×320. **f.** Skeletal muscle fibers cut in cross section. ×220.

■ IDENTIFYING TISSUES

Recognition of tissues is based on the presence of specific components within cells and on specific cellular relationships.

Keeping these few basic facts and concepts about the fundamental four tissues in mind can facilitate the task of examining and interpreting histologic slide material. The first goal is to recognize aggregates of cells as tissues and to determine the special characteristics that are present. Are the cells present at a surface? Are they in contact with their neighbors, or are they separated by definable intervening material? Do they belong to a group with special properties such as muscle or nerve?

The structure and function of each fundamental tissue are examined in subsequent chapters. In focusing on a single specific tissue, we are, in a sense, artificially separating the constituent tissues of organs. However, this separation is necessary to understand and appreciate the histology of the various organs of the body and the means by which they operate as functional units and integrated systems.

101 HISTOLOGY NOTEBOOK

TISSUES: CONCEPT AND CLASSIFICATION

OVERVIEW OF TISSUES

- **Tissues** are aggregates or groups of cells organized to perform one or more specific functions.
- All **organs** are made up of only **four basic tissue types**: epithelium (epithelial tissue), connective tissue, muscle tissue, and nerve tissue.

EPITHELIAL TISSUE

- **Epithelium** is characterized by close cell apposition and location at a free surface.
- Epithelial tissue covers body surfaces, lines body cavities and tubes, and forms **glands.**
- Epithelium is classified based on morphologic characteristics: **number of cell layers** (simple or stratified) and **shape of cells** (squamous, cuboidal, or columnar).
- Free surfaces of epithelial cells exhibit **surface modifications** (microvilli, stereocilia, or cilia).
- Epithelial cells rest on the **basal lamina.**

CONNECTIVE TISSUE

- **Connective tissue** is characterized on the basis of its **extracellular matrix**. It underlies and supports (structurally and functionally) the other three basic tissues.
- Connective tissue is classified into **three categories** based on the content of its extracellular matrix and the characteristics of individual cells: **embryonic, proper connective tissue** (loose and dense), and **specialized connective tissues.**
- Examples of specialized connective tissue include **bone, cartilage, adipose tissue**, and **blood.**

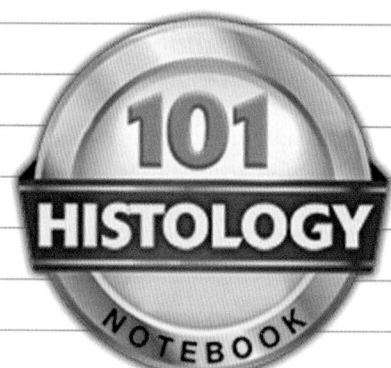

MUSCLE TISSUE

- **Muscle tissue** is categorized based on the ability of its cells to contract.
- All types of **muscle cells** contain the contractile proteins **actin** and **myosin**, which are arranged in myofilaments and are responsible for muscle contraction.
- **Skeletal muscle** and **cardiac muscle** cells have cross-striations that are formed by a specific arrangement of myofilaments. **Smooth muscle** cells do not exhibit striations.

NERVE TISSUE

- **Nerve tissue** receives, transmits, and integrates information from outside and inside the body.
- **Nerve cells (neurons)** are highly specialized to transmit electrical impulses. A typical neuron is made up of a cell body, a single long **axon** to carry impulses away from the cell body, and multiple **dendrites** to receive impulses and carry them toward the cell body.
- Neurons are found in both the **central nervous system (CNS)**, which comprises the brain and spinal cord, and the **peripheral nervous system (PNS)**, which comprises the nerves and ganglia.
- In the CNS, the supporting cells are called **neuroglial cells.** In the PNS, the supporting cells are called **Schwann (neurilemmal) cells** and **satellite cells.**

HISTOGENESIS OF TISSUES

- Three **germ layers** that give rise to all tissues and organs include the **ectoderm, mesoderm,** and **endoderm.**
- Ectodermal-derived structures develop from either surface ectoderm or neuroectoderm.
- **Surface ectoderm** gives rise to the epidermis (and its derivatives), cornea and lens epithelia of the eye, enamel of the teeth, components of the internal ear, adenohypophysis, and mucosa of the oral cavity and lower part of the anal canal.
- **Neuroectoderm** gives rise to the neural tube, neural crest, and both their derivatives.
- **Mesoderm** gives rise to connective tissue; muscle tissue; heart, blood, and lymphatic vessels; spleen; kidneys and gonads with genital ducts and their derivatives; mesothelium, which lines body cavities; and the adrenal cortex.
- **Endoderm** gives rise to alimentary canal epithelium; extramural digestive gland epithelium (liver, pancreas, and gallbladder); epithelium of the urinary bladder and most of the urethra; respiratory system epithelium; thyroid, parathyroid, and thymus glands; parenchyma of the tonsils; and epithelium of the tympanic cavity and auditory (Eustachian) tubes.

5 EPITHELIAL TISSUE

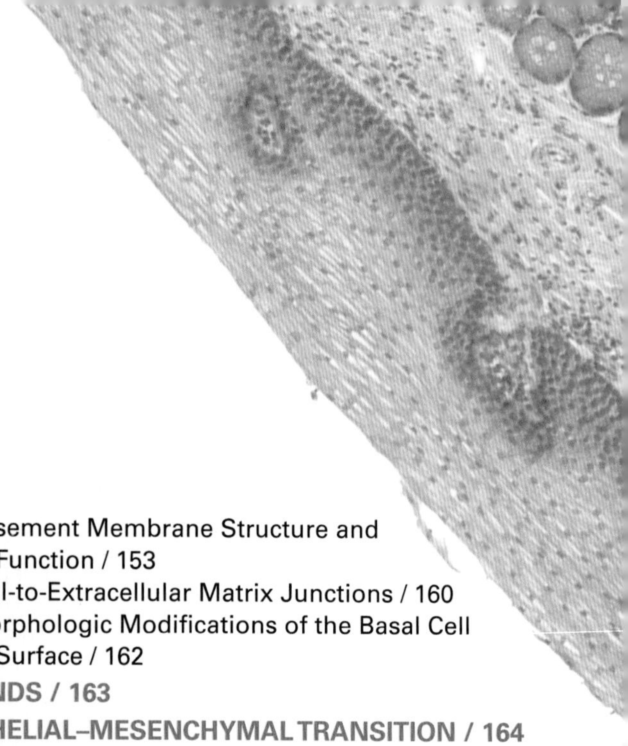

■ OVERVIEW OF EPITHELIAL STRUCTURE AND FUNCTION

Epithelium covers body surfaces, lines body cavities, and constitutes glands.

Epithelium is an avascular tissue composed of cells that cover the **exterior body surfaces** and line **internal closed cavities** (including the vascular system) and **body tubes** that communicate with the exterior (the alimentary, respiratory, and genitourinary tracts). Notable exceptions are the joint cavities that are lined by mesenchymally derived connective tissue cells. Epithelium also forms the **secretory portion (parenchyma) of glands** and their ducts. In addition, specialized epithelial cells function as **receptors for the special senses** (smell, taste, hearing, and vision).

The cells that make up epithelium have three principal characteristics:

- They are closely apposed and adhere to one another by means of specific cell-to-cell adhesion molecules (C-CAMs) that form specialized **cell junctions** (Fig. 5.1).
- They exhibit functional and morphologic polarity. In other words, different functions are associated with three distinct morphologic surface domains: a **free surface** or **apical domain**, a **lateral domain**, and a **basal domain**. The properties of each domain are determined by specific lipids and integral membrane proteins.
- Their basal surface is attached to an underlying **basement membrane**, a noncellular, protein–polysaccharide-rich layer demonstrable at the light microscopic (LM) level by histochemical methods (see Fig. 1.2, page 6).

In special situations, epithelial cells lack a free surface (epithelioid tissues).

In some locations, cells are closely apposed to one another but lack a free surface. Although the close apposition of these cells and the presence of a basement membrane would classify them as epithelium, the absence of a free surface more appropriately classifies such cell aggregates as **epithelioid tissues**. The epithelioid cells are derived from progenitor mesenchymal cells (nondifferentiated cells of embryonic origin found in connective tissue).

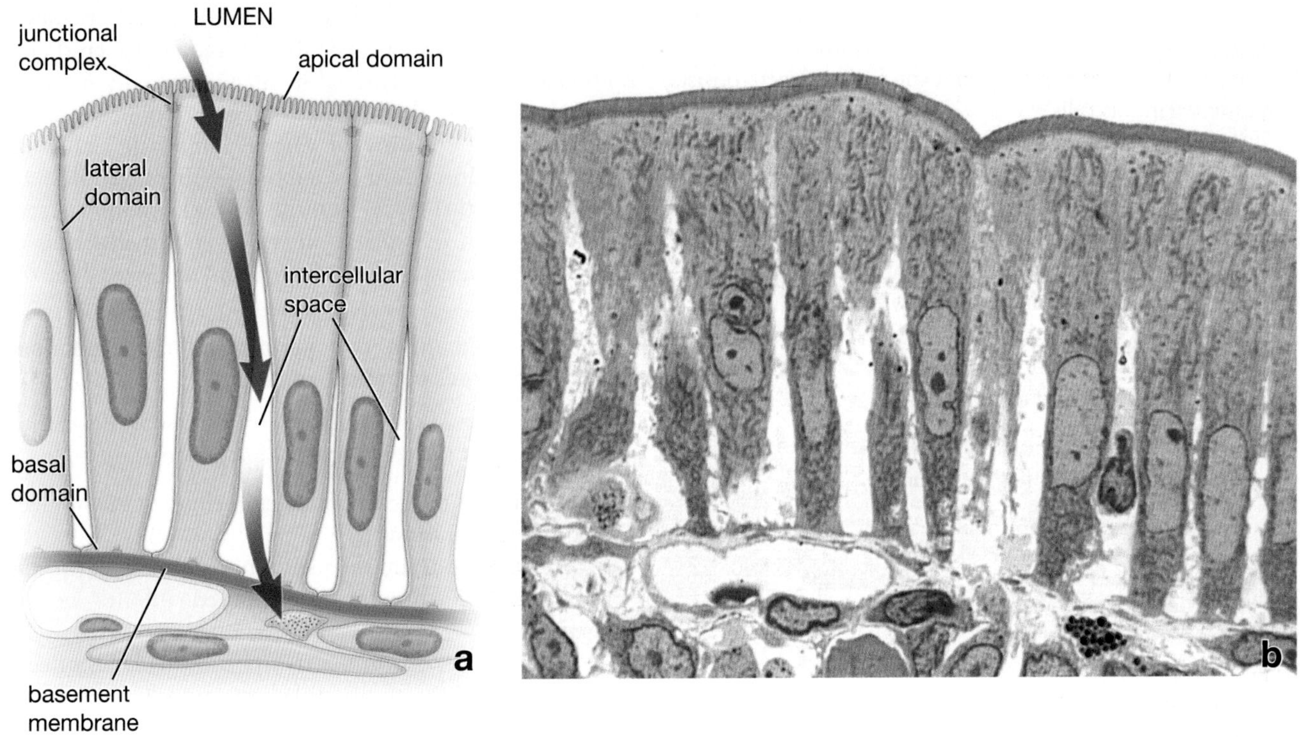

FIGURE 5.1. Diagram of small intestine absorptive epithelial cells. a. All three cellular domains of a typical epithelial cell are indicated on the diagram. The junctional complex provides adhesion between adjoining cells and separates the luminal space from the intercellular space, limiting the movement of fluid between the lumen and the underlying connective tissue. The intracellular pathway of fluid movement during absorption (*arrows*) is from the intestinal lumen into the cell, then across the lateral cell membrane into the intercellular space, and, finally, across the basement membrane to the connective tissue. **b.** This photomicrograph of a plastic-embedded, thin section of intestinal epithelium, stained with toluidine blue, shows cells actively engaged in fluid transport. Like the adjacent diagram, the intercellular spaces are prominent, reflecting fluid passing into this space before entering the underlying connective tissue. ×1,250.

Although the progenitor cells of these epithelioid tissues may have arisen from a free surface or the immature cells may have had a free surface at some time during development, the mature cells lack a surface location or surface connection. Epithelioid organization is typical of most endocrine glands; examples of such tissue include the interstitial cells of Leydig in the **testis** (Plate 5.3, page 174), the lutein cells of the **ovary**, the islets of Langerhans in the **pancreas**, the parenchyma of the **adrenal gland**, and the anterior lobe of the **pituitary gland**. Epithelioreticular cells of the **thymus** may also be included in this category. Epithelioid patterns are also formed by accumulations of connective tissue macrophages in response to certain types of injury and infections as well as by many tumors derived from epithelium.

Epithelium creates a selective barrier between the external environment and the underlying connective tissue.

Covering and lining epithelium forms a sheet-like cellular investment that separates underlying or adjacent connective tissue from the external environment, internal cavities, or fluid connective tissue, such as the blood and lymph. Among other roles, this epithelial investment functions as a **selective barrier** that facilitates or inhibits the passage of specific substances between the exterior (including the body cavities) environment and the underlying connective tissue compartment.

■ CLASSIFICATION OF EPITHELIUM

The traditional classification of epithelium is descriptive and based on two factors: the number of cell layers and the shape of the surface cells. This terminology, therefore, reflects only structure, not function. Thus, epithelium is described as

- **simple** when it is one cell layer thick and
- **stratified** when it has two or more cell layers.

The individual cells that compose an epithelium are described as

- **squamous** when the width of the cell is greater than its height;
- **cuboidal** when the width, depth, and height are approximately the same; and
- **columnar** when the height of the cell appreciably exceeds the width (the term *low columnar* is often used when a cell's height only slightly exceeds its other dimensions).

By describing the number of cell layers (i.e., simple or stratified) and the surface cell shape, the various configurations of epithelia are easily classified. The cells in some exocrine glands are more or less **pyramidal**, with their apices directed toward a lumen. However, these cells are still classified as either cuboidal or columnar, depending on their height relative to their width at the base of the cell.

In a **stratified epithelium**, the shape and height of the cells usually vary from layer to layer, but *only the shape of the* *cells that form the surface layer is used in classifying the epithelium.* For example, a stratified squamous epithelium consists of more than one layer of cells, and the surface layer consists of flat or squamous cells.

In some instances, a third factor—**specialization of the apical cell surface domain**—can be added to this classification system. For example, some simple columnar epithelia are classified as simple columnar ciliated when the apical surface domain possesses cilia. The same principle applies to stratified squamous epithelium, in which the surface cells may be keratinized or nonkeratinized. Thus, epidermis would be designated as stratified squamous keratinized epithelium because of the keratinized cells at the surface.

Pseudostratified epithelium and transitional epithelium are special classifications of epithelium.

Two special categories of epithelium are pseudostratified and transitional.

- **Pseudostratified epithelium** appears stratified, although some of the cells do not reach the free surface; all rest on the basement membrane (Plate 5.2, page 172). Thus, it is actually a **simple epithelium**. The distribution of pseudostratified epithelium is limited in the body. Also, it is often difficult to discern whether all of the cells contact the basement membrane. For these reasons, identification of pseudostratified epithelium usually depends on knowing where it is normally found.
- **Transitional epithelium (urothelium)** is a term applied to the epithelium lining the lower urinary tract, extending from the minor calyces of the kidney down to the proximal part of the urethra. Urothelium is a **stratified epithelium** with specific morphologic characteristics that allow it to distend (Plate 5.3, page 174). This epithelium is described in Chapter 20, Urinary System, pages 795-797.

The cellular configurations of the various types of epithelia and their appropriate nomenclature are illustrated in Table 5.1.

Endothelium and mesothelium are the simple squamous epithelia lining the vascular system and body cavities.

Specific names are given to epithelium in certain locations:

- **Endothelium** is the epithelial lining of the blood and lymphatic vessels. Because of its strategic location between the blood and tissue, the endothelium of blood vessels is often called the **vascular endothelium**. It consists of highly specialized simple squamous cells that regulate and monitor cellular transport, vascular smooth muscle tone, immune responses, and synthesis and secretion of a variety of hormones and active metabolites (for details, see Chapter 13, Cardiovascular System, pages 452-456).
- **Endocardium** is the epithelial lining of the ventricles and atria of the heart.
- **Mesothelium** is the epithelium that lines the walls and covers the contents of the closed cavities of the body (i.e., the abdominal, pericardial, and pleural cavities; Plate 5.1, page 170).

Both endothelium and endocardium, as well as mesothelium, are almost always simple squamous epithelia. Epithelial cells are polygonal in shape, generally oriented along the axis of the vessel. An exception is found in **postcapillary venules** of certain lymphatic tissues in which the endothelium is cuboidal. These venules are called **high endothelial venules (HEV)**. Another exception is found in the spleen, in which endothelial cells of the venous sinuses are rod shaped and arranged like the staves of a barrel.

A specific epithelium can perform different functions based on the types of cells it contains.

An epithelium may serve one or more functions, depending on the activity of the cell types that are present:

- **Secretion**, as in the columnar epithelium of the stomach and the gastric glands
- **Absorption**, as in the columnar epithelium of the intestines and proximal convoluted tubules in the kidney
- **Transportation**, as in the transport of materials or cells along the surface of an epithelium propelled by motile cilia (transport of dust particles in the bronchial tree) or transport of materials across an epithelium (pinocytosis or endocytosis) to and from the connective tissue
- **Mechanical protection**, as in the stratified squamous epithelium of the skin (epidermis) and the transitional epithelium of the urinary bladder
- **Receptor function** to receive and transduce external stimuli, as in the taste buds of the tongue, olfactory epithelium of the nasal mucosa, and the retina of the eye

Epithelia involved in secretion or absorption are typically simple or, in a few cases, pseudostratified. The height of the cells often reflects the level of secretory or absorptive activity. Simple squamous epithelia are compatible with a high rate of transepithelial transport. Stratification of the epithelium usually correlates with transepithelial impermeability. Finally, in some pseudostratified epithelia, basal cells are the **stem cells** that give rise to the mature functional cells of the epithelium, thus balancing cell turnover.

■ CELL POLARITY

Epithelial cells exhibit distinct **polarity**. They have an **apical domain**, a **lateral domain**, and a **basal domain**. Specific biochemical characteristics are associated with each cell surface. These characteristics and the geometric arrangements of the cells in the epithelium determine the functional polarity of all three cell domains.

The free or apical domain is always directed toward the exterior surface or the lumen of an enclosed cavity or tube. The lateral domain communicates with adjacent cells and is characterized by specialized attachment areas. The basal domain rests on the basal lamina, anchoring the cell to underlying connective tissue.

The molecular mechanism responsible for establishing polarity in epithelial cells is required to create a fully functional

TABLE 5.1 Types of Epithelium

Classification		Some Typical Locations	Major Function
Simple squamous	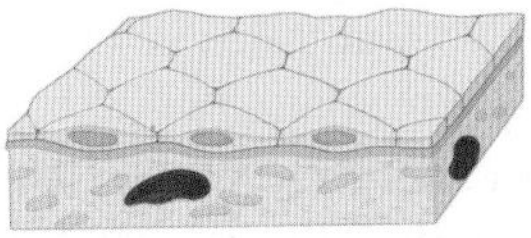	Vascular system (endothelium) Body cavities (mesothelium) Bowman capsule (kidney) Respiratory spaces in lung	Exchange, barrier in central nervous system Exchange and lubrication
Simple cuboidal	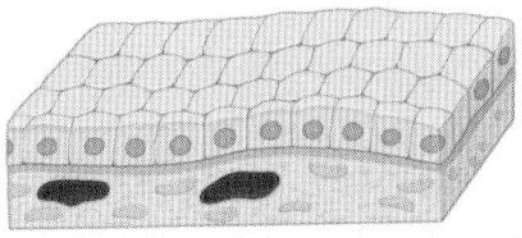	Small ducts of exocrine glands Surface of ovary (germinal epithelium) Kidney tubules Thyroid follicles	Absorption and conduit Barrier Absorption and secretion
Simple columnar	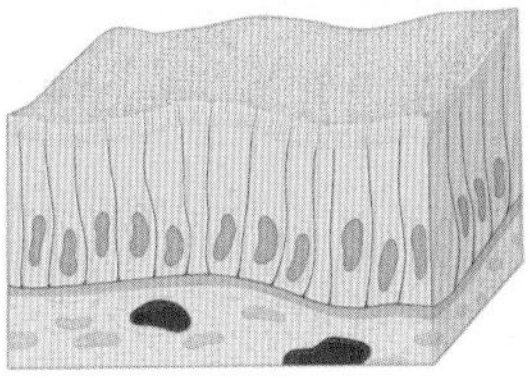	Small intestine and colon Stomach lining and gastric glands Gallbladder	Absorption and secretion Secretion Absorption
Pseudostratified	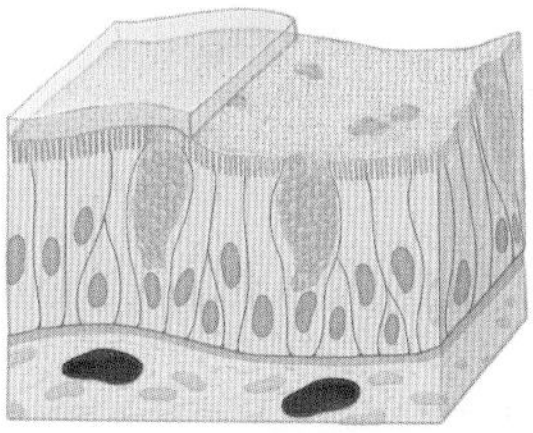	Trachea and bronchial tree Ductus deferens Efferent ductules of epididymis	Secretion and conduit Absorption and conduit
Stratified squamous	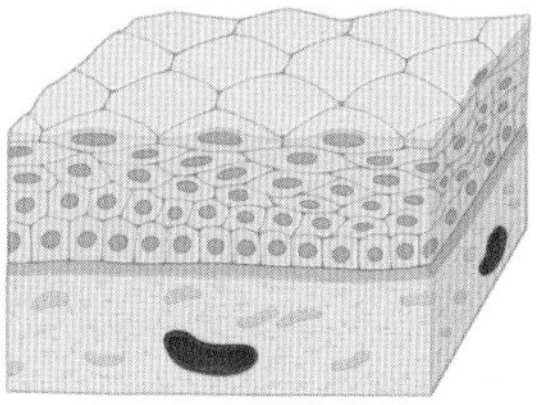	Epidermis Oral cavity and esophagus Vagina	Barrier and protection
Stratified cuboidal	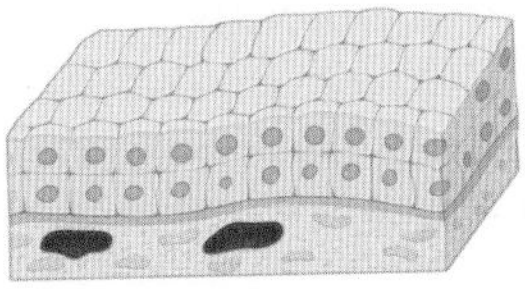	Sweat gland ducts Large ducts of exocrine glands Anorectal junction	Barrier and conduit
Stratified columnar	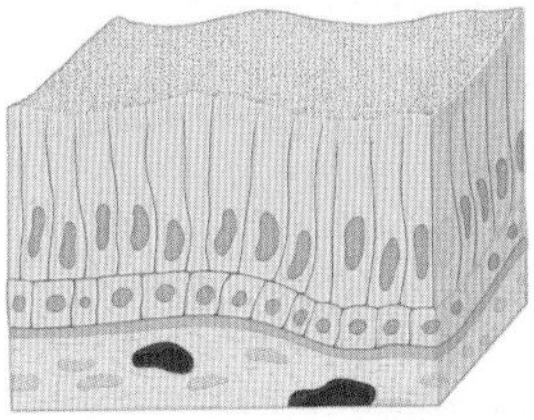	Largest ducts of exocrine glands Anorectal junction	Barrier and conduit
Transitional (urothelium)	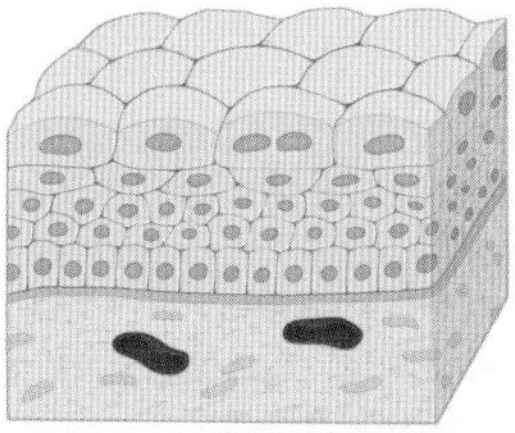	Renal calyces Ureters Bladder Urethra	Barrier, distensible property

barrier between adjacent cells. Junctional complexes (which are discussed later in this chapter) are formed in the apical parts of the epithelial cells. These specialized attachment sites not only are responsible for tight cell adhesions but also allow epithelia to regulate paracellular movements of solutes down their electroosmotic gradients. In addition, junctional complexes separate the apical plasma membrane domain from basal and lateral domains and allow them to specialize and recognize different molecular signals.

■ THE APICAL DOMAIN AND ITS MODIFICATIONS

In many epithelial cells, the **apical domain** exhibits special structural surface modifications to carry out specific functions. In addition, the apical domain may contain specific enzymes (e.g., hydrolases), ion channels, and carrier proteins (e.g., glucose transporters). The structural surface modifications include the following:

- **Microvilli**, cytoplasmic processes containing a core of actin filaments
- **Stereocilia (stereovilli)**, microvilli of unusual length
- **Cilia**, cytoplasmic processes containing a bundle of microtubules

Microvilli

Microvilli are finger-like cytoplasmic projections on the apical surface of most epithelial cells.

As observed with the electron microscope (EM), **microvilli** vary widely in appearance. In some cell types, microvilli are short, irregular, bleb-like projections. In other cell types, they are tall, closely packed, uniform projections that greatly increase the free cell surface area. In general, the number and shape of the microvilli of a given cell type correlate with the cell's absorptive capacity. Thus, cells that principally transport fluid and absorb metabolites have many closely packed, tall microvilli. Cells in which transepithelial transport is less active have smaller, more irregularly shaped microvilli.

Among the fluid-transporting epithelia (e.g., those of the intestine and kidney tubules), a distinctive border of vertical striations at the apical surface of the cell, representing an astonishing number of 15,000 close-packed microvilli, is easily seen in the LM. In intestinal absorptive cells, this surface structure was originally called the **striated border**; in the kidney tubule cells, it is called the **brush border**. Where there is no apparent surface modification based on LM observations, any microvilli present are usually short and not numerous, which explains why they may

FOLDER 5.1

CLINICAL CORRELATION: EPITHELIAL METAPLASIA

Epithelial metaplasia is a reversible conversion of one mature epithelial cell type to another mature epithelial cell type. Metaplasia is generally an adaptive response to stress, chronic inflammation, or other abnormal stimuli. The original cells are substituted by cells that are better suited to the new environment and more resistant to the effects of abnormal stimuli. Metaplasia results from reprogramming of epithelial stem cells that changes the patterns of their gene expression.

The most common epithelial metaplasia is **columnar to squamous** and occurs in the glandular epithelium, where the columnar cells become replaced by the stratified squamous epithelium. For example, **squamous metaplasia** frequently occurs in the pseudostratified respiratory epithelium of the trachea and bronchi in response to prolonged exposure to cigarette smoke. It also occurs in the cervical canal in women with chronic infections (e.g., human papillomavirus infection). In this example, simple columnar epithelium of the cervical canal is replaced by stratified squamous nonkeratinized epithelium (Fig. F5.1.1). In addition, squamous metaplasia is noticeable in the urothelium (transitional epithelium) and is associated with chronic parasitic infections, such as schistosomiasis.

Squamous-to-columnar epithelial metaplasia may also occur. For example, as a result of gastroesophageal reflux, the stratified squamous nonkeratinized epithelium of the lower part of the esophagus can undergo metaplastic transformation into an intestinal-like simple columnar epithelium containing goblet cells, a condition known as *Barrett esophagus*.

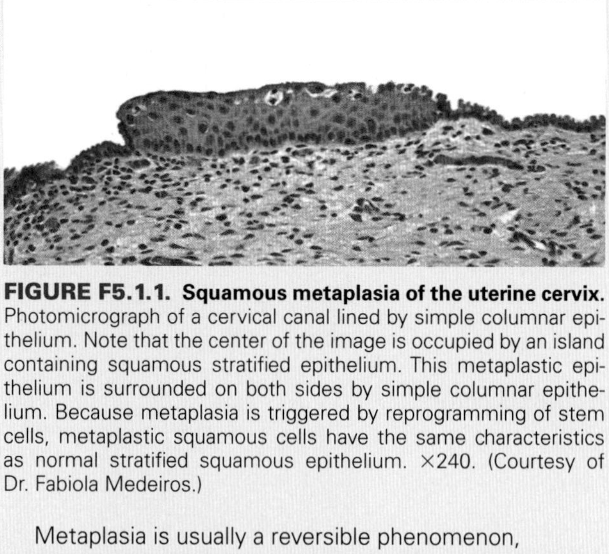

FIGURE F5.1.1. Squamous metaplasia of the uterine cervix. Photomicrograph of a cervical canal lined by simple columnar epithelium. Note that the center of the image is occupied by an island containing squamous stratified epithelium. This metaplastic epithelium is surrounded on both sides by simple columnar epithelium. Because metaplasia is triggered by reprogramming of stem cells, metaplastic squamous cells have the same characteristics as normal stratified squamous epithelium. ×240. (Courtesy of Dr. Fabiola Medeiros.)

Metaplasia is usually a reversible phenomenon, and if the stimulus that caused metaplasia is removed, tissues often return to their normal pattern of differentiation. If abnormal stimuli persist for a long time, squamous metaplastic cells may transform into squamous cell carcinoma. Cancers of the lung, cervix, and bladder often originate from squamous metaplastic epithelium. Squamous-to-columnar transformed epithelium may give rise to **glandular adenocarcinomas**.

Treatment of metaplasia involves removing the pathogenic stimulus (i.e., cessation of smoking, eradication of infectious agents, etc.) and monitoring the metaplastic site with periodic tissue sampling to ensure that cancerous changes do not develop.

escape detection in the LM. The variations seen in microvilli of various types of epithelia are shown in Figure 5.2. The microvilli of the intestinal epithelium (striated border) are the most highly ordered and are even more uniform in appearance than those that constitute the brush border of kidney cells.

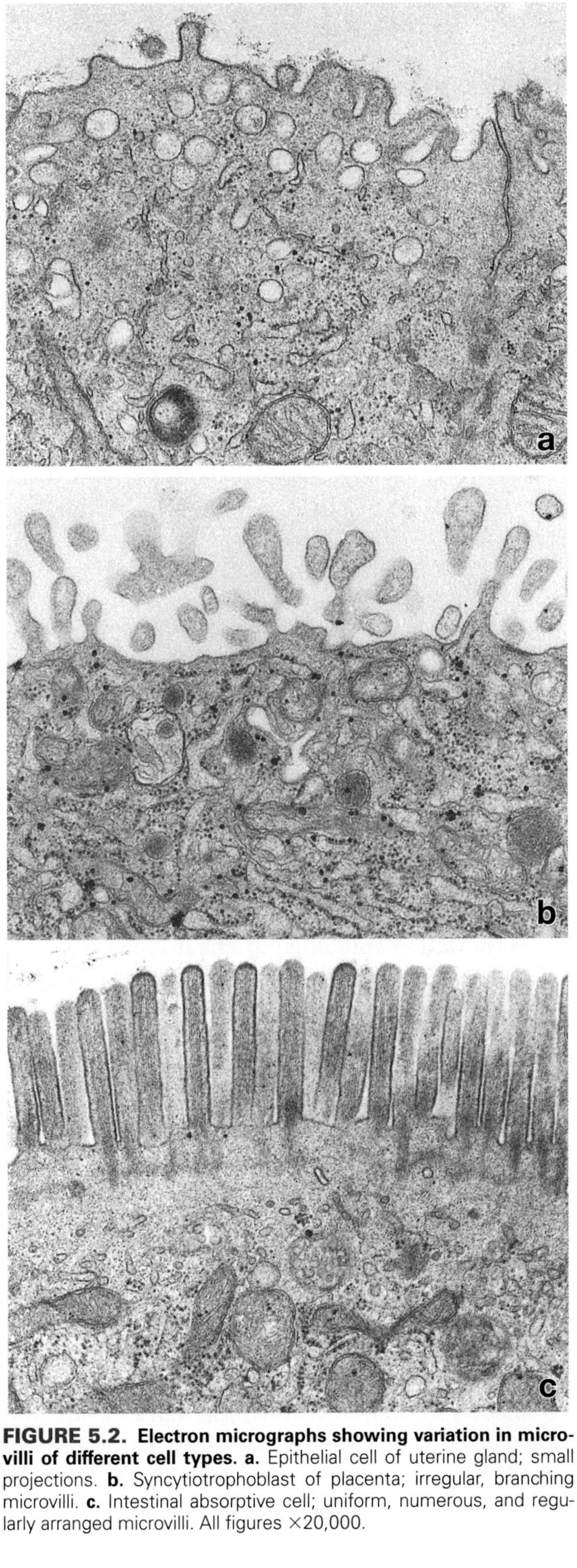

FIGURE 5.2. Electron micrographs showing variation in microvilli of different cell types. a. Epithelial cell of uterine gland; small projections. **b.** Syncytiotrophoblast of placenta; irregular, branching microvilli. **c.** Intestinal absorptive cell; uniform, numerous, and regularly arranged microvilli. All figures ×20,000.

The internal structure of microvilli contains a core of actin filaments that are cross-linked by several actin-bundling proteins.

Microvilli contain a conspicuous core of about 20–30 **actin filaments**. Their barbed (plus) ends are anchored to **villin**, a 95-kDa actin-bundling protein located at the tip of the microvillus. The actin bundle extends down into the apical cytoplasm. Here, it interacts with a horizontal network of actin filaments, the **terminal web**, which lies just below the base of the microvilli (Fig. 5.3a). The actin filaments inside the microvillus are cross-linked at 10-nm intervals by other **actin-bundling proteins**, such as **fascin** (57 kDa), **espin** (30 kDa), and **fimbrin** (68 kDa). This cross-linkage provides support and gives rigidity to the microvilli. In addition, the core of actin filaments is associated with **myosin I**, a molecule that binds the actin filaments to the plasma membrane of the microvillus. The addition of villin to epithelial cells growing in cultures induces the formation of microvilli on the free apical surface.

The **terminal web** is composed of **actin filaments** stabilized by **spectrin** (468 kDa), which also anchors the terminal web to the apical cell membrane (Fig. 5.3b). The presence of **myosin II** and **tropomyosin** in the terminal web explains its contractile ability; these proteins decrease the diameter of the apex of the cell, causing the microvilli, whose stiff actin cores are anchored into the terminal web, to spread apart and increase the intermicrovillus space.

The functional and structural features of microvilli are summarized in Table 5.2.

Stereocilia

Stereocilia are unusually long, immotile microvilli.

Stereocilia are not widely distributed among epithelia. They are, in fact, limited to the **epididymis**, the proximal part of the **ductus deferens** of the male reproductive system, and the **sensory (hair) cells of the inner ear**. They are included in this section because this unusual surface modification is traditionally treated as a separate structural entity.

Stereocilia of the genital ducts are extremely long processes that extend from the apical surface of the cell and facilitate absorption. Unique features include an apical cell protrusion from which they arise and thick stem portions that are interconnected by cytoplasmic bridges. Because EM reveals their internal structure to be that of unusually long microvilli, some histologists now use the term **stereovilli** (Fig. 5.4a). Seen in the LM, these processes frequently resemble the hairs of a paintbrush because of the way they aggregate into pointed bundles.

Like microvilli, stereocilia are supported by internal bundles of **actin filaments** that are cross-linked by **fimbrin**. The actin filaments' barbed (plus) ends are oriented toward the tips of the stereocilia and the pointed (minus) ends at the base. This organization of the actin core within stereocilia shares many construction principles with the microvilli, although the filaments can be as long as 120 μm.

Stereocilia develop from microvilli by the lateral addition of actin filaments to the actin bundle as well as by elongation of the actin filaments. Unlike microvilli, an

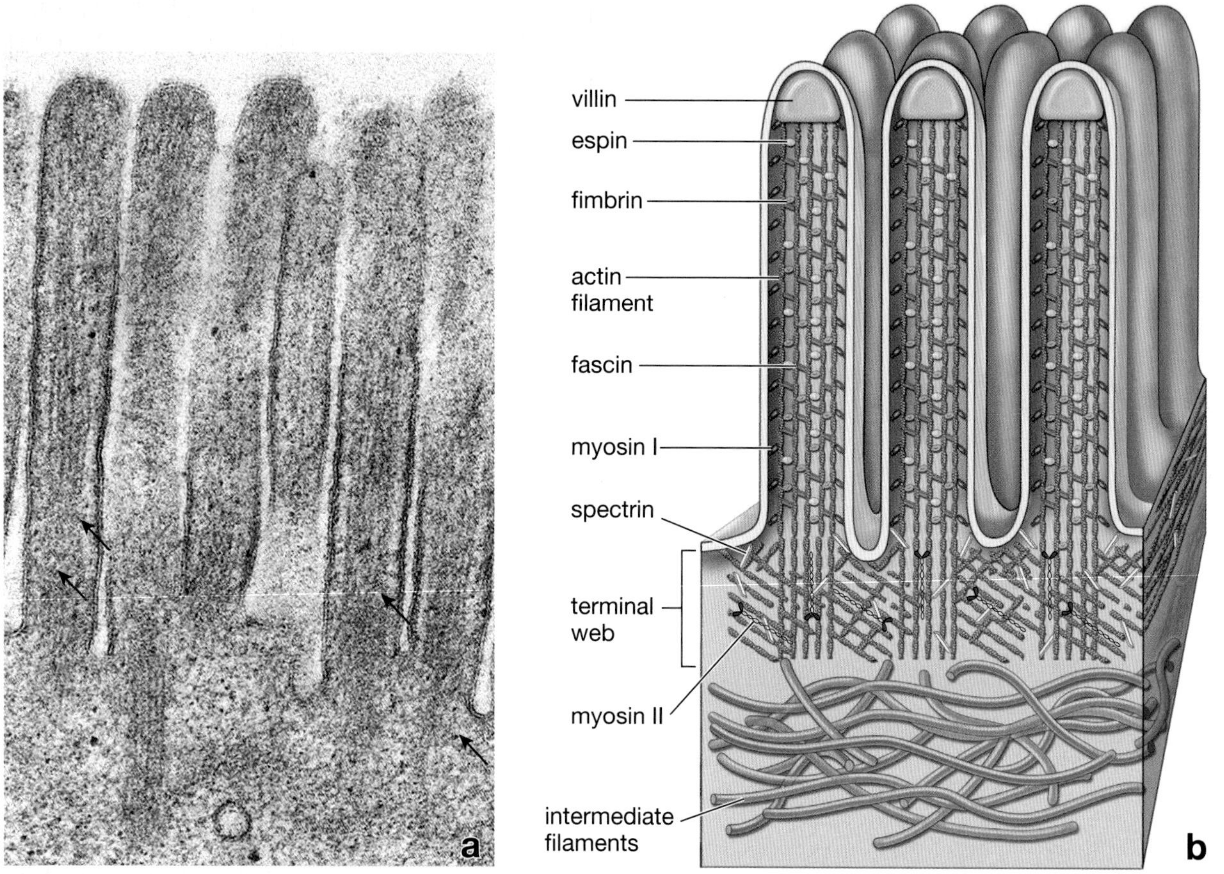

FIGURE 5.3. Molecular structure of microvilli. a. High magnification of microvilli from Figure 5.2c. Note the presence of the actin filaments in the microvilli (*arrows*), which extend into terminal web in the apical cytoplasm. ×80,000. **b.** Schematic diagram showing molecular structure of microvilli and the location of specific actin filament–bundling proteins (fimbrin, espin, and fascin). Note the distribution of myosin I within the microvilli and myosin II within the terminal web. The spectrin molecules stabilize the actin filaments within the terminal web and anchor them into the apical plasma membrane.

80-kDa actin-binding protein, **ezrin**, closely associated with the plasma membrane of stereocilia, anchors the actin filaments to the plasma membrane. The stem portion of the stereocilium and the apical cell protrusion contain the cross-bridge–forming molecule **α-actinin** (Fig. 5.4b). A striking difference between microvilli and stereocilia, other than size and the presence of ezrin, is the absence of villin at the tip of the stereocilium.

Stereocilia of the sensory epithelium of the ear have some unique characteristics.

Stereocilia of the sensory epithelium of the ear also derive from microvilli. They are exquisitely sensitive to mechanical vibration and serve as **sensory mechanoreceptors** rather than absorptive structures. They are uniform in diameter and organized into ridged bundles of increasing heights, forming characteristic staircase patterns (Fig. 5.5a). Their internal structure is characterized by the high density of **actin filaments** extensively cross-linked by **espin**, which is critical to the normal structure and function of stereocilia. Stereocilia of sensory epithelia lack both ezrin and α-actinin.

Because stereocilia can be easily damaged by overstimulation, they have a molecular mechanism to continuously renew their structure, which needs to be maintained in proper working condition for a lifetime. Using fluorescent-labeled actin molecules, researchers have found that actin monomers are constantly added at the tips and removed from the base of the stereocilia, whereas the entire bundle of actin filaments moves toward the base of the stereocilium (Fig. 5.5b, c). This **treadmilling effect** of the actin core structure is highly regulated and depends on the length of the stereocilium.

The functional and structural features of stereocilia in comparison to microvilli and cilia are summarized in Table 5.2.

Cilia

Cilia are common surface modifications present on nearly every cell in the body. They are hair-like extensions of the apical plasma membrane containing an **axoneme**, the microtubule-based internal structure. The axoneme extends from the **basal body**, a centriole-derived, **microtubule-organizing center (MTOC)** located in the apical region of a ciliated cell. The basal bodies are associated with several accessory structures that assist them with anchoring into cell cytoplasm. Cilia, including basal bodies and basal body–associated structures, form the **ciliary apparatus** of the cell.

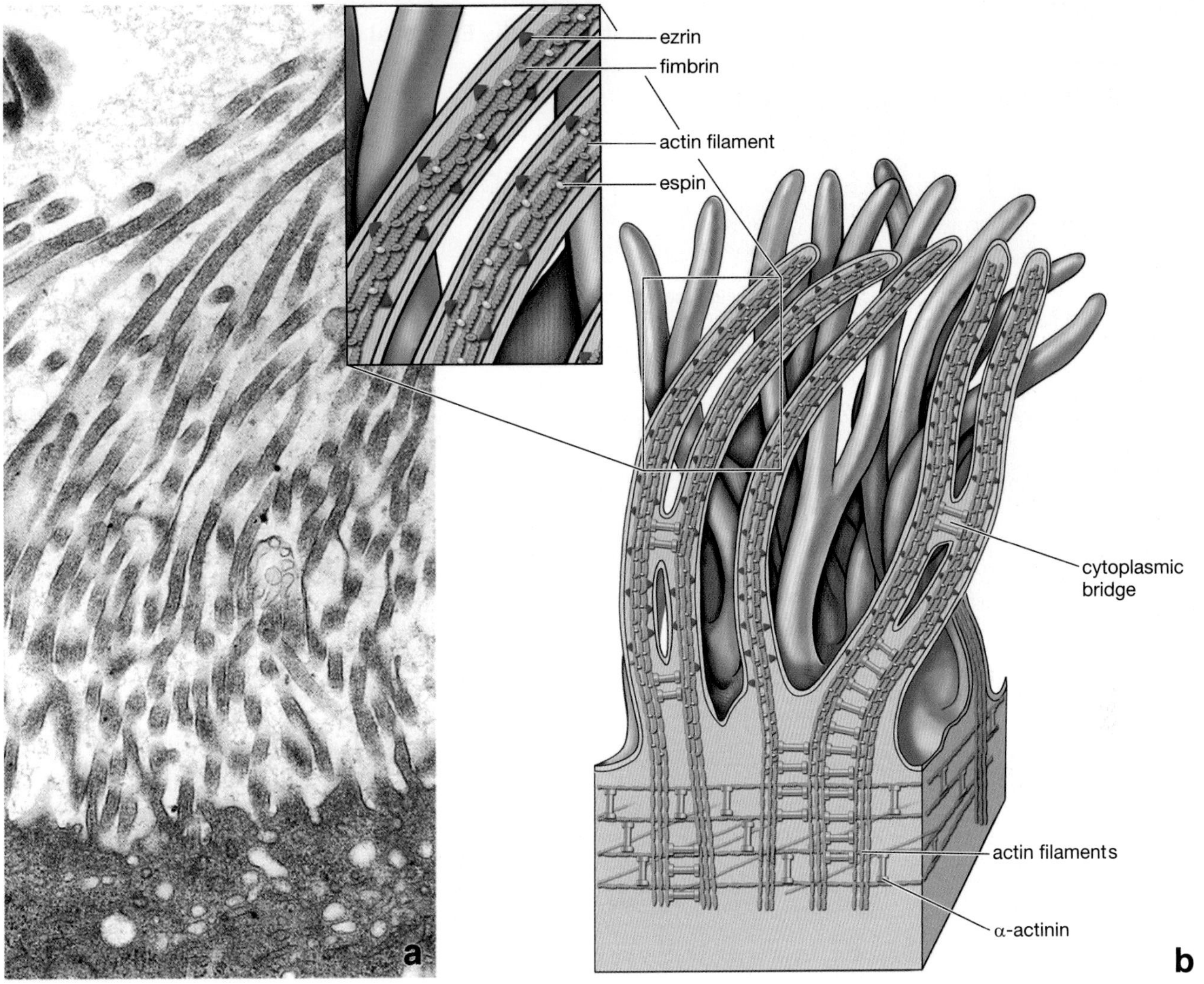

FIGURE 5.4. Molecular structure of stereocilia. a. Electron micrograph of stereocilia from the epididymis. The cytoplasmic projections are similar to microvilli, but they are extremely long. ×20,000. **b.** Schematic diagram showing the molecular structure of stereocilia. They arise from the apical cell protrusions, having thick stem portions that are interconnected by cytoplasmic bridges. Note the distribution of actin filaments within the core of the stereocilium and the actin-associated proteins, fimbrin and espin, in the elongated portion (**inset**); and α-actinin in the terminal web, apical cell protrusion, and occasional cytoplasmic bridges between neighboring stereocilia.

In general, cilia are classified as motile, primary, or nodal.

Based on their functional characteristics, cilia are classified into three basic categories:

- **Motile cilia** have been historically the most studied of all cilia. They are found in large numbers on the apical domain of many epithelial cells. Motile cilia and their counterparts, **flagella**, possess a **typical 9 + 2 axonemal organization** with microtubule-associated motor proteins that are necessary for the generation of forces needed to induce motility.
- **Primary cilia (monocilia)** are solitary projections found on almost all eukaryotic cells. The term *monocilia* implies that only a single cilium per cell is usually present. Primary cilia are immotile because of different arrangements of microtubules in the axoneme and lack of microtubule-associated motor proteins. They function as **chemosensors, osmosensors**, and **mechanosensors**, and they mediate light sensation, odorant, and sound perception in multiple organs in the body. It is now widely accepted that the primary cilia of cells in developing tissues are essential for normal tissue morphogenesis.
- **Nodal cilia** are found in the embryo on the **bilaminar embryonic disc** at the time of gastrulation. They are concentrated in the area that surrounds the **primitive node**, hence their name nodal cilia. They have an axonemal internal architecture similar to that of primary cilia; however, they are distinct in their ability to perform clockwise **rotational movement**. They play an important role in early embryonic development.

The functional and structural features of all three types of cilia are summarized in Table 5.2.

TABLE 5.2 Summary of Apical Domain Modifications in the Epithelial Cells

	General Structure	Cross Section	Motion Trajectory	Localization and Function
Microvilli	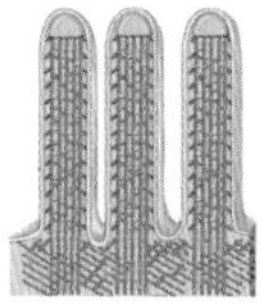 Average 1–3 μm in length, bundle of actin filament anchored in the terminal web	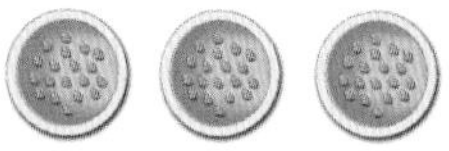 Core of actin filaments cross-linked by actin-bundling proteins; diameter 50–100 nm	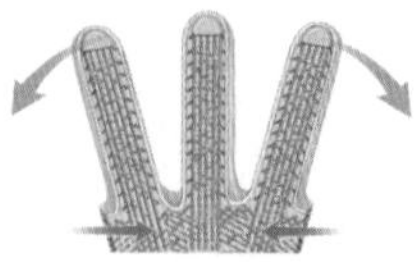 Passive movement owing to contraction of terminal web	• Present in many epithelial cells • Increase absorptive surface of the cell • Visible in LM as striated border (intestinal absorptive cells) or brush border (kidney tubule cells)
Stereocilia	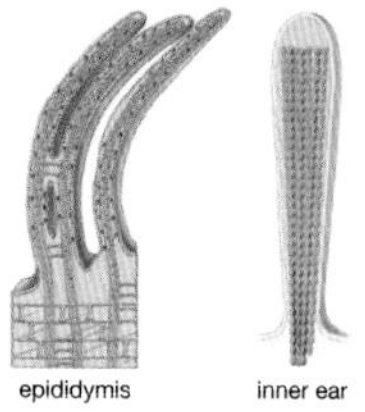 Considerably longer; up to 120 μm, actin filament bundle anchored in the terminal web; capable of regeneration (inner ear)	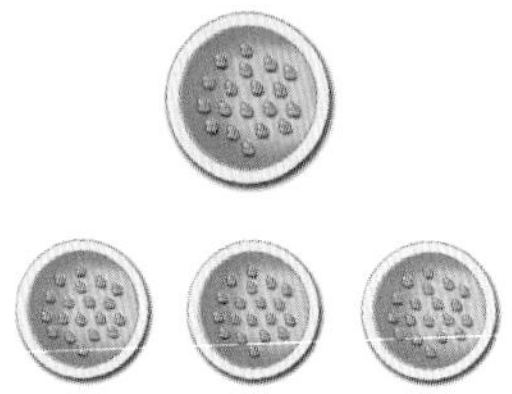 Core of actin filaments cross-linked by actin-bundling proteins; diameter 100–150 nm	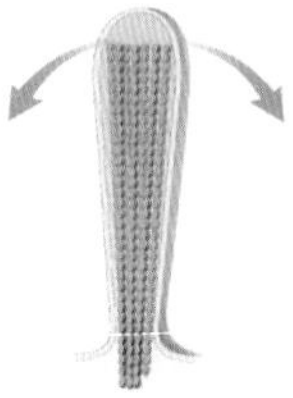 Passive movement owing to fluid flow (genital system) or vibration of endolymph (inner ear)	• Limited distribution • In male reproductive system (epididymis, proximal part of ductus deferens) have absorptive function • In sensory hair cells in the inner ear function as mechanoreceptors
Cilia – **Motile**	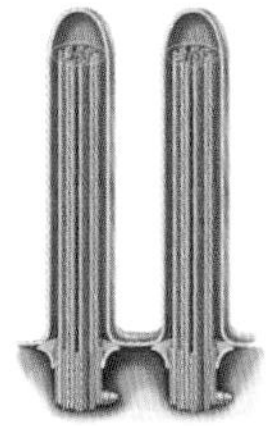 From 5 to 10 μm in length (flagella in sperm cells much longer, 50–100 μm), possess axoneme, basal bodies with basal body–associated structures; specific intraflagellar transport system for cilia development and normal function	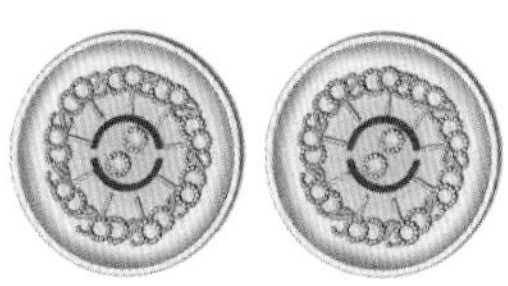 Core of microtubules arranged in 9 + 2 pattern with associated motor proteins; diameter about 250 nm	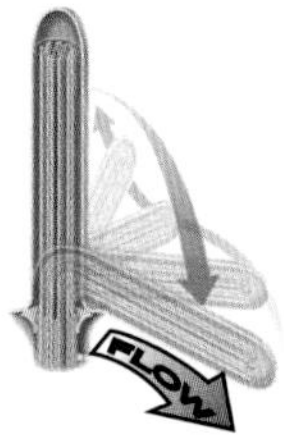 Active movement; rapid forward movement with slow recovery stroke (half-cone trajectory)	• Most commonly found on epithelia, which function in transporting secretions, proteins, foreign bodies, or cells on their surface (oviduct, trachea and bronchial tree, brain ependyma, and olfactory epithelium) • Present on sperm cells as flagella; provide a forward movement to the sperm cell
Cilia – **Primary**	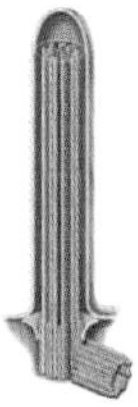 Average 2–3 μm in length; possess axoneme, basal bodies; have specialized plasma membrane with calcium entry channels and intraflagellar transport system	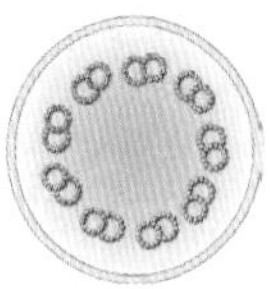 Core of microtubules arranged in 9 + 0 pattern; lack of ciliary dyneins, central pair of microtubules, and radial spokes; diameter about 250 nm	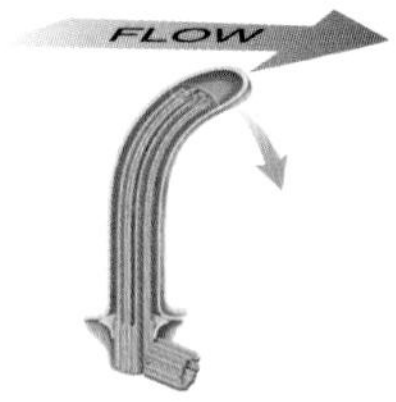 No active movement; passively bend due to flow of fluid	• Found in almost all cells in the body • Well documented in kidney ducts, bile duct epithelium, thyroid gland, thymus, neurons, Schwann cells, chondrocytes, fibroblasts, adrenal cortex, and pituitary cells • Function as sensory antennae • Generate and transmit signals from extracellular space into the cell
Cilia – **Nodal**	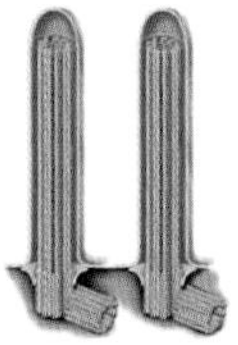 About 5–6 μm in length; have structure similar to primary cilia, except that they have an ability for active movement	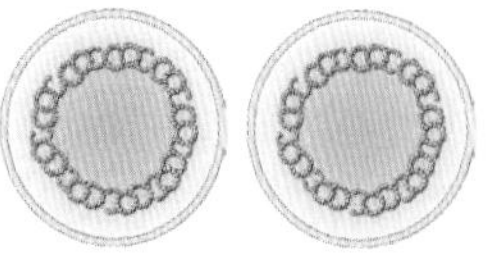 Core of microtubules arranged in 9 + 0 pattern with associated motor proteins (ciliary dyneins); central pair of microtubules and radial spokes are missing; diameter about 250 nm	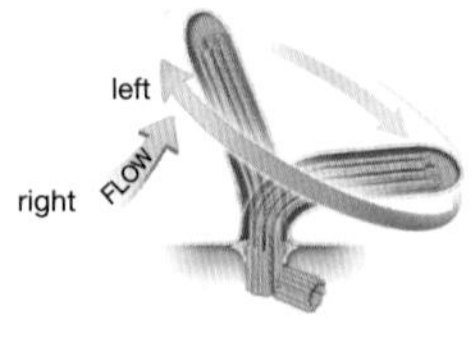 Active rotational clockwise movement (full cone trajectory)	• Found in the embryo during gastrulation on the bilaminar disc near the area of primitive node • Essential in developing left–right asymmetry of internal organs

LM, light microscope.

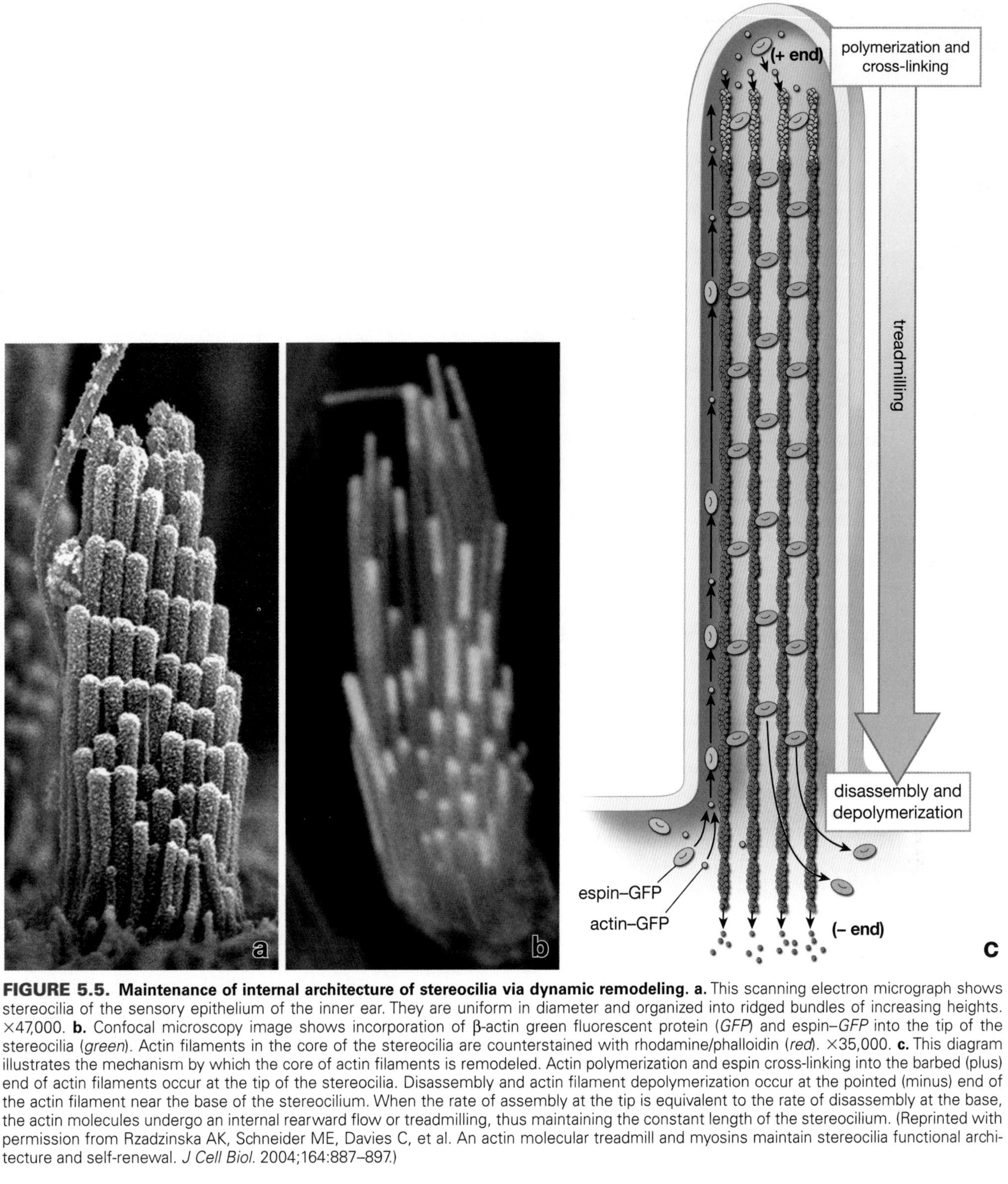

FIGURE 5.5. Maintenance of internal architecture of stereocilia via dynamic remodeling. a. This scanning electron micrograph shows stereocilia of the sensory epithelium of the inner ear. They are uniform in diameter and organized into ridged bundles of increasing heights. ×47,000. **b.** Confocal microscopy image shows incorporation of β-actin green fluorescent protein (*GFP*) and espin–*GFP* into the tip of the stereocilia (*green*). Actin filaments in the core of the stereocilia are counterstained with rhodamine/phalloidin (*red*). ×35,000. **c.** This diagram illustrates the mechanism by which the core of actin filaments is remodeled. Actin polymerization and espin cross-linking into the barbed (plus) end of actin filaments occur at the tip of the stereocilia. Disassembly and actin filament depolymerization occur at the pointed (minus) end of the actin filament near the base of the stereocilium. When the rate of assembly at the tip is equivalent to the rate of disassembly at the base, the actin molecules undergo an internal rearward flow or treadmilling, thus maintaining the constant length of the stereocilium. (Reprinted with permission from Rzadzinska AK, Schneider ME, Davies C, et al. An actin molecular treadmill and myosins maintain stereocilia functional architecture and self-renewal. *J Cell Biol.* 2004;164:887–897.)

Motile cilia are capable of moving fluid and particles along epithelial surfaces.

Motile cilia possess an internal structure that allows them to move. In most ciliated epithelia, such as the trachea, bronchi, or oviducts, cells may have as many as several hundred cilia arranged in orderly rows. In the tracheobronchial tree, the cilia sweep mucus and trapped particulate material toward the oropharynx where it is swallowed with saliva and eliminated from the body. In the oviducts, cilia help transport ova and fluid toward the uterus.

Cilia give a "crew-cut" appearance to the epithelial surface.

In the LM, **motile cilia** appear as short, fine, hair-like structures, approximately 0.25 µm in diameter and 5–10 µm in length, that emanate from the free surface of the cell (Fig. 5.6). A thin, dark-staining band is usually seen extending across the cell at the base of the cilia. This dark-staining band represents structures known as **basal bodies.** These structures take up stain and appear as a continuous band when viewed in the LM. When viewed with the EM, however, the basal body of each cilium appears as a distinct individual structure.

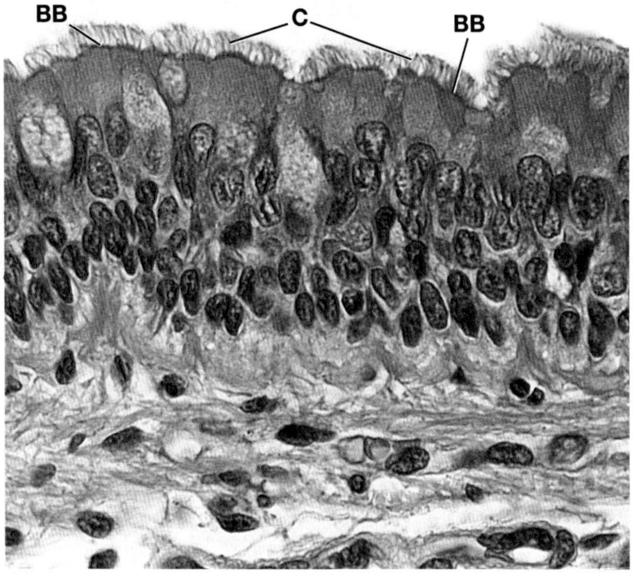

FIGURE 5.6. Ciliated epithelium. Photomicrograph of a hematoxylin and eosin (H&E)-stained specimen of tracheal pseudostratified ciliated epithelium. The cilia (*C*) appear as hair-like processes extending from the apical surface of the cells. The dark line immediately below the ciliary processes is produced by the basal bodies (*BB*) associated with the cilia. ×750.

Motile cilia contain an axoneme, which represents an organized core of microtubules arranged in a 9 + 2 pattern.

EM of a cilium in longitudinal profile reveals an **internal core of microtubules** called the **axoneme** (Fig. 5.7a). A cross-sectional view reveals the characteristic configuration of nine pairs or doublets of circularly arranged microtubules surrounding two central microtubules (Fig. 5.7b).

The microtubules composing each doublet are constructed so that the wall of one microtubule, designated the **B microtubule**, is actually incomplete; it shares a portion of the wall of the other microtubule of the doublet, the **A microtubule**. The A microtubule is composed of **13 tubulin protofilaments**, arranged in a side-by-side configuration, whereas the B microtubule is composed of **10 tubulin protofilaments**. Tubulin molecules incorporated into ciliary microtubules are tightly bound together and post-translationally modified in the process of acetylation and polyglutamylation. Such modifications ensure that the microtubules are highly stable and resist depolymerization.

When seen in cross section at high resolution, each doublet exhibits a pair of "arms" that contain **ciliary dynein**, a microtubule-associated motor protein. This motor protein uses the energy of adenosine triphosphate (ATP) hydrolysis to move along the surface of the adjacent microtubule (see Fig. 5.7). The dynein arms occur at 24-nm intervals along the length of the A microtubule and extend out to form temporary cross-bridges with the B microtubule of the adjacent doublet. A passive elastic component formed by **nexin** (165 kDa) permanently links the A microtubule with the B microtubule of adjacent doublets at 86-nm intervals. The **two central microtubules** are separate but partially enclosed by a **central sheath projection** at 14-nm intervals along the length of the cilium (see Fig. 5.7). **Radial spokes** extend from each of the nine doublets toward the two central microtubules at 29-nm intervals. The proteins forming the radial spokes and the nexin connections between the outer doublets make large-amplitude oscillations of the cilia possible.

Basal bodies and basal body–associated structures firmly anchor cilia in the apical cell cytoplasm.

The **9 + 2 microtubule array** courses from the tip of the cilium to its base, whereas the outer paired microtubules join the **basal body**. The basal body is a modified centriole. It functions as an MTOC consisting of nine short **microtubule triplets** arranged in a ring. Each of the paired microtubules of the ciliary axoneme (A and B microtubules) is continuous with two of the triplet microtubules of the basal body. The third incomplete **C microtubule** in the triplet extends from the bottom to the **transitional zone** at the top of the basal body near the transition between the basal body and the axoneme. The **two central microtubules** of the cilium originate at the transitional zone and extend to the top of the axoneme (see Fig. 5.7b). A cross section of the basal body would reveal nine circularly arranged microtubule triplets, but not the two central single microtubules of the cilium.

Basal bodies are associated with several **basal body–associated structures**, such as alar sheets (transitional fibers), basal feet, and striated rootlets (see Figs. 5.7 and 5.8).

- The **alar sheet** (transitional fiber) is a collar-like extension between the transitional zone of a basal body and the plasma membrane. It originates near the top end of the basal body C microtubule and inserts into the cytoplasmic domain of the plasma membrane. It tethers the basal body to the apical plasma membrane (see Fig. 5.7).
- The **basal foot** is an accessory structure that is usually found in the midregion of the basal body (see Fig. 5.8). Because in typical epithelial ciliated cells, all basal feet are oriented in the same direction (Fig. 5.9), it has been hypothesized that they function in coordinating ciliary movement. They are most likely involved in adjusting basal bodies by rotating them to the desired position. Localization of myosin molecules associated with basal feet supports this hypothesis.
- The **striated rootlet** is composed of longitudinally aligned protofilaments containing **rootletin** (a 220-kDa protein). The striated rootlet projects deep into the cytoplasm and firmly anchors the basal body within the apical cell cytoplasm (see Fig. 5.8).

Cilia movement originates from the sliding of microtubule doublets, which is generated by the ATPase activity of the dynein arms.

Ciliary activity is based on the movement of the doublet microtubules in relation to one another. Ciliary movement is initiated by the dynein arms (see Fig. 5.7b). The **ciliary dynein** located in the arms of the A microtubule forms temporary cross-bridges with the B microtubule of the adjacent doublet. Hydrolysis of ATP produces a **sliding**

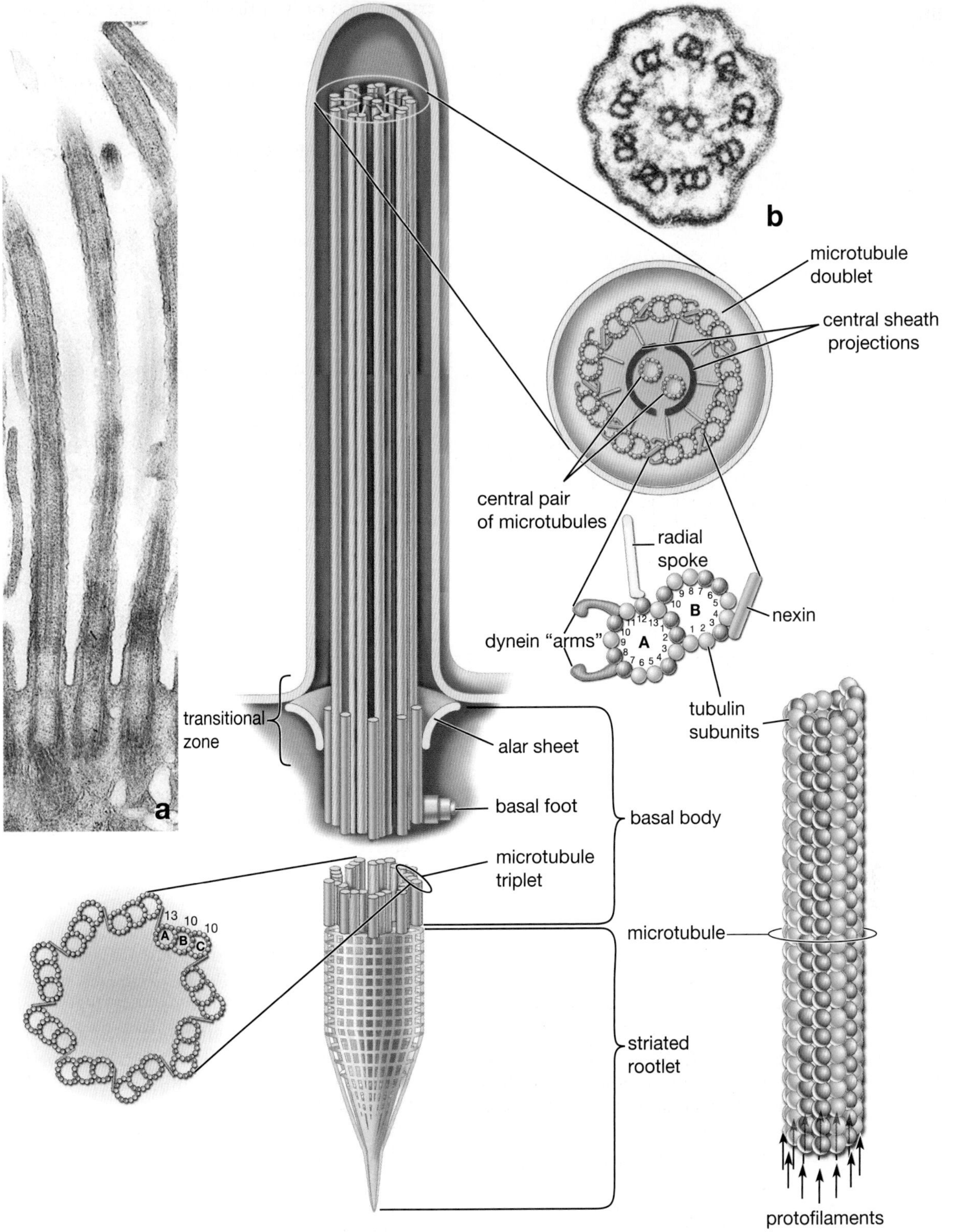

FIGURE 5.7. Molecular structure of cilia. This figure shows the three-dimensional arrangement of microtubules within the cilium and the basal body. A cross section of the cilium (*right*) illustrates the pair of central microtubules and the nine surrounding microtubule doublets (9 + 2 configuration). The molecular structure of the microtubule doublet is shown below the cross section. Note that the A microtubule of the doublet is composed of 13 tubulin dimers arranged in a side-by-side configuration (*lower right*), whereas the B microtubule is composed of 10 tubulin dimers and shares the remaining dimers with those of the A microtubule. The dynein arms extend from the A microtubule and make temporary cross-bridges with the B microtubule of the adjacent doublet. The basal body is anchored by the striated rootlet within the cell cytoplasm. Note the presence of the basal foot in the midsection of the basal body. A cross section of the basal body (*lower left*) shows the arrangement of nine microtubule triplets. These structures form a ring connected by nexin molecules. Each microtubule doublet of the cilium is an extension of two inner A and B microtubules of the corresponding triplet. The C microtubule is shorter and extends only to the transitional zone. **Inset a.** Electron micrograph of longitudinally sectioned cilia from the oviduct. The internal structures within the cilia are microtubules. The basal bodies appear empty because of the absence of the central pair of microtubules in this portion of the cilium. ×20,000. **Inset b.** Electron micrograph of cross section of the cilium showing corresponding structures with drawing below. ×180,000.

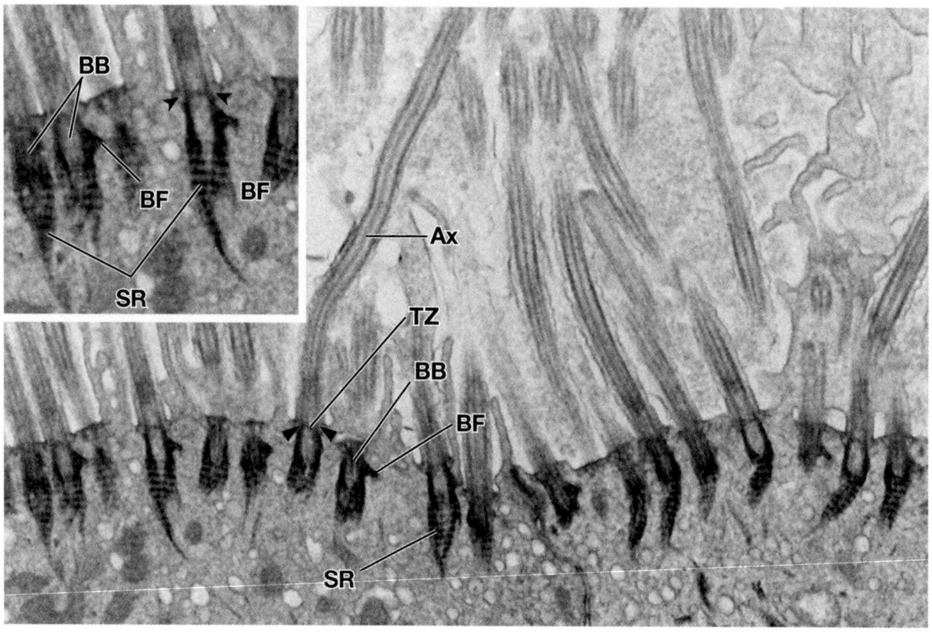

FIGURE 5.8. Ciliated surface of the respiratory mucosa. Electron micrograph shows a longitudinally sectioned cilium from the respiratory epithelium of the nasal cavity. At this magnification, most of the basal bodies (*BB*) appear empty because of the absence of the central pair of microtubules in this portion of the cilium. Structural details of the basal body and basal body–associated structures are easily visible in this section as well as in the higher magnification insert. Note that almost all *BB* in this section possess striated rootlets (*SR*). They anchor the *BB* deep within the apical cell cytoplasm. Each basal body has a single asymmetric basal foot (*BF*) projecting laterally; several are visible in this section. The transitional zone (*TZ*) extends from the upper end of the basal body into the axoneme (*Ax*), which is formed by a 9 + 2 microtubular arrangement. A central pair of microtubules is present in most of these sections. In addition, an alar sheath (*arrowheads*) provides a wing-like extension between the *TZ* and plasma membrane. The first and second *BB* from the *right* have well-preserved alar sheaths. ×15,000. *Inset* ×25,000. (Courtesy of Dr. Jeffrey L. Salisbury.)

movement of the bridge along the B microtubule. The dynein molecules produce a continuous shear force during this sliding directed toward the ciliary tip. Because of this ATP-dependent phase, a cilium that remains rigid exhibits a rapid forward movement called the **effective stroke.**

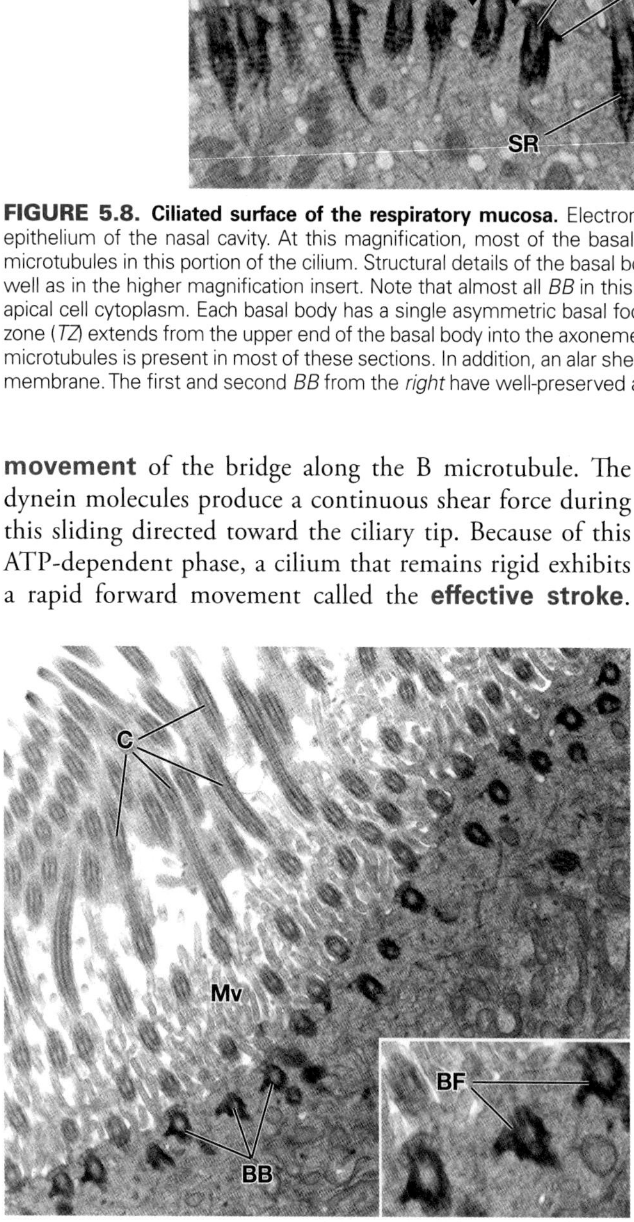

FIGURE 5.9. Basal bodies and cilia. This diagnostic electron micrograph obtained during biopsy of the nasal mucosa from a child undergoing evaluation for primary ciliary dyskinesia shows a normal appearance of basal bodies (*BB*) and cilia (*C*). It is an oblique section through the apical part of ciliated cells. *BB* seen in cross section appear as more dense structures than the longitudinal profiles of the *C* that appear in the oblique section above. Several profiles of microvilli (*Mv*) are visible at the apical cell surface. ×11,000. **Inset.** Three *BB* sectioned at the level of basal feet (*BF*). Note that all basal feet are oriented in the same direction. They most likely rotate the basal body to a desired angle in an effort to coordinate ciliary movement. ×24,000. (Courtesy of Patrice C. Abell-Aleff.)

At the same time, the passive elastic connections provided by the protein nexin and the radial spokes accumulate the energy necessary to bring the cilium back to the straight position. Cilia then become flexible and bend toward the lateral side on the slower return movement, the **recovery stroke.**

However, if all dynein arms along the length of the A microtubules in all nine doublets attempted to form temporary cross-bridges simultaneously, no effective stroke of the cilium would result. Thus, regulation of the active shear force is required. Current evidence suggests that the central pair of microtubules in 9 + 2 cilia undergo rotation with respect to the nine outer doublets. This rotation may be driven by another motor protein, kinesin, which is associated with the central pair of microtubules. The central microtubule pair can act as a "distributor" that progressively regulates the sequence of interactions of the dynein arms to produce an effective stroke.

Cilia beat in a synchronous pattern.

Motile cilia with a 9 + 2 pattern display a precise and synchronous undulating movement. Cilia in successive rows start their beat so that each row is slightly more advanced in its cycle than the following row, thus creating a wave that sweeps across the epithelium. As previously discussed, basal feet of basal bodies are most likely responsible for synchronization of ciliary movement. During the process of **cilia formation**, all basal feet become oriented in the same direction of effective stroke by rotating basal bodies. This orientation allows cilia to achieve a **metachronal rhythm** that is responsible for moving mucus over epithelial surfaces or facilitating the flow of fluid and other substances through tubular organs and ducts.

Primary cilia are nonmotile and contain a 9 + 0 pattern of microtubules.

In contrast to motile cilia with the 9 + 2 pattern of microtubules, **primary cilia** or monocilia display a **9 + 0 microtubule arrangement**. They are called *primary cilia* or *monocilia* because a cell usually possesses only one such cilium (Fig. 5.10). Cilia with this pattern have the following characteristics:

- They are nonmotile and passively bend by the flow of the fluid.
- They lack microtubule-associated motor proteins (dynein arms) needed to generate motile force.
- The central pair of microtubules and radial spokes at the center of the axoneme with surrounding them proteins are missing.
- The axoneme originates from a basal body that resembles a mature centriole positioned orthogonally in relation to its immature counterpart.
- Primary cilium formation is synchronized with cell cycle progression and centrosome duplication events.

Primary cilia are present in most cells of epithelial, connective, muscle, and nervous tissues. They are also present in **stem cells** and in almost all cells during **embryogenesis** and fetal development. Examples of cells possessing primary cilia in epithelium include the epithelial cells of the rete testis and efferent ductules in the **male reproductive tract**, epithelial cells lining the uterine tube (uterus [endometrium]) and vagina in the **female reproductive tract**, epithelial cells lining the **biliary tract**, epithelial cells of **kidney** tubules (Fig. 5.10b), epithelial-like ependymal cells lining the fluid-filled cavities of the **central nervous system**, photoreceptor cells in the **retina**, and the vestibular hair cells of the **ear**. Table 5.3 summarizes the location of primary cilia in various tissues and organs in the body.

Primary cilia were formerly classified as nonfunctional vestigial developmental abnormalities of 9 + 2 motile cilia. Experimental studies have elevated the status of primary cilia to the level of important **cellular signaling devices**. Acting similarly to an antenna on a global positioning system (GPS) device, which receives signals from a satellite to pinpoint the user's location, primary cilia receive chemical, osmotic, light, and mechanical stimuli from the extracellular environment. In response to these stimuli, primary cilia generate signals that are transmitted into the cell to modify cellular processes in response to changes in the external environment. In many mammalian cells, signaling through the primary cilia seems to be essential for controlled cell division, cell migration during tissue regeneration, and subsequent gene expression.

Primary cilia containing a 9 + 0 pattern of microtubules function as signal receptors that sense the flow of fluid in organs.

Primary cilia function in secretory organs such as the kidneys, liver, or pancreas as sensors of fluid flow. They extend from the surface of epithelial cells lining secretory ducts into the extracellular lumen (Fig. 5.11). For instance, primary cilia found in the glomerulus and tubular cells of the kidney function as **mechanoreceptors**; fluid flow through the renal corpuscle and tubules causes them to bend, which initiates an influx of calcium into the cell (see Fig. 5.11). In humans, mutations in **PKD1**, **PKD2**, and **PKHD1** genes appear to affect the development of these primary cilia, leading to **polycystic kidney disease (PKD)**. The proteins **polycystin-1** and **polycystin-2** encoded by PKD1 and PKD2 genes, respectively, are essential in the formation of the **calcium channels** associated with **primary cilia** (see Fig. 5.10b). The PKHD1 gene encodes the large protein **fibrocystin/polyductin** that targets the polycystin-2–binding domain.

There are two major forms of PKD that are distinguished by the age of onset and its inheritance pattern. The **autosomal dominant form (ADPKD)** affects 1 in 500–1,000

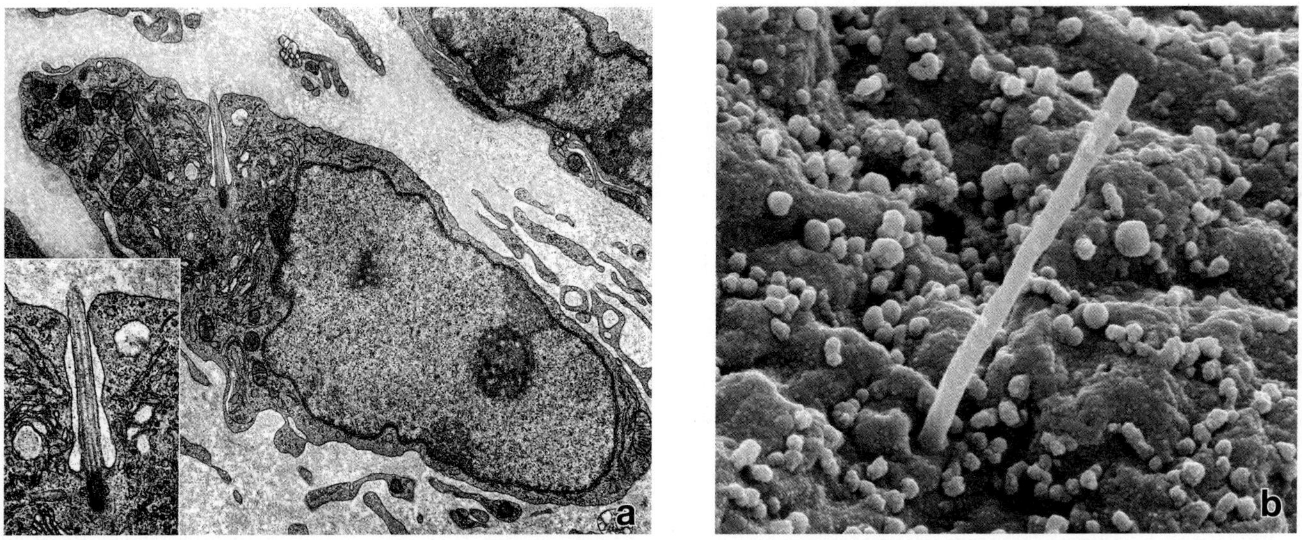

FIGURE 5.10. Primary cilia in the connective tissue and the kidney tubule. a. Electron micrograph shows a fibroblast surrounded by the extracellular matrix from the uterine connective tissue containing a primary cilium. The primary cilium is characterized by a 9 + 0 pattern microtubule arrangement. ×45,000. The *inset* shows the cilium at a higher magnification. Note the visible basal body and doublets of microtubules emerging from the basal body. ×90,000. **b.** This scanning electron micrograph shows a single primary cilium projecting into the lumen of the collecting tubule of the kidney. Primary cilia are prominent on the free surface of the collecting tubule cells and function as mechanoreceptors that are activated by fluid flow through the tubules. Passive bending of cilia opens calcium channels, allowing an influx of calcium into the cell cytoplasm that initiates signaling cascades. ×65,000. (Courtesy of Dr. Tetyana V. Masyuk.)

TABLE 5.3 Examples of Tissues and Organs Containing Cells With Primary Cilia

Tissue	Example of Cells
Epithelial tissue	Epithelial cells lining the following structures: Blood and lymphatic vessels (endothelium) Air passages (respiratory and olfactory epithelium) Oral cavity (oral mucosa) Renal tubules Biliary tree (cholangiocytes) Pancreatic ducts Female reproductive tract (uterine tube, uterus, vagina) Male reproductive tract (prostate glands, efferent ductules, rete testis, seminal vesicles, myoid cells) Mammary gland ducts (including myoepithelial cells)
Connective tissue	Fibroblasts in all types of connective tissues Tendinocytes in tendons Osteoblasts and osteocytes in bone Chondroblasts and chondrocytes in cartilage Ameloblasts and odontoblasts in developing teeth Synovial cells (synoviocytes) in joint capsule
Muscle tissue	Smooth muscle cells Skeletal muscle cells
Nerve tissue	Neurons Schwann cells Ependymal cells
Organ	**Example of Cells**
Skin	Basal cells Keratinocytes Melanocytes Fibroblasts (in dermis)
Kidney	Podocytes Mesangial cells Interstitial cells Endothelium of blood vessels Epithelial cells of renal tubules and Bowman capsule
Testis	Leydig cells Myoid cells Epithelial cells of rete testis and efferent ductules
Ovary	Germinal epithelium Follicular cells Theca interna cells Stromal cells
Spleen	Reticular cells
Liver	Cholangiocytes Hepatic stellate cells
Endocrine glands	Secretory cells of adrenal glands, thyroid gland, parathyroid gland, pituitary gland, and islets of Langerhans (endocrine pancreas)
Sensory organs	Photoreceptor cells in retina Olfactory epithelium Taste buds Internal ear

people and usually begins in adulthood. It is characterized by multiple expanding cysts in both kidneys, which ultimately destroy the renal cortex and lead to renal failure. The **autosomal recessive form (ARPKD)** is much less common (estimated 1 in 20,000–40,000 people) and begins after birth or in early infancy. This form is often lethal early in life.

Individuals with ADPKD often exhibit other pathologies not associated with the kidney that are attributed to ciliary abnormalities. These include **cysts in the pancreas and liver** that are accompanied by enlargement and dilatation of the biliary tree system. Other changes include **retinitis pigmentosa** (abnormalities of the photoreceptors cells of the retina that cause progressive vision loss), sensorineural hearing loss, diabetes, and learning disabilities. Gaining a deeper understanding of the roles that primary cilia play in the body may help explain many of the pathologic conditions that can affect vital internal organs.

During early embryonic development, nodal cilia containing a 9 + 0 pattern of microtubules establish the left–right asymmetry of internal organs.

Internal organs in the body show a **left–right asymmetry** with regard to their position and morphology. Such morphologic asymmetries are essential for the proper function of

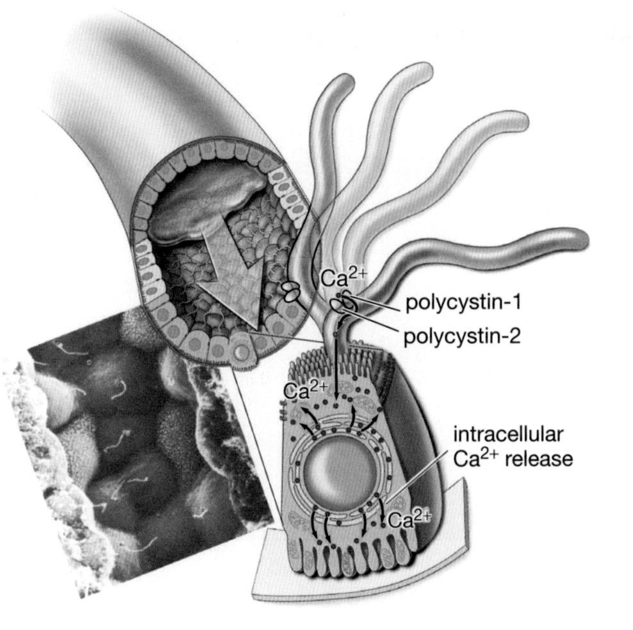

FIGURE 5.11. Primary cilia as fluid-flow sensors. Primary cilia in the kidney act as receptors to sense the flow of fluid through the tubules. Deflection of the primary cilium opens mechanoreceptor calcium channels, which are formed by the polycystin-1 and polycystin-2 proteins. This subsequently initiates the influx of calcium into the cell, releasing additional intracellular calcium from the endoplasmic reticulum. The scanning electron micrograph *inset* shows primary cilia projecting into the lumen of the collecting tubule. ×27,000. (Courtesy of Dr. C. Craig Tisher.)

internal organs and are controlled by a genetic pathway that operates in the developing embryo.

Cilia play an essential role in breaking the left–right symmetry seen in the early stages of embryo development. This process begins on the ventral surface of the bilaminar embryonic disc in the area near the **primitive (ventral) node**, a transient midline structure formed during gastrulation. A specialized type of motile cilium (one per cell) has been observed in cells of this area that are similar in appearance to the primary cilia. However, despite their 9 + 0 architectural pattern, they are motile and capable of producing a **unidirectional clockwise rotation**. Owing to their presence near the primitive node, these cilia are called **nodal cilia**. In contrast to nonmotile primary cilia, they contain dynein arms (motor protein complexes) that cause the A microtubule to slide relative to the B microtubule in the adjacent microtubule doublet. In addition, the absence of the central pair of microtubules and stabilizing radial spokes keeps the nodal cilia rotating clockwise instead of beating along a plane. The trajectory of nodal cilia movement resembles a full cone in contrast to the half-cone trajectory traceable in the conventional motile 9 + 2 cilia (see Table 5.2).

During gastrulation, the clockwise rotation of nodal cilia generates a leftward **unidirectional flow (nodal flow) of the extraembryonic fluid**. The nodal flow transports small signaling molecules (e.g., lipoproteins) to the left side of the embryo, triggering left-specific signaling pathways. Also, shear resistance and mechanical stimuli generated by the flow are sensed by cells. For instance, nonmotile primary cilia surrounding the primitive node react to the stronger fluid flow on the left side by opening mechanoreceptor calcium channels and initiating specific signaling mechanisms that differ from those on the right side of the embryo. This leads to **asymmetric left-sided gene expression** later in development.

When nodal cilia are immotile or absent, nodal flow does not occur, leading to random placement of internal body organs. **Primary ciliary dyskinesia** (immotile cilia syndrome) often results in **situs inversus**, a condition in which the position of the heart and abdominal organs is reversed. For details, see Folder 5.2 (page 139).

The first stage of ciliogenesis includes generation of centrioles.

The first stage of **ciliary apparatus formation (ciliogenesis)** in differentiating cells involves the generation of multiple centrioles. This process occurs via the **centriolar pathway**, in which pairs of existing centrioles are duplicated (see pages 78-79 in Chapter 2, Cell Cytoplasm), or more commonly via the **acentriolar pathway** in which centrioles are formed de novo without involvement of existing centrioles. Both pathways give rise to multiple **procentrioles**, the immediate precursors of centrioles. Procentrioles mature (elongate) to **form centrioles**, one for each cilium, and migrate to the apical surface of the cell. After perpendicularly aligning themselves and securing to the apical cell membrane by alar sheets (transitional fibers), centrioles assume the function of **basal bodies**. The next stage of ciliary apparatus formation involves the formation of the remaining basal body–associated structures that include basal feet and striated rootlets. From each of the nine triplets that make up the basal body, a microtubule doublet grows upward by polymerization of α- and β-tubulin molecules. A growing projection of the apical cell membrane becomes visible and contains the nine doublets found in the mature cilium. During the **elongation stage** of motile cilia formation, the assembly of two single, central microtubules begins in the transitional zone from γ-tubulin rings. The subsequent polymerization of tubulin molecules occurs within the ring of doublet microtubules, thus yielding the characteristic axonemal 9 + 2 arrangement. Subsequently, the axoneme grows upward from the basal body, pushing the cell membrane outward to form the **mature cilium**.

Ciliogenesis depends on the bidirectional intraflagellar transport mechanism that supplies precursor molecules to the growing cilium.

During the growth and elongation of the cilium, precursor molecules are delivered from the cell body to the most distal end of the elongating axoneme by **intraflagellar transport (IFT)**. Because cilia lack the molecular machinery for protein synthesis, the IFT is the only mechanism for delivering proteins required for cilia assembly and growth. In some ways, the IFT can be compared to the vertical lift assembly used at a construction site to move building materials and tools up and down a building. As the building increases in height, the track of the lift extends as well. Similarly, the IFT utilizes **raft-like platforms** assembled from approximately 17 different **intraflagellar transport proteins** that move up and down the growing axoneme between the outer doublets of microtubules and the plasma membrane of the elongating cilium (Fig. 5.12). Cargo molecules (including inactive cytoplasmic dynein molecules) are loaded onto the IFT platform while it is docked near the base of the cilium. Utilizing **kinesin II** as a motor protein, the fully loaded platform is moved upward toward the tip of the cilium (anterograde transport). The "building materials" are then unloaded at the tip of the cilium (the site

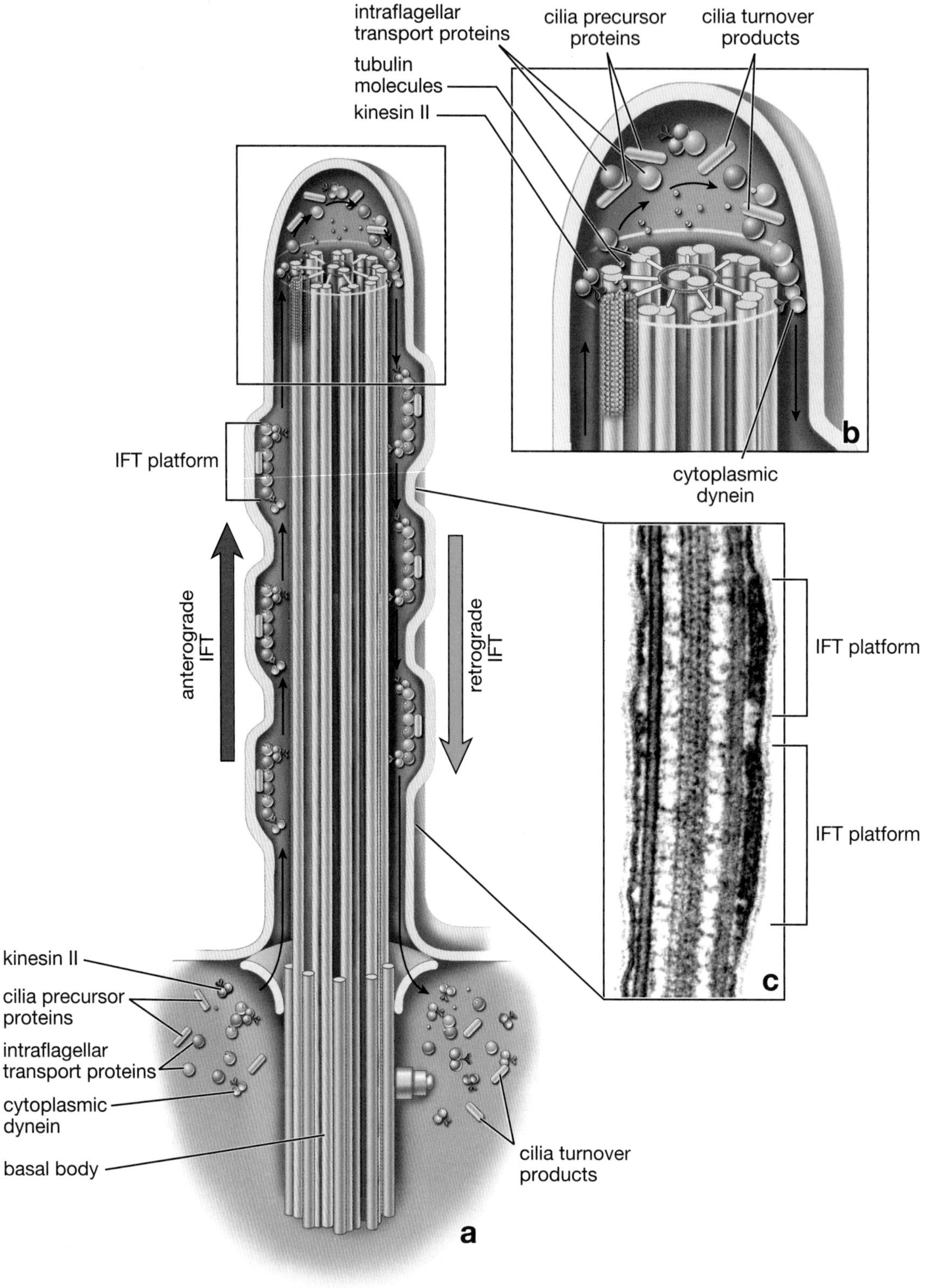

FIGURE 5.12. Intraflagellar transport mechanism within the cilium. a. Assembly and maintenance of cilia depend on the intraflagellar transport (*IFT*) mechanism that utilizes raft-like platforms. The *IFT* platforms move up and down between the outer doublets of microtubules and plasma membrane of the elongating cilium. Cargo molecules (including inactive cytoplasmic dynein) are loaded onto the *IFT* platform while it is docked near the base of the cilium. Using kinesin II as a motor protein, the fully loaded platform is moved upward toward the plus ends of the microtubules at the tip of the cilium (anterograde transport). **b.** The cargo is then unloaded at the tip of the cilium (the site of axoneme assembly). Here, particles turn around, and the platform powered by cytoplasmic dynein heads back to the base of the cilium (retrograde transport) after picking up turnover products (including inactivated kinesin II). **c.** Electron micrograph of a longitudinal section of a *Chlamydomonas* flagellum with two groups of *IFT* platforms. ×55,000. (Reprinted with permission from Pedersen LB, Veland IR, Schrøder JM, et al. Assembly of primary cilia. *Dev Dyn.* 2008;237:1993–2006.)

FOLDER 5.2

CLINICAL CORRELATION: PRIMARY CILIARY DYSKINESIA (IMMOTILE CILIA SYNDROME)

Cilia are present in almost all organs and play a significant role in the human body. There is increasing evidence that ciliary dysfunction is involved in many human disorders. Several hereditary disorders grouped under the general name of **primary ciliary dyskinesia (PCD)**, also known as **immotile cilia syndrome**, affect the function of cilia. PCD represents a group of autosomal recessive hereditary disorders affecting 1 in 20,000 individuals at birth.

The clinical features of PCD reflect the distribution of motile cilia. For instance, the mucociliary transport that occurs in the respiratory epithelium is one of the important mechanisms protecting the body against invading bacteria and other pathogens. Motile cilia covering the epithelium of the respiratory tract are responsible for the clearance of the airway. Failure of the mucociliary transport system occurs in **Kartagener syndrome**, which is caused by a structural abnormality that results in absence of dynein arms (Fig. F5.2.1). In addition, electron microscopy (EM) examination of basal bodies from individuals with Kartagener syndrome often reveals misoriented basal feet pointing in different directions. **Young syndrome**, which is characterized by malformation of the radial spokes and dynein arms, also affects ciliary function in the respiratory tract. The most prominent symptoms of PCD are chronic respiratory disorders (including bronchitis and sinusitis), otitis media (inflammation of the middle ear cavity), persistent cough, and asthma. Respiratory problems are caused by severely impaired or absent ciliary motility that results in reduced or absent mucociliary transport in the tracheobronchial tree.

The flagellum of sperm, cilia of the efferent ductules in the testis, and cilia of the female reproductive system share the same organization (9 + 2) pattern with the cilia of the respiratory tract. Therefore, males with PCD are sterile because of immotile flagella. In contrast, some females with the syndrome may be fertile; however, there is an increased incidence of ectopic pregnancy. In such individuals, the ciliary movement may be sufficient, although impaired, to permit transport of the ovum through the oviduct to the uterus.

Some individuals with PCD may also develop symptoms of **hydrocephalus internus** (accumulation of fluid in the brain) or transient dilatation of inner brain ventricles. The ependymal cells lining the cerebrospinal fluid–filled space in the brain possess motile cilia with a 9 + 2 pattern. These cilia may be important for the circulation of cerebrospinal fluid through the narrow spaces between the brain ventricles.

About 50% of patients with PCD have **situs inversus** (a condition in which the organs of the viscera are transposed through the sagittal plane), providing a link between left–right asymmetry and nodal cilia.

Diagnosis of PCD in individuals with clinical syndromes compatible with PCD can be established by EM (see Fig. F5.2.1).

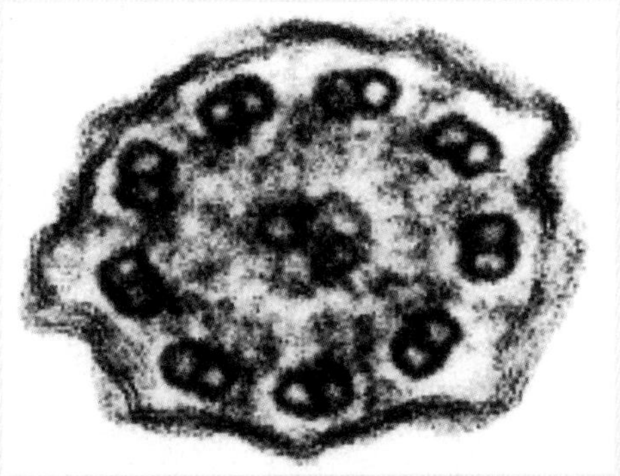

FIGURE F5.2.1. Electron micrograph of a cilium from an individual with primary ciliary dyskinesia. In this cross section, note the absence of dynein arms on microtubule doublets. ×180,000. (Courtesy of Patrice Abell-Aleff.)

of axoneme assembly). Here, the platform turns around and heads back to the base of the cilium (retrograde transport) after picking up turnover products (including inactivated kinesin II). During this process, **cytoplasmic dynein** is activated and utilized as a motor protein to return the platform to the base of the cilium (see Fig. 5.12). Several proteins, including IFT raft proteins (kinesis, cytoplasmic dynein, polaris, IFT20, etc.), are important to ciliogenesis and subsequent maintenance of the functional cilium. Mutations in genes encoding these proteins result in the loss of cilia or ciliary dysfunctions. For instance, the IFT20 raft protein transports cargo proteins for sperm flagella formation. A mutation in this gene can affect male fertility and spermiogenesis.

■ THE LATERAL DOMAIN AND ITS SPECIALIZATIONS IN CELL-TO-CELL ADHESION

The **lateral domain** of epithelial cells is in close contact with the opposed lateral domains of neighboring cells. Like the other domains, the lateral domain is characterized by the presence of unique proteins, in this case, the **cell adhesion molecules (CAMs)** that are part of junctional specializations. The molecular composition of the lipids and proteins that form the lateral cell membrane differs significantly from the composition of those that form the apical cell membrane. In addition, the lateral cell surface membrane in some epithelia may form folds and processes, invaginations, and evaginations that create interdigitating and interleaving tongue-and-groove margins between neighboring cells.

Viewed with the LM, terminal bars represent epithelial cell-to-cell attachment sites.

Before the advent of EM, the close apposition of epithelial cells was attributed to the presence of a viscous adhesive substance referred to as *intercellular cement.* This cement is stained deeply at the apicolateral margin of most cuboidal and columnar epithelial cells. When viewed in a plane perpendicular to the epithelial surface, the stained material appears as a dot-like structure. When the plane of section passes parallel to and includes the epithelial surface, however, the dot-like component is seen as a dense bar or line between the apposing cells (Fig. 5.13). The bars, in fact, form a polygonal structure (or band) that encircles each cell to bind them together. Arrangement of this band can be compared to the plastic rings that hold together a six-pack of canned beverages.

Because of its location in the terminal or apical portion of the cell and its bar-like configuration, the stainable material visible in LM was called the **terminal bar**. It is now evident that intercellular cement as such does not exist. The terminal bar, however, does represent a significant structural complex. EM has shown that it includes a specialized site that joins epithelial cells (Fig. 5.14a). It is also the site of a considerable barrier to the passage (diffusion) of substances between adjacent epithelial cells. The specific structural components that make up the barrier and the attachment device are readily identified with the EM and are collectively referred to as a **junctional complex** (see Table 5.5, page 152). These complexes are responsible for

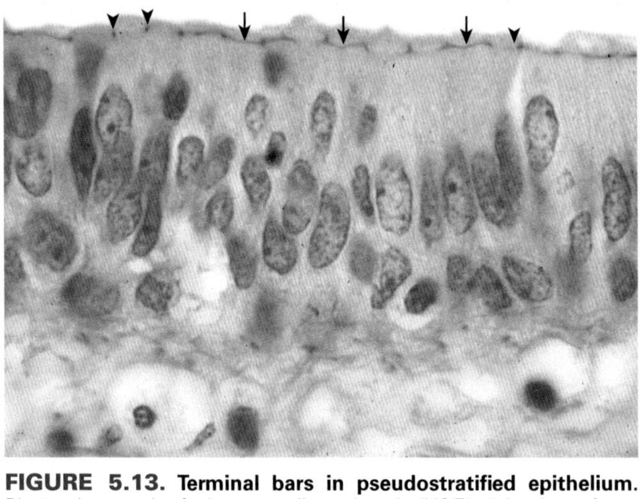

FIGURE 5.13. Terminal bars in pseudostratified epithelium. Photomicrograph of a hematoxylin and eosin (H&E)-stained specimen showing the terminal bars in a pseudostratified epithelium. The bar appears as a dot (*arrowheads*) when seen on its cut edge. When the bar courses parallel to the cut surface and lie within the thickness of the section, it is seen as a linear or bar-like profile (*arrows*). ×550.

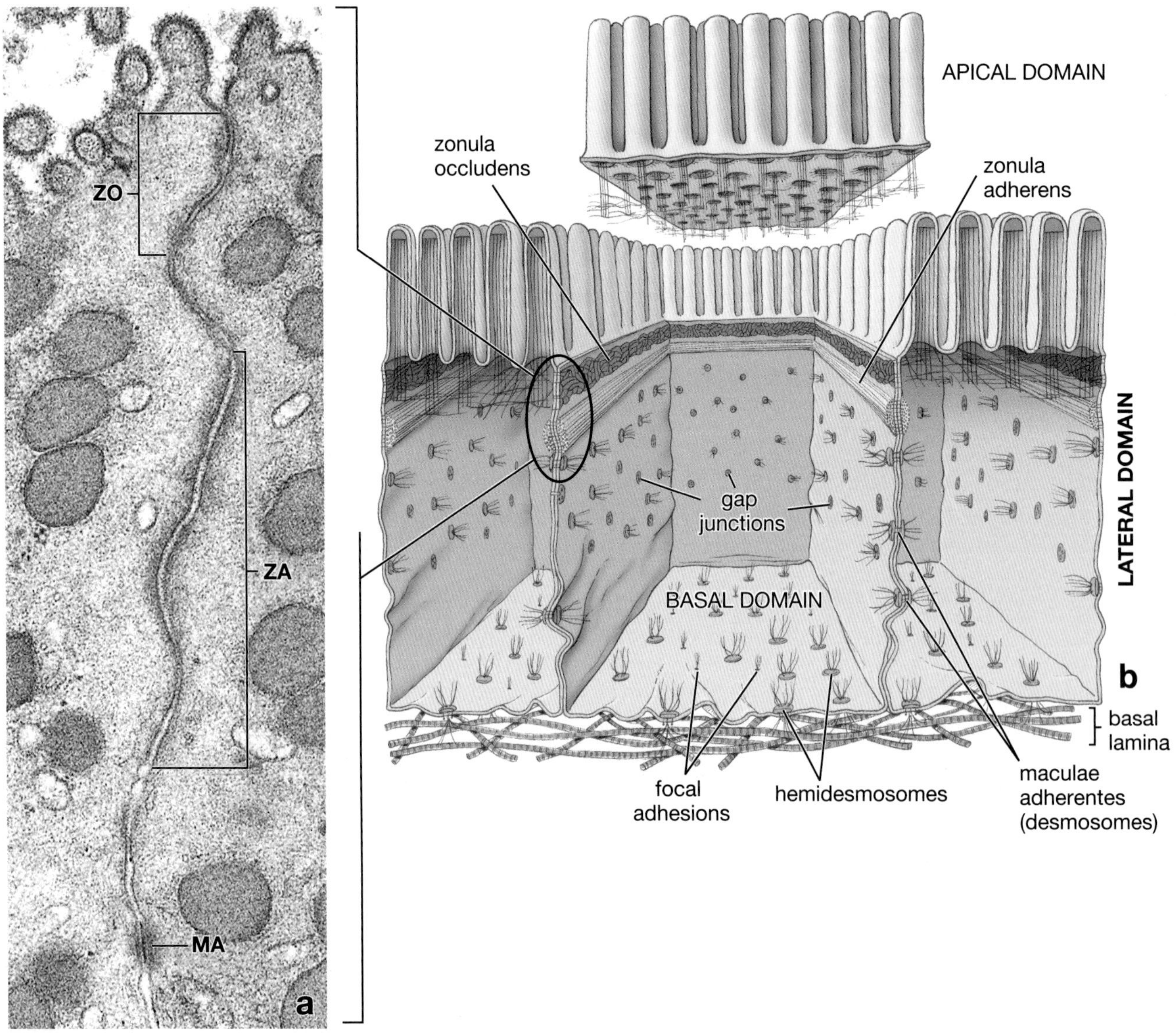

FIGURE 5.14. Junctional complex. a. Electron micrograph of the apical portion of two adjoining epithelial cells of the gastric mucosa showing the junctional complex. It consists of the zonula occludens (*ZO*), zonula adherens (*ZA*), and macula adherens (*MA*). ×30,000. **b.** Diagram showing the distribution of cell junctions in the three cellular domains of columnar epithelial cells. The apical domain with microvilli has been lifted to better illustrate the spatial arrangements of junctional complexes within the cell.

joining individual cells together. There are three types of junctional complexes (Fig. 5.14b):

- **Occluding junctions**, also called **tight junctions**, are essential for establishing a barrier between different compartments of the body and allow epithelial cells to function as a barrier. Occluding junctions form the primary **paracellular diffusion barrier** between adjacent cells. By limiting the movement of ions, water, and other macromolecules through the intercellular space, they maintain the physicochemical separation of tissue compartments. Because they are located at the most apical point between adjoining epithelial cells, occluding junctions act as fences to prevent the migration of lipids and specialized membrane proteins between the apical and lateral surfaces, thus maintaining **cell polarity** and integrity of these two domains. In addition, occluding junctions recruit various signaling molecules to the cell surface and link them to the **actin filaments** of the cell cytoskeleton.
- **Anchoring junctions** provide mechanical stability to epithelial cells by linking the cytoskeleton of one cell to the cytoskeleton of an adjacent cell. These junctions are important in creating and maintaining the structural unity of the epithelium. Anchoring junctions interact with both **actin** and **intermediate filaments** and can be found not only on the lateral cell surface but also on the basal domain of the epithelial cell. Through their signal transduction capability, anchoring junctions also play important roles in cell-to-cell recognition, morphogenesis, and differentiation.
- **Communicating junctions** allow direct communication between adjacent cells by diffusion of small (<1.2 kDa) molecules (e.g., ions, amino acids, sugars, nucleotides, second messengers, metabolites). This type of intercellular communication permits the coordinated cellular activity that is important for maintaining organ homeostasis.

Occluding Junctions

The **zonula occludens** (pl., *zonulae occludentes*) represents the most apical component in the junctional complex between epithelial cells.

The zonula occludens is created by localized sealing of the plasma membrane between two adjacent cells.

Examination of the **zonula occludens** or **tight junction** with the transmission electron microscope (TEM) reveals a narrow region in which the plasma membranes of two adjoining cells come in close contact to seal off the intercellular space (Fig. 5.15a). At high resolution, the zonula occludens appears not only as a continuous seal but also as a series of focal fusions between the cells. These focal fusions are created by transmembrane proteins of adjoining cells that join in the intercellular space (Fig. 5.15b). The arrangement of these proteins in forming the seal is best visualized by the freeze-fracture technique (Fig. 5.15c). When the plasma membrane is fractured at the site of the zonula occludens, the junctional proteins are observed on the P-face of the membrane, where they appear as ridge-like structures. The opposing

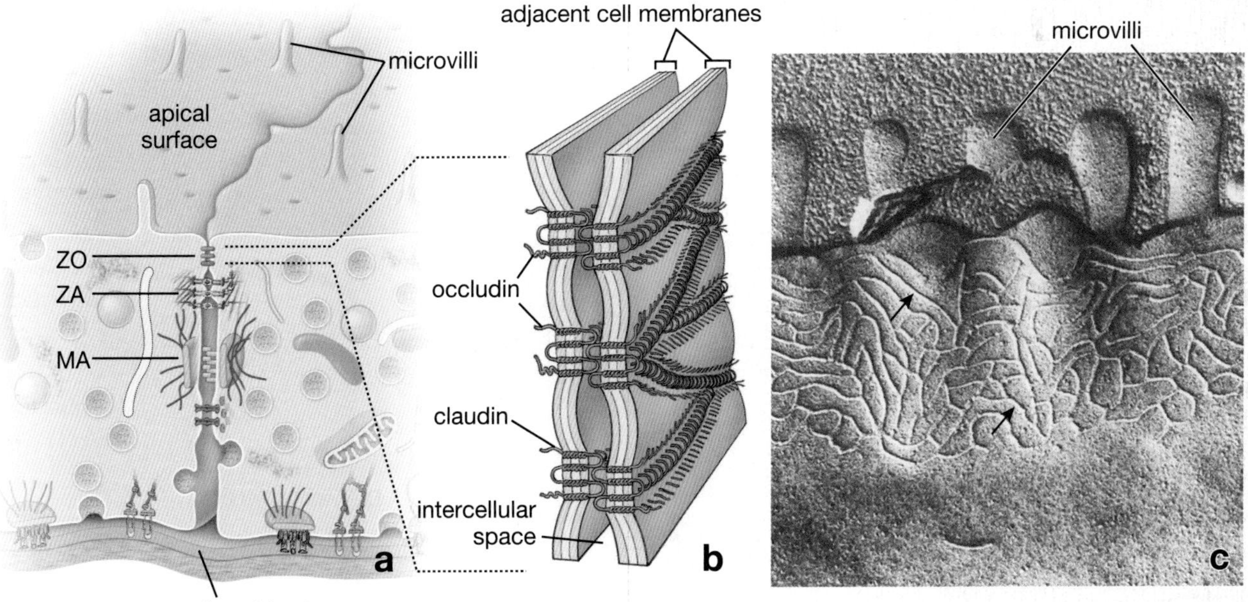

FIGURE 5.15. Junctional complex. a. This diagram shows the location of anchoring cell-to-cell junctions in the epithelial cell. The junctional complex near the apical (luminal) surface comprises zonula occludens (*ZO*), zonula adherens (*ZA*), and macula adherens (*MA*), also called *desmosome*. Below the *MA*, note the communicating junctions. Also, cell-to-extracellular matrix junctions (hemidesmosomes and focal adhesions) are visible on the basal cell membrane. **b.** Diagram showing the organization and pattern of distribution of the transmembrane proteins within the occluding junction. Compare the linear pattern of grooves with the ridges detected in the freeze-fracture preparation on the right side. **c.** Freeze-fracture preparation of zonula occludens shown here reveals an anastomosing network of ridges (*arrows*) located on the fractured membrane surface near the apical part of the cell (note the presence of microvilli at the cell surface). This is the P-face of the membrane. (The E-face of the fractured membrane would show a complementary pattern of grooves.) The ridges represent linear arrays of transmembrane proteins (most likely occludins) involved in the formation of the zonula occludens. The membrane of the opposing cell contains a similar network of proteins, which is in register with the first cell. The actual sites of protein interaction between the cells form the anastomosing network. ×100,000. (Reprinted with permission from Hull BE, Staehelin LA. Functional significance of the variations in the geometrical organization of tight junction networks. *J Cell Biol.* 1976;68:688–704.)

surface of the fractured membrane, the E-face, reveals complementary grooves resulting from detachment of the protein particles from the opposing surface. The ridges and grooves are arranged as a honeycomb-like network of anastomosing **intramembranous particle strands**, creating a belt of junctions that surrounds each cell and seals the whole intercellular space within the epithelial sheets. The number of strands as well as the degree of anastomosis vary in different cells.

The zonula occludens undergoes modification in areas where the corners of three epithelial cells meet together.

The **zonula occludens** has been classically described as a **bicellular contact** structure because it only seals the space between two adjacent cells. However, because most apical domains of epithelial cells are polygonal in shape, only the sides of these cells form a zonula occludens with this classically bicellular contact with neighboring cells. Their vertices form a modified **tricellular zonula occludens** junction at a **tricellular contact**, where the corners of three epithelial cells meet together (Fig. 5.16). As the zonula occludens approaches a tricellular contact region, apical extensions of the intramembranous particle strands that have run horizontally turn vertically to run along the lateral domain at the corner of each epithelial cell, thus forming a pair of vertical strands. These two vertical strands are referred to as **central sealing elements** (see Fig 5.16) and contain unique proteins, different than those found in bilateral contacts. These elements are more effective in maintaining the epithelial barrier in the specific areas of tricellular contacts. The corners of the plasma membranes from all three cells never completely seal the extracellular space at their meeting points. Their corners containing central sealing elements border a long and narrow space called the **central tube**, which is an integral part of the extracellular space. Because the central tube represents a weak point for the epithelial barrier, unique proteins (i.e., **tricellulin**) are required to seal this area and maintain the epithelial permeability barrier.

Several proteins are involved in the formation of zonula occludens strands.

Zonula occludens strands correspond to the location of the rows of transmembrane proteins. Four major groups of transmembrane proteins are found in the zonula occludens (Fig. 5.17; Table 5.4):

- **Claudins** constitute a family of proteins (20–27 kDa) that form the backbone of tight junctions and are integral components of zonula occludens strands. In addition, claudins (especially claudin-2 and claudin-16) are able to form **extracellular aqueous channels** for the paracellular passage of ions and other small molecules. About 24 different members of the claudin family have been characterized to date. Mutations in the gene encoding **claudin-14** have been linked to human **hereditary deafness**. A mutated form of claudin-14 causes an increased permeability of zonula occludens in the organ of Corti (receptor of hearing), affecting the generation of action potentials.
- **Occludin**, a 60-kDa protein, participates in forming and maintaining the barrier between adjacent cells and acts as a fence to restrict the movement of lipids and proteins between the apical and lateral domains. Occludin is present in most occluding junctions. However, several types of epithelial cells do not have occludin within their strands but still possess well-developed and fully functional zonulae occludentes. Multiple viruses exploit tight junctions to

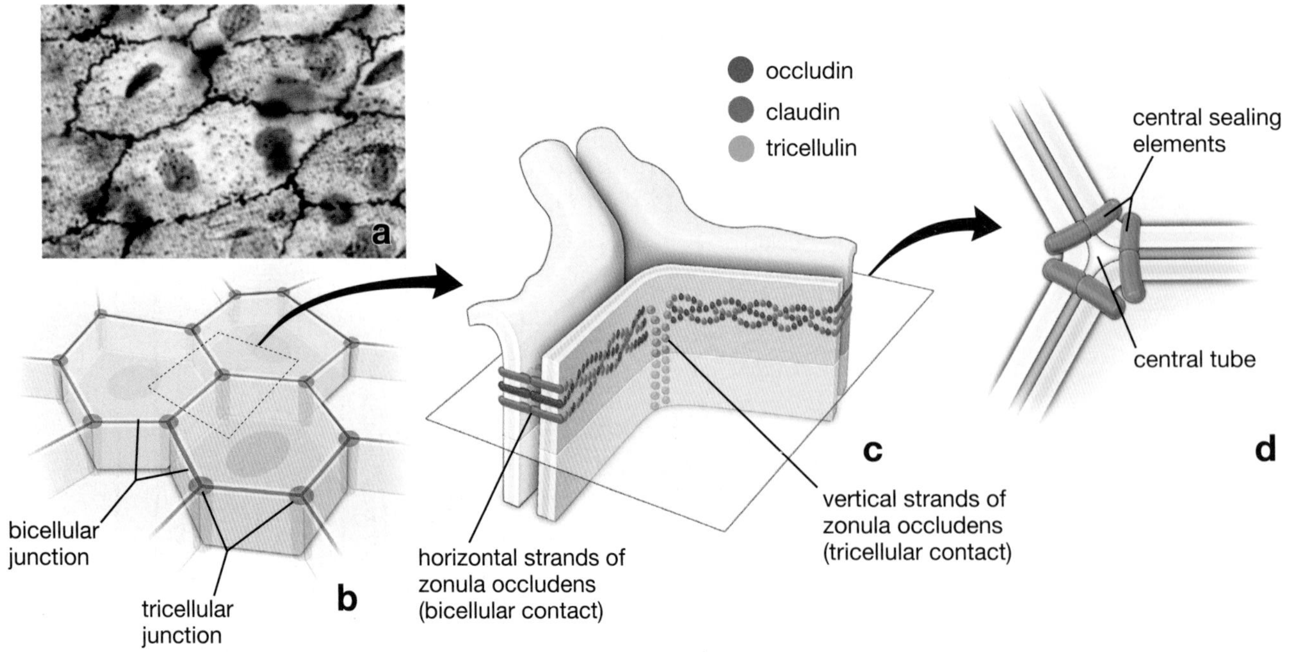

FIGURE 5.16. Tricellular zonula occludens junctions. a. This image of the apical surface of mesothelial cells impregnated with silver salts clearly shows the polygonal shape of epithelial cells. Their boundaries are delineated by black lines marked by the precipitated silver. Note that in addition to regions where the cells are in close apposition to one another, there are also regions where three cells come together to form tricellular contacts. ×700. **b.** This schematic drawing shows the polygonal shape of epithelial cells and areas of tricellular and bicellular contacts. **c.** The horizontal strands of zonula occludens (formed by occludins and claudins) seal only the space between two adjacent cells. In corners where three epithelial cells meet, the zonula occludens is modified to form a tricellular junction. The horizontal strands of the zonula occludens approaching this tricellular contact turn vertically to run along the corner of each epithelial cell. A pair of these vertical strands is composed of unique proteins that include tricellulin. **d.** In this cross section of a tricellular junction, note the central sealing elements formed by vertical strands of tricellulins that border a narrow space between all three cells. This space, called the *central tube*, represents a potential place for intercellular (paracellular) passage of water and solutes.

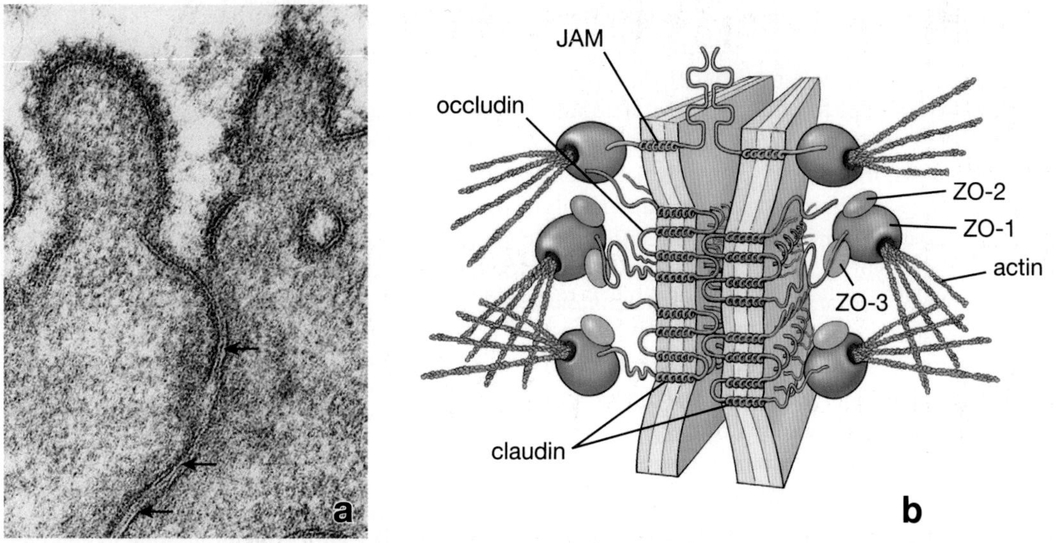

FIGURE 5.17. Zonula occludens. a. Electron micrograph of the zonula occludens (*ZO*) showing the close approximation of the outer lamellae of adjoining plasma membranes. The extracellular domains of proteins involved in the formation of this junction (occludins) appear as single, electron-dense lines (*arrows*). ×100,000. **b.** Diagram showing three transmembrane proteins involved in the formation of zonula occludens: occludin, claudin, and junctional adhesion molecule (*JAM*). Occludin and claudin have four transmembrane domains with two extracellular loops, but *JAM* has only a single transmembrane domain, and its extracellular portion possesses two immunoglobulin-like loops. Several major associated proteins of the occluding junction and their interactions are also shown. Note that one of the associated proteins, ZO-1, interacts with the cell cytoskeleton by binding actin filaments.

TABLE 5.4 Major Proteins Localized Within the Zonula Occludens Junction

Zonula Occludens Protein	Associated Protein Partners	Function
Claudin	Claudin, ZO-1, JAM	Forms backbone of ZO strands; forms and regulates aqueous channels used for paracellular diffusion
Occludin	Occludin, ZO-1, ZO-2, ZO-3, Vap33, actin	Is present in most occluding junctions; maintains a barrier between apical and lateral cell surface
JAM	JAM, ZO-1, claudin	Present in occluding junctions in endothelial cells; mediates interactions between endothelial cells and monocyte adhesions
Tricellulin	Tricellulin, angulins, claudin, occludin	Present in specific areas of ZO at tricellular contacts
ZO-1	ZO-2, ZO-3, occludin, claudin, JAM, cingulin, actin, ZONAB, ASIP, AF-6, afadin, α-catenin	Important link in transduction of signals from all transmembrane proteins; interacts with actin filaments; has tumor suppressor action
ZO-2	ZO-1, occludin, cingulin, 4.1R	Required in the epidermal growth factor–receptor signaling mechanism
ZO-3	ZO-1, occludin, actin	Interacts with ZO-1, occludin, and actin filaments of cell cytoskeleton
AF-6	RAS, ZO-1	Small protein involved in molecular transport system and signal transduction
Cingulin	ZO-1, ZO-2, ZO-3, cingulin, myosin II	Acidic, heat-stable protein that cross-links actin filaments into sedimentable complexes
Symplekin	CPSF-100	Dual-location protein: localized in ZO and the interchromatin particles of the karyoplasm
ASIP/Par3	PKC-ζ	Controls relocation of asymmetrically distributed proteins
Rab3b	GTPase	Members of the RAS oncogene family of proteins; control the assembly of protein complexes for docking of transport vesicles
Rab13	δ-PDE	
Rab8	G/C kinase, Sec4	
Sec4	Rab8	GTPase required for polarized delivery of cargo vesicles to plasma membrane
Sec6	Sec8	Participates in fusion of Golgi vesicle with the plasma membrane
Sec8	Sec6	Inhibits basolateral translocation of LDLP receptors after formation of ZO

AF, antisecretory factor; *ASIP*, agouti signaling protein; *CPSF*, cleavage and polyadenylation specificity factor; *G/C*, germinal center; *GTPase*, guanosine triphosphatase; *JAM*, junctional adhesion molecule; *LDLP*, low-density lipoprotein; *PDE*, phosphodiesterases; *PKC*, protein kinase C; *RAS*, rat sarcoma; *ZO*, zonula occludens; *ZONAB*, zonula occludens-1–associated nucleic acid binding.

invade cells and tissues by binding to zonula occludens proteins (e.g., hepatitis C virus, adenovirus). For example, a viral envelope protein of **hepatitis C** virus binds to occludin to disrupt the integrity of the zonula occludens, allowing the virus to invade the cell.

- **Junctional adhesion molecule (JAM)** is a 40-kDa protein that belongs to the immunoglobulin superfamily (IgSF). JAM does not itself form a zonula occludens strand but is instead associated with claudins. It is responsible for increasing the electrical resistance of the cell membrane, thereby reducing paracellular permeability. JAM is involved in the formation of occluding junctions in endothelial cells as well as between endothelial cells and monocytes migrating from the vascular space to the connective tissue.
- **Tricellulin**, a 64-kDa protein, is localized in specific areas of the zonula occludens at tricellular contacts. Tricellulin is a component of the junction and is recruited to this junction by the **angulin family of proteins** (angulin-1, angulin-2, and angulin-3), whose members are also expressed in the corners where three epithelial cells meet. Tricellulin plays a critical role in maintaining the epithelial barrier and organizing actin filaments in tricellular contacts, forming crucial points that support the tensile forces generated by the actin cytoskeleton.

The extracellular portions of these transmembrane proteins function as a zipper and seal the intercellular space between adjacent cells, thus creating a barrier against paracellular diffusion. The cytoplasmic portions of all four proteins contain a unique amino acid sequence that attracts regulatory adaptor and signaling proteins called **PDZ domain proteins**. These proteins include the **zonula occludens proteins ZO-1, ZO-2**, and **ZO-3** (see Fig. 5.17). Occludin, claudins, and tricellulins interact with the actin cytoskeleton through ZO-1 and ZO-3. The ZO-1 protein binds the zonula adherens junction proteins afadin and α-catenin, thus providing an important link between the zonula occludens and zonula adherens junctions. Regulatory functions during the formation of the zonula occludens have been suggested for all ZO proteins. In addition, ZO-1 is a tumor suppressor, and ZO-2 is required in the epidermal growth factor–receptor signaling mechanism. The ZO-3 protein interacts with ZO-1 and the cytoplasmic domain of occludins. The proteins localized in the region of the zonula occludens are summarized in Table 5.4. Many pathogenic agents, such as cytomegalovirus, dengue virus, and cholera toxins, act on ZO-1 and ZO-2, causing the junction to become permeable.

The zonula occludens separates the luminal space from the intercellular space and connective tissue compartment.

It is now evident that the **zonula occludens** plays an essential role in the selective passage of substances from one side of an epithelium to the other. The ability of epithelia to create a diffusion barrier is controlled by two distinct pathways for the transport of substances across the epithelia (Fig. 5.18a):

- The **transcellular pathway** occurs across the plasma membrane of the epithelial cell. In most of these pathways, transport is active and requires specialized energy-dependent membrane **transport proteins** and **channels**. These proteins and channels move selected substances across the apical plasma membrane into the cytoplasm and then across the lateral membrane below the level of the occluding junction into the intercellular compartment.

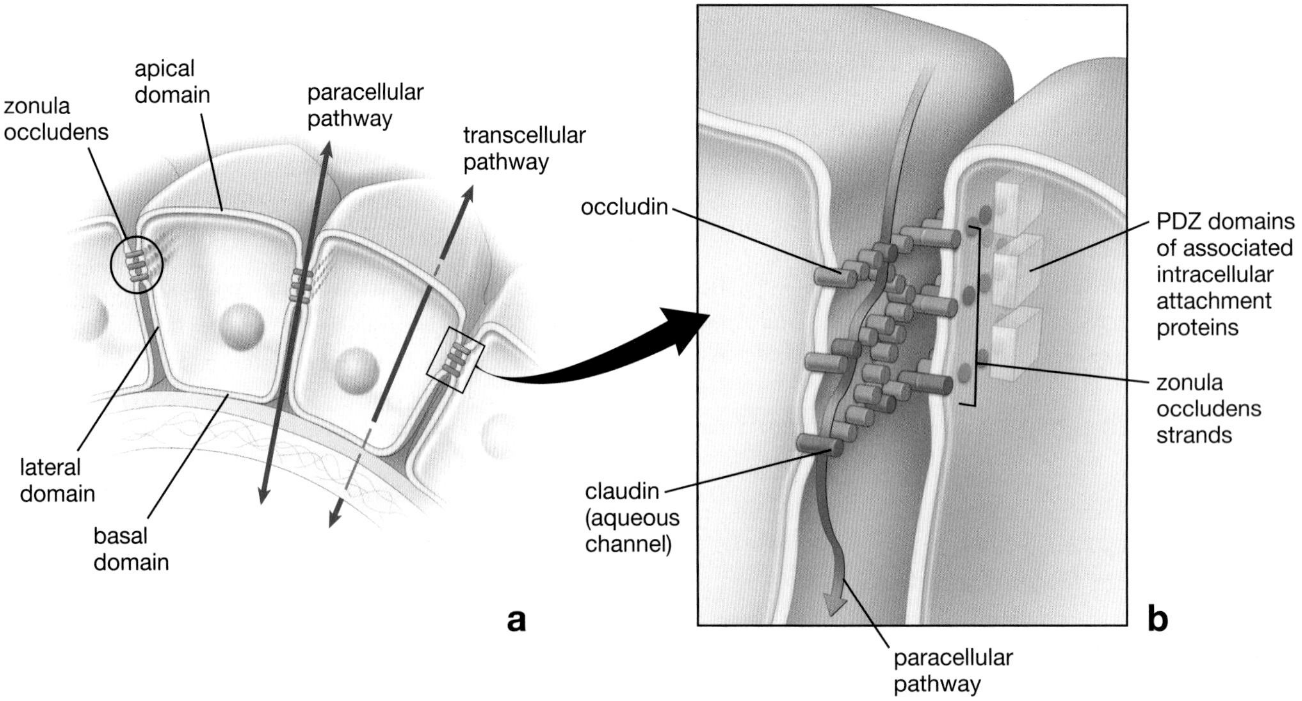

FIGURE 5.18. Two transcellular and paracellular pathways for transport of substances across the epithelia. a. The transcellular pathway occurs across the plasma membrane of the epithelial cell and represents an active transport system that requires specialized energy–dependent membrane transport proteins and channels. The paracellular pathway occurs across the zonula occludens between two epithelial cells. The amount of water, electrolytes, and other small molecules transported through this pathway is contingent on the tightness of the zonula occludens. **b.** Structure of the extracellular and cytoplasmic portions of tight junction strands. Two zonula occludens strands from neighboring cells fuse in a zipper-like manner and create a barrier to movement between the cells. Aqueous pores allow water to move between the cells. The permeability of the barrier depends on the mixture of claudins and occludins in the zipper seal. The cytoplasmic portion of the strand attracts PDZ domain proteins that function in cell signaling.

- The **paracellular pathway** occurs across the zonula occludens between two epithelial cells. The amount of water, electrolytes, and other small molecules transported through this pathway is contingent on the **tightness** of the **zonula occludens** and **tricellular zonula occludens** junctions. The permeability of an occluding junction depends on the molecular composition of the zonula occludens strands and thus the number of active aqueous channels in the seal (see the following section). Under physiologic conditions, substances transported through this pathway may be regulated or coupled to transcellular transport.

Permeability of the zonula occludens depends not only on the complexity and number of strands but also on the characteristics of proteins involved in their formation.

Microscopic observations of different kinds of epithelia reveal that the complexity and number of strands forming the zonulae occludentes varies. In epithelia in which anastomosing strands or fusion sites are sparse, such as certain kidney tubules, the intercellular pathway is partially permeable to water and solutes. In contrast, in epithelia in which the strands are numerous and extensively intertwined, such as intestinal and urinary bladder epithelia, the intercellular region is highly impermeable.

However, in some epithelial cells, the number of strands does not directly correlate with the tightness of the seal. Differences in tightness between different zonulae occludentes could be explained by the presence of aqueous pores within individual zonula occludens strands (Fig. 5.18b). **Claudins** not only form the backbone of the individual zonula occludens strand but also are responsible for the formation of **extracellular aqueous channels**. For instance, claudin-16 functions as an aqueous Mg^{2+} channel between specific kidney epithelial cells. Similarly, claudin-2 is responsible for the presence of high-conductance aqueous pores in kidney tubule epithelium. Therefore, the combinations and ratios of claudins to occludins and other proteins found within individual paired zonula occludens strands determine tightness and selectivity of the seal between cells.

Tricellular zonula occludens junctions are uniquely placed permeability barriers formed at the corners of epithelial cells. As discussed earlier, the central tube at these junctions represents a weak point for the epithelial barrier and a potential conduit for paracellular passage of water and solutes. Tightness of these junctions is regulated by **tricellulin** and other structural proteins found in central sealing elements (see pages 142-144). Recent experimental studies involving epithelia that do not express tricellulin molecules (tricellulin-knockdown cells) found decreased transepithelial electrical resistance and increased permeability of water, solutes, and other macromolecules in these tricellulin-free cells.

The zonula occludens establishes functional domains in the plasma membrane.

As a junction, the **zonula occludens** not only controls the passage of substances across the epithelial layer but also **restricts the movement of lipid rafts** containing specific proteins within the plasma membrane itself. The cell segregates certain internal membrane proteins on the apical (free) surface and restricts others to the lateral or basal surfaces. In the intestine, for instance, the enzymes for terminal digestion of peptides and saccharides (dipeptidases and disaccharidases) are localized in the membrane of the microvilli of the apical surface. The Na^+/K^+-ATPase that drives salt and transcellular water transport, as well as amino acid and sugar transport, is restricted to the lateral plasma membrane below the zonula occludens.

Anchoring Junctions

Anchoring junctions provide lateral adhesions between epithelial cells using proteins that link into the cytoskeleton of adjacent cells. Two types of anchoring cell-to-cell junctions can be identified on the lateral cell surface:

- **Zonula adherens** (pl., *zonulae adherentes*), which interacts with the network of actin filaments inside the cell
- **Macula adherens** (pl., *maculae adherentes*) or **desmosome**, which interacts with intermediate filaments

In addition, two other types of anchoring junctions can be found where epithelial cells rest on the connective tissue matrix. These **focal adhesions** (focal contacts) and **hemidesmosomes** are discussed in the section on the basal domain (see pages 145-150).

Cell adhesion molecules play important roles in cell-to-cell and cell-to-extracellular matrix adhesions.

Transmembrane proteins known as **cell adhesion molecules (CAMs)** form an essential part of every anchoring junction on both lateral and basal cell surfaces. The extracellular domains of CAMs interact with similar domains belonging to CAMs of neighboring cells. If the binding occurs between different types of CAMs, it is described as **heterotypic binding; homotypic binding** occurs between CAMs of the same type (Fig. 5.19). CAMs have a selective adhesiveness of relatively low strength, which allows cells to easily join and dissociate.

The **cytoplasmic domains** are linked through a variety of intracellular proteins to components of the **cell cytoskeleton**. Through the cytoskeleton connection, CAMs are able to control and regulate diverse intracellular processes associated with cell adhesion, cell proliferation, and cell migration. In addition, CAMs are implicated in many other cellular functions, such as intercellular and intracellular communications, cell recognition, regulation of intercellular diffusion barrier, generation of immune responses, and apoptosis. From early embryonic development, every type of tissue at every stage of differentiation is defined by the expression of specific CAMs. Changes in the expression pattern of one or several CAMs may lead to pathologic changes during tissue differentiation or maturation. To date, about 60 CAMs have been identified, and they are classified on the basis of their molecular structure into five major families: cadherins, nectins, integrins, selectins, and the IgSF (see Fig. 5.19).

- **Cadherins** are represented by the family of transmembrane **Ca^{2+}-dependent CAMs** localized mainly within the zonula adherens. At these sites, cadherins maintain homotypic interactions with similar proteins from the neighboring cell. They are associated with a group of intracellular proteins (catenins) that link cadherin molecules to **actin filaments** of the cell cytoskeleton. Through this interaction, cadherins convey signals that regulate

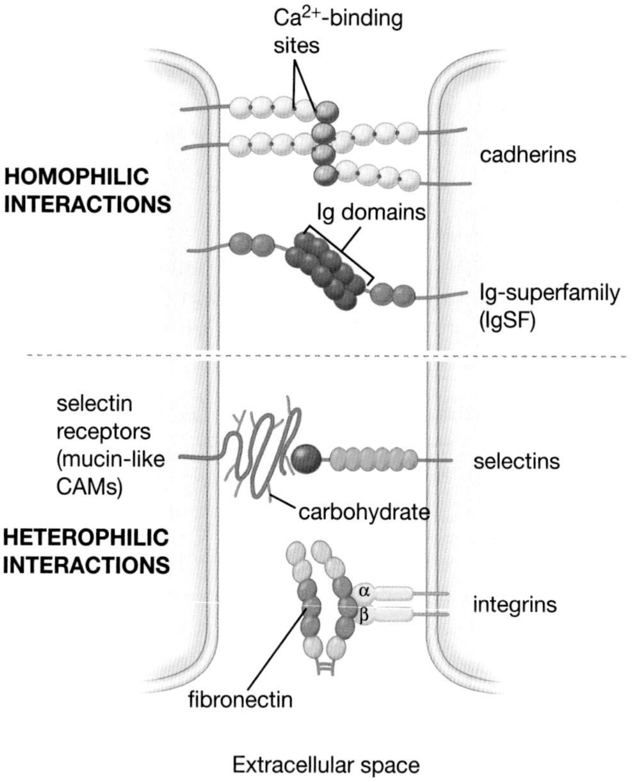

FIGURE 5.19. Cell adhesion molecules (*CAMs*). Cadherin and immunoglobulin superfamily (*IgSF*) CAMs exhibit homotypic binding in which two identical molecules from the neighboring cells interact. Binding that occurs between different types of CAMs (e.g., selectins and integrins) is considered heterotypic binding (no identical pair of molecules reacts with each other). Note that integrins bind to the extracellular matrix proteins (e.g., fibronectin). For simplicity of this drawing, the associated intracellular attachment proteins are not shown.

mechanisms of growth and cell differentiation. Cadherins control cell-to-cell interactions and participate in cell recognition and embryonic cell migration. **Epithelial,** or **E-cadherin**, the most studied member of this family, maintains the zonula adherens junction between epithelial cells. It also acts as an important suppressor of epithelial tumor cells.

- **Nectins** are represented by a family of transmembrane **Ca^{2+}-independent immunoglobulin-like CAMs.** In contrast with cadherins, nectins are able to establish homophilic interactions with the same family member and heterophilic interactions with related nectin family members. They are also unable to establish strong adhering junctions. These types of weaker junctions might be favorable to the dynamic regulation of cell-to-cell adhesion during embryologic development, rapid tissue remodeling, and regeneration.
- **Integrins** are represented by two **transmembrane glycoprotein** subunits consisting of 15 α- and 9 β-chains. This composition allows for the formation of different combinations of integrin molecules that are able to interact with various proteins (heterotypic interactions). Integrins interact with **extracellular matrix molecules** (such as collagens, laminin, and fibronectin) and with **actin** and **intermediate filaments** of the cell cytoskeleton. Through these interactions, integrins regulate cell adhesion, control cell movement and shape, and participate in cell growth and differentiation.
- **Selectins** are expressed on white blood cells (leukocytes) and endothelial cells and **mediate neutrophil–endothelial cell recognition.** This heterotypic binding initiates neutrophil migration through the endothelium of blood vessels into the extracellular matrix. Selectins are also involved in directing lymphocytes into accumulations of lymphatic tissue (a process called **lymphocyte homing**).
- **Immunoglobulin superfamily (IgSF).** Many molecules involved in immune reactions share a common precursor element in their structure. However, several other molecules with no known immunologic function also share this same repeat element. Together, the genes encoding these related molecules have been defined as the **immunoglobulin gene superfamily.** It is one of the largest gene families in the human genome, and its glycoproteins perform a wide variety of important biological functions. IgSF members mediate homotypic cell-to-cell adhesions and are represented by the intercellular cell adhesion molecule (ICAM), C-CAM, vascular cell adhesion molecule (VCAM), Down syndrome cell adhesion molecule (DSCAM), platelet endothelial cell adhesion molecules (PECAM), JAMs, and many others. These proteins play key roles in cell adhesion and differentiation, cancer and tumor metastasis, angiogenesis (new vessel formation), inflammation, immune responses, and microbial attachment as well as many other functions.

The zonula adherens provides lateral adhesion between epithelial cells.

The integrity of epithelial surfaces depends, in large part, on the lateral adhesion of the cells with one another and their ability to resist separation. Although the zonula occludens involves close contact with adjoining cell membranes, their resistance to mechanical stress is limited. Reinforcement of this region depends on a strong bonding site below the zonula occludens. Like the zonula occludens, this lateral adhesion device occurs in a continuous band- or belt-like configuration around the cell; thus, the adhering junction is referred to as a **zonula adherens**.

Zonula adherens is composed of two families of transmembrane proteins: the cadherins and the nectins.

The zonula adherens in most epithelial cells is composed of the transmembrane family of CAMs, the **cadherins**. On the cytoplasmic side, the tail of E-cadherin is bound to **catenin proteins (α- and β-catenin)** (Fig. 5.20a). The resulting **E-cadherin–catenin complex** binds to **vinculin** and **α-actinin** and is required for the interaction of cadherins with the actin filaments of the cytoskeleton. The extracellular components of the E-cadherin molecules from adjacent cells are linked by **Ca^{2+} ions** or an additional extracellular link protein. E-cadherin–catenin complexes form strong adhering junctions; however, their morphologic and functional integrity is calcium dependent. Removal of Ca^{2+} leads to the dissociation of E-cadherin molecules and disruption of the junction. In addition, the E-cadherin–catenin complex functions as a **master molecule** in regulating not only cell adhesion but also polarity, differentiation, migration, proliferation, and survival of epithelial cells.

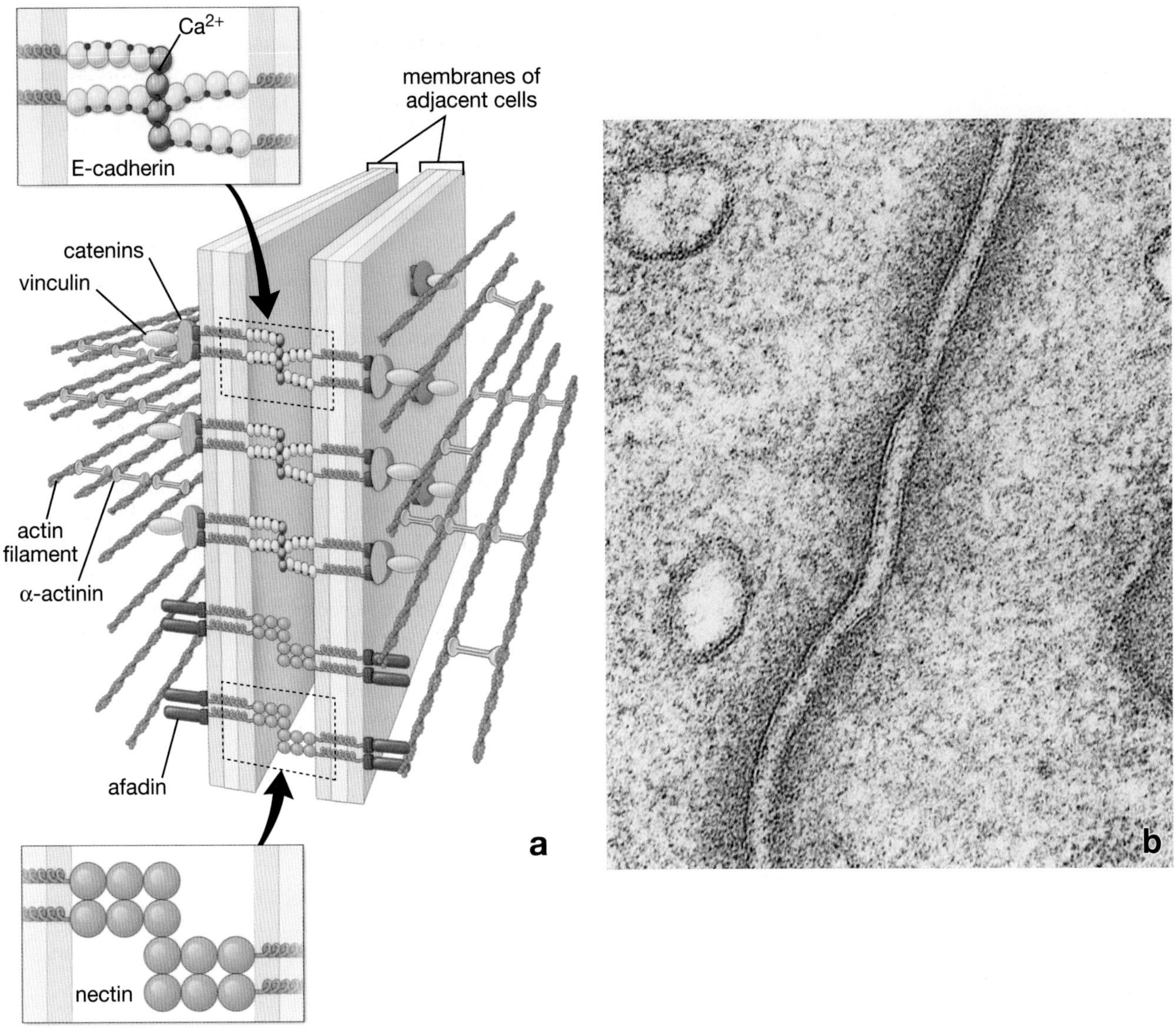

FIGURE 5.20. Zonula adherens. a. Molecular organization of zonula adherens. Actin filaments of adjacent cells are attached to the E-cadherin–catenin complex by α-actinin and vinculin. The E-cadherin–catenin complex interacts with identical molecules embedded in the plasma membrane of the adjacent cell. Interactions between transmembrane proteins are mediated by calcium ions. Nectin proteins shown in the lower part of the junction are members of a calcium-independent family of transmembrane proteins. Their interactions are not as strong as that between cadherins; thus, they mediate much weaker adhering junctions found in specialized areas exposed to dynamic changes and rapid tissue remodeling. **b.** Electron micrograph of the zonula adherens from Figure 5.15a at higher magnification. The plasma membranes are separated by a relatively uniform intercellular space. This space appears clear, showing only a sparse amount of a diffuse electron-dense substance, which represents the extracellular domains of E-cadherin. The cytoplasmic side of the plasma membrane exhibits a moderately electron-dense material containing actin filaments. ×100,000.

As described earlier, in most of the epithelial cells, zonula adherens is formed by E-cadherin–catenin complexes; however, in many instances, these junctions often contain additional CAMs belonging to the **nectin family** (nectin-1, nectin-2, nectin-3, and nectin-4). Nectins are transmembrane proteins, and their extracellular domains develop both homophilic and heterophilic associations with proteins from the adjacent plasma membrane. The cytoplasmic tail of nectin binds **afadin**, a large (206-kDa) actin-binding protein that anchors the nectin to the **actin cytoskeleton** (see Fig. 5.20a). In some specialized cell-to-cell adhesion sites, cadherins are absent and nectins function as the primary CAM. Nectin-based zonulae occludentes are fundamentally different from those based on cadherin. Nectin molecules are unable to provide strong cell-to-cell adhesions. These **weak nectin-based adhering junctions** are formed in specialized areas where junctions are exposed to dynamic regulation and rapid tissue remodeling. Such junctions include Sertoli-to-spermatid junctions in the testis, junctions between pigmented and nonpigmented cells in the ciliary epithelium of the eye, and junctions within dental papilla and the neural tube during embryonic development. Recent research studies indicate that the **nectin–afadin complex** is an essential target protein for the **measles virus** (MV) to enter the respiratory epithelium. MV uses the paracellular pathway and by binding to nectin creates an opening on the lateral domain of epithelial cell for rapid spread in the airway epithelium.

Electron microscopy features of the zonula adherens include a clear intercellular space and fuzzy plaques along the cytoplasmic side of plasma membranes.

When examined with the TEM, the zonula adherens is characterized by a uniform 15- to 20-nm space between the opposing cell membranes (Fig. 5.20b). The **intercellular space**

FOLDER 5.3
CLINICAL CORRELATION: JUNCTIONAL COMPLEXES AS A TARGET OF PATHOGENIC AGENTS

Epithelia form a physical barrier that allows the body to maintain internal homeostasis while protecting the organism from harmful pathogenic agents from the external environment. The easiest way for many viruses, bacteria, and parasites to successfully compromise the protective functions of the epithelial layer is to destroy the junctional complexes between epithelial cells. Several proteins found in junctional specializations of the cell membrane are affected by molecules produced or expressed by these pathogenic agents.

Bacteria

A common bacterium that causes food poisoning, *Clostridium perfringens*, attacks the zonula occludens junction. This microorganism is widely distributed in the external environment and is found within the intestinal flora of humans and many domestic animals. Food poisoning symptoms are characterized by intense abdominal pain and diarrhea that begins 8–22 hours after eating foods contaminated by these bacteria. Symptoms usually abate within 24 hours. The enterotoxin produced by *C. perfringens* is a small 35-kDa protein whose carboxy-terminus binds specifically to the claudin-3 and claudin-4 molecules of the zonula occludens. Its amino-terminus forms pores within the apical domain of the plasma membrane. Binding to claudins prevents their incorporation into the zonula occludens strands and leads to malfunction and breakdown of the junction. Dehydration that occurs with this type of food poisoning is a result of a massive movement of fluids via paracellular pathways into the lumen of the intestines.

Helicobacter pylori, another bacterium, resides within the stomach and binds to the extracellular domains of zonula occludens proteins. During this process, the CagA surface-exposed 128-kDa protein produced by the bacteria is translocated from the microorganism into the cytoplasm, where it targets both ZO-1 and JAM proteins. As a result, the zonula occludens barrier becomes disrupted, and its capacity for tyrosine kinase signaling diminishes, causing cytoskeletal rearrangements. *H. pylori* causes injury to the protective barrier of the stomach that may lead to the development of gastric ulcers and gastric carcinomas.

Viruses

The specific group of RNA viruses responsible for infant enteritis (inflammation of the intestines) uses the intracellular JAM signaling pathway. The attachment and endocytosis of the reovirus is initiated by the interaction of its viral attachment protein with a JAM molecule. This interaction activates nuclear factor-κB protein (NF-κB), which migrates into the nucleus and triggers a cascade of cellular events, leading to apoptosis. This finding suggests that JAMs are used as signal transduction molecules to convey impulses from the external environment to the cell nucleus.

Zonula occludens–associated proteins that express the PDZ domain sequence are targets of oncogenic adenoviruses and papillomaviruses. The viral oncoproteins produced by these viruses bind via their PDZ-binding domains to ZO-2 and multi-PDZ–containing protein-1 (MUPP-1). The oncogenic effect of these interactions is attributed, in part, to the sequestration and degradation of the zonula occludens and the tumor suppressor proteins associated with the viruses.

Parasites

The common house dust mite, *Dermatophagoides pteronyssinus*, also destroys zonula occludens junctions. It belongs to the Arachnid family, which includes spiders, scorpions, and ticks. When its fecal pellets are inhaled with dust particles, serine and cysteine peptidases present in the pellets cleave occludin and ZO-1 protein, resulting in the breakdown of zonula occludens junctions in the respiratory epithelium. The loss of the protective epithelial barrier in the lung exposes the lung to inhaled allergens and initiates an immune response that can lead to severe asthma attacks.

is of low electron density, appearing almost clear, but it is evidently occupied by extracellular components of adjacent E-cadherin or nectin molecules and Ca^{2+} ions. Within the confines of the zonula adherens, a moderately electron-dense material called **fuzzy plaque** is found along the cytoplasmic side of the membrane of each cell. This material corresponds to the location of the cytoplasmic component of the **E-cadherin–catenin complex** and its associated proteins (α-actinin, catenins, vinculin, and afadin) into which actin filaments attach. Evidence also suggests that the fuzzy plaque represents the stainable substance in LM, the terminal bar. Associated with the electron-dense material is an array of 6-nm **actin filaments** that stretch across the apical cytoplasm of the epithelial cell, the terminal web.

The fascia adherens is a sheet-like junction that stabilizes nonepithelial tissues.

Physical attachments that occur between cells in tissues other than epithelia are usually not prominent, but there is at least one notable exception. **Cardiac muscle cells** are arranged end to end, forming thread-like contractile units. The cells are attached to each other by a combination of typical desmosomes, or maculae adherentes, and **broad adhesion plates** that morphologically resemble the zonula adherens of epithelial cells. Because the attachment is not ring like but rather has a broad face, it is called the **fascia adherens** (Fig. 5.21). At the molecular level, the structure of the fascia adherens is similar to that of the zonula adherens; it also contains the **zonula occludens ZO-1** protein found in the tight junctions of epithelial cells.

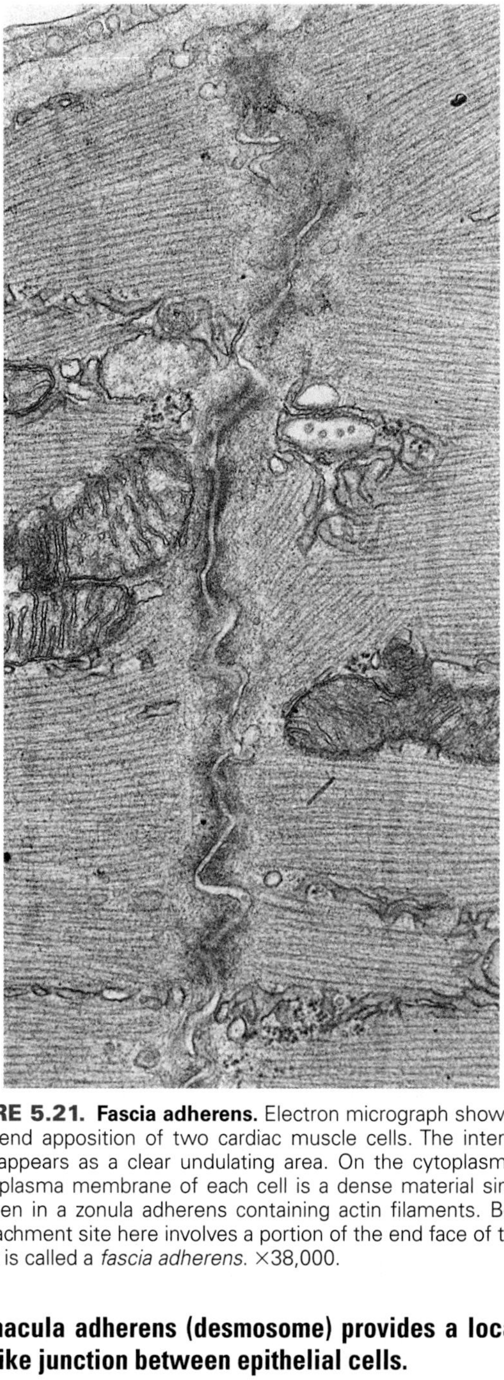

FIGURE 5.21. Fascia adherens. Electron micrograph showing the end-to-end apposition of two cardiac muscle cells. The intercellular space appears as a clear undulating area. On the cytoplasmic side of the plasma membrane of each cell is a dense material similar to that seen in a zonula adherens containing actin filaments. Because the attachment site here involves a portion of the end face of the two cells, it is called a *fascia adherens*. ×38,000.

The macula adherens (desmosome) provides a localized spot-like junction between epithelial cells.

The **macula adherens** *[L., macula, spot]* represents a major anchoring cell-to-cell junction that provides a particularly strong attachment, as shown by microdissection studies. The macula adherens was originally described in epidermal cells and was called a **desmosome** *[Gr., desmo, bond; Gr., soma, body]*. These junctions are localized on the lateral domain of the cell, much like a series of spot welds (see Fig. 5.14a), and they mediate direct cell-to-cell contact by providing anchoring sites for intermediate filaments. Increasing evidence suggests that the macula adherens, in addition to its structural function, participates in tissue morphogenesis and differentiation.

In simple epithelium formed by cuboidal or columnar cells, the macula adherens is found in conjunction with occluding (zonula occludens) and adhering (zonula adherens) junctions. Because the macula adherens occupies small, localized sites on the lateral cell surface, it is not a continuous structure around the cell, as is the zonula adherens. Thus, a section perpendicular to the surface of a cell that cuts through the entire lateral surface will often not include a macula adherens. The section will always, however, include the zonula adherens.

In the area of the macula adherens, desmogleins and desmocollins provide the linkage between the plasma membranes of adjacent cells.

EM reveals that the macula adherens has a complex structure. On the cytoplasmic side of the plasma membrane of each of the adjoining cells is a disc-shaped structure consisting of very dense material called the **desmosomal attachment plaque**. This structure measures about 400 nm × 250 nm × 10 nm and anchors **intermediate filaments** (Fig. 5.22a). The filaments appear to loop through the attachment plaques and extend back out into the cytoplasm. They are thought to play a role in dissipating physical forces throughout the cell from the attachment site. At the molecular level, each attachment plaque is composed of several constitutive proteins, mainly **desmoplakins** and **plakoglobins**, which are capable of anchoring the intermediate filaments (Fig. 5.22b).

The **intercellular space** of the macula adherens is conspicuously wider (up to 30 nm) than that of the zonula adherens and is occupied by a dense medial band, the **intermediate line**. This line represents extracellular portions of transmembrane glycoproteins, the **desmogleins** and **desmocollins**, which are members of the cadherin family of Ca^{2+}-dependent CAMs. In the presence of Ca^{2+}, extracellular portions of desmogleins and desmocollins bind adjacent identical molecules of neighboring cells (homotypic binding). X-ray crystallographic studies suggest that the extracellular binding domain of proteins from one cell interacts with two adjacent cadherin domains in an antiparallel orientation, thus forming a continuous **cadherin zipper** in the area of the desmosome (see Fig. 5.22b). The cytoplasmic portions of desmogleins and desmocollins are integral components of the desmosomal attachment plaque. They interact with the **plakoglobins** and **desmoplakins** that are involved in desmosome assembly and the anchoring of **intermediate filaments**.

The cells of different epithelia require different types of attachments.

In epithelia that serve as physiologic barriers, the junctional complex is particularly significant because it serves to create a long-term barrier, allowing the cells to compartmentalize and restrict the free passage of substances across the epithelium. Although it is the zonula occludens of the junctional complex that principally affects this function, it is the adhesive properties of the zonulae and maculae adherentes that guard against the physical disruption of the barrier. In other epithelia, there is a need for substantially stronger attachment between cells in several planes. In the stratified epithelial cells of the epidermis, for example, numerous maculae adherentes maintain adhesion between adjacent cells. In cardiac muscle, where there is a similar need for strong adhesion, a combination of the macula adherens and the fascia adherens serves this function.

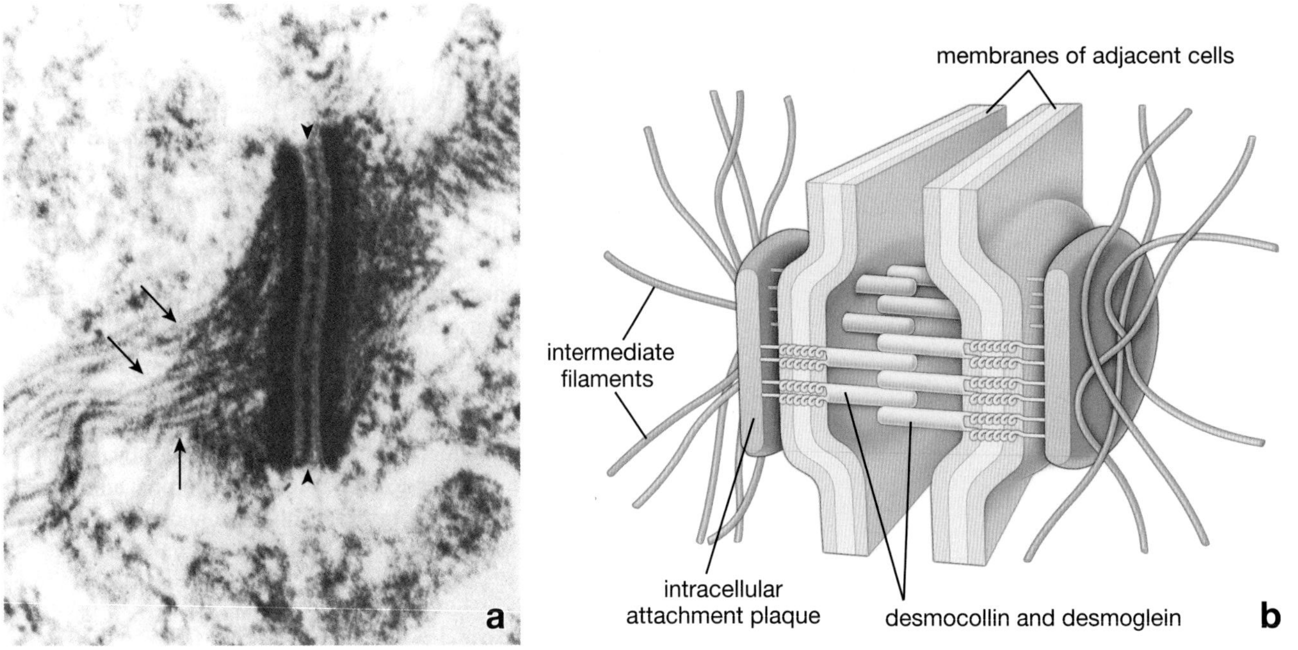

FIGURE 5.22. Molecular structure of the macula adherens (desmosome). a. Electron micrograph of a macula adherens showing the intermediate filaments (*arrows*) attaching to a dense, intracellular attachment plaque located on the cytoplasmic side of the plasma membrane. The intercellular space is also occupied by electron-dense material (*arrowheads*) containing desmocollins and desmogleins. The intercellular space above and below the macula adherens is not well defined because of the extraction of the plasma membrane to show components of this structure. ×40,000. (Courtesy of Dr. Ernst Kallenbach.) **b.** Schematic diagram showing the structure of a macula adherens. Note the intracellular attachment plaque with anchored intermediate filaments. The extracellular portions of desmocollins and desmogleins from opposing cells interact with each other in the localized area of the desmosome, forming the "cadherin zipper."

Communicating Junctions

Communicating junctions, also called **gap junctions** or **nexuses**, are the only known cellular structures that permit the direct passage of signaling molecules from one cell to another. They are present in a wide variety of tissues, including epithelia, smooth and cardiac muscle, and nerves. Gap junctions are important in tissues in which the activity of adjacent cells must be coordinated, such as epithelia engaged in fluid and electrolyte transport, vascular and intestinal smooth muscle, and heart muscle. A gap junction consists of an **accumulation of transmembrane channels** or **pores** in a tightly packed array. Cells exchange ions, regulatory molecules, and small metabolites through these pores. The number of pores in a gap junction can vary widely, as can the number of gap junctions between adjacent cells.

A variety of methods are used to study the structure and function of gap junctions.

Various procedures have been used to study gap junctions, including the injection of dyes and fluorescent or radiolabeled compounds and the measurement of **electric current flow** between cells. In dye studies, a fluorescent dye is injected with a micropipette into one cell. After a short period, the dye can be readily visualized in immediately adjacent cells. Electrical conductance studies show that neighboring cells joined by gap junctions exhibit a low electrical resistance between them when current flow is high; therefore, gap junctions are also called **low-resistance junctions**.

Current molecular biology techniques allow for isolation of complementary DNA clones encoding a family of gap junction proteins (connexins) and expressing them in tissue culture cells. Connexins expressed in transfected cells produce gap junctions, which can be isolated and studied by molecular and biochemical methods as well as by the improved imaging techniques of electron crystallography and atomic force microscopy (AFM).

Gap junctions are formed by 12 subunits of the connexin protein family.

When viewed with the TEM, the **gap junction** appears as an area of contact between the plasma membranes of adjacent cells (Fig. 5.23a). High-resolution imaging techniques such as cryoelectron microscopy have been used to examine the structure of gap junctions. These studies reveal groups of tightly packed **channels**, each formed by **two half-channels** called **connexons** embedded in the facing membranes. These channels are represented by pairs of connexons that bridge the extracellular space between adjacent cells. As the name implies, the connexon in one cell membrane is precisely aligned to dock with a corresponding connexon on the membrane of an adjacent cell, allowing communication between the cells.

Each connexon contains six symmetrical subunits of an integral membrane protein called **connexin (Cx)** that is paired with a similar structure from the adjacent membrane; thus, each channel consists of 12 subunits. The subunits are configured in a circular arrangement to surround a 10-nm-long cylindrical transmembrane channel with a diameter of 2.8 nm (Fig. 5.23b).

Currently, 21 members of the connexin family of proteins have been identified. All traverse the lipid bilayer 4 times (i.e., they have four transmembrane domains). Most connexons pair with identical connexons (homotypic interaction) on the adjacent plasma membrane. These channels allow molecules to pass evenly in both directions; however, heterotypic channels can be asymmetrical in function, passing certain molecules faster in one direction than in another.

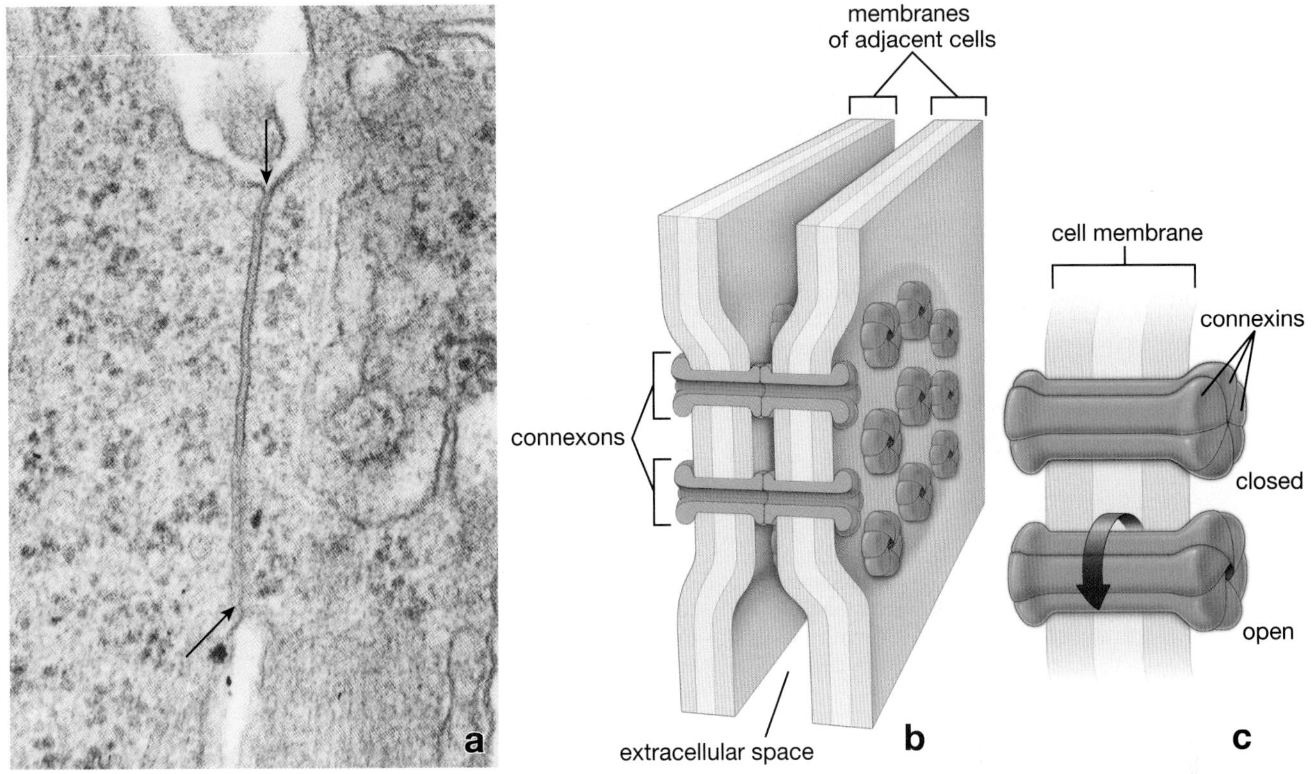

FIGURE 5.23. Structure of a gap junction. a. Electron micrograph showing the plasma membranes of two adjoining cells forming a gap junction. The unit membranes (*arrows*) approach one another, narrowing the intercellular space to produce a 2-nm-wide gap. ×76,000. **b.** Drawing of a gap junction showing the membranes of adjoining cells and the structural components of the membrane that form channels or passageways between the two cells. Each passageway is formed by a circular array of six subunits, dumbbell-shaped transmembrane proteins that span the plasma membrane of each cell. These complexes, called *connexons*, have a central opening of about 2 nm in diameter. The channels formed by the registration of the adjacent complementary pairs of connexons permit the flow of small molecules through the channel, but not into the intercellular space. Conversely, substances in the intercellular space can permeate the area of a gap junction by flowing around the connexon complexes, but they cannot enter the channels. **c.** The diameter of the channel in an individual connexon is regulated by reversible changes in the conformation of the individual connexins.

Atomic force microscopy reveals conformational changes in connexins that cause gap junction channels to open or close.

Earlier EM studies of isolated gap junctions suggested that the gap junction channels open and close by twisting of the connexin subunits (Fig. 5.23c). Recent AFM studies provide a dynamic view of the conformational changes that take place in connexons. Channels in gap junctions fluctuate rapidly between an open and a closed state through reversible changes in the conformation of individual connexins. The conformational change in connexin molecules that triggers the closure of gap junction channels at their extracellular surface appears to be induced by Ca^{2+} ions (Fig. 5.24). However, other calcium-independent gating mechanisms responsible for closing and opening of the cytoplasmic domains of gap junction channels have also been identified.

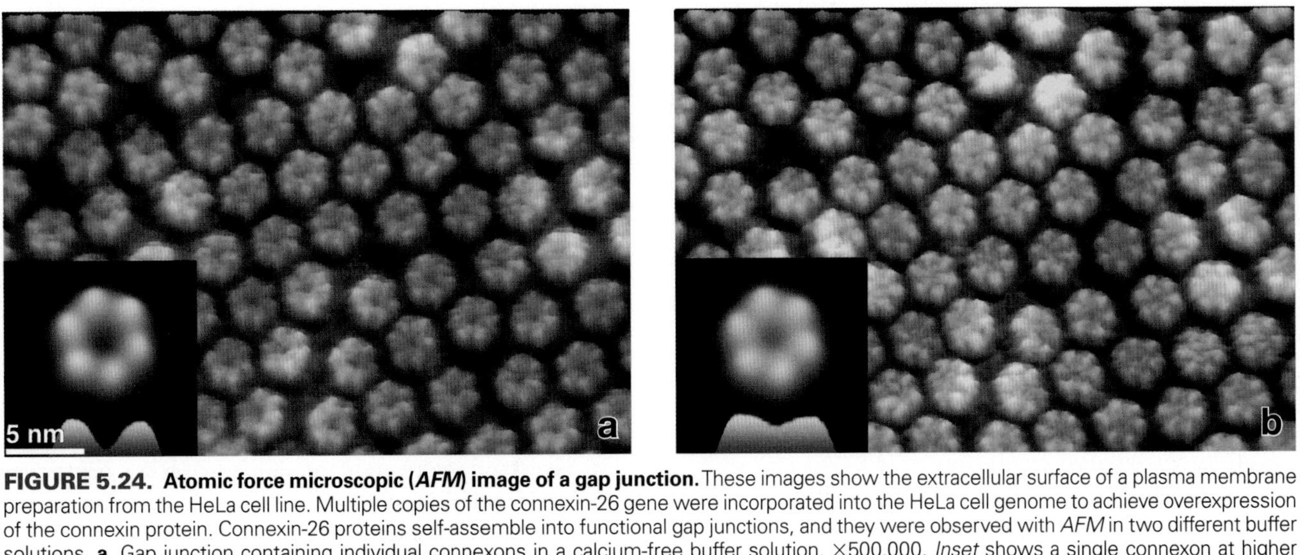

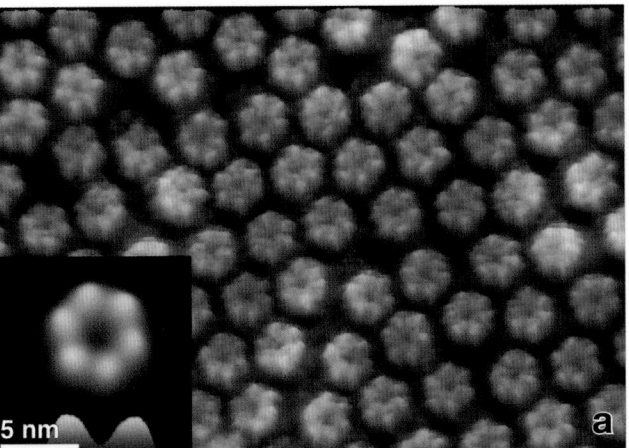

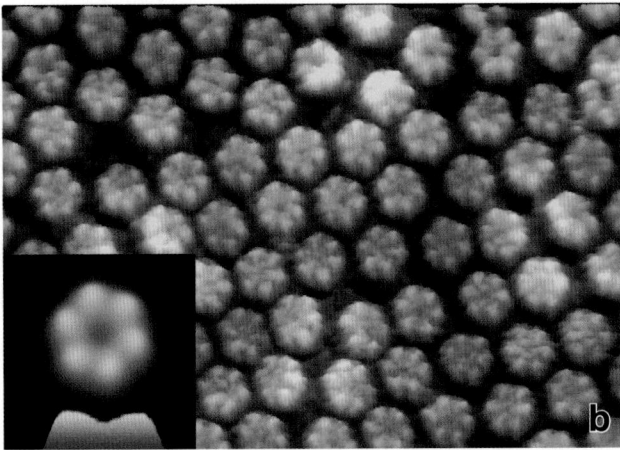

FIGURE 5.24. Atomic force microscopic (*AFM*) image of a gap junction. These images show the extracellular surface of a plasma membrane preparation from the HeLa cell line. Multiple copies of the connexin-26 gene were incorporated into the HeLa cell genome to achieve overexpression of the connexin protein. Connexin-26 proteins self-assemble into functional gap junctions, and they were observed with *AFM* in two different buffer solutions. **a.** Gap junction containing individual connexons in a calcium-free buffer solution. ×500,000. *Inset* shows a single connexon at higher magnification. Note the clear profiles of individual connexin molecules assembled into the connexon. The open profile of the channel is also visible. ×2,000,000. **b.** The same preparation of connexons in a buffer containing Ca^{2+}. ×500,000. **Inset.** Note that the conformational change of the connexin molecules has caused the channel to close and has reduced the height of the connexon. ×2,000,000. (Courtesy of Dr. Gina E. Sosinsky.)

TABLE 5.5 Summary of Junctional Features

	Classification		Major Link Proteins	Extracellular Ligands	Cytoskeleton Components	Associated Intracellular Attachment Proteins	Functions
Occluding junction *(cell to cell)*	**Zonula occludens (tight junction)**	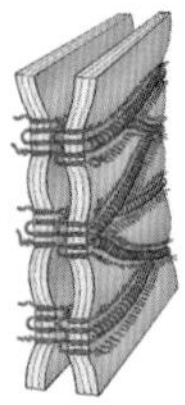	Occludins, claudins, JAMs, tricellulin (in tricellular junctions)	Occludins, claudins, JAMs, tricellulin in adjacent cell	Actin filaments	ZO-1, ZO-2, ZO-3, angulins, AF-6, cingulin, symplectin, ASIP/Povr 3, Rab36, 13, 8, Sec4, 6, 8	Seals adjacent cells together, controls passage of molecules between them (permeability), defines apical domain of plasma membrane, involved in cell signaling
Anchoring junction *(cell to cell)*	**Zonula adherens**	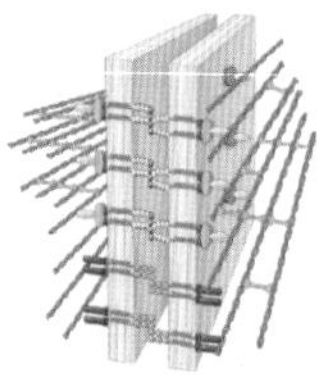	E-cadherin–catenin complex, nectins	E-cadherin–catenin complex, nectins in adjacent cell	Actin filaments	α-Actinin, vinculin, catenins, afadin	Couples the actin cytoskeleton to the plasma membrane at regions of cell–cell adhesion
	Macula adherens (desmosome)	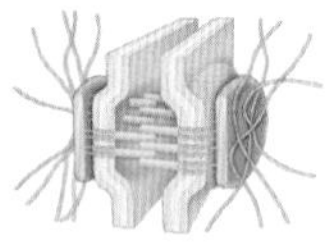	Cadherins (e.g., desmogleins, desmocollins)	Desmogleins, desmocollins in adjacent cell	Intermediate filaments	Desmoplakins, plakoglobins	Couples the intermediate filaments to the plasma membrane at regions of cell–cell adhesion
Anchoring junction *(cell to extracellular matrix)*	**Focal adhesion**	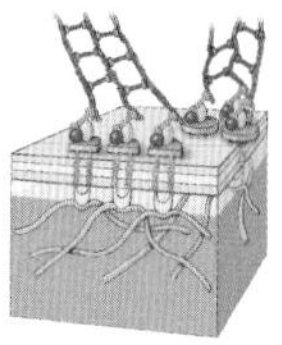	Integrins	Extracellular matrix proteins (e.g., fibronectin)	Actin filaments	Vinculin, talin, α-actinin, paxillin	Anchors the actin cytoskeleton to the extracellular matrix, detects and transduces signals from outside the cell
	Hemidesmosome	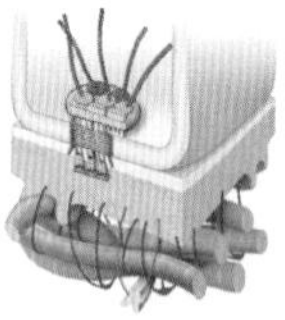	Integrins ($\alpha_6\beta_4$ integrin), collagen XVII	Extracellular matrix protein (e.g., laminin-332, collagen IV)	Intermediate filaments (possible microtubules and actin filaments via interaction with plectin)	Desmoplakin-like proteins, BP230 plectin, erbin	Anchors the intermediate filaments to the extracellular matrix
Communicating junction *(cell to cell)*	**Gap junction (nexus)**	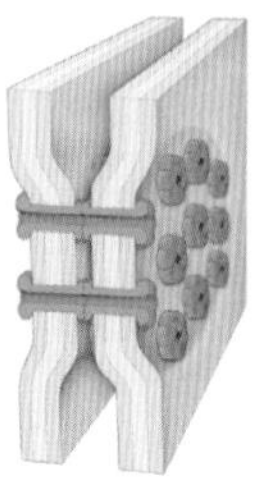	Connexin	Connexin in adjacent cell	None	Not known	Creates a conduit between two adjacent cells for passage of small ions and informational micromolecules

AF, antisecretory factor; *ASIP*, agouti signaling protein; *BP*, bullous pemphigoid; *JAM*, junctional adhesion molecule; *ZO*, zonula occludens.

Mutations in connexin genes are major pathogenic factors in several diseases. For instance, a mutation in the gene encoding **connexin-26 (Cx26)** is associated with **congenital deafness.** The gap junctions formed by Cx26 are found in the inner ear and are responsible for recirculating K^+ in the cochlear sensory epithelium. Other mutations affecting **Cx46** and **Cx50** genes have been identified in individuals with inherited **cataracts.** Both proteins are localized within the lens of the eye and form extensive gap junctions between the epithelial cells and the lens fibers. These gap junctions play a crucial role in delivering nutrients to and removing metabolites from the avascular environment of the lens.

A summary of the features of all of the junctions discussed in this chapter is found in Table 5.5 (page 152).

Morphologic Modifications of the Lateral Cell Surface

Lateral cell surface folds (plicae) create interdigitating cytoplasmic processes of adjoining cells.

The **lateral surfaces** of certain epithelial cells show a tortuous boundary as a result of **infoldings** or **plicae** along the border of each cell with its neighbor (Fig. 5.25). These infoldings increase the lateral surface area of the cell and are particularly prominent in epithelia that transport fluids and electrolytes, such as the intestinal and gallbladder epithelium. In active fluid transport, sodium ions are pumped out of the cytoplasm at the lateral plasma membrane by Na^+/K^+-ATPase localized in that membrane. Anions then diffuse across the membrane to maintain electrical neutrality, and water diffuses from the cytoplasm into the intercellular space, driven by the osmotic gradient between the sodium concentration in the intercellular space and the concentration in the cytoplasm. The **intercellular space** distends because of the accumulating fluid moving across the epithelium, but the degree of distension is limited by junctional attachments in the apical and basal portions of the cell. Hydrostatic pressure gradually builds up in the intercellular space and drives an essentially isotonic fluid from the space into the underlying connective tissue. The occluding junction at the apical end of the intercellular space prevents fluid from moving in the opposite direction. As the action of the sodium pump depletes the cytoplasm of sodium and water, they are replaced by diffusion across the apical plasma membrane. The surface area of the apical plasma membrane is greatly increased by the presence of microvilli, thus allowing the continuous movement of fluid from the lumen (i.e., intestines or gallbladder) to the connective tissue as long as the Na^+/K^+-ATPase is active.

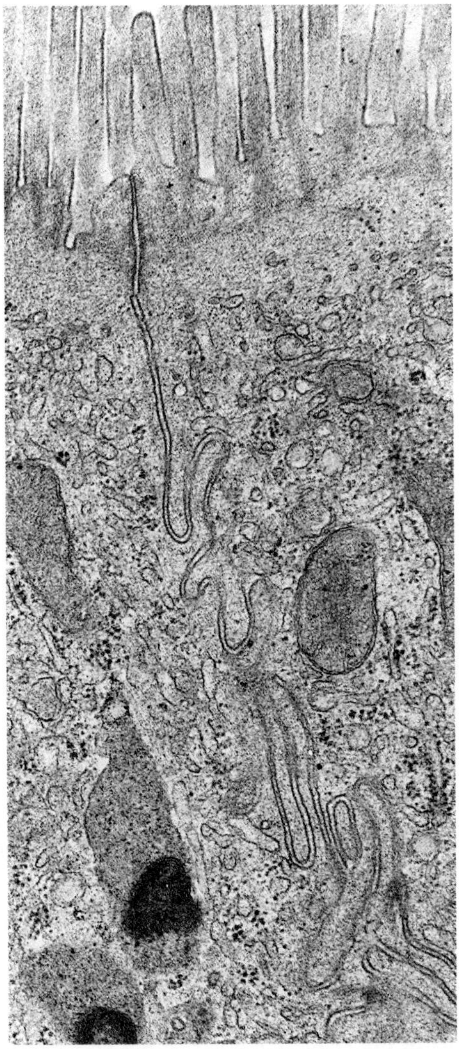

FIGURE 5.25. Lateral interdigitations. This electron micrograph shows infoldings or interdigitations at the lateral surfaces of two adjoining intestinal absorptive cells. ×25,000.

■ THE BASAL DOMAIN AND ITS SPECIALIZATIONS IN CELL-TO-EXTRACELLULAR MATRIX ADHESION

The basal domain of epithelial cells is characterized by several features:

- The **basement membrane** is a specialized structure located next to the basal domain of epithelial cells and the underlying connective tissue stroma.
- **Cell-to-extracellular matrix junctions** anchor the cell to the extracellular matrix; they are represented by focal adhesions and hemidesmosomes.
- **Basal cell membrane infoldings** increase the cell surface area and facilitate morphologic interactions between adjacent cells and extracellular matrix proteins.

Basement Membrane Structure and Function

The term **basement membrane** was originally given to an amorphous, dense layer of variable thickness at the basal surfaces of epithelia. Although a prominent structure referred to as *basement membrane* is observed with hematoxylin and eosin (H&E) stain in a few locations such as the trachea (Fig. 5.26) and, occasionally, the urinary bladder and ureters, basement membrane requires special staining to be seen in the LM. This requirement is caused, in part, by its thinness and by the effect of the eosin stain, which makes it indistinguishable from the immediately adjacent connective tissue. In the trachea, the structure that is often described as a basement membrane includes not only the true basement membrane but also an additional layer of closely spaced and aligned collagen fibrils that belong to the connective tissue.

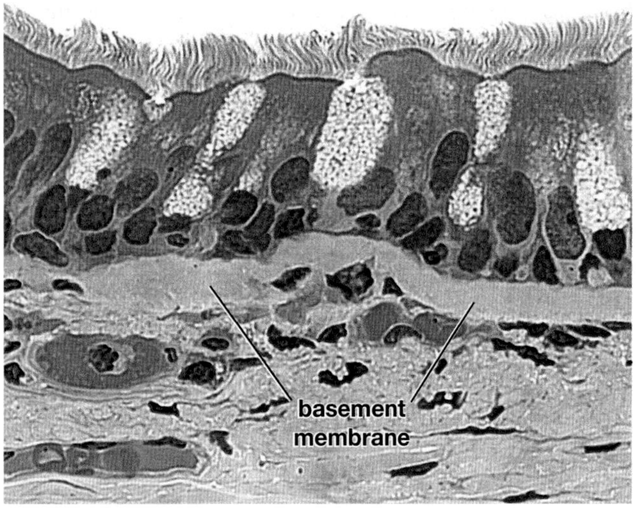

FIGURE 5.26. Tracheal basement membrane. Photomicrograph of an hematoxylin and eosin (H&E)-stained section of the pseudostratified ciliated epithelium of the trachea. The basement membrane appears as a thick homogeneous layer immediately below the epithelium. It is actually a part of the connective tissue and is composed largely of densely packed collagen fibrils. ×450.

In contrast to H&E (Fig. 5.27a), the **periodic acid–Schiff (PAS) staining technique** (Fig. 5.27b) results in a **positive reaction** at the site of the basement membrane. It appears as a thin, well-defined magenta layer between the epithelium and the connective tissue. The stain reacts with the sugar moieties of proteoglycans, accumulating in sufficient amounts and density to make the basement membrane visible in the LM. Techniques involving the reduction of silver salts by the sugars blacken the basement membrane and are also used to demonstrate this structure. Although the **basement membrane** is classically described as exclusively associated with epithelia, similar **PAS-positive** and **silver-reactive** sites can be demonstrated surrounding peripheral nerve–supporting cells, adipocytes, and muscle cells (Fig. 5.28); this feature helps delineate them from the surrounding connective tissue in histologic sections. Connective tissue cells other than adipocytes do not show a similar PAS-positive or silver reaction. That most connective tissue cells are not surrounded by basement membrane material is consistent with their lack of adhesion to connective tissue fibers. In fact, they must migrate within the tissue under appropriate stimuli to function.

The basal lamina is the structural attachment site for overlying epithelial cells and underlying connective tissue.

Former descriptions of basal lamina were based on the investigation of specimens routinely prepared for EM. The examination of the site of epithelial **basement membranes** with the EM reveals a discrete layer of electron-dense matrix material 40- to 60-nm thick between the epithelium and the adjacent connective tissue (Fig. 5.29) called the **basal lamina** or, sometimes, **lamina densa**. When observed at high resolution, this layer exhibits a network of fine, 3- to 4-nm filaments composed of **laminins**, a **type IV collagen molecule**, and various associated **proteoglycans** and **glycoproteins**. Between the basal

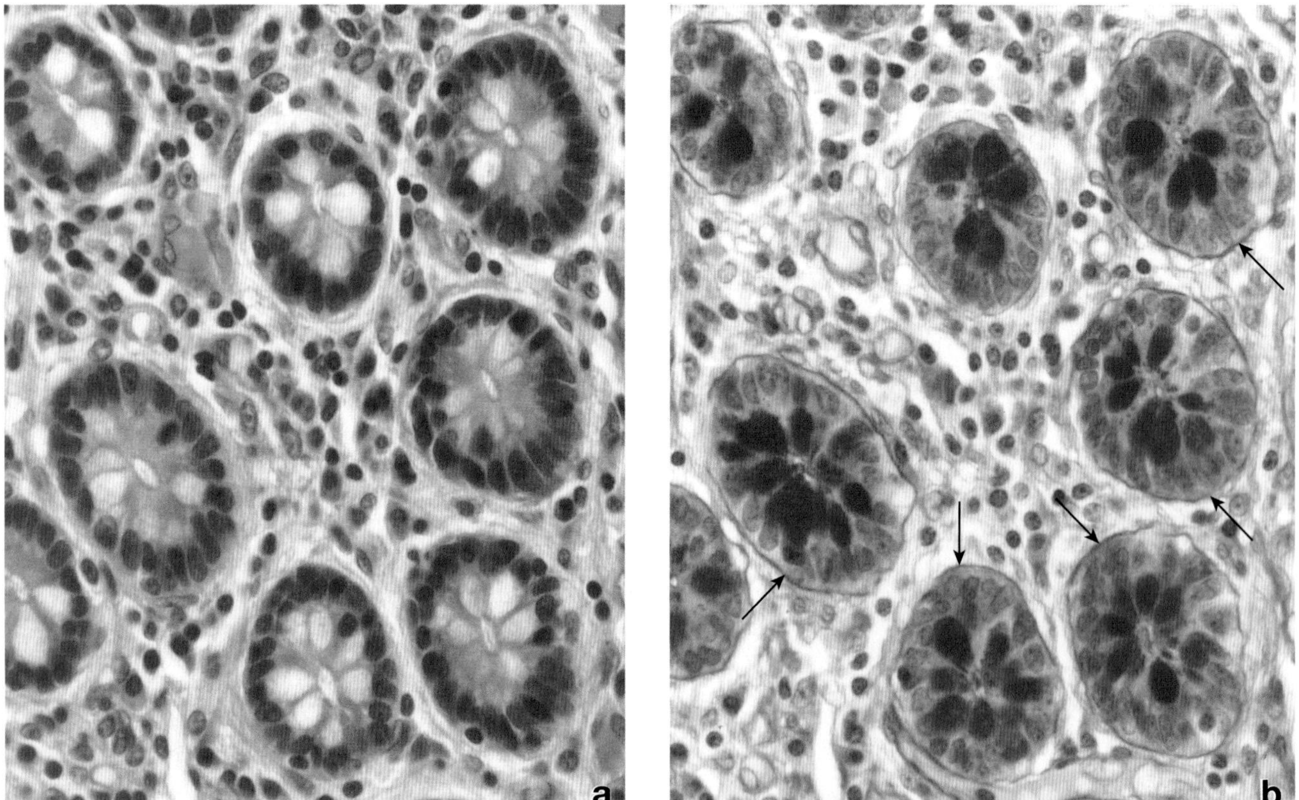

FIGURE 5.27. Photomicrographs showing serial sections of intestinal glands of the colon. The glands in this specimen have been cross-sectioned and appear as round profiles. **a.** This specimen was stained with hematoxylin and eosin (H&E). Note that neither the basement membrane nor the mucin that is located within the goblet cells is stained. ×550. **b.** This section was stained by the periodic acid–Schiff (PAS) method. It reveals the basement membrane as a thin, magenta layer (*arrows*) between the base of the epithelial cells of the glands and the adjacent connective tissue. The mucin within the goblet cells is also PAS positive. ×550.

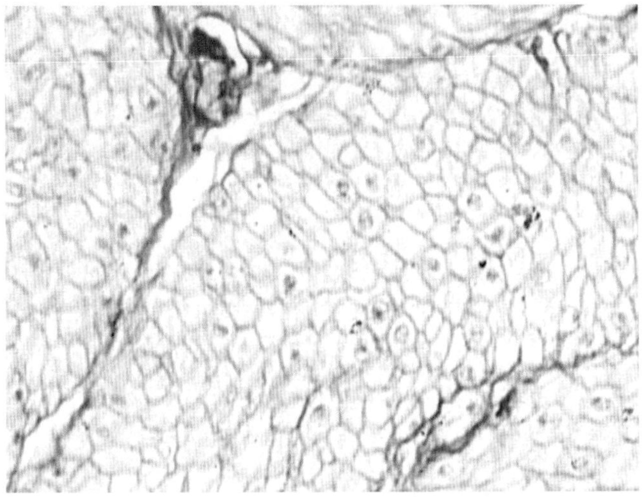

FIGURE 5.28. Smooth muscle external lamina. This photomicrograph is stained by the periodic acid–Schiff (PAS) method and counterstained with hematoxylin (pale nuclei). The muscle cells have been cut in cross section and appear as polygonal profiles because of the presence of PAS-positive basement membrane material surrounding each cell. The cytoplasm is not stained. As the plane of section passes through each smooth muscle cell, it may or may not pass through the portion of the cell that includes the nucleus. Therefore, in some of the polygonal profiles, nuclei can be seen; in other profiles, no nuclei are seen. ×850.

lamina and the cell is a relatively clear or electron-lucent area, the **lamina lucida** (also about 40 nm wide). The area outlined by the lamina lucida contains extracellular portions of CAMs, mainly **fibronectin** and **laminin receptors**. These receptors are members of the integrin family of transmembrane proteins.

With the development of new EM preparation techniques, the lamina lucida appears to be an artifact of fixation; in the living state, the basal lamina is composed of a single layer of the lamina densa.

If the tissue specimen for EM is fixed using low-temperature, high-pressure freezing (HPF) methods (without chemical fixatives), it retains much more of the tissue than specimens routinely fixed with glutaraldehyde. EM examination of such specimens reveals that the basal lamina is composed only of the lamina densa. No lamina lucida is detected. The lamina lucida may thus be an artifact of chemical fixation that appears as the epithelial cells shrink away from a high concentration of macromolecules deposited next to the basal domain of the epithelial cells. It probably results from the rapid dehydration that occurs during tissue processing for EM. Other structures visible with traditional EM are also not visible when tissues are prepared by the HPF method (Fig. 5.30).

The basal lamina in nonepithelial cells is referred to as the external lamina.

Muscle cells, adipocytes, and **peripheral nerve–supporting cells** exhibit an extracellular electron-dense material that resembles the basal lamina of epithelium. This material also corresponds to a PAS-positive staining reaction, as described earlier (see Fig. 5.28). Although the term **basement membrane** is not ordinarily applied to the extracellular stainable material of these nonepithelial cells in LM, the term **basal lamina** or **external lamina** is typically used at the EM level.

The basal lamina contains molecules that come together to form a sheet-like structure.

Analyses of basal laminae derived from epithelia in many locations (kidney glomeruli, lung, cornea, lens of the eye) indicate that they consist of approximately 50 proteins that can be classified into four groups: collagens, laminins, glycoproteins, and proteoglycans. These proteins are synthesized and secreted by the epithelial cells and other cell types that possess an external lamina.

- **Collagens.** At least three types of collagen species are present in the basal lamina; they represent a fraction of the approximately 28 types of collagen found in the body. The major component, comprising 50% of all basal lamina

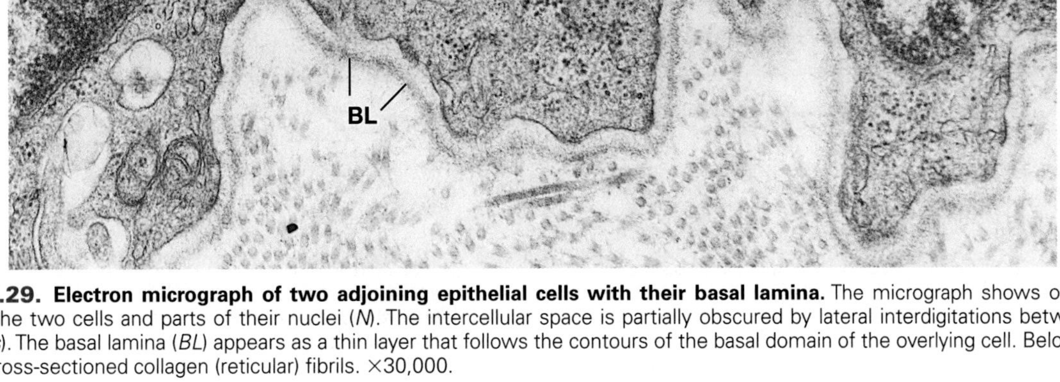

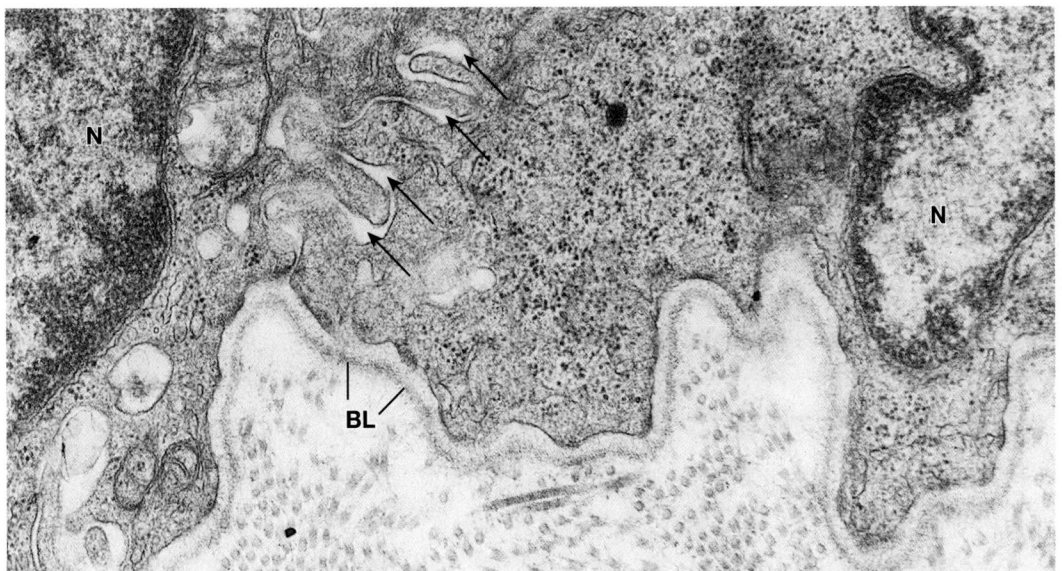

FIGURE 5.29. Electron micrograph of two adjoining epithelial cells with their basal lamina. The micrograph shows only the basal portions of the two cells and parts of their nuclei (*N*). The intercellular space is partially obscured by lateral interdigitations between the two cells (*arrows*). The basal lamina (*BL*) appears as a thin layer that follows the contours of the basal domain of the overlying cell. Below the *BL* are numerous cross-sectioned collagen (reticular) fibrils. ×30,000.

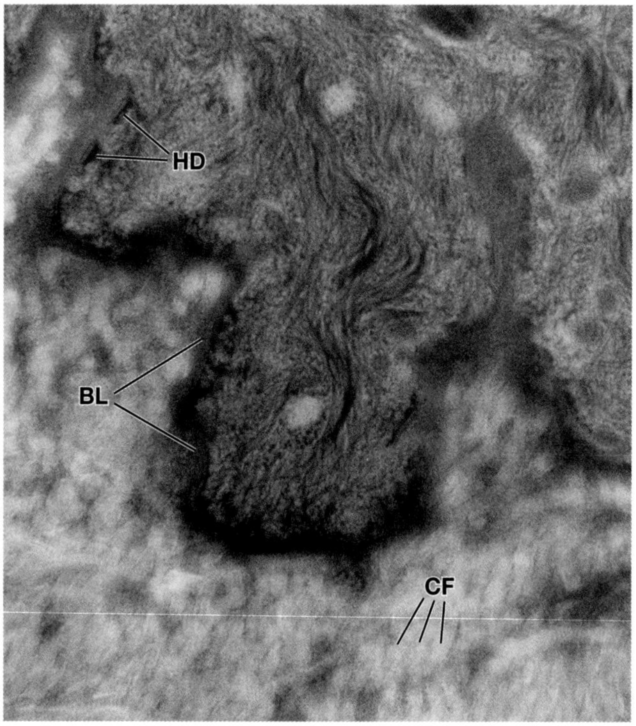

FIGURE 5.30. Electron micrograph of epithelial cells preserved by low-temperature, high-pressure freezing. This electron micrograph shows the basal domain of an epithelial cell obtained from human skin. The specimen was prepared by low-temperature, high-pressure freezing, which retains more tissue components than does chemical fixation. Note that a separate lamina densa or lamina lucida is not seen in this preparation. The lamina lucida is most likely an artifact that appears as the epithelial cell shrinks away from a high concentration of macromolecules just beneath the epithelial cell. This region of highly concentrated macromolecules precipitates into the artifact known as the *lamina densa*. *BL*, basal lamina; *HD*, hemidesmosome; *CF*, collagen fibrils. ×55,000. (Courtesy of Douglas R. Keene.)

proteins, is **type IV collagen**. The molecular characteristics and function of type IV collagen in forming a scaffold of basal lamina are described in the next section. The presence of different type IV collagen isoforms provides specificity to the basal lamina associated with different tissues. Two nonfibrillar types of collagens, **type XV collagen** and **type XVIII collagen**, are also found in the basal lamina. Type XV collagen plays an important role in stabilizing the structure of the external lamina in skeletal and cardiac muscle cells, whereas type XVIII collagen is mainly present in vascular and epithelial basal laminae and is believed to function in angiogenesis. In addition, **type VII collagen** forms anchoring fibrils that link the basal lamina to the underlying reticular lamina (described later).

- **Laminins.** These cross-shaped glycoprotein molecules (140–400 kDa) are composed of three polypeptide chains. They are essential in initiating the assembly of the basal lamina. Laminins possess binding sites for different **integrin receptors** in the basal domain of the overlying epithelial cells. They are involved in many **cell-to-extracellular matrix interactions.** They also play roles in the development, differentiation, and remodeling of epithelium. There are approximately 15 different variations of laminin molecules.
- **Entactin/nidogen.** This small, rod-like sulfated glycoprotein (150 kDa) serves as a link between **laminin** and the **type IV collagen network** in almost all basal laminae. Each entactin molecule is organized into distinct domains that bind calcium, support cell adhesion, promote neutrophil chemotaxis and phagocytosis, and interact with laminin, perlecan, fibronectin, and type IV collagen.
- **Proteoglycans.** Most of the volume of the basal lamina is probably attributable to its proteoglycan content. Proteoglycans consist of a **protein core** to which **heparan sulfate** (e.g., perlecan, agrin), **chondroitin sulfate** (e.g., bamacan), or **dermatan sulfate side chains** are attached. Because of their highly anionic character, these molecules are extensively hydrated. They also carry a **high negative charge**; this quality suggests that proteoglycans play a role in regulating the passage of ions across the basal lamina. The most common heparan sulfate proteoglycan found in all basal laminae is the large multidomain proteoglycan **perlecan** (400 kDa). It provides additional cross-links to the basal lamina by binding to laminin, type IV collagen, and entactin/nidogen. **Agrin** (500 kDa) is another important molecule found almost exclusively in the glomerular basement membrane of the kidney. It plays a major role in renal filtration as well as in cell-to-extracellular matrix interactions.

The molecular structure of type IV collagen determines its role in the formation of the basal lamina network suprastructure.

The **type IV collagen molecule** is similar to other collagens in that it contains three polypeptide chains. Each chain has a short **amino-terminus domain (7S domain)**, a long middle **collagenous helical domain** (which interacts with the remaining two chains in the fully assembled molecule), and a **carboxy-terminus globular noncollagenous**

FOLDER 5.4

FUNCTIONAL CONSIDERATIONS: BASEMENT MEMBRANE AND BASAL LAMINA TERMINOLOGY

The terms **basement membrane** and **basal lamina** are used inconsistently in the literature. Some authors use *basement membrane* when referring to both light (LM) and electron microscopic (EM) images. Others dispense with the term *basement membrane* altogether and use *basal lamina* in both LM and EM. Because the term *basement membrane* originated with the LM, it is used in this book only in the context of LM descriptions and only in relation to epithelia. The EM term *basal lamina* is reserved for the ultrastructural content to denote the layer present at the interface of connective tissue with epithelial cells. In this context, the LM term *basement membrane* actually describes basal lamina and the underlying reticular lamina combined. The term **external lamina** is used to identify *basal lamina* when it forms a peripheral cellular investment, as in muscle cells and peripheral nerve–supporting cells.

domain (NC1 domain). The six known chains of type IV collagen molecules ($\alpha1$–$\alpha6$) form three sets of triple helical molecules known as **collagen protomers**. They are designated as $[\alpha1(\text{IV})]_2\ \alpha2(\text{IV})$, $\alpha3(\text{IV})\ \alpha4(\text{IV})\ \alpha5(\text{IV})$, and $[\alpha5(\text{IV})]_2\ \alpha6(\text{IV})$ protomers (see Table 6.2).

Protomer assembly begins when the three NC1 domains assemble to form an **NC1 trimer** (Fig. 5.31). The next step in the assembly of the basal lamina structure is the formation of **type IV collagen dimer** molecules. This is achieved when two NC1 trimers interact to form an **NC1 hexamer**. Next, four dimers join in the region of the 7S domain to form a **tetramer.** The 7S domain of the tetramer (called the *7S box*) determines the geometry of the tetramer. Finally, the **type IV collagen scaffold** is formed when other collagen tetramers interact end to end with each other. This scaffold forms the suprastructure of the basal lamina. Assembly of this suprastructure is genetically determined. Those containing $[\alpha1(\text{IV})]_2\ \alpha2(\text{IV})$ protomers are found in all basal laminae. Those containing $\alpha3(\text{IV})\ \alpha4(\text{IV})\ \alpha5(\text{IV})$ protomers occur mainly in the kidney and lungs, and those containing $[\alpha5(\text{IV})]_2\ \alpha6(\text{IV})$ protomers are restricted to the skin, esophagus, and Bowman capsule in the kidney.

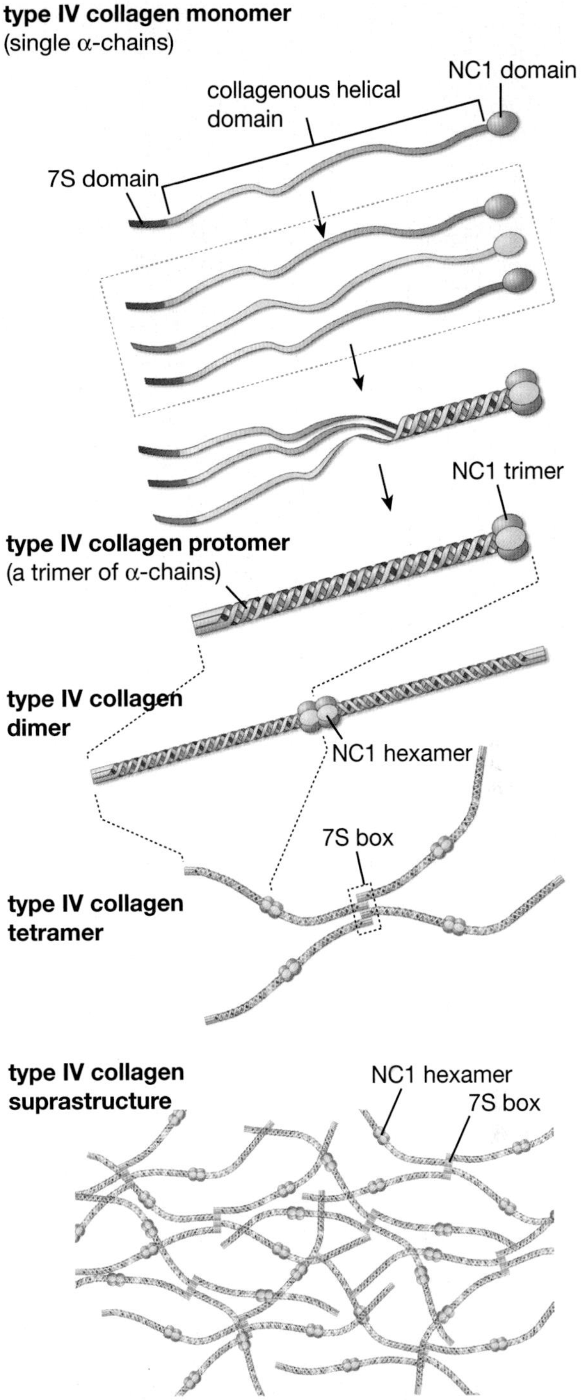

FIGURE 5.31. Formation of the type IV collagen suprastructure. Each type IV collagen molecule has three domains: an amino-terminus (7S domain), a middle collagenous helical domain, and a carboxy-terminus (NC1 domain). The NC1 domain initiates the assembly of the type IV collagen protomer, which consists of three molecules. Protomer formation proceeds like a zipper from the NC1 domain toward the 7S domain, resulting in a fully assembled protomer. The next step in assembly is the dimerization of type IV collagen protomers. Two type IV collagen protomers become connected via their NC1 domains, and their two NC1 trimers join to form an NC1 hexamer. Next, four dimers join at their 7S domains to form tetramers connected by the 7S box. These tetramers interact to form the type IV collagen suprastructure via their interactions with the 7S domains of other tetramers and also by lateral associations between type IV collagen protomers.

Basal lamina self-assembly is initiated by the polymerization of laminins on the basal cell domain and interaction with the type IV collagen suprastructure.

The constituents of the basal lamina come together in a **process of self-assembly** to form a sheet-like structure. This process is initiated by both **type IV collagen** and **laminins.** The primary sequence of these molecules contains information for their self-assembly (other molecules of the basal lamina are incapable of forming sheet-like structures by themselves). Studies using cell lines have shown that the first step in the self-assembly of the basal lamina is **calcium-dependent polymerization** of laminin molecules on the basal cell surface domain (Fig. 5.32). This process is aided by CAMs (integrins). At the same time, the type IV collagen suprastructure becomes associated with laminin polymers. These two structures are joined primarily by entactin/nidogen bridges and are additionally secured by other proteins (perlecan, agrin, fibronectin, etc.). The scaffold of type IV collagen and laminins provides the site for other basal lamina molecules to interact and form the fully functional basal lamina.

A layer of reticular fibers underlies the basal lamina.

There is still a lack of agreement about the extent to which the basal lamina seen with the EM corresponds to the structure described as the basement membrane in the LM. Some investigators contend that the **basement membrane** includes not only the **basal lamina** but also a secondary layer of small unit fibrils of **type III collagen (reticular fibers)** that forms the reticular lamina. The reticular lamina, as such, belongs to the connective tissue and is not a product of the epithelium. The reticular lamina was once regarded as the component that reacted with silver, whereas the polysaccharides of the basal lamina and the ground substance associated with the reticular fibers were thought to be the components stained with the PAS reaction. However, convincing arguments can be made for the basal lamina reacting with both PAS and silver in several sites. In normal kidney glomeruli, for example, no collagen (reticular) fibers are associated with the basal lamina of the epithelial cells (Fig. 5.33), although a positive reaction occurs with both PAS staining and silver impregnation. Also, in the spleen, where the basal lamina of the venous sinuses forms a unique pattern of ring-like bands rather than a thin, sheath-like layer around

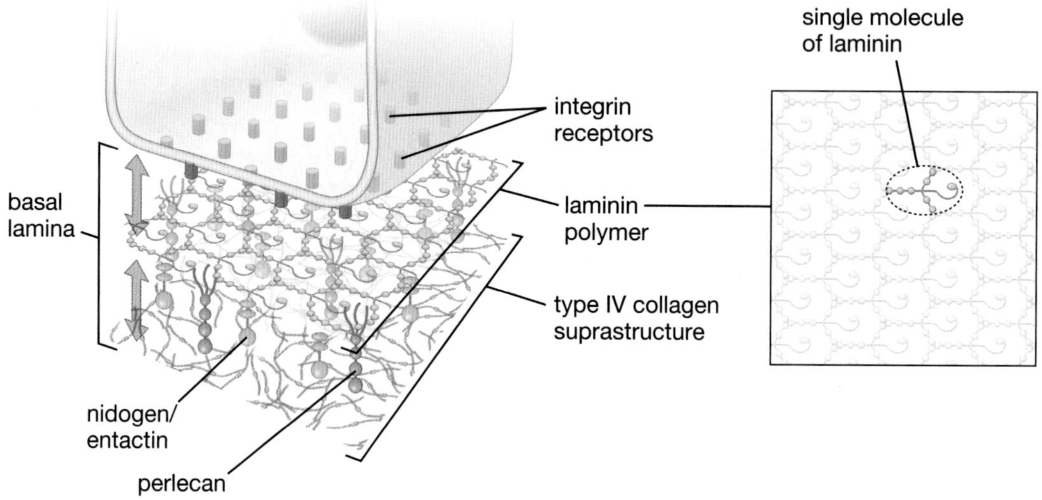

FIGURE 5.32. Molecular components of the basal lamina. To produce a basal lamina, each epithelial cell must first synthesize and secrete its molecular components. The assembly of the basal lamina occurs outside the cell at its basal domain. The calcium-dependent polymerization of laminin molecules that occurs at the basal cell surface initiates basal lamina formation. Laminin polymers are next anchored to the cell surface by integrin receptors. At the same time, the type IV collagen suprastructure is assembled (see Fig. 5.31) in close proximity to laminin polymers. These two structures are connected by entactin or nidogen bridges and are additionally secured by other proteins (i.e., perlecan). The primary scaffold of type IV collagen connected to laminin polymers provides the site for other basal lamina molecules to interact and form the fully functional basal lamina.

the vessel, exactly corresponding images are seen with the PAS and silver techniques as well as with the EM (Fig. 5.34).

Several structures are responsible for attachment of the basal lamina to the underlying connective tissue.

On the opposite side of the basal lamina, the connective tissue side, several mechanisms provide attachment of the basal lamina to the underlying connective tissue:

- **Anchoring fibrils (type VII collagen)** are usually found in close association with hemidesmosomes. They either extend from the basal lamina to the structures called **anchoring plaques** in the connective tissue matrix or loop back to the basal lamina (Fig. 5.35). The anchoring fibrils entrap **type III collagen** (reticular) fibers in the underlying connective tissue, which ensures sound epithelial anchorage. Anchoring fibrils are critical to the

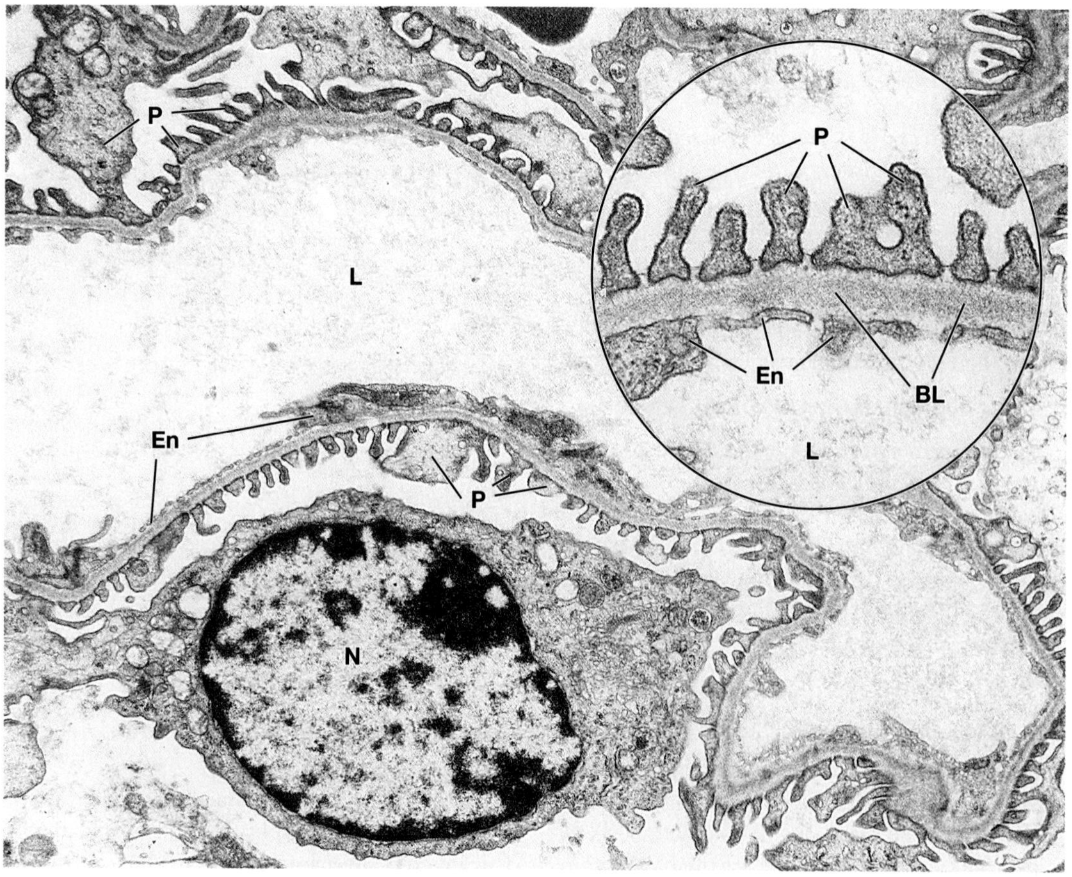

FIGURE 5.33. Basal lamina in the kidney glomerulus. Electron micrograph of a kidney glomerular capillary showing the basal lamina (*BL*) interposed between the capillary endothelial cell (*En*) and the cytoplasmic processes (*P*, podocytes) of epithelial cells. The epithelial cell is located on the outer (abluminal) surface of the endothelial cell. ×12,000. **Inset.** Relationship at higher magnification. Note that the endothelial cells and epithelial cells are separated by the shared basal lamina and that no collagen fibrils are present. *L*, lumen of capillary; *N*, nucleus of epithelial cell. ×40,000.

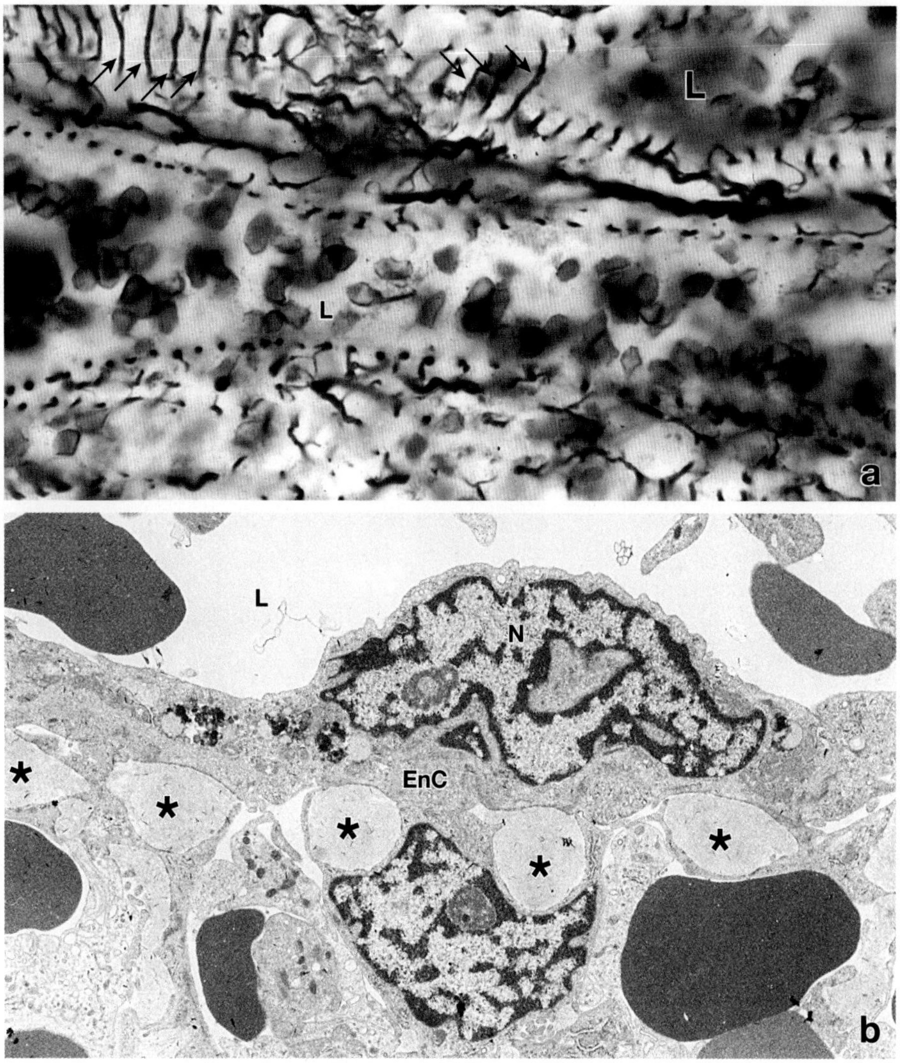

FIGURE 5.34. Demonstration of basement membrane material in splenic vessels. a. Photomicrograph of a silver preparation revealing two longitudinally sectioned venous sinuses in the spleen. These blood vessels are surrounded by a modified basement membrane, which takes the form of a ring-like structure, much like the hoops of a barrel, rather than a continuous layer or lamina. The rings are blackened by the silver and appear as bands where the walls of the vessel have been tangentially sectioned (*arrows*). To the right, the cut has penetrated deeper into the vessel and shows the lumen (*L*). Here, the cut edges of the rings are seen on both sides of the vessel. In the lower vessel, the cut rings have been sectioned in a virtually perpendicular plane, and the rings appear as a series of dots. ×400. **b.** Electron micrograph of the wall of a venous sinus, showing a longitudinally sectioned endothelial cell (*EnC*). The nucleus (*N*) of the cell is protruding into the lumen (*L*). The basal lamina material (*asterisks*) has the same homogeneous appearance as seen by electron microscopy in other sites, except that it is aggregated into ring-like structures rather than into a flat layer or lamina. Moreover, its location and plane of section correspond to the silver-reactive, dot-like material in the panel above. ×25,000.

function of the anchoring junctions; mutations in the collagen VII gene result in **dystrophic epidermolysis bullosa**, an inherited blistering skin disease in which the epithelium is detached below the basement membrane.

- **Fibrillin microfibrils** are 10–12 nm in diameter and attach the lamina densa to elastic fibers. Fibrillin microfibrils are known to have elastic properties. A mutation in the fibrillin gene (FBN1) causes **Marfan syndrome** and other related connective tissue disorders.
- **Discrete projections of the lamina densa** on its connective tissue side interact directly with the reticular lamina to form an additional binding site with type III collagen.

Organ-specific molecules within the basal lamina perform a variety of functions.

In recent years, the **basal lamina** has been recognized as an important regulator of cell behavior rather than just a structural feature of the epithelial tissue. Organ-specific molecules have been identified in the basal lamina. Although morphologically all basal laminae appear similar, their molecular composition and functions are unique to each tissue. The following are various functions now attributed to the basal lamina:

- **Structural attachment**. As noted, the basal lamina serves as an intermediary structure in the attachment of cells to the adjacent connective tissue. Epithelial cells are anchored into the basal lamina by cell-to-extracellular matrix junctions, and the basal lamina is attached to underlying connective tissue by anchoring fibrils and fibrillin microfibrils.
- **Compartmentalization**. Structurally, basal and external laminae separate or isolate the connective tissue from epithelia, nerve, and muscle tissues. Connective tissue—including all of its specialized tissues, such as bone and cartilage (with the exception of adipose tissue, in that its cells possess an external lamina)—can be viewed as a single, continuous compartment. In contrast, epithelia, muscles, and nerves are separated from adjacent connective tissue by intervening basal or external laminae. For any substance to move from one tissue to another (e.g., from one compartment to another), it must cross such a lamina.
- **Filtration**. The movement of substances to and from the connective tissue is regulated in part by the basal lamina, mainly through ionic charges and integral spaces. Filtration is well characterized in the kidney, in which the plasma filtrate must cross the compound basal laminae of capillaries and adjacent epithelial cells to reach the urinary space within the renal corpuscle.
- **Tissue scaffolding**. The basal lamina serves as a guide or scaffold during regeneration. Newly formed cells or growing processes of a cell use the basal lamina that remains after cell loss, thus helping to maintain the original tissue architecture. For example, when nerves are damaged, new neuromuscular junctions from a growing axon will be established only if the external lamina

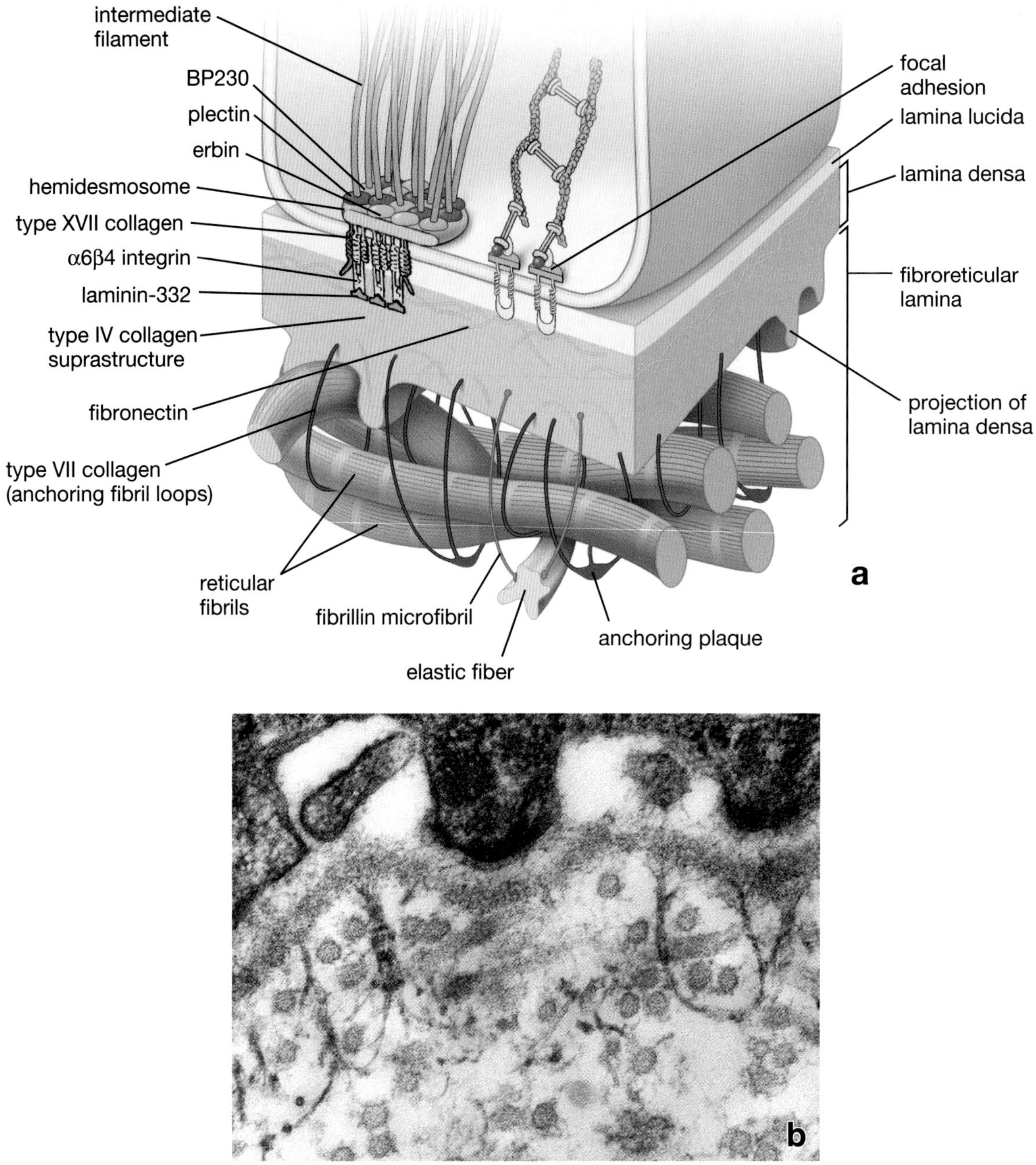

FIGURE 5.35. Schematic diagram and electron micrograph of the basal portion of epithelial cell. a. This diagram shows the cellular and extracellular components that provide attachment between epithelial cells and the underlying connective tissue. On the connective tissue side of the basal lamina, anchoring fibrils extend from the basal lamina to the collagen (reticular) fibrils of the connective tissue, providing structural attachment at this site. On the epithelial side, laminin (*green*), collagen XVII (*red*), and integrins (*yellow*) are present in the lamina lucida and lamina densa and provide adhesion between the basal lamina and the intracellular attachment plaques of hemidesmosomes. **b.** This high-magnification electron micrograph of human skin shows the basal portion of human epithelial cells with underlying basal lamina. The electron-lucent space, the lamina lucida located just below the basal cell membrane, is occupied by anchoring filaments formed by laminin and type XVII collagen molecules. Anchoring filaments are responsible for attaching the basal cell membrane to the basal lamina. The loop-like fibers originating from the basal lamina represent anchoring fibrils of type VII collagen that link the basal lamina with the reticular fibers (type III collagen) and with anchoring plaques located within the extracellular matrix. ×200,000. (Courtesy of Douglas R. Keene.)

remains intact after injury. The basal laminae also allow cells to migrate under physiologic conditions but act as barriers against tumor cell invasion.

- **Regulation and signaling.** Many molecules that reside in the basal lamina interact with cell surface receptors, influencing epithelial cell behavior during morphogenesis, fetal development, and wound healing by regulating cell shape, proliferation, differentiation, and motility as well as gene expression and apoptosis. For instance, the basal lamina of endothelial cells has recently been found to be involved in the regulation of tumor angiogenesis.

Cell-to-Extracellular Matrix Junctions

The organization of cells in epithelium depends on the support provided by the extracellular matrix on which the basal surface of each cell rests. **Anchoring junctions** maintain the morphologic integrity of the epithelium–connective tissue interface. The two major anchoring junctions are

- **focal adhesions**, which anchor actin filaments of the cytoskeleton into the basal lamina, and
- **hemidesmosomes**, which anchor the intermediate filaments of the cytoskeleton into the basement membrane

In addition, transmembrane proteins located in the basal cell domain (mainly related to the integrin family of adhesion molecules) interact with the basal lamina.

Focal adhesions create a dynamic link between the actin cytoskeleton and extracellular matrix proteins.

Focal adhesions form a structural link between the actin cytoskeleton and extracellular matrix proteins. They are responsible for attaching long bundles of actin filaments (stress fibers) into the basal lamina (Fig. 5.36a). Focal adhesions play a prominent role during **dynamic changes that occur in epithelial cells** (e.g., migration of epithelial cells in wound repair). Coordinated remodeling of the actin cytoskeleton and the controlled formation and dismantling of focal adhesions provide the **molecular bases for cell migration**. Focal adhesions are also found in other nonepithelial cells, such as fibroblasts and smooth muscle cells.

In general, **focal adhesions** consist of a cytoplasmic face to which **actin filaments** are bound, a transmembrane connecting region, and an extracellular face that binds to the proteins of the extracellular matrix. The **integrin** family is the main type of transmembrane protein found in focal adhesions. Integrins are concentrated in clusters within the areas where the junctions can be detected. On the cytoplasmic face, integrins interact with **actin-binding proteins** (α-actinin, vinculin, talin, paxillin) as well as many regulatory proteins, such as **focal adhesion kinase** or **tyrosine kinase** (Fig. 5.36b). On the extracellular side, integrins bind to extracellular matrix glycoproteins, usually laminin and fibronectin.

Focal adhesions play an important role in sensing and transmitting signals from the extracellular environment into the interior of the cell.

Focal adhesions are also important sites for **signal detection** and **transduction**. They are able to detect contractile forces or mechanical changes in the extracellular matrix and convert them into biochemical signals. This phenomenon, known as **mechanosensitivity**, allows cells to alter their adhesion-mediated functions in response to external mechanical stimuli. Integrins transmit these signals to the interior of the cell, where they affect cell migration, differentiation, and growth. Recent studies indicate that focal adhesion proteins also serve as a common point of entry for signals resulting from stimulation of various classes of growth factor receptors.

Hemidesmosomes occur in epithelia that require strong, stable adhesion to the connective tissue.

A variant of the anchoring junction similar to the desmosome is found in certain epithelia subject to abrasion and mechanical shearing forces that would tend to separate the epithelium from the underlying connective tissue. Typically, this junction occurs in the cornea, the skin, and the mucosa of the oral cavity, esophagus, and vagina. In these locations, it appears as if half the desmosome is present, hence the name **hemidesmosome**. Hemidesmosomes are found on the **basal cell surface**, where they provide increased adhesion to the basal lamina (Fig. 5.37a). When observed with the EM, the hemidesmosome exhibits an **intracellular attachment plaque** on the cytoplasmic side of the basal plasma membrane. The protein composition of this structure is similar to that of the desmosomal plaque, as it contains a **desmoplakin-like family of proteins** capable of anchoring intermediate filaments of the cytoskeleton. Three major proteins have been identified in the plaque:

- **Plectin** (450 kDa) functions as a cross-linker of the intermediate filaments that bind them to the hemidesmosome attachment plaque. Recent studies indicate that plectin also interacts with microtubules, actin filaments, and myosin II. Thus, plectin cross-links and integrates all elements of the cytoskeleton.

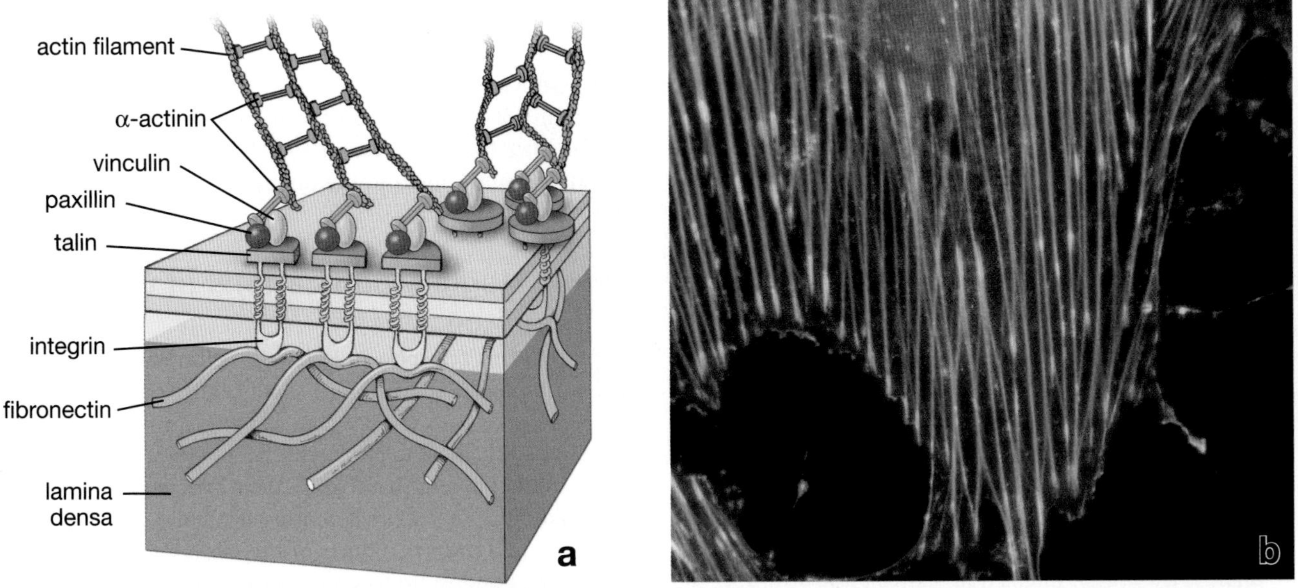

FIGURE 5.36. Molecular structure of focal adhesions. a. Diagram showing the molecular organization of focal adhesions. On the cytoplasmic side, note the arrangement of different actin-binding proteins. These proteins interact with integrins, the transmembrane proteins, the extracellular domains of which bind to proteins of the extracellular matrix (e.g., fibronectin). **b.** This image was obtained from the fluorescence microscope and shows cells cultured on the fibronectin-coated surface stained with fluorescein-labeled phalloidin to visualize actin filaments (stress fibers) in *green*. Next, using indirect immunofluorescence techniques, focal adhesions were labeled with primary monoclonal antibody against phosphotyrosine and visualized with secondary rhodamine-labeled antibody (*red*). The phosphotyrosine is a product of the tyrosine kinase reaction in which tyrosine molecules of the associated proteins are phosphorylated by this enzyme. Tyrosine kinase is closely associated with focal adhesion molecules, so the area where focal adhesions are formed is labeled *red*. Note the relationship of focal adhesions and actin filaments at the periphery of the cell. ×3,000. (Courtesy of Dr. Keith Burridge.)

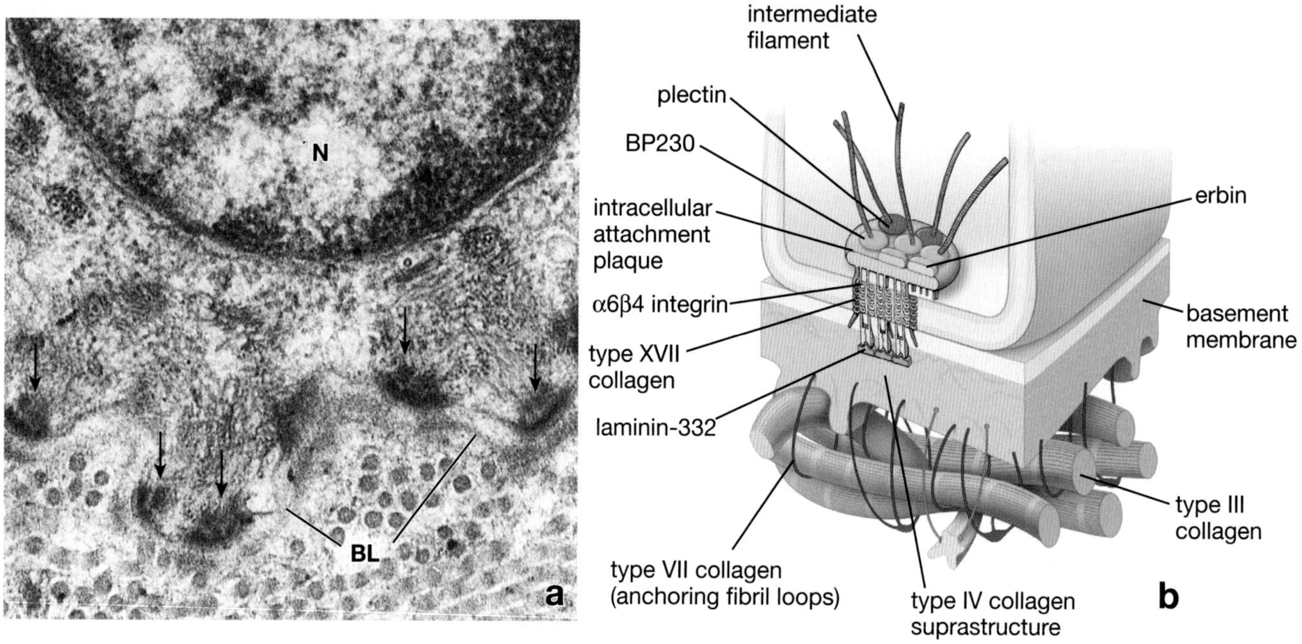

FIGURE 5.37. Molecular structure of hemidesmosome. a. Electron micrograph of the basal aspect of a gingival epithelial cell. Below the nucleus (*N*), intermediate filaments are seen converging on the intracellular attachment plaques (*arrows*) of the hemidesmosome. Below the plasma membrane are the basal lamina (*BL*) and collagen (reticular) fibrils (most of which are cut in cross section) of the connective tissue. ×40,000. **b.** Diagram showing the molecular organization of a hemidesmosome. The intracellular attachment plaque is associated with transmembrane adhesion molecules, such as those of the integrin family and transmembrane type XVII collagen, and contains plectin, BP230, and erbin. Note that the intermediate filaments seem to originate or terminate in the intracellular attachment plaque. Extracellular portions of integrins bind to laminin-332 and type IV collagen. With the help of anchoring fibrils (type VII collagen), laminin, and integrin, the attachment plaque is secured to the reticular fibers (type III collagen) of the extracellular matrix.

- **BP230** (230 kDa) attaches intermediate filaments to the intercellular attachment plaque. The absence of functional BP230 causes **bullous pemphigoid**, a disease characterized clinically by blister formation. High levels of antibodies directed against components of the hemidesmosome, including antibodies against BP230 and type XVII collagen, are detected in people with this disease. For this reason, BP230 is called **bullous pemphigoid antigen 1 (BPAG1)**, and the collagen XVII molecule is called **bullous pemphigoid antigen 2 (BPAG2)** or **BP 180**.
- **Erbin** (180 kDa) mediates an association of BP230 with integrins.

In contrast to the desmosome, whose transmembrane proteins belong to the cadherin family of calcium-dependent molecules, the majority of transmembrane proteins found in the **hemidesmosome** belong to the **integrin class of cell matrix receptors.** These include the following:

- **$\alpha_4\beta_6$ integrin**, a heterodimer molecule containing two polypeptide chains. Its extracellular domain enters the basal lamina and interacts with the type IV collagen suprastructure containing laminins (laminin-332), entactin/nidogen, or perlecan. On the extracellular surface of the hemidesmosome, laminin molecules form thread-like **anchoring filaments** that extend from the integrin molecules to the structure of the basement membrane (Fig. 5.37b). Interaction between **laminin-332** and **$\alpha_6\beta_4$ integrin** stabilizes the hemidesmosome and is essential for hemidesmosome formation and for the maintenance of epithelial adhesion. Mutation of the genes encoding laminin-332 chains results in **junctional epidermolysis bullosa**, another hereditary blistering skin disease.
- **Type XVII collagen (BPAG2, BP 180)**, a transmembrane molecule (180 kDa) that regulates the expression and function of laminin. In experimental models, type XVII collagen inhibits the migration of endothelial cells during angiogenesis and regulates keratinocyte migration in the skin (see Fig. 5.37b).
- **CD151** (32 kDa), a glycoprotein that participates in the clustering of integrin receptors to facilitate cell-to-extracellular matrix interactions

Despite their similarity in names, the terms *anchoring filaments* and *anchoring fibrils* do not describe the same structure. **Anchoring filaments** are formed mainly by **laminin** and **type XVII collagen** molecules. They attach the basal cell membrane of epithelial cells to the underlying basal lamina. **Anchoring fibrils** are formed by **type VII collagen** and attach the basal lamina to the underlying reticular fibers (see pages 158-159).

Morphologic Modifications of the Basal Cell Surface

Many cells that transport fluid have **infoldings** at the **basal cell surface.** These infoldings significantly increase the surface area of the basal cell domain, allowing for more transport proteins and channels to be present. Basal surface modifications are prominent in cells that participate in the active transport of molecules (e.g., in proximal and distal tubules of the kidney; Fig. 5.38) and in certain ducts of the salivary glands. In addition, mitochondria are typically concentrated at this basal site to provide the energy requirements for active transport. The mitochondria are usually oriented vertically within the folds. The orientation of the mitochondria, combined with the basal membrane infoldings, results in a striated appearance along the basal aspect of the cell when observed in the LM. Because of this phenomenon, the salivary gland ducts that possess these cells are referred to as **striated ducts**.

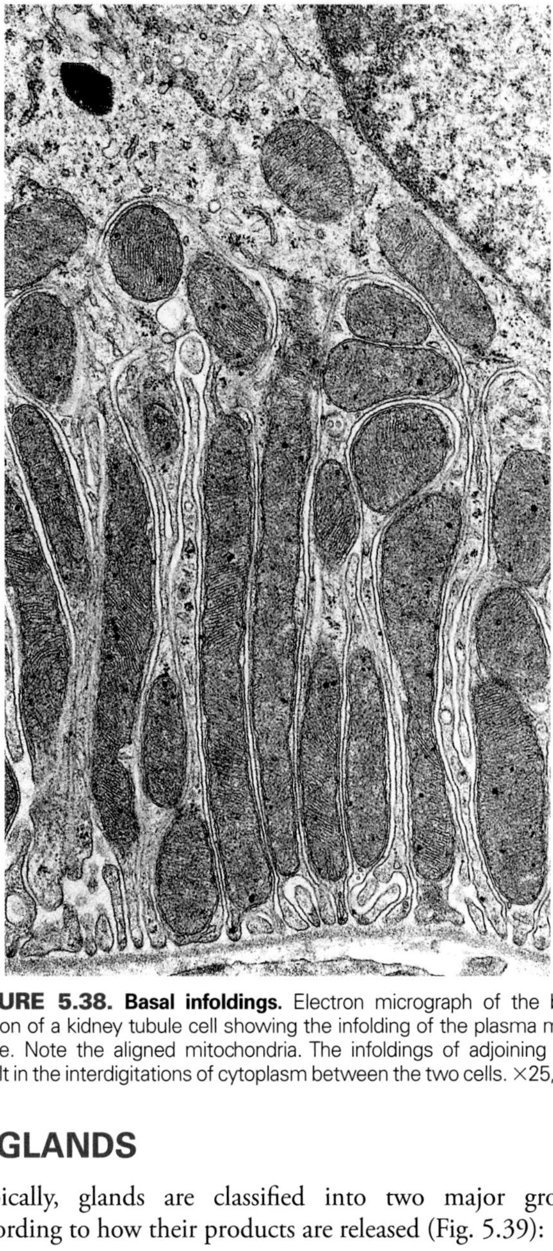

FIGURE 5.38. Basal infoldings. Electron micrograph of the basal portion of a kidney tubule cell showing the infolding of the plasma membrane. Note the aligned mitochondria. The infoldings of adjoining cells result in the interdigitations of cytoplasm between the two cells. ×25,000.

■ GLANDS

Typically, glands are classified into two major groups according to how their products are released (Fig. 5.39):

- **Exocrine glands** secrete their products onto a surface directly or through epithelial ducts or tubes that are connected to a surface. Ducts may convey the secreted material in an unaltered form or may modify the secretion by concentrating it or adding or reabsorbing constituent substances.
- **Endocrine glands** lack a duct system. They secrete their products into the connective tissue, from which they enter the bloodstream to reach their target cells. The products of endocrine glands are called **hormones**.

In some epithelia, individual cells secrete substances that do not reach the bloodstream but rather affect other nearby cells. Such secretory activity is referred to as **paracrine signaling** (see Fig. 5.39). Cells that produce paracrine substances (paracrines) release them into the subjacent extracellular matrix. Paracrine substances have a very limited signaling range; they reach the target cells by diffusion. For example, endothelial cells of blood vessels affect vascular smooth muscle cells by releasing multiple factors that cause either contraction or relaxation of the vascular wall.

In addition, a cell may secrete molecules that bind to receptors that are present on the same cell. This type of messaging is called **autocrine signaling** (see Fig. 5.39). In many cases, signaling molecules (autocrines) initiate negative feedback pathways to modulate their own secretion. This signaling mechanism is frequently used by cells of the immune system and involves the family of interleukin signaling molecules.

Cells of exocrine glands exhibit different mechanisms of secretion.

The cells of exocrine glands have three basic release mechanisms for secretory products (see Fig. 5.39):

- **Merocrine secretion.** This secretory product is delivered in **membrane-bound vesicles** to the apical surface of the cell. Here, vesicles fuse with the plasma membrane and extrude their contents by exocytosis. This is the most common mechanism of secretion and is found, for example, in pancreatic acinar cells.
- **Apocrine secretion.** The secretory product is released in the apical portion of the cell, surrounded by a thin layer of cytoplasm within an envelope of plasma membrane. This mechanism of secretion is found in the **lactating mammary gland**, where it is responsible for releasing large lipid droplets into the milk.
- **Holocrine secretion.** The secretory product accumulates within the maturing cell, which simultaneously undergoes destruction orchestrated by **programmed cell death** pathways. Both secretory products and cell debris are discharged into the lumen of the gland. This mechanism is found in the **sebaceous glands of skin** and the **tarsal (meibomian) glands of the eyelid**.

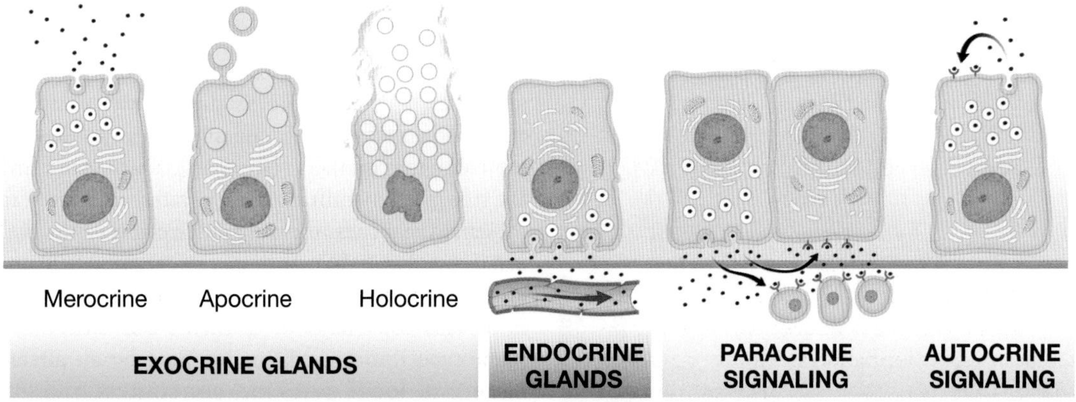

FIGURE 5.39. Types of glands and their mechanism of secretion. This diagram shows two types of glands (exocrine and endocrine) and two types of signaling mechanisms (paracrine and autocrine) that are used to influence the behavior of nearby cells. Note that the three basic types of secretions are shown in cells of the exocrine glands. Merocrine secretion is the most common and involves exocytosis of the vesicle content at the apical cell membrane. The best example of holocrine secretion causing disintegration of secretory cells is seen in sebaceous glands of hair follicles, whereas apocrine secretion is best observed in mammary gland cells that secrete lipid droplets into milk.

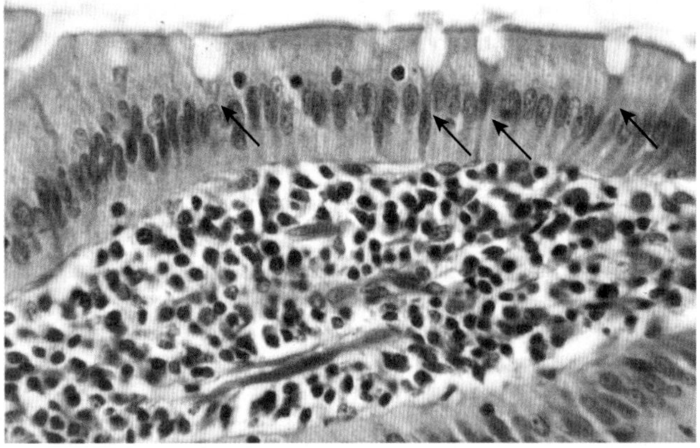

FIGURE 5.40. Unicellular glands. Photomicrograph of intestinal epithelium showing single goblet cells (*arrows*) dispersed among absorptive cells. Each goblet cell may be regarded as a unicellular gland—the simplest exocrine-type gland. ×350.

Exocrine glands are classified as either unicellular or multicellular.

Unicellular glands are the simplest in structure. In unicellular exocrine glands, the secretory component consists of single cells distributed among other nonsecretory cells. A typical example is the **goblet cell**, a mucus-secreting cell positioned among other columnar cells (Fig. 5.40). Goblet cells are located in the surface lining and glands of the intestines and in certain passages of the respiratory tract.

Multicellular glands are composed of more than one cell. They exhibit varying degrees of complexity. Their structural organization allows subclassification according to the arrangement of the secretory cells (parenchyma) and the presence or absence of branching of the duct elements.

The simplest arrangement of a multicellular gland is a cellular sheet in which each surface cell is a secretory cell. For example, the lining of the stomach and its gastric pits is a sheet of mucus-secreting cells (Fig. 5.41).

Other multicellular glands typically form tubular invaginations from the surface. The end pieces of the gland contain the secretory cells; the portion of the gland connecting the secretory cells to the surface serves as a duct. If the duct is unbranched, the gland is called **simple**; if the duct is branched, it is called **compound**. If the secretory portion is shaped like a tube, the gland is **tubular**; if it is shaped like a flask or grape, the gland is **alveolar** or **acinar**; if the tube ends in a sac-like dilation, the gland is **tubuloalveolar**. Tubular secretory portions may be straight, branched, or coiled; alveolar portions may be single or branched. Various combinations of duct and secretory portion shapes are found in the body. Classification and description of exocrine glands may be found in Table 5.6.

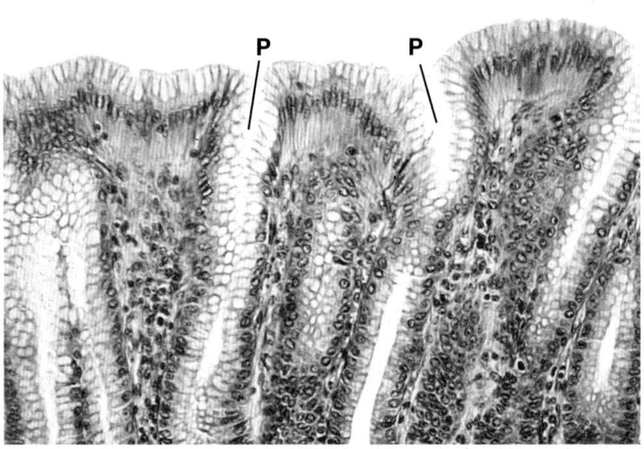

FIGURE 5.41. Mucus-secreting surface cells of stomach. Photomicrograph of stomach surface. The epithelial cells lining the surface are all mucus-secreting cells, as are the cells lining the gastric pits (*P*). The cells of the gastric pit form simple tubular glands. ×260.

Mucous and serous glands are so named for the type of secretion produced.

The secretory cells of exocrine glands associated with the various body tubes (e.g., the alimentary canal, respiratory passages, and urogenital system) are often described as being *mucous* or *serous* or both.

Mucous secretions are viscous and slimy, whereas **serous secretions** are watery. Goblet cells, secretory cells of the sublingual salivary glands, and surface cells of the stomach are examples of mucus-secreting cells. The mucous nature of the secretion results from extensive glycosylation of the constituent proteins with anionic oligosaccharides. The **mucinogen granules**, the secretory product within the cell, are, therefore, **PAS positive** (see Fig. 5.27a). However, they are water soluble and lost during routine tissue preparation. For this reason, the cytoplasm of mucous cells appears to be empty in H&E-stained paraffin sections. Another characteristic feature of a mucous cell is that its nucleus is usually flattened against the base of the cell by accumulated secretory product (Fig. 5.42).

In contrast to mucus-secreting cells, **serous cells** produce poorly glycosylated or nonglycosylated **protein secretions**. The nucleus is typically round or oval (Fig. 5.43). The apical cytoplasm is often intensely stained with eosin if its secretory granules are well preserved. The perinuclear cytoplasm often appears basophilic because of an extensive rough endoplasmic reticulum, a characteristic of protein-synthesizing cells.

Serous cell–containing acini (sing., *acinus*) are found in the parotid gland and pancreas. Acini of some glands, such as the submandibular gland, contain both mucous and serous cells. In routine tissue preparation, the serous cells are more removed from the lumen of the acinus and are shaped as crescents or **demilunes (half-moons)** at the periphery of the mucous acinus.

■ EPITHELIAL–MESENCHYMAL TRANSITION

Epithelial cells can undergo an epithelial–mesenchymal transition in which they lose their characteristics and acquire mesenchymal cell features.

The **epithelial–mesenchymal transition (EMT)** is a process in which an epithelial cell loses its characteristics and acquires a mesenchymal cell phenotype. Epithelial cells' cell-to-cell junctions, apical and basal domain specializations, and epithelial markers are lost during this transition, and newly transformed cells acquire cell motility, a spindle cell shape, and mesenchymal markers (Fig. 5.44). During the EMT process, the basement membrane disintegrates, and newly transformed mesenchymal cells migrate away from their epithelial layer of origin (see Fig. 5.44). They increase resistance to apoptosis and anoikis (cell detachment–induced apoptosis). The reprogramming and conversion of epithelial cells into a mesenchymal phenotype during EMT is initiated by an alteration in the balance of **local cytokine concentrations** (e.g., TGF-β, FGF, EGF) that upregulate specific transcription factors called **EMT-TFs** (e.g., Snail family, Twist1, and Zeb1).

EMT is a reversible process. During the **mesenchymal–epithelial transition (MET)** process, some mesenchymal

TABLE 5.6 Classification of Multicellular Glands

	Classification		Typical Location	Features
Simple glands	**Simple tubular**	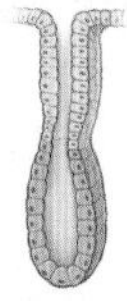	Large intestine: Intestinal glands of the colon	Secretory portion of the gland is a straight tube formed by the secretory cells (goblet cells).
	Simple coiled tubular	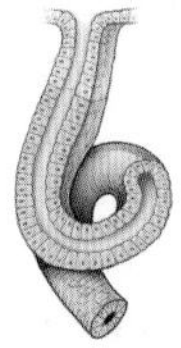	Skin: Eccrine sweat gland	Coiled tubular structure is composed of the secretory portion located deep in the dermis.
	Simple branched tubular	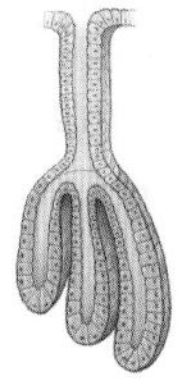	Stomach: Mucus-secreting glands of the pylorus Uterus: Endometrial glands	Branched tubular glands with wide secretory portion are formed by the secretory cells and produce a viscous mucous secretion.
	Simple acinar	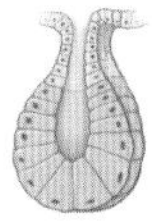	Urethra: Paraurethral and periurethral glands	Simple acinar glands develop as an outpouching of the transitional epithelium and are formed by a single layer of secretory cells.
	Branched acinar	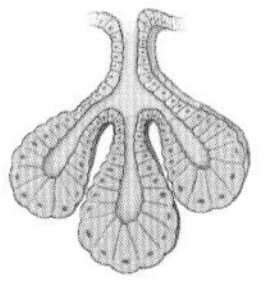	Stomach: Mucus-secreting glands of cardia Skin: Sebaceous glands	Branched acinar glands with secretory portions are formed by mucus-secreting cells; the short, single-duct portion opens directly into the lumen.
Compound glands	**Compound tubular**	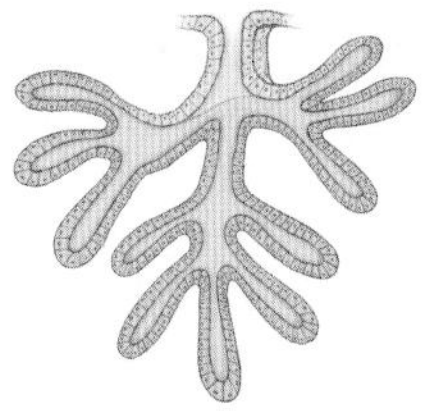	Duodenum: Submucosal glands of Brunner	Compound tubular glands with coiled secretory portions are located deep in the submucosa of the duodenum.
	Compound acinar	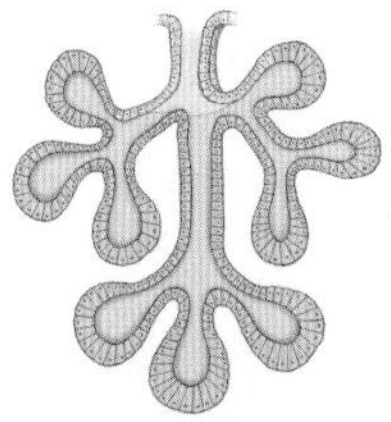	Pancreas: Exocrine portion	Compound acinar glands with alveolar-shaped secretory units are formed by pyramid-shaped serous-secreting cells.
	Compound tubuloacinar	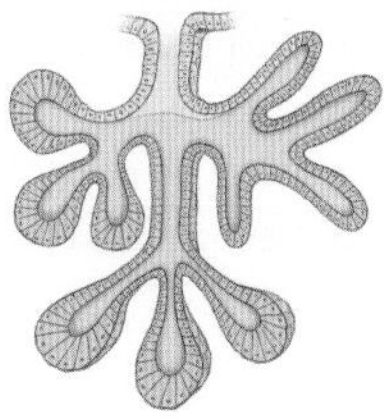	Neck region and oral cavity: Submandibular salivary gland	Compound tubuloacinar glands can have both mucous-branched tubular and serous-branched acinar secretory units; they have serous end-caps (demilunes).

cells can return to the epithelial cell phenotype (see Fig. 5.44). EMT-TFs are regulated by miRNA and other post-translational regulators (e.g., miR-200 family, miR-34). These factors can downregulate EMT-TFs to repress the EMT process and influence MET transformation.

EMT and MET processes can be classified into three categories taking into account the environment in which the transition occurs:

- **Type 1** occurs during **embryonic development.** A classic example of EMT can be seen during gastrulation in the early embryo, where epithelial cells of the epiblast (in the bilaminar germ disc) invaginate into the space between the epiblast and the hypoblast, giving rise to **mesoderm** (of the trilaminar germ disc). Mesodermal cells have mesenchymal cell characteristics acquired in the EMT process and migrate to generate intermediate mesoderm, paraxial

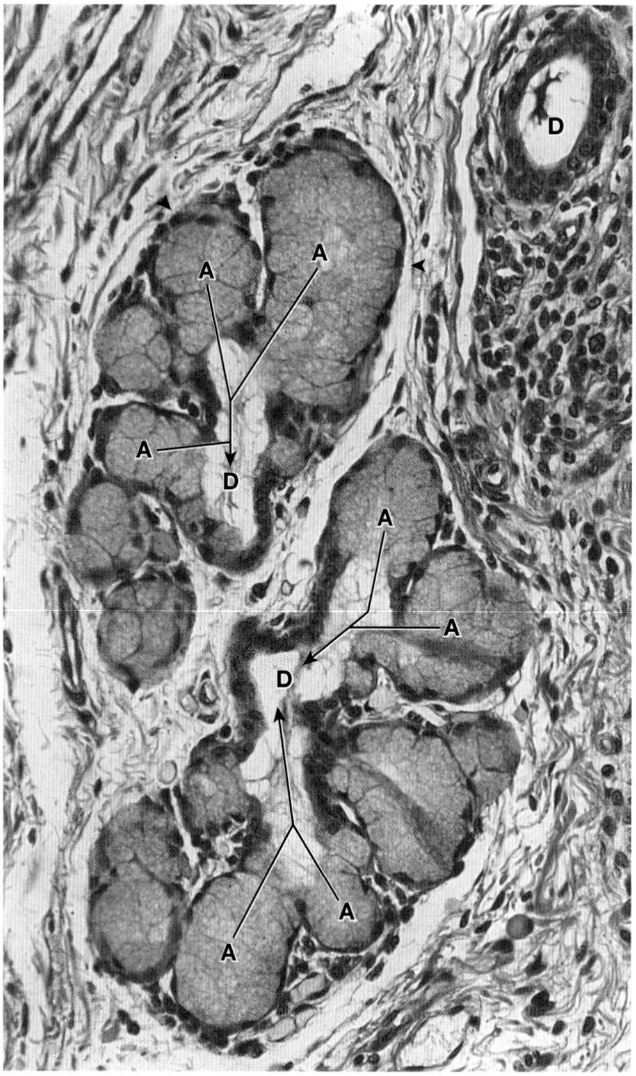

FIGURE 5.42. Mucus-secreting compound gland. Photomicrograph showing two small lobes of a mucus-secreting gland associated with the larynx. Each displays the beginning of a duct (*D*) into which mucin is secreted (*arrows*). The individual secretory cells that form the acinus (*A*) are difficult to define. Their nuclei (*arrowheads*) are flattened and located in the very basal portion of the cell, a feature typical of mucus-secreting glands. The cytoplasm is filled with mucin that has been retained during preparation of the tissue and appears stained. ×350.

mesoderm, and lateral plate mesoderm. These mesodermal cells then undergo MET to give rise to the organs in the urogenital system, notochord, somites, body walls of the abdomen and thorax, and the wall of the gut tube. During further embryonic development, cells may sequentially undergo several rounds of EMT and MET (e.g., during somite formation or heart development).

- **Type 2** occurs during the **wound healing** after injury. During the healing process, a connective tissue scar is formed due to EMT, cell reprogramming, and cell differentiation. Thus, the healing process can be regarded as **reparative fibrosis**. Most fibroblasts within the interstitial tissue are believed to originate through the EMT mechanism. In pathologic conditions, the abnormal formation of connective tissue causes excessive deposition of fibers (**progressive fibrosis**) in the extracellular matrix, leading to organ damage. EMT is associated with uncontrolled fibrosis in the kidney, liver, lung, intestine, and other organs, where the major source of fibroblasts and myofibroblasts comes from transformed epithelial cells following the EMT process. The sequential transitions of EMT to MET were also observed during somatic cell differentiation and transdifferentiation. For example, several rounds of EMT and MET are essential for the differentiation of human embryonic stem cells into liver hepatocytes.
- **Type 3** occurs during the **malignant process**, where neoplastic epithelial cells are transformed during the EMT process into cells with a mesenchymal phenotype. These transformed cancer cells can invade the surrounding tissues and migrate to **distal metastatic sites** via lymphatic or blood vessels. Recent studies indicate that enzymes involved in metabolic reprogramming during EMT malignant tumor progression can be used as biomarkers to therapeutically target cancers.

■ EPITHELIAL CELL RENEWAL

Most epithelial cells have a finite life span of less than that of the whole organism.

Surface epithelia and epithelia of many simple glands belong to the category of **continuously renewing cell populations**. The rate of cell turnover (i.e., the replacement rate) is characteristic of a specific epithelium. For example, the cells lining the small intestine are renewed every 4–6 days in humans. The replacement cells are produced by the mitotic activity of self-maintaining **adult stem cells**. They are located in sites called **niches**. In the small intestine, niches of adult stem cells are located in the lower portion of the intestinal glands. They then migrate and differentiate into four principal cell types. Enterocytes (columnar absorptive cells), goblet cells (mucus secreting), and enteroendocrine cells (regulatory and hormone secreting) continue to differentiate and mature while they migrate up along the villi to the surface of the intestinal lumen. The migration of these new cells continues until they reach the tips of the villi, where they undergo apoptosis and slough off into the lumen. The fourth cell type, the Paneth cell, migrates downward and resides at the bottom of the crypt. The **transcription factor Math1** expressed in the intestinal epithelium determines the fate of the cell. The cells committed to the secretory lineage (i.e., they will differentiate into goblet, enteroendocrine, or Paneth cells) have increased expression of Math1. Inhibition of Math1 expression characterizes the default developmental pathway into absorptive intestinal cells (enterocytes).

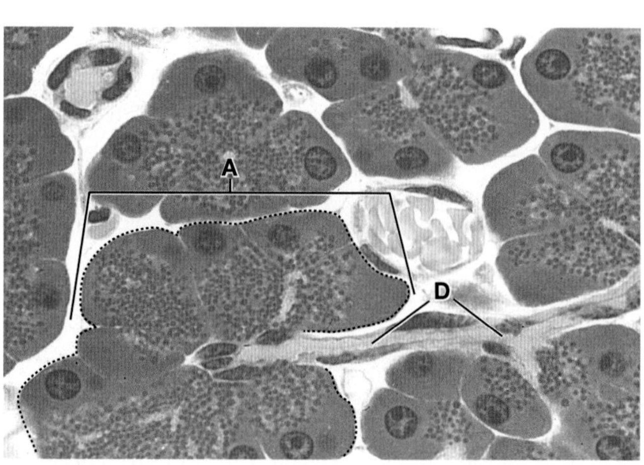

FIGURE 5.43. Serous-secreting compound gland. Photomicrograph of pancreatic acinus (*A*; outlined by the *dotted line*) with its duct (*D*). The small round objects within the acinar cells represent the zymogen granules, the stored secretory precursor material. ×320.

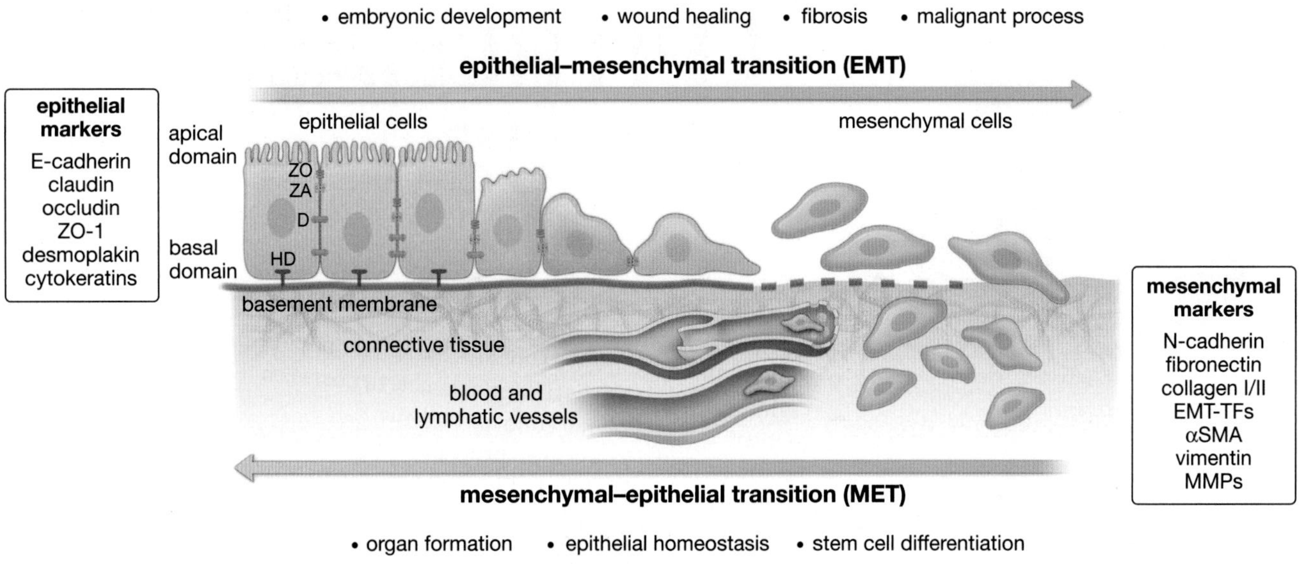

FIGURE 5.44. The epithelial–mesenchymal transition process. This diagram shows the sequential changes that occur during the process of epithelial–mesenchymal transition (*EMT*), in which epithelial cells (*pink* cells on the left) lose their epithelial characteristics and acquire mesenchymal cell features (*green* cells on the right). During the transition process, specific transmembrane proteins involved in junctional complexes, which define the functional polarity of epithelial cells, are gradually lost. The apical domain and its modifications (e.g., microvilli) disappear, along with the zonula occludens (*ZO*), zonula adherens (*ZA*), desmosomes (*D*), and hemidesmosome (*HD*). The basal domain detaches from the extracellular matrix and the newly transformed cells acquire motility, a spindle cell shape, and mesenchymal cell markers. Note that during *EMT*, the basement membrane disintegrates, and newly transformed mesenchymal cells migrate away from the epithelial layer of their origin to invade underlying connective tissue. In the case of transformed cancer cells, they obtain access to lymphatic and blood vessels, which allows them to migrate to distal metastatic sites. *EMT* is a reversible process, meaning that some mesenchymal cells may eventually return to the epithelial cell phenotype. *αSMA*, α-smooth muscle actin; *EMT-TFs*, epithelial–mesenchymal transition transcription factors (Snail, Twist1, and Zeb1); MMPs, matrix metalloproteinases; *ZO-1*, zonula occludens-1 protein.

Similarly, the **stratified squamous epithelium of skin** is replaced in most sites during a period of approximately 47 days (see Chapter 15, Integumentary System, page 544). Cells in the basal layer of the epidermis, appropriately named the **stratum basale (germinativum)**, undergo mitosis to provide for cell renewal. As these cells differentiate, they are pushed toward the surface by new cells in the basal layer. Ultimately, the cells become keratinized and slough off. In both of the abovementioned examples, a steady state is maintained within the epithelium, with new cells normally replacing exfoliated cells at the same rate. The discovery and generation of **induced pluripotent stem (iPS) cells** from human keratinocytes demonstrates that somatic adult cells can be reprogrammed to a pluripotent state by the enforced expression of several embryonic transcription factors. Keratinocyte-derived iPS cells appear to have morphologic and functional characteristics that are identical to human embryonic stem cells. In the future, iPS cells may play an important role in both custom-tailored cell therapy (homologous cell recombination and transplantation) and disease modeling. This involves generating iPS cells from a patient's epidermis, which can be further differentiated in vitro into disease-affected cell types and tested for responses to novel drug therapies.

In other epithelia, particularly in more complex glands, individual cells may live for a long time, and cell division is rare after the mature state is reached. These epithelial cells are characteristic of **stable cell populations** in which relatively little mitotic activity occurs, such as in the liver. However, loss of significant amounts of liver tissue through physical trauma or acute toxic destruction is accommodated by the active proliferation of undamaged liver cells. The liver tissue is essentially restored by the stimulated mitotic activity of healthy liver tissue.

FOLDER 5.5

FUNCTIONAL CONSIDERATIONS: MUCOUS AND SEROUS MEMBRANES

In two general locations, **surface epithelium** and its underlying **connective tissue** are regarded as a functional unit called a **membrane**. The two types of membrane are **mucous membrane** and **serous membrane**. The term *membrane* as used here should not be confused with the biological membranes of cells or should the designations *mucous* and *serous* be confused with the nature of the gland secretion as discussed earlier.

Mucous membrane, also called **mucosa**, lines those cavities that connect with the outside of the body, namely, the alimentary canal, the respiratory tract, and the genitourinary tract. It consists of surface epithelium (with or without glands), a supporting connective tissue called the **lamina propria**, a basement membrane separating the epithelium from the lamina propria, and sometimes a layer of smooth muscle called the **muscularis mucosae** as the deepest layer.

Serous membrane, also called **serosa**, lines the peritoneal, pericardial, and pleural cavities. These cavities are usually described as closed cavities of the body, although, in the female, the peritoneal cavity communicates with the exterior via the genital tract. Structurally, the serosa consists of a lining epithelium, the **mesothelium**, a supporting connective tissue, and a basement membrane between the two. Serous membranes do not contain glands, but the fluid on their surface is watery.

HISTOLOGY 101 NOTEBOOK

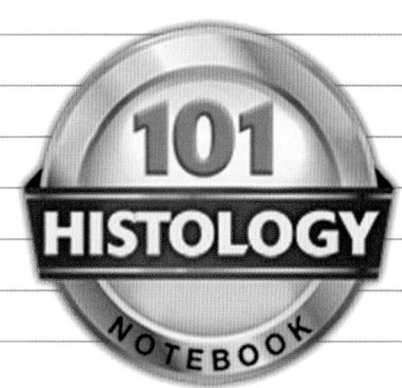

EPITHELIAL TISSUE

OVERVIEW OF EPITHELIAL STRUCTURES

- **Epithelium** is an avascular tissue that covers body surfaces, lines body cavities, and forms glands. It creates a barrier between the external environment and underlying connective tissue.
- **Epithelial cells** have three principal characteristics: They are closely **apposed to each other** and bound together by specific **cell junctions**, they exhibit functional and morphologic **polarity** (different functions are associated with apical, lateral, and basal domains), and their basal surface is attached to an underlying **basement membrane.**

CLASSIFICATION OF EPITHELIUM

- **Epithelium** that is one cell layer thick and rests on the basement membrane is called a **simple epithelium**. The cells of simple epithelia vary in height and width (squamous, cuboidal, and columnar).
- Epithelia that are two or more cell layers thick are called **stratified epithelia**. The shape of cells on the free surface determines its classification.
- **Pseudostratified epithelium** appears stratified. It is a simple epithelium with all cells resting on the basement membrane but not all extending to the free epithelial surface.
- **Transitional epithelium (urothelium)** is stratified and lines the lower part of the urinary tract. Cells on its free surface layer transition from large, round, dome-shaped cells to squamous cells depending on the degree of distention of the urinary organ.

APICAL DOMAIN

- The **apical domain** exhibits surface modifications to carry out specific functions.
- **Microvilli** are small, finger-like cytoplasmic processes containing a core of actin filaments. They increase the apical surface area for absorption and are visible in light microscope (LM) as **striated** or **brush borders.**
- **Stereocilia (stereovilli)** are long microvilli with limited distribution to the male reproductive system (absorption) and sensory epithelium of the inner ear (**sensory mechanoreceptors**).
- **Motile cilia** are hair-like extensions of apical plasma membrane containing an **axoneme,** a core of microtubules in a 9 + 2 arrangement. Cilia movement originates from the coordinated sliding of microtubule doublets generated by the activity of **dynein**, a microtubule-based motor protein.
- **Primary cilia (monocilia)** have a 9 + 0 microtubule arrangement, are immotile, and function as chemosensors, osmosensors, and mechanosensors. They are present in almost all eukaryotic cells.

LATERAL DOMAIN: CELL-TO-CELL ADHESIONS

- The **lateral domain** is characterized by the presence of **cell adhesion molecules (CAMs)** that form **junctional complexes (occluding, anchoring, or communicating junctions)** between the apposed lateral domains of neighboring cells.
- The **zonula occludens** (tight) junction is located at the most apical ends of the lateral membrane of adjacent cells and restricts the passage of substances between these cells (paracellular passage).
- **Anchoring junctions** (**zonula adherens** and **macula adherens**) provide adhesions between epithelial cells using **CAMs** that are linked to the cytoskeleton of adjacent cells. Majority of anchoring junctions utilize calcium-dependent **cadherins** family of proteins. Some specialized cell-to-cell adhesions utilize calcium-independent **nectins** as the primary CAM.
- The **zonula adherens** encircles the cell just below its tight junction and is composed of **E-cadherin–catenin complexes** that interact with actin filaments. The **macula adherens (desmosome)** provides a scattered, localized, spot-like junction and is composed of **desmogleins** and **desmocollins** that attach to the desmosomal plaques anchoring the intermediate filaments.
- **Communicating (gap) junctions** consist of an accumulation of transmembrane channels (formed by two half-channels, the **connexons**) in a tightly packed array. They allow for the exchange of ions, regulatory molecules, and small metabolites between cells.

BASAL DOMAIN: BASEMENT MEMBRANE AND CELL-TO-EXTRACELLULAR MATRIX ADHESION

- The **basal domain** is characterized by the presence of a **basement membrane, cell-to-extracellular matrix junctions** (focal adhesions and hemidesmosomes), and **basal cell membrane infoldings**.
- The **basement membrane** (periodic acid–Schiff [PAS] positive in LM) is a dense layer of specialized extracellular matrix proteins that consists of a **basal lamina** (visible in EM) and a **reticular lamina**.
- The **basal lamina** consists of a scaffold of **laminin polymers** with an underlying **type IV collagen suprastructure** that provides an interaction site for many CAMs.
- The **basal lamina** is attached to the underlying **reticular lamina** (type III collagen) via anchoring fibrils (type VII collagen) and to elastic fibers via fibrillin microfibrils.
- The **basement membrane** serves as an attachment site of epithelia to connective tissue, compartmentalizes connective tissue, filters substances that pass to and from the epithelium, provides a scaffold during tissue regeneration, and is involved in cell signaling.
- **Focal adhesions** are integrin-based, dynamic anchoring junctions that anchor **actin filaments** to the basement membrane. Their fast formation and dismantling provide the molecular bases for cell migration.
- **Hemidesmosomes** are integrin-based, stable anchoring junctions that anchor the **intermediate filaments** to the basement membrane via intercellular plaques.

GLANDS

- **Glands** are classified into two groups according to how their secretory products are released: **exocrine** and **endocrine glands**.
- **Exocrine glands** secrete their products directly onto a surface or through epithelial ducts that may modify their secretion (concentrating, removing, or adding substances).
- **Exocrine glands** are classified as either **mucous glands**, which produce mucous secretions, or **serous glands**, which produce protein-rich watery secretions.
- Cells of exocrine glands have three mechanisms of secretion: **merocrine** (in which secretory product is released by exocytosis), **apocrine** (in which secretory product is released in vesicles containing a thin layer of cytoplasm), and **holocrine** (in which secretory product is accompanied by cell debris from the dying secretory cell).
- **Endocrine glands** lack a duct system. They secrete their products (hormones) into the bloodstream to reach a specific receptor on distant target cells.

EPITHELIAL-MESENCHYMAL TRANSITION

- **Epithelial cells** can undergo **epithelial–mesenchymal transition (EMT)** in which they lose their epithelial characteristics and acquire mesenchymal cell features. The reverse process is called **mesenchymal–epithelial transition (MET)**. Both processes occur in the embryonic development, wound healing, fibrosis, and malignant transformation of cancer cells.

EPITHELIAL CELL RENEWAL

- **Epithelial cells** belong to the category of **continuously renewing cell populations**. The replacement cells are produced by the mitotic division of **adult stem cells** residing in different sites (**niches**) in various epithelia.

PLATE 5.1 ■ SIMPLE SQUAMOUS AND SIMPLE CUBOIDAL EPITHELIA

Epithelium consists of a diverse group of cell types, each of which possesses specific functional characteristics. The cells that comprise an epithelium are arranged in close apposition with one another and typically are located at what may be described as the free surfaces of the body. Such free surfaces include the exterior of the body, the outer surface of many internal organs, and the lining of body cavities, tubes, and ducts.

Epithelium is classified on the basis of the arrangement of the cells that it contains and their shape. If the cells are present in a single layer, they constitute a **simple epithelium**. If they are present in multiple layers, they constitute a **stratified epithelium**. The shape of the cells is typically described as **squamous** if the cell is wider than it is tall, **cuboidal** if its height and width are approximately the same, or **columnar** if the cell is taller than it is wide.

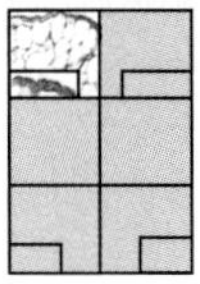

Simple squamous epithelium, mesovarium, human, hematoxylin and eosin (H&E), ×350; inset ×875.

This micrograph shows the surface epithelium of the mesovarium covered by **mesothelium**, a name given to the **simple squamous epithelium** that lines the internal cavities of the body. **Mesothelial cells** (*MC*) are recognized by their nuclei at this low magnification. Beneath the mesothelial cells is a thin layer of connective tissue (*CT*) and adipose cells (*A*). The *inset* reveals at higher magnification the nuclei (*N*) of the mesothelial cells.

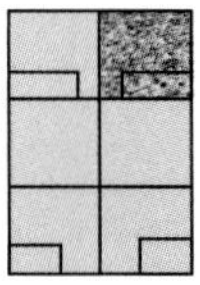

Simple squamous epithelium, mesentery, rat, silver impregnation, ×350; inset ×700.

This is an intermediate magnification of a whole mount of a piece of mesentery. The mesentery was placed on the slide and prepared for microscopic examination. The microscope was focused on the surface of the mesentery. By this method, the boundaries of the surface **mesothelial cells** are delineated as black lines by the precipitated silver. Note that the cells are in close apposition to one another and that they have a polygonal shape. The *inset* reveals several mesothelial cells, each of which exhibits a nucleus (*N*) that has a round or oval profile. Because of the squamous shape of the mesothelial cells, the nuclei are not spherical but rather are disc like.

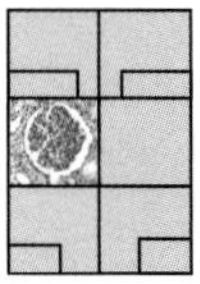

Simple squamous epithelium, kidney, human, H&E, ×350.

This micrograph shows a kidney renal corpuscle. The wall of the renal corpuscle, known as the *parietal layer of Bowman capsule*, is a spherical structure that consists of a **simple squamous epithelium** (*SSE*). The interior of the corpuscle contains a capillary network from which fluid is filtered to enter the urinary space (*US*) and then into the proximal convoluted tubule (*PCT*). Nuclei (*N*) of the **squamous cells** of the parietal layer of Bowman capsule are ovoid and appear to protrude slightly into the urinary space. The free surface of this simple squamous epithelium faces the urinary space, whereas the basal surface of the epithelial cells rests on a layer of connective tissue (*CT*).

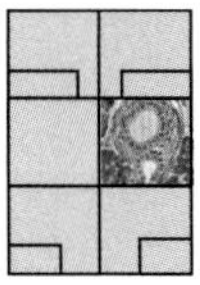

Simple cuboidal epithelium, pancreas, human, H&E, ×700.

This photomicrograph shows two pancreatic ducts (*PD*) that are lined by a **simple cuboidal epithelium.** The duct cell nuclei (*N*) tend to be spherical, a feature consistent with the cuboidal shape of the cell. The free surface of the epithelial cells faces the lumen of the duct, and the basal surface rests on connective tissue (*CT*). Careful examination of the free surface of the epithelial cells reveals some of the terminal bars (*TB*) between adjacent cells.

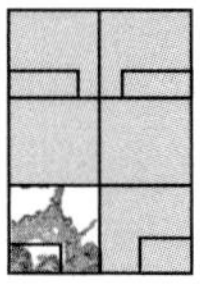

Simple cuboidal epithelium, lung, human, H&E, ×175; inset ×525.

This photomicrograph shows the epithelium of the smallest conducting bronchioles of the lung. The **simple cuboidal epithelium** consists of cuboidal cells (*CC*). The *inset* shows a higher magnification of the **cuboidal cells** (*CC*). Note the spherical nuclei. These small cells have relatively little cytoplasm, thus the nuclei appear close to one another. The free surface of the epithelial cells faces the airway (*AW*), whereas the basal surface of these cells rests on its basement membrane and underlying dense connective tissue (*CT*).

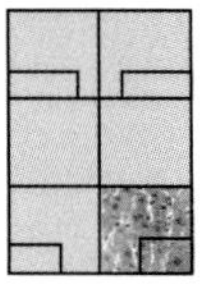

Simple cuboidal epithelium, liver, human, H&E, ×450; inset ×950.

This micrograph reveals cords of **hepatocytes** (*H*), **simple cuboidal cells** that make up the liver parenchyma. The hepatic epithelial cell cords are mostly separated from one another by blood sinusoids (*S*). The *inset* shows a higher magnification of a hepatic cell and reveals an unusual feature in that several surfaces of these cells possess a groove representing the free surface of the cell. Where the groove of one cell faces a groove of the adjacent cell, a small canal-like structure, the canaliculus (*C*), is formed. Bile is secreted from the cell into the canaliculus.

A, adipose cells
AW, airway
C, canaliculus
CC, cuboidal cells
CT, connective tissue
H, hepatocytes
MC, mesothelial cells
N, nucleus
PCT, proximal convoluted tubule
PD, pancreatic duct
S, sinusoid
SSE, simple squamous epithelium
TB, terminal bar
US, urinary space

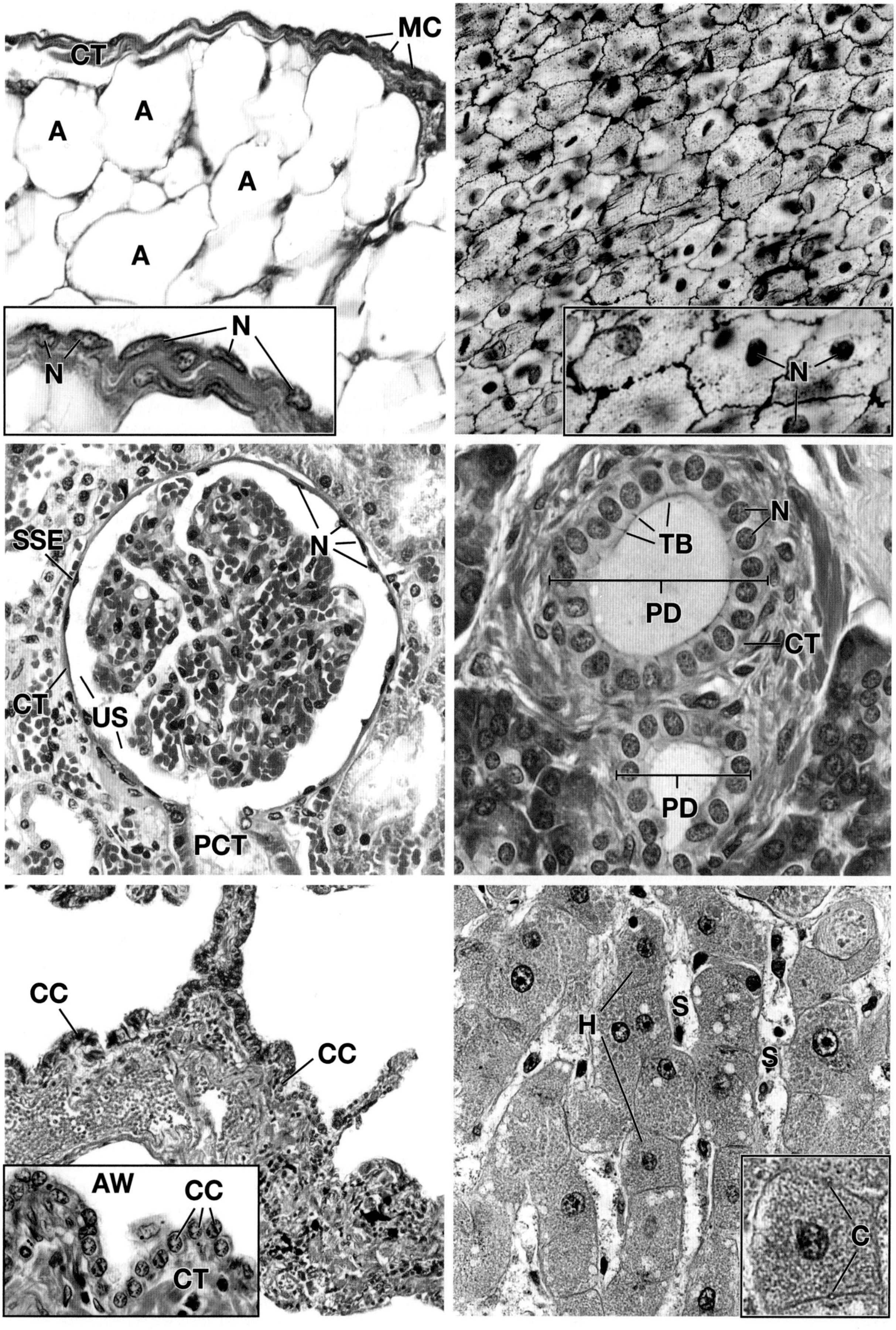
MC
CT
A
A
A
A
N
N
N
N
SSE
N
CT
US
PCT
N
TB
PD
CT
PD
CC
CC
AW
CC
CT
H
S
S
C

PLATE 5.2 ■ SIMPLE AND STRATIFIED EPITHELIA

Simple epithelia are only one cell layer thick. They are characteristic of organ systems primarily involved in transport, absorption, and secretion, such as the intestine, vascular system, digestive glands and other exocrine glands, and kidney. **Stratified epithelia** have more than one layer and are typical of surfaces that are subject to frictional stress, such as skin, oral mucosa and esophagus, and vagina.

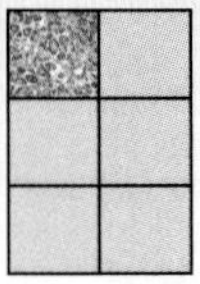

Simple epithelium, exocrine pancreas, monkey, hematoxylin and eosin (H&E) ×450.

This micrograph shows three types of epithelium forms. In the *circle* is a well-oriented acinus, a functional group of secretory cells, each of which is pyramidal in shape. The secretory cells form a spherical or tubular structure. The free surface of the cells and the lumen are located in the center of the *circle*. The lumen is not evident here but is evident in a similar cell arrangement in the middle right image below (see *circle*). Because the height of the cells (the distance from the edge of the *circle* to the lumen) is greater than the width, the epithelium is **simple columnar**. The second epithelial type is represented by a small, longitudinally sectioned duct (*arrows*) extending across the field. It is composed of flattened cells (note the nuclear shape), and on this basis, the epithelium is classified as **simple squamous**. Finally, there is a larger cross-sectioned duct (*asterisk*) into which the smaller duct enters. The nuclei of this larger duct tend to be round, and the cells tend to be square in profile. Thus, these duct cells are a **simple cuboidal epithelium**.

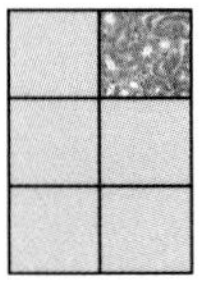

Simple cuboidal epithelium, kidney, human, H&E ×450.

This section shows cross-sectioned tubules of several types. Those labeled with *arrows* provide another example of a **simple cuboidal epithelium**. The *arrows* point to the lateral cell boundaries; note that cell width approximates cell height. The cross-sectioned structures marked with *asterisk* are another type of tubule; they are smaller in diameter but are also composed of a simple cuboidal epithelium.

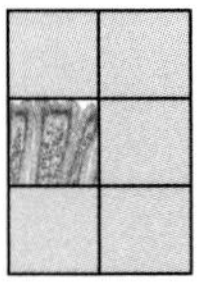

Simple columnar epithelium, colon, human, H&E ×350.

The **simple columnar epithelium** of the colon shown here consists of a single layer of absorptive cells and mucus-secreting cells (goblet cells). The latter can be recognized by the light-staining "goblet" (*arrows*) that contains the cell's secretory product. The epithelium lines the lumen of the colon and extends down into the connective tissue to form the intestinal glands (*GL*). Both cell types are tall with their nuclei located at the base of the cell. The connective tissue (*CT*) contains numerous cells, many of which are lymphocytes and plasma cells.

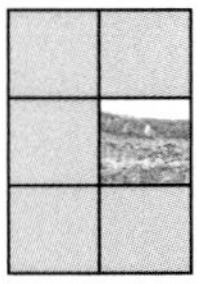

Pseudostratified epithelium, trachea, monkey, H&E ×450.

In addition to the tall **columnar cells** (*CC*) in this columnar epithelium, there is a definite layer of **basal cells** (*BC*). The columnar cells, which contain elongated nuclei and possess cilia (*C*), extend from the surface to the basement membrane, clearly visible in the trachea as a thick, acellular, homogeneous region that is part of the connective tissue (*CT*). The basal cells are interspersed between the columnar cells. Because all of the cells rest on the basement membrane, they are regarded as a single layer, as opposed to two discrete layers, one over the other. Because the epithelium appears to be stratified but is not, it is called **pseudostratified columnar epithelium**. The *circle* in the micrograph delineates a tracheal gland similar to the acinus in exocrine pancreas (*circle*). Note that the lumen of the gland is clearly visible and the cell boundaries are also evident. The gland epithelium is simple columnar.

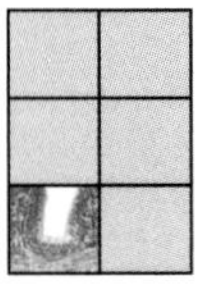

Pseudostratified epithelium, epididymis, human, H&E ×450.

This is another example of **pseudostratified columnar epithelium**. Again, two layers of nuclei are evident, those of basal cells (*BC*) and those of columnar cells (*CC*). As in the previous example, however, although not evident, the columnar cells rest on the basement membrane; thus, the epithelium is pseudostratified. Note that where the epithelium is vertically oriented, on the *right* of the micrograph, there appear to be more nuclei, and the epithelium is thicker. This is a result of a tangential plane of section. As a rule, the thinnest area of an epithelium should always be examined to visualize its true organization.

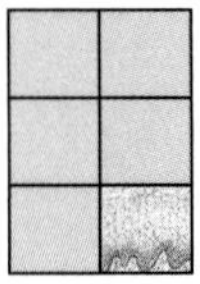

Stratified squamous epithelium, vagina, human, H&E ×225.

This is the **stratified squamous epithelium** of the vaginal wall. The deeper cells, particularly those of the basal layer, are small, with little cytoplasm, and thus, the nuclei appear closely packed. As the cells become larger, they tend to flatten out, forming disc-like squames. Cytoplasm of epithelial cells above the basal layer appears empty because of the large amounts of accumulated glycogen that is lost during slide preparation. Because the surface cells retain a flattened shape, the epithelium is called *stratified squamous*. Underlying connective tissue (*CT*) contains numerous fibroblasts.

BC, basal cell
C, cilia
CC, columnar cell
CT, connective tissue
GL, intestinal gland
arrows, *upper left,* duct composed of simple squamous epithelium; *upper right,* lateral boundaries of cuboidal tubule cells; *middle left,* mucus cups of goblet cells
asterisk, duct or tubule of simple cuboidal epithelium

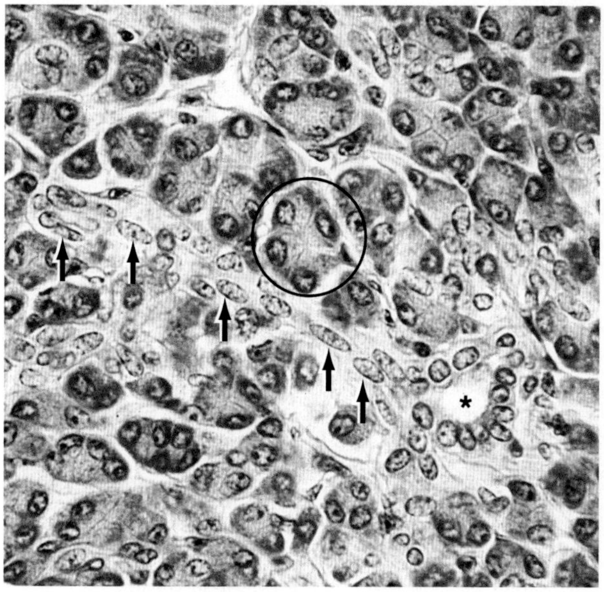
*

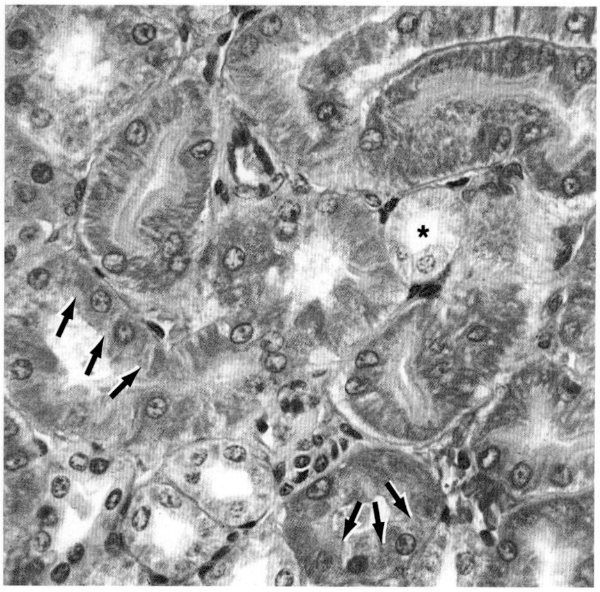
*

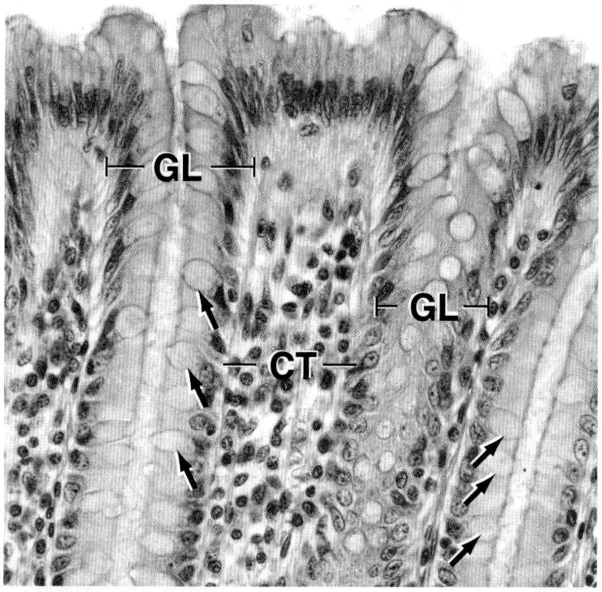
GL
GL
CT

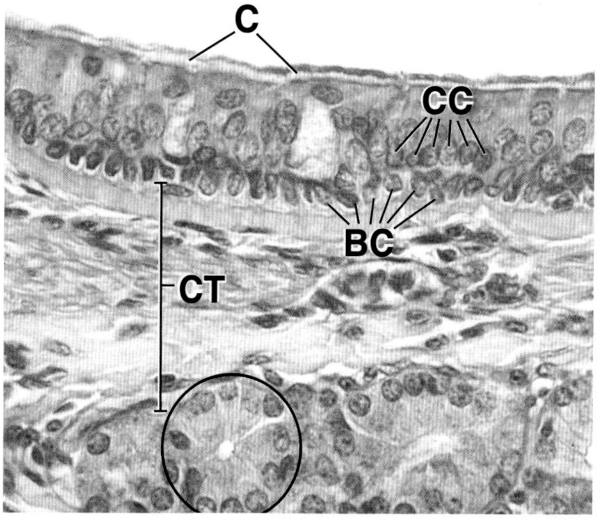
C
CC
BC
CT

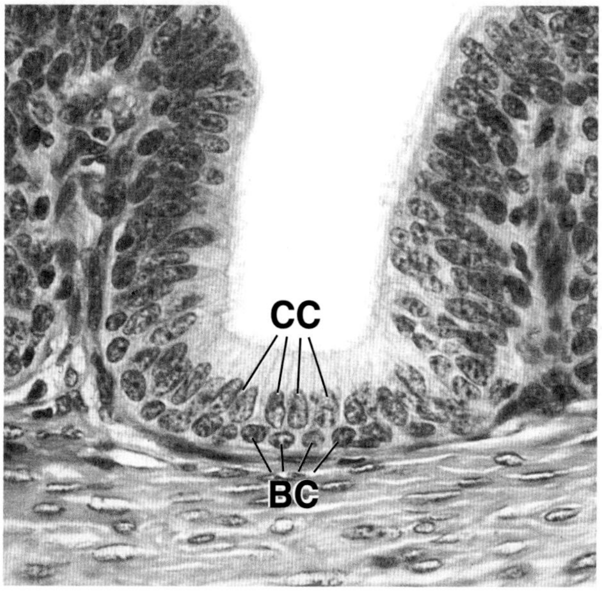
CC
BC

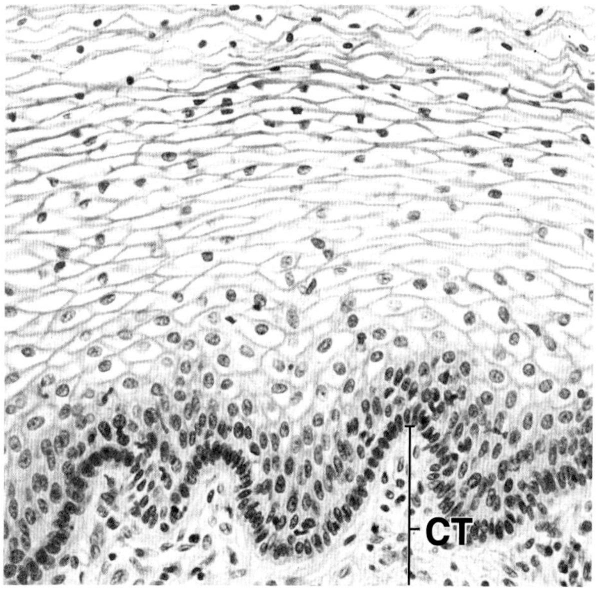
CT

PLATE 5.3 ■ STRATIFIED EPITHELIA AND EPITHELIOID TISSUES

Tissues that resemble epithelia but lack the characteristic free surface are designated **epithelioid tissues**. This structure is characteristic of the endocrine organs, which develop from typical epithelia but lose their connection to a surface during development.

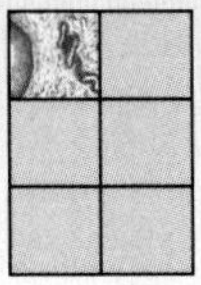

Stratified epithelia, esophagus, monkey, hematoxylin and eosin (H&E) ×250.

This part of the wall of the esophagus reveals two different epithelia. On the *left* is the lining epithelium of the esophagus. It is multilayered with squamous surface cells; therefore, it is a **stratified squamous epithelium** (*SS*). On the *right* is the duct of an esophageal gland cut in several planes. By examining a region where the plane of section is at a right angle to the surface, the true character of the epithelium becomes apparent. In this case, the epithelium consists of two cell layers with cuboidal surface cells; thus, it is **stratified cuboidal epithelium** (*StCu*).

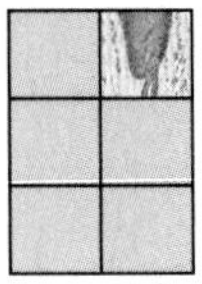

Stratified epithelia, skin, human, H&E ×450.

This section shows a portion of the duct of a sweat gland just before the duct enters the **stratified squamous epithelium** (*SS*) of the skin. The *dashed line* traces the duct within the epidermis. This duct also consists of a **stratified cuboidal epithelium** (*StCu*) in two layers; the cells of the inner layer (the surface cells) appear more or less square. Because the epidermal surface cells are not included in the field, the designation stratified squamous cannot be made from the information offered by the micrograph.

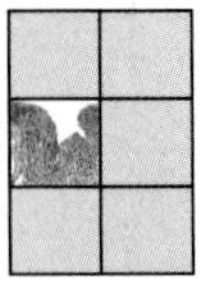

Epithelial transition, anorectal junction, human, H&E ×300.

The area shown here is the terminal part of the large intestine. The luminal epithelium on the *left* is typical **simple columnar epithelium** (*SCol*) of the colon. This epithelium undergoes an abrupt transition (*arrowhead*) to a **stratified cuboidal epithelium** (*StCu*) at the anal canal. Note the general cuboidal shape of most of the surface cells (*arrows*) and the underlying layers of cells. The simple columnar epithelium on the *left* is part of an intestinal gland that is continuous with the **simple columnar epithelium** at the intestinal luminal surface. The connective tissue (*CT*) at this site is heavily infiltrated with lymphocytes, giving it an appearance unlike the connective tissue of other specimens on this plate.

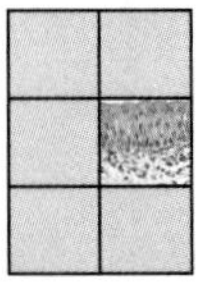

Transitional epithelium (urothelium), urinary bladder, monkey, H&E ×400.

The epithelium of the urinary bladder is called **transitional epithelium**, a stratified epithelium that changes in appearance according to the degree of distention of the bladder. In the nondistended state, as here, it is about four or five cells deep. The surface cells are large and dome shaped (*asterisks*). The cells immediately under the surface cells are pear shaped and slightly smaller. The deepest cells are the smallest, and their nuclei appear more crowded. When the bladder is distended, the superficial cells are stretched into squamous cells, and the epithelium is reduced in thickness to about three cells deep. The bladder wall usually contracts when it is removed, unless special steps are taken to preserve it in a distended state. Thus, its appearance is usually like that in this image. A large number of fibroblasts are visible in the underlying connective tissue (*CT*).

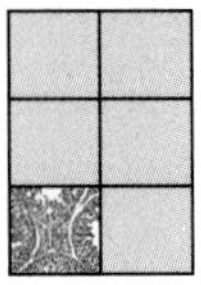

Epithelioid tissues, testis, monkey, H&E ×350.

This section shows the **interstitial (Leydig) cells** of the testis (*IC*). These cells possess certain epithelial characteristics. They do not possess a free surface, however, nor do they develop from a surface; instead, they develop from mesenchymal cells. They are referred to as **epithelioid cells** because they contact similar neighboring cells in much the same way that epithelial cells contact each other. Leydig cells are endocrine in nature, and they are surrounded by a rich network of capillaries (*C*) and lymphatic channels.

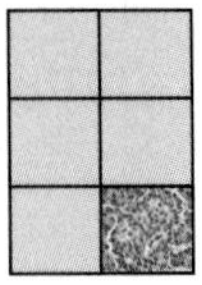

Epithelioid tissues, endocrine pancreas, human, H&E ×450.

Cells of the **endocrine islet (of Langerhans)** (*En*) of the pancreas also have an **epithelioid arrangement**. The cells are in contact but lack a free surface, although they have developed from an epithelial surface by invagination. In contrast, the surrounding alveoli of the exocrine pancreas (*Ex*), which developed from the same epithelial surface, are made up of cells with a free surface onto which the secretory product is discharged. Capillaries (*C*) are prominent in endocrine tissues. Similar examples of epithelioid tissue are seen in the adrenal and the parathyroid and pituitary glands, all of which are endocrine glands.

C, capillary
CT, connective tissue
En, endocrine cells
Ex, exocrine cells
IC, interstitial (Leydig) cells
SCol, simple columnar epithelium
SS, stratified squamous epithelium
StCu, stratified cuboidal epithelium
arrowhead, transition site of simple stratified epithelium to stratified cuboidal
arrows, surface cuboidal cells
asterisks, dome-shaped cells

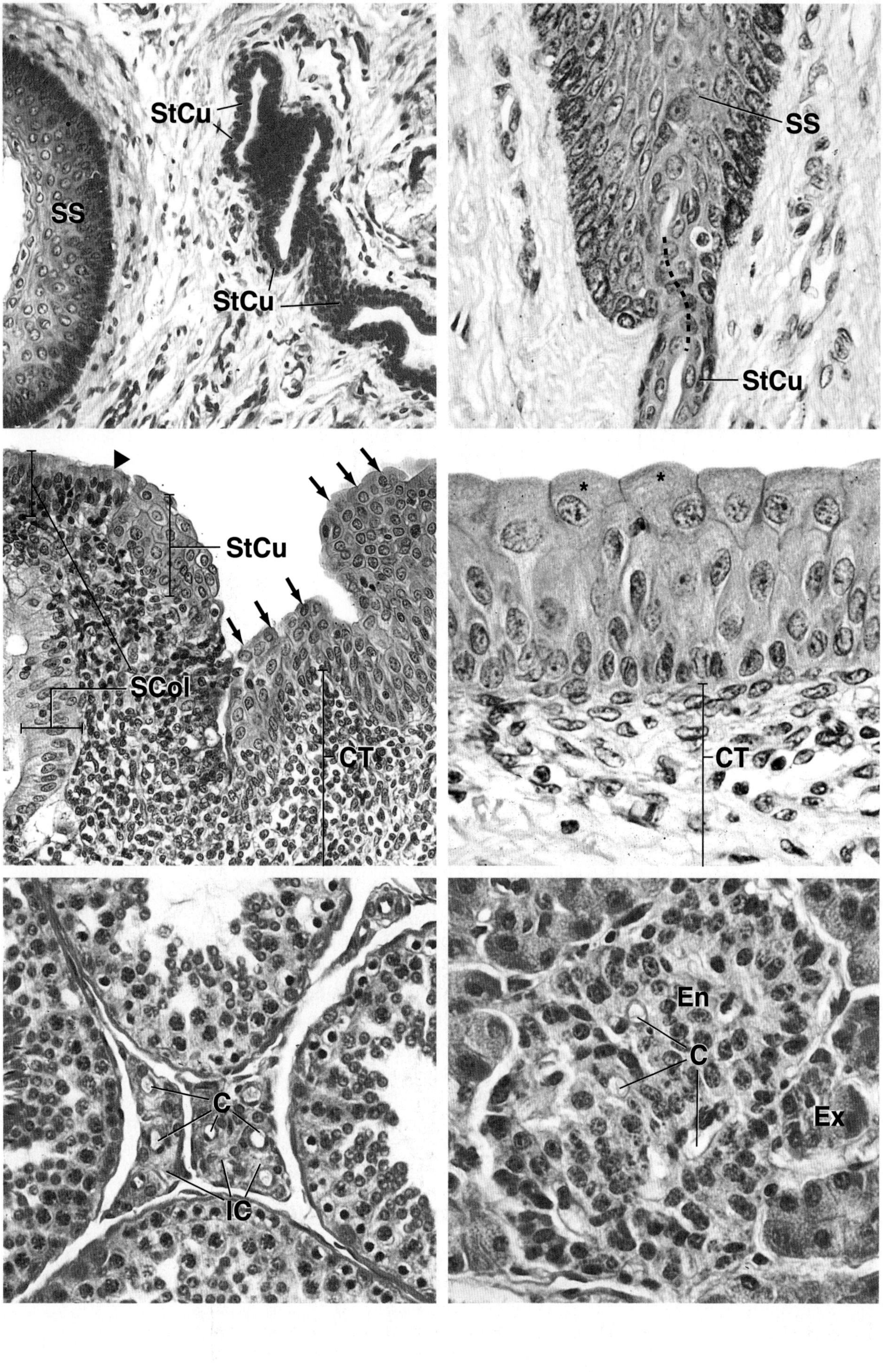
StCu
SS
StCu
SS
StCu
StCu
SCol
CT
*
*
CT
C
IC
En
C
Ex

6 CONNECTIVE TISSUE

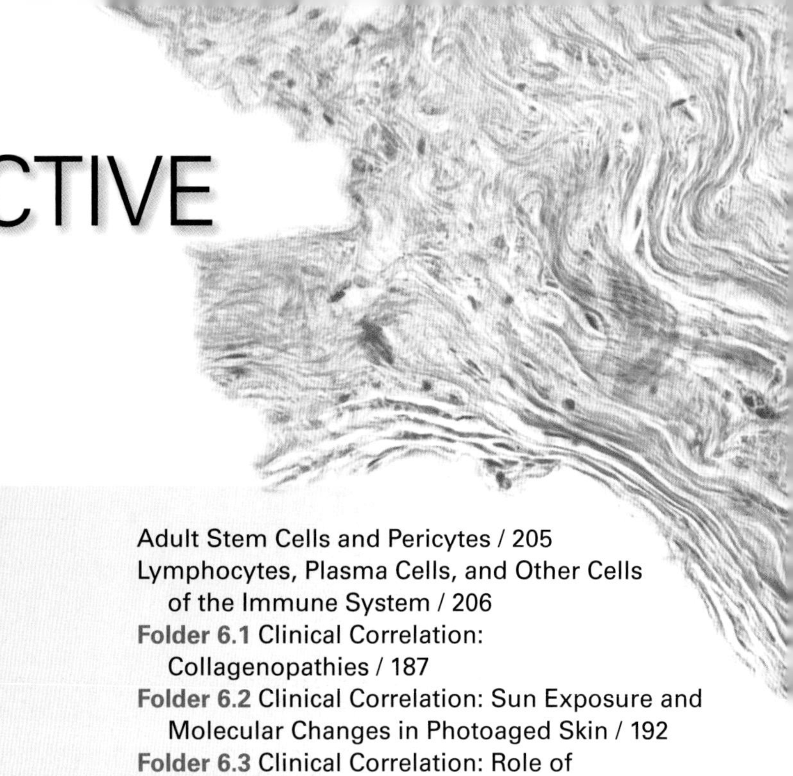

■ OVERVIEW OF CONNECTIVE TISSUE

Connective tissue comprises a diverse group of cells within a tissue-specific extracellular matrix.

In general, **connective tissue** consists of **cells** and an **extracellular matrix (ECM)**. ECM includes protein fibers (collagen, elastic, and reticular) and an amorphous component containing specialized molecules (proteoglycans, multiadhesive glycoproteins, and glycosaminoglycans [GAGs]) that constitute the **ground substance**. Connective tissue forms a vast and continuous compartment throughout the body, bounded by the basal laminae of the various epithelia and by the basal or external laminae of muscle cells and nerve-supporting cells.

Different types of connective tissue are responsible for a variety of functions.

The functions of the various connective tissues are reflected in the types of cells and fibers present within the tissue and the composition of the ground substance in the ECM. For example, in loose connective tissue, many cell types are present (Fig. 6.1). One type, the fibroblast, produces the extracellular fibers that serve a structural role in the tissue. Fibroblasts also produce and maintain the ground substance. Other cell types, such as lymphocytes, plasma cells, macrophages, and eosinophils, are associated with the body's defense system; they function within the ECM of the tissue. In contrast, bone tissue, another form of connective tissue, contains only a single cell type, the osteocyte. This cell produces the fibers that make up the bulk of bone tissue. A unique feature of bone is that its fibers are organized in a specific pattern and become calcified to create the hardness associated with this tissue. Similarly, in tendons and ligaments, fibers are the prominent feature of the tissue. These fibers are arranged in parallel array and are densely packed to impart maximum strength.

Classification of connective tissue is primarily based on the composition and organization of its extracellular components and on its functions.

Connective tissue encompasses a variety of tissues with differing functional properties but with certain common characteristics that allow them to be grouped together. For convenience, they are classified in a manner that reflects these features. Table 6.1 presents the classification of connective tissues, including subtypes.

■ EMBRYONIC CONNECTIVE TISSUE

Embryonic mesenchyme gives rise to the various connective tissues of the body.

Mesoderm, the middle embryonic germ layer, gives rise to almost all of the connective tissues of the body. An exception is

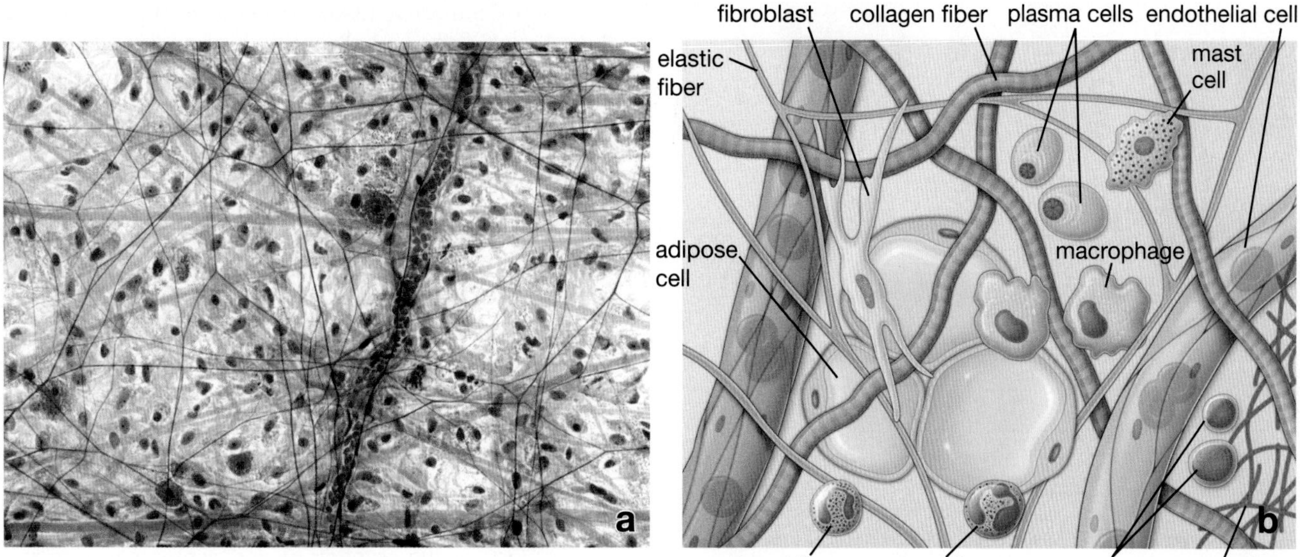

FIGURE 6.1. Loose connective tissue. a. Photomicrograph of a mesentery spread stained with Verhoeff hematoxylin to show nuclei and elastic fibers; it has been counterstained with safranin for identification of mast cell granules and with orange G for identification of other proteins (mainly collagen fibers). The elastic fibers appear as *blue-black*, thin, long, and branching threads without discernible beginnings or endings. Collagen fibers appear as *orange*-stained, long, straight profiles and are considerably thicker than the elastic fibers. Most of the visible nuclei are presumed to be those of fibroblasts. Nuclei of other cell types (e.g., lymphocytes, plasma cells, and macrophages) are also present, but not identifiable. Mast cells are identified by the *bright reddish* granules within their cytoplasm. Eosinophils and neutrophils (when present) can be identified by their unique segmented nuclei and the presence of specific granules (*reddish* in the case of eosinophils). Note the presence of small blood vessel filled with red blood cells. ×150. **b.** Schematic diagram illustrating the components of loose connective tissue. Note the different cell types most frequently found in the loose connective tissue with the surrounding extracellular matrix, which contains blood vessels and three different types of fibers. The *pink* homogeneous background of this diagram represents ground substance.

the head region, where specific progenitor cells are derived from ectoderm by way of the neural crest cells. Through proliferation and migration of the mesodermal and specific neural crest cells, a **primitive connective tissue** referred to as **mesenchyme** (in the head region, it is sometimes called **ectomesenchyme**) is established in the early embryo. Maturation and proliferation of the mesenchyme give rise not only to the various connective tissues of the adult but also to muscle, the vascular and urogenital systems, and the serous membranes of the body cavities. The manner in which the mesenchymal cells proliferate and organize sets the stage for the type of mature connective tissue that will form at any specific site.

TABLE 6.1 Classification of Connective Tissue

Embryonic Connective Tissue	
Mesenchyme	Mucous connective tissue
Connective Tissue Proper	
Loose connective tissue	Dense connective tissue
	Regular
	Irregular
Specialized Connective Tissue[a]	
Cartilage (see Chapter 7, Cartilage)	Blood (see Chapter 10, Blood)
Bone (see Chapter 8, Bone)	Hemopoietic tissue (see Chapter 10, Blood)
Adipose tissue (see Chapter 9, Adipose Tissue)	Lymphatic tissue (see Chapter 14, Immune System and Lymphatic Tissues and Organs)

[a]In the past, the designations elastic tissue and reticular tissue have been listed as separate categories of specialized connective tissue. The tissues usually cited as examples of elastic tissue are certain ligaments associated with the spinal column and the tunica media of elastic arteries. The identifying feature of reticular tissue is the presence of reticular fibers and reticular cells together forming a three-dimensional stroma. Reticular tissue serves as the stroma for hemopoietic tissue (specifically the red bone marrow) and lymphatic tissue organs (lymph nodes and spleen, but not the thymus).

Embryonic connective tissue is present in the embryo and within the umbilical cord.

Embryonic connective tissue is classified into two subtypes:

- **Mesenchyme** is primarily found in the embryo. It contains small, spindle-shaped cells of relatively uniform appearance (Fig. 6.2a). Processes extend from these cells and contact similar processes of neighboring cells, forming a three-dimensional cellular network. Gap junctions are present where the processes make contact. The extracellular space is occupied by a viscous ground substance. Collagen and reticular fibers are present; they are very fine and relatively sparse. The paucity of collagen fibers is consistent with the limited physical stress on the growing fetus.
- **Mucous connective tissue** is present in the umbilical cord. It consists of a specialized, almost gelatin-like ECM composed mainly of hyaluronan; its ground substance is frequently referred to as **Wharton jelly**. The spindle-shaped cells are widely separated and appear much like fibroblasts in the near-term umbilical cord (e.g., the cytoplasmic processes are thin and difficult to visualize in routine hematoxylin and eosin [H&E] preparation). Wharton jelly occupies large intercellular spaces located between thin, wispy collagen fibers (Fig. 6.2b). Some of the cells isolated from Wharton jelly express significant amounts of mesenchymal stem cell markers and have the ability to differentiate under certain conditions into osteocytes, chondrocytes, adipocytes, and neural-like cells. These cells are called **Wharton jelly mesenchymal stem cells** and may have potential therapeutic application in the future.

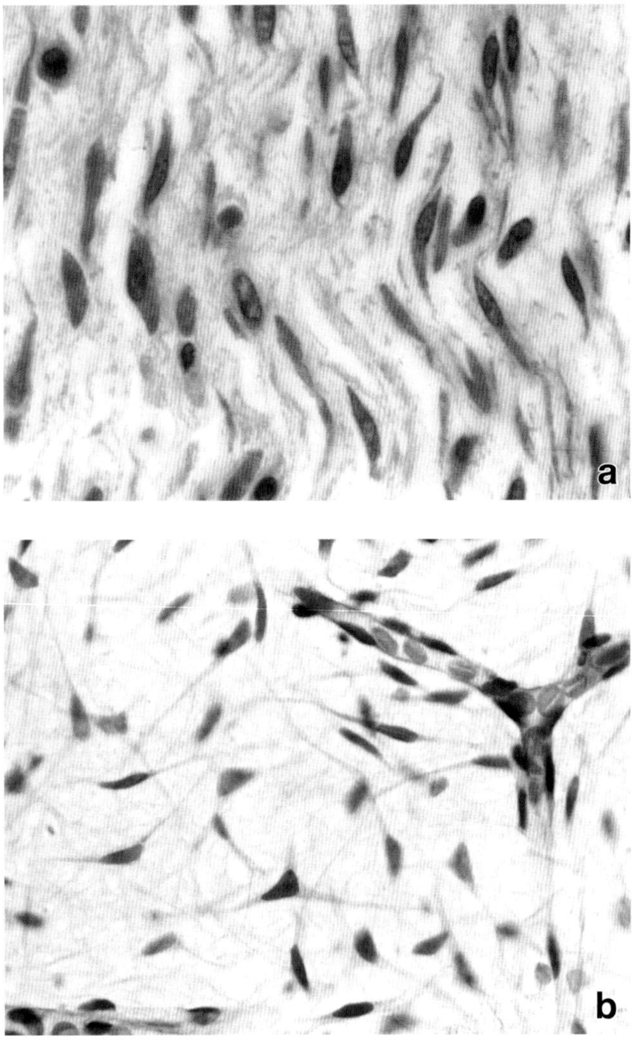

FIGURE 6.2. Embryonic connective tissue. a. Photomicrograph of mesenchymal tissue from a developing fetus stained with hematoxylin and eosin (H&E). Although morphologically the mesenchymal cells appear as a homogeneous population, they give rise to cells that will differentiate into various cell types. Their cytoplasmic processes often give the cell a tapering or spindle appearance. The extracellular component of the tissue contains a sparse arrangement of reticular fibers and abundant ground substance. ×480. **b.** Photomicrograph of Wharton jelly from the umbilical cord stained with H&E. Wharton jelly consists of a specialized, almost gelatin-like ground substance that occupies large intercellular spaces located between the spindle-shaped mesenchymal cells. ×480.

■ CONNECTIVE TISSUE PROPER

Connective tissues that belong to this category are divided into two general subtypes:

- **Loose connective tissue**, sometimes called **areolar tissue**
- **Dense connective tissue**, which can be further subcategorized into two basic types based on the organization of its collagen fibers: **dense irregular connective tissue** and **dense regular connective tissue**

Loose connective tissue is characterized by loosely arranged fibers and abundant cells of various types.

Loose connective tissue is a cellular connective tissue with thin and relatively sparse collagen fibers (Fig. 6.3). The ground substance, however, is abundant; in fact, it occupies more volume than the fibers do. It has a viscous to gel-like consistency and plays an important role in the diffusion of oxygen and nutrients from the small vessels that course through this connective tissue as well as in the diffusion of carbon dioxide and metabolic wastes back to the vessels.

Loose connective tissue is primarily located beneath the epithelia that cover the body surfaces and line the internal surfaces of the body. It is also associated with the epithelium of glands and surrounds the smallest blood vessels (Plate 6.1, page 210). This tissue is thus the initial site where pathogenic agents, such as bacteria that have breached an epithelial surface, are challenged and destroyed by cells of the immune system. Most cell types in loose connective tissue are transient wandering cells that migrate from local blood vessels in response to specific stimuli. Loose connective tissue, therefore, is the site of **inflammatory and immune reactions**. During these reactions, loose connective tissue can swell considerably. In areas of the body where foreign substances are continually present, large populations of immune cells are maintained. For example, the **lamina propria**, the loose connective tissue of mucous membranes, such as those of the respiratory and alimentary systems, contains large numbers of these cells.

Dense irregular connective tissue is characterized by abundant fibers and few cells.

Dense irregular connective tissue contains mostly collagen fibers. Cells are sparse and typically of a single type, the fibroblast. This tissue also contains relatively little ground substance (Plate 6.1, page 210). Because of its high proportion of collagen fibers, dense irregular connective tissue provides significant strength. Typically, the fibers are arranged in bundles oriented in various directions (thus, the term *irregular*) that can withstand stresses on organs or structures. Skin contains a relatively thick layer of dense irregular connective tissue called the **reticular layer** (or **deep layer**) of the dermis. The reticular layer provides resistance to tearing as a consequence of stretching forces from different directions. Similarly, hollow organs (e.g., the intestinal tract) possess a distinct layer of dense irregular connective tissue called the **submucosa** in which

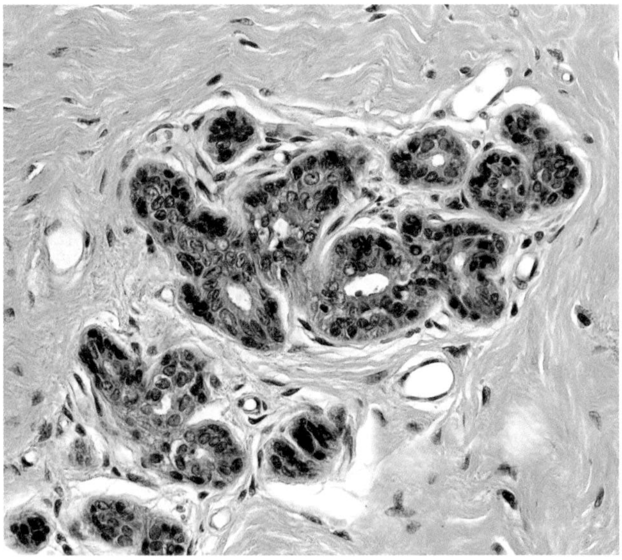

FIGURE 6.3. Loose and dense irregular connective tissue. Photomicrograph comparing loose and dense irregular connective tissue from the mammary gland stained with Masson trichrome. In the *center*, loose connective tissue surrounds the glandular epithelium. The loose connective tissue is composed of a wispy arrangement of collagen fibers with many cells. Note the large number of nuclei visible at this low magnification. On the *upper left* and *lower right* of the figure is dense irregular connective tissue. In contrast, few nuclei are revealed in the dense connective tissue. However, collagen is considerably more abundant and is composed of very thick fibers. ×100.

the fiber bundles course in varying planes. This arrangement allows the organ to resist excessive stretching and distension.

Dense regular connective tissue is characterized by ordered and densely packed arrays of fibers and cells.

Dense regular connective tissue is the main functional component of tendons, ligaments, and aponeuroses. As in dense irregular connective tissue, the fibers of dense regular connective tissue are the prominent feature, and there is little ground substance. However, in dense regular connective tissue, the fibers are arranged in parallel array and are densely packed to provide maximum strength. The cells that produce and maintain the fibers are packed and aligned between fiber bundles.

- **Tendons** are cord-like structures that attach muscle to bone. They consist of parallel bundles of collagen fibers. Situated between these bundles are rows of fibroblasts called **tendinocytes** (Fig. 6.4 and Plate 6.2, page 212). Tendinocytes are surrounded by a specialized ECM that separates them from the load-bearing collagen fibrils. In H&E-stained cross sections of tendon, the tendinocytes appear stellate. In transmission electron micrograph (TEM) sections parallel to the long axis of tendons, the cytoplasmic projections of the cell lie between the fibers and appear as thin cytoplasmic sheets. In most H&E-stained longitudinal sections, however, tendinocytes appear only as rows of typically flattened basophilic nuclei. The cytoplasmic sheets that extend from the body of the tendinocytes are not usually evident in longitudinal H&E-stained sections because they blend in with the collagen fibers. The substance of the tendon is surrounded by a thin connective tissue capsule, the **epitendineum**, in which the collagen fibers are not nearly as orderly (Plate 6.2, page 212). Typically, the tendon is subdivided into fascicles by **endotendineum**, a connective tissue extension of the epitendineum. It contains the small blood vessels and nerves of the tendon.
- **Ligaments**, like tendons, consist of fibers and fibroblasts arranged in parallel. The fibers of ligaments, however, are less regularly arranged than those of tendons. Ligaments

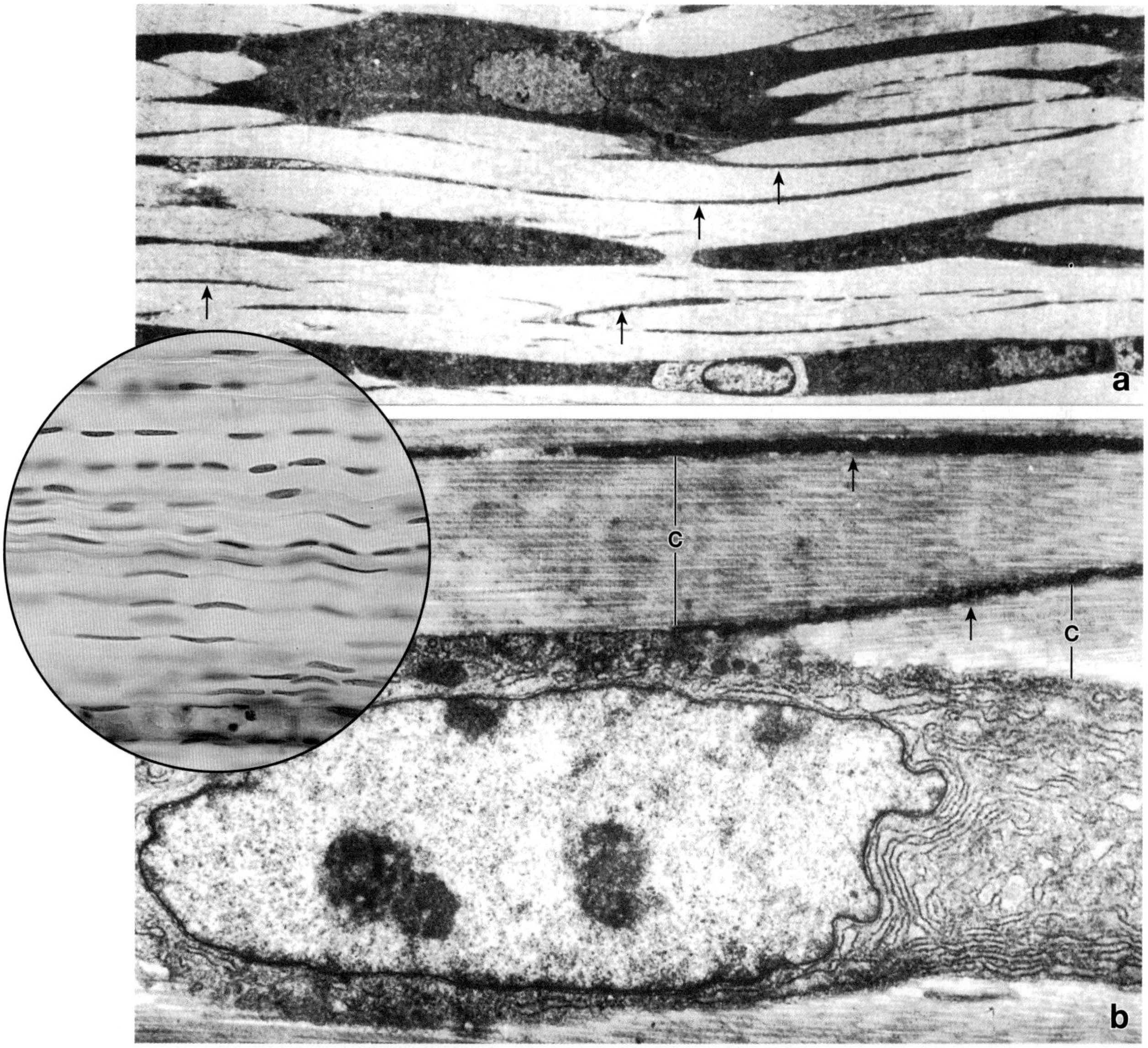

FIGURE 6.4. Dense regular connective tissue—tendon. a. Electron micrograph of a tendon at low magnification showing tendinocytes (fibroblasts) and their thin processes (*arrows*) lying between the collagen bundles. ×1,600. **b.** A tendinocyte with prominent profiles of rough endoplasmic reticulum (*rER*) is shown at higher magnification. The collagen fibers (*C*) can be resolved as consisting of very tightly packed collagen fibrils. The *arrows* indicate processes of tendinocytes. ×9,500. **Inset.** Photomicrograph of a tendon. Note the orderly and regular alignment of the bundles of collagen fibers. Tendinocytes are aligned in rows between the collagen fibers. ×200. (Electron micrographs modified from Rhodin J. *Histology*. Oxford University Press; 1974.)

join bone to bone, which, in some locations, such as in the spinal column, require some elasticity. Although collagen is the major extracellular fiber of most ligaments, some of the ligaments associated with the spinal column (e.g., ligamenta flava) contain many more elastic fibers and fewer collagen fibers. These ligaments are called **elastic ligaments**.

- **Aponeuroses** resemble broad, flattened tendons. Instead of fibers lying in parallel arrays, the fibers of aponeuroses are arranged in multiple layers. The bundles of collagen fibers in one layer tend to be arranged at a 90-degree angle to those in the neighboring layers. The fibers within each of the layers are arranged in regular arrays; thus, aponeurosis is a dense regular connective tissue. This **orthogonal array** is also found in the cornea of the eye and is responsible for its transparency.

■ CONNECTIVE TISSUE FIBERS

There are three principal types of connective tissue fibers.

Connective tissue fibers are present in varying amounts, depending on the structural needs or function of the connective tissue. Each type of fiber is produced by fibroblasts and is composed of protein consisting of long peptide chains. The three types of connective tissue fibers are

- **collagen fibers**,
- **reticular fibers**, and
- **elastic fibers**.

Collagen Fibers and Fibrils

Collagen fibers are the most abundant type of connective tissue fiber.

Collagen fibers are the most abundant structural components of connective tissue. They are flexible and have a remarkably high-tensile strength. In the light microscope, collagen fibers typically appear as wavy structures of variable width and indeterminate length. They stain readily with eosin and other acidic dyes. They can also be colored with the aniline blue dye used in Mallory trichrome connective tissue stain or with the light green dye used in Masson trichrome stain.

When examined with the TEM, collagen fibers appear as bundles of fine, thread-like subunits. These subunits are **collagen fibrils** (Fig. 6.5). Within an individual fiber, the collagen fibrils are relatively uniform in diameter. In different locations and at different stages of development, however, the fibrils differ in size. In developing or immature tissues, the fibrils may be as small as 15 or 20 nm in diameter. In dense regular connective tissue in tendons or other tissues that are subject to considerable stress, they may measure up to 300 nm in diameter.

Collagen fibrils have a 68-nm banding pattern.

Collagen fibrils stained with osmium or other heavy metals examined with the TEM exhibit a sequence of closely spaced transverse bands that repeat every 68 nm along the length of the fibril (Fig. 6.5, *inset*). This regular banding pattern can also be observed on the surface of the collagen fibrils when they are examined with the atomic force microscope (AFM; Fig. 6.6). This banding pattern reflects the fibril's subunit structure, specifically the size and shape of the collagen molecule and the arrangement of the molecules that form the fibril (Fig. 6.7). The **collagen molecule** (formerly called *tropocollagen*) measures about 300 nm long by 1.5 nm thick and has a head and a tail. Within each fibril, the collagen molecules align head to tail in overlapping rows with a gap between the molecules in each row and a one-quarter-molecule stagger between adjacent rows. These gaps are clearly visible with the AFM (see Fig. 6.6). The tensile strength of the fibril is created by the covalent bonds between the collagen molecules of adjacent rows, not the head-to-tail attachment of the molecules in a row. The banding pattern observed with the TEM (see Fig. 6.5, *inset*) is caused largely by osmium deposition in the space between the heads and tails of the molecules in each row.

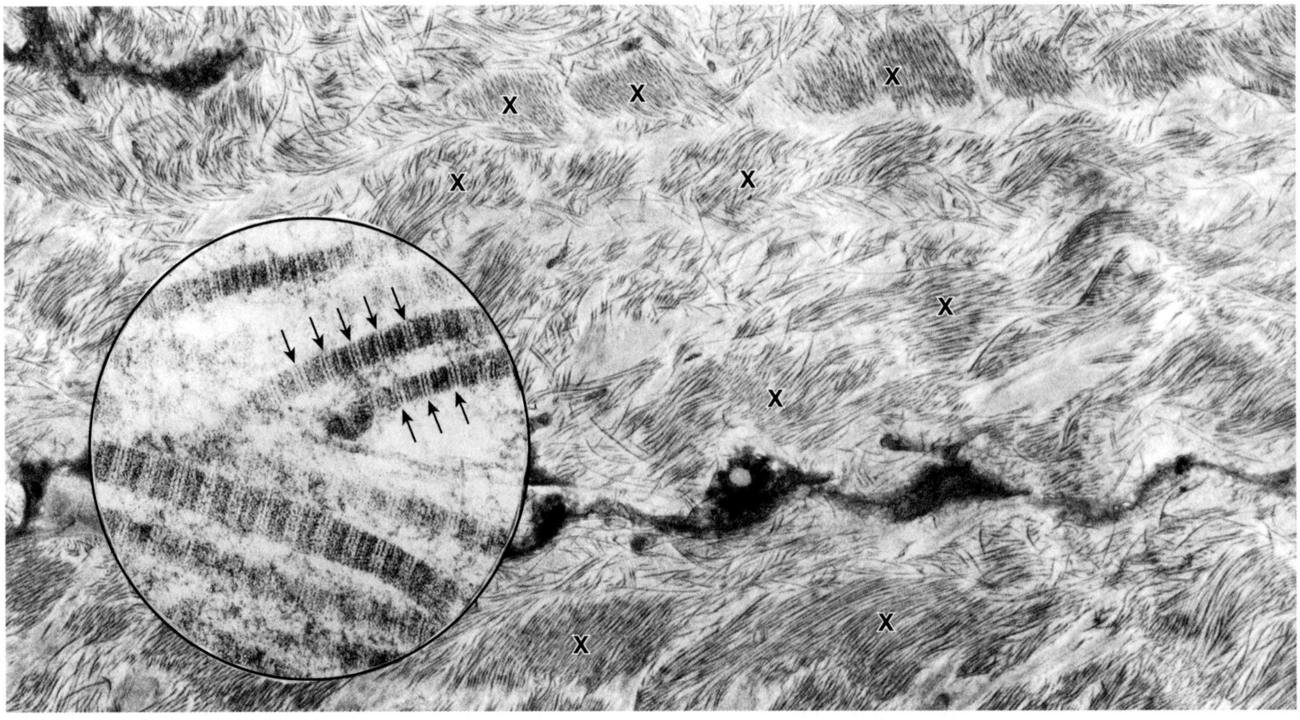

FIGURE 6.5. Collagen fibrils in dense irregular connective tissue. Electron micrograph of dense irregular connective tissue from the capsule of the testis of a young male. The thread-like collagen fibrils are aggregated in some areas (*X*) to form relatively thick bundles; in other areas, the fibrils are more dispersed. ×9,500. **Inset.** A longitudinal array of collagen fibrils from the same specimen seen at higher magnification. Note the banding pattern. The spacing of the *arrows* indicates the 68-nm repeat pattern. ×75,000.

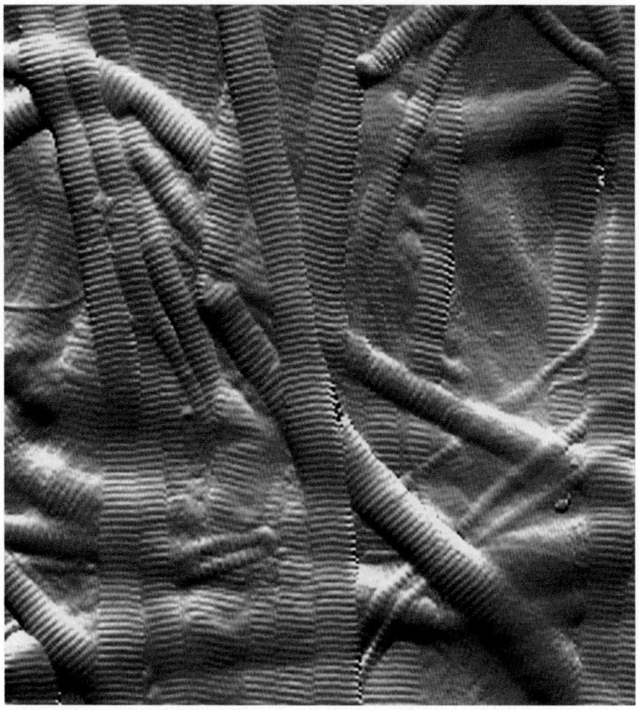

FIGURE 6.6. Collagen fibrils in dense irregular connective tissue. This atomic force microscopic image of type I collagen fibrils in the connective tissue shows the banding pattern on the surface of collagen fibrils. Note the random orientation of collagen fibrils that overlie and crisscross each other in the connective tissue matrix. ×65,000. (Courtesy of Dr. Gabriela Bagordo, JPK Instruments AG, Berlin, Germany.)

Each collagen molecule is a triple helix composed of three intertwined polypeptide chains.

A single **collagen molecule** consists of three polypeptides known as **α-chains**. The α-chains intertwine, forming a right-handed triple helix (Fig. 6.7d). Every third amino acid in the chain is a **glycine** molecule, except at the ends of the α-chains. A **hydroxyproline** or **hydroxylysine** frequently precedes each glycine in the chain, and a **proline** frequently follows each glycine in the chain. The ring structure of proline and hydroxyproline residues allows for sharp turns of the α-chain necessary for the assembly of the tight triple-helix structure. Along with proline and hydroxyproline, glycine is essential for the triple-helix conformation—it is the only amino acid small enough to fit into the center of the triple helix (Fig. 6.7e). Associated with the helix are sugar groups that are joined to hydroxylysyl residues. Because of these sugar groups, collagen is properly described as a **glycoprotein**.

The α-chains that constitute the helix are not all alike. They vary in size from 600 to 3,000 amino acids. To date, at least 46 types of α-chains encoded by different collagen genes have been identified and mapped to loci on several different chromosomes. As many as 29 different types of collagens have been categorized on the basis of the combinations of α-chains they contain. These various collagens are classified by Roman numerals I–XXIX according to the chronology of their discovery. In contrast, the nomenclature of genes encoding collagen chains is written as a combination of capital letters "COL" (for collagen) with numerical digits describing collagen type and α-chain number preceding capital letter A (for α). For example, gene encoding type I collage α1-chain is identified as COL1A1, where COL1 indicates collagen type I and A1 indicates α1-chain. Therefore, gene COL9A3 would be responsible for encoding α3-chain in the collagen type IX molecule.

A collagen molecule may be **homotrimeric** (consisting of three identical α-chains) or **heterotrimeric** (consisting of two or even three genetically distinct α-chains). For example, **type I collagen** found in loose and dense connective tissue is heterotrimeric. Two of the α-chains, identified as α1 (encoded by COL1A1 gene), are identical, and one, identified as α2, (encoded by COL1A2 gene), is different. Thus, in collagen nomenclature, it is designated $[\alpha1(I)]_2\ \alpha2(I)$ (Table 6.2). **Type II collagen** is homotrimeric and present in hyaline and elastic cartilage, where it occurs as very fine fibrils. The collagen molecules of type II collagen are composed of three identical α1-chains (encoded by COL2A1 gene). Because these α-chains differ from those of other collagens, type II collagen is designated $[\alpha1(II)]_3$.

Several classes of collagens are identified on the basis of their polymerization pattern.

Most of the collagen molecules polymerize into supramolecular aggregates, such as fibrils or networks, and they are

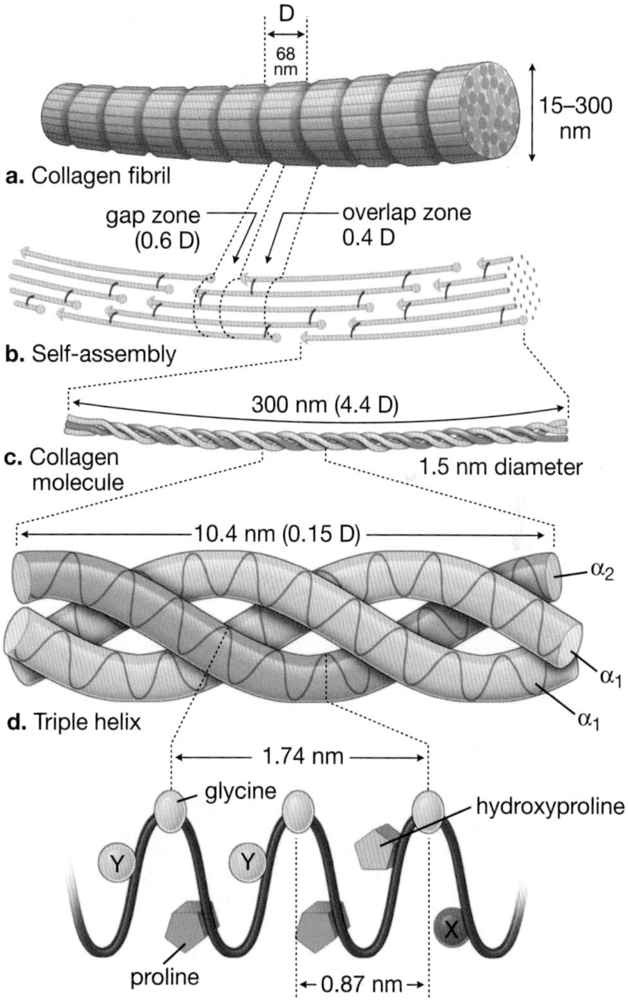

FIGURE 6.7. Diagram showing the molecular character of a type I collagen fibril in increasing order of structure. a. A collagen fibril displays periodic banding with a distance (*D*) of 68 nm between repeating bands. **b.** Each fibril is self-assembled from staggered collagen molecules, which are covalently cross-linked with lysine and hydroxylysine residues in adjacent molecules (*purple links*). **c.** Each molecule is about 300 nm long and 1.5 nm in diameter. **d.** The collagen molecule is a triple-helix cross-linked by numerous hydrogen bonds between prolines and glycines. **e.** The triple helix consists of three α-chains. Every third amino acid of the α-chain is a glycine. The *X* position following glycine is frequently a proline, and the *Y* position preceding the glycine is frequently a hydroxyproline. Some amino acids (e.g., glutamic acid, leucine, phenylalanine) prefer the *X* position and others prefer the *Y* position (e.g., arginine, glutamine, lysine, methionine, threonine).

TABLE 6.2 Types of Collagen, Composition, Location, and Function

Type	Composition[a]	Location	Functions
I	$[\alpha1(I)]_2\ \alpha2(I)$	Connective tissue of skin, bone, tendon, ligaments, dentin, sclera, fascia, and organ capsules (accounts for 90% of body collagen)	Provides resistance to force, tension, and stretch
II	$[\alpha1(II)]_3$	Cartilage (hyaline and elastic), notochord, and intervertebral disc	Provides resistance to intermittent pressure
III	$[\alpha1(III)]_3$	Prominent in loose connective tissue and organs (uterus, liver, spleen, kidney, lung, etc.), smooth muscle, endoneurium, blood vessels, and fetal skin	Forms reticular fibers; arranged in a loose meshwork of thin fibers that provides a supportive scaffolding for the specialized cells of various organs and blood vessels
IV	$[\alpha1(IV)]_2\ \alpha2(IV)$ or $\alpha3(IV)\ \alpha4(IV)\ \alpha5(IV)$ or $[\alpha5(IV)]_2\ \alpha6(IV)$	Found in all basal laminae of epithelial cells (i.e., epidermis, GI tract lining, kidney glomeruli, etc.), external laminae of nonepithelial cells (i.e., muscle cells, adipocytes, Schwann cells, etc.), and lens capsule	Provides support and aids in attachment of cells to connective tissue; in the kidney, contributes to filtration barrier
V	$[\alpha1(V)]_2\ \alpha2(V)$ or $\alpha1(V)\ \alpha2(V)\ \alpha3(V)$	Distributed uniformly throughout connective tissue stroma; may be related to reticular network; localized in reticular fibers of the splenic red pulp	Localized at the surface of type I collagen fibrils along with types XII and XIV collagen to modulate biomechanical properties of the fibril
VI	$[\alpha1(VI)]_2\ \alpha2(VI)$ or $\alpha1(VI)\ \alpha2(VI)\ \alpha3(VI)$ or other combinations with $\alpha4(VI)$, $\alpha5(VI)$ and $\alpha6(VI)$ that substitute for $\alpha3(VI)$ chain	Forms part of the cartilage matrix immediately surrounding the chondrocytes. Expressed in external lamina of skeletal muscles (α1, α2, α2), myotendinous junctions (α5), and both the perimysium and the endomysium (α6).	Attaches the chondrocytes and skeletal muscle cells to the matrix; covalently bound to type I collagen fibrils
VII	$[\alpha1(VII)]_3$	Present in anchoring fibrils of skin, eye, uterus, and esophagus	Secures basal lamina to connective tissue fibers
VIII	$[\alpha1(VIII)]_2\ \alpha2(VIII)$	Produced by endothelial cells	Facilitates movement of endothelial cells during angiogenesis
IX	$\alpha1(IX)\ \alpha2(IX)\ \alpha3(IX)$	Found in cartilage associated with type II collagen fibrils	Stabilizes network of cartilage type II collagen fibers by interaction with proteoglycan molecules at their intersections
X	$[\alpha1(X)]_3$	Produced by chondrocytes in the zone of hypertrophy of normal growth plate	Contributes to the bone mineralization process by forming hexagonal lattices necessary to arrange types II, IX, and XI collagen within cartilage
XI	$[\alpha1(XI)]_2\ \alpha2(XI)$ or $\alpha1(XI)\ \alpha2(XI)\ \alpha3(XI)$	Produced by chondrocytes; associated with type II collagen fibrils; forms the core of type I collagen fibrils	Regulates size of type II collagen fibrils; essential for cohesive properties of cartilage matrix
XII	$[\alpha1(XII)]_3$	Isolated from skin and placenta; abundant in tissues in which mechanical strain is high	Localized at the surface of type I collagen fibrils along with types V and XIV collagen to modulate biomechanical properties of the fibril
XIII	$[\alpha1(XIII)]_3$	Detected in bone, cartilage, intestine, skin, placenta, and striated muscles	An unusual transmembrane collagen associated with the basal lamina along with type VII collagen
XIV	$[\alpha1(XIV)]_3$	Isolated from placenta; also detected in the bone marrow	Localized at the surface of type I collagen fibrils along with types V and XII collagen to modulate biomechanical properties of the fibril; has a strong cell–cell-binding property
XV	$[\alpha1(XV)]_3$	Present in tissues derived from mesenchyme; expressed in heart and skeletal muscles	Involved in adhesion of basal lamina to the underlying connective tissue
XVI	$[\alpha1(XVI)]_3$	Broad tissue distribution; associated with fibroblasts and arterial smooth muscle cells but not associated with type I collagen fibrils	Contributes to structural integrity of connective tissue
XVII	$[\alpha1(XVII)]_3$	Another unusual transmembrane collagen found in epithelial cell membranes	Interacts with integrins to stabilize hemidesmosome structure
XVIII	$[\alpha1(XVIII)]_3$	Found in epithelial and vascular basement membrane	Represents a basement membrane heparan sulfate proteoglycan thought to inhibit endothelial cell proliferation and angiogenesis
XIX	$[\alpha1(XIX)]_3$	Discovered from the sequence of human rhabdomyosarcoma cDNA; present in fibroblasts and liver	Pronounced vascular and stromal interaction suggests involvement in angiogenesis.
XX	$[\alpha1(XX)]_3$	Discovered in chick embryonic tissue; also in corneal epithelium, sternal cartilage, and tendons	Binds to the surface of other collagen fibrils
XXI	$[\alpha1(XXI)]_3$	Found in human gingiva, heart and skeletal muscle, and other tissues containing type I collagen fibrils	Plays a role in maintaining a three-dimensional architecture of dense connective tissues

Type	Composition[a]	Location	Functions
XXII	$[\alpha1(XXII)]_3$	Found in myotendinous junction, skeletal and heart muscle, articular cartilage–synovial fluid junction, and at the border between hair follicle and dermis	Belongs to FACIT family; expressed at tissue junctions in skin; influences epithelial–mesenchymal interactions during hair follicle morphogenesis and cycling
XXIII	$[\alpha3(XXIII)]_3$	Discovered in metastatic tumor cells; also expressed in heart, retina, and metastatic prostate cancer cells	Transmembrane collagen that interacts with ECM proteins (collagens XIII and XXV, fibronectin, heparin); increased expression in metastatic prostate cancer
XXIV	$[\alpha1(XXIV)]_3$	Found coexpressed with type I collagen in the developing bone and eye	Fibrillar-like collagen; regarded as an ancient molecule that regulates type I collagen fibrillogenesis in bone and eye during fetal development
XXV	$[\alpha1(XXV)]_3$	A brain-specific transmembrane collagen; discovered in amyloid plaques in brains of patients with Alzheimer disease; overexpressed in neurons	Binds to fibrillized β-amyloid peptide of amyloid plaques in Alzheimer disease
XXVI	$[\alpha1(XXVI)]_3$	Found in neonatal and adult testes and ovaries;	Interacts with HSP47, a specific collagen-binding molecular chaperone; required for collagen maturation
XXVII	$[\alpha1(XXVII)]_3$	Expressed in human fetal epiphyseal cartilages	Plays a role in the transition of cartilage to bone during endochondral bone formation
XXVIII	$[\alpha1(XXVIII)]_3$	Expressed in peripheral nerves originating from dorsal root ganglia; its structure is similar to that of collagen VI	Most likely plays a role in assembly of basement membranes in peripheral nerve fiber–supporting cells
XXIX	$[\alpha1(XXIX)]_3$	Found in epidermis	Implicated in epidermal integrity and function. Lack of this collagen is characteristic of atopic dermatitis.

[a]Each collagen molecule is composed of three polypeptide α-chains intertwined in a helical configuration. The Roman numerals in the parentheses in the "Composition" column indicate that the α-chains have a distinctive structure that differs from the chains with different numerals. Thus, collagen type I has two identical α1-chains and one α2-chain; collagen type II has three identical α1-chains.

■ fibrillar collagen; ■ FACITs; ■ basement membrane–forming collagen; ■ hexagonal network–forming collagen; □ transmembrane collagens; ■ multiplexins.

cDNA, complementary DNA; *ECM*, extracellular matrix; *FACIT*, fibril-associated collagens with interrupted triple helix.

divided into several subgroups on the basis of their structural or amino acid sequence similarities:

- **Fibrillar collagens** include types I, II, III, V, and XI collagen molecules. These types are characterized by uninterrupted glycine–proline–hydroxyproline repeats and aggregate to form 68-nm-banded fibrils (as diagramed in Fig. 6.7a).
- **Fibril-associated collagens with interrupted triple helices (FACITs)** have interruptions in their triple helices that provide flexibility to the molecule. They are located on the surface of different fibrils and are represented by types IX, XII, XIV, XVI, XIX, XX, XXI, XXII, XXVI, XXVII, and XXIX collagens. For instance, type IX collagen binds and interacts with type II collagen in the cartilage at the intersections of the fibrils. This collagen interaction serves to stabilize this tissue by binding type II collagen fibrils with proteoglycans of the ECM.
- **Hexagonal network–forming collagens** are represented by collagen types VIII and X.
- **Transmembrane collagens** are represented by types XIII (found in focal adhesions), XVII (found within hemidesmosomes), XXIII (found in metastatic cancer cells), and XXV (a brain-specific collagen).
- **Multiplexins** are collagens with multiple triple-helix domains and interruptions. They comprise collagen types XV and XVIII, which reside in the basement membrane zones. These collagen molecules possess multiple short triple–helical domains connected by unique non–triple-helical regions that impart flexibility to the collagen molecule.
- **Basement membrane–forming collagens** include type IV collagen, which is responsible for the collagen suprastructure in the basement membrane of epithelial cells (see pages 155-158); type VI collagen, which forms beaded filaments; type VII collagen, which forms anchoring fibrils that attach the basement membrane to the ECM; and type XXVIII collagen, which, in peripheral nerves, plays a role in the assembly of basement membranes of supporting cells.

Table 6.2 lists the collagens that have been characterized to date (I–XXIX), including their structural variations and some of the roles presently ascribed to them.

Biosynthesis and Degradation of Collagen Fibers

Collagen fiber formation involves events that occur both within and outside the fibroblast.

The production of **fibrillar collagen** (I, II, III, V, and XI) involves a series of events within the fibroblast that leads to the production of **procollagen**, the precursor of the collagen molecule. These events take place in membrane-bound organelles within the cell. Production of the actual fibril occurs outside the cell and involves enzymatic activity at the plasma membrane to produce the collagen molecule, followed by assembly of the molecules into fibrils in the ECM under guidance by the cell (Fig. 6.8).

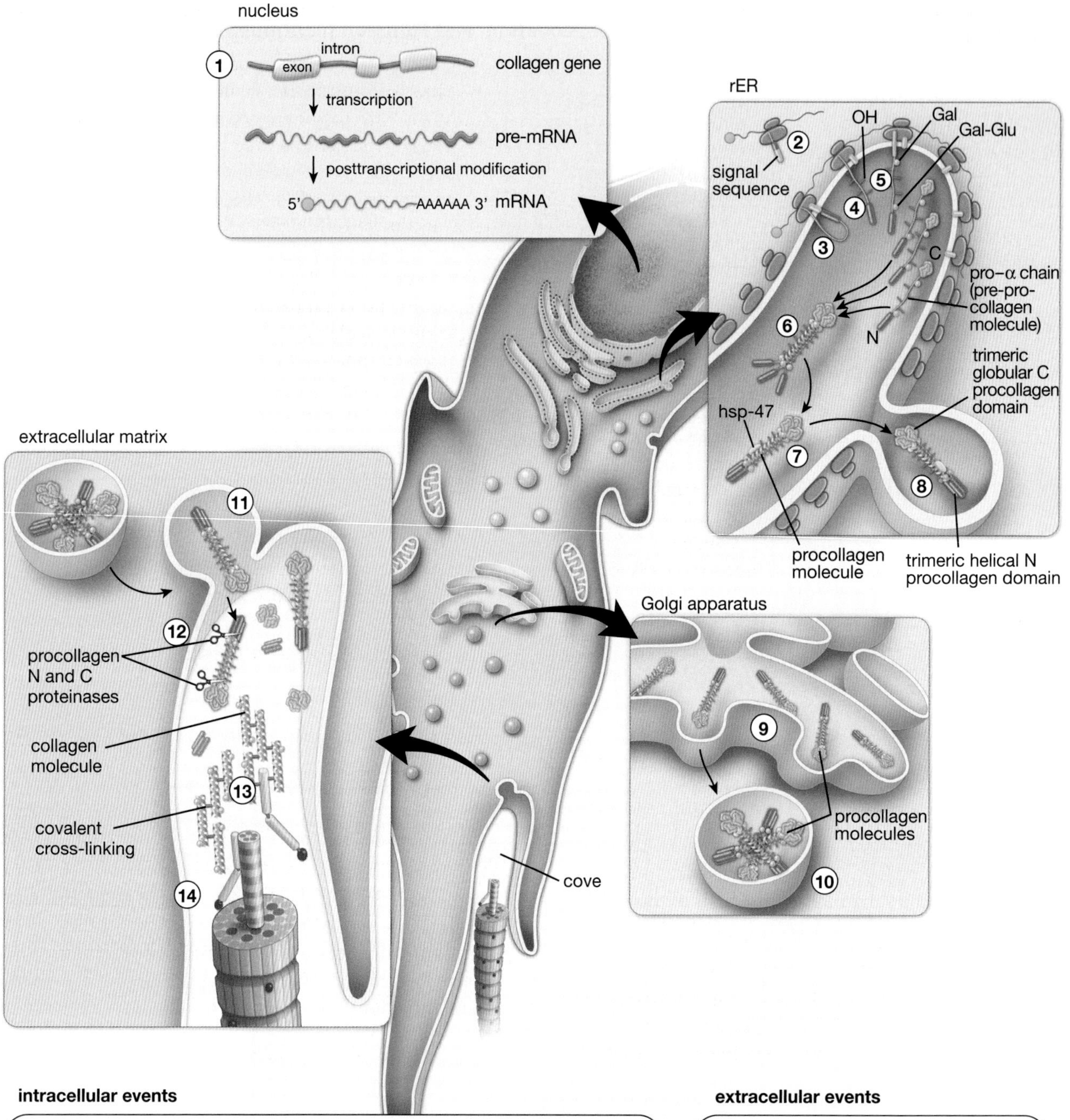

intracellular events

1. Formation of mRNA in the nucleus
2. Initiation of synthesis of pro–α chains with signal sequences by ribosomes
3. Synthesis of pro–α chains on the rER
4. Hydroxylation of proline and lysine residues (vitamin C required) and cleavage of signal sequence from pro–α chain
5. Glycosylation of specific hydroxylysyl residues in the rER
6. Formation of procollagen triple helix molecules from a C terminus toward the N terminus in a zipper-like manner
7. Stabilization of the triple helix by formation of intra- and interchain hydrogen and disulfide bounds and chaperone proteins (e.g., hsp-47)
8. Transport of procollagen molecules to Golgi apparatus
9. Packaging of procollagen molecules by Golgi into secretory vesicles
10. Movement of vesicles to plasma membrane, assisted by molecular motor proteins associated with microtubules

extracellular events

11. Exocytosis of procollagen molecules
12. Cleavage of trimeric globular C- and helical N-procollagen domains by procollagen N- and C-proteinases
13. Polymerization (self-assembly) of collagen molecules into collagen fibrils (in cove of fibroblast) with development of covalent cross-linking initiated by copper-dependent lysyl oxidase (LOX)
14. Incorporation of other collagens (e.g., type V, FACITs, etc.) into collagen fibrils

FIGURE 6.8. Collagen biosynthesis. Schematic representation of the biosynthetic events and organelles participating in collagen synthesis. Bold numbers correspond to the numbered events in collagen biosynthesis listed at the *bottom*.

Collagen molecule biosynthesis involves a number of intracellular events.

The steps in biosynthesis of almost all fibrillar collagens are similar, but **type I collagen** has been studied in the most detail. In general, the synthetic pathway for collagen molecules is similar to other constitutive secretory pathways used by the cell. The unique features of **collagen biosynthesis** are expressed in multiple post-translational processing steps that are required to prepare the molecule for the extracellular assembly process. Intracellular processing events are as follows:

- Collagen α-chains are synthesized in the rough endoplasmic reticulum (rER) as long precursors containing large globular amino- and carboxy-terminus propeptides called **pro–α-chains** (**preprocollagen molecules**). The newly synthesized polypeptides are simultaneously discharged into the cisternae of the rER, where intracellular processing begins.
- Within the cisternae of the rER, a number of **post-translational modifications** of the preprocollagen molecules occur, including the following:
  - The amino-terminus signal sequence is cleaved.
  - **Proline** and **lysine residues are hydroxylated**, whereas the polypeptides are still in the nonhelical conformation. **Ascorbic acid (vitamin C)** is a required cofactor for the addition of hydroxyl groups to proline and lysine residues in pro–α-chains by the enzymes prolylhydroxylase and lysylhydroxylase; without hydroxylation of proline and lysine residues, the hydrogen bonds essential to the final structure of the collagen molecule cannot form. This explains why wounds fail to heal and bone formation is impaired in **scurvy** (vitamin C deficiency).
  - *O*-Linked sugar groups are added to some hydroxylysine residues (glycosylation), and *N*-linked sugars are added to the two terminal positions.
  - The **globular structure** is formed at the carboxy-terminus, which is stabilized by disulfide bonds. Formation of this structure ensures the correct alignment of the three α-chains during the formation of the triple helix.
  - A **triple helix** (beginning from the carboxy-terminus) is formed by three α-chains, except at the terminals where the polypeptide chains remain uncoiled.
  - Intrachain and interchain hydrogen and disulfide bonds form that influence the shape of the molecule.
  - The triple-helix molecule is stabilized by the binding of the **chaperone heat-shock protein 47 (hsp47)**, which also prevents the premature aggregation of the trimers within the cell. The resultant molecule is **procollagen**.
- The folded procollagen molecules pass to the Golgi apparatus and begin to associate into small bundles. This bundling is achieved by the lateral associations between uncoiled terminals of the procollagen molecules. Free and small aggregates of procollagen molecules are packaged into secretory vesicles and transported to the cell surface.

Formation of collagen fibrils (fibrillogenesis) involves the following extracellular events.

- As procollagen is secreted from the cell, it is converted into a mature **collagen molecule** by procollagen peptidases associated with the cell membrane, which cleave the uncoiled ends of the procollagen (Fig. 6.9). Serum levels of **procollagen type I N-terminal propeptide (PINP)** can be measured and used as indicators for collagen type I metabolism. An elevated level of PINP is indicative of increased production of collagen type I, which is associated with bone metastases in breast and prostate cancer.
- The aggregated collagen molecules then align to form the final **collagen fibrils** in a process known as **fibrillogenesis**. The cell controls the orderly array of the newly formed fibrils by directing the secretory vesicles to a localized surface site for discharge. The cell simultaneously creates specialized collagen assembly sites called **coves**. These invaginations of the cell surface allow molecules to accumulate and assemble (see Fig. 6.8). Within the cove, the collagen molecules align in rows and self-assemble longitudinally in a head-to-tail manner. They also aggregate laterally in a quarter-staggered pattern (see Fig. 6.7).

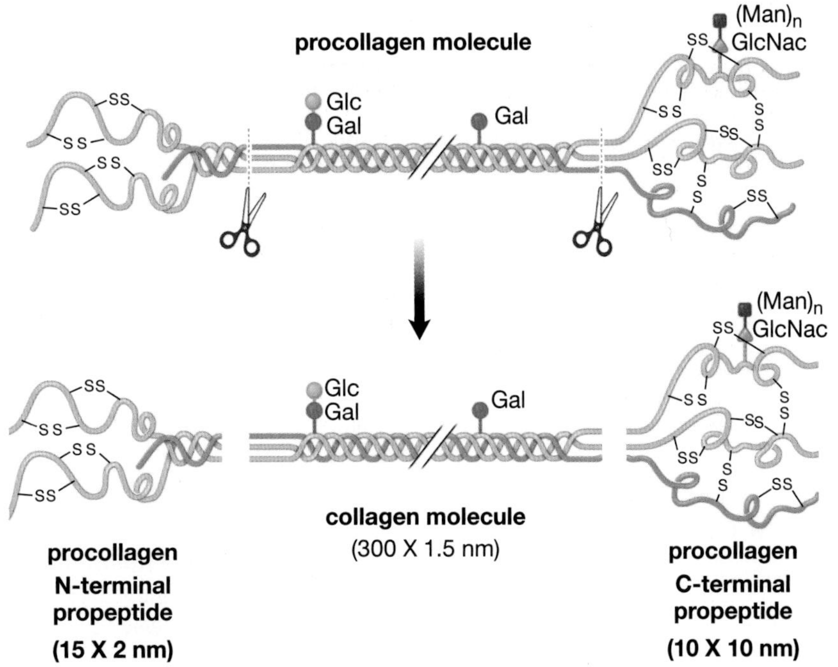

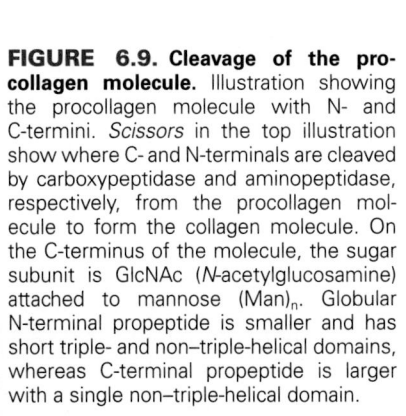

FIGURE 6.9. Cleavage of the procollagen molecule. Illustration showing the procollagen molecule with N- and C-termini. *Scissors* in the top illustration show where C- and N-terminals are cleaved by carboxypeptidase and aminopeptidase, respectively, from the procollagen molecule to form the collagen molecule. On the C-terminus of the molecule, the sugar subunit is GlcNAc (*N*-acetylglucosamine) attached to mannose $(Man)_n$. Globular N-terminal propeptide is smaller and has short triple- and non–triple-helical domains, whereas C-terminal propeptide is larger with a single non–triple-helical domain.

The collagen molecules are then cross-linked by covalent bonds formed between the lysine and hydroxylysine aldehyde groups. These covalent cross-links are catalyzed by a copper-dependent lysyl oxidase (LOX). Collagen biogenesis results in the formation of highly organized polymers called **fibrils.** The fibrils further associate with each other to form larger **collagen fibers**, which, on a per weight basis, have a tensile strength comparable to that of steel. For example, collagen type I fiber of 1 mm in diameter can withstand a load of 10–40 kg before it breaks.

Menkes syndrome (Menkes kinky hair syndrome) is an X-linked recessive disorder caused by mutations in genes coding for the **copper-transport protein** (ATP7A), leading to a systemic deficit of copper and subsequent dysfunction of copper-dependent enzymes. Because **lysyl oxidase** requires copper for proper function, its deficiency will affect cross-linking of collagen and elastin molecules during the final steps of fibrillogenesis. The defective collagen and elastin fibers contribute to the many connective tissue manifestations of this disease, including premature rapture of fetal membranes, poor growth, abnormal skeletal development, loose skin and joints, arterial aneurysms, poor wound healing, and characteristic short, fragile, brittle, and twisted hair (pili torti; *Lat. pili, hair* and *Lat. torti, twisted*) with a low amount of pigment.

Collagen fibrils often consist of more than one type of collagen.

Usually, different types of fibrillar collagens assemble into fibrils composed of more than one type of collagen molecule. For example, **type I collagen fibrils** often contain small amounts of types II, III, V, and XI. Current studies indicate that assembly of type I collagen fibrils is preceded by the formation of a fibrillar core containing type V and type XI molecules. Subsequently, type I collagen molecules are deposited and polymerized on the surface of the fibrillar core (Fig. 6.10). In addition, small amounts of types II and III collagen molecules are incorporated into type I collagen fibrils. Collagen types V and XI are important regulators of fibrillogenesis. They control the thickness of type I fibrils by limiting the deposition of collagen molecules after the fibril has reached the desired diameter.

Fully mature collagen fibers are usually associated with the FACIT family of collagen molecules that reside on their surfaces. For example, type I fibrils are associated with type XII and type XIV collagens. These collagens contribute to the three-dimensional organization of fibers within the ECM. Type II collagen fibrils, which are abundant within the cartilage, are usually smaller in diameter than type I fibrils. However, these fibrils are also associated with type IX collagen (another member of the FACIT subgroup). Collagen type IX resides on the surface of the type II fibril and anchors it to proteoglycans and other components of the cartilaginous ECM (Fig. 6.11).

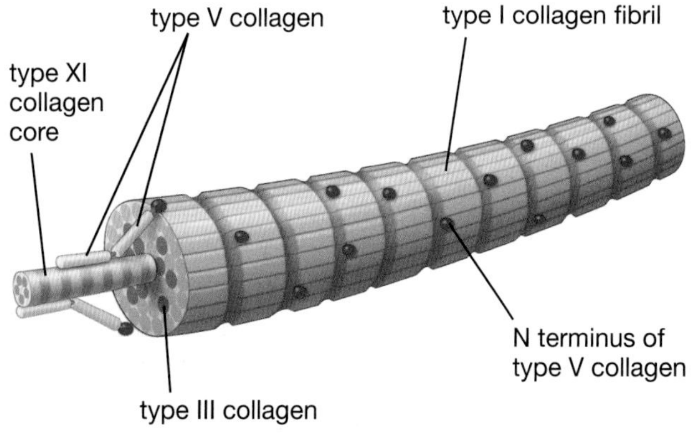

FIGURE 6.10. Type I collagen fibril. The type I collagen fibril contains small amounts of other collagen types such as types II, III, V, and XI. Note that the core of the fibril contains collagen types V (which has a role in type I fibril assembly and regulating fibril diameter) and XI (which help initiate the assembly of the type I fibril).

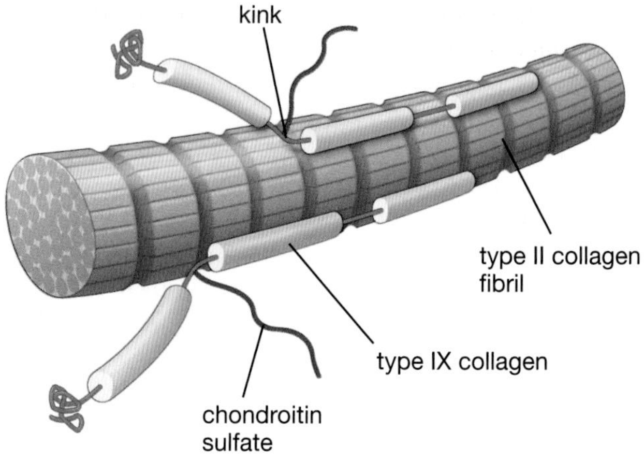

FIGURE 6.11. Type II collagen fibril. This diagram illustrates the interaction between type II collagen fibrils and type IX collagen molecules in the cartilaginous matrix. Collagen type IX provides the link between the collagen fibrils and *GAG* molecules, which stabilizes the network of cartilage fibers.

Collagen molecules are synthesized by various types of connective tissue and epithelial cells.

Collagen molecules are largely synthesized by connective tissue cells. These cells include fibroblasts in a variety of tissues (e.g., chondrocytes in cartilage, osteoblasts in bone, and pericytes in blood vessels). In addition, the collagen molecules of the basement membrane (see pages 155-158) are produced by epithelial cells. The synthesis of collagen is regulated by complex interactions among growth factors, hormones, and cytokines. For example, transforming growth factor β (TGF-β) and platelet-derived growth factor (PDGF) stimulate collagen synthesis by fibroblasts, whereas steroid hormones (glucocorticoids) inhibit its synthesis.

Collagen fibers are degraded by either proteolytic or phagocytic pathways.

All proteins in the body are being continually degraded and resynthesized. These processes allow tissues to grow and remodel. Collagen fibers also undergo constant but slow turnover. The half-life of collagen molecules varies from days to several years (e.g., in skin and cartilage). Initial fragmentation of insoluble collagen molecules occurs through mechanical wear, the action of free radicals, or proteinase cleavage. Further degradation is continued by specific enzymes called **proteinases.** The resulting collagen fragments are then phagocytosed by cells and degraded by their lysosomal enzymes. **Excessive collagen degradation** is observed in several diseases (e.g., degradation of cartilage collagen in **rheumatoid arthritis** or bone collagen in **osteoporosis**). Secreted collagen molecules are degraded mainly by two different pathways:

- **Proteolytic degradation** occurs outside the cells through the activity of enzymes called **matrix metalloproteinases (MMPs).** These enzymes are synthesized and secreted into the ECM by a variety of connective tissue cells (fibroblasts, chondrocytes, monocytes, neutrophils, and macrophages), some epithelial cells (keratinocytes in the epidermis), and cancer cells. The MMPs include **collagenases** (which degrade types I, II, III, and X collagens), **gelatinases** (which degrade most types of denatured collagens, laminin, fibronectin, and elastin), **stromelysins** (which degrade proteoglycans, fibronectin, and denatured collagens), **matrilysins** (which degrade type IV collagen and proteoglycans), **membrane-type MMPs** (which are produced by cancer cells and have a potent pericellular fibrinolytic activity), and **macrophage metalloelastases** (which degrade elastin, type IV collagen, and laminin).

In general, triple-helical undenatured forms of collagen molecules are resistant to degradation by MMPs. In contrast, damaged or denatured collagen (gelatin) is degraded by many MMPs, with gelatinases playing a prominent role. MMP activity can be specifically inhibited by **tissue inhibitors of metalloproteinases (TIMPs)**. Because MMPs are secreted by invasive (migrating) cancer cells, researchers are investigating synthetic therapeutic agents that inhibit the activity of MMPs to control the spread of cancer cells.

- **Phagocytic degradation** occurs intracellularly and involves macrophages to remove components of the ECM. Fibroblasts are also capable of phagocytosing and degrading collagen fibrils within the lysosomes of the cell.

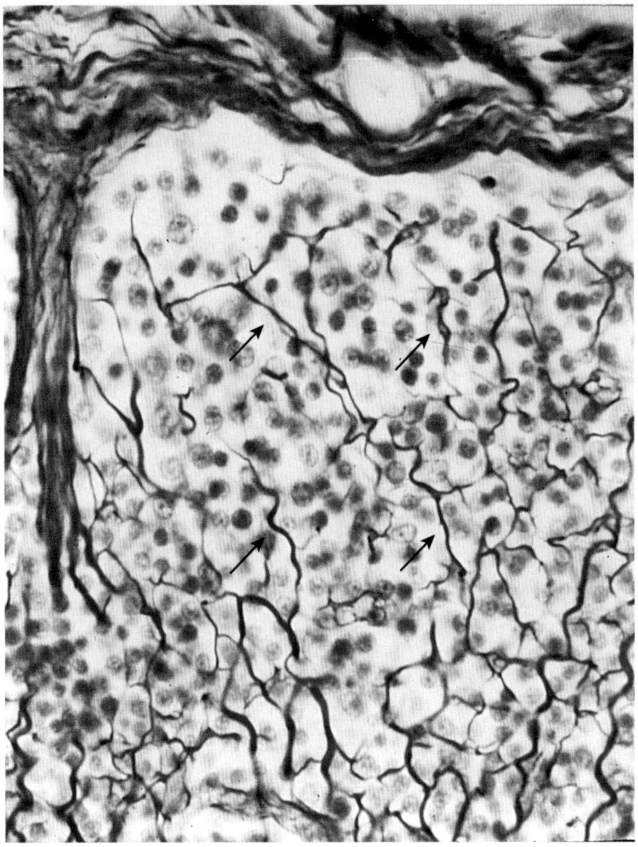

FIGURE 6.12. Reticular fibers in a lymph node. Photomicrograph of a lymph node silver preparation showing the connective tissue capsule at the *top* and a trabecula extending from it at the *left*. The reticular fibers (*arrows*) form an irregular anastomosing network. ×650.

Reticular Fibers

Reticular fibers provide a supporting framework for the cellular constituents of various tissues and organs.

Reticular fibers and collagen type I fibers share a prominent feature in that they both consist of collagen fibrils. Unlike collagen fibers, however, reticular fibers are composed of **type III collagen**. The individual fibrils that constitute a reticular fiber exhibit a 68-nm banding pattern (the same as the fibrils of type I collagen). The fibrils have a narrow diameter (about 20 nm), exhibit a branching pattern, and typically do not bundle to form thick fibers.

In routinely stained H&E preparations, reticular fibers cannot be identified positively. When visualized in the light microscope with special techniques, reticular fibers have a thread-like appearance. Because they contain a much greater relative concentration of sugar groups than do collagen type I fibers, reticular fibers are readily displayed by means of the **periodic acid–Schiff (PAS) reaction.** They are also revealed with special silver-staining procedures, such as the Gomori and Wilder methods. After silver treatment, the fibers appear black; thus, they are said to be **argyrophilic** (Fig. 6.12). The thicker collagen fibers in such preparations are colored brown.

FOLDER 6.1
CLINICAL CORRELATION: COLLAGENOPATHIES

The important role of collagens in the body can be illustrated by **collagenopathies** (collagen diseases), which are caused by a deficit or abnormality in the production of specific collagens. Most collagenopathies are attributed to mutations in genes encoding the α-chains in the various collagens. Mutation of collagen (COL) genes produces a wide variety of genetic disorders that range from mild to lethal, depending on the mutation of the collagen gene and its subsequent effect on the molecular structure of the collagen and its function in the body.

For instance, mutations of type I collagen genes (COL1A1 and COL1A2) are responsible for **osteogenesis imperfecta**, a disorder of bone fragility. Some mutations in less severe types of osteogenesis imperfecta result in the production of abnormal messenger RNA (mRNA). which is either captured and retained in the nucleus, or degraded in the cytoplasm, before it can be fully translated into the rough endoplasmic reticulum (rER). As a result, only half the normal amount of procollagen molecules are synthesized. In the more severe types of this disease, missense mutations can substitute an alternate amino acid for a glycine residue, resulting in abnormal triple-helix and procollagen formation, which affects self-assembly and cross-linking of collagen fibrils. In addition to COL1A1 and COL1A2 mutations, there are at least 13 other genes linked to osteogenesis imperfecta that are involved in post-translational modification of collagen. In the future, gene therapy could potentially be used to either control deposition of faulty collagen or reverse the disease process caused by the mutated genes. The following table lists the most common collagenopathies that occur in humans.

(*continued*)

FOLDER 6.1
CLINICAL CORRELATION: COLLAGENOPATHIES (*continued*)

The Most Common Collagenopathies in Humans

Type of Collagen	Disease	Symptoms
I	Osteogenesis imperfecta	Repeated fractures after minor trauma, brittle bones, lax ligaments, abnormal teeth, thin skin, weak tendons, blue sclerae, and progressive hearing loss. Genes affected are COL1A1 and COL1A2.
II	Kniest dysplasia; achondrogenesis, type 2	Short stature, restricted joint mobility, ocular changes leading to blindness, wide metaphyses, and joint abnormality seen in radiographs. Gene affected is COL2A1.
III	Hypermobile Ehlers–Danlos syndrome (hEDS), type 3 (has an additional mutation of tenascin X gene); Vascular Ehlers–Danlos syndrome (vEDS), type 4	Type 3: Hypermobility of all joints, dislocations, deformity of finger joints, and early onset of osteoarthritis; owing to clinical presentation and mutation of tenascin X gene, hEDS is included in this group. (However, to date, no collagen gene mutation was found.) Type 4: Pale, translucent, thin skin; severe bruising, and early morbidity and mortality (resulting from rupture of vessels and internal organs); vEDS is caused by mutation of α1-chain of collagen III gene (COL3A1).
IV	Alport syndrome	Hematuria resulting from structural changes in the glomerular basement membrane of the kidney, progressive hearing loss, and ocular lesions Different mutations in type IV collagen genes are responsible for Alport syndrome (COL4A3), benign familial hematuria (COL4A4), X-linked Alport syndrome (COL4A5), and diffuse leiomyomatosis with Alport syndrome (COL4A6).
V	Classic Ehlers–Danlos syndrome (cEDS), types 1 and 2 (includes additional rare mutations of α1-chain of type I collagen gene)	Symptoms similar to type 3 (hypermobility of joints) but with additional skin involvement (fragility, hyperelasticity, delayed wound healing cause atrophic scarring); type 1 manifests with more severe skin abnormalities than type 2. More than 90% of cEDS is caused by mutation of α1- and α2-chains of collagen V gene (COL5A1 and COL5A2, respectively).
VI	Bethlem myopathy; Ullrich congenital muscular dystrophy	Symptoms include slowly progressive muscle weakness with contractures and hypermobility in wrist and ankle joints. Caused by mutation of COL6A1, COL6A2, COL6A3, and, recently found, COL6A4, COL6A5, and COL6A6 genes.
VII	Kindler syndrome	Severe blistering and scarring of the skin after minor trauma, resulting from the absence of anchoring fibrils encoded within COL7A1 gene.
IX	Multiple epiphyseal dysplasia (MED) types 2, 3, and 4	Skeletal deformations resulting from impaired endochondral ossification and dysplasia (MED), premature degenerative joint disease. Mutations affect genes encoding different chains of type IX collagen: COL9A1 (MED type 4), COL9A2 (MED type 2), and COL9A3 (MED type 3).
X	Schmid metaphyseal chondrodysplasia	Skeletal deformations characterized by modifications of the vertebral bodies and chondrodysplasia metaphyses of the long bone (mutation of COL10A1 gene).
XI	Weissenbacher–Zweymüller syndrome, Stickler syndrome (includes additional mutations of type II collagen gene)	Similar clinical features to type II collagenopathies in addition to craniofacial and skeletal deformations, severe myopia, retinal detachment, and progressive hearing loss (mutations of COL11A1 and COL11A2 genes).
XVII	Generalized atrophic benign epidermolysis bullosa (GABEB)	Blistering skin disease with mechanically induced dermal–epidermal separation, epidermolysis bullosa resulting from faulty hemidesmosomes, skin atrophy, nail dystrophy, and alopecia (mutations of COL17A1 gene).
XVIII	Knobloch syndrome	Abnormality in basement membrane formation; characterized by eye abnormality (retinal detachment, myopia, cataracts, lens dislocation) and skull defects. Caused by mutation of α1-chain of collagen XVIII gene (COL18A1).

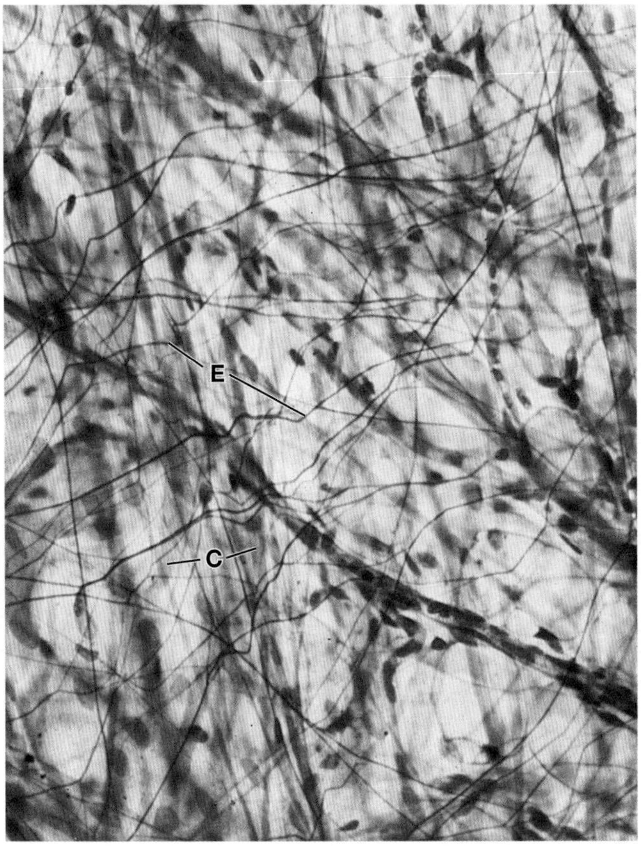

FIGURE 6.13. Collagen and elastic fibers. Photomicrograph of a mesentery spread stained with resorcin-fuchsin. The mesentery is very thin, and the microscope can be focused through the entire thickness of the tissue. The delicate thread-like branching strands are the elastic fibers (*E*). Collagen fibers (*C*) are also evident. They are much thicker; although they cross one another, they do not branch. ×200.

Reticular fibers are named for their arrangement in a mesh-like pattern or network.

In loose connective tissue, networks of **reticular fibers** are found at the boundary of connective tissue and epithelium as well as surrounding adipocytes, small blood vessels, nerves, and muscle cells. They are also found in embryonic tissues. The prevalence of reticular fibers is an indicator of tissue maturity. They are prominent in the initial stages of wound healing and scar tissue formation, where they provide early mechanical strength to the newly synthesized ECM. As embryonic development or wound healing progresses, reticular fibers are gradually replaced by the stronger type I collagen fibers. Reticular fibers also function as a supporting stroma in hemopoietic and lymphatic tissues (but not in the thymus). In these tissues, a special cell type, the **reticular cell**, produces the collagen of the reticular fiber. This cell maintains a unique relationship to the fiber. It surrounds the fiber with its cytoplasm, thus isolating the fiber from other tissue components.

In most other locations, reticular fibers are produced by fibroblasts. Important exceptions to this general rule include the endoneurium of peripheral nerves, where Schwann cells secrete reticular fibers; tunica media of blood vessels; and muscularis of the alimentary canal, where smooth muscle cells secrete reticular and other collagen fibers.

Elastic Fibers

Elastic fibers allow tissues to respond to stretch and distension.

Elastic fibers are typically thinner than collagen fibers and are arranged in a branching pattern to form a three-dimensional network. Because elastin is roughly 1,000 times more flexible than collagen, elastic fibers are interwoven with collagen fibers to limit the distensibility of the tissue and prevent tearing from excessive stretching (Plate 6.3, page 214). Elastic fibers are produced by many of the same cells that produce collagen and reticular fibers, particularly fibroblasts, smooth muscle cells, endothelial cells, and chondrocytes.

Elastic fibers stain with eosin but not well, so they cannot always be distinguished from collagen fibers in routine H&E preparations. Because elastic fibers become somewhat refractile with certain fixatives, they may be distinguished from collagen fibers in specimens stained with H&E when they display this characteristic. Elastic fibers can also be selectively stained with special dyes, such as orcein or resorcin-fuchsin, as shown in Figure 6.13.

Elastic material is a major extracellular substance in vertebral ligaments, larynx, and elastic arteries.

In elastic ligaments, the elastic material consists of thick fibers interspersed with collagen fibers. Examples of this material are found in the **ligamenta flava** of the vertebral column and the **ligamentum nuchae** of the neck. Finer fibers are present in elastic ligaments of the **vocal folds** of the larynx.

In elastic arteries, the elastic material is present as fenestrated lamellae, which are sheets of elastin with gaps or openings. The

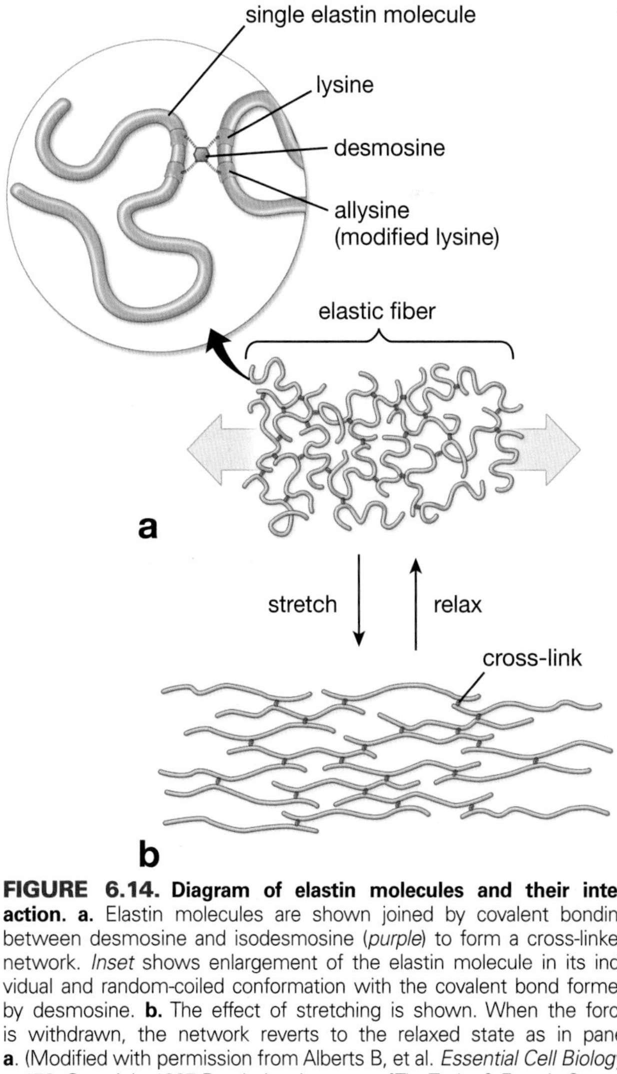

FIGURE 6.14. Diagram of elastin molecules and their interaction. a. Elastin molecules are shown joined by covalent bonding between desmosine and isodesmosine (*purple*) to form a cross-linked network. *Inset* shows enlargement of the elastin molecule in its individual and random-coiled conformation with the covalent bond formed by desmosine. **b.** The effect of stretching is shown. When the force is withdrawn, the network reverts to the relaxed state as in panel **a**. (Modified with permission from Alberts B, et al. *Essential Cell Biology*, p. 153. Copyright 1997. Routledge, Inc., part of The Taylor & Francis Group.)

lamellae are arranged in concentric layers between layers of smooth muscle cells. Like the collagen fibers in the tunica media of blood vessel walls, the elastic material of arteries is produced by smooth muscle cells, not by fibroblasts. In contrast to elastic fibers, microfibrils are not found in the lamellae. Only the amorphous elastin component is seen in electron micrographs.

The elastic property of the elastin molecule is related to its unusual polypeptide backbone, which causes random coiling.

Elastin (tropoelastin, 72 kDa) is one of the most hydrophobic proteins in the body. It is characterized by the presence of hydrophobic regions (which comprise >80% of the entire protein structure) alternating with hydrophilic regions. Like collagen, elastin is rich in proline and glycine; however, unlike collagen, it is poor in hydroxyproline and completely lacks hydroxylysine. The distribution of nonpolar amino acids such as glycine, valine, proline, and leucine, often arranged in repetitive motifs, makes the elastin molecule hydrophobic and allows for random coiling of its fibers. This permits elastic fibers to "slide" over one another or to be stretched and then recoil to their original state. The hydrophilic domains of elastin are rich in lysine and alanine, and they participate in cross-linking.

Elastin also contains **desmosine** and **isodesmosine**, two large amino acids unique to elastin, which are also responsible for the covalent bonding of elastin molecules to one another. These covalent bonds link four sites on elastin molecules into either desmosine or isodesmosine cross-links (Fig. 6.14). Elastin forms fibers of variable thicknesses, or lamellar layers (as in elastic arteries).

Elastin is encoded by one of the largest genes in the human genome. The **elastin (ELN) gene** consists of approximately 48 kilobases of genomic DNA on chromosome 7. Analysis of the human ELN gene has revealed that functionally distinct hydrophobic and hydrophilic domains of the elastin are encoded in separate exons that alternate in the genes. The ELN gene has 34 exons with an exon/intron ratio of approximately 1:20; therefore, less than 10% of the kilobases carry the sequence that encodes elastin.

Because the introns of the elastin gene contain large amounts of repetitive sequences, the likelihood of replication errors is increased. These errors may lead to diseases such as supravalvular aortic stenosis (SVAS) and cutis laxa syndrome. In **supravalvular aortic stenosis (SVAS)**, mutated elastin forms thinner elastic fibers and disorganized elastic lamellae in the wall of the ascending aorta. This triggers a compensation reaction in which increased production and deposition of smooth muscle in the aortic wall thickens the artery wall and progressively narrows the lumen. **Cutis laxa** is an inherited or acquired disease characterized by wrinkled, redundant, sagging, and inelastic skin caused by defective dermal elastic fibers synthesis. Most inherited forms of cutis laxa cause associated multiple organ systems abnormalities owing to the prevalence of mutated elastin in the body.

Elastic fibers are composed of cross-linked elastin molecules and a network of fibrillin microfibrils with associated proteins.

Fibrillin-1 (350 kDa) is a glycoprotein that polymerizes in the extracellular space in a head-to-tail arrangement to form fine **fibrillin microfibrils** measuring 10–12 nm in diameter. In electron microscopy, a fibrillin microfibril exhibits regular densities (beads) in 56-nm intervals, which are most likely attributed to the three-dimension molecular structure of fibrillin-1. During polymerization, the tail domain (C-terminus) of one fibrillin-1 molecule is folded back when it is cross-linked to the head domain (N-terminus) of another molecule (Fig. 6.15). During the early stages of elastogenesis, fibrillin microfibrils function as substrates for the assembly of elastic fibers. The microfibrils are formed first; elastin molecules are then deposited on the surface of the microfibrils. With both the TEM and scanning electron micrograph (SEM), elastin appears as an amorphous structure of low electron density. In contrast, fibrillin microfibrils are electron dense and are readily apparent even within the elastin matrix (Fig. 6.16). In mature fibers, fibrillin microfibrils are located within the elastic fiber and at its periphery. The presence of microfibrils within the fiber is associated with the growth process; thus, as the fiber is formed and thickens, the microfibrils become entrapped within the newly deposited elastin.

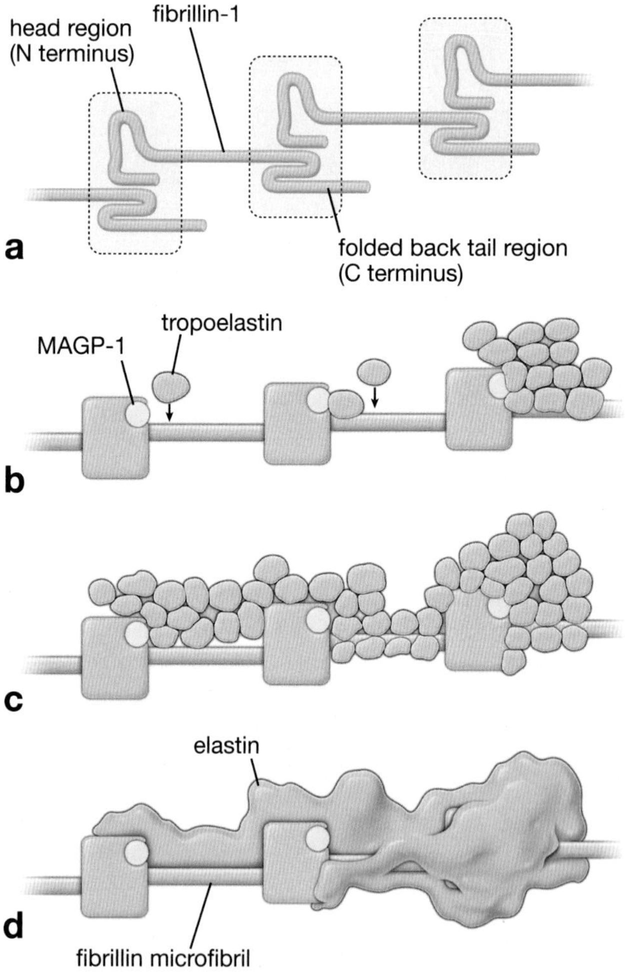

FIGURE 6.15. Diagram of elastogenesis. a. Elastic fibers are formed in the extracellular matrix of connective tissue. This model shows the molecular structure of fibrillar microfibrils. The fibrillin-1 molecule polymerizes in a head-to-tail arrangement to form fibrillin microfibrils. The regular densities (*beads*) are formed by the interactions between the folded-back C-terminus tail domain of one fibrillin-1 molecule with the head domain (N-terminus) of another molecule. **b.** Formation of the elastin fiber is initiated by MAGP-1 molecules, which are associated with microfibrils at the bead region. The presence of MAGP-1 allows the tropoelastin molecule to be deposited on the microfibril, cross-linked to the fibrillin microfibril and MAGP-1. **c.** Tropoelastin molecules are laid down in small clumps. They are cross-linked by lysyl oxidase. **d.** Mature elastin fibers show a gradual fusion of tropoelastin molecules to form amorphous elastin fibers incorporating fibrillin microfibrils in its structure.

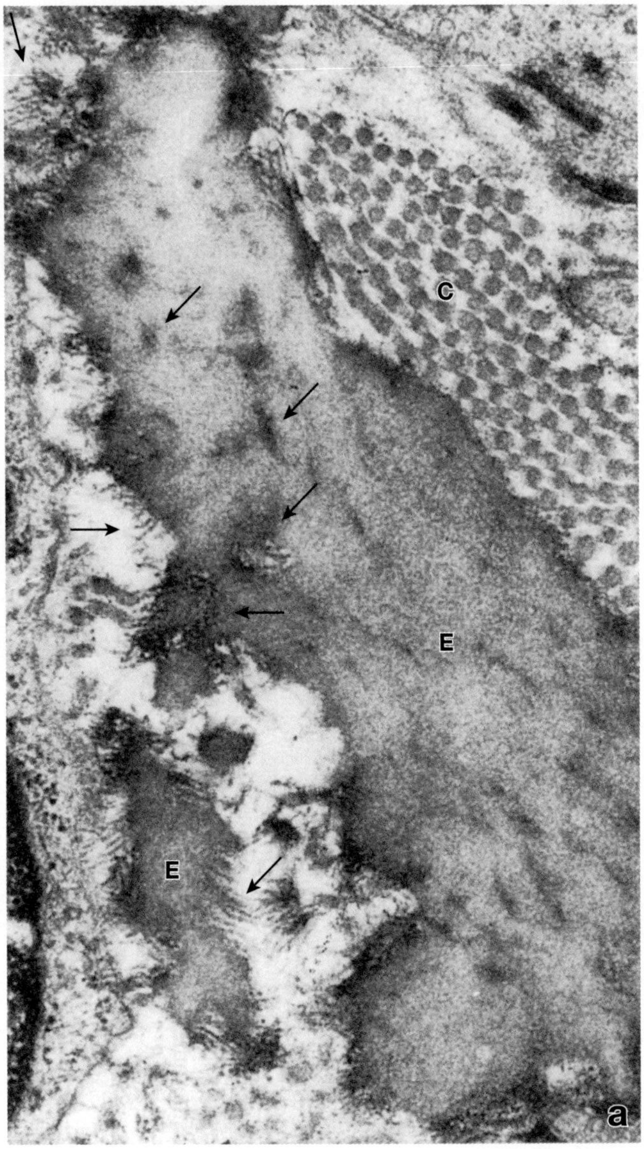

FIGURE 6.16. a. Transmission electron micrograph of an elastic fiber. The elastin (*E*) of the fiber has a relatively amorphous appearance. The fibrillin microfibrils (*arrows*) are present at the periphery and within the substance of the fiber. A number of collagen fibrils (*C*) are also present in this electron micrograph. ×40,000. **b. Scanning electron micrograph of an elastic fiber.** This scanning electron micrograph of the human dense irregular connective tissue from the dermis shows structure of elastic fiber (*E*) and illustrates its relative size in comparison to surrounding collagen fibrils (*C*). Note the presence of small fibrillin microfibrils (*arrows*) at the surface of elastic fiber. ×40,000. (Courtesy of Douglas R. Keene.)

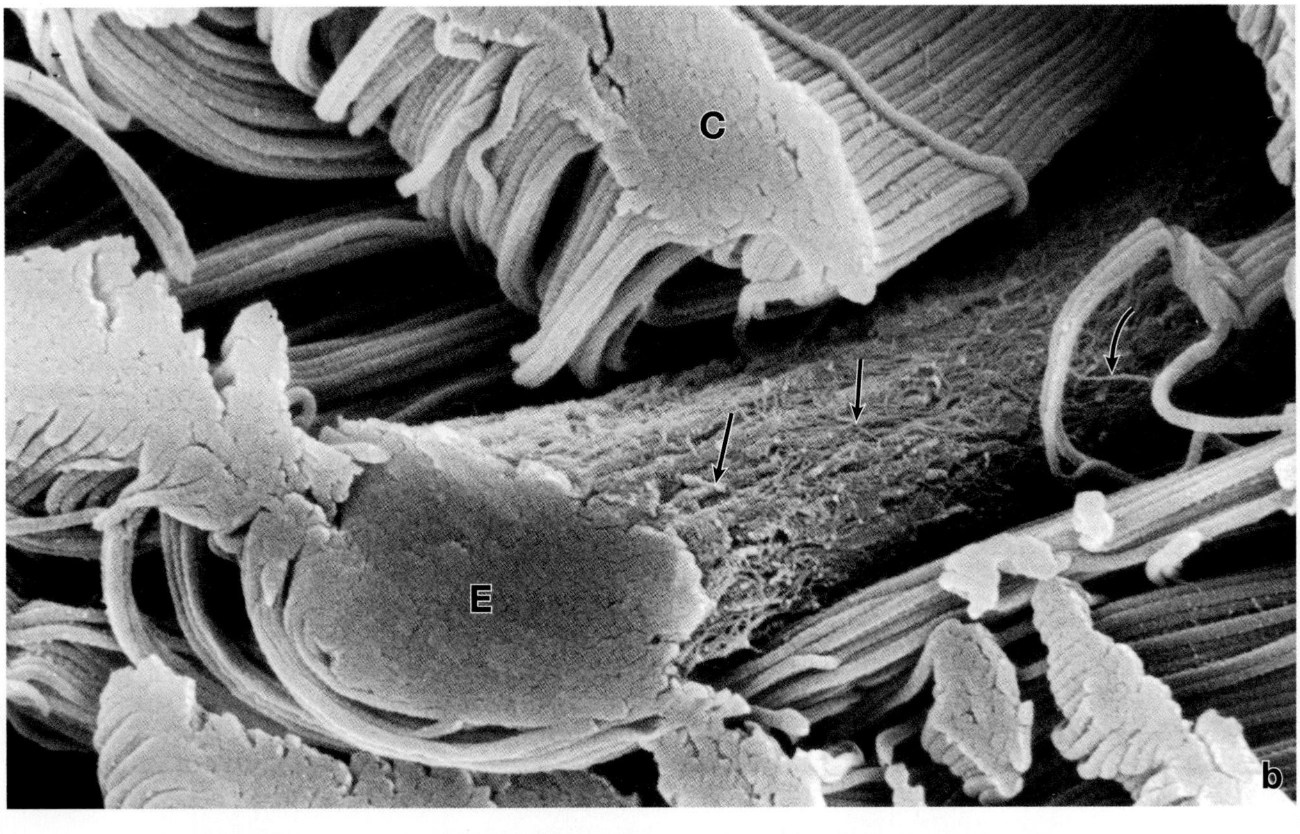

FOLDER 6.2

CLINICAL CORRELATION: SUN EXPOSURE AND MOLECULAR CHANGES IN PHOTOAGED SKIN

Chronologic aging of the skin is a complex process that is associated with functional and structural changes within the stratified squamous epithelium (epidermis) as well as the underlying connective tissue of the dermis. When these changes are intensified by prolonged exposure to solar or ultraviolet (UV) radiation, the process is referred to as **photoaging**. Chronic sun exposure ages the skin at an accelerated rate, especially in exposed areas of the body such as the face, neck, dorsal surface of the hands, and forearms. Clinical signs associated with photoaging include dyspigmentation, freckles, deep wrinkles, increased laxity, and increased risk for cutaneous cancers.

The most prominent changes in the dermis of photoaged skin are associated with connective tissue fibers. Decreased production of type I and type III collagen fibers is observed in normal-aged skin; however, these changes are more pronounced in sun-exposed regions. Sunlight exposure affects collagen biogenesis by altering the cross-linking that occurs between collagen molecules during fibrillogenesis (see pages 185-186). These alterations result in the formation of collagen fibers with abnormal stability and decreased resistance to enzymatic degradation.

The overall number of **elastic fibers** also decreases with age; however, in photoaged skin, the number of abnormally thick and nonfunctional elastic fibers increases. Studies of **fibrillin microfibrils** from photoaged skin reveal that the microfibrillar network is affected by solar radiation. Excessive sun exposure causes the fibrillin microfibrils to undergo extensive changes. They become sparse and truncated, leading to the formation of abnormal extracellular matrix (ECM) characterized by aberrant nonfunctional elastic fibers that eventually degenerate into homogeneous and amorphous elastin-containing masses.

Photoaging is also characterized by abnormal degradation of the connective tissue matrix associated with accumulation of nonfunctional matrix components. Fibroblasts and neutrophils residing in radiation-damaged areas of the skin secrete matrix metalloproteinases (MMP-1 and MMP-9), elastases, and other proteases (cathepsin G). These enzymes are modulated by tissue inhibitors of metalloproteinases (TIMPs) that protect extracellular proteins from endogenous degradation. In photoaged skin, TIMP levels are significantly reduced, which further contributes to photodamage of the skin.

The best strategy to prevent photodamage caused by solar and UV radiation is the use of physical and chemical sunscreens to prevent UV penetration into the skin. Other methods are also used in treating damaged skin, including reducing skin inflammatory reactions with anti-inflammatory medications, inhibiting activities of elastase and other MMPs to prevent degradation of ECM, and stimulating natural or applying synthetic inhibitors of MMPs activities to control destruction of connective tissue ECM.

In addition to fibrillin microfibrils, several associated proteins are involved in the regulation and assembly of elastin fibers, including:

- **EMILIN-1** (elastin microfibril interface-located protein, 106 kDa) is a glycoprotein found at the elastin–fibrillin microfibril interface that most likely regulates the production of elastin aggregates during the formation of fibers.
- **MAGP-1** (microfibril-associated glycoprotein, 20–30 kDa), another glycoprotein, is a component of almost all elastin-associated fibrillin microfibrils. It binds to elastin molecules, fibrillin-1, and various ECM proteins. Both EMILIN-1 and MAGP-1 play a major role in regulating elastogenesis.

Absence of **fibrillin microfibrils** during elastogenesis results in the formation of elastin sheets or lamellae, as found in blood vessels. Abnormal expression of the **fibrillin gene (FBN1)** is linked to **Marfan syndrome**, a complex, autosomal dominant connective tissue disorder. Immunofluorescence of a skin biopsy specimen from a person with this syndrome shows an absence of elastin-associated fibrillin microfibrils. One of the consequences of this disease is abnormal elastic tissue. In addition, mutation in the **EMILIN-1 gene locus** results in alterations of the fine structure of elastic fibers and of cell morphology in the elastic arteries.

Biosynthesis of elastin fibers is similar to that of collagen.

As noted, **elastic fibers** are produced by **fibroblasts** in connective tissue, **chondrocytes** in elastic cartilage, and **smooth muscle** and **endothelial cells** within the walls of the vessels.

Translation of messenger RNA (mRNA) takes place on the surface of rER, and polypeptide chains of tropoelastin are released into the rER lumen. Tropoelastin is then transported to the Golgi apparatus, where it undergoes very little post-translational modification, and is subsequently secreted to the extracellular space. Secretion of tropoelastin occurs only at specific regions of the plasma membrane. These regions correspond to extracellular accumulation of fibrillin microfibrils that form a scaffold upon which elastin is deposited. In the presence of MAGP-1, tropoelastin is laid down in small clumps that gradually fuse to form amorphous elastin fibers incorporating fibrillin microfibrils in its structure (see Fig. 6.15).

Elastin synthesis parallels collagen production; in fact, both processes can occur simultaneously in a cell. The orderly modification and assembly of procollagen and proelastin, as well as the synthesis of other connective tissue components, are controlled by signal sequences that are incorporated into the beginning of the polypeptide chains of each of the molecules. This signal sequence ensures that the components of procollagen and proelastin remain separate and are properly identified as they pass through the organelles of the cell.

■ EXTRACELLULAR MATRIX

The **extracellular matrix (ECM)** is a complex and intricate structural network that surrounds and supports cells within the connective tissue. It contains a variety of fibers such as **collagen** and **elastic fibers** that are formed from different types of structural proteins. In addition, the ECM contains a variety of **proteoglycans** (e.g., aggrecan, syndecan-1), **multiadhesive glycoproteins** (such as fibronectin and laminin), and **glycosaminoglycans** (e.g., dermatan sulfate, keratan sulfate, hyaluronan). The last three groups of molecules constitute the **ground substance**.

All molecules found in the ECM share common domains, and the function of the ECM relies largely on the interactions between these molecules. Each connective tissue cell secretes a different ratio of ECM molecules that contribute to the formation of many different architectural arrangements; therefore, the ECM possesses specific mechanical and biochemical properties characteristic of the tissue in which it is present. For instance, the properties of the ECM in loose connective tissue are different from those of the ECM in cartilage or bone.

The extracellular matrix not only provides mechanical and structural support for tissue but also influences extracellular communication.

The ECM provides mechanical and structural support as well as tensile strength for the tissue. It also functions as a biochemical barrier and plays a role in regulating the metabolic functions of the cells surrounded by the matrix. The ECM anchors cells within tissues through cell-to-ECM adhesion molecules and provides pathways for cell migration (e.g., during wound repair). Recent studies indicate that the ECM exerts a regulatory effect on embryonic development and cell differentiation. The matrix is capable of binding and retaining growth factors, which, in turn, modulate cell growth. With the aid of cell adhesion molecules, the ECM also influences the transmission of information across the plasma membrane of the connective tissue cells. Thus, the current view of ECM components (fibers and ground substance molecules) is that they form a dynamic and interactive system that informs cells about the biochemical and mechanical changes in their extracellular environment.

Ground substance is part of the extracellular matrix that occupies the spaces between the cells and fibers; it consists of glycosaminoglycans, proteoglycans, and multiadhesive glycoproteins.

Ground substance is a viscous, clear substance with a slippery feel and high water content. In the light microscope, ground substance appears amorphous in sections of tissue preserved by freeze drying or in frozen sections stained with basic dyes or by the PAS method. In routine H&E preparations, ground substance is always lost because of its extraction during fixation and dehydration of the tissue. The result is an empty background; only cells and fibers are evident. Thus, in most histologic preparations, the appearance of ground substance—or its lack of appearance—belies its functional importance. Ground substance consists predominately of three groups of molecules: **proteoglycans**, which are very large macromolecules composed of a core protein; **glycosaminoglycan (GAG) molecules**, which are covalently bound to the proteoglycans; and **multiadhesive glycoproteins**. The size and structure of the three groups of molecules vary enormously.

GAGs are responsible for the physical properties of ground substance.

GAGs are the most abundant heteropolysaccharide components of ground substance. These molecules represent long-chain unbranched polysaccharides composed of repeating disaccharide units. The disaccharide units contain one of

TABLE 6.3 Glycosaminoglycans

Name	Molecular Weight (kDa)	Disaccharide Composition	Localization	Function
Hyaluronan	100–10,000	D-Glucuronic acid + *N*-acetylglucosamine	Synovial fluid, vitreous humor, ECM of connective tissues	Large polymers of hyaluronan can displace a large volume of water. Thus, this polymer is an excellent lubricant and shock absorber.
Chondroitin 4-sulfate	25	D-Glucuronic acid + *N*-acetylgalactosamine 4-sulfate	Cartilage, bone, heart valves	Chondroitin sulfates and hyaluronan are fundamental components of aggrecan found in articular cartilage. Aggrecan confers on articular cartilage shock-absorbing properties.
Chondroitin 6-sulfate	25	D-Glucuronic acid + *N*-acetylgalactosamine 6-sulfate		
Dermatan sulfate	35	L-Iduronic acid + *N*-acetylgalactosamine 4-sulfate	Skin, blood vessels, heart valves	Dermatan sulfate proteoglycans have been implicated in cardiovascular disease, tumorigenesis, infection, wound repair, fibrosis, and as a modulator in cell behavior.
Keratan sulfate	10	Galactose or galactose 6-sulfate + *N*-acetylglucosamine 6-sulfate	Bone, cartilage, cornea	Keratan sulfate proteoglycans function in cellular recognition of protein ligands, axonal guidance, cell motility, corneal transparency, and embryo implantation
Heparan sulfate	15	Glucuronic acid or L-iduronic acid 2-sulfate + *N*-sulfamyl-glucosamine or *N*-acetylglucosamine	Basal lamina; normal component of cell surface	Facilitates interactions with fibroblast growth factor (FGF) and its receptor
Heparin	40	Glucuronic acid or L-iduronic acid 2-sulfate + *N*-sulfanyl-glucosamine or *N*-acetylglucosamine 6-sulfate	Limited to granules of mast cells and basophils	Functions as an anticoagulant; facilitates interactions with FGF and its receptor

ECM, extracellular matrix.

two modified sugars enzymes—***N*-acetylgalactosamine (GalNAc) transferase** or ***N*-acetylglucosamine (GlcNAc) transferase**—and a uronic acid such as **glucuronate** or **iduronate**. GAGs (except hyaluronan) are synthesized by connective tissue cells as a covalent, post-translational modification of proteins called **proteoglycans**. For example, heparin is formed by enzymatic cleavage of heparan sulfate; dermatan sulfate is similarly modified from chondroitin sulfate.

GAGs are **highly negatively charged** because of the sulfate and carboxyl groups located on many of the sugars, hence their propensity for staining with basic dyes. The high density of the negative charge (polyanions) also attracts water, forming a hydrated gel. The gel-like composition of ground substance permits rapid diffusion of water-soluble molecules. At the same time, the rigidity of the GAGs provides a structural framework for the cells. GAGs are located primarily within the ground substance as well as on the surface of cells within the ECM. On the basis of differences in specific sugar residues, the nature of their linkages, and the degree of their sulfation, a family of seven distinct GAGs is recognized. They are listed and partially characterized in Table 6.3.

Hyaluronan is always present in the extracellular matrix as a free carbohydrate chain.

The GAG **hyaluronan (hyaluronic acid)** deserves special note because it differs from the other GAGs in several respects. It is an exceedingly long, rigid molecule composed of a carbohydrate chain of thousands of sugars rather than the several hundred or fewer sugars found in other GAGs. Hyaluronan molecules are very large (100–10,000 kDa) and can hold a large volume of water. They are synthesized by enzymes on the cell surface; therefore, they are not post-translationally modified like all other GAGs. Hyaluronan is also unique among the GAGs in that it does not contain sulfate.

Each hyaluronan molecule is always present in the form of a free carbohydrate chain; in other words, it is not covalently bound to protein, so it does not form proteoglycans. By means of special **link proteins**, however, proteoglycans indirectly bind to hyaluronan, forming giant macromolecules called **proteoglycan aggregates** (Fig. 6.17). These molecules are abundant in the ground substance of cartilage. The pressure, or turgor, that occurs in these giant hydrophilic proteoglycan aggregates accounts for the ability of cartilage to resist compression without inhibiting flexibility, making them excellent shock absorbers.

Another important function of **hyaluronan** is to immobilize certain molecules in the desired location of the ECM. For instance, ECM contains binding sites for several growth factors, such as TGF-β. The binding of growth factors to proteoglycans may cause either their local aggregation or dispersion, which, in turn, either inhibits or enhances the movement of migrating macromolecules, microorganisms, or metastatic cancer cells in the extracellular environment. In addition, hyaluronan molecules act as efficient insulators because other macromolecules have difficulty diffusing through the dense hyaluronan network. With this property, hyaluronan (and other polysaccharides) regulates the distribution and transport of plasma proteins within the connective tissue.

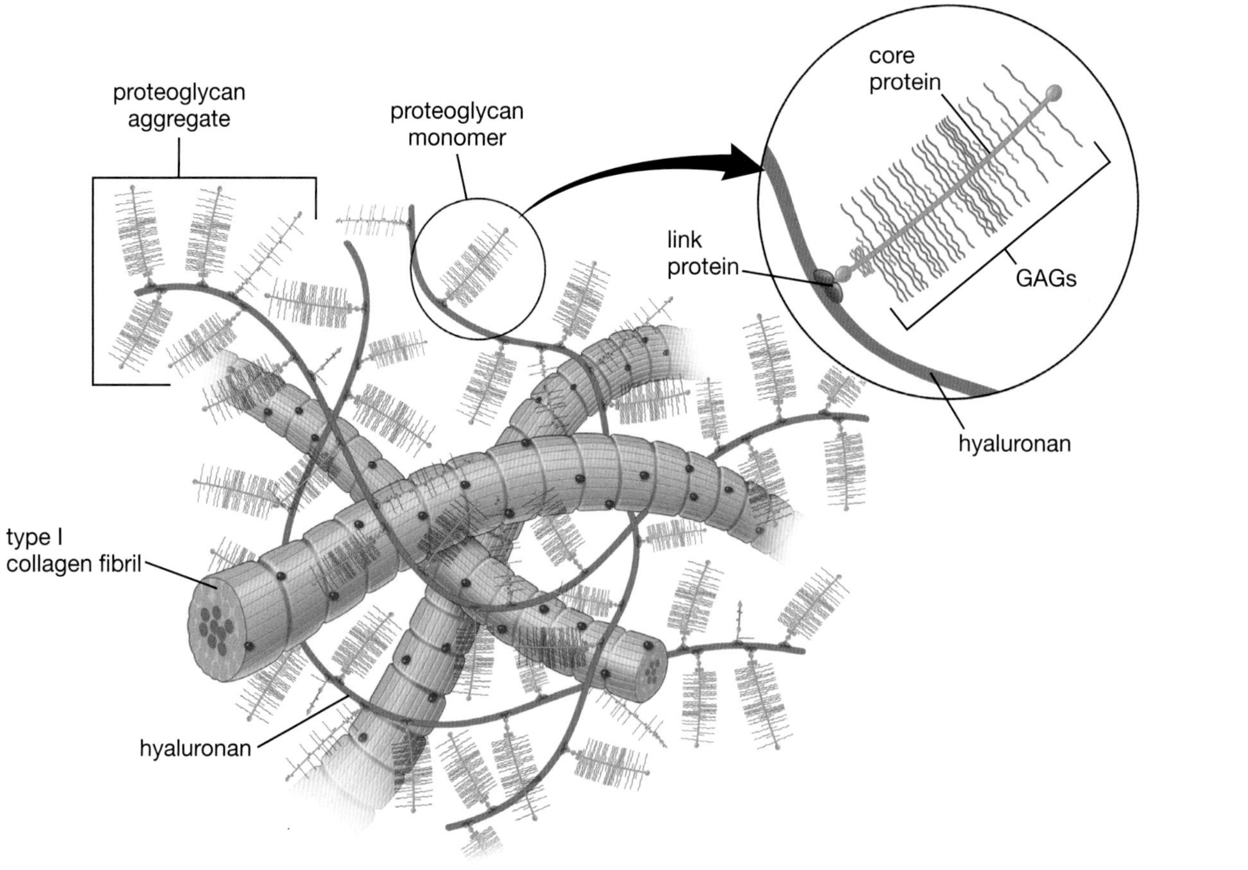

FIGURE 6.17. Proteoglycan structure. This schematic drawing shows, on the *right*, a proteoglycan monomer and its relationship to the hyaluronan molecule as represented in the ground substance of cartilage. The proteoglycan monomer consists of different numbers of *GAGs* covalently bound to the core protein. The end of the core protein of the proteoglycan monomer interacts with a link protein, which attaches the monomer to the hyaluronan forming the proteoglycan aggregate. On the *left*, hyaluronan molecules forming linear aggregates, each with many proteoglycan monomers, are interwoven with a network of collagen fibrils.

Proteoglycans are composed of GAGs covalently attached to core proteins.

The majority of GAGs in the connective tissue are linked to core proteins, forming **proteoglycans**. The GAGs extend perpendicularly from the core in a brush-like structure. The linkage of GAGs to the protein core involves a specific trisaccharide composed of two galactose residues and a xylulose residue. The trisaccharide linker is coupled through an *O*-glycosidic bond to the protein core that is rich in serine and threonine residues, allowing multiple GAG attachments. Proteoglycans are remarkable for their diversity (Fig. 6.18). The number of GAGs attached to the protein core varies from 1 (i.e., decorin) to more than 200 (i.e., aggrecan). A core protein may have identical GAGs attached to it (as in the case of fibroglycan or versican) or different GAG molecules (as in the case of aggrecan or syndecan-1).

Proteoglycans are found in the ground substance of all connective tissues and also as membrane-bound molecules on the surface of many cell types. Transmembrane proteoglycans, such as **syndecan-1**, link cells to ECM molecules (see Fig. 6.18). Syndecan-1 carries 3–5 heparan sulfate and chondroitin sulfate chains that allow for interaction with a large variety of ligands including fibroblast growth factors (FGFs), vascular endothelial growth factor (VEGF), TGF-β, and ECM molecules, such as fibronectin. As an example of this function, syndecan-1 is expressed on the surface of B lymphocytes at two different phases of their development. Syndecan-1 molecules are first expressed during early development when lymphocytes are attached to the matrix protein of the bone marrow as they undergo differentiation. The loss of expression of this proteoglycan coincides with the release of the B lymphocyte into the circulation. The second time B lymphocytes express syndecan-1 is during its differentiation into a plasma cell within the connective tissue. Syndecan-1 anchors the plasma cell to the ECM proteins of the connective tissue.

Aggrecan (1,000–2,500 kDa) is another important extracellular proteoglycan. Its molecules are noncovalently bound to the long molecule of hyaluronan (like bristles to the backbone in a bottle brush); this binding is facilitated by linking proteins. To each aggrecan core protein, multiple chains of chondroitin sulfate and keratan sulfate are covalently attached through the trisaccharide linker. The most common proteoglycans are summarized in Table 6.4. Aggrecan is a cartilage-specific proteoglycan and a critical component in cartilage structure and the function of joints.

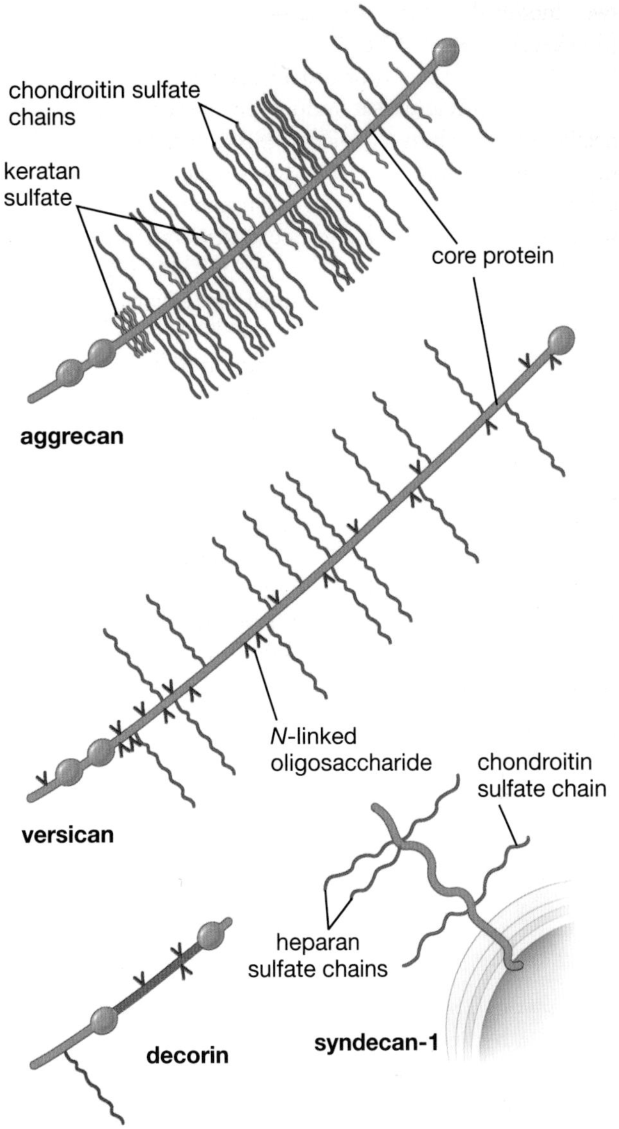

FIGURE 6.18. Common proteoglycan monomers of the connective tissue matrix. Note the diversity of proteoglycan molecules; the number of glycosaminoglycans (*GAGs*) attached to the protein core varies from one in decorin to >200 in aggrecan. Note also that versican has identical *GAG* molecules (chondroitin sulfate) attached to the core molecule, whereas aggrecan has a mixture of chondroitin sulfate and keratan sulfate attached to the core protein. Syndecan-1 is a transmembrane proteoglycan that attaches the cell membrane to the extracellular matrix.

Multiadhesive glycoproteins play an important role in stabilizing the ECM and linking it to cell surfaces.

Multiadhesive glycoproteins represent a small but important group of proteins residing in the ECM. They are multidomain and multifunctional molecules that play an important role in stabilizing the ECM and linking it to the cell surface. They possess binding sites for a variety of ECM proteins, such as collagens, proteoglycans, and GAGs; they also interact with cell surface receptors, such as integrin and laminin receptors (Fig. 6.19). Multiadhesive glycoproteins regulate and modulate functions of the ECM related to cell movement and cell migration as well as stimulate cell proliferation and differentiation. Among the best characterized multiadhesive glycoproteins are the following:

- **Fibronectin** (250–280 kDa) is the most abundant glycoprotein in connective tissue. Fibronectins are dimer molecules formed from two similar peptides linked by disulfide bonds at a carboxy-terminus to form 50-nm-long arms (see Fig. 6.19). Each molecule contains several binding domains that interact with different ECM molecules (e.g., heparan sulfate; collagen types I, II, and III; fibrin; hyaluronan; and fibronectin) and integrin, a cell surface receptor. Binding to a cell surface receptor activates fibronectin, which then assembles into fibrils. Fibronectin plays an important role in cell attachment to the ECM. At least 20 different fibronectin molecules have been identified to date.
- **Laminin** (140–400 kDa) is present in basal and external laminae. It possesses binding sites for collagen type IV molecules, heparan sulfate, heparin, entactin, laminin, and the laminin receptor on the cell surface. The process of basal lamina assembly and the role of the laminin in this process are described in Chapter 5, Epithelial Tissue (see pages 155-158).

TABLE 6.4 Proteoglycans

Name	Molecular Weight (kDa)	Molecular Composition	Localization	Function
Aggrecan	2,500	Linear molecule; binds via a link protein to hyaluronan; contains ~100 molecules of keratan sulfate and ~60 chondroitin sulfate chains	Cartilage, chondrocytes	Responsible for hydration of extracellular matrix of cartilage
Decorin	38	Small protein that contains only one chondroitin sulfate or dermatan sulfate chain	Connective tissue, fibroblasts, cartilage, and bone	Functions in collagen fibrillogenesis; by attaching to neighboring collagen molecules, helps to orient fibers; regulates thickness of the fibril and interacts with transforming growth factor β (TGF-β)
Versican	260	Associated with a link protein; contains 12–15 chains of chondroitin sulfate attached to a core protein	Fibroblasts, skin, smooth muscle, brain, and mesangial cells of the kidney	Possesses EGF-like domains on the core protein; participates in cell-to-cell and cell-to-extracellular matrix interactions; binds to fibulin-1
Syndecan-1	33	Family of at least four different types of transmembrane proteoglycans, containing varying amounts of both heparan sulfate and chondroitin sulfate molecules	Embryonic epithelia, mesenchymal cells, developing lymphatic tissue cells, lymphocytes, and plasma cells	The extracellular domain binds collagens, heparin, tenascin, and fibronectin; intracellular domain binds to cytoskeleton via actin

EGF, epithelial growth factor.

- **Tenascin** (280 kDa per monomer) appears during embryogenesis, but its synthesis is switched off in mature tissues. It reappears during wound healing and is also found within musculotendinous junctions and malignant tumors. Tenascin is a disulfide-linked dimer molecule that consists of six chains joined at their amino-terminus (see Fig. 6.19). It has binding sites for fibrinogen, heparin, and EGF-like growth factors; thus, it participates in cell attachment to the ECM.
- **Osteopontin** (44 kDa) is present in the ECM of bone. It binds to osteoclasts and attaches them to the underlying bone surface. Osteopontin plays an important role in sequestering calcium and promoting calcification of the ECM.

Important multiadhesive glycoproteins found in the ECM of connective tissue are summarized in Table 6.5.

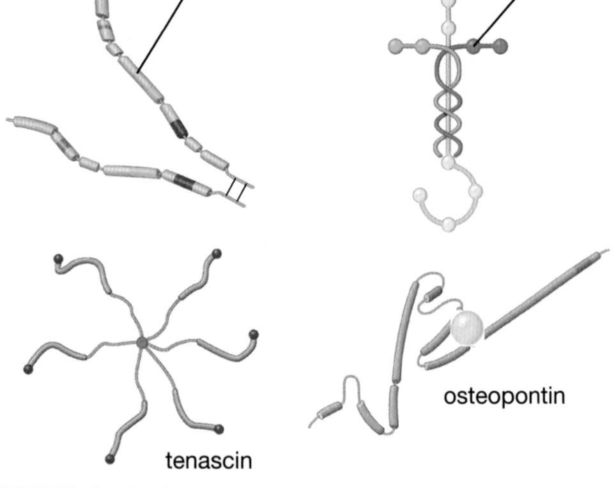

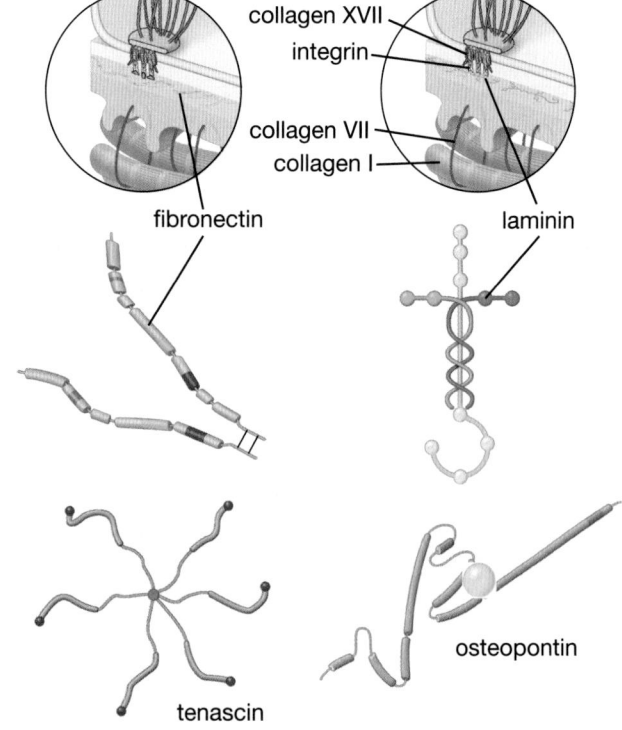

FIGURE 6.19. Common multiadhesive glycoproteins. These proteins reside in the extracellular matrix and are important in stabilizing the matrix and linking it to the cell surface. They are multifunctional molecules of different shapes and possess multiple binding sites for a variety of extracellular matrix proteins, such as collagens, proteoglycans, and GAGs. Note that multiadhesive proteins interact with basal membrane receptors, such as integrin and laminin receptors.

■ CONNECTIVE TISSUE CELLS

Connective tissue cells can be resident or wandering.

The cells that make up the **resident cell population** are relatively stable; they typically exhibit little movement and can be regarded as permanent residents of the tissue. These resident cells include

- **fibroblasts** and a closely related cell type, the **myofibroblast**;
- **macrophages**;
- **adipocytes**;
- **mast cells**; and
- **adult stem cells**.

TABLE 6.5 Multiadhesive Glycoproteins

Name	Molecular Weight (kDa)	Molecular Composition	Localization	Function
Fibronectin	250–280	Dimer molecule formed from two similar peptides linked by a disulfide bond	Present in the ECM of many tissues	Responsible for cell adhesion and mediates migration; possesses binding sites for integrins, type IV collagen, heparin, and fibrin
Laminin	140–400	Cross-shaped molecule formed from three polypeptides (α-chain and two β-chains)	Present in basal laminae of all epithelial cells and external laminae of muscle cells, adipocytes, and Schwann cells	Anchors cell surfaces to the basal lamina; possesses binding sites for collagen type IV, heparan sulfate, heparin, entactin, laminin, and integrin receptors on the cell surface
Tenascin	1,680	Giant protein formed from six chains connected by disulfide bonds	Embryonic mesenchyme, perichondrium, periosteum, musculotendinous junctions, wounds, tumors	Modulates cell attachments to the ECM; possesses binding sites for fibronectin, heparin, EGF-like growth factors, integrins, and CAMs
Osteopontin	44	Single-chain glycosylated polypeptide	Bone	Binds to osteoclasts; possesses binding sites for calcium, hydroxyapatite, and integrin receptors on the osteoclast membrane
Entactin/nidogen	150	Single-chain rod-like–sulfated glycoprotein	Basal lamina–specific protein	Links laminin and type IV collagen; has binding sites for perlecan and fibronectin

CAM, cell adhesion molecule; *ECM*, extracellular matrix; *EGF*, epithelial growth factor.

The **wandering cell population** or **transient cell population** consists primarily of cells that have migrated into the tissue from the blood in response to specific stimuli. These include

- **lymphocytes**,
- **plasma cells**,
- **neutrophils**,
- **eosinophils**,
- **basophils**, and
- **monocytes**.

Fibroblasts and Myofibroblasts

The fibroblast is the principal cell of connective tissue.

Fibroblasts are responsible for the synthesis of collagen, elastic, and reticular fibers and the complex carbohydrates of the ground substance. Research suggests that a single fibroblast is capable of producing all of the ECM components.

Fibroblasts reside in close proximity to collagen fibers. In routine H&E preparations, however, often, only the nucleus is visible. It appears as an elongated or disc-like structure, sometimes with a nucleolus evident. The thin, pale-staining, flattened processes that form the bulk of the cytoplasm are usually not visible, largely because they blend with the collagen fibers. In some specially prepared specimens, it is possible to distinguish the cytoplasm of the cell from the fibrous components (Fig. 6.20a). When ECM material is produced during active growth or in wound repair (in **activated fibroblasts**), the cytoplasm of the fibroblast is more extensive and may display basophilia as a result of increased amounts of rER associated with protein synthesis (Fig. 6.20b). When examined with the TEM, the fibroblast cytoplasm exhibits profiles of rER and a prominent Golgi apparatus (Fig. 6.21).

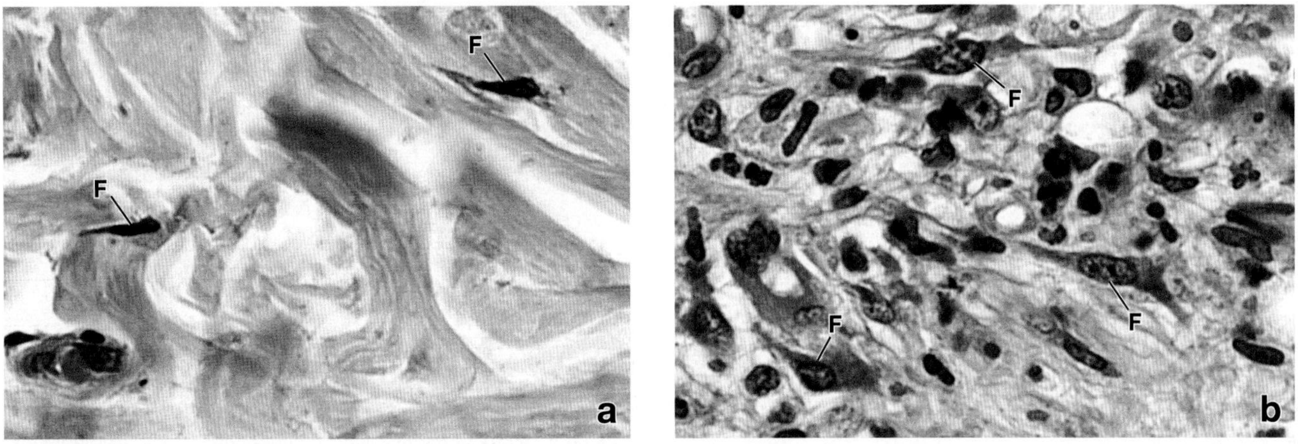

FIGURE 6.20. Fibroblasts in connective tissue. a. Photomicrograph of a connective tissue specimen in a routine hematoxylin and eosin (H&E)-stained, paraffin-embedded preparation shows nuclei of fibroblasts (*F*). ×600. **b.** During wound repair, the activated fibroblasts (*F*) exhibit more basophilic cytoplasm, which is readily observed with the light microscope. ×500.

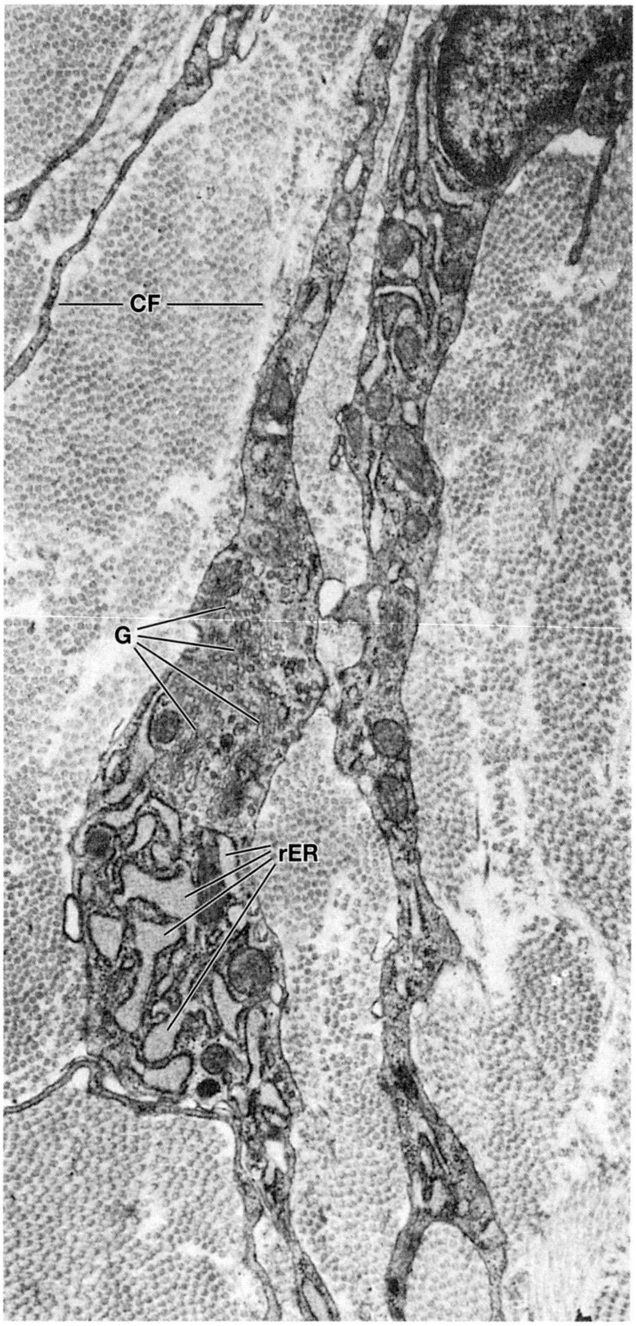

FIGURE 6.21. Electron micrograph of fibroblasts. The processes of several fibroblasts are shown. The nucleus of one fibroblast is in the *upper right* of the micrograph. The cytoplasm contains conspicuous profiles of rough endoplasmic reticulum (*rER*). The cisternae of the reticulum are distended, indicating active synthesis. The membranes of the Golgi apparatus (*G*) are seen in proximity to the *rER*. Surrounding the cells are collagen fibrils (*CF*), almost all of which have been cut in cross section and thus appear as *small dots* at this magnification. ×11,000.

The myofibroblast displays properties of both fibroblasts and smooth muscle cells.

The **myofibroblast** is an elongated, spindly connective tissue cell not readily identifiable in routine H&E preparations. It is characterized by the presence of bundles of actin filaments with associated actin motor proteins such as nonmuscle myosin (page 76). Expression of **α-smooth muscle actin** (α-SMA; actin isoform found in vascular smooth muscles) in myofibroblasts is regulated by TGF-β1. The actin bundles transverse the cell cytoplasm, originating and terminating on the opposite sides of the plasma membrane. The site where actin fibers attach to the plasma membrane also serves as a cell-to-ECM anchoring junction and is called a **fibronexus**; it resembles the focal adhesion found in epithelial cells (see pages 160-162). The arrangement of actin bundles and their attachment sites form a **mechanotransduction system**, in which forces generated by the contraction of intracellular actin bundles are transmitted to the ECM.

With the TEM, the myofibroblast displays characteristics typical of a fibroblast along with characteristics of smooth muscle cells. In addition to rER and Golgi profiles, the myofibroblast contains bundles of longitudinally disposed actin filaments and dense bodies similar to those observed in smooth muscle cells (Fig. 6.22). As in the smooth muscle

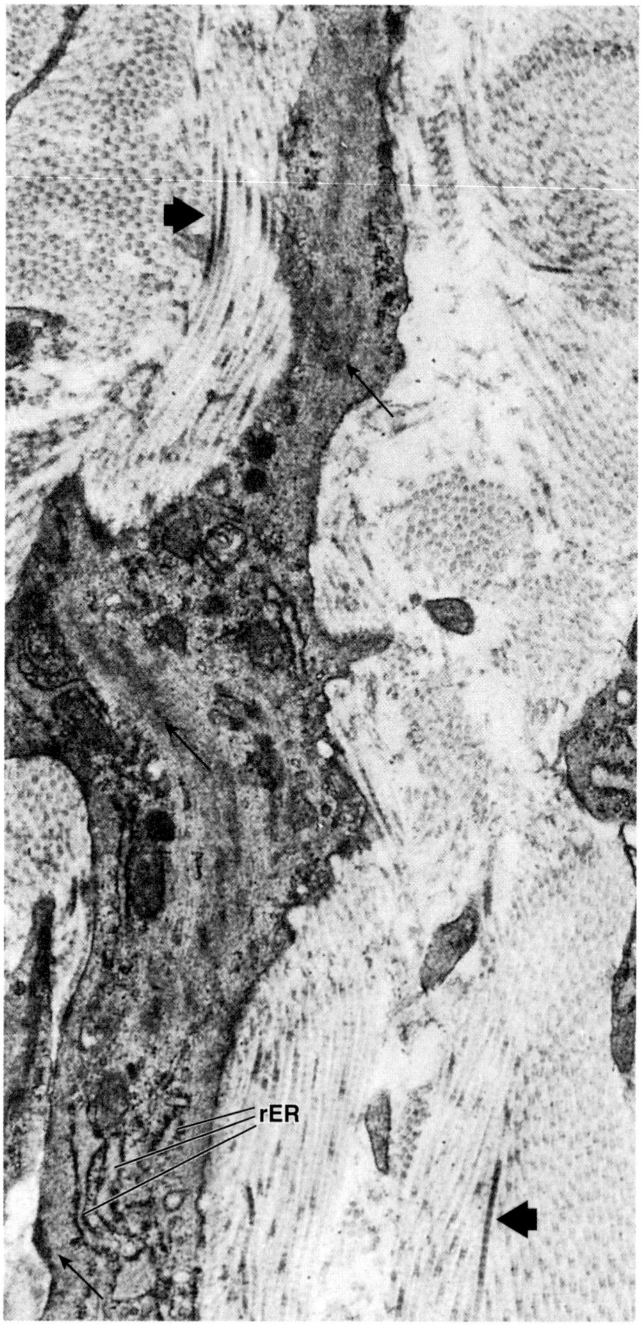

FIGURE 6.22. Electron micrograph of a myofibroblast. The cell exhibits some features of a fibroblast, such as areas with a moderate amount of rough endoplasmic reticulum (*rER*). Compare with Figure 6.21. Other areas, however, contain aggregates of thin filaments and cytoplasmic densities (*arrows*), features that are characteristic of smooth muscle cells. The *arrowheads* indicate longitudinal profiles of collagen fibrils. ×11,000.

cell, the nucleus often shows an undulating surface profile, a phenomenon associated with cell contraction. The myofibroblast differs from the smooth muscle cell in that it lacks a surrounding basal lamina (smooth muscle cells are surrounded by a basal or external lamina). Also, it usually exists as an isolated cell, although its processes may contact the processes of other myofibroblasts. Such points of contact exhibit gap junctions, indicating intercellular communication.

Macrophages

Macrophages are phagocytic cells derived from monocytes that contain an abundant number of lysosomes.

Connective tissue **macrophages**, also known as tissue **histiocytes**, are derived from blood cells called **monocytes**. Monocytes migrate from the bloodstream into the connective tissue, where they differentiate into macrophages.

In the light microscope and with conventional stains, tissue macrophages are difficult to identify unless they display obvious evidence of **phagocytic activity**—for example, visible ingested material within their cytoplasm. Another feature that assists in identifying macrophages is an indented or kidney-shaped nucleus (Fig. 6.23a). Lysosomes are abundant in the cytoplasm and can be revealed by staining for acid phosphatase activity (both in the light microscope and with the TEM); a positive reaction is a further aid in the identification of the macrophage. With the TEM, the surface of the macrophage exhibits numerous folds and finger-like projections (Fig. 6.23b). The surface folds engulf the substances to be phagocytosed. The lysosomes of the macrophage, along with the surface cytoplasmic projections, are the structures most indicative of the specialized phagocytic capability of the cell. The macrophage may also contain endocytotic vesicles, phagolysosomes, and other evidence of phagocytosis (e.g., residual bodies).

The rER, smooth ER (sER), and Golgi apparatus support the synthesis of proteins involved in the cell's phagocytic and digestive functions, as well as its secretory functions. Secretory products leave the cell by both the constitutive and regulated exocytotic pathways. Regulated secretion can be activated by phagocytosis, immune complexes, complement, and signals from lymphocytes (including the release of

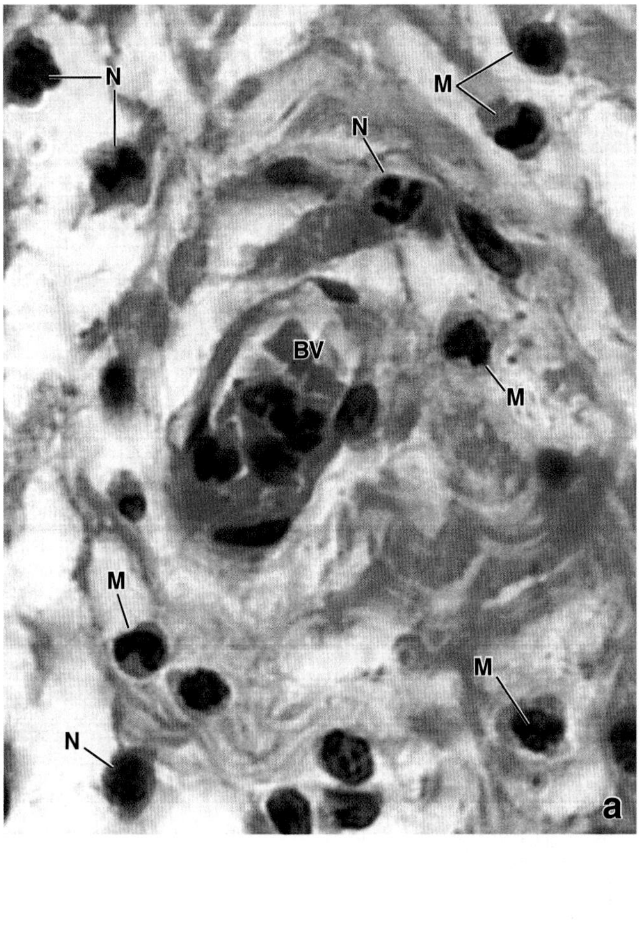

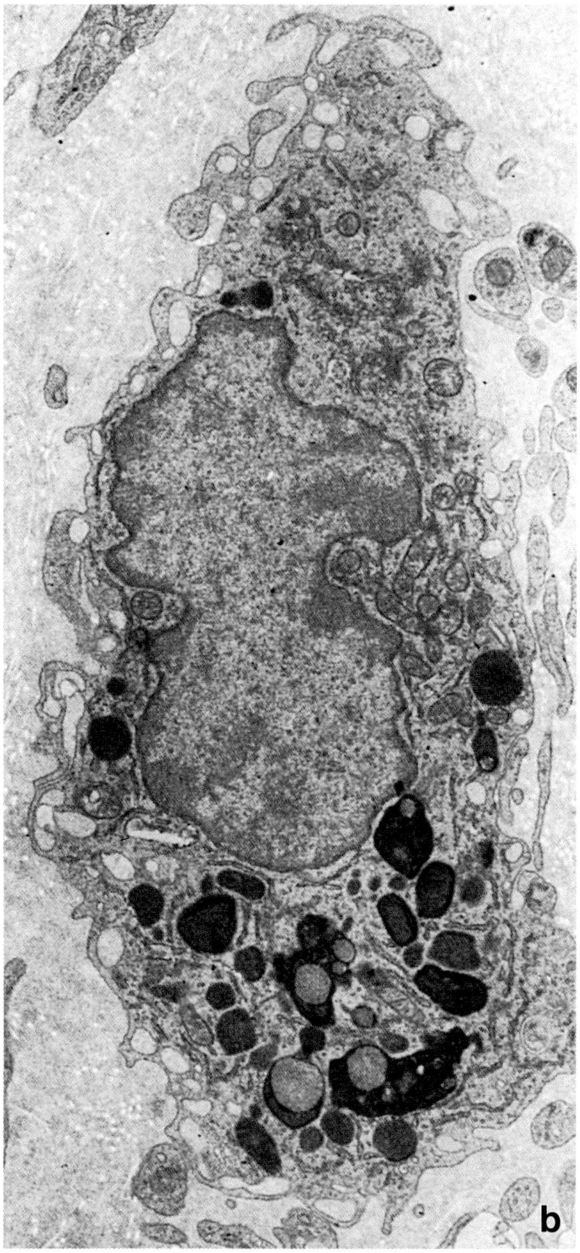

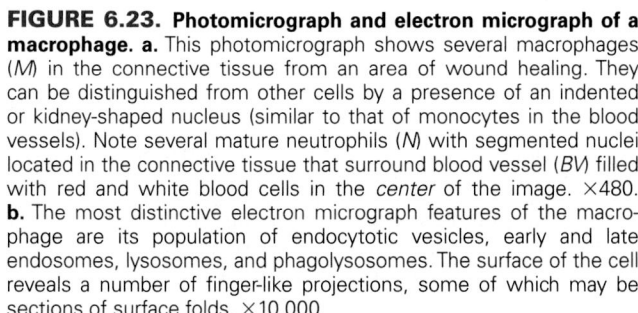

FIGURE 6.23. Photomicrograph and electron micrograph of a macrophage. a. This photomicrograph shows several macrophages (*M*) in the connective tissue from an area of wound healing. They can be distinguished from other cells by a presence of an indented or kidney-shaped nucleus (similar to that of monocytes in the blood vessels). Note several mature neutrophils (*N*) with segmented nuclei located in the connective tissue that surround blood vessel (*BV*) filled with red and white blood cells in the *center* of the image. ×480. **b.** The most distinctive electron micrograph features of the macrophage are its population of endocytotic vesicles, early and late endosomes, lysosomes, and phagolysosomes. The surface of the cell reveals a number of finger-like projections, some of which may be sections of surface folds. ×10,000.

lymphokines, biologically active molecules that influence the activity of other cells). The secretory products released by the macrophage include a wide variety of substances related to the immune response, anaphylaxis, and inflammation. The release of neutral proteases and GAGases (enzymes that break down GAGs) facilitates the migration of macrophages through the connective tissue.

Macrophages are antigen-presenting cells and play an important role in immune response reactions.

Although the main function of the macrophage is phagocytosis, either as a defense activity (e.g., phagocytosis of bacteria) or as a cleanup operation (e.g., phagocytosis of cell debris), it also plays an important role in immune response reactions.

Macrophages have specific proteins on their surface known as **major histocompatibility complex II (MHC II)** molecules that allow them to interact with **helper CD4$^+$ T lymphocytes**. When macrophages engulf a foreign cell, antigens—short polypeptides (7–10 amino acids long) from the foreign cell—are displayed on the surface of the MHC II molecules. If a CD4$^+$ T lymphocyte recognizes the displayed antigen, it becomes activated, triggering an immune response (see Chapter 14, Immune System and Lymphatic Tissues and Organs, pages 492-493). Because macrophages "present" antigens to helper CD4$^+$ T lymphocytes, they are known as **antigen-presenting cells (APCs)**.

Macrophages arrive after neutrophils at the site of tissue injury and undergo differentiation.

At the site of tissue injury, the first cells to reach the injured area are neutrophils. They are the first cells to recognize foreign organisms or infectious agents and initiate destruction by either reactive oxygen intermediates or oxygen-independent killing mechanisms (see pages 310-311). During this destruction process, large amounts of secretory products and cellular debris are generated at the site of injury. In addition, microorganisms that survived the action of neutrophils may also be present. After 24 hours, monocytes from blood vessels enter the site of injury and differentiate into macrophages, where they remain until inflammation resolves. Initially, the macrophage's objective is to kill microorganisms that have survived the attack of neutrophils. Simultaneously, macrophages are activated by the interaction with several molecules produced by neutrophils and invading microorganisms. During this process, macrophages undergo a series of functional, morphologic, and biochemical modifications triggered by various gene activations.

Classically activated macrophages (M1 macrophages) promote inflammation, the destruction of ECM, and apoptosis.

Activation by interferon γ (IFN-γ), tumor necrosis factor α (TNF-α), or by bacterial lipopolysaccharide (LPS) creates the **classically activated macrophage** or **M1 macrophage**. These macrophages have the capacity, through the production of nitric oxide (NO) and other intermediates, to destroy microorganisms at the site of inflammation. They also secrete interleukin (IL)-12, which stimulates helper CD4$^+$ T lymphocytes. In turn, helper T cells secrete IL-2, which stimulates cytotoxic CD8$^+$ T lymphocytes to arrive at the site of inflammation. In summary, M1 macrophages elicit **chronic inflammation** and **tissue injury**. When macrophages encounter large foreign bodies, they may fuse to form a large cell with as many as 100 nuclei that engulfs the foreign body. These multinucleated cells are called **foreign-body giant cells (Langhans cells)**.

Alternatively activated macrophages (M2 macrophages) assist in the resolution of inflammation and promote rebuilding of ECM, cell proliferation, and angiogenesis.

When the inflammatory stimulus is removed from the site of tissue injury, the body switches into a repair mode that includes the removal of cell debris, synthesis of components of new ECM, and revascularization of the injured tissue. During this period, macrophages are activated by cytokines IL-4, IL-5, IL-10, or IL-13. These types of cells are called **alternatively activated macrophages or M2 macrophages**. M2 macrophages are anti-inflammatory in that they assist in **resolution of inflammation**. They secrete IL-4 to promote differentiation of B lymphocytes into plasma cells and VEGF to stimulate angiogenesis. M2 macrophages also secrete ECM components (e.g., fibronectin and other multiadhesive glycoproteins). They promote **wound repair** owing to their anti-inflammatory, proliferative, and angiogenic activities. M2 macrophages are also efficient at combating parasitic infections (i.e., schistosomiasis). In addition to their beneficial activities, M2 macrophages are involved in pathogenesis of **allergy** and **asthma**.

Mast Cells

Mast cells develop in the bone marrow and differentiate in connective tissue.

Mast cells are large, ovoid, connective tissue cells (20–30 μm in diameter) with a spherical nucleus and cytoplasm filled with large, intensely basophilic granules. They are not easily identified in human tissue sections unless special fixatives are used to preserve the granules. After glutaraldehyde fixation, mast cell granules can be displayed with basic dyes, such as toluidine blue. It stains the granules intensely and metachromatically because they contain heparin, a highly sulfated proteoglycan (Fig. 6.24a). The cytoplasm displays small amounts of rER, mitochondria, and a Golgi apparatus. The cell surface contains numerous microvilli and folds.

The **mast cell** is related, but not identical, to the basophil, a white blood cell that contains similar granules (Table 6.6). They both arise from a pluripotential **hemopoietic stem cell (HSC)** in the bone marrow. **Mast cell progenitors** (MCPs) initially circulate in the peripheral blood as agranular cells of monocytic appearance. After migrating into the connective tissue, these immature cells differentiate and produce their characteristic granules (Fig. 6.24b). In contrast, **basophil progenitors** (BaPs) differentiate and remain within the circulatory system. The surface of mature mast cells expresses a large number of **high-affinity F_c receptors (FcεRI)** to which immunoglobulin E (IgE) antibodies are attached. Binding of a specific antigen to exposed IgE antibody molecules on the mast cell surface leads to an aggregation of F_c receptors. This triggers mast cell activation, which results in granule exocytosis (degranulation) and the release of granule content into the ECM. Mast cells can also be activated by an IgE-independent mechanism during complement protein activation.

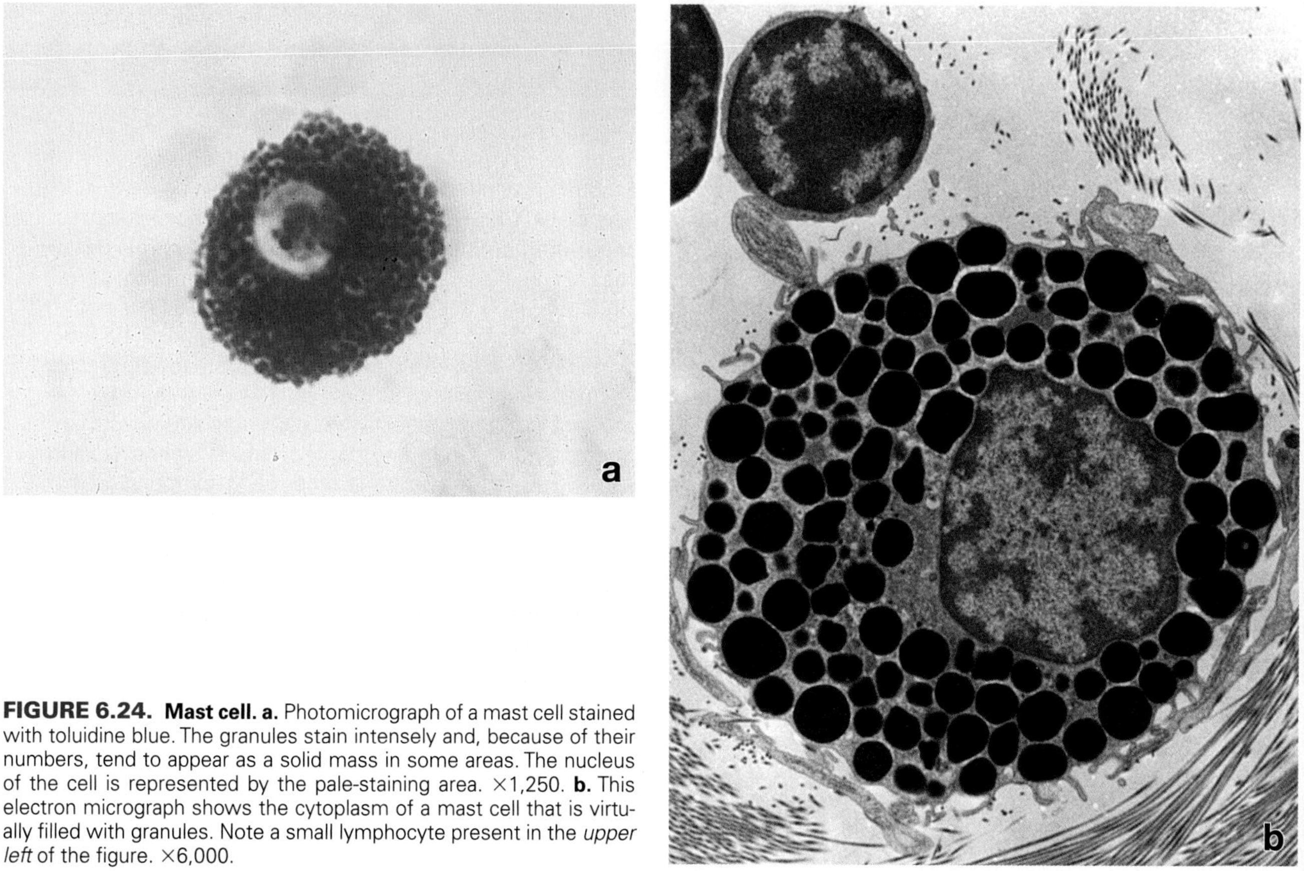

FIGURE 6.24. Mast cell. a. Photomicrograph of a mast cell stained with toluidine blue. The granules stain intensely and, because of their numbers, tend to appear as a solid mass in some areas. The nucleus of the cell is represented by the pale-staining area. ×1,250. **b.** This electron micrograph shows the cytoplasm of a mast cell that is virtually filled with granules. Note a small lymphocyte present in the *upper left* of the figure. ×6,000.

Two types of human mast cells have been identified based on morphologic and biochemical properties. Most mast cells in the connective tissue of the skin, intestinal submucosa, mammary glands, and axillary lymph nodes contain cytoplasmic granules with a lattice-like internal structure. These cells contain granule-associated tryptase and chymase and are referred to as **MC_{TC} mast cells or connective tissue mast cells**. In contrast, mast cells in the lungs and intestinal mucosa have granules with a scroll-like internal structure. These cells produce only tryptase and are termed **MC_T mast cells or mucosal mast cells**. Nearly equivalent concentrations of each type are found in nasal mucosa.

Mast cells are especially numerous in the connective tissues of skin and mucous membranes but are not present in the brain and spinal cord.

Connective tissue mast cells (**MC_{TC} mast cells**) are distributed chiefly in the connective tissue of skin in the vicinity of small blood vessels, hair follicles, sebaceous glands, and sweat glands. Mast cells are also present in the capsules of organs and the connective tissue that surrounds the blood vessels of internal organs. A notable exception is the central nervous system. Although the **meninges** (sheets of connective tissue that surround the brain and spinal cord) contain mast cells, the connective tissue around the small

TABLE 6.6 Comparison of Features Characteristic of Mast Cells and Basophils

Characteristic Features	Mast Cells	Basophils
Origin	Hemopoietic stem cell	Hemopoietic stem cell
Site of differentiation	Connective tissue	Bone marrow
Cell divisions	Yes (occasionally)	No
Cells in circulation	No	Yes
Life span	Weeks to months	Days
Size	20–30 μm	7–10 μm
Shape of nucleus	Round	Segmented (usually bilobar)
Granules	Many, large, metachromatic	Few, small, basophilic
High-affinity surface receptors for IgE antibodies (FcεRI)	Present	Present
Marker of cellular activity	Tryptase	Not yet established

IgE, immunoglobulin E; *FcεRI*, Fc receptors.

FOLDER 6.3

CLINICAL CORRELATION: ROLE OF MYOFIBROBLASTS IN WOUND REPAIR

An important role of myofibroblasts occurs during the process of **wound healing**. A clean surgical skin incision begins the healing process when a **blood clot** containing fibrin and blood cells fills the narrow space between the edges of the incision. The **inflammatory process**, which begins as early as 24 hours after the initial injury, contains the damage to a small area, aids in the removal of injured and dead tissues, and initiates the deposition of new ECM proteins. During the initial phases of inflammation, neutrophils and monocytes infiltrate the injury (maximum infiltration by neutrophils occurs in the first 1–2 days after injury). Monocytes transform into macrophages (they usually replace neutrophils by day 3 after injury; page 312). At the same time, in response to local growth factors, fibroblasts and vascular endothelial cells begin to proliferate and migrate into the delicate fibrin matrix of the blood clot, forming the **granulation tissue**, a specialized type of tissue characteristic of the repair process. Usually by day 5 after injury, the fully developed granulation tissue bridges the incision gap. It is composed mainly of large numbers of small vessels, fibroblasts, and myofibroblasts and variable numbers of other inflammatory cells.

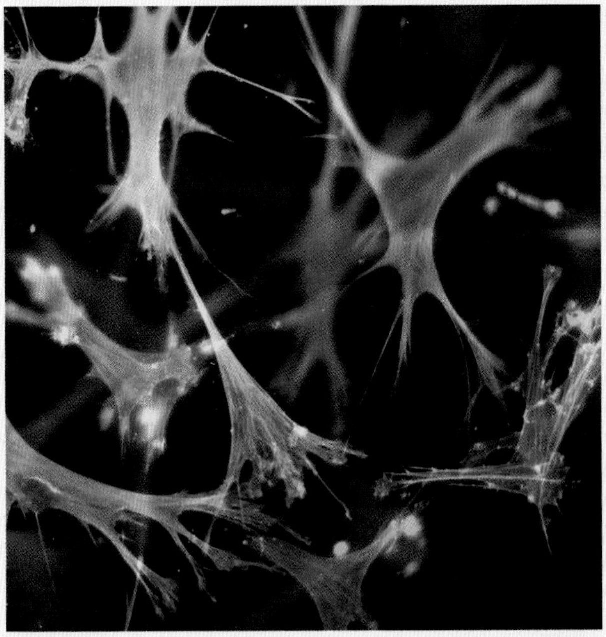

FIGURE F6.3.1. Fibroblasts and myofibroblasts in culture. This immunofluorescence image shows wild-type 3T3 fibroblasts cultured on a collagen lattice. Under the stimulation of certain growth factors such as TGF-β1, some fibroblasts differentiate to myofibroblasts, expressing α-SMA, the marker of myofibroblast differentiation. Cells were stained with fluorescein-labeled phalloidin to visualize F-actin filaments (*green*), and α-SMA were labeled with primary antibodies against α-SMA and visualized with secondary goat anti-mouse antibodies conjugated with FITC (*red*). Co-localization of α-SMA with F-actin is indicated by the *yellow* color. Note that some cells have completed their differentiation, and others are in the early stages. ×1,000. *α-SMA*, α smooth muscle actin; *TGF-β1*, tumor growth factor β1. (Courtesy of Dr. Boris Hinz.)

Migrating fibroblasts exert tractional forces on the ECM, reorganizing it along lines of stress. Under the influence of growth factors such as transforming growth factor β1 (TGF-β1) and mechanical forces, fibroblasts undergo differentiation into **myofibroblasts**. This process can be visualized by monitoring the synthesis of α smooth muscle actin (α-SMA). This type of actin is not present in the cytoplasm of fibroblasts (Fig. F6.3.1). The myofibroblasts generate and maintain a steady contractile force (similar to that of smooth muscle cells) that causes shortening of the connective tissue fibers and wound closure. At the same time, myofibroblasts synthesize and lay down collagen fibers and other ECM components that are responsible for tissue remodeling.

During the second week of wound healing, the number of cells in tissue undergoing repair decreases; most of the myofibroblasts undergo apoptosis and disappear, resulting in a **connective tissue scar** that has very few cellular elements. In some pathologic conditions, myofibroblasts persist and continue the process of remodeling. This continued remodeling causes **hypertrophic scar** formation, resulting in excessive connective tissue contracture. Extensive numbers of myofibroblasts are found in most contractive diseases of connective tissue (fibromatoses). For example, **palmar fibromatosis (Dupuytren disease)** is characterized by the thickening of palmar aponeurosis, which leads to progressive flexion contracture of the fourth and fifth digits of the hand (Fig. F6.3.2). If scar tissue grows beyond the boundaries of the original wound and does not regress, it is called a **keloid**. Its formation is more common among African Americans than other ethnic groups.

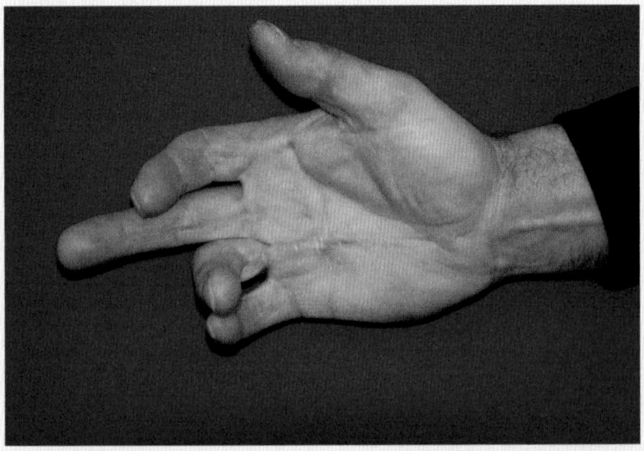

FIGURE F6.3.2. Hand of a patient with Dupuytren disease. Dupuytren disease is an example of a contractive disease of connective tissue of the palm. The most commonly affected areas—near the crease of the hand close to the base of the ring and small fingers—form contracted fibrous cords, which are infiltrated by an extensive number of myofibroblasts. Most patients report problems when they try to place the affected hand on a flat surface. In severe cases, the fingers are permanently flexed and interfere with everyday activities, such as washing hands or placing the hand into a pocket. (Courtesy of Dr. Richard A. Berger.)

FOLDER 6.4

FUNCTIONAL CONSIDERATIONS: THE MONONUCLEAR PHAGOCYTE SYSTEM

The originally proposed classification of macrophages, monocytes, and their precursors into the **mononuclear phagocyte system (MPS)** was based on their common morphology, function, origin, and cell kinetics. Recent studies challenging the classic MSP concept that all macrophages are derived from monocytes propose that resident macrophages are instead maintained entirely by self-renewal.

MPS cells represent a network of phagocytic cells primarily involved in phagocytosis and antigen processing and antigen presentation. MSP cells are composed of monocytes, macrophages, and dendritic cells and are classified depending on their physical and functional characteristics. **Monocytes** are circulating cells and can easily travel from the blood into the tissue compartment where they differentiate into macrophages. Directed by signaling molecules, **macrophages** migrate within target tissues toward a destination point, where they react with foreign substances, pathogens, and microorganisms to initiate an immune response. They also secrete chemokines and cytokines and express various receptors, such as pattern recognition receptors (PRRs), receptors for complement, and receptors for F_c fragments of immunoglobulins (Ig). **Dendritic cells** are antigen-presenting cells with phagocytic functions in the adaptive immune response

As mentioned earlier, the original classification was built on the presumption that all macrophages are derived from monocytes that originate from bone marrow hematopoietic stem cells. It is now accepted that cells of the MPS arise from two distinct populations of progenitor cells in separate waves during hematopoiesis. The early population derives from the **erythro-myeloid progenitor cells** originating from the **yolk sac** (extraembryonic primitive hematopoietic wave). These embryonic macrophages are first seen at 3–4 weeks of gestation and develop independently from blood monocytes. They migrate to developing tissues and organs and become **resident macrophages**. The second population originates from **bone marrow hematopoietic stem cells** (definitive hematopoietic wave) and represents **monocyte-derived macrophages.** Monocytes first appear in the circulation much later in development, at about the 17th week of gestation. Therefore, it is important to understand that MPS cells represent a mixed type of cell population with different embryologic origins. Both populations of macrophages are antigen-presenting cells; however, they demonstrate different phenotypes and divergent functionality. Yolk sac–derived resident macrophages are self-sustaining and represent a resident self-renewing phagocytic population in the tissues, whereas monocyte-derived macrophages are replenished from an influx of circulating monocytes.

Resident tissue macrophages also adapt to each tissue environment to perform specific functions. For example, **microglia cells** represent small, stellate cells located primarily along the capillaries of the central nervous system that function as phagocytic cells. They arise from erythro-myeloid progenitor cells in the yolk sac and migrate and differentiate in the central nervous system during the embryonic and perinatal stages of development. Similarly, macrophages of the liver (**Kupffer cells**), lungs (**alveolar macrophages**), and skin (**Langerhans cells**) are also yolk sac derived; their acquisition of tissue-specific macrophage phenotypes correlates with the development and maturation of organs where they reside. Microglial cells in the brain and Langerhans cells in the skin cannot be replenished by bone marrow–derived monocytes.

Similarly, **osteoclasts** derived from the fusion of granulocyte/macrophage progenitor cells (GMP) are also included in the MPS. Also, fibroblasts of the subepithelial sheath of the lamina propria of the intestine and uterine endometrium have been shown to differentiate into cells with morphologic, enzymatic, and functional characteristics of resident connective tissue macrophages.

The various cells of the MPS are listed in the following table.

Cells of the Mononuclear Phagocyte System

Cells	Location
Monocytes and their precursors in bone marrow: monoblasts and promonocytes	Blood and bone marrow
Resident macrophages	Connective tissue, spleen, lymph nodes, bone marrow, adipose tissue, and thymus
Dendritic cells	Lymph nodes, spleen
Stellate sinusoidal macrophages (Kupffer cell)	Liver
Alveolar macrophages	Lungs
Mesangial cells	Kidney
Placental macrophages (Hofbauer cell)	Placenta
Pleural and peritoneal macrophages	Serous cavities
Microglia	Central nervous system
Langerhans cells	Epidermis of skin, oral mucosa, foreskin, female genital epithelium
Intestinal macrophages	Gastrointestinal tract: submucosa and lamina propria
Peritubular and interstitial macrophages	Testis
Osteoclasts (originate from hemopoietic progenitor cells)	Bone
Fibroblast-derived macrophages (originate from mesenchymal cells)	Lamina propria of intestine, endometrium of uterus
Multinucleated giant cells (e.g., foreign-body giant cells, Langhans giant cells; originate from fusion of several macrophages)	Pathologic granulomas: suture granuloma, tuberculosis

blood vessels within the brain and spinal cord is devoid of mast cells. The absence of mast cells protects the brain and spinal cord from the potentially disruptive effects of the edema caused by allergic reactions. Mast cells are also numerous in the thymus and, to a lesser degree, in other lymphatic organs, but they are not present in the spleen.

Most mast cell secretory products (mediators of inflammation) are stored in granules and released at the time of mast cell activation.

Mast cells contain intensely basophilic granules that store chemical substances known as **mediators of inflammation**. Mediators produced by mast cells are divided into two categories: **preformed mediators** that are stored in secretory granules and released upon cell activation and **newly synthesized mediators** (mostly lipids and cytokines) that are often absent in the resting cells, although they are produced and secreted by activated mast cells.

Preformed mediators found inside mast cell granules are the following:

- **Histamine** is a biogenic amine that increases the permeability of small blood vessels, causing edema in the surrounding tissue and a skin reaction demonstrated by an itching sensation. In addition, it increases mucus production in the bronchial tree and prompts contraction of smooth muscle in the pulmonary airways. Histamine's effects can be blocked by **antihistaminic agents**. These competitive inhibitors have a similar chemical structure and bind to histamine receptors without initiating histamine's effects.
- **Heparin** is a sulfated GAG that is an anticoagulant. Its expression is limited essentially to the granules of mast cells and basophils. When heparin unites with antithrombin III and platelet factor IV, it can block numerous coagulation factors. On the basis of its anticoagulant properties, heparin is useful for the treatment of **thrombosis**. It also interacts with FGF and its receptor to induce signal transduction in the cells.
- **Serine proteases** (tryptase and chymase). **Tryptase** is selectively concentrated in the secretory granules of human mast cells (but not basophils). It is released by mast cells together with histamine and serves as a marker of mast cell activation. **Chymase** plays an important role in generating angiotensin II in response to vascular tissue injury. Mast cell chymase also activates MMPs and induces apoptosis of vascular smooth muscle cells, particularly in the area of atherosclerotic lesions.
- **Eosinophil chemotactic factor (ECF)** and **neutrophil chemotactic factor (NCF)**, which attract eosinophils and neutrophils, respectively, to the site of inflammation. The secretions of eosinophils counteract the effects of histamine and leukotrienes.

Newly synthesized mediators include the following:

- **Leukotriene C (LTC_4)** is released from the mast cell and then cleaved in the ECM, yielding two active leukotrienes—**D (LTD_4)** and **E (LTE_4)**. They represent a family of modified lipids conjugated to glutathione (LTC_4) or cysteine (LTD_4 and LTE_4). Leukotrienes are released from mast cells during anaphylaxis (see Folder 6.5 for a description of anaphylaxis) and promote inflammation, including eosinophil migration and the increase in vascular permeability. Similar to histamine, leukotrienes trigger prolonged constriction of smooth muscle in the pulmonary airways, causing **bronchospasm**. The bronchoconstrictive effects of leukotrienes develop more slowly and last much longer than the effects of histamine. Bronchospasm caused by leukotrienes can be prevented by **leukotriene receptor antagonists** (blockers), but not by antihistaminic agents. The leukotriene receptor antagonists are among the most prescribed drugs for the management of **asthma**; they are used for both the treatment and prevention of acute asthma attacks.
- **Tumor necrosis factor α (TNF-α)** is a major cytokine produced by mast cells. It increases expression of adhesion molecules in endothelial cells and has antitumor effects.
- Several **interleukins (IL-4, IL-3, IL-5, IL-6, IL-8, and IL-16), growth factors (GM-CSF), and prostaglandin D_2 (PGD_2)** are also released during mast cell activation. These mediators are not stored in granules but are synthesized by the cell and released immediately into the ECM.

Mediators released during mast cell activation as a result of interactions with allergens are responsible for a variety of symptoms and signs that are characteristic of **allergic reactions**.

Basophils

Basophils that develop and differentiate in the bone marrow share many features with mast cells.

Basophils are granulocytes that circulate in the bloodstream and comprise less than 1% of peripheral white blood cells (leukocytes). Developmentally, they represent a separate lineage from mast cells, despite sharing a common precursor cell in the bone marrow. Basophils develop and mature in the **bone marrow** and are released into the circulation as mature cells. They also have many other common features with mast cells, such as **basophilic secretory granules**, an ability to secrete similar mediators, and an abundance of **high-affinity F_c receptors for IgE antibodies** on their cell membranes. They participate in allergic reactions (see Folder 6.5) and, together with mast cells, release histamine, heparin, heparan sulfate, ECF, NCF, and other mediators of inflammation. In contrast to mast cells, basophils do not produce PGD_2 and IL-5. Basophils and their features are discussed in more detail in Chapter 10, Blood (pages 313-314).

Adipocytes

The adipocyte is a connective tissue cell specialized to store neutral fat and produce a variety of hormones.

Adipocytes differentiate from mesenchymal stem cells and gradually accumulate fat in their cytoplasm. They are located throughout loose connective tissue as individual cells and groups of cells. When they accumulate in large numbers, they are called **adipose tissue**. Adipocytes are also involved in the synthesis of a variety of hormones, inflammatory mediators, and growth factors. This specialized connective tissue is discussed in Chapter 9, Adipose Tissue, page 280.

FOLDER 6.5

CLINICAL CORRELATION: THE ROLE OF MAST CELLS AND BASOPHILS IN ALLERGIC REACTIONS

Exposure to a specific antigen (allergen) that reacts with IgE antibodies bound to the surface of mast cells or basophils via their high-affinity receptors (FcεRI) initiates mast cell activation. This type of IgE-dependent activation triggers a cascade of events, resulting in an **allergic reaction**. These reactions can occur as immediate hypersensitivity reactions (usually within seconds to minutes after exposure to an allergen), late-phase reactions, or chronic allergic inflammations.

The **immediate hypersensitivity reaction** involves IgE-mediated release of histamine and other mediators from mast cells and also from basophils. The clinical symptoms caused by these mediators vary, depending on which organ system is affected.

The release of mediators in the superficial layers of the skin can manifest as erythema (redness), swelling and itching, or pain sensations. Respiratory symptoms include sneezing, rhinorrhea (runny nose), increased production of mucus, coughing, bronchospasm (constriction of bronchi), and pulmonary edema. Individuals with these symptoms often complain of tightness in the chest, shortness of breath, and wheezing. The gastrointestinal tract can also be affected with symptoms of nausea, vomiting, diarrhea, and abdominal cramping.

In highly sensitive individuals, the antigen injected by an insect can trigger a massive discharge of mast cells and basophil granules that affect more than one system. This condition is known as **anaphylaxis**. Dilation and increased permeability of systemic blood vessels can cause **anaphylactic shock**. This often-explosive, life-threatening reaction is characterized by significant hypotension (decreased blood pressure), decreased circulating blood volume (leaky vessels), and smooth muscle cell constriction in the bronchial tree. The individual has difficulty breathing and may exhibit a rash as well as nausea and vomiting. Symptoms of anaphylactic shock usually develop within 1–3 minutes, and immediate treatment with vasoconstrictors such as epinephrine is required. Clinical assessment of the activation of basophils in systemic anaphylactic reactions is not possible because an assay for a specific cellular marker released by basophils (and not by other cells such as mast cells) has not yet been developed.

Following resolution of the signs or symptoms of an immediate hypersensitivity reaction, an affected individual may develop a **late-phase allergic reaction** 6–24 hours later. The symptoms of these reactions may include redness, persistent swelling of the skin, nasal discharge, sneezing, and coughing, usually accompanied by an elevated white blood cell count. These symptoms usually last a few hours and then disappear within 1–2 days of the initial allergen exposure. In the respiratory system, the late-phase reaction is believed to be responsible for the development of persistent asthma.

If the exposure to an allergen is persistent (for instance, by a dog-owning patient who is allergic to dogs), it can result in **chronic allergic inflammation**. Tissues in such individuals accumulate a variety of immune cells such as eosinophils and T lymphocytes that cause more tissue damage and prolong inflammation. This can lead to permanent structural and functional changes in the affected tissue.

Adult Stem Cells and Pericytes

Niches of adult stem cells are located in various tissues and organs.

Many tissues in mature individuals contain reservoirs of stem cells called **adult stem cells**. Compared with embryonic stem cells, adult stem cells cannot differentiate into multiple lineages. They are usually capable of differentiating only into lineage-specific cells. Adult stem cells are found in many tissues and organs, residing in specific sites referred to as **niches**. Cells residing within niches in various tissues and organs (excluding the bone marrow) are called **tissue stem cells**. They have been identified in the gastrointestinal tract—for instance, in the stomach (isthmus of the gastric gland), small and large intestines (base of the intestinal gland), and many other areas. Bone marrow represents a unique reservoir of stem cells. In addition to containing **hemopoietic stem cells (HSCs)** (see Chapter 10, Blood, see pages 321-322), bone marrow also contains at least two other populations of stem cells: a heterogeneous population of **multipotent adult progenitor cells (MAPCs)** that appear to have broad developmental capabilities and **bone marrow stromal cells (BMSCs)** that can generate chondrocytes, osteoblasts, adipocytes, muscle cells, and endothelial cells. MAPCs are adult counterparts of embryonic stem cells. Niches of adult stem cells, called **mesenchymal stem cells**, are found in the loose connective tissue of adults. These cells give rise to differentiated cells that function in the repair and formation of new tissue, such as in wound healing and the development of new blood vessels (neovascularization).

The vascular pericytes that partially wrap around capillaries and venules are mesenchymal stem cells.

Pericytes, also called **adventitial cells** or **perivascular cells**, are typically wrapped, at least partially, around capillaries and venules (Fig. 6.25). Their nuclei are shaped similarly to that of endothelial cells (i.e., flattened but curved to conform to the tubular shape of the vessel). Several observations support the interpretation that vascular pericytes are indeed mesenchymal stem cells. Experimental studies show that in response to external stimuli, pericytes express a cohort of proteins similar to those of stem cells in the bone marrow. Pericytes are surrounded by basal lamina material that is continuous with the basal lamina of the capillary endothelium; thus, they are not truly located in the connective tissue compartment. The role of pericytes as **mesenchymal stem cells** has been confirmed experimentally in studies that demonstrate the ability of cultured pericytes from retinal capillaries to differentiate into a variety of cells, including osteoblasts, adipocytes, chondrocytes, and fibroblasts.

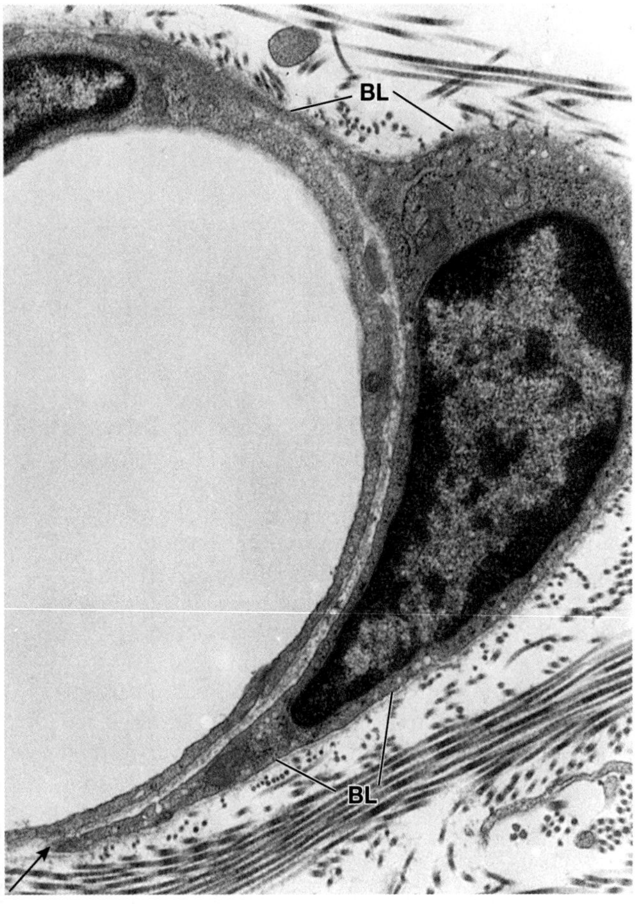

FIGURE 6.25. Electron micrograph of a small blood vessel. The nucleus at the *upper left* belongs to the endothelial cell that forms the wall of the vessel. At the *right* is another cell, a pericyte, which is in intimate relation to the endothelium. Note that the basal lamina (*BL*) covering the endothelial cell divides (*arrow*) to surround the pericyte. ×11,000.

TEM studies demonstrate that pericytes surrounding the smallest venules have cytoplasmic characteristics almost identical to those of the endothelial cells of the same vessel. Pericytes associated with larger venules have characteristics of smooth muscle cells of the tunica media of small veins. In fortuitous sections cut parallel to the long axis of venules, the distal portion and proximal portion of the same pericyte exhibit characteristics of endothelial cells and smooth muscle cells, respectively. These studies suggest that during the development of new vessels, cells with characteristics of **pericytes** may differentiate into smooth muscle found in the vessel wall.

The fibroblasts and blood vessels within healing wounds develop from mesenchymal stem cells associated with the tunica adventitia of venules.

Autoradiographic studies of wound healing using parabiotic (crossed-circulation) pairs of animals have established that mesenchymal stem cells located in the tunica adventitia of venules and small veins are the primary source of new cells in healing wounds. In addition, fibroblasts, pericytes, and endothelial cells in portions of the connective tissue adjacent to the wound divide and give rise to additional cells that form new connective tissue and blood vessels.

Lymphocytes, Plasma Cells, and Other Cells of the Immune System

Lymphocytes are principally involved in immune responses.

Connective tissue **lymphocytes** are the smallest of the wandering cells in the connective tissue (see Fig. 6.24b). They have a thin rim of cytoplasm surrounding a deeply staining, heterochromatic nucleus. Often, the cytoplasm of connective tissue lymphocytes may not be visible. Normally, small numbers of lymphocytes are found in the connective tissue throughout the body. The number increases dramatically, however, at the sites of tissue **inflammation** caused by pathogenic agents. Lymphocytes are most numerous in the lamina propria of the respiratory and gastrointestinal tracts, where they are involved in immunosurveillance against pathogens and foreign substances that enter the body by crossing the epithelial lining of these systems.

Lymphocytes are a heterogeneous population of at least three major functional cell types: T cells, B cells, and natural killer (NK) cells.

At the molecular level, **lymphocytes** are characterized by the expression of specific molecules on the plasma membrane known as a **cluster of differentiation (CD) proteins**. CD proteins recognize specific ligands on target cells. Because some CD proteins are present only on specific types of lymphocytes, they are considered specific marker proteins. On the basis of these specific markers, lymphocytes can be classified into three functional cell types.

- **T lymphocytes** are characterized by the presence of the CD2, CD3, CD5, and CD7 marker proteins and **T-cell receptors (TCRs)**. These cells have a long life span and are effectors in **cell-mediated immunity**.
- **B lymphocytes** are characterized by the presence of CD9, CD19, and CD20 proteins and attached IgM and IgD. These cells recognize antigens, have a variable life span, and are effectors in **antibody-mediated (humoral) immunity**.
- **NK lymphocytes** are non–T, non–B lymphocytes that express CD16a, CD56, and CD94 proteins not found in other lymphocytes. These cells neither produce Igs nor express TCR on their surface. Thus, NK lymphocytes are not antigen specific. Similar in action to T lymphocytes, however, they destroy virus-infected cells and some tumor cells by a cytotoxic mechanism.

In response to the presence of antigens, lymphocytes become activated and may divide several times, producing clones of themselves. In addition, clones of B lymphocytes mature into plasma cells. A description of lymphocytes and their functions during immune response reactions is presented in Chapter 14, Immune System and Lymphatic Tissues and Organs (see pages 487-491).

Plasma cells are antibody-producing cells derived from B lymphocytes.

Plasma cells are a prominent constituent of loose connective tissue at sites where antigens tend to enter the body (e.g., the gastrointestinal and respiratory tracts). They are also a normal component of salivary glands, lymph nodes, and hematopoietic tissue. Once derived from its **B-lymphocyte**

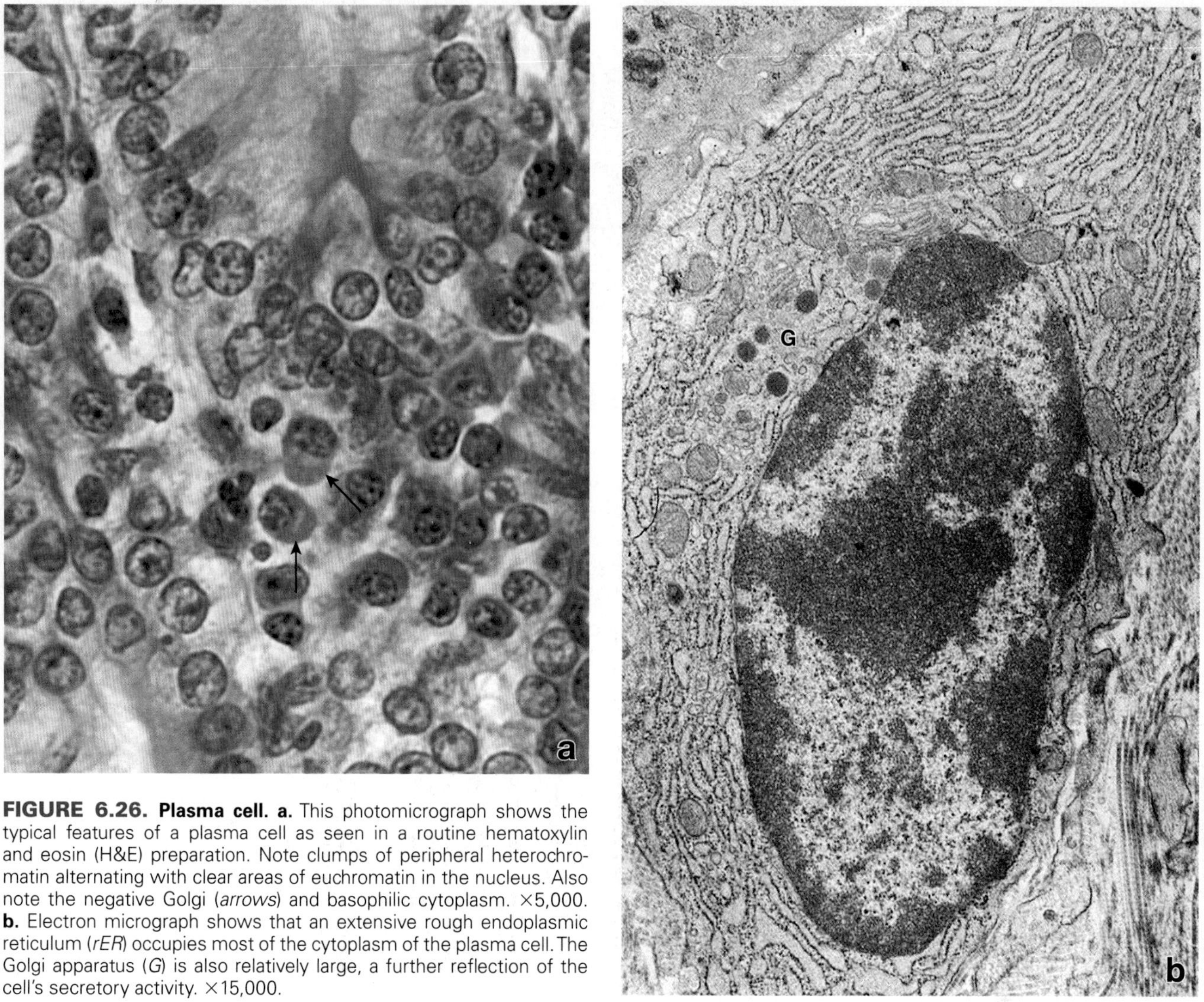

FIGURE 6.26. Plasma cell. a. This photomicrograph shows the typical features of a plasma cell as seen in a routine hematoxylin and eosin (H&E) preparation. Note clumps of peripheral heterochromatin alternating with clear areas of euchromatin in the nucleus. Also note the negative Golgi (*arrows*) and basophilic cytoplasm. ×5,000. **b.** Electron micrograph shows that an extensive rough endoplasmic reticulum (*rER*) occupies most of the cytoplasm of the plasma cell. The Golgi apparatus (*G*) is also relatively large, a further reflection of the cell's secretory activity. ×15,000.

precursor, a plasma cell has only limited migratory ability and a somewhat short life span of 10–30 days.

The plasma cell is a relatively large, ovoid cell (20 μm) with a considerable amount of cytoplasm. The cytoplasm displays strong basophilia because of an extensive rER (Fig. 6.26a). The Golgi apparatus is usually prominent because of its relatively large size and lack of staining. It appears in light microscope preparations as a clear area in contrast to the basophilic cytoplasm.

The **nucleus** is spherical and typically offset or eccentrically positioned. It is small—not much larger than the nucleus of the lymphocyte. It exhibits large clumps of peripheral heterochromatin alternating with clear areas of euchromatin. This arrangement has traditionally been described as resembling a **cartwheel** or **analog clock face**, with the heterochromatin resembling the spokes of the wheel or the numbers on a clock (Fig. 6.26b). The heterochromatic nucleus of the plasma cell is somewhat surprising, given the cell's function in synthesizing large amounts of protein. However, because the cells produce large amounts of only one type of protein—a **specific antibody**—only a small segment of the genome is exposed for transcription.

Eosinophils, monocytes, and neutrophils are also observed in connective tissue.

Certain cells rapidly migrate from the blood to enter the connective tissue, particularly neutrophils and monocytes in response to tissue injury. Their presence generally indicates an acute inflammatory reaction. In these reactions, neutrophils migrate into the connective tissue in substantial numbers, followed by large numbers of monocytes. As noted, the monocytes then differentiate into macrophages. A description of these cells and their roles is found in Chapter 10, Blood (see pages 305-314). The **eosinophil**, which functions in **allergic reactions** and **parasitic infections**, is also described. Eosinophils may be observed in normal connective tissue, particularly the lamina propria of the intestine, as a result of chronic immunologic responses that occur in these tissues.

HISTOLOGY 101 NOTEBOOK

CONNECTIVE TISSUE

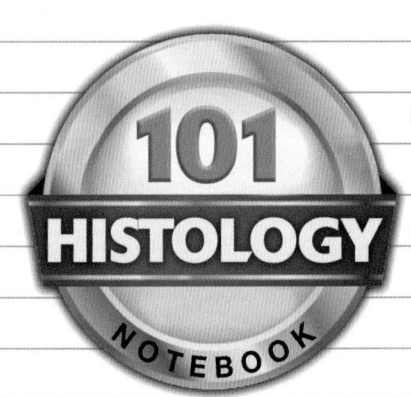

OVERVIEW OF CONNECTIVE TISSUE

- **Connective tissue** forms a continuous compartment throughout the body that connects and supports other tissue. It is bounded by the basal laminae of various epithelia and by the external laminae of muscle cells and nerve-supporting cells.
- Connective tissue comprises a diverse group of **cells** within a tissue-specific **extracellular matrix (ECM)**. ECM contains protein fibers and **ground substance.**
- Classification of connective tissue is primarily based on the composition and organization of its extracellular components and on its functions: **embryonic, connective tissue proper**, and **specialized connective tissue.**

EMBRYONIC CONNECTIVE TISSUES

- **Mesenchyme** is derived from embryonic mesoderm and gives rise to various connective tissues of the body. It contains a loose network of spindle-shaped cells that are suspended in a viscous ground substance containing fine collagen and reticular fibers.
- **Mucous connective tissue** is present in the umbilical cord. It contains widely separated spindle-shaped cells embedded in a gelatin-like, hyaluronan-rich ECM; its ground substance is called **Wharton jelly.**

CONNECTIVE TISSUE PROPER

- **Connective tissue proper** is divided into **loose** and **dense** connective tissue. Dense connective tissue is further subdivided into **dense irregular** and **dense regular** connective tissue.
- **Loose connective tissue** is characterized by large numbers of cells of various types embedded in an abundant gel-like ground substance with loosely arranged fibers. It typically surrounds glands, various tubular organs, and blood vessels and is found beneath the epithelia that cover internal and external body surfaces.
- **Dense irregular connective tissue** contains few cells (primary fibroblasts), randomly distributed bundles of collagen fibers, and relatively little ground substance. It provides significant strength and allows organs to resist excessive stretching and distension.
- **Dense regular connective tissue** is characterized by densely packed, parallel arrays of collagen fibers with cells (tendinocytes) aligned between the fiber bundles. It is the main functional component of tendons, ligaments, and aponeuroses.

CONNECTIVE TISSUE FIBERS

- There are three principal types of **connective tissue fibers**: collagen, reticular, and elastic fibers.
- **Collagen fibers** are the most abundant structural components of connective tissue. They are flexible, have a high-tensile strength, and are formed from **collagen fibrils** that exhibit a characteristic 68-nm banding pattern.
- **Collagen fiber formation** involves events that occur both within the fibroblasts (production of procollagen molecules) and outside the fibroblasts in the ECM (polymerization of collagen molecules into fibrils, which are assembled into larger collagen fibers).
- **Reticular fibers** are composed of **type III collagen** and provide a supporting framework for cells in various tissues and organs (abundant in lymphatic tissues).
- In the lymphatic and hemopoietic tissues, reticular fibers are produced by specialized **reticular cells**. In most other tissues, reticular fibers are produced by fibroblasts.
- **Elastic fibers** are produced by fibroblasts, chondrocytes, endothelial cells, and smooth muscle cells. They allow tissues to respond to stretch and distension.
- Elastic fibers are composed of cross-linked **elastin** molecules associated with a network of **fibrillin microfibrils**, which are made of fibrillin and fibrillin-associated proteins (EMILINs and MAGPs).

EXTRACELLULAR MATRIX

- The **ECM** provides mechanical and structural support for connective tissue, influences extracellular communication, and provides pathways for cell migration. In addition to protein fibers, the ECM contains ground substance that is rich in **proteoglycans**, hydrated **glycosaminoglycans (GAGs)**, and **multiadhesive glycoproteins**.
- **GAGs** are the most abundant heteropolysaccharide components of ground substance. These molecules are composed of long-chain unbranched polysaccharides containing many sulfate and carboxyl groups. They covalently bind to core proteins to form **proteoglycans** that are responsible for the physical properties of ground substance.
- The largest and longest GAG molecule is **hyaluronan**. By means of special **link proteins**, proteoglycans indirectly bind to hyaluronan, forming giant macromolecules called **proteoglycan aggregates**.
- The binding of water and other molecules (e.g., growth factors) to proteoglycan aggregates regulates the movement and migration of macromolecules, microorganisms, and metastatic cancer cells in the ECM.
- **Multiadhesive glycoproteins** (e.g., fibronectin, laminin, and tenascin) are multifunctional molecules that possess binding sites for a variety of ECM proteins (e.g., collagens, proteoglycans, and GAGs). They also interact with cell surface receptors, such as integrin and laminin receptors.

CONNECTIVE TISSUE CELLS

- Connective tissue cells are classified as part of the **resident cell population** (relatively stable, nonmigratory) or the **wandering** (or **transient**) **cell population** (primarily cells that have migrated from blood vessels).
- **Resident cells** include fibroblasts (and myofibroblasts), macrophages, adipocytes, mast cells, and adult stem cells. **Wandering (transient) cells** include lymphocytes, plasma cells, neutrophils, eosinophils, basophils, and monocytes (described in Chapter 10, Blood, see pages 305-314).
- **Fibroblasts** are the principal cells of connective tissue. They are responsible for the synthesis of collagen and other components of the ECM.
- Fibroblasts that express actin filaments and associated actin motor proteins such as nonmuscle myosin are called **myofibroblasts.**
- **Macrophages** are phagocytic cells derived from **monocytes** that contain an abundant number of lysosomes and play an important role in immune response reactions.
- **Adipocytes** are specialized connective tissue cells that store neutral fat and produce a variety of hormones (see Chapter 9, Adipose Tissue, page 280).
- **Mast cells** develop in the bone marrow and differentiate in connective tissue. They contain basophilic granules that store mediators of inflammation. Upon activation, mast cells synthesize leukotrienes, interleukins, and other inflammation-promoting cytokines.
- **Adult stem cells** reside in specific locations (called **niches**) in various tissues and organs. They are difficult to distinguish from other cells of connective tissue.

PLATE 6.1 ■ LOOSE AND DENSE IRREGULAR CONNECTIVE TISSUE

Loose and dense irregular connective tissue represents two of the several types of connective tissue. The others are namely cartilage, bone, blood, adipose tissue, and reticular tissue. **Loose connective tissue** is characterized by a relatively high proportion of cells within a matrix of thin and sparse collagen fibers. In contrast, **dense irregular connective tissue** contains few cells, almost all of which are fibroblasts that are responsible for the formation and maintenance of the abundant collagen fibers that form the matrix of this tissue. The cells that are typically associated with loose connective tissue are **fibroblasts**, the collagen-forming cells, and those cells that function in the immune system and those of the body's general defense system. Thus, in loose connective tissue, there are, to varying degrees, lymphocytes, macrophages, eosinophils, plasma cells, and mast cells.

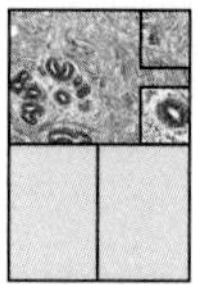

Loose and dense irregular connective tissue, mammary gland, human, hematoxylin and eosin (H&E) ×175; insets ×350.

This micrograph shows at low magnification both loose connective tissue (*LCT*) and dense irregular connective tissue (*DICT*) for comparative purposes. The **loose connective tissue** surrounds the glandular epithelium (*GE*). The **dense irregular connective tissue** consists mainly of thick bundles of collagen fibers with few cells present, whereas the loose connective tissue has a relative paucity of fibers and a considerable number of cells. The *upper inset* is a higher magnification of the dense connective tissue. Note that only a few cell nuclei are present relative to the larger expanse of collagen fibers. The *lower inset*, revealing the glandular epithelium and surrounding loose connective tissue, shows very few fibers but large numbers of cells. Typically, the cellular component of loose connective tissue contains a relatively small proportion of fibroblasts but large numbers of lymphocytes, plasma cells, and other connective tissue cell types.

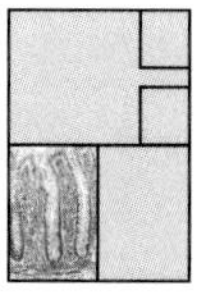

Loose connective tissue, colon, monkey, Mallory trichrome ×250.

This micrograph reveals an extremely cellular **loose connective tissue** (*LCT*), also called lamina propria, which is located between the intestinal glands of the colon. The simple, columnar, mucus-secreting epithelial cells seen here represent the glandular tissue. The Mallory stain colors cell nuclei *red* and collagen *blue*. Note how the cells are surrounded by a framework of blue-stained collagen fibers. Also shown in this micrograph is a band of smooth muscle, the muscularis mucosa (*MM*) of the colon and below that, seen in part, is **dense irregular connective tissue** (*DICT*) that forms the submucosa of the colon. Typically, the collagen fibers (*CF*) that lie just below the epithelial cells (*Ep*) at the luminal surface are more concentrated and thus appear prominently in the micrograph.

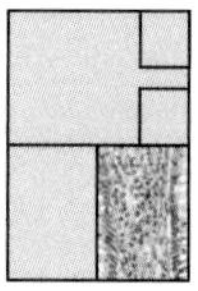

Loose connective tissue, colon, monkey, Mallory trichrome ×700.

Shown at higher magnification is the *boxed* area in the adjacent figure. The base of the epithelial cells (*Ep*) is seen on each side of the micrograph. The **collagen fibers** (*CF*) appear as thin threads that form a stroma surrounding the cells. The mixture of cells that are present here consists of **lymphocytes** (*L*), **plasma cells** (*P*), fibroblasts, smooth muscle cells, macrophages (*M*), and occasional mast cells.

CF, collagen fibers
DICT, dense irregular connective tissue
Ep, epithelial cells
GE, glandular epithelium
L, lymphocyte
LCT, loose connective tissue
M, macrophage
MM, muscularis mucosa
P, plasma cells

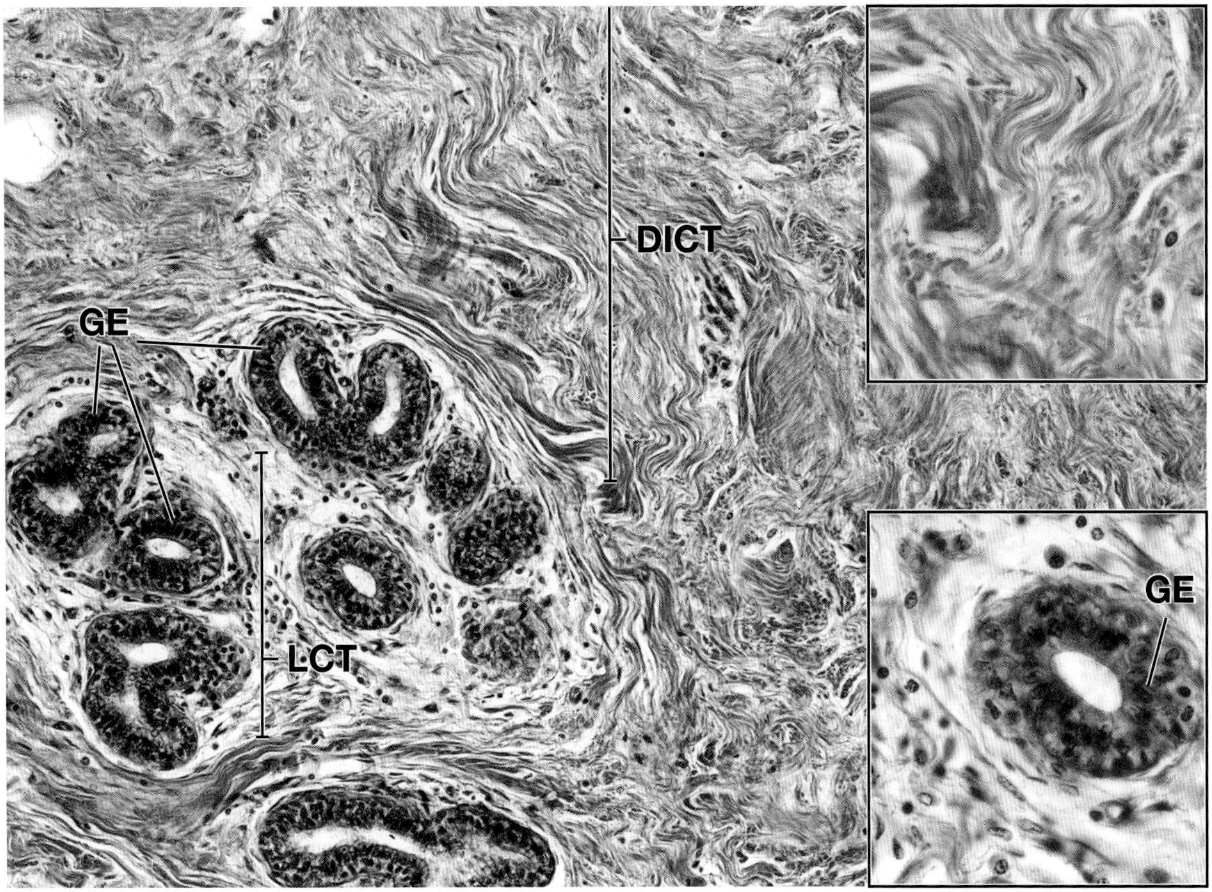
DICT
GE
LCT
GE

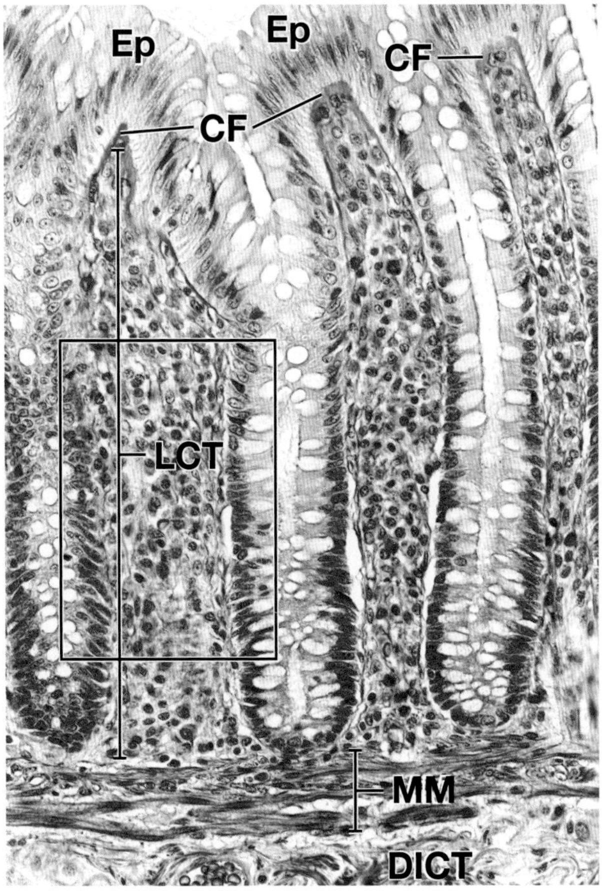
Ep
Ep
CF
CF
LCT
MM
DICT

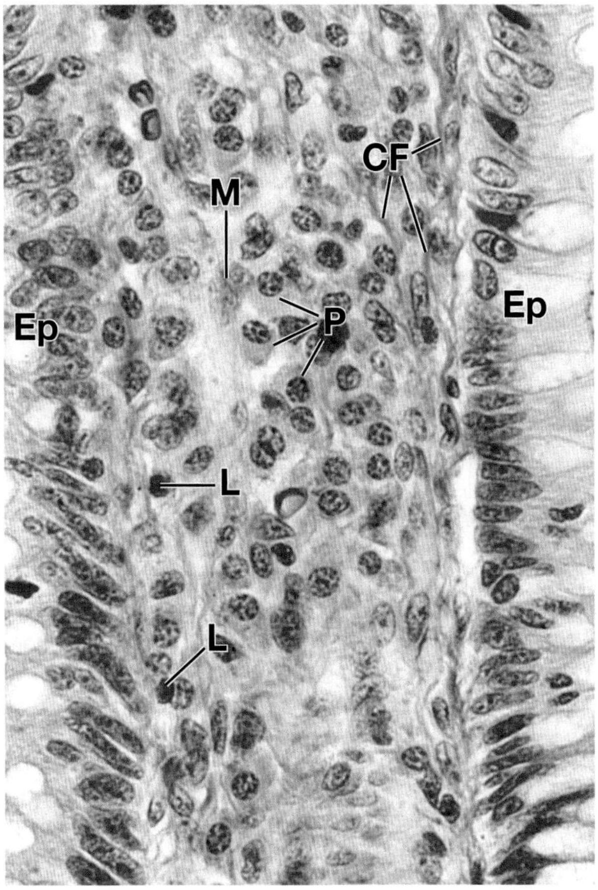
CF
M
Ep
P
Ep
L
L

PLATE 6.2 ■ DENSE REGULAR CONNECTIVE TISSUE, TENDONS, AND LIGAMENTS

Dense regular connective tissue is distinctive in that its fibers are very densely packed and are organized in parallel array into fascicles. The collagen fibrils that make up the fibers are also arranged in an ordered parallel array. **Tendons,** which attach muscle to bone, and **ligaments**, which attach bone to bone, are examples of this type of tissue. Ligaments are similar to tendons in most respects, but their fibers and the organization of the fascicles tend to be less ordered.

In tendons as well as ligaments, the fascicles are separated from one another by dense irregular connective tissue, the **endotendineum**, through which travel vessels and nerves. Also, a fascicle may be partially divided by connective tissue septa that extend from the endotendineum and contain the smallest vessels and nerves. Some of the fascicles may be grouped into larger functional units by a thicker, surrounding connective tissue, the **peritendineum**. Finally, the fascicles and groups of fascicles are surrounded by dense irregular connective tissue, the **epitendineum**.

The fibroblasts, also called *tendinocytes* in tendons, are elongated cells that possess exceedingly thin, sheet-like cytoplasmic processes that reside between and embrace adjacent fibers. The margins of the cytoplasmic processes contact those of neighboring tendon cells, thus forming a syncytium-like cytoplasmic network.

The most regular dense connective tissue is that of the stroma of the cornea of the eye (see Chapter 24, Eye, see pages 983-987). In this tissue, the collagen fibrils are arranged in parallel in lamellae that are separated by large, flattened fibroblasts. Adjacent lamellae are arranged at approximately right angles to one another, thus forming an **orthogonal array**. The extreme regularity of fibril size and fibril spacing in each lamella, in conjunction with the orthogonal array of the lamellae, is believed to be the basis of corneal transparency.

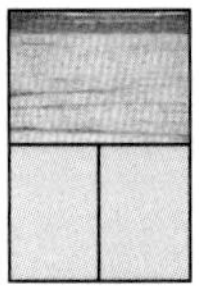

Dense regular connective tissue, tendon, longitudinal section, human, hematoxylin and eosin (H&E) ×100.

This specimen includes the surrounding dense irregular connective tissue of the tendon, the **epitendineum** (*Ept*). The **tendon fascicles** (*TF*) that make up the tendon are surrounded by a less dense connective tissue than that associated with the epitendineum. In longitudinal sections such as this, the connective tissue that surrounds the individual fascicles, the **endotendineum** (*Ent*), seems to disappear at certain points, with the result that one fascicle appears to merge with a neighboring fascicle. This is due to an obliqueness in the plane of section rather than an actual merging of fascicles. The collagen that makes up the bulk of the tendon fascicle has a homogeneous appearance as a result of the orderly packing of the individual collagen fibrils. The nuclei of the tendinocytes appear as elongate profiles arranged in linear rows. The cytoplasm of these cells blends in with the collagen, leaving only the nuclei as the representative feature of the cell.

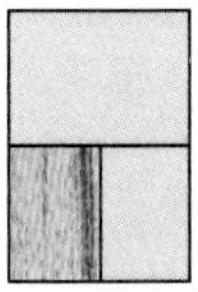

Dense regular connective tissue, tendon, longitudinal section, human, H&E ×400.

This higher magnification micrograph shows the ordered single-file array of the **tendinocyte nuclei** (*TC*) along with the intervening collagen. The latter has a homogeneous appearance. The cytoplasm of the cells is indistinguishable from the collagen, as is typical in H&E paraffin specimens. The variation in nuclear appearance is due to the plane of section and the position of the nuclei within the thickness of the section. A small blood vessel (*BV*) coursing within the endotendineum is also present in the specimen.

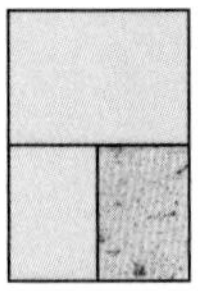

Dense regular connective tissue, tendon, cross section, human, H&E ×400.

This specimen is well preserved, and the densely packed collagenous fibers appear as a homogeneous field, even though the fibers are viewed on their cut ends. The nuclei appear irregularly scattered, as opposed to their more uniform pattern in the longitudinal plane. This is explained by examining the *dashed line* in the *lower left* figure, which is meant to represent an arbitrary cross-sectional cut of the tendon. Note the irregular spacing of the nuclei that are in the plane of the cut. Lastly, several small blood vessels (*BV*) are present within the **endotendineum** (*Ent*) within a fascicle.

BV, blood vessel
Ent, endotendineum
Ept, epitendineum
TC, tendinocyte nuclei
TF, tendon fascicle
dashed line, arbitrary cross-sectional cut of tendon

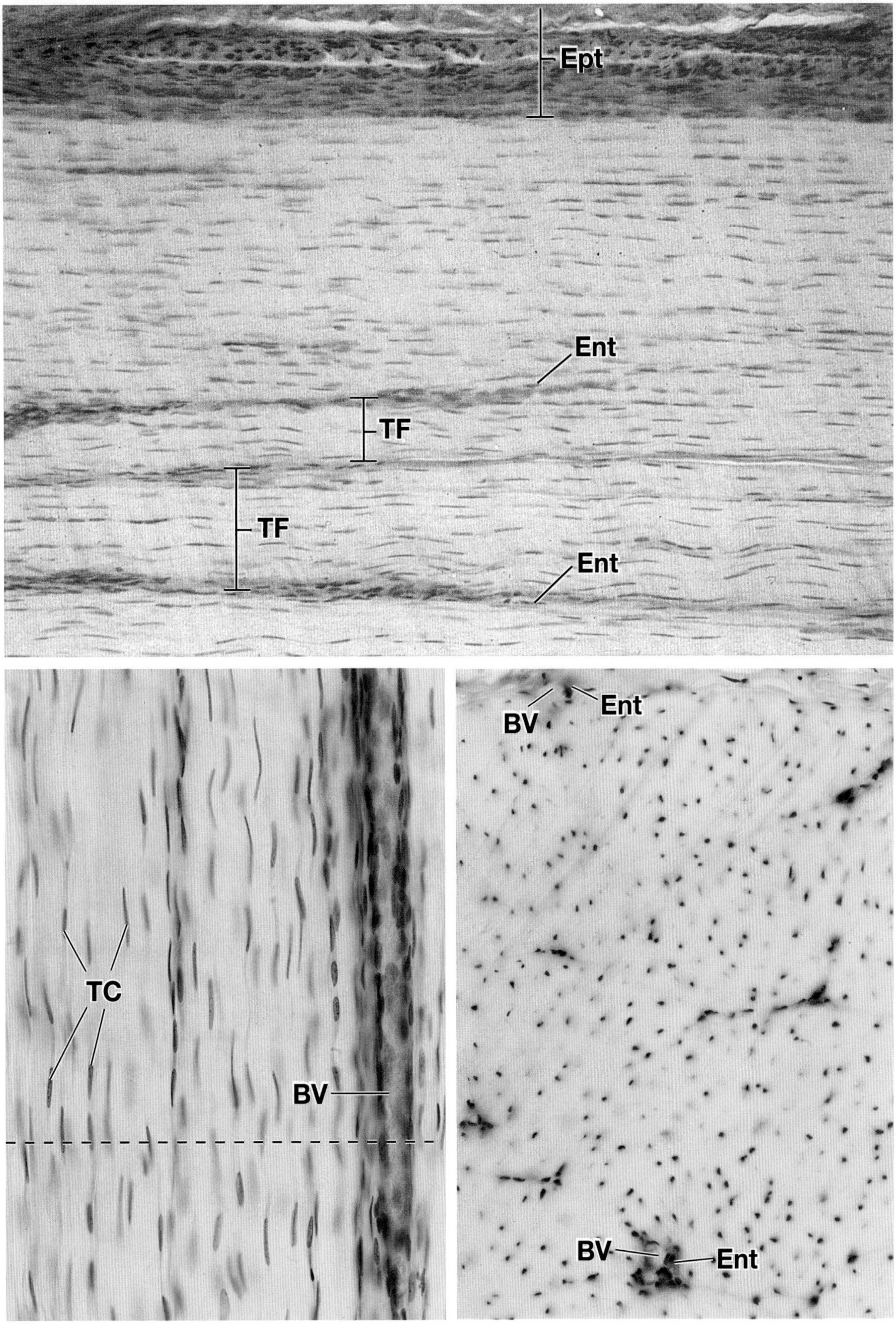
Ept
Ent
TF
TF
Ent
TC
BV
BV
Ent
BV
Ent

PLATE 6.3 ■ ELASTIC FIBERS AND ELASTIC LAMELLAE

Elastic fibers are present in loose and dense connective tissue throughout the body but in lesser amounts than collagenous fibers. Elastic fibers are not conspicuous in routine hematoxylin and eosin (H&E) sections but are visualized readily with special staining methods. (The following selectively color elastic material: Weigert elastic tissue stain, *purple-violet*; Gomori aldehyde fuchsin stain, *blue-black*; Verhoeff hematoxylin elastic tissue stain, *black*; and modified Taenzer-Unna orcein stain, *red-brown*.) By using a combination of the special elastic stains and counterstains, such as H&E, not only the elastic fibers but also the other tissue components may be revealed, thus allowing to study the relationships between the elastic material and other connective tissue components.

Elastic material occurs in both fibrous and lamellar forms. In loose and dense connective tissue and elastic cartilage (see Plate 7.3, page 234), the elastic material is in fibrous form. Similarly, the elastic ligaments that connect the cervical vertebrae and that are particularly prominent in grazing animals have a mixture of elastic and collagenous fibers in a tightly packed array. In the major, largest diameter arteries (e.g., aorta, pulmonary, common carotid, and other primary branches of the aorta), the *tunica media* consists of fenestrated layers of elastic tissue alternating with layers containing smooth muscle cells and collagenous tissue. This allows stretching and elastic rebound to assist in the propulsion of the blood. All arteries and most large arterioles have an *internal elastic membrane* that supports the delicate endothelium and its immediately subjacent connective tissue. It should be noted that both the collagen and elastic components of the tunica media are produced by the smooth muscle cells of this layer.

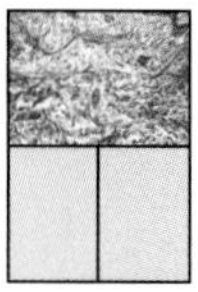

Elastic fibers, dermis, monkey, Weigert ×160.

This shows the connective tissue of the skin, referred to as the *dermis*, stained to show the nature and distribution of the **elastic fibers** (*E*), which appear *purple*. The **collagen fibers** (*C*) have been stained by eosin, and the two fiber types are easily differentiated. The connective tissue at the *top* of the figure, close to the epithelium (the papillary layer of the dermis), contains thin elastic fibers (see *upper left*) as well as less coarse collagen fibers. The *lower portion* shows considerably heavier elastic and collagen fibers. Also note that many of the elastic fibers appear as short rectangular profiles. These profiles simply represent fibers traveling through the thickness of the section at an oblique angle to the path of the knife. Careful examination will also reveal a few fibers that appear as dot-like profiles. They represent cross-sectioned elastic fibers. Overall, the elastic fibers of the dermis have a three-dimensional interlacing configuration, thus showing a variety of forms.

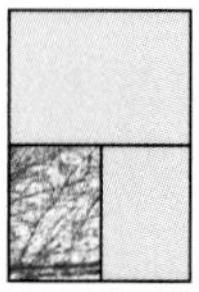

Elastic fibers, mesentery, rat, Weigert ×160.

This is a whole mount specimen of mesentery prepared to show the connective tissue elements and differentially stained to reveal elastic fibers. The **elastic fibers** (*E*) appear as thin, long, crisscrossing, and branching threads without discernible beginnings or endings and with a somewhat irregular course. Again, the **collagen fibers** (*C*) are contrasted by their eosin staining and appear as long, straight profiles that are considerably thicker than the elastic fibers.

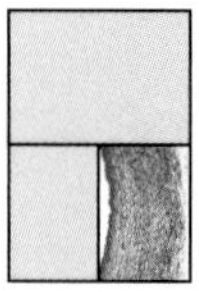

Elastic lamellae, elastic artery, monkey, Weigert ×80.

Elastic material also occurs in sheets or lamellae rather than string-like fibers. This figure shows the wall of an elastic artery (pulmonary artery) that was stained to show the elastic material. Each of the *wavy lines* is a **lamella of elastic material** that is organized in the form of a fenestrated sheet or membrane. The plane of section is such that the elastic membranes are seen on the edge. This specimen was not subsequently stained with H&E. The empty-appearing spaces between elastic layers contain collagen fibers and smooth muscle cells, but they remain essentially unstained. In the muscular layer of blood vessel, both elastin and collagen are secreted by the smooth muscle cells.

Tissues of the body containing large amounts of elastic material are limited in distribution to the walls of elastic arteries and some ligaments that are associated with the spinal column.

BV, blood vessel
C, collagen fibers
D, duct of sweat gland
E, elastic fibers

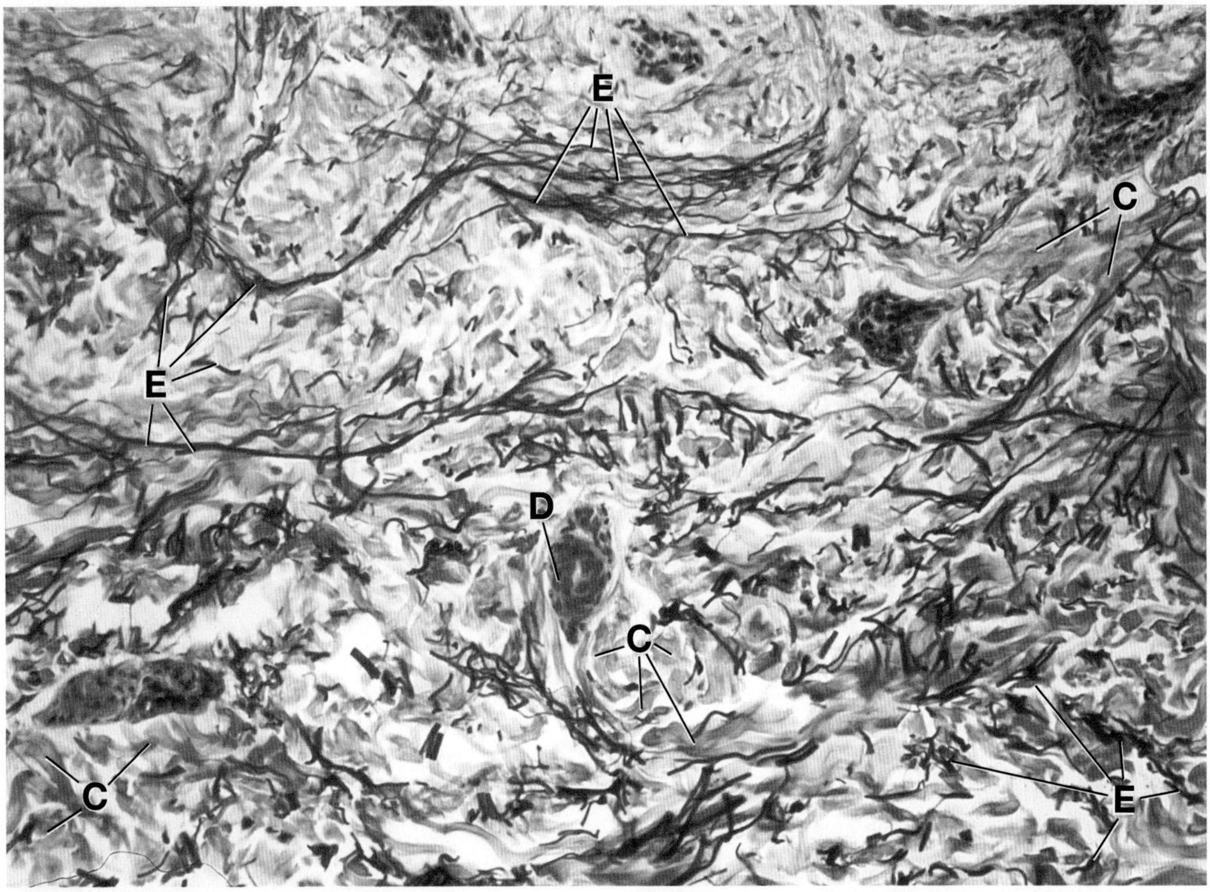
E
C
E
D
C
C
E

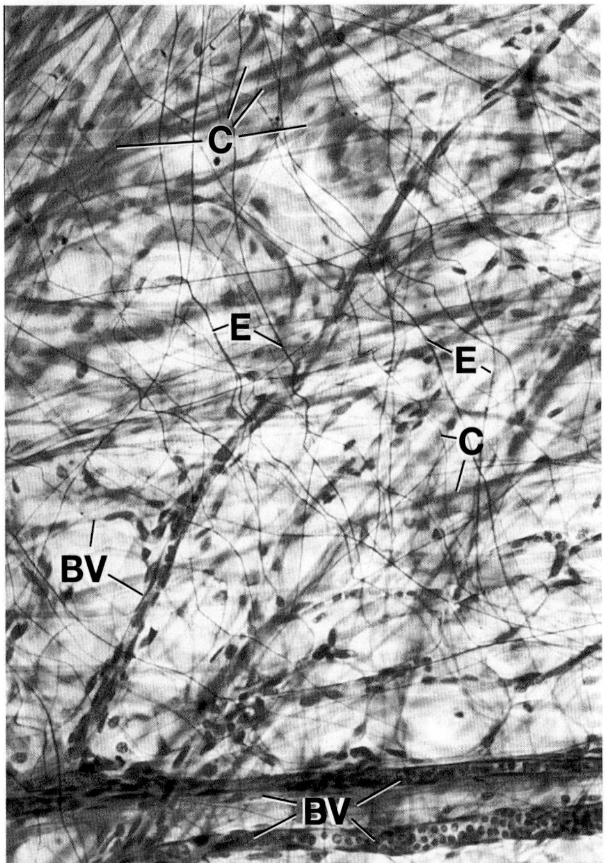
C
E
E
C
BV
BV

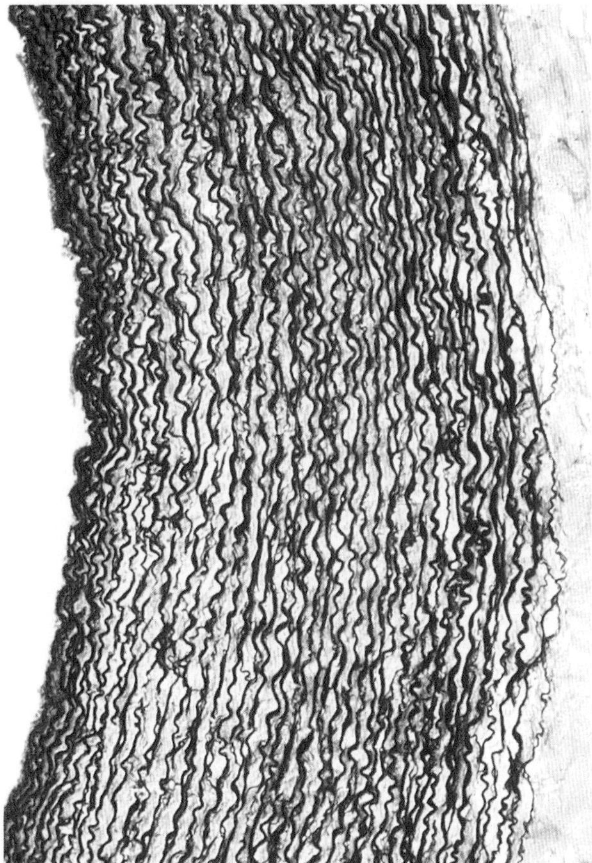

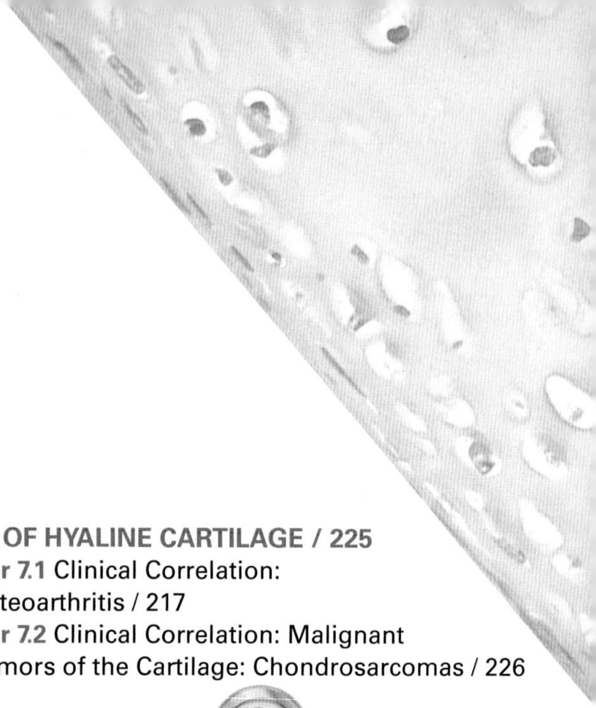

7 CARTILAGE

■ OVERVIEW OF CARTILAGE

Cartilage is a form of connective tissue composed of cells called chondrocytes and a highly specialized extracellular matrix.

Cartilage is an avascular tissue that consists of **chondrocytes** and an extensive **extracellular matrix**. More than 95% of cartilage volume consists of extracellular matrix, which is a functional element of this tissue. The chondrocytes are sparse but essential participants in the production and maintenance of the matrix (Fig. 7.1).

The extracellular matrix in cartilage is not only solid and firm but also somewhat pliable, which accounts for its resilience. Because there is no vascular network within cartilage, the composition of the extracellular matrix is crucial to the survival of the chondrocytes. The large ratio of **glycosaminoglycans (GAGs)** to **type II collagen fibers** in the cartilage matrix permits diffusion of substances between blood vessels in the surrounding connective tissue and the chondrocytes dispersed within the matrix, thus maintaining the viability of the tissue. Close interactions are seen between two classes of structural molecules that possess contrasting biophysical characteristics: the meshwork of tension-resisting collagen fibrils and the large amounts of heavily hydrated proteoglycan aggregates. The latter are extremely weak in shear and allow the cartilage to bear weight, especially at points of movement such as synovial joints. Because it maintains this property even while growing, cartilage is a key tissue in the development of the fetal skeleton and in most growing bones.

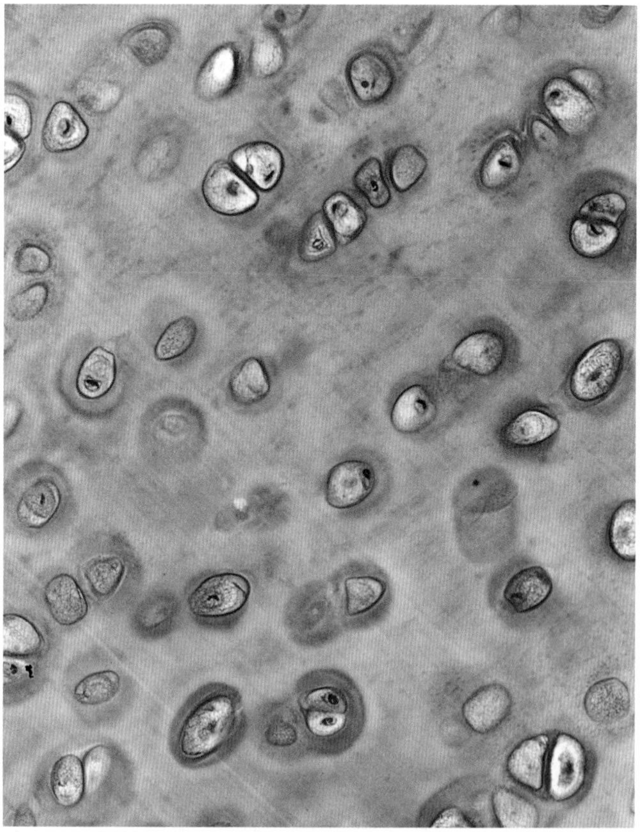

FIGURE 7.1. General structure of hyaline cartilage. This photomicrograph of a routine hematoxylin and eosin (H&E) preparation of hyaline cartilage shows its general features. Note the extensive extracellular matrix that separates a sparse population of chondrocytes. ×450.

Three types of cartilage that differ in appearance and mechanical properties are distinguished on the basis of the characteristics of their matrix:

- **Hyaline cartilage** is characterized by matrix-containing type II collagen fibers, GAGs, proteoglycans, and multiadhesive glycoproteins.
- **Elastic cartilage** is characterized by elastic fibers and elastic lamellae in addition to the matrix material of hyaline cartilage.
- **Fibrocartilage** is characterized by abundant type I collagen fibers as well as the matrix material of hyaline cartilage. Table 7.1 lists the locations, functions, and features of each type of cartilage.

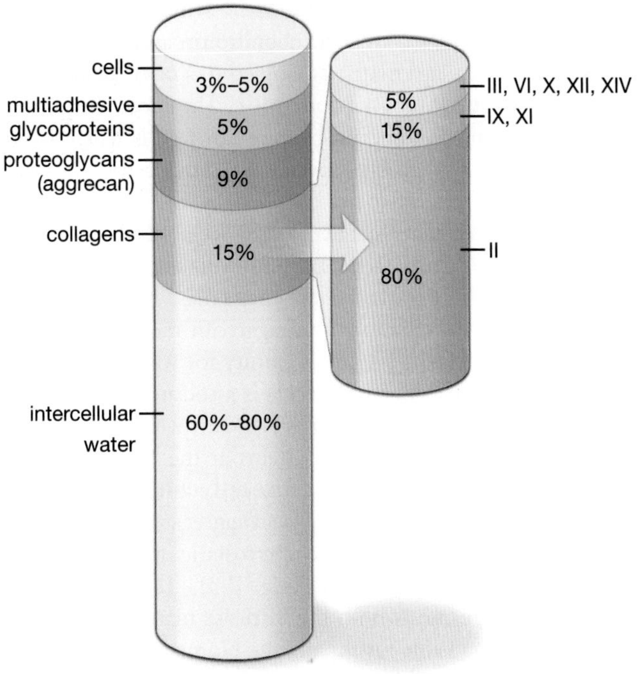

FIGURE 7.2. Molecular composition of hyaline cartilage. Cartilage's net weight is 60%–80% intercellular water, which is bound by proteoglycan aggregates. About 15% of the total weight is attributed to collagen molecules, of which type II collagen is the most abundant. Chondrocytes occupy only 3%–5% of the total cartilage mass.

■ HYALINE CARTILAGE

Hyaline cartilage is distinguished by a homogeneous, amorphous matrix.

The matrix of hyaline cartilage appears glassy in the living state, hence the name *hyaline* [*Gr. hyalos, glassy*]. Throughout the **cartilage matrix** are spaces called **lacunae**. Located within these lacunae are the **chondrocytes**. Hyaline cartilage is not a simple, inert, homogeneous substance but a complex living tissue. It provides a low-friction surface, participates in lubricating synovial joints, and distributes applied forces to the underlying bone. Although its capacity for repair is limited, under normal circumstances, it shows no evidence of abrasive wear over a lifetime. An exception is articular cartilage, which, in many individuals, breaks down with age (Folder 7.1). The macromolecules of hyaline cartilage matrix consist of collagen (predominantly type II fibrils and other cartilage-specific collagen molecules), proteoglycan aggregates containing GAGs, and multiadhesive glycoproteins (noncollagenous proteins). Figure 7.2 illustrates the relative distribution of the various components that constitute cartilage matrix.

Hyaline cartilage matrix is produced by chondrocytes and contains three major classes of molecules.

Three classes of molecules exist in hyaline cartilage matrix:

- **Collagen molecules.** Collagen is the major matrix protein. Four types of collagen participate in the formation of a three-dimensional meshwork of relatively thin (20-nm diameter) and short matrix fibrils. **Type II collagen** constitutes the bulk of the fibrils (see Fig. 7.2), **type IX collagen** facilitates fibril interaction with the matrix proteoglycan molecules, **type XI collagen** regulates the fibril size, and **type X collagen** organizes the collagen fibrils into a three-dimensional hexagonal lattice that is crucial to its successful mechanical function. In addition, **type VI collagen** is also found in the matrix, mainly at the periphery of the chondrocytes where it helps to attach these cells to the matrix framework. Because types II, VI, IX, X, and XI are found in significant amounts only in the cartilage matrix, they are referred to as **cartilage-specific collagen molecules.** (Review the types of collagen in Table 6.2.)
- **Proteoglycans.** The ground substance of hyaline cartilage contains three kinds of GAGs: **hyaluronan,**

FOLDER 7.1

CLINICAL CORRELATION: OSTEOARTHRITIS

Osteoarthritis, a degenerative joint disease, is one of the most common types of joint diseases. The pathogenesis of osteoarthritis is unknown, but it is related to aging and injury of articular cartilage. Most individuals show some evidence of this disease by age 65. The disease is characterized by **chronic joint pain** with various degrees of **joint deformity** and **destruction of the articular cartilage**. Osteoarthritis commonly affects weight-bearing joints: hips, knees, lower lumbar vertebra, and joints of the hand and foot. There is a decrease in proteoglycan content, which reduces the intercellular water content in the cartilage matrix. Chondrocytes also play an important role in the pathogenesis of osteoarthritis. Interleukin-1 (IL-1) and tumor necrosis factor α (TNF-α) stimulate the production of metalloproteinases and inhibit synthesis of type II collagen and proteoglycans by chondrocytes. In the early stages of the disease, the superficial layer of the articular cartilage is disrupted. Eventually, destruction of the cartilage extends to the bone, where the exposed subchondral bone becomes a new articular surface. These changes result in a progressive reduction of mobility and increased pain with joint movement. There is no cure for osteoarthritis, and treatment focuses on relieving pain and stiffness to allow a greater range of joint movement. Osteoarthritis may stabilize with age, but more often, it slowly progresses with eventual long-term disability.

chondroitin sulfate, and **keratan sulfate**. As in loose connective tissue matrix, the chondroitin and keratan sulfate of the cartilage matrix are joined to a **core protein** to form a **proteoglycan monomer**. The most important proteoglycan monomer in hyaline cartilage is **aggrecan**, also known as cartilage-specific proteoglycan core protein, which in humans is encoded by the ACAN gene. It has a molecular weight of 250 kDa. Each molecule contains approximately 100 chondroitin sulfate chains and as many as 60 keratan sulfate molecules. Because of the presence of the sulfate groups, aggrecan molecules have a large negative charge with an affinity for water molecules. Each linear hyaluronan molecule is associated with a large number of aggrecan molecules (>300), which are bound to the hyaluronan by link proteins at the N-terminus of the molecule to form large **proteoglycan aggregates**. These highly charged proteoglycan aggregates are bound to the collagen matrix fibrils by electrostatic interactions and multiadhesive glycoproteins (Fig. 7.3). The entrapment of these aggregates within the intricate matrix of collagen fibrils is responsible for the unique biomechanical properties of hyaline cartilage. Cartilage matrix also contains other proteoglycans (e.g., decorin, biglycan, and fibromodulin). These proteoglycans do not form aggregates but bind to other molecules and help stabilize the matrix.

- **Multiadhesive glycoproteins**, also referred to as *noncollagenous* and *nonproteoglycan-linked glycoproteins*, influence interactions between the chondrocytes and the matrix molecules. Examples of such proteins are **anchorin CII** (cartilage annexin V), a small 34-kDa molecule that functions as a collagen receptor on chondrocytes, and **tenascin** and **fibronectin** (see Table 6.5, page 197), which also help anchor chondrocytes to the matrix. Multiadhesive glycoproteins have clinical value as markers of cartilage turnover and degeneration.

Hyaline cartilage matrix is highly hydrated to provide resilience and diffusion of small metabolites.

Like other connective tissue matrices, cartilage matrix is highly hydrated. Between 60% and 80% of the net weight of hyaline cartilage is intercellular water (see Fig. 7.2). Much of this water is bound tightly to the **aggrecan–hyaluronan aggregates**, which create a high osmotic swelling pressure. These large hydrodynamic domains in the matrix are accountable for imparting resilience to the cartilage. The network of collagen type II fibers is not only responsible for the shape and tensile strength of hyaline cartilage but also provides a framework to resist the swelling pressure from aggrecan molecules. Some of the water is bound loosely enough to allow diffusion of small metabolites to and from the chondrocytes.

In articular cartilage, both transient and regional changes occur in water content during joint movement and when the joint is subjected to pressure. The high degree of hydration and the movement of water in the matrix allow the cartilage matrix to respond to varying pressure loads and contribute to the cartilage's weight-bearing capacity. Throughout life,

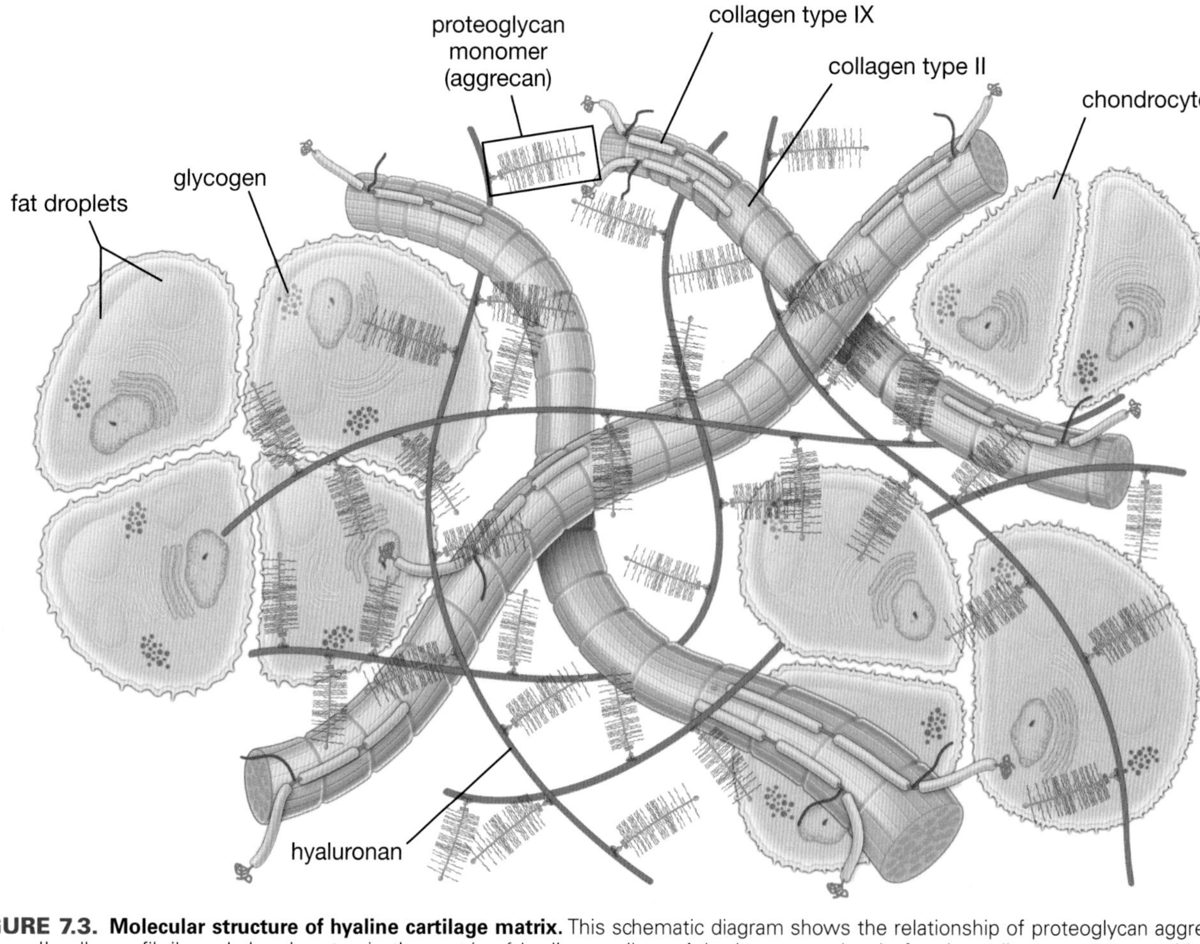

FIGURE 7.3. Molecular structure of hyaline cartilage matrix. This schematic diagram shows the relationship of proteoglycan aggregates to type II collagen fibrils and chondrocytes in the matrix of hyaline cartilage. A hyaluronan molecule forming a linear aggregate with many proteoglycan monomers is interwoven with a network of collagen fibrils. The proteoglycan monomer (such as aggrecan) consists of ~180 glycosaminoglycans joined to a core protein. The end of the core protein contains a hyaluronan-binding region that is joined to the hyaluronan by a link protein. Isogenous groups of chondrocytes are dispersed in extracellular matrix.

cartilage undergoes continuous **internal remodeling** as the cells replace matrix molecules lost through degradation. Normal matrix turnover depends on the ability of the chondrocytes to detect changes in matrix composition. The chondrocytes respond by synthesizing appropriate types of new molecules. In addition, the matrix acts as a signal transducer for the embedded chondrocytes. Thus, pressure loads applied to the cartilage, as in synovial joints, create mechanical, electrical, and chemical signals that help direct the synthetic activity of the chondrocytes. As the body ages, however, the composition of the matrix changes, and the chondrocytes lose their ability to respond to these stimuli.

Chondrocytes are specialized cells that produce and maintain the extracellular matrix.

In **hyaline cartilage**, chondrocytes are distributed either singularly or in clusters called **isogenous groups** (Fig. 7.4).

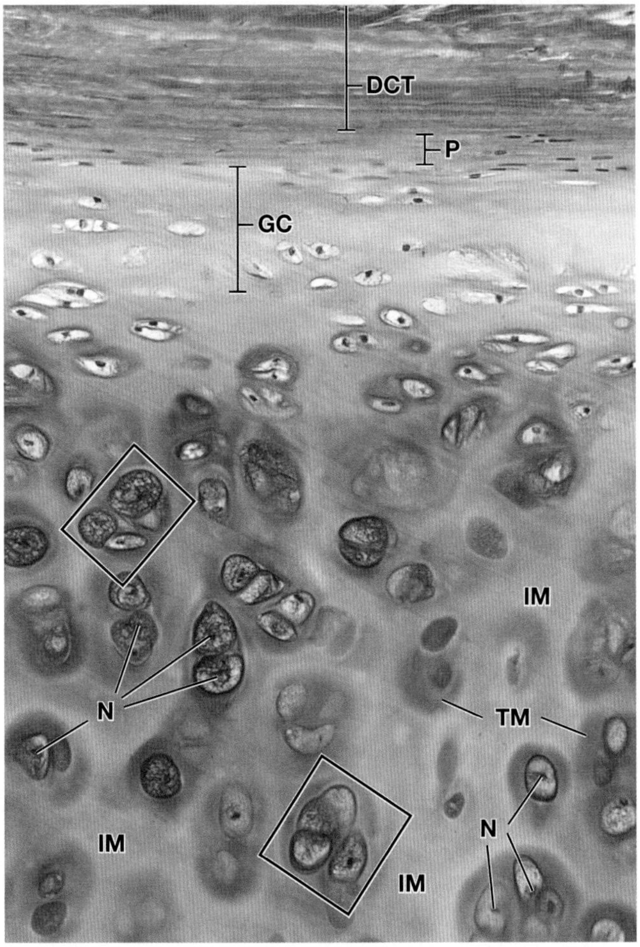

FIGURE 7.4. Photomicrograph of a typical hyaline cartilage specimen stained with hematoxylin and eosin. The *upper* portion of the micrograph shows dense connective tissue (*DCT*) overlying the perichondrium (*P*), from which new cartilage cells are derived. A slightly basophilic layer of growing cartilage (*GC*) underlying the perichondrium contains chondroblasts and immature chondrocytes that display little more than the nucleus residing in an empty-appearing lacuna. This layer represents deposition of new cartilage (appositional growth) on the surface of the existing hyaline cartilage. Mature chondrocytes with clearly visible nuclei (*N*) reside in the lacunae and are well preserved in this specimen. They produce the cartilage matrix that shows the dark-staining capsule or territorial matrix (*TM*) immediately surrounding the lacunae. The interterritorial matrix (*IM*) is more removed from the immediate vicinity of the chondrocytes and is less intensely stained. Growth from within the cartilage (interstitial growth) is reflected by the chondrocyte pairs and clusters that are responsible for the formation of isogenous groups (*rectangles*). ×480.

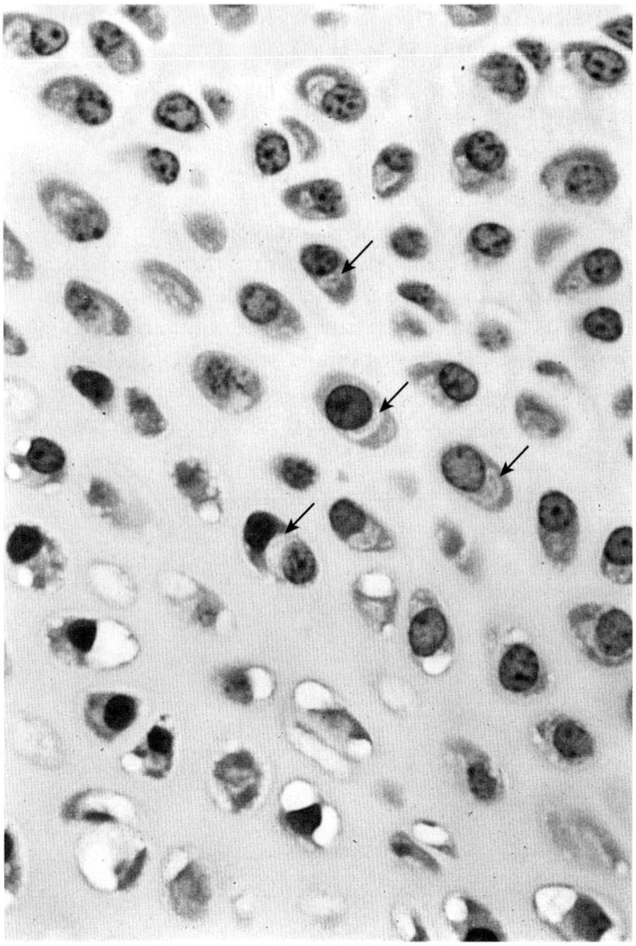

FIGURE 7.5. Photomicrograph of young, growing cartilage. This specimen was preserved in glutaraldehyde, embedded in plastic, and stained with hematoxylin and eosin (H&E). The chondrocytes, especially those in the *upper* part of the photomicrograph, are well preserved. The cytoplasm is deeply stained, exhibiting a distinct and relatively homogeneous basophilia. The clear areas (*arrows*) represent sites of the Golgi apparatus. ×520.

When the chondrocytes are present in isogenous groups, they represent cells that have recently divided. As the newly divided chondrocytes produce the matrix material that surrounds them, they are dispersed. They also secrete metalloproteinases (MMPs), enzymes that degrade cartilage matrix, allowing the cells to expand and reposition themselves within the growing isogenous group.

The appearance of chondrocyte cytoplasm varies according to chondrocyte activity. Chondrocytes that are active in matrix production display areas of cytoplasmic basophilia, which are indicative of protein synthesis, and clear areas, which indicate their large Golgi apparatus (Fig. 7.5). Chondrocytes secrete not only the collagen present in the matrix but also all of the GAGs and proteoglycans. In older, less active cells, the Golgi apparatus is smaller; clear areas of cytoplasm, when evident, usually indicate sites of extracted lipid droplets and glycogen stores. In such specimens, chondrocytes also display considerable distortion resulting from shrinkage after the glycogen and lipid are lost during the preparation of the tissue. In the transmission electron microscope (TEM), the active chondrocyte displays numerous profiles of rough-surfaced endoplasmic reticulum (rER), a large Golgi apparatus, secretory granules, vesicles, intermediate filaments, microtubules, and actin microfilaments (Fig. 7.6).

Components of the hyaline cartilage matrix are not uniformly distributed.

Because the proteoglycans of hyaline cartilage contain a high concentration of bound sulfate groups, ground substance stains with basic dyes and hematoxylin (Plate 7.1, page 230). Thus, the basophilia and metachromasia seen in stained sections of cartilage provide information about the distribution and relative concentration of sulfated proteoglycans. However, under closer examination, the matrix does not stain uniformly. Rather, three different regions are described based on the staining property of the matrix (Fig. 7.7).

- The **capsular (pericellular) matrix** is a ring of more densely staining matrix located immediately around the chondrocyte (see Fig. 7.4). It contains the highest concentration of sulfated proteoglycans, hyaluronan, biglycans, and several multiadhesive glycoproteins (e.g., fibronectin, decorin, and laminin). The capsular matrix contains almost exclusively type VI collagen that forms a tightly woven enclosure around each chondrocyte. Type VI collagen binds to integrin receptors on the cell surface and anchors the chondrocytes to the matrix. A higher concentration of type IX collagen is also present in the capsular matrix.
- The **territorial matrix** is a region that is more removed from the immediate vicinity of the chondrocytes. It surrounds the isogenous group and contains a randomly arranged network of type II collagen fibrils with smaller quantities of type IX collagen. It also has a lower concentration of sulfated proteoglycans and stains less intensely than the capsular matrix.
- The **interterritorial matrix** is a region that surrounds the territorial matrix and occupies the space between groups of chondrocytes.

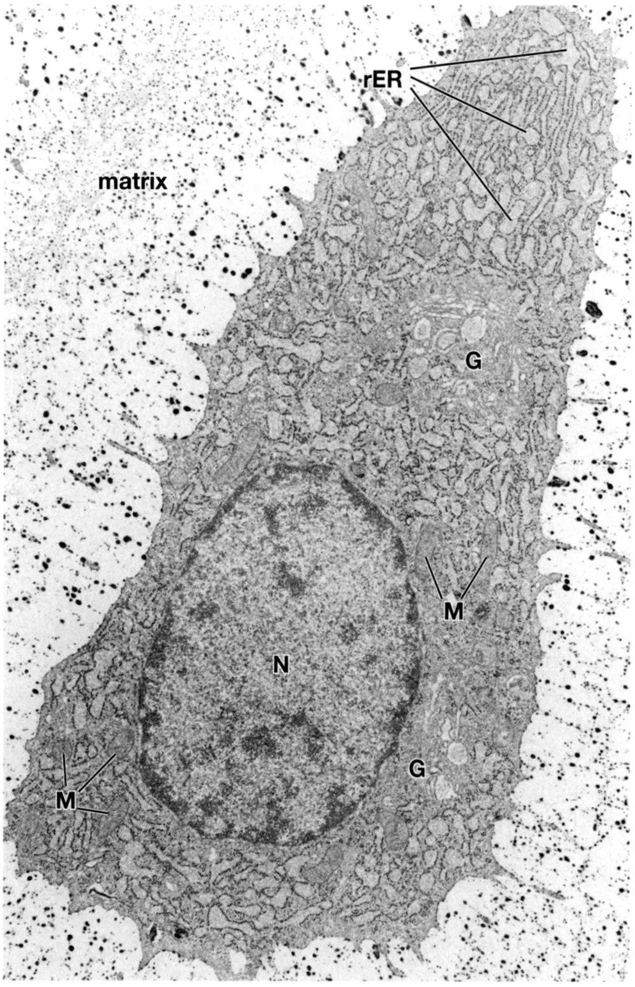

FIGURE 7.6. Electron micrograph of a young, active chondrocyte and surrounding matrix. The nucleus (*N*) of the chondrocyte is eccentrically located, like those in Figure 7.5, and the cytoplasm displays numerous and somewhat dilated profiles of rough-surfaced endoplasmic reticulum (*rER*), Golgi apparatus (*G*), and mitochondria (*M*). The large amount of *rER* and the extensive Golgi apparatus indicate that the cell is actively engaged in the production of cartilage matrix. The numerous dark particles in the matrix contain proteoglycans. The particularly large particles adjacent to the cell are located in the region of the matrix that is identified as the capsule or territorial matrix. ×15,000. (Courtesy of Dr. H. Clarke Anderson.)

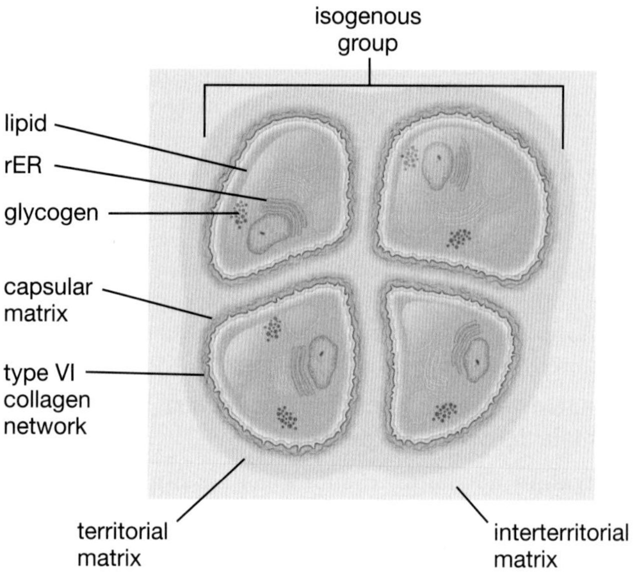

FIGURE 7.7. Diagram of cartilage matrices. Note the areas of capsular, territorial, and interterritorial matrices. The characteristics of each are described in the text. *rER*, rough-surfaced endoplasmic reticulum.

In addition to these regional differences in the concentration of sulfated proteoglycans and distribution of collagen fibrils, there is a decrease in proteoglycan content that occurs as cartilage ages, which is also reflected by staining differences.

Hyaline cartilage provides a model for the developing skeleton of the fetus.

In early fetal development, hyaline cartilage is the precursor of bones that develop by the process of **endochondral ossification** (Fig. 7.8). Initially, most long bones are represented by cartilage models that resemble the shape of the mature bone (Plate 7.2, page 232). During the developmental process, in which most of the cartilage is replaced by bone, residual cartilage at the proximal and distal ends of the bone serves as growth sites called **epiphyseal growth plates (epiphyseal discs)**. This cartilage remains functional as long as the bone grows in

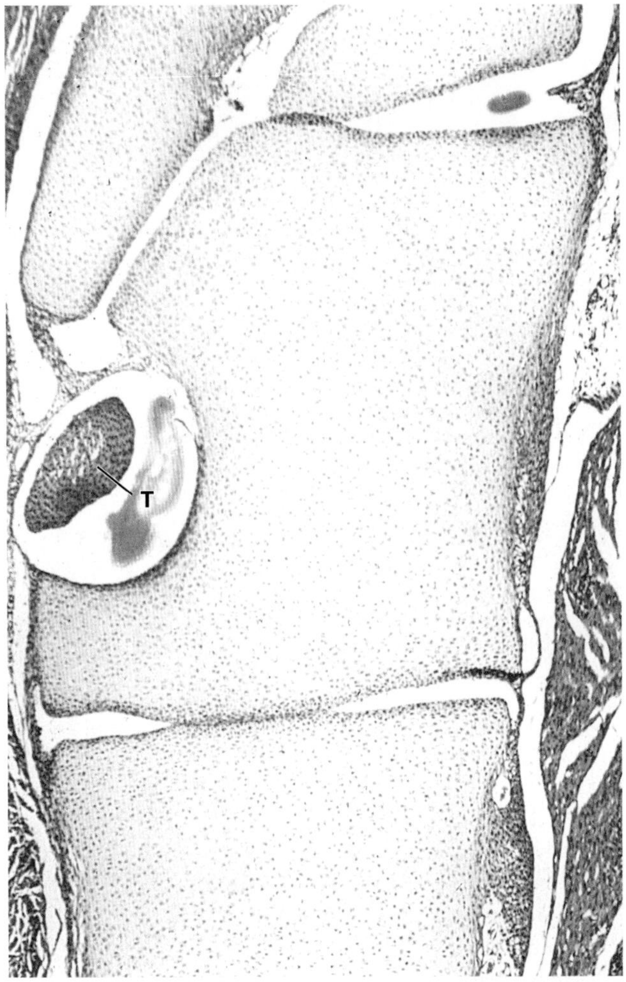

FIGURE 7.8. Photomicrograph of several cartilages that form the initial skeleton of the foot. The hyaline cartilage of developing tarsal bones will be replaced by bone as endochondral ossification proceeds. In this early stage of development, synovial joints are being formed between developing tarsal bones. Note that nonarticulating surfaces of the hyaline cartilage models of tarsal bones are covered by perichondrium, which also contributes to the development of joint capsules. Also, a developing tendon (*T*) is evident in the indentation of the cartilage seen on the *left* side of the micrograph. ×85.

length (Fig. 7.9). In a fully grown individual, a remnant of cartilage from the developing skeleton is found on the articular surface of joints (articular cartilage) and in the rib cage (costal cartilages). Hyaline cartilage also exists in the adult as the skeletal unit in the trachea, bronchi, larynx, and nose.

A firmly attached connective tissue, the perichondrium, surrounds hyaline cartilage.

The **perichondrium** is a dense irregular connective tissue composed of cells that are indistinguishable from fibroblasts. In many respects, the perichondrium resembles the capsule that surrounds glands and many organs. It also serves as the source of new cartilage cells. When actively growing, the perichondrium appears divided into an inner cellular layer, which gives rise to new cartilage cells, and an outer fibrous layer. This division is not always evident, especially in perichondrium that is not actively producing new cartilage or in very slow-growing cartilage. The changes that occur during the differentiation of new chondrocytes in growing cartilage are illustrated in Figure 7.4.

Hyaline cartilage of articular joint surfaces does not possess a perichondrium.

Hyaline cartilage that covers the articular surfaces of movable joints is termed **articular cartilage.** In general, the structure of articular cartilage is similar to that of hyaline cartilage. However, the free, or articular, surface has no perichondrium. Also, on the opposite surface, the cartilage contacts the bone, and there is no perichondrium. Articular cartilage is a remnant of the original hyaline cartilage template of the developing bone, and it persists throughout adult life. In adults, the articular cartilage is 2- to 5-mm thick and is divided into four zones (Figs. 7.10 and 7.11):

- The **superficial (tangential) zone** is a pressure-resistant region closest to the articular surface. It contains numerous

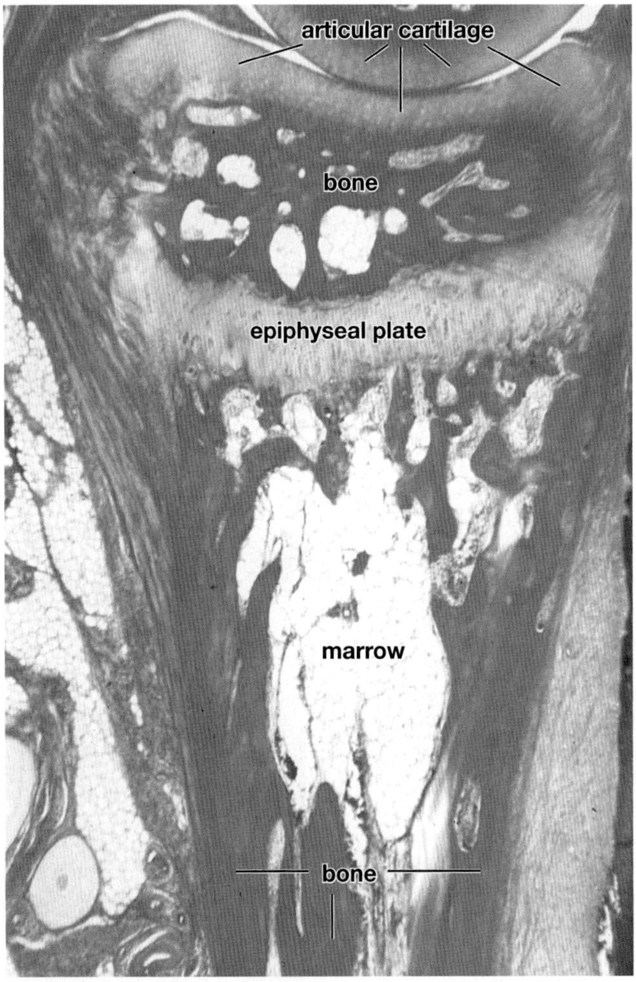

FIGURE 7.9. Photomicrograph of the proximal end of a growing long bone. A disc of hyaline cartilage—the epiphyseal plate—separates the more proximally located epiphysis from the funnel-shaped diaphysis located distal to the plate. The articular cartilage on the surface of the epiphysis contributes to the synovial joint and is also composed of hyaline cartilage. The cartilage of the epiphyseal plate disappears when lengthwise growth of the bone is completed, but the articular cartilage remains throughout life. The spaces within the bone are occupied by marrow. ×85.

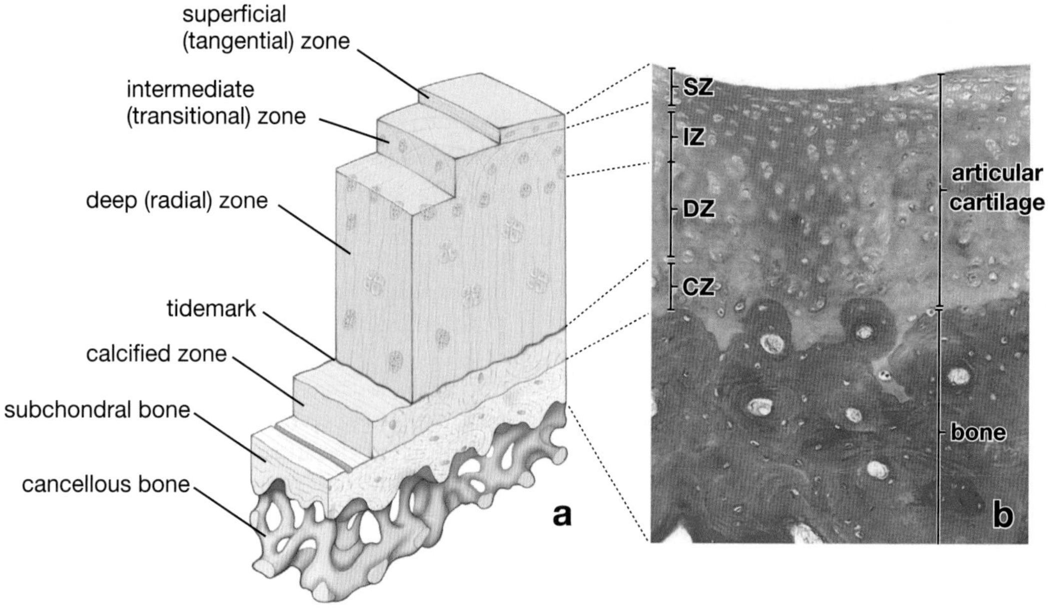

FIGURE 7.10. Diagram and photomicrograph of articular cartilage. a. This diagram shows the organization of the collagen network and chondrocytes in the various zones of articular cartilage. **b.** Photomicrograph of normal articular cartilage from an adult. The superficial zone (*SZ*) exhibits elongated and flattened chondrocytes. The intermediate zone (*IZ*) contains round chondrocytes. The deep zone (*DZ*) contains chondrocytes arranged in short columns. The calcified zone (*CZ*), which borders the subchondral bone, exhibits small chondrocytes surrounded by the calcified matrix. Also, this zone is lighter staining than the matrix of the more superficial zones. The *tidemark* separates calcified zone from subchondral bone. ×160.

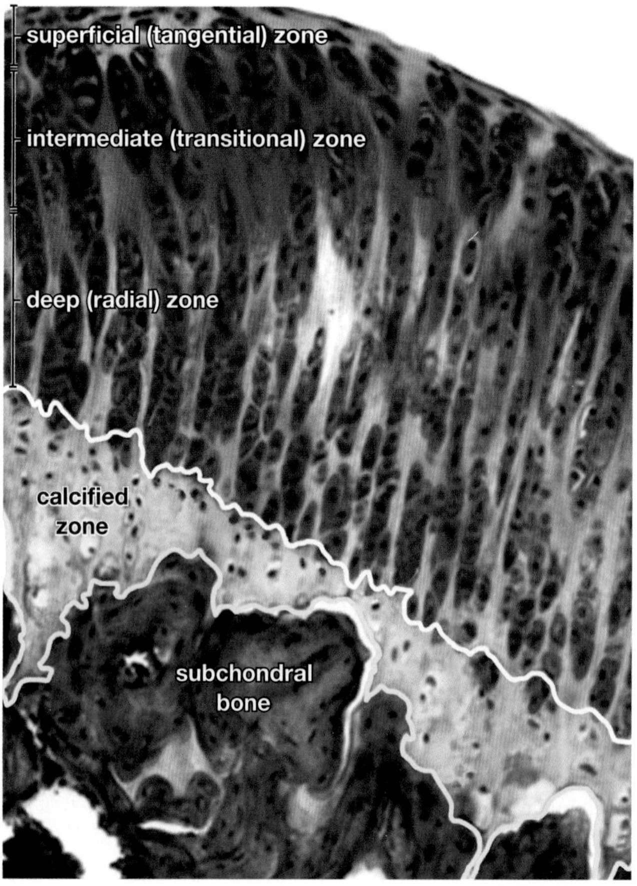

FIGURE 7.11. Photomicrograph of articular cartilage obtained from a tibial surface of a 12-week-old rat knee joint. This specimen is stained with safranin-O, Fast Green, and hematoxylin that are commonly used in histologic articular cartilage examination. The superficial (tangential) zone is stained light green due to a high condensation of type II collagen fibrils that are arranged in fascicles parallel to the free surface. Both intermediate (transitional) and deep (radial) zones are stained intensely red by safranin-O due to a high concentration of cartilage-specific proteoglycans (mainly sulfated glycosaminoglycans). The calcified zone is stained light green and contains collagen fibrils embedded in calcified matrix with a few small chondrocytes. Note that the calcified zone is separated from the deep zone by the tidemark (chondro-osseus junction) that is traced by the *white line* and by the cement line from subchondral bone, which is indicated by the *yellow line*. Subchondral bone that exhibits a typical osteonal pattern is stained deep blue. ×240. (Reprinted with permission from Schultz M, Molligan J, Schon L, et al. Pathology of the calcified zone of articular cartilage in post-traumatic osteoarthritis in rat knees. *PLoS One*. 2015;10[3]:e0120949.)

elongated and flattened chondrocytes surrounded by a condensation of type II collagen fibrils that are arranged in fascicles parallel to the free surface.

- The **intermediate (transitional) zone** lies below the superficial zone and contains round chondrocytes randomly distributed within the matrix. Collagen fibrils are less organized and are arranged in a somewhat oblique orientation to the surface.
- The **deep (radial) zone** is characterized by small, round chondrocytes that are arranged in short columns perpendicular to the free surface of the cartilage. The collagen fibrils are positioned between columns parallel to the long axis of the bone (see Fig 7.11).
- The **calcified zone** is characterized by a calcified matrix with the presence of small chondrocytes. This zone is separated from the deep (radial) zone by a smooth, undulating, heavily calcified line called the **tidemark (chondro-osseus junction)**. Above this line, proliferation of chondrocytes within the cartilage lacunae provides new cells for interstitial growth. In articular cartilage renewal, chondrocytes migrate from this region toward the joint surface. The calcified zone rests on the **subchondral bone** (a layer of bone just below the articular cartilage), and its junction is clearly defined by the **cement line** (see Fig 7.11). In response to **joint injury**, active calcification is triggered in the subchondral bone, resulting in the formation of a thicker subchondral bone plate.

The renewal process of mature articular cartilage is very slow. This slow growth is a reflection of the highly stable type II collagen network and the long half-life of its proteoglycan molecules. Also, in healthy articular cartilage, metalloproteinase (MMP-1 and MMP-13) activity is low.

■ ELASTIC CARTILAGE

Elastic cartilage is distinguished by the presence of elastin in the cartilage matrix.

In addition to containing the normal components of hyaline cartilage matrix, **elastic cartilage matrix** also contains a dense network of branching and anastomosing elastic fibers and interconnecting sheets of elastic material (Fig. 7.12 and Plate 7.3, page 234). These fibers and lamellae are best demonstrated in paraffin sections with special stains, such as resorcin-fuchsin and orcein. The elastic material gives the cartilage elastic properties in addition to the resilience and pliability that are characteristic of hyaline cartilage.

Elastic cartilage is found in the external ear, walls of the external acoustic meatus, auditory (Eustachian) tube, and epiglottis of the larynx. The cartilage in all of these locations is surrounded by a perichondrium similar to that found around most hyaline cartilage. Unlike hyaline cartilage, which calcifies with aging, the matrix of elastic cartilage does not calcify during the aging process.

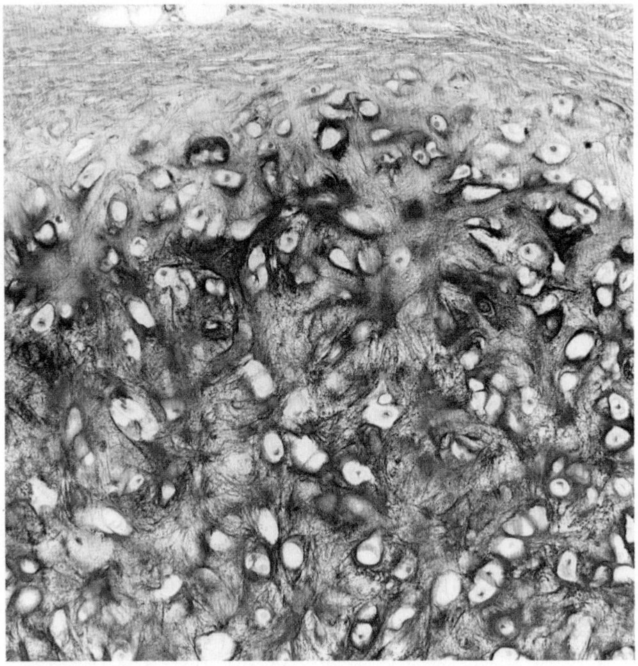

FIGURE 7.12. Photomicrograph of elastic cartilage from the epiglottis. This specimen was stained with orcein and reveals elastic fibers, stained brown, within the cartilage matrix. The elastic fibers are of various sizes and constitute a significant part of the cartilage. Chondrocyte nuclei are evident in many of the lacunae. The perichondrium is visible at the *top* of the photomicrograph. ×180.

■ FIBROCARTILAGE

Fibrocartilage consists of chondrocytes and their matrix material in combination with dense connective tissue.

Fibrocartilage is a combination of dense regular connective tissue and hyaline cartilage. The chondrocytes are dispersed among the collagen fibers singularly, in rows, and in isogenous groups (Fig. 7.13 and Plate 7.4, page 236). These chondrocytes appear similar to the chondrocytes of hyaline cartilage, but they have considerably less cartilage matrix material. There is also no surrounding perichondrium as in hyaline and elastic cartilage. In a section containing fibrocartilage, a population of cells with rounded nuclei and a small amount of surrounding amorphous matrix material can typically be seen. These nuclei belong to chondrocytes. Within the fibrous areas are nuclei that are flattened or elongated. These are fibroblast nuclei.

Fibrocartilage is typically present in intervertebral discs, the pubic symphysis, articular discs of the sternoclavicular and temporomandibular joints, menisci of the knee joint, triangular fibrocartilage complex of the wrist, and certain places where tendons attach to bones. The presence of fibrocartilage in these sites indicates that resistance to both compression and shearing forces is required of the tissue. The cartilage serves much like a shock absorber. The degree to which such forces occur is reflected in the amount of cartilage matrix material present.

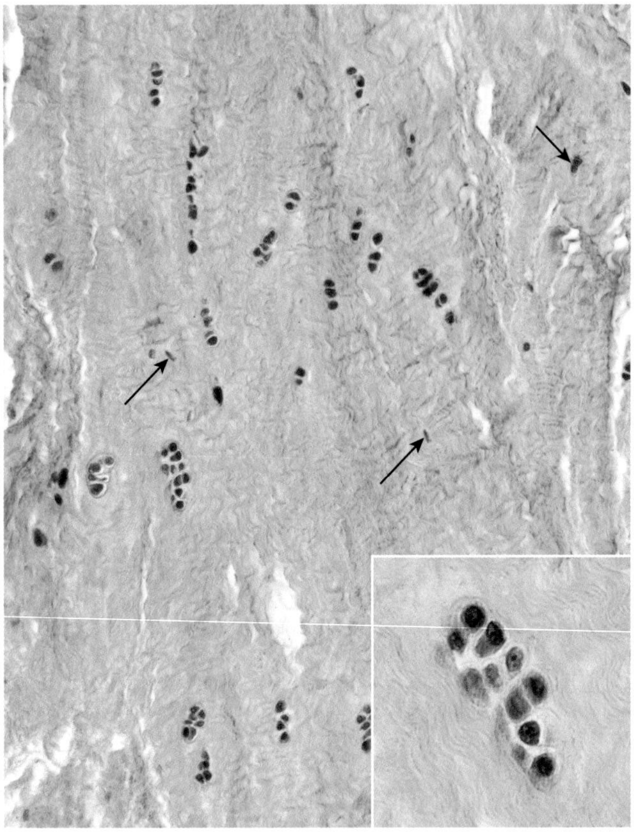

FIGURE 7.13. Photomicrograph of fibrocartilage from an intervertebral disc. The collagen fibers are stained green in this Gomori trichrome preparation. The tissue has a fibrous appearance and contains a relatively small number of fibroblasts with elongated nuclei (*arrows*) as well as more numerous chondrocytes with dark round nuclei. The chondrocytes exhibit close spatial groupings and are arranged either in rows among the collagen fibers or in isogenous groups. ×60. **Inset.** Higher magnification of an isogenous group. Chondrocytes are contained within lacunae. Typically, there is little cartilage matrix surrounding the chondrocytes. ×700.

Extracellular matrix of fibrocartilage is characterized by the presence of both type I and type II collagen fibrils.

The cells in fibrocartilage synthesize a wide variety of extracellular matrix molecules not only during its development stage but also during its mature, fully differentiated state. This allows the fibrocartilage to respond to changes in the external environment (such as mechanical forces, nutritional changes, and changing levels of hormones and growth factors). The **extracellular matrix of fibrocartilage** contains significant quantities of both **type I collagen** (characteristic of connective tissue matrix) and **type II collagen** (characteristic of hyaline cartilage).

The relative proportions of these collagens can vary. For example, menisci of the knee joint contain only a small quantity of type II collagen, whereas the intervertebral disc contains equal amounts of type I and type II collagen fibers. The ratio of type I to type II collagen in fibrocartilage changes with age. In older individuals, there is more type II collagen because of the metabolic activity of chondrocytes, which continuously produce and discharge type II collagen fibrils into the surrounding matrix. In addition, the extracellular matrix of fibrocartilage contains larger amounts of **versican** (a proteoglycan monomer secreted by fibroblasts) than aggrecan (produced by chondrocytes). Versican can also bind to hyaluronan to form highly hydrated proteoglycan aggregates (see Table 6.4, page 196). **Intervertebral disc degeneration** is associated with proteolytic degradation of proteoglycan aggregates present within the extracellular matrix of the fibrocartilage.

■ CHONDROGENESIS AND CARTILAGE GROWTH

Most cartilage arises from mesenchyme during chondrogenesis.

Chondrogenesis, the process of cartilage development, begins with the aggregation of chondroprogenitor mesenchymal cells to form a mass of rounded, closely apposed cells. In the head, most of the cartilage arises from aggregates of ectomesenchyme derived from neural crest cells. The site of hyaline cartilage formation is recognized initially by an aggregate of mesenchymal or ectomesenchymal cells known as a **chondrogenic nodule**. Expression of **transcription factor SOX-9** triggers differentiation of these cells into **chondroblasts**, which then secrete cartilage matrix (expression of SOX-9 coincides with secretion of type II collagen). The chondroblasts progressively move apart as they deposit matrix. When they are completely surrounded by matrix material, the cells are called **chondrocytes**. The mesenchymal tissue immediately surrounding the chondrogenic nodule gives rise to the perichondrium.

Chondrogenesis is regulated by many molecules, including extracellular ligands, nuclear receptors, transcription factors, adhesion molecules, and matrix proteins. Specifically, aggrecan, a cartilage matrix proteoglycan, plays an important role during chondrogenesis. Experimental studies reveal that aggrecan is required for chondrocyte differentiation from chondroprogenitor cells. Mutations of the **aggrecan gene (ACAN)** in humans cause early growth cessation of epiphyseal cartilages in long bones (despite normally timed puberty). This condition is linked to **spondyloepimetaphyseal dysplasia**, a skeletal disorder characterized by severe short stature (dwarfism) with advanced bone maturation and early onset of osteoarthritis (see Folder 7.1). Furthermore, the growth and development of the cartilage skeleton are influenced by biomechanical forces. These forces not only regulate the shape, regeneration, and aging of cartilage but also modify cell-to-extracellular matrix interactions within the cartilage.

Cartilage is capable of two kinds of growth: appositional and interstitial.

With the onset of matrix secretion, cartilage growth continues via a combination of two processes:

- **Appositional growth**, the process that forms new cartilage at the surface of existing cartilage
- **Interstitial growth**, the process that forms new cartilage within an existing cartilage mass

New cartilage cells produced during appositional growth are derived from the inner portion of the surrounding perichondrium. The cells resemble fibroblasts in form and function, producing the collagen component of the perichondrium

TABLE 7.1 Summary of Cartilage Features

Features	Hyaline Cartilage	Elastic Cartilage	Fibrocartilage
	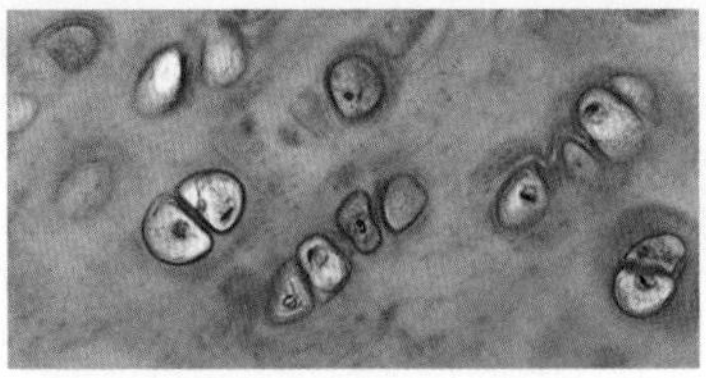	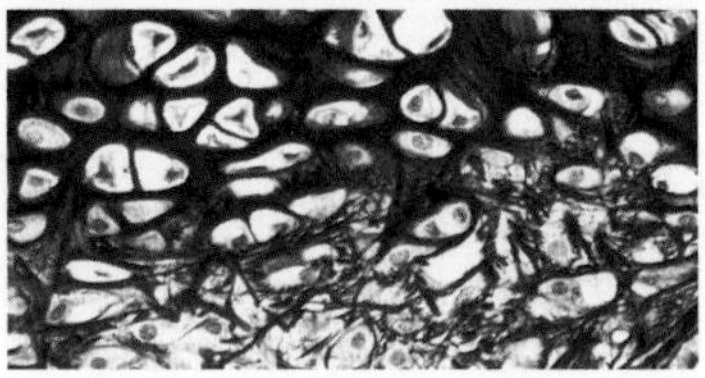	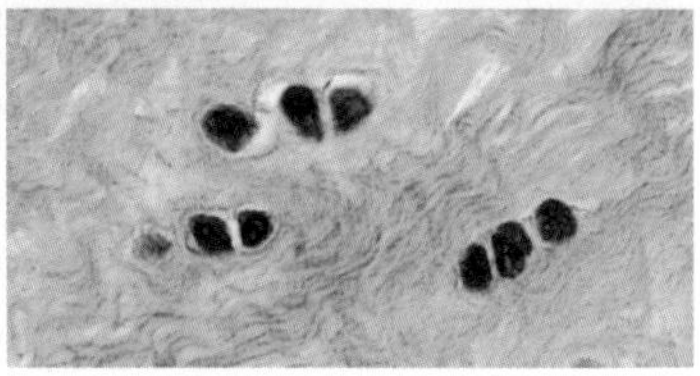
Location	Fetal skeletal tissue, epiphyseal plates, articular surface of synovial joints, costal cartilages of rib cage, cartilages of nasal cavity, larynx (thyroid, cricoid, and arytenoids), rings of trachea, and plates in bronchi	Pinna of external ear, external acoustic meatus, auditory (Eustachian) tube, and cartilages of larynx (epiglottis, corniculate, and cuneiform cartilages)	Intervertebral discs, pubic symphysis, articular discs (sternoclavicular and temporomandibular joints), menisci (knee joint), triangular fibrocartilage complex (wrist joint), and insertion of tendons
Function	• Resists compression • Provides cushioning, smooth, and low-friction surface for joints • Provides structural support in respiratory system (larynx, trachea, and bronchi) • Forms foundation for development of fetal skeleton and further endochondral bone formation and bone growth	Provides flexible support for soft tissues	Resists deformation under stress
Presence of perichondrium	Yes (except articular cartilage and epiphyseal plates)	Yes	No
Undergoes calcification	Yes (e.g., during endochondral bone formation, during aging process)	No	Yes (e.g., calcification of fibrocartilaginous callus during bone repair)
Main cell types present	Chondroblasts and chondrocytes	Chondroblasts and chondrocytes	Chondrocytes and fibroblasts
Characteristic features of extracellular matrix	Type II collagen fibrils and aggrecan monomers (the most important proteoglycan)	Type II collagen fibrils, elastic fibers, and aggrecan monomers	Types I and II collagen fibers Proteoglycan monomers: aggrecan (secreted by chondrocytes) and versican (secreted by fibroblasts)
Growth	Interstitially and appositionally, very limited in adults		
Repair	Very limited capability, commonly forms a scar, resulting in fibrocartilage formation		

(type I collagen). When cartilage growth is initiated, however, the cells undergo a differentiation process guided by expression of the transcription factor SOX-9. The cytoplasmic processes disappear, the nucleus becomes rounded, and the cytoplasm increases in amount and prominence. These changes result in the cell becoming a chondroblast. Chondroblasts function in cartilage matrix production, including secretion of type II collagen. The new matrix increases the cartilage mass, whereas new fibroblasts are produced simultaneously to maintain the cell population of the perichondrium.

New cartilage cells produced during interstitial growth arise from the division of chondrocytes within their lacunae (see Fig. 7.4). This is possible only because the chondrocytes retain the ability to divide and the surrounding matrix is distensible, thus permitting further secretory activity. Initially, the daughter cells of the dividing chondrocytes occupy the same lacuna. As a new matrix is secreted, a partition is formed between the daughter cells; at this point, each cell occupies its own lacuna. With continued secretion of matrix, the cells move even farther apart from each other. The overall growth of cartilage thus results from the interstitial secretion of new matrix material by chondrocytes and by the appositional secretion of matrix material by newly differentiated chondroblasts (Folder 7.2).

■ REPAIR OF HYALINE CARTILAGE

Cartilage has a limited ability for repair.

Cartilage can tolerate considerably intense and repetitive stress. However, when damaged, cartilage manifests a striking inability to heal, even in the most minor injuries. This lack of response to injury is attributable to the avascularity of cartilage, the immobility of the chondrocytes, and the limited ability of mature chondrocytes to proliferate. Some repair can occur but only if the defect involves the perichondrium.

FOLDER 7.2

CLINICAL CORRELATION: MALIGNANT TUMORS OF THE CARTILAGE: CHONDROSARCOMAS

Chondrosarcomas are generally slow-growing malignant tumors characterized by secretion of cartilage matrix. Approximately 3.6% of primary bone tumors diagnosed in the United States each year are chondrosarcomas. These tumors are the second most common matrix-producing tumors of bone after osteosarcomas (malignant bone-forming tumors). They occur more commonly in men than women and usually affect individuals aged 45 years and older.

Chondrosarcomas originate predominantly in the axial skeleton (and most commonly involve vertebrae, pelvic bones, ribs, scapulae, and sternum) and in the metaphyses of the proximal ends of long bones (most often, the femur and humerus). The most common symptom reported by patients is a deep pain, often present for months and typically dull in character. Because cartilaginous tissue is compressed inside the bone, in most cases, the initial growth of a tumor cannot be palpated. Radiographs, computed tomography (CT), and magnetic resonance imaging (MRI) scans are essential for the initial diagnosis and later for the evaluation of the extent of deep intramedullary tumors.

Chondrosarcomas are classified by grades that strongly correlate with prognosis. Microscopically, grade 1 represents the least aggressive and grade 3 represents the most aggressive tumor. Most chondrosarcomas (90%) are pathologically classified as conventional (grades 1 and 2); they rarely metastasize and are composed of hyaline cartilage that infiltrates the bone marrow cavity and surrounds existing bony trabeculae (Fig. F7.2.1). Multiple chondroblasts that are often binucleated with pleomorphic and hyperchromatic nuclear patterns are frequently seen in a single lacuna. The cartilaginous matrix may also undergo mineralization and subsequent endochondral ossification. Metastatic spread to lungs and lymph nodes is more frequently associated with grade 3 lesions.

Immunohistochemical localization of collagen types can be used to determine the stage of tissue differentiation, which may be a prognostic indicator, and confirm the diagnosis. The presence of **collagen types II and X** and the proteoglycan **aggrecan** in biopsies indicates mature tumors associated with good prognosis. Conversely, the presence of **collagen type I** indicates changes in the extracellular matrix toward dedifferentiated (fibrous) types of tumor with poorer prognosis. In addition, **transcription factor SOX-9**, which is essential for differentiation of mesenchymal cells into chondroblasts during normal fetal development, is expressed in chondrosarcomas.

Treatment of chondrosarcoma is primarily surgical: The tumor is widely excised. Chemotherapy and radiation play limited roles in treatment. Patients with adequately resected low-grade tumors have an excellent survival rate.

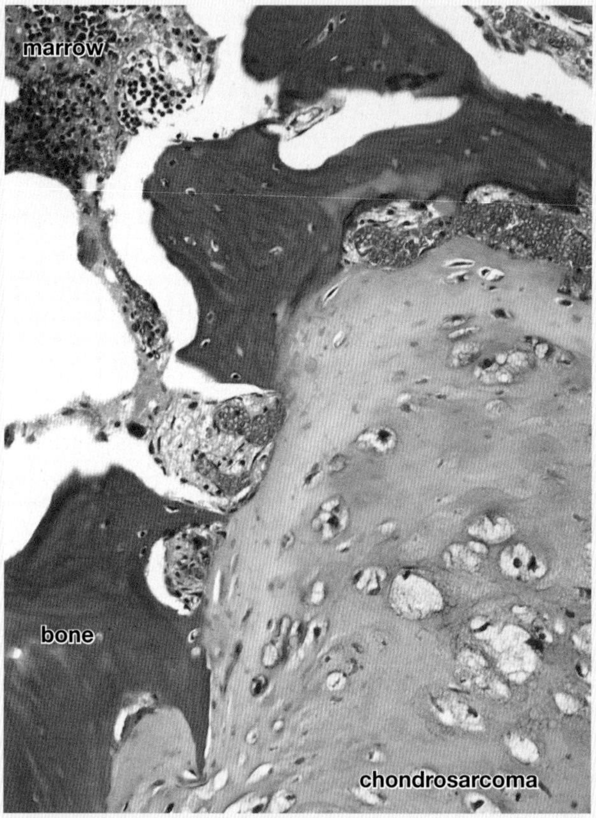

FIGURE F7.2.1. Photomicrograph of a chondrosarcoma (grade 1) from the epiphysis of the long bone stained with hematoxylin and eosin (H&E). This photomicrograph shows a tissue mass of chondrosarcoma infiltrating intertrabecular spaces of the bone marrow. Note the presence of malignant chondrocytes in various stages of maturity. Small area of active bone marrow is visible in the *upper left* corner of the image. ×240. (Courtesy of Dr. Fabiola Medeiros.)

In these injuries, repair results from the activity of the **pluripotential progenitor cells** located in the perichondrium. Even then, however, few cartilage cells, if any, are produced. Repair mostly involves the production of dense connective tissue.

At the molecular level, cartilage repair is a tentative balance between deposition of **type I collagen** in the form of scar tissue and repair by expression of **cartilage-specific collagens**. However, in adults, new blood vessels commonly develop at the site of the healing wound that stimulates the growth of bone rather than actual cartilage repair. The limited ability of cartilage to repair itself can cause significant problems in cardiothoracic surgery, such as coronary artery bypass graft surgery, when costal cartilage must be cut to enter the chest cavity. A variety of treatments may improve the healing of articular cartilage, including perichondrial grafts, autologous cell transplantation, insertion of artificial matrices, and application of growth factors.

When hyaline cartilage calcifies, it is replaced by bone.

Hyaline cartilage is prone to **calcification**, a process in which calcium phosphate crystals become embedded in the cartilage matrix. The matrix of hyaline cartilage undergoes calcification as a regular occurrence in three well-defined situations:

- The portion of articular cartilage that is in contact with bone tissue in growing and adult bones, but not the surface portion, is calcified.
- Calcification always occurs in cartilage that is about to be replaced by bone (endochondral ossification) during an individual's growth period.
- Hyaline cartilage in the adult calcifies with time as part of the aging process.

In most situations, given sufficient time, cartilage that calcifies is replaced by bone. For example, in older individuals, portions of the cartilage rings in the trachea are often replaced by bone tissue (Fig. 7.14). Chondrocytes normally derive all of their nutrients and dispose of wastes by diffusion of materials through the matrix. When the matrix becomes heavily calcified, diffusion is impeded and the chondrocytes swell and die. The ultimate consequence of this event is the removal of the calcified matrix and its replacement by bone.

Many investigators believe the process of cartilage removal involves a specific cell type designated as a **chondroclast**. This cell is described as resembling an osteoclast in both morphology and lytic function. Early studies of chondroclast structure and function were carried out on the developing mandible, in which the resorption of Meckel cartilage is not followed by bone replacement (endochondral ossification). **Chondroclasts** have also been observed on the deep surface of resorbed articular cartilage in some joint diseases. For instance, these multinucleated cells have been identified on both calcified and noncalcified articular cartilage erosions in **rheumatoid arthritis**. Recent immunocytochemical studies on chondroclasts obtained from pathologic joint specimens revealed that chondroclasts express the **osteoclast-type phenotype**. It is likely that **chondroclasts are mature osteoclasts**, which are capable to resorb cartilage and are found wherever cartilage is being removed.

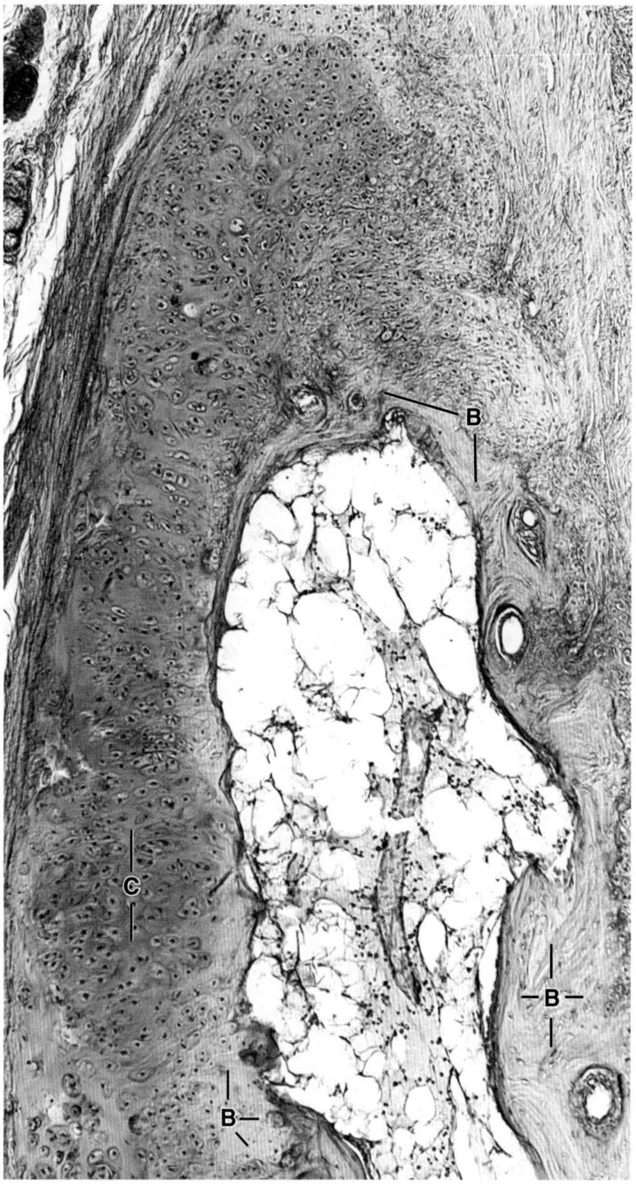

FIGURE 7.14. Photomicrograph of a tracheal ring from an elderly individual, stained with hematoxylin and eosin (H&E). The darker, somewhat basophilic areas on the *left* side of the micrograph represent normal cartilage matrix (*C*). The lighter and more eosinophilic areas represent bone tissue (*B*) that has replaced the original cartilage matrix. A large marrow cavity has formed within the cartilage structure and is visible in the *center* of the micrograph. ×75.

HISTOLOGY 101 NOTEBOOK

CARTILAGE

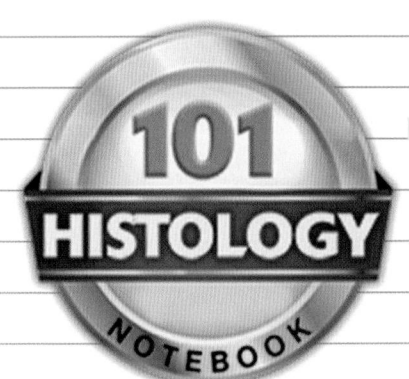

OVERVIEW OF CARTILAGE

- **Cartilage** is a solid, firm, and somewhat pliable form of connective tissue composed of **chondrocytes** and a highly specialized **extracellular matrix** (comprises 95% of cartilage volume).
- Chondrocytes reside within **lacunae** surrounded by extracellular matrix.
- Cartilage is an **avascular structure**; therefore, the composition of the extracellular matrix is essential for diffusion of substances between chondrocytes and blood vessels in the surrounding connective tissue.
- There are three major types of cartilage: **hyaline cartilage, elastic cartilage,** and **fibrocartilage.**

HYALINE CARTILAGE

- The homogeneous, amorphous **extracellular matrix** of hyaline cartilage is produced by chondrocytes and appears glassy.
- **Hyaline cartilage matrix** contains three classes of molecules: **collagen molecules** (mainly type II and other cartilage-specific collagens, e.g., types VI, IX, X, XI); **proteoglycan aggregates**, which contain glycosaminoglycans (GAGs); and **multiadhesive glycoproteins.**
- The ground substance of hyaline cartilage contains three types of GAGs: **hyaluronan, chondroitin sulfate**, and **keratan sulfate.** The last two bind to a core protein to form a **proteoglycan monomer**. Aggrecan is the most abundant proteoglycan monomer in hyaline cartilage.
- **Hyaluronan** molecules interact with a large number of aggrecan molecules to form large **proteoglycan aggregates.** Their negative charges bind and hold large amounts of water molecules.
- **Chondrocytes** are distributed either singularly or in clusters called **isogenous groups.**
- Extracellular matrix surrounding individual chondrocytes (**capsular matrix**) or the isogenous group (**territorial matrix**) varies in collagen content and staining properties. The **interterritorial matrix** surrounds the territorial matrix and occupies the space between isogenous groups.
- A firmly attached connective tissue, the **perichondrium**, surrounds hyaline cartilage. It is not present on the free, or articular, surfaces of articular cartilage in synovial joints.
- Hyaline cartilage is a key tissue in the development of the fetal skeleton (**endochondral ossification**) and in most growing bones (**epiphyseal growth plates**).

ELASTIC CARTILAGE

- **Elastic cartilage** contains normal components of hyaline cartilage matrix with the addition of a dense network of **elastic fibers** and **interconnecting sheets of elastic material**.
- The presence of **elastin** in the extracellular matrix gives elastic cartilage great flexibility to endure repeated bending.
- Elastic cartilage is found in the **external ear, middle ear** (auditory tube), and **larynx**. It is always surrounded by the perichondrium.
- The elastic cartilage matrix **does not calcify** during the aging process.

FIBROCARTILAGE

- **Fibrocartilage** is a combination of dense regular connective tissue and hyaline cartilage.
- Fibrocartilage is typically present in intervertebral discs, the pubic symphysis, insertion of tendons, and structures within certain joints (e.g., menisci of the knee joint).
- The **extracellular matrix** of fibrocartilage contains varying amounts of both **type I** and **type II collagen fibrils**. In addition, ground substance contains larger amounts of **versican** than aggrecan molecules.

CHONDROGENESIS AND CARTILAGE GROWTH

- Most cartilage arises from mesenchyme during **chondrogenesis**. Expression of **transcription factor SOX-9** triggers differentiation of mesenchymal cells into cartilage-producing cells called **chondroblasts**.
- Cartilage is capable of two kinds of growth: **appositional growth** (forms new cartilage at the surface of an existing cartilage) and **interstitial growth** (forms new cartilage by mitotic division of chondrocytes within an existing cartilage mass).

REPAIR OF HYALINE CARTILAGE

- Owing to its avascular nature, cartilage has **limited ability for repair**. Repair mostly involves the production of dense connective tissue.
- In the aging process, hyaline cartilage is prone to **calcification** and is replaced by bone.

PLATE 7.1 ■ HYALINE CARTILAGE

Hyaline cartilage is an avascular form of connective tissue composed of cells called **chondrocytes** and a highly specialized homogeneous-appearing extracellular matrix. The hyaline matrix contains **type II collagen** molecules, **proteoglycan aggregates**, and **multiadhesive glycoproteins**. In addition to type II collagen that constitutes the bulk of the fibrils, the hyaline matrix contains sufficient amounts of type VI, IX, X, and XI collagens called **cartilage-specific collagens**. All collagen molecules interact with each other in a three-dimensional felt-like arrangement. The matrix is highly hydrated—>60% of its net weight consists of water, most of which is bound to proteoglycan aggregates (aggrecan monomers bound to a long hyaluronan molecule).

Hyaline cartilage is found in the adult as the structural framework for the larynx, trachea, and bronchi; it is found on the articular ends of the ribs and on the surfaces of synovial joints. In addition, hyaline cartilage constitutes much of the fetal skeleton and plays an important role in the growth of most bones. At most sites in the body, except for synovial joint surfaces, hyaline cartilage is surrounded by dense irregular connective tissue called the **perichondrium**.

Hyaline cartilage displays both **appositional growth**, the addition of new cartilage at its surface by chondroblasts, and **interstitial growth**, the division and differentiation of chondrocytes within its extracellular matrix. The newly divided cells produce a new cartilage matrix, thus expanding the volume of the cartilage from inside. Therefore, the overall growth of cartilage results from the interstitial secretion of new matrix by chondrocytes and by the appositional secretion of matrix by newly differentiated chondroblasts.

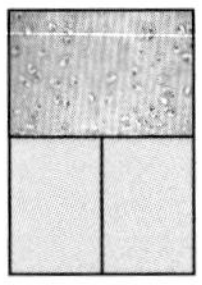

Hyaline cartilage, trachea, human, hematoxylin and eosin (H&E) ×450.

This micrograph reveals hyaline cartilage from the trachea as seen in a routinely prepared specimen. The cartilage appears as an avascular expanse of matrix material and a population of cells called **chondrocytes** (*Ch*). The chondrocytes produce the matrix; the space each chondrocyte occupies is called a **lacuna** (*L*). Surrounding the cartilage and in immediate apposition to it is a cover of connective tissue, the **perichondrium** (*P*). The perichondrium serves as a source of new chondrocytes during **appositional growth** of the cartilage. Often, the perichondrium reveals two distinctive layers: an outer, more fibrous layer and an inner, more cellular layer. The inner, more cellular layer, containing chondroblasts and chondroprogenitor cells, provides for external growth.

Cartilage matrix contains collagenous fibrils masked by ground substance in which they are embedded; thus, the fibrils are not evident. The matrix also contains, among other components, sulfated glycosaminoglycans that exhibit basophilia with hematoxylin or other basic dyes. Also, the matrix material immediately surrounding a lacuna tends to stain more intensely with basic dyes. This region is referred to as a **capsule** (*Cap*). Not uncommonly, the matrix may appear to stain more intensely in localized areas (*asterisks*) that look much like the capsule matrix. This results from the inclusion of a capsule within the thickness of the section, but not the lacuna it surrounds.

Frequently, two or more chondrocytes are located extremely close to one another, separated by only a thin partition of matrix. These are isogenous cell clusters that arise from a single predecessor cell. The proliferation of new chondrocytes by this means with the consequent addition of matrix results in **interstitial growth** of the cartilage.

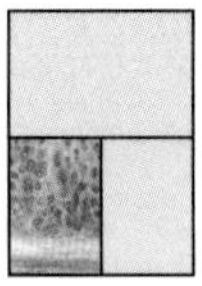

Hyaline cartilage, trachea, human, H&E ×160.

The hyaline cartilage in this micrograph is from a specimen obtained shortly after death and kept cool during fixation. The procedure reduces the loss of its negatively charged sulfate groups; thus, the matrix is stained more heavily with hematoxylin. Also, note the very distinct and deeply stained capsules (*arrows*) surrounding the chondrocytes. The capsule represents the site where the sulfated glycosaminoglycans are most concentrated. In contrast to the basophilia of the cartilage matrix, the **perichondrium** (*P*) is stained with eosin. The lightly stained region between the perichondrium and the deeply stained matrix is the matrix that has not yet matured. It has fewer sulfate groups.

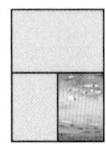

Hyaline cartilage, trachea, human, H&E ×850.

This higher magnification micrograph reveals the area within the *rectangle* in the *lower left* figure. The chondrocytes (*Ch*) in the *upper part* of the micrograph represent an isogenous group and are producing matrix material for interstitial growth. A prominent capsule is not yet evident. The lightly stained basophilic area reveals immature chondrocytes (*arrows*) within the perichondrium (*P*). Closest to the cartilage matrix, within the **perichondrium** (*P*), are several chondrocytes that exhibit just barely detectable cytoplasm and elongated nuclei (*FCh*). These cells are formative chondrocytes that are just beginning to, or will shortly, produce matrix material. In contrast, the nuclei near the *bottom edge* of the micrograph are fibroblast nuclei (*Fib*); they belong to the outer layer of the perichondrium. Note how attenuated their nuclei are compared with the formative chondroblast nuclei of the inner perichondrial layer.

Cap, capsule
Ch, chondrocytes
FCh, formative chondrocytes
Fib, fibroblasts
L, lacuna
P, perichondrium
arrows, immature chondrocytes
asterisk, capsule of a lacuna (lacuna and its chondrocyte not included within the thickness of the section)

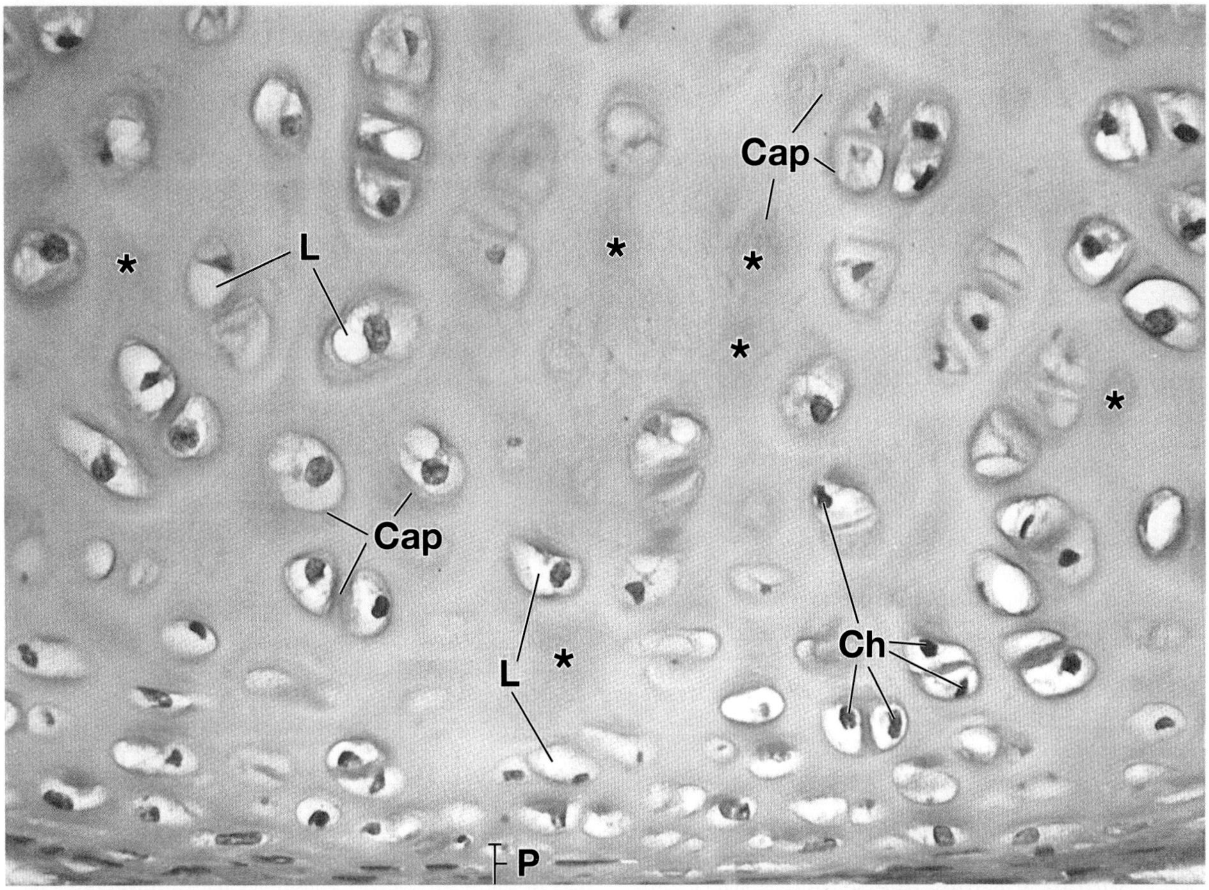
Cap
L
*
Cap
Ch
P

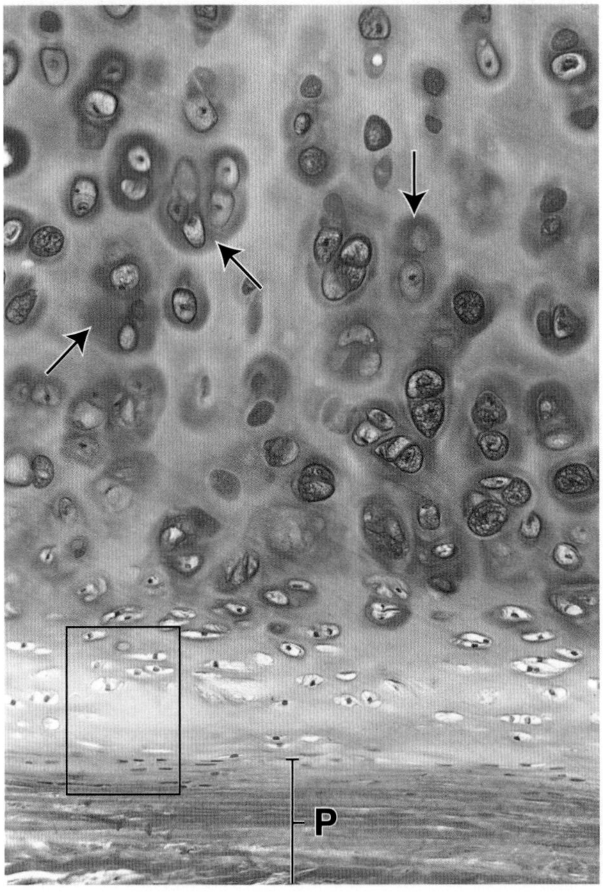
P

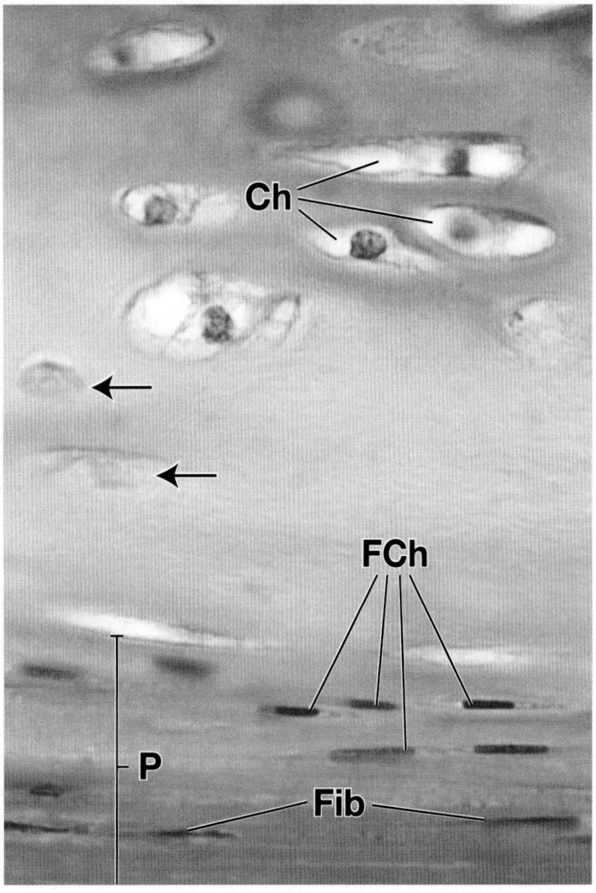
Ch
FCh
P
Fib

PLATE 7.2 ■ HYALINE CARTILAGE AND THE DEVELOPING SKELETON

Hyaline cartilage is present as a precursor to bones that develop in the fetus by the process of endochondral ossification. This cartilage is replaced by bone tissue, except where one bone contacts another, as in a movable joint. In these locations, cartilage persists and covers the end of each bone as articular cartilage, providing a smooth, well-lubricated surface against which the end of one bone moves on the other in the joint. In addition, cartilage, being capable of interstitial growth, persists in weight-supporting bones and other long bones as a growth plate as long as growth in length occurs. The role of hyaline cartilage in bone growth is considered briefly here and in more detail in Plates 8.3 and 8.4.

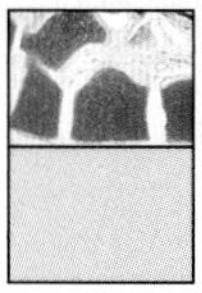

Developing skeleton, fetal foot, rat, hematoxylin and eosin (H&E) ×85.

This section shows the **cartilages** (*C*) that will ultimately become the bones of the foot. In several places, developing ligaments (*L*) can be seen where they join the cartilages. The nuclei of the fibroblasts within the ligaments are just barely perceptible. They are aligned in rows and are separated from other rows of fibroblasts by collagenous material. The hue and intensity of the color of the cartilage matrix, except at the periphery, are due to the combined uptake of the H&E. The collagen of the matrix stains with eosin; however, the presence of sulfated glycosaminoglycans results in staining by hematoxylin. The matrix of cartilage that is about to be replaced by bone, such as that shown here, becomes impregnated with calcium salts, and the calcium is also receptive to staining with hematoxylin. The many enlarged lacunae (seen as light spaces within the matrix where the chondrocytes have fallen out of the lacunae) are due to hypertrophy of the chondrocytes, an event associated with calcification of the matrix. Thus, where these large lacunae are present, that is, in the center region of the cartilage, the matrix is heavily stained.

This figure also shows that the cartilage is surrounded by perichondrium, except where it faces a **joint cavity** (*JC*). Here, the bare cartilage forms a surface. Note that the joint cavity is a space between the cartilages whose boundaries are completed by **connective tissue** (*CT*). The connective tissue at the surface of the cavity constitutes the synovial membrane in the adult and contributes to the formation of a lubricating fluid (synovial fluid) that is present in the joint cavity. All surfaces that will enclose the adult joint cavity are derived originally from the mesenchyme. Synovial fluid is a viscous substance containing, among other things, hyaluronan and glycosaminoglycans; it can be considered an exudate of interstitial fluid. The synovial fluid could be considered an extension of the extracellular matrix, as the joint cavity is not lined by an epithelium.

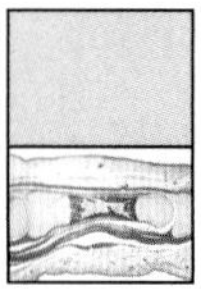

Developing skeleton, fetal finger, human, thionine–picric acid ×30.

This photomicrograph shows a developing long bone of the finger and its articulation with the distal and proximal bones. Before the stage shown here, each bone consisted entirely of a hyaline cartilaginous structure similar to the cartilages seen in the previous figure but shaped like the long bones into which they would develop. Here, only the ends, or epiphyses, of the bone remain as cartilage, the **epiphyseal cartilage** (*C*). The shaft, or diaphysis, has become a cylinder of bone tissue (*B*) surrounding the **marrow cavity** (*MC*). The dark region at the ends of the marrow cavity is calcified cartilage (*arrowhead*) that is being replaced by bone. The bone at the ends of the marrow cavity constitutes the **metaphysis**. With this staining method, the calcified cartilage appears *dark brown*. The newly formed metaphyseal bone is admixed with the degenerating calcified cartilage and is difficult to define at this low magnification; it has the same *yellow-brown* color as the diaphyseal bone. With the continued proliferation of cartilage, the bone grows in length. Later, the cartilage becomes calcified; bone is then produced and occupies the site of the resorbed cartilage. With the cessation of cartilage proliferation and its replacement by bone, growth of the bone stops, and only the cartilage at the articular surface remains. The details of this process are explained in Plates 8.3 and 8.4 that depict endochondral bone formation.

B, bone
C, cartilage
CT, connective tissue
JC, joint cavity
L, ligament
MC, marrow cavity
arrowhead, calcified cartilage

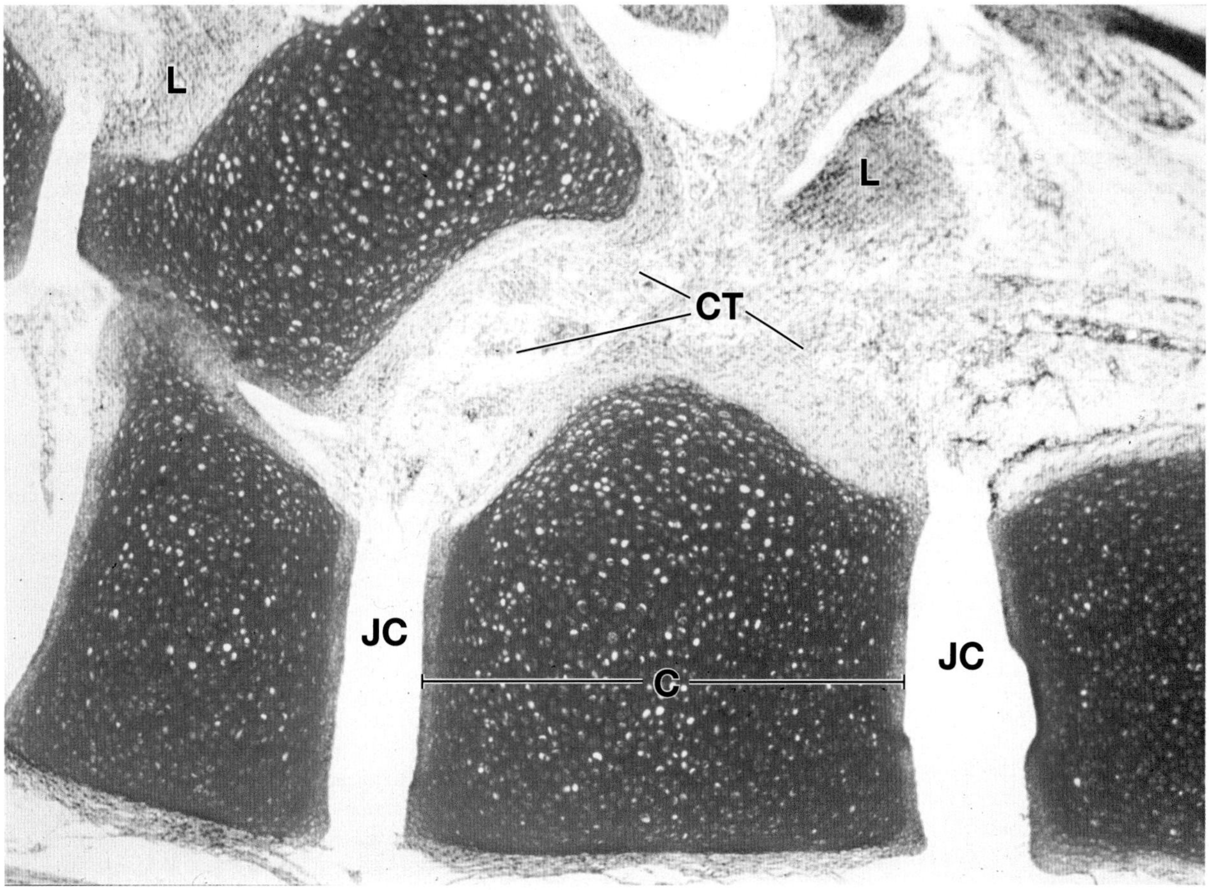
L
L
CT
JC
C
JC

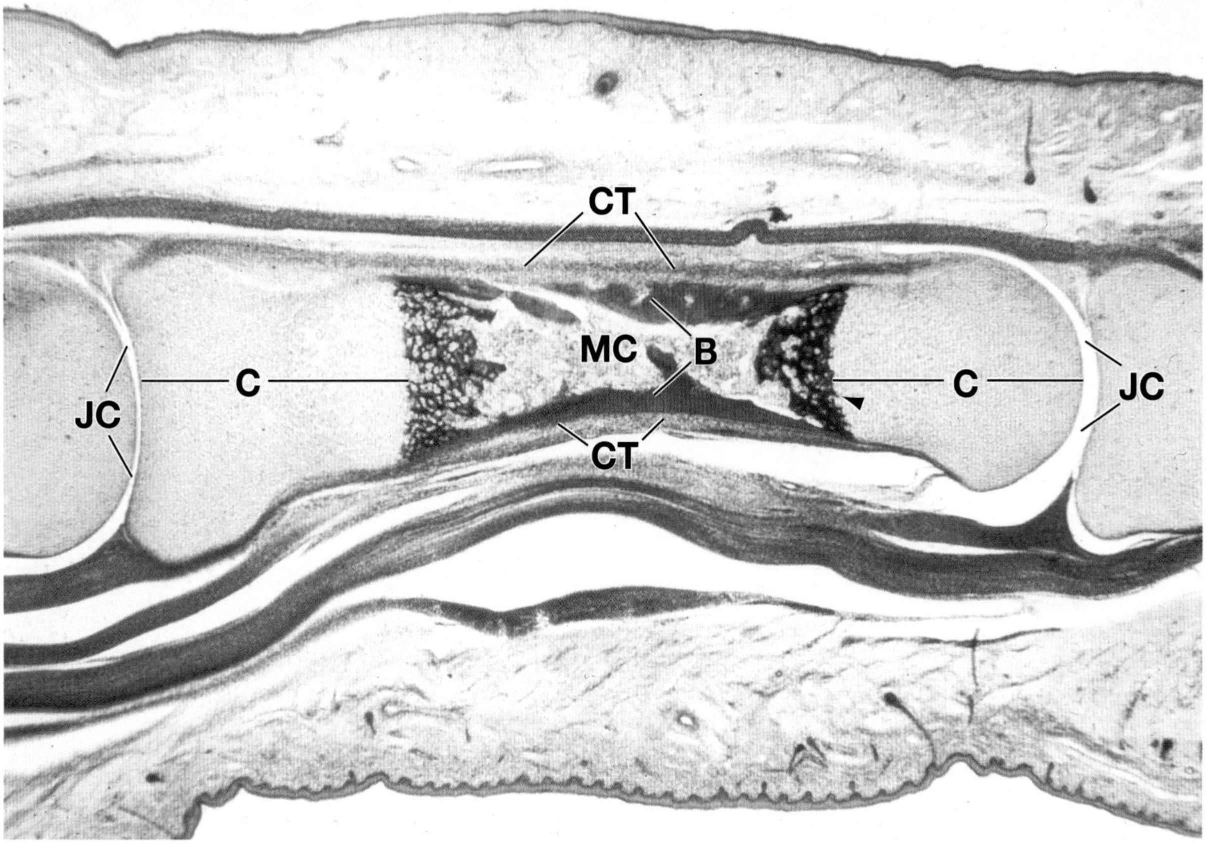
CT
MC
B
JC
C
C
JC
CT

PLATE 7.3 ■ ELASTIC CARTILAGE

Elastic cartilage has a matrix containing elastic fibers and elastic lamellae in addition to type II collagen and other components found in the extracellular matrix of hyaline cartilage. It is found in the auricle of the external ear, auditory tube, epiglottis, and other parts of the larynx (i.e., cuneiform cartilages, vocal processes of arytenoid cartilages). The elastic material imparts properties of elasticity, as distinguished from resiliency, which are not shared by hyaline cartilage. Elastic cartilage is surrounded by perichondrium, and it, too, increases in size by both appositional and interstitial growth. Unlike hyaline cartilage, however, elastic cartilage does not normally undergo the calcification process.

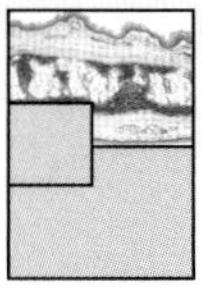

Elastic cartilage, epiglottis, human, hematoxylin and eosin (H&E) and orcein stains ×80.

This section of the epiglottis contains **elastic cartilage** (*EC*) as the centrally located, purple-stained tissue. The essential components of the cartilage, namely, the matrix containing elastic fibers, which stains *purple*, and the light, unstained lacunae surrounded by matrix, are evident in this low-magnification micrograph. The perimeter of the cartilage is covered by **perichondrium** (*PC*); its fibrous character is just barely visible in this figure. The epiglottis contains many small perforations (epiglottic foramina); note the presence of adipose tissue (*AT*) within these openings. Adipose tissue in this micrograph is visible within the boundaries of the elastic cartilage.

Above and below the elastic cartilage is connective tissue, and each surface of the epiglottis is formed by stratified squamous nonkeratinized epithelium (*SE*). Mucous glands (*MG*) can be seen in the connective tissue at the *bottom* of this figure.

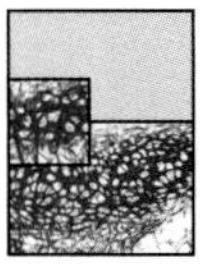

Elastic cartilage, epiglottis, human, H&E and orcein stains ×250; inset ×400.

This shows an area of the **elastic cartilage** at higher magnification. The elastic fibers appear as *purple*, elongated profiles within the matrix. They are most evident at the edges of the cartilage, but they are obscured in some deeper parts of the matrix, where they blend with the elastic material that forms a honeycomb about the lacunae. **Elastic fibers** (*E*) are also apparent in the adipose tissue (*AT*), between the adipocytes.

Some of the lacunae in the cartilage are arranged in pairs separated by a thin plate of matrix. The plate of matrix appears as a bar between the adjacent lacunae. This is a reflection of interstitial growth by the cartilage, in that the adjacent cartilage cells are derived from the same parent cell. They have moved away from each other and secreted a plate of cartilage matrix between them to form two lacunae. Most **chondrocytes** (*Ch*) shown in this figure occupy only part of the lacuna. This is, in part, due to shrinkage, but it is also due to the fact that older chondrocytes contain large lipid droplets that are lost during tissue preparation. The shrinkage of chondrocytes within the lacunae or their loss during preparation causes the lacunae to stand out as light, unstained areas against the darkly stained matrix.

The *inset* shows the elastic cartilage at still higher magnification. Here, the elastic fibers (*E*) are again evident as elongated profiles, chiefly at the edges of the cartilage. Most chondrocytes in this part of the specimen show little shrinkage. Many of the cells display a typically rounded nucleus, and the cytoplasm is evident. Note, again, that some lacunae contain two chondrocytes, indicating interstitial growth.

AT, adipose tissue
Ch, chondrocytes
E, elastic fiber
EC, elastic cartilage
MG, mucous gland
PC, perichondrium
SE, stratified squamous nonkeratinized epithelium

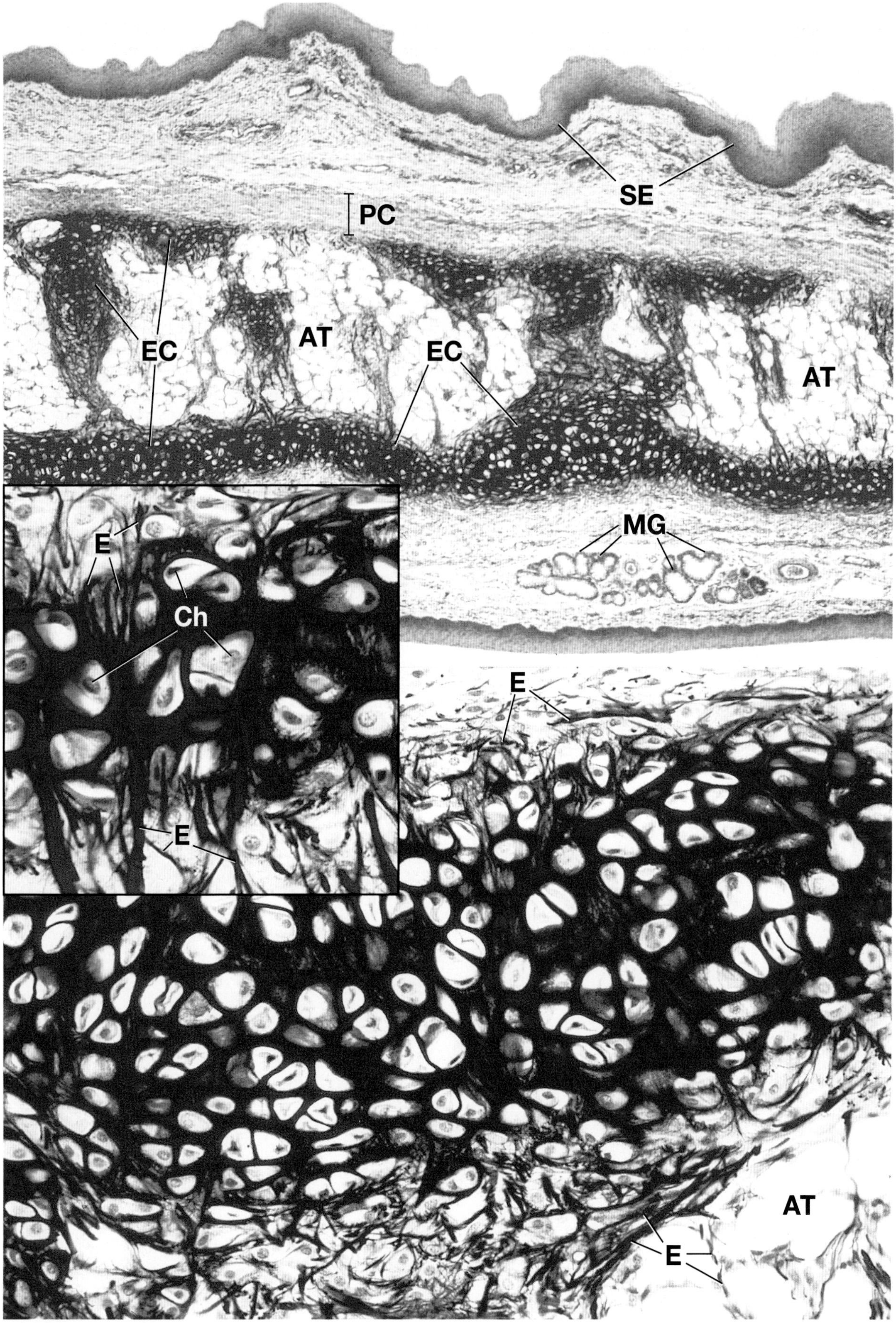
SE
PC
EC
AT
EC
AT
MG
E
Ch
E
E
AT
E

PLATE 7.4 ■ FIBROCARTILAGE

Fibrocartilage is a combination of dense irregular connective tissue and hyaline cartilage. It has a matrix with large bundles of type I collagen in addition to type II collagen. The amount of cartilage varies, but in most locations, the cartilage cells and their matrix occupy a lesser portion of the tissue mass. Fibrocartilage is found at the intervertebral discs, pubic symphysis, knee joint, mandibular joint, sternoclavicular joint, and shoulder joint. It may also be present along the grooves or insertions for tendons and ligaments. Its presence is associated with sites where resilience is required in dense connective tissue to help absorb sudden physical impact, that is, where resistance to both compressive and shearing forces is required in the tissue. Histologically, fibrocartilage appears as small fields of cartilage blending almost imperceptibly with regions of dense fibrous connective tissue. It is usually identified by the presence of aggregates of rounded chondrocytes (isogenous groups) among bundles of collagen fibers and by the basophilic staining of the capsular matrix material and territorial matrix secreted by these cells. No perichondrium is present.

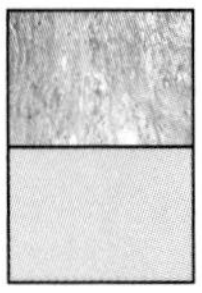

Fibrocartilage, intervertebral disc, human, Mallory trichrome ×160.

This is a low-magnification view of **fibrocartilage**. The Mallory method stains collagen *light blue*. The tissue has a fibrous appearance, and at this low magnification, the nuclei of the **fibroblasts** (*F*) appear as small, elongated, or spindle-shaped bodies. There are relatively few fibroblasts present, as is characteristic of dense connective tissue. The **chondrocytes** (*Ch*) are more numerous and exhibit close spatial groupings, that is, **isogenous groups**. Some of the chondrocytes appear as elongated clusters of cells, whereas others appear in single-file rows. The matrix material immediately surrounding the chondrocytes has a homogeneous appearance and is thereby distinguishable from the fibrous connective tissue.

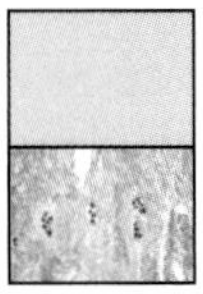

Fibrocartilage, intervertebral disc, human, Mallory trichrome ×700.

This figure shows the area circumscribed by the *rectangle* in the micrograph above at higher magnification. The chondrocytes are contained within lacunae (*arrows*), and their cytoplasm stains deeply. The surrounding **cartilage matrix** material is scant and blends into the dense connective tissue. Cartilage matrix material can be detected best by observing the larger group of chondrocytes at the *left* of this figure and then observing this same area in the previous figure. Note the light homogeneous area around the cell nest in the lower power view. This is the region of cartilage matrix. At the greater magnification of this figure, it is possible to see that some of the collagen fibers are incorporated in the matrix, where they appear as wispy bundles.

Ch, chondrocytes	**F,** fibroblast	**arrows,** lacunae

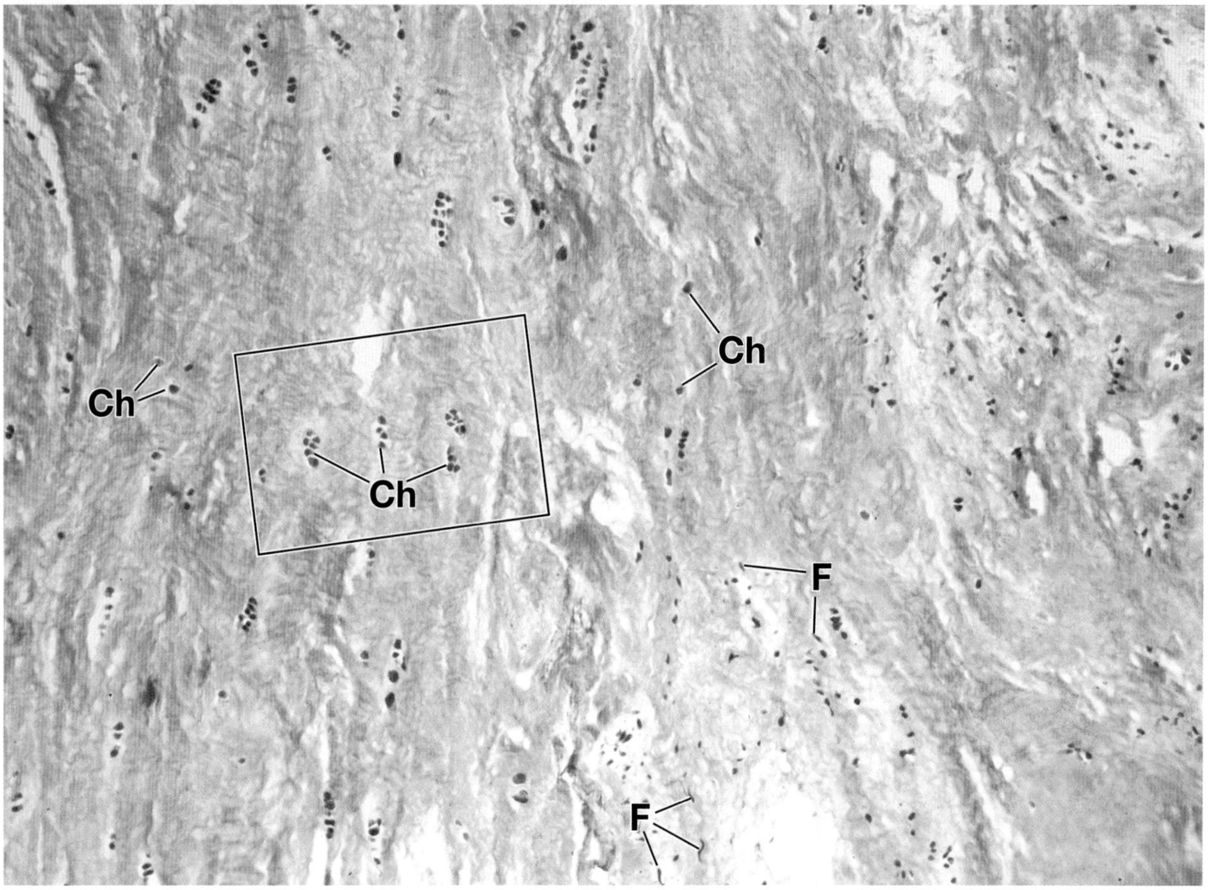
Ch
Ch
Ch
F
F

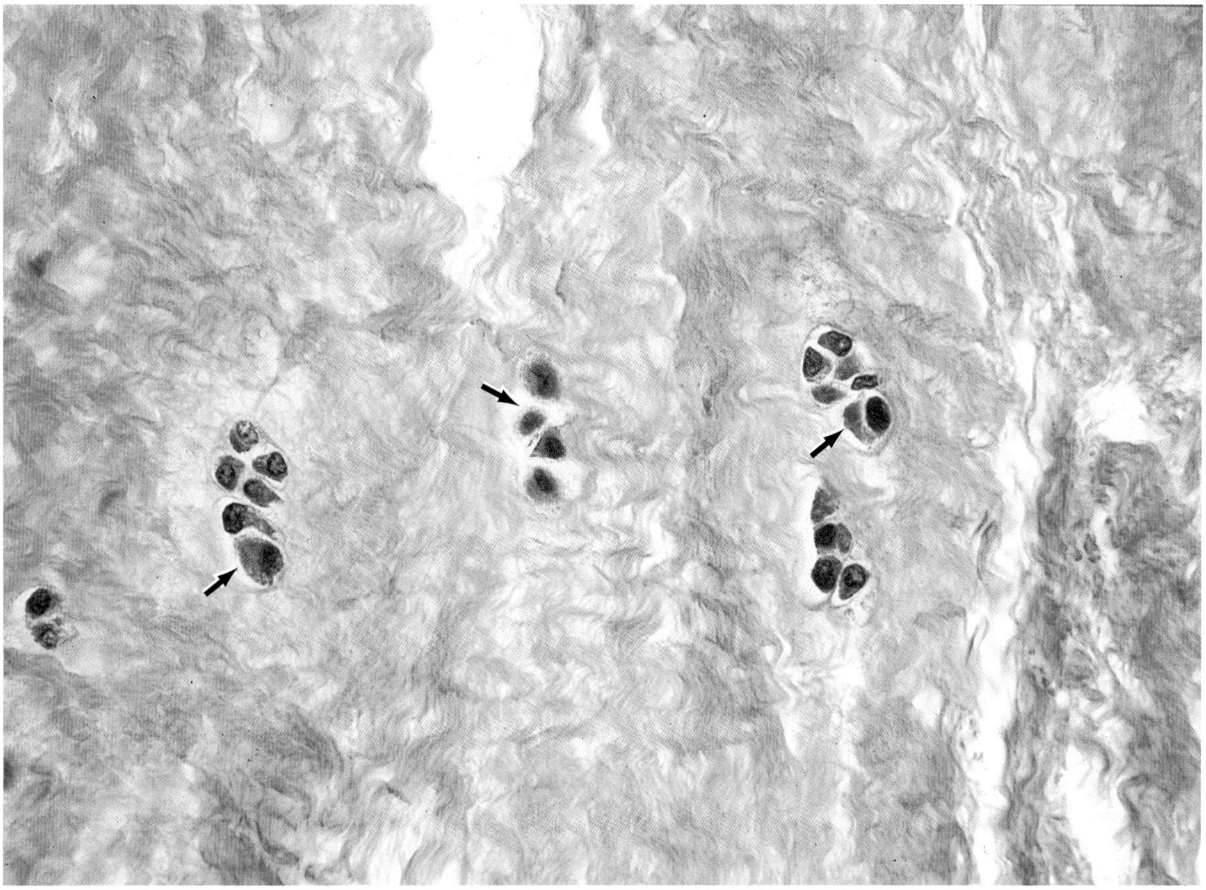

8 BONE

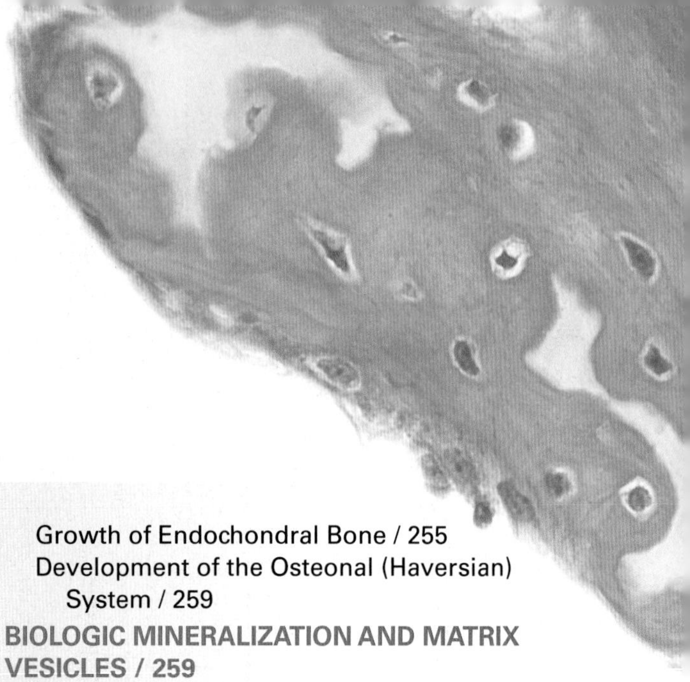

■ OVERVIEW OF BONE

Bone is a connective tissue characterized by a mineralized extracellular matrix.

Bone is a specialized form of connective tissue that, like other connective tissues, consists of cells and extracellular matrix. The feature that distinguishes bone from other connective tissues is the mineralization of its matrix, which produces an extremely hard tissue capable of providing *support* and *protection*. The mineral is calcium phosphate in the form of **hydroxyapatite crystals** $[Ca_{10}(PO_4)_6(OH)_2]$.

By virtue of its mineral content, bone also serves as a **storage site for calcium and phosphate**. Both calcium and phosphate can be mobilized from the bone matrix and taken up by the blood as needed to maintain appropriate levels throughout the body. Thus, in addition to support and protection, bone plays an important secondary role in the homeostatic regulation of blood calcium levels.

Bone matrix contains mainly type I collagen along with other matrix (noncollagenous) proteins.

The major structural component of **bone matrix** is **type I collagen** and, to a lesser extent, **type V collagen**. Trace amounts of other types such as type III, XI, and XIII collagens have also been found in the matrix. All collagen molecules constitute about 90% of the total weight of the bone matrix proteins.

The matrix also contains other matrix (noncollagenous) proteins that constitute the **ground substance** of bone. As a minor component of bone, constituting only 10% of the total weight of bone matrix proteins, they are essential to bone development, growth, remodeling, and repair. Both the collagen and the ground substance become mineralized to form bone tissue. The four main groups of noncollagenous proteins found in the bone matrix are the following:

- **Proteoglycan macromolecules** contain a core protein with various numbers of covalently attached side chains of **glycosaminoglycans** (hyaluronan, chondroitin sulfate, and keratan sulfate). Some proteoglycans, such as keratan sulfate, contain **osteoadherin**, a bone-specific protein that strongly binds to hydroxyapatite crystals. Proteoglycans contribute to the compressive strength of bone. They are also responsible for binding growth factors, and in certain conditions, they may inhibit mineralization. Proteoglycans are described in detail in Chapter 6, Connective Tissue (Table 6.3, page 193).
- **Multiadhesive glycoproteins** are responsible for attachment of bone cells and collagen fibers to the mineralized

ground substance. Some important **glycoproteins** are **osteonectin**, which serves as a glue between the collagen and hydroxyapatite crystals; **podoplanin (E11)**, which is produced exclusively by osteocytes in response to mechanical stress; **dentin matrix protein (DMP)**, which is critical for bone matrix mineralization; **bone sialoproteins**, such as **osteopontin** (also known as **BSP-1**), which mediates attachment of cells to bone matrix; and **BSP-2**, which mediates cell attachment and initiates calcium phosphate formation during the mineralization process.
- **Bone-specific, vitamin K–dependent proteins** serve a variety of functions and include **osteocalcin**, which captures calcium from the circulation and attracts and stimulates osteoclasts in bone remodeling; **protein S**, which assists in the removal of cells undergoing apoptosis; and **matrix Gla-protein (MGP)**, which participates in the development of vascular calcifications.
- **Growth factors** and **cytokines** are small regulatory proteins and include insulin-like growth factors (IGFs), tumor necrosis factor α (TNF-α), transforming growth factor β (TGF-β), platelet-derived growth factors (PDGFs), **bone morphogenic proteins (BMPs)**, **sclerostin** (a BMP antagonist), and **interleukins (IL-1, IL-6)**. BMPs are unique because they induce the differentiation of mesenchymal cells into osteoblasts, the bone-producing cells. Recombinant human **BMP-7**, also known as **osteogenic protein-1 (OP-1)**, is now used clinically to induce bone growth after bone surgery involving large bone defects, spinal fusions, or implantation of graft materials.

Bone matrix contains lacunae connected by a network of canaliculi.

Within the bone matrix are spaces called **lacunae** (sing., *lacuna*), each of which contains a bone cell or **osteocyte**. The osteocyte extends numerous processes into small tunnels called **canaliculi**. Canaliculi course through the mineralized matrix, connecting adjacent lacunae and allowing contact between the cell processes of neighboring osteocytes (Plate 8.1, page 270). In this manner, a continuous network of canaliculi and lacunae-containing cells and their processes is formed throughout the entire mass of mineralized tissue. Electron micrographs show that osteocyte processes communicate by gap junctions. Bone tissue depends on the osteocytes to maintain viability.

In addition to osteocytes, four other cell types are associated with bone:

- **Osteoprogenitor cells** are derived from mesenchymal stem cells; they give rise to osteoblasts.
- **Osteoblasts** secrete the extracellular matrix of bone; once the cell is surrounded by its secreted matrix, it is referred to as an **osteocyte**.
- **Bone-lining cells** remain on the bone surface when there is no active growth. They are derived from those osteoblasts that remain after bone deposition ceases.
- **Osteoclasts** resorb bone and are present on bone surfaces where bone is being removed or remodeled (reorganized) or where bone has been damaged.

Osteoprogenitor cells and osteoblasts are developmental precursors of the osteocyte. Osteoclasts are phagocytotic cells derived from fusion of hemopoietic progenitor cells in bone marrow that give rise to the neutrophilic granulocyte and monocyte lineages. Each of these cells is described in more detail later.

GENERAL STRUCTURE OF BONES

Bone as an Organ

Bones are the principal organs of the musculoskeletal system; bone tissue is the structural component of bones.

Typically, a **bone** consists of bone tissue and other specialized connective tissues, including cartilage, hemopoietic tissue, fat tissue, and associated blood vessels and nerves. Bones, muscles, and joints form the musculoskeletal system. Its primary functions include supporting the body, allowing motion, and protecting vital organs. The musculoskeletal system is made up of bones (the adult human skeletal comprises ~206 bones), skeletal muscles, tendons, cartilages, ligaments, joints, and other connective tissue components that support and connect these elements.

Bones are classified according to shape; the location of spongy and compact bone varies with bone shape.

Spongy and compact bone tissues are located in specific parts of bones. The distribution of these tissues within bones contributes to their shape and is therefore an important factor in how bones are classified. On the basis of shape, bones can be classified into four groups:

- **Long bones** are longer in one dimension than other bones and consist of a shaft and two ends (e.g., the tibia and the metacarpals). A schematic diagram of a long bone sectioned longitudinally through the shaft is shown in Figure 8.1.

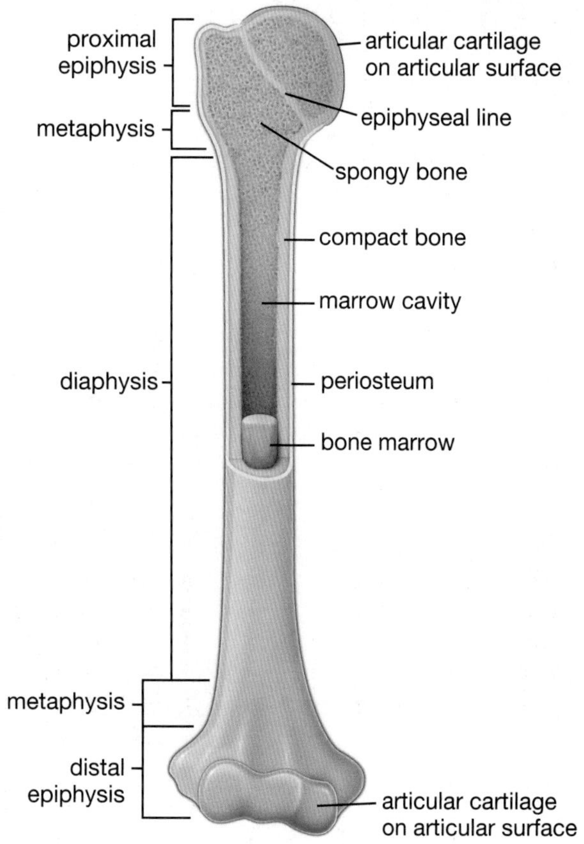

FIGURE 8.1. Structure of a typical long bone. The diaphysis (shaft) of a long bone in the adult contains yellow bone marrow in a large marrow cavity surrounded by a thick-walled tube of compact bone. A small amount of spongy bone may line the inner surface of the compact bone. The proximal and distal ends, or epiphyses, of the long bone consist chiefly of spongy bone with a thin outer shell of compact bone. The expanded or flared part of the diaphysis nearest the epiphysis is referred to as the metaphysis. Except for the articular surfaces that are covered by hyaline (articular) cartilage, indicated in *blue*, the outer surface of the bone is covered by a fibrous layer of connective tissue called the periosteum.

- **Short bones** are nearly equal in length and diameter (e.g., the carpal bones of the hand).
- **Flat bones** are thin and plate-like (e.g., the bones of the calvaria [skullcap], scapula, and the sternum). A flat bone consists of two layers of relatively thick compact bone with an intervening layer of spongy bone.
- **Irregular bones** have a shape that does not fit into any one of the three groups just described; the shape may be complex (e.g., a vertebra), or the bone may contain air spaces or sinuses (e.g., the ethmoid bone).

Long bones have a shaft, called the **diaphysis**, and two expanded ends, each called an **epiphysis** (Fig. 8.2). The articular surface of the epiphysis is covered with hyaline cartilage. The flared portion of the bone between the diaphysis and the epiphysis is called the **metaphysis**. It extends from the diaphysis to the **epiphyseal line**. A large cavity filled with bone marrow, called the **marrow** or **medullary cavity**, forms the inner portion of the bone. In the shaft, almost the entire thickness of the bone tissue is compact; at most, only a small amount of spongy bone faces the marrow cavity. At the ends of the bone, the reverse is true. Here, the spongy bone is extensive, and the compact bone consists of little more than a thin outer shell (see Fig. 8.2).

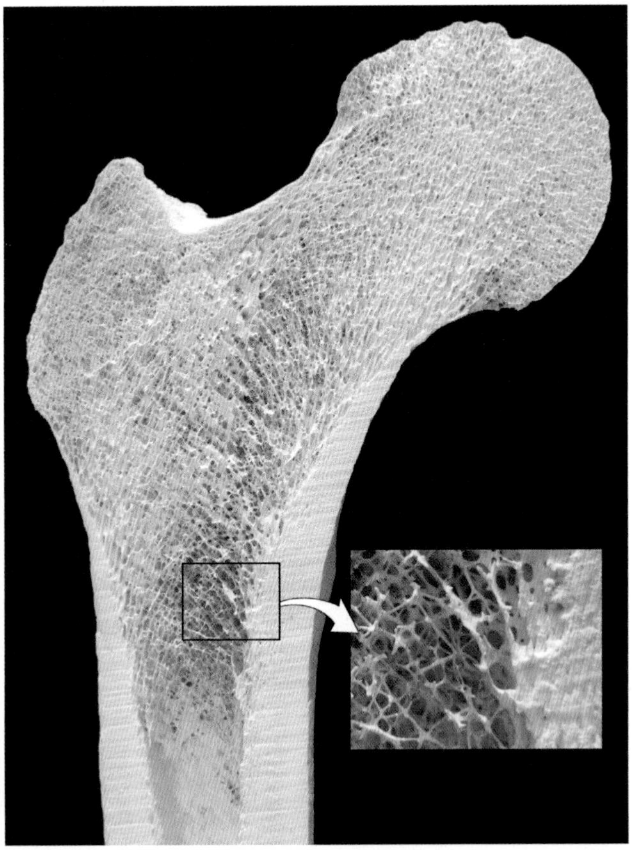

FIGURE 8.2. Epiphysis of an adult long bone. This photograph shows a longitudinally sectioned proximal epiphysis of the femur after the bone was processed by alkaline hydrolysis. The interior of the bone exhibits a spongy configuration and represents spongy (cancellous) bone. It consists of numerous interconnecting bony trabeculae separated by a labyrinth of interconnecting marrow spaces. The three-dimensional orientation of bony trabeculae is not random but is correlated with the magnitude and directionality of hip joint loads (forces acting on the hip joint and transmitted on the head of the femur). The outer portion of the bone has a solid structure and represents compact (dense) bone. It is particularly well visualized in the diaphysis, which encloses the bone marrow cavity. *Inset* from the rectangular area shows enlargement of the boundary between spongy and compact bone.

Short bones possess a shell of compact bone and have spongy bone and a marrow space on the inside. Short bones usually form movable joints with their neighbors; like long bones, their articular surfaces are covered with hyaline cartilage. Elsewhere, **periosteum**, a fibrous connective tissue capsule, covers the outer surface of the bone.

To allow movement and stability during locomotion, different bones are connected by different types of joints.

If the bone forms a freely **movable joint** (also called a **synovial joint**), the contact areas of the two bones are referred to as articular surfaces. The articular surfaces are covered by hyaline cartilage, also called **articular cartilage**, because of its location and function. The space between articulating bones is called the joint cavity; it contains a lubricating fluid (synovial fluid). Articular cartilage is not covered with perichondrium. The details of articular cartilage are discussed in Chapter 7, Cartilage (pages 221-223) and Folder 8.1 (page 241).

The **articular capsule** that surrounds the joint cavity is composed of an outer fibrous layer of dense irregular connective tissue and inner layer of **synovial membrane** that is attached to the edges of **articular cartilages**. Although the synovial membrane lines the joint cavity, it is not considered an epithelium. The synovial membrane consists of two types of mesenchymally derived synoviocytes: type A, macrophage-like cells, and type B, fibroblast-like cells. In most synovial joints, the articular capsule is reinforced from the exterior by ligaments. Some synovial joints have fibrocartilaginous structures superimposed between the articulating surfaces (i.e., menisci in the knee joint or the intraarticular disc in the temporomandibular joint).

In addition to movable joints, bones can be connected by **slightly movable** or **immovable joints**. These joints have no joint cavity and are held together by either fibrocartilage (i.e., intervertebral discs or pubic symphysis permitting slight movements), irregular connective tissue (i.e., sutures of the skull), or cartilage (between certain bones of the rib cage). The ability of the bone to perform its skeletal function is attributable to the bone tissue, regular and irregular connective tissue (i.e., ligaments, joint capsule), and the articular (hyaline) cartilage in the synovial joints.

The surgical replacement of joints due to **osteoarthritis**, the most frequent idiopathic disease of joints characterized by degeneration of articular cartilage, is called an **arthroplasty**. During this procedure, the damaged articular surface with underlying bone tissue is removed and replaced with an artificial joint (called a **prosthesis**) made of metal, plastic, or ceramic materials designed to mimic the normal anatomic structures of the joint. Due to excellent biocompatibility, a titanium metal prosthesis (often coated with hydroxyapatite crystals, growth factors, or both) is commonly used. They develop a strong structural and functional connection (osseointegration) between living bone and the surface of the implant.

Outer Surface of Bones

Bones are covered by periosteum, a sheath of dense fibrous connective tissue containing osteoprogenitor cells.

Bones are covered by a **periosteum** except in areas where they articulate with another bone. In the latter case, the articulating surface is covered by cartilage. The periosteum

FOLDER 8.1

CLINICAL CORRELATION: JOINT DISEASES

Inflammation of the joints or **arthritis** can be caused by many factors and can produce varying degrees of pain and disability. Arthritis is caused by a pathologic response of articular cartilage to injury.

Simple trauma to a joint by a single incident or by repeated insult can damage the articular cartilage, causing it to calcify. Eventually, the cartilage is replaced by bone. This process can lead to **ankylosis** (i.e., bony fusion in the joint and subsequent loss of motion). The foot and knee joints of runners and football players and hand and finger joints of stringed-instrument players are especially vulnerable to this condition.

Immune responses or infectious processes that localize in joints, as in **rheumatoid arthritis** or **tuberculosis**, can also damage the articular cartilages, producing both severe joint pain and gradual ankylosis. Surgical replacement of the damaged joint with a prosthetic joint can often relieve the pain and restore joint motion in seriously debilitated individuals.

Another common cause of damage to articular cartilages is the deposition of crystals of uric acid in the joints, particularly those of the toes and fingers. This condition is known as **gouty arthritis** or, more simply, **gout**. Gout has become more common due to the widespread use of thiazide diuretics in the treatment of hypertension. In genetically predisposed individuals, gout is the most common side effect of these drugs. Gout causes severe pain due to the presence of sharp, needle-like uric acid crystals in the joint. Damage to the cartilage also causes the formation of calcareous deposits that deform the joint and limit its motion.

that covers an actively growing bone consists of an outer fibrous layer that resembles other dense irregular connective tissues and an inner, more cellular layer that is in direct contact with bone. The cellular layer contains **skeletal stem cells**, including osteoprogenitor cells. If active bone formation is not in progress on the bone surface, the fibrous layer is the main component of the periosteum, and the inner layer is not well defined. The relatively few cells that are present, the **periosteal cells**, are, however, capable of undergoing division and becoming osteoblasts under the appropriate stimulus. **Periostin**, a 90-kDa extracellular matrix protein secreted by periosteal cells, is a key regulator of periosteal responses to mechanical stress, injury, and bone repair.

In general, the collagen fibers of the periosteum are arranged parallel to the surface of the bone in the form of a capsule. The character of the periosteum is different where ligaments and tendons attach to the bone. Collagen fibers from these structures extend obliquely or at right angles to the long axis of the bone, where they are continuous with the collagen fibers of the extracellular matrix. These fibers are called **perforating** or **Sharpey fibers**. They extend into the outer circumferential and interstitial lamellae but usually do not enter the osteons.

Bone Cavities

Bone cavities are lined by endosteum, a layer of connective tissue cells that contains osteoprogenitor cells.

The **lining tissue** of both the compact bone facing the marrow cavity and the trabeculae of spongy bone within the cavity is referred to as **endosteum**. The endosteum is often only one cell layer thick and consists of osteoprogenitor cells that can differentiate into bone matrix–secreting cells (osteoblasts) and bone-lining cells. Osteoprogenitor cells and bone-lining cells are difficult to distinguish at the microscopic level. They are both flattened in shape with elongated nuclei and indistinguishable cytoplasmic features. Because of their location within the bone cavities, they are frequently called **endosteal cells**.

The marrow cavity and the spaces in spongy bone contain bone marrow.

Red bone marrow consists of blood cells in different stages of development and a network of reticular cells and fibers that serve as a supporting framework for the developing blood cells and vessels. As an individual grows, the amount of red marrow does not increase proportionately with bone growth. In later stages of growth and in adults, when the rate of blood cell formation has diminished, the tissue in the marrow cavity consists mostly of fat cells; it is then called **yellow marrow**. In response to appropriate stimuli, such as extreme blood loss, yellow marrow can revert to red marrow. In the adult, red marrow is normally restricted to the spaces of spongy bone in a few locations, such as the sternum and the iliac crest. Diagnostic bone marrow samples and marrow for transplantation are obtained from these sites.

■ TYPES OF BONE TISSUE

Bone tissue is classified as either compact (dense) or spongy (cancellous).

If a bone is cut, two distinct structural arrangements of bone tissue can be recognized (see Fig. 8.2 and Plate 8.2, page 272). A compact, dense layer forms the outside of the bone (**compact bone**); a sponge-like meshwork consisting of **trabeculae** (thin, anastomosing spicules of bone tissue) forms the interior of the bone (**spongy bone**). The spaces within the meshwork are continuous and, in a living bone, are occupied by marrow and blood vessels.

Mature Bone

Mature bone is composed of structural units called osteons (Haversian systems).

Mature bone is largely composed of cylindrical units called **osteons** or **Haversian systems** (Fig. 8.3). The osteons consist of **concentric lamellae** (sing., *lamella*) of bone matrix surrounding a central canal, the **osteonal (Haversian) canal**, which contains the vascular and nerve supply of the

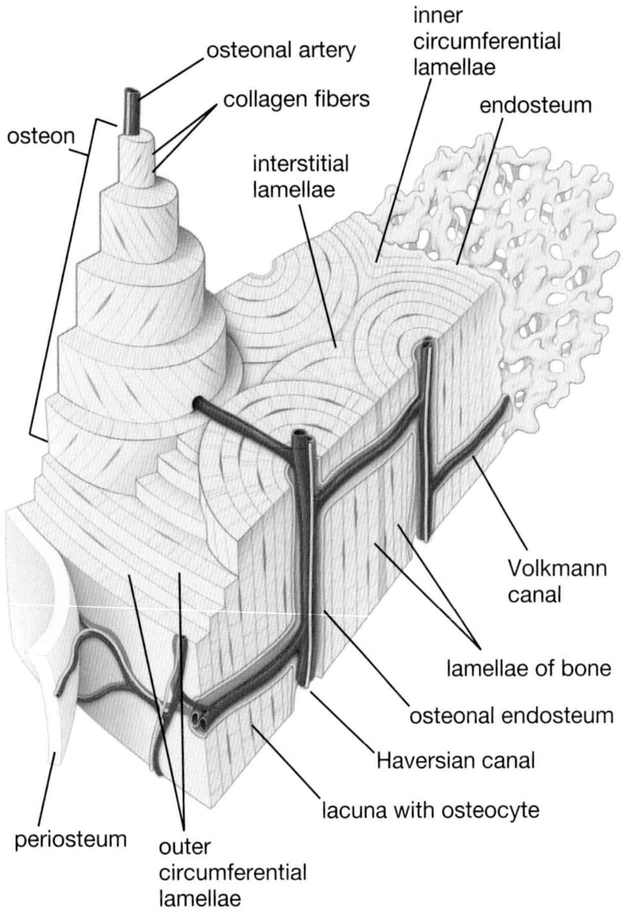

FIGURE 8.3. Diagram of a section of compact bone removed from a long bone. The concentric lamellae and the Haversian canal that they surround constitute an osteon (Haversian system). One of the Haversian systems in this diagram is drawn as an elongated cylindrical structure rising above the plane of the bone section. It consists of several concentric lamellae that have been partially removed to show the perpendicular orientation of collagen fibers in adjacent layers. Interstitial lamellae result from bone remodeling and formation of new Haversian systems. The inner and outer surfaces of the compact bone in this diagram show additional lamellae—the outer and inner circumferential lamellae—arranged in broad layers. Both the inner circumferential lamellae and the spongy bone on the internal surface of the compact bone are covered by a thin layer of endosteum, which faces the bone marrow spaces. The outer surface of the bone is covered by periosteum that contains a thicker layer of connective tissue. Branches of nutritional arteries and small veins accompanied by nerves are shown within the Haversian and Volkmann canals. These vessels and nerves also supply the periosteum and endosteum.

osteon. Canaliculi containing the processes of osteocytes are generally arranged in a radial pattern with respect to the canal (Plate 8.1, page 270). The system of canaliculi that opens to the osteonal canal also serves for the passage of substances between the osteocytes and blood vessels. Between the osteons are remnants of previous concentric lamellae called **interstitial lamellae** (see Fig. 8.3). Because of this organization, mature bone is also called **lamellar bone**.

The long axis of an osteon is usually parallel to the long axis of the bone. The collagen fibers in the concentric lamellae in an osteon are laid down parallel to one another in any given lamella but in different directions in adjacent lamellae. This arrangement gives the cut surface of lamellar bone the appearance of plywood and imparts great strength to the osteon.

Lamellar bone is also found at sites other than the osteon. **Circumferential lamellae** follow the entire inner and outer circumferences of the shaft of a long bone, appearing much like the growth rings of a tree (see Fig. 8.3). **Perforating (Volkmann) canals** are channels in lamellar bone through which blood vessels and nerves travel from the periosteal and endosteal surfaces to reach the osteonal (Haversian) canal; they also connect osteonal canals to one another (Fig. 8.4). They usually run at approximately right angles to the long axis of the osteons and of the bone (see Fig. 8.3). Volkmann canals are not surrounded by concentric lamellae, a key feature in their histologic identification.

Mature spongy bone is structurally similar to mature compact bone.

Mature **spongy bone** is similar in structure to mature compact bone except that the tissue is arranged as **trabeculae** or **spicules**; numerous interconnecting marrow spaces of various sizes are present among the bone tissue. The matrix of the bone is lamellated.

Arteries that enter the marrow cavity through the nutrient foramina supply blood to the shaft of long bones.

Nutrient foramina are openings in the bone through which blood vessels pass to reach the marrow. The greatest numbers of nutrient foramina are found in the diaphysis and epiphysis (Fig. 8.5). Metaphyseal arteries supplement the blood supply to the bone. Veins that drain the blood from bone exit through the nutrient foramina or through the bone tissue of the shaft and continue out through the periosteum.

The **nutrient arteries** that supply the diaphysis and epiphysis arise developmentally as the principal vessels of the periosteal buds. The metaphyseal arteries, in contrast, arise developmentally from periosteal vessels that become incorporated into the metaphysis during the growth process (i.e., through the widening of the bone).

The blood supply to bone tissue is essentially centrifugal.

The blood that nourishes bone tissue moves from the marrow cavity into and through the bone tissue and out via periosteal veins; thus, its flow is in a centrifugal direction. With respect to nourishment of the bone tissue itself, Volkmann canals provide the major route of entry for vessels to pass through the compact bone. The smaller blood vessels enter the Haversian canals, which contain a single arteriole and a venule or a single capillary. A lesser blood supply to the outermost portions of the compact bone is provided by the branches of periosteal arteries (see Fig. 8.5). Bone tissue lacks lymphatic vessels; lymphatic drainage occurs only from the periosteum.

Immature Bone

Bone tissue initially formed in the skeleton of a developing fetus is called **immature bone**. It differs from mature bone in several respects (Fig. 8.6):

- Immature bone does not display an organized lamellated appearance. On the basis of its collagen fiber arrangement, such bone is designated **nonlamellar**. Nonlamellar bone is also referred to as **bundle bone** or **woven bone** because of the interlacing arrangement of the collagen fibers.
- Immature bone contains relatively more cells per unit area than does mature bone.
- The cells in immature bone tend to be randomly arranged, whereas cells in mature bone are usually arranged with their long axes in the same direction as the lamellae.

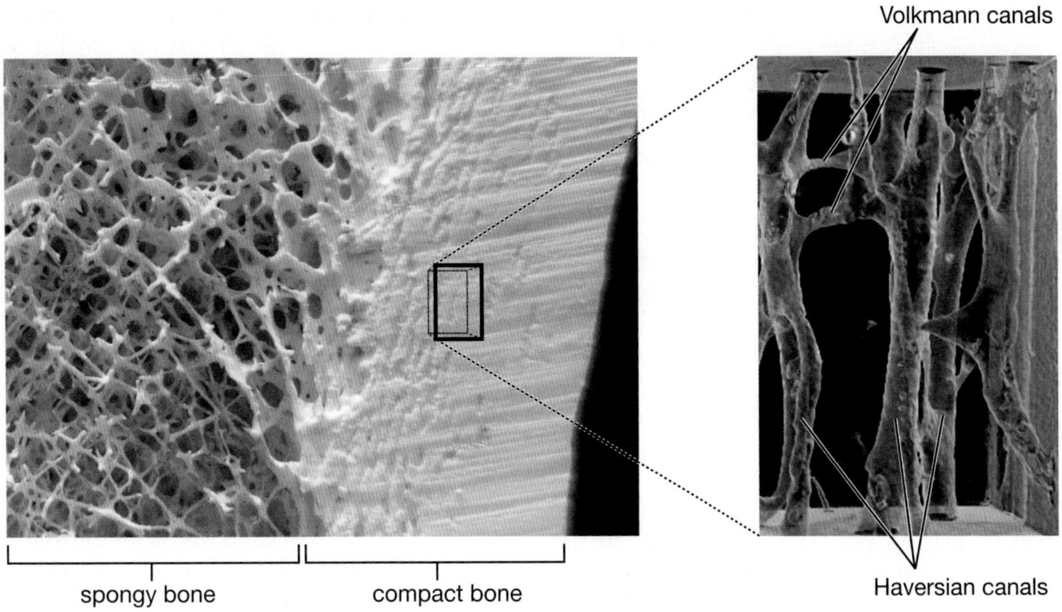

FIGURE 8.4. Three-dimensional reconstruction of Haversian and Volkmann canals from a compact bone. a. This photograph shows enlargement of the interphase between compact and spongy bone from a diaphysis of the femur. **b.** Using high-resolution quantitative computed tomography (CT), a three-dimensional reconstruction of the Haversian and Volkmann canals was obtained from a small area of the compact bone indicated on the adjacent photograph. Note that all Haversian canals run parallel to each other in the same direction and are interconnected by perpendicularly oriented Volkmann canals. ×180. (Courtesy of Dr. Mark Knackstedt, Australian National University.)

- The matrix of immature bone has more ground substance than does the matrix of mature bone. The matrix in immature bone stains more intensely with hematoxylin, whereas the matrix of mature bone stains more intensely with eosin.

Although not evident in typical histologic sections (Fig. 8.7), immature bone is not heavily mineralized when it is initially formed, whereas mature bone undergoes prolonged secondary mineralization. The secondary mineralization of mature bone is evident in microradiographs of ground sections that show younger Haversian systems to be less mineralized than older Haversian systems (see Fig. 8.25).

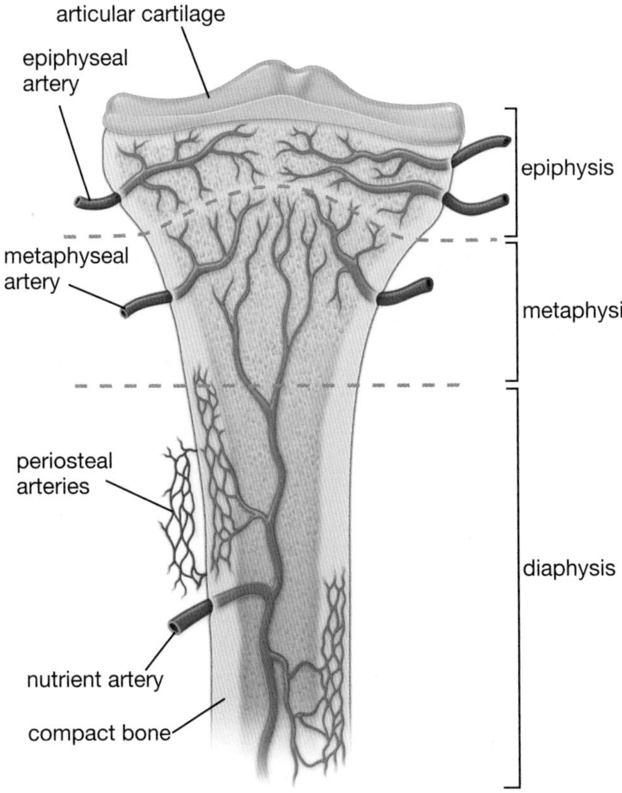

FIGURE 8.5. Diagram showing the blood supply of an adult long bone. The nutrient artery and the epiphyseal arteries enter the bone through nutrient foramina. These openings in the bone arise developmentally as the pathways of the principal vessels of periosteal buds. Metaphyseal arteries arise from periosteal vessels that become incorporated into the metaphysis as the bone grows in diameter.

Immature bone forms more rapidly than mature bone. Although mature bone is clearly the major bone type in the adult and immature bone is the major bone type in the fetus, areas of immature bone are present in adults, especially where bone is being remodeled. Areas of immature bone are common in the alveolar sockets of the adult oral cavity and where tendons insert into bones. It is this immature bone in the alveolar sockets that makes orthodontic corrections possible in adults.

■ CELLS OF BONE TISSUE

As noted previously, five designated cell types are associated with bone tissue: osteoprogenitor cells, osteoblasts, osteocytes, bone-lining cells, and osteoclasts. With the exception of the osteoclast, each of these cells may be regarded as a differentiated form of the same basic cell type (Fig. 8.8). Each undergoes transformation from a less mature form to a more mature form in relation to functional activity (growth of bone). In contrast, the osteoclast originates from a different cell line and is responsible for bone resorption, an activity associated with bone remodeling.

Osteoprogenitor Cells

The osteoprogenitor cell is derived from mesenchymal stem cells.

Osteogenesis, the process of new bone formation, is essential to normal bone function. It requires a population of renewable **osteoprogenitor cells** (osteoblast precursor cells) that are responsive to molecular stimuli that transform them into bone-forming cells. Osteoprogenitor cells are derived from **mesenchymal stem cells** in the bone marrow that have

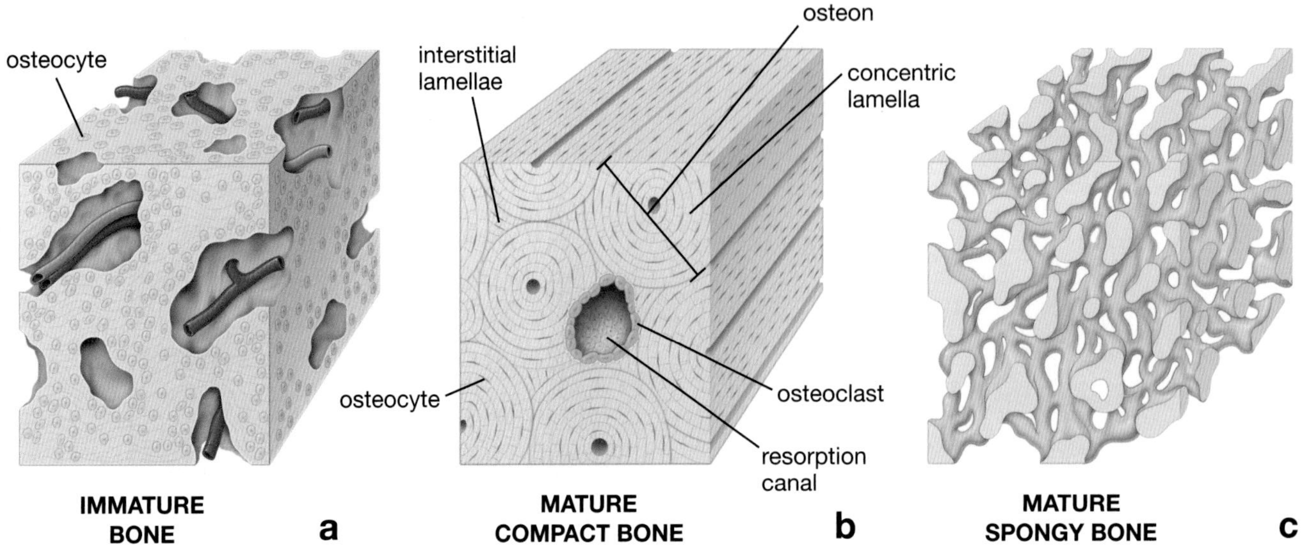

FIGURE 8.6. Diagram of immature and mature compact and spongy bone. a. Immature (woven) bone does not display an organized lamellar appearance because of the interlacing arrangement of the collagen fibers. The cells tend to be randomly arranged. **b.** The cells in mature compact bone are organized in a circular manner that reflects the lamellar structure of the Haversian system. Resorption canals in mature bone are lined by osteoclasts (in cutting cones) and have their long axes oriented in the same direction as the Haversian canals. **c.** Mature spongy bone represents a meshwork of trabeculae (thin, anastomosing spicules of bone tissue). The spaces within the meshwork are continuous and, in a living bone, are occupied by bone marrow.

the potential to differentiate into many different cell types, including fibroblasts, osteoblasts, adipocytes, chondrocytes, and muscle cells. The key factor that triggers differentiation of osteoprogenitor cells is a transcription factor called **core binding factor alpha-1 (CBFA1)**, also called **runt-related transcription factor 2 (RUNX2)**. This protein prompts the expression of genes that are characteristic of the phenotype of the osteoblast. IGF-1 and IGF-2 stimulate osteoprogenitor cell proliferation and differentiation into osteoblasts. As noted on page 239, BMPs also play a role in the differentiation into osteoblasts. Several clinical studies have demonstrated that **pulsed electromagnetic field stimulation (PEMF)** assists in the healing of bone fractures by increasing bone tissue regeneration. This effect is related to increased cellular

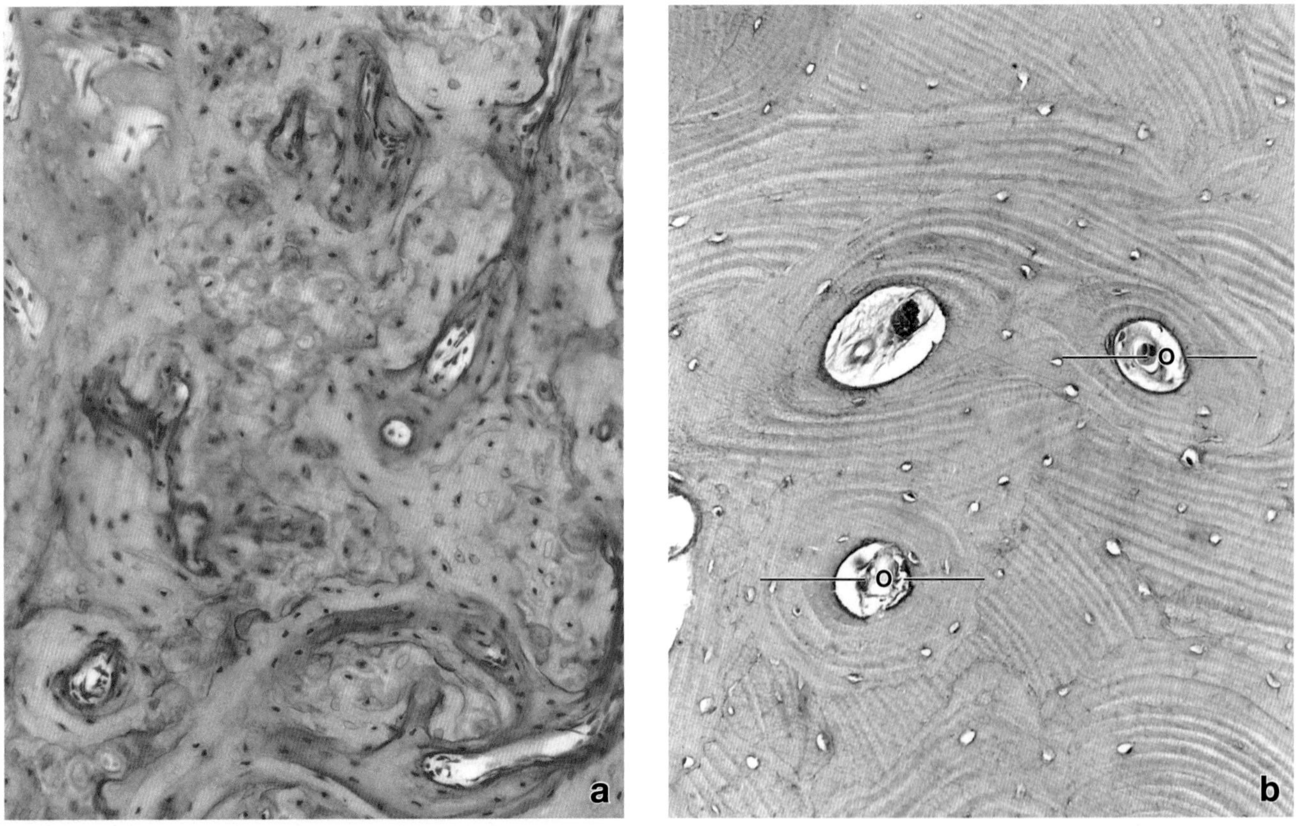

FIGURE 8.7. Photomicrographs of decalcified immature and mature bone. a. Decalcified immature bone, stained with H&E, showing the relationship of cells to the extracellular matrix. The immature bone has more cells, and the matrix is not layered in osteonal arrays. ×130. **b.** This cross section of decalcified mature compact bone stained with H&E shows several osteons (*O*) with concentric lamellae. The Haversian canals contain blood vessels, nerve, and connective tissue. Osteocytes undergo considerable shrinkage during routine slide preparation, revealing empty lacunae with a small nucleus attached to their walls. Mature bone has fewer osteocytes per unit area than immature bone. Note the presence of interstitial lamellae between neighboring osteons. ×160.

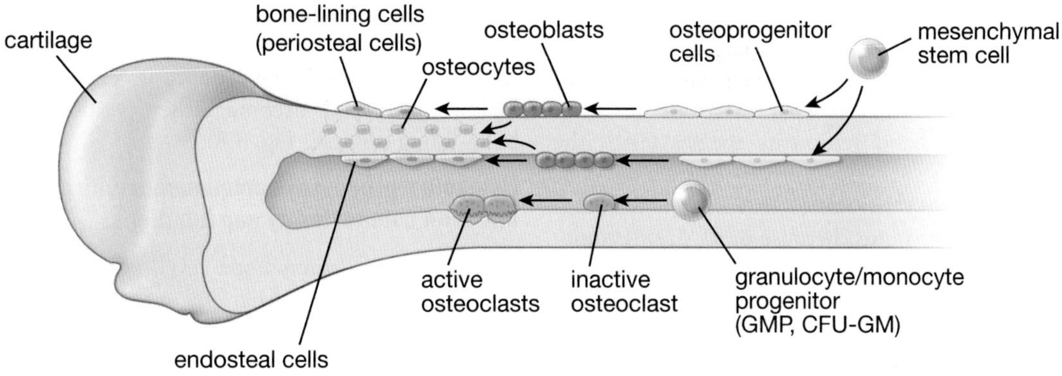

FIGURE 8.8. Schematic drawing of cells associated with bone. All cells except osteoclasts originate from the mesenchymal stem cells, which differentiate into osteoprogenitor cells, osteoblasts, and finally osteocytes and bone-lining cells. Bone-lining cells on external bone surfaces are part of the periosteum, hence the term *periosteal cells*. Bone-lining cells on internal bone surfaces are frequently called endosteal cells. Note that osteoprogenitor cells and bone-lining cells have a similar microscopic appearance and are often difficult to distinguish from each other. Osteoclasts originate from hemopoietic progenitor cells, which differentiate into bone-resorbing cells. The specific details of osteoclast differentiation are illustrated in Figure 8.15.

differentiation of osteoprogenitor cells after stimulation with an electromagnetic field. This approach is now being used as an effective tissue-engineering strategy to treat bone defects, accelerate fracture repair, and help vertebrae fuse after spinal fusion surgery.

The osteoprogenitor cell is a resting cell that can differentiate into an osteoblast and secrete bone matrix.

Osteoprogenitor cells are found on the external and internal surfaces of bones and may also reside in the microvasculature supplying bone. Morphologically, they resemble the **periosteal cells** that form the innermost layer of the periosteum and the **endosteal cells** that line the marrow cavities, the osteonal (Haversian) canals, and the perforating (Volkmann) canals. In growing bones, osteoprogenitor cells appear as flattened or squamous cells with lightly staining, elongated, or ovoid nuclei and inconspicuous acidophilic or slightly basophilic cytoplasm. Electron micrographs reveal profiles of rough-surfaced endoplasmic reticulum (rER) and free ribosomes as well as a small Golgi apparatus and other organelles.

Osteoblasts

The osteoblast is the differentiated bone-forming cell that secretes bone matrix.

Like its close relatives, the fibroblast and the chondroblast, the **osteoblast** is a versatile secretory cell that retains the ability to divide. It secretes both **type I collagen** (which constitutes 90% of the protein in bone) and **bone matrix proteins**, which constitute the initial unmineralized bone, or **osteoid**. Bone matrix proteins produced by the osteoblast include **calcium-binding proteins**, such as osteocalcin and osteonectin; **multiadhesive glycoproteins**, such as bone sialoproteins (BSP-1 [osteopontin] and BSP-2); thrombospondins; various **proteoglycans** and their aggregates; and **tissue nonspecific alkaline phosphatase (TNAP)**. Circulating levels of TNAP and osteocalcin are used clinically as markers of osteoblast activity.

The osteoblast is also responsible for the calcification of bone matrix. The calcification process appears to be initiated by the osteoblast through the secretion into the matrix of small, 50- to 250-nm, membrane-limited **matrix vesicles**. The vesicles are actively secreted only during the period in which the cell produces the bone matrix. The structure and function of these vesicles are discussed later in this chapter (pages 259-263).

Osteoblasts are recognized in the light microscope by their cuboidal or polygonal shape and their aggregation into a single layer of cells lying in apposition to the forming bone (Fig. 8.9). The newly deposited matrix is not immediately

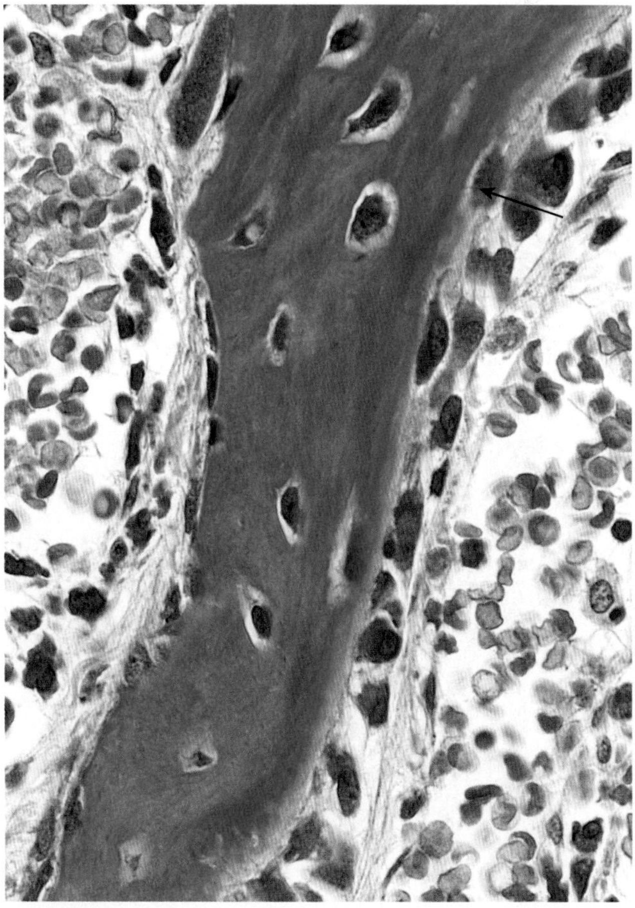

FIGURE 8.9. Photomicrograph of a growing bone spicule stained with Mallory-Azan. Osteocytes are embedded within the bone matrix of the spicule, which is stained *dark blue*. These cells are metabolically active, laying down the unmineralized bone matrix (osteoid). A number of osteoblasts are aligned on the right side of the spicule. Between these cells and the calcified bone spicule is a thin, light blue–stained layer of osteoid. This is the uncalcified matrix material produced by the osteoblasts. One of the cells (*arrow*) has virtually surrounded itself by its osteoid product; thus, it can now be called an osteocyte. On the left side of the spicule, the nongrowing part, are inactive osteoblasts. The cells exhibit flattened nuclei and attenuated cytoplasm. ×550.

calcified. It stains lightly or not at all compared with the mature mineralized matrix, which stains heavily with eosin. Because of this unique staining property of the newly formed matrix, osteoblasts appear to be separated from the bone by a light band. This band represents the **osteoid**, the nonmineralized matrix.

The cytoplasm of an **active osteoblast** is markedly basophilic, and the Golgi apparatus, because of its size, is sometimes observed as a clear area adjacent to the nucleus. Small, periodic acid–Schiff (PAS)-positive granules are observed in the cytoplasm, and a strong alkaline phosphatase reaction associated with the cell membrane can be detected by appropriate histochemical staining.

In contrast to the secreting osteoblasts found in active matrix deposition, **inactive osteoblasts** are flat or attenuated cells that cover the bone surface. These cells resemble osteoprogenitor cells. Osteoblasts respond to mechanical stimuli to mediate the changes in bone growth and bone remodeling. As osteoid deposition occurs, the osteoblast is eventually surrounded by osteoid matrix and thereby becomes an osteocyte.

Not every osteoblast is designated to become an osteocyte. Only 10% to 20% of osteoblasts differentiate into osteocytes. Most osteoblasts undergo apoptosis. Others transform into inactive cells and become either periosteal or endosteal bone-lining cells (see Fig. 8.8).

Osteoblast processes communicate with other osteoblasts and with osteocytes by gap junctions.

At the electron microscope level, osteoblasts exhibit thin cytoplasmic processes that penetrate the adjacent osteoid produced by the cell and are joined to similar processes of adjacent osteocytes by gap junctions. This early establishment of junctions between an osteoblast and adjacent osteocytes (as well as between adjacent osteoblasts) allows neighboring cells within the bone tissue to communicate.

The osteoblast cytoplasm is characterized by abundant rER and free ribosomes (Fig. 8.10). These features are consistent with its basophilia observed in the light microscope as well as with its role in the production of collagen and proteoglycans for the extracellular matrix. The Golgi apparatus and surrounding regions of the cytoplasm contain numerous

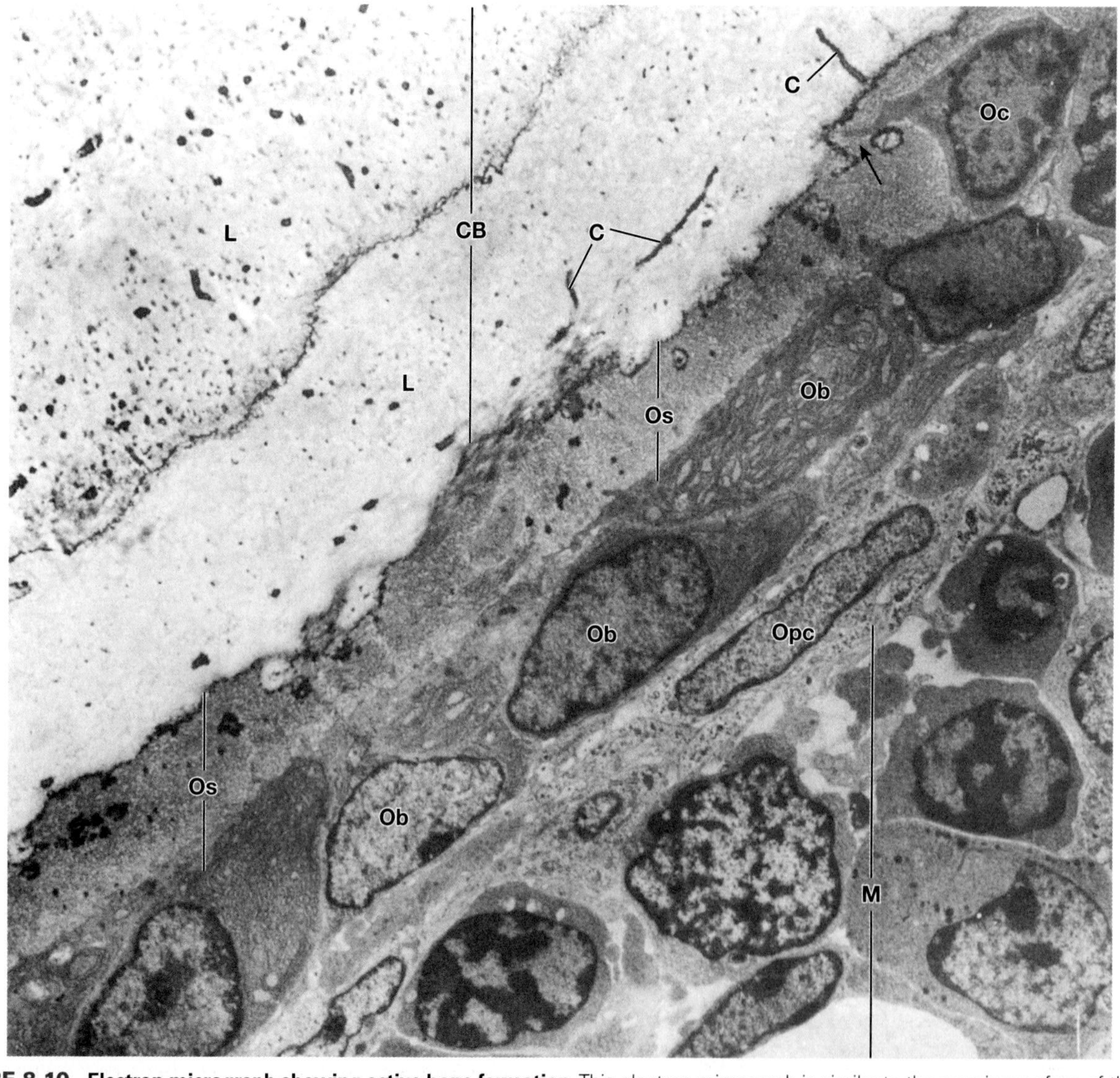

FIGURE 8.10. Electron micrograph showing active bone formation. This electron micrograph is similar to the growing surface of the bone spicule in the preceding light micrograph (see Fig. 8.9). The marrow cavity (*M*) with its developing blood cells is seen in the *lower right* corner. Osteoprogenitor cells (*Opc*) are evident between the marrow and the osteoblasts (*Ob*). They exhibit elongated or ovoid nuclei. The osteoblasts are aligned along the growing portion of the bone, which is covered by a layer of osteoid (*Os*). In this same region, one of the cells (*upper right* corner) embedded within the osteoid exhibits a small process (*arrow*). This cell, because of its location within the osteoid, can now be called an osteocyte (*Oc*). The remainder of the micrograph (*upper left*) is composed of calcified bone matrix (*CB*). Within the matrix are canaliculi (*C*) containing osteocyte processes. The boundary between two adjacent lamellae (*L*) of previously formed bone is evident as an irregular dark line. ×9,000.

vesicles with a flocculent content that is presumed to consist of matrix precursors. These vesicles are the PAS-staining granules seen in light microscopy. The matrix vesicles, also produced by the osteoblast, appear to arise by an ectosomal pathway, originating as sphere-like outgrowths that pinch off from the apical plasma membrane or microvilli to become free in the matrix. Other cell organelles include numerous rod-shaped mitochondria and occasional dense bodies and lysosomes.

Osteocytes

The osteocyte is the mature bone cell enclosed by bone matrix that was previously secreted as an osteoblast.

When completely surrounded by osteoid or bone matrix, the osteoblast is referred to as an **osteocyte** (see Fig. 8.9). The process of transformation from osteoblast to osteocyte takes approximately 3 days. During this time, the osteoblast produces a large amount of extracellular matrix (nearly 3 times its own cellular volume), reduces its cell volume by roughly 70% in comparison to the volume of the original osteoblast, decreases size and number of organelles, and develops long cell processes that radiate from its cell body. Each osteocyte develops on average about 50 cell processes. Following bone matrix mineralization, each osteocyte occupies a space, or **lacuna**, that conforms to the shape of the cell. Osteocytes' cytoplasmic processes are enclosed by **canaliculi** within the matrix (Fig. 8.11). They communicate with processes of neighboring osteocytes and bone-lining cells by means of **gap junctions** formed by a family of bone-expressed connexins. Osteocytes also communicate indirectly with distant osteoblasts, endothelial cells of bone marrow vasculature, pericytes of blood vessels, and other cells through the expression of various signaling molecules, such as nitric oxide or glutamate transporters. In addition to typical cell-to-cell communication (gap junctions are discussed in Chapter 5, Epithelial Tissue, pages 150-151), osteocyte processes contain **hemichannels** (the unopposed half of gap junction channels) that provide communication between cells and extracellular matrix.

In hematoxylin and eosin (H&E)-stained sections, the canaliculi and their processes are not discernible. However, in

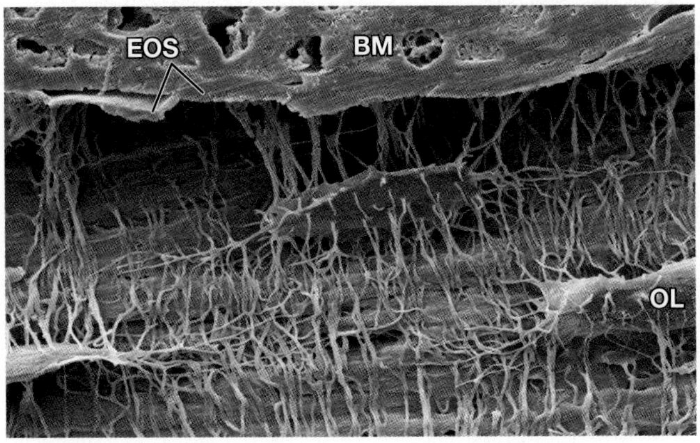

FIGURE 8.11. Osteocyte lacunae with extensive network of canaliculi. This scanning electron micrograph of an acid-etched, resin-embedded sample of bone from a 4-month-old mouse shows a network of canaliculi interconnecting three osteocyte lacunae (*OL*) and endosteal cells. In this method, resin fills the osteocyte lacunae, canaliculi, osteoid, and bone marrow spaces but does not penetrate mineralized bone matrix. Phosphoric acid is usually used to remove the mineral, leaving behind a resin cast. The *upper part* of the image is occupied by bone marrow cells (*BM*), which are separated from bone tissue by the endosteum (*EOS*). ×2,000. (Courtesy of Dr. Lynda Bonewald.)

ground sections, the canaliculi are readily evident (Plate 8.1, page 270). Osteocytes are typically smaller than their precursor cells because of their reduced perinuclear cytoplasm. Often, in routinely prepared microscopic specimens, the cell is highly distorted by shrinkage and other artifacts that result from decalcification of the matrix prior to sectioning the bone. In such instances, the nucleus may be the only prominent feature. In well-preserved specimens, osteocytes exhibit less cytoplasmic basophilia than osteoblasts, but little additional cytoplasmic detail can be seen (Plate 8.2, page 272).

Osteocytes are metabolically active and multifunctional cells that respond to mechanical forces applied to the bone.

In the past, osteocytes were considered passive cells responsible only for maintaining the bone matrix. Recent discoveries show that osteocytes are metabolically active and multifunctional cells. They are involved in the process of **mechanotransduction** in which they respond to mechanical forces applied to the bone. Decreased mechanical stimuli (e.g., immobilization, muscle weakness, weightlessness in space) cause bone loss, whereas increased mechanical stimuli promote bone formation.

Due to the slight flexibility of bone, mechanical forces applied to the bone (e.g., to the femur or tibia during walking) cause interstitial fluid to flow out of the canaliculi and lacunae on the compressed side of the bone. Movement of interstitial fluid through the canalicular system generates a **transient electrical potential (streaming potential)** at the moment when the stress is applied. The streaming potential opens voltage-gated calcium channels in the membranes of the osteocytes over which the tissue fluid flows. Resulting increases in intracellular calcium, adenosine triphosphate (ATP), nitric oxide concentration, and prostaglandin E_2 (PGE_2) synthesis alter expression of *c-fos* and *cox-2* genes responsible for bone formation. The shear stress of the fluid flow also induces the opening of **hemichannels** that allow release of accumulated intracellular molecules into the extracellular space of the canaliculi. In addition, expression of the IGF-1 gene results in the increased production of IGF-1, which promotes conversion of osteoprogenitor cells into osteoblasts. Thus, the regions of a bone under the most stress will have the largest deposition of new bone. The osteocyte also has primary cilium that recent studies suggest may play a possible role in detecting the flow of interstitial fluid within the lacuna and may be involved in mechanosensation and molecular signaling (see Chapter 5, Epithelial Tissue, pages 135-136 for detailed information about the primary cilium's structure and function).

An osteocyte responds to reduced mechanical stress by secreting **matrix metalloproteinases (MMPs)**. The empty space surrounding osteocytes is the result of enzymatic degradation of bone matrix by MMP. Increased mechanical stress activates molecular mechanisms similar to those found in the matrix-producing osteoblasts. Thus, the osteocytes are responsible for reversible remodeling of their pericanalicular and perilacunar bone matrix. This process is called **osteocytic remodeling**.

Osteocytes appear in different functional states during the osteocytic remodeling of their perilacunar and pericanalicular microenvironment.

Electron microscopy has revealed osteocytes in various functional states related to the **osteocytic remodeling** process. Indeed, there is histologic and microradiographic evidence (i.e., enlarged lacunae and reduced radiodensity) that the osteocyte can remodel the surrounding bone matrix. As mentioned earlier, osteocytes can modify their microenvironment (the volume of their lacunae or diameter of their canaliculi) in response to environmental stimuli. Because the surface area of lacunae and canaliculi inside the bone is several orders of magnitude greater than the surface area of the bone itself, removal of minute amounts of mineralized matrix by each osteocyte would have significant effects on circulating levels of calcium and phosphates.

Three functional states, each with a characteristic morphology, have been identified based on the appearance of osteocytes in electron micrographs:

- **Quiescent osteocytes** exhibit a paucity of rER and a markedly diminished Golgi apparatus (Fig. 8.12a). An osmiophilic lamina representing mature calcified matrix is seen in close apposition to the cell membrane.
- **Formative osteocytes** show evidence of matrix deposition and exhibit certain characteristics similar to those of osteoblasts. Thus, the rER and Golgi apparatus are more abundant, and there is evidence of osteoid in the pericellular space within the lacuna (Fig. 8.12b).
- **Resorptive osteocytes**, like formative osteocytes, contain numerous profiles of endoplasmic reticulum and a well-developed Golgi apparatus. Moreover, lysosomes are conspicuous (Fig. 8.12c). The concept of degradation of bone by the resorptive osteocytes (previously called **osteocytic osteolysis**) has fallen out of favor because it is not the dominant form of bone resorption. However, some osteocytic perilacunar and canalicular remodeling has been observed, and it may act as a backup system for calcium and phosphate ion homeostasis, especially during lactation, stress, and reproductive cycles. It is also possible that changes in the size of the lacunae and canaliculi or surrounding extracellular matrix might modulate mechanotransduction and osteoblasts' responses to mechanical forces applied to bone.

Osteocytes are long-living cells and their deaths are attributed to apoptosis, degeneration/necrosis, senescence (old age), or bone remodeling activity of the osteoclasts. The natural **life span of osteocytes** in humans is estimated to be about **10–20 years**. The percentage of dead osteocytes in bone increases with age, from 1% at birth to 75% in the eighth decade of life. It is hypothesized that when the age of an individual exceeds the upper limit of the life span of the osteocyte, these cells may die (senescence) and their lacunae and canaliculi may fill with mineralized tissue.

Bone-Lining Cells

Bone-lining cells are derived from osteoblasts and cover bone that is not remodeling.

In sites where remodeling is not occurring, the bone surface is covered by a layer of flat cells with attenuated cytoplasm and a paucity of organelles beyond the perinuclear region (Fig. 8.13a). These cells are designated simply as **bone-lining**

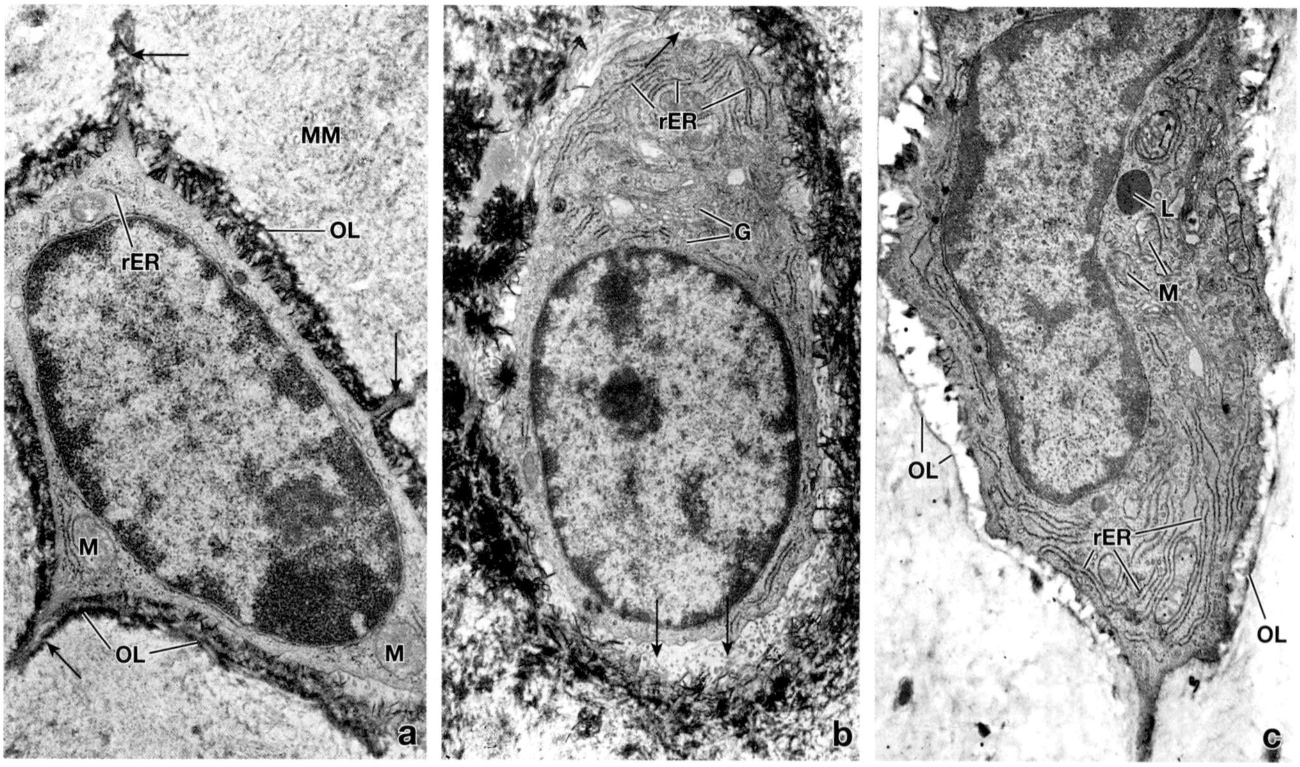

FIGURE 8.12. Electron micrographs of three different functional stages of an osteocyte. a. Relatively quiescent osteocyte that contains only a few profiles of rough endoplasmic reticulum (*rER*) and a few mitochondria (*M*). The cell virtually fills the lacuna that it occupies; the *arrows* indicate where cytoplasmic processes extend into canaliculi. Hydroxyapatite crystals have been lost from the matrix, which is ordinarily mineralized (*MM*), but some hydroxyapatite crystals fill the pericellular space. The hydroxyapatite crystals obscure the other substances within the pericellular space. The dark band marking the boundary of the lacuna is the osmiophilic lamina (*OL*). ×25,000. **b.** A formative osteocyte containing larger amounts of rER and a large Golgi apparatus (*G*). Of equal importance is the presence of a small amount of osteoid in the pericellular space within the lacuna. The osteoid shows profiles of collagen fibrils (*arrows*) not yet mineralized. The lacuna of a formative osteocyte is not bounded by an osmiophilic lamina. ×25,000. **c.** A resorptive osteocyte containing a substantial amount of rER, a large Golgi apparatus, mitochondria (*M*), and lysosomes (*L*). The pericellular space is devoid of collagen fibrils and may contain some flocculent material. The lacuna containing a resorptive osteocyte is bounded by a less conspicuous osmiophilic lamina (*OL*). ×25,000.

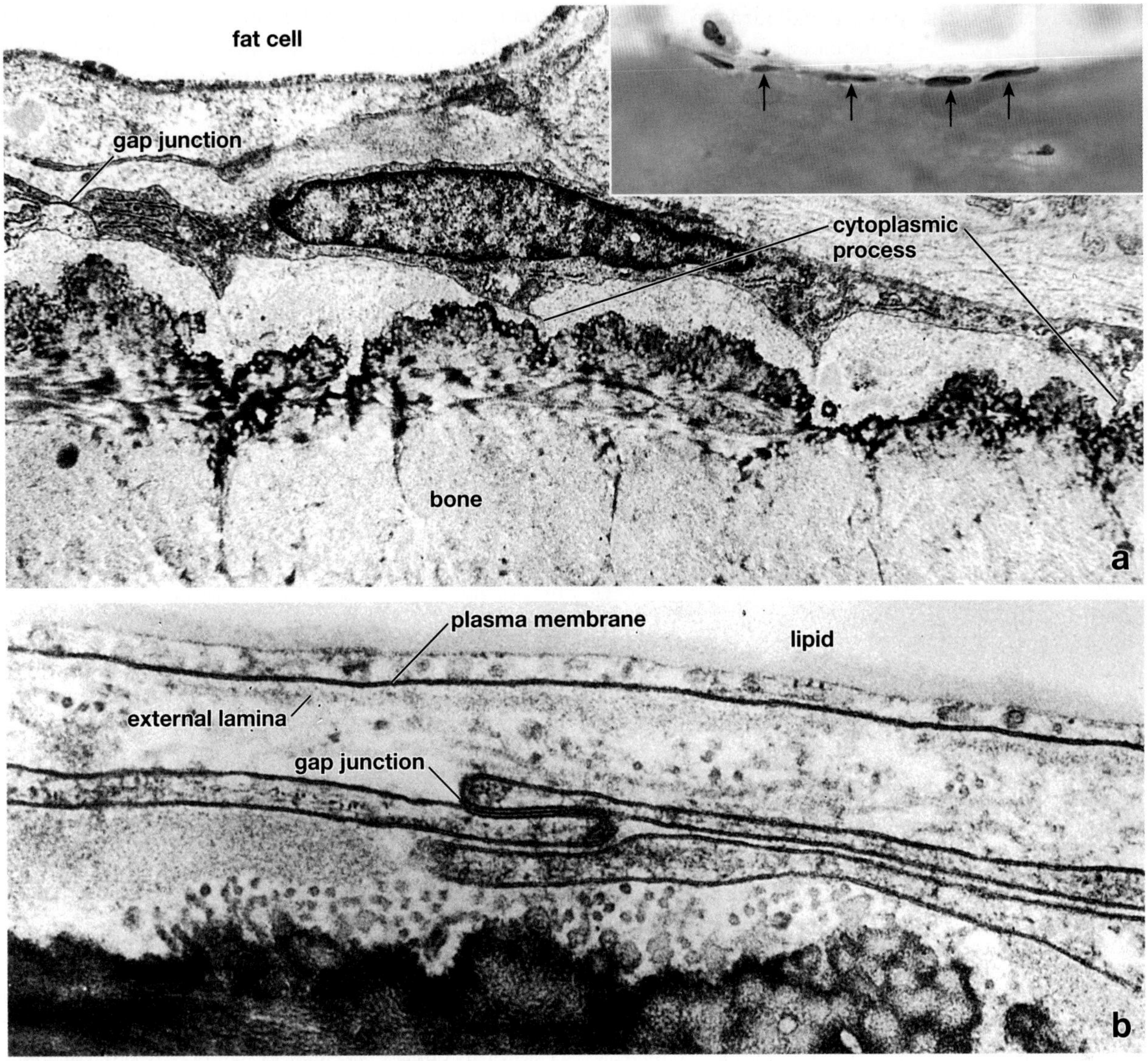

FIGURE 8.13. Electron micrograph of bone-lining cells. a. The cytoplasm of a bone-lining cell located on the surface of a spicule of mature bone is very attenuated and contains small amounts of rough endoplasmic reticulum (*rER*) and free ribosomes. A gap junction is seen between the two adjacent bone-lining cells. In addition, cytoplasmic processes are clearly seen where they pass through the matrix of unmineralized bone (osteoid). A fat cell of the marrow is also present. ×8,900. (Reprinted with permission from Miller SC, Bowman BM, Smith JM, et al. Characterization of endosteal bone-lining cells from fatty marrow bone sites in adult beagles. *Anat Rec*. 1980;198:163–173.) **Inset.** High-magnification photomicrograph of a similar bone spicule stained with H&E, included for orientation purposes. The bone-lining cells (endosteal cells) on the surface of the spicule are indicated by the *arrows*. ×350. **b.** Electron micrograph of the cytoplasm of two bone-lining cells observed at higher magnification. The gap junction is clearly seen where the two cells are in apposition. The edge of a fat cell is seen at the *top* of the electron micrograph; its lipid, thin rim of cytoplasm, plasma membrane, and external lamina are also evident. ×27,000.

cells. Bone-lining cells on external bone surfaces are called **periosteal cells**, and those lining internal bone surfaces are often called **endosteal cells** (see Fig. 8.8). Gap junctions are present where the bone-lining cell processes contact one another (Fig. 8.13b).

Bone-lining cells represent a population of cells that are derived from osteoblasts. They are thought to function in the maintenance and nutritional support of the osteocytes embedded in the underlying bone matrix and regulate the movement of calcium and phosphate into and out of the bone. These suggested roles are based on the observation that the cell processes of bone-lining cells extend into the canalicular channels of the adjacent bone (see Fig. 8.13b) and communicate by means of gap junctions with osteocytic processes. In these respects, bone-lining cells are somewhat comparable to osteocytes.

Osteoclasts

The osteoclast is responsible for bone resorption.

Osteoclasts are large, multinucleated cells found at sites where bone is being removed. They rest directly on the bone tissue where resorption is taking place (Fig. 8.14). As a result of osteoclast activity, a shallow bay called a **resorption bay (Howship lacuna)** can be observed in the bone directly under the osteoclast. The cell is conspicuous not only because of its large size but also because of its marked acidophilia. It also exhibits a strong histochemical reaction for acid phosphatase because of the numerous lysosomes that it contains. One of these enzymes, the 35-kDa iron-containing **tartrate-resistant acid phosphatase (TRAP)**, is used clinically as a marker of osteoclast activity and differentiation.

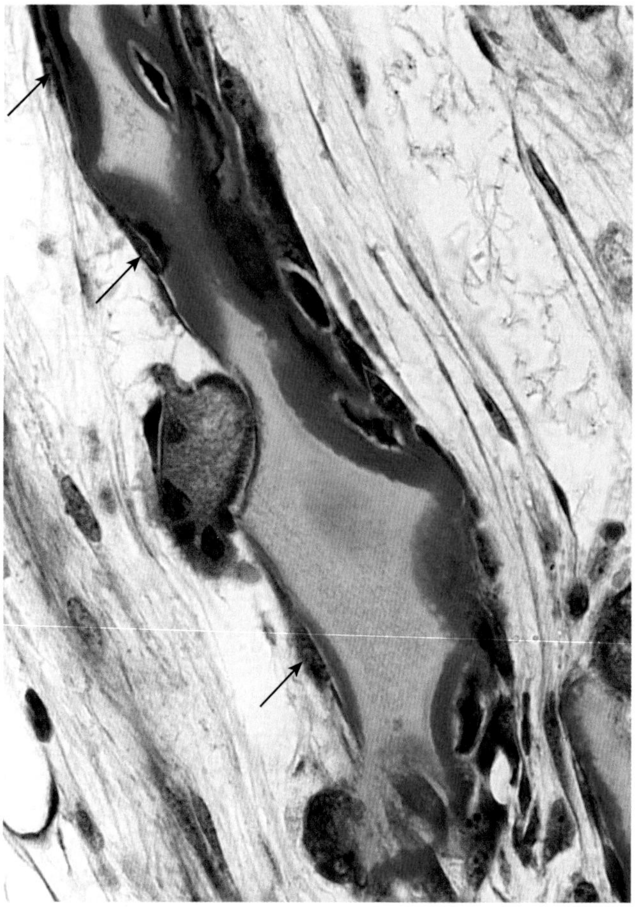

FIGURE 8.14. Photomicrograph of an osteoclast on a bone spicule. This Mallory-stained specimen shows a spicule made of calcified cartilage (stained *light blue*) and a covering of bone tissue (stained *dark blue*). An osteoclast on the left side of the spicule has resorbed bone tissue and lies in a depression (Howship lacuna) in the spicule. The light band between the osteoclast and the bone spicule corresponds to the ruffled border of the osteoclast. The *arrows* on the nongrowing surface indicate cytoplasm of inactive bone-lining cells (osteoprogenitor cells). In contrast, bone is being deposited on the opposite side of the spicule, as evidenced by the presence of osteoblasts on this surface and newly formed osteocytes just below the surface of the spicule. ×550.

Osteoclasts are derived from the fusion of mononuclear hemopoietic progenitor cells under the influence of multiple cytokines.

Contrary to what was once thought, **osteoclasts** are not related to osteoblasts. They are derived from the fusion of mononuclear hemopoietic cells, namely, **granulocyte/macrophage progenitor cells (GMP, CFU-GM)** that give rise to granulocyte and monocyte cell lineages (see Fig. 10.19). Osteoclast formation occurs in close association with stromal cells in bone marrow. These cells secrete essential cytokines for differentiation of both osteoclasts and macrophages from GMP progenitor cells, including monocyte colony-stimulating factor (M-CSF), tumor necrosis factor (TNF), and several interleukins. Initially, cells committed to become osteoclasts (osteoclast precursors) express two important transcription factors, **c-fos** and **NF-κB**; later, a receptor molecule called **receptor activator of nuclear factor-κB (RANK)** is expressed on their surface. The RANK receptor interacts with the **RANK ligand (RANKL) molecule** produced and expressed on the stromal cell surface (Fig. 8.15). The **RANK–RANKL signaling mechanism** is essential for osteoclast differentiation and maturation. Alternatively, during **inflammation**, activated T lymphocytes can produce both membrane-bound and soluble RANKL molecules. Therefore, inflammatory processes can stimulate osteoclast-mediated bone resorption. This pathway can be blocked by **osteoprotegerin (OPG)**, which serves as a "decoy" receptor for RANKL. Lack of available ligand affects the RANK–RANKL signaling pathway and acts as a potent inhibitor of osteoclast formation. OPG is produced mainly by osteoblasts and is regulated by many bone metabolic regulators, such as IL-1, TNF, TGF-β, and vitamin D. PGE_2 is secreted by stressed osteocytes and stimulates the production of RANKL; however, active osteoblasts in the region of bone deposition produce OPG that inactivates RANKL. Thus, regions where osteoblasts are depositing new bone will have little or no osteoclastic activity in contrast to surrounding regions with higher osteoclastic activity. All substances that promote bone remodeling by osteoclast differentiation and bone resorption act through the OPG/RANKL system in the bone marrow. Both OPG and RANKL are detected in free form in the blood, and their concentrations can be measured for diagnostic purposes and to monitor therapy of many bone diseases.

Newly formed osteoclasts undergo an activation process to become bone-resorbing cells.

The newly formed **osteoclast** must be activated to become a bone-resorbing cell. During this process, it becomes highly polarized. When actively resorbing bone, osteoclasts exhibit three specialized regions:

- The **ruffled border** is the part of the cell in direct contact with bone. Its numerous deep plasma membrane infoldings form microvillous-type structures that increase the surface area available for exocytosis of hydrolytic enzymes and secretion of protons by ATP-dependent proton pumps as well as endocytosis of degradation products and bone debris. The ruffled border stains less intensely than the remainder of the cell and often appears as a light band adjacent to the bone at the resorption site (see Fig. 8.14). At the electron microscopic level, hydroxyapatite crystals from the bone substance are observed between the processes of the ruffled border (Fig. 8.16). Internal to the ruffled border and in close proximity are numerous mitochondria and lysosomes. The nuclei are typically located in the part of the cell more removed from the bone surface. In this same region are profiles of rER, multiple stacks of Golgi apparatus, and many vesicles.
- The **clear zone** (sealing zone) is a ring-like perimeter of cytoplasm adjacent to the ruffled border that demarcates the bone area being resorbed. Essentially, the clear zone is a compartment at the site of the ruffled border where resorption and degradation of the matrix occurs. It contains abundant actin filaments but essentially lacks other organelles. The actin filaments are arranged in a ring-like structure surrounded on both sides by actin-binding proteins such as vinculin and talin (Fig. 8.17). The plasma membrane at the site of the clear zone contains cell and **extracellular matrix adhesion molecules** that provide a tight seal between the plasma membrane and mineralized matrix of the bone. Several classes of **integrin extracellular receptors** (i.e., $\alpha_v\beta_3$ vitronectin receptor, $\alpha_2\beta_1$ type I collagen receptor, or $\alpha_v\beta_1$ vitronectin/fibrinogen receptor) help maintain the seal.

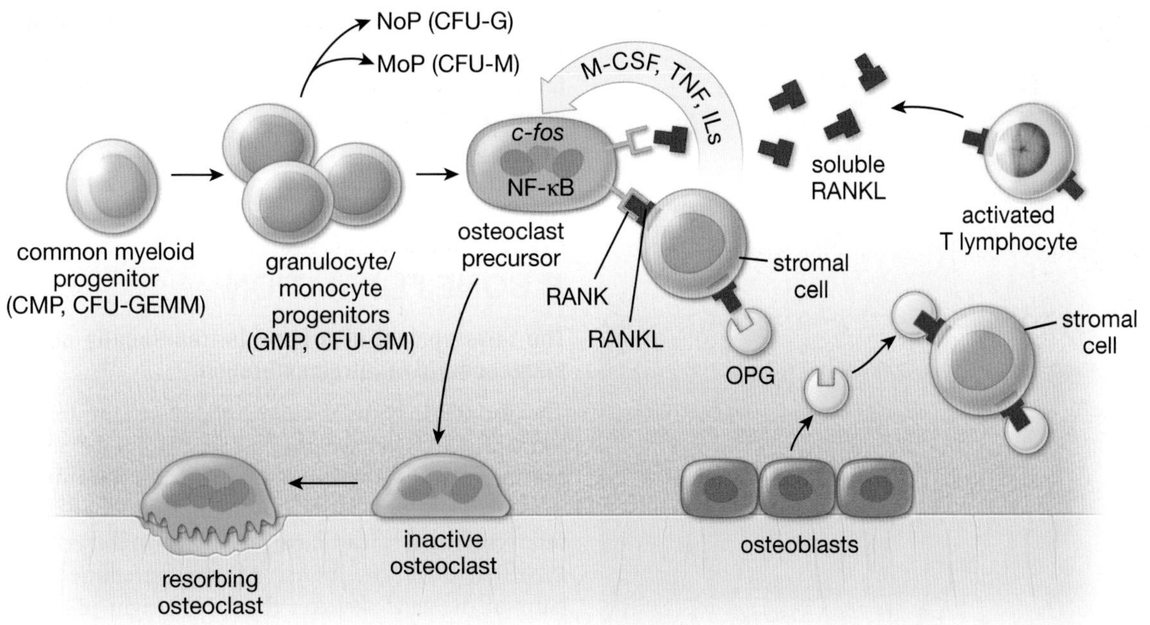

FIGURE 8.15. The origin of osteoclasts. Osteoclasts are derived from fusion of *granulocyte/monocyte progenitor cells* (*GMP, CFU-GM*), which originate from multipotential common myeloid progenitor cells (*CMP, CFU-GEMM*). GMP cells also give rise to the granulocyte and monocyte cell lineages such as neutrophil progenitor (*NoP, CFU-G*) and monocyte progenitor (*MoP, CFU-M*) cells. Osteoclast formation occurs in close association with stromal cells in bone marrow, which secrete monocyte colony-stimulating factor (*M-CSF*), tumor necrosis factor (*TNF*), and several interleukins (*ILs*). Osteoclast precursors express *c-fos*, NFκB, and receptor molecules called *RANK* (*receptor activator of nuclear factor-κB*). The signal generated by the interaction of the RANK receptor with the *RANK ligand* (*RANKL*) *molecule* is essential for osteoclast differentiation and maturation. During inflammation, T lymphocytes produce both soluble and membrane-bound RANKL molecules, which increase bone resorption. These pathways can be blocked by *osteoprotegerin* (*OPG*). Note that activated T lymphocytes can stimulate formation of osteoclasts by producing both membrane-bound and soluble RANKL molecules.

- The **basolateral region** functions in the exocytosis of digested material (see Fig. 8.17). Transport vesicles containing degraded bone material endocytosed at the ruffled border fuse here with the cell membrane to release their contents. TRAP has been found within these vesicles, suggesting its role in the fragmentation of endocytosed material.

Osteoclasts resorb bone tissue by releasing protons and lysosomal hydrolases into the constricted microenvironment of the extracellular space.

Some, if not most, of the vesicles in the **osteoclast** are lysosomes. Their contents are released into the extracellular space in the clefts between the cytoplasmic processes of the ruffled border, a clear example of **lysosomal enzymes** functioning outside the cell. Once liberated, these hydrolytic enzymes, which include **cathepsin K** (a cysteine protease) and **matrix metalloproteinases**, degrade collagen and other proteins of the bone matrix.

Before digestion can occur, however, the bone matrix must be decalcified through acidification of the bony surface, which initiates dissolution of the mineral matrix. The cytoplasm of the osteoclast contains **carbonic anhydrase II**, which produces carbonic acid (H_2CO_3) from carbon dioxide and water. Subsequently, the carbonic acid dissociates to bicarbonate (HCO_3) and a proton (H^+). With the help of **ATP-dependent proton pumps**, protons are transported through the ruffled border, generating a low pH (4–5) in the microenvironment of the resorption bay. This local acidic environment created in the extracellular space between the bone and the osteoclast is protected by the clear zone. **Chloride channels** coupled with **proton pumps** facilitate the electroneutrality of the ruffled border membrane (see Fig. 8.17). Excess bicarbonate is removed by passive exchange with chloride ions via **chloride–carbonate protein** exchangers located at the basolateral membrane.

The acidic environment initiates the degradation of the mineral component of bone (composed primarily of hydroxyapatites) to calcium ions, soluble inorganic phosphates, and water. When resorption of designated bone tissue is complete, osteoclasts undergo apoptosis. Recent studies indicate that many drugs used to inhibit bone resorption in osteoporosis (i.e., bisphosphonates and estrogens) promote **osteoclast apoptosis** (Folder 8.2).

Osteoclast function is regulated by many factors.

Digested materials from the resorbed bone are transported in endocytic vesicles across the osteoclast. The content of the endocytic vesicles that originate at the ruffled border is released at the basolateral region (see Fig. 8.17), which is usually in contact with blood vessels. Therefore, numerous coated pits and coated vesicles are present at the ruffled border. Osteoclasts are observed at sites where bone remodeling is in progress. (The process of remodeling is described in more detail later in this chapter.) Thus, at sites where osteons are being altered or where bone is undergoing change during the growth process, osteoclasts are relatively numerous.

Parathyroid hormone (PTH) secreted by the principal (chief) cells of the parathyroid glands is the most important regulator of calcium and phosphate levels in the extracellular fluid. Because osteoclasts do not have PTH receptors, PTH exerts only an indirect effect on osteoclasts. In contrast, osteocytes, osteoblasts, and T lymphocytes all have **PTH receptors** that activate adenyl cyclase, increasing intracellular levels of cyclic adenosine monophosphate (cAMP). Brief intermittent exposure to PTH increases bone mass through

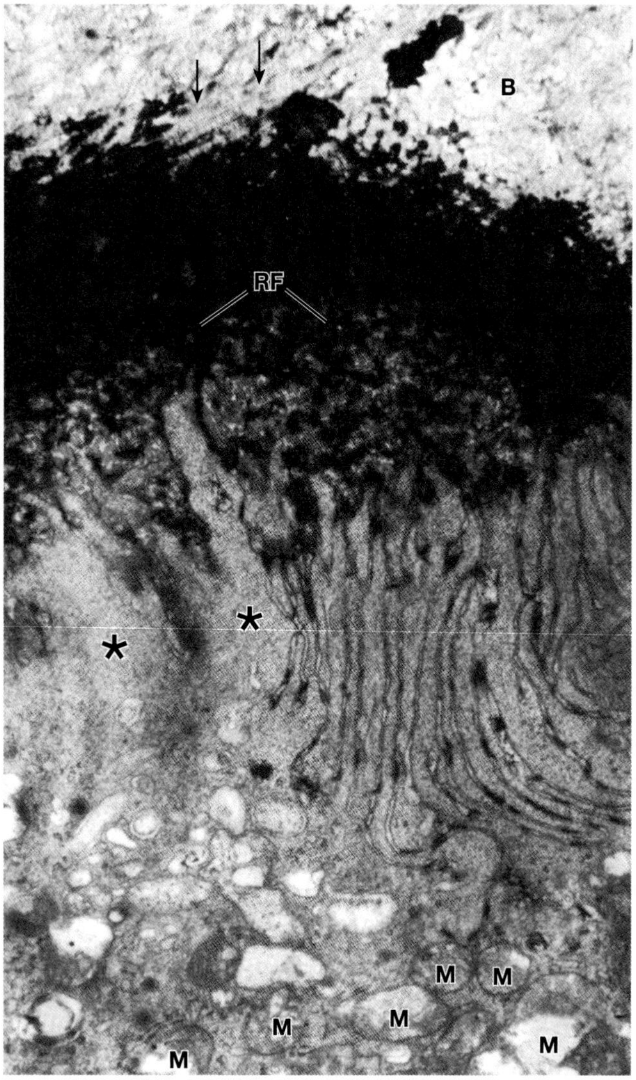

FIGURE 8.16. Electron micrograph of an osteoclast. This micrograph shows a segment of bone surface (*B*) and a portion of an osteoclast that is in apposition to the partially digested bone. The resorption front (*RF*) of the osteoclast possesses numerous infoldings of the plasma membrane. When viewed in the light microscope, these infoldings are evident as the ruffled border. When the plane of section is parallel to the infoldings (*asterisks*), a broad, nonspecialized expanse of cytoplasm is seen. The cytoplasm of the osteoclast contains numerous mitochondria (*M*), lysosomes, and Golgi apparatus, all of which are functionally linked with the resorption and degradation of the bone matrix. In the *upper part* of the figure, some collagen fibrils are evident; the *arrows* indicate where 68-nm cross-banding is visible. ×10,000.

the cAMP/IGF-1 pathway in osteocytes and osteoblasts. However, prolonged, continuous exposure to PTH increases the production of RANKL by T lymphocytes (see Fig. 8.15) and osteoblasts, leading to osteoclastic hyperactivity and eventually osteoporosis. Estrogen suppresses RANKL production by T lymphocytes. **Calcitonin**, secreted by the parafollicular cells of the thyroid gland, has the singular effect of reducing osteoclastic activity.

Other molecules that play an important role in regulating osteoclast activity include cathepsin K, carbonic anhydrase II, and proteins encoding the proton pump (TCIRG1). Deficiency of these proteins causes **osteopetrosis**, a rare congenital disease characterized by increased bone density and defective osteoclast function. In individuals with osteopetrosis, osteoclasts do not function properly, which causes bones to appear dense on X-ray; however, they are actually very fragile and break easily.

Recent research indicates that both healthy and dying osteocytes communicate with osteoclasts to recruit them for bone remodeling. Osteocyte death through apoptosis occurring at sites of bone damage generates apoptotic bodies that express RANKL molecules. These molecules, acting through RANK–RANKL signaling pathways, increase osteoclastic activity (Table 8.1).

■ BONE FORMATION

The development of a bone is traditionally classified as endochondral or intramembranous.

The distinction between endochondral and intramembranous formation rests on whether a cartilage model serves as the precursor of the bone (**endochondral ossification**) or whether the bone is formed by a simpler method, without the intervention of a cartilage precursor (**intramembranous ossification**). The bones of the extremities and those parts of the axial skeleton that bear weight (e.g., vertebrae) develop by endochondral ossification. The flat bones of the skull and face, the mandible, and the clavicle develop by intramembranous ossification.

The existence of two distinct types of ossification does not imply that existing bone is either membranous bone or endochondral bone. These names refer *only* to the mechanism by which a bone is initially formed. Because of the remodeling that occurs later, the initial bone tissue laid down by endochondral formation or by intramembranous formation is soon replaced. The replacement bone is established on the preexisting bone by appositional growth and is identical in both cases. Although the long bones are classified as being formed by endochondral formation, their continued growth involves the histogenesis of both endochondral and intramembranous bone, with the latter occurring through the activity of the periosteal (membrane) tissue.

Intramembranous Ossification

In intramembranous ossification, bone formation is initiated by condensation of mesenchymal cells that differentiate into osteoblasts.

The first evidence of intramembranous ossification is seen around the eighth week of human development within embryonic connective tissue, the mesenchyme. Some of the spindle-shaped, pale-staining **mesenchymal cells** migrate and aggregate in specific areas (e.g., the region of flat bone development in the head), forming **ossification centers**. This condensation of cells within the mesenchymal tissue initiates the process of intramembranous ossification (Fig. 8.18a). Mesenchymal cells in these ossification centers elongate and differentiate into **osteoprogenitor cells**. These cells express **CBFA1 transcription factor**, which is essential for osteoblast differentiation and the expression of genes necessary for both intramembranous and endochondral ossification. The osteoprogenitor cell cytoplasm changes from eosinophilic to basophilic, and a clear Golgi area becomes evident. These cytologic changes result in the differentiated **osteoblast**, which then secretes collagens (mainly type I collagen molecules), bone sialoproteins, osteocalcin, and other components of the bone matrix (osteoid). The osteoblasts accumulate at the periphery of the ossification center and

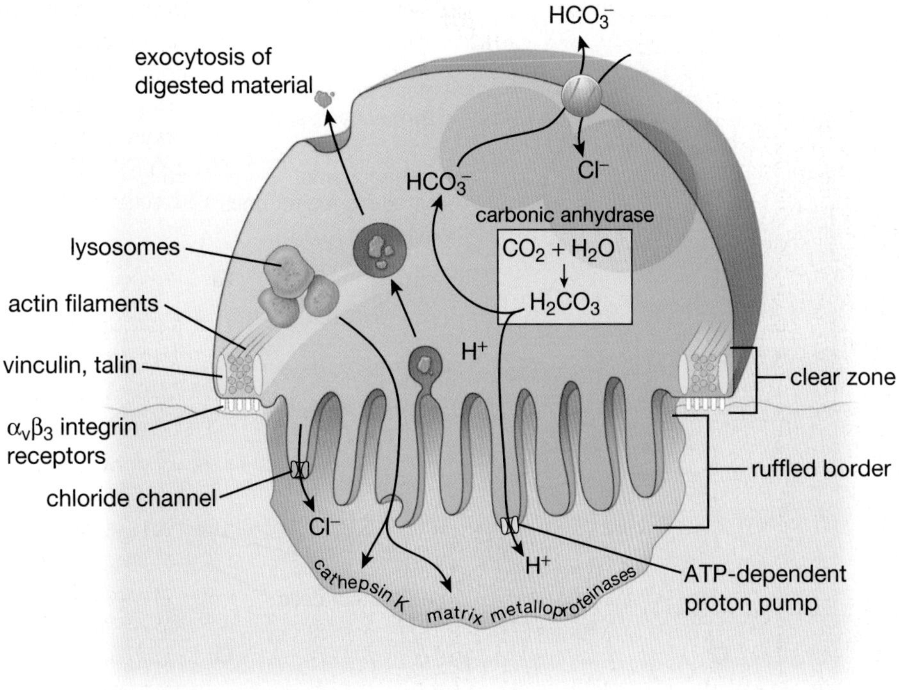

FIGURE 8.17. Schematic drawing of an osteoclast. This drawing shows the structure of the osteoclast and its three regions: the ruffled border, clear zone, and basolateral region. Note that the clear zone contains abundant actin filaments arranged in a ring-like structure surrounded on both sides by actin-binding proteins such as vinculin and talin. The plasma membrane at the site of the clear zone contains cell-to-extracellular matrix adhesion molecules (integrin receptors) that provide a tight seal between the plasma membrane and mineralized matrix of the bone. The pathways for proton and chloride transport are described in the text.

TABLE 8.1 Summary Features of Osteoblasts, Osteocytes, and Osteoclasts

Features	Osteoblast	Osteocyte	Osteoclast
	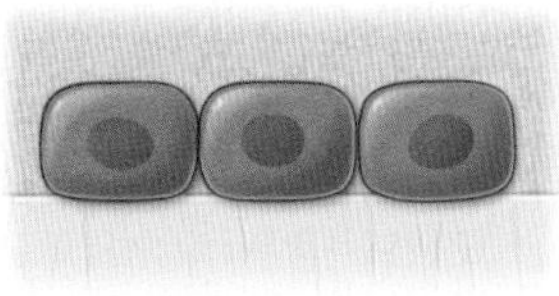	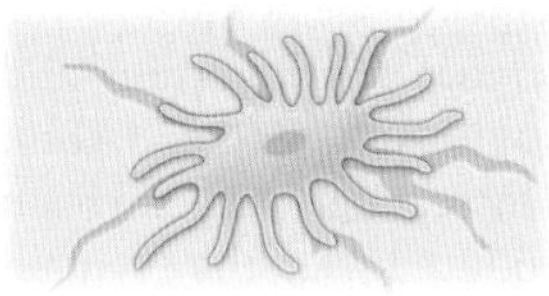	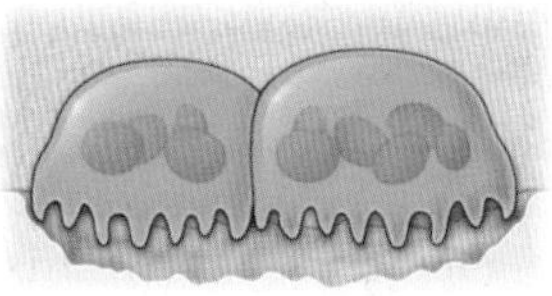
Location	Bone surface; closing cone of resorption canals	Lacunae and canaliculi of bone matrix	Bone surface; cutting cone of resorption canals
Percentage of all cells in the bone	>5%	~95%	>1%
Function	Deposits bone matrix; initiates mineralization by releasing matrix vesicles	Maintains bone matrix; senses mechanical stress; regulates calcium and phosphate homeostasis	Resorbs bone by enzymatic hydrolysis of the mineralized bone matrix
Cell morphology	Cuboidal or polygonal, mononuclear cell; basophilic cytoplasm; negative Golgi	Small, oval, mononuclear cell; pale cytoplasm; long cell processes	Large, multinuclear cell; acidophilic cytoplasm; ruffled border; underlying Howship lacuna
Precursor cells	Osteoprogenitor cell	Osteoblast	Hemopoietic cells (GMP, CFU-GM)
Differentiation process/ transcription factors	CBFA1 (RUNX2); IGF-1	Selection process from osteoblasts not known	c-fos; NF-κB; RANK–RANKL signaling
Major hormonal/regulatory receptors	RANKL, PTH receptors	RANKL, PTH receptors	RANK, calcitonin receptors; tartrate-resistant acid phosphatase (TRAP) receptors
Life span	Weeks (~12 days)	Years (~10–20 years)	Days (~3 days)
Biochemical markers	Osteocalcin; bone sialoprotein (BSP-2)	Dentin matrix protein-1 (DMP-1); podoplanin (E11 protein); sclerostin; fibroblastic growth factor-23 (FGF-23)	Tartrate-resistant acid phosphatase (TRAP); cathepsin K; matrix metalloproteinase-9 (MMP-9)

CBFA1, core binding factor alpha-1; GMP/CFU-GM, granulocyte/macrophage progenitor cells; IGF-1, insulin-like growth factor 1; NF-κB, nuclear factor-κB; PTH, parathyroid hormone; RANK, receptor activator of nuclear factor-κB; RANKL, RANK ligand molecule; RUNX2, runt-related transcription factor 2.

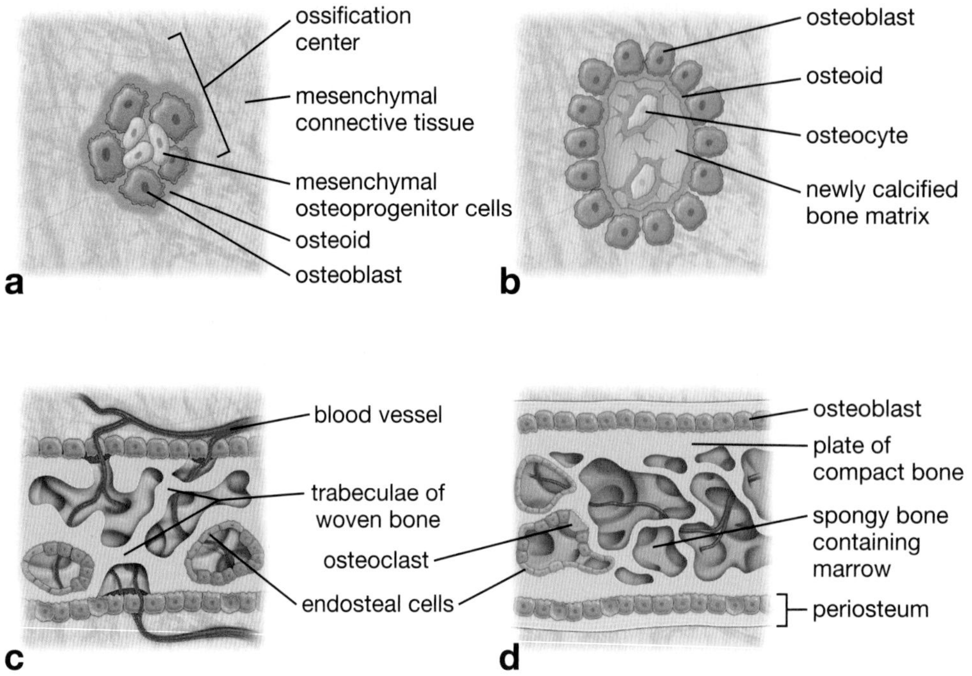

FIGURE 8.18. Intramembranous ossification. a. An ossification center appears in the mesenchymal connective tissue. It consists of aggregated mesenchymal-derived osteoprogenitor cells that further differentiate into bone-secreting cells, the osteoblasts. They begin to deposit unmineralized bone matrix, the osteoid. **b.** The osteoblasts accumulate at the periphery of the ossification center and continue to secrete osteoid toward the center of the nodule. As the process continues, osteoid undergoes mineralization and trapped osteoblasts become osteocytes. Osteocytes exhibit processes that communicate with each other and with osteoblasts. **c.** The newly formed tissue has a microscopic structure of immature (woven) bone with thick trabeculae lined by osteoblasts and endosteal cells. **d.** Further growth and remodeling of the bone results in replacement of woven bone by the inner and outer layers of compact bone with spongy bone between them. Spaces between trabeculae become occupied by bone marrow cells that arrive with blood vessels. Note that one space is lined by inactive endosteal cells and the other is lined by osteoblasts, osteoclasts, and endosteal cells, an indication of the active remodeling process.

continue to secrete osteoid at the center of the nodule. As the process continues, the osteoid undergoes mineralization, and the entrapped osteoblasts become **osteocytes** (Fig. 8.18b). Within the bony matrix, osteocytes increasingly separate from one another as more matrix is produced, but they remain attached by thin cytoplasmic processes. With time, the matrix becomes mineralized, and the interconnecting cytoplasmic processes of osteocytes are contained within canaliculi.

Initially, newly formed bone matrix appears in histologic sections as small, irregularly shaped spicules and trabeculae.

Bone matrix appears in histologic sections as small, irregularly shaped spicules and trabeculae, which are characteristic of spongy bone. A number of the osteoprogenitor cells come into apposition with the initially formed spicules, become osteoblasts, and add more matrix (Fig. 8.19 and Plate 8.5, page 278). During this process, called **appositional growth**, the spicules enlarge and become joined in a trabecular network with the general shape of the developing bone. Through continued mitotic activity, the osteoprogenitor cells maintain their numbers and thus provide a constant source of osteoblasts for growth of the bone spicules. The new osteoblasts, in turn, lay down bone matrix in successive layers, giving rise to **woven bone** (Fig. 8.18c). This immature bone, discussed on pages 242-243, is characterized internally by interconnecting spaces occupied by connective tissue and blood vessels. Further growth and remodeling result in replacement of woven bone by compact bone in the periphery and spongy bone in the center of the newly formed bone (Fig. 8.18d). Spaces between trabeculae become occupied by bone marrow cells that arrive with blood vessels. Bone tissue formed by the process just described is referred to as **membrane bone** or **intramembranous bone**.

Endochondral Ossification

Endochondral ossification also begins with the proliferation and aggregation of mesenchymal cells at the site of the future bone. Under the influence of different growth factors and bone morphogenic proteins (BMPs) (see page 239), the mesenchymal cells initially express type II collagen and differentiate into chondroblasts that, in turn, produce cartilage matrix.

Initially, a hyaline cartilage model with the general shape of the bone is formed.

Once established, the **cartilage model** (a miniature version of the future definitive bone) grows by interstitial and appositional growth (Plate 8.3, page 274). The increase in the length of the cartilage model is attributed to interstitial growth. The increase in its width is largely the result of the addition of cartilage matrix produced by new chondrocytes that differentiate from the chondrogenic layer of the perichondrium surrounding the cartilage mass. Illustration *1* of Figure 8.20 shows an early cartilage model.

The first sign of ossification is the appearance of a cuff of bone around the cartilage model.

At this stage, the perichondrial cells in the midregion of the cartilage model no longer give rise to chondrocytes. Instead, **osteoblasts** are produced. Thus, the connective tissue

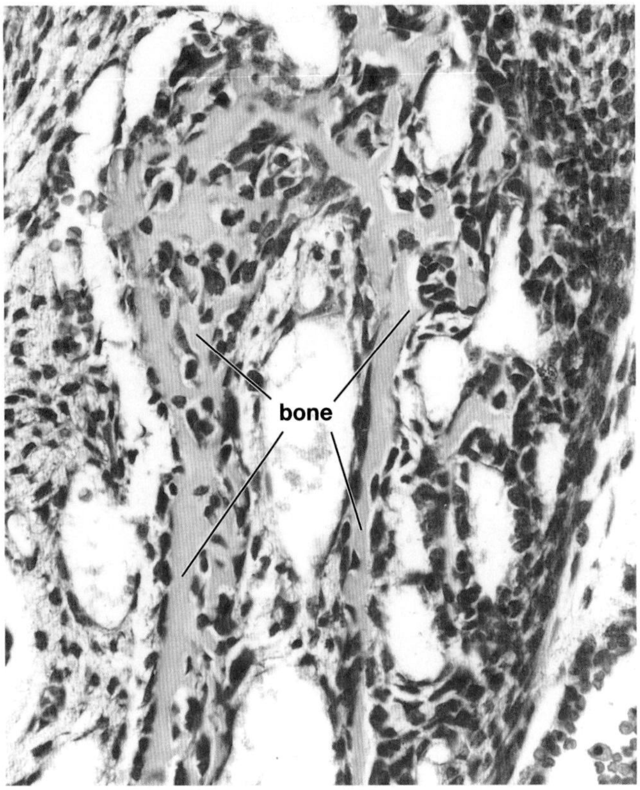

FIGURE 8.19. Section of mandible developing by the process of intramembranous ossification. This photomicrograph shows a section from a developing mandible stained with H&E. In this relatively early stage of development, the mandible consists of bone spicules of various sizes and shapes. The bone spicules interconnect with each other and form trabeculae, providing the general shape of the developing bone (no cartilage model is present). The numerous osteoblasts responsible for this growing region of spicules are seen at the surface of the newly deposited bone. The older, calcified portion of spicules contains osteocytes surrounded by bone matrix. In the *right portion* of the figure, adjacent to the bone spicules, the connective tissue is very cellular and is developing into the early periosteum. ×250.

surrounding this portion of the cartilage is *no longer functionally a perichondrium*; rather, because of its altered role, it is now called the **periosteum**. Moreover, because the cells within this layer are differentiating into osteoblasts, an **osteogenic layer** can now be identified within the periosteum. Because of these changes, a layer of bone is formed around the cartilage model (Plate 8.3, page 274). This bone can be classified as either periosteal bone, because of its location, or intramembranous bone, because of its method of development. In the case of a long bone, a distinctive cuff of periosteal bone, the **bony collar**, is established around the cartilage model in the diaphyseal portion of the developing bone. The bony collar is shown in illustration *2* of Figure 8.20.

With the establishment of the periosteal bony collar, the chondrocytes in the midregion of the cartilage model become hypertrophic.

As the chondrocytes enlarge, their surrounding cartilage matrix is resorbed, forming thin irregular cartilage plates between the **hypertrophic cells**. The hypertrophic cells begin to synthesize TNAP, RANKL, and vascular endothelial growth factor (VEGF); concomitantly, the surrounding **cartilage matrix** undergoes **calcification** (see illustration *3* of Fig. 8.20). The calcification of the cartilage matrix should not be confused with mineralization that occurs in bone tissue.

The calcified cartilage matrix inhibits diffusion of nutrients, causing the degeneration, death, and possible transdifferentiation of the chondrocytes in the cartilage model.

With the degeneration, death, and possible transdifferentiation of the chondrocytes, much of the matrix breaks down, and neighboring lacunae become confluent, producing an increasingly large cavity. While these events are occurring, one or several blood vessels grow through the thin diaphyseal bony collar to vascularize the cavity (see illustration *4* of Fig. 8.20).

Mesenchymal stem cells migrate into the cavity along the growing blood vessels.

Mesenchymal stem cells residing in the developing periosteum migrate along the penetrating blood vessels and differentiate into osteoprogenitor cells in the bone marrow cavity. **Hemopoietic stem cells (HSCs)** also gain access to the cavity via the new vasculature, leaving the circulation to give rise to the marrow, which includes all blood cell progenitors. As the calcified cartilage breaks down and is partially removed, some remains as irregular spicules. When the osteoprogenitor cells come in apposition to the remaining calcified cartilage spicules, they become osteoblasts and begin to deposit bone matrix (osteoid) on the spicule framework. In addition, some osteoblasts may derive from the pool of reprogrammed hypertrophic chondrocytes that underwent chondrocyte-to-osteoblast transdifferentiation. Thus, bone formed in this manner may be described as endochondral bone. This initial site where bone begins to form in the diaphysis of a long bone is called the **primary ossification center** (see illustration *5* of Fig. 8.20). The combination of bone, which is initially only a thin layer, and the underlying calcified cartilage is described as a **mixed spicule**.

Histologically, mixed spicules can be recognized by their staining characteristics. Calcified cartilage tends to be basophilic, whereas bone is distinctly eosinophilic. With the Mallory stain, bone stains a deep blue, and calcified cartilage stains light blue (Fig. 8.21). Also, calcified cartilage no longer contains cells, whereas the newly produced bone may reveal osteocytes in the bone matrix. Such spicules persist for a short time before the calcified cartilage component is removed. The remaining bone component of the spicule may continue to grow by appositional growth, thus becoming larger and stronger, or it may undergo resorption as new spicules are formed.

Growth of Endochondral Bone

Endochondral bone growth begins in the second trimester of pregnancy and continues into early adulthood.

The events described previously represent the early stage of endochondral bone formation that occurs in the fetus, beginning at about the 12th week of development. The continuing growth process that lasts into early adulthood is described in the following section.

Growth in length of long bones depends on the presence of epiphyseal cartilage.

As the diaphyseal marrow cavity enlarges (see illustration *6* of Fig. 8.20), a distinct zonation can be recognized in the cartilage at both ends of the cavity. This remaining cartilage,

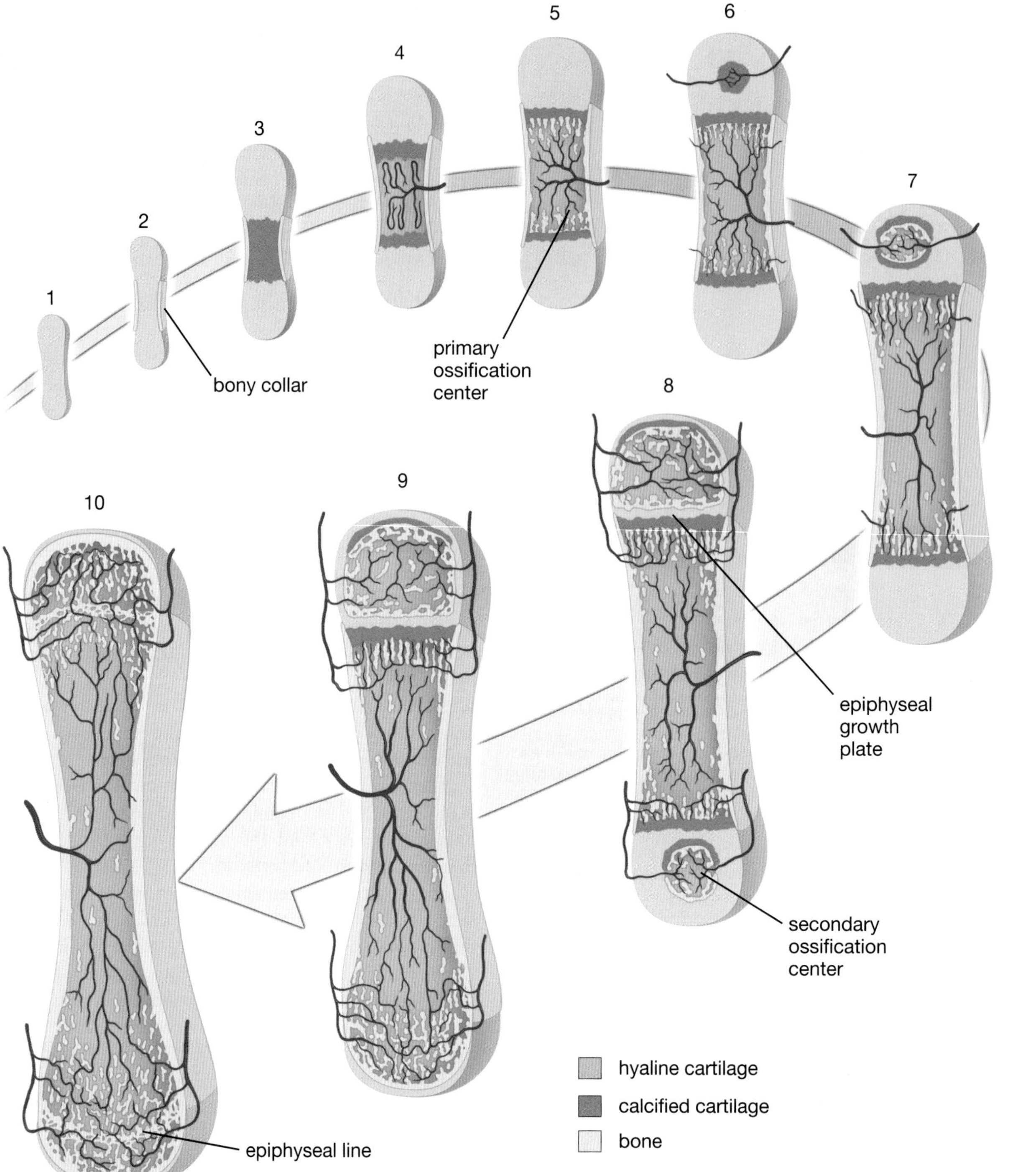

FIGURE 8.20. Schematic diagram of developing long bone. Illustrations *1* to *10* depict longitudinal sections through the long bone. The process begins with the formation of a cartilage model (*1*); next, a periosteal (perichondrial) collar of bone forms around the diaphysis (shaft) of the cartilage model (*2*); next, the cartilaginous matrix in the shaft begins to calcify (*3*). Blood vessels and connective tissue cells then erode and invade the calcified cartilage (*4*), creating a primitive marrow cavity in which remnant spicules of calcified cartilage remain at the two ends of the cavity. As a primary center of ossification develops, the endochondral bone is formed on spicules of calcified cartilage. The bone at the ends of the developing marrow cavity constitutes the metaphysis. Periosteal bone continues to form as a result of intramembranous ossification (*5*); it can be recognized histologically because it is not accompanied by local cartilage erosion, or is the bone deposited on spicules of calcified cartilage. Blood vessels and perivascular cells invade the proximal epiphyseal cartilage (*6*), and a secondary center of ossification is established in the proximal epiphysis (*7*). A similar epiphyseal (secondary) ossification center forms at the distal end of the bone (*8*), and epiphyseal cartilage is thus formed between each epiphysis and the diaphysis. With continued growth of the long bone, the distal epiphyseal cartilage disappears (*9*), and finally, with cessation of growth, the proximal epiphyseal cartilage disappears (*10*). The metaphysis then becomes continuous with the epiphysis. Epiphyseal lines remain where the epiphyseal plate last existed.

referred to as **epiphyseal cartilage**, exhibits distinct zones as illustrated in Figure 8.22 and Plate 8.4, page 276. During endochondral bone formation, the avascular cartilage is gradually replaced by vascularized bone tissue. This replacement is initiated by **vascular endothelial growth factor (VEGF)** and is accompanied by expression of genes responsible for production of type X collagen and matrix metalloproteases (enzymes responsible for degradation of cartilage matrix). The **zones in the epiphyseal cartilage**, beginning with the zone most distal to the

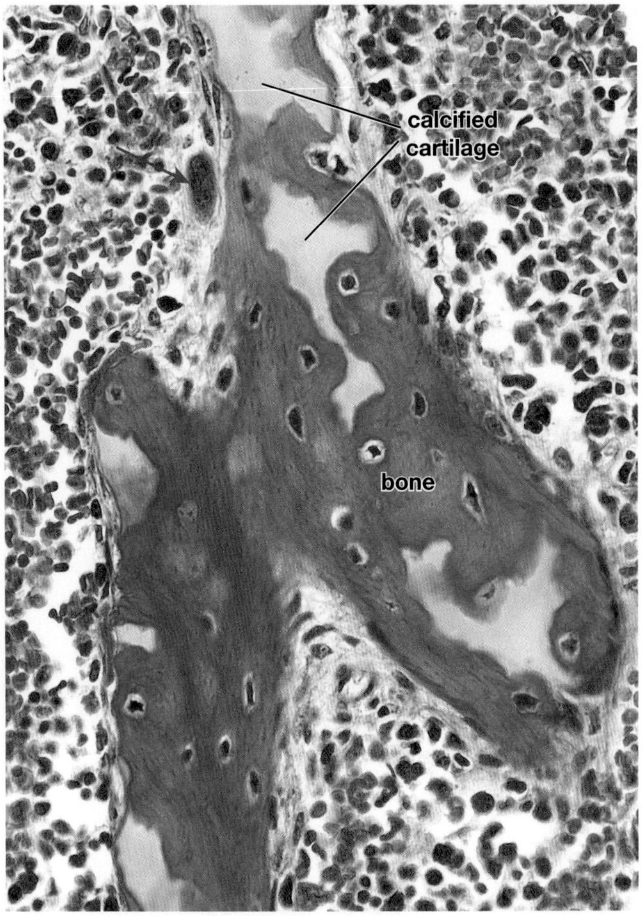

FIGURE 8.21. Photomicrograph of a mixed bone spicule formed during endochondral bone formation. In this Mallory-Azan–stained section, bone has been deposited on calcified cartilage spicules. In the *center* of the photomicrograph, the spicules have already grown to create an anastomosing trabecula. The initial trabecula still contains remnants of calcified cartilage, as shown by the *light-blue* staining of the calcified matrix compared with the *dark-blue* staining of the bone. In the *upper part* of the spicule, note a lone osteoclast (*arrow*) aligned near the surface of the spicule, where remodeling is about to be initiated. ×275.

diaphyseal center of ossification and proceeding toward that center, are as follows:

- The **zone of reserve cartilage** exhibits no cellular proliferation or active matrix production.
- The **zone of proliferation** is adjacent to the zone of reserve cartilage in the direction of the diaphysis. In this zone, the cartilage cells undergo divisions and organize into distinct columns. These cells are larger than those in the reserve zone and actively produce collagen (mainly types II and XI) and other cartilage matrix proteins.
- The **zone of hypertrophy** contains 10- to 20-fold enlarged (hypertrophic) cartilage cells. The cytoplasm of these cells is clear, a reflection of the glycogen that they normally accumulate (which is lost during tissue preparation). Chondrocytes in this zone remain metabolically active; they continue to secrete type II collagen while increasing their secretion of type X collagen. Hypertrophic chondrocytes also secrete VEGF, which initiates vascular invasion, and RANKL, which affects osteoclast development to maintain a balance between bone resorption and bone formation (see pages 250-251). The cartilage matrix is compressed to form linear bands between the columns of hypertrophied cartilage cells.
- In the **zone of calcified cartilage**, the hypertrophied cells begin to degenerate and the cartilage matrix becomes calcified. The calcified cartilage then serves as an initial scaffold for deposition of new bone. In the past, hypertrophic chondrocytes positioned in the more proximal part of this zone have been considered the terminal state of growth plate chondrocytes, having undergone degenerative maturation resulting in nuclear condensation and apoptosis. However, programmed cell death by apoptosis is not the only fate of hypertrophic chondrocytes. Recent research findings show that some hypertrophic chondrocytes may undergo chondrocyte-to-osteoblast transdifferentiation and directly become osteoblasts.
- The **zone of resorption** is the zone nearest the diaphysis. The calcified cartilage here is in direct contact with the connective tissue of the marrow cavity. In this zone, small blood vessels and accompanying osteoprogenitor cells invade the region previously occupied by the dying chondrocytes. They form a series of spearheads (see Fig. 8.22), leaving the calcified cartilage as longitudinal spicules. In cross section, the calcified cartilage resembles a honeycomb because of the absence of the cartilage cells. The invading blood vessels are the source of osteoprogenitor cells, which will differentiate into osteoblasts.

Bone deposition occurs on the cartilage spicules in the same manner as described for the formation of the initial ossification center.

As bone is laid down on the calcified spicules, the cartilage is resorbed, ultimately leaving primary spongy bone. This spongy bone undergoes reorganization through osteoclastic activity and addition of new bone tissue, thus accommodating the continued growth and physical stresses placed on the bone.

Shortly after birth, a **secondary ossification center** develops in the proximal epiphysis. The cartilage cells undergo hypertrophy and degenerate. As in the diaphysis, calcification of the matrix occurs, and blood vessels and osteogenic cells from the perichondrium invade the region, creating a new marrow cavity (see illustration *7* of Fig. 8.20). Later, a similar epiphyseal ossification center forms at the distal end of the bone (see illustration *8* of Fig. 8.20). This center is also regarded as a secondary ossification center, although it develops later. With the development of the secondary ossification centers, the only cartilage that remains from the original model is the articular cartilage at the ends of the bone and a transverse disc of cartilage, known as the **epiphyseal growth plate**, which separates the epiphyseal and diaphyseal cavities (Plate 8.3, page 274).

Cartilage of the epiphyseal growth plate is responsible for maintaining the growth process.

For a bone to retain proper proportions and its unique shape, both external and internal remodeling must occur as the bone grows in length. The proliferative zone of the epiphyseal plate gives rise to the cartilage on which bone is later laid down. In reviewing the growth process, it is important to realize the following:

- The thickness of the epiphyseal plate remains relatively constant during growth.
- The amount of new cartilage produced (zone of proliferation) equals the amount resorbed (zone of resorption).
- The resorbed cartilage is, of course, replaced by spongy bone.

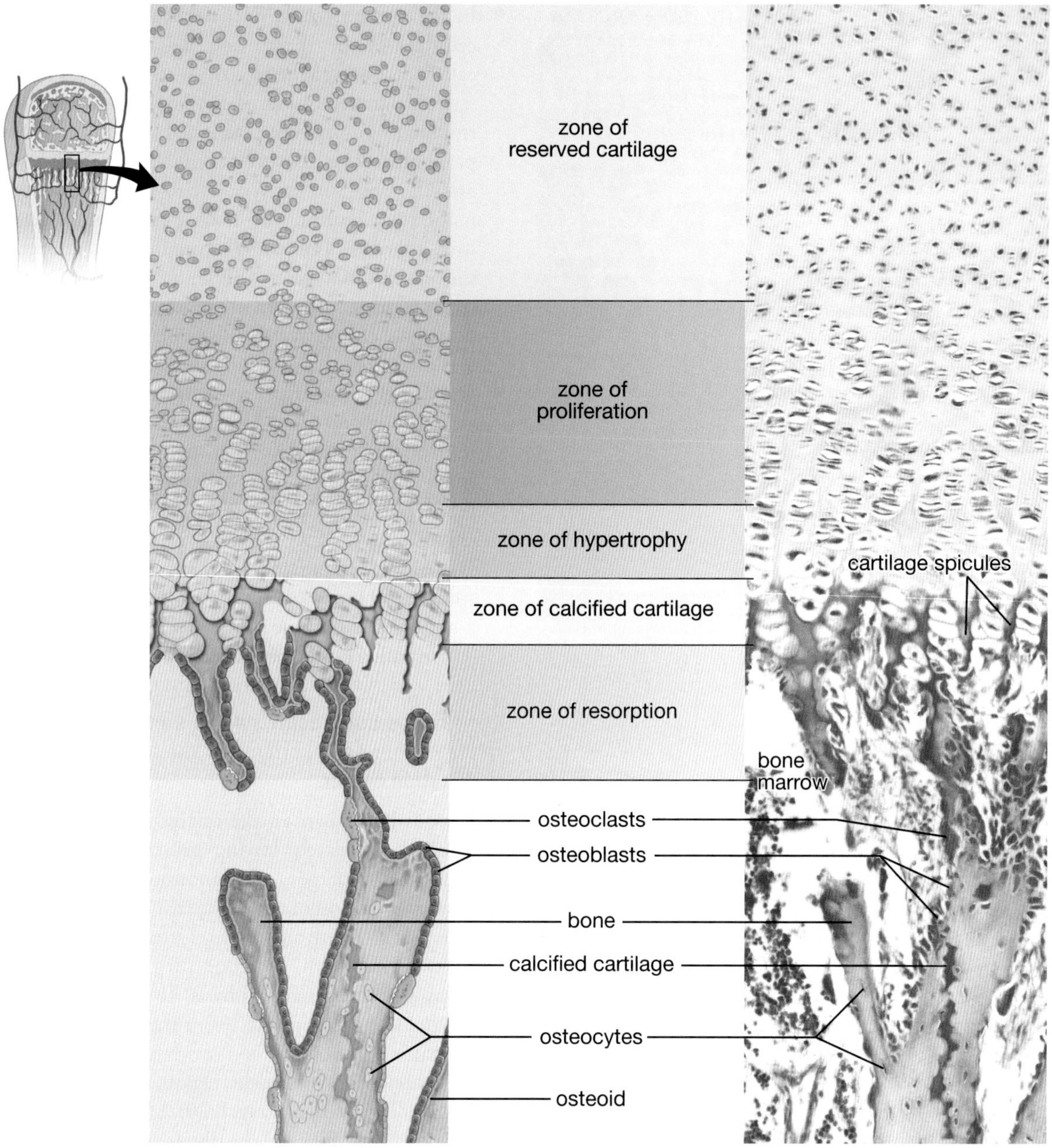

FIGURE 8.22. Longitudinal section through the diaphyseal side of the epiphyseal growth plate from a fetal metacarpal bone. Photomicrograph on the *right* shows active bone formation on the diaphyseal side of the epiphyseal growth plate. The zonation is apparent in this H&E-stained specimen (×180) because chondrocytes undergo divisions, hypertrophy, and eventually apoptosis, leaving room for invading bone-forming cells. In the corresponding diagram on the *left*, bone marrow cells have been removed, leaving osteoblasts, osteoclasts, and endosteal cells lining the internal surfaces of the bone. Note that calcified cartilage (*blue*) is present in the bone spicules.

Actual lengthening of the bone occurs when new cartilage matrix is produced at the epiphyseal plate. Production of new cartilage matrix pushes the epiphysis away from the diaphysis, elongating the bone. This incremental growth is followed by the same processes—namely, hypertrophy, calcification, resorption, and ossification—by which newly formed cartilage is replaced by bone tissue during fetal development.

Bone increases in width or diameter when appositional growth of new bone occurs between the cortical lamellae and the periosteum. The marrow cavity then enlarges by resorption of bone on the endosteal surface of the cortex of the bone. As bones elongate, remodeling is required. It consists of preferential resorption of bone in some areas and deposition of bone in other areas, as described previously and as outlined in Figure 8.23.

When an individual achieves maximal growth, proliferation of new cartilage within the epiphyseal plate terminates.

When the proliferation of new cartilage ceases, the cartilage that has already been produced in the epiphyseal plate continues to undergo the changes that lead to the deposition of new bone until, finally, there is no remaining cartilage. At this point, the epiphyseal and diaphyseal marrow cavities become confluent. The elimination of the epiphyseal plate is referred to as **epiphyseal closure**. In illustration *9* of Figure 8.20, the lower epiphyseal cartilage is no longer present; in illustration *10*, both epiphyseal cartilages are gone. Growth is now complete, and the only remaining cartilage is found on the articular surfaces of the bone. Vestigial evidence of the site of the epiphyseal plate is reflected by an **epiphyseal line** consisting of bone tissue (see Fig. 8.2).

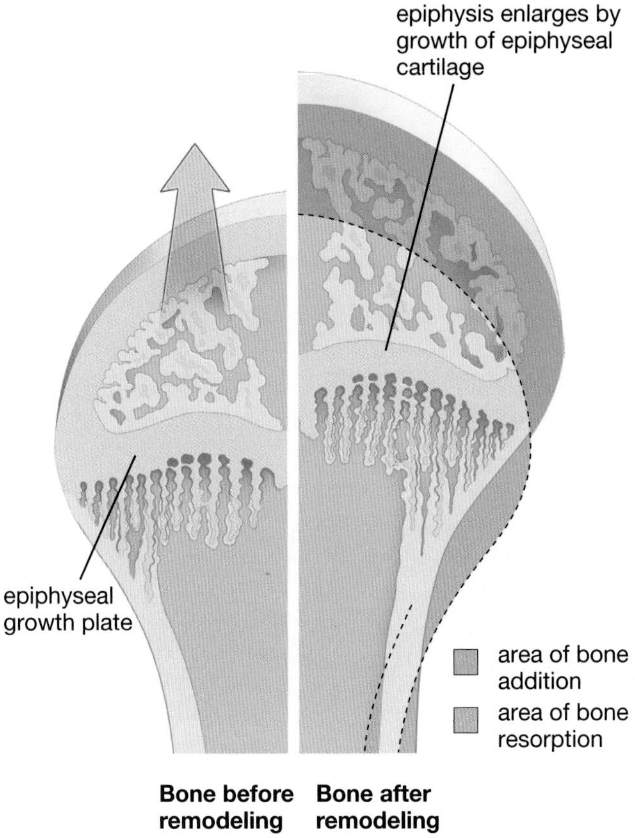

FIGURE 8.23. Diagram of external remodeling of a long bone. This diagram shows two periods during the growth of the bone. The younger bone profile (before remodeling) is shown on the *left*; the older (after remodeling) on the *right*. Superimposed on the *right side* of the figure is the shape of the bone (*right half* only) as it appeared at an earlier time. The bone is now longer, but it has retained its general shape. To grow in length and retain the general shape of the particular bone, bone resorption occurs on some surfaces, and bone deposition occurs on other surfaces, as indicated in the diagram. (Based on Ham AW, Some histophysiological problems peculiar to calcified tissues. *J Bone Joint Surg Am.* 1952;24A:701–728.)

Development of the Osteonal (Haversian) System

Osteons typically develop in preexisting compact bone.

Compact bone can take several different forms. Compact bone may be formed from fetal spongy bone by continued deposition of bone on the spongy bone spicules; it may be deposited directly as adult compact bone (e.g., the circumferential lamellae of an adult bone); or it might be older compact bone consisting of osteons and interstitial lamellae. The process in which new osteons are formed is referred to as **internal remodeling**.

During the development of new osteons, osteoclasts bore a tunnel, the resorption cavity, through compact bone.

Formation of new osteons in compact bone initially involves the creation of a tunnel-like space, the resorption cavity, by osteoclast activity. This resorption cavity will have the dimensions of the new osteon. When osteoclasts have produced an appropriately sized cylindrical tunnel by resorption of compact bone, blood vessels and their surrounding connective tissue occupy the tunnel. As the tunnel is occupied, new bone deposition on its wall begins almost immediately. These two aspects of cellular activity—namely, osteoclast resorption and osteoblast synthesis—constitute a **bone-remodeling** unit. A bone-remodeling unit consists of two distinct parts: an advancing **cutting cone** (also called a **resorption canal**) and a **closing cone** (Fig. 8.24).

The tip of the cutting cone consists of advancing osteoclasts closely followed by an advancing capillary loop and pericytes. It also contains numerous dividing cells that give rise to osteoblasts, additional pericytes, and endothelial cells. (Recall that osteoclasts are derived from mononuclear hemopoietic progenitor cells.) The osteoclasts drill a canal about 200 μm in diameter. This canal establishes the diameter of the future osteonal (Haversian) system. The cutting cone constitutes only a small fraction of the length of the bone-remodeling unit; thus, it is seen much less frequently than the closing cone.

After the diameter of the future Haversian system is established, osteoblasts begin to fill the canal by depositing the organic matrix of bone (osteoid) on its walls in successive lamellae. This process is depicted in bone section in Figure 8.25 as the result of sequential injections of different fluorescent dyes into experimental animals to examine rate of bone remodeling. With time, the bone matrix in each of the lamellae becomes mineralized. As the successive lamellae of bone are deposited, *from the periphery inward*, the canal ultimately attains the relatively narrow diameter of the adult osteonal canal (see Fig. 8.25).

Compact adult bone contains Haversian systems of varying age and size.

Microradiographic examination of a ground section of bone reveals that younger Haversian systems are less completely mineralized than older systems (Fig. 8.26). They undergo a progressive secondary mineralization that continues (up to a point) even after the osteon has been fully formed. Figure 8.26 also illustrates the dynamic internal remodeling of compact bone. In the adult, deposition balances resorption. In an older person, resorption often exceeds deposition. If this imbalance becomes excessive, **osteoporosis** develops (see Folder 8.2).

■ BIOLOGIC MINERALIZATION AND MATRIX VESICLES

Biologic mineralization is a cell-regulated extracellular event under the control of osteoblasts.

The organic matrix of bone, the **osteoid**, is produced by bone-forming cells: osteoblasts in bone and ameloblasts and odontoblasts in developing teeth. Once osteoid is laid down, osteoblasts initiate the **mineralization** process, which occurs in the **extracellular matrix** of bone, cartilage, and in the dentin, cementum, and enamel of teeth. Except for enamel, the matrices of these structures contain collagen fibrils and ground substance. At the same time, mineralization is initiated within the collagen fibrils and in the ground substance surrounding them. In enamel, mineralization occurs within the extracellular matrix secreted by the enamel organ.

Osteoblasts synthesize the majority of extracellular matrix components and control the mineralization process by secreting **regulatory proteins** such as osteocalcin, bone sialoproteins, and osteoadherin. Osteoblasts also modulate the local concentration of phosphate ions by regulating the activity of **tissue nonspecific alkaline phosphatase (TNAP)**, which hydrolyzes phosphate groups from a variety

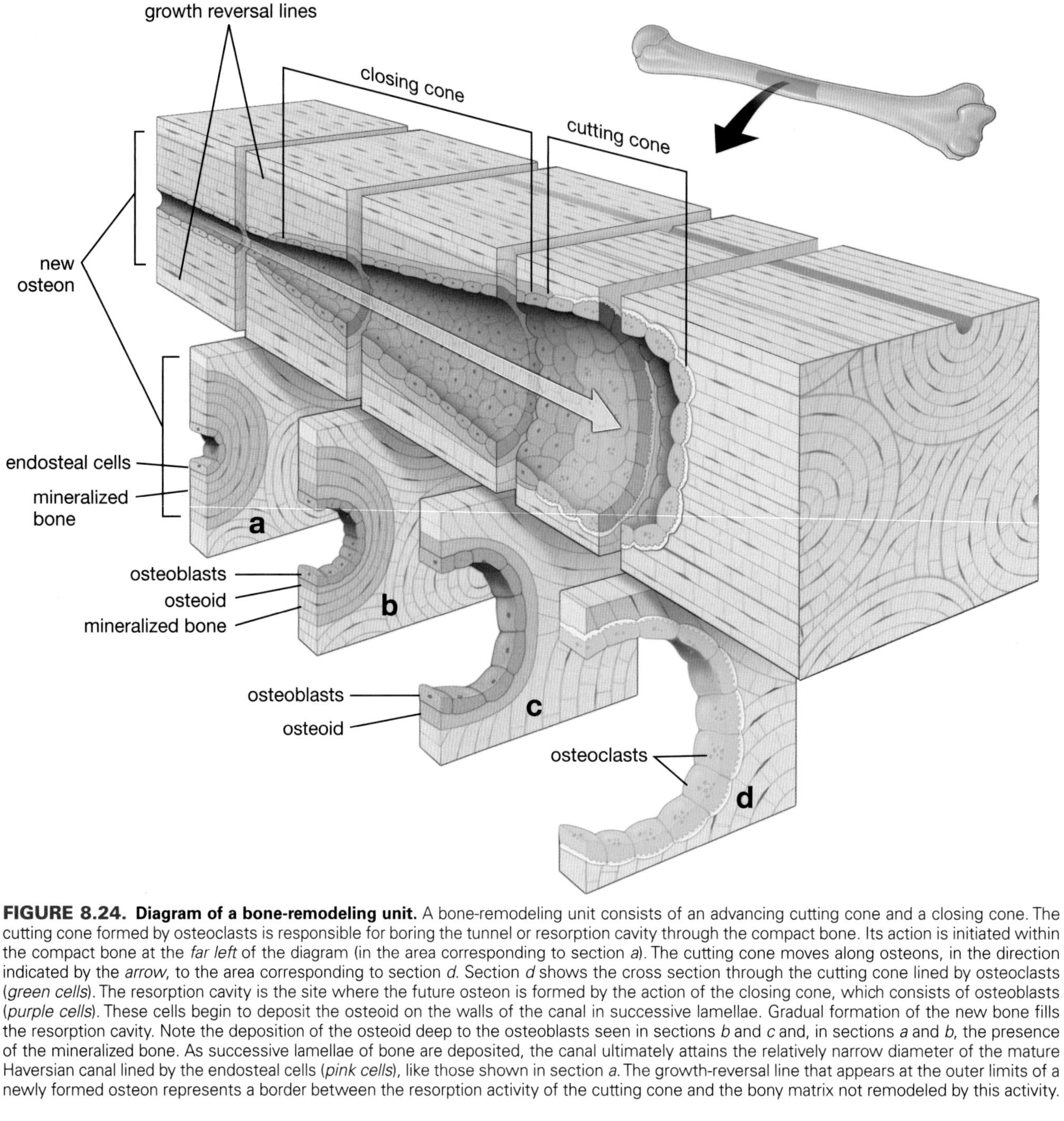

FIGURE 8.24. Diagram of a bone-remodeling unit. A bone-remodeling unit consists of an advancing cutting cone and a closing cone. The cutting cone formed by osteoclasts is responsible for boring the tunnel or resorption cavity through the compact bone. Its action is initiated within the compact bone at the *far left* of the diagram (in the area corresponding to section *a*). The cutting cone moves along osteons, in the direction indicated by the *arrow*, to the area corresponding to section *d*. Section *d* shows the cross section through the cutting cone lined by osteoclasts (*green cells*). The resorption cavity is the site where the future osteon is formed by the action of the closing cone, which consists of osteoblasts (*purple cells*). These cells begin to deposit the osteoid on the walls of the canal in successive lamellae. Gradual formation of the new bone fills the resorption cavity. Note the deposition of the osteoid deep to the osteoblasts seen in sections *b* and *c* and, in sections *a* and *b*, the presence of the mineralized bone. As successive lamellae of bone are deposited, the canal ultimately attains the relatively narrow diameter of the mature Haversian canal lined by the endosteal cells (*pink cells*), like those shown in section *a*. The growth-reversal line that appears at the outer limits of a newly formed osteon represents a border between the resorption activity of the cutting cone and the bony matrix not remodeled by this activity.

of physiologic substrates. Despite the extracellular location of biologic mineralization, this process is controlled by osteoblasts and is regulated by membrane transporters, enzymes, and surrounding extracellular matrix proteins.

Local accumulation of Ca^{2+} and PO_4 ions in the extracellular matrix is essential for initiation of mineralization.

In places where the mineralization of bone, cartilage, dentin, and cementum is initiated, the local concentration of Ca^{2+} and PO_4 ions in the matrix must exceed the normal threshold level. Several events are responsible for this increase. The binding of extracellular Ca^{2+} by **osteocalcin** and other bone sialoproteins creates a high local concentration of this ion. In turn, the high Ca^{2+} concentration stimulates the osteoblasts to secrete **TNAP**, which increases the local concentration of PO_4 ions. The high PO_4 ions concentration stimulates further increases in Ca^{2+} concentration in areas where mineralization will be initiated.

Formation of hydroxyapatite crystals is initiated in the lumen of matrix vesicle and next spreads into extracellular matrix.

In areas with a high extracellular Ca^{2+} and PO_4 ions concentration, osteoblasts begin the **mineralization** process by releasing small (50- to 200-nm) **matrix vesicles**. These matrix vesicles represent **ectosomes** that are released from the apical plasma membrane or microvilli of the osteoblast near the osteoblast–osteoid interface. The plasma membrane of matrix vesicles contains several membrane transporters and enzymes, and their lumen provides a nurturing microenvironment for calcium phosphate nucleation and subsequent crystal growth. Matrix vesicles contain **annexins**, **TNAPs**,

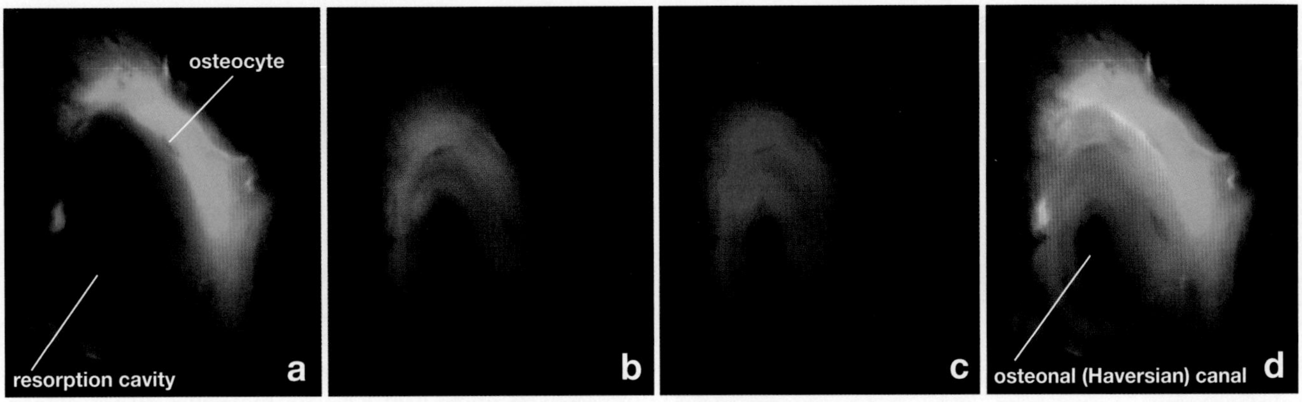

FIGURE 8.25. Osteon formation during bone remodeling. Bone remodeling was examined in an experimental animal (rat) by daily intraperitoneal injections of three different fluorescent dyes (calcein, xylenol orange, and alizarin complexone) every 9 days for 27 days. These stains have a high affinity for calcium ions and are incorporated into the bone matrix during the mineralization process. The bone tissue was fixed in paraformaldehyde solution and sectioned using a precision saw. To limit light scattering and absorption, the tissue was embedded in the optical clearing reagent 2,2′-thiodiethanol (TDE). Each fluorescent marker has a different emission wavelength, as shown in panels a, b, and c. The overlay image of the entire newly formed osteon is shown in panel d. This sequence of fluorescent labeling shows the centripetal (directed toward the center) formation of the osteon from the periphery toward the osteonal canal. **a.** For the first 9 days, calcein was injected. This image shows green fluorescence (light emission between 497 and 557 nm) of the newly deposited bone matrix at the periphery of the resorption cavity (closing cone). **b.** Following calcein treatment, xylenol orange was injected for the second 9-day period. The orange color indicates fluorescence of the second wave of bone deposition that narrows the original resorption cavity. This image shows fluorescent light emission between 545 and 625 nm. **c.** Alizarin complexone was injected during the third 9-day period to label the newly calcified matrix. This image shows the layer of bone matrix deposition (*red*; light emission between 610 and 690 nm) that outlines the boundary of the osteonal (Haversian) canal in the center of the newly formed osteon. **d.** This image shows an overlay of all three fluorescent zones extending from the earliest deposited outer (peripheral) lamellae of the osteon (*green label*) through the middle lamellae (*orange label*) and to the most recently deposited inner lamellae (*red label*) near the osteonal canal. ×380. (Courtesy of Dr. Barış Baykal, University of Health Sciences, Gülhane Faculty of Medicine, Ankara, Türkiye).

carbonic anhydrases, and pyrophosphatases. TNAP and annexin A5 expressed on the surface of the matrix vesicle bind to type I collagen, which anchors the vesicle to the extracellular matrix. Annexin A5 is a channel protein for Ca^{2+} entry into the matrix vesicles. Influx of Ca^{2+} into the matrix vesicle is accompanied by simultaneous transport of PO_4 ions via the **Na^+-phosphate cotransporter 3 (NPT3)**.

The initial **matrix vesicle–mediated mineralization phase** takes place within the matrix vesicles (Fig. 8.27). In this phase, the following events occur:

- The **matrix vesicles** accumulate Ca^{2+} and PO_4 ions that cause the local isoelectric point to increase, which results in formation of small (10 nm), noncrystalline spheroidal particles of **amorphous calcium phosphate** [$Ca_9(HPO_4)(PO_4)_5(OH)$], also called calcium-deficient hydroxyapatite.
- Amorphous calcium phosphate undergoes further crystallization to **octacalcium phosphate** [$Ca_8H_2(PO_4)_6 \cdot 5H_2O$].
- In the presence of a high concentration of Ca^{2+} and PO_4 ions, the octacalcium phosphate crystal grows within the matrix vesicle into insoluble, needle-like **hydroxyapatite crystals** [$Ca_{10}(PO_4)_6(OH)_2$]. Hydroxyapatite crystals accumulate within the matrix vesicle.
- Phospholipases punch holes in the plasma membrane of the matrix vesicles through which elongating hydroxyapatite crystals exit and begin to emerge from the lumen into the surrounding extracellular matrix.

In the second **collagen mineralization phase** that takes place outside matrix vesicle, the hydroxyapatite crystals form **mineralized nodules** (Fig. 8.28). In this phase, the following events occur:

- High levels of Ca^{2+}, PO_4 ions, and Ca^{2+}-binding proteins (including osteopontin [BSP-1], osteocalcin, and osteonectin) in the extracellular matrix provide a favorable environment for continuing **nucleation of hydroxyapatite crystals**.
- The hydroxyapatite crystals grow rapidly between collagen fibrils and proteoglycan ground substance molecules until they join neighboring crystals produced by other mineralized nodules. In this way, a **wave of mineralization** sweeps through the osteoid.
- Complete rupture and **disintegration of matrix vesicles** occur later in this phase.

■ BONE AS A TARGET OF ENDOCRINE HORMONES AND AS AN ENDOCRINE ORGAN

Bone serves as a reservoir for body calcium.

The maintenance of normal blood calcium levels is critical to health and life. Because bone serves as a reservoir for body calcium, its release and retrieval from the blood is closely monitored by endocrine hormones such as parathyroid hormone and calcitonin. Calcium may be delivered from the bone matrix to the blood if the circulating blood levels of calcium fall below a critical point (physiologic calcium concentration ranges from 8.9 to 10.1 mg/dL). Conversely, excess blood calcium may be removed from the blood and stored in bone.

These processes are regulated by **parathyroid hormone (PTH)**, secreted by the principal (chief) cells of the parathyroid glands, and **calcitonin**, secreted by the parafollicular cells of the thyroid gland (Folder 8.4).

- **PTH** acts on the bone to *increase low blood calcium levels* to normal. PTH release results in the rapid mobilization of Ca^{2+} from bone.
- **Calcitonin** acts on the bone to *decrease elevated blood calcium levels* to normal.

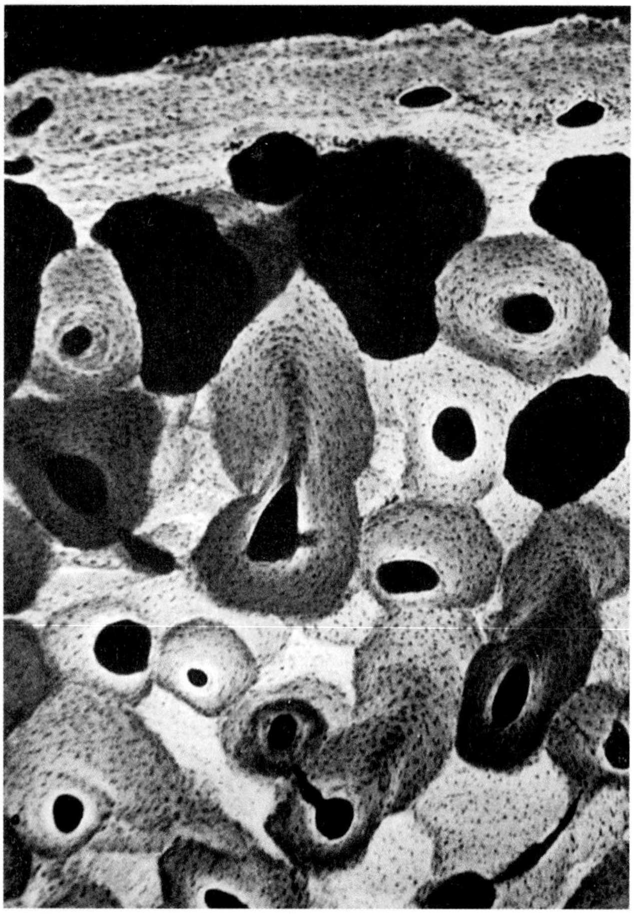

FIGURE 8.26. Microradiograph of the cross section of a bone. This 200-μm-thick cross section of bone from a healthy 19-year-old male shows various degrees of mineralization in different osteons. Mature compact bone is actively replacing immature bone, which is seen on the periosteal (*upper*) surface. The degree of mineralization is reflected by the shade of light and dark in the microradiograph. Thus, *very light areas* represent the highly mineralized tissue that deflects the X-rays and prevents them from striking the photographic film. Conversely, *dark areas* contain less mineral and, thus, are less effective in deflecting the X-rays. Note that the interstitial lamellae (the older bone) are very light, whereas some of the osteons are very dark (these are the most newly formed). The Haversian canals appear *black*, as they represent only soft tissue. ×157. (Courtesy of Dr. Jenifer Jowsey.)

PTH regulates the distribution of total body Ca^{2+}. It stimulates both osteocytes and osteoclasts (indirectly via RANK–RANKL signaling pathways because osteoclasts do not have PTH receptors) to resorb bone, thereby releasing calcium into the blood. As described previously (see pages 247-248), resorption of bone by osteocytes occurs during osteocytic remodeling. PTH also reduces excretion of calcium by the kidney and stimulates absorption of calcium by the small intestine. PTH further acts to maintain homeostasis by stimulating the kidney to excrete the excess phosphate produced by bone resorption.

Calcitonin inhibits bone resorption, specifically inhibiting the effects of PTH on osteoclasts. It is highly active in young individuals but decreases in activity as individuals age.

The mechanisms by which PTH helps regulate serum calcium levels and bone resorption are more complex. PTH has an **anabolic action** (it increases bone formation) as well as a **catabolic action** (it causes bone resorption). Clinical trials in which PTH was administered in intermittent subcutaneous doses to postmenopausal women with osteoporosis have shown significant increases in bone formation and bone mineral density. Increases in the density of spongy (cancellous) bone due to PTH treatment were shown in the ilium, vertebral bodies, and the shafts of radial and femoral bones (see Folder 8.2). The possible mechanisms behind this counterintuitive anabolic action of PTH are most likely related to its dosing. Brief or intermittent treatment with PTH is anabolic; it stimulates bone deposition through cAMP/IGF-1 pathways in osteocytes and osteoblasts. Conversely, prolonged and continuous treatment is catabolic; it increases production of RANKL molecules by osteoblasts and T lymphocytes, leading to activation of osteoclasts and bone resorption.

Bone cells produce endocrine hormones that are involved in regulating phosphate and glucose metabolism.

Several newly discovered hormones produced by osteoblasts and osteocytes contribute to mineral and nutrient homeostasis. These hormones include the following:

- **Fibroblast growth factor 23 (FGF-23)**, which is produced by osteocytes, regulates serum phosphate levels by altering the levels of active vitamin D and the activity of specific phosphate transporters in the kidney. FGF-23 is an important factor in aiding PTH in the disposal of excess phosphate released from hydroxyapatites during bone resorption.
- **Osteocalcin**, which is produced by osteoblasts, is linked to a pathway regulating energy and glucose metabolism. It targets adipocytes and insulin-producing cells in the pancreas. In addition, osteocalcin has been shown to induce testosterone production in Leydig cells of the testes.

Both FGF-23 and osteocalcin function as classic endocrine hormones; that is, they are produced exclusively in bone tissue and act on distant target organs through a regulatory feedback mechanism. Understanding the endocrine role of bone tissue will improve diagnosis and management of osteoporosis, diabetes mellitus, and other metabolic disorders.

■ BIOLOGY OF BONE REPAIR

Bone can repair itself after injury either by a direct (primary) or indirect (secondary) bone healing process.

Repair of **bone fracture** occurs by two processes: direct or indirect bone healing. **Direct (primary) bone healing** occurs when the fractured bone is surgically stabilized with compression plates, thereby completely restricting movement between fractured fragments of bone. In this process, bone undergoes internal remodeling similar to that of mature bone. The cutting cones formed by the osteoclasts cross the fracture line and generate longitudinal resorption canals that are later filled by bone-producing osteoblasts residing in the closing cones (see pages 259-261 for details). This process results in the simultaneous generation of a bony union and the restoration of Haversian systems.

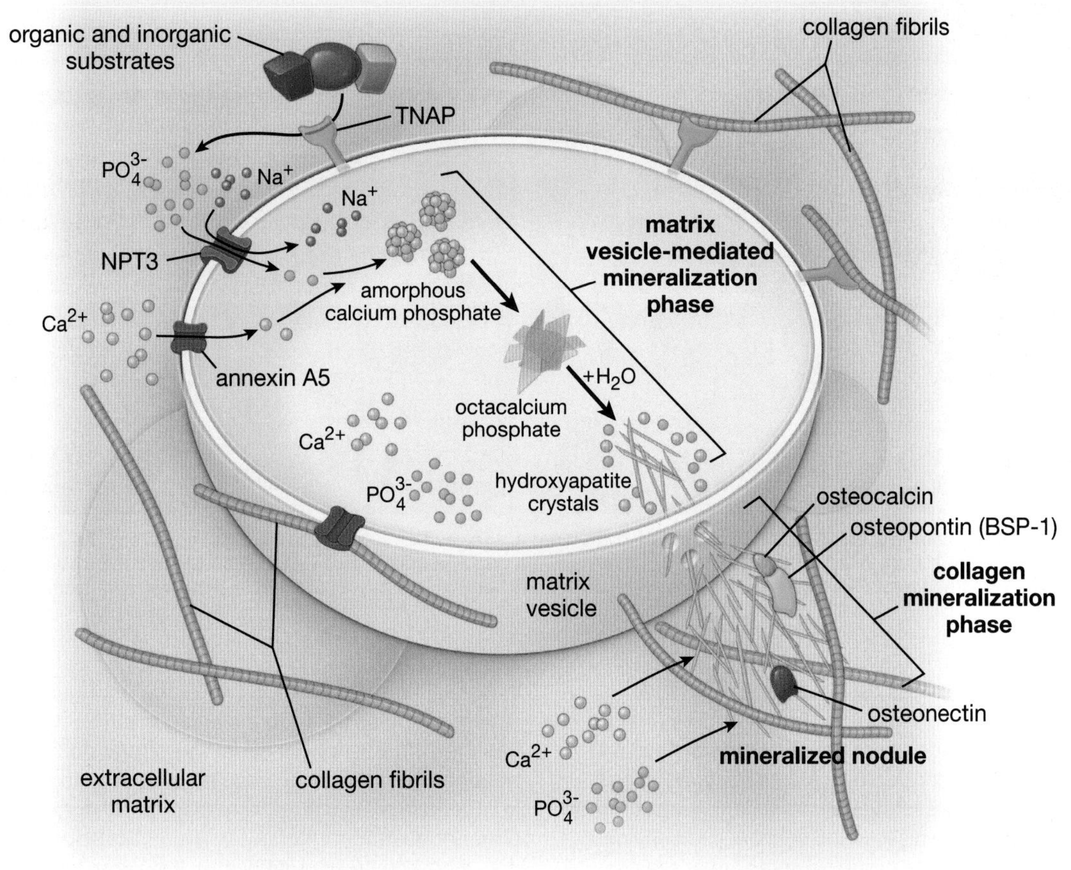

FIGURE 8.27. Schematic representation of the mineralization processes and the role of matrix vesicles. Matrix vesicles are released from the osteoblast at the osteoblast–osteoid interface. The plasma membrane of matrix vesicles contains several proteins, including Ca^{2+} channels (annexins), Na+–phosphate cotransporters (*NPT3*), and tissue nonspecific alkaline phosphatases (*TNAP*). TNAP increases the extracellular concentration of PO_4 ions, which are transported into the vesicle via NPT3 cotransporters. Annexin A5 allows for influx of Ca^{2+}. In the matrix vesicle–mediated mineralization phase, both Ca^{2+} and PO_4 ions accumulate in the vesicle lumen and initiate a stepwise process of hydroxyapatite crystals formation. Hydroxyapatite crystals emerge from the lumen into the extracellular matrix through holes punched in the vesicle membrane by phospholipases. Next, the collagen mineralization phase takes place outside the matrix vesicle, which results in the organization of hydroxyapatite crystals into mineralized nodules. High concentrations of Ca^{2+}, PO_4 ions, and Ca^{2+}-binding proteins in the extracellular matrix provide a favorable environment for hydroxyapatite crystals growth. They rapidly expand into spaces between collagen fibrils until they join neighboring crystals produced by other mineralized nodules. In this way, a wave of mineralization sweeps through the osteoid. *BSP*, bone sialoprotein.

FOLDER 8.2

CLINICAL CORRELATION: OSTEOPOROSIS

Osteoporosis, which literally means porous bone, is the most common bone disease, affecting an estimated 75 million people in the United States, Europe, and Japan. It is characterized by progressive loss of normal bone density accompanied by the deterioration of its microarchitecture. Osteoporosis is caused by an imbalance between osteoclast-mediated bone resorption and osteoblast-mediated bone deposition, resulting in decreased bone mass, enhanced bone fragility, and increased risk of fracture. In healthy individuals, osteoclast activity is primarily regulated by PTH and to a lesser degree by IL-1 and TNF. In addition, differentiation of osteoclast precursors is influenced by M-CSF and IL-6. Female hormones known as *estrogens* (especially estradiol) not only inhibit formation of these cytokines but also modulate the expression of RANKL, therefore limiting the activity of osteoclasts. In postmenopausal women in whom estrogen levels are reduced, secretion of these cytokines is increased, resulting in enhanced activity of osteoclasts leading to intensified bone resorption. Osteoporosis is estimated to be present in one-third of postmenopausal women and most of the elderly population. It results in more than 1.3 million fractures annually in the United States.

There are three general types of osteoporosis.

- **Type I primary osteoporosis** occurs in postmenopausal women. Because this type appears at an earlier stage of life than type II, its long-term effect is usually more severe than osteoporosis that develops in the later years of life.
- **Type II primary osteoporosis** occurs in elderly individuals in their seventh or eighth decade of life and is the leading cause of serious morbidity and functional loss in this age group.
- **Secondary osteoporosis** develops as a result of drug therapy (i.e., corticosteroids) or disease processes that may affect bone remodeling, including malnutrition, prolonged immobilization, weightlessness (i.e., with space travel), and metabolic bone diseases (i.e., hyperparathyroidism, metastatic cancers).

(*continued*)

FOLDER 8.2

CLINICAL CORRELATION: OSTEOPOROSIS (*continued*)

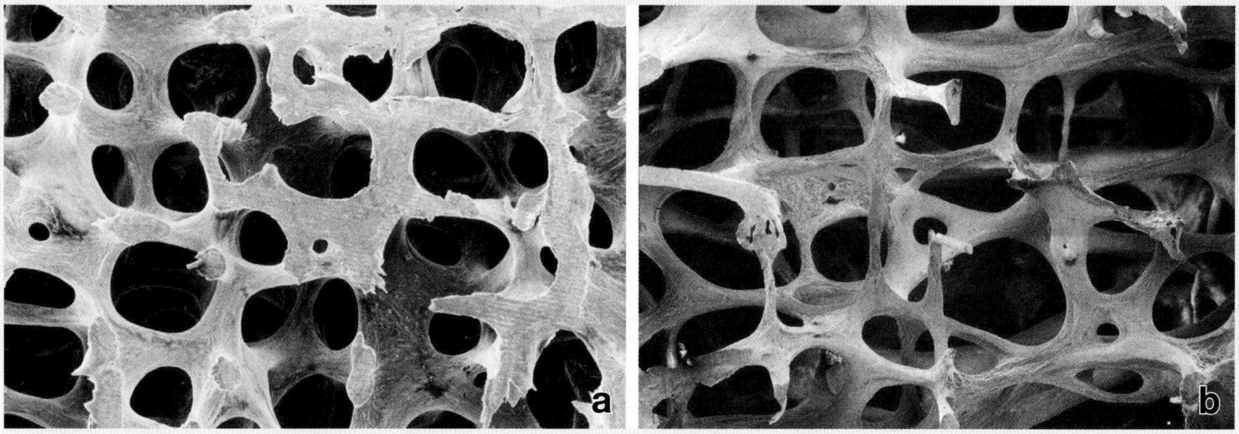

FIGURE F8.2.1. Scanning electron micrograph of trabecular bone. a. This image shows a section from the trabecular bone obtained from a vertebral body of a healthy individual. **b.** This specimen was obtained from a vertebral body of an elderly woman showing extensive signs of osteoporosis. Compare the pattern of trabecular architecture in osteoporosis with normal vertebral bone. (Courtesy of Dr. Alan Boyd.)

Osteoporotic bone has a normal histologic structure; however, there is less tissue mass (Fig. F8.2.1), which results in weakened bones that are more prone to fractures following even minor trauma. Femoral head and neck fractures (commonly known as *hip fractures*), wrist fractures, and compressed vertebrae fractures are common injuries that frequently disable and confine an elderly person to a wheelchair. Individuals with fractures are at greater risk for death, not directly from the fracture, but from the complications immobilization, which included an increased risk of pneumonia, pulmonary thrombosis, and embolism.

Treatment of individuals with osteoporosis includes an improved diet with vitamin D and calcium supplementation and moderate exercise to help slow further bone loss. In addition to diet and exercise, pharmacologic therapy directed toward slowing down bone resorption is often used.

For postmenopausal women, several treatment options are available. **Hormone replacement therapy** (HRT) with estrogen and progesterone is approved for the prevention of osteoporotic fractures in postmenopausal women, but it is not considered a first-line therapy because of its association with an increased risk of cardiovascular disease, blood clots, and breast cancer. HRT is recommended for fracture prevention if a woman also has severe symptoms of menopause (such as hot flashes) or if she cannot tolerate other therapies and she does not have risk factors for or a history of cardiovascular disease or breast cancer.

Selective estrogen receptor modulators (SERMs), such as raloxifene, bind to estrogen receptors and act as an estrogen agonist (mimicking estrogen action) in bone; in other tissues, it blocks the estrogen receptor action (acting as an estrogen antagonist). SERM therapy has the same beneficial effect as estrogen on bone tissue but does not cause the same adverse effects as estrogen in other tissues (such as increased risk of breast cancer). Other nonestrogen therapies include **bisphosphonates** (i.e., alendronate or risedronate), which inhibit osteoclastic activity by inducing apoptosis of osteoclasts.

Hormonal therapy in osteoporosis includes the use of **human parathyroid hormone recombinant** (i.e., teriparatide), which has the same physiologic action on bone and kidneys as the hormone. In intermittent doses, it promotes bone formation by increasing osteoblastic activity and improving thickness of trabecular bone. Release of PTH is modified by physical exercise and depends on the intensity and duration of exercise. Short-duration, high-intensity exercise and long-duration, low-intensity exercise seem to have no impact on PTH secretion.

Therapies targeting RANK, RANKL, and OPG molecules that control the development, commitment, differentiation, and function of cells in the osteoclast lineage are also available for patients with osteoporosis. Denosumab, a human **monoclonal antibody**, mimics the action of osteoprotegerin (OPG) which serves as a soluble decoy receptor for RANKL. Denosumab blocks RANK–RANKL signaling pathway, reduces the number of differentiating osteoclasts by inhibiting their activation and survival, thus preventing bone resorption.

Indirect (secondary) bone healing involves responses from periosteum and surrounding soft tissues as well as endochondral and intramembranous bone formation. This type of bone repair occurs in fractures that are treated with nonrigid or semirigid bone fixation (i.e., treatment with casts, fracture braces, external fixation, intramedullary nailing, or application of metal plates over the fracture gap). The major stages of indirect bone healing are shown in Figure 8.29.

Bone fracture initiates an acute inflammatory response that is necessary for bone healing.

The initial response to **bone fracture** is similar to the response to any injury that produces tissue destruction and hemorrhage. Initially, a **fracture hematoma** (a collection of blood that surrounds the fracture ends of the bones) is formed (Fig. 8.29b), and bone necrosis is seen at the ends

FOLDER 8.3
CLINICAL CORRELATION: NUTRITIONAL FACTORS IN BONE FORMATION

Both nutritional and hormonal factors affect the degree of bone mineralization. **Calcium deficiency** during growth causes **rickets**, a condition in which the bone matrix does not calcify normally. Rickets may be caused by insufficient amounts of dietary calcium or insufficient vitamin D (a steroid prohormone), which is needed for absorption of calcium by the intestines. An X-ray of a child with advanced rickets presents classic radiologic symptoms: bowed lower limbs (outward curve of long bones of the leg and thighs) and a deformed chest and skull (often having a distinctive "square" appearance). If rickets is not treated while a child is still growing, skeletal deformities and short stature may be permanent. In adults, the same nutritional or vitamin deficiency leads to **osteomalacia**. Although rickets and osteomalacia are no longer major health problems in populations where nutrition is adequate, they are among the most frequent childhood diseases in many developing countries.

In addition to its influence on intestinal absorption of calcium, vitamin D is needed for normal calcification. Other vitamins known to affect bone are vitamins A and C. Vitamin A deficiency suppresses endochondral growth of bone; vitamin A excess leads to fragility and subsequent fractures of long bones. Vitamin C is essential for synthesis of collagen, and its deficiency leads to **scurvy**. The matrix produced in scurvy is unable to calcify. Another form of insufficient bone mineralization often seen in postmenopausal women is the condition known as **osteoporosis** (see Folder 8.2).

of the fractured bone fragments. Injury to nearby soft tissues and degranulation of platelets from the blood clot secrete cytokines (e.g., TNF-α, IL-1, IL-6, IL-11, IL-18) and initiate an acute inflammatory response. This process is reflected by the infiltration of neutrophils followed by the migration of macrophages. Fibroblasts and capillaries subsequently proliferate and grow into the site of the injury. Also, specific mesenchymal stem cells arrive at the site of injury from the surrounding soft tissues and bone marrow. The fracture hematoma, which initially contained entrapped erythrocytes within a network of fibrin, is gradually replaced by **granulation tissue**, a type of newly formed loose connective tissue containing collagen type III and type II fibers. Both fibroblasts and periosteal cells participate in this phase of healing.

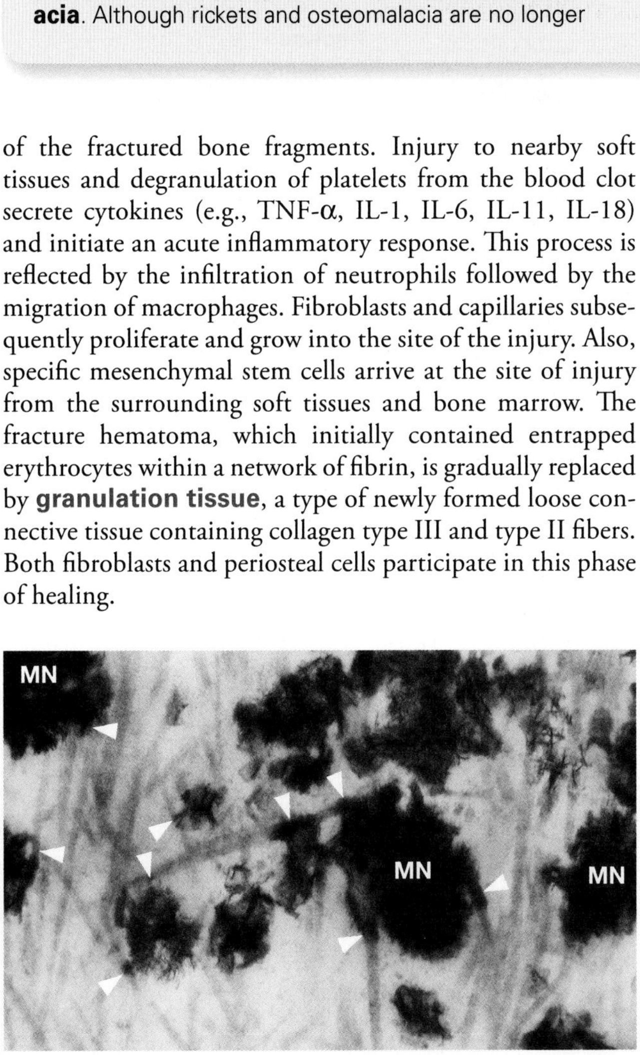

FIGURE 8.28. Electron micrograph of osteoid with mineralized nodules. This micrograph shows several mineralized nodules (*MN*) in different stages of formation surrounded by collagen fibrils in the collagen mineralization phase of the osteoid. Mineralized nodules are formed by hydroxyapatite crystals that exited the lumen of matrix vesicles and continue to grow in size between collagen fibrils. Note that mineralized nodules have multiple connections with collagen fibrils (*arrowheads*), which are remnants of the collagen binding sites of proteins (i.e., tissue nonspecific alkaline phosphatases [*TNAP*] and annexin A5) expressed on the surface of matrix vesicles. × 30,000. (Reprinted with permission from Amizuka N, Li M, Kobayashi M, et al. Vitamin K2, a gamma-carboxylating factor of gla-proteins, normalizes the bone crystal nucleation impaired by Mg-insufficiency. *Histol Histopathol.* 2008;23:1353–1366.)

Granulation tissue transforms into a fibrocartilaginous soft callus, which gives the fracture site a stable, semirigid structure.

As the granulation tissue becomes denser, chondroblasts differentiate from the skeletal stem cells residing in periosteal lining. The newly produced cartilage matrix invades the periphery of granulation tissue. The dense connective tissue and newly formed cartilage grows and covers the bone at the fracture site, producing a **soft callus** (Fig. 8.29c). This callus will form even if the fractured parts are not in immediate apposition to each other, and it helps stabilize and bind together the fractured bone (Fig. 8.30).

A bony callus replaces fibrocartilage at the fracture site and allows for weight bearing.

While the callus is forming, osteoprogenitor cells of the periosteum divide and differentiate into osteoblasts. The newly formed osteoblasts begin to deposit osteoid on the outer surface of the callus (intramembranous process) at a distance from the fracture. This new bone formation progresses toward the fracture site until new bone forms a bony sheath over the fibrocartilaginous callus. Osteogenic buds from the new bone invade the callus and begin to deposit bone within the callus, gradually replacing the original fibrous and cartilaginous callus with a **hard callus** (Fig. 8.29d). In addition, endosteal proliferation and differentiation occur in the marrow cavity, and bone grows from both ends of the fracture toward the center. When this bone unites, the bony union of the fractured bone, produced by the osteoblasts and derived from both the periosteum and endosteum, consists of spongy bone. As in normal endochondral bone formation, the spongy bone is gradually replaced by compact bone. The hard callus becomes more solid and mechanically rigid.

The remodeling process restores the original shape of the bone.

Although the hard callus is a rigid structure providing mechanical stability to the fracture site, it does not fully restore the properties of normal bone. Bone remodeling of the hard

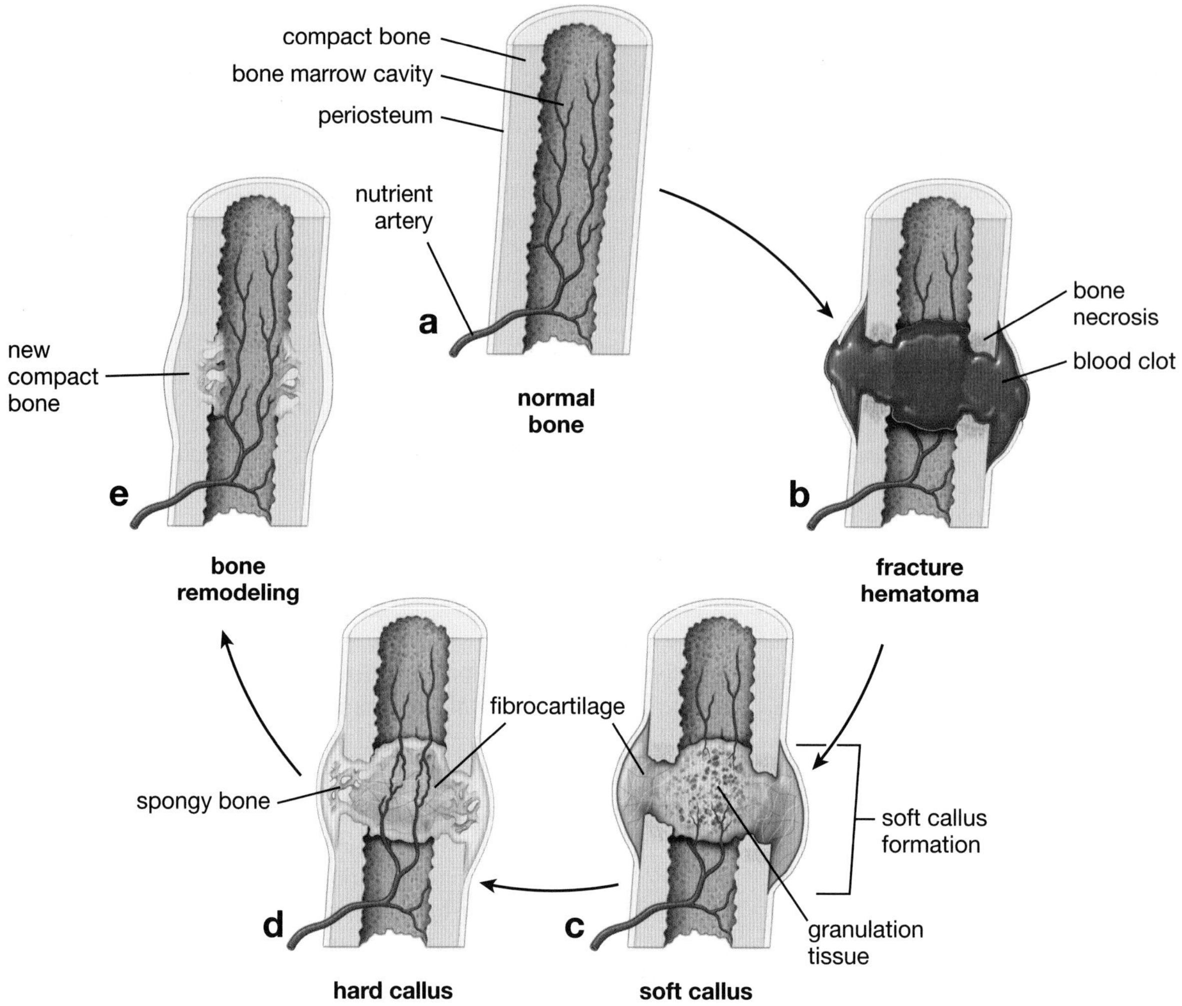

FIGURE 8.29. Bone fracture and stages of bone healing process. a. View of healthy bone before fracture. **b.** The initial response to the injury produces a fracture hematoma that surrounds the ends of the fractured bone. The ends of bone fragments undergo necrosis. An acute inflammatory reaction develops and is manifested by infiltration of neutrophils and macrophages, activation of fibroblasts, and proliferation of capillaries. The fracture hematoma is gradually replaced by granulation tissue. **c.** Fibrocartilage matrix is deposited. Newly formed fibrocartilage fills the gap at the fracture site producing a soft callus. This stabilizes and binds together the fractured ends of the bone. **d.** The osteoprogenitor cells from the periosteum differentiate into osteoblasts and begin to deposit new bone on the outer surface of the callus (intramembranous process) until new bone forms a bony sheath over the fibrocartilaginous soft callus. The cartilage in the soft callus calcifies and is gradually replaced by bone as in endochondral ossification. Newly deposited woven bone forms a bony hard callus. **e.** Bone remodeling of the hard callus transforms woven bone into the lamellar mature structure with a central bone marrow cavity. The hard callus is gradually replaced by compact bone through the action of osteoclasts and osteoblasts, which restores bone to its original shape.

FOLDER 8.4

FUNCTIONAL CONSIDERATIONS: HORMONAL REGULATION OF BONE GROWTH

Hormones other than PTH and calcitonin have major effects on bone growth. One such hormone is **pituitary growth hormone** (GH, somatotropin). This hormone stimulates growth in general and, especially, growth of epiphyseal cartilage and bone. It acts directly on osteoprogenitor cells, stimulating them to divide and differentiate. Chondrocytes in epiphyseal growth plates are regulated by insulin-like growth factor I (IGF-1), which is primarily produced by the liver in response to GH. In addition to IGF-1, insulin and thyroid hormones stimulate chondrocyte activity. Oversecretion in childhood, caused by a defect in the mechanism regulating GH secretion or a GH-secreting tumor in the pituitary gland, leads to **gigantism**, an abnormal increase in the length of bones. Absence or hyposecretion of GH in childhood leads to failure of growth of the long bones, resulting in **pituitary dwarfism**. Absence or severe hyposecretion of thyroid hormone during development and infancy leads to failure of bone growth and dwarfism, a condition known as **congenital hypothyroidism**. When oversecretion of GH occurs in an adult, bones do not grow in length as a result of epiphyseal closure. Instead, abnormal thickening and selective overgrowth of hands, feet, mandible, nose, and intramembranous bones of the skull occurs. This condition, known as **acromegaly**, is caused by increased activity of osteoblasts on bone surfaces.

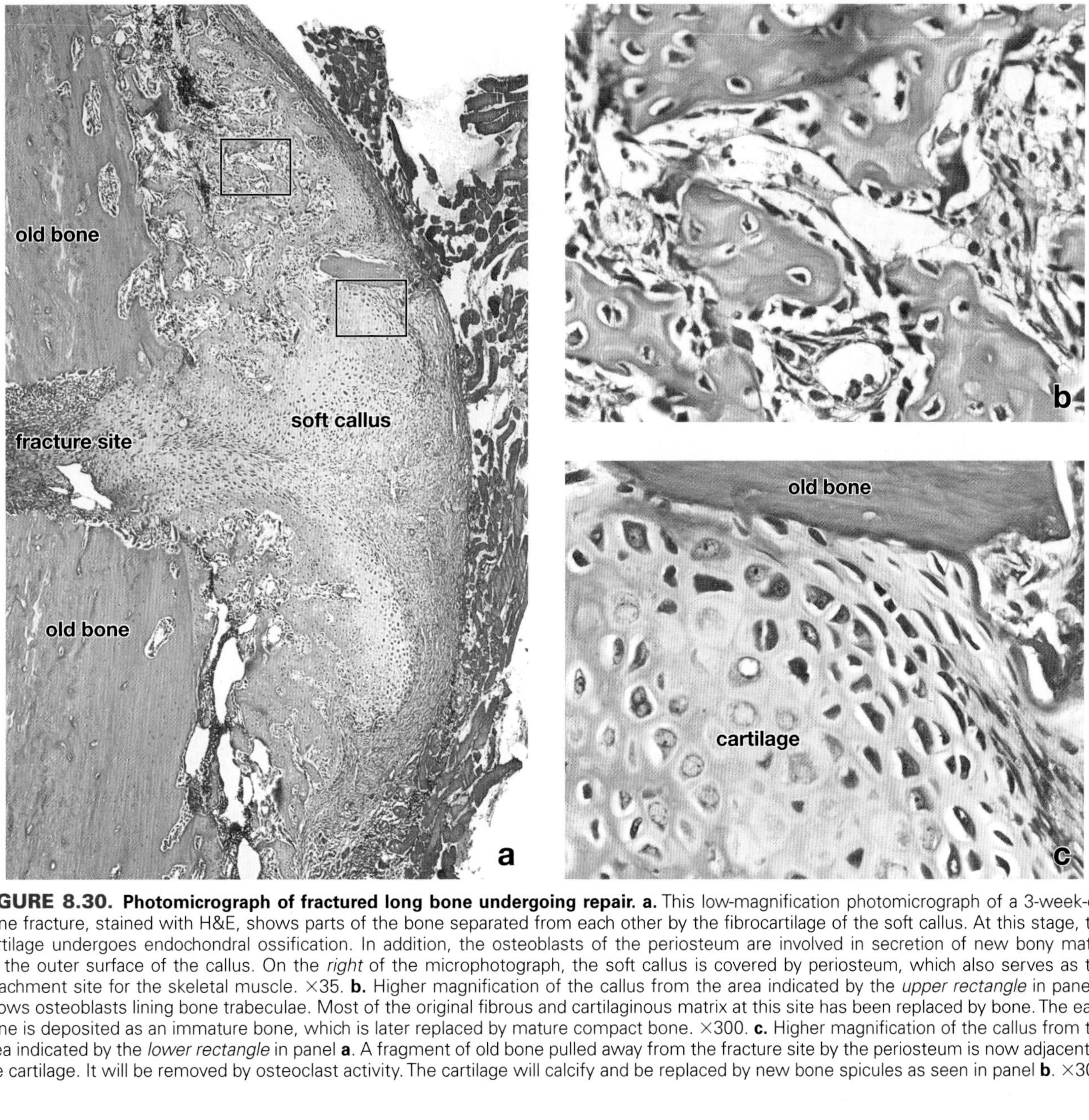

FIGURE 8.30. Photomicrograph of fractured long bone undergoing repair. a. This low-magnification photomicrograph of a 3-week-old bone fracture, stained with H&E, shows parts of the bone separated from each other by the fibrocartilage of the soft callus. At this stage, the cartilage undergoes endochondral ossification. In addition, the osteoblasts of the periosteum are involved in secretion of new bony matrix on the outer surface of the callus. On the *right* of the microphotograph, the soft callus is covered by periosteum, which also serves as the attachment site for the skeletal muscle. ×35. **b.** Higher magnification of the callus from the area indicated by the *upper rectangle* in panel **a** shows osteoblasts lining bone trabeculae. Most of the original fibrous and cartilaginous matrix at this site has been replaced by bone. The early bone is deposited as an immature bone, which is later replaced by mature compact bone. ×300. **c.** Higher magnification of the callus from the area indicated by the *lower rectangle* in panel **a**. A fragment of old bone pulled away from the fracture site by the periosteum is now adjacent to the cartilage. It will be removed by osteoclast activity. The cartilage will calcify and be replaced by new bone spicules as seen in panel **b**. ×300.

callus must occur in order to transform the newly deposited woven bone into a lamellar mature bone. Subsequently, the bone marrow cavity must be restored. While compact bone is being formed, remnants of the hard callus are removed by the action of osteoclasts, and gradual **bone remodeling** restores the bone to its original shape (Fig. 8.29e).

In healthy individuals, **bone healing** usually takes 6–12 weeks, depending on the severity of the break and the specific bone that is fractured. The inflammatory process lasts approximately 1 week. It is typically accompanied by pain and swelling, and it leads to granulation tissue formation. The soft callus is formed approximately 2–3 weeks after fracture. The hard callus in which the fractured fragments are firmly united by new bone requires 3–4 months to develop. The process of bone remodeling may last from a few months to several years until the bone has completely returned to its original shape. Setting the bone (i.e., reapproximating the normal anatomic configuration) and holding the parts in place by internal fixation (by pins, screws, or plates) or by external fixation (by casts or by pins and screws) expedites the healing process.

BONE

OVERVIEW OF BONE

- **Bone** is a specialized type of connective tissue characterized by a **mineralized extracellular matrix** that stores calcium and phosphate.
- Bone contributes to the **skeleton**, which supports the body, protects vital structures, provides the mechanical basis for body movement, and harbors bone marrow.

GENERAL STRUCTURE OF BONES

- **Bones** are classified according to shape into long, short, flat, or irregular bones.
- **Long bones** are tubular in shape and consist of two ends (**proximal** and **distal epiphyses**) and a long shaft **(diaphysis)**. **Metaphysis** is the junction between the diaphysis and the epiphysis.
- Bone is covered by **periosteum**, a connective tissue membrane that attaches to the outer surface by **Sharpey fibers**. Periosteum contains a layer of osteoprogenitor (periosteal) cells that can differentiate into osteoblasts.
- **Bone cavities** are lined by **endosteum**, a single layer of cells that contains osteoprogenitor (endosteal) cells, osteoblasts, and osteoclasts.
- Bones articulate with neighboring bones by **synovial joints**, a movable connection. The articular surfaces that form contact areas between two bones are covered by **hyaline (articular) cartilage.**

GENERAL STRUCTURE OF BONE TISSUE

- **Bone tissue** formed during development is called **immature (woven) bone**. It differs from **mature (lamellar) bone** in its collagen fiber arrangement.
- Bone tissue is classified as either **compact** (dense) or **spongy** (cancellous). Compact bone lies outside and beneath the periosteum, whereas an internal, sponge-like meshwork of trabeculae forms spongy bone.
- **Mature (lamellar) bone** is mostly composed of **osteons (Haversian systems)**. These concentric lamellar structures are organized around an **osteonal (Haversian) canal** that contains the vascular and nerve supply of the osteon. **Perforating (Volkmann) canals** are perpendicularly arranged and connect osteonal canals to one another.
- The **lacunae** between concentric lamellae contain **osteocytes** that are interconnected with other osteocytes and the osteonal canal via **canaliculi.**

CELLS AND EXTRACELLULAR MATRIX

- **Osteoprogenitor cells** derive from mesenchymal stem cells in the bone marrow. They differentiate under the influence of the core binding factor alpha-1 (CBFA1) transcription factor (RUNX2) into osteoblasts.
- **Osteoblasts** differentiate from osteoprogenitor cells and secrete **osteoid**, an unmineralized bone matrix that undergoes mineralization triggered by matrix vesicles.
- **Osteocytes** are mature bone cells enclosed within **lacunae** of bone matrix. They communicate with other osteocytes by a network of long cell processes occupying **canaliculi**, and they respond to mechanical forces applied to the bone.
- **Osteoclasts** differentiate from hemopoietic progenitor cells; they resorb bone matrix during bone formation and remodeling. They differentiate and mature under the control of the **RANK–RANKL signaling mechanism.**
- **Bone matrix** contains mainly type I collagen along with other noncollagenous proteins and regulatory proteins.

BONE FORMATION

- The development of bone is classified as **endochondral** (a cartilage model serves as the precursor of the bone) or **intramembranous ossification** (without involvement of a cartilage precursor).
- Flat bones of the skull, mandible, and clavicle develop by **intramembranous ossification**; all other bones develop by endochondral ossification.
- In **endochondral ossification**, the **hyaline cartilage model** is formed. Next, osteoprogenitor cells surrounding this model differentiate into bone-forming cells that initially deposit bone on the cartilage surface (periosteal **bony collar**) and later penetrate the diaphysis to form the **primary ossification center**.
- **Secondary ossification centers** develop later within the epiphyses.
- Primary and secondary ossification centers are separated by the **epiphyseal growth plate**, seen in children and adolescents, that provides a source for new cartilage involved in bone growth.
- The **epiphyseal growth plate** has several zones (reserve cartilage, proliferation, hypertrophy, calcified cartilage, and resorption). Resorbed calcified cartilage is replaced by bone.

BONE GROWTH, REMODELING, AND REPAIR

- Elongation of endochondral bone depends on **the interstitial growth of cartilage** on the epiphyseal growth plate.
- Bone increases in width (diameter) by **appositional growth** of new bone that occurs between the compact bone and the periosteum.
- Bone is constantly being remodeled throughout life by **bone-remodeling units** composed of osteoclasts and osteoblasts. This process allows bone to change shape in response to mechanical load.
- Bone can repair itself after injury either by a **direct (primary)** or **indirect (secondary)** bone healing process.
- After injury, periosteal cells become activated to produce a **soft (fibrocartilage) callus**, which is subsequently replaced by a **hard (bony) callus**.

PHYSIOLOGIC ASPECTS OF BONE

- Bone serves as a **reservoir for Ca^{2+}** in the body. Ca^{2+} may be removed from bone if the circulating level of Ca^{2+} in the blood falls below the critical value. Likewise, excess Ca^{2+} may be removed from the blood and stored in bone.
- Maintenance of blood Ca^{2+} levels is regulated by **parathyroid hormone (PTH)**, secreted by the parathyroid glands, and **calcitonin**, secreted by the thyroid gland.
- **PTH** stimulates both osteocytes and osteoclasts (indirectly via RANK–RANKL signaling pathways because osteoclasts do not have PTH receptors) to resorb bone, thereby increasing Ca^{2+} levels in the blood.
- **Calcitonin** inhibits bone resorption by inhibiting the effects of PTH on osteoclasts, thereby lowering blood Ca^{2+} levels.

PLATE 8.1 ■ BONE, GROUND SECTION

Bone is a specialized connective tissue characterized by a mineralized extracellular matrix. Calcium phosphate, in the form of **hydroxyapatite crystals** [$Ca_{10}(PO_4)_6OH_2$], is deposited along the collagen fibrils and in the proteoglycan ground substance. Bone serves as a storage site for calcium and phosphate, which can be released to the blood to maintain homeostatic levels. **Osteocytes** reside in lacunae in the bone matrix and extend fine cellular processes into canaliculi that connect the lacunae, thus forming a continuous network of cells within the mineralized tissue. Bones are organs of the skeletal system; bone tissue is the structural component of bones.

Ground sections of bone are prepared from bone that has not been fixed but merely allowed to dry. Thin slices of the dried bone are then cut with a saw and further ground to a thinness that allows viewing in a light microscope. Slices may be treated with India ink to fill spaces that were formerly occupied by organic matter, for example, cells, blood vessels, and unmineralized matrix. A simpler method is to mount the ground specimen on a slide with a viscous medium that traps air in some of the spaces, as in the specimen in this plate. Here, some of the osteonal canals and a perforating canal are filled with the mounting medium, making them translucent instead of black. Specimens prepared in this manner are of value chiefly to display the architecture of the compact bone.

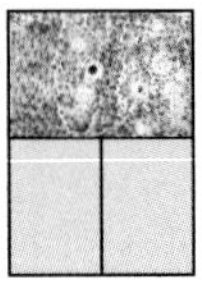

Ground bone, long bone, human, ×80.

This figure reveals a cross-sectioned area of a long bone at low magnification and includes the outer or peripheral aspect of the bone, identified by the presence of **circumferential lamellae** (*CL*). (The exterior or periosteal surface of the bone is not included in the micrograph.) To their *right* are the **osteons** (*O*) or Haversian systems that appear as circular profiles. Between the osteons are **interstitial lamellae** (*IL*), the remnants of previously existing osteons.

Osteons are essentially cylindrical structures. In the shaft of a long bone, the long axes of the osteons are oriented parallel to the long axis of the bone. Thus, a cross section through the shaft of a long bone would reveal the osteons in cross section, as in this figure. At the center of each osteon is an **osteonal (Haversian) canal** (*HC*) that contains blood vessels, connective tissue, and cells lining the surface of the bone material. Because the organic material is not retained in ground sections, the Haversian canals and other spaces will appear black, as they do here, if filled with India ink or air. Concentric layers of mineralized substance, the concentric lamellae, surround the Haversian canal and appear much the same as growth rings of a tree. The canal is also surrounded by concentric arrangements of lacunae. These appear as the small, dark, elongate structures.

During the period of bone growth and during adult life, there is constant internal remodeling of bone. This involves the destruction of osteons and formation of new ones. The breakdown of an osteon is usually not complete; however, part of the osteon may remain intact. Moreover, portions of adjacent osteons may also be partially destroyed. The space created by the breakdown process is reoccupied by a new osteon. The remnants of the previously existing osteons become the interstitial lamellae.

Blood vessels reach the Haversian canals from the marrow through other tunnels called **perforating (Volkmann) canals** (*VC*). In some instances, as here, Volkmann canals travel from one Haversian canal to another. Volkmann canals can be distinguished from Haversian canals in that they pass through lamellae, whereas Haversian canals are surrounded by concentric rings of lamellae.

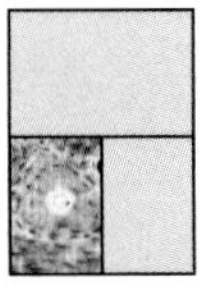

Ground bone-osteon, long bone, human, ×300.

This figure shows a higher magnification micrograph of the labeled **osteon** from the *upper* figure. It includes Haversian canal (*HC*) surrounded by concentric lamellae and some of the interstitial lamellae (*IL*) that are now seen at the *bottom* of the micrograph (the micrograph has been reoriented). Note the **lacunae** (*L*) and the fine thread-like profiles emanating from the lacunae. These thread-like profiles represent the canaliculi, spaces within the bone matrix that contain cytoplasmic processes of the osteocyte. The canaliculi of each lacuna communicate with canaliculi of neighboring lacunae to form a three-dimensional channel system throughout the bone.

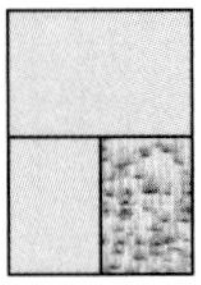

Ground bone, long bone, human, ×400.

In a still higher magnification, the **circumferential lamellae** are found around the shaft of the long bone at the outer as well as the inner surface of the bone. The osteoblasts that contribute to the formation of circumferential lamellae at these sites come from the periosteum and endosteum, respectively, whereas the osteons are constructed from osteoblasts in the canal of the developing Haversian system. This figure reveals not only the lacunae (*L*) and canaliculi but also the lamellae of the bone. The latter are just barely defined by the faint lines (*arrows*) that extend across the micrograph. Collagenous fibers in neighboring lamellae are oriented in different directions. This change in orientation accounts for the faint line or interface between adjacent lamellae.

CL, circumferential lamellae
HC, Haversian canal
IL, interstitial lamellae
L, lacuna
O, osteon
VC, Volkmann canal
arrows, lamellar boundary

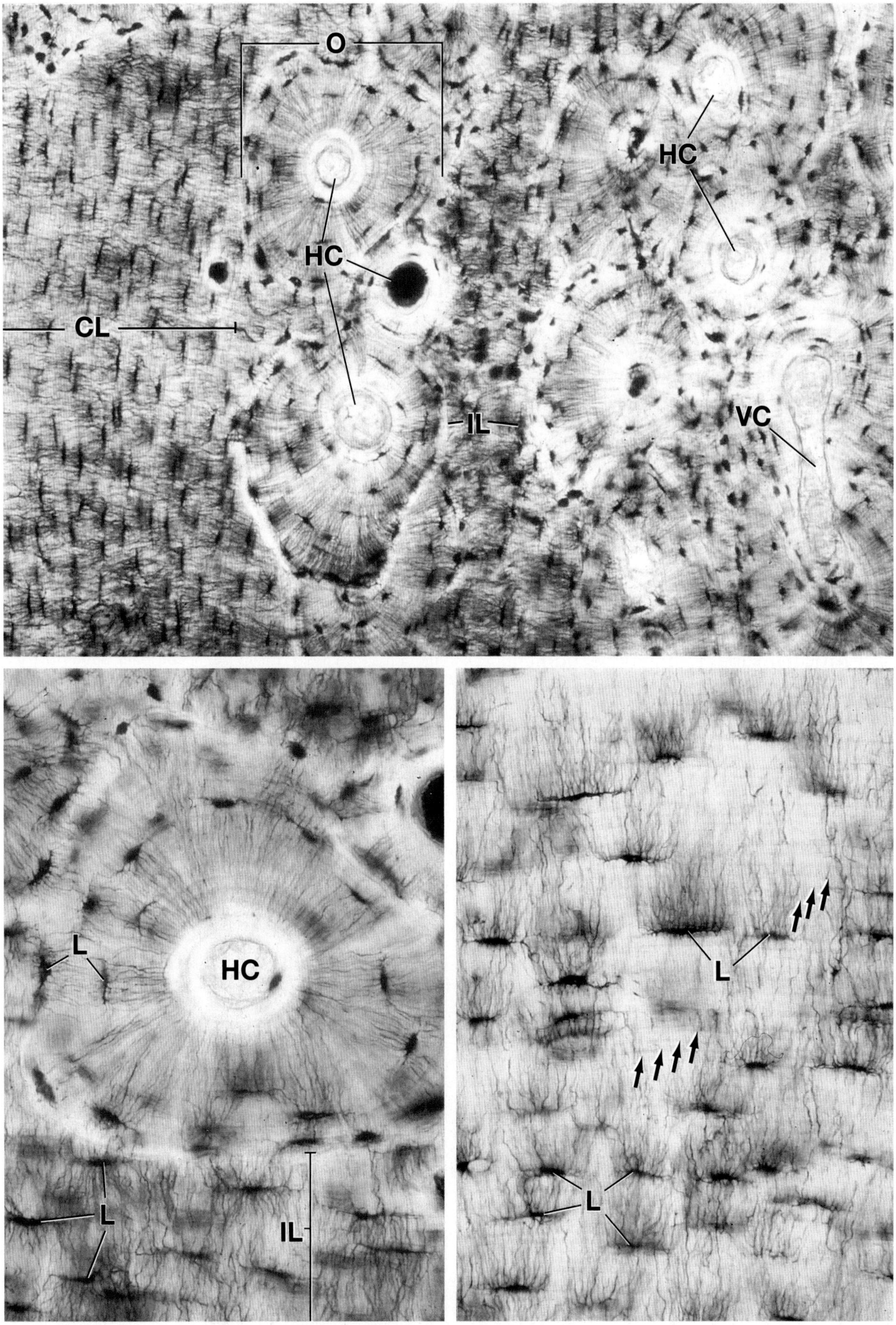
O
HC
HC
CL
IL
VC
L
HC
L
IL
L
L

PLATE 8.2 ■ BONE AND BONE TISSUE

Bone represents one of the specialized connective tissues. It is characterized by a mineralized extracellular matrix. It is the mineralization of the matrix that sets bone tissue apart from the other connective tissues and results in an extremely hard tissue that is capable of providing support and protection to the body. The mineral is calcium phosphate in the form of hydroxyapatite crystals. Bone also provides a storage site for calcium and phosphate. Both can be mobilized from the bone matrix and taken up by the blood as needed to maintain normal levels. Bone matrix contains type I collagen and, in small amounts, a number of other types of collagen, that is, types V, III, XI, and XIII. Other matrix proteins that constitute the ground substance of bone such as proteoglycan macromolecules, multiadhesive glycoproteins, growth factors, and cytokines are also present. Bone is typically studied in histologic preparations by removing the calcium content of the bone (decalcified bone), thus allowing it to be sectioned like other soft tissues.

ORIENTATION MICROGRAPH: The orientation micrograph shows the proximal end of a decalcified humerus from an infant. The interior of the head of the bone, the **epiphysis** (*E*), consists of spongy (cancellous) bone made up of an anastomosing network of **trabeculae** (*T*) in the form of bone spicules. The outer portion consists of a dense layer of bone tissue known as **compact bone** (*CB*). Its thickness varies in different parts of the bone. The wider portion of the bone adjacent to the **epiphyseal growth plate** (*EGP*) known as **metaphysis** (*M*) contains **spongy bone** (*SB*). The shaft of this bone, the **diaphysis** (*D*), is also made up of compact bone (*CB*) and contains bone marrow cavity filled with **bone marrow** (*BM*), which at this stage of life is in the form of active hemopoietic tissue. Cartilage is also a component of the bone, present as **articular cartilage** (*AC*) and as an epiphyseal growth plate (*EGP*) in growing bones.

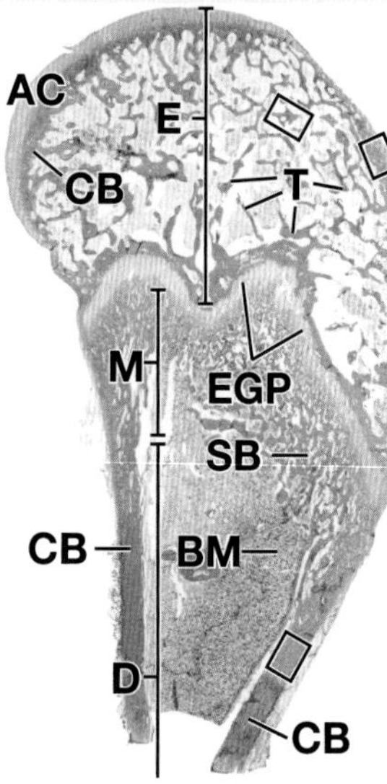

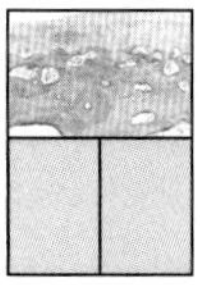

Articular surface, long bone, human, H&E ×178.

The articular surface of the epiphysis within the *top right box* on the orientation micrograph containing articular cartilage and the underlying bone tissue is shown here at higher magnification. The lighter staining area is the **articular cartilage** (*AC*) of the glenohumeral (shoulder) joint. Note the presence of isogenous groups of **chondrocytes** (*Ch*), a characteristic feature of growing cartilage. Below the cartilage is a darker staining area of **compact bone** (*CB*). It can be distinguished from the cartilage by the presence of **Haversian canals** (*HC*) and arrangement of the **osteocytes** (*Oc*). The osteocytes lie within the bone matrix but are typically recognized only by their nuclei. Because bone matrix is laid down in layers (lamellae), bone characteristically shows linear or circular patterns surrounding HCs. The irregular spaces seen within the bone tissue are **resorption canals** (*RC*) that contain, in addition to blood vessels, the osteoclasts and osteoblasts. Presence of resorption canals indicates an active process of bone remodeling.

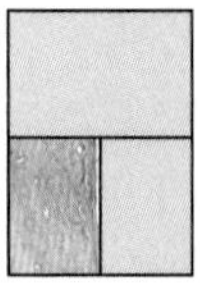

Compact bone, long bone, human, H&E ×135.

Bone from the diaphysis within the *bottom right box* on the orientation micrograph is shown here at higher magnification. The outer surface of the bone is covered by dense connective tissue known as **periosteum** (*P*). The remaining tissue in the micrograph is **compact bone** (*CB*). **Haversian canals** (*HC*) are surrounded by the **osteocytes** (*Oc*) and are recognized by their nuclei within the bone matrix. Another feature worth noting in this growing bone is the presence of bone-resorbing cells known as **osteoclasts** (*Ocl*). They are large multinucleated cells found at sites in bone where remodeling is taking place (see Plate 8.4).

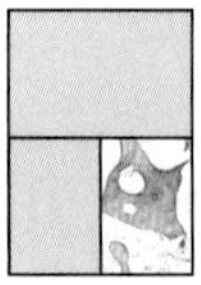

Spongy bone, long bone, human, H&E ×135.

The area in the *top left box* in the orientation micrograph containing spongy bone in the epiphysis is shown here at higher magnification. Although the bone tissue at this site forms a three-dimensional structure consisting of branching trabeculae, its structural organization and components are the same as that seen in compact bone. Note the nuclei of **osteocytes** (*Oc*). As bone matures, the bone tissue becomes reorganized and forms **osteons** (*O*), which consist of **Haversian canals** (*HC*) and surrounding layers (lamellae) of bone matrix. The two circular spaces are the **resorption canals** (*RC*), in which bone tissue has been removed and will be replaced by new tissue in the form of osteons. The spaces surrounding the spongy bone contain bone marrow consisting mainly of adipocytes. Other cells that have the capacity to form bone or hemopoietic tissue are also present.

AC, articular cartilage
BM, bone marrow
CB, compact bone
Ch, chondrocytes
D, diaphysis
E, epiphysis
EGP, epiphyseal growth plate
HC, Haversian canal
M, metaphysis
O, osteons
Oc, osteocytes
Ocl, osteoclasts
P, periosteum
RC, resorption canal
SB, spongy bone
T, trabeculae

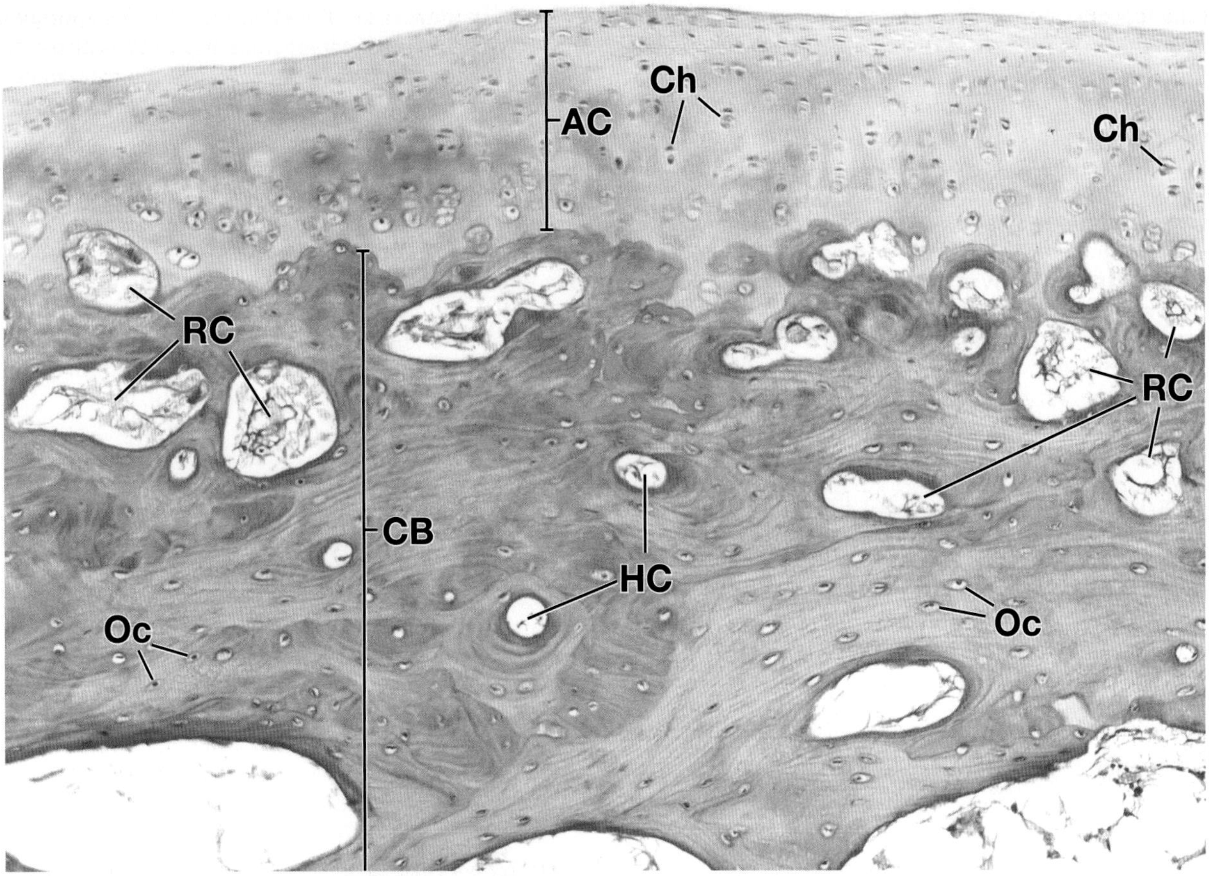
Ch
AC
Ch
RC
RC
CB
HC
HC
Oc
Oc

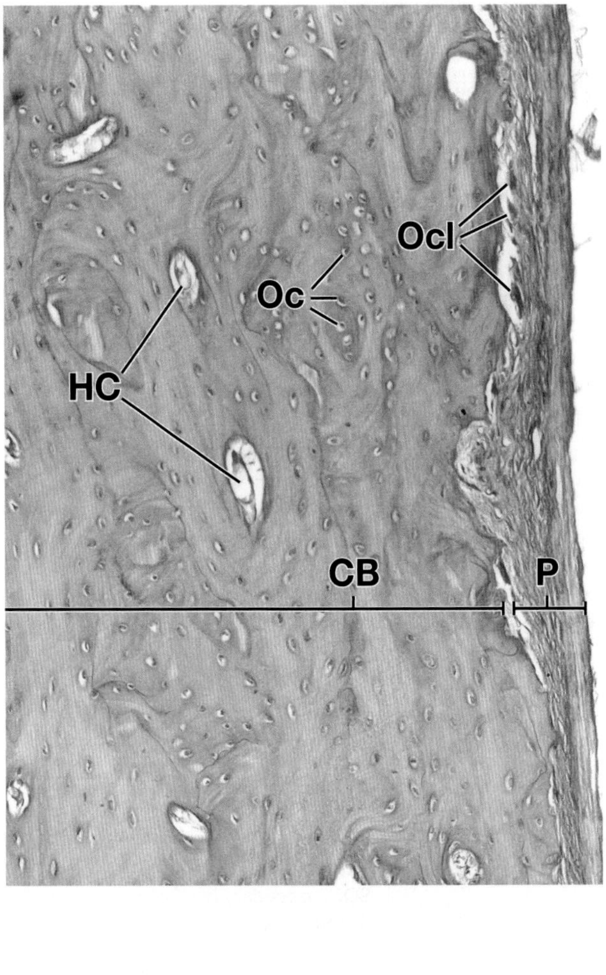
Ocl
Oc
HC
CB
P

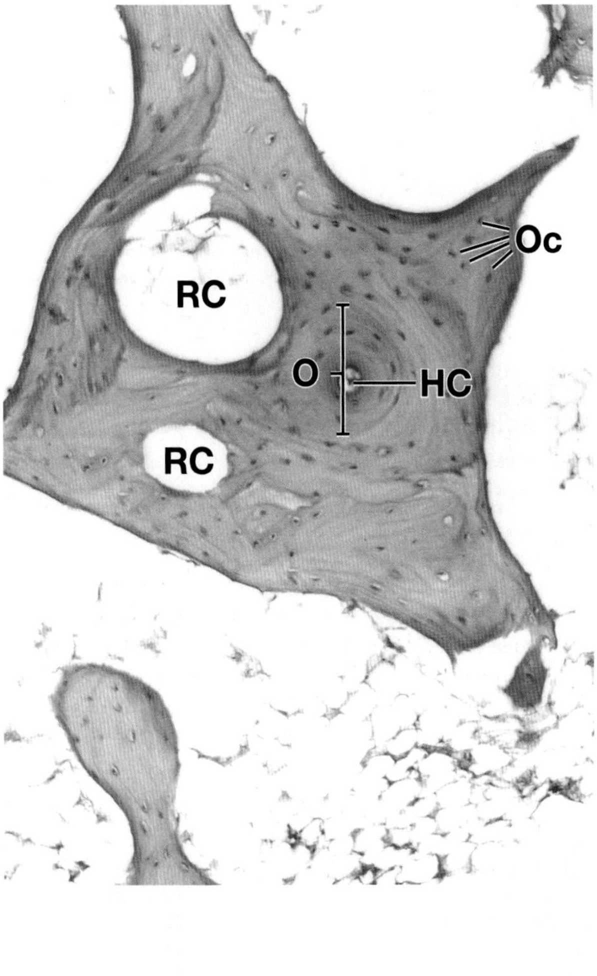
Oc
RC
O
HC
RC

PLATE 8.3 ■ ENDOCHONDRAL BONE FORMATION I

Endochondral bone formation involves a cartilage model that represents a cartilage precursor to the newly formed bone. The cartilage model appears as a miniature version of the future bone. Bone that arises through this process is formed by the simultaneous removal of the cartilage model and its replacement with bone tissue. The first sign of bone formation is the appearance of bone-forming cells around the shaft (diaphysis) of the cartilage model. The bone-forming cells, known as **osteoblasts**, are derived from osteoprogenitor cells in surrounding mesenchyme. They secrete collagens, bone sialoproteins, osteocalcin, and other components of the bone matrix. The initial deposition of these products is referred to as a *periosteal bony collar* and contains osteoid (unmineralized bone), which later becomes mineralized. With the initial establishment of this periosteal bony collar, the chondrocytes in the center of the cartilage model become hypertrophic (see *upper figure*), which leads to their death (or transdifferentiation into osteoblasts), and the cartilage matrix in this region becomes calcified. At the same time, blood vessels grow through the thin bony collar and vascularize the center of the bone diaphysis, allowing infiltration of precursor cells of bone marrow. Osteoprogenitor cells enter the bone marrow cavity with blood vessels and differentiate into osteoblasts. In long bones, this process is repeated in the epiphyses of the cartilage model (see lower micrograph). The process of the actual deposition of bone is described and illustrated in the next plate.

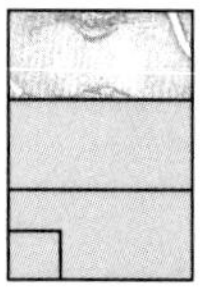

Developing bone, fetal finger, monkey, H&E ×240.

An early stage in the process of endochondral bone formation in the fetal digit is shown in this micrograph. Proximal and distal **epiphyses** (*E*) of this developing bone are made of cartilage. This bone of the fetal digit is connected by joints with other bones; note **joint cavities** (*JC*) on both edges of this micrograph. The midregion of this long bone reveals **chondrocytes** that have undergone marked **hypertrophy** (*HCh*). The cytoplasm of these chondrocytes appears very clear or washed out. Their nuclei, when included in the plane of section, appear as small, condensed basophilic bodies. Note how the cartilage matrix in this region is calcified and has been compressed into narrow linear bands of tissue surrounding the chondrocytes. The **calcified cartilage matrix** (*CCM*) stains more intensely with hematoxylin in routine H&E preparation and appears darker. At this stage of development, bone tissue has been produced to form the early periosteal **bony collar** (*BC*) around the cartilage model. This bone tissue is produced by appositional growth from bone-forming cells that were derived from the mesenchyme in the tissue surrounding the cartilage. This process represents intramembranous bone formation, which will be described later.

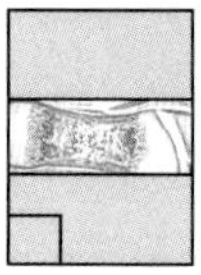

Developing bone, fetal finger, human, H&E ×60.

The bone shown in this micrograph represents a later stage of development. Most of the diaphysis of the bone contains the **bone marrow cavity** (*Cav*) filled with marrow, part of which is highly cellular and represents accumulations of hemopoietic **bone marrow cells** (*BMC*). The nonstaining areas consist of adipose tissue, which occupies much of the remainder of the bone marrow cavity. The thin bony collar seen earlier has now developed into a relatively thicker mass of **diaphyseal bone** (*DB*). The part of the bone in which bone tissue is being deposited by **endochondral bone** (*EB*) formation is seen at both ends of the bone marrow cavity. Note that its eosinophilic character is similar to the diaphyseal bone. As these processes continue in the shaft of the bone, **cartilages** (*C*) on both proximal and distal epiphyses are invaded by blood vessels and connective tissue from the periosteum (periosteal bud), and it undergoes the same changes that occurred earlier in the shaft (except that no periosteal bony collar is formed).

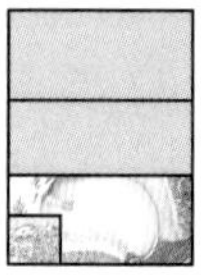

Developing bone, proximal epiphysis of long bone, human, H&E ×60; inset ×200.

This micrograph shows considerable developmental advancement beyond that of the bone in the above micrograph. A **secondary ossification center** (*SOC*) has been established in the proximal epiphysis of this long bone. At a slightly later time, a similar epiphyseal ossification center will form at the distal end of the bone. The process of endochondral bone formation occurs the same way as in the diaphysis. With time, these epiphyseal centers of ossification will increase in size to form much larger cavities (*dashed line*). The consequence of this activity is that an **epiphyseal growth plate** (*EGP*) is formed. As visible on this micrograph, the epiphyseal growth plate, consisting of cartilage, separates the SOCs at the proximal end of the bone from the primary ossification center formed in the shaft of the bone. This cartilaginous plate is essential for the longitudinal growth of the bone and will persist until bone growth ceases. The *inset* shows the secondary ossification center at higher magnification. Within this area, new **endochondral bone** (*EB*) is already being produced. The new bone appears eosinophilic in contrast to the more basophilic appearance of the surrounding **cartilage** (*C*). Note that its staining pattern of endochondral bone in the SOC is identical to the more abundant endochondral bone (*EB*) that replaces **calcified cartilage** (*CC*) at the upper end of the diaphysis.

BC, bony collar
BMC, bone marrow cells
C, cartilage
Cav, bone marrow cavity
CC, calcified cartilage
CCM, calcified cartilage matrix
DB, diaphyseal bone
E, epiphysis
EB, endochondral bone
EGP, epiphyseal growth plate
HCh, hypertrophic chondrocytes
JC, joint cavity
SOC, secondary ossification center
dashed line, epiphyseal center of ossification

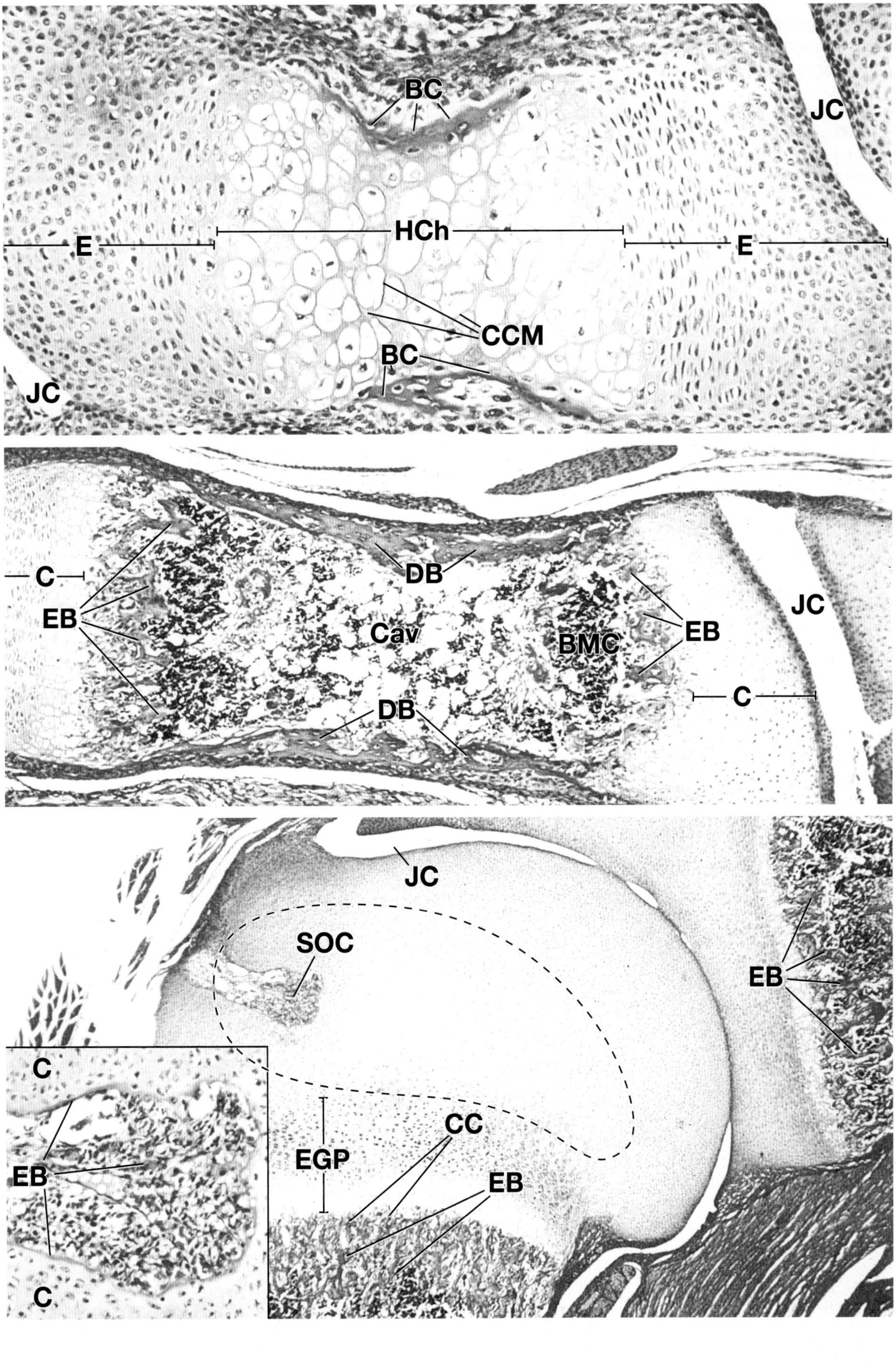
BC
JC
E
HCh
E
CCM
BC
JC
C
EB
DB
Cav
BMC
EB
JC
C
DB
JC
SOC
EB
C
EB
C
EGP
CC
EB

PLATE 8.4 ■ ENDOCHONDRAL BONE FORMATION II

Endochondral bone formation is the principal process by which the long bones (e.g., the bones of the appendages and digits) increase in length to achieve their adult dimensions. As long as an **epiphyseal growth plate** exists between the primary (diaphyseal) and secondary (epiphyseal) ossification centers, the bone will continue to grow in length. During bone growth, distinct zoning can be recognized in the epiphyseal growth plate at both ends of the early formed marrow cavity. In the part of the cartilage that is farthest away from the bone marrow cavity at both ends of the growing bone, individual chondrocytes, separated by cartilage matrix, have not yet began to participate in the bone-forming process. This region is called the zone of reserve cartilage. As these chondrocytes immerse in changes leading to their proliferation, hypertrophy, and eventual death (or transdifferentiation to osteoblasts), their microscopic appearance and changes in extracellular matrix define different functional zones of endochondral bone formation.

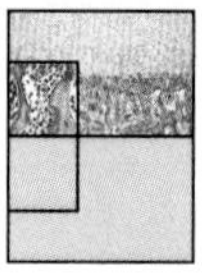

Endochondral bone formation, epiphysis of long bone, human, H&E ×80; inset ×380.

This is a photomicrograph of an epiphysis at higher magnification than that seen in Plate 8.3. Different zones of the cartilage of the epiphyseal plate reflect the progressive changes that occur in active growth of endochondral bone. These zones are not sharply delineated, and the boundaries between them are somewhat arbitrary. They lead toward the bone marrow (*BM*) cavity, so that the first zone is furthest from the cavity. There are five zones:

- **Zone of reserve cartilage** (*ZRC*): The cartilage cells of this zone have not yet begun to participate in the growth of the bone; thus, they are reserve cells. These cells are small, usually only one to a lacuna, and not grouped. At some point, some of these cells will proliferate and undergo the changes outlined for the next zone.
- **Zone of proliferation** (*ZP*): The cells of this zone undergo divisions and are increasing in number; they are slightly larger than the chondrocytes in the zone of reserve cartilage and are close to their neighbors; they begin to form rows.
- **Zone of hypertrophy** (*ZH*): The cells of this zone are aligned in rows and are significantly larger than the cells in the preceding zone.
- **Zone of calcified cartilage** (*ZCC*): In this zone, the cartilage matrix is impregnated with calcium salts. The calcified cartilage will serve as an initial scaffold for the deposition of the new bone. Chondrocytes positioned in the more proximal part of this zone undergo apoptosis.
- **Zone of resorption** (*ZR*): This zone is represented by eroded cartilage that is in direct contact with the connective tissue of the marrow cavity. Small blood vessels and accompanying osteoprogenitor cells invade the region previously occupied by the dying chondrocytes. They form a series of spearheads, leaving on both sides the **calcified cartilage** (*CC*) as longitudinal spicules. Osteoprogenitor cells give rise to osteoblasts that begin lining the surfaces of exposed spicules. **Endochondral bone** (*EB*) is then deposited on the surfaces of these calcified cartilage spicules by osteoblasts, thus forming **mixed spicules** as seen in the *inset*. Note the **osteoblasts** (*Ob*), some of which are just beginning to produce bone in apposition to the calcified cartilage (*CC*). The lower right of the *inset* shows mixed spicules containing endochondral bone (*EB*) and calcified cartilage (*CC*). Several osteoblasts (*Ob*), and an osteoclast (*Ocl*) are present on the surface of the spicules. An osteocyte (*Oc*) already embedded in the bone matrix is also visible.

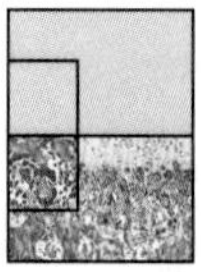

Endochondral bone formation, epiphysis of long bone, human, H&E ×150; inset ×380.

This is a higher magnification of the lower area from the above figure. It shows **calcified cartilage spicules** on which bone has been deposited. In the *lower* portion of the figure, the spicules have already grown to create anastomosing bone **trabeculae** (*T*). These initial trabeculae still contain remnants of calcified cartilage, as shown by the bluish color of the cartilage matrix (compared with the red staining of the bone). **Osteoblasts** (*Ob*) are aligned on the surface of the spicules, where bone formation is active. Several **osteocytes** (*Oc*) already embedded in the bone matrix are also visible. The *inset* reveals several **osteoclasts** (*Ocl*) in higher magnification. They are in apposition to the spicules, which are mostly made of calcified cartilage. A small amount of bone is evident, based on the red-stained material. The light area (*arrow*) represents the **ruffled border** of the osteoclast.

BM, bone marrow	**Ocl,** osteoclast	**ZR,** zone of resorption
CC, calcified cartilage	**T,** trabeculae	**ZRC,** zone of reserve cartilage
EB, endochondral bone	**ZCC,** zone of calcified cartilage	**arrow,** ruffled border of osteoclast
Ob, osteoblast	**ZH,** zone of hypertrophy	
Oc, osteocyte	**ZP,** zone of proliferation	

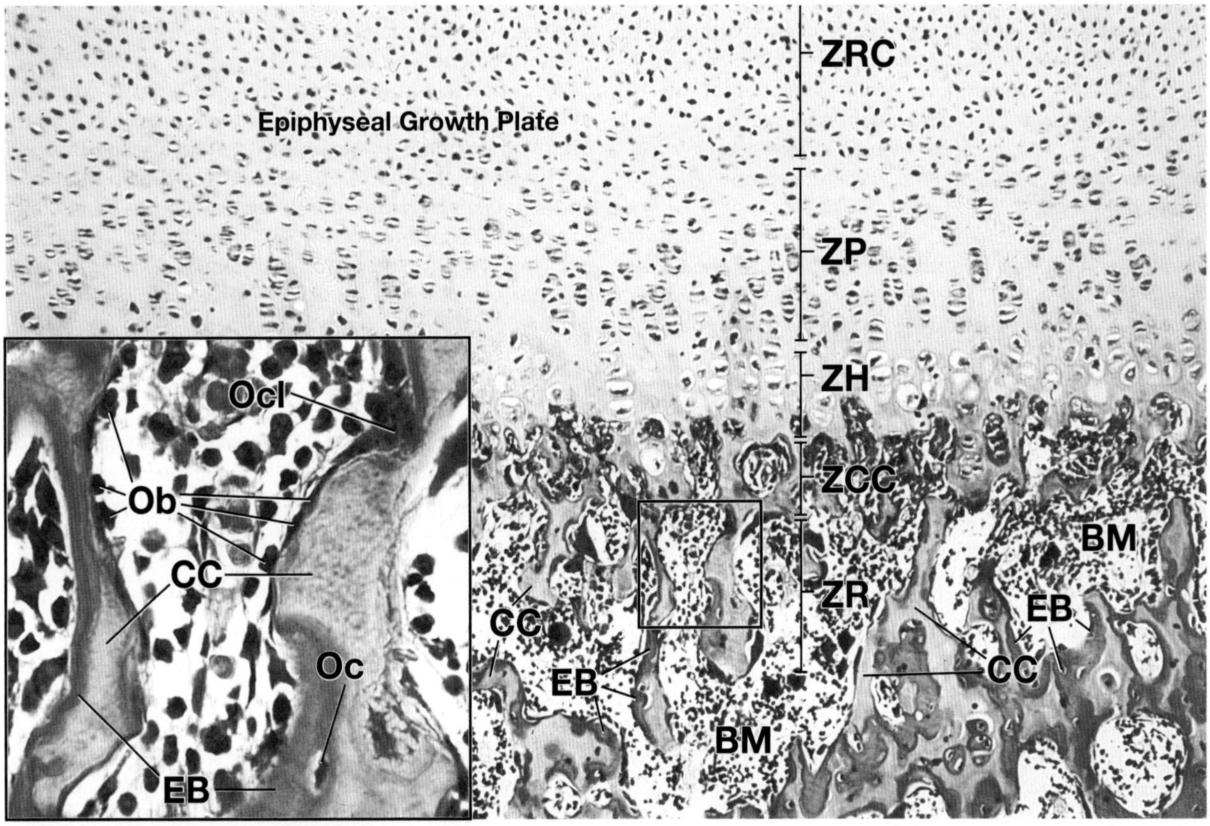
ZRC
Epiphyseal Growth Plate
ZP
ZH
ZCC
ZR
BM
EB
CC
CC
EB
BM
Ocl
Ob
CC
Oc
EB

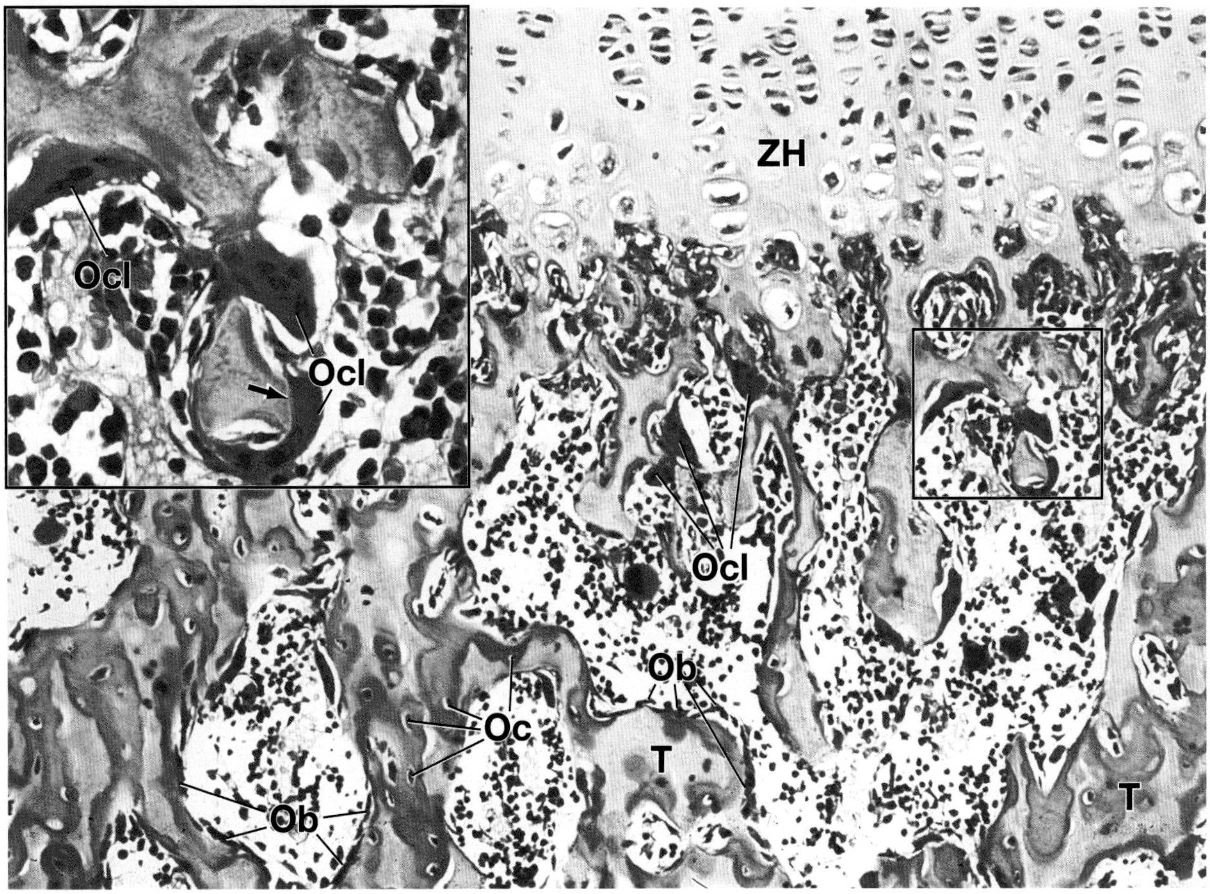
ZH
Ocl
Ocl
Ocl
Ob
Oc
T
Ob
T

Intramembranous bone formation is limited to those bones that are not required to perform an early supporting function, for example, the flat bones of the skull. This process requires the proliferation and differentiation of cells of the mesenchyme to become **osteoblasts**, the bone-forming cells. They produce bone-specific extracellular matrix. This initial matrix, called **osteoid**, undergoes mineralization to form bone.

As the osteoblasts continue to secrete their product, some are entrapped within their matrix and are then known as **osteocytes**. They are responsible for maintenance of the newly formed bone tissue. The remaining osteoblasts continue the bone deposition process at the bone surface. They are capable of reproducing to maintain an adequate population for continued growth.

This newly formed bone appears first as **spicules** that enlarge and interconnect as growth proceeds, creating a three-dimensional trabecular structure similar in shape to the future mature bone. The interstices contain blood vessels and connective tissue (mesenchyme). As the bone continues to grow, remodeling occurs. This involves resorption of localized areas of bone tissue by **osteoclasts** in order to maintain appropriate shape in relation to size and to permit vascular nourishment during the growth process.

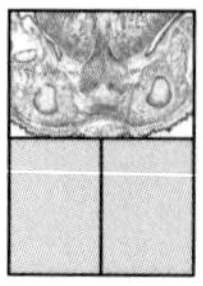

Intramembranous bone formation, fetal head, human, Mallory trichrome ×45.

A cross section of the developing mandible, as seen at this relatively early stage of development, consists of **bone spicules** (*BS*) of various sizes and shapes. The bone spicules interconnect and, in three dimensions, have the general shape of the mandible. Other structures present that will assist in orientation include **developing teeth** (*DT*), **Meckel cartilage** (*MC*), seen on the *left side*, and the **oral cavity** (*OC*). The *bottom surface* of the specimen shows the **epidermis** (*Ep*) of the submandibular region of the neck. A large portion of the developing tongue is seen in the *upper half* of the figure. The tongue consists largely of developing striated visceral muscle fibers arranged in a three-dimensional orthogonal array that is characteristic of this organ.

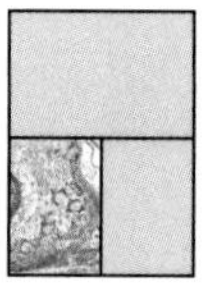

Intramembranous bone formation, fetal head, human, Mallory trichrome ×175.

This higher magnification view of the *boxed area* in the *upper* micrograph shows the interconnections of the **bone spicules** (*BS*) of the developing mandible. Within and around the spaces enclosed by the developing spicules is mesenchymal tissue. These mesenchymal cells contain stem cells that will form the vascular components of the bone as well as the osteoprogenitor cells that will give rise to new osteoblasts. The denser connective tissue (*CT*) will differentiate into the periosteum on one side of the developing mandible. Other structures shown in the field include numerous blood vessels (*BV*) and the enamel organ of a **developing tooth** (*DT*).

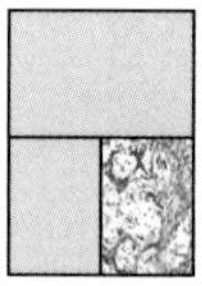

Intramembranous bone formation, fetal head, human, Mallory trichrome ×350.

This higher magnification micrograph of a portion of the field in the *lower left* micrograph shows the distinction between newly deposited osteoid, which stains *blue*, and mineralized bone, which stains *red*. **Osteoblasts** are seen in two different levels of activity. Osteoblasts that are relatively inactive (*IOb*) and are in apposition to well-formed osteoid exhibit elongate nuclear profiles and appear to be flattened on the surface of the osteoid. Those osteoblasts that are actively secreting new osteoid (*AOb*) appear as tall, columnar-like cells adjacent to the osteoid. One of the spicules shows a cell completely surrounded by bone matrix; this is an osteoblast that has become trapped in its own secretions and is now an **osteocyte** (*Oc*). At this magnification, the embryonic tissue characteristics of the mesenchyme and the sparseness of the **mesenchymal cells** (*MeC*) are well demonstrated. The highly cellular connective tissue (*CT*) on the *right margin* of the micrograph is the developing perichondrium. Some of its cells have osteoprogenitor cell characteristics and will develop into osteoblasts to allow growth of the bone at its surface.

AOb, active osteoblast
BS, bone spicules
BV, blood vessels
CT, connective tissue
DT, developing teeth
Ep, epidermis
IOb, inactive osteoblast
MC, Meckel cartilage
MeC, mesenchymal cells
Oc, osteocyte
OC, oral cavity

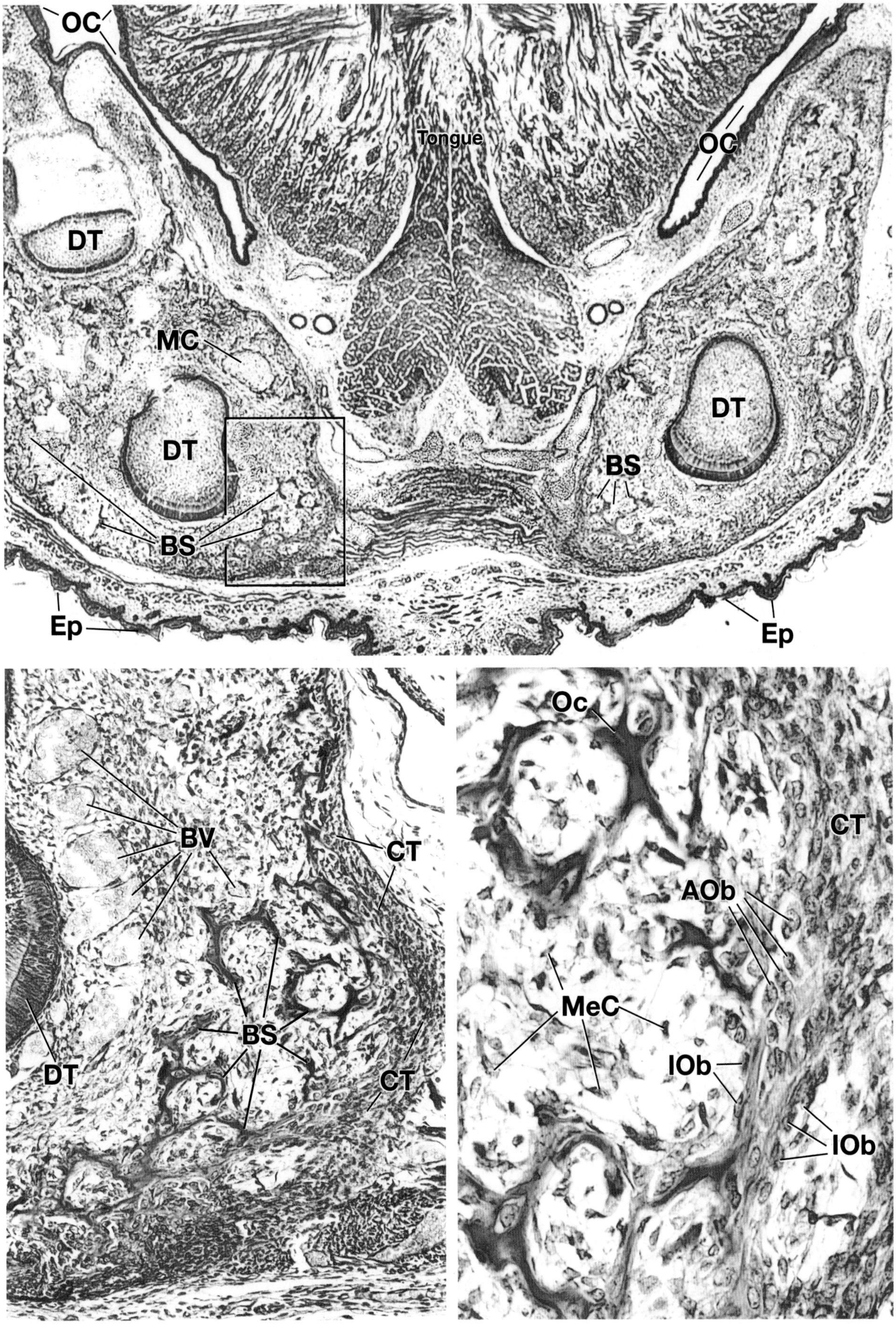
OC
Tongue
OC
DT
MC
DT
DT
BS
BS
Ep
Ep
BV
CT
BS
DT
CT
Oc
CT
AOb
MeC
IOb
IOb

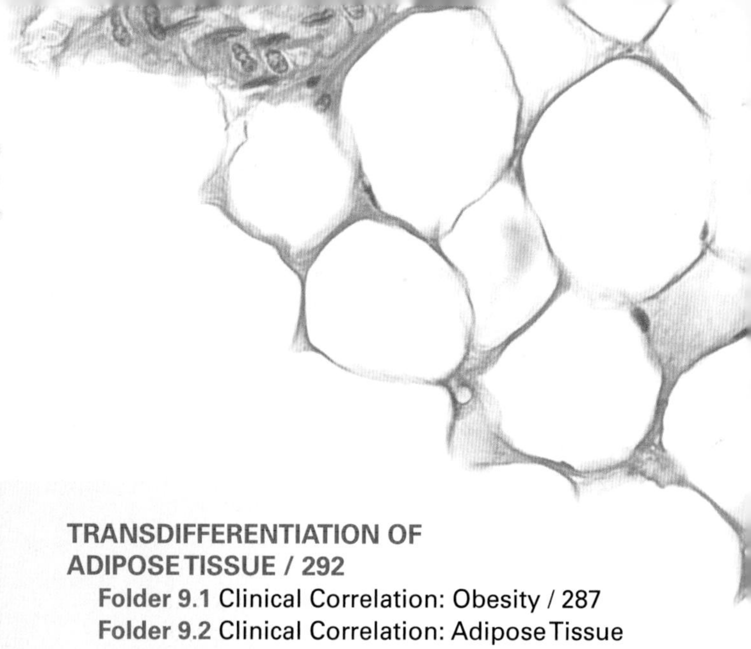

9 ADIPOSE TISSUE

■ OVERVIEW OF ADIPOSE TISSUE

Adipose tissue is a specialized connective tissue that plays an important role in energy homeostasis.

Individual fat cells, or **adipocytes**, and groups of adipocytes are found throughout loose connective tissue. Tissues in which adipocytes are the primary cell type are designated **adipose tissue**. Adipocytes play a key role in energy homeostasis.

For its survival, the body needs to ensure continuous delivery of energy despite highly variable supplies of nutrients from the external environment. To meet the body's energy demands when nutrient supplies are low, adipose tissue efficiently stores excess energy. The body has a limited capacity to store carbohydrate and protein; therefore, energy reserves are stored within **lipid droplets** of adipocytes in the form of **triglycerides**. Triglycerides represent a dynamic form of **energy storage** that is added when food intake is greater than energy expenditure and is tapped when energy expenditure is greater than food intake. The energy stored in adipocytes can be rapidly released for use at other sites in the body.

Triglycerides are the most concentrated form of metabolic energy storage available to humans. Because triglycerides lack water, they have about twice the energy density of carbohydrates and proteins. The energy density of triglycerides is approximately 37.7 kJ/g (9 cal/g), whereas the density of carbohydrates and proteins is 16.8 kJ/g (4 cal/g). In the event of food deprivation, triglycerides are an essential source of water and energy. Some animals can rely solely on metabolic water obtained from fatty acid oxidation for the maintenance of their water balance. For instance, the hump of a camel consists largely of adipose tissue and is a source of water and energy for this desert animal.

Adipocytes perform other important functions in addition to their role as fat storage containers. They also regulate energy metabolism by secreting autocrine, paracrine, and endocrine substances. Adipose tissue is considered a major **endocrine organ**. Considerable evidence links increased endocrine activity of adipocytes to the metabolic and cardiovascular complications associated with **obesity**.

Historically, there were only two major types of adipose tissue identified: white (unilocular) and brown (multilocular); however, recent classifications include a third type: beige (paucilocular) adipose tissue.

The three types of adipose tissue, white adipose tissue, brown adipose tissue, and beige adipose tissue, are so named because of their color in the living state, which is attributable to their high mitochondrial density and high vascularization:

- **White adipose tissue** is the predominant type in adult humans.
- **Brown adipose tissue** is present in large amounts in humans during fetal life. It diminishes during the first decade after birth but continues to be present in varying amounts, mainly around internal organs.
- **Beige adipose tissue** or "brite" (brown-in-white) adipose tissue consists of an accumulation of brown-like adipocytes within the subcutaneous white adipose tissue deposits in adult humans.

In general, white adipose tissue stores excess energy in lipids; in contrast, brown and beige adipose tissues dissipate energy through the production of heat. All adipose tissues produce biologically active substances to regulate energy homeostasis.

■ WHITE ADIPOSE TISSUE

White (unilocular) adipose tissue represents at least 10% of the body weight of a normal healthy individual.

Function of White Adipose Tissue

Functions of white adipose tissue include energy storage, insulation, cushioning of vital organs, and secretion of hormones.

White adipose tissue forms a fatty layer of the **subcutaneous (superficial) fascia** called the *panniculus adiposus [Lat. panniculus, a little garment; adipatus, fatty]* in the connective tissue beneath the skin. Because the thermal conductivity of adipose tissue is only about one-half that of skeletal muscle, the subcutaneous fascia provides significant thermal insulation against the cold by reducing the rate of heat loss. Concentrations of adipose tissue are found in the connective tissue under the skin of the abdomen, buttocks, axilla, and thigh. Sex differences in the thickness of this fatty layer in the skin of different parts of the body account, in part, for the differences in body contour between females and males. In both sexes, the **mammary fat pad** is a preferential site for accumulation of adipose tissue; the nonlactating female **mammary gland** is composed primarily of this tissue. In the lactating female, the mammary fat pad plays an important role in supporting breast function. It provides lipids and energy for milk production, but it is also a site for the synthesis of growth factors that modulate responses to steroid hormones and proteins that regulate mammary gland function.

Internally, adipose tissue is preferentially located in the greater omentum, mesentery, and retroperitoneal space and is usually abundant around the kidneys. It is also found in the **bone marrow** and between other tissues, where it fills in spaces. Adipose tissue functions as a cushion in the palms of the hands and the soles of the feet, beneath the visceral pericardium (around the outside of the heart), and in the orbits around the eyeballs. It retains this structural function even during reduced caloric intake; when adipose tissue elsewhere becomes depleted of lipid, this structural adipose tissue remains undiminished.

White adipose tissue secretes a variety of adipokines, which include hormones, growth factors, and cytokines.

White adipocytes actively synthesize and secrete **adipokines**, a group of biologically active substances, which include hormones, growth factors, and cytokines (Fig. 9.1). For this reason, adipose tissue is regarded as an important player in energy homeostasis, adipogenesis, steroid metabolism, angiogenesis, and immune responses.

A notable adipokine is **leptin** *[Gr. leptos, thin]*, a 16-kDa peptide hormone discovered in 1994. Leptin is involved in the regulation of energy homeostasis and is primarily secreted by adipocytes. Small amounts of leptin are also produced in other organs (e.g., stomach, placenta, mammary glands, and ovaries). Leptin inhibits food intake and stimulates metabolic rate and loss of body weight. Thus, leptin fulfills the criteria for a **circulating satiety factor** that controls food intake when the body's store of energy is sufficient. Leptin participates in an endocrine signaling pathway that communicates the energy state of adipose tissue to brain centers that regulate food uptake. It acts on the central nervous system by binding

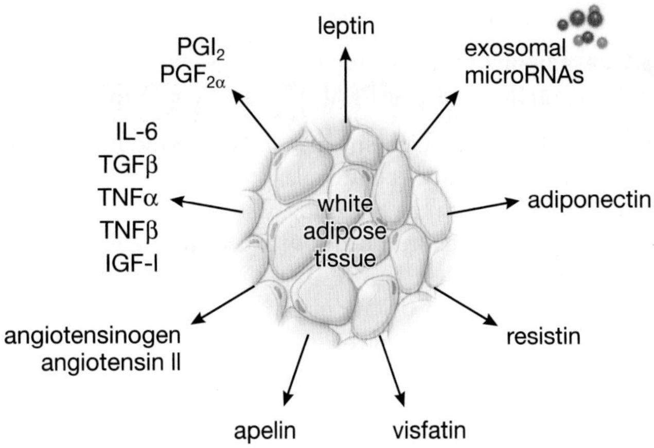

FIGURE 9.1. Major adipokines secreted by white adipose tissue. This schematic drawing shows various types of adipokines secreted by white adipose tissue, including hormones (e.g., leptin), cytokines (e.g., insulin-like growth factor 1), and other molecules with specific biological functions (e.g., prostaglandins). Note secretion of exosomes, extracellular nanovesicles that facilitate intercellular communication. They contain small fragments of adipocyte RNA (microRNAs) responsible for the regulation of gene expression in distant organs, which, in turn, affects whole-body metabolism. IGF-1, insulin-like growth factor 1; IL-6, interleukin-16; PGI_1, prostaglandin I_1; TGF-β, transforming growth factor β; TNF-α, tumor necrosis factor α; TNF-β, tumor necrosis factor β.

to specific receptors, mainly in the **hypothalamus**. Leptin also regulates the production of **steroid hormones** (testosterone, estrogens, and glucocorticoids). In addition, leptin communicates the fuel state of adipocytes from fat storage sites to other metabolically active tissues (i.e., from adipose tissue to muscle at a different site).

In addition to leptin, adipose tissue secretes a variety of other adipokines, such as **adiponectin**, **resistin**, retinol-binding protein 4 (RBP-4), visfatin, apelin, plasminogen activator inhibitor 1 (PAI-1), tumor necrosis factors (TNFs), interleukin-6 (IL-6), monocyte chemotactic protein 1 (MCP-1), **angiotensinogen (AGE)**, and others. Some adipokines are also synthesized in other tissues. For example, AGE is synthesized in the liver; increased production of this peptide by adipose tissue contributes to hypertension (elevation of blood pressure), a frequent complication of obesity.

Recently, **microRNAs (miRNAs)** were found in circulating intact exosomes (membrane-bound extracellular vesicles) secreted by white adipocytes. These miRNAs represent small (about 22 nucleotides) RNA molecules that contain intact genetic information specific to adipocytes. Exosomal miRNAs participate in various metabolic processes, such as glucose/lipid metabolism, insulin signaling, inflammation, and differentiation of white and brown adipocytes in various tissues.

Adipocytes also help regulate the synthesis of sex hormones and glucocorticoids. Specific enzymes expressed in adipocytes convert the inactive forms of these hormones to their active forms. In this way, these enzymes influence the sex steroid profiles of obese individuals. Obesity associated with increased secretion of **growth factors** (tumor necrosis factor α [TNF-α], transforming growth factor β [TGF-β], insulin-like growth factor 1 [IGF-1]) and **cytokines** (IL-6 and prostaglandins) may be linked to metabolic abnormalities and development of diabetes. Table 9.1 presents a summary of the most important adipokines produced by white adipocytes and their functions.

Differentiation of Adipocytes

White adipocytes differentiate from mesenchymal stem cells under the control of PPARγ/RXR transcription factors.

During embryonic development, **white adipocytes** derive from undifferentiated perivascular **mesenchymal stem cells** associated with the adventitia of small venules (Fig. 9.2). A transcription factor called **peroxisome proliferator–activated receptor γ (PPARγ)**, in complex with the **retinoid X receptor (RXR)**, plays a critical role in adipocyte differentiation and initiation of lipid metabolism. This complex induces the maturation of **early lipoblasts (adipoblasts)** or preadipocytes into mature fat cells of white adipose tissue. Most of the PPARγ target genes in adipose tissue influence lipogenic pathways and initiate the storage of triglycerides. Therefore, **PPARγ/RXR** is regarded as the **"master-switch"** regulator in differentiation of white adipocytes.

White adipose tissue begins to form midway through fetal development.

Lipoblasts initially develop from stromal–vascular cells along the small blood vessels in the fetus and are free of lipids. These cells are committed to becoming adipocytes at this early stage by expressing PPARγ/RXR transcription factors. Collections of such cells are sometimes called **primitive fat organs**. They are characterized by proliferating early lipoblasts and proliferating capillaries. Lipid accumulation in lipoblasts produces the typical morphology of adipocytes.

Early lipoblasts look like fibroblasts but develop small lipid inclusions and a thin external lamina.

Transmission electron microscopy (TEM) studies reveal that **early lipoblasts** have an elongated configuration, multiple cytoplasmic processes, and abundant endoplasmic reticulum and Golgi apparatus. As lipoblastic differentiation begins, vesicles increase in number, with a corresponding decrease in rough-surfaced endoplasmic reticulum (rER). Small **lipid inclusions** appear at one pole of the cytoplasm. Pinocytotic vesicles and an **external lamina** also appear. The presence of an external lamina is a feature that further distinguishes adipocytes from proper connective tissue cells.

Midstage lipoblasts become ovoid as lipid accumulation changes the cell dimensions.

With continued development, the early lipoblasts assume an oval configuration. The most characteristic feature at this stage is an extensive concentration of vesicles and **small lipid droplets** around the nucleus and extending toward both poles of the cell. Glycogen particles appear at the periphery of the lipid droplets, and pinocytotic vesicles and basal lamina become more apparent. These cells are designated **midstage lipoblasts**.

The mature adipocyte is characterized by a single large lipid inclusion surrounded by a thin rim of cytoplasm.

In the late stage of differentiation, the cells increase in size and become more spherical. Small lipid droplets coalesce to form a **single large lipid droplet** that occupies the central portion of the cytoplasm. Smooth-surfaced endoplasmic reticulum (sER) is abundant, whereas rER is less prominent. These cells are designated **late lipoblasts**. Eventually, the lipid mass compresses the nucleus to an eccentric position,

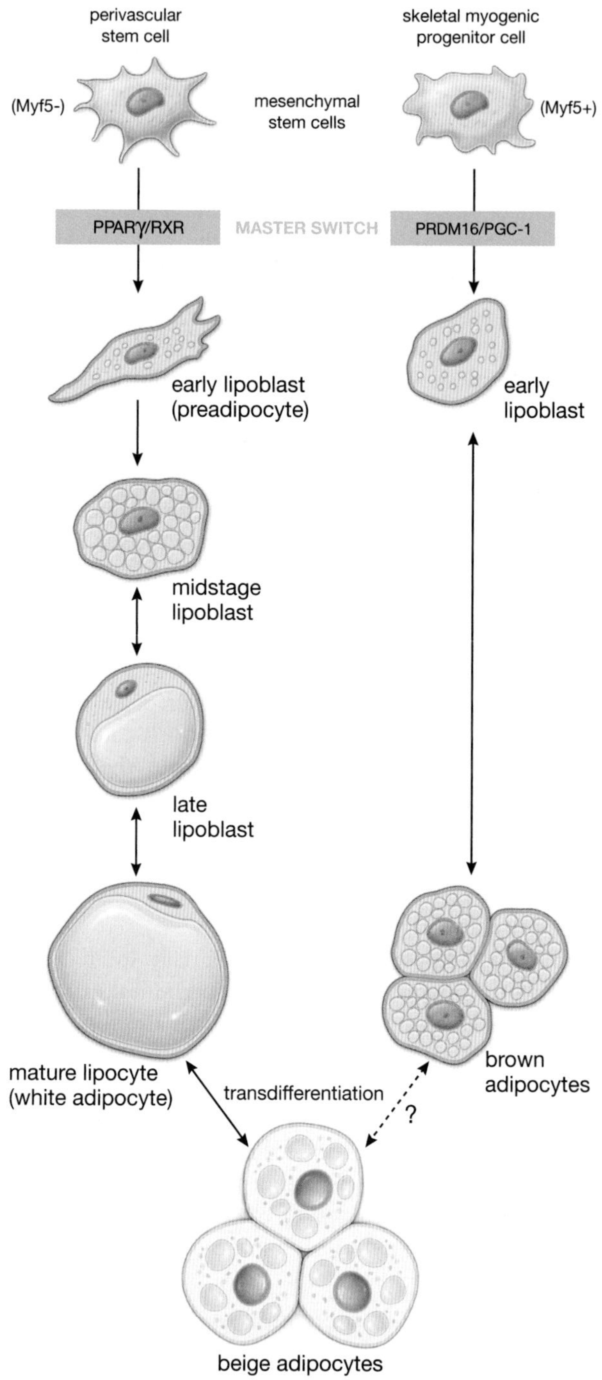

FIGURE 9.2. Development of white and brown adipose tissue cells. Brown and white adipose cells arise from distinctly different cellular lineages. White adipocytes derive from undifferentiated perivascular mesenchymal stem cells associated with the adventitia of small venules. By expressing PPARγ/RXR transcription factors, these cells will differentiate into early lipoblasts (preadipocytes) committed to white adipocyte lineage development. Brown adipocytes also have a mesenchymal origin; however, they derive from common skeletal myogenic progenitor stem cells expressing myogenic factor 5 (Myf5) protein found in dermatomyotomes of developing embryos. By expressing PRDM16/PGC-1 transcription factors, these cells will differentiate into early lipoblasts committed to the brown adipocyte lineage development. Note that the developmental lineage of white adipocytes does not express myogenic factor and is Myf5 negative. Lipoblasts develop an external (basal) lamina and begin to accumulate numerous lipid droplets in their cytoplasm. In white adipose tissue, these droplets fuse to form a single large lipid droplet that eventually fills the mature cell, compressing the nucleus, cytoplasm, and cytoplasmic organelles into a thin rim around the droplet. In brown adipose tissue, the individual lipid droplets remain separate. Beige adipocytes are shown here arising from white adipocytes. Beige adipocytes also develop from progenitor cells as shown in Figure 9.9; however, transdifferentiation from white adipocytes is the most common developmental pathway.

producing a *signet-ring* appearance in hematoxylin and eosin (H&E) preparations. Because these cells have a single lipid droplet, they are designated **unilocular** *[Lat. unus, single; loculus, a little place]* **adipocytes** or mature lipocytes.

Structure of Adipocytes and Adipose Tissue

Unilocular adipocytes are large cells, sometimes 100 μm or more in diameter.

When isolated, **white adipocytes** are spherical, but they may appear polyhedral or oval when crowded together in adipose tissue. Their large size is due to the accumulated lipid in the cell. The nucleus is flattened and displaced to one side of the lipid mass; the cytoplasm forms a thin rim around the lipid. In routine histologic sections, the lipid is lost through extraction by organic solvents, such as xylene; consequently, adipose tissue appears as a delicate meshwork of polygonal profiles (Fig. 9.3). The thin strand of meshwork that separates adjacent adipocytes represents the cytoplasm of both cells and the extracellular matrix. The strand is usually so thin, however, that it is not possible to resolve its component parts in the light microscope.

Adipose tissue is richly supplied with blood vessels, and capillaries are found at the angles of the meshwork where adjacent adipocytes meet. Silver stains show that adipocytes are surrounded by reticular fibers (type III collagen), which are secreted by the adipocytes. Special stains also reveal the presence of unmyelinated nerve fibers and numerous mast cells. A summary of white adipose tissue features is listed in Table 9.2.

The lipid mass in the adipocyte is not membrane bound.

TEM reveals that the interface between the contained lipid and surrounding cytoplasm of the adipocyte is composed of a 5-nm-thick condensed layer of lipid reinforced by parallel **vimentin filaments** measuring 5–10 nm in diameter. This layer separates the hydrophobic contents of the lipid droplet from the hydrophilic cytoplasmic matrix.

The perinuclear cytoplasm of the adipocyte contains a small Golgi apparatus, free ribosomes, short profiles of rER, microfilaments, and intermediate filaments. Filamentous forms of mitochondria and multiple profiles of sER are also found in the thin rim of cytoplasm surrounding the lipid droplet (Fig. 9.4).

Regulation of Adipose Tissue

It is almost impossible to separate regulation of adipose tissue from digestive processes and functions of the central nervous system. These interconnected hormonal and neural signals emanating from the adipose tissue, alimentary tract, and central nervous system form the **brain–gut–adipose axis** that regulates appetite, hunger, satiety, and energy homeostasis (Fig. 9.5).

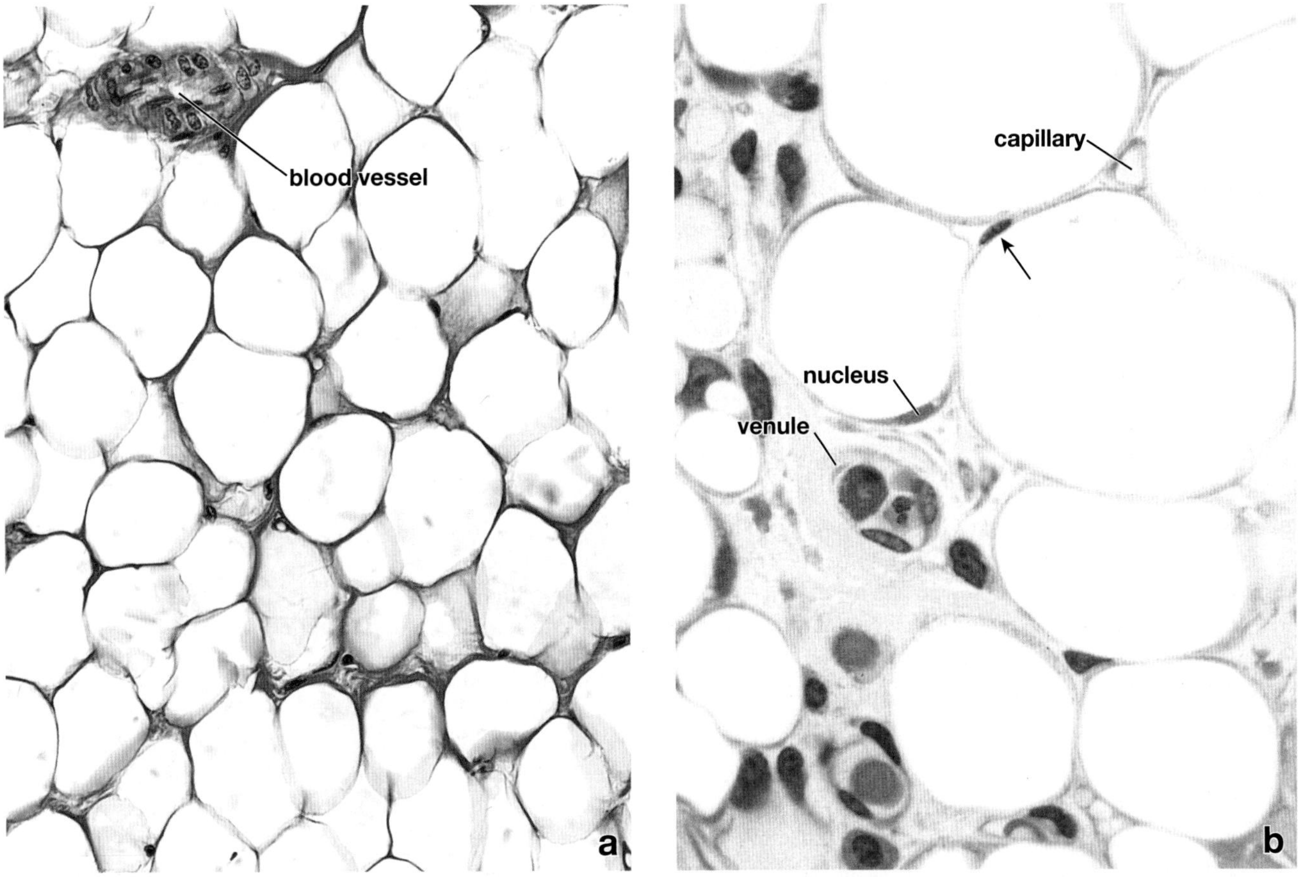

FIGURE 9.3. White adipose tissue. a. Photomicrograph of white adipose tissue showing its characteristic meshwork in a hematoxylin and eosin (H&E)-stained paraffin preparation. Each space represents a single large drop of lipid before its dissolution from the cell during tissue preparation. The surrounding eosin-stained material represents the cytoplasm of the adjoining cells and some intervening connective tissue. ×320. **b.** High-power photomicrograph of a glutaraldehyde-preserved, plastic-embedded specimen of white adipose tissue. The cytoplasm of the individual adipose cells is recognizable in some areas, and part of the nucleus of one of the cells is included in the plane of section. A second nucleus (*arrow*), which appears intimately related to one of the adipose cells, may actually belong to a fibroblast; it is difficult to tell with assurance. Because of the large size of adipose cells, the nucleus is infrequently observed in a given cell. A capillary and a small venule are also evident in the photomicrograph. ×950.

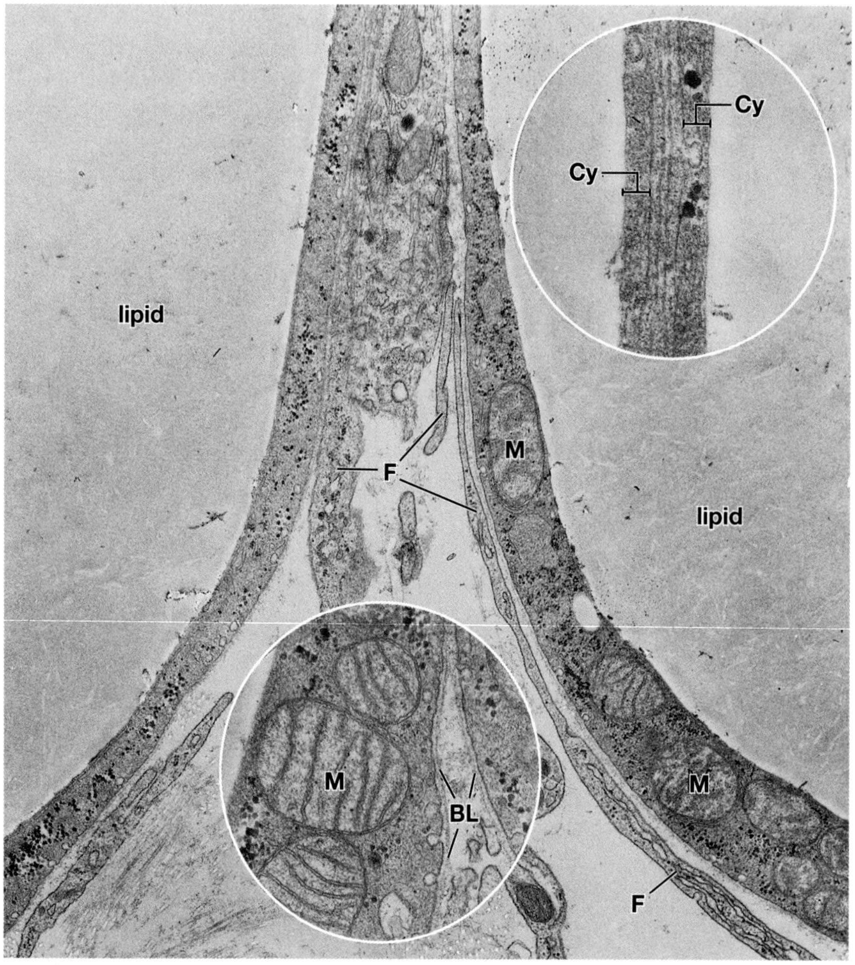

FIGURE 9.4. Electron micrograph showing portions of two adjacent adipose cells. The cytoplasm of the adipose cells reveals mitochondria (*M*) and glycogen (the latter appears as very dark particles). ×15,000. **Upper inset.** Attenuated cytoplasm (*Cy*) of two adjoining adipose cells. Each cell is separated by a narrow space containing external (basal) lamina and an extremely attenuated process of a fibroblast. ×65,000. **Lower inset.** The external (basal) lamina (*BL*) of the adipose cells appears as a discrete layer by which the cells are adequately separated from one another. *F*, fibroblast processes. ×30,000.

The amount of an individual's adipose tissue is determined by two physiologic systems: one associated with short-term weight regulation and the other with long-term weight regulation.

The amount of adipose tissue in an individual is regulated by two physiologic systems. The first system, which is associated with **short-term weight regulation**, controls appetite and metabolism on a daily basis. Two small peptide hormones produced in the gastrointestinal tract—**ghrelin**, an appetite stimulant, and **peptide YY (PYY)**, an appetite suppressant—have been linked to this system. The second system, which is associated with **long-term weight regulation**, controls appetite and metabolism on a continual basis (over months and years). Two major hormones influence this system, **leptin** and **insulin**, along with other hormones, including thyroid hormone, glucocorticoids, and hormones of the pituitary gland (see Fig. 9.5).

Ghrelin and peptide YY control appetite as part of the short-term weight control system.

Ghrelin is a small, 28-amino-acid polypeptide produced by gastric epithelial cells. In addition to its appetite stimulatory role, it acts on the anterior lobe of the pituitary gland to release growth hormone. In humans, ghrelin functions through receptors located in the **hypothalamus**, increasing the sense of hunger. As such, it is considered a "meal-initiator" factor. A mutation of a gene located on chromosome 15 causes **Prader–Willi syndrome**, in which an overproduction of ghrelin leads to morbid obesity. In individuals with this syndrome, compulsive eating and an obsession with food usually arise at an early age. The urge to eat in these individuals is physiologic, overwhelming, and very difficult to control. If not treated, these individuals often die before age 30 of complications attributable to obesity.

The small, 36-amino-acid long gastrointestinal hormone **peptide YY** is produced by the small intestine and plays an important role in promoting and maintaining weight loss by inducing a greater sense of fullness soon after a meal. It also acts through receptors in the **hypothalamus** that **suppress appetite**. It decreases food intake in individuals by inducing satiety or a sense of fullness and the desire to stop eating. In experimental clinical studies, the infusion of PYY into humans has been shown to reduce food intake by 33% over a period of 24 hours.

Two hormones, leptin and insulin, are responsible for long-term regulation of body weight.

The discovery of **leptin** and its **Ob(Lep) gene**, which, in human, resides on chromosome 7, has given some insight into the mechanism of **energy homeostasis**, provided a framework for studying the pathogenesis of **obesity**, the biological response to **starvation**, and helped with understanding of the neural mechanisms that **control feeding**.

Leptin (a 16-kDa protein) is an adipose tissue hormone that plays a critical role in energy homeostasis, metabolism, and regulation of neuroendocrine functions. Leptin circulation in the body reflects on the adipose tissue mass and the amount of stored energy. It also guides the central nervous system to maintain the balance between the ingestion of food and the expenditure of energy. Leptin has an immediate effect on the brain for appetite regulation by binding with leptin

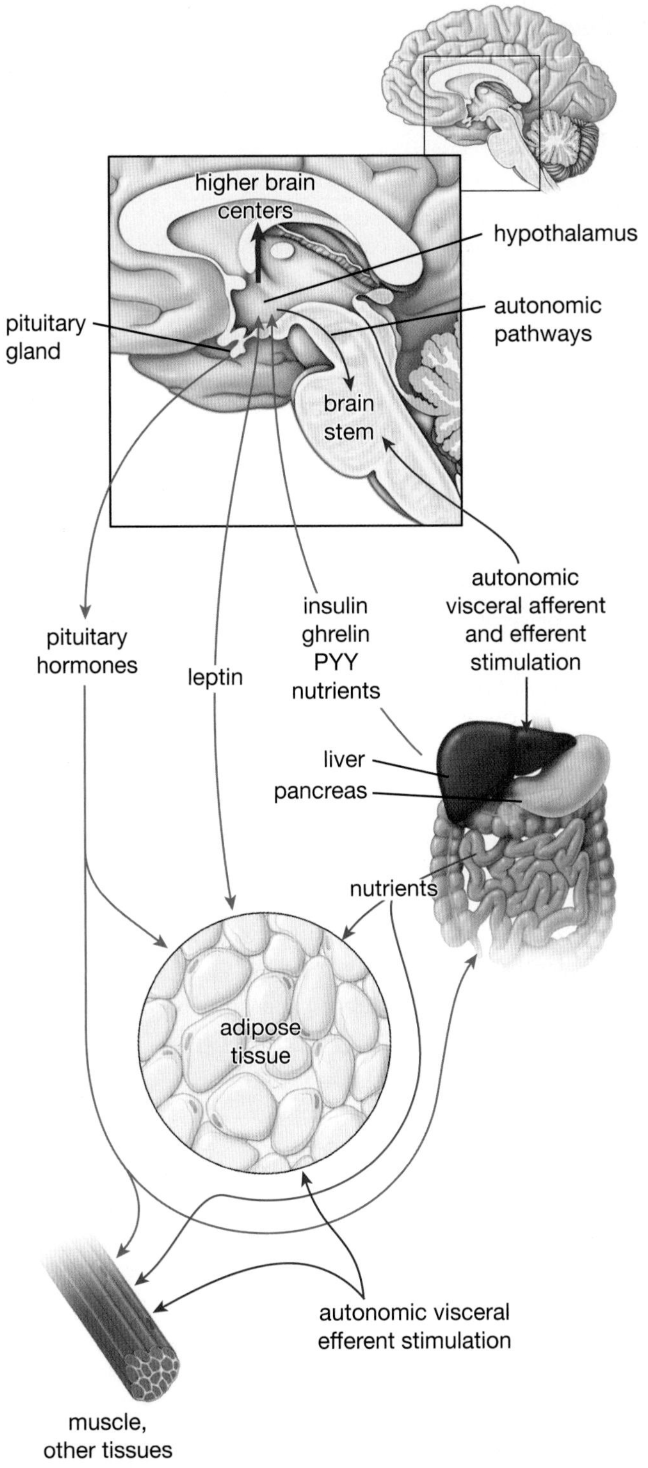

FIGURE 9.5. Regulation of energy homeostasis. This schematic diagram shows the relationship of adipose tissue to the central nervous system and gastrointestinal system within the brain–gut–adipose axis that is responsible for regulating energy homeostasis.

receptors in the hypothalamus. This neuroendocrine system protects individuals from the risks associated with starvation or obesity. In addition, leptin stimulates fatty acid oxidation and reduces body fat accumulation in nonadipose tissues, resulting in improved insulin sensitivity. Leptin levels fall during starvation (i.e., individuals with **anorexia nervosa**) and elicit adaptive responses, leading to reduced energy expenditure (e.g., cessation of menstruation, insulin resistance, and alterations of immune function). Most obese individuals have high endogenous levels of leptin. Mutations in the genes encoding leptin or its receptor cause **morbid obesity** in mice and humans, and leptin can effectively treat obesity in leptin-deficient patients.

Insulin, the pancreatic hormone that **regulates blood glucose levels**, is also involved in the regulation of adipose tissue metabolism. It enhances the conversion of glucose into the triglycerides of the lipid droplet by the adipocyte. Like leptin, insulin **regulates weight** by acting on brain centers in the hypothalamus. In contrast to leptin, insulin is required for the accumulation of adipose tissue. Antiobesity drug research is currently focusing on substances that can inhibit insulin and leptin signaling in the hypothalamus.

Deposition and mobilization of lipid are influenced by neural and hormonal factors.

One of the major metabolic functions of adipose tissue involves the **uptake of fatty acids** from the blood and their **conversion to triglycerides** within the adipocyte. Triglycerides are then stored within the cell's lipid droplet. When adipose tissue is stimulated by neural or hormonal mechanisms, triglycerides are broken down into glycerol and fatty acids, a process called **mobilization**. The fatty acids pass through the adipocyte cell membrane to enter a capillary. Here, they are bound to the carrier protein **albumin** and transported to other cells, which use fatty acids as metabolic fuel.

Neural mobilization is particularly important during periods of fasting and exposure to severe cold. During the early stages of experimental starvation in rodents, adipose cells in a denervated fat pad continue to deposit fat. Adipose cells in the intact contralateral fat pad mobilize fat. It is now known that **norepinephrine** (which is liberated by the endings of nerve cells of the sympathetic nervous system) initiates a series of metabolic steps that lead to the activation of **lipase**. This enzyme splits triglycerides, which constitute more than 90% of the lipids stored in the adipocyte. This enzymatic activity is an early step in the mobilization of lipids.

Hormonal mobilization involves a complex system of hormones and enzymes that control fatty acid release from adipocytes. These include insulin, glucagon, growth hormone, thyroid hormones, and adrenal steroids. **Insulin** is an important hormone that promotes lipid synthesis by stimulating lipid synthesis enzymes (fatty acid synthase, acetyl-CoA carboxylase) and suppresses lipid degradation by inhibiting the action of hormone-sensitive lipase and thus blocking the release of fatty acids. **Glucagon**, another pancreatic hormone, and **growth hormone** from the pituitary gland both increase lipid utilization (lipolysis). **Thyroid hormones** increase lipogenesis (formation of lipids) followed by promoting lipolytic enzymes, which break down the stored lipids in adipocytes into free fatty acids. **Adrenal steroids**, such as cortisol, stimulate lipolysis in adipocytes to liberate free fatty acids and triglycerides for energy utilization. In addition, elevated levels of **tumor necrosis factor** α **(TNF-**α**)** have been implicated as a causative factor in the development of insulin resistance associated with obesity and diabetes.

■ BROWN ADIPOSE TISSUE

Brown adipose tissue, abundant in newborns, is markedly reduced in adults.

Brown adipose tissue, a key thermogenic tissue, is present in large amounts in the newborn, which helps to offset the extensive heat loss that results from the newborn's high

TABLE 9.1 **Summary of Molecules Synthesized and Secreted by White Adipose Tissue and Their Functions**

Molecule	Major Function or Effect
Acylation-stimulating protein (ASP)	Influences the rate of triglyceride synthesis in adipose tissue
Adiponectin	Stimulates fatty acid oxidation in liver and muscles Decreases plasma triglycerides and glucose concentrations and increases insulin sensitivity in cells Plays a role in the pathogenesis of familial combined hyperlipidemia Correlated with insulin resistance and hyperinsulinemia
Adipophilin	Serves as a specific marker for lipid accumulation in cells
Adipsin	Regulates adipose tissue metabolism by facilitating fatty acid storage and stimulating triglyceride synthesis
Angiotensinogen (AGE) and angiotensin II (AngII)	AGE: Precursor of vasoactive AngII, which regulates blood pressure and electrolyte levels in the serum and is also involved in the metabolism and differentiation of adipose tissue AngII: During development, inhibits differentiation of lipoblasts; in mature adipocytes, it regulates lipid storage
Apelin	Increases cardiac muscle contractility Decreases blood pressure
Insulin-like growth factor 1 (IGF-1)	Stimulates proliferation of a wide variety of cells and mediates many of the effects of growth hormone
Interleukin-6 (IL-6)	Interacts with cells of immune system and regulates glucose and lipid metabolism Decreases activity of adipose tissue in cancer and other wasting disorders
Leptin	Regulates appetite and body energy expenditure Signals to the brain about body fat stores Increases formation of new vessels (angiogenesis) Involved in blood pressure control by regulating vascular tone Potent inhibitor of bone formation
Plasminogen activator inhibitor 1 (PAI-1)	Inhibits fibrinolysis (a process that degrades blood clots)
Prostaglandins I_2 and $F_{2\alpha}$ (PGI_2 and $PGF_{2\alpha}$)	Helps regulate inflammation, blood clotting, ovulation, menstruation, and acid secretion
Resistin	Increases insulin resistance Linked to obesity and type 2 diabetes
Retinol-binding protein 4 (RBP-4)	Produced mainly by visceral adipose tissue Decreases insulin sensitivity and alters glucose homeostasis
Transforming growth factor β (TGF-β)	Regulates a wide variety of biological responses, including proliferation, differentiation, apoptosis, and development
Tumor necrosis factor α and β (TNF-α, TNF-β)	Interferes with insulin receptor signaling and is a possible cause of development of insulin resistance in obesity
Visfatin	Produced by visceral adipose tissue; its level correlates with visceral adipose tissue mass Involved in regulation of body mass index Decreases blood glucose levels

Modified from Vázquez-Vela ME, Torres N, Tovar AR. White adipose tissue as endocrine organ and its role in obesity. *Arch Med Res.* 2008;39:715–728.

surface-to-mass ratio and to avoid lethal hypothermia (a major risk of death for preterm babies). In newborns, brown adipose tissue makes up about 5% of the total-body mass and is located on the back, along the upper half of the spine, and toward the shoulders. The amount of brown adipose tissue gradually decreases as the body grows, but it remains widely distributed throughout the first decade of life in the cervical, axillary, paravertebral, mediastinal, sternal, and abdominal regions of the body. It then disappears from most sites, except for regions around the kidney, adrenal glands, large vessels (e.g., aorta), and regions of the neck (deep cervical and supraclavicular), back (interscapular and paravertebral), and thorax (mediastinum). **Positron emission tomography (PET)** used to detect cancer cells based on their uptake of large amounts of radioactively labeled glucose (^{18}F-FDG) is able to detect patterns characteristic of brown adipose tissue within the region of the adult body described above (see Folder 9.3, page 293). These findings have been confirmed with tissue biopsies.

Adipocytes of brown, multilocular adipose tissue contain numerous fat droplets.

The cells of **brown (multilocular) adipose tissue** are smaller than those of white adipose tissue. The cytoplasm of each cell contains many small lipid droplets, hence the name *multilocular*. In contrast, white *unilocular* adipocytes

FOLDER 9.1

CLINICAL CORRELATION: OBESITY

Obesity is epidemic in the United States. According to current estimates by the National Institutes of Health (NIH), about two-thirds of Americans are considered to be obese, and 300,000 die annually from obesity-related metabolic diseases (i.e., diabetes, hypertension, cardiovascular diseases, and cancer). An individual is considered obese when the percentage of body fat exceeds the average percentage for the individual's age and sex. The prevalence of obesity has increased in the past decade from 12% to 18%. The increases are seen in both sexes and at all socioeconomic levels, with the greatest increase reported in the 18- to 29-year-old age group.

The **body mass index (BMI)**, expressed as weight (kg)/height (m)^2, is closely correlated with the total amount of body fat and is commonly used to classify overweight and obesity among adults. A BMI of 18.5–24.9 kg/m^2 is considered normal. A BMI of 25–29.9 kg/m^2 is considered overweight, and a BMI of ≥30 kg/m^2 is considered obese. Obesity is associated with an increased risk of mortality as well as with many diseases such as hypertension, cardiovascular diseases, diabetes, and cancer. It is a chronic condition related to both a person's genetic makeup and their environment.

Obesity genes encode the molecular components of the short- and long-term weight regulation systems, which include leptin, ghrelin, and other factors that regulate energy balance. In addition, several of these factors modulate glucose metabolism by adipose tissue and contribute to the development of insulin resistance, which is associated with **type 2 diabetes**. Intensive research directed toward adipocyte-derived proteins may in the future provide potential drugs for reducing obesity and overcoming insulin resistance.

Microscopic examination of adipose tissue from an obese individual shows hypertrophic adipocytes with a gigantic lipid droplet. Debris from damaged or dead adipocytes is often seen dispersed among hypertrophic adipocytes. Dead adipocytes are found ~30 times more often in obese than in nonobese individuals. Large macrophages are seen to infiltrate the obese adipose tissue; their roles are to remove damaged cells and cellular debris and to alter secretion of adipokines (Fig. F9.1.1). In addition, macrophages inhibit differentiation of adipocytes from their progenitor cells, leading to hypertrophy of the existing fat cells. Owing to the large size of the macrophages, as well as the length of time required for the removal of cellular debris, the obese adipose tissue shows signs of **chronic low-grade inflammation**. The number of macrophages positively correlates to the size of adipocytes and coincides with the emergence of insulin resistance.

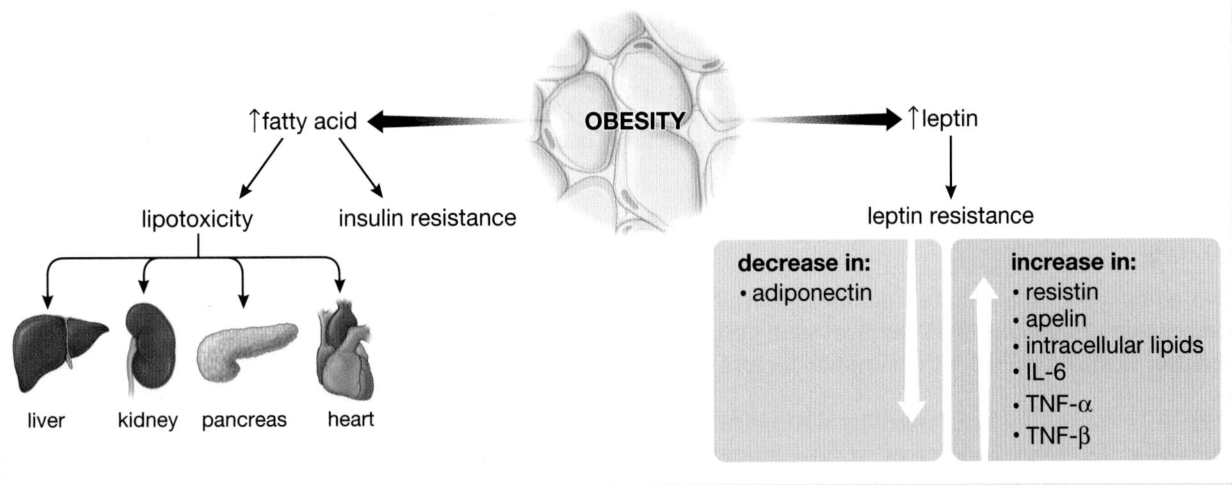

FIGURE F9.1.1. Changes in adipocyte metabolism in obesity. Adipocytes from obese individuals are hypertrophic and produce more leptin. Increased leptin secretion causes nonadipose tissue to become resistant to leptin. Hypertrophic adipocytes also secrete high amounts of fatty acids and adipokines that promote insulin resistance. This leads to pathologic accumulation of lipids in organs, such as the kidney (renal lipotoxicity), liver (nonalcoholic fatty liver disease), pancreas, and heart. (Modified from Vázquez-Vela ME, Torres N, Tovar AR. White adipose tissue as endocrine organ and its role in obesity. *Arch Med Res.* 2008;39:715–728.)

contain only one large lipid droplet, and *paucilocular [Lat. paucus, having few]* adipocytes contain fewer lipid droplets. The nucleus of a mature brown adipocyte is typically located in an eccentric position within the cell, but it is not flattened like the nucleus of a white adipocyte. In routine H&E-stained sections, the cytoplasm of the brown adipocyte consists largely of empty vacuoles because the lipid that ordinarily occupies the vacuolated spaces is lost during preparation (Fig. 9.6). Brown adipocytes depleted of their lipid more closely resemble epithelial cells than connective tissue cells. The brown adipocyte contains numerous large spherical mitochondria with numerous cristae, a small Golgi apparatus, and only small amounts of rER and sER. The mitochondria contain large amounts of cytochrome oxidase, which imparts the brown color to the cells.

Brown adipose tissue is subdivided into lobules by partitions of connective tissue, but the connective tissue stroma between individual cells within the lobules is sparse. The tissue has a rich supply of capillaries that enhance its color. Numerous unmyelinated, noradrenergic sympathetic nerve fibers are present among the fat cells. Brown adipose tissue features are listed in Table 9.2.

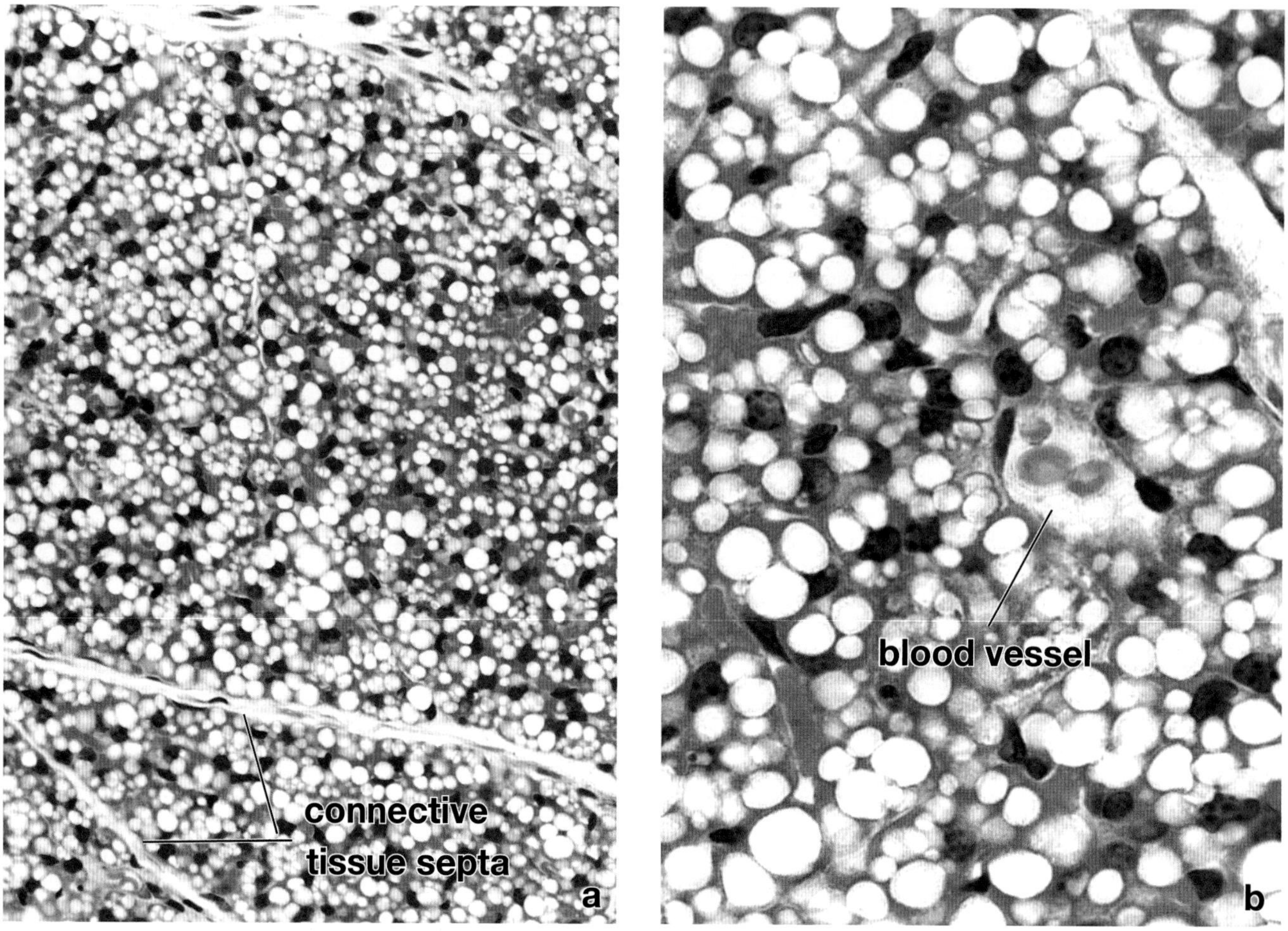

FIGURE 9.6. Brown adipose tissue. a. Photomicrograph of brown adipose tissue from a newborn in a hematoxylin and eosin (H&E)-stained paraffin preparation. The cells contain fat droplets of varying size. ×150. **b.** This photomicrograph, obtained at a higher magnification, shows the brown adipose cells with round and often centrally located nuclei. Most of the cells are polygonal and closely packed, with numerous lipid droplets. In some cells, large lipid droplets displace nuclei toward the cell periphery. A network of collagen fibers and capillaries surrounds the brown adipose cells. ×320.

Brown adipocytes differentiate from mesenchymal skeletal myogenic progenitor (Myf5 positive) stem cells under the control of PRDM16/PGC-1 transcription factors.

Brown adipocytes are also derived from **mesenchymal stem cells** but from a different cellular lineage than those differentiating into white adipocytes. Lineage tracing experiments show that brown adipose tissue and skeletal muscle derive from common **skeletal myogenic progenitor stem cells** found in dermatomyotomes of the developing embryo. These cells are characterized by expression of the myogenic lineage marker **myogenic factor 5 (Myf5)**, which remains detectable in mature brown adipocytes and in all stages of their differentiation. In contrast to white adipocytes, differentiation of brown adipocytes is influenced by a different pair of transcription factors. When the zinc-finger protein known as **PR domain containing 16 (PRDM16)** is activated, myogenic progenitor cells synthesize several members of the **PPARγ coactivator 1 (PGC-1)** family of transcription factors, activating brown adipocyte differentiation and suppressing skeletal muscle development. Loss of PRDM16 from brown adipocyte precursors causes a loss of brown fat characteristics and promotes skeletal muscle differentiation. Therefore, **PRDM16/PGC-1** is regarded as a "**master-switch**" regulator in differentiation of brown adipocytes. These factors, in turn, regulate the expression of genes that encode a specific mitochondrial protein called **uncoupling protein (UCP-1)** or **thermogenin** (a 33-kDa inner mitochondrial membrane protein), which is essential for brown adipocyte metabolism (thermogenesis). Clinical observations confirm that under normal conditions, brown adipose tissue can expand in response to increased blood levels of **norepinephrine**. This becomes evident in patients with **pheochromocytoma**, an endocrine tumor of the adrenal medulla that secretes excessive amounts of epinephrine and norepinephrine. In these individuals, the UCP-1 gene is activated by norepinephrine stimulation, which also protects brown adipocytes by inhibiting apoptosis. In the past, it was thought that uncoupling proteins were expressed only in brown adipose tissue. Several similar uncoupling protein homologs are present in other tissues. UCP-2 is linked to hyperinsulinemia and obesity and may be involved in the regulation of body weight. UCP-3 is expressed in skeletal muscles and may account for the thermogenic effects of thyroid hormone. UCP-4 and UCP-5 are brain mitochondria–specific molecules.

FOLDER 9.2

CLINICAL CORRELATION: ADIPOSE TISSUE TUMORS

The study of the numerous varieties of benign and malignant **adipose tissue tumors** provides further insight into, and confirmation of, the sequence of adipose tissue differentiation described earlier. As with epithelial tumors and tumors of fibroblast origin, the variety of adipose tissue tumors reflects the normal pattern of adipose tissue differentiation; that is, discrete tumor types can be described that consist primarily of cells resembling a given stage in normal adipose tissue differentiation.

Lipoma is the most common benign tumor of adipose tissue in adulthood. It is more common than all other soft-tissue tumors combined. Lipomas are subclassified by the morphology of the predominant cell in the tumor. For instance, **conventional lipomas** consist of mature white adipocytes. **Fibrolipomas** have adipocytes surrounded by an excess of fibrous tissue, and **angiolipomas** contain adipocytes separated by an unusually large number of vascular channels. Most lipomas show structural chromosome aberrations that include balanced rearrangements, often involving chromosome 12. Lipomas are usually found in subcutaneous tissues in middle-aged and elderly individuals. They are characterized as well-defined, soft, and painless masses of mature adipocytes and are most often located in the subcutaneous fascia of the back, thorax, and proximal parts of the upper and lower limbs. Treatment of lipomas usually involves a simple surgical excision.

Malignant tumors of adipose tissue, called **liposarcomas**, are rare. They are typically detected in older individuals and are mainly found in the deep adipose tissues of the lower limbs, abdomen, and shoulder area. Liposarcomas may contain both well-differentiated, mature adipocytes and early, undifferentiated cells (Fig. F9.2.1). Tumors containing more cells in earlier stages of differentiation are more aggressive and more frequently metastasize. Typically, liposarcomas are surgically removed, but if a tumor has already metastasized, chemotherapy and radiation therapy can be utilized as presurgical or postsurgical treatments.

Although the term *lipoma* relates primarily to white adipose tissue tumors, tumors of brown adipose tissue are also found. Not surprisingly, these are called **hibernomas**. They are rare, benign, and slow-growing soft-tissue tumors of brown fat most commonly arising in the periscapular region, axillary fossa, neck, or mediastinum. Most hibernomas contain a mixture of white and brown adipose tissue; pure hibernomas are very rare.

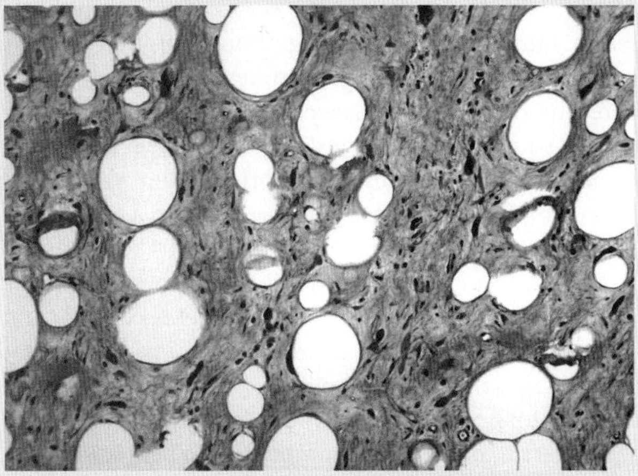

FIGURE F9.2.1. Well-differentiated liposarcoma. This photomicrograph was obtained from a tumor surgically removed from the retroperitoneal space of the abdomen. Well-differentiated liposarcoma is characterized by a predominance of mature adipocytes that vary in size and shape. They are interspersed between broad fibrous septa of connective tissue containing cells (most are fibroblasts) with atypical hyperchromatic nuclei. Relatively few scattered spindle cells with hyperchromatic and pleomorphic nuclei are found within the connective tissue. ×340. (Courtesy of Dr. Fabiola Medeiros.)

Metabolism of lipid in brown adipose tissue generates heat in a process known as thermogenesis.

Hibernating animals have large amounts of **brown adipose tissue**. The tissue serves as a ready source of lipid. When oxidized, it produces heat to warm the blood flowing through the brown fat on arousal from hibernation and in the maintenance of body temperature in the cold. This type of heat production is known as **nonshivering thermogenesis**.

Brown adipose tissue is also present in nonhibernating animals and humans and again serves as a source of heat. As in the mobilization of lipid in white adipose tissue, lipid is mobilized and heat is generated by brown adipocytes when they are stimulated by the sympathetic nervous system. This process, known as the **human adaptive thermogenesis** response, is a target of current obesity research. Mechanisms to increase brown fat differentiation may potentially be an attractive treatment in both diet-induced and genetically acquired obesity.

Thermogenic activity of brown adipose tissue is facilitated by UCP-1 that is found in the inner mitochondrial membrane.

The mitochondria in eukaryotic cells produce and store energy as an electrochemical proton gradient across the inner mitochondrial membrane. As described earlier (see pages 61-64), this energy is used to synthesize adenosine triphosphate (ATP) when the protons return to the mitochondrial matrix through the ATP synthase enzyme located at the inner mitochondrial membrane.

The unique large, round **mitochondria** in the cytoplasm of brown adipose tissue cells contain **uncoupling protein (UCP-1)**, which uncouples the oxidation of fatty acids from the production of ATP. As a result, protons are allowed to travel from the intermembrane space back to the mitochondrial matrix along the gradient without passing through ATP synthase and thus without producing ATP. This can occur because an alternative pathway for the protons' return is available through UCP-1 that facilitates proton transport across the inner mitochondrial membrane. The movement of protons from the inner mitochondrial compartment dissipates the mitochondrial proton gradient, thus uncoupling respiration from ATP synthesis. The energy produced by the mitochondria is then dissipated as heat in a process known as **thermogenesis**.

The metabolic activity of brown adipose tissue is regulated by the sympathetic nervous system and is related to ambient outdoor temperature.

The **metabolic activity** of brown adipose tissue is largely regulated by **norepinephrine** released from sympathetic nerve terminals, which stimulates lipolysis and hydrolysis of triglycerides as well as increases mitochondrial expression and activity of **UCP-1** molecules. In experimental animals, UCP-1 activity has been shown to increase during cold stress. In humans, UCP-1 is responsible for the adaptive thermogenesis response, a regulated heat production that is triggered by changes in the external environment. In addition, cold stimulates glucose utilization in brown adipocytes by overexpression of glucose transporters (Glut-4). Clinical studies using **PET scans** in adults have shown a direct relationship between ambient temperature and the amount of brown fat accumulated in the body. An increase in the amount of brown adipose tissue has been reported on the neck and supraclavicular regions during the winter months, especially in lean individuals. This is supported by autopsy findings of larger amounts of brown fat in outdoor workers exposed to cold. Modern molecular imaging techniques now allow clinicians to precisely locate where brown fat is distributed in the body, which is essential for proper differential diagnosis of cancerous lesions (see Folder 9.3, page 293).

Brown adipose tissue secretes active substances called batokines that contribute to the regulation of various body functions.

Like white adipose tissue, brown adipose tissue actively synthesizes and secretes biologically active substances collectively called **batokines** (Fig. 9.7). They contribute to the regulation of various functions, such as thermogenic activity, immune activity, vascularization, substrate utilization, and other functions related to whole-body energy expenditure and glucose homeostasis.

Several batokines act locally (via autocrine and paracrine mechanisms) to promote hypertrophy and hyperplasia of brown adipose tissue, including its vascularization and innervation, to enhance their own thermogenic activity. Examples of these molecules include nerve growth factor (NGF) and fibroblast growth factor 21 (FGF21) that increase sympathetic innervation and trigger cell division, and vascular endothelial growth factor A (VEGF-A) that promotes vascularization of brown adipose tissue.

Some batokines act as endocrine factors to target peripheral tissues, such as white adipose tissue, lymphatic tissue, liver, pancreas, heart, and bone. These include FGF21, neuregulin-4 (NRG4), VEGF-A, myostatin, and bone morphogenetic protein 8B (BMP-8B). In addition, exosomal miRNA molecules secreted by brown adipocytes have systemic effects on body metabolism by acting on distant organs, such as the liver, skeletal muscles, heart, and others.

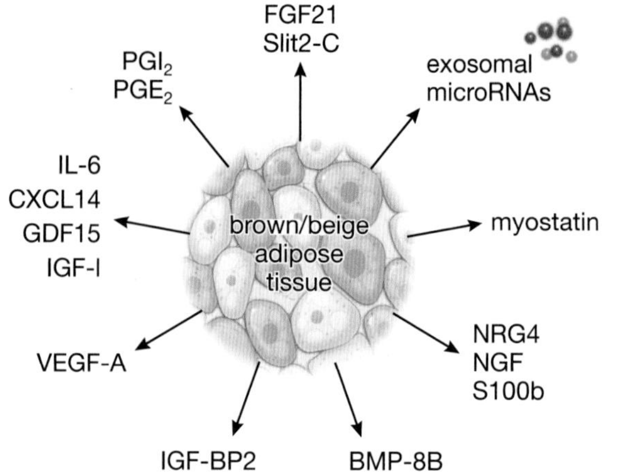

FIGURE 9.7. Major batokines secreted by brown/beige adipose tissue. This schematic drawing shows various types of batokines secreted by brown and beige adipose tissue that contribute to the regulation of various functions, such as thermogenic activity, immune activity, vascularization, substrate utilization, and other functions. These include fibroblast growth factor-21 (FGF21), which stimulates transdifferentiation of adipose tissue; C-terminal fragment of the Slit 2 protein (Slit2-C), which stimulates adipose thermogenesis; insulin-like growth factor–binding protein 2 (IGF-BP2), which influences bone growth; neuregulin-4 (NRG4), which promotes neuronal processes outgrowth; nerve growth factor (NGF) and S100b protein, which target sympathetic nervous endings promoting innervation; vascular endothelial growth factor A (VEGF-A), which induces vascularization of adipose tissue; bone morphogenetic protein 8B (BMP-8B), which acts locally on brown adipose tissue, enhancing thermogenesis and in the hypothalamus, activating the sympathetic nervous system; myostatin, which decreases performance of skeletal muscles; interleukin-6 (IL-6), insulin-like growth factor 1 (IGF-1), chemokine (C-X-C motif) ligand-14 (CXCL14), and growth/differentiation factor-15 (GDF15) that acts on immune system; prostaglandins (PGI2 and PGE2), which promote development of brown adipocytes; and exosomal microRNAs, which regulate gene expression in distant organs, thus affecting whole-body metabolism.

■ BEIGE ADIPOSE TISSUE

Beige adipose tissue exhibit cellular and molecular features that are intermediate between white and brown adipose tissue.

Recently, a new type of adipose tissue has been identified within the subcutaneous white adipose tissue throughout the body. This adipose tissue consists of pockets of brown-like adipocytes that were named **beige adipocytes** or *"brite"* *(brown-in-white)* adipocytes. The morphology of these paucilocular cells is intermediate between that of white and brown adipocytes (they contain fewer lipid droplets than brown adipocytes). They have a thermogenic ability owing to the expression of the UCP-1 protein, although this activity is not completely UCP-1 dependent. When compared to brown adipocytes, beige adipocytes have much lower levels of UCP-1 protein expression in their mitochondria, but their UCP-1 is highly inducible in response to cold exposure or hormonal (norepinephrine) stimulation. It is postulated that increases in intracellular Ca^{2+} activate ATP synthesis for ATP-dependent metabolic thermogenesis to generate heat and increase energy expenditure. The comparison between all three types of adipose tissues and their UCP-1 distribution is shown in Figure 9.8.

Beige adipocytes are genetically different from brown adipocytes. They develop from white adipocyte precursor stem cells; thus, they do not have the same skeletal myogenic

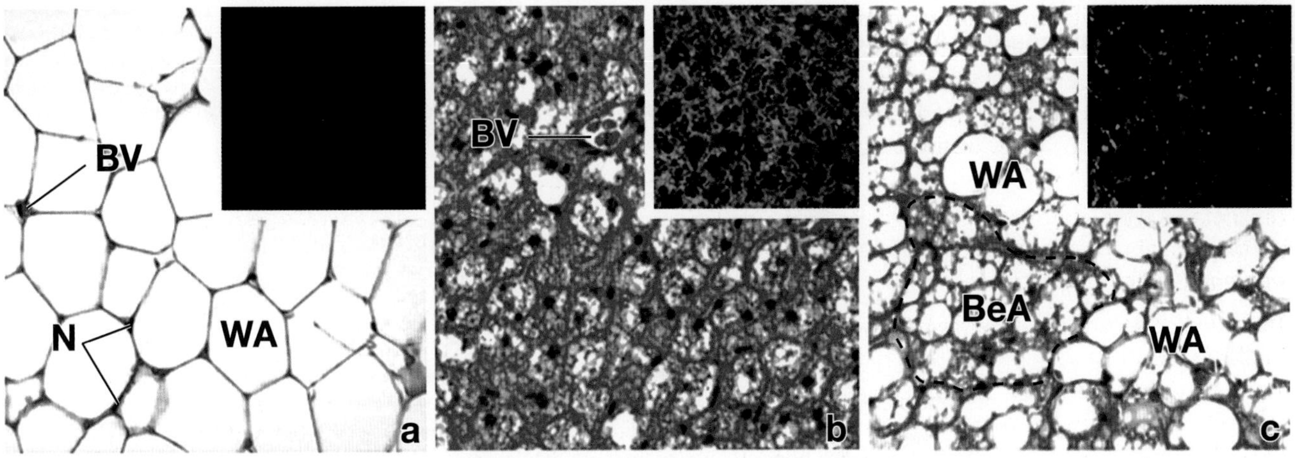

FIGURE 9.8. Three types of adipose tissue with UCP-1 immunofluorescence. Photomicrographs of three different adipose tissues were obtained from C57BL/6 mice and routinely processed for hematoxylin and eosin (H&E) preparation. **a.** White adipose tissue from the subcutaneous fat pad. White adipocytes (*WA*) are tightly packed together and appear polyhedral in shape with large lipid droplets (represented by *white* spaces because lipids are washed out in routine slide preparation). Note a narrow rim of cytoplasm with flattened nuclei (*N*). A few blood vessels (*BV*) and smaller capillaries can be found in this section. **b.** Brown adipose tissue from the interscapular region. Brown adipocytes are polygonal and closely packed, with numerous lipid droplets. Note that nuclei are round and typically pushed to the cell periphery by lipid droplets. Brown tissue has an extensive blood vessel (*BV*) network. **c.** Beige adipose tissue from the subcutaneous fat pad. Beige adipocytes (*BeA*) form a pocket inclusion (see area indicated by *dashed line*) within the white adipose tissue (*WA*). Corresponding insets provide pattern of UCP-1 distributions in each tissue. Note that white adipose tissue does not exhibit UCP-1 activity (no staining), brown tissue has an abundance of UCP-1, and beige adipose tissue exhibits staining in the area of accumulation of brown-like adipocytes (dispersed between white adipocytes [*WA*]). UCP-1 was visualized using an indirect immunofluorescence technique that utilizes primary goat polyclonal antibodies against the UCP-1 protein, followed by secondary anti-goat antibodies conjugated with Alexa Fluor 488 fluorescent stain. ×180. (Courtesy of Prof. Dr. Carlos A. Mandarim-de-Lacerda, Universidade do Estado do Rio de Janeiro, Brazil.)

pregenital cells origin as brown adipocytes (Fig. 9.9). Beige adipocytes are **Myf5 negative** and express specific beige markers, such as t-box transcription factor-1 (tBX1) and transmembrane protein-26 (TMEM26). Research has shown that beige adipocytes are generated in two independent coexisting pathways:

- **White-to-brown transdifferentiation** pathway (note that precursor cells for white adipose cells are Myf5 negative; see page 282). The vast majority (80%–95%) of newly formed beige adipocytes arise through this pathway.
- **De novo differentiation** from the specific white adipose precursor cells that reside within white adipose tissue. White adipocyte precursor cells, especially those expressing tBX1 and TMEM26 markers, have a greater ability to proliferate and differentiate into beige adipocytes. PRDM16 seems to be a key transcriptional co-regulator in this process.

Beige adipocytes actively synthesize and secrete batokines, biologically active substances similar to brown adipocytes (see Fig. 9.7).

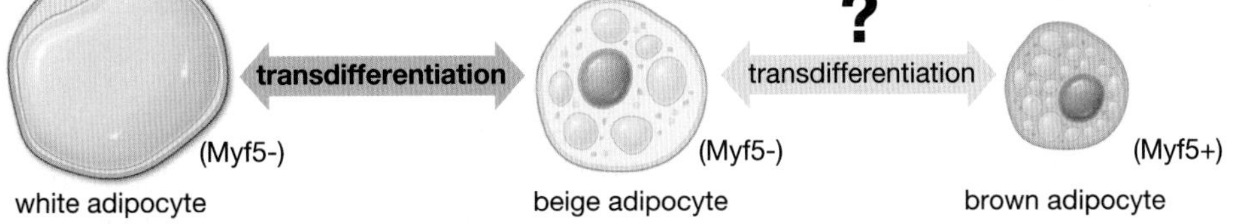

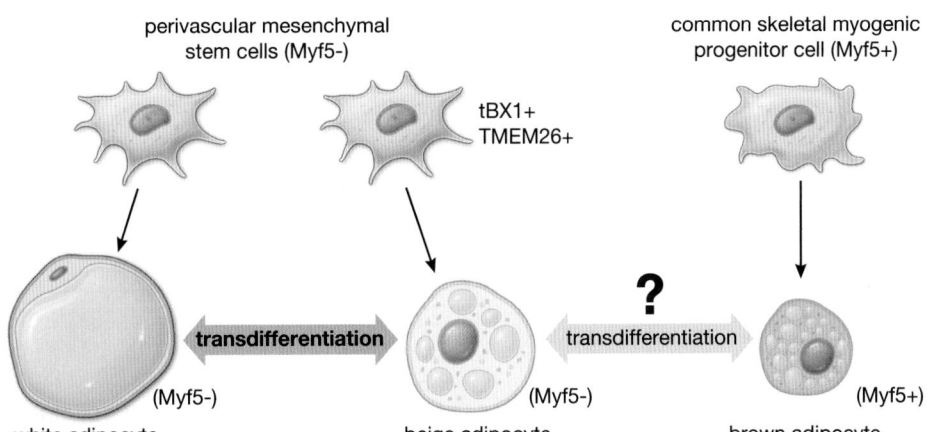

FIGURE 9.9. Development of beige adipocytes. Beige adipocytes are genetically different from brown adipocytes. There are two pathways by which they develop. The first and most common is the white-to-brown transdifferentiation pathway, which accounts for 80%–95% of beige adipocyte development. This process is induced after exposure to cold or norepinephrine stimulation. The second pathway includes de novo differentiation from perivascular mesenchymal stem cells (specific white adipose precursors) that reside within white adipose tissue. Precursor cells, especially those expressing tBX1 and TMEM26 markers, have a greater propensity to proliferate and differentiate into beige adipocytes. Note that both white and beige adipocytes are myogenic factor 5 (Myf5) negative. The development of brown adipocytes progresses from common skeletal myogenic pregenital cells; therefore, they express Myf5 protein markers. Transdifferentiation of brown-to-beige adipocytes is questionable; there are only a few reports of Myf5 markers on beige adipocytes.

TABLE 9.2 Summary of Adipose Tissue Features

Features	White Adipose Tissue	Brown Adipose Tissue	Beige Adipose Tissue
	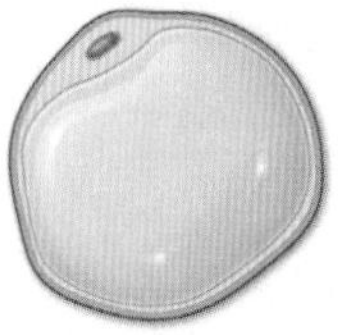	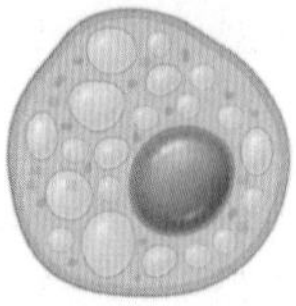	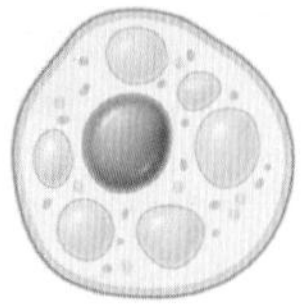
Location	Subcutaneous layer, mammary gland, greater omentum, mesenteries, retroperitoneal space, visceral pericardium, orbits (eye sockets), bone marrow cavity	Large amounts in newborns Remnants in adults at the retroperitoneal space, deep cervical and supraclavicular regions of the neck, interscapular, paravertebral regions of the back, mediastinum	Distributed throughout the body in various deposits of subcutaneous white adipose tissue
Function	Metabolic energy storage, insulation, cushioning, hormone production (adipokines), source of metabolic water	Heat production (thermogenesis UCP-1 dependent), hormone production (batokines)	Heat production (thermogenesis), hormone production (batokines)
Adipocyte morphology	Unilocular, spherical, flattened nucleus, rim of cytoplasm Large diameter (15–150 μm)	Multilocular, spherical, round eccentric nucleus Smaller diameter (10–25 μm)	Paucilocular, spherical, round nucleus Smaller diameter (10–25 μm)
Precursor cells	Perivascular mesenchymal stem cells (Myf5 negative)	Common skeletal myogenic progenitor cells (Myf5 positive)	Perivascular mesenchymal stem cells (Myf5 negative)
Specific cellular markers	Ob (leptin), HOXC8, and HOXC9	LHX8 and ZIC1	TMEM26 and TBX1
Transcription factors "master switch" in differentiation	PPARγ/RXR	PRDM16/PGC-1	Low expression of PRDM16
UCP-1 gene expression	No	Yes	Yes
Thermogenesis mechanism	No existing	UCP-1 dependent	Not completely UCP-1 dependent, utilize ATP-Ca^{2+} cycling
Mitochondria	Few, elongated, filamentous with poorly developed cristae	Many, large, round, with well-developed cristae	Many, but less than in brown adipocytes, large, round, with well-developed cristae
Innervation	Few sympathetic nerve fibers	High density of noradrenergic sympathetic nerve fibers	High density of noradrenergic sympathetic nerve fibers
Vascularization	Few blood vessels	Highly vascularized tissue	Highly vascularized tissue
Response to environmental stress (i.e., cold exposure)	Decreased lipogenesis Increased lipoprotein lipase activity Transdifferentiation to brown adipose tissue	Increased lipogenesis Decreased lipoprotein lipase activity Increased heat production	Increased lipogenesis Decreased lipoprotein lipase activity Increased heat production
Growth and differentiation	Throughout entire life from stromal perivascular cells	During fetal period from common skeletal myogenic progenitor cells Decreases in adult life	Throughout entire life from white-to-brown transdifferentiation and de novo from precursor cells Induced in individuals with pheochromocytoma, hibernoma, or chronic cold exposure

■ TRANSDIFFERENTIATION OF ADIPOSE TISSUE

Adipocytes undergo white-to-brown and brown-to-white transformation in response to the thermogenic needs of an organism.

Exposure to chronic cold temperatures increases the thermogenic demands of an organism. Studies have shown that in cold conditions, mature white adipocytes can transform into brown-like adipocytes to generate body heat. Conversely, brown-like adipocytes transform into white adipocytes when the energy balance is positive and the body requires an increase in triglyceride storage capacity. This phenomenon, known as **transdifferentiation**, has been observed in experimental animals and humans. After 3–5 days of cold exposure, white adipose tissue in mice undergoes a "**browning phenomenon**" to produce pockets of paucilocular, UCP-1–positive **beige adipocytes** within the white adipose

FOLDER 9.3

CLINICAL CORRELATION: PET SCANNING AND BROWN ADIPOSE TISSUE INTERFERENCE

Positron emission tomography, also called a "PET scan," is a diagnostic tool that can locate malignant cells in the body. PET is based on the detection of high-energy γ rays created when positrons (subatomic particles of antimatter), produced during decay of radioactive materials, are encountered by electrons. The procedure requires the injection of a radioactive tracer, most commonly **18-fluorine-2-fluoro-2-deoxy-d-glucose (^{18}F-FDG)**. This radioactive glucose isotope is used in PET imaging because malignant cells metabolize glucose at a greater rate than normal cells. After injection of the isotope, a detector scans the entire body and records radiation emitted by the ^{18}F-FDG tracer as it becomes incorporated within the body's cells. A computer reassembles the signals into images, which are, in effect, biological maps of ^{18}F-FDG distribution in the body. Recently, owing to greater diagnostic accuracy and improved biopsy methods, combined PET and computed tomography (CT) scanners are utilized more frequently.

One drawback to PET imaging is that many normal tissues and benign lesions also show increased glucose metabolism and can thus be misinterpreted as malignant. For example, brown and beige adipose tissues, with its increased glucose uptake mediated by increased activity of glucose transporters, can be a potential source of **false-positive interpretation** of PET scans. Because both brown and beige adipose tissues are present in the neck, supraclavicular regions, and mediastinum (see pages 285-286), it is commonly observed on PET scans, especially in underweight patients and during winter months, when beige adipose tissue is more predominant. This ^{18}F-FDG uptake most likely represents activated brown adipose tissue during increased sympathetic nerve activity related to cold stress.

A typical PET image of brown/beige fat is usually bilateral and symmetrical; however, in the mediastinum, the image may be asymmetrical or focal and can mimic malignancy. False-positive results from brown/beige fat ^{18}F-FDG uptake in these areas have been reported in young women undergoing scans for diagnosis and staging of breast cancer. Therefore, understanding that brown and beige fat can show increased radioactive tracer uptake is crucial for establishing an accurate diagnosis and avoiding false-positive results (Fig. F9.3.1).

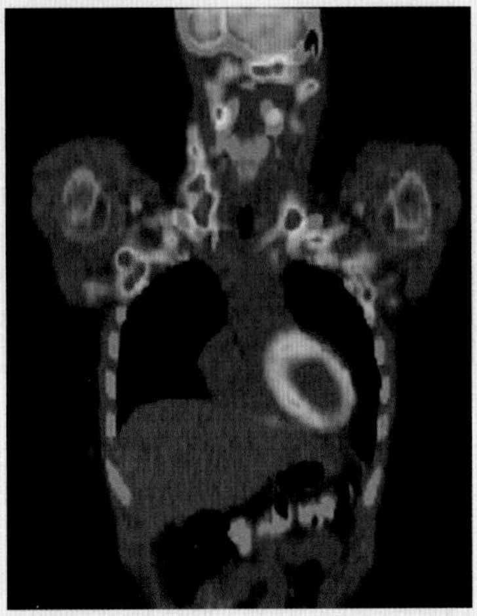

FIGURE F9.3.1. Coronal positron emission tomography/computed tomography (PET/CT) image of a healthy young woman. This *upper part* of the coronal section of a whole-body PET/CT scan shows extensive bilateral increased ^{18}F-FDG uptake (*red color*) in the neck, supraclavicular, and upper axillary regions. Note that moderate increase in radioactive tracer uptake is also detectable in the myocardium (*yellow color*). Regions of extensive metabolic activity correlate with the distribution pattern of low-density brown adipose tissue. PET/CT imaging allows for precise localization of increased ^{18}F-FDG uptake areas and differentiation between brown adipose tissue tracer uptake and malignant tumor findings. (Courtesy of Dr. Jolanta Durski.)

tissue. This change in the phenotype of adipocytes occurs in the absence of cell division (no increase in DNA content) or apoptosis, suggesting that white adipocytes transform directly into brown-like (beige) adipocytes. These findings are also supported by observations of differential gene expression. In addition, mice with abundant natural or induced brown adipose tissue are resistant to obesity, whereas genetically modified mice without functional brown adipocytes are prone to **obesity** and **type 2 diabetes.** The putative genome reprogramming mechanism that drives the browning phenomenon could be used for future therapeutic strategies aimed at controlling the amount of brown adipose tissue in the body. This discovery may lead to the control of obesity and type 2 diabetes.

White-to-brown transdifferentiation of adipose tissue is induced by cold exposure and physical activity.

Cold exposure and physical activity induce conversion of white-to-brown adipocytes via several molecular pathways. Cold temperatures are sensed by the central nervous system, causing increased stimulation of the noradrenergic sympathetic nerve system. Increased amounts of brown/beige adipose tissue have been found in outdoor workers in northern countries and in individuals with pheochromocytoma (a noradrenaline-secreting tumor). Recent studies indicate that the density of the sympathetic nerves innervating white adipose tissue is one of the most important factors in white-to-brown transdifferentiation. Physical exercise stimulation is more complex and involves secretion of atrial and ventricular natriuretic peptides in the heart that act on the kidney, which, in turn, activate transcription factors essential for brown adipocyte differentiation. Other triggers of transdifferentiation include reprograming of adipose tissue genes by activating specific transcription factors ("master regulators") and growth factors, such as FGF21. Many epidemiologic studies demonstrated an inverse correlation between the presence or amount of brown/beige adipose tissue and body weight as well as obesity-associated complications. In the future, signaling pathways and molecules involved in adipocyte transdifferentiation may open new avenues in pharmacologic treatment of obesity, diabetes, and other metabolic diseases.

ADIPOSE TISSUE

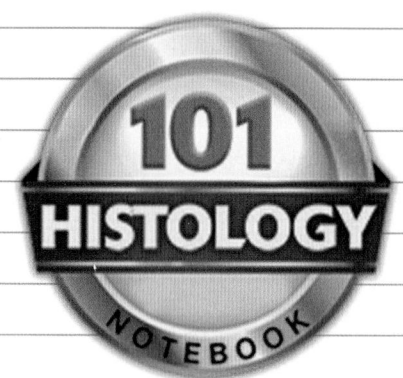

OVERVIEW OF ADIPOSE TISSUE

- **Adipose tissue** is a specialized connective tissue that plays an important role in energy homeostasis (stores energy in lipid droplets in the form of triglycerides) and hormone production (adipokines and batokines).
- There are three types of adipose tissue: **white (unilocular)**, **brown (multilocular)**, and **beige (paucilocular)** adipose tissue.

WHITE ADIPOSE TISSUE

- **White adipose tissue** represents at least 10% of body weight in a normal healthy adult. White adipose tissue with supporting collagen and reticular fibers forms the **subcutaneous fascia**, is concentrated in the mammary fat pads, and surrounds several internal organs.
- **White adipocytes** are very large cells ($\geq$100 μm in diameter) with a single large lipid droplet (unilocular), a thin rim of cytoplasm, and a flattened, peripherally displaced nucleus.
- A single large lipid droplet within the white adipocyte represents cytoplasmic inclusion and is not membrane bound.
- White adipose tissue secretes a variety of **adipokines**, which include hormones (e.g., leptin), growth factors, cytokines, and exosomal microRNAs (miRNAs).
- White adipocytes differentiate from perivascular mesenchymal stem (myogenic factor 5 [Myf5] negative) cells under the control of **PPARγ/RXR transcription factors** ("master switch" for white adipocyte differentiation).
- The amount of adipose tissue is regulated by two hormonal pathways: **short-term weight regulation** pathway (**peptide YY** and **ghrelin**) and **long-term weight regulation** pathway (**leptin** and **insulin**).
- **Triglycerides** stored in adipocytes are released by lipases that are activated during **neural mobilization** (which involves **norepinephrine** released from sympathetic nerves) and/or **hormonal mobilization** (which involves **glucagon** and **growth hormone**).

BROWN ADIPOSE TISSUE

- **Brown adipose tissue** is abundant in newborns (5% of total-body mass) but is markedly reduced in adults.
- **Brown adipocytes** are smaller than white adipocytes and contain many lipid droplets (multilocular) and cytoplasm with a round nucleus and abundance of mitochondria.
- Brown adipose tissue secretes a variety of **batokines**, which include growth factors, cytokines, and exosomal miRNAs.
- Brown adipocytes differentiate from skeletal myogenic mesenchymal (Myf5 positive) stem cells under the control of **PRDM16/PGC-1 transcription factors** (the "master switch" for brown adipocyte differentiation).
- Brown adipocytes express a specific mitochondrial protein called **uncoupling protein (UCP-1)** or **thermogenin**, which is essential for brown adipocyte metabolism.
- Metabolism of lipids in brown adipose tissue generates heat (**thermogenesis**) by uncoupling the oxidation of fatty acids in the mitochondria from ATP production.
- The **metabolic activity** of brown adipose tissue is regulated by **norepinephrine** released from sympathetic nerves and is related to ambient outdoor temperature (cold weather increases the amount of brown adipose tissue).

BEIGE ADIPOSE TISSUE

- **Beige adipose tissue** is widely distributed throughout the body in the form of brown-like adipocytes pockets within white adipose tissue
- **Beige adipocytes** have intermediate features between white and brown adipocytes, containing fewer lipid droplets (paucilocular) than brown adipocytes.
- Beige adipose tissue secretes a variety of **batokines** similar to that of brown adipose tissue.
- White adipocytes can undergo white-to-brown **transdifferentiation** in response to the thermogenic needs of the body. Transdifferentiation is a major source of beige adipocytes in the body.
- Cold exposure, hormonal activity (norepinephrine), and physical activity induce white-to-brown transdifferentiation that increases the number of beige adipocytes in white adipose tissue.
- Beige adipocytes also express the **uncoupling protein (UCP-1)**; however, thermogenic activity is not completely UCP1 dependent.

PLATE 9.1 ■ ADIPOSE TISSUE

Adipose tissue is widely distributed throughout the body and in varying amounts in different individuals. It is a specialized connective tissue consisting of **triglyceride**-storing cells called **adipocytes**. Adipose tissue is also considered an endocrine organ that secretes **adipokines** and **batokines** that include many factors with autocrine, paracrine, and endocrine functions. Adipose tissue has a rich blood supply, which complements its metabolic and endocrine functions. Three types of adipose tissue are now recognized. The most common and abundant is referred to as **white adipose tissue.** White adipocytes catabolize triglycerides, and when energy expenditure exceeds energy intake, **fatty acids** are released into circulation. In addition, **glycerol** and fatty acids released from the adipocytes participate in glucose metabolism. White adipocytes are very large cells whose cytoplasm contains a single large vacuole in which the fat is stored in the form of triglycerides. When observed in a typical hematoxylin and eosin (H&E) section, white adipose tissue appears as a mesh-like structure (see Orientation Micrograph). The second type is **brown adipose tissue**. It consists of smaller cells. Their cytoplasm is characterized by numerous vesicles that occupy much of the cells' volume. It also is very richly vascularized. Brown adipose tissue is found in human newborns where it assists in maintaining body temperature. The third type is **beige adipose tissue.** Beige adipocytes represent pockets of brown-like adipocytes within white adipose tissue. They exhibit morphology intermediate between that of white and brown adipocytes and contain fewer vesicles filled with lipids than brown adipocytes. In general, white adipose tissue stores energy reserves in lipid droplets, whereas the metabolic function of brown and beige adipose tissue is lipid oxidation to produce heat.

ORIENTATION MICROGRAPH: Shown here is white adipose tissue from the hypodermis of skin. It consists of numerous adipocytes closely packed in lobules. Dense irregular connective tissue (*DICT*) surrounds the adipose tissue. The loss of the fat within the cell during routine H&E slide preparation gives the adipose tissue a mesh-like appearance. Note the small blood vessels (*BV*) observed at the periphery of the tissue. They provide a rich capillary network within the adipose tissue. Several sweat gland ducts (*SGD*) are also present in the dense connective tissue.

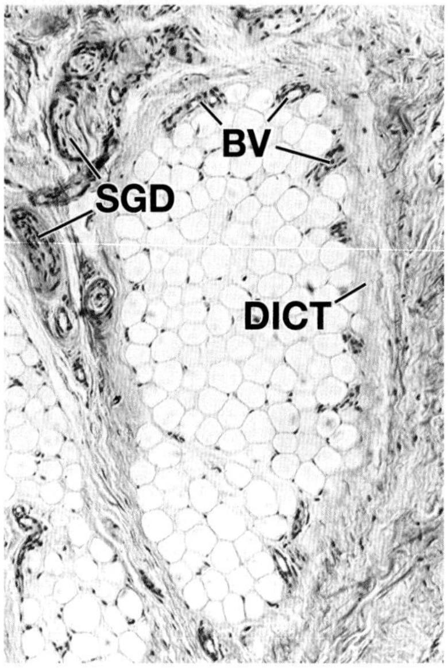

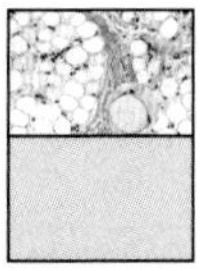

White adipose tissue, human, H&E ×363; inset ×700.

This is a higher magnification micrograph of **white adipose tissue** from the specimen shown in the orientation micrograph. It reveals portions of several lobules of adipose cells. Dense irregular connective tissue (*DICT*) separates the lobules from surrounding structures. In well-preserved specimens, the **adipocytes** (*A*) have a spherical profile in which they exhibit a very thin rim of cytoplasm surrounding a single large fat-containing vacuole. Because the fat is lost during tissue preparation, one only sees the rim of cytoplasm and an almost clear space. Between the cells, there is an extremely thin, delicate connective tissue stroma holding the adipocytes together, and within this stroma are small blood vessels (*BV*), mostly capillaries and venules. Most of the nuclei that are observed within the adipose tissue belong to fibroblasts, adipocytes, or cells of small blood vessels. However, distinguishing between fibroblast nuclei and adipocyte nuclei is often difficult. The *inset* shows a white adipocyte whose nucleus (*N*) is relatively easy to identify. It appears to reside within the rim of cytoplasm (*Cy*), giving the adipocyte the classic "signet-ring" appearance. A second nucleus (*N′*), partially out of the plane of section, appears to reside between the cytoplasmic rims of two adjacent cells. This is probably the nucleus of a fibroblast. Because of the relatively large size of the adipocyte, it is very infrequent that the nucleus of the cell is included in the plane of section of a given cell. Other cells that may be seen within the delicate connective tissue stroma are mast cells (*MC*).

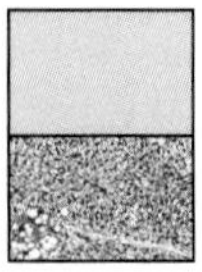

Brown adipose tissue, human, hematoxylin and eosin (H&E) ×450; inset ×1,100.

The **brown adipose tissue** shown here consists of small fat cells that are very closely packed with minimal intercellular space. Because of this arrangement, it is hard to define individual cells at this magnification. At higher magnification (not shown), it is possible to identify some individual cells. One cell, whose boundaries could be identified at higher magnification, is circumscribed by a *dotted line*. Each cell contains many small, fat-containing vacuoles surrounded by cytoplasm. Included in this cell is its nucleus (*N*). As noted, brown adipose tissue is highly vascularized, and in this specimen, one can see numerous blood vessels (*BV*) as evidenced by the red blood cells that they contain. It is even more difficult to distinguish fibroblasts within the lobule from nuclei of the fat cells. Even at higher magnification (*inset*), it is difficult to determine which nuclei belong to which cells. A capillary (*C*) can be identified in the *inset*. Again, it is recognized by the presence of red blood cells. Where the lobules are slightly separated from one another (*arrows*), small elongate nuclei of fibroblasts in the connective tissue septa can be recognized. These belong to fibroblasts in the connective tissue forming the septa.

A, adipocytes
BV, blood vessels
C, capillary
Cy, cytoplasm
DICT, dense irregular connective tissue
MC, mast cells
N, nucleus of adipocyte
N′, nucleus of fibroblast
SGD, sweat gland ducts
arrows, connective tissue septa

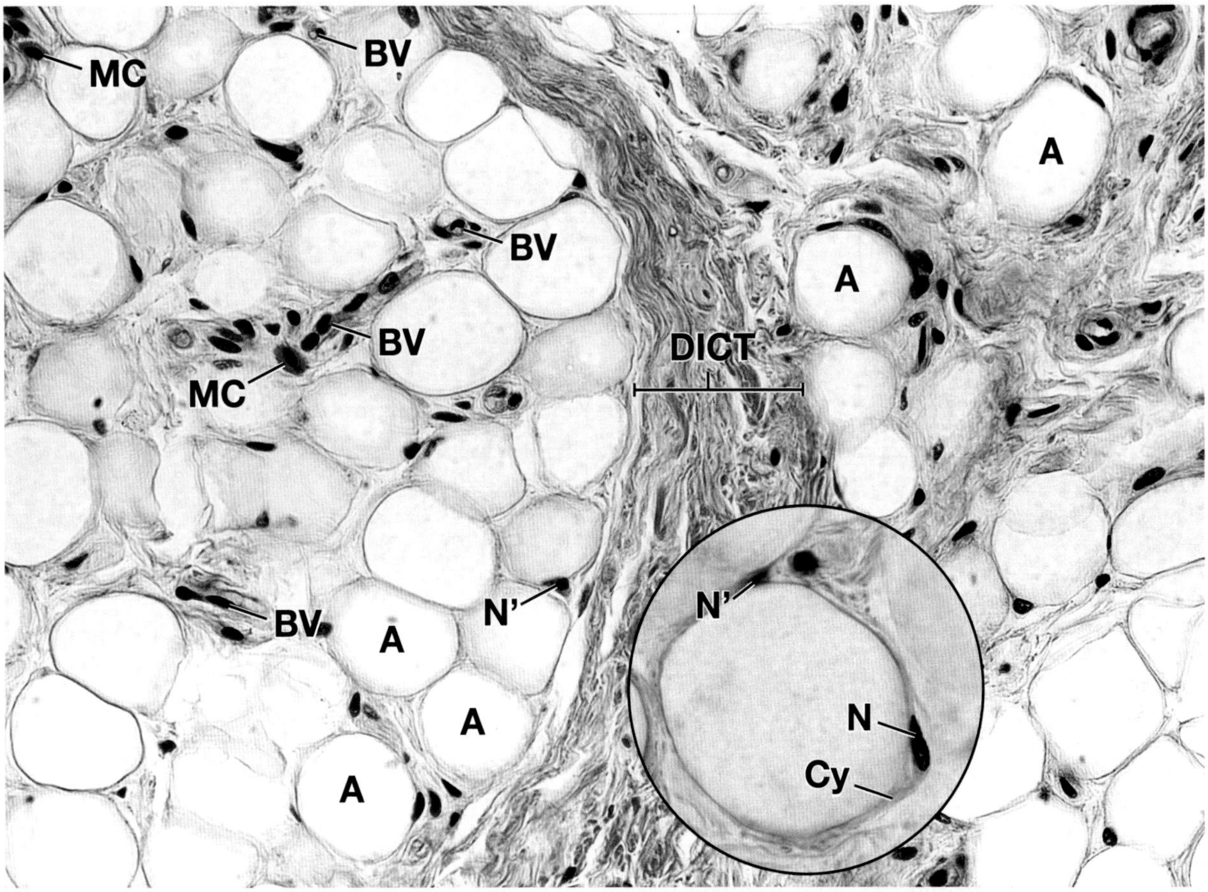
MC
BV
BV
BV
MC
DICT
A
A
BV
A
N'
A
A
N'
N
Cy

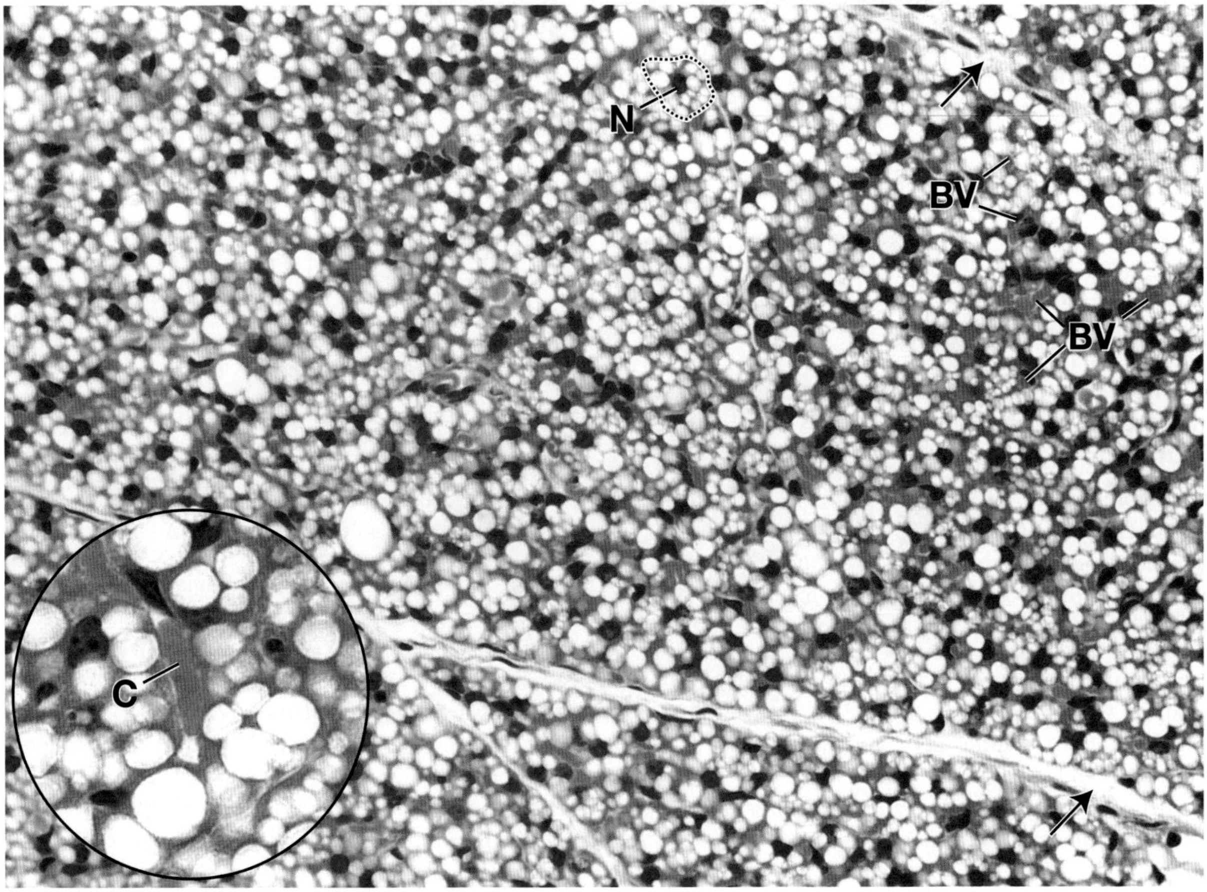
N
BV
BV
C

10 BLOOD

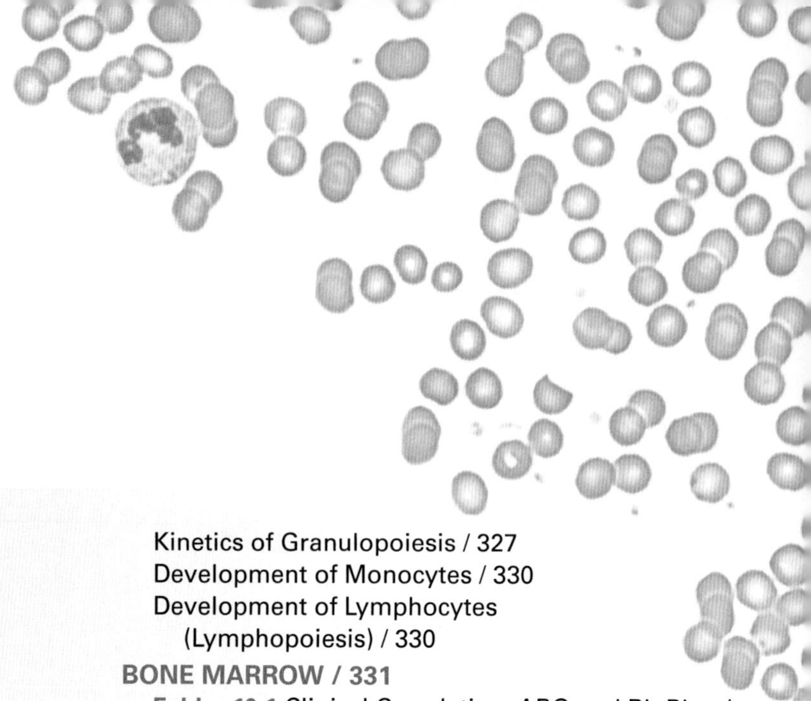

■ OVERVIEW OF BLOOD

Blood is a fluid connective tissue that circulates through the cardiovascular system.

Like other connective tissues, **blood** consists of cells and an extracellular component. Total blood volume in the average adult is approximately 6 L or 7%–8% of total body weight. The heart's pumping action propels blood through the cardiovascular system to the body tissues. Blood's many functions include the following:

- Delivery of nutrients and oxygen directly or indirectly to cells
- Transport of wastes and carbon dioxide away from cells
- Delivery of hormones and other regulatory substances to and from cells and tissues
- Maintenance of homeostasis by acting as a buffer and participating in coagulation and thermoregulation
- Transport of humoral agents and cells of the immune system that protect the body from pathogenic agents, foreign proteins, and transformed cells (e.g., cancer cells)

Blood consists of cells and their derivatives and a protein-rich fluid called plasma.

Blood cells and their derivatives include the following:

- **Erythrocytes**, also called **red blood cells**
- **Leukocytes**, also known as **white blood cells**
- **Thrombocytes**, also termed **platelets**

Plasma is the liquid extracellular material that imparts fluid properties to blood. The relative volume of cells and plasma in whole blood is approximately 45% and 55%, respectively. The volume of packed erythrocytes in a sample of blood is called the **hematocrit (HCT)** or **packed cell volume (PCV)**. The HCT is measured by centrifuging a blood sample to which anticoagulants have been added and then calculating the percentage of the centrifuge tube volume occupied by the erythrocytes compared with that of the whole blood (Fig. 10.1). A **normal hematocrit** is 39%–50% in men and 35%–45% in women; thus, 39%–50% and 35%–45% of the blood volume for men and women, respectively,

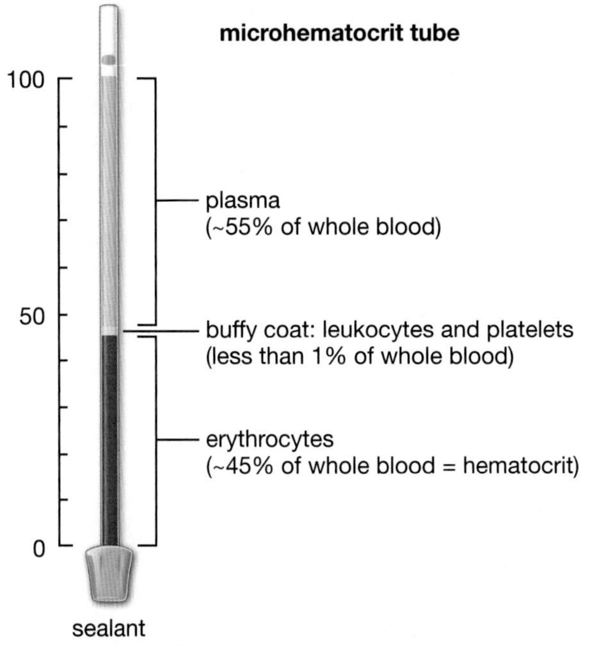

FIGURE 10.1. Blood composition. Blood composition is clearly apparent after centrifuging a small volume of blood in a microhematocrit tube. The volume of packed erythrocytes occupies about 45% of whole blood (this fraction is called *hematocrit*). The thin layer between erythrocytes and plasma contains leukocytes and platelets; it is often referred to as a *buffy coat*. The remaining volume (about 55%) consists of a *pale yellow*, opaque fluid and represents protein-rich blood plasma.

consist of erythrocytes. Low hematocrit values often reflect reduced numbers of circulating erythrocytes (a condition called **anemia**) and may indicate significant blood loss caused by internal or external bleeding.

Leukocytes and **platelets** constitute 1% of the blood volume. In a blood sample that has been centrifuged, the cell fraction (the part of the sample that contains the cells) consists mainly of packed erythrocytes (~99%). The leukocytes and platelets are contained in a narrow, light-colored layer between the erythrocytes and plasma called the **buffy coat** (see Fig. 10.1). As Table 10.1 indicates, there are nearly 1,000 times more erythrocytes (~5×10^{12} cells/L of blood) than leukocytes (~7×10^{9}/L of blood).

TABLE 10.1 Formed Elements of the Blood

Formed Elements	Cells/L in Adults		
	Male	Female	%
Erythrocytes	$4.3–5.7 \times 10^{12}$	$3.9–5.0 \times 10^{12}$	
Leukocytes	$3.5–10.5 \times 10^{9}$	$3.5–10.5 \times 10^{9}$	100
Agranulocytes			
Lymphocytes	$0.9–2.9 \times 10^{9}$	$0.9–2.9 \times 10^{9}$	25.7–27.6[a]
Monocytes	$0.3–0.9 \times 10^{9}$	$0.3–0.9 \times 10^{9}$	8.6[a]
Granulocytes			
Neutrophils	$1.7–7.0 \times 10^{9}$	$1.7–7.0 \times 10^{9}$	48.6–66.7[a]
Eosinophils	$0.05–0.5 \times 10^{9}$	$0.05–0.5 \times 10^{9}$	1.4–4.8[a]
Basophils	$0–0.3 \times 10^{9}$	$0–0.3 \times 10^{9}$	0–0.3[a]
Thrombocytes (platelets)	$150–450 \times 10^{9}$	$150–450 \times 10^{9}$	

[a]Percentage of leukocytes.

■ PLASMA

Although blood cells are of major interest in histology, a brief examination of plasma is also useful. The composition of **plasma** is summarized in Table 10.2. More than 90% of plasma by weight is water, which serves as the solvent for a variety of **solutes**, including proteins, dissolved gases, electrolytes, nutrients, regulatory substances, and waste materials. The solutes in the plasma help maintain **homeostasis**, a steady state that provides optimal pH and osmolarity for cellular metabolism.

Plasma proteins consist primarily of albumin, globulins, and fibrinogen.

Albumin is the main protein constituent of plasma, accounting for approximately one-half of the total plasma proteins. It is the smallest plasma protein (about 70 kDa) and is made in the liver. Albumin is responsible for exerting the concentration gradient between blood and extracellular tissue fluid. This major osmotic pressure on the blood vessel wall, called the **colloid osmotic pressure**, maintains the correct proportion of blood to tissue fluid volume. If a significant amount of albumin leaks out of the blood vessels into the loose connective tissue or is lost from the blood to urine in the kidneys, the colloid osmotic pressure of the blood decreases and fluid accumulates in the tissues. This increase in tissue fluid is most readily noted by swelling of the ankles at the end of the day. Albumin also acts as a carrier protein; it binds and transports hormones (thyroxine), metabolites (bilirubin), and drugs (barbiturates).

Globulins include **immunoglobulins (γ-globulins)**, the largest component of the globulin fraction, and **nonimmune globulins (α-globulin** and **β-globulin)**. Immunoglobulins are antibodies, a class of functional immune system molecules secreted by plasma cells. (Antibodies are discussed in Chapter 14, Immune System and Lymphatic Tissues and Organs, pages 488-490).

Nonimmune globulins are secreted by the liver. They help maintain the osmotic pressure within the vascular system and also serve as carrier proteins for various substances, such as copper (by ceruloplasmin), iron (by transferrin), and the protein **hemoglobin** (by haptoglobin). Nonimmune globulins also include fibronectin, lipoproteins, coagulation factors, and other molecules that are transferred between the blood and the extravascular connective tissue.

Fibrinogen, the largest plasma protein (340 kDa), is made in the liver. In a series of cascade reactions with other coagulation factors, soluble fibrinogen is transformed into insoluble protein **fibrin** (323 kDa). During the conversion of fibrinogen to fibrin, fibrinogen chains are broken to produce fibrin monomers that rapidly polymerize to form long fibers. These fibers become cross-linked to form an impermeable net at the site of damaged blood vessels, thereby preventing further blood loss.

With the exception of these large plasma proteins and regulatory substances, which are small proteins or polypeptides, most plasma constituents are small enough to pass through the blood vessel wall into the extracellular spaces of the adjacent connective tissue.

In general, plasma proteins react with common fixatives; they are often retained within the blood vessels in tissue

TABLE 10.2 Composition of Blood Plasma

Component	%
Water	91–92
Protein (albumin, globulins, fibrinogen)	7–8
Other solutes:	1–2
Electrolytes (Na^+, K^+, Ca^{2+}, Mg^{2+}, Cl^-, HCO^{3-}, PO_4^{3-}, SO_4^{2-})	
Nonprotein nitrogen substances (urea, uric acid, creatine, creatinine, ammonium salts)	
Nutrients (glucose, lipids, amino acids)	
Blood gases (oxygen, carbon dioxide, nitrogen)	
Regulatory substances (hormones, enzymes)	

sections. Plasma proteins do not possess a structural form above the molecular level; thus, when they are retained in blood vessels in the tissue block, they appear as a homogeneous substance that stains evenly with eosin in hematoxylin and eosin (H&E)-stained sections.

Serum is the same as blood plasma, except that clotting factors have been removed.

For laboratory purposes, samples of blood are often drawn from a vein (a procedure called **venipuncture**). When blood is removed from the circulation, it immediately clots. A **blood clot** consists mostly of erythrocytes entangled in a network of fine fibers composed of fibrin. To prevent clotting of a blood sample, an **anticoagulant** such as citrate or heparin is added to the blood specimen as it is obtained. Citrate binds calcium ions, which are essential for triggering the cascade of coagulation reactions; heparin deactivates the clotting factors in the plasma. Plasma that lacks coagulation factors is called **serum**. For many biochemical laboratory tests, plasma and blood serum can be used interchangeably. Serum is preferred for several specific tests because the anticoagulants in plasma can interfere with the results. However, tests of clotting ability require that all coagulation factors be preserved; therefore, serum is inappropriate for these tests.

The interstitial fluid of connective tissues is derived from blood plasma.

The fluid that surrounds tissue cells, called **interstitial fluid**, has an electrolyte composition that reflects that of blood plasma, from which it is derived. The composition of interstitial fluid in nonconnective tissues, however, is subject to considerable modification by the absorptive and secretory activities of epithelia. Epithelia may create special microenvironments conducive to their function. For example, a blood–brain barrier exists between the blood and the nerve tissue. Barriers also exist between the blood and the parenchymal tissue in the testis, thymus gland, eye, and other epithelial compartments. Fluids, barriers, and their functions are discussed in subsequent chapters that describe these particular organs.

Examination of blood cells requires special preparation and staining.

The preparation method that best displays the cell types of peripheral blood is the **blood smear**. This method differs from usual histologic preparations in that the specimen is not embedded in paraffin and sectioned. Rather, a drop of blood is placed directly on a slide and spread thinly over the surface of the slide (i.e., "pulled" with the edge of another slide) to produce a monolayer of cells (Fig. 10.2a). The preparation is then air dried and stained. Another difference in the preparation of a blood smear is that instead of H&E, special mixtures of dyes are used to stain the blood cells. The resulting preparation may then be examined with a high-power oil-immersion lens, with or without a coverslip (Fig. 10.2b and Plate 10.1, page 336).

The modified Romanowsky-type stain commonly used for blood smears consists of a mixture of methylene blue (a basic dye), related azures (also basic dyes), and eosin (an acidic dye). On the basis of their appearance after staining,

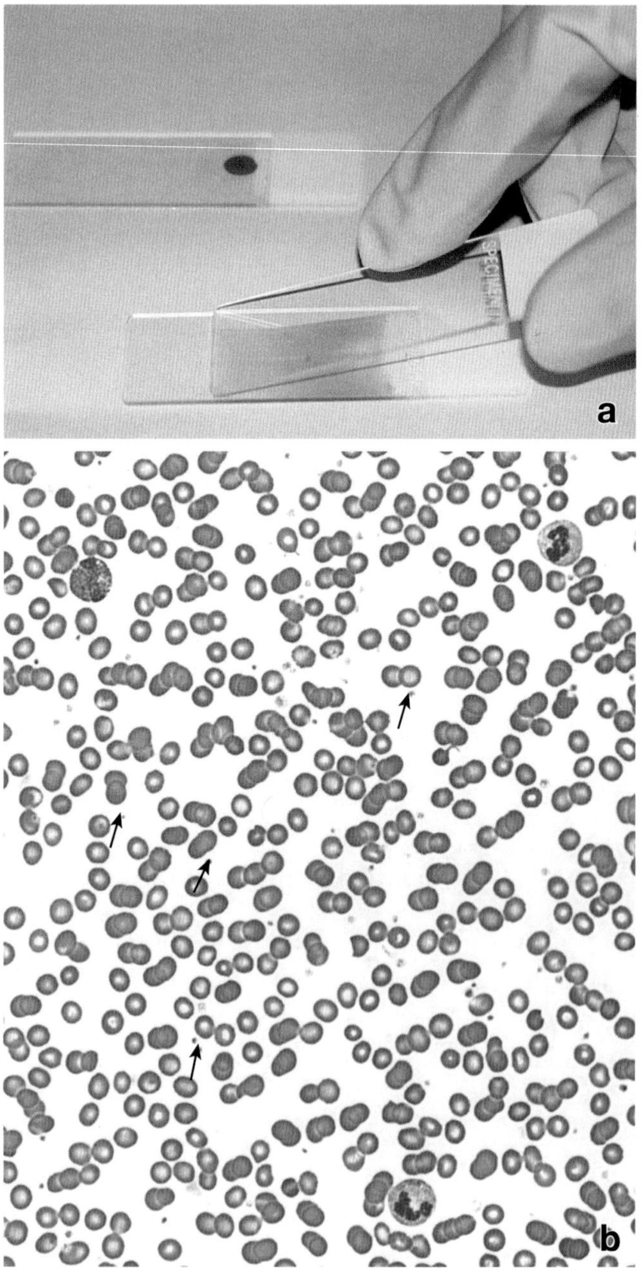

FIGURE 10.2. Blood smear: preparation technique and overview photomicrograph. a. Photograph showing the method of producing a blood smear. A drop of blood is placed directly on a glass slide and spread over its surface with the edge of another slide. **b.** Photomicrograph of smear from peripheral blood stained with Wright stain showing the cells evenly distributed. The cells are mainly erythrocytes. Three leukocytes are present. Platelets are indicated by *arrows*. ×350.

leukocytes are traditionally divided into **granulocytes** (neutrophils, eosinophils, and basophils) and **agranulocytes** (lymphocytes and monocytes). Although both cell types may contain granules, granulocytes possess obvious, specifically stained granules in their cytoplasm. In general, the basic dyes stain nuclei, granules of basophils, and RNA in the cytoplasm, whereas the acidic dye stains the erythrocytes and the granules of eosinophils. Scientists originally thought that the fine neutrophil granules were stained by a "neutral dye" that formed when methylene blue and its related azures were combined with eosin. The mechanism by which the specific neutrophil granules are stained is still not clearly understood. Some of the basic dyes (the azures) are metachromatic and may impart a violet to red color to the material they stain.

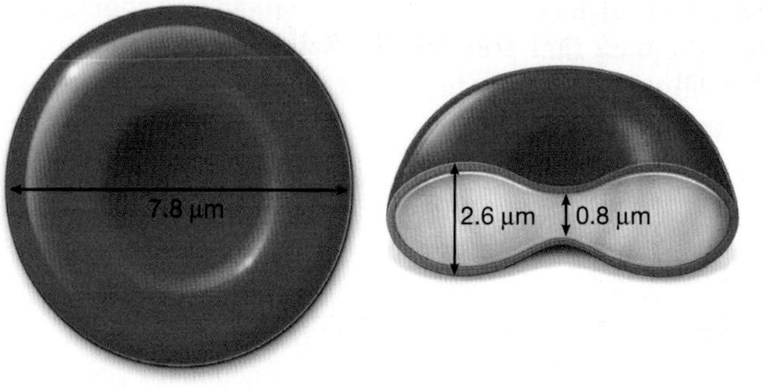

FIGURE 10.3. Erythrocyte. The erythrocyte is an anucleated cell in a shape of a biconcave disc containing hemoglobin. The surface area of an erythrocyte is about 140 μm^2, and its mean corpuscular (cell) volume ranges from 80 to 99 fL (1 fL = 10^{-15} L).

■ ERYTHROCYTES

Erythrocytes are anucleate, biconcave discs.

Erythrocytes or **red blood cells** are anucleate cells devoid of typical organelles. They function only within the bloodstream to bind oxygen for delivery to the tissues and, in exchange, bind carbon dioxide for removal from the tissues. Their shape is that of a biconcave disc with a **diameter of 7.8 µm**, an edge thickness of 2.6 µm, and a central thickness of 0.8 µm (Fig. 10.3). This shape maximizes the cell's surface area (~140 μm^2), an important attribute in gas exchange.

The life span of erythrocytes is approximately **120 days.** In a healthy individual, approximately 1% of erythrocytes are removed from the circulation each day because of senescence (aging); however, the bone marrow continuously produces new erythrocytes to replace those lost. The majority of aged erythrocytes (~90%) are phagocytosed by macrophages in the spleen, bone marrow, and liver. The remaining aged erythrocytes (~10%) break down intravascularly, releasing insignificant amounts of hemoglobin (Hgb) into the blood.

In H&E-stained sections, erythrocytes are usually 7–8 µm in diameter. Because their size is relatively consistent in fixed tissue, they can be used to estimate the size of other cells and structures in tissue sections; in this role, erythrocytes are appropriately referred to as the "**histologic ruler.**"

Because both living and preserved erythrocytes usually appear as biconcave discs, they can give the impression that their form is rigid and inelastic (Fig. 10.4). They are, in fact, extremely deformable. They pass easily through the narrowest capillaries by folding over on themselves. They stain uniformly with eosin. In thin sections viewed with the transmission electron microscope (TEM), the contents of an erythrocyte appear as a dense, finely granular material.

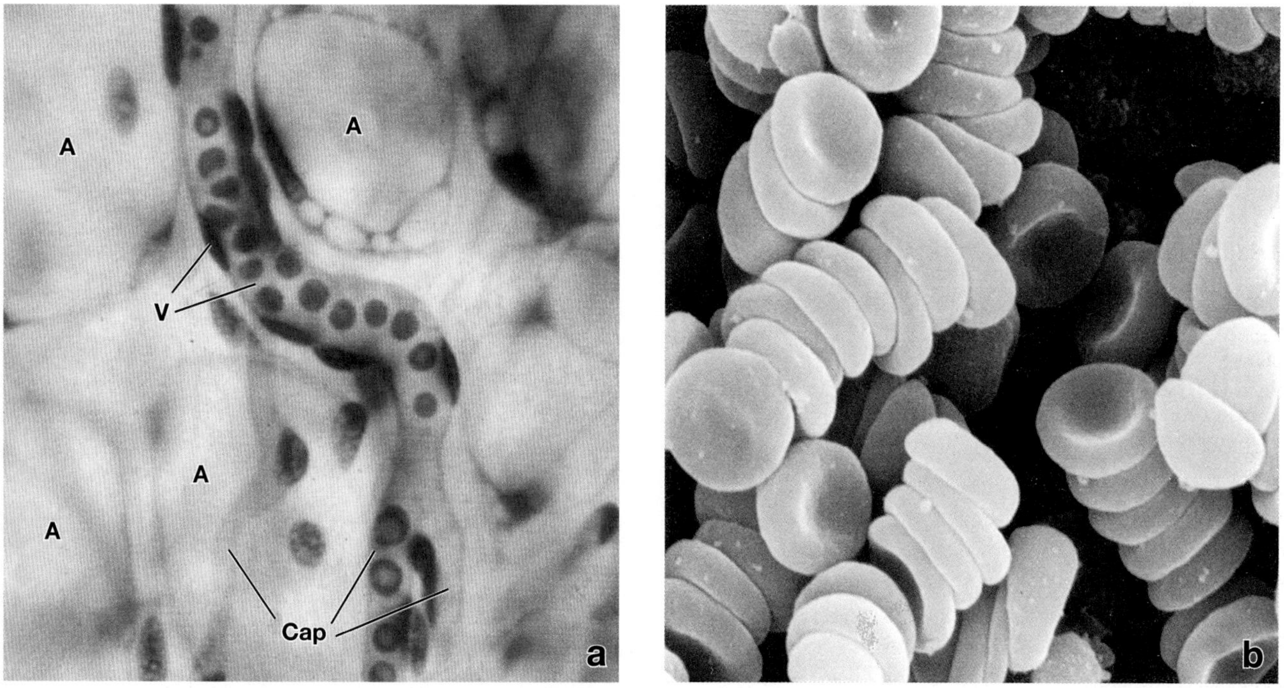

FIGURE 10.4. Erythrocyte morphology. a. Photomicrograph of three capillaries (*Cap*) joining to form a venule (*V*), as observed in adipose tissue within a full-thickness mesentery spread. The erythrocytes appear in a single file in one of the capillaries (the other two are empty). The *light center* area of some of the erythrocytes results from their biconcave shape. Erythrocytes are highly plastic and can fold on themselves when passing through very narrow capillaries. The large round structures are adipose cells (*A*). ×470. **b.** Scanning electron micrograph of erythrocytes collected in a blood tube. Note the biconcave shape of the cells. The stacks of erythrocytes in these preparations are not unusual and are referred to as *rouleau*. Such formations in vivo indicate an increased level of plasma immunoglobulin. ×2,800.

The shape of the erythrocyte is maintained by a specialized cytoskeleton that provides the mechanical stability and flexibility necessary to withstand forces experienced during circulation.

As erythrocytes in circulation navigate through a small network of capillaries, they are exposed to high amounts of shear force that cause them to undergo rapid and reversible deformations. To cope with this stress, the erythrocyte cell membrane has a unique cytoskeletal structure. In addition to a typical lipid bilayer, it contains two functionally significant groups of proteins.

- **Integral membrane proteins** represent most of the proteins in the lipid bilayer. They consist of two major families: glycophorins and band 3 proteins. The extracellular domains of these integral membrane proteins are glycosylated and express specific blood group antigens. **Glycophorin C**, a member of the glycophorin family of transmembrane proteins, assists in attaching the underlying cytoskeletal protein network to the cell membrane. **Band 3 protein** is the most abundant transmembrane protein in the erythrocyte cell membrane. It binds Hgb and acts as an anchoring site for cytoskeletal proteins (Fig. 10.5).
- **Peripheral membrane proteins** reside on the inner surface of the cell membrane. They are organized into a two-dimensional hexagonal lattice network that laminates the inner layer of the membrane. The lattice itself, which is positioned parallel to the membrane, is composed mainly of cytoskeletal proteins, including **α-spectrin** and **β-spectrin** molecules. They assemble to form an antiparallel heterodimer held together by multiple lateral bonds. Dimers then associate in a head-to-head formation to produce long and flexible tetramers. The spectrin filaments are anchored to the lipid bilayer by two large protein complexes. The first is the **band 4.1 protein complex** containing band 4.1, actin, tropomyosin, tropomodulin, adducin, and dematin (see Fig. 10.5); this complex interacts with glycophorin C and other transmembrane proteins. The second complex is the **ankyrin protein complex** containing ankyrin and band 4.2 protein; this complex interacts with band 3 and other integral membrane proteins (see Fig. 10.5).

This unique cytoskeletal arrangement contributes to the shape of the erythrocyte and imparts elastic properties and stability to the membrane. The cytoskeleton is not static. For example, molecular bonds along the length of spectrin molecules dissociate and reassociate as the erythrocyte undergoes deformation in response to various physical factors and chemical stimuli. Therefore, flexible interactions within spectrin dimers, ankyrin, and band 4.1 complexes are key regulators of membrane elasticity and mechanical stability. Any change in the expression of genes that encode these cytoskeleton proteins can result in abnormally shaped and fragile erythrocytes. For example, **hereditary spherocytosis** is an autosomal dominant genetic disorder affecting

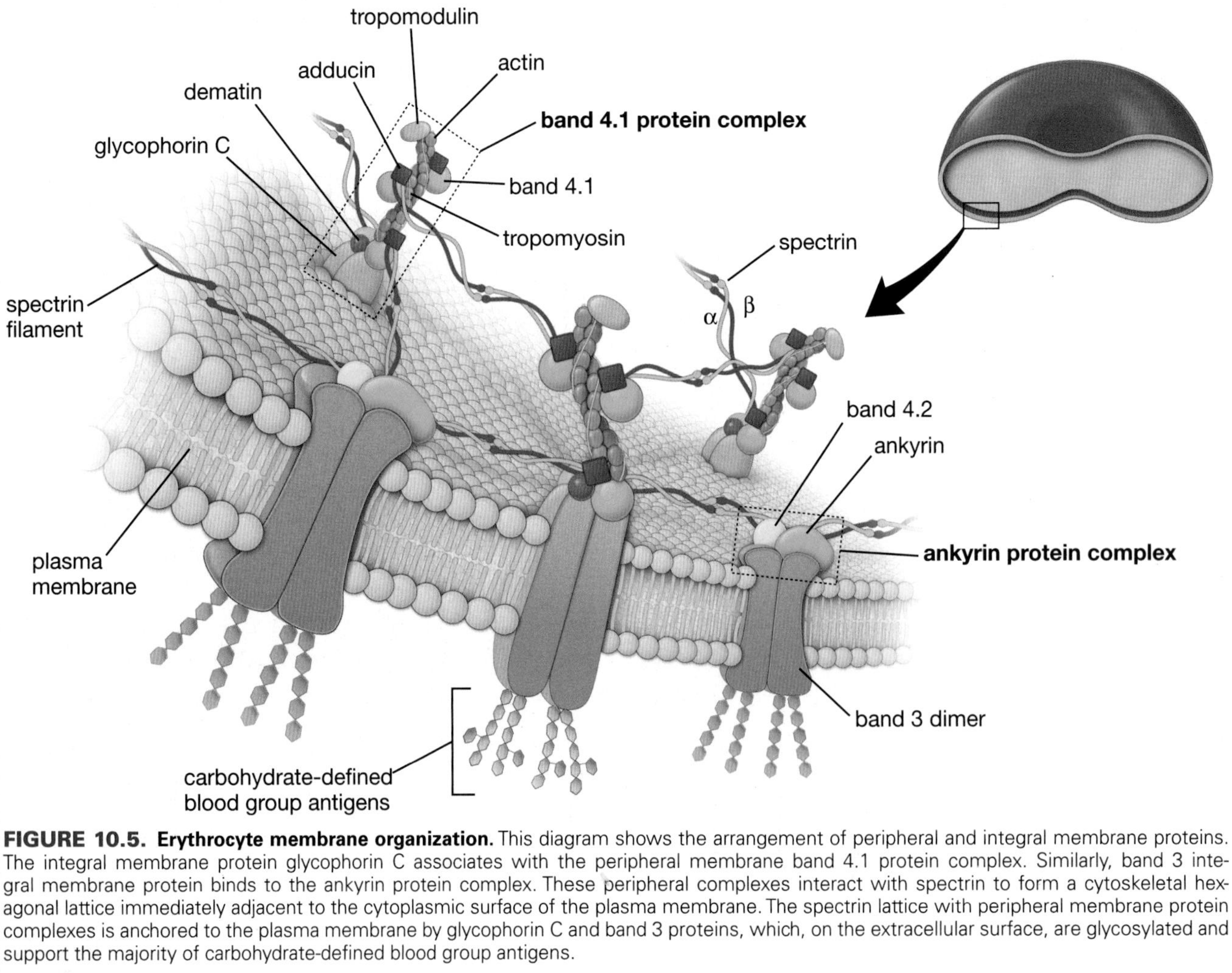

FIGURE 10.5. Erythrocyte membrane organization. This diagram shows the arrangement of peripheral and integral membrane proteins. The integral membrane protein glycophorin C associates with the peripheral membrane band 4.1 protein complex. Similarly, band 3 integral membrane protein binds to the ankyrin protein complex. These peripheral complexes interact with spectrin to form a cytoskeletal hexagonal lattice immediately adjacent to the cytoplasmic surface of the plasma membrane. The spectrin lattice with peripheral membrane protein complexes is anchored to the plasma membrane by glycophorin C and band 3 proteins, which, on the extracellular surface, are glycosylated and support the majority of carbohydrate-defined blood group antigens.

ankyrin complex proteins (band 3, band 4.2, spectrin, and other erythrocyte integral membrane proteins) that function in anchoring the erythrocyte plasma membrane to the cytoplasm. Defects in these anchoring proteins cause the erythrocyte's plasma membrane to detach and peel off from the cytoplasm and result in spherical erythrocytes. Another erythrocyte membrane abnormality, **hereditary elliptocytosis**, is caused by one of several autosomal dominant mutations affecting spectrin molecules. In this mutation, spectrin-to-spectrin lateral bonds and spectrin–ankyrin–band 4.1 protein junctions are defective. The plasma membrane in the affected cells fails to rebound from deformations and progressively elongates, resulting in the formation of elliptical erythrocytes. In both conditions, erythrocytes are unable to adapt to changes in the environment (e.g., osmotic pressure and mechanical deformations), which results in premature destruction of the cells or **hemolysis**.

Erythrocytes contain hemoglobin, a protein specialized for the transport of oxygen and carbon dioxide.

Erythrocytes transport oxygen and carbon dioxide bound to the protein **hemoglobin** (68 kDa). Hgb binds to oxygen molecules in the lung (which requires a high oxygen affinity) and, after transporting it through the circulatory system, unloads oxygen in the tissues (which requires a low oxygen affinity). A monomer of Hgb is similar in composition and structure to myoglobin, the oxygen-binding protein found in striated muscle. The disc shape of the erythrocyte facilitates gas exchange because more Hgb molecules fit more closely to the plasma membrane than they would be in a spherical cell. Thus, gases have less distance to diffuse within the cell to reach a binding site on the Hgb. A high concentration of Hgb is present within erythrocytes and is responsible for their uniform staining with eosin and the cytoplasmic granularity seen with the TEM.

FOLDER 10.1

CLINICAL CORRELATION: ABO AND RH BLOOD GROUP SYSTEMS

ABO Blood Group System

An important factor in blood transfusion is the **ABO blood group system**, which essentially involves three antigens called *A*, *B*, and *O* (Table F10.1.1). These antigens are glycoproteins and glycolipids and differ only slightly in their composition. They are present on the surface of erythrocytes and are attached to the extracellular domains of integral membrane proteins called **glycophorins** and **band 3 proteins**. The presence of A, B, or O antigens determines the four primary **blood groups: A, B, AB,** and **O**. All humans have enzymes that catalyze the synthesis of the O antigen. Blood is described as a specific type depending on the presence or absence of AB group antigens. Individuals with type A blood have an additional enzyme (***N*-acetylgalactosamine transferase** or **N-Acetylglucosamine transferase**) that adds *N*-acetylgalactosamine to the O antigen. Individuals with type B blood have an enzyme (**galactose transferase** or B-glycosyltransferase) that adds galactose to the O antigen (Fig. F10.1.1). Individuals with type AB blood express both enzymes, whereas individuals who lack both enzymes have type O blood. In humans, **ABO genes** consist of at least seven exons, and they are located on chromosome 9. The O allele is recessive, whereas A and B alleles are codominant.

The differences in the carbohydrate molecules of these antigens are detected by specific antibodies against either A or B antigen. Individuals with type A blood possess serum anti-B antibodies that are directed against the B antigen. Individuals with type B blood possess serum anti-A antibodies that are directed against the A antigen. Individuals with type AB blood do not have antibodies directed against A or B antigen. Thus, they are **universal acceptors** of any blood type. Individuals with type O blood have both anti-A and anti-B antibodies in their serum and neither A nor B antigen on their erythrocytes. Thus, these individuals are **universal blood donors**.

If an individual is transfused with blood of an incompatible type, the recipient's antibodies will attack the donor erythrocytes, causing a **hemolytic transfusion reaction** or destruction of the transfused erythrocytes. To prevent such a life-threatening complication, blood for transfusion must be always cross-matched to the blood of a recipient. In this procedure, serum from the recipient is tested against the donor's erythrocytes. If there is no reaction to this cross-match test, then the donor's blood can be used for the transfusion.

TABLE F10.1.1 ABO Blood Group System

Blood Type	Erythrocyte Surface Antigen	Serum Antibody	Can Give Blood to	Can Receive Blood From
A	A antigen	Anti-B	A and AB	A and O
B	B antigen	Anti-A	B and AB	B and O
AB	A and B antigens	No antibodies	Only AB	A, B, AB, and O (universal blood recipient)
O	O antigen (no A or B antigen)	Anti-A and anti-B	A, B, AB, and O (universal blood donor)	Only O

(*continued*)

FOLDER 10.1

CLINICAL CORRELATION: ABO AND RH BLOOD GROUP SYSTEMS (*continued*)

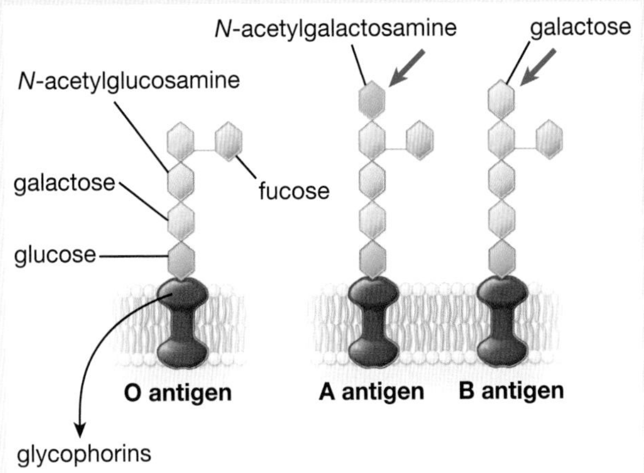

FIGURE F10.1.1. ABO blood group antigens. The ABO antigens are not primary gene products but are instead products of enzymatic reactions (glycosylations). This schematic drawing shows the differences between the three major antigens responsible for the ABO blood group system. The immunodominant structure of antigen O is depicted as it attaches to an extracellular domain of glycophorins, the integral membrane proteins of erythrocyte cell membranes. Note that differences between O antigen and A antigen are due to the presence of an additional sugar molecule, *N*-acetylgalactosamine (*blue arrow middle*), which is added by genetically encoded functional *N*-acetylgalactosamine transferase expressed in individuals with type A blood. Similarly, individuals with type B blood have a galactose molecule (*blue arrow right*) attached by the enzyme galactose transferase. Individuals with type AB blood express both enzymes (thus, both A and B antigens are present) and individuals with type O blood lack both functional enzymes, thus possessing only the immunodominant core structure of antigen O.

Rh Blood Group System

The other important blood group system, the **Rh system**, is based on the **Rhesus (Rh) antigen**. In humans, this system is represented by a 40-kDa transmembrane nonglycosylated **Rh30 polypeptide** that shares antigenic sites with rhesus monkey erythrocytes. Rh30 polypeptide is a component of a larger (90-kDa) erythrocyte integral membrane protein complex that includes **Rh50 glycoprotein**. Although the Rh30 polypeptide expresses many antigen sites on its extracellular domain, only five of them—**D**, **C**, **c**, **E**, and **e antigens**—have clinical significance. Interactions between Rh30 and Rh50 molecules are essential for the expression of D, C, c, E, and e antigens. Only one D antigen determines Rh status. Therefore, an individual who possesses D antigen is referred to as **Rh positive (Rh+)**, and an individual who lacks expressed D antigen is referred to as **Rh negative (Rh–)**. All antigens stimulate the production of anti-Rh antibodies in individuals without the same antigens.

Rh incompatibility—in which a pregnant individual is **Rh(D–)** and the fetus is Rh(D+)—can become a major clinical issue in pregnancy if it is not detected early and preventive measures are taken. If an individual is Rh(D−) and becomes pregnant with an Rh(D+) fetus, anti-D antibodies will be produced in response to the D antigen expressed on fetal erythrocytes. This is called **Rh(D+) sensitization**. Fetal erythrocytes can leak into the circulation during pregnancy, childbirth, or following a miscarriage or abortion. Usually, there are not enough antibodies produced during a first pregnancy to cause a reaction in the fetus. However, if a sensitized individual becomes pregnant again with an Rh(D+) fetus, the antibodies may cross the placenta and attack the Rh(D+) antigens on the fetal red blood cells, triggering a hemolytic transfusion reaction in the fetus called **erythroblastosis fetalis**. Administration of **anti-D immunoglobulin (RhoGAM)** to any Rh(D−) person during and following each pregnancy or following a miscarriage destroys any circulating Rh(D+) fetal erythrocytes that persist in the person's blood, thus preventing Rh-incompatibility reactions in future pregnancies.

Hemoglobin consists of four polypeptide chains of globin: α, β, δ, and γ. Each polypeptide chain is bound to an iron-containing heme group (Fig. 10.6). During oxygenation, each of the four iron-containing heme groups can reversibly bind one oxygen molecule. During gestational and postnatal periods, the synthesis of Hgb polypeptide chains varies, resulting in different Hgb types (Fig. 10.7). Depending on the activation of different globin genes and the particular globin chain being synthesized, the following types of Hgb can be distinguished:

- **HbA** is most prevalent in adults, accounting for about 96% of total hemoglobin. It is a tetramer with two α-chains and two β-chains (α2β2).
- **HbA$_2$** accounts for 1.5%–3% of total Hgb in adults. It consists of two α-chains and two δ-chains (α2δ2).
- **HbF** accounts for less than 1% of total Hgb in adults. It contains two α-chains and two γ-chains (α2γ2) and is the principal form of Hgb in the fetus. HbF production falls dramatically after birth; however, some individuals produce HbF throughout their lives. Although HbF persists in slightly higher percentages than normal in those with **sickle cell disease** and **thalassemia**, it does not appear to have a pathologic role.

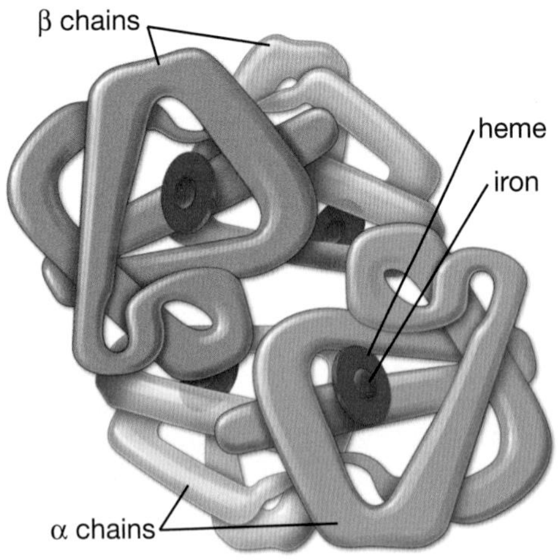

FIGURE 10.6. Structural diagram of the hemoglobin molecule. Each hemoglobin molecule is composed of four subunits. Each subunit contains a heme, the iron-containing portion of hemoglobin, embedded in a hydrophobic cleft of a globin chain. The folding of the globin chain places the heme near the surface of the molecule, where it is readily accessible to oxygen. There are four different types of globin chains: α, β, δ, and γ, occurring in pairs. The types of globin chains present in the molecules determine the type of hemoglobin. The figure illustrates hemoglobin A (HbA), which is composed of two α-chains and two β-chains.

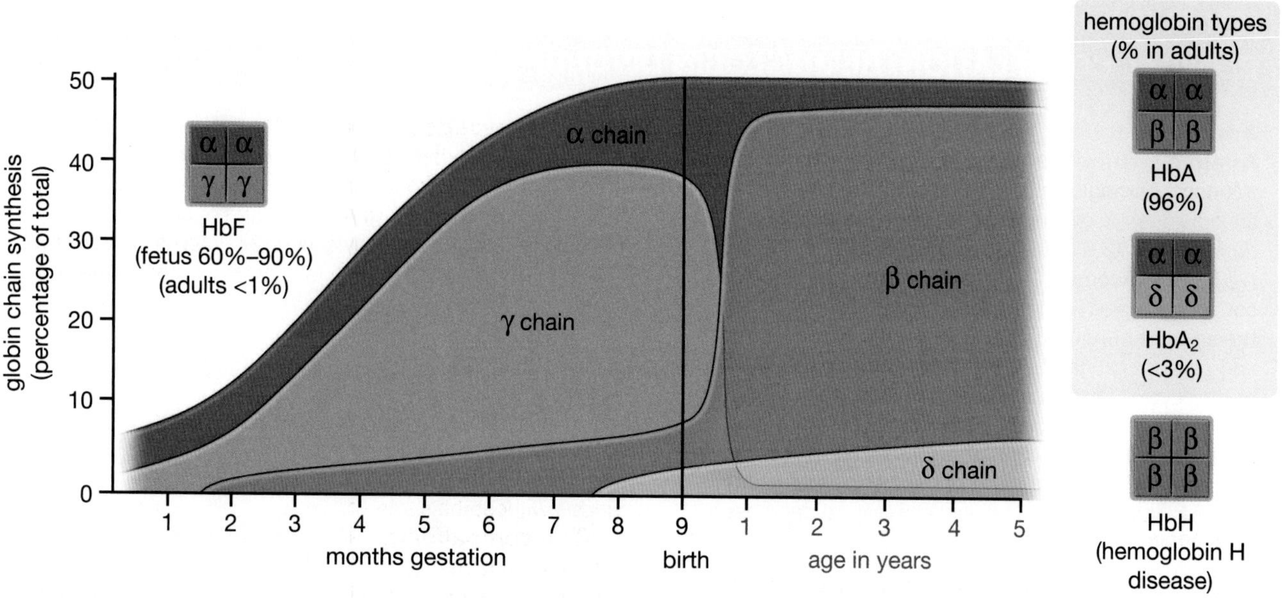

FIGURE 10.7. Major globin chain synthesis and hemoglobin composition in prenatal and postnatal periods. The type of hemoglobin differs in the gestational and postnatal periods. This diagram represents a timeline for the synthesis of the four major globin chains (α, β, δ, and γ) and for hemoglobin composition. In the early stages of development, α- and γ-chains form fetal hemoglobin (HbF), which predominates at birth. In the second month of gestation, synthesis of β-chains gradually increases. After birth, it drastically escalates to form with α-chains, predominately adult hemoglobin (HbA). During this time, γ-chain synthesis declines. During the eighth month of prenatal development, δ-chain production is initiated to form hemoglobin containing two δ-chains and two α-chains (HbA_2). Adult hemoglobin types HbA (96%) and HbA_2 (<3%) within the *light blue box* are regarded as normal hemoglobin types. Traces of HbF are considered normal in levels <1%. An example of the pathologic hemoglobin shown in this diagram is HbH, which is formed as a tetramer of β-chains.

Mutations in the genes encoding the globin chains can cause disorders in hemoglobin production. One example is **hemoglobin H (HbH) disease**, which is caused by molecular defects of the globin α-chain genes in which expression of the globin α-chain is decreased. On the molecular level, HbH disease is characterized by the accumulation of excess β-chains that form tetramers (β2β2; see Fig. 10.7). Clinically, it is characterized by mild chronic hemolytic anemia with high reticulocyte counts (5%–10%). Another example is a mutation in the gene encoding the globin β-chain that causes **sickle cell disease** (see Folder 10.3). Interestingly, more than 550 types of abnormal hemoglobin molecules have been identified, but most have no clinical significance.

■ LEUKOCYTES

Leukocytes are subclassified into two general groups. The basis for this division is the presence or absence of prominent **specific granules** in the cytoplasm. As previously noted, cells containing specific granules are classified as **granulocytes** (neutrophils, eosinophils, and basophils) (Plate 10.1, page 336), and cells that lack specific granules are classified as **agranulocytes** (lymphocytes and monocytes) (Plate 10.2, page 338). However, both agranulocytes and granulocytes possess a small number of nonspecific **azurophilic granules**, which are lysosomes. The relative number of the various leukocytes is given in Table 10.1.

FOLDER 10.2

CLINICAL CORRELATION: HEMOGLOBIN IN PATIENTS WITH DIABETES

As mentioned in the text, about 96% of total hemoglobin in adults is represented by **hemoglobin type HbA**. Approximately 8% of HbA consists of several subtypes that display slight chemical differences. These subtypes are HbA1a1, HbA1a2, HbA1b, and HbA1c. Of these subtypes, **hemoglobin type A1c** is of clinical significance because it binds irreversibly to glucose. It is referred to as **glycated** or **glycosylated hemoglobin**. Levels of this hemoglobin subtype are used to monitor an individual's blood glucose levels over the previous 2–3 months (clinically referred to as an **A1c test**). Individuals with diabetes have increased levels of glycated HbA1c in the blood because of their elevated blood glucose level. Because the normal life span of erythrocytes is about 120 days (see page 301), glycated hemoglobin can only be eliminated when the red blood cells containing it are destroyed. Thus, HbA1c values are directly proportional to the concentration of glucose in the blood over the entire life span of the erythrocyte. In healthy individuals and in those with diabetes that is being effectively controlled, HbA1c levels should not be >7% of the total hemoglobin. Because HbA1c values are not subject to short-term fluctuations in blood glucose levels, this measurement can be performed at any time and does not require fasting.

FOLDER 10.3

CLINICAL CORRELATION: HEMOGLOBIN DISORDERS

Anemia

Anemia is defined clinically as a decrease in the concentration of hemoglobin in the blood for the age and sex of an individual. A low hemoglobin concentration is generally defined as <13.5 g/dL (135 g/L) for men and <12 g/dL (120 g/L) for women. In certain anemias, the decreased concentration of hemoglobin is caused by a decrease in the amount of hemoglobin in each cell. However, most anemias are caused by a reduction in the number of erythrocytes. Causes of anemia include loss of blood (hemorrhage), insufficient production of erythrocytes, or accelerated destruction of erythrocytes in the circulation. Insufficient dietary iron or deficiencies of vitamins such as vitamin B_{12} or folic acid can lead to decreased production of erythrocytes. Gastric atrophy, as a result of autoimmune disease, with concomitant destruction of the parietal cells that secrete **intrinsic factor**, a molecule essential for absorption of vitamin B_{12} by cells in the ileum, is the cause of a form of anemia called **pernicious anemia**. The clinical symptoms of anemia vary, depending on the type of anemia, the underlying cause, and other associated medical conditions. The common symptoms of even mild anemia include weakness, fatigue, and loss of energy. The other symptoms associated with anemia are shortness of breath, frequent headaches, difficulty concentrating, mental confusion, loss of sexual drive, dizziness, leg cramps, insomnia, and pale skin.

Sickle Cell Disease

Sickle cell disease is caused by a single-point mutation in the gene that encodes the **β-globin chain of hemoglobin A (HbA)**. The result of this mutation is an abnormal β-globin chain in which the amino acid valine is substituted for glutamic acid in position 6. Hemoglobin containing this abnormal β-globin chain is designated **sickle hemoglobin (HbS)**. The substitution of the hydrophobic valine for the hydrophilic glutamic acid causes HbS molecules during conditions of low oxygen saturation to aggregate and grow in length beyond the diameter of the erythrocyte. Instead of the normal biconcave disc shape, many of the erythrocytes become sickle shaped, hence the name of this disease (Fig. F10.3.1). The sickling process is reversible and begins when oxygen saturation is reduced to <85% in homozygous individuals and <40% in heterozygous individuals. Sickled erythrocytes are more rigid than normal cells and adhere more readily to the endothelial surface. Thus, the blood becomes more viscous and sickled erythrocytes may pile up in the smallest capillaries, depriving portions of tissues and organs of oxygen and nutrients. Large-vessel obstruction may also occur, which, in children, frequently leads to stroke. Sickled erythrocytes are also more fragile and break down or are destroyed more quickly (after 20 days) than normal erythrocytes.

Sickle cell disease is a homozygous recessive genetic disorder. However, heterozygous individuals with sickle cell trait may occasionally have clinical consequences at high altitude or when under extreme physical stress.

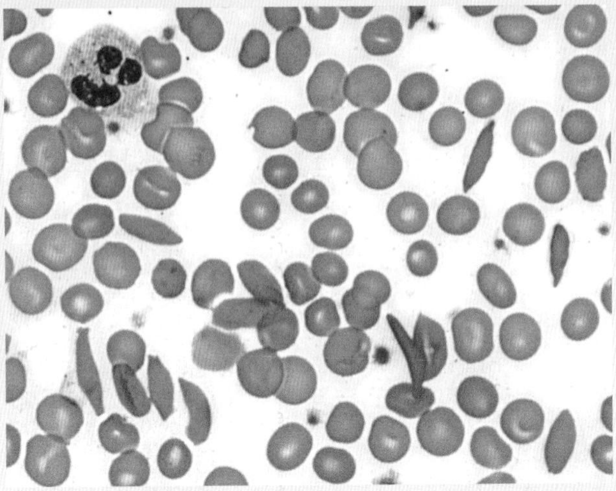

FIGURE F10.3.1. Photomicrograph of a sickle cell anemia blood smear. Blood smear stained with Wright stain shows abnormal "boat" and "sickle" shaped cells from an individual with sickle cell anemia. ×400.

Neutrophils

Neutrophils are the most numerous white blood cells as well as the most common granulocytes.

Neutrophils measure 10–12 μm in diameter in blood smears and are obviously larger than erythrocytes. Although named for their lack of characteristic cytoplasmic staining, they are also readily identified by their multilobal nucleus; thus, they are also called **polymorphonuclear neutrophils** or polymorphs. Mature neutrophils possess two to four lobes of nuclear material joined by thinner nuclear strands (Plate 10.1, page 336). The arrangement is not static; rather, in living neutrophils, the lobes and connecting strands change their shape, position, and even number.

The chromatin of the neutrophil has a characteristic arrangement. Wide regions of heterochromatin are located chiefly at the periphery of the nucleus and are in contact with the nuclear envelope. Regions of euchromatin are located primarily at the center of the nucleus, with relatively smaller regions contacting the nuclear envelope (Fig. 10.8). In women, the **Barr body** (the condensed, single, inactive X chromosome) forms a drumstick-shaped appendage on one of the nuclear lobes.

Neutrophils contain three types of granules.

The cytoplasm of a neutrophil contains three kinds of granules. The different types of granules reflect the various phagocytotic functions of the cell:

- **Azurophilic granules (primary granules)** are larger and less numerous than specific granules. They arise early in granulopoiesis and occur in all granulocytes as well as in monocytes and lymphocytes. The azurophilic granules are the lysosomes of the neutrophil and contain **myeloperoxidase (MPO)** (a peroxidase enzyme), which appears as a finely stippled material with the TEM. MPO

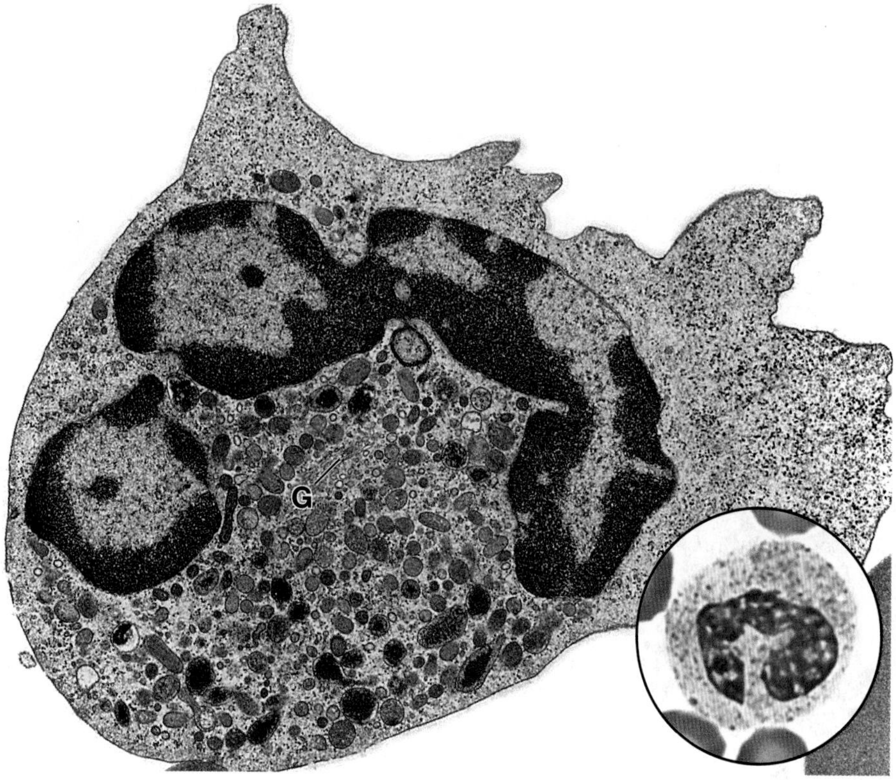

FIGURE 10.8. Electron micrograph of a human mature neutrophil. The nucleus shows the typical multilobed configuration with the heterochromatin at the periphery and the euchromatin more centrally located. A small Golgi apparatus (*G*) is present; other organelles are sparse. The punctate appearance of the cytoplasm adjacent to the convex aspect of the nuclear profile is caused by glycogen particles. Adjacent to the concave aspect of the nuclear profile are numerous granules. Specific granules appear less dense and more rounded than azurophilic granules. The latter are fewer in number and are extremely electron dense. ×22,000. (Courtesy of Dr. Dorothea Zucker-Franklin.) For comparison, the *inset* shows a neutrophil from a blood smear observed in the light microscope. ×1,800.

helps to generate highly reactive bactericidal hypochlorite and chloramines. In addition to containing a variety of the typical **acid hydrolases**, azurophilic granules also contain cationic proteins called **defensins**, which function similarly to antibodies, and the antimicrobial peptide **cathelicidin** to kill pathogens.

- **Specific granules (secondary granules)** are the smallest granules and are at least twice as numerous as azurophilic granules. They are barely visible in the light microscope; in electron micrographs, they are ellipsoidal (see Fig. 10.8). Specific granules contain various **enzymes** (i.e., type IV collagenase, gelatinase, phospholipase) as well as **complement activators** and other **antimicrobial peptides** (i.e., lysozymes, lactoferrins).
- **Tertiary granules** are of two types. One type contains **phosphatases** (enzymes that remove a phosphate group from a substrate) and is sometimes called a **phosphasome**. The other type contains **metalloproteinases**, such as gelatinases and collagenases, which are thought to facilitate the migration of the neutrophil through the connective tissue.

Aside from these granules, membrane-bound organelles are sparse. A small Golgi apparatus is evident in the center of the cell, and mitochondria are relatively few in number (see Fig. 10.8).

Neutrophils are motile cells; they leave the circulation and migrate to their site of action in the connective tissue.

Neutrophils are the first cells to arrive at the infection site and are characterized by their potent antimicrobial and antifungal capacity. This capacity reflects their cellular components and processes, such as the synthesis of antimicrobial peptides and neutrophil-specific proteolytic enzymes, production of reactive oxygen intermediates (ROIs) used in the respiratory burst reaction, and formation of neutrophil extracellular traps (NETs).

An important property of neutrophils and other leukocytes is their **motility**. In order to perform their immune functions of patrolling for and eliminating pathogens, leukocytes must continually move throughout all compartments of the body. The blood and lymphatic vessels serve as the main conduits for the movement of neutrophils and other leukocytes. These cells repeatedly cross the endothelium of these vessels in a highly regulated process called **diapedesis** as they enter (**intravasation**) and exit (**extravasation**) the circulation. Neutrophils are the most numerous of the first wave of cells to enter an area of tissue damage. Diapedesis occurs in the specialized postcapillary venules (HEV or high endothelial venules) of secondary lymphatic organs (see pages 509-510), the endothelium of postcapillary venules in most inflamed/damaged peripheral tissues, and capillaries in inflamed lung and liver. Their migration to the area of tissue damage is controlled by the expression of **adhesion molecules** on the neutrophil surface that interact with corresponding ligands on endothelial cells (Fig. 10.9).

Interaction of circulating neutrophils with the luminal surface of the endothelium initiates diapedesis.

The **initial phase** of neutrophil migration occurs in the postcapillary venules and is regulated by a mechanism involving neutrophil–endothelial cell recognition. **E-selectin** and **P-selectin** (types of cell adhesion molecules) are found on the surface of endothelial cells of the postcapillary venule; they both interact with circulating neutrophils that express relatively high numbers of Sialyl-Lewis^x (s-Le^x) carbohydrates on their surface. Owing to the brief, reversible binding of E-selectin and P-selectin with s-Le^x carbohydrates, the neutrophil becomes partially tethered to the endothelial cell (see Fig. 10.9). This interaction causes the neutrophils to slow down and roll on the surface of the endothelium. The neutrophil–endothelial interaction can be compared to a rolling

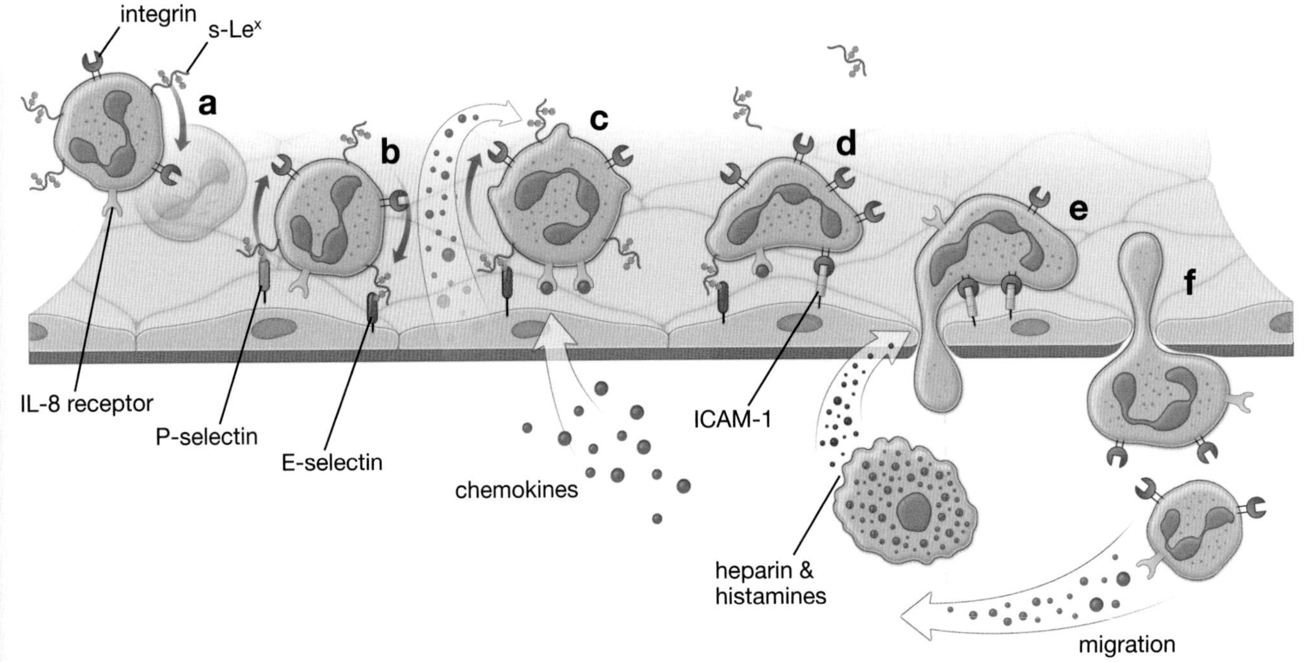

FIGURE 10.9. Diagram of events in the migration of a neutrophil from a postcapillary venule into the connective tissue utilizing paracellular diapedesis pathway. a. A neutrophil traveling in a blood vessel expresses a high number of cell-to-cell recognition molecules, such as Sialyl-Lewis^x (s-Le^x) carbohydrates, integrin, and interleukin receptors. **b.** Circulating neutrophils are slowed down by the interaction of their surface s-Le^x molecules with E- and P-selectins expressed on the endothelium of the postcapillary venule. **c.** As a result of this interaction, the cell rolls on the surface of the endothelium. The neutrophil then adheres to the endothelium and responds to chemokines (e.g., interleukin-8) secreted by the endothelial cells. **d.** These chemokines induce the expression of other adhesion molecules on the surface of the neutrophil, such as integrins (e.g., VLA-5), which provide tight bonds with the immunoglobulin superfamily of adhesion molecules (e.g., intercellular adhesion molecule 1 [ICAM-1]) expressed on the surface of the endothelium. These interactions provide firm adhesion of the neutrophil to the endothelial surface. **e.** The neutrophil then extends a pseudopod to an intercellular junction, which undergoes disassembly process to create paracellular gap. Histamine and heparin released from the mast cells in the connective tissue facilitate neutrophil migration through the vessel wall. **f.** Once the neutrophil leaves the circulation and enters the connective tissue, its further migration is directed by chemoattractant molecules that interact with specific receptors on its surface.

tennis ball (the neutrophil) on a tilted surface covered with Velcro (the endothelial surface). As the ball rolls, miniature hooks (representing selectins) on the Velcro surface catch the fibrous, felt-covered ball. This interaction slows and eventually stops the movement of the tennis ball.

In the **second phase**, the tight binding of neutrophils to the endothelial surface is achieved by another group of adhesion molecules, called **integrins** (i.e., VLA-5), which are expressed on the neutrophil surface. They are activated by chemokine signals from endothelial cells. Integrins expressed on the neutrophil surface bind to **immunoglobulin superfamily** adhesion molecules residing on endothelial cells (e.g., intercellular adhesion molecule 1 [ICAM-1], vascular cell adhesion molecule 1 [VCAM-1]). Some chemokines, such as **interleukin-8** (IL-8), bind to receptors located on neutrophils, facilitating their migration toward a designated site of inflammation. These interactions secure stable adhesion of the neutrophil to the endothelial surface, allowing the process of diapedesis to begin.

Diapedesis proceeds along either transcellular or paracellular pathways.

Diapedesis proceeds as the neutrophils or other leukocytes extend their pseudopods either through the **paracellular gap** that is formed between two endothelial cells (**paracellular pathway**) or into the **transcellular pore** created within the endothelial cell (**transcellular pathway**). Both pathways require energy. Formation of a transcellular pore requires extensive remodeling of the endothelial plasma membrane with reorganization of the cytoskeleton and displacement of intracellular organelles. Similarly, opening of a paracellular gap also requires energy for the disassembly of intercellular junctions.

The diapedesis pathway taken by individual cells is most likely the "path of least resistance," which is determined by several factors associated with the specific endothelium, type of migrating leukocyte, and migratory/inflammatory stimuli. In several organs, **transcellular diapedesis** is predominant. For instance, the extravasation of newly differentiated cells from the bone marrow occurs via the transcellular pathway as they cross the endothelium of bone marrow sinusoids (see pages 331-332). In pathologic conditions, migration of leukocytes (extravasation) across the blood–brain barrier and blood–retinal barrier exclusively depends on the transcellular pathway.

In the paracellular pathway, diapedesis proceeds as the neutrophil extends a pseudopod to an intercellular junction. Disassembly of intercellular junctions is necessary to create the paracellular gap. Histamines and heparin released at the injury site by perivascular mast cells contribute to this migration process. Proteases secreted by the migrating neutrophil breach the basement membrane, thereby allowing the neutrophil to enter the underlying connective tissue.

With the TEM, the cytoplasmic contents of a neutrophil pseudopod appear as a stretch of finely granular cytoplasmic matrix with no membranous organelles (see Fig. 10.8). The finely granular appearance is attributable to the presence of actin filaments, some microtubules, and glycogen. These are involved in the extension of the cytoplasm to form the pseudopod and the subsequent contraction that pulls the cell forward. Once the neutrophil enters the connective tissue, further migration to the injury site is directed by a process known as **chemotaxis**, the binding of chemoattractant molecules and extracellular matrix proteins to specific receptors on the surface of the neutrophil.

Neutrophils are active phagocytes that use a variety of surface receptors to recognize bacteria and other infectious agents at the site of inflammation.

Once at the site of tissue injury, the neutrophil must first recognize any foreign substances before phagocytosis can occur. Like most phagocytic cells, **neutrophils** have a variety of receptors on their cell membranes that recognize and bind to bacteria, foreign organisms, and other infectious agents (Fig. 10.10). Some of these organisms and agents bind directly to neutrophils (no modifications of their surfaces are required), whereas others must be opsonized (coated with antibodies or complement) to make them more attractive to the neutrophil. The most common receptors used by neutrophils during phagocytosis include the following:

- **F_c receptors** on the neutrophil surface bind to the exposed F_c region of immunoglobulin G (IgG) antibodies that coat bacterial surfaces (see Fig. 10.10). Binding of IgG-coated bacteria activates the neutrophil's phagocytic activity and causes a rapid surge in intracellular metabolism.
- **Complement receptors (CRs)** facilitate binding and uptake of immune complexes that are opsonized by active C3 complement proteins, namely, C3b. Binding of bacteria or other C3b-coated antigens to CRs triggers phagocytosis, resulting in the activation of a neutrophil's lytic pathways and respiratory burst reactions.
- **Scavenger receptors (SRs)** are a structurally diverse group of transmembrane glycoproteins that bind to modified (acetylated or oxidized) forms of low-density lipoproteins (LDLs), polyanionic molecules that are often found on the surface of both Gram-positive and Gram-negative bacteria and apoptotic bodies. Binding of these receptors increases the phagocytic activity of neutrophils.
- **Toll-like receptors**, also known as **pattern recognition receptors (PRRs)**, are neutrophil receptors that recognize pathogenic molecules such as endotoxins, lipopolysaccharides, peptidoglycans, and lipoteichoic acids that are arranged in predictable **pathogen-associated molecular patterns (PAMPs)** and are commonly expressed on bacterial surfaces and other infectious agents. Like other phagocytic cells, neutrophils possess a variety of toll-like receptors that recognize PAMPs. Binding of bacterial antigens to these receptors causes phagocytosis and the release of cytokines, such as **interleukin-1 (IL-1)**, **interleukin-3 (IL-3)**, and **tumor necrosis factor α (TNF-α)** from the neutrophil. IL-1, historically known as a **pyrogen** (fever-causing agent), induces the synthesis of prostaglandins, which, in turn, act on the thermoregulatory center of the hypothalamus to produce **fever**. Therefore, fever is a consequence of acute reaction to invading pathogens that cause a massive neutrophilic response.

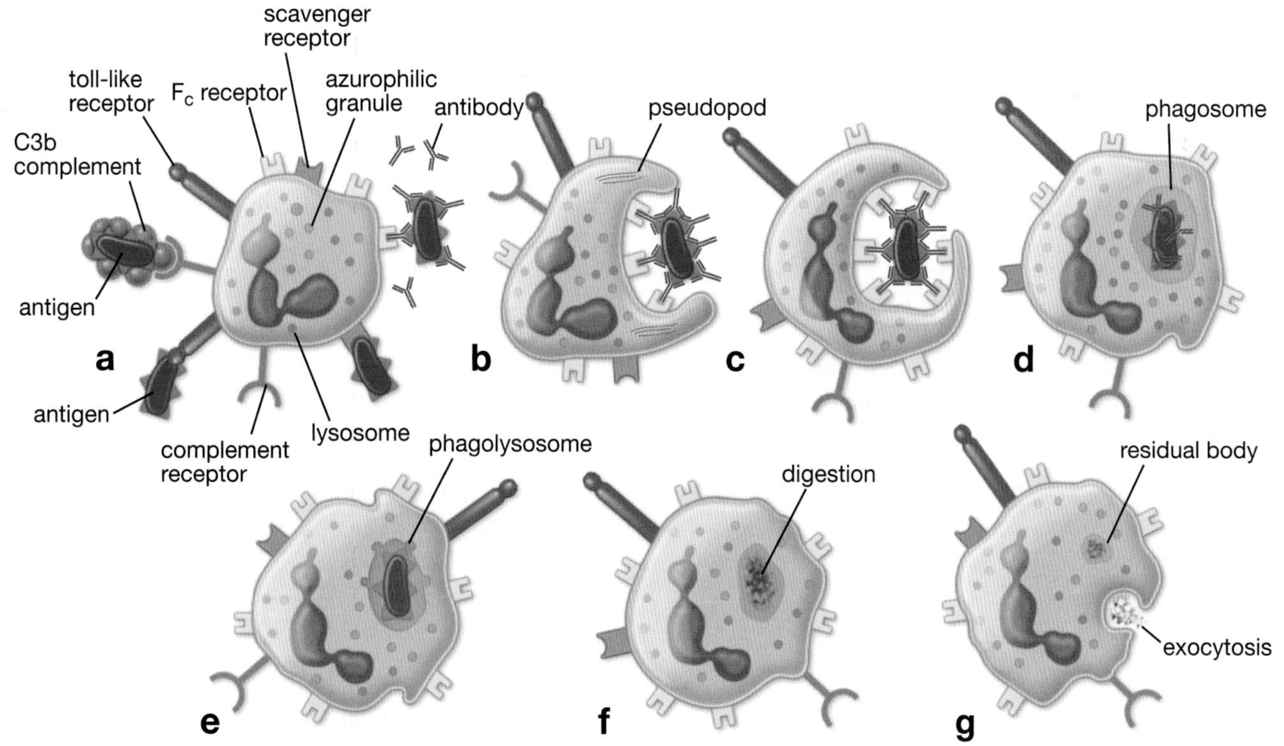

FIGURE 10.10. Neutrophil phagocytosis. a. Antibody-dependent phagocytosis begins with recognition and attachment of immune complexes formed between foreign material (antigen) and antibodies. In this process, F_c receptors on the neutrophil surface interact with the F_c region of antibodies bound to the antigen. **b.** The antigen is then engulfed by pseudopods of the neutrophil. **c.** As the pseudopods come together and fuse, the antigen is internalized. **d.** Once the phagosome is formed, digestion is initiated by activation of membrane-bound oxidases of the phagosome. **e.** Both specific and azurophilic granules fuse with the phagosome and release their contents, forming a phagolysosome. This fusion and release of granules is called *degranulation*. **f.** The enzymatic contents of the granules are responsible for killing and digesting the microorganism. The entire digestive process occurs within the phagolysosome, which protects the cell from self-injury. **g.** The digested material is either exocytosed into the extracellular space or stored as residual bodies within the neutrophil.

Phagocytosed bacteria are killed within phagolysosomes by the toxic reactive oxygen intermediates produced during a respiratory burst.

Phagocytosis begins when the neutrophil recognizes and attaches to the antigen. Extended pseudopods of the neutrophil engulf the antigen and internalize it to form a **phagosome** (see Fig. 10.10). Specific and azurophilic granules fuse with the phagosome membrane, and the lysosomal hydrolases of the azurophilic granules digest the foreign material. During phagocytosis, the neutrophil's glucose and oxygen utilization increases noticeably and is referred to as the **respiratory burst**. It results in the synthesis of several oxygen-containing compounds called **reactive oxygen intermediates (ROIs)**. They include free radicals such as oxygen and hydroxyl radicals that are used to immobilize and kill live bacteria within the phagolysosomes. By definition, free radicals possess an unpaired electron within their chemical structure, which makes them highly reactive and, therefore, capable of damaging intracellular molecules, including lipids, proteins, and nucleic acids.

The process by which microorganisms are killed within neutrophils is termed **oxygen-dependent intracellular killing**. In general, two biochemical pathways are involved in this process: The first is the **phagocyte oxidase (phox) system** that utilizes the phagocyte's **nicotinamide adenine dinucleotide phosphate (NADPH) oxidase complex** in the phagolysosome membrane; the second is associated with the lysosomal enzyme **myeloperoxidase (MPO)** found in the azurophilic granules of neutrophils (Fig. 10.11).

The phox system produces NADPH that ultimately generates free radicals.

Within the phagocyte oxidase pathway, or **phox system**, phagocytosis proceeds by signaling the cell to produce sufficient amounts of NADPH needed to generate superoxide anions. Increased glucose uptake and shunting of NADPH metabolism are achieved via the pentose phosphate pathway (also known as *pentose shunt*). The cytosolic NADPH becomes an electron donor: The NADPH oxidase enzyme complex transports electrons across the membrane to molecular O_2 inside the phagolysosome to generate the free radical **superoxide anions (O_2^-)**. These superoxide anions are converted into ROIs. The superoxide dismutase converts superoxide anions to singlet oxygen ($^1O_2$) and hydrogen peroxide (H_2O_2), which further reacts with superoxide anions to

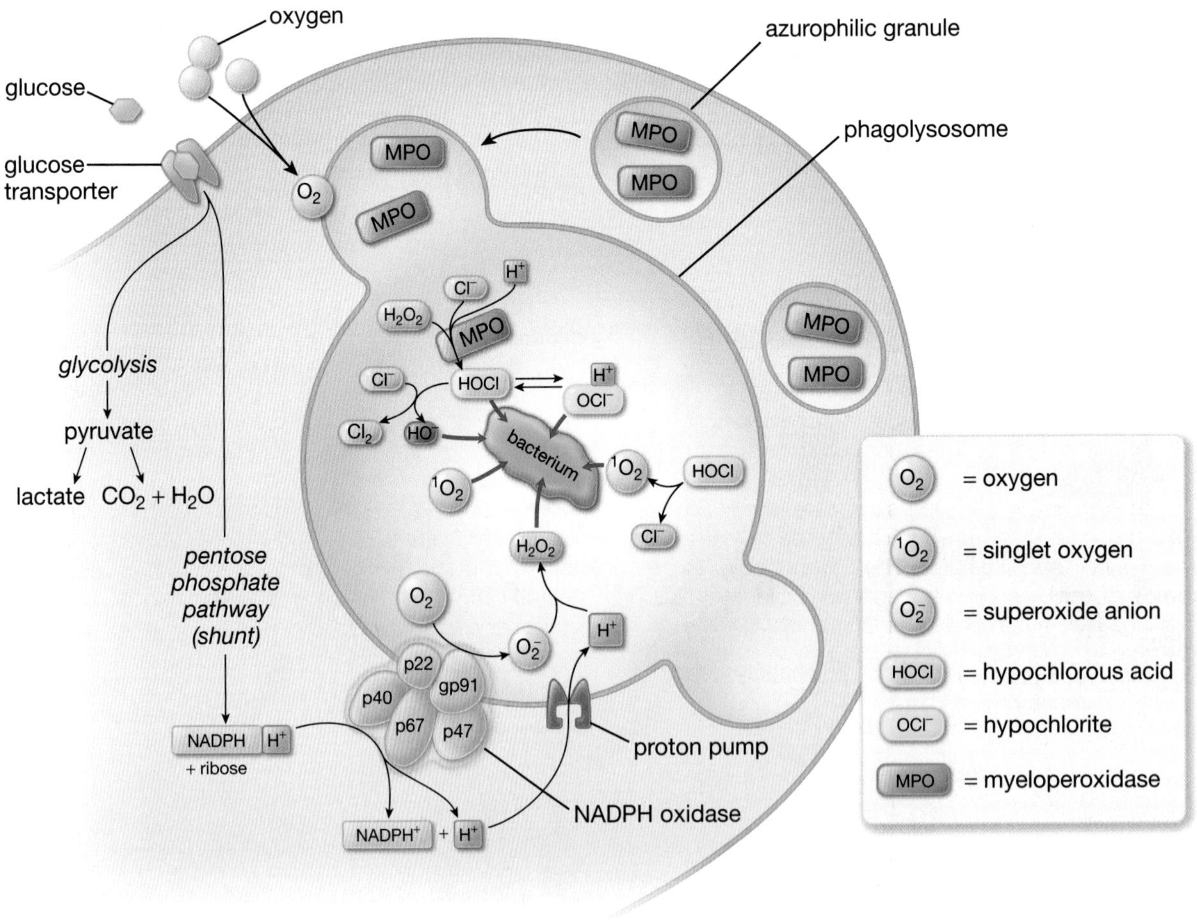

FIGURE 10.11. Pathways leading to synthesis of reactive oxygen intermediates during neutrophil's respiratory burst reactions. This schematic diagram shows a phagolysosome that contains an already phagocytosed bacterium. Two oxygen-dependent killing mechanisms are depicted in this drawing. The first mechanism depends on the phagocyte oxidase (phox) system that utilizes the NADPH oxidase complex (which contains five subunits). This complex transports excess electrons across the membrane of the phagolysosome, where they interact with molecular oxygen to generate free superoxide anions. These anions are converted into reactive oxygen intermediates. Another enzyme superoxide dismutase converts superoxide anions to singlet oxygen and hydrogen peroxide, which further reacts with superoxide anions to produce bactericidal hydroxyl radicals and more singlet oxygen molecules. The second mechanism involves lysosomal enzyme myeloperoxidase (*MPO*) found in the azurophilic granules of neutrophils. MPO catalyzes the production of hypochlorous acids from hydrogen peroxide and chloride anions. Hypochlorous acid is further metabolized to a highly toxic hypochlorite (bleach) and chlorine. Some of the hypochlorite anions may spontaneously break down to yield toxic singlet oxygen and chloride ions. All molecules produced during oxygen bursts in neutrophils (associated with *red arrows*) are highly effective in killing ingested bacteria.

produce bactericidal **hydroxyl radicals (OH^-)** (the neutral form of the hydroxyl ion) and more singlet oxygen molecules (see Fig. 10.11).

The myeloperoxidase-associated system uses heme as a cofactor.

Oxygen-dependent killing with **myeloperoxidase (MPO)** involvement occurs when azurophilic granules containing MPO fuse with phagosomes containing phagocytosed bacteria. During the neutrophil's respiratory burst, MPO, using heme as a cofactor, catalyzes a reaction that produces **hypochlorous acid (HOCl)** from hydrogen peroxide (H_2O_2) and a chloride anion (Cl^-). Hypochlorous acid, which is about 1,000 times more effective in bacterial killing than hydrogen peroxide, is further metabolized to a highly toxic hypochlorite OCl^- (bleach) and chlorine (Cl_2). Some of the hypochlorite may spontaneously break down to yield toxic singlet oxygen ($^1O_2$) and chloride ions (Cl^-) (see Fig. 10.11).

Nitric oxide also participates in intracellular killing mechanisms but is not found in humans.

In addition, **nitric oxide (NO)** and other **reactive nitrogen intermediates (RNIs)** have also been implicated in intracellular microbial killing mechanisms. NO has been found in neutrophils; however, it is believed that RNI-mediated killing mechanisms do not appear to have a critical role in humans. The main role of neutrophil-derived NO is to induce vasodilatation, which, in turn, facilitates the migration of neutrophils from the blood vessels to surrounding connective tissue.

Phagocytosed bacteria can also be killed by a diverse arsenal of oxygen-independent killing mechanisms utilizing bacteriolytic enzymes and antimicrobial peptides.

In addition to the oxygen-dependent respiratory burst reactions, microorganisms can be killed by bacteriolytic enzymes and cationic antimicrobial peptides that are stored within the granules of the neutrophil's cytoplasm. These **oxygen-independent killing mechanisms** are directed toward the bacterial cell membrane, causing its breakdown and leakage. Neutrophils contain particularly large amounts of cationic antimicrobial proteins such as defensins and antimicrobial peptides called **cathelicidins**. Similar to lysozymes and cathepsins stored in the specific granules, these cationic antimicrobial proteins break down the bacterial wall. In addition, lysosomal hydrolytic enzymes that digest bacterial proteins and lactoferrins that chelate iron from nutritional bacterial pathways contribute to the destruction of the invading bacteria. These mechanisms are not as efficient as oxygen-dependent killing pathways. Neutrophils from patients with defects in oxygen-dependent pathways, such as those with **chronic granulomatous disease** (see Folder 10.4), are still able to destroy phagocytosed bacteria to some degree. However, because of the low efficiency of these processes, individuals with these defects are more susceptible to serious infections.

Following intracellular digestion by the neutrophil, the remnants of degraded material are stored in residual bodies or exocytosed. Most neutrophils die in this process; the accumulation of dead bacteria and dead neutrophils constitutes the thick exudate called **pus**. The yellow-green

FOLDER 10.4

CLINICAL CORRELATION: INHERITED DISORDERS OF NEUTROPHILS; CHRONIC GRANULOMATOUS DISEASE

A primary example of a genetic immunodeficiency disorder that affects oxygen-dependent killing mechanisms is **chronic granulomatous disease (CGD)**. This inherited disorder of neutrophils and other phagocytic cells is caused by the mutation or absence of one of the components of the **NADPH oxidase complex (phox system)**. As a result, neutrophils cannot produce reactive oxygen intermediates (ROIs). The NADPH oxidase complex consists of five molecules. Two of them, **glycoprotein 91 (gp91)** and **protein 22 (p22)**, are part of a membrane-bound cytochrome called **cytochrome B558** (see Fig. 10.11). Three other cytosolic components—**protein 47 (p47), protein 67 (p67)**, and **protein 40 (p40)**—are components of **Rac-2 GTPase**, which is required for oxidase activity. Neutrophil activation and stimulation from phagocytosis cause cytosolic proteins to translocate to the plasma membrane of the phagolysosome to assemble the active NADPH oxidase complex. The assembled enzyme transports electrons from cytosolic NADPH across the membrane to molecular O_2 residing inside the phagolysosome, generating bactericidal superoxide anions O_2^- and other ROIs.

Approximately 50%–70% of all CGD cases are caused by a mutation in the **CYBB (cytochrome B, b subunit) gene** located on the X chromosome. This gene encodes glycoprotein 91 (gp91), which is necessary for proper function of the NADPH oxidase complex. Because **gp91 deficiency** is an X-linked disease, CGD caused by this mutation is often referred to as **X91 disease**. Another 20%–40% of those with CGD have mutations in the **NCF1 gene** on chromosome 7 that codes for protein 47. Mutations in genes NCF2 (which encodes protein 67) and CYBA (which encodes protein 22) are rare, accounting for <10% of all cases of CGD. Mutations in the NCF1, NCF2, and CYBA genes produce autosomal recessive forms of CGD.

CGD hampers the ability of neutrophils to kill certain types of bacteria and fungi. Individuals with this disease are frequently affected by recurrent life-threatening bacterial and fungal infections and chronic inflammatory conditions. The most common pathologic changes occur in tissues and organs that form barriers against the entry of microorganisms from the external environment. They include skin (skin infections), gingiva (swollen inflamed gums), lungs (pneumonia), lymph nodes (lymphadenitis), gastrointestinal tract (enteritis, diarrhea), liver, and spleen. Another characteristic feature of CGD is the development of enlarged, tumor-like masses called **granulomas**. The presence of granulomas may cause serious problems in the gastrointestinal tract by obstructing the passage of food and in the genitourinary tract by blocking the flow of urine from the kidneys and bladder.

color of the pus and mucus secretions (e.g., from infected lungs) comes from the heme pigment of the MPO enzyme in azurophilic granules of neutrophils.

NETosis is the formation of neutrophil extracellular traps (NETs) that represents an alternative route of bacterial killing.

Neutrophil extracellular trap–associated cell death (NETosis) is a unique form of microorganism killing that is usually associated with neutrophil death known as "**suicidal NETosis**" (see pages 107-109). Upon recognizing phagocytosed pathogens, neutrophils modify their nuclear histone structures, resulting in chromatin decondensation and disruption of their nuclear and cellular membranes. Cytoplasm, which is now dispersed among extracellular chromatin, forms a large web of extracellular strands that allow antimicrobial proteins to contact the microorganisms. The extracellular net functions as a trap for immobilizing and killing microorganisms and preventing their dispersion through the tissues. Signals generated by microorganismal destruction induce inflammation that results in the recruitment of immune response cells to the infection site.

Inflammation and wound healing also involve monocytes, lymphocytes, eosinophils, basophils, and fibroblasts.

Monocytes also enter the connective tissue as a secondary response to tissue injury. At the site of tissue injury, they transform into **macrophages** that phagocytose cell and tissue debris, fibrin, remaining bacteria, and dead neutrophils. Normal wound healing depends on the participation of macrophages in the inflammatory response; they become the major cell type in the inflammatory site after the neutrophils are spent. Simultaneously, fibroblasts near the site and undifferentiated mesenchymal cells in the adventitia of small vessels at the site begin to divide and differentiate into fibroblasts and myofibroblasts that then secrete the fibers and ground substance of the healing wound. Like neutrophils, monocytes are attracted to the inflammatory site by chemotaxis. Lymphocytes, eosinophils, and basophils also play a role in **inflammation**, but they are more involved in the immunologic aspects of the process (see Chapter 14, Immune System and Lymphatic Tissues and Organs, page 482). Eosinophils and lymphocytes are more commonly found at sites of chronic inflammation.

Eosinophils

Eosinophils are about the same size as neutrophils, and their nuclei are typically bilobed (Fig. 10.12 and Plate 10.1, page 336). As in neutrophils, the compact heterochromatin of eosinophils is chiefly adjacent to the nuclear envelope, whereas the euchromatin is located in the center of the nucleus.

Eosinophils are named for the large, eosinophilic, refractile granules in their cytoplasm.

The cytoplasm of eosinophils contains two types of granules: numerous, large, elongated specific granules and azurophilic

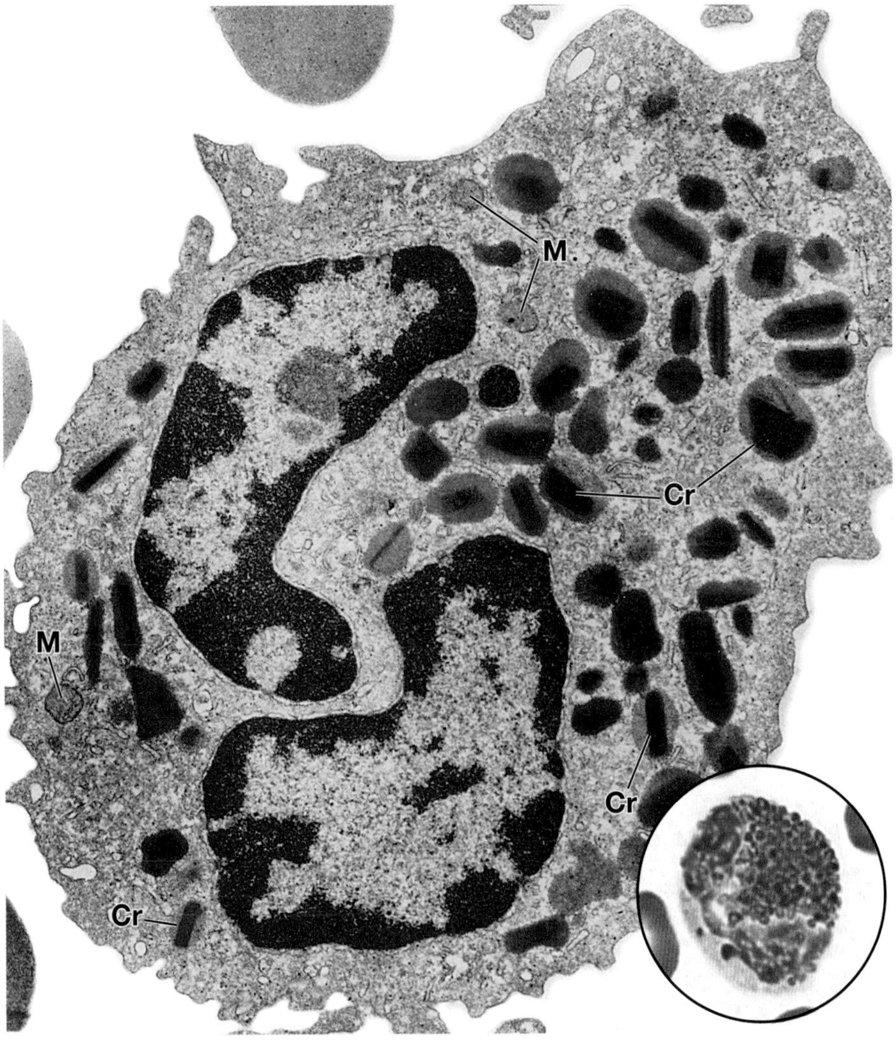

FIGURE 10.12. Electron micrograph of a human eosinophil. The nucleus is bilobed, but the connecting segment is not within the plane of section. The granules are of moderate size, compared with those of the basophil, and show a crystalline body (*Cr*) within the less electron-dense matrix of the granule. *M*, mitochondria. ×26,000. (Courtesy of Dr. Dorothea Zucker-Franklin.) **Inset.** Light microscopic image of an eosinophil from a blood smear. ×1,800.

FOLDER 10.5

CLINICAL CORRELATION: HEMOGLOBIN BREAKDOWN AND JAUNDICE

If the conjugation of bilirubin or its excretion into bile by the liver cells is inhibited, or if blockage of the bile duct system occurs, **bilirubin** may reenter the blood, causing a yellow appearance of the sclera of the eye and the skin. This condition is called **jaundice**. Jaundice can be caused by the destruction of circulating erythrocytes. An example of such a condition is a **hemolytic transfusion reaction** when ABO-incompatible blood is administered to a patient, usually because of a clerical error. Massive hemolysis of the transfused erythrocytes may be associated with severe systemic complications, such as hypotension (decreased blood pressure), renal failure, and even death.

Jaundice also occurs in a variety of **hemolytic anemias** that result from either inherited defects of erythrocytes (e.g., hereditary spherocytosis) or external factors such as pathogenic microorganisms, animal venoms, chemicals, and drugs. Mild jaundice is common in newborn infants (**physiologic jaundice**) because of the inefficiency of the bilirubin-conjugating system in the newborn liver. Excessive levels (>30 mg/dL) of unconjugated bilirubin in the blood (hyperbilirubinemia) during infancy may cause **kernicterus**, a rare neurologic disorder in which toxic levels of bilirubin may accumulate in the brain.

granules (otherwise, the eosinophil contains only a sparse representation of membranous organelles).

- **Azurophilic granules (primary granules)** are lysosomes. They contain a variety of the usual **lysosomal acid hydrolases** and other hydrolytic enzymes that function in the destruction of parasites and hydrolysis of antigen–antibody complexes internalized by the eosinophil.
- **Specific granules (secondary granules)** of eosinophils contain a **crystalloid body** that is readily seen with the TEM, surrounded by a less electron-dense matrix. These crystalloid bodies are responsible for the refractivity of the granules in the light microscope. They contain four major proteins: an arginine-rich protein called **major basic protein (MBP)**, which accounts for the intense acidophilia of the granule; **eosinophil cationic protein (ECP)**; **eosinophil peroxidase (EPO)**; and **eosinophil-derived neurotoxin (EDN)**. MBP is localized in the crystalloid body; the other three proteins are found in the granule matrix. MBP, ECP, and EPO have a strong cytotoxic effect on protozoans and helminthic parasites; EDN causes nervous system dysfunction in parasitic organisms; histaminase neutralizes the activity of histamine; and arylsulfatase neutralizes leukotrienes secreted by basophils and mast cells (see Chapter 6, Connective Tissue, pages 200-204). Specific granules also contain **histaminase**, **arylsulfatase**, **collagenase**, and **cathepsins**.

Eosinophils are associated with allergic reactions, parasitic infections, and chronic inflammation.

Eosinophils develop and mature in the bone marrow. Once released from the bone marrow, they circulate in peripheral blood and then migrate to the connective tissue. Eosinophils are activated by interactions with IgG, IgA, or secretory IgA antibodies. The release of **arylsulfatase** and **histaminase** by eosinophils at the sites of allergic reaction moderates the potentially deleterious effects of inflammatory vasoactive mediators. The eosinophil also participates in other immunologic responses and phagocytoses antigen–antibody complexes. Thus, the number of eosinophils in blood samples of individuals with **allergic reactions** and **parasitic infections** is usually high (**eosinophilia**). Eosinophils play a major role in host defense against helminthic parasites. They are also found in large numbers in the lamina propria of the intestinal tract and at other sites of potential chronic inflammation (i.e., lung tissues in patients with asthma).

Basophils

Basophils are similar in size to neutrophils and are so named because the numerous large granules in their cytoplasm stain with basic dyes (Plate 10.1, page 336).

Basophils are the least numerous of the white blood cells, accounting for less than 0.5% of total leukocytes.

Often, several hundred white blood cells must be examined in a blood smear before one **basophil** is found. The lobed basophil nucleus is usually obscured by the granules in stained blood smears, but its characteristics are evident in electron micrographs (Fig. 10.13). Heterochromatin is chiefly in a peripheral location, and euchromatin is chiefly centrally located; typical cytoplasmic organelles are sparse. The basophil plasma membrane possesses numerous high-affinity **F_c receptors** for IgE antibodies. In addition, a specific 39-kDa protein called **CD40L** is expressed on the basophil's surface. CD40L interacts with a CR (CD40) on B lymphocytes, which results in increased synthesis of IgE.

The basophil cytoplasm contains two types of granules: specific granules, which are larger than the specific granules of the neutrophil, and nonspecific azurophilic granules.

- **Azurophilic granules (primary granules)** are the lysosomes of basophils and contain a variety of lysosomal acid hydrolases similar to those in other leukocytes.
- **Specific granules (secondary granules)** exhibit a grainy texture and myelin figures when viewed with the TEM. These granules contain a variety of substances, namely, heparin, histamine, heparan sulfate, leukotrienes, IL-4, and IL-13. **Heparin**, a sulfated glycosaminoglycan, is an anticoagulant. **Histamine** and **heparan sulfate** are vasoactive agents that among other actions cause dilation of small blood vessels. **Leukotrienes** are modified lipids that trigger prolonged constriction of smooth muscles in the pulmonary airways (see page 204). **Interleukin-4 (IL-4)** and **interleukin-13 (IL-13)** promote synthesis of IgE antibodies. The intense basophilia of these specific granules correlates with the high concentration of sulfates within the glycosaminoglycan molecules of heparin and heparan sulfate.

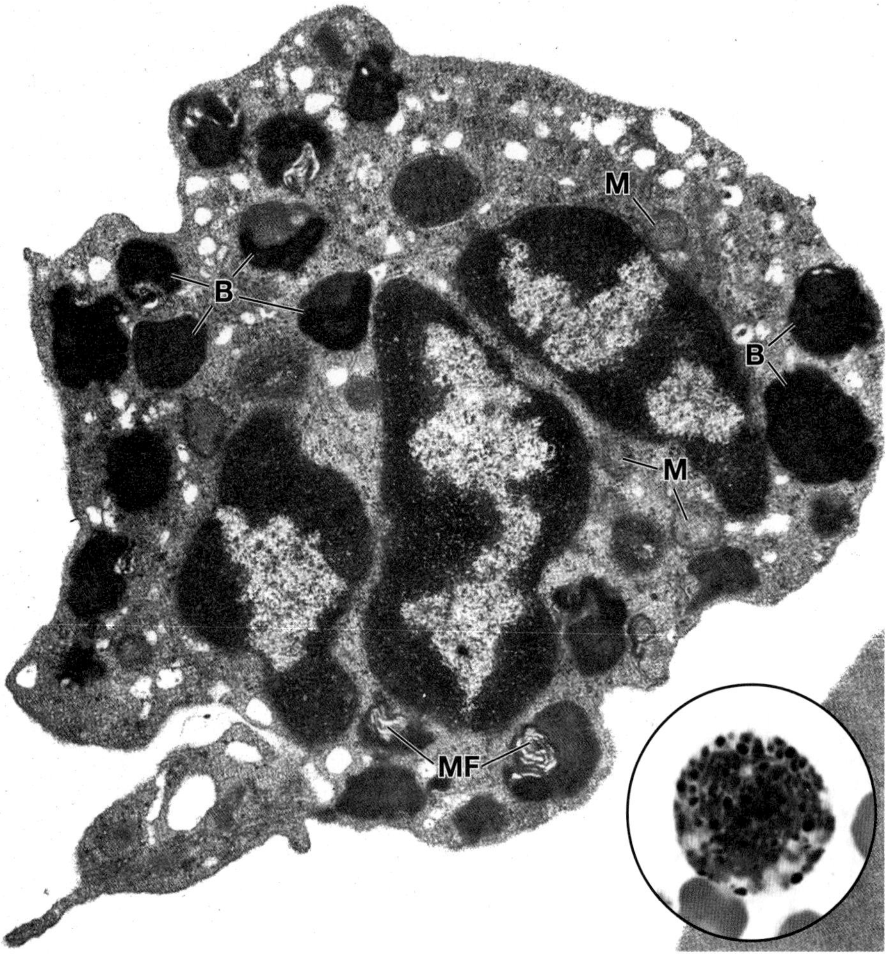

FIGURE 10.13. Electron micrograph of a human basophil. The nucleus appears as three separate bodies; the connecting strands are not in the plane of section. The basophil granules (*B*) are very large and irregularly shaped. Some granules reveal myelin figures (*MF*). *M*, mitochondria. ×26,000. (Courtesy of Dr. Dorothea Zucker-Franklin.) **Inset.** Light microscopic appearance of a basophil from a blood smear. ×1,800.

The function of basophils is closely related to that of mast cells.

Basophils are functionally related to, but not identical with, mast cells of the connective tissue (see Table 6.6, page 201). Both mast cells and basophils bind an antibody secreted by plasma cells, **IgE**, through high-affinity F_c receptors expressed on their cell surface. The subsequent exposure to, and reaction with, the antigen (allergen) specific for IgE triggers the activation of basophils and mast cells and the release of vasoactive agents from cell granules. These substances are responsible for the severe vascular disturbances associated with **hypersensitivity reactions** and **anaphylaxis**.

Furthermore, both basophils and mast cells are derived from the same **basophil–mast cell progenitor (BMCP) cell**. If a specific BMCP expresses the granulocyte-related transcription factor **CCAAT/enhancer-binding protein α (C/EBPα)**, the cell becomes committed to differentiate into a **basophil progenitor (BaP) cell**. Basophils develop and differentiate in the bone marrow and are released into the peripheral blood as mature cells. In the absence of C/EBPα transcription factor, a BMCP cell migrates to the spleen and, after further differentiation, travels as a **mast cell progenitor (MCP)** to the intestine, where it becomes a mature mast cell.

Lymphocytes

Lymphocytes are the main functional cells of the lymphatic or immune system.

Lymphocytes are the most common agranulocytes and account for about 30% of the total blood leukocytes. In understanding the function of the lymphocytes, one must realize that most lymphocytes found in blood or lymph represent recirculating **immunocompetent cells** (i.e., cells that have developed the capacity to recognize and respond to antigens and are in transit from one lymphatic tissue to another). Therefore, lymphocytes are different in several aspects from other leukocytes:

- Lymphocytes are not terminally differentiated cells. When stimulated, lymphocytes divide and differentiate into other types of effector cells.
- Lymphocytes can exit from the lumen of blood vessels into tissues and subsequently can recirculate back into blood vessels.
- Despite the fact that common lymphoid progenitor (CLP) cells (see pages 321-323) originate in the bone marrow, lymphocytes are capable of developing outside the bone marrow in tissues associated with the immune system (see Chapter 14, Immune System and Lymphatic Tissues and Organs, page 482).

In tissues associated with the immune system, three groups of lymphocytes can be identified according to size: small, medium, and large lymphocytes, ranging in diameter from 6 to 30 μm. The large lymphocytes are either **activated lymphocytes**, which possess surface receptors that interact with a specific antigen, or **natural killer (NK) lymphocytes**. In the bloodstream, most lymphocytes are small or medium sized, 6–15 μm in diameter. The majority—more than 90%—are small lymphocytes.

In blood smears, the mature lymphocyte approximates the size of an erythrocyte.

When observed in the light microscope in a blood smear, small lymphocytes have an intensely staining, slightly indented, spherical nucleus (Plate 10.1, page 336). The cytoplasm appears as a very thin, pale blue rim surrounding the nucleus. In general, there are no recognizable cytoplasmic organelles other than an occasional fine azurophilic granule. The TEM reveals that the cytoplasm primarily contains free ribosomes and a few mitochondria. Other organelles are so sparse that they are usually not seen in a thin section. Small, dense lysosomes that correspond to the azurophilic granules seen in the light microscope are occasionally observed; a pair of centrioles and a small Golgi apparatus are located in the cell center, the area of the indentation of the nucleus.

In the medium lymphocyte, the cytoplasm is more abundant, the nucleus is larger and less heterochromatic, and the Golgi apparatus is somewhat more developed (Fig. 10.14). Greater numbers of mitochondria and polysomes and small profiles of rough endoplasmic reticulum (rER) are also seen in these medium-sized cells. The ribosomes are the basis for the slight basophilia displayed by lymphocytes in stained blood smears.

Three functionally distinct types of lymphocytes are present in the body: T lymphocytes, B lymphocytes, and NK cells.

The characterization of lymphocyte types is based on their function, not on their size or morphology. **T lymphocytes (T cells)** are so named because they undergo differentiation in the thymus. **B lymphocytes (B cells)** are so named because they were first recognized as a separate population in the bursa of Fabricius in birds or bursa-equivalent organs (e.g., bone marrow) in mammals. **Natural killer (NK) cells** develop from the same precursor cell as B and T cells and are so named because they are programmed to kill certain types of transformed cells.

- **T cells** have a long life span and are involved in cell-mediated immunity. T cells are characterized by the presence of cell surface recognition proteins called **T-cell receptors (TCRs)**, which, in most T cells, comprise two glycoprotein chains called α- and β-TCR chains. They express CD2, CD3, CD5, and CD7 marker proteins on their surface; however, they are subclassified on the basis of the presence or absence of CD4 and CD8 proteins. **$CD4^+$ T lymphocytes** possess the CD4 marker and recognize antigens bound to major histocompatibility complex II (MHC II) molecules. **$CD8^+$ T lymphocytes** possess the CD8 marker and recognize antigen bound to MHC I molecules.

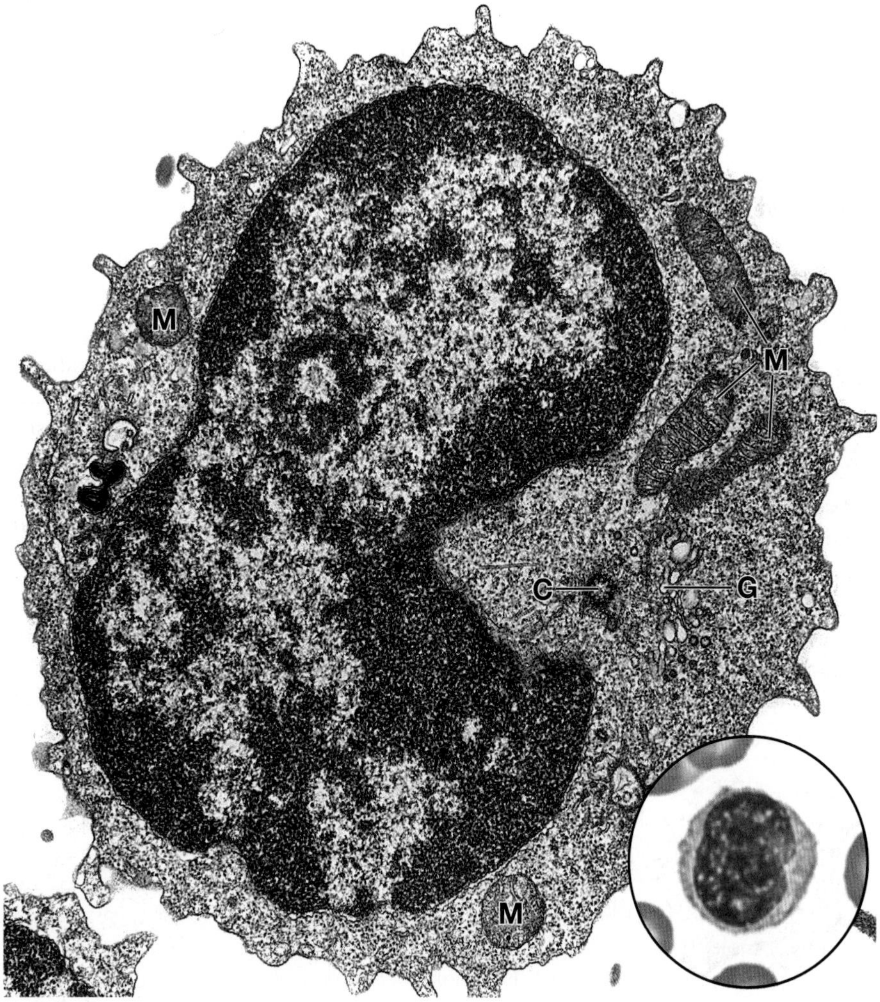

FIGURE 10.14. Electron micrograph of a medium-sized lymphocyte. The punctate appearance of the cytoplasm is caused by the presence of numerous free ribosomes. Several mitochondria (*M*) are evident. The cell center or centrosphere region of the cell (the area of the nuclear indentation) also shows a small Golgi apparatus (*G*) and a centriole (*C*). ×26,000. (Courtesy of Dr. Dorothea Zucker-Franklin.) **Inset.** Light microscopic appearance of a medium-sized lymphocyte from a blood smear. ×1,800.

- **B cells** have variable life spans and are involved in the production of circulating antibodies. Mature B cells in blood express **IgM** and **IgD**, and **MHC II** molecules on their surface. Their specific markers are CD9, CD19, and CD20.
- **NK cells** are programmed during their development to kill certain virus-infected cells and some types of tumor cells. They also secrete an antiviral agent, **interferon-γ (IFN-γ)**. NK cells are larger than B and T cells (~15 μm in diameter) and have a kidney-shaped nucleus. Because NK cells have several large cytoplasmic azurophilic granules easily seen by light microscopy, they are also called large granular lymphocytes (LGLs). Their specific markers include CD16a, CD56, and CD94.

T and B cells are indistinguishable in blood smears and tissue sections; immunocytochemical staining for different types of markers and receptors on their cell surface must be used to identify them. NK lymphocytes can be identified in the light microscope by size, nuclear shape, and presence of cytoplasmic granules; however, immunocytochemical staining for their specific markers is used to confirm microscopic identification.

T lymphocytes, B lymphocytes, and natural killer lymphocytes (NK cells) express different surface molecules.

Although T and B cells cannot be distinguished on the basis of their morphology, their distinctive surface proteins (CD proteins) can be used to identify the cells with immunolabeling techniques. In addition, immunoglobulins are expressed on the surface of **B cells** that function as antigen receptors. In contrast, **T cells** do not have antibodies but express TCRs. These recognition proteins appear during discrete stages in the maturation of the cells within the thymus. In general, the surface molecules mediate or augment specific T-cell functions and are required for the recognition or binding of T cells to antigens displayed on the surface of target cells.

In human blood, 60%–80% of lymphocytes are mature T cells, and 20%–30% are mature B cells. Approximately 5%–15% of the cells do not demonstrate the surface markers associated with neither T nor B cells. These are **NK cells** that are part of nonspecific (innate) immunity. NK cells have the ability to kill certain types of target cells in a similar manner to that of cytotoxic $CD8^+$ T cells. After activation, NK cells release perforins and granzymes (fragmentins), substances that create channels in the cell's plasma membrane and induce fragmentation of DNA.

Several different subsets of T lymphocytes have been identified: cytotoxic, helper, suppressor, gamma/delta ($\gamma\delta$), mucosa-associated invariant T (MAIT), and resident memory T cells (Trm).

The activities of cytotoxic, helper, suppressor, and $\gamma\delta$ T lymphocytes are mediated by molecules located on their surface. Immunolabeling techniques have made it possible to identify specific subsets of T cells and study their function:

- **Cytotoxic $CD8^+$ T lymphocytes (CTLs)** serve as the primary effector cells in cell-mediated immunity. $CD8^+$ cells are specifically sensitized T lymphocytes that recognize antigens through the TCRs on viral or neoplastic host cells. Cytotoxic $CD8^+$ T cells only recognize antigens bound to MHC I molecules. After the TCR binds the antigen–MHC I complex, the CTL cells secrete lymphokines and perforins that produce ion channels in the membrane of the infected or neoplastic cell, leading to its lysis (see Chapter 14, Immune System and Lymphatic Tissues and Organs, see pages 494-495). Cytotoxic CTL cells play a significant role in rejection of allografts and tumor immunology.
- **Helper $CD4^+$ T (TH) cells** are critical for induction of an immune response to a foreign antigen. Antigen bound to MHC II molecules is presented by antigen-presenting cells such as macrophages to a helper $CD4^+$ T lymphocyte. Binding of the TCR to the antigen–MHC II complex activates the helper $CD4^+$ T cells. The activated helper $CD4^+$ T lymphocytes then produce ILs, which act in an autocrine mode to simulate the proliferation and differentiation of more helper $CD4^+$ T lymphocytes. Newly differentiated cells synthesize and secrete lymphokines that affect function as well as differentiation of macrophages, eosinophils, mast cells, B cells, T cells, and NK cells. B cells differentiate into plasma cells and synthesize antibody. Several subsets of helper $CD4^+$ T cells have been identified (i.e., TH1, TH2, and TH17 cells). For details, see Chapter 14, Immune System and Lymphatic Tissues and Organs (page 488).
- **Regulatory (suppressor) T cells** represent a phenotypically diverse population of T lymphocytes that can functionally suppress an immune response to foreign and self-antigen by influencing the activity of other cells in the immune system. **$CD4^+CD25^+FOXP3^+$ regulatory (suppressor) T cells** are representative examples of these cells that can downregulate the ability of T lymphocytes to initiate immune responses. The FOXP3 marker indicates an expression of the forkhead-box family of transcription factors that are characteristic of many T cells. Furthermore, tumor-associated **$CD8^+CD45RO^+$ T suppressor cells** secrete IL-10 and also suppress T-cell activation. The suppressor T cells may also function in suppressing B-cell differentiation and in regulating erythroid cell maturation in the bone marrow.
- **Gamma/delta ($\gamma\delta$) T cells** represent a small population of T cells that possess a distinct TCR on their surface. In contrast to most T cells, which have a TCR composed of two glycoprotein chains, namely, α- and β-TCR chains, $\gamma\delta$ T cells possess TCRs made up of one γ-chain and one δ-chain. These cells develop in the thymus and migrate into various epithelial tissues (e.g., skin, oral mucosa, intestine, and vagina). Once they colonize an epithelial tissue, they do not recirculate between blood and lymphatic organs. They are also known as **intraepithelial lymphocytes**. Their location within the skin and mucosa of internal organs allows them to function as a first line of defense against invading organisms.
- **Mucosa-associated invariant T (MAIT) cells** represent a subset of T cells that express receptors composed of two invariant α- and β-TCR chains. These cells recognize metabolites of that riboflavin (vitamin B_2) synthesis pathway present in fungi and bacteria. After activation, MAIT cells secrete IFN-γ and TNF-α and are capable of destroying the infected cells.
- **Resident memory T cells (Trm)** represent a new subset of non-recirculating memory T lymphocytes. These cells are generated after exposure to antigen in peripheral tissues (i.e., gastrointestinal tract, lung, skin, and reproductive tract) and provide immunological memory at the site of initial exposure. Trm cells express specific markers of residency **CD69**, **CD103**, **CD49a**, but lack molecules enabling them to leave the peripheral tissues and migrate to lymph nodes.

Monocytes

Monocytes are the precursors of the cells of the mononuclear phagocyte system.

Monocytes are the largest of the white blood cells in a blood smear (average diameter is 18 μm). They travel from the bone marrow to the body tissues, where they differentiate into the various phagocytes of the mononuclear phagocyte system—that is, connective tissue macrophages, osteoclasts, alveolar macrophages, perisinusoidal macrophages in the liver (Kupffer cells), and macrophages of lymph nodes, spleen, and bone marrow, among others (see Chapter 6, Connective Tissue, page 203). Monocytes remain in the blood for only about 3 days.

The nucleus of the monocyte is typically more indented than that of the lymphocyte (Fig. 10.15 and Plate 10.2, page 338). The indentation is the site of the cell center where the well-developed Golgi apparatus and centrioles are located. Monocytes also contain smooth endoplasmic reticulum, rER, and small mitochondria. Although these cells are classified as agranular, they contain small, dense, azurophilic granules. These granules contain typical lysosomal enzymes similar to those found in the azurophilic granules of neutrophils.

Monocytes transform into macrophages, which function as antigen-presenting cells in the immune system.

During inflammation, monocytes leave the blood vessel at the site of inflammation, transform into tissue macrophages, and phagocytose bacteria, other cells, and tissue debris. The monocyte–macrophage is an **antigen-presenting cell** and plays an important role in immune responses by partially degrading antigens and presenting their fragments on the MHC II molecules located on the macrophage surface of helper $CD4^{+}$ T lymphocytes for recognition.

■ THROMBOCYTES

Thrombocytes are small, membrane-bound, anucleate cytoplasmic fragments derived from megakaryocytes.

Thrombocytes (platelets) are derived from large polyploid cells (cells whose nuclei contain multiple sets of chromosomes) in the bone marrow called **megakaryocytes** (Fig. 10.16). Megakaryocyte differentiation is regulated by transcription factors and by interactions with hormones (mainly thrombopoietin), chemokines, cytokines, and molecules of the extracellular matrix. In platelet formation, small bits of cytoplasm are separated from the peripheral regions of the megakaryocyte by extensive **platelet demarcation channels**. The membrane that lines these channels arises by invagination of the plasma membrane; therefore, the channels are in continuity with the extracellular space. The continued development and fusion of the platelet demarcation membranes result in the complete partitioning of cytoplasmic fragments to form individual platelets. Mature megakaryocytes migrate to the endothelial cell of bone marrow sinusoids and extend long, branched protrusions, termed **proplatelets**, into the lumen of the sinusoid, where they release large numbers of platelets from their ends.

Human platelets circulate for 7–10 days, and they are removed from the circulation by the liver.

After entering the vascular system from the bone marrow, the platelets circulate as discoid structures about 2–3 μm in diameter. If unused in hemostatic events or pathologic processes, life span of a human platelet is about 7–10 days. Recent studies show that stellate sinusoidal macrophages (Kupffer cells) residing in the hepatic sinusoids continually scan circulating platelets with touch-and-go interactions as these pass through the liver. During aging, platelets expose galactose residues on their surface that mediate platelet binding to hepatocytes and

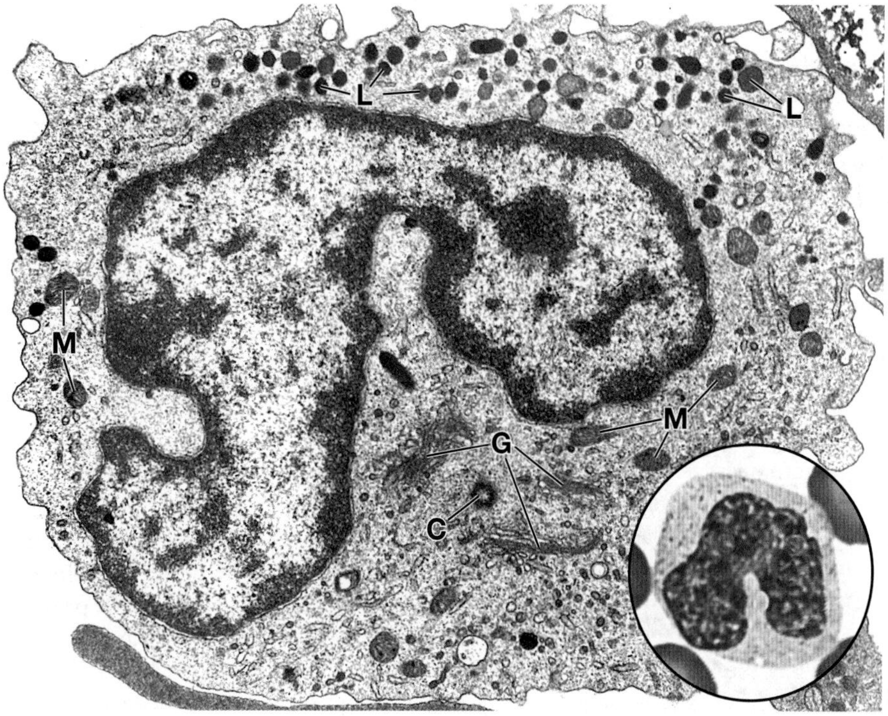

FIGURE 10.15. Electron micrograph of a human mature monocyte. The nucleus is markedly indented, and adjacent to this site, a centriole (*C*) and several Golgi profiles (*G*) are evident. The small dark granules are azurophilic granules, the lysosomes (*L*) of the cell. The slightly larger and less dense profiles are mitochondria (*M*). ×22,000. (Courtesy of Dr. Dorothea Zucker-Franklin.) **Inset.** Light microscopic appearance of a monocyte from a blood smear. ×1,800.

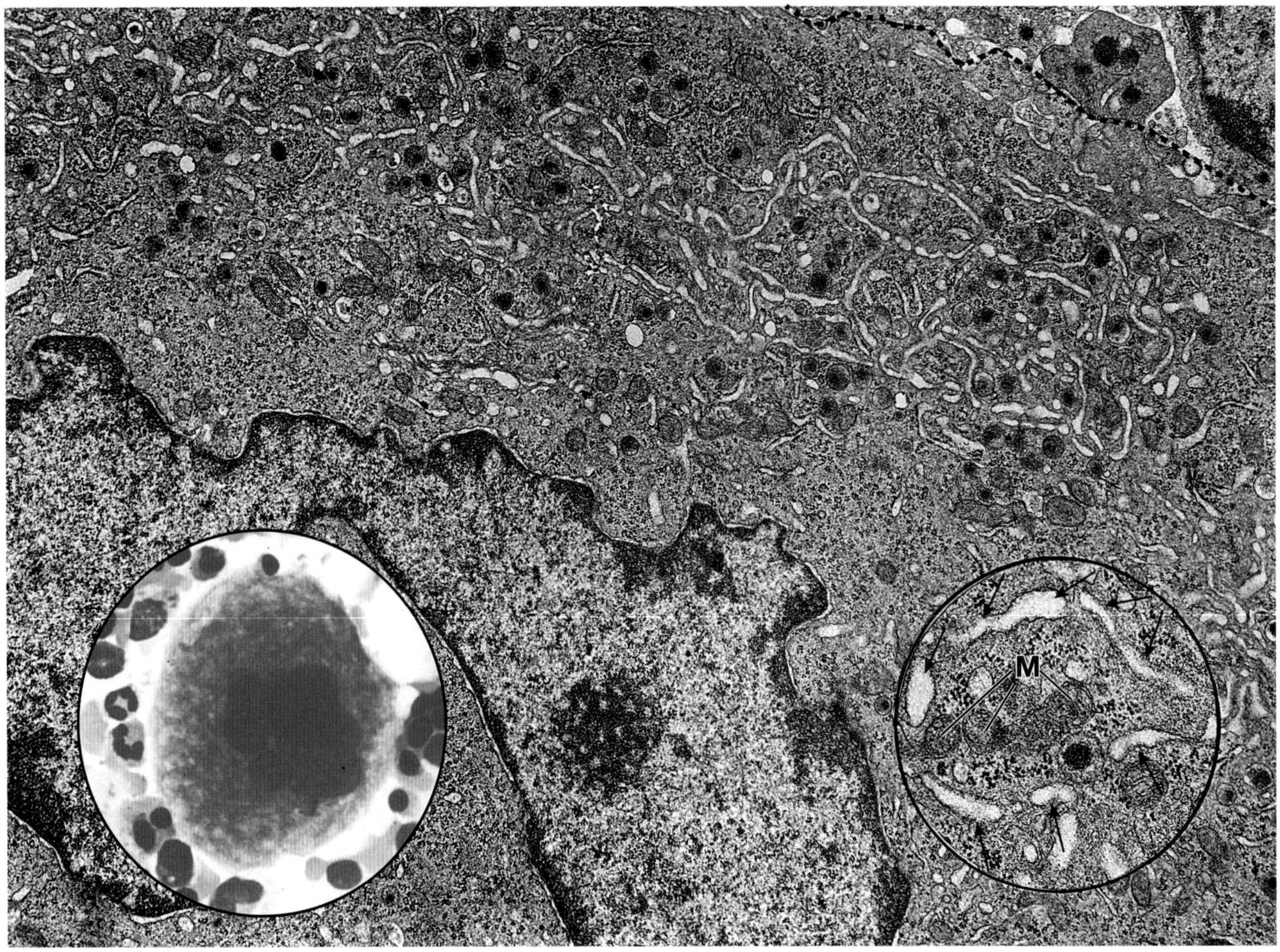

FIGURE 10.16. Electron and light micrographs of a megakaryocyte. This electron micrograph shows a portion of a megakaryocyte from a bone marrow section. Two lobes of the nucleus and the surrounding cytoplasm are visible. The cell border is indicated by the *dotted line* (*upper right*). The cytoplasm reveals evidence of platelet formation as indicated by the extensive platelet demarcation channels. ×13,000. **Left inset.** Light micrograph showing an entire megakaryocyte from a marrow smear. Its nucleus is multilobed and folded on itself, giving an irregular outline. The "foamy" peripheral cytoplasm of the megakaryocyte represents areas in which segmentation to form platelets is occurring. The smaller surrounding cells are developing blood cells. ×1,000. **Right inset.** Higher power electron micrograph showing a section of cytoplasm that is almost fully partitioned by platelet demarcation channels (*arrows*). It also shows mitochondria (*M*), a very dense γ granule, and glycogen particles. For comparison, Figure 10.17a shows a mature circulating platelet. ×30,000.

Kupffer cells. Aged platelets are removed from the circulation by the phagocytic action of Kupffer cells (see pages 700-702).

Structurally, platelets may be divided into four zones based on organization and function.

The TEM reveals a structural organization of the thrombocyte cytoplasm that can be categorized into the following four zones (Fig. 10.17):

- The **peripheral zone** consists of the cell membrane covered by a thick surface coat of glycocalyx. The glycocalyx consists of glycoproteins, glycosaminoglycans, and several coagulation factors adsorbed from the plasma. The integral membrane glycoproteins function as receptors in platelet function.
- The **structural zone**, near the periphery, comprises microtubules, actin filaments, myosin, and actin-binding proteins that form a network supporting the plasma membrane. The marginal band containing 8–24 coiled microtubules resides as a bundle immediately below the actin filament network. These multiple microtubule coils are circumferentially arranged and are responsible for maintaining the platelet's discoid shape.
- The **organelle zone** occupies the center of the platelet. It consists of mitochondria, peroxisomes, glycogen particles, and at least three types of granules dispersed within the cytoplasm. The most numerous granules are **alpha (α) granules** (300–500 nm in diameter) that contain mainly fibrinogen, coagulation factors (factors V and XI, protein S, and antithrombin), plasminogen, plasminogen activator inhibitor, metalloproteinase 4 (MMP-4), tissue inhibitor of metalloproteinase 4 (TIMP-4), and a variety of growth factors, including platelet-derived growth factor (PDGF), endothelial growth factor (EGF), vascular endothelial growth factor (VEGF), insulin-like growth factor 1 (IGF-1), and transforming growth factor β (TGF-β). The contents of these granules play an important role in the initial phase of vessel repair, blood coagulation, and platelet aggregation. Based on proteomic studies, more than 300 soluble proteins are released by an alpha (α) granule during platelet activation. The smaller, denser, and less numerous **gamma (γ) granules**, also known as *dense or delta* (δ) *granules*, mainly contain nucleotides such as adenosine diphosphate (ADP), adenosine triphosphate (ATP), uridine triphosphate (UTP), and guanosine triphosphate (GTP); bioactive amines (serotonin and histamine); and

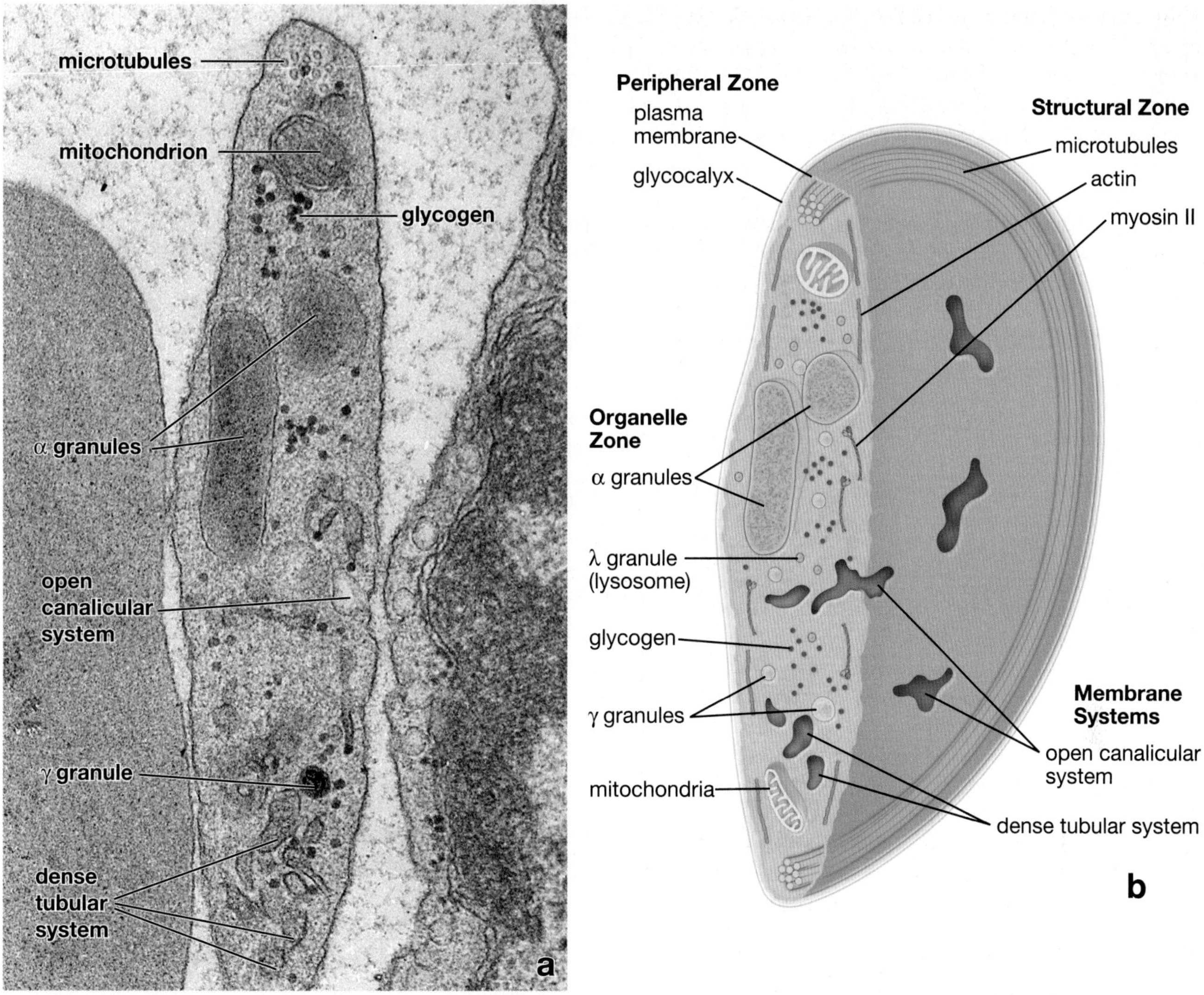

FIGURE 10.17. Platelet electron micrograph and diagram. a. High-magnification electron micrograph of a platelet situated between an erythrocyte on the *left* and an endothelial cell on the *right*. Visible organelles include a mitochondrion, microtubules, a single profile of the surface-connected open canalicular system, profiles of the dense tubular system, moderately dense α granules, a single very dense γ granule, and glycogen particles. The microfilaments are not evident against the background matrix of the platelet. **b.** Diagram of a platelet showing the components of the four structural zones.

cations of Ca^{+2}, Mg^{+2}, and K^{+}. Gamma (γ) granules facilitate platelet adhesion and vasoconstriction around the injured vessel. **York platelet syndrome (YPS)** is caused by mutations in Ca^{+2} channel proteins in platelets and is characterized by thrombocytopenia and deficiency of platelet Ca^{+2} storage in gamma (γ) granules. Platelets from individuals with YPS are abnormally large and exhibit giant electron-opaque organelles. The **lambda (λ) granules** are similar to lysosomes found in other cells and contain several hydrolytic enzymes. The contents of lambda (λ) granules function in clot resorption during the later stages of vessel repair.

- The **membrane zone** consists of two types of membrane channels: (1) the **open canalicular system (OCS)** and (2) the **dense tubular system (DTS)**. The OCS is a developmental remnant of the platelet demarcation channels and is simply a membrane that did not participate in subdividing the megakaryocyte cytoplasm. In effect, open canaliculi are invaginations into the cytoplasm from the plasma membrane. The DTS contains an electron-dense material originating from the rER of the megakaryocyte, which serves as a storage site for calcium ions. DTS channels do not connect with the surface of the platelet; however, both OCS and DTS fuse in various areas of the platelet to form membrane complexes that are important in the regulation of the intraplatelet calcium concentration.

Platelets function in continuous surveillance of blood vessels, blood clot formation, and repair of injured tissue.

Platelets are involved in several aspects of **hemostasis** (control of bleeding). They continuously survey the endothelial lining of blood vessels for gaps and breaks. When a blood vessel wall is injured or broken, the exposed connective tissue at the damaged site promotes platelet adhesion. Adhesion of the platelets at the damaged site triggers their degranulation and release of serotonin, adenosine diphosphate (ADP), and thromboxane A_2.

Serotonin is a potent vasoconstrictor that causes vascular smooth muscle cells to contract, thereby reducing local blood flow at the site of injury. **Adenosine diphosphate (ADP)**, a nucleotide, and the signaling molecule **thromboxane A_2** are responsible for the further aggregation of platelets into a **primary hemostatic plug**. The mass of aggregated platelets stops the extravasation of blood.

At the same time, the activated platelets release their alpha (α) and gamma (γ) granules and participate in the intrinsic pathway of blood coagulation known as **platelet thromboplastin factor (PF_3)**. As recent cellular and molecular studies indicate, this is not a true "factor" or detectable molecule but rather an activity of the platelet plasma membrane. The glycocalyx on the plasma membrane of activated platelets supplies a catalytic lipoprotein surface for converting **soluble fibrinogen** into **fibrin** and interactions with other plasma coagulation factors at the site of platelet aggregation. Fibrin then forms a loose mesh over the initial plug and is further stabilized by covalent cross-links that produce a dense aggregation of fibers (Fig. 10.18). Platelets and red blood cells become trapped in this mesh. The initial platelet plug is transformed into a definitive clot called a **secondary hemostatic plug** by additional tissue factors secreted by the damaged blood vessel.

After the definitive clot is formed, platelets cause clot retraction, probably as a function of the actin and myosin found in the structural zone of the platelet. Contraction of the clot permits the return of normal blood flow through the vessel. Finally, after the clot has served its function, it is lysed by plasmin, a fibrinolytic enzyme that circulates in the plasma in an inactive form known as **plasminogen**. The hydrolytic enzymes released from the λ granules assist in this process. The activator for plasminogen conversion, **tissue plasminogen activator (TPA)**, is derived principally from endothelial cells. A synthetic form of **TPA** is used as an emergency treatment to minimize the damage caused by clots that lead to strokes. The current standard of care based on safety and efficacy for **acute ischemic stroke** is an intravenous injection of TPA within 3–4.5 hours of the onset of symptoms. The goals of the TPA treatment are recanalization of the occluded cerebral arteries and the reperfusion of ischemic areas of the brain to decrease or prevent morbidity and mortality.

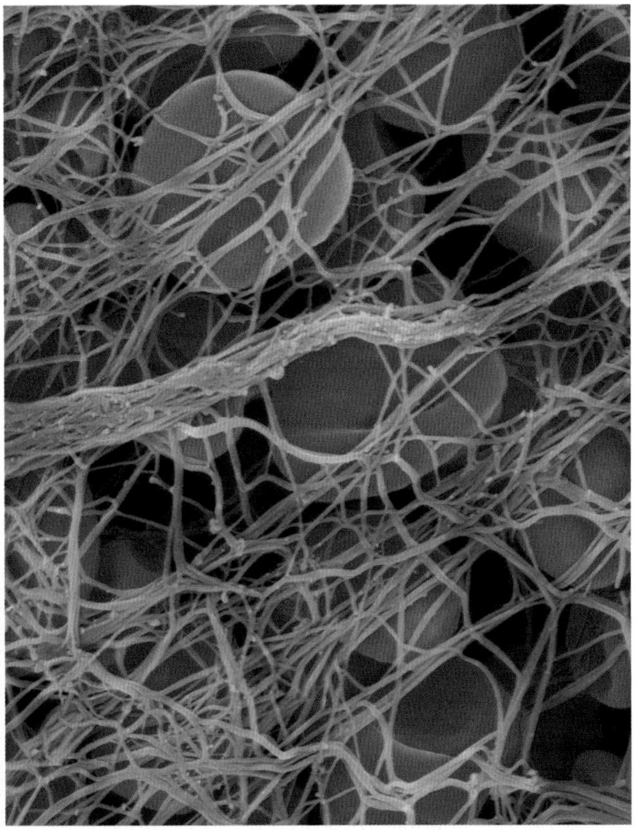

FIGURE 10.18. Scanning electron micrograph of blood clot. High-magnification scanning electron micrograph shows initial stage of blood clot formation. Red blood cells are entrapped in a loose mesh of fibrin fibers that are extensively cross-linked to form an impermeable hemostatic plug that prevents movement of cells and fluids from the lumen of the injured vessel. ×1,600. (Copyright Dennis Kunkel Microscopy, Inc.)

An additional role of platelets is to help repair the injured tissues beyond the vessel itself. PDGF released from the α granules stimulates smooth muscle cells and fibroblasts to divide and allow tissue repair.

■ COMPLETE BLOOD COUNT

A **complete blood count (CBC)** is one of the most commonly ordered laboratory test panels. It provides relative numbers and calculations obtained from the cells (erythrocytes and leukocytes) and formed elements (thrombocytes) in the blood sample. These calculations are usually performed by automated blood cell counters that analyze different components of blood using the principle of **flow cytometry** design.

In preparation for counting, the blood sample is diluted in a suspension fluid. As a thin stream of fluid with suspended cells flows through the narrow tubing of the cell counter, the light detector and electrical impedance sensor identify different cell types based on their size and electrical resistance. Data obtained from automatic blood analyzers are usually very accurate owing to the large number of cells counted (~10,000) in each category. Computer-assisted blood cell analysis systems use cameras and image-processing technologies to automatically count and analyze cells. However, in some cases, manual cell count under a light microscope is still necessary. A typical CBC laboratory panel includes the following:

- **Leukocyte (white blood cell) count.** An elevated count of leukocytes (leukocytosis) may indicate an inflammatory reaction response (i.e., infections, burns, bone fractures, other body injuries). The leukocyte count can also be elevated after strenuous exercise because of stress or in pregnancy and labor. Hyperleukocytosis (leukocyte count $>100 \times 10^9$ cells/L) is commonly an indication of leukemia (a type of blood cancer). A decreased leukocyte count (leukopenia) is usually associated with radiation and chemotherapy, autoimmune diseases, bone marrow diseases (aplastic anemia), the use of specific drugs (antipsychotic, antiepileptic, immunosuppressive), HIV, and AIDS.
- **Leukocyte types (white blood cell differential).** The major types of white blood cells reported are neutrophils, eosinophils, basophils, lymphocytes, and monocytes. Immature neutrophils (band cells) are also reported. Each type of leukocyte plays a different role in protecting the body, and percentages of their distribution in the blood sample give important information about the status of the immune system. Refer to the appropriate sections of this chapter for descriptions and functions of these cells.
- **Erythrocytes (red blood cell) count.** An elevated erythrocyte count (polycythemia) may be related to intrinsic factors affecting erythrocyte production in the bone marrow (primary polycythemia) or as a response to stimuli (e.g., hormones) produced by other organs in the body that promote erythropoiesis. Examples of primary polycythemia may include genetic diseases such as polycythemia vera or

primary familiar and congenital polycythemia (PFCP). Secondary polycythemia is usually due to increased production of erythropoietin in response to chronic hypoxia, high altitude, or an erythropoietin-secreting tumor. A decreased erythrocyte count (anemia) may be caused by blood loss (external or internal bleeding), iron or vitamin B_{12} deficiencies, poor nutrition, pregnancy, chronic diseases, and genetic disorders (e.g., sickle cell anemia).

- **Hematocrit (HCT**; also called **packed cell volume [PCV])** measures the percentage of erythrocyte volume in the blood sample.
- **Hemoglobin (Hgb)**. The Hgb concentration in the blood reflects an erythrocyte's ability to carry oxygen. Normal Hgb values are 13.5–17.5 g/dL (140–180 g/L) in men and 12–15.5 g/dL (120–150 g/L) in women. HCT and Hgb values are the two major tests that are used to evaluate for anemia or polycythemia.
- **Erythrocyte indices**. Usually, four erythrocyte indices are included in the CBC: **mean corpuscular volume (MCV)**, which relates to the size of the red blood cells; **mean corpuscular hemoglobin (MCH)**, which shows the amount of Hgb in an average erythrocyte; **mean corpuscular hemoglobin concentration (MCHC)**, which provides the percentage of Hgb concentration in an average erythrocyte; and the **red blood cell distribution width (RDW)**, which shows if the erythrocytes are all the same or if they are different in sizes or shapes. These indices are automatically calculated from other measurements and are useful in differential diagnosis.
- **Thrombocyte (platelet) count**. Thrombocytes are important in blood clotting, and their elevation (thrombocythemia) may be related to proliferative disorders of the bone marrow, inflammation, decreased function of the spleen, or as a result of splenectomy. Low thrombocyte count (thrombocytopenia) may be related to decreased production of thrombocytes in the bone marrow (i.e., hereditary syndromes, leukemia, infections, vitamin B_{12} deficiency) or increased destruction of thrombocytes in the peripheral tissues (i.e., autoimmune diseases, genetic disorders, disseminated intravascular coagulation). Destruction of thrombocytes also may be induced by medications. In addition, the **mean platelet volume (MPV)** can be calculated to provide the average size of platelets in the volume of examined blood.

■ FORMATION OF BLOOD CELLS (HEMOPOIESIS)

Hemopoiesis (hematopoiesis) includes both **erythropoiesis** and **leukopoiesis** (development of red and white blood cells, respectively) as well as **thrombopoiesis** (development of platelets; Fig. 10.19). Blood cells have a limited life span; they are continuously produced and destroyed. The ultimate objective of hemopoiesis is to maintain a constant level of the different cell types found in the peripheral blood. Both the human erythrocyte (life span of 120 days) and the platelet (life span of 10 days) spend their entire life in the circulating blood. Leukocytes, however, migrate out of the circulation shortly after entering it from the bone marrow and spend most of their variable life spans (and perform all of their functions) in the tissues.

In the adult, erythrocytes, granulocytes, monocytes, and platelets are formed in the **red bone marrow**; lymphocytes are also formed in the red bone marrow and the lymphatic tissues. To study the stages of blood cell formation, a sample of bone marrow aspirate (see page 333) is prepared as a stained smear in a manner similar to that of a smear of blood.

Hemopoiesis is initiated in early embryonic development.

During fetal life, both erythrocytes and leukocytes are formed in several organs before the differentiation of the bone marrow. The first or **yolk-sac phase** of hemopoiesis begins in the third week of gestation and is characterized by the formation of "blood islands" in the wall of the yolk sac of the embryo. In the second, or **hepatic phase**, early in fetal development, hemopoietic centers appear in the liver (Fig. 10.20). Blood cell formation in these sites is largely limited to erythroid cells, although some leukopoiesis occurs in the liver. The liver is the major blood-forming organ in the fetus during the second trimester. The third or **bone marrow phase** of fetal hemopoiesis and leukopoiesis involves the bone marrow (and other lymphatic tissues) and begins during the second trimester of pregnancy. After birth, hemopoiesis takes place only in the red bone marrow and some lymphatic tissues, as in the adult (Fig. 10.21). The precursors of both blood cells and germ cells arise in the yolk sac.

Monophyletic Theory of Hemopoiesis

Blood cells are derived from a common hemopoietic stem cell.

The common hemopoietic stem cell in the monophyletic theory of hemopoiesis is called the **hemopoietic stem cell (HSC)**, also known as the pluripotential stem cell (PPSC). This stem cell is capable not only of differentiating into any blood cell lineage but also of renewing itself (i.e., the pool of stem cells is self-sustaining). HSCs also have the potential to differentiate into multiple non–blood cell lineages and contribute to the cellular regeneration of various tissues and multiple organs. During embryonic development, HSCs are present in the circulation and undergo tissue-specific differentiation in different organs. Human HSCs have been isolated from umbilical cord blood, fetal liver, and fetal and adult bone marrow. In the adult, HSCs have the potential to repair tissues under pathologic conditions (e.g., ischemic injury, organ failure). Human HSCs express specific molecular marker proteins such as CD34 and CD90 but do not express lineage-specific markers (Lin^-) that are found on lymphocytes, granulocytes, monocytes, megakaryocytes, and erythroid cells. Human HSC can be identified by the presence or absence of the specific **Lin^-**, **$CD34^+$**, **$CD38^-$**, **$CD90^+$**, and **$CD45RA^-$** cell surface markers. HSCs are not identifiable in routine preparations of blood cells; however, they can be identified and isolated using immunocytochemical methods.

A hemopoietic stem cell (HSC) in the bone marrow gives rise to multiple colonies of progenitor stem cells.

In the bone marrow, descendants of the HSC differentiate into two major colonies of multipotential progenitor cells: the common myeloid progenitor (CMP) cells and the common lymphoid progenitor (CLP) cells.

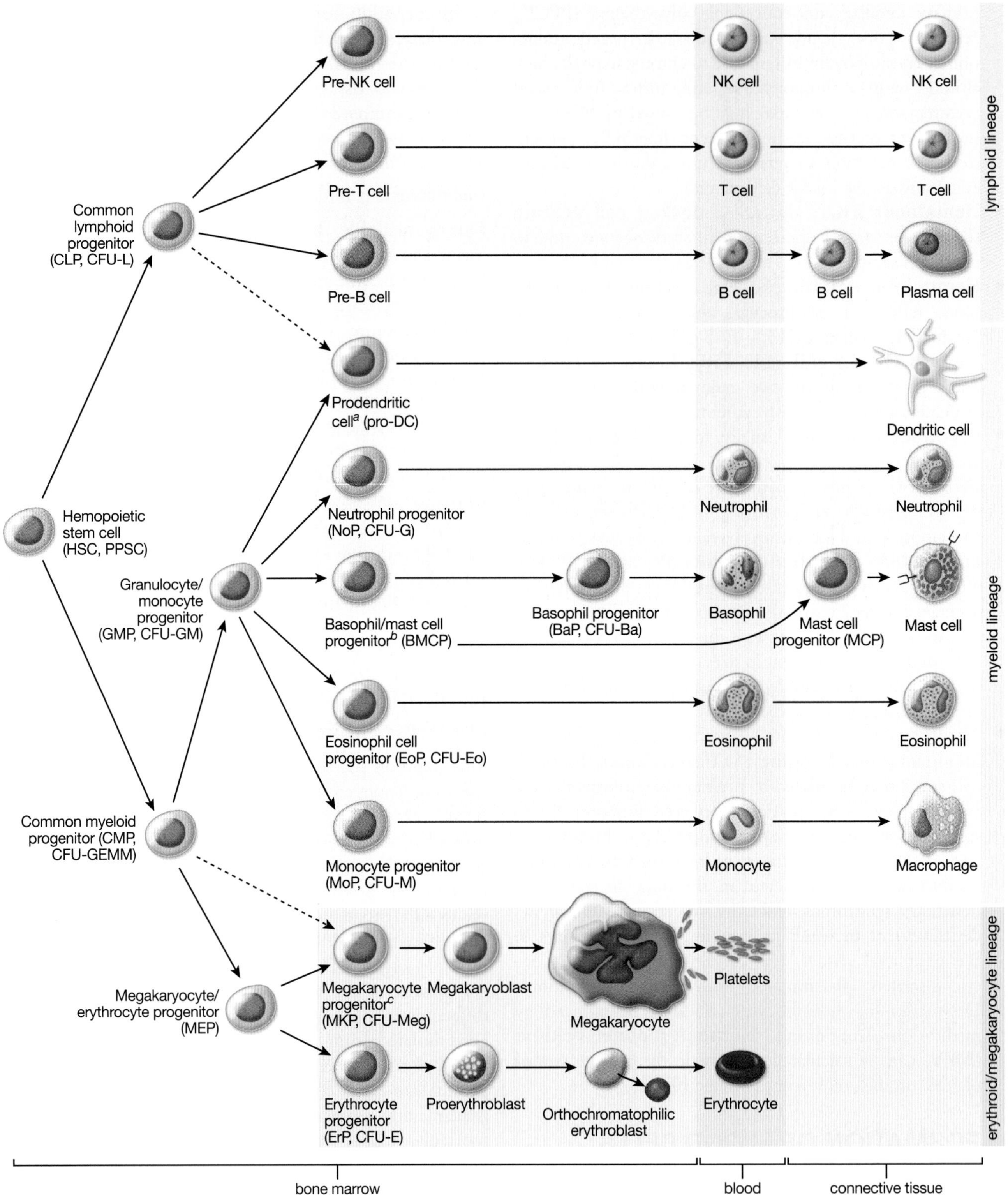

FIGURE 10.19. Hemopoiesis. This chart is based on the most recent concepts in hemopoiesis. It shows blood cells' development from hemopoietic stem cells in the bone marrow to mature cells and their distribution in the blood and connective tissue compartments. In all lineages, extensive proliferation occurs during differentiation. Cytokines (including hemopoietic growth factors) act individually and together at all stages in the process, from development of the first stem cell to mature blood or connective tissue cell. Note that the second acronym listed in parenthesis with a name of the progenitor cell refers to previously used nomenclature: CFU-Ba, colony-forming units—basophil; CFU-E, colony-forming units—erythrocyte; CFU-Eo, colony-forming units—eosinophil; CFU-G, colony-forming units—neutrophil; CFU-GEMM, colony-forming units—granulocyte, erythrocyte, monocyte, megakaryocyte; CFU-GM, colony-forming units—granulocyte/monocyte; CFU-L, colony-forming units—lymphoid; CFU-M, colony-forming units—monocyte; CFU-Meg, colony-forming units—megakaryocyte; PPSC, pluripotential stem cell. For clarity of reading these acronyms are not used in the text.

[a]Prodendritic cells can differentiate from common lymphoid progenitor cells.
[b]If committed to enter the mast cell lineage, the basophil/mast cell progenitor cell migrates to the spleen where it differentiates into a mast cell progenitor cell. After further differentiation in the spleen, it migrates to the intestine to become a mast cell precursor.
[c]A megakaryocyte progenitor cell may also differentiate directly from a common myeloid progenitor cell.

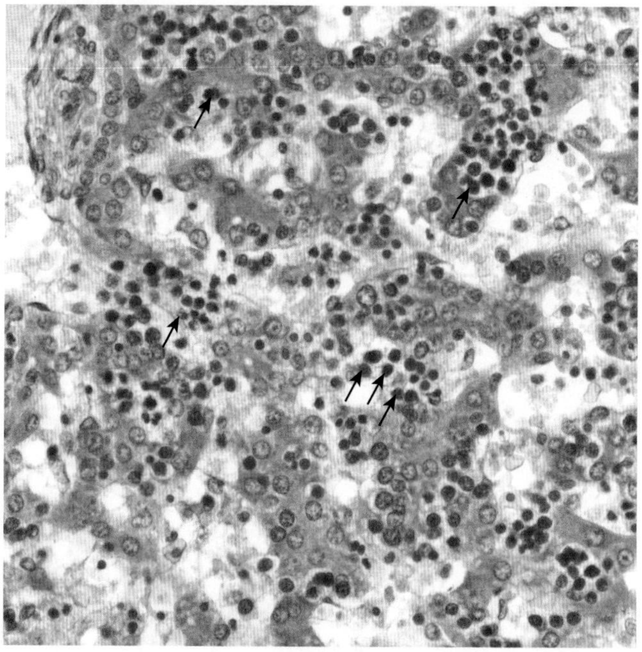

FIGURE 10.20. Hepatic stage of hemopoiesis. Photomicrograph of the fetal liver stained with hematoxylin and eosin (H&E) shows active hemopoiesis. The small round bodies (*arrows*) are mostly nuclei of developing erythrocytes. Although it is difficult to discern, these cells are located between developing liver cells and the wall of the vascular sinus. ×350.

Ultimately, **common myeloid progenitor (CMP) cells**, differentiate into the following specific **lineage-restricted progenitors** (Table 10.3):

- **Megakaryocyte/erythrocyte progenitor (MEP) cells.** These bipotential stem cells give rise to monopotent **megakaryocyte-committed progenitor cells (MKP)** and other monopotent **erythrocyte-committed progenitor cells (ErP)** that give rise to the erythrocyte lineage.
- **Granulocyte/monocyte progenitor (GMP) cells.** Development of GMP cells requires expression of high levels of **PU-1 transcription factor**. These cells then give rise to **neutrophil progenitors (NoP)**, which differentiate into the neutrophilic lineage; **eosinophil progenitors (EoPs)**, which give rise to eosinophils; **basophil/mast cell progenitors (BMCPs)**, which give rise to either **basophil progenitor cells (BaP)** in the bone marrow or **mast cell progenitors (MCPs)**, which migrate via spleen to the gastrointestinal mucosa; and, finally, **monocyte progenitors (MoP)** that develop toward monocyte lineages. In addition to the specific lineage progenitors, GMP cells can give rise to **dendritic cells (DCs)**, which are professional antigen-presenting cells. Dendritic cells are discussed in Chapter 14, Immune System and Lymphatic Tissues and Organs (page 506).

Common lymphoid progenitor (CLP) cells are multipotential cells capable of differentiating into T cells, B cells, and NK cells. NK cells are thought to be the prototype of T cells; both possess a similar capability to destroy other cells. Lymphocytes are discussed in Chapter 14, Immune System and Lymphatic Tissues and Organs, pages 487-491. Dendritic cells can also develop from CLP cells.

Figure 10.22 shows the stages of blood cell development in which characteristic cell types can be identified in the light microscope in a tissue section or bone marrow smear. Hemopoiesis is initiated in an apparently random manner when individual HSCs begin to differentiate into one of the lineage-restricted progenitor cells. Progenitor cells have surface receptors for specific cytokines and growth factors, including **colony-stimulating factors (CSFs)** that influence their proliferation and maturation into a specific lineage.

Development of Erythrocytes (Erythropoiesis)

Erythrocyte development starts from CMP cells that, under the influence of erythropoietin, IL-3, and IL-4, differentiate into MEP cells. Expression of **transcription factor GATA-1** is required for the terminal differentiation of MEP cells into definitive erythroid cell lineage. Under GATA-1 influence, MEP cells transform into **erythropoietin-sensitive**

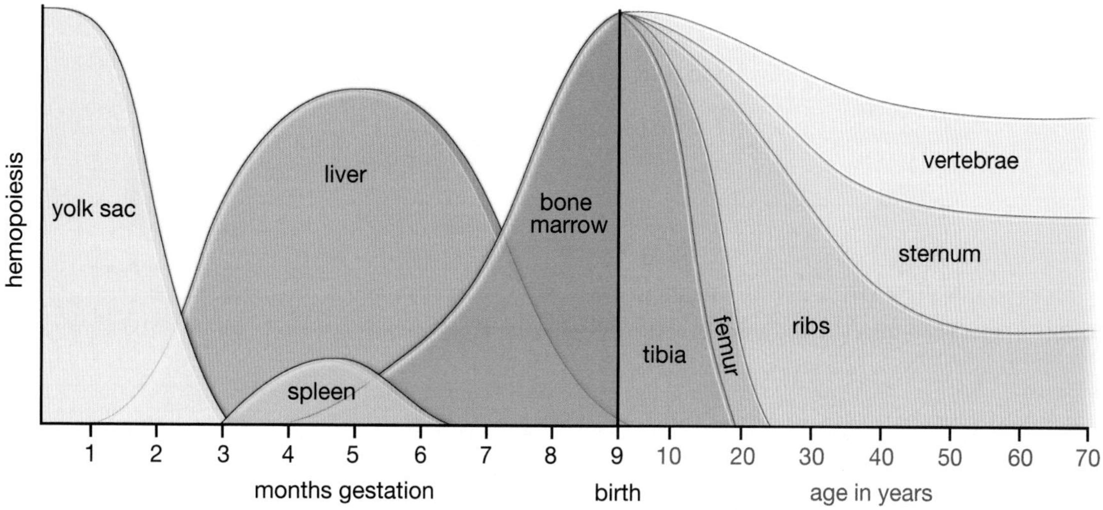

FIGURE 10.21. Dynamics of hemopoiesis from embryonic through adult life. During embryonic and fetal life, erythrocytes are formed in several organs. Essentially, three major organs involved in hemopoiesis can be sequentially identified: the yolk sac in the early developmental stages of the embryo, the liver during the second trimester of pregnancy, and the bone marrow during the third trimester. The spleen participates to a very limited degree during the second trimester of pregnancy. At birth, most hemopoiesis occurs in the red bone marrow. In children and young adults, hemopoiesis occurs in the red bone marrow of all bones, including long bones such as the femur and tibia. In adults, hemopoiesis is maintained primarily in flat bones (e.g., pelvic bones, sacrum, ribs, sternum, cranium) and vertebrae.

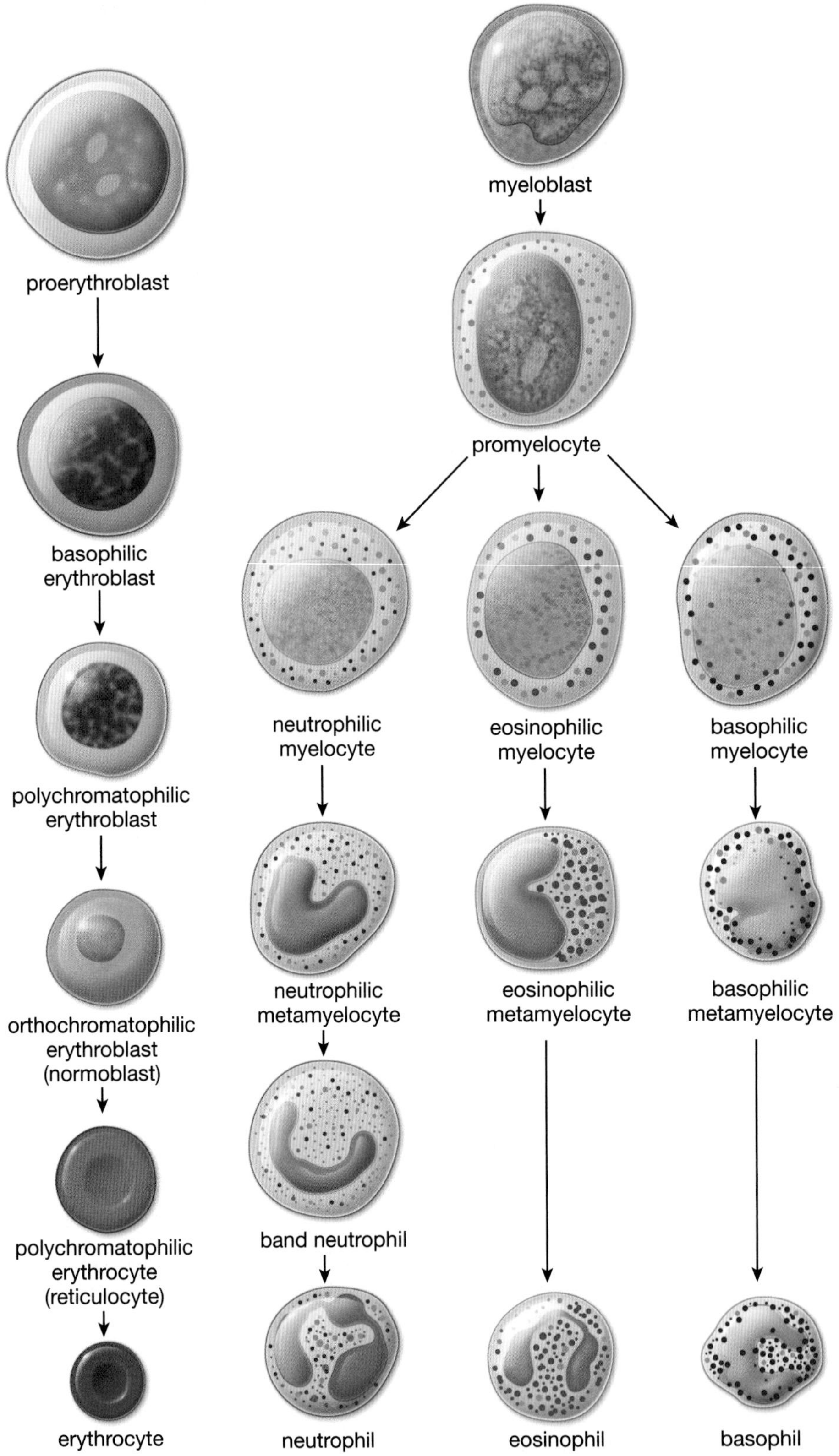

FIGURE 10.22. Stages of erythrocytic and granular leukocytic differentiation. Shown here are normal human bone marrow cells as they would typically appear in a smear.

erythrocyte-committed progenitors (ErPs) that give rise to the **proerythroblast.**

The first microscopically recognizable precursor cell in erythropoiesis is called the proerythroblast.

The **proerythroblast** is a relatively large cell measuring 12–20 μm in diameter. It contains a large, spherical nucleus with one or two visible nucleoli. The cytoplasm shows mild basophilia because of the presence of free ribosomes. Within the proerythroblast, components necessary for Hgb production begin to accumulate. This stage lasts approximately 24 hours. Although recognizable, the proerythroblast is not easily identified in routine bone marrow smears.

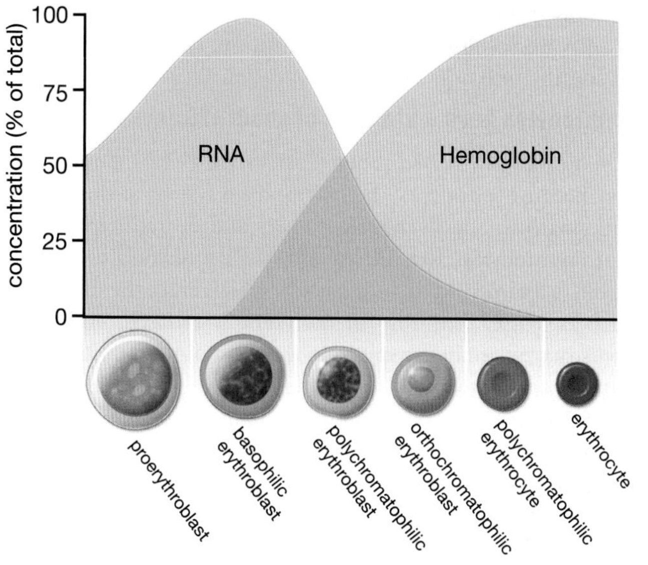

FIGURE 10.23. **Timeline of relative RNA and hemoglobin concentration during erythropoiesis.**

The basophilic erythroblast is smaller than the proerythroblast, from which it arises by mitotic division.

The nucleus of the **basophilic erythroblast** is smaller (10–16 μm in diameter) and progressively more heterochromatic with repeated mitoses. The cytoplasm shows strong basophilia because of the large number of free ribosomes (polyribosomes) that synthesize Hgb (Fig. 10.23). The accumulation of Hgb in the cell gradually changes the staining reaction of the cytoplasm so that it begins to stain with eosin. This stage lasts approximately 24 hours. At the stage when the cytoplasm displays both acidophilia, because of the staining of Hgb, and basophilia, because of the staining of the ribosomes, the cell is called a **polychromatophilic erythroblast**.

The polychromatophilic erythroblast shows both acidophilic and basophilic staining of cytoplasm.

The staining reactions of the **polychromatophilic erythroblast** may blend to give an overall gray or lilac color to the cytoplasm, or distinct pink (acidophilic) and purple (basophilic) regions may be resolved in the cytoplasm. The nucleus of the cell is smaller than that of the basophilic erythroblast, and coarse heterochromatin granules form a checkerboard pattern that helps identify this cell type. This is the last stage in which the polychromatophilic erythroblast is capable of undergoing mitosis and cell division to produce two daughter cells at the same stage of maturation and development. This stage lasts approximately 30 hours.

The orthochromatophilic erythroblast is recognized by its increased acidophilic cytoplasm and dense nucleus.

The next named stage in erythropoiesis is the **orthochromatophilic erythroblast (normoblast)**. This cell has a small, compact, densely stained nucleus. The cytoplasm is eosinophilic because of the large amount of Hgb (Fig. 10.24). It is only slightly larger than a mature erythrocyte. At this stage, the orthochromatophilic erythroblast is no longer capable of division. Late in this stage, the nucleus is ejected from the cell. Often, small fragments of the nucleus are left behind; these are called *Howell–Jolly bodies*. This stage lasts approximately 48 hours.

The polychromatophilic erythrocyte has extruded its nucleus.

The orthochromatophilic erythroblast loses its nucleus by extruding it from the cell; it is then ready to pass into the blood sinusoids of the red bone marrow. Some polyribosomes that can still synthesize Hgb are retained in the cell. These polyribosomes impart a slight basophilia to the otherwise eosinophilic cells; for this reason, these new cells are called **polychromatophilic erythrocytes** (Fig. 10.25). The polyribosomes of the new erythrocytes can also be demonstrated with special stains that cause the polyribosomes to clump and form a reticular network. Consequently, polychromatophilic erythrocytes are also (and more commonly) called **reticulocytes**. Typically, polychromatophilic erythrocytes reside in the bone marrow for 24 hours and then move into the peripheral circulation for an additional 24 hours. After this short period in the peripheral circulation, they are retained by the spleen. Reticulocytes normally constitute about 1%–2% of the total erythrocyte count. However, if increased numbers of erythrocytes enter the bloodstream (as during increased erythropoiesis to compensate for blood loss), the number of reticulocytes increases.

The stage of maturation of red blood cells can be determined by a careful examination of the nucleus and cytoplasm.

As erythrocytes mature, several visible trends can be recognized (see Fig. 10.22), including the following:

- Change in the overall **size of the cell**. As the proerythroblast differentiates into the erythroblast, its cell diameter decreases from 12–20 to 7.8 μm.
- Change in the **size of the nucleus**. During differentiation, the size of the nucleus decreases to a more significant degree than the size of the cell. As a result, the nucleus-to-cytoplasm

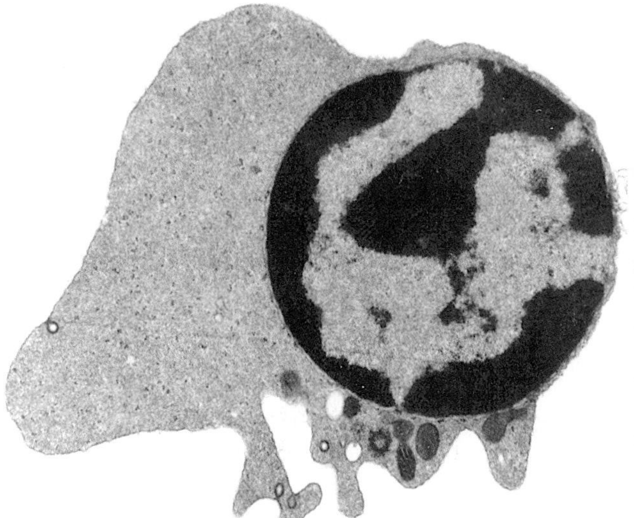

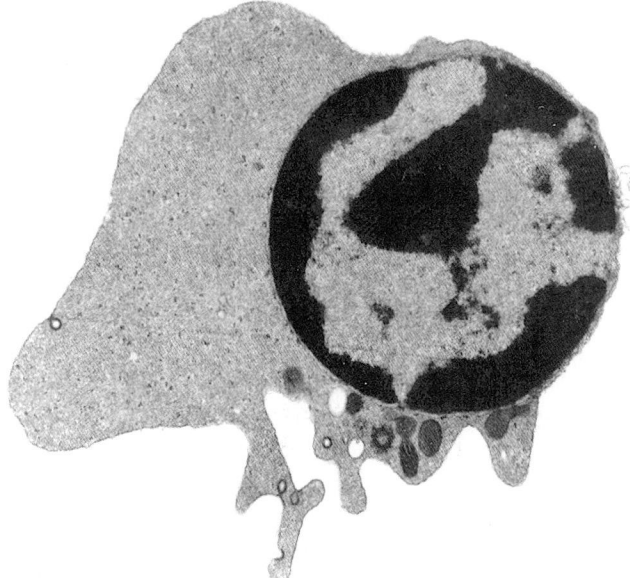

FIGURE 10.24. **Electron micrograph of an orthochromatophilic erythroblast (normoblast).** The cell is shown just before extrusion of the nucleus. The cytoplasm contains a group of mitochondria located below the nucleus and small cytoplasmic vacuoles. The cytoplasm is relatively dense because of its hemoglobin content. The fine, dense particles scattered in the cytoplasm are ribosomes. ×10,000. (Courtesy of Dr. Dorothea Zucker-Franklin.)

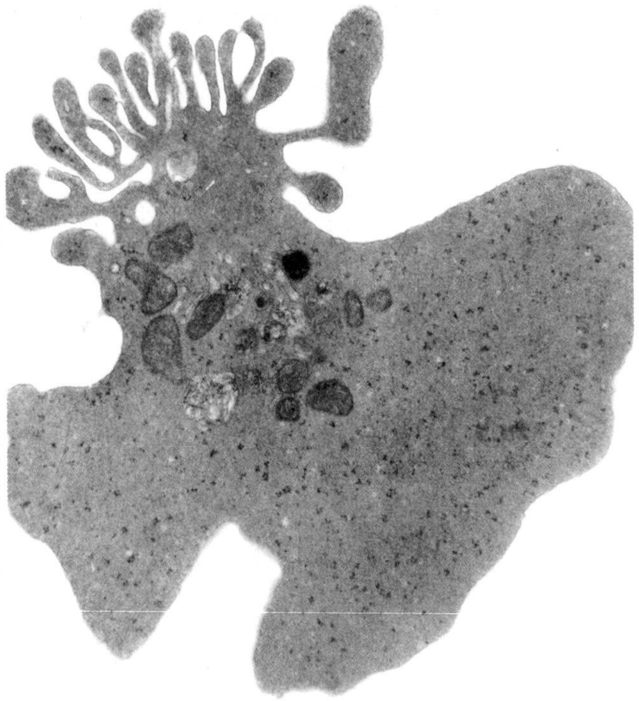

FIGURE 10.25. Electron micrograph of a polychromatophilic erythrocyte (reticulocyte). The nucleus is no longer present, and the cytoplasm shows the characteristic fimbriated processes that occur just after nuclear extrusion. Mitochondria are still present, as are early and late endosomes and ribosomes. ×16,500. (Courtesy of Dr. Dorothea Zucker-Franklin.)

ratio increases from 1:8 in the proerythroblast to 1:2 in the orthochromatophilic erythroblast.

- Change in the **number of nucleoli**. Because nucleoli represent sites of active relative RNA (rRNA) synthesis, nucleoli disappear with maturation as the cells cease their synthesis of Hgb and other proteins.
- Change in the **nuclear chromatin pattern**. As the proerythroblast undergoes differentiation, the heterochromatin becomes coarser, clumped, and condensed. Ultimately, the nucleus in the orthochromatophilic erythroblast becomes so condensed that no visible chromatin pattern can be seen.
- Change in **staining appearance** of the cytoplasm. As cells undergo differentiation, the appearance of their cytoplasm changes from dark blue (basophilic) to gray and pink (eosinophilic). Cytoplasmic basophilia correlates with the amount of RNA and the number of organelles present in cytoplasm (i.e., mitochondria, rER, polyribosomes, and ribosomes) in the early stages of development. As the amount of RNA and number of organelles decline in developing erythroblasts (see Fig. 10.23), the cytoplasmic basophilia fades and is gradually replaced by eosinophilia, which correlates with the amount of Hgb accumulated within the maturing cell.

Kinetics of Erythropoiesis

Mitoses occur in proerythroblasts, basophilic erythroblasts, and polychromatophilic erythroblasts.

At each of these stages of development, the erythroblast divides several times. It takes about a week for the progeny of a newly formed basophilic erythroblast to reach the circulation. Nearly all erythrocytes are released into the circulation as soon as they are formed; bone marrow is not a storage site for erythrocytes. Erythrocyte formation and release are regulated by **erythropoietin**, a 34-kDa glycoprotein hormone synthesized and secreted by the kidney in response to decreased blood oxygen concentration. Erythropoietin acts on specific receptors expressed on the surface of ErP.

Erythrocytes have a life span of about 120 days in humans.

When erythrocytes are about **4 months (~120 days) old**, they become senescent. The macrophage system of the spleen, bone marrow, and liver phagocytoses and degrades the senescent erythrocytes. The **heme** and **globin** dissociate, and the globin is hydrolyzed to amino acids, which enter the metabolic pool for reuse. The iron on the heme is released, enters the iron storage pool in the spleen in the form of **hemosiderin** or **ferritin**, and is stored for reuse in Hgb synthesis. The remainder of the heme moiety of the Hgb molecule is partially degraded to **bilirubin**, bound to albumin, released into the bloodstream, and transported to the liver where it is conjugated and excreted via the gallbladder as the **bilirubin glucuronide** of bile.

Development of Thrombocytes (Thrombopoiesis)

Each day, the bone marrow of a healthy adult produces about 1×10^{11} platelets, a number that can increase 10-fold in times of increased demand. **Thrombocytopoiesis** from bone marrow progenitors is a complex process of cell divisions and differentiation that requires the support of ILs, CSFs, and hormones.

Thrombocytes (platelets) develop from a bipotent megakaryocyte/erythrocyte progenitor (MEP) cell that differentiates into a megakaryocyte-committed progenitor (MKP) cell and finally into a megakaryocyte.

Platelets are produced in the bone marrow from the same **common myeloid progenitor (CMP) cell** as the erythroid and myeloid lineage. Under the influence of granulocyte–macrophage colony-stimulating factor (GM-CSF) and IL-3, a CMP stem cell differentiates into a bipotent **megakaryocyte/erythrocyte progenitor (MEP) cell**. Further development proceeds toward a unipotent **megakaryocyte-committed progenitor (MKP) cell**, which further develops into the **megakaryoblast**. The megakaryoblast that develops from this MKP is a large cell (about 30 μm in diameter) with a nonlobed nucleus. No evidence of platelet formation is seen at this stage. Successive **endomitoses** occur in the megakaryoblast (i.e., chromosomes replicate), but neither karyokinesis nor cytokinesis occurs. Under stimulation by **thrombopoietin**, a 30-kDa glycoprotein hormone produced by the liver and kidney, ploidy increases from $8n$ to $64n$ before chromosomal replication ceases. The cell then becomes a platelet-producing megakaryocyte that measures 50–70 μm in diameter and contains a complex multilobed nucleus and scattered azurophilic granules. Both the nucleus and the cell increase in size in proportion to the ploidy of the cell. With the TEM, multiple centrioles and multiple Golgi apparatus are also seen in these cells.

When bone marrow is examined in a smear, platelet fields are seen to fill much of the peripheral cytoplasm of the megakaryocyte. When examined with the TEM, the peripheral cytoplasm of the megakaryocyte appears to be divided into small compartments by invagination of the plasma membrane. As described earlier, these invaginations are the platelet demarcation channels (see Fig. 10.16). **Thrombocytopenia** (a decrease in the number of blood platelets) is an important clinical problem in the management of patients with immune system disorders and cancer (i.e., leukemia). It increases the risk of bleeding and, in cancer patients, often limits the dose of chemotherapeutic agents.

Development of Granulocytes (Granulopoiesis)

Granulocytes originate from the multipotential **common myeloid progenitor (CMP)** stem cell, which differentiates into **granulocyte/monocyte progenitors (GMPs)** under the influence of cytokines, such as GM-CSF, granulocyte colony-stimulating factor (G-CSF), and IL-3. GM-CSF is a cytokine secreted by endothelial cells, T cells, macrophages, mast cells, and fibroblasts. It stimulates GMP cells to produce granulocytes (neutrophils, eosinophils, and basophils) and monocytes. The **neutrophil progenitor (NoP)** undergoes six morphologically identifiable stages in the process of maturation: myeloblast, promyelocyte, myelocyte, metamyelocyte, band (immature) cell, and mature neutrophil. Eosinophils and basophils undergo a morphologic maturation similar to that of neutrophils. GMP cells, when induced by GM-CSF, IL-3, and IL-5, differentiate into **eosinophil progenitors (EoPs)** and eventually become eosinophils. Lack of IL-5 causes the GMP cells to differentiate into **basophil progenitors (BaPs)**, which produce basophils. Eosinophilic and basophilic precursors cannot be differentiated from neutrophilic precursors morphologically in the light microscope until the cells reach the myelocytic stage when the specific granules appear.

Myeloblasts are the first recognizable cells that begin the process of granulopoiesis.

The **myeloblast** is the earliest microscopically recognizable neutrophil precursor cell in the bone marrow. It has a large, euchromatic, spherical nucleus with three to five nucleoli. It measures 14–20 μm in diameter and has a large nuclear-to-cytoplasmic volume. The small amount of agranular cytoplasm stains intensely basophilic. A Golgi area is often seen where the cytoplasm is unstained. The myeloblast matures into a promyelocyte.

Promyelocytes are the only cells that produce azurophilic granules.

The **promyelocyte** has a large spherical nucleus with azurophilic (primary) granules in the cytoplasm. Azurophilic granules are produced only in promyelocytes; cells in subsequent stages of granulopoiesis do not make azurophilic granules. For this reason, the number of azurophilic granules is reduced, with each division of the promyelocyte and its progeny. Promyelocytes do not exhibit subtypes. Recognition of the neutrophil, eosinophil, and basophil lines is possible only in the next stage—the myelocyte—when specific (secondary) and tertiary granules begin to form.

Myelocytes first exhibit specific granules.

Myelocytes begin with a more or less spherical nucleus that becomes increasingly heterochromatic and acquires a distinct indentation during subsequent divisions. Specific granules begin to emerge from the convex surface of the Golgi apparatus, whereas azurophilic granules are seen on the concave side. The significance of this separation is unclear. Myelocytes continue to divide and give rise to metamyelocytes.

The metamyelocyte is the stage at which neutrophil, eosinophil, and basophil lines can be clearly identified by the presence of numerous specific granules.

A few hundred granules are present in the cytoplasm of each **metamyelocyte**, and the specific granules of each variety outnumber the azurophilic granules. In the neutrophil, this ratio of specific to azurophilic granules is about 2:1. The nucleus becomes more heterochromatic, and the indentation deepens to form a kidney bean–shaped structure. Theoretically, the metamyelocyte stage in granulopoiesis is followed by the band stage and then the segmented stage. Although these stages are obvious in the neutrophil line, they are rarely, if ever, observed in the eosinophil and basophil lines in which the next easily recognized stages of development are the **mature eosinophil** and **mature basophil**, respectively.

In the neutrophil line, the band (stab) cell precedes the development of the first distinct nuclear lobes.

The nucleus of the **band (stab) cell** is elongated and of nearly uniform width, giving it a horseshoe-like appearance. Nuclear constrictions then develop in the band neutrophil and become more prominent until two to four nuclear lobes are recognized; the cell is then considered a **mature neutrophil**, also called a **polymorphonuclear neutrophil** or **segmented neutrophil**. Although the percentage of band cells in the circulation is almost always low (0%–3%), it may increase in acute or chronic inflammation and infection.

Kinetics of Granulopoiesis

Granulopoiesis in the bone marrow takes about 2 weeks. The **mitotic (proliferative) phase** of granulopoiesis lasts about 1 week and stops at the late myelocyte stage. The **postmitotic phase**, characterized by cell differentiation—from metamyelocyte to mature granulocyte—also lasts about 1 week. Neutrophil homeostasis, which includes a balance of neutrophil production, release from the bone marrow, circulation in peripheral blood, and clearance from the circulation, is discussed later.

Neutrophil homeostasis is controlled by CXCL12, a chemokine produced by stromal cells that signals CXCR4 receptors expressed on neutrophils.

Normally, the bone marrow produces more than 10^{11} neutrophils each day. A large storage pool of mature neutrophils is retained within the bone marrow for up to 4–6 days, constituting the bone marrow reserve. Under normal conditions, neutrophils are retained in the bone marrow because of the presence of the chemokine **CXCL12**, also known as stromal derived factor 1 (SDF-1), that is produced by stromal cells. The binding of CXCL12 to the receptor **CXCR4**, expressed on neutrophils, generates the **retention signal** that arrests mature neutrophils in the bone marrow. In response to tissue injury or infection, this pool of neutrophils can be rapidly mobilized to increase circulating levels in under 1 hour. This rapid release of neutrophils results from the loss of the retention signal. Inflammatory cytokines, such as **granulocyte colony-stimulating factor (G-CSF)** or **interferons (IFN-α, IFN-γ)** produced remotely at the sites of inflammation, act systemically on the bone marrow. Neutrophil mobilization from the bone marrow is achieved by lowering levels of CXCL12 in the bone marrow and possibly downregulating the expression of CXVR4 receptors on neutrophils.

The relevance of the CXL12-CXCR4 axis has also been demonstrated experimentally by introducing a CXCR4 competitive antagonist chemical compound called **AMD3100,** which stimulates neutrophil release from the bone marrow. This chemical compound is currently an approved drug (Plerixafor) used when neutrophil mobilization from the bone marrow is necessary, such as autologous stem cell transplantation.

When in the blood, neutrophils have the shortest life span of any circulating cells. A given neutrophil may circulate for only a few minutes or as long as 16 hours before entering the perivascular connective tissue (the measured half-life of circulating human neutrophils is only 8–12 hours). The mechanisms regulating the number of neutrophils in the blood are unknown. However, they most likely leave the blood randomly by diapedesis across the endothelium of blood vessels. It takes about 6–8 hours for one-half of the circulating neutrophils to leave the peripheral blood.

Neutrophils live for 1–2 days in the connective tissue. As they age, neutrophils upregulate CXCR4 expression, facilitating their migration back to the bone marrow and other organs (i.e., liver and spleen). There they are destroyed by apoptosis and are subsequently engulfed by macrophages. **CXCR4** is thus a **master regulator** of neutrophil homeostasis by acting as a signal for neutrophil release from the bone marrow as well as a signal for removing senescent neutrophils from the blood circulation.

Large numbers of neutrophils are also lost by migration into the lumen of the gastrointestinal tract, from which they are discharged with feces.

Mutations of the gene encoding CXCR4 receptor in neutrophils results in **WHIM syndrome**. WHIM is an acronym for clinical symptoms such as warts, hypogammaglobulinemia, infections, and myelokathexis (chronic leukopenia and neutropenia). In this autosomal dominant disorder, **defective CXCR4 receptors** on neutrophils cannot be internalized, resulting in enhanced and prolonged signaling. Neutrophils are retained in the bone marrow, resulting in chronic **neutropenia** (lack of neutrophils in circulation). Despite having normal numbers of mature neutrophils in the bone marrow, patients with WHIM exhibit a very low blood count of neutrophils (neutropenia) and are more susceptible to potentially life-threatening bacterial infections. Treatment with AMD3100 is beneficial for these patients; a single dose can increase neutrophil numbers for 1–9 hours, which lasts up to 24 hours in some patients.

Bone marrow maintains a large reserve of fully functional neutrophils ready to replace or supplement circulating neutrophils at times of increased demand.

As a result of CXL12-CXCR4 axis retention and regulated release of neutrophils from the bone marrow, approximately 5–30 times as many mature and near-mature neutrophils are normally present in the bone marrow than are present in the circulation. This **bone marrow reserve pool** releases neutrophils into the circulation and is replenished by maturing cells. The reserve neutrophils can be quickly released in response to inflammation, infection, or strenuous exercise as described in the section on neutrophil homeostasis.

A reservoir of neutrophils is also present in the vascular compartment. This reserve consists of a freely **circulating pool** and a **marginated pool**, with the latter contained within small blood vessels. The neutrophils adhere to the endothelium much as they do before leaving the vasculature at the sites of injury or infection (see pages 307-309). The normally marginated neutrophils, however, loosely adhere to the endothelium through the action of selectin and can be recruited very quickly. They are in dynamic equilibrium with the circulating pool, which is approximately equal to the size of the marginated pool.

The size of the reserve pool in the bone marrow and vascular compartment depends on the rate of granulopoiesis, the life span of the neutrophils, and the rates of migration into the bloodstream and connective tissue. The entire hemopoietic process is summarized in Table 10.3.

Transcription factors control the fate of hemopoietic cells, whereas cytokines and local mediators regulate all stages of hemopoiesis.

Chemical interactions between HSCs and their bone marrow microenvironment play an important role in defining the fate of these multipotential stem cells by activating specific differentiation pathways. Signaling molecules from a variety of bone marrow cells initiate intracellular pathways that ultimately target a select group of synergistic and inhibitory proteins known as **transcription factors**. These factors specifically bind to promoter or enhancer regions located on the bone marrow cell's DNA. By controlling the transcription of the specific genes downstream, these transcription factors trigger a cascade of genetic changes that ultimately determines the fate of the cells during differentiation.

In addition to identifying the various intracellular transcription factors, recent studies have identified and begun to characterize numerous **signaling molecules** found in the bone marrow. These include glycoproteins that act as both circulating hormones and local mediators to regulate the progress of hemopoiesis and the rate of differentiation of other cell types (Table 10.4). Specific hormones such as **erythropoietin** or **thrombopoietin**, discussed in a previous section, regulate erythrocyte and thrombocyte development, respectively. Other factors, collectively called **colony-stimulating factors (CSFs)**, are subclassified according to the specific cell or group of cells that they affect. Among the most completely characterized factors are several that stimulate granulocyte and monocyte formation, including GM-CSF, G-CSF, and macrophage colony-stimulating factor (M-CSF). **Interleukins**, produced by lymphocytes, act on other leukocytes and their progenitors. IL-3 is a cytokine that appears to affect most progenitor cells and even terminally differentiated cells. Any particular cytokine may act at one or more stages in hemopoiesis, affecting cell division, differentiation, or cell function. These factors are synthesized by many different cell types, including kidney cells (erythropoietin), liver hepatocytes (thrombopoietin), T lymphocytes (IL-3), endothelial cells (IL-6), adventitial cells in the bone marrow (IL-7), and macrophages (the CSFs that affect granulocyte and macrophage development).

The isolation, characterization, manufacture, and clinical testing of **cytokines** in the treatment of human disease are major activities of the rapidly growing biotechnology industry. Several hemopoietic and lymphopoietic cytokines have been manufactured by recombinant DNA technology

TABLE 10.3 **Summary of Features During Maturation of Common Myeloid Progenitor Cell**

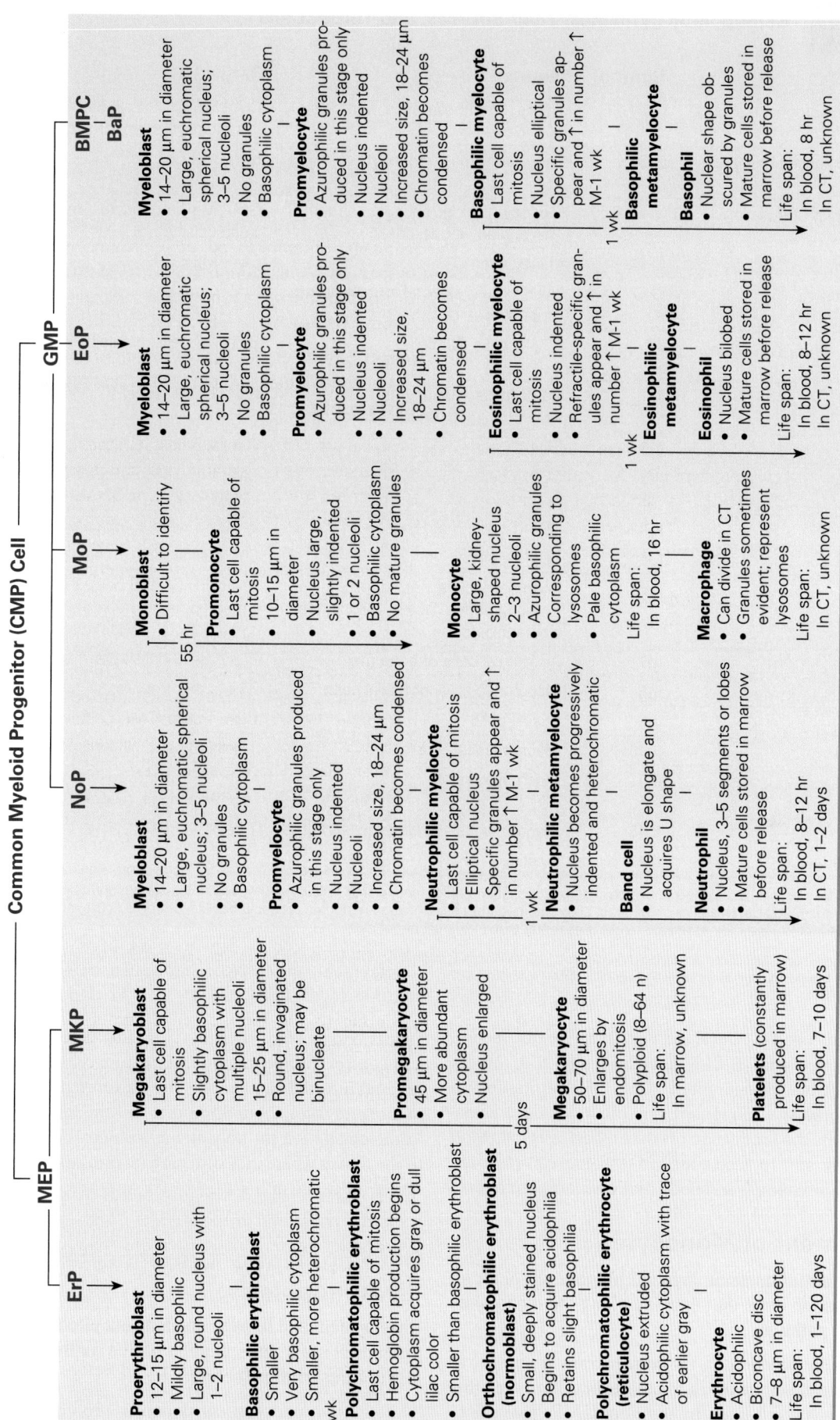

Common Myeloid Progenitor (CMP) Cell → MEP (ErP, MKP); GMP (NoP, MoP, EoP, BMPC – BaP)

ErP	MKP	NoP	MoP	EoP	BMPC – BaP
Proerythroblast • 12–15 μm in diameter • Mildly basophilic • Large, round nucleus with 1–2 nucleoli	**Megakaryoblast** • Last cell capable of mitosis • Slightly basophilic cytoplasm with multiple nucleoli • 15–25 μm in diameter • Round, invaginated nucleus; may be binucleate	**Myeloblast** • 14–20 μm in diameter • Large, euchromatic spherical nucleus; 3–5 nucleoli • No granules • Basophilic cytoplasm	**Monoblast** • Difficult to identify 55 hr	**Myeloblast** • 14–20 μm in diameter • Large, euchromatic spherical nucleus; 3–5 nucleoli • No granules • Basophilic cytoplasm	**Myeloblast** • 14–20 μm in diameter • Large, euchromatic spherical nucleus; 3–5 nucleoli • No granules • Basophilic cytoplasm
Basophilic erythroblast • Smaller • Very basophilic cytoplasm • Smaller, more heterochromatic 1 wk	5 days **Promegakaryocyte** • 45 μm in diameter • More abundant cytoplasm • Nucleus enlarged	**Promyelocyte** • Azurophilic granules produced in this stage only • Nucleus indented • Nucleoli • Increased size, 18–24 μm • Chromatin becomes condensed	**Promonocyte** • Last cell capable of mitosis • 10–15 μm in diameter • Nucleus large, slightly indented • 1 or 2 nucleoli • Basophilic cytoplasm • No mature granules	**Promyelocyte** • Azurophilic granules produced in this stage only • Nucleus indented • Nucleoli • Increased size, 18–24 μm • Chromatin becomes condensed	**Promyelocyte** • Azurophilic granules produced in this stage only • Nucleus indented • Nucleoli • Increased size, 18–24 μm • Chromatin becomes condensed
Polychromatophilic erythroblast • Last cell capable of mitosis • Hemoglobin production begins • Cytoplasm acquires gray or dull lilac color • Smaller than basophilic erythroblast	**Megakaryocyte** • 50–70 μm in diameter • Enlarges by endomitosis • Polyploid (8–64 n) Life span: In marrow, unknown	**Neutrophilic myelocyte** • Last cell capable of mitosis • Elliptical nucleus • Specific granules appear and ↑ in number ↑ M-1 wk 1 wk	**Monocyte** • Large, kidney-shaped nucleus • 2–3 nucleoli • Azurophilic granules • Corresponding to lysosomes • Pale basophilic cytoplasm Life span: In blood, 16 hr	**Eosinophilic myelocyte** • Last cell capable of mitosis • Nucleus indented • Refractile-specific granules appear and ↑ in number ↑ M-1 wk 1 wk	**Basophilic myelocyte** • Last cell capable of mitosis • Nucleus elliptical • Specific granules appear and ↑ in number ↑ M-1 wk 1 wk
Orthochromatophilic erythroblast (normoblast) • Small, deeply stained nucleus • Begins to acquire acidophilia • Retains slight basophilia	**Platelets** (constantly produced in marrow) Life span: In blood, 7–10 days	**Neutrophilic metamyelocyte** • Nucleus becomes progressively indented and heterochromatic	**Macrophage** • Can divide in CT • Granules sometimes evident; represent lysosomes Life span: In CT, unknown	**Eosinophilic metamyelocyte**	**Basophilic metamyelocyte**
Polychromatophilic erythrocyte (reticulocyte) • Nucleus extruded • Acidophilic cytoplasm with trace of earlier gray		**Band cell** • Nucleus is elongate and acquires U shape		**Eosinophil** • Nucleus bilobed • Mature cells stored in marrow before release Life span: In blood, 8–12 hr In CT, unknown	**Basophil** • Nuclear shape obscured by granules • Mature cells stored in marrow before release Life span: In blood, 8 hr In CT, unknown
Erythrocyte • Acidophilic • Biconcave disc • 7–8 μm in diameter Life span: In blood, 1–120 days		**Neutrophil** • Nucleus, 3–5 segments or lobes • Mature cells stored in marrow before release Life span: In blood, 8–12 hr In CT, 1–2 days			

This table summarizes the maturation of blood cells with histologic characteristics at the various stages, maturation time, and life span after leaving the marrow. Times indicated along vertical lines are the approximate time between recognizable stages. M-1 wk indicates an increase in number by mitosis for 1 wk before differentiation begins.

BaP, basophil progenitor; *BMCP*, basophil/mast cell progenitor; *CT*, connective tissue; *EoP*, eosinophil progenitor; *ErP*, erythrocyte progenitor; *GMP*, granulocyte/monocyte progenitor; *MEP*, megakaryocyte/erythrocyte progenitor; *MKP*, megakaryocyte progenitor; *MoP*, monocyte progenitor; *NoP*, neutrophil progenitor.

TABLE 10.4 Hemopoietic Cytokines, Their Sources, and Target Cells

Cytokine[a]	Symbol	Source	Target
Granulocyte–macrophage colony-stimulating factor	GM-CSF	T cells, endothelial cells, fibroblasts	CMP, ErP, GMP, EoP, BaP, MKP, all granulocytes, erythrocytes
Granulocyte colony-stimulating factor	G-CSF	Endothelial cells, monocytes	ErP, GMP, EoP, BaP, MKP
Monocyte colony-stimulating factor	M-CSF	Monocytes, macrophages, endothelial and adventitial cells	GMP, MoP, monocytes, macrophages, osteoclasts
Erythropoietin	EPO	Kidney, liver	CMP, MEP, ErP
Thrombopoietin	TPO	Liver, kidney, skeletal muscle, bone marrow	MKP, megakaryocytes
Interferon-γ	IFN-γ	$CD4^+$ T cells, NK cells	B cells, T cells, NK cells, neutrophils, monocytes
Interleukin-1	IL-1	Neutrophils, monocytes, macrophages, endothelial cells	$CD4^+$ T cells, B cells
Interleukin-2	IL-2	$CD4^+$ T cells	T cells, B cells, NK cells
Interleukin-3	IL-3	$CD4^+$ T cells	CMP, ErP, GMP, EoP, BaP, MKP, all granulocytes, erythroid cells
Interleukin-4	IL-4	$CD4^+$ T cells, mast cells	B cells, T cells, mast cells
Interleukin-5	IL-5	$CD4^+$ T cells	EoP, eosinophils, B cells
Interleukin-6	IL-6	Endothelial cells, neutrophils, macrophages, T cells, adipocytes, osteoblasts	CMP, ErP, GMP, B cells, T cells, macrophages, hepatocytes, osteocytes, osteoclasts, adipocytes
Interleukin-7	IL-7	Adventitial cells of bone marrow	Early pre–B cells , pre–T cells
Interleukin-8	IL-8	Macrophages, endothelial cells	T cells, neutrophils
Interleukin-9	IL-9	$CD4^+$ T cells	$CD4^+$ T cells, CMP, ErP
Interleukin-10	IL-10	Macrophages, T cells	T cells, B cells, NK cells
Interleukin-11	IL-11	Macrophages	CMP, ErP, GMP, T cells, B cells, macrophages, megakaryocytes
Interleukin-12	IL-12	Macrophages, dendritic cells, B cells	T cells
Interleukin-13	IL-13	T cells	B cells

[a]Hemopoietic cytokines include colony-stimulating factors (CSFs), interleukins, and inhibitory factors. They are almost all glycoproteins with a basic polypeptide chain of about 20 kDa. Nearly all of them act on progenitor stem cells, lineage-restricted progenitor cells, committed cells, and maturing and mature cells. Therefore, the targets listed are target lines rather than individual target cells.

BaP, basophil progenitor; CMP, common myeloid progenitor; EoP, eosinophil progenitor; ErP, erythrocyte-committed progenitor; GMP, granulocyte/monocyte progenitor; MEP, megakaryocyte/erythrocyte progenitor; MKP, megakaryocyte-committed progenitor; MoP, monocyte progenitor; NK, natural killer.

and are already used in clinical settings. These include **recombinant erythropoietin**, **G-CSF**, **GM-CSF**, and **IL-3**; others are under active development. GM-CSF (sargramostim [Leukine], filgrastim [Neupogen], and others) is used clinically to stimulate the production of white blood cells following chemotherapy and to accelerate white blood cell recovery following chemotherapy and bone marrow transplantation.

Development of Monocytes

The multipotential common myeloid progenitor stem cell also gives rise to cells that develop along the monocyte–macrophage pathway.

Monocytes are produced in the bone marrow from a GMP stem cell that can mature into a monocyte or cells of the other three granulocytic cell lines. In addition, GMPs give rise to DCs. The proliferation and differentiation of a CMP into a committed GMP is controlled by IL-3. Further differentiation of the **monocyte progenitor (MoP) cell** lineage depends on the continued presence of PU.1 and Egr-1 transcription factors and is stimulated by IL-3 and GM-CSF. GM-CSF also controls differentiation into mature cells, which are then released into the circulation. The transformation of MoPs to monocytes takes about 55 hours, and the monocytes remain in the circulation for only about 16 hours before emigrating to the tissues where they differentiate into tissue macrophages under influence of both GM-CSF and M-CSF. Their subsequent life span is not yet fully understood.

Development of Lymphocytes (Lymphopoiesis)

Development and lineage commitment of common lymphoid progenitor stem cells depend on the expression of a variety of transcription factors.

Although lymphocytes continuously proliferate in the peripheral lymphatic organs, the bone marrow remains the primary site of lymphopoiesis in humans. Members of the **Ikaros family of transcription factors** play major roles in the differentiation of pluripotent HSCs into **common**

lymphoid progenitor (CLP) cells. CLP differentiation is summarized as follows:

- **T lymphocytes** are derived from CLP progeny that expresses **GATA-3 transcription factor**. These cells leave the bone marrow as pre–T lymphocytes and travel to the thymus, where they complete their differentiation and thymic cell education (see Chapter 14, Immune System and Lymphatic Tissues and Organs, pages 514-516). They then enter the circulation as long-lived, small T lymphocytes.
- **B lymphocytes** are derived from CLP cells in which B-cell–specific genes have been activated by a transcription factor called **Pax5**. They develop in the so-called **bursa-equivalent organs**, such as the bone marrow, gut-associated lymphatic tissue, and spleen.
- **NK cells** most likely differentiate under the influence of IL-2 and IL-15 into immature pre–NK cells and, after acquisition of NK cell effector functions (ability to secrete IFN and cytotoxicity), become mature NK cells. However, little is known about factors that may influence the development and lineage commitment of NK cells. The bone marrow is the main NK cell–producing organ. However, recent studies suggest that lymph nodes or the fetal thymus may also contain NK progenitor cells. Lymphocytes constitute as much as 30% of all nucleated cells in the bone marrow. The development and differentiation of lymphocytes are discussed in more detail in Chapter 14, Immune System and Lymphatic Tissues and Organs, pages 487-492.

■ BONE MARROW

Red bone marrow lies entirely within the spaces of bone, medullary cavity of young long bones, and spaces of spongy bone.

Bone marrow consists of blood vessels, specialized units of blood vessels called **sinusoids**, and a sponge-like network of hemopoietic cells (Fig. 10.26). The bone marrow sinusoids provide the barrier between the hemopoietic compartment and the peripheral circulation. In sections, the cells in hemopoietic compartment appear to lie in "cords" between sinusoids or between sinusoids and bone.

The sinusoid of red bone marrow is a unique vascular unit. It occupies the position normally occupied by a capillary; that is, it is interposed between arteries and veins. It is believed to be derived from vessels that have just nourished the cortical bone tissue. The sinusoids arise from these vessels at the corticomedullary junction. The sinusoid wall consists of an endothelial lining, a discontinuous basement membrane, and an incomplete covering of adventitial cells. The endothelium is a simple squamous epithelium.

The **adventitial cell**, also called a **reticular cell**, sends sheet-like extensions into the substance of the hemopoietic cords, which provide some support for the developing blood cells. In addition, adventitial cells produce reticular fibers. They also play a role in stimulating the differentiation of developing progenitor cells into blood cells by secreting several cytokines (e.g., CSFs, IL-5, IL-7). When blood cell

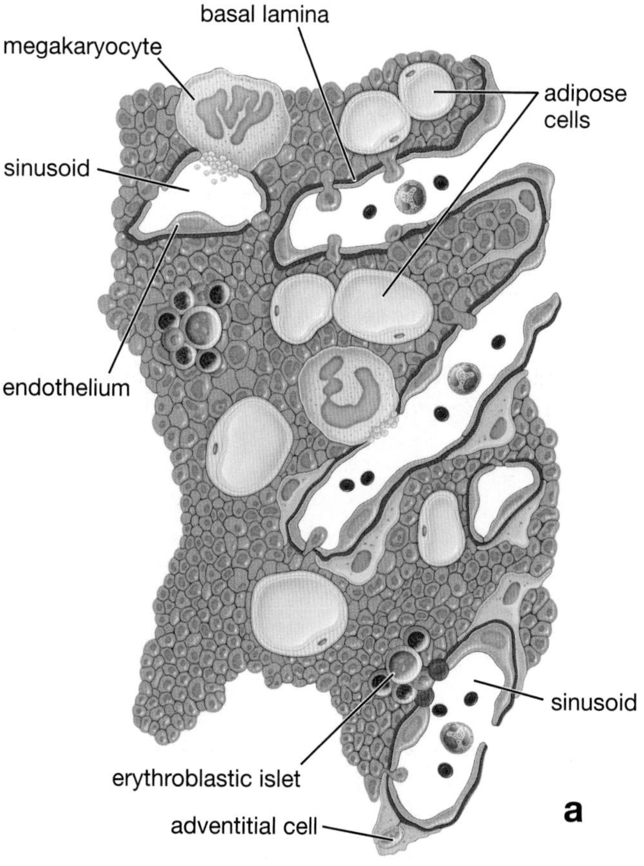

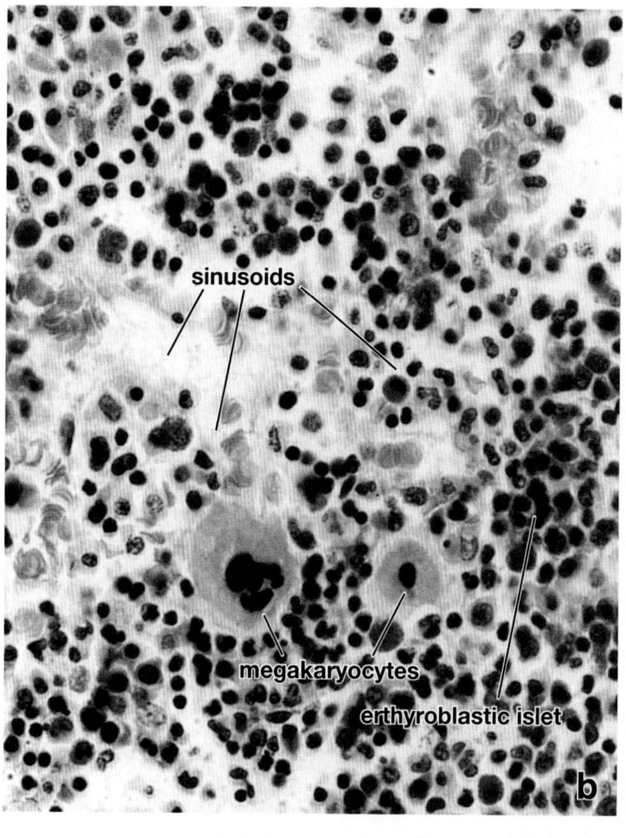

FIGURE 10.26. Bone marrow with active hemopoiesis. a. Schematic drawing of bone marrow shows several features: erythroblastic islets engaged in the formation of erythrocytes, megakaryocytes discharging platelets into the sinusoids, endothelial cells (*pink*) resting on a basal lamina (*dark red*) that is absent where blood cells are entering the sinusoids, adventitial or reticular cells (*blue*) extending from the basal lamina into the hemopoietic compartment, and dispersed adipose cells. **b.** Photomicrograph of bone marrow section stained with hematoxylin and eosin (H&E) showing active hemopoietic centers in close proximity to bone marrow sinusoids. ×420.

formation and the passage of mature blood cells into the sinusoids are active, adventitial cells and the basal lamina become displaced by mature blood cells as they approach the endothelium to enter the sinusoid from the bone marrow cavity.

The bone marrow sinusoidal system is a closed circulation system; newly formed blood cells use transcellular diapedesis pathway to penetrate the endothelium to enter the circulation.

As a maturing blood cell or megakaryocyte process pushes against an endothelial cell, the abluminal plasma membrane is pressed against the luminal plasma membrane until they fuse, thus forming a transitory **transcellular diapedesis pore**. Active cis-SNARE complexes facilitate fusion of both endothelial plasma membranes in a process similar to fusion of a transport vesicle with its target membrane (pages 42-44). The migrating cell or megakaryocyte process literally pierces the endothelial cell. Transcellular pores tend to form predominantly in close proximity to intact intercellular junctions where the endothelium is thinnest. Thus, a cell migrating across the bone marrow endothelium primarily uses the transcellular rather than the paracellular pathway. Each blood cell must squeeze through a transcellular pore to enter the lumen of a sinusoid. Similarly, a megakaryocyte process must protrude through a pore so that the platelets can be released directly into the sinusoid lumen. During transcellular passage, the pore contracts, maintaining the integrity of the endothelial cell. Also, interactions of endothelial surface adhesion molecules (e.g., ICAM-1 and VICAM-1) with leukocyte integrins minimize disruption of the endothelial barrier. The transcellular pore closes as the blood cell completes its passage into the sinusoid lumen or the megakaryocyte process that has been extruded is subsequently withdrawn.

In active **red bone marrow**, the cords of hemopoietic cells contain predominately developing blood cells and megakaryocytes. The cords also contain macrophages, mast cells, and some adipose cells. Although the cords of hemopoietic tissue appear to lack organization, specific types of blood cells develop in nests or clusters. Each nest in which

FOLDER 10.6

CLINICAL CORRELATION: CELLULARITY OF THE BONE MARROW

Bone marrow cellularity is one of the most important factors in evaluating the function of the bone marrow. The assessment of bone marrow cellularity is semiquantitative and represents the ratio of hemopoietic cells to adipocytes. The most reliable evaluation of cellularity is obtained from the microscopic examination of a sample of bone marrow that preserves the organization of the marrow. Smear preparations are not accurate preparations with which to assess bone marrow cellularity.

Bone marrow cellularity decreases with age. The range of normal bone marrow cellularity for a specific age can be calculated by subtracting an individual's age from 100 and then adding (for the higher range) and subtracting (for the lower range) 10%. Thus, a 30-year-old individual's bone marrow contains between 60% and 80% of active bone marrow cells ($100 - 30 = 70 \pm 10\%$); in contrast, a 70-year-old individual's marrow contains active cells in the range of 20%–40% ($100 - 70 = 30 \pm 10\%$). Bone marrow with a normal age–specific index is called **normocellular bone marrow**. Deviation from age-specific normal indices indicates a pathologic change in the marrow.

In **hypocellular bone marrow**, which occurs in aplastic anemia or after chemotherapy, only a small number of blood-forming cells are present in a marrow sample (Fig. F10.6.1a). Thus, a 50-year-old individual with this condition might have a bone marrow cellularity index of 10%–20%. In the same-aged individual with acute myelogenous leukemia, the bone marrow cellularity index might be 80%–90%. **Hypercellular bone marrow** is characteristic of bone marrow affected by tumors originating from hemopoietic cells (Fig. F10.6.1b).

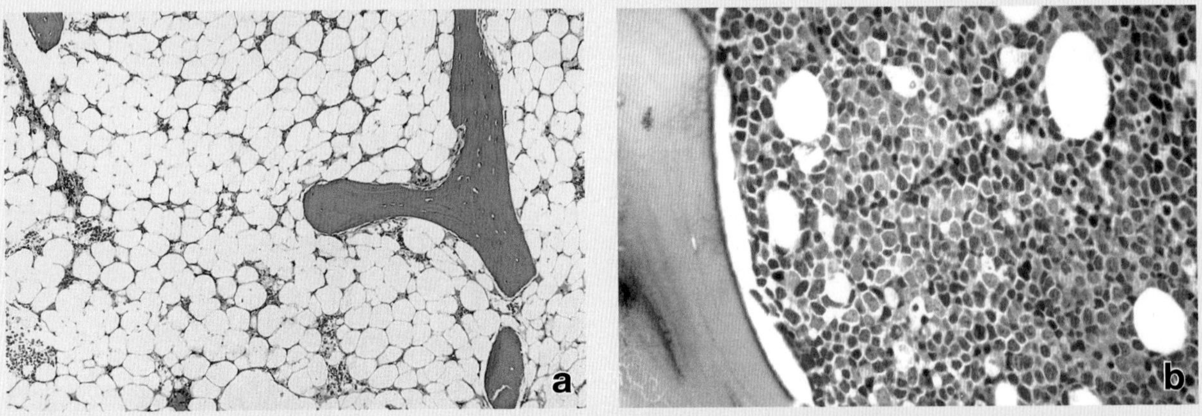

FIGURE F10.6.1. Cellularity of the bone marrow. a. This photomicrograph of a bone marrow section from an individual with aplastic anemia shows hypocellular bone marrow. It consists largely of adipose cells and lacks normal hemopoietic activity. ×120. **b.** This photomicrograph of bone marrow section from an individual with acute myelogenous leukemia shows hypercellular bone marrow. Note that the entire field of view next to the bony trabecula is filled with tightly packed myeloblasts. Only a few adipose cells are visible in this image. ×280. (Reprinted with permission from Rubin E, Gorstein F, Schwarting R, et al. *Rubin's Pathology* [4th ed.]. Lippincott Williams & Wilkins; 2004, Fig. 20-12, Fig. 20-54.)

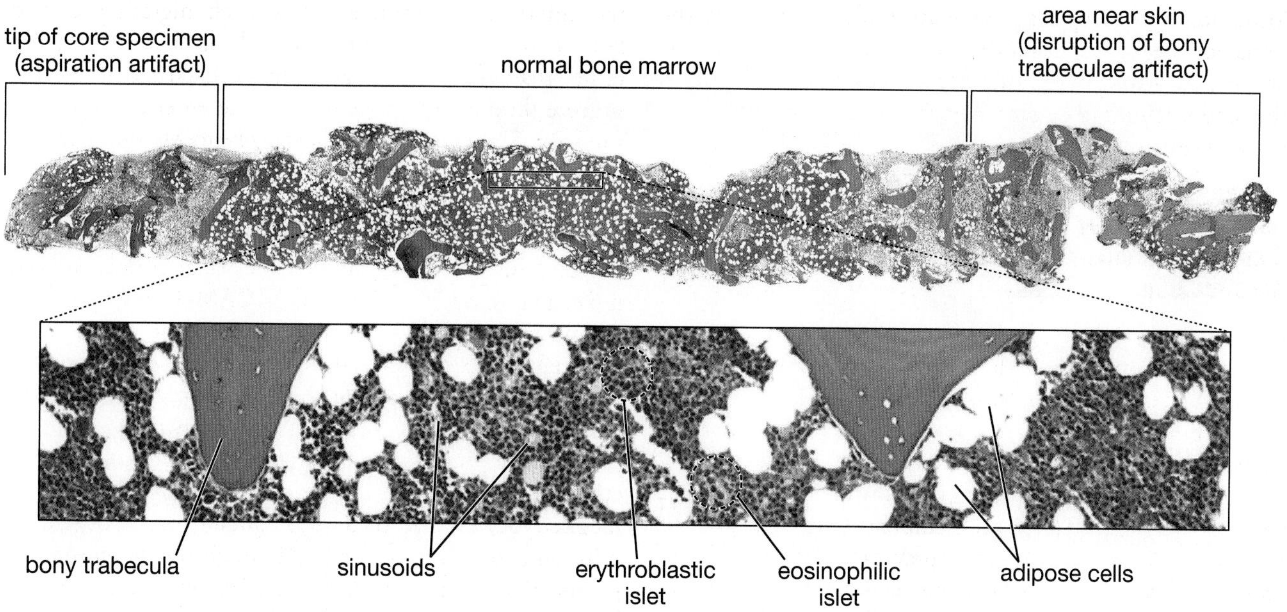

FIGURE 10.27. Core specimen from a bone marrow biopsy. The low-magnification photomicrograph (*top*) shows the entire length of a bone marrow core biopsy specimen obtained from the posterior part of the iliac crest of a 25-year-old woman with a short history of fever, night sweats, fatigue, leukocytosis with absolute lymphocytosis, splenomegaly, a positive polymerase chain reaction (PCR) for cytomegalovirus, and a clonal $CD8^+$ T-lymphocyte proliferation. The *right side* of the image shows disruption of the bony trabeculae, an indication of an artifact from needle insertion in the area close to the skin surface. The lighter, more eosinophilic area near the tip of the core specimen without an evident bone marrow pattern represents aspiration artifact. ×12. Photomicrograph (*bottom*) showing a higher magnification of the area indicated by the *rectangle*. The bone marrow in this patient appears to be normocellular (70% cellularity) with normal hemopoiesis (see Folder 10.6 for an explanation of bone marrow cellularity). ×110. (Courtesy of Dr. Gabriel C. Caponetti, Creighton University.)

erythrocytes develop contains a macrophage. These nests are located near the sinusoid wall. Megakaryocytes are also located adjacent to the sinusoid wall, and they discharge their platelets directly into the sinusoid through transcellular pores in the endothelium. Granulocytes develop in cell nests farther from the sinusoid wall. When mature, the granulocyte migrates to the sinusoid and enters the bloodstream.

Bone marrow not active in blood cell formation contains predominately adipose cells, giving it the appearance of adipose tissue.

Inactive bone marrow is called **yellow bone marrow**. It is the chief form of bone marrow in the medullary cavity of adult bones that are no longer hemopoietically active, such as the long bones of the arms, legs, fingers, and toes. In these bones, the red bone marrow has been replaced completely by fat. Even in hemopoietically active bone marrow in adult humans—such as that in the ribs, vertebrae, pelvis, and shoulder girdle—about one-half of the bone marrow space is occupied by adipose tissue and half by hemopoietic tissue. The yellow bone marrow retains its hemopoietic potential; when necessary, such as after severe loss of blood, it can revert to red bone marrow, both by extension of the hemopoietic tissue into the yellow bone marrow and by repopulation of the yellow bone marrow by circulating stem cells.

Bone marrow examination is essential for the diagnosis and management of many disorders of the blood and bone marrow.

Examination of bone marrow aspirate and bone marrow core needle (trephine) biopsy is essential for the diagnosis of bone marrow disorders. When used together, both methods provide a comprehensive evaluation of the bone marrow. Indications for **bone marrow examination** include unexplained anemia (low erythrocyte counts), abnormal peripheral blood smear morphology, diagnosis and staging of hematologic malignant disorders (e.g., leukemia), and suspected bone marrow metastases. Usually, the final diagnosis is based on both clinical findings and results of several diagnostic procedures, including peripheral blood examination, bone marrow aspirate and core biopsy, and other specific tests (e.g., immunophenotyping, molecular genetic studies).

In **bone marrow aspiration**, a needle is inserted through the skin until it penetrates the bone. The preferred anatomic site for a bone marrow biopsy is the posterior part of the iliac crest (hip bone). A small amount of bone marrow is obtained by applying negative pressure with a syringe attached to the needle. The aspirate is then spread as a smear on a glass slide, and the specimen is examined with a microscope to examine individual cell morphology. In **bone marrow core biopsy**, intact bone marrow is obtained for laboratory analysis. Usually, a small incision is made in the skin to allow the biopsy needle to pass into the bone. The biopsy needle is advanced through the bone with a rotating motion (similar to a corkscrew movement through a cork) and then withdrawn with a small, solid piece of bone marrow inside. After the needle is withdrawn, the core sample is removed from the needle and processed for routine H&E slide preparation. The core biopsy specimen obtained in this procedure allows analysis of bone marrow architecture (Fig. 10.27). It is typically used to diagnose and stage different types of cancer or monitor the results of chemotherapy.

101 HISTOLOGY NOTEBOOK

BLOOD

OVERVIEW OF BLOOD

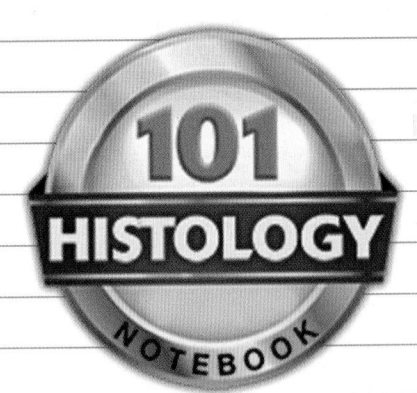

- **Blood** is a fluid connective tissue that circulates through the cardiovascular system. It consists of protein-rich liquid extracellular matrix called **plasma** and formed elements (**white blood cells, red blood cells,** and **platelets**).
- The volume of **red blood cells (erythrocytes)** in whole blood is called the **hematocrit (HCT)** or **packed cell volume (PCV)**; HCT is ~45% in men and women.
- **White blood cells (leukocytes)** constitute about 1% of blood volume.

PLASMA

- Plasma proteins consist primarily of **albumin** (responsible for **colloid osmotic pressure**), **globulins** (including **immunoglobulins** and **nonimmune globulins**), and **fibrinogen** (involved in blood clotting). All plasma proteins are secreted by the liver.
- **Serum** is blood plasma from which clotting factors have been removed.

ERYTHROCYTES (RED BLOOD CELLS)

- **Erythrocytes** are anucleate, biconcave discs (7.8 μm in diameter) that are packed with Hgb and are designed to withstand shear forces experienced during circulation. Their normal life span is about 120 days.
- **Hemoglobin** is a specialized protein that consists of four chains of globins with iron-containing heme groups for binding, transporting, and releasing O_2 and CO_2.
- There are three major types of **hemoglobin** in adult humans: **HbA** (~96% of total Hgb), **HbA_2** (~3%), and **HbF** (>1% but prevalent in the fetus).

LEUKOCYTES (WHITE BLOOD CELLS)

- **Leukocytes** are subclassified into two groups based on the presence or absence of **specific granules** in the cytoplasm: **granulocytes** (neutrophils, eosinophils, basophils) or **agranulocytes** (lymphocytes, monocytes).
- **Neutrophils** (47%–67% of all leukocytes) have polymorphic, multilobed nuclei. Their specific granules contain various enzymes, complement activators, and antimicrobial peptides (i.e., lysozymes, lactoferrins) for destroying microorganisms at sites of inflammation.
- Neutrophils leave circulation via **postcapillary venules** in a process of neutrophil–endothelial cell recognition. This involves cell adhesion molecules (**selectins and integrins**) and subsequent diapedesis (transendothelial migration) of neutrophils.
- **Eosinophils** (1%–4% of all leukocytes) have bilobed nuclei and eosinophilic-specific granules containing proteins that are cytotoxic to protozoans and helminthic parasites. Eosinophils are associated with allergic reactions, parasitic infections, and chronic inflammation.
- **Basophils** (<0.5% of all leukocytes) have irregular lobed nuclei obscured by large, basophilic-specific granules containing heparin, histamine, heparan sulfate, and leukotrienes. These substances play an important role in allergic reactions and chronic inflammations.
- **Lymphocytes** (26%–28% of all leukocytes) are the main functional cells of the immune system. They vary in size and have dense spherical nuclei surrounded by a thin rim of cytoplasm.
- There are three major types of lymphocytes: **T lymphocytes** (**T cells**; involved in cell-mediated immunity), **B lymphocytes** (**B cells**; involved in antibody production), and **natural killer (NK) cells** (programmed to kill certain virus-infected and cancer cells).
- **Monocytes** (3%–9% of all leukocytes) have indented nuclei. After migration from the vascular system, they transform into **macrophages** and other cells of the mononuclear phagocyte system. They function as **antigen-presenting cells** in the immune system.

THROMBOCYTES (PLATELETS)

- **Thrombocytes** are small, membrane-bounded, anucleate cytoplasmic fragments derived from megakaryocytes.
- Thrombocytes are divided into four zones (**peripheral**, **structural**, **organelle**, and **membrane**) based on their organization and function.

FORMATION OF BLOOD CELLS (HEMOPOIESIS)

- **Hemopoiesis** (hematopoiesis) is initiated in early embryonic development and includes **erythropoiesis** (development of red blood cells), **leukopoiesis** (development of white blood cells), and **thrombopoiesis** (development of platelets).
- In adults, **hemopoietic stem cells (HSCs)** reside in the bone marrow. Under the influence of cytokines and growth factors, they differentiate into **common myeloid progenitor (CMP) cells** (which give rise to megakaryocytes, erythrocytes, neutrophils, eosinophils, basophils and/or mast cells, and monocytes) and **common lymphoid progenitor (CLP) cells** (which give rise to T cells, B cells, and NK cells).
- During **erythropoiesis**, erythrocytes evolve from **proerythroblasts** and **basophilic, polychromatophilic,** and **orthochromatophilic erythroblasts** to **polychromatophilic** and mature **erythrocytes.**
- Developing red blood cells become smaller, change their cytoplasm appearance (from blue to red) due to intense accumulation of Hgb, and extrude their nuclei.
- During **thrombopoiesis**, thrombocytes (platelets) are produced in the bone marrow by **megakaryocytes** (large polyploid cells of the red bone marrow) that develop from the same CMP stem cells as the erythroblasts.
- During **granulopoiesis**, granulocytes originate from the CMP stem cell, which differentiates into **granulocyte/monocyte progenitors (GMPs)**. CMP stem cells also give rise to monocytes.
- **Neutrophil progenitor (NoP)** cells undergo six morphologically identifiable stages in development: **myeloblast, promyelocyte, myelocyte** (first to exhibit specific granules), **metamyelocyte**, **band (immature) cell**, and **mature neutrophil**. The development of other granulocytes follows a similar path.
- During **lymphopoiesis**, lymphocytes develop from the CLP stem cell and their fate depends on expression of specific transcription factors. They differentiate in the bone marrow and other lymphatic tissues.

BONE MARROW

- **Red bone marrow** contains cords of active hemopoietic cells that lie within the medullary cavity in children and within the spaces of spongy bone in adults.
- Bone marrow contains specialized blood vessels (**sinusoids**) into which newly developed blood cells and platelets are released.
- Bone marrow not active in hemopoiesis consists of predominately adipose cells and is called **yellow bone marrow**.

PLATE 10.1 ■ ERYTHROCYTES AND GRANULOCYTES

Blood is a connective tissue, fluid in character, and consists of formed elements and plasma. **Red blood cells** (erythrocytes), **white blood cells** (leukocytes), and **thrombocytes (platelets)** constitute the formed elements. Collectively, they make up 45% of the blood volume. Red blood cells transport and exchange oxygen and carbon dioxide. They constitute 99% of the blood cells. White blood cells are categorized as agranulocytes and granulocytes. The **agranulocytes** are further classified as lymphocytes and monocytes. The **granulocytes**, so named for the character of the granules that they contain in their cytoplasm, consist of neutrophils, eosinophils, and basophils. Each type of white blood cell plays a specific role in immune and protective responses in the body. They typically leave the circulation and enter the connective tissue to perform their specific roles. In contrast, red blood cells function only within the vascular system. Blood platelets are responsible for blood clotting and consequently have an essential role in incidents of small vessel damage.

Blood smears are utilized for microscopic examination and identification of relative numbers of white blood cells in circulating blood. The blood smear is prepared by placing a small drop of blood on a microscope slide and then smearing it across the slide with the edge of another slide. When properly executed, this method provides a uniform, single layer of blood cells that is allowed to air dry and then stained. Wright stain, a modified Romanowsky stain, is generally utilized. In examining the specimen under the microscope, it is useful to use a low magnification to find areas in which the blood cells have a uniform distribution like that seen in the smear on the adjacent page. Once this is accomplished, by switching to a higher magnification, one can identify the various types of white blood cells and, in fact, determine the relative number of each cell type. A normal cell count is as follows: neutrophils, 48.6%–66.7%; eosinophils, 1.4%–4.8%; basophils, 0%–0.3%; lymphocytes, 25.7%–27.6%; and monocytes, 8.6%–9.0%.

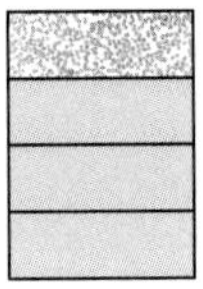

Blood smear, human, Wright stain ×200.

This low-magnification photomicrograph shows part of a blood smear in which the blood cells are uniformly distributed. The majority of cells are **red blood cells**. Because of their biconcave shape, most of the red blood cells appear donut shaped. Two white cells, both granulocytes, are evident. One cell is a **neutrophil** (*N*), the other granulocyte is an **eosinophil** (*E*). However, at this magnification, the major distinction is in the staining of their cytoplasm. Higher magnification, as in next figures, allows for a more precise characterization of each cell type.

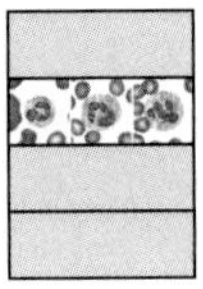

Neutrophils, blood smear, human, Wright stain ×2,200.

Neutrophils exhibit variation in size and nuclear morphology that is associated with the age of the cell. The nucleus seen on the *left* is that of a neutrophil that has just passed the band stage and has recently entered the bloodstream. The cell is relatively small; its cytoplasm exhibits distinctive, fine granules. The *middle* neutrophil is considerably larger, and its cytoplasm contains more fine granules. The nucleus still exhibits a U shape, but lobulation (*arrows*) is becoming apparent with the constriction of the nucleus at several points. The neutrophil to the *right* shows greater maturity as evidenced by its distinctive lobulation. Here, the lobules are connected by a very thin nuclear "bridge." A very distinctive feature associated with the nucleus of this cell is the presence of a Barr body (*arrow*), indicative of blood that has been drawn from a female.

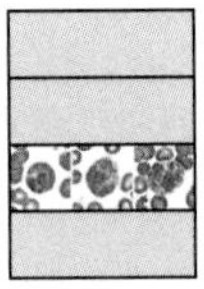

Eosinophils, blood smear, human, Wright stain ×2,200.

The **eosinophils** seen in these micrographs similarly represent different stages of maturity. The eosinophil at the *left* is relatively small and is just beginning to show lobulation. The cytoplasm is almost entirely filled with eosinophilic granules that characterize this cell type. The lighter stained area, devoid of granules, probably represents the site of the Golgi apparatus (*arrow*). The eosinophil shown in the *middle* is larger, and its nucleus is now distinctively bilobed. At one site, three distinct granules (*arrows*) are evident. Note their spherical shape and relative uniform size. The eosinophil at the *right* is more mature in that it displays at least three lobes. By going through focus, the eosinophil granules often appear to "light up" owing to their crystalline structure.

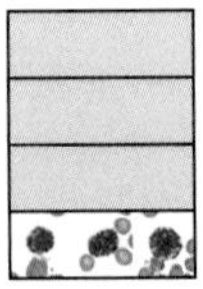

Basophils, blood smear, human, Wright stain ×2,200.

The cells shown here are **basophils** and also represent different stages of maturation. The basophil at the *left* is relatively young and small. The basophilic granules are variable in size and tend to obscure the morphology of the nucleus. Also, they are less plentiful than the granules seen in the eosinophil. The nucleus of the *middle* basophil appears to be bilobed, but the granules that lie over the nucleus again tend to obscure the precise shape. The basophil at the *right* is probably more mature. The granules almost entirely obscure the nuclear shape. A few blood platelets (*arrowheads*) are seen in several of the micrographs. Typically, they appear as small, irregular-shaped bodies.

E, eosinophil | **N,** neutrophil | **arrowheads,** platelets

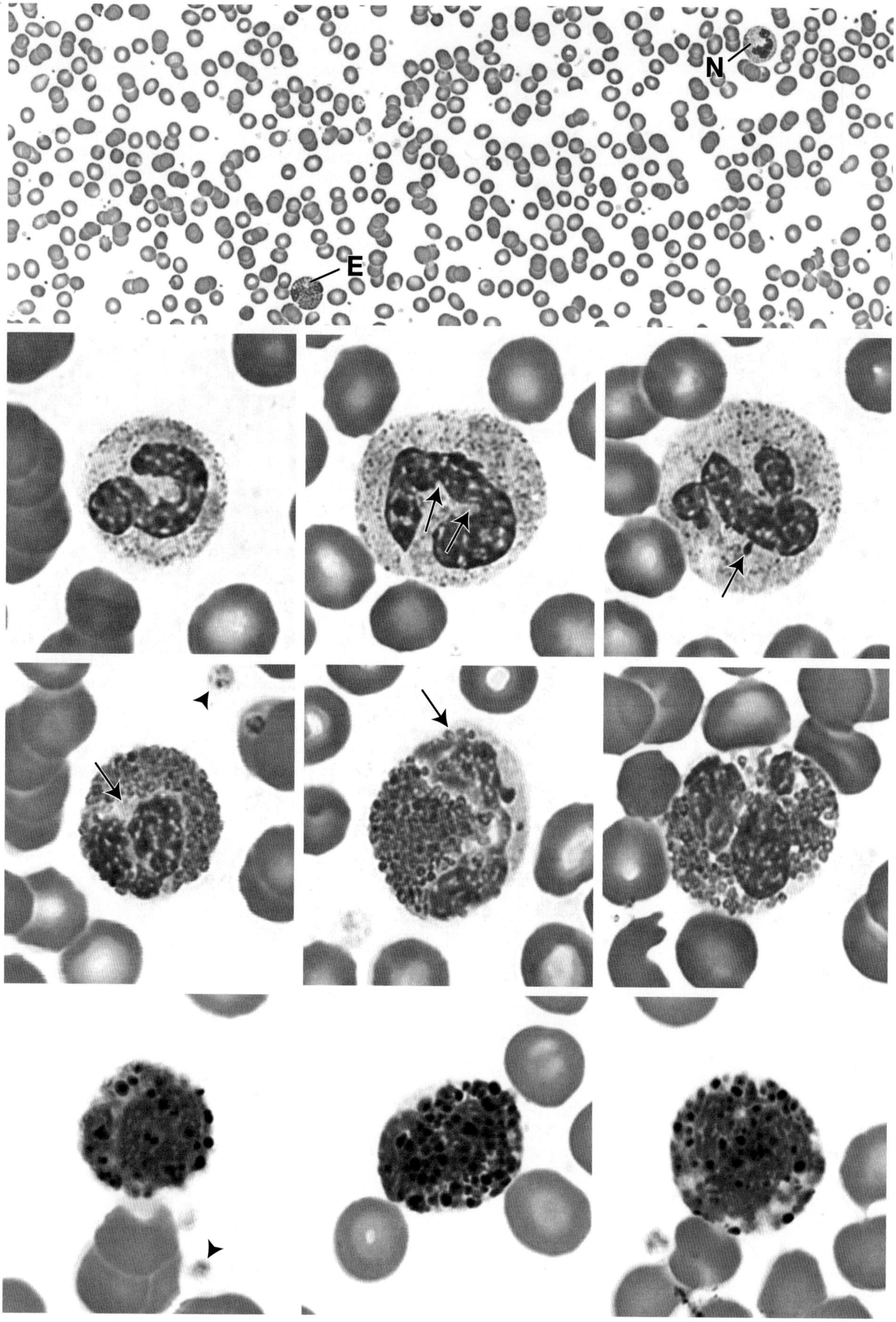
N
E

PLATE 10.2 ■ AGRANULOCYTES AND RED MARROW

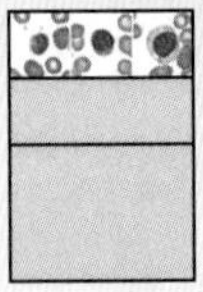

Lymphocytes, blood smear, human, Wright stain ×2,150.

The **lymphocytes** shown here vary in size, but each represents a mature cell. Circulating lymphocytes are usually described as small, medium, and large. A small lymphocyte is shown in the *left panel*. Lymphocytes in this category range in size from 7 to 9 μm. A large lymphocyte is seen in the *right panel*. These cells may be as large as 16 μm. The lymphocyte in the *middle panel* is intermediate in size. The difference in lymphocyte size is attributable mostly to the amount of cytoplasm present. However, the nucleus also contributes to the size of the cell but to a lesser degree. In differential counts, lymphocyte size is disregarded. Two **platelets** (*arrows*) are evident in the *left panel*.

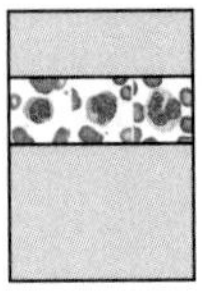

Monocytes, blood smear, human, Wright stain ×2,150.

The white blood cells in these panels are mature **monocytes**. Their size ranges from ~13 to 20 μm, with the majority falling in the upper size range. The nucleus exhibits the most characteristic feature of the monocyte, namely, an indentation, which is sometimes so prominent that it exhibits a U shape as is evident in the *right panel*. The cytoplasm is very weakly basophilic. Small, azurophilic granules (lysosomes) are also characteristic of the cytoplasm and are similar to those seen in neutrophils. Platelets (*arrows*) are present in the *left* and *middle panels*.

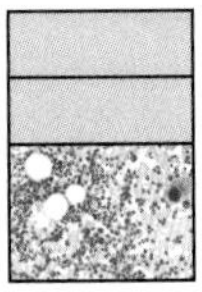

Bone marrow smear, human, Giemsa ×180.

This low-magnification photomicrograph shows a **bone marrow smear**. This type of preparation allows for the examination of developing red and white blood cells. A marrow smear is made in a manner similar to that of a peripheral blood smear. A sample of bone marrow is aspirated from a bone and simply placed on a slide and spread into a thin monolayer of cells. A wide variety of cell types are present in the marrow smear. Most of the cells are developing granulocytes and developing erythrocytes. Mature **erythrocytes** (*Ey*) are also present in large numbers. They are readily identified by their lack of a nucleus and eosinophilic staining. Often intermixed with these red cells are small groups of reticulocytes. These are very young erythrocytes that contain residual ribosomes in their cytoplasm. The presence of ribosomes slightly alters the color of the reticulocyte, giving it a slightly blue coloration in comparison to the mature eosinophilic erythrocyte. The reticulocytes are best distinguished at higher magnifications. In addition, **adipocytes** (*A*) are found in variable numbers. In preparations such as this, the lipid content is lost during preparation, and recognition of the cell is based on a clear or unstained round space. Another large cell that is typically present is the **megakaryocyte** (*M*), which produces platelets. The megakaryocyte is a polyploid cell that exhibits a large and irregular nuclear profile.

At this low magnification, it is difficult to distinguish the earlier stages of the developing cell types. However, examples of each stage of development in both cell lines are presented in the following plates. In contrast, many cells in their late stage of development, particularly in the granulocyte series, can be identified with some degree of assuredness at low magnification. For example, some band **neutrophils** (*BN*) and young **eosinophils** (*E*) can be identified by their morphology and staining characteristics.

A, adipocytes
BN, band neutrophil
E, eosinophils
Ey, erythrocytes
M, megakaryocyte
arrows, platelets

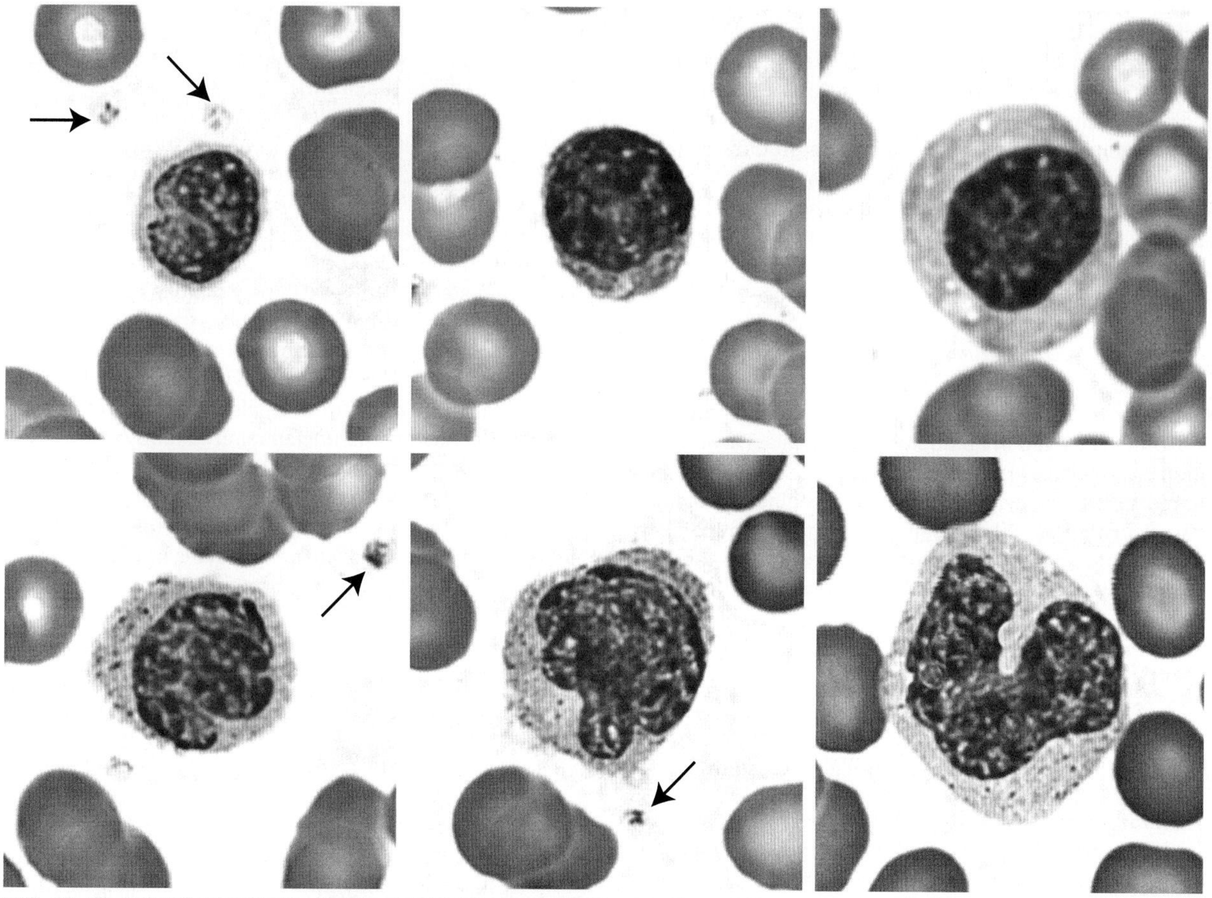

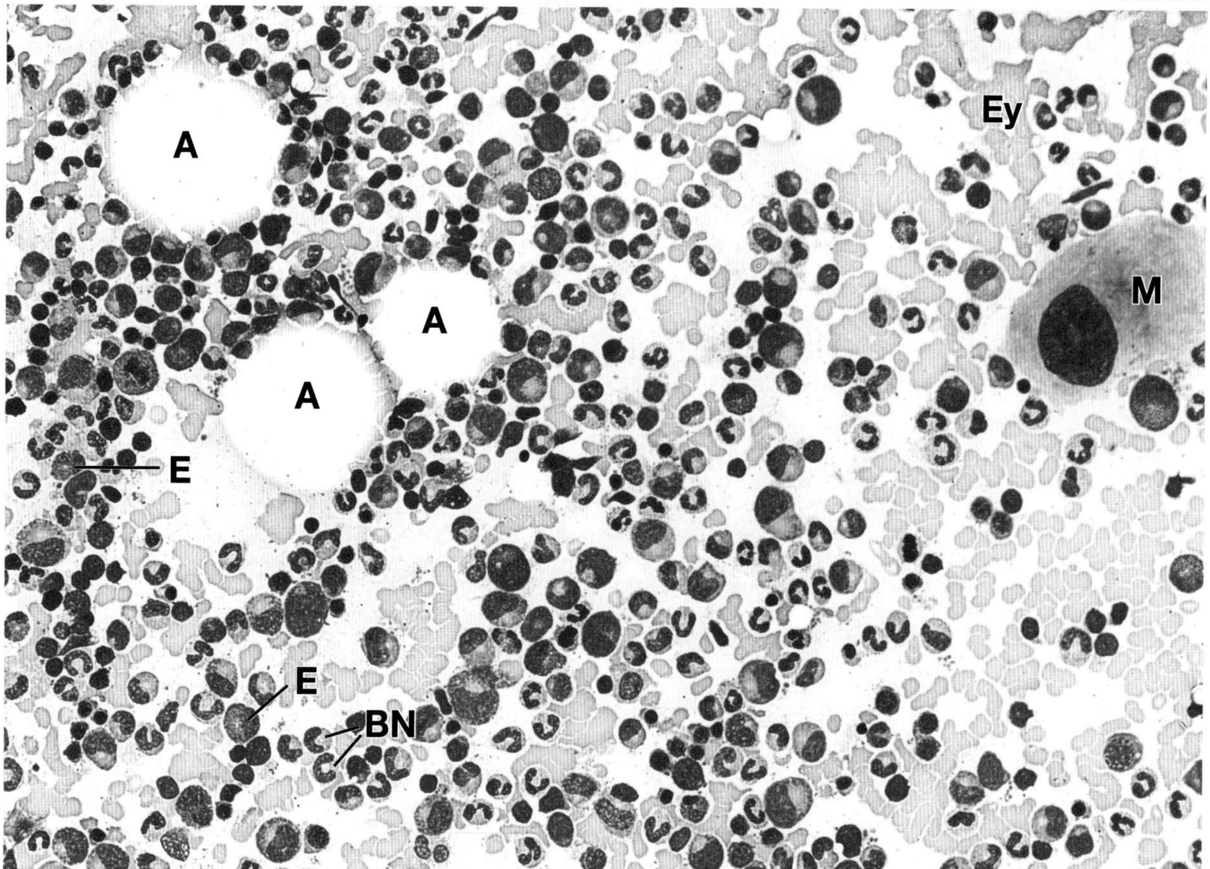
A
A
A
E
E
BN
Ey
M

PLATE 10.3 ■ ERYTHROPOIESIS

Erythropoiesis is the process by which the concentration of erythrocytes in the peripheral bloodstream is maintained under normal conditions in a steady state. Stimulation of erythroid stem cells (ErP) by hormonal action results in proliferation of precursor cells that undergo differentiation and maturation in the bone marrow. The earliest recognizable precursor of the red blood cell is the proerythroblast. These cells lack hemoglobin. Their cytoplasm is basophilic, and the nucleus exhibits a dense chromatin structure and several nucleoli. The Golgi apparatus, when evident, appears as a light staining area. The basophilic erythroblast is smaller than the proerythroblast, from which it arises by mitotic division. Its nucleus is smaller. The cytoplasm shows strong basophilia owing to the increasing number of ribosomes involved in hemoglobin synthesis. The accumulation of hemoglobin in the cell gradually changes the staining reaction of the cytoplasm so that it begins to stain with eosin. The recognizable presence of hemoglobin in the cell by virtue of its staining signifies its transition to the polychromatophilic erythroblast. The cytoplasm in the earlier part of this stage may exhibit a blue-gray color. Over time, increasing amounts of hemoglobin are synthesized and concomitantly, decreasing the numbers of ribosomes are present. The nucleus of the cell is smaller than that of the basophilic erythroblast, and the heterochromatin is much coarser. At the end of this stage, the nucleus has become much smaller and the cytoplasm more eosinophilic. This is the last stage in which mitosis occurs. The next definable stage is the orthochromatophilic erythroblast, also called a *normoblast*. Its nucleus is smaller than earlier stages and is extremely condensed. The cytoplasm is considerably less blue, leaning more to a pink or eosinophilic coloration. It is slightly larger than a mature erythrocyte. At this stage, it is no longer capable of division. In the next stage, the polychromatophilic erythrocyte, also more commonly called a *reticulocyte*, has lost its nucleus and is ready to pass into the blood sinusoids of the red bone marrow. Some ribosomes that can still synthesize hemoglobin are present in the cell. These ribosomes create a very slight basophilia in the cell. Comparison of this cell to typical mature erythrocytes in the marrow smear reveals a slight difference in coloration.

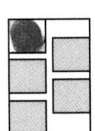

Proerythroblast, bone marrow smear, human, Giemsa ×2,200.

The **proerythroblast** shown here is a large cell, larger than the cells that follow in the developmental process. Note the very large size of the nucleus that occupies most of the cell volume. Several nucleoli (*N*) are evident. The cytoplasm is basophilic. Division of this cell results in the basophilic erythroblast.

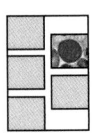

Basophilic erythroblast, bone marrow smear, human, Giemsa ×2,200.

The **basophilic erythroblast** shown here is smaller than its predecessor. The nuclear-to-cytoplasmic ratio is decreased. The greater abundance of cytoplasm is deeply basophilic compared to that of the proerythroblast. Typically, nucleoli are absent. As maturation continues, the cell decreases in size.

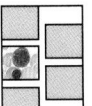

Polychromatophilic erythroblast, bone marrow smear, human, Giemsa ×2,200.

Two **polychromatophilic erythroblasts** are seen in this micrograph. The larger and less mature cell exhibits a pronounced clumping of its chromatin. The cytoplasm is basophilic but is considerably lighter in color than that of the basophilic erythroblast. The cytoplasm also exhibits some eosinophilia, which is indicative of hemoglobin production. The smaller cell represents a later stage of a polychromatophilic erythroblast. Note how much denser the chromatin appears as well as how much smaller the nucleus has become. Also, the cytoplasm now favors eosinophilia. However, some basophilia is still evident.

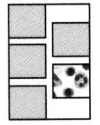

Orthochromatophilic erythroblast, bone marrow smear, human, Giemsa ×2,200.

Two **orthochromatophilic erythroblasts** are seen in this micrograph. Their nuclei have become even smaller, and the nucleus exhibits a compact, dense staining. The cytoplasm is predominantly eosinophilic but still possesses a degree of basophilia. Overall, the cell is only slightly larger than a mature erythrocyte. At this stage, the cell is no longer capable of division.

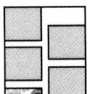

Polychromatophilic erythrocyte, bone marrow smear, human, Giemsa ×2,200.

A **polychromatophilic erythrocyte** (*PE*) is seen in this micrograph. Its nucleus has been extruded, and the cytoplasm exhibits a slight basophilia. In proximity are a number of **mature erythrocytes** (*E*). Compare the coloration of the polychromatophilic erythrocyte with that of the mature red blood cells. Polychromatophilic erythrocytes can also be readily demonstrated with special stains that cause the remaining ribosomes in the cytoplasm to clump and form a visible reticular network; hence, the polychromatophilic erythrocyte is also commonly called a *reticulocyte*.

E, erythrocytes | **N,** nucleoli | **PE,** polychromatophilic erythrocyte

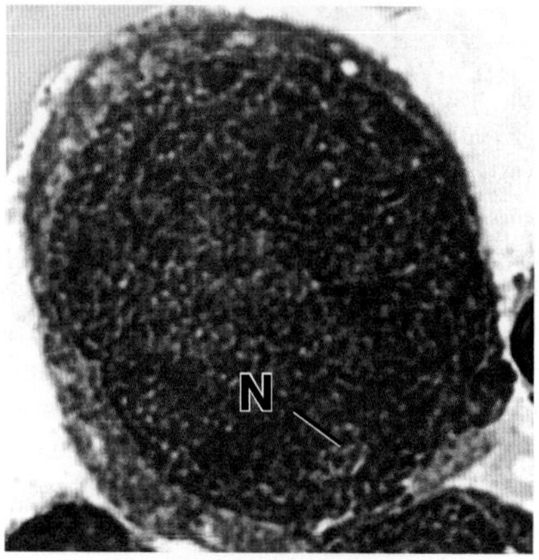

proerythroblast
(pronormoblast)

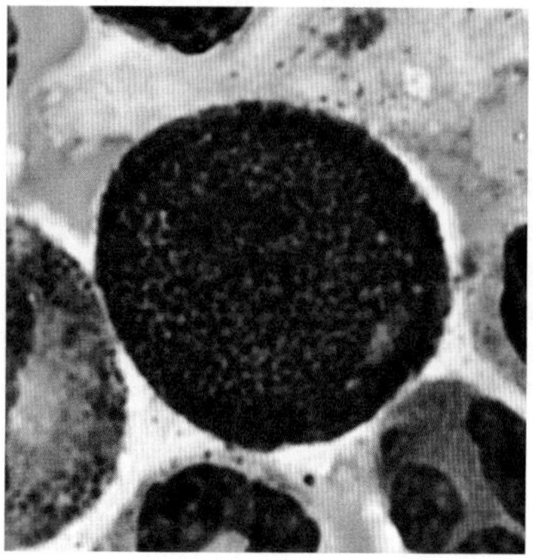

basophilic erythroblast
(basophilic normoblast)

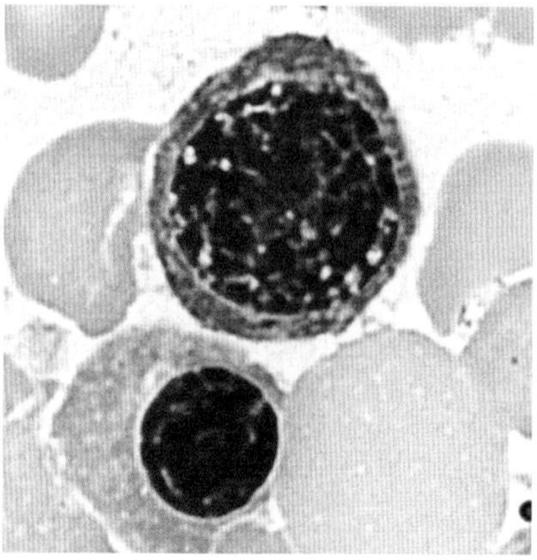

polychromatophilic erythroblast
(polychromatophilic normoblast)

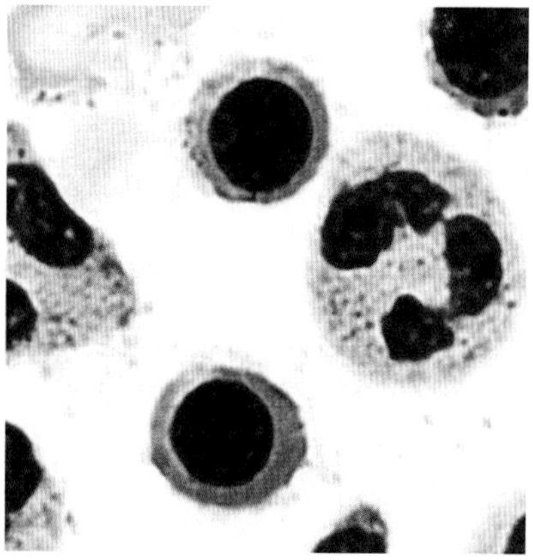

orthochromatophilic erythroblast
(normoblast)

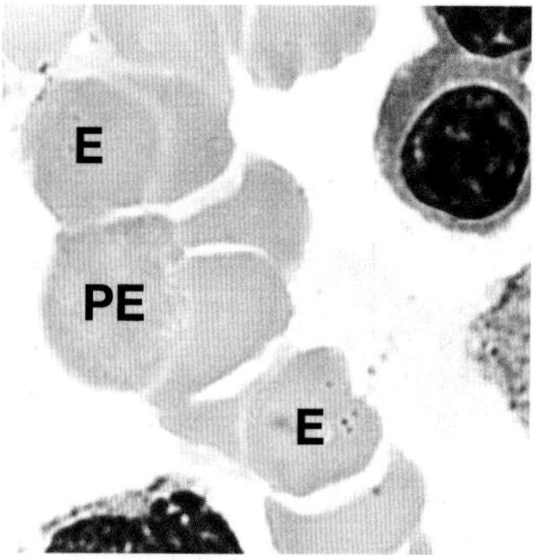

polychromatophilic erythrocyte
(reticulocyte)

PLATE 10.4 ■ GRANULOPOIESIS

Granulopoiesis is the process by which granulocytes (neutrophils, eosinophils, and basophils) differentiate and mature in the bone marrow. The earliest recognizable stage is the myeloblast, which is followed consecutively by the promyelocyte, myelocyte, metamyelocyte, band cell, and, finally, the mature granulocyte. It is not possible to differentiate eosinophil, basophil, or neutrophil precursors morphologically until the myelocyte stage is reached—when specific granules characteristic of each cell type appear. The cells of the basophil lineage are extremely difficult to locate in a marrow smear because of the minimal number of these cells in the marrow.

The **myeloblast** is characterized by a large, euchromatic, spherical nucleus with three to five nucleoli. The cell measures 14–20 μm in diameter. The cytoplasm stains deeply basophilic. The presence of a light or poorly staining area indicates a Golgi apparatus. The **promyelocyte** exhibits a similar size range, 15–21 μm; nucleoli are present. Promyelocyte cytoplasm stains similarly to that of the myeloblast, but it is distinguished by the presence of large, blue-black, primary azurophilic granules, also called *nonspecific granules*. The **myelocyte** ranges from 16 to 24 μm. Its chromatin is more condensed than its precursor, and nucleoli are absent. The cytoplasm of the neutrophilic myelocyte is characterized by small, pink-to-red specific granules with some azurophilic granules present. The eosinophilic lineage has a similar-appearing nucleus, but its specific granules are large. The **metamyelocyte** ranges from 12 to 18 μm. The nuclear-to-cytoplasmic ratio is further decreased, and the nucleus assumes a kidney shape. There are few azurophilic granules at this stage in cells, and there is a predominance of small, pink-to-red specific granules. The eosinophilic metamyelocyte shows an increased number of specific granules compared to the neutrophilic metamyelocyte. The **band cells** are further reduced in size, 9–15 μm. The chromatin of the nucleus exhibits further condensation and has a horseshoe shape. In the neutrophilic band cell, the small, pink-to-red specific granules are the only granule type present. The eosinophilic band cell shows little or no change relative to the specific granules, but the nucleus exhibits a kidney shape. Mature granulocytes are shown in Plate 10.1.

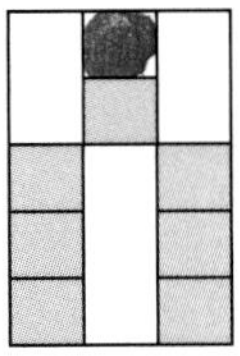

Myeloblast, bone marrow smear, human, Giemsa ×2,200.

The myeloblast shown here exhibits a deep blue cytoplasm with a lighter region that represents the Golgi area (*G*). The nucleus is round. Several nucleoli (*N*) are evident.

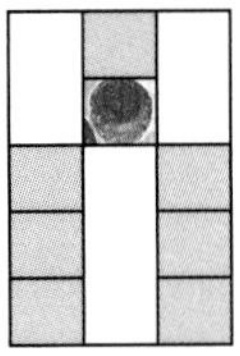

Promyelocyte, bone marrow smear, human, Giemsa ×2,200.

The promyelocyte exhibits a round nucleus with one or more nucleoli (*N*) present. The cytoplasm is basophilic and exhibits relatively large blue-black azurophilic granules (*AG*).

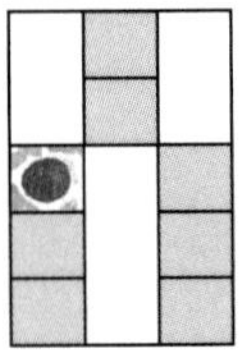

Eosinophilic myelocyte, bone marrow smear, human, Giemsa ×2,200.

The eosinophilic myelocyte exhibits a nucleus the same as that described for the neutrophilic myelocyte. The cytoplasm, however, contains the large specific granules characteristic of eosinophils, but they are fewer in number.

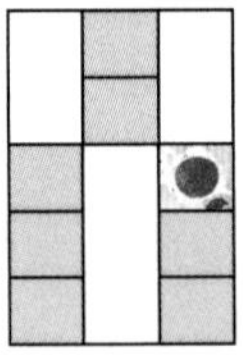

Neutrophilic myelocyte, bone marrow smear, human, Giemsa ×2,200.

The neutrophilic myelocyte retains the round nucleus, but nucleoli are now absent. The cytoplasm exhibits its small, pink-to-red specific granules.

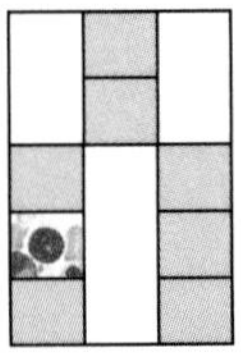

Eosinophilic metamyelocyte, bone marrow smear, human, Giemsa ×2,200.

The eosinophilic metamyelocyte exhibits a kidney- or bean-shaped nucleus. The cytoplasm exhibits numerous characteristic eosinophilic granules that are present throughout the cytoplasm.

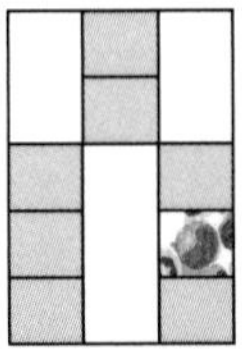

Neutrophilic metamyelocyte, bone marrow smear, human, Giemsa ×2,200.

The neutrophilic metamyelocyte differs from its precursor by the presence of a kidney- or bean-shaped nucleus. The small, pink-to-red specific granules are now seen in the cytoplasm, and few or no azurophilic granules are present.

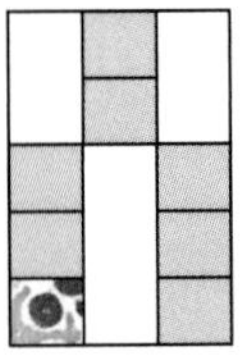

Eosinophilic band cell, bone marrow smear, human, Giemsa ×2,200.

The eosinophilic band cell exhibits a horseshoe-shaped nucleus. Its cytoplasm is filled with the eosinophilic granules.

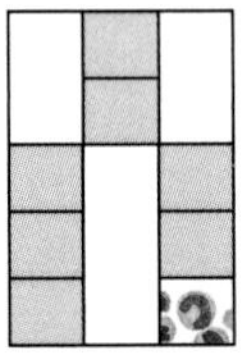

Neutrophilic band cell, bone marrow smear, human, Giemsa ×2,200.

The band or nonsegmented neutrophil exhibits a horseshoe-shaped nucleus with abundant small, pink-to-red specific granules in the cytoplasm.

AG, azurophilic granules | **G,** Golgi apparatus | **N,** nucleoli

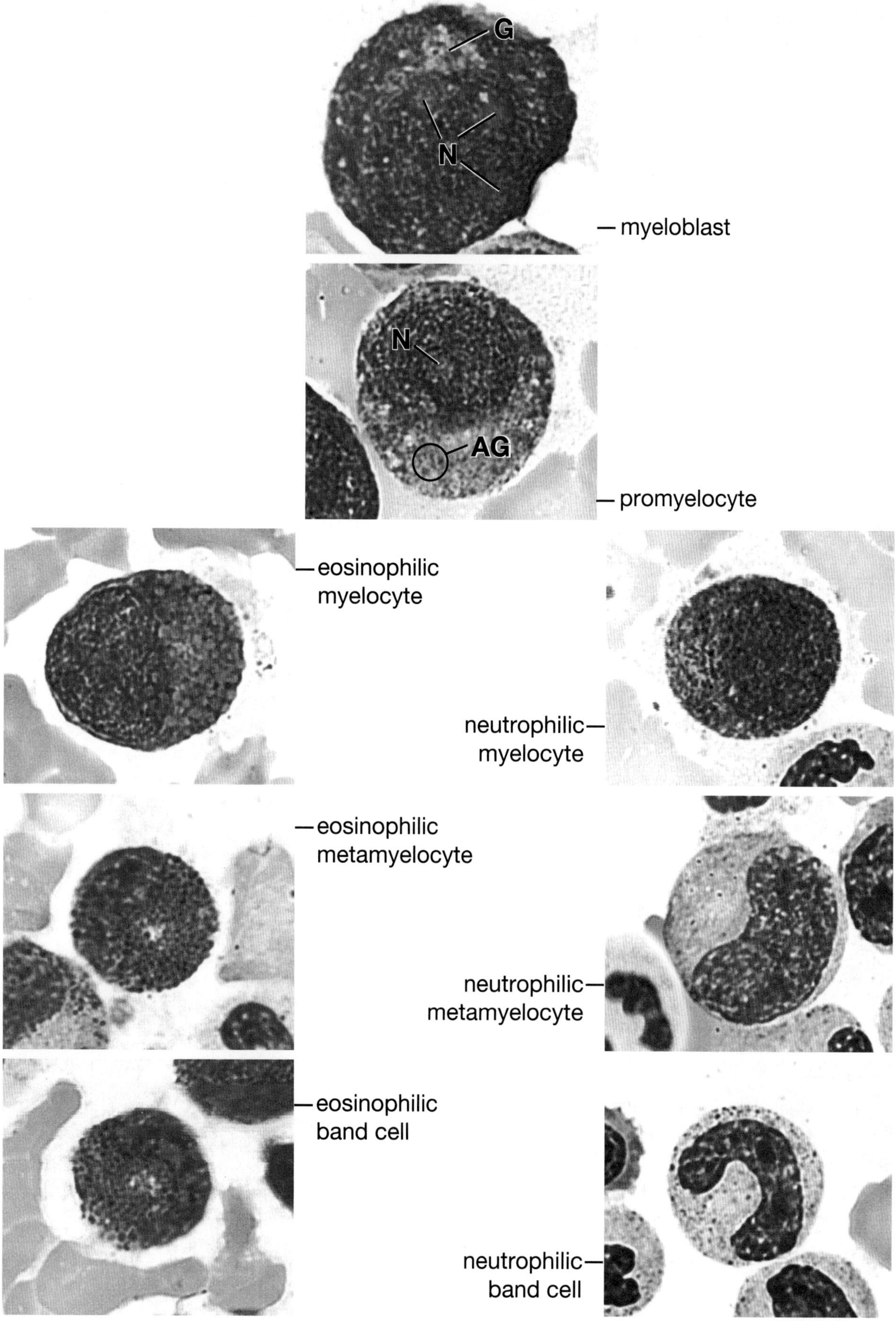
G
N
myeloblast
N
AG
promyelocyte
eosinophilic myelocyte
neutrophilic myelocyte
eosinophilic metamyelocyte
neutrophilic metamyelocyte
eosinophilic band cell
neutrophilic band cell

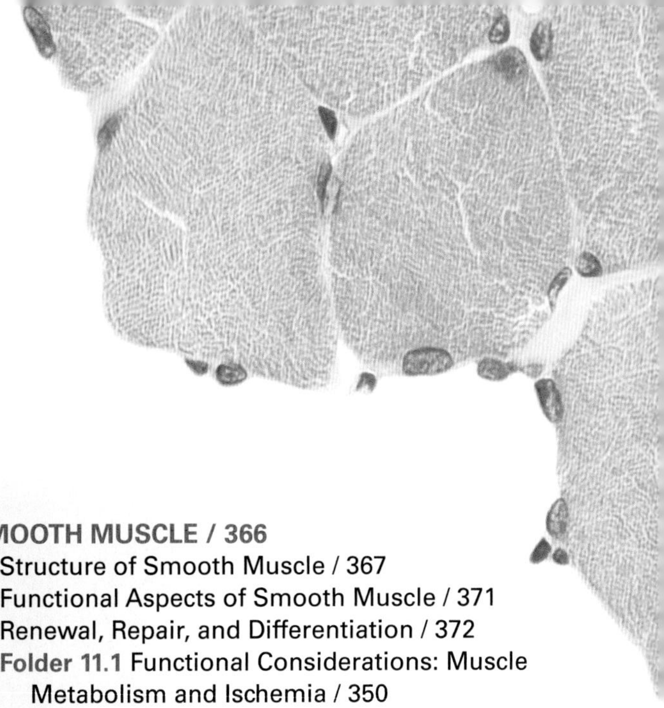

11 MUSCLE TISSUE

OVERVIEW AND CLASSIFICATION OF MUSCLE

Muscle tissue is responsible for movement of the body and its parts and for changes in the size and shape of internal organs. This tissue is characterized by aggregates of specialized, elongated cells arranged in parallel array that have the primary role of **contraction** (Fig. 11.1).

Myofilament interaction is responsible for muscle cell contraction.

Two types of **myofilaments** are associated with cell contraction:

- **Thin filaments** (6–8 nm in diameter, 1.0 μm long) are composed primarily of the protein **actin**. Each thin filament of fibrous actin (**F-actin**) is a polymer primarily formed from globular actin molecules (**G-actin**).
- **Thick filaments** (~15 nm in diameter, 1.5 μm long) are composed primarily of the protein **myosin II**. Each thick filament consists of 200–300 myosin II molecules. The long, rod-shaped tail portion of each molecule aggregates in a regular parallel but staggered array, whereas the head portions project out in a regular helical pattern.

The two types of myofilaments occupy the bulk of the cytoplasm, which, in muscle cells, is called **sarcoplasm** *[Gr. sarcos, flesh; plasma, thing]*. Muscle cells contain a large number of aligned contractile filaments that the cells use for the single purpose of producing mechanical work. Actin and myosin are also present in most other cell types (although in considerably smaller amounts), where they play a role in cellular activities, such as cytokinesis, exocytosis, and cell migration.

Muscle is classified according to the appearance of the contractile cells.

Two principal types of muscle are recognized:

- **Striated muscle**, in which the cells exhibit cross-striations at the light microscope level
- **Smooth muscle**, in which the cells do not exhibit cross-striations

Striated muscle tissue is further subclassified on the basis of its location:

- **Skeletal muscle** is attached to bone and is responsible for movement of the axial and appendicular skeleton and maintenance of body position and posture. In addition, skeletal muscles of the eye (extraocular muscles) provide precise eye movement.
- **Visceral striated muscle** is morphologically identical to skeletal muscle but is restricted to the soft tissues, namely, the tongue, pharynx, lumbar part of the diaphragm, and upper part of the esophagus. These muscles play essential roles in speech, breathing, and swallowing.

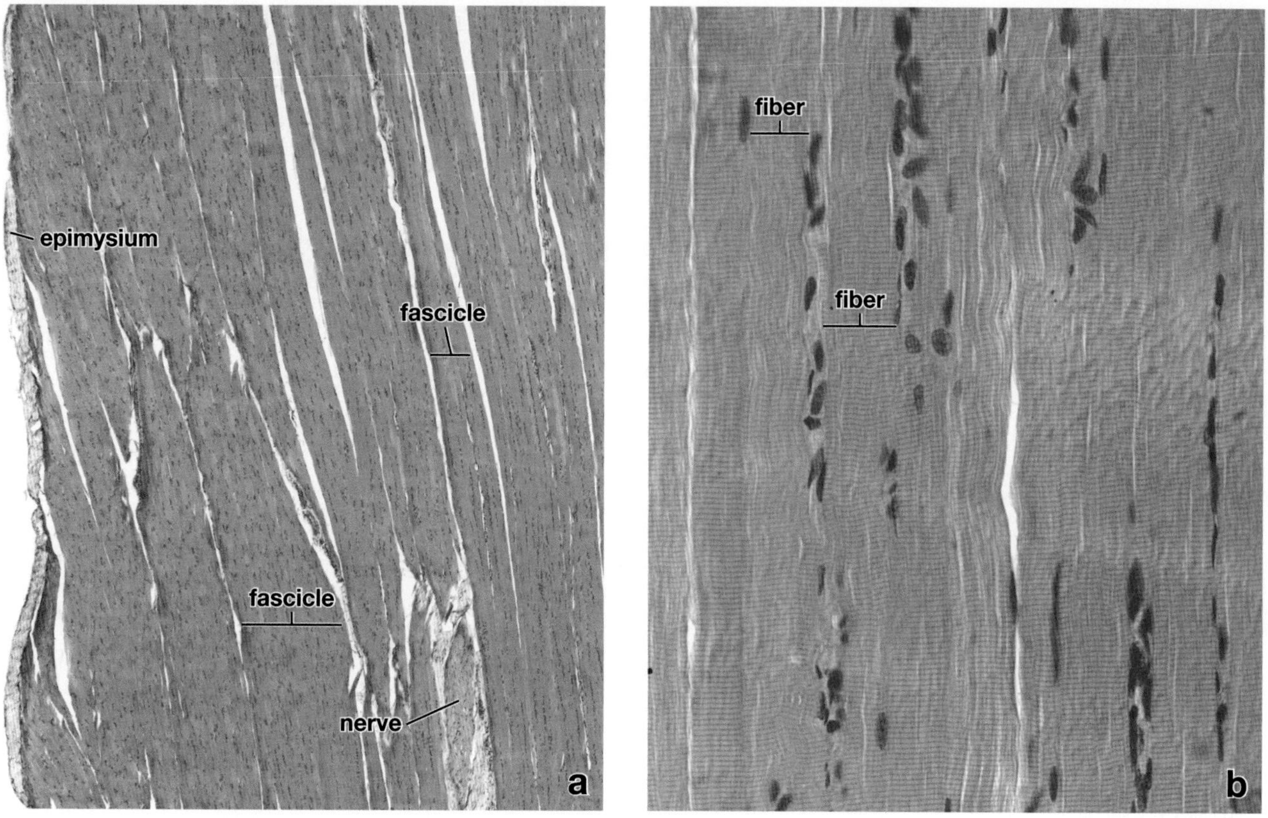

FIGURE 11.1. Photomicrograph of a skeletal muscle. a. This low-magnification photomicrograph shows skeletal muscle in longitudinal section. Muscle fibers (cells) are arranged in parallel fascicles; they are vertically oriented, and the length of each fiber extends beyond the *upper* and *lower edge* of the micrograph. The fascicles appear to be of different thicknesses. This is largely a reflection of the plane of section through the muscle. Note on the *left* the epimysium, the sheath of dense connective tissue surrounding the muscle. ×160. **b.** At higher magnification, cross-striations of the muscle fibers are readily seen. The nuclei of skeletal muscle fibers are located in the cytoplasm immediately beneath the plasma membrane. ×360.

- **Cardiac muscle** is a type of striated muscle found in the wall of the heart and in the base of the large veins that empty into the heart.

The cross-striations in striated muscle are produced largely by the specific cytoarchitectural arrangement of both thin and thick myofilaments. This arrangement is the same in all types of striated muscle cells. The main differences between skeletal muscle cells and cardiac muscle cells are in their size, shape, and organization relative to one another.

Smooth muscle cells do not exhibit cross-striations because the myofilaments do not achieve the same degree of order in their arrangement. In addition, the myosin-containing myofilaments in smooth muscle are highly labile. Smooth muscle is restricted to the viscera and vascular system, the arrector pili muscles of the skin, and the intrinsic muscles of the eye.

■ SKELETAL MUSCLE

A skeletal muscle cell is a multinucleated syncytium.

In skeletal muscle, each muscle cell, more commonly called a **muscle fiber**, is actually a multinucleated **syncytium**. A muscle fiber is formed during development by the fusion of small, individual muscle cells called **myoblasts** (see page 360). When viewed in cross section, a mature multinucleated muscle fiber reveals a polygonal shape with a diameter of 10–100 μm (Plate 11.1, page 376). Their length varies from almost a meter, as in the sartorius muscle of the lower limb, to as little as a few millimeters, as in the stapedius muscle of the middle ear. (*Note:* A muscle fiber should not be confused with a connective tissue fiber; muscle fibers are skeletal muscle cells, whereas connective tissue fibers are extracellular products of connective tissue cells.)

The nuclei of a skeletal muscle fiber are located in the cytoplasm immediately beneath the plasma membrane, also called the **sarcolemma**, which consists of the plasma membrane of the muscle cell, its external lamina, and the surrounding reticular lamina.

A skeletal muscle consists of striated muscle fibers held together by connective tissue.

The connective tissue that surrounds both individual muscle fibers and bundles of muscle fibers is essential for force transduction (Fig. 11.2). At the end of the muscle, the connective tissue continues as a tendon or other arrangement of collagen fibers that attaches the muscle, usually to bone. A rich supply of blood vessels and nerves travels in the connective tissue.

The connective tissue associated with muscle is named according to its relationship with the muscle fibers:

- **Endomysium** is the delicate layer of reticular fibers that immediately surrounds individual muscle fibers (see Fig. 11.2a). Only small-diameter blood vessels and the finest neuronal branches are present within the endomysium, running parallel to the muscle fibers.
- **Perimysium** is a thicker connective tissue layer that surrounds a group of fibers to form a **bundle** or **fascicle**. Fascicles are functional units of muscle fibers that tend to work together to perform a specific function. Larger blood vessels and nerves travel in the perimysium.
- **Epimysium** is the sheath of dense connective tissue that surrounds a collection of fascicles that constitutes the

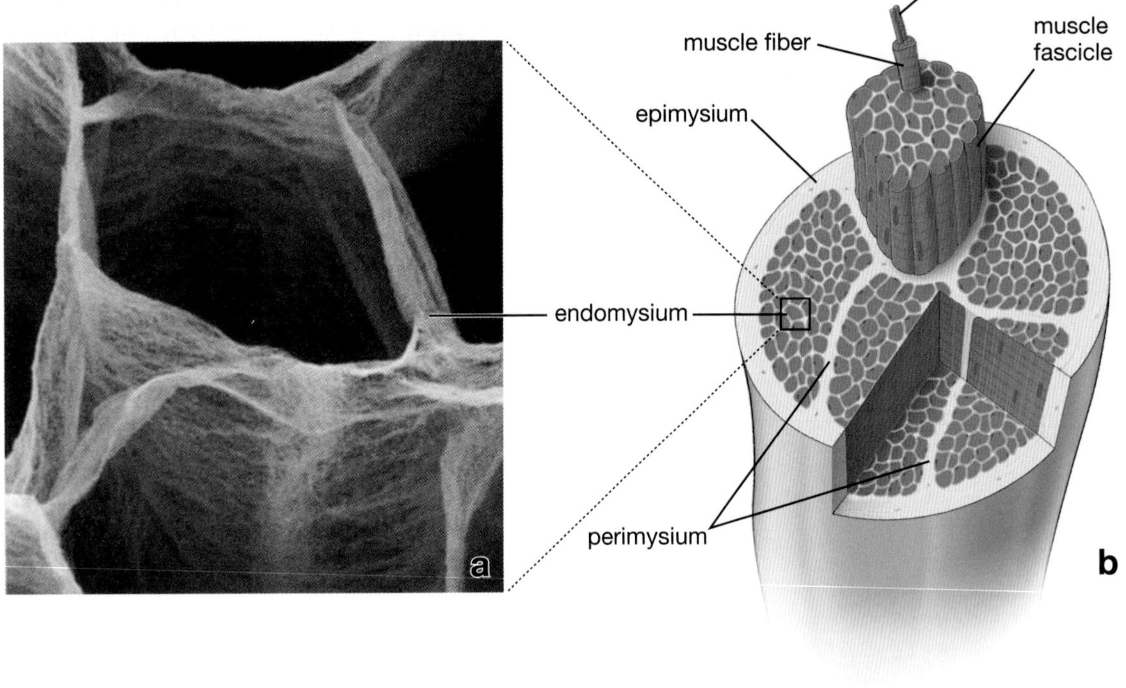

FIGURE 11.2. General organization of skeletal muscle. a. This freeze-fracture scanning electron micrograph (SEM) of an intramuscular connective tissue was obtained from the bovine semitendinosus muscle. The specimen was routinely fixed for SEM and subsequently treated according to the cell maceration method with sodium hydroxide to remove muscle cells. Note the delicate honeycomb structure of the endomysium surrounding individual muscle cells. ×480. **b.** This schematic diagram shows the general organization of skeletal muscle and its relation to the surrounding connective tissue. Note the organization of the endomysium that surrounds individual muscle cells (fibers), the perimysium that surrounds a muscle bundle, and the epimysium that surrounds the entire muscle. (Reprinted with permission from Nishimura T, Hattori A, Takahashi K. Structural changes in intramuscular connective tissue during the fattening of Japanese black cattle: effect of marbling on beef tenderization. *J Anim Sci.* 1999;77:93–104.)

muscle (see Fig. 11.1a). In gross anatomy, it is also called **deep investing fascia**, which can surround not only individual muscles but also groups of muscles to form compartments. The major vascular and nerve supply of the muscle penetrates the epimysium.

Skeletal muscle fibers are characterized by speed of contraction, enzymatic velocity, and metabolic activity.

The current classification of skeletal muscle fibers is based on **contractile speed**, **enzymatic velocity** of the fiber's myosin ATPase reaction, and **metabolic profile**. The contractile speed determines how fast the fiber can contract and relax. Velocity of the myosin ATPase reaction determines the rate at which this enzyme is capable of breaking down adenosine triphosphate (ATP) molecules during the contraction cycle. The **metabolic profile** indicates the capacity for ATP production by oxidative phosphorylation or glycolysis. Fibers characterized by **oxidative metabolism** contain large amounts of myoglobin and an increased number of mitochondria, with their constituent cytochrome electron transport complexes. **Myoglobin** is a small, globular, 17.8-kDa oxygen-binding protein that contains a ferrous form of iron (Fe^{+2}). It resembles hemoglobin in the erythrocytes and is found in various amounts in muscle fibers. Myoglobin functions primarily to store oxygen in muscle fibers and provides a ready source of oxygen for muscle metabolism. **Traumatic injuries** to skeletal muscles (e.g., crash injuries) cause breakdown (rhabdomyolysis) and release of **myoglobin** from the injured muscle cells into the circulation. The myoglobin is removed from the bloodstream by kidneys; however, large amounts of myoglobin are toxic to the renal tubular epithelium, causing acute **renal failure**. Detection of myoglobin in the blood is a sensitive but nonspecific test for muscle injury.

Three types of skeletal muscle fibers—red, white, and intermediate—can be identified by color in vivo.

It has long been known that skeletal muscle fibers differ in diameter and in their natural color in vivo. The color differences are not apparent in hematoxylin and eosin (H&E)-stained sections. However, histochemical reactions based on oxidative enzyme activity, specifically the **succinic dehydrogenase** and **nicotinamide adenine dinucleotide–tetrazolium reductase (NADH-TR)** as well as **myosin ATPase** reactions, confirm the observations seen in fresh tissue and reveal several types of skeletal muscle fibers (Fig. 11.3). The most obvious nomenclature to describe these differences is division into red, white, and intermediate fibers.

Based on enzymatic activities, skeletal muscle fibers are classified into type I (slow oxidative), type IIa (fast oxidative glycolytic), and type IIb (fast glycolytic) fibers.

Three types of fiber are typically found in any given skeletal muscle; the proportion of each type varies according to the functional role of the muscle.

- **Type I fibers** or **slow oxidative fibers** are small fibers that appear red in fresh specimens and contain many mitochondria and large amounts of myoglobin and cytochrome complexes. Their high levels of mitochondrial oxidative enzymes are demonstrated by their strong succinic dehydrogenase and NADH-TR histochemical staining reactions as described previously (see Fig. 11.3). Type I fibers are **slow-twitch, fatigue-resistant motor units** (a twitch is a single, brief contraction of the muscle). These fibers have great resistance to fatigue but generate less tension than other fibers. Their

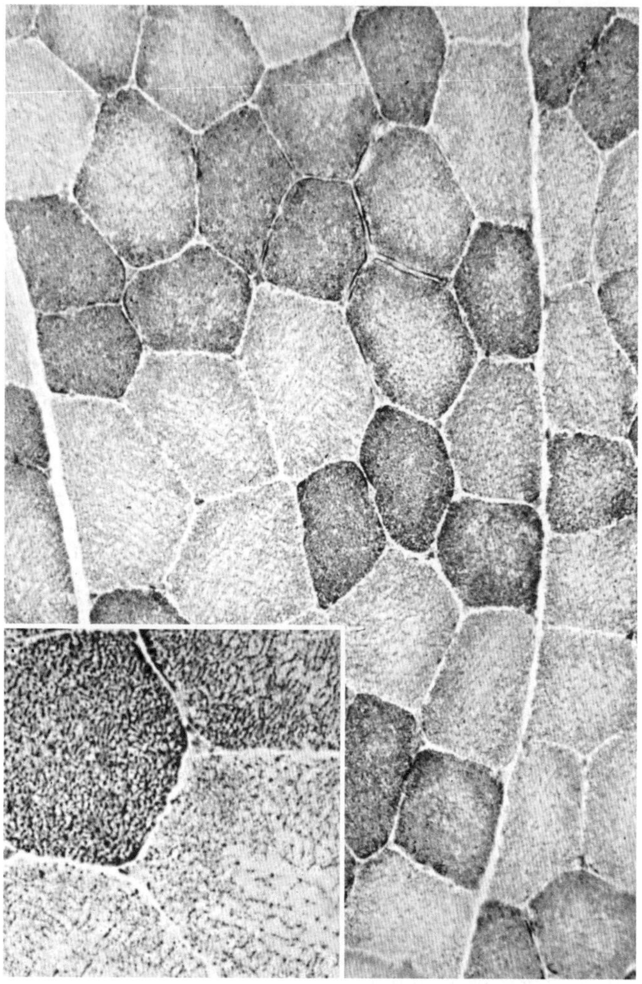

FIGURE 11.3. Cross section of skeletal muscle fibers. This cross section of muscle fibers stained with the nicotinamide adenine dinucleotide–tetrazolium reductase (NADH-TR) demonstrates two fiber types. The deeply stained, smaller muscle fibers exhibit strong oxidative enzyme activity and correspond to the type I slow oxidative fibers. The lighter staining, larger fibers correspond to the type IIb fast glycolytic fibers. ×280. **Inset.** Portions of the two fiber types at higher magnification. The reaction also reveals the mitochondria that contain the oxidative enzymes. The contractile components, the myofibrils, are unstained. ×550. (Original slide specimen courtesy of Dr. Scott W. Ballinger.)

myosin ATPase reaction velocity is the slowest of all of the fiber types. Type I fibers are typically found in the limb muscles of mammals and the breast muscle of migrating birds. More importantly, they are the principal fibers of the long **erector spinae muscles** of the back in humans, where they are particularly adapted to the long, slow contraction needed to maintain an erect posture. A high percentage of these fibers make up the muscles of high-endurance athletes, such as marathon runners.

- **Type IIa fibers** or **fast oxidative glycolytic fibers** are the intermediate fibers seen in fresh tissue. They are of medium size with many mitochondria and high myoglobin content. In contrast to type I fibers, type IIa fibers contain large amounts of glycogen and are capable of anaerobic glycolysis. Their myosin ATPase reaction velocity is high. They make up **fast-twitch, fatigue-resistant motor units** that generate high-peak muscle tension. Athletes who have a high percentage of these fast oxidative glycolytic fibers include 400- and 800-m sprinters, middle-distance swimmers, and hockey players.
- **Type IIb fibers** or **fast glycolytic fibers** are large fibers that appear light pink in fresh specimens and contain less myoglobin and fewer mitochondria than type I and type IIa fibers. They have a low level of oxidative enzymes but exhibit high anaerobic enzyme activity and store a considerable amount of glycogen. These fibers are **fast-twitch, fatigue-prone motor units** and generate high-peak muscle tension. Their myosin ATPase velocity is the fastest of all the fiber types. They also fatigue rapidly as a result of the production of lactic acid. Thus, type IIb fibers are adapted for rapid contraction and precise, fine movements. They constitute most fibers of the **extraocular muscles** and the muscles that control the **movements of the digits**. These muscles have a greater number of neuromuscular junctions than do type I fibers, thus allowing more precise neuronal control of movements in these muscles. Short-distance sprinters, weight lifters, and other field athletes have a high percentage of type IIb fibers.

Myofibrils and Myofilaments

The structural and functional subunit of the muscle fiber is myofibril.

A **muscle fiber** is filled with longitudinally arrayed structural subunits called **myofibrils** (Fig. 11.4). Myofibrils are

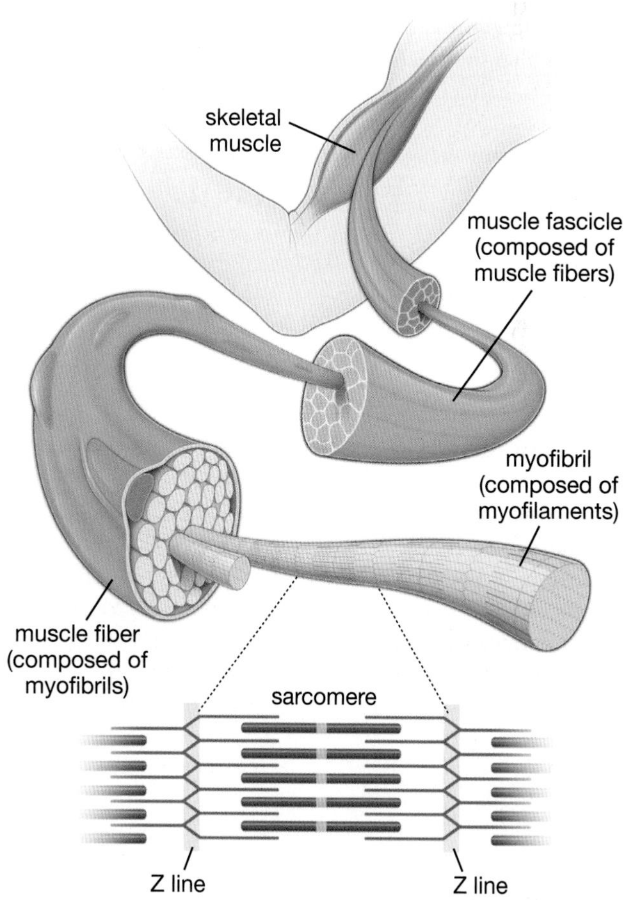

FIGURE 11.4. Organization of a skeletal muscle. A skeletal muscle consists of bundles of muscle fibers called *fascicles.* In turn, each fascicle consists of a bundle of elongated muscle fibers (cells). The muscle fiber represents a collection of longitudinal units, the myofibrils, which, in turn, are composed of myofilaments of two types: thick (myosin) filaments and thin (actin) filaments. The myofilaments are organized in a specific manner that imparts a cross-striated appearance to the myofibril and fiber. The functional unit of the myofibril is the sarcomere; it extends in both directions from one Z line to the next Z line. The A band marks the extent of the myosin filaments. Actin filaments extend from the Z line into the region of the A band, where they interdigitate with the myosin filaments as shown.

visible in favorable histologic preparations and are best seen in cross sections of muscle fibers. In these sections, they give the fiber a stippled appearance. Myofibrils extend the entire length of the muscle cell.

Myofibrils are composed of bundles of myofilaments.

Myofilaments are the individual filamentous polymers of myosin II (thick filaments) and actin and its associated proteins (thin filaments). Myofilaments are the actual contractile elements of striated muscle. The bundles of myofilaments that make up the myofibril are surrounded by a well-developed, smooth-surfaced endoplasmic reticulum (sER), also called the **sarcoplasmic reticulum**. This reticulum forms a highly organized tubular network around the contractile elements in all striated muscle cells. Mitochondria and glycogen deposits are located between the myofibrils in association with the sER.

Cross-striations are the principal histologic feature of striated muscle.

Cross-striations are evident in H&E-stained preparations of longitudinal sections of muscle fibers (Plate 11.2, page 378). They may also be seen in unstained preparations of living muscle fibers examined with a phase-contrast or polarizing microscope, in which they appear as alternating light and dark bands. These bands are termed the **A band** and the **I band** (see Fig. 11.4).

In polarizing microscopy, the dark bands are birefringent (i.e., they alter the polarized light in two planes). Therefore, the dark bands, being doubly refractive, are **anisotropic** and are given the name **A band**. The light bands are monorefringent (i.e., they do not alter the plane of polarized light). Therefore, they are **isotropic** and are given the name **I band**.

Both the A and I bands are bisected by narrow regions of contrasting density (see Fig. 11.4). The light I band is bisected by a dense line, the **Z line**, also called the **Z disc** *[Ger. zwischenscheibe, between discs]*. The dark A band is bisected by a less dense, or light, region called the **H band** *[Ger. hell, light]*. Furthermore, bisecting the light H band is a narrow dense line called the **M line** *[Ger. mitte, middle]*. The M line is best demonstrated in electron micrographs (Fig. 11.5), although in ideal H&E preparations, it can be detected in the light microscope.

As noted earlier, the cross-banding pattern of striated muscle is a result of the arrangement of the two kinds of myofilaments. To understand the mechanism of contraction, this banding pattern must be considered in functional terms.

The functional unit of the myofibril is sarcomere, the segment of the myofibril between two adjacent Z lines.

The **sarcomere** is the basic contractile unit of striated muscle. It is the portion of a myofibril between two adjacent Z lines. A sarcomere measures 2–3 μm in relaxed mammalian muscle. It may be stretched to more than 4 μm and, during extreme contraction, may be reduced to as little as 1 μm in length (Fig. 11.6). The entire muscle cell exhibits cross-striations because sarcomeres in adjacent myofibrils are arranged with their Z lines in alignment.

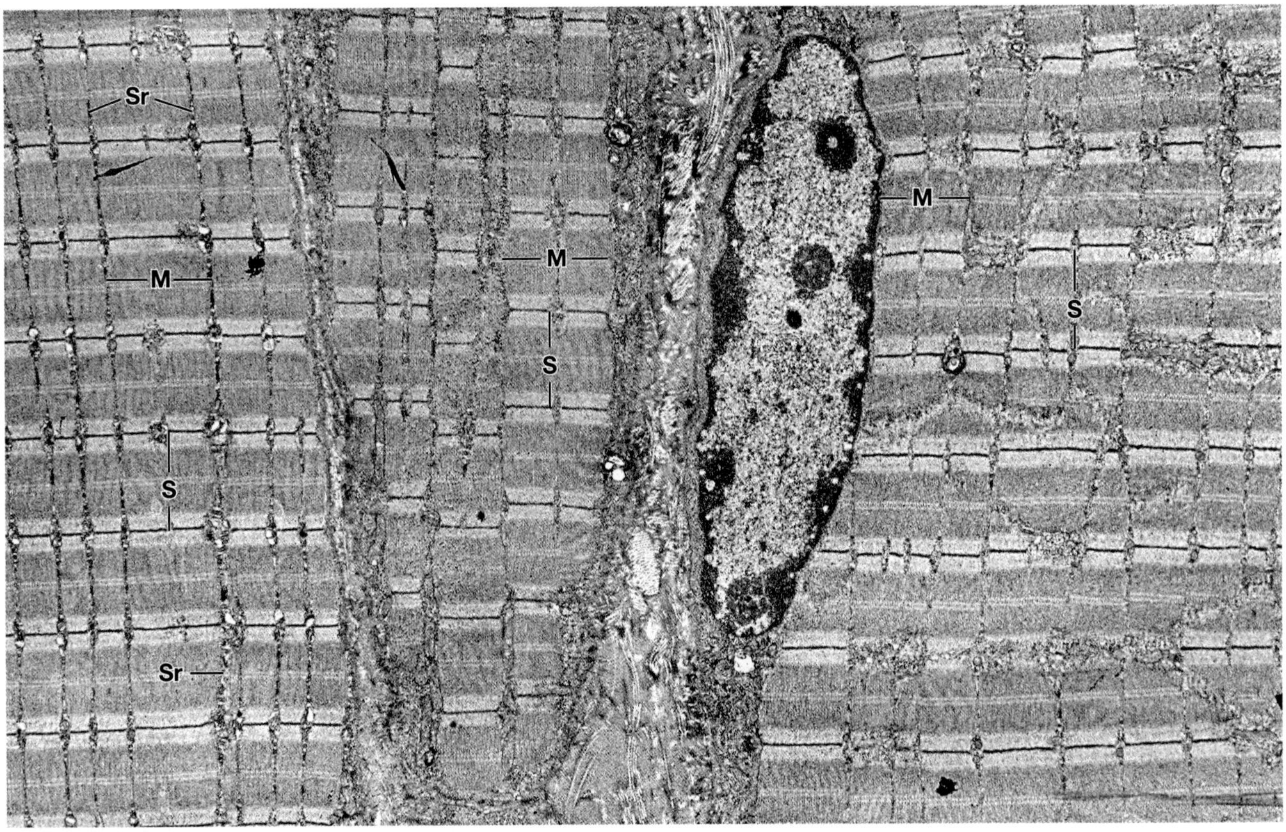

FIGURE 11.5. Electron micrograph of skeletal muscle fiber. This low-magnification electron micrograph shows the general organization of skeletal muscle fibers. Small portions of three muscle fibers in longitudinal profile are included in this micrograph. The muscle fiber on the *right* reveals a nucleus at its periphery. Two fibers—one in the *middle* and another on the *left*—exhibit regular profiles of myofibrils separated by a thin layer of surrounding sarcoplasm (*Sr*). Each repeating part of the myofibril between adjacent Z lines is a sarcomere (*S*). The cross-banded pattern visible on this micrograph reflects the arrangement, in register, of the individual myofibrils (*M*); a similar pattern found in the myofibril reflects the arrangement of myofilaments. The detailed features of a sarcomere are shown at higher magnification in Figure 11.10a. The presence of connective tissue in the extracellular space between the fibers constitutes the endomysium of the muscle. ×6,500.

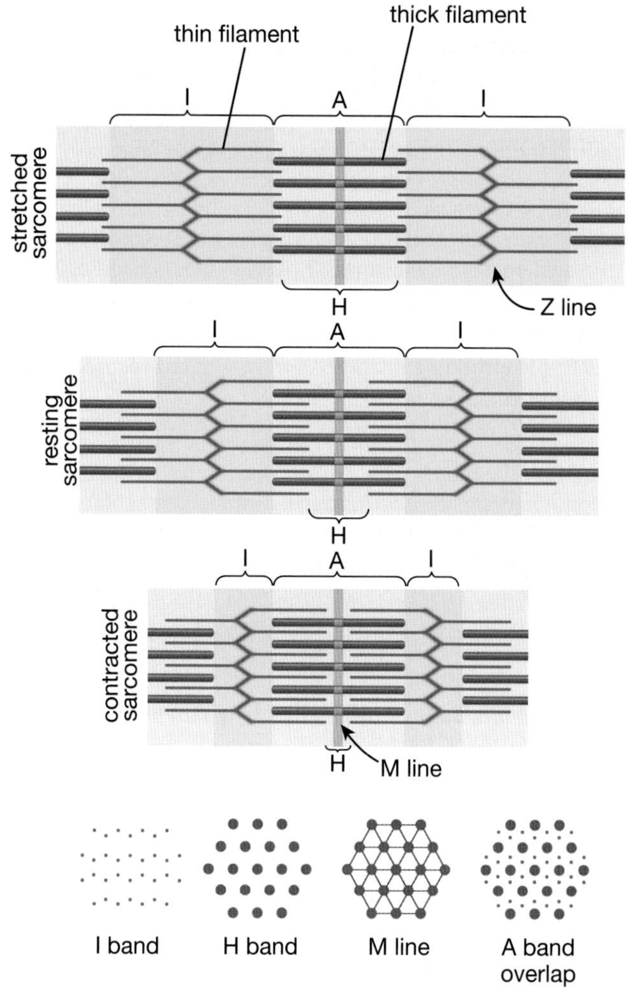

FIGURE 11.6. Sarcomeres in different functional stages. In the resting state (*middle*), interdigitation of thin (actin) and thick (myosin) filaments is not complete; the H and I bands are relatively wide. In the contracted state (*bottom*), the interdigitation of the thin and thick filaments is increased according to the degree of contraction. In the stretched state (*top*), the thin and thick filaments do not interact; the H and I bands are very wide. The length of the A band always remains the same and corresponds to the length of the thick filaments; the lengths of the H and I bands change, again in proportion to the degree of sarcomere relaxation or contraction. The cross sections through different regions of the sarcomere are also shown (*from left to right*): through thin filaments of the I band; through thick filaments of the H band; through the center of the A band where adjacent thick filaments are linked to form the M line; and through the A band, where thin and thick filaments overlap. Note that each thick filament is within the center of a hexagonal array of thin filaments.

The arrangement of thick and thin filaments gives rise to the density differences that produce the cross-striations of the myofibril.

The **myosin-containing thick filaments** are about 1.6 μm long and are restricted to the central portion of the sarcomere (i.e., the A band). The **actin-containing thin filaments** attach to the Z line and extend into the A band to the edge of the H band. Portions of two sarcomeres, on either side of a Z line, constitute the I band and contain only thin filaments. In a longitudinal section of a sarcomere, the Z line appears as a zigzag structure, with matrix material, the Z matrix, bisecting the zigzag. The **Z line** and its matrix material anchor the thin filaments from adjacent sarcomeres to the angles of the zigzag by **α-actinin**, an actin-binding protein. The **Z matrix** includes a number of proteins (e.g., telethonin, talin, desmin, myotilin, filamin C) that anchor Z lines to that of neighboring myofibrils and adjacent cell membrane (see Figs. 11.4 and 11.6).

Thin filaments primarily consist of polymerized actin molecules coupled with regulatory proteins and other thin filament–associated proteins that are entwined together.

A typical **thin filament** is 5–6 nm in diameter and consists of a double-stranded helix of polymerized actin monomers (Fig. 11.7). Each thin filament measures approximately 1.0–1.3 μm in length, depending on muscle type. The two important regulatory proteins in striated muscles, tropomyosin and troponin, are entwined with two actin strands. Other thin filament–associated proteins include tropomodulin and nebulin.

- **G-actin** is a small, 42-kDa molecule that polymerizes to form a double-stranded helix, the F-actin filament. These actin filaments are polar; all G-actin molecules are oriented in the same direction. The plus (barbed) end of each filament is bound to the Z line by α-actinin with nebulin assistance; the minus (pointed) end extends toward the M line and is protected by tropomodulin, an actin-capping protein (see Fig. 11.7). Each G-actin molecule of the thin filament has a binding site for myosin. In resting muscle, this binding site is protected by the tropomyosin molecule.

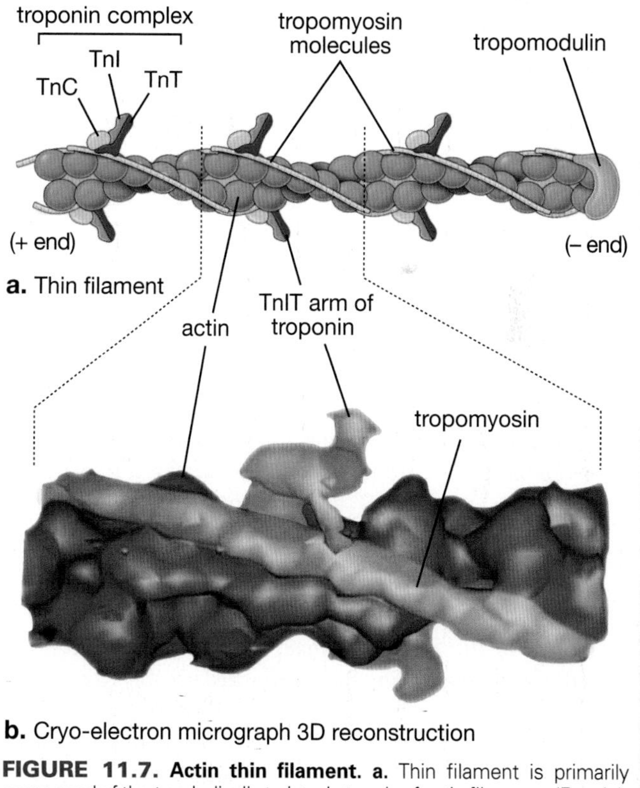

FIGURE 11.7. Actin thin filament. a. Thin filament is primarily composed of the two helically twisted strands of actin filaments (F-actin). Each actin molecule contains binding sites for myosin, which is physically blocked by tropomyosin to prevent muscle contraction. Troponin complex is a key regulatory protein; its TnC component binds calcium. This initiates a conformational shift in the troponin complex resulting in the repositioning of tropomyosin and troponin off the myosin binding sites on actin molecules. **b.** This three-dimensional reconstruction of a 10-actin–long stretch segment of the thin filament is based on the crystal structures of actin, tropomyosin, and troponin filtered to 25-Å resolution. Note the asymmetric shape of the troponin molecule with its extended TnIT arm and elongated, rod-shaped tropomyosin. *TnC*, troponin-C; *TnT*, troponin-T; *TnI*, troponin-I. (Reprinted with permission from Pirani A, Xu C, Hatch V, et al. Single particle analysis of relaxed and activated muscle thin filaments. *J Mol Biol.* 2005;346:761–772.)

FOLDER 11.1

FUNCTIONAL CONSIDERATIONS: MUSCLE METABOLISM AND ISCHEMIA

Like all cells, muscle cells depend on the energy source contained in the high-energy phosphate bonds of adenosine triphosphate (ATP) and phosphocreatine. The energy stored in these high-energy phosphate bonds comes from the metabolism of **fatty acids** and **glucose**. Glucose is the primary metabolic substrate in actively contracting muscle. It is derived from the general circulation as well as from the breakdown of glycogen, which is normally stored in the muscle fiber cytoplasm. As much as 1% of the dry weight of skeletal and cardiac muscle may be glycogen.

In rapidly contracting muscles, such as the leg muscles in running or the extraocular muscles, most of the energy for contraction is supplied by anaerobic glycolysis of stored glycogen. The buildup of intermediary metabolites from this pathway, particularly lactic acid, can produce an oxygen deficit that contributes to ischemic pain (cramps) in cases of extreme muscular exertion. However, recent studies indicate that lactic acid production alone is insufficient to trigger ischemic pain because the pH change caused by lactic acid in the muscle is so small. It was found that ATP released from ischemic muscle works in concert with lactic acid by increasing the pH sensitivity of the acid-sensing ion channel 3 (ASIC3) that is used by sensory neurons to detect lactic acidosis and convey this message in the form of ischemic pain.

Most of the energy used by muscle recovering from contraction or by resting muscle is derived from oxidative phosphorylation. This process closely follows the β-oxidation of fatty acids in mitochondria that liberates two carbon fragments. The oxygen needed for oxidative phosphorylation and other terminal metabolic reactions is derived from hemoglobin in circulating erythrocytes and from oxygen bound to myoglobin stored in the muscle cells.

- **Tropomyosin** is a 64-kDa protein that also consists of a double helix of two polypeptides. It forms filaments that run in the groove between the F-actin molecules in the thin filament. In resting muscle, tropomyosin and its regulatory protein, the troponin complex, mask the myosin-binding site on the actin molecule.
- **Troponin complex** consists of three globular subunits. Each tropomyosin molecule contains one troponin complex.
    - **Troponin-C (TnC)** is the smallest subunit of the troponin complex (18 kDa). It binds Ca^{2+}, an essential step in the initiation of contraction.
    - **Troponin-T (TnT)**, a 30-kDa subunit, binds to tropomyosin, anchoring the troponin complex.
    - **Troponin-I (TnI)**, also a 30-kDa subunit, binds to actin, thus inhibiting actin–myosin interaction.

Both the TnT and TnI subunits join together to form an asymmetrical TnIT arm, which is visible in a three-dimensional reconstruction of the troponin complex (see Fig. 11.7). In cardiac muscle, TnI and TnT are present as specific cardiac isoforms not expressed in other tissues. Therefore, these subunits can be used as highly specific markers of cardiac muscle cell damage (see pages 365-366).

- **Tropomodulin** is a small, approximately 40-kDa actin-binding protein that is attached to the free (negative) end of the thin filament. This actin-capping protein maintains and regulates the length of the actin filament in the sarcomere. Variations in thin filament length (such as those in type I and type IIb muscle fibers) affect the length–tension relationship during muscle contraction and, therefore, influence the physiologic properties of the muscle.
- **Nebulin** is an elongated, inelastic, 600-kDa protein attached to the Z lines that spans most of the length of the thin filament, except for its minus-pointed end. Nebulin acts as a "molecular ruler" for the length of the thin filament because the molecular weight of different nebulin isoforms correlates to the length of thin filaments during muscle development. In addition, nebulin adds stability to the thin filaments anchored by the α-actinin in Z lines.

Thick filaments consist primarily of myosin molecules.

The major component of **thick filaments** is myosin II, a member of the myosin superfamily of motor proteins that produces motility by cyclic interaction with actin subunits in striated muscle. This actomyosin cross-bridge cycle causes the thick and thin filaments to slide past each other, producing movement.

Myosin II, a 510-kDa, rod-shaped, actin-associated motor protein is a dimer composed of two **heavy polypeptide chains** (222 kDa each) and four **light chains.** Myosin has two globular heads (S1 region) that are connected via lever arms (S2 region) with a long tail (Fig. 11.8). Each myosin monomer contains one 18-kDa **essential light chain (ELC)** and one 22-kDa **regulatory light chain (RLC)** that are wrapped around the lever arm region just below the myosin head (see Fig. 11.8).

The regulatory light chain stabilizes the lever arm. Interaction between the heavy and light chains determines the

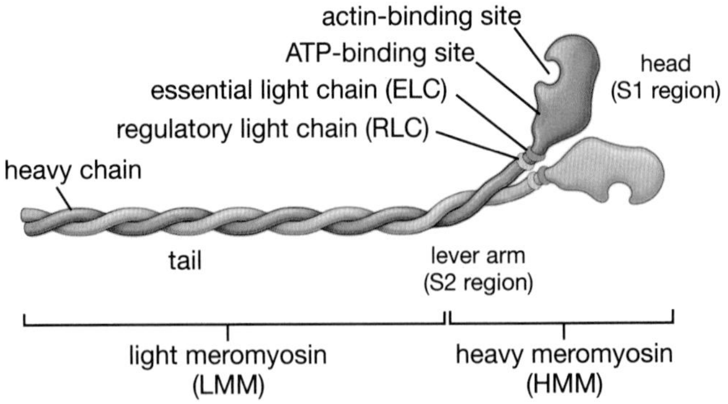

FIGURE 11.8. Schematic diagram of myosin II molecule. A complete myosin molecule has two globular heads (S1 region), lever arms (S2 region), and a long tail. It is characterized by the presence of two heavy chains and two pairs of light chains. Further subdivision of the myosin molecule is based on myosin degradation by two protease enzymes, α-chymotrypsin and papain. Enzymatic cleavage with α-chymotrypsin produces long, tail-like fragments called *light meromyosin* (*LMM*) and *heavy meromyosin* (*HMM*), which may be further cleaved with papain into the head (S1) and lever arm (S2) regions. The head contains both the adenosine triposphate (ATP)-binding site expressing ATPase activity and the actin-binding site.

speed and strength of muscle contraction. Each globular myosin head represents a heavy-chain **motor domain** that projects at an approximate right angle at one end of the myosin molecule. The myosin head has **two specific binding sites**, one for ATP with **ATPase activity** and one for actin. Enzymatic digestion of myosin produces two fragments, a heavy meromyosin (HMM) and light meromyosin (LMM). The HMM consists of the heads, lever arms, and both pairs of light chains, whereas the LMM consists of the tail (see Fig. 11.8).

Myosin molecules in striated muscle aggregate tail to tail to form bipolar **thick myosin filaments**; the tail segments overlap so that the globular heads project from the thick filament (Fig. 11.9). The "**bare zone**" in the middle of the filament does not have globular projections. Thick filaments are connected to each other at their bare zones by a family of M-line proteins (Fig. 11.10).

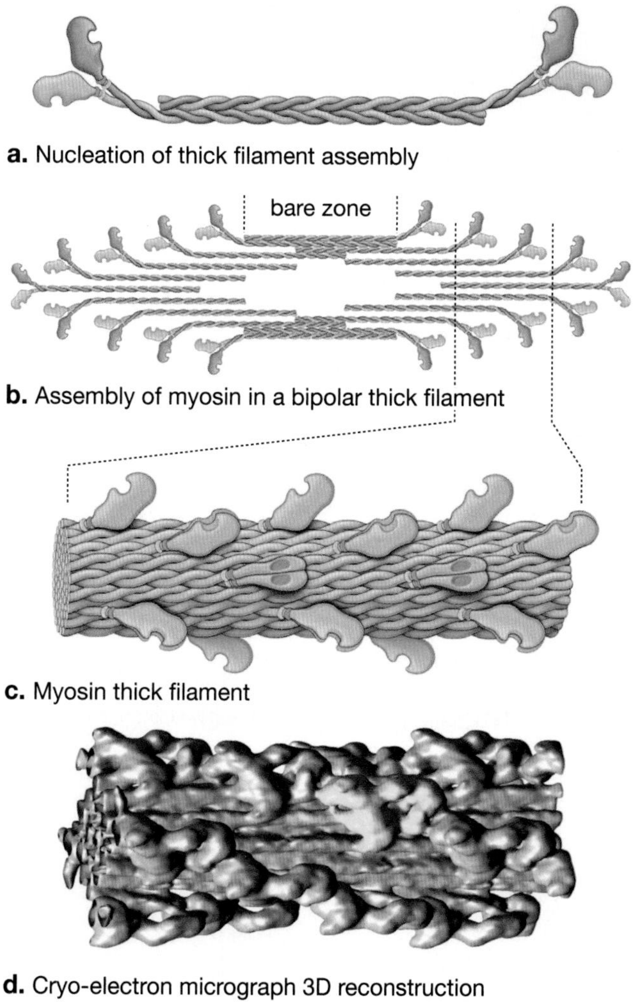

FIGURE 11.9. Nucleation, assembly, and structure of a bipolar myosin II thick filament. a. Thick filament assembly is initiated by the two tails of myosin molecules that bind together in an antiparallel manner. **b.** Diagram showing further assembly of myosin molecules into a thick bipolar filament. The myosin heads point away from the bare zone, which is free of myosin heads. Note that myosin tails in the bare zone have both antiparallel and parallel arrangements, but in the distal portion of the filament, they overlap only in a parallel manner. **c.** Diagram of a section of a myosin bipolar thick filament. Note the spiral arrangement of myosin heads. **d.** Three-dimensional reconstruction of a frozen–hydrated tarantula thick filament, filtered to 2-nm resolution. It shows several myosin heads (one highlighted in *yellow*) and tails of myosin molecules in parallel arrangement. (Reprinted with permission from Alamo L, Wriggers W, Pinto A, et al. Three-dimensional reconstruction of tarantula myosin filaments suggests how phosphorylation may regulate myosin activity. *J Mol Biol.* 2008;384:780–975.)

Accessory proteins maintain precise alignment of thin and thick filaments within the sarcomere.

To maintain the efficiency and speed of muscle contraction, both thin and thick filaments in each myofibril must be aligned precisely and kept at an optimal distance from one another. Proteins known as **accessory proteins** are essential in regulating the spacing, attachment, and alignment of the myofilaments. These structural protein components of skeletal muscle fibrils constitute less than 25% of the total protein of the muscle fiber. They include the following (see also Fig. 11.10):

- **Titin**, a large (2,500-kDa) protein, spans half of the sarcomere. Titin extends from the Z line and thin filament at its N-terminus toward the thick filament and M line at its C-terminus. Between the thick and thin filaments, two spring-like portions of titin help center the thick filament in the middle between the two Z lines. Owing to the presence of molecular "springs," titin prevents excessive stretching of the sarcomere by developing a passive restoring force that helps with its shortening.
- **α-Actinin**, a short, bipolar, rod-shaped, 190-kDa actin-binding protein, bundles thin filaments into parallel arrays and anchors them at the Z line. It also cross-links titin's N-terminus embedded in the Z line.
- **Desmin**, a type of 53-kDa intermediate filament, forms a lattice that surrounds the sarcomere at the level of the Z lines, attaching them to one another and to the plasma membrane via linkage protein ankyrin, thus forming stabilizing cross-links between neighboring myofibrils.
- **M-line proteins** include several myosin-binding proteins that hold thick filaments in register at the M line and attach titin molecules to the thick filament. M-line proteins include **myomesin** (185 kDa), **M-protein** (165 kDa), **obscurin** (700 kDa), and **muscle creatine phosphatase** (MM-CK, 81 kDa).
- **Myosin-binding protein C (MyBP-C)**, a 140- to 150-kDa protein, contributes to normal assembly and the stabilization of thick filaments. It forms several distinct transverse stripes on both sides of the M line that interact with titin molecules.
- **Dystrophin**, a large, 427-kDa protein, is thought to link laminin, which resides in the external lamina of the muscle cell, to actin filaments. The absence of this protein is associated with progressive muscular weakness, a genetic condition called **Duchenne muscular dystrophy**. Dystrophin is encoded on the X chromosome; for this reason, it affects only males. Research into gene therapy to restore normal functioning in individuals with this disorder is ongoing (Folder 11.2).

When a muscle contracts, each sarcomere shortens, but the myofilaments remain the same length.

During contraction, the sarcomere and I band shorten, whereas the A band remains the same length. To maintain the myofilaments at a constant length, the shortening of the sarcomere must be caused by an increase in the overlap of the thick and thin filaments. This overlap can readily be seen by comparing electron micrographs of resting and contracted muscle. The H band narrows and the thin filaments penetrate the H band during contraction. These observations indicate that the thin filaments slide past the thick filaments during contraction.

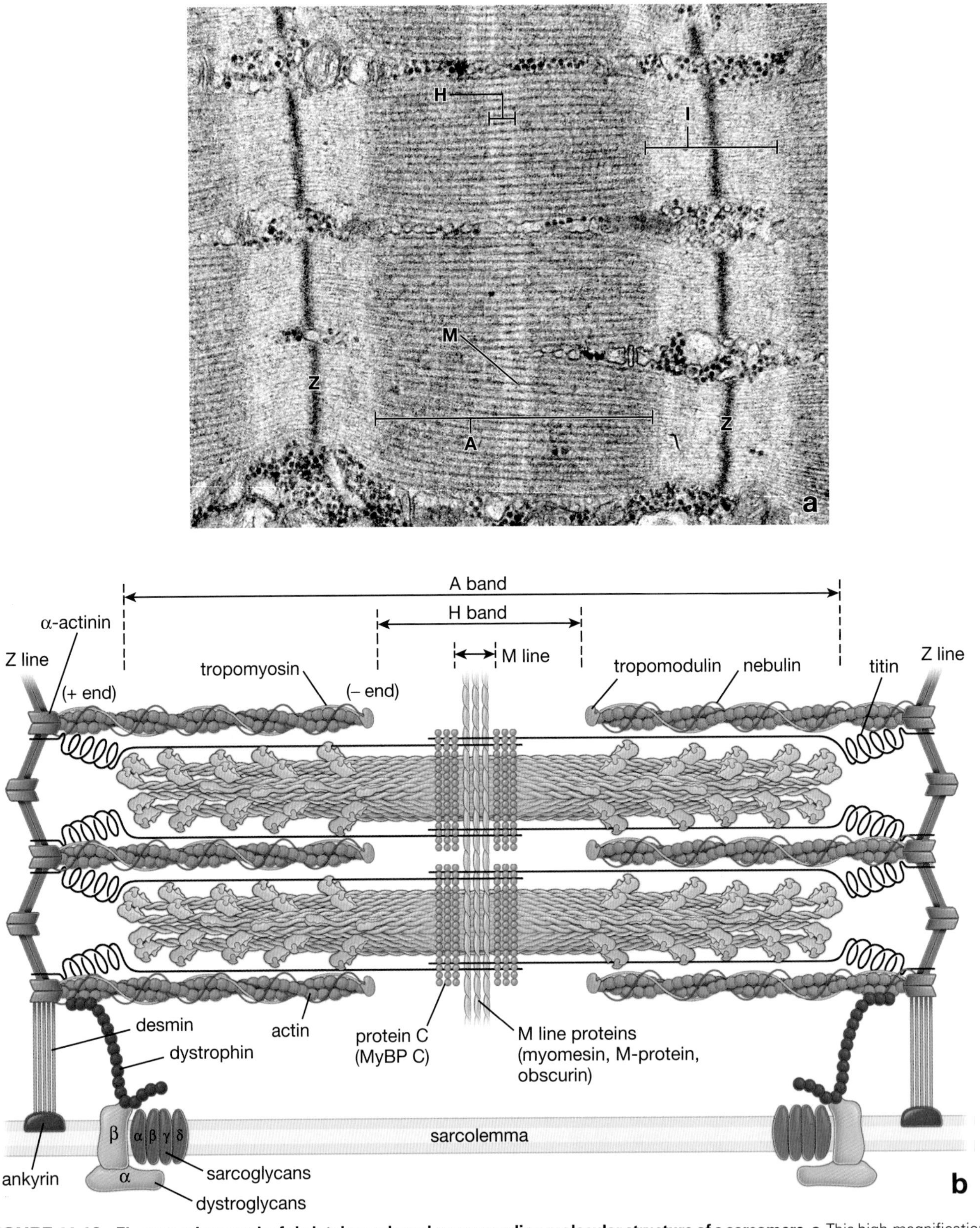

FIGURE 11.10. Electron micrograph of skeletal muscle and corresponding molecular structure of a sarcomere. a. This high-magnification electron micrograph shows a longitudinal section of the myofibrils. The I band, which is bisected by the Z line, is composed of barely visible, thin (actin) filaments. They are attached to the Z line and extend across the I band into the A band. The thick filaments, composed of myosin, account for the full width of the A band. Note that in the A band, there are additional bands and lines. One of these, the M line, is seen at the middle of the A band; another, the less electron-dense H band, consists only of thick filaments. The lateral parts of the A band are more electron dense and represent areas where the thin filaments interdigitate with the thick filaments. ×35,000. **b.** Diagram illustrating the distribution of myofilaments and accessory proteins within a sarcomere. The accessory proteins are titin, a large elastic molecule that anchors the thick (myosin) filaments to the Z line; α-actinin, which bundles thin (actin) filaments into parallel arrays and anchors them at the Z line; nebulin, an elongated inelastic protein attached to the Z lines that wraps around the thin filaments and assists α-actinin in anchoring the thin filament to Z lines; tropomodulin, an actin-capping protein that maintains and regulates the length of the thin filaments; tropomyosin, which stabilizes thin filaments and, in association with troponin, regulates binding of calcium ions; M-line proteins (myomesin, M-protein, obscurin), which hold thick filaments in register at the M line; myosin-binding protein C, which contributes to normal assembly of thick filaments and interacts with titin; and two proteins (desmin and dystrophin), which anchor sarcomeres into the plasma membrane. The interactions of these various proteins maintain the precise alignment of the thin and thick filaments in the sarcomere and the alignment of sarcomeres within the cell.

FOLDER 11.2

CLINICAL CORRELATION: MUSCULAR DYSTROPHIES—DYSTROPHIN AND DYSTROPHIN-ASSOCIATED PROTEINS

Dystrophin is a rod-shaped cytoskeletal protein with a short head and a long tail that is located just beneath the skeletal muscle cell membrane. F-actin is bound at the end portion of the tail. Two groups of transmembrane proteins—α- and β-dystroglycans and α-, β-, γ-, and δ-sarcoglycans—participate in a **dystrophin–glycoprotein complex** that links dystrophin to the extracellular matrix proteins laminin and agrin. Dystroglycans form the actual link between dystrophin and laminin; sarcoglycans are merely associated with the dystroglycans in the membrane. Distribution of dystrophin in healthy individuals is visualized using immunostaining methods (Fig. F11.2.1).

Several forms of muscular dystrophy are attributed to mutations of single genes encoding several proteins of the dystrophin–glycoprotein complex. **Duchenne muscular dystrophy (DMD)** and **Becker muscular dystrophy (BMD)** are associated with mutations that affect dystrophin expression (Fig. F11.2.2); different forms of **limb-girdle muscular dystrophy (LGMD)** are caused by mutations in the genes found on the short arm of the X chromosome encoding the four different sarcoglycans, and another form of **congenital muscular dystrophy (CMD)** is caused by a mutation in the gene encoding the α2-chain of muscle laminin. Most cases of DMD are caused by a high frequency of gene deletions that create frame shifts, resulting in the absence of dystrophin in the affected muscle fibers. Characterization of the dystrophin gene and its products has allowed direct genetic testing and prenatal diagnosis for this disorder.

Because of its inheritance as an X-linked recessive trait, DMD primarily affects boys (an estimated 1 in 3,500 boys worldwide). Onset of DMD is between 3 and 5 years of age and progresses rapidly. Most boys become unable to walk by age 12, and by age 20, they must use a respirator to breathe. BMD is similar to DMD, except that it progresses at a much slower rate. Symptoms usually appear at about age 12, and the ability to walk is lost at an average age of 25–30. At the current time, there is no known cure for muscular dystrophies, and available treatment is aimed at controlling symptoms to maximize the quality of life. Intensive research efforts are being directed to implement gene therapy for the treatment of affected patients. The general approach is to replace defective dystrophin genes within muscle cells using a specially engineered virus that would carry "normal" genes, infect muscle cells, and induce cells to express dystrophin. Another method is transplantation of "healthy" satellite (muscle stem) cells that can divide and differentiate into normal muscle cells. Stem cell therapy has been tested in laboratory animals and yielded encouraging results.

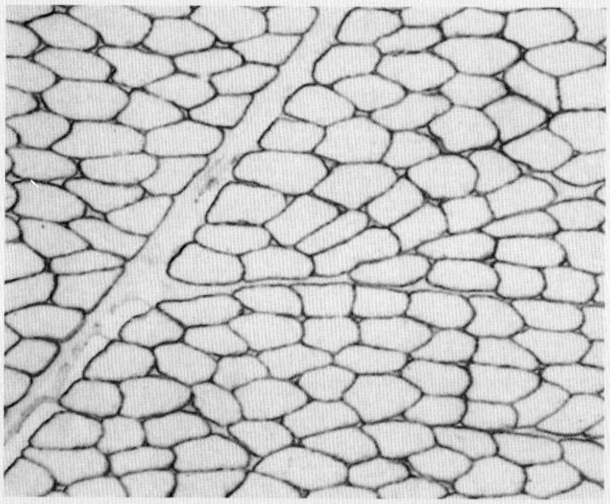

FIGURE F11.2.1. Distribution of dystrophin in human skeletal muscle. This cross section of skeletal muscle fibers from a healthy individual was immunostained with goat polyclonal antibody against dystrophin using the immunoperoxidase method. Because dystrophin and associated dystrophin–glycoprotein complexes connect the muscle cytoskeleton to the surrounding extracellular matrix through the cell membrane, the localization of dystrophin outlines cell membrane. Note the regular shape of skeletal muscle cells and pattern of dystrophin distribution. ×480. (Courtesy of Dr. Andrew G. Engel.)

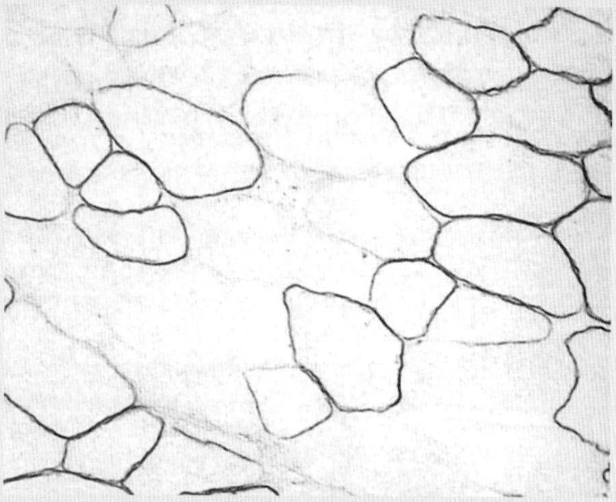

FIGURE F11.2.2. Distribution of dystrophin in a patient with Duchenne muscular dystrophy (DMD). This cross section of skeletal muscle was obtained from a patient with DMD. Slide preparation was similar to that of Figure F11.2.1. Compare the pattern and intensity of the dystrophin distribution within the affected muscle fibers to that of the normal individual. This muscle shows signs of hypertrophy. Some fibers do not express any dystrophin; others express variable levels of dystrophin. ×480. (Courtesy of Dr. Andrew G. Engel.)

The Actomyosin Cross-Bridge Cycle

In resting muscle, myosin heads are prevented from binding with actin molecules by tropomyosin, which covers myosin-binding sites on actin molecules (Fig. 11.11a). Following nerve stimulation, Ca^{2+} is released into the sarcoplasm and binds to troponin, which then acts on the tropomyosin to expose the myosin-binding sites on actin molecules (Fig. 11.11b). Once the binding sites are exposed, the myosin heads are able to interact with actin molecules and form cross-bridges, and the two filaments slide over one another.

Shortening of a muscle involves rapid, repeated interactions between actin and myosin molecules that move the thin filaments along the thick filament.

The cross-bridge cycle in skeletal muscle is referred to as the **actomyosin cross-bridge cycle** and is often described as a

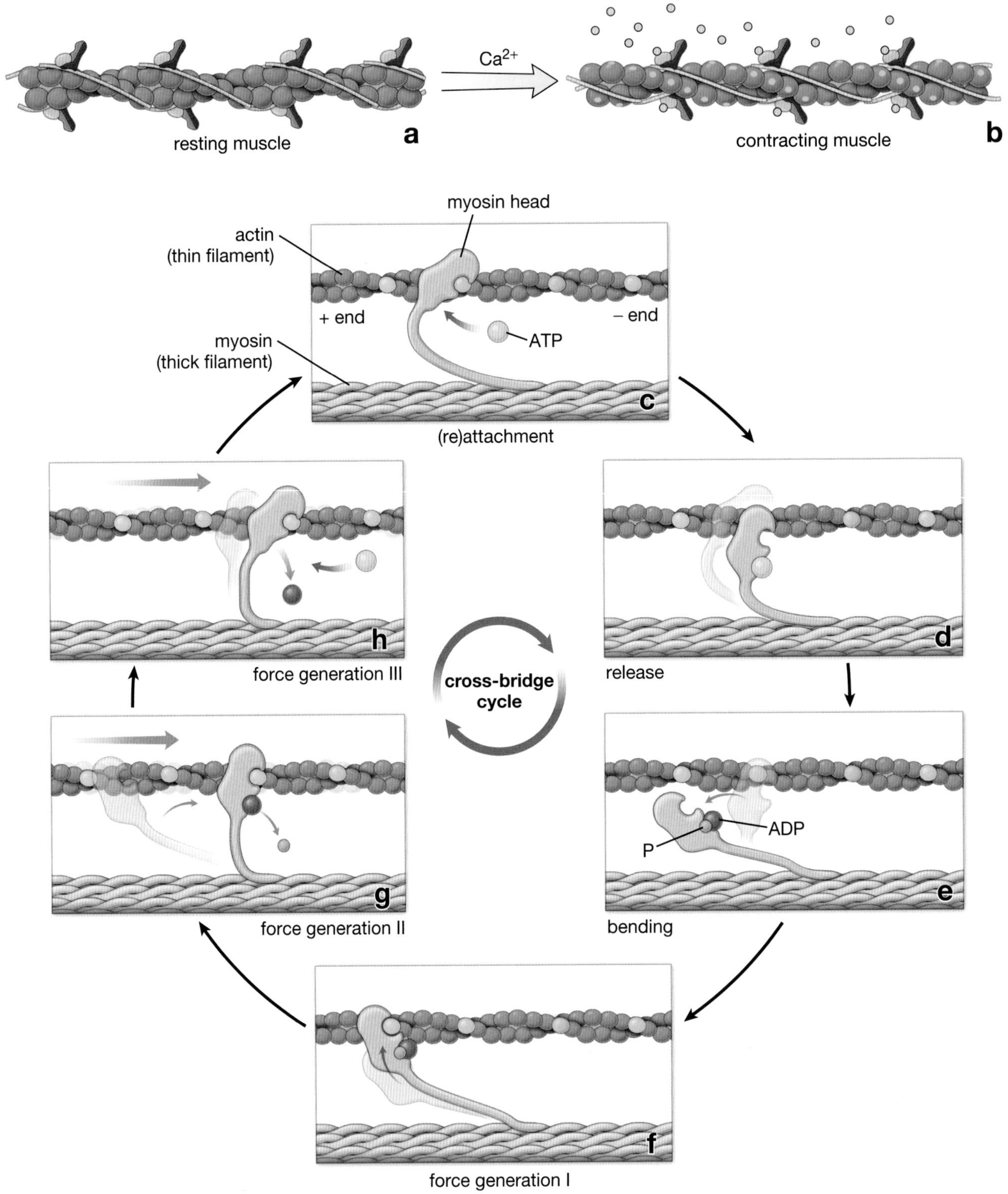

FIGURE 11.11. Actomyosin cross-bridge cycle. For a detailed description of the cross-bridge cycle, refer to the chapter text that corresponds to each depicted stage. **a.** and **b.** Only tropomyosin and troponin complexes are shown for clarity. **c–h.** The thin filament is shown without any actin accessory proteins. *ADP*, adenosine diphosphate; *ATP*, adenosine triphosphate; *P*, inorganic phosphate.

series of coupled biochemical and mechanical events. Myosin, as an actin-associated motor protein with ATPase activity, converts chemical energy into mechanical force by cycling between actin-attached and actin-detached states during its ATPase cycle. Each cross-bridge cycle consists of **five stages**: attachment, release, bending, force generation, and reattachment. In cardiac or smooth muscle, relative durations of individual stages may be altered by changes in the molecular composition of tissue-specific myosin molecules. However, the basic cycle is believed to be the same for all myosin–actin interactions.

Attachment is the initial stage of the cross-bridge cycle; the myosin head is tightly bound to the actin molecule of the thin filament.

At the beginning of the cross-bridge cycle, the **myosin head is strongly bound to the actin molecule** of the thin filament, and ATP is absent (Fig. 11.11c). Position of the myosin head in this stage is referred to as an *original* or **unbent conformation**. This very short-lived arrangement is known as the **rigor configuration**. The muscular stiffening and rigidity that begins at the moment of death is caused by a lack of ATP and is known as **rigor mortis**. In an actively contracting muscle, this step ends with the binding of ATP to the myosin head.

Release is the second stage of the cross-bridge cycle; the myosin head is uncoupled from the thin filament.

In this stage of the cross-bridge cycle, **ATP binds to the myosin head** and induces conformational changes of the actin-binding site. This change reduces the affinity of the myosin head for the actin molecule of the thin filament, causing the **myosin head to uncouple from the thin filament** (Fig. 11.11d).

Bending is the third stage of the cross-bridge cycle and "resets" the motor of the myosin; the myosin head, as a result of hydrolysis of ATP, assumes its prepower stroke position.

The ATP-binding site on the myosin head undergoes further conformational changes, causing the **myosin head to bend** by rotating the lever arm of myosin to assume its prepower stroke position. This movement is initiated by the breakdown of ATP into adenosine diphosphate (ADP) and inorganic phosphate (P_i); both products, however, remain bound to the myosin head (Fig. 11.11e). In this stage of the cycle, the **linear displacement of the myosin head** relative to the thin filament is approximately 5 nm. This stage is sometimes referred to as a "**recovery stroke**."

Force generation is the fourth stage of the cross-bridge cycle; the myosin head releases inorganic phosphate, and the power stroke occurs.

The myosin head binds weakly to its new binding site on the actin molecule of the thin filament (Fig. 11.11f), causing the release of P_i (Fig. 11.11g). This release has two effects. First, the binding affinity between the myosin head and its new attachment site increases. Second, the **myosin head generates a force** as it returns to its original unbent position. Thus, as the myosin head straightens, it forces movement of the thin filament along the thick filament. This is the "**power stroke**" of the cycle. During this stage, ADP is lost from the myosin head (Fig. 11.11h).

Reattachment is the fifth and last stage of the cross-bridge cycle; the myosin head binds tightly to a new actin molecule.

The **myosin head is again tightly bound to a new actin molecule** of the thin filament (rigor configuration), and the cycle can repeat (see Fig. 11.11c).

The two heads of the myosin molecule work together in a productive and coordinated manner. Although an individual myosin head may detach from the thin filament during the cycle, heads of other myosins in the same thick filament will attach to actin molecules, thereby resulting in movement. Because the myosin heads are arranged as mirror images on either side of the H band (antiparallel arrangement), this action pulls the thin filaments into the A band, thus shortening the sarcomere.

Regulation of Muscle Contraction

Regulation of contraction involves Ca^{2+}, sarcoplasmic reticulum, and the transverse tubular system.

Ca^{2+} must be available for the reaction between actin and myosin. After contraction, Ca^{2+} must be removed. This rapid delivery and removal of Ca^{2+} is accomplished by the sarcoplasmic reticulum and the transverse tubular system.

The **sarcoplasmic reticulum** forms a membranous compartment of flattened cisternae and anastomosing channels that serves as a reservoir for calcium ions. It occupies 1%–5% of the total volume of muscle fiber and is arranged as a repeating series of networks around the myofibrils. Each network of the reticulum extends from one A–I junctions to the next A–I junctions within a sarcomere. The adjacent network of sarcoplasmic reticulum continues from the A–I junctions to the next A–I junctions of the neighboring sarcomere. Therefore, one network of sarcoplasmic reticulum surrounds the A band, and the adjacent network surrounds the I band (Fig. 11.12). Where the two networks meet, at the junction between A and I bands, the sarcoplasmic reticulum forms slightly enlarged and more regular ring-like channels that encircle the sarcomere. These enlargements, called **terminal cisternae**, are the Ca^{2+} reservoirs.

The plasma membrane of the terminal cisternae contains an abundance of **gated Ca^{2+}-release channels** called

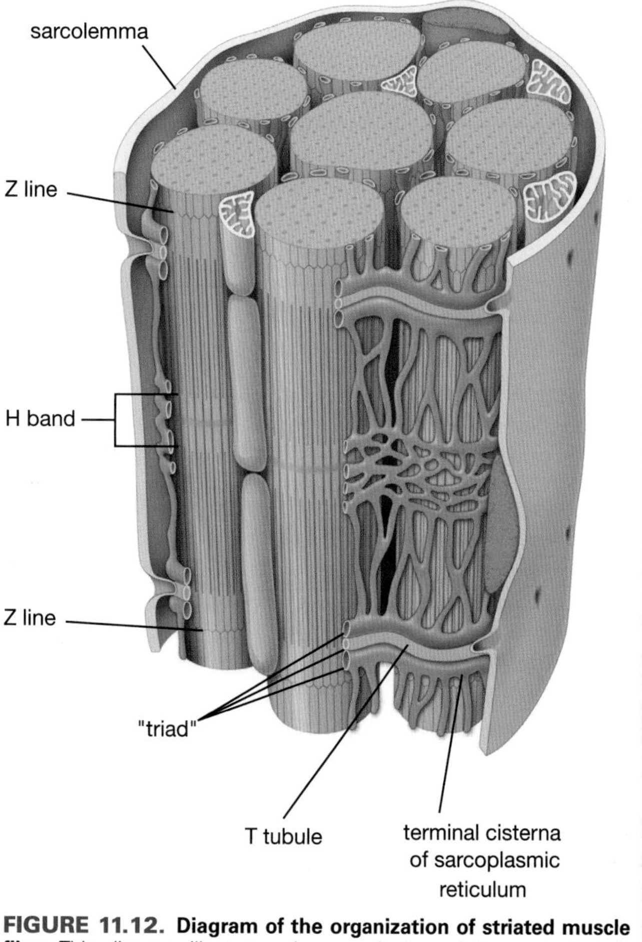

FIGURE 11.12. Diagram of the organization of striated muscle fiber. This diagram illustrates the organization of the sarcoplasmic reticulum and its relationship to the myofibrils. Note that in striated muscle fibers, two transverse (*T*) tubules supply a sarcomere. Each T tubule is located at an A–I band junction and is formed as an invagination of the sarcolemma of striated muscle. It is associated with two terminal cisternae of the sarcoplasmic reticulum that surrounds each myofibril, one cisterna on either side of the T tubule. The triple structure as seen in cross section, where the two terminal cisternae flank a transverse tubule at the A–I band junction, is called a *triad*. Depolarization of the T-tubule membrane initiates the release of calcium ions from the sarcoplasmic reticulum and eventually triggers muscle contraction.

ryanodine receptors (**RyR1** is the primary isoform in the skeletal muscle), which are involved in releasing Ca^{2+} into the sarcoplasm. Also located around the myofibrils in association with the sarcoplasmic reticulum are large numbers of mitochondria and glycogen granules, both of which are involved in providing the energy necessary for the reactions needed for contraction. The luminal surface of the sarcoplasmic reticulum contains **calsequestrin**, a highly acidic calcium–binding protein capable of binding up to 50 internalized Ca^{2+} ions. Calsequestrin allows the Ca^{2+} required for initiation of muscle contraction to be stored at high concentration (up to 20 mM), whereas the free Ca^{2+} concentration within the lumen of sarcoplasmic reticulum remains very low (<1 mM). This significantly reduces the concentration gradient against which the Ca^{2+}-activated ATPase pumps must transport Ca^{2+} into the lumen of the sarcoplasmic reticulum.

The **transverse tubular system**, or **T system**, consists of numerous tubular invaginations of the plasma membrane; each one is called a **T tubule**. T tubules penetrate to all levels of the muscle fiber and are located between adjacent terminal cisternae at the A–I junctions (see Fig. 11.12). They contain **voltage-sensor proteins** called **dihydropyridine-sensitive receptors (DHSRs)**, which are depolarization-sensitive transmembrane channels that are activated when the plasma membrane depolarizes. Conformational changes of these proteins directly affect gated Ca^{2+}-release channels (RyR1 isoform of ryanodine receptors) located in the adjacent plasma membrane of the terminal cisternae.

The complex of **one T tubule** and **two adjacent terminal cisternae** is called a **triad** structure. These structures are found in skeletal muscle at the level of A–I junctions. Triads are important elements for coupling extracellular events (e.g., nerve stimulation) with intracellular responses (e.g., Ca^{2+} release) that lead to muscle contraction.

The depolarization of the T-tubule membrane triggers the release of Ca^{2+} from the terminal cisternae to initiate muscle contraction by changes in the thin filaments.

When a nerve impulse arrives at the neuromuscular junction, the release of neurotransmitter (acetylcholine [ACh]) from the nerve ending triggers a localized plasma membrane depolarization of the muscle cell. The depolarization, in turn, causes **voltage-gated Na^+ channels** in the plasma membrane to open, allowing an influx of Na^+ from the extracellular space into the muscle cell. The influx of Na^+ results in general depolarization, which spreads rapidly over the entire plasma membrane of the muscle fiber. When the depolarization encounters the opening of the T tubule, it is transmitted along the membranes of the T system into the interior of the cell. Electrical charges activate **voltage-sensor proteins (DHSRs)** located in the membrane of the T tubule. These proteins have the structural and functional properties of Ca^{2+} channels; however, in skeletal muscle, their short-lasting activation is not sufficient to open Ca^{2+} channels, and Ca^{2+} transport from the lumen of the T tubule into the sarcoplasm does not occur. Instead, activation of voltage-sensor proteins opens **gated Ca^{2+}-release channels (ryanodine receptors)** in the adjacent terminal sacs of the sarcoplasmic reticulum that store high concentrations of Ca^{2+} molecules. Opening of gated Ca^{2+}-release channels in the sarcoplasmic reticulum causes a rapid and massive release of Ca^{2+} into the sarcoplasm. The increased concentration of Ca^{2+} in the sarcoplasm initiates contraction of the myofibril by binding to the TnC portion of the troponin complex on the thin filaments (see pages 353-355). The change in molecular conformation of TnC causes the TnI to dissociate from the actin molecules, allowing the troponin complex to uncover myosin-binding sites on the actin molecules. The myosin heads are now free to interact with actin molecules to initiate the muscle contraction cycle.

Muscle relaxation results from the decrease in cytosolic-free Ca^{2+} concentration.

Simultaneously, a **Ca^{2+}-activated ATPase pump** in the membrane of the sarcoplasmic reticulum transports Ca^{2+} back into the sarcoplasmic storage site. Low concentration of free Ca^{2+} within the sarcoplasmic reticulum is maintained by calsequestrin, a calcium-binding protein, which aids in the efficiency of Ca^{2+} uptake. Binding of Ca^{2+} to calsequestrin within the sarcoplasmic reticulum thus reduces the free Ca^{2+} concentration gradient against which Ca^{2+}-activated ATPase pumps must work. The resting concentration of Ca^{2+} is restored in the cytosol in less than 30 milliseconds. This restoration of resting Ca^{2+} concentration near the myofilaments normally relaxes the muscle and causes the contraction to stop. Contraction will continue, however, as long as nerve impulses continue to depolarize the plasma membrane of the T tubules.

Motor Innervation

Skeletal muscle fibers are richly innervated by motor neurons that originate in the spinal cord or brainstem. The axons of the neurons branch as they near the muscle, giving rise to twigs or terminal branches that end on individual muscle fibers (Fig. 11.13).

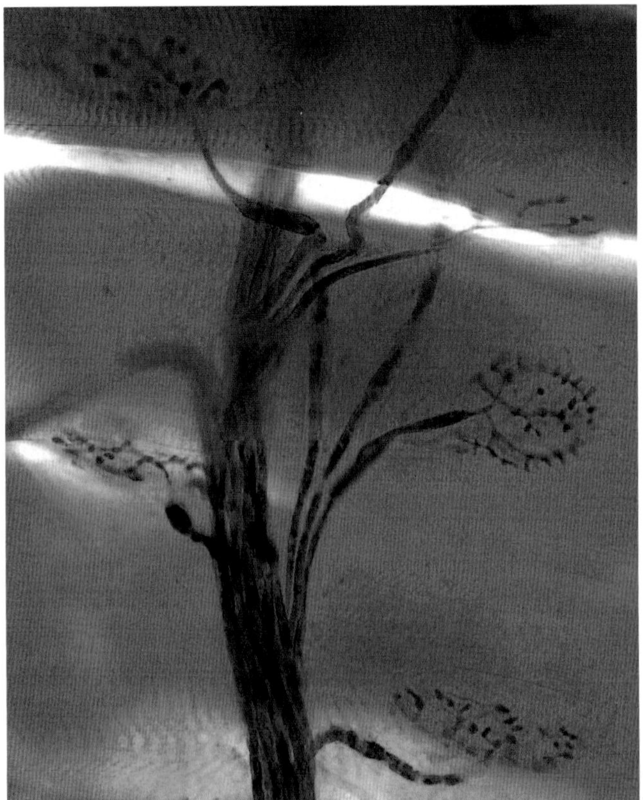

FIGURE 11.13. Photomicrograph of a neuromuscular junction. This silver preparation shows a motor nerve and its final branches that lead to the neuromuscular junctions (motor end plates). The skeletal muscle fibers are oriented horizontally in the field and are crossed perpendicularly by the motor nerve fibers. Note that these fibers distally lose their myelin sheath and divide extensively into small swellings, forming a cluster of neuromuscular junctions. ×620.

The neuromuscular junction is the contact made by the terminal branches of the axon with the muscle fiber.

At the **neuromuscular junction** (motor end plate), the myelin sheath of the axon ends, and the terminal portion of the axon is covered by only a thin portion of the **nonmyelinating (terminal) Schwann cell** with its external lamina. The end of the axon ramifies into a number of end branches, each of which lies in a shallow depression on the surface of the muscle fiber, the receptor region (Fig. 11.14). The axon ending is a typical presynaptic structure and contains numerous mitochondria and synaptic vesicles that contain the neurotransmitter **acetylcholine (ACh)**.

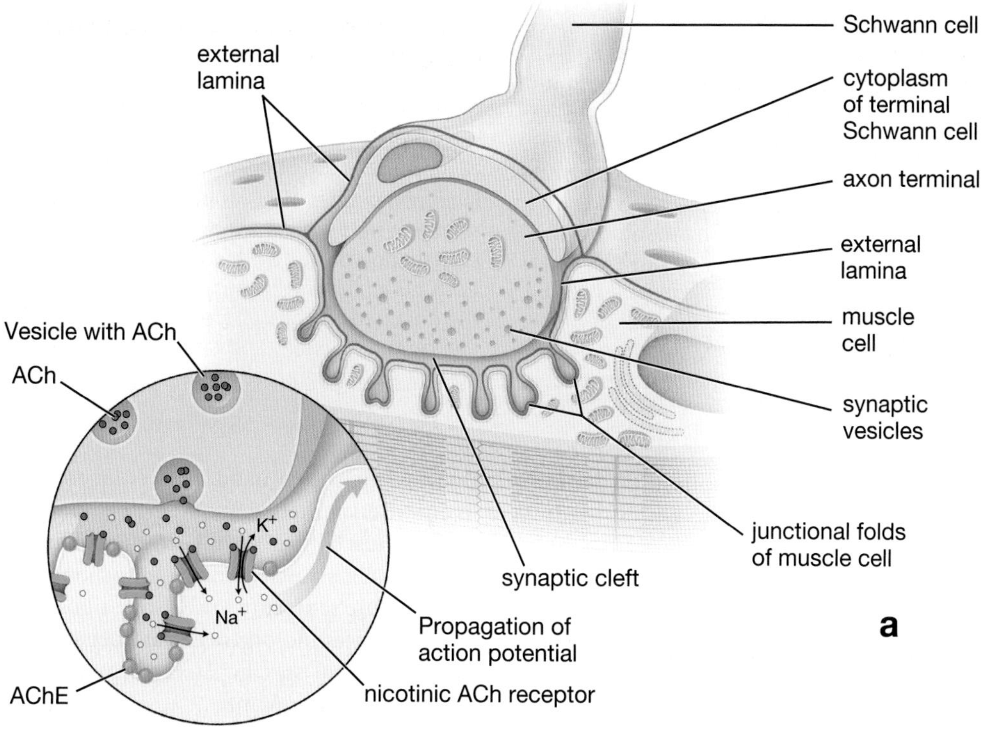

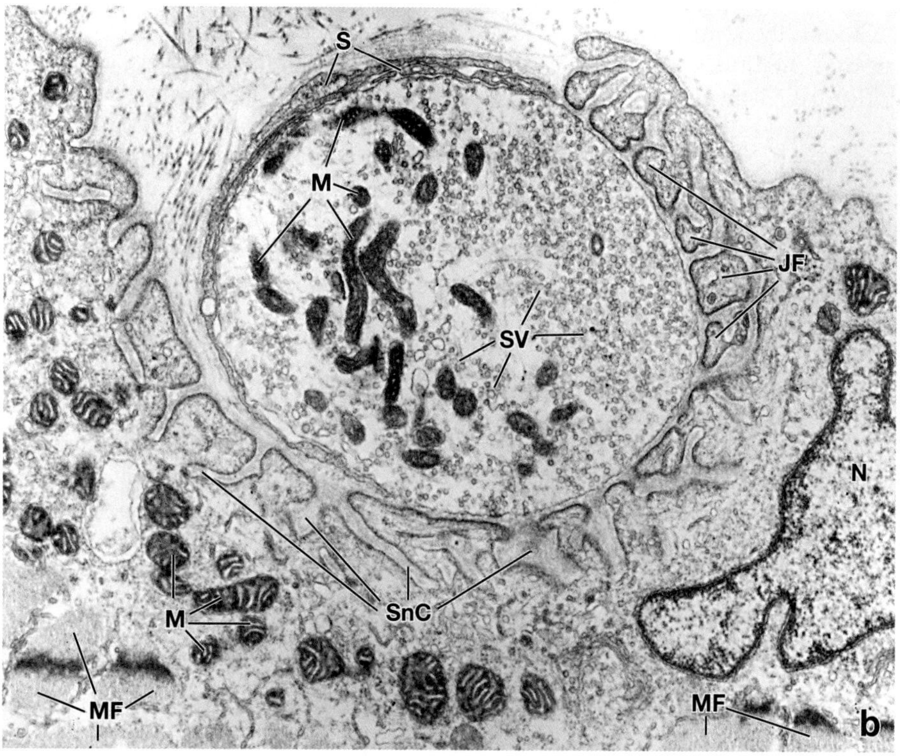

FIGURE 11.14. Neuromuscular junction. a. Diagram of a neuromuscular junction. An axon is shown making contact with a muscle cell. Note how the junctional folds of the muscle cell augment the surface area within the synaptic cleft. The external lamina extends throughout the cleft area. The cytoplasm of the terminal Schwann cell is shown covering the axon terminal. The circular *inset* shows nicotinic acetylcholine receptors in a junctional fold that open after stimulation by acetylcholine (*ACh*), allowing sodium and potassium ions to enter and exit the cell, respectively. Acetylcholinesterase (*AChE*) breaks down the *ACh*, preventing continuous stimulation. **b.** Electron micrograph of a neuromuscular junction shows the axon ending within the synaptic cleft of a skeletal muscle fiber. An aggregation of mitochondria (*M*) and numerous synaptic vesicles (*SV*) is visible. The portion of the motor axon ending that is not in opposition to the muscle fiber is covered by terminal Schwann cell cytoplasm (*S*), but no myelin is present. The muscle fiber shows the junctional folds (*JF*) and the subneural clefts (*SnC*) between them. The external lamina of the muscle fiber is barely evident within the subneural clefts. Other structures present are the aggregated mitochondria (*M*) of the muscle fiber in the region of the neuromuscular junction, the nucleus (*N*) of the muscle fiber, and some myofibrils (*MF*). ×32,000. (Courtesy of Dr. George D. Pappas.)

FOLDER 11.3

CLINICAL CORRELATION: MYASTHENIA GRAVIS

During normal function, **acetylcholine (ACh) molecules** released into the synaptic cleft at the neuromuscular junction bind to the nicotinic ACh receptors on the sarcolemma of the skeletal muscle cell. As discussed earlier, these receptors represent *transmitter-gated Na^+ channels* that control the influx of Na^+ necessary for generating an action potential, leading to initiation of muscle contraction. After stimulating their own receptors, ACh molecules are quickly degraded by the enzyme *acetylcholinesterase (AChE)* into acetic acid and choline, which is taken up by the axon terminal and reused for ACh synthesis (see page 403).

In **myasthenia gravis**, nicotinic ACh receptors are blocked by antibodies directed against the body's own receptor proteins. Thus, myasthenia gravis is an autoimmune disease caused by the reduced number of functional ACh receptor sites. In addition, other abnormalities within the synaptic cleft (e.g., widening of the synaptic cleft, disappearance of junctional folds) also occur, further reducing the effectiveness of the muscle fibers. Myasthenia gravis is characterized by noticeable weakening of the muscle fiber response to a nerve stimulus. Initially, weakness begins with extraocular muscles and causes drooping eyelids, double vision, and generalized muscular weakness. Other somatic musculature might be affected, including respiratory muscles. As the disease progresses, the number of neuromuscular junctions is reduced. An effective pharmacologic treatment for myasthenia gravis is administration of AChE inhibitors. These substances reinforce neuromuscular transmission by preventing the degradation of ACh within the synaptic cleft. In addition to AChE inhibitors, immunosuppression and resection of the enlarged thymus (if present) may reduce the activity of the immune system and rate of production of antibodies against ACh receptors.

Release of acetylcholine into the synaptic cleft initiates depolarization of the plasma membrane, which leads to muscle cell contraction.

The muscle fiber plasma membrane that underlies the synaptic cleft has many deep **junctional folds** (subneural folds). Specific **cholinergic receptors** for ACh are limited to the plasma membrane immediately bordering the cleft and at the top of the folds. The external lamina extends into the junctional folds (see Fig. 11.14a). The synaptic vesicles of the axon terminal release ACh into the cleft, which then binds to **nicotinic ACh receptors (nAChR)** on the sarcolemma of the striated muscle. The nAChR in striated muscles is a **transmitter-gated Na^+ channel**. Binding of ACh opens Na^+ channels, causing an influx of Na^+ into striated muscle cell. This influx results in a localized membrane depolarization, which, in turn, leads to the events described earlier (see Fig. 11.14a). An enzyme called **acetylcholinesterase (AChE)** quickly breaks down the ACh to prevent continued stimulation. For a more detailed description of ACh function, see Chapter 12, Nerve Tissue (page 401).

Neuromuscular transmission can be blocked by bacterial toxins and pharmacologic agents. For example, **botulinum toxin**, produced by the anaerobic bacteria *Clostridium botulinum*, blocks the release of ACh from the axon terminal. Botulinum toxin cleaves specific **soluble *N*-ethylmaleimide–sensitive factor attachment protein receptor (SNARE)** proteins that are essential for binding and fusion of the synaptic vesicles with the presynaptic membrane (see page 42). Transmission at the neuromuscular junction can also be inhibited by the postsynaptic blockade by various poisons and pharmacologic agents. Derivatives of **curare**, a paralyzing poison used on arrow tips in South America, bind to **nicotinic ACh receptors** without opening the ion channels. This poison causes paralysis of skeletal muscles (including the diaphragm) without directly affecting the contraction of cardiac muscle. Other pharmacologic compounds, such as **succinylcholine**, bind to the nAChR, causing ion channels to open. Succinylcholine is used as a short-term muscle relaxant in emergency medicine and during surgical procedures.

The muscle fiber cytoplasm that underlies the junctional folds contains nuclei, many mitochondria, rough-surfaced endoplasmic reticulum (rER), free ribosomes, and glycogen. These cytoplasmic organelles are believed to be involved in the synthesis of specific ACh receptors in the membrane of the cleft as well as AChE.

A neuron along with the specific muscle fibers that it innervates is called a *motor unit*.

There are more muscle fibers than motor neurons; thus, a single neuron may innervate several to a hundred or more muscle fibers. A **motor unit** consists of a **single motor neuron** and the **group of skeletal muscle fibers** that it innervates. Muscles capable of the most delicate movements have a low ratio of muscle fibers per motor neuron in their motor units. For example, in eye muscles, the innervation ratio is about one neuron to three muscle fibers; in the postural muscles of the back and lower limbs, a single neuron may innervate hundreds of muscle fibers. In the gastrocnemius, a leg muscle, the innervation ratio is one motor neuron to approximately 1,000–2,000 muscle fibers. Thus, depolarization generated in relatively few motor units can generate substantial forces needed for sudden changes in body position.

The nature of muscle contraction is determined by the number of motor neuron endings as well as by the number of specific types of muscle fibers that are depolarized. Although depolarization of a muscle fiber at a single neuromuscular junction is characterized as an "all-or-none" phenomenon, not all nerve terminals discharge at once, which allows a graded response to the contractile stimulus.

Innervation is necessary for muscle cells to maintain their structural integrity.

The motor nerve cell not only instructs the muscle cells to contract but also exerts a trophic influence on the muscle cells. If the nerve supply to a muscle is disrupted, the muscle cell undergoes regressive changes known as **tissue atrophy**. The most conspicuous indication of this atrophy is thinning of the muscle and its cells. If innervation is reestablished surgically or by the slower process of natural regeneration of the nerve, the muscle can regain normal shape and strength.

The events leading to contraction of skeletal muscle can be summarized as a series of steps.

The events involved in contraction can be summarized as follows (the *numbers* refer to the numbers in Fig. 11.15):

1. The contraction of a skeletal muscle fiber is initiated when a nerve impulse traveling along the axon of a motor neuron arrives at the neuromuscular junction.
2. The nerve impulse prompts the release of ACh into the synaptic cleft that binds into ACh-gated Na^+ channels, causing local depolarization of sarcolemma.
3. Voltage-gated Na^+ channels open, and Na^+ enters the cell.
4. General depolarization spreads over the plasma membrane of the muscle cell and continues via membranes of the T tubules.
5. Voltage-sensor proteins (DHSRs) in the plasma membrane of T tubules change their conformation.
6. At the muscle cell triads, the T tubules are in close contact with the lateral enlargements of the sarcoplasmic reticulum, where gated Ca^{2+}-release channels (RyR1) are activated by conformational changes of voltage-sensor proteins (DHSRs).
7. Ca^{2+} is rapidly released from the sarcoplasmic reticulum into the sarcoplasm.
8. Accumulated Ca^{2+} diffuses to the myofilaments, where it binds to the TnC portion of the troponin complex.
9. The actomyosin cross-bridge cycle is initiated.
10. Ca^{2+} is returned to the terminal cisternae of the sarcoplasmic reticulum, where it is concentrated and captured by calsequestrin, a Ca^{2+}-binding protein.

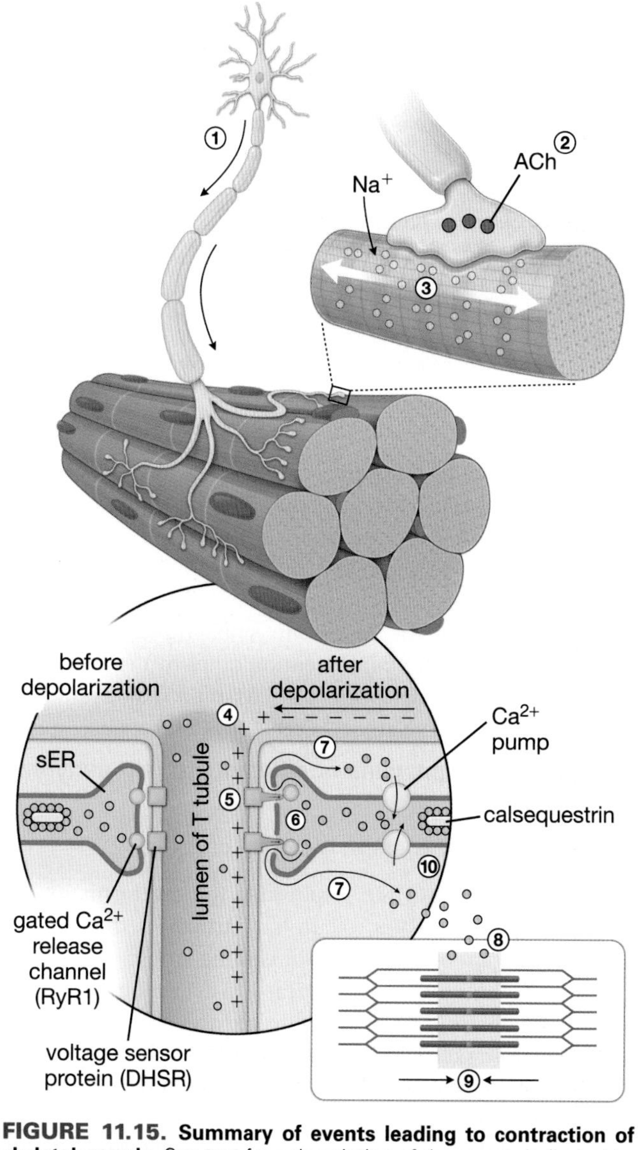

FIGURE 11.15. Summary of events leading to contraction of skeletal muscle. See text for a description of the events indicated by the *numerals*. *ACh*, acetylcholine.

Sensory Innervation

Encapsulated sensory receptors in muscles and tendons are examples of **proprioceptors**. These receptors are part of the somatic sensory system that provides information about the degree of stretching and tension in a muscle. Proprioceptors inform the central nervous system about the body's position and movement in space.

The muscle spindle is a specialized stretch receptor located within the skeletal muscle.

The **muscle spindle** is a specialized stretch receptor found in all skeletal muscles; it consists of two types of modified muscle fibers called **spindle cells** and **neuron terminals** (Fig. 11.16). Both types of modified muscle fibers are surrounded by an **internal capsule**. A fluid-filled space separates the internal capsule from an outer **external capsule**. One type of spindle cell, the **nuclear bag fiber**, contains an aggregation of nuclei in an expanded midregion; the other type, called a **nuclear chain fiber**, has many nuclei arranged in a chain. A typical muscle spindle is composed of two to four nuclear bag fibers and approximately six to eight nuclear chain fibers. The muscle spindle transmits information about the degree of stretching in a muscle. The two types of **sensory afferent nerve fibers (Ia and II)** carry information from the muscle spindle. Type Ia fibers have annulospiral endings that are spirally arranged around the midregion of both types of spindle cells, and type II fibers have flower-spray endings over the striated portions of the bag fibers.

When skeletal muscle is stretched, nerve endings of sensory nerves become activated and convey sensory information about muscle length and velocity of stretch. In addition, spindle cells receive motor (efferent) innervation from the spinal cord and brain via two types of **motor efferent (type γ) nerve fibers**, which are thought to regulate the sensitivity of the stretch receptors. **Dynamic γ fibers (γ-D)** and **static γ fibers (γ-S)** provide innervation to the spindle cells either during the dynamic phase of muscle stretching or during the static phase when the stretch is not affecting the muscle length. Muscle spindles convey their impulses to the central nervous system, which, in turn, modulates the activity of motor neurons innervating that particular muscle.

Similar encapsulated receptors, **Golgi tendon organs**, are found in the tendons of muscle and respond to increased tension in the muscle. These receptors contain only **sensory (afferent, Ib) nerve fibers**, and they monitor muscle tension (or the force of contraction) within an optimal range.

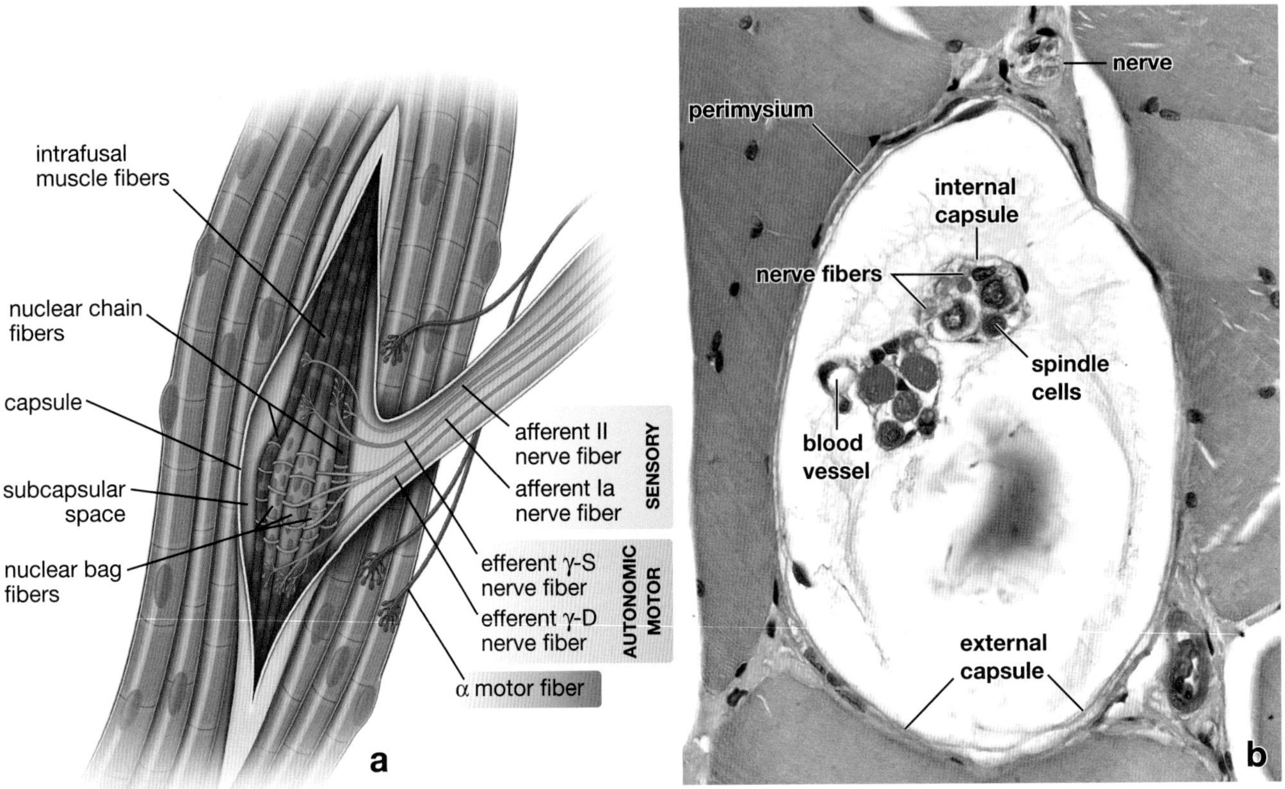

FIGURE 11.16. Muscle spindle. a. Schematic diagram of a muscle spindle. The diameter of the spindle is expanded to illustrate structural details. Each spindle contains approximately two to four nuclear bag fibers and six to eight nuclear chain fibers. In the nuclear bag fibers, the muscle fiber nuclei are clumped in the expanded central portion of the fiber, hence the name *bag*. In contrast, the nuclei concentrated in the central portion of the nuclear chain fibers are arranged in a chain. Both afferent II and Ia (sensory) and γ efferent (motor) nerve fibers supply muscle spindle cells. The afferent nerve fibers respond to excessive stretching of the muscle, which, in turn, inhibits the somatic motor stimulation of the muscle. The efferent nerve fibers regulate the sensitivity of the afferent endings in the muscle spindle. **b.** Photomicrograph of a cross section of a muscle spindle showing two bundles of spindle cells in the encapsulated, fluid-filled receptor. In one bundle, several of the spindle cells are cut at the level that reveals their nuclei. An internal capsule surrounds the spindle cells. The external capsule of the muscle spindle and the adjacent perimysium can be seen as a faint double-layer boundary of the receptor. Immediately above and outside the muscle spindle is a nerve that may be supplying the spindle. The types of nerves associated with the spindle cells as well as the type of spindle cells cannot be distinguished in this hematoxylin and eosin (H&E)-stained section. Located near one of the bundles of spindle cells is a small blood vessel. The flocculent material within the capsule consists of precipitated proteoglycans and glycoproteins from the fluid that filled the spindle before fixation. ×550.

Development, Repair, Healing, and Renewal

Development of the myogenic stem cell lineage depends on expression of various myogenic regulatory factors.

Myoblasts are derived from a self-renewing population of multipotential myogenic stem cells that originate in the embryo from unsegmented paraxial mesoderm (cranial muscle progenitors) or segmented mesoderm of somites (epaxial and hypaxial muscle progenitors). Early in embryonic development, these cells express **MyoD transcription factor**, which, along with other myogenic regulatory factors (MRFs), plays a key role in activation of muscle-specific gene expressions and differentiation of all skeletal muscle lineages. A balancing effect on skeletal–muscle development is achieved by the expression of the **myostatin gene**, which leads to the synthesis of **myostatin**, a 26-kDa protein belonging to the bone morphogenetic protein/transforming growth factor β (BMP/TGF-β) protein superfamily. Myostatin exerts an inhibitory effect on muscle growth and differentiation. It is thought that MyoD preferentially upregulates myostatin gene expression and controls myogenesis during not only the embryonic and fetal periods but also postnatal stages of development. The **hypermuscular phenotypes** observed on inactivation of the **myostatin gene** in animals and humans have confirmed the role of myostatin as a negative regulator of skeletal muscle development. Experimental studies have demonstrated that muscle mass increases through myostatin inhibition and that the myostatin signaling pathway may be a potent therapeutic intervention point in the treatment of **muscle-wasting diseases**, such as muscular dystrophy, amyotrophic lateral sclerosis (ALS), AIDS, and cancer.

Skeletal muscle progenitors differentiate into early and late myoblasts.

Developing muscle contains two types of myoblasts:

- **Early myoblasts** are responsible for the formation of **primary myotubes**, chain-like structures that extend between tendons of the developing muscle. Primary myotubes are formed by a nearly synchronous fusion of early myoblasts. Myotubes undergo further differentiation into mature skeletal muscle fibers. In the light microscope, primary myotubes exhibit a chain of multiple central nuclei surrounded by myofilaments.
- **Late myoblasts** give rise to **secondary myotubes**, which are formed in the innervated zone of developing

muscle where the myotubes have direct contact with nerve terminals. Secondary myotubes continue to be formed by sequential fusion of myoblasts into the already formed secondary myotubes at random positions along their length. Secondary myotubes are characterized by a smaller diameter, more widely spaced nuclei, and an increased number of myofilaments (Fig. 11.17). In the mature multinucleated muscle fiber, the nuclei are located exclusively in the peripheral sarcoplasm, just inside the plasma membrane.

Some nuclei that appear to belong to the skeletal muscle fiber are nuclei of satellite cells.

Late in fetal development, the multipotential **myogenic stem cell** population generates **satellite cells**, which are characterized by the expression of paired box transcription factor family member **Pax7**. Therefore, in a developing muscle, a pool of undifferentiated cells that have the potential to undergo myogenic differentiation is preserved. These satellite cells are interposed between the plasma membrane of the muscle fiber and its external lamina. Satellite cells are small with scant cytoplasm, and they make up 2%–7% of all nuclei associated with a single muscle fiber. The cytoplasm typically blends in with the muscle cell sarcoplasm when viewed in the light microscope, thus making them difficult to identify. Each satellite cell has a single nucleus with a chromatin network denser and coarser than that of muscle cell nuclei.

Satellite cells are responsible for the skeletal muscle's ability to regenerate, but their regenerative capacity is limited. They are normally mitotically quiescent, and because they express Pax7 transcription factor, they can be identified using immunofluorescence methods (Fig. 11.18). However, after muscle tissue injury, some satellite cells are activated and become **myogenic precursors of muscle cells**; they reenter the cell cycle and begin to coexpress **Pax7** with **MyoD**, which is a key transcription factor for myogenic differentiation. Myogenic precursor cells then downregulate Pax7 and differentiate, giving rise to new myoblasts. As long as the external lamina remains intact, the myoblasts fuse within the external lamina to form myotubes, which then mature into a new fiber. In contrast, if the external lamina is disrupted, fibroblasts repair the injured site, with subsequent scar tissue formation.

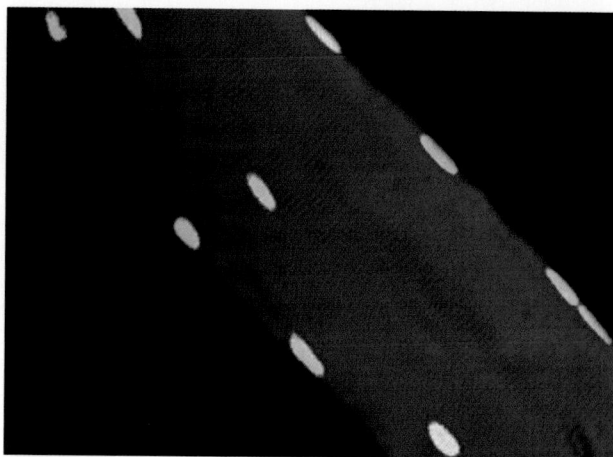

FIGURE 11.18. Confocal microscopy image of satellite cells. This confocal image of a single skeletal muscle fiber from a diaphragm shows striations on the surface of cell membrane. The striation pattern is visible owing to staining with the voltage-sensitive lipophilic styryl dye RH414 (*orange-red*) and coincides with the distribution of the T tubules in muscle fiber. Nuclei of skeletal muscles are stained with propidium iodide (*green*). Two nuclei stained *white* represent satellite cells; they are stained for the presence of Pax7 transcription factor. ×550. (Courtesy of Dr. Garry C. Sieck, Mayo Clinic.)

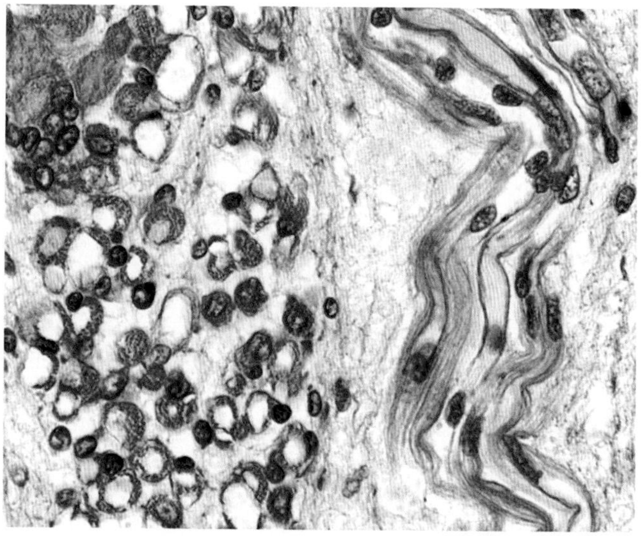

FIGURE 11.17. Photomicrograph of developing skeletal muscle myotubes. This photomicrograph shows a cross section (on the *left*) and a longitudinal section (on the *right*) of developing skeletal muscle fibers in the stage of secondary myotubes. These myotubes are formed by sequential fusion of myoblasts, forming elongated tubular structures. Note that the myotubes have a small diameter and widely spaced, centrally positioned nuclei that gradually become displaced into the cell periphery by the increased number of newly synthesized myofilaments. In the mature multinucleated muscle fiber (*upper left*), all nuclei are positioned in the peripheral sarcoplasm, just inside the cell plasma membrane (sarcolemma). ×220.

Muscular dystrophies are characterized by progressive degeneration of skeletal muscle fibers, which places a constant demand on the satellite cells to replace the degenerated fibers. Ultimately, the satellite cell pool is exhausted. New experimental data indicate that, during this process, additional myogenic cells are recruited from the bone marrow to supplement the available satellite cells. The rate of degeneration exceeds the rate of regeneration, however, resulting in loss of muscle function. Treatment strategies for muscular dystrophies may include the transplantation of satellite cells or their myogenic bone marrow counterparts into damaged muscle or finding ways to restore their function.

■ CARDIAC MUSCLE

Cardiac muscle has the same types and arrangement of contractile filaments as skeletal muscle. Therefore, cardiac muscle cells and the fibers they form exhibit cross-striations, evident in routine histologic sections. In addition, cardiac muscle fibers exhibit densely staining cross-bands, called **intercalated discs**, that cross the fibers in a linear manner or frequently in a way that resembles the risers of a stairway (Fig. 11.19 and Plate 11.4, page 382). The intercalated discs represent highly specialized attachment sites between adjacent cells. This linear cell-to-cell attachment of the cardiac muscle

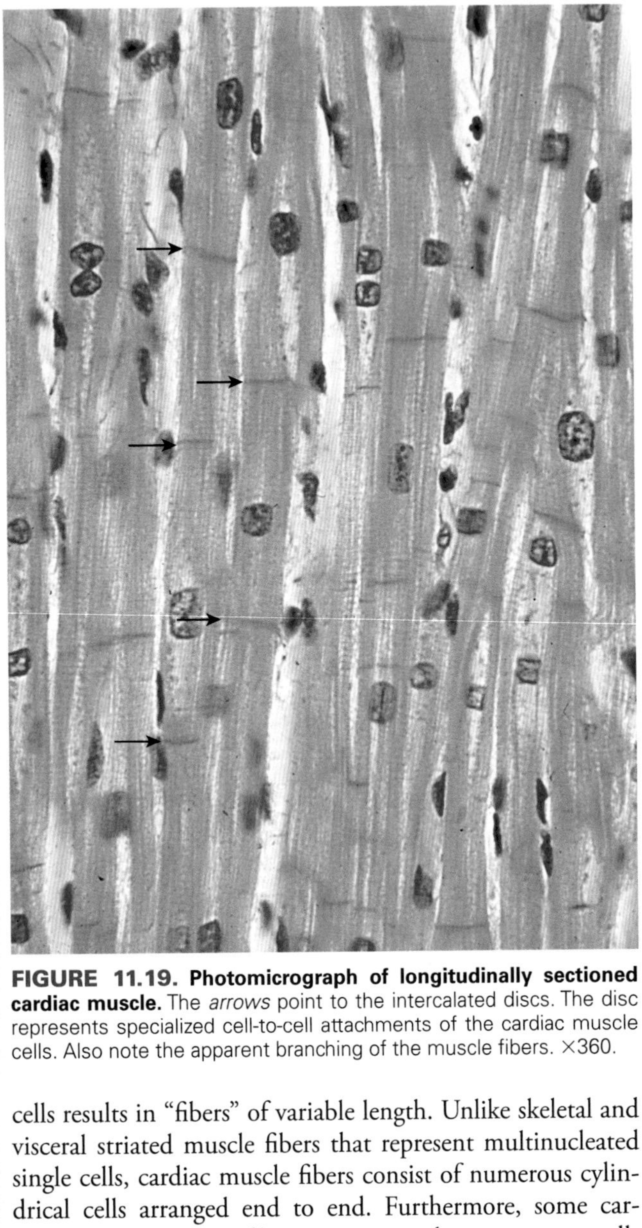

FIGURE 11.19. Photomicrograph of longitudinally sectioned cardiac muscle. The *arrows* point to the intercalated discs. The disc represents specialized cell-to-cell attachments of the cardiac muscle cells. Also note the apparent branching of the muscle fibers. ×360.

cells results in "fibers" of variable length. Unlike skeletal and visceral striated muscle fibers that represent multinucleated single cells, cardiac muscle fibers consist of numerous cylindrical cells arranged end to end. Furthermore, some cardiac muscle cells in a fiber may join with two or more cells through intercalated discs, thus creating a branched fiber. Cardiac muscle fibers are surrounded by a thin layer of connective tissue **endomysium** that contains a rich network of blood capillaries.

Structure of Cardiac Muscle

The cardiac muscle nucleus lies in the center of the cell.

Cardiac muscle cells are approximately 15 μm in diameter and 80 μm in length, which may vary depending on the stage of muscle contraction. Each cardiac muscle cell exhibits a single nucleus; however, it is not unusual to find binucleated cardiac muscle cells (see page 366). The central location of the nucleus in cardiac muscle cells is one feature that helps distinguish them from multinucleated skeletal muscle fibers, whose nuclei lie immediately beneath the plasma membrane. The transmission electron microscope (TEM) reveals that the myofibrils of cardiac muscle separate to pass around the nucleus, thus outlining a biconical **juxtanuclear region** in which the cell organelles are concentrated. This region is rich in mitochondria and contains the Golgi apparatus, lipofuscin pigment granules, and glycogen. In the **atria** of the heart, **atrial granules** measuring 0.3–0.4 μm in diameter are also concentrated in the juxtanuclear cytoplasm. These granules contain two polypeptide hormones: **atrial natriuretic factor (ANF)** *[L. natrium, sodium]* and **brain natriuretic factor (BNF)**. Both hormones are diuretics, affecting urinary excretion of sodium. They inhibit renin secretion by the kidney and aldosterone secretion by the adrenal gland. They also inhibit contractions of vascular smooth muscle. In congestive heart failure, the levels of circulating BNF increase.

Numerous large mitochondria and glycogen stores are adjacent to each myofibril.

In addition to the juxtanuclear mitochondria, cardiac muscle cells are characterized by large mitochondria that are densely packed between the myofibrils. These **large mitochondria** often extend the full length of a sarcomere and contain numerous, closely packed cristae (Fig. 11.20). Concentrations of **glycogen granules** are also located between the myofibrils. Thus, the structures that store energy (glycogen granules) and the structures that release and recapture energy (mitochondria) are located adjacent to the structures (myofibrils) that use the energy to drive contraction.

The intercalated discs represent junctions between cardiac muscle cells.

As previously noted, the **intercalated disc** represents the attachment site between cardiac muscle cells. In the light microscope, the disc appears as a densely staining linear structure that is oriented transversely to the muscle fiber. Often, it consists of short segments arranged in a step-like manner (Fig. 11.21). When the site of the intercalated disc is examined with the TEM, the densely staining structure seen in the light microscope can be attributed to the presence of a **transverse component** that crosses the fibers at a right angle to the myofibrils. The transverse component is analogous to the risers of the stairway. A **lateral component** (not visible in the light microscope) occupies a series of surfaces perpendicular to the transverse component and lies parallel to the myofibrils. The lateral component is analogous to the steps of the stairway. Both components of the intercalated disc contain **specialized cell-to-cell junctions** between adjoining cardiac muscle cells:

- **Fascia adherens** (adhering junction) is the major constituent of the transverse component of the intercalated disc and is responsible for its staining in routine H&E preparations. It holds the cardiac muscle cells at their ends to form the functional cardiac muscle fiber (see Fig. 5.21, page 149). It always appears as a transverse boundary between the cardiac muscle cells. The TEM reveals an intercellular space between the adjacent cells that is filled with electron-dense material, resembling the material found in the zonula adherens of epithelia. The fascia adherens serves as the site at which the **thin filaments in the terminal sarcomere anchor onto the plasma membrane**. In this way, the fascia adherens is functionally similar to the epithelial zonula adherens, where actin filaments of the terminal web are also anchored.
- **Maculae adherentes** (desmosomes) bind the individual muscle cells to one another. Maculae adherentes

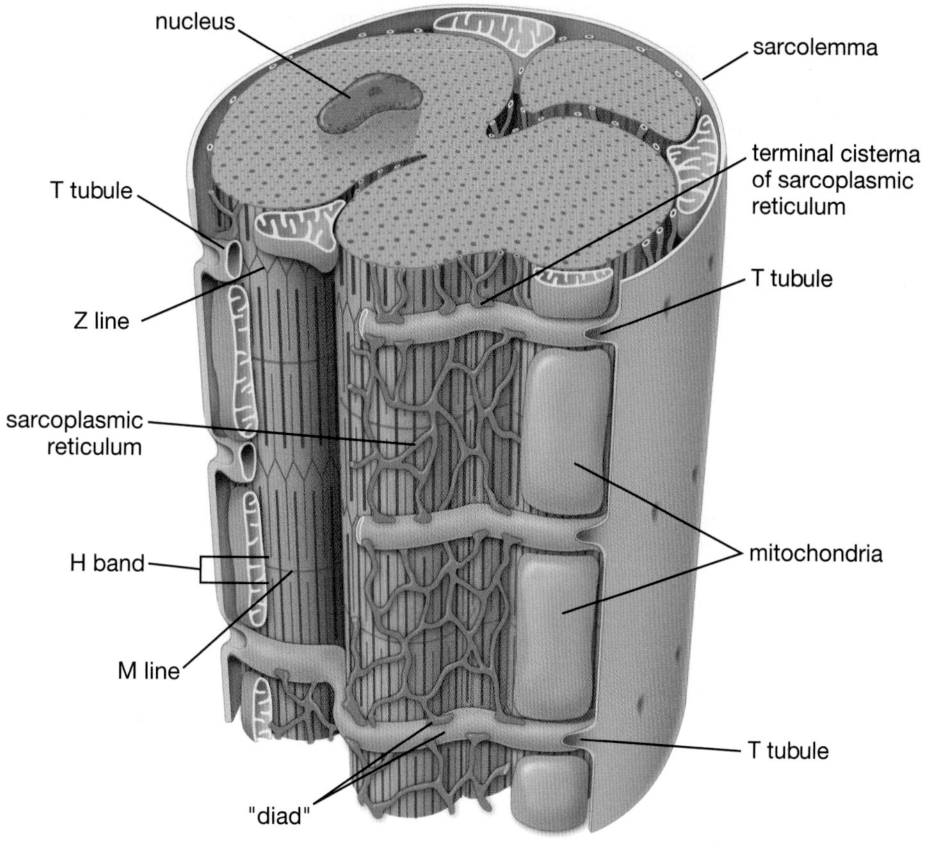

FIGURE 11.20. Diagram of the organization of cardiac muscle fiber. The T tubules of cardiac muscle are much larger than the T tubules of skeletal muscle and carry an investment of external lamina material into the cell. They also differ in that they are located at the level of the Z line. The portion of the sarcoplasmic reticulum adjacent to the T tubule is not in the form of an expanded cisterna but rather is organized as a "diad" anastomosing network.

help prevent the cells from pulling apart under the strain of regular repetitive contractions. They reinforce the fascia adherens and are found in both the transverse and lateral components of the intercalated discs.

- **Gap junctions** (communicating junctions) constitute the major structural element of the lateral component of the intercalated disc. Gap junctions provide ionic continuity between the adjacent cardiac muscle cells, thus allowing informational macromolecules to pass from cell to cell. This exchange permits cardiac muscle fibers to behave as a syncytium while retaining cellular integrity and individuality. The position of the gap junctions on the lateral surfaces of the intercalated disc protects them from the forces generated during contraction.

The sER in cardiac muscle cells is organized into a single network along the sarcomere, extending from Z line to Z line.

The sER of cardiac muscle is not as well organized as that of skeletal muscle. It does not separate bundles of myofilaments into discrete myofibrils. The T tubules in cardiac muscle penetrate the myofilament bundles at the level of the Z line, between the ends of the sER network. Thus, there is **only one T tubule per sarcomere** in cardiac muscle. **Small terminal cisternae of the sER** are in close proximity to the **T tubules** to form a **diad** structure at the level of the Z line (see Fig. 11.20). The external lamina adheres to the invaginated plasma membrane of the T tubule as it penetrates into the cytoplasm of the muscle cell. The T tubules are larger and more numerous in cardiac ventricular muscle than in skeletal muscle. They are less numerous, however, in cardiac atrial muscle.

Passage of Ca^{2+} from the lumen of the T tubule to the sarcoplasm of a cardiac muscle cell is essential to initiate the contraction cycle.

As discussed in the section on skeletal muscle, depolarization of the T-tubule membrane activates **voltage-sensor proteins (DHSRs)** that are similar in structure and function to Ca^{2+} channels. In contrast to skeletal muscle, long-lasting depolarization in cardiac muscle activates DHSRs and prompts their slow conformational change into functional Ca^{2+} channels (Fig. 11.22). Thus, in the first stage of the cardiac muscle contraction cycle, Ca^{2+} from the lumen of the T tubule is transported to the sarcoplasm of cardiac muscle cell, which then opens **gated Ca^{2+}-release channels** in the adjacent terminal sacs of the sarcoplasmic reticulum. Gated Ca^{2+}-release channels in cardiac muscle sarcoplasmic reticulum are composed of **RyR2 isoform of ryanodine receptors**, which is the primary isoform in the cardiac muscle. This **calcium-triggered calcium-release mechanism** causes a rapid release of additional Ca^{2+} that initiates subsequent steps of the contraction cycle, which are identical to those in skeletal muscle.

The differences between initiation of cardiac and skeletal muscle contractions—the longer lasting membrane

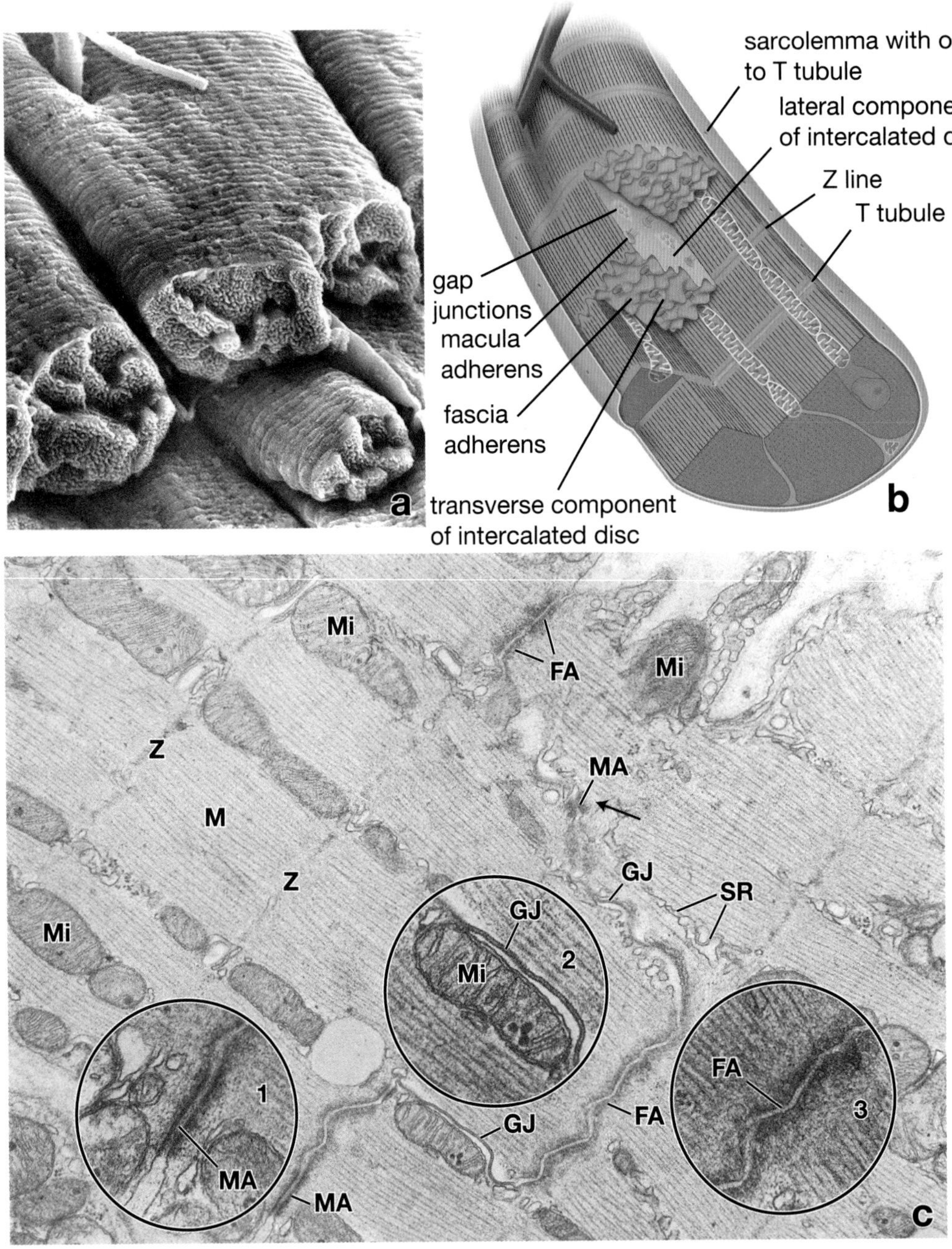

FIGURE 11.21. Structure of cardiac muscle fiber. a. This scanning electron micrograph shows the heart muscle tissue preparation obtained from a monkey right ventricle. The sample was ultrasonicated within sodium hydroxide, resulting in digestion of collagen fibers and separation of cardiac myocytes at the intercalated discs. Note the branching pattern of myocytes and clearly visible transverse and lateral components of the intercalated discs. ×32,000. **b.** Three-dimensional drawing of an intercalated disc, which represents a highly specialized attachment site between adjacent cardiac muscle cells. The intercalated disc is composed of the transverse component that crosses the fibers at a right angle to the myofibrils (analogous to the risers of a stairway) and a lateral component that occupies a series of surfaces perpendicular to the transverse component and parallel to the myofibrils (analogous to the steps of a stairway). The fascia adherens (*FA*) is the major constituent of the transverse component. It holds the cardiac muscle cells at their ends and serves as the attachment site for thin filaments. The maculae adherentes reinforce the FA and are also found in the lateral components. The gap junctions are found only in the lateral component of the intercalated disc. **c.** This electron micrograph reveals portions of two cardiac muscle cells joined by an intercalated disc. The line of junction between the two cells takes an irregular, step-like course, making a number of nearly right-angle turns. In its course, different parts of the intercalated disc are evident. These include the transverse components (FA and maculae adherentes) and lateral components (gap junctions and maculae adherentes). The macula adherens (*MA*) is enlarged in *inset 1* (×62,000). The FA is more elongated than the MA. In contrast to the MA, the FA occupies a much larger area along the irregular outline of the transverse component of the intercalated disc. The gap junction (*GJ*) is enlarged in *inset 2* (×62,000). The FA is enlarged in *inset 3* (×62,000). The FA of the intercalated disc corresponds to the zonula adherens of epithelial tissues. Other features typical of cardiac muscle are also present: mitochondria (*Mi*), sarcoplasmic reticulum (*SR*), and components of the sarcomere, including Z lines (*Z*), M line (*M*), and myofilaments. This particular specimen is in a highly contracted state, and consequently, the I band is practically obscured. ×30,000. (**Part a** reprinted with permission from Zhang L, Ina K, Kitamura H, et al. The intercalated discs of monkey myocardial cells and Purkinje fibers as revealed by scanning electron microscopy. *Arch Histol Cytol.* 1996;59:453–465.)

depolarization and activation of voltage-sensitive Ca^{2+} channels in the wall of the T tubule—account for an approximately 200-millisecond delay from the start of depolarization in a cardiac muscle twitch (see Fig. 11.22). In addition, in contrast to skeletal muscle, release of Ca^{2+} from the sarcoplasmic reticulum alone is insufficient to initiate cardiac muscle contraction.

Mutations in the gene encoding RyR2 receptors are associated with stress-induced **polymorphic ventricular tachycardia** (torsades de pointes). This type of tachycardia (fast resting heart rate) is characterized by an abnormal heart rate that can range from 150 to 250 beats/min accompanied by unique ECG findings. These findings include a series of twisted QRS complexes in relation to the isoelectric baseline from positive to net negative and back again. Polymorphic ventricular tachycardia is often associated with prolonged QT intervals on ECG. Individuals with this syndrome can experience brief, self-terminating episodes of tachycardia or have recurrent persistent episodes that may lead to ventricular fibrillation and sudden cardiac death.

Specialized cardiac-conducting muscle cells (Purkinje fibers) exhibit a spontaneous rhythmic contraction.

The intrinsic spontaneous contraction or beat of cardiac muscle is evident in embryonic cardiac muscle cells as well as in cardiac muscle cells in tissue culture. The heartbeat is initiated, locally regulated, and coordinated by specialized, modified cardiac muscle cells called **cardiac-conducting cells** (Plate 11.5, page 384). These cells are organized into the **conducting system of the heart.** Cardiac-conducting cells form **nodes** (local accumulation of cells in the right atrium of the heart) and specialized conducting fibers called **Purkinje fibers** that generate and rapidly transmit the contractile impulse to various parts of the myocardium in a precise sequence.

Cells in Purkinje fibers differ from cardiac muscle cells in that they are larger and their myofibrils are located mostly at the periphery of the cell. The cytoplasm between the nucleus and the peripherally located myofibrils stains poorly owing to the large amount of glycogen present in this part of the cell. Purkinje fibers mostly lack T tubules. Occasionally, T tubules can be found, and their frequency depends on the size of the heart.

Both parasympathetic and sympathetic nerve fibers terminate in the nodes. Sympathetic stimulation accelerates the heartbeat by increasing the frequency of impulses to the cardiac-conducting cells. Parasympathetic stimulation slows the heartbeat by decreasing the frequency of the impulses. The impulses carried by these nerves do not initiate contraction but only modify the rate of intrinsic cardiac muscle contraction by their effect at the nodes. The structure and functions of the conducting system of the heart are described in Chapter 13, Cardiovascular System (pages 448-449).

The events leading to contraction of cardiac muscle can be summarized as a series of steps.

The events involved in contraction of cardiac muscle are as follows (the *numbers* refer to Fig. 11.22):

1. Contraction of a cardiac muscle fiber initiates when the cell membrane depolarization traveling along Purkinje fibers reaches its destination in cardiac myocytes.
2. General depolarization spreads over the plasma membrane of the muscle cell, causing the opening of voltage-gated Na^+ channels. Na^+ enters the cell.
3. General depolarization continues via membranes of the T tubules.
4. Voltage-sensor proteins (DHSRs) in the plasma membrane of T tubules change their conformation into functional Ca^{2+} channels.
5. An increase in the cytoplasmic Ca^{2+} concentration opens RyR2-gated Ca^{2+}-release channels in the sarcoplasmic reticulum.
6. Ca^{2+} is rapidly released from the sarcoplasmic reticulum and increases the pool of Ca^{2+} that enters the sarcoplasm through the calcium channels in the plasma membrane.
7. Accumulated Ca^{2+} diffuses to the myofilaments, where it binds to the TnC portion of the troponin complex.
8. The actomyosin cross-bridge cycle similar to that of skeletal muscle is initiated.
9. Ca^{2+} is returned to the terminal cisternae of the sarcoplasmic reticulum, where it is concentrated and captured by calsequestrin, a Ca^{2+}-binding protein.

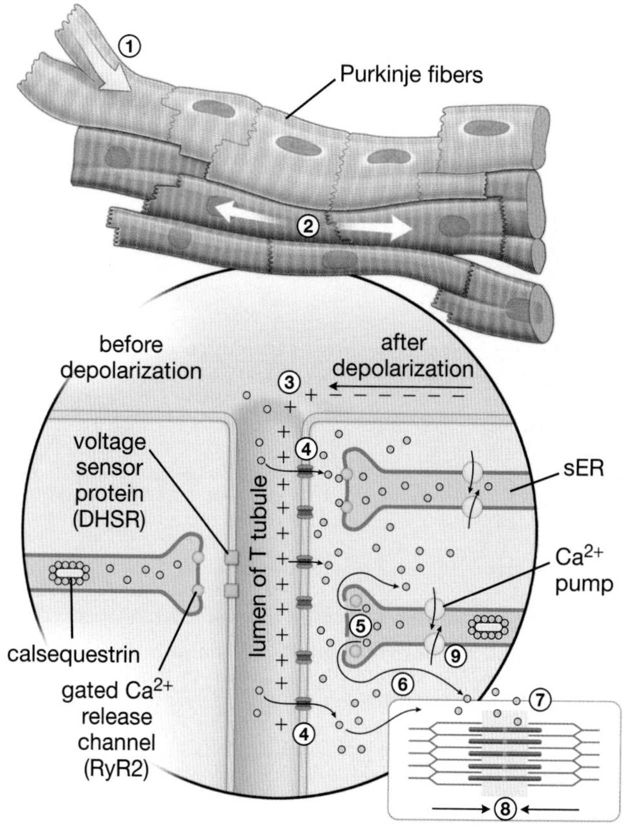

FIGURE 11.22. Summary of events leading to contraction of cardiac muscle. See text for a description of the events indicated by the *numerals. DSHR,* dihydropyridine-sensitive receptor; *RyR2,* ryanodine receptor 2; *sER,* smooth-surfaced endoplasmic reticulum.

Injury and Repair

One of the most common reasons for death of heart muscle cells (necrosis) is **myocardial infarction (MI)** induced by inadequate blood supply (ischemia) of the myocardium.

Localized injury to cardiac muscle tissue that results in the death of cells is repaired by replacement with fibrous connective tissue. Consequently, cardiac function is lost at the site of injury. This pattern of injury and repair is seen in nonfatal MI. Confirmation of suspected MI can be made through the detection of specific markers in the blood. These markers are the structural subunits **TnI** and **TnT** of the **cardiac troponin complex**. These intracellular proteins are usually released from dying cardiac muscle cells into the bloodstream within 3–12 hours after an MI. TnI levels remain elevated for up to 2 weeks from the time of the initial injury; thus, it is regarded as an excellent marker for diagnosing MI that has recently occurred.

Regeneration of heart muscle after destruction of cardiac cells may be possible.

The death of cardiac muscle cells results in loss of cardiac function and blood pumping capacity. In the past, it was thought that once cardiac muscle cells were destroyed, they could not be replaced by new muscle cells. However, research performed in the past decade has revealed that the cardiac muscle cell retains some capacity for division. In addition, several studies have identified endogenous **cardiac muscle progenitor cells** in the heart and bone marrow.

Studies of hearts removed from individuals who had received heart transplants reveal nuclei of cardiac muscle cells **undergoing mitosis**. Although the number of dividing nuclei in these hearts was low (0.1%), it suggests that damaged cardiac muscle cells can potentially reenter the cell cycle and synthesize DNA, followed by mitosis and cytokinesis resulting in cell division. Recent studies that used carbon isotope (^{14}C) to date the age of cardiac muscle cells show that the adult heart contains a small population of cardiac muscle cells generated during the human life span. These studies estimated an approximate turnover rate in cardiac muscle cells of 1% per year in younger individuals that declines by one-half with aging.

Most of the DNA synthesis that occurs in the cardiac muscle cells does not lead to new muscle cell formation. Cardiac muscle cells are able to complete mitosis without cell division, resulting in **binucleated cells**. It is estimated that 25%–57% of all human cardiac muscle cells are binucleated.

In addition, cardiac muscle cells can undergo chromosomal replication without completing either mitosis or cytokinesis, resulting in **polyploid nuclei** containing multiple sets of chromosomes. In the adult heart, it is estimated that most cardiac muscle cell nuclei are polyploid. They are formed by undergoing at least one additional (4n: tetraploid) or two additional (8n: octoploid) rounds of chromosomal replication. Polyploidy in cardiac muscle cells increases with myocardial hypertrophy or other cardiac muscle cell injuries and could be mistaken for cell divisions.

Research has revealed the presence of **cardiac muscle progenitor cells** in adults that are capable of limited differentiation into cardiac muscle cells and other cells found in the heart (i.e., endothelial and smooth muscle cells). Efforts are now focused on defining the mechanisms that trigger progenitors to differentiate to induce human cardiac muscle to regenerate into healthy tissue.

■ SMOOTH MUSCLE

Smooth muscle generally occurs as bundles or sheets of elongated fusiform cells with finely tapered ends (Fig. 11.23 and Plate 11.6, page 386). The smooth muscle cells, also called **fibers**, do not contain highly arranged thick and thin filament; thus, they lack the striated pattern found in skeletal and cardiac muscle. They range in length from 20 μm in the walls of small blood vessels to about 200 μm in the wall of the intestine; they may be as large as 500 μm in the wall of the uterus during pregnancy. Smooth muscle cells are interconnected by **gap junctions**, the specialized communication junctions between the cells (Fig. 11.24). Small molecules or ions can pass from cell to cell via these junctions and provide communication links that regulate contraction of the entire bundle or sheet of smooth muscle.

Smooth muscle cytoplasm stains rather evenly with eosin in routine H&E preparations because of the concentrations of actin and myosin within these cells. The nuclei of smooth muscle cells are located in the center of the cell and often have a corkscrew appearance in longitudinal section. This characteristic is a result of contraction of the cell during fixation and is often useful in distinguishing smooth muscle cells from

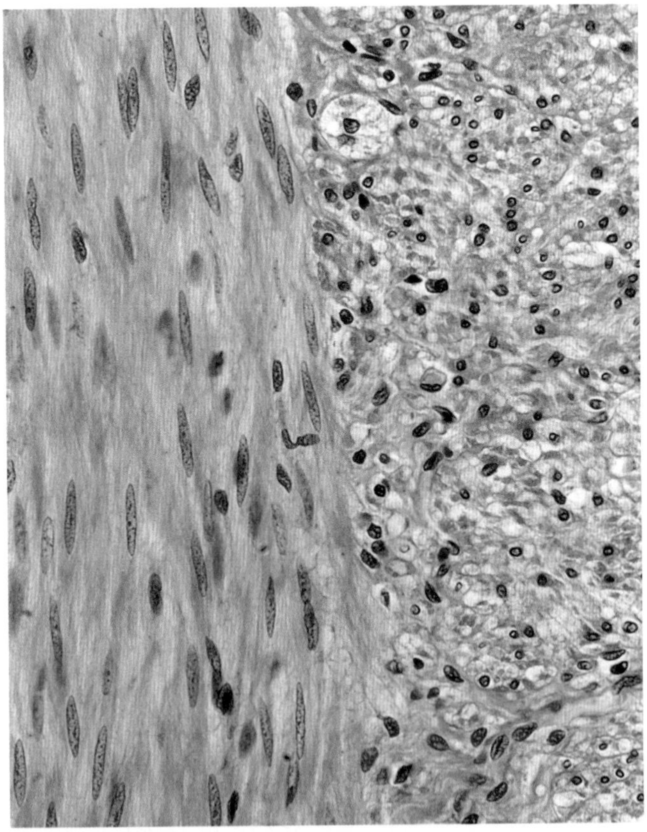

FIGURE 11.23. Photomicrograph of smooth muscle from a human colon. The smooth muscle shown in this micrograph is arranged in two layers. On the *left*, the muscle cells are cut in longitudinal section; on the *right*, they are cut in cross section. Smooth muscle cells are elongated and have tapering ends. Note that the nuclei in the longitudinally sectioned muscle cells appear elongated and also exhibit tapering ends, thus matching the shape of the cell. In contrast, the nuclei in the cross-sectioned muscle cells are circular in profile. Also, some of the cross-sectioned cells appear to lack a nucleus, which reflects that fact that the section passed through one of the ends of the cell. Also note that the longitudinally sectioned muscle cells are not easily delineated from one another because of the way they lie one over the other within the thickness of the section. ×400.

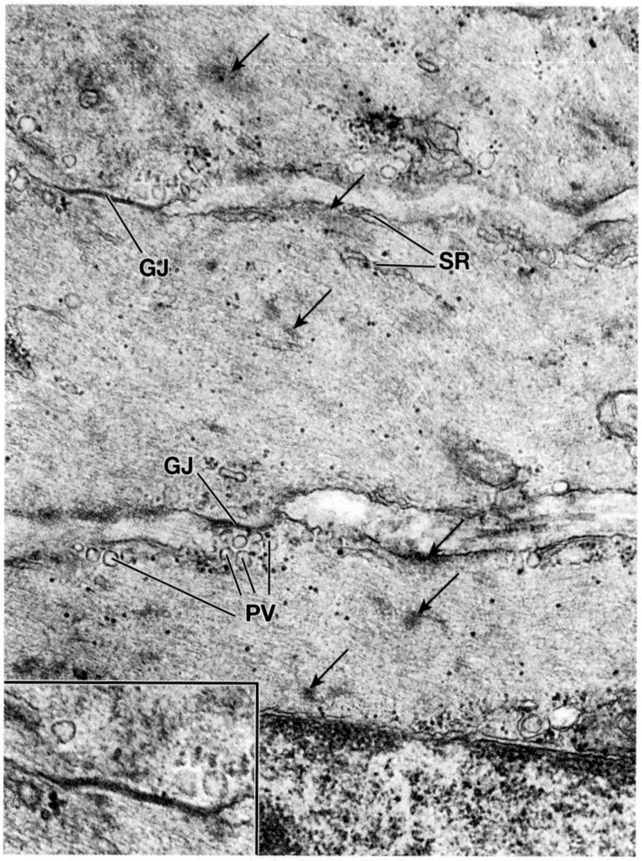

FIGURE 11.24. Electron micrograph of smooth muscle cells. This electron micrograph shows parts of three smooth muscle cells. The nucleus of one cell is in the *lower part* of the micrograph. The bulk of the cytoplasm is occupied by thin (actin) filaments, which are just recognizable at this magnification. The α-actinin–containing cytoplasmic densities, or dense bodies, are visible among the myofilaments (*arrows*). Elements of the sarcoplasmic reticulum (*SR*) and the pinocytotic vesicles (*PV*) are also indicated. The other two cells in the *middle* and *upper part* of the micrograph possess visible gap junctions (*GJ*) that allow communication between adjacent cells. The *small dark particles* are glycogen. ×25,000. **Inset.** Enlargement of the gap junction. Note the presence of pinocytotic vesicles. ×35,000.

fibroblasts in routine histologic sections. In the noncontracted cell, the nucleus appears as an elongated structure with tapering ends, lying in the center axis of the cell. When the nucleus is included in a cross section of a smooth muscle fiber, it appears as a round or circular profile whether the cell is contracted or relaxed. The TEM shows that most of the cytoplasmic organelles are concentrated at each end of the nucleus. These include numerous mitochondria, some cisternae of the rER, free ribosomes, glycogen granules, and a small Golgi apparatus.

Structure of Smooth Muscle

Smooth muscle cells possess a contractile apparatus of thin and thick filaments and a cytoskeleton of desmin and vimentin intermediate filaments.

The remaining sarcoplasm is filled with **thin filaments** that form a part of the contractile apparatus. **Thick myosin filaments** are scattered throughout the sarcoplasm of a smooth muscle cell. They are extremely labile and tend to be lost during tissue preparation. Special techniques can be used, however, to retain the structural integrity of the thick filaments and thus demonstrate them with the TEM. The thin filaments in a smooth muscle cell are attached to **cytoplasmic densities** or **dense bodies** that are visible among the filaments (Fig. 11.25). These structures are distributed throughout the sarcoplasm in a network of intermediate filaments containing the protein **desmin**. Intermediate filaments are part of the cytoskeleton of the cell. Note that vascular smooth muscle contains **vimentin** filaments in addition to desmin filaments.

The components of the contractile apparatus in smooth muscle cells are as follows:

- **Thin filaments** contain **actin**, the smooth muscle isoform of **tropomyosin**, and two smooth muscle–specific proteins, **caldesmon** and **calponin**. No troponin is associated with smooth muscle tropomyosin. Actin is involved in the force-generating interaction with smooth muscle myosin (SMM) molecules. Research suggests that the tropomyosin position on the actin filament is regulated by phosphorylation of myosin heads. Caldesmon (120–150 kDa) and calponin (34 kDa) are actin-binding proteins that block the myosin-binding site. The action of these proteins is Ca^{2+} dependent and is also controlled by the phosphorylation of myosin heads.
- **Thick filaments** containing **smooth muscle myosin (SMM)** differ slightly from those found in skeletal muscle. They, too, are composed of two polypeptide **heavy chains** and four **light chains**. However, the structure of thick filaments in smooth muscle is different than in skeletal muscle. Rather than a bipolar arrangement, SMM molecules are oriented in one direction on one side of the filament and in an opposite direction on the other side of the filament. In this arrangement, myosin molecules are staggered in parallel between two immediate neighbors and are also bound to an antiparallel partner via a short overlap at the very tip of their tails (Fig. 11.26). The polarity of the myosin heads is the same along the entire length of one side of the filament and the opposite on the opposite side. This **side-polar myosin filament** also has no central "bare zone" but instead has asymmetrically tapered bare ends. This organization maximizes the interaction between thick and thin filaments, allowing the overlapped thin filaments to be pulled over the entire length of the thick filaments.

Several more proteins are associated with the contractile apparatus and are essential to initiation or regulation of smooth muscle contractions.

- **Myosin light-chain kinase (MLCK)** is a 130- to 150-kDa enzyme that is important in the mechanism of contraction in smooth muscle. It initiates the contraction cycle after its activation by Ca^{2+}–calmodulin complex. Active MLCK phosphorylates one of the myosin regulatory light chains, enabling it to form a cross-bridge with actin filaments.
- **Calmodulin**, a 17-kDa Ca^{2+}-binding protein, is related to the TnC found in skeletal muscle, which regulates the intracellular concentration of Ca^{2+}. A **Ca^{2+}–calmodulin complex** binds to MLCK to activate this enzyme. It may also, with caldesmon, regulate its phosphorylation and release from F-actin.
- **α-Actinin**, a 31-kDa protein, provides structural component to dense bodies.

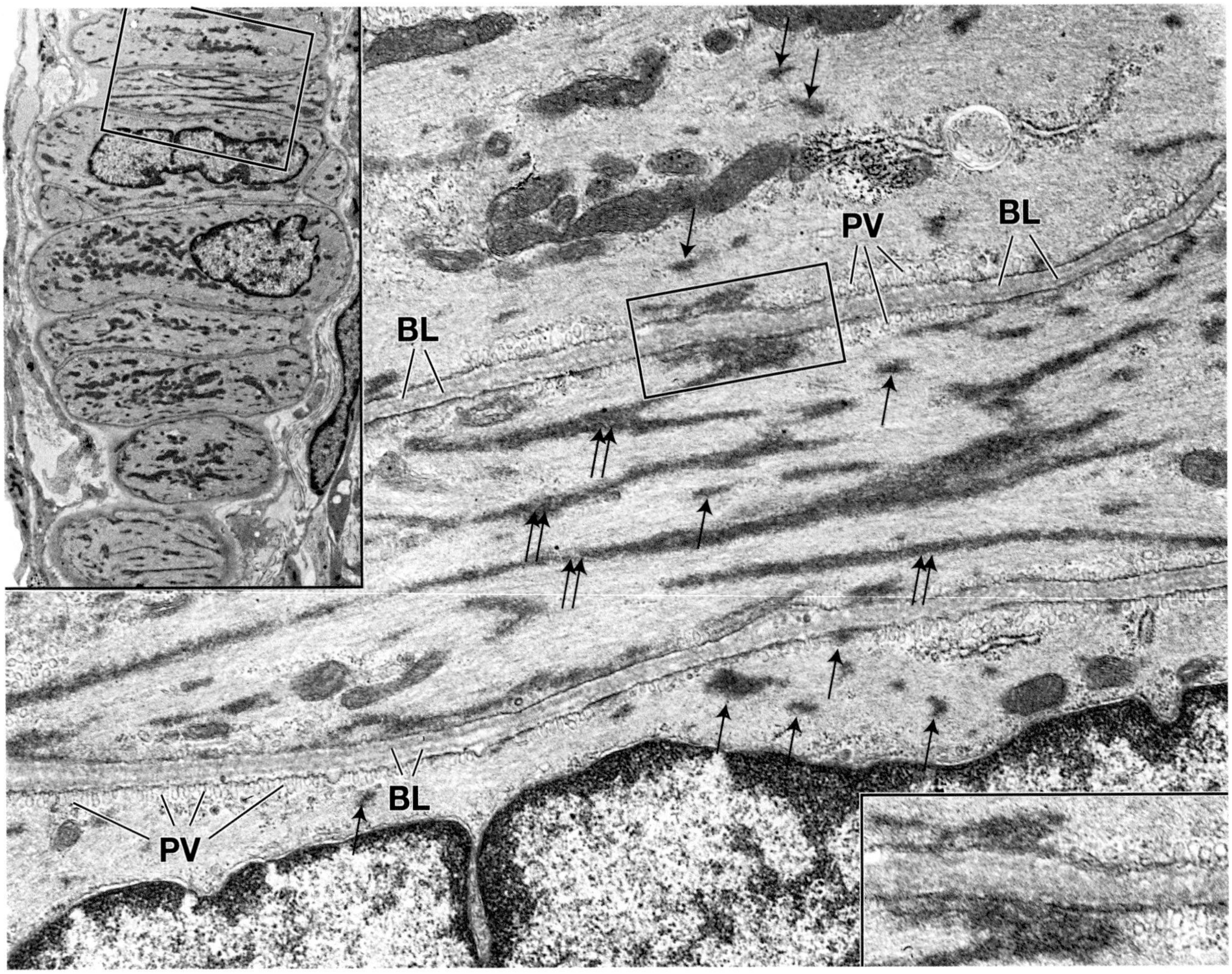

FIGURE 11.25. Electron micrographs showing the cytoplasmic densities in vascular smooth muscle cells. Upper inset. The plane of section includes only the smooth muscle cells in the vascular wall. The *rectangle* in the *inset* shows portions of three smooth muscle cells that appear at higher magnification in the large electron micrograph. The α-actinin–containing cytoplasmic densities (*single arrows*) usually appear as irregular masses, some of which are in contact with, and attached to, the plasma membrane. The cell in the *center* of the micrograph has been cut in a plane closer to the cell surface and reveals these same densities as a branching structure (*double arrows*). A three-dimensional model of the cytoplasmic densities would reveal an anastomosing network. *BL*, basal (external) lamina; *PV*, pinocytotic vesicles. ×27,000. **Lower inset.** Higher magnification of cytoplasmic densities attached to the plasma membrane from the area indicated by the *rectangle*. Note that each cell possesses a basal (external) lamina. In addition, the pinocytotic vesicles can be observed in different stages of their formation. ×49,500.

Dense bodies provide an attachment site for thin filaments and intermediate filaments.

Dense bodies contain a variety of attachment plaque proteins, including **α-actinin**, which anchors both thin filaments and intermediate filaments either directly or indirectly to the sarcolemma. They play an important role in transmitting contractile forces generated inside the cell to the cell surface, altering the cell's shape (Fig. 11.27). Two intermediate filament proteins, **desmin** and **vimentin**, are highly expressed in smooth muscle cells. Intermediate filaments formed from these proteins are essential for providing links between dense bodies, cell cytoskeleton, and sarcolemma.

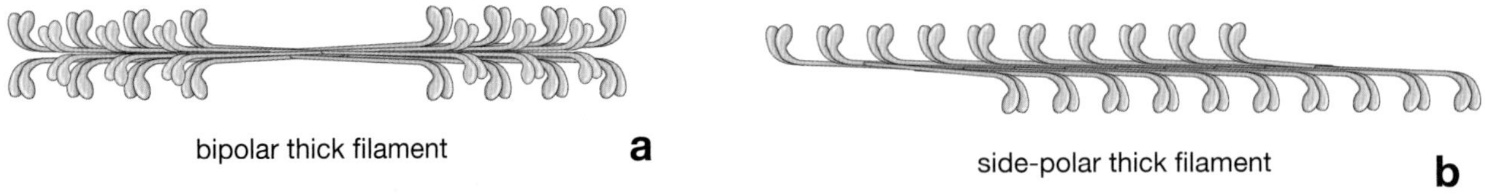

FIGURE 11.26. Comparison of myosin filaments of skeletal muscle and smooth muscle. This drawing shows the different arrangements of myosin thick filaments. **a.** Bipolar thick filaments are present in skeletal and cardiac muscles. They have a helical parallel–antiparallel arrangement of myosin molecules with their globular heads projecting from both ends of the filament. This filament has a "bare zone" in the middle of the filaments that does not have globular heads. **b.** Side-polar nonhelical thick filaments are present in smooth muscle. In these filaments, smooth muscle myosin II molecules are staggered in parallel by two immediate neighbors and are also bound to an antiparallel partner via a short overlap at the very tip of their tails. The polarity of the myosin heads is the same along the entire length of one side of the filament and the opposite on the opposite side. There is no central "bare zone"; instead, the filament has asymmetrically tapered bare ends.

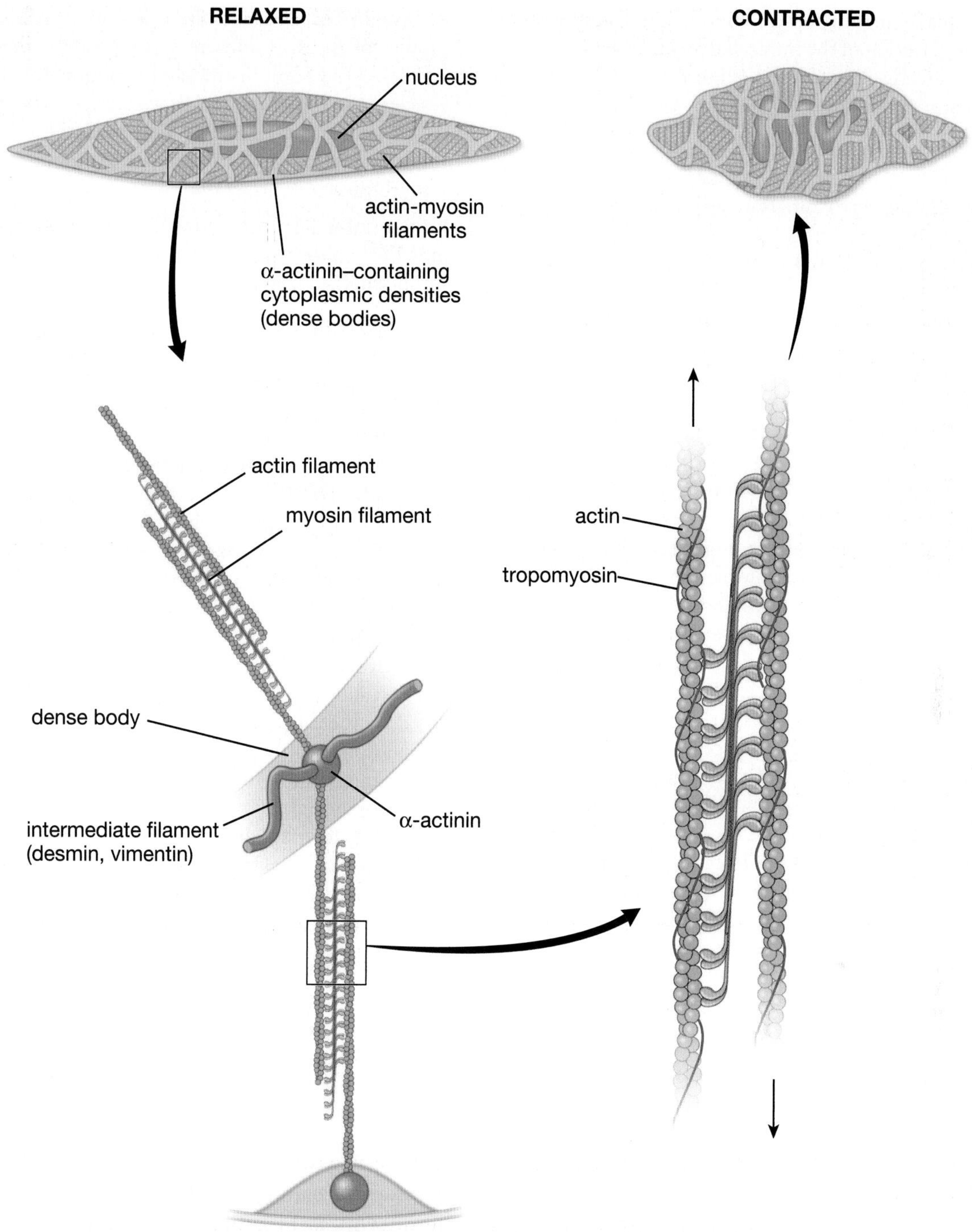

FIGURE 11.27. A suggested model for smooth muscle cell contraction. Bundles of smooth muscle myofilaments containing thin and thick filaments are shown as thin lines (*dark brown*) anchored to a network of interconnected thicker lines (*beige*) that represent cytoplasmic densities (dense bodies). They are visible in both relaxed and contracted muscle cells in the *upper part* of this figure. By following the *arrow* from relaxed cells down, the enlargement of two filaments shows the detailed arrangement of side-polar thick filaments interacting with actin thin filaments. Both myofilaments are anchored into cytoplasmic densities that are considered intracellular analogs of striated muscle Z lines. They contain the actin-binding protein α-actinin and binding sites for intermediate filaments. These densities, in turn, are anchored on the sarcolemma. Note the enlarged fragment of side-polar thick myosin filament and its interaction with actin filaments *on the right*. During the contraction cycle, both actin filaments slide in opposite directions on the myosin filament, shortening the length of the entire myofilament. Because most of the contractile myofilament bundles are oriented obliquely to the long axis of the cell, their contraction shortens the length of the cell and produces the "corkscrew" shape of the nucleus.

These links help in contraction of smooth muscle cell by stabilizing position of dense bodies and allowing inward movement of the surrounding cell membrane (altering cell shape).

Dense bodies are intracellular analogs of the striated muscle's Z lines. In support of this concept is the finding that dense bodies, although frequently appearing as small, isolated, irregular, electron-dense bodies, may also appear as irregular linear structures. In fortuitous sections, they exhibit a branching configuration consistent with a three-dimensional anastomosing network that extends from the sarcolemma into the interior of the cell (see Fig. 11.25).

Contraction in smooth muscle is initiated by a variety of impulses, including mechanical, electrical, and chemical stimuli.

The mechanisms that cause the contraction of smooth muscle cells are very different from those of striated muscle. Smooth muscle has diverse signal transduction pathways that initiate and modulate smooth muscle contraction. These pathways all lead to elevation of the intracellular concentration of Ca^{2+}, which is directly responsible for muscle contraction. Thus, muscle contraction can be triggered by the following:

- **Mechanical impulses**, such as passive stretching of vascular smooth muscle, that activate mechanosensitive ion channels, leading to initiation of spontaneous muscle contraction (myogenic reflex)
- **Electrical depolarizations**, such as those during neural stimulation of smooth muscle, that prompt the release of the neurotransmitters ACh and norepinephrine from their synaptic nerve endings and stimulate receptors located in the sarcolemmal plasma membrane, which changes the membrane potential. This causes opening of **voltage-dependent Ca^{2+} channels (VDCC)** (see later).
- **Hormonal or chemical stimuli**, such as those elicited by angiotensin II, vasopressin, or thromboxane A_2, act on specific cell membrane receptors, leading to their activation and muscle contraction. When cell membrane receptors such as **G-protein–coupled receptors (GPCR)** or **tyrosine kinase receptors (TKR)** are activated by extracellular ligands, they stimulate the synthesis of **inositol 1,4,5-trisphosphate (IP_3)**, and **diacylglycerol (DAG)**, two important second messengers in smooth muscle cells. These substances use **second messenger pathways** that do not require the generation of an action potential and cell depolarization to trigger muscle contraction. DAG opens receptor-operated Ca^{2+} channels (ROC) on the cell membrane, leading to Ca^{2+} influx. IP_3 can activate IP_3 receptors (IP_3R) on the sER membranes, stimulating Ca^{2+} release from the sER into the cytosol. The other second messenger pathway used by smooth muscle is the **nitric oxide (NO)-cGMP** pathway.

Instead of a T system, smooth muscle cells have caveolae that contain several proteins involved in the regulation of intracellular Ca^{2+}

A characteristic feature of smooth muscle cells is the presence of large numbers of **caveolae** (see Fig. 11.24). Caveolae represent invaginated microdomains of the plasma membrane rich in cholesterol and glycosphingolipids. They contain various signaling proteins and are often described as "invaginated lipid rafts." They differ from similar invaginations (i.e., coated pits that form endocytic vesicles) by the presence of **caveolin**, a 22-kDa integral membrane protein that inserts into the inner leaflet of the plasma membrane. Rather than a clathrin basket-like cage to generate vesicle-like invagination of the plasma membrane, caveolae oligomerize a caveolin scaffold to achieve the same invagination effect. In addition to numerous signaling proteins, caveolae in smooth muscle cells contain various **Ca^{2+} channels**, such as the transient receptor potential canonical (**TRPC**) channel, which allows the influx of Ca^{2+}; Na^+/Ca^{2+} exchanger (**NCX**), which removes Ca^{2+} from the cell; and **GPCR** that are involved in ligand-mediated regulation of intracellular Ca^{2+}.

Invaginated caveolae are often in proximity to sparse profiles of the sER and are surrounded by the cytoplasmic vesicles. The cell membrane invaginations, underlying vesicles, and sER function in a manner analogous to the T system of striated muscle to deliver Ca^{2+} to the cytoplasm. Intracellular Ca^{2+} concentrations are important in regulating smooth muscle contraction.

Intracellular Ca^{2+} regulation in smooth muscles involves both Ca^{2+} influx from extracellular space and sarcoplasmic reticulum Ca^{2+} release.

Several systems control intracellular Ca^{2+} concentration by regulating Ca^{2+} entry into the cell and Ca^{2+} release from sER storage sites. An influx of Ca^{2+} from the extracellular space in smooth muscle is achieved both by depolarizing the cell membrane with subsequent activation of **voltage-dependent Ca^{2+} channels (VDCC)** and by **receptor-operated Ca^{2+} channels (ROCC)** in the cell membrane. Ca^{2+} release from the sER is achieved through direct activation by second messenger molecules of **gated Ca^{2+}-release channels**, such as modified **ryanodine receptors (RyR)** and **IP_3 receptors (IP_3 R)**, both located in the sER. In the noncontracted cell, the amount of Ca^{2+} entering the cell after activation of the VDCCs is usually insufficient to initiate smooth muscle contraction and must be supplemented by the release of Ca^{2+} from the sER. The Ca^{2+} then binds to **calmodulin**, which activates the phosphorylation of **myosin light-chain kinase** to initiate contraction. After the contraction cycle commences, Ca^{2+} is removed from the sarcoplasm by **ATP-dependent calcium pumps** and sequestered in the sER or delivered to the extracellular environment.

Contraction of smooth muscle is initiated by a Ca^{2+}-mediated change in thick filaments using the calmodulin–myosin light-chain kinase system.

A modified version of the sliding filament model can explain contraction in both the striated and smooth muscles (see Fig. 11.27). As in striated muscle, contraction is initiated by an increase in the Ca^{2+} concentration in the cytosol, but the contraction does not act through a troponin–tropomyosin complex on the thin filament. Rather, in smooth muscle, an increase in Ca^{2+} concentration stimulates a **myosin light-chain kinase (MLCK)** to phosphorylate one of the two **regulatory light chains** of the **smooth muscle myosin** molecule. The Ca^{2+} binds to calmodulin to form the **Ca^{2+}–calmodulin complex**, which, in turn, binds to MLCK to activate the phosphorylation reaction of the regulatory light chain of myosin (Fig. 11.28). When the light chain is phosphorylated, smooth muscle myosin changes its conformation from inactive (folded) to active (unfolded) configuration that can assemble into **side-polar myosin filaments**.

Phosphorylation also activates the actin-binding site of the myosin head, allowing for attachment to the actin filament. In the presence of ATP, the myosin head bends, producing contraction. When it is dephosphorylated, the myosin head dissociates from actin. This phosphorylation occurs slowly, with maximum contraction often taking up to a second to achieve. In addition, dephosphorylation promotes disassembly of myosin filaments and return of myosin to its folded inactive state (see Fig. 11.28).

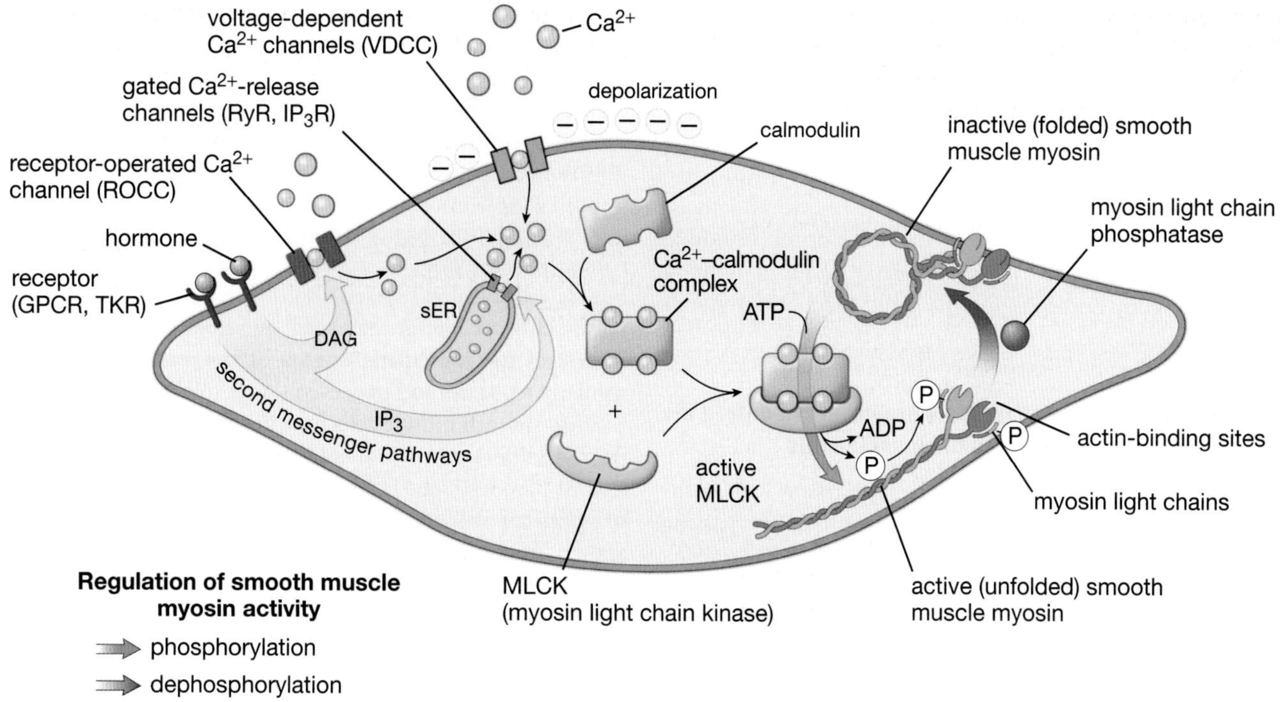

FIGURE 11.28. Schematic diagram illustrating steps leading to initiation of smooth muscle contraction. An increase in the Ca^{2+} concentration within the cytosol is necessary to initiate smooth muscle contraction. This increase is achieved either by initial depolarization of the cell membrane and activation of voltage-dependent Ca^{2+} channels (*VDCC*) or by hormonal stimulation of cell surface G-protein–coupled receptors (*GPCR*) and/or tyrosine kinase receptors (*TKR*). Activation of receptors stimulates the synthesis of inositol 1,4,5-trisphosphate (*IP_3*) and diacylglycerol (*DAG*), two important second messengers in smooth muscle cells. DAG opens receptor-operated Ca^{2+} channels (*ROC*) on the cell membrane, leading to an influx of extracellular Ca^{2+}. *IP_3* activates gated Ca^{2+}-release channels (*RyR* or *IP_3R*) on the sER membranes, stimulating Ca^{2+} release from the smooth-surfaced endoplasmic reticulum (sER) into the cytosol. Intracellular Ca^{2+} binds to calmodulin (four Ca^{2+} molecules per one molecule of calmodulin) to form the Ca^{2+}–calmodulin complex. This complex then binds to myosin light-chain kinase (*MLCK*) to phosphorylate one of the two regulatory light chains of the smooth muscle myosin molecule. When phosphorylated, the myosin changes its conformation from inactive (folded) to active (unfolded), which allows its assembly into side-polar filaments. The actin-binding site on the myosin head is activated, allowing it to attach to the actin filament. In the presence of adenosine triphosphate (ATP), the myosin head bends, producing contraction. Dephosphorylation of smooth muscle myosin molecules by myosin light chain promotes disassembly of myosin filaments. *ADP*, adenosine diphosphate.

Smooth muscle myosin hydrolyzes ATP at about 10% of the rate of skeletal muscle, producing a slow cross-bridging cycle that results in slow contraction of these cells. Thus, smooth muscle cells and nonmuscle cells that contract by this same mechanism are capable of sustained contractions over long periods of time while using only 10% of the ATP that would be used by a striated muscle cell performing the same work.

The force of smooth muscle contraction may be maintained for long periods in a "latch state."

In addition to normal phosphorylation of the regulatory light chains of myosin, smooth muscle cells possess a secondary mechanism that allows them to maintain long-term contraction with minimal expenditure of ATP. This mechanism is detected in vascular smooth muscles, for example, and is used to maintain the force of contraction (tone of blood vessels) for an extended time. This so-called **latch state** of smooth muscle contraction occurs after the initial Ca^{2+}-dependent myosin phosphorylation. The myosin head attached to the actin molecule becomes dephosphorylated, causing its ATPase activity to decrease. As a result of the decrease in ATPase activity, the myosin head is unable to detach from the actin filament, which maintains the contracted state. The latch state is comparable in many ways to rigor mortis in striated muscle.

Functional Aspects of Smooth Muscle

Smooth muscle is specialized for slow, prolonged contraction.

As noted previously, smooth muscle cells may enter the latch state and remain contracted for long periods of time without fatiguing. They may contract in a wave-like manner, producing peristaltic movements such as those in the gastrointestinal tract and the male genital tract, or contraction may occur along the entire muscle, producing extrusive movements (e.g., those in the urinary bladder, gallbladder, and uterus). Smooth muscle exhibits a **spontaneous contractile activity** in the absence of nerve stimuli.

Contraction of smooth muscle is usually regulated by postsynaptic neurons of the **autonomic nervous system (ANS)**; most smooth muscle is directly innervated by both sympathetic and parasympathetic nerves. In the gastrointestinal tract, the third component of the ANS, the **enteric division**, is the primary source of nerves to the muscular layers.

Although Ca^{2+} enters the cytoplasm during depolarization by **voltage-dependent Ca^{2+} channels (VDCC)**, some Ca^{2+} channels, called **receptor-operated Ca^{2+} channels (RyR, IP_3R)**, are activated by hormones via their second messenger pathways (see Fig. 11.28). Thus, smooth muscle contraction may also be initiated by certain hormones secreted from the posterior pituitary gland (e.g., oxytocin and, to a lesser extent, antidiuretic hormone [ADH]). **Oxytocin** is a potent stimulator of smooth muscle contraction, and its release by the posterior lobe of the pituitary gland plays an essential role in uterine contraction during parturition. It is often used to induce or enhance labor. In addition to oxytocin, smooth muscle cells may be stimulated or inhibited by hormones secreted by the adrenal medulla (e.g., epinephrine and norepinephrine). Various peptide secretions from enteroendocrine cells also stimulate or inhibit smooth muscle contraction, particularly in the alimentary canal and its associated organs.

Nerve terminals in smooth muscle are observed only in the connective tissue adjacent to the muscle cells.

Nerve fibers pass through the connective tissue within the bundles of smooth muscle cells; enlargements in the passing nerve fiber, or **boutons en passant** (see page 397), occur adjacent to the muscle cells to be innervated. The enlargements contain synaptic vesicles with neuromuscular transmitters. However, the neuromuscular site is not comparable to the neuromuscular junction of striated muscle. Rather, a considerable distance, usually 10–20 μm (in some locations, up to 200 μm), may separate the nerve terminal and the smooth muscle. The neurotransmitter released by the nerve terminal must diffuse across this distance to reach the muscle.

Not all smooth muscle cells are exposed directly to the neurotransmitter, however. As discussed earlier, smooth muscle cells make contact with neighboring cells by **gap junctions**. As in cardiac muscle, contraction is propagated from cell to cell via gap junctions, thus producing coordinated activity within a smooth muscle bundle or layer. The gap junction between two smooth muscle cells was originally designated a **nexus**, a term still in use.

Smooth muscle cells also secrete connective tissue matrix.

Smooth muscle cells have organelles typical of secretory cells. A well-developed rER and Golgi apparatus are found in the perinuclear zone. Smooth muscle cells synthesize both **type IV (basal lamina) collagen and type III (reticular) collagen** as well as elastin, proteoglycans, and multiadhesive glycoproteins. Except at the gap junctions, smooth muscle cells are surrounded by an **external lamina**. In some locations, such as the walls of blood vessels and the uterus, smooth muscle cells secrete large amounts of both type I collagen and elastin.

Renewal, Repair, and Differentiation

Smooth muscle cells are capable of dividing to maintain or increase their numbers.

Smooth muscle cells may respond to injury by undergoing mitosis. In addition, smooth muscle contains regularly replicating populations of cells. Smooth muscle in the uterus proliferates during the normal menstrual cycle and during pregnancy; both activities are under hormonal control. The smooth muscle cells of blood vessels also divide regularly in the adult, presumably to replace damaged or senile cells; the smooth muscle of the muscularis externa of the stomach and colon regularly replicates and may even slowly thicken during life.

New smooth muscle cells have been shown to differentiate from undifferentiated mesenchymal stem cells in the adventitia of blood vessels. **Differentiation of smooth muscle progenitor cells** is regulated by a variety of intracellular and environmental stimuli, and developing muscles exhibit a wide range of different phenotypes at different stages of their development. To date, no transcription factors have been identified that are characteristic for the smooth muscle cell lineage. However, **serum response factor (RF)**, a member of the MADS–box transcription factor family, has been shown to regulate most smooth muscle differentiation marker genes. Smooth muscle cells have also been shown to develop from the division and differentiation of endothelial cells and pericytes during the repair process after vascular injury.

Vascular pericytes are located within the basal lamina of capillaries and postcapillary venules. They function as multipotential mesenchymal progenitor cells. In capillaries, their cytoplasmic morphology is difficult to distinguish from that of the endothelial cell. In postcapillary venules and pericytic venules, they may form a nearly complete investment of the vessel with cells that resemble smooth muscle cells (see Chapter 6, Connective Tissue, pages 205-206 and Chapter 13, Cardiovascular System, pages 465-466).

Fibroblasts in healing wounds may develop morphologic and functional characteristics of smooth muscle cells (**myofibroblasts**; see page 198). Epithelial cells in numerous locations, particularly sweat glands, mammary glands, salivary glands, lacrimal glands, and the iris of the eye, may acquire the characteristics of smooth muscle cells (**myoepithelial cells**). **Myoid cells** of the testis have a contractile function in the seminiferous tubules, and cells of the **perineurium**, a concentric layer of connective tissue that surrounds groups of nerve fibers and partitions peripheral nerves into distinct fascicles, function as contractile cells as well as transport barrier cells.

FOLDER 11.4

FUNCTIONAL CONSIDERATIONS: COMPARISON OF THE THREE MUSCLE TYPES

Cardiac muscle shares structural and functional characteristics with skeletal muscle and smooth muscle. In both cardiac and skeletal muscles, the contractile elements—thick and thin filaments—are organized into sarcomeres surrounded by smooth-surfaced endoplasmic reticulum (sER) and mitochondria. Both cardiac and smooth muscle cells retain their individuality, although both are in functional communication with their neighbors through gap junctions. In addition, cardiac and smooth muscle cells have a spontaneous beat that is regulated, but not initiated, by autonomic or hormonal stimuli. Both have centrally located nuclei and perinuclear organelles. These common characteristics suggest that cardiac muscle may have evolved in the direction of skeletal muscle from the smooth muscle of primitive circulatory systems. A summary of major characteristics of all three muscle types is provided in the following table.

FOLDER 11.4

FUNCTIONAL CONSIDERATIONS: COMPARISON OF THE THREE MUSCLE TYPES (*continued*)

Comparison of the Three Muscle Types

	Skeletal 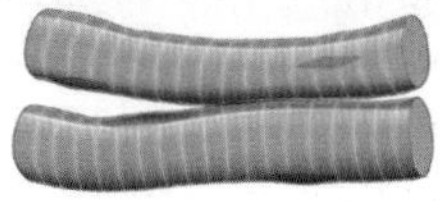	**Cardiac** 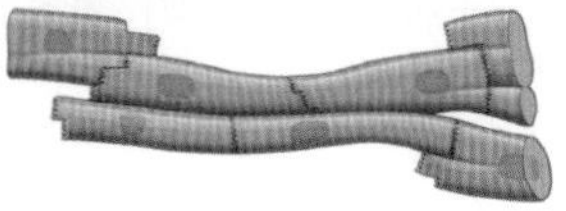	**Smooth** 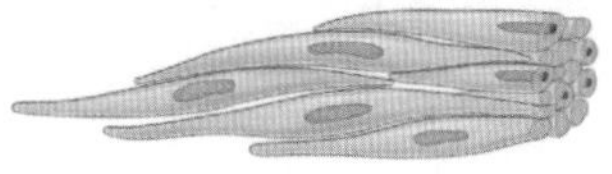
Structural features			
Muscle cell	Large, elongated cell, 10–100 μm in diameter, up to 100 cm in length (sartorius muscle)	Short, narrow cell, 10–100 μm in diameter, 80–100 μm in length	Short, elongated, fusiform cell, 0.2–2 μm in diameter, 20–200 μm in length
Location	Muscles of skeleton, visceral striated (e.g., tongue, esophagus, diaphragm)	Heart, superior and inferior venae cavae, pulmonary veins	Vessels, organs, and viscera
Structural features			
Connective tissue components	Epimysium, perimysium, endomysium	Endomysium, subendocardial and subpericardial connective tissue	Endomysium, sheaths, and bundles
Fiber	Single skeletal muscle cell	Linear branched arrangement of several cardiac muscle cells	Single smooth muscle cell
Sarcomere	Present	Present	None
Striation	Present	Present	None
Nucleus	Many peripheral	Single central, surrounded by juxtanuclear region	Single central
T tubules	Present at A–I junction (triad: with two terminal cisternae), two T tubules/sarcomere	Present at Z lines (diad: with small terminal cisternae), one T tubule/sarcomere; Purkinje fibers have less number of T tubules.	None, well-developed sER, many invaginations (caveolae) and cytoplasmic vesicles
Cell-to-cell junctions	None	Intercalated discs containing 1. Fasciae adherentes 2. Macula adherens (desmosome) 3. Gap junctions	Gap junctions (nexus)
Special features	Well-developed sER and T tubules	Intercalated discs, Purkinje fibers	Dense bodies, desmin and vimentin filaments, caveolae, and cytoplasmic vesicles
Functions			
Type of innervation	Voluntary	Involuntary	Involuntary
Efferent innervation	Somatic	Autonomic	Autonomic
Type of contraction	"All or none" (type I and type II fibers)	"All or none" rhythmic (pacemakers, conductive system of the heart)	Slow, partial, rhythmic, spontaneous contractions (pacemakers of stomach)
Regulation of contraction	By binding of Ca^{2+} to TnC, causes tropomyosin movement and exposes myosin-binding sites on actin filaments	By binding of Ca^{2+} to TnC, causes tropomyosin movement and exposes myosin-binding sites on actin filaments	By phosphorylation of myosin light chain by myosin light-chain kinase in the presence of Ca^{2+}–calmodulin complex
Growth and regeneration			
Mitosis	None	None (in normal condition)	Present
Response to demand	Hypertrophy	Hypertrophy	Hypertrophy and hyperplasia
Regeneration	Limited (satellite cells and myogenic cells from bone marrow)	None (in normal condition)	Present

sER, smooth-surfaced endoplasmic reticulum; *TnC*, troponin-C.

HISTOLOGY 101 NOTEBOOK

MUSCLE TISSUE

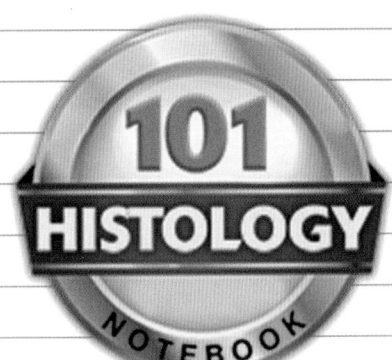

OVERVIEW OF MUSCLE TISSUE

- **Muscle tissue** is responsible for movement of the body and produces changes in the size and shape of internal organs.
- There are three major types of muscle tissue: **skeletal**, **cardiac**, and **smooth muscle**.

SKELETAL MUSCLE

- **Skeletal muscle** cells called skeletal muscle **fibers** are long, cylindrical, multinucleated syncytia with diameters from 10 to 100 μm.
- Skeletal muscle fibers are held together by connective tissue. **Endomysium** surrounds individual fibers, **perimysium** surrounds a group of fibers to form a **fascicle**, and **epimysium** is dense connective tissue that surrounds the entire muscle.
- Three **types of skeletal muscle fibers** are distinguished based on contractile speed, enzymatic velocity, and metabolic profile. The three types of fibers are **red (type I, slow oxidative)**, **intermediate (type IIa, fast oxidative glycolytic)**, and **white (type IIb, fast glycolytic)**.
- The structural and functional subunit of the muscle fiber is **myofibril**. It is composed of precisely aligned **myofilaments**: myosin-containing **thick filaments** and actin-containing **thin filaments**. The smallest contractile unit of striated muscle is **sarcomere**.
- The arrangement of **thick** and **thin filaments** gives rise to the density differences that produce the cross-striations of the myofibril. The light-staining isotropic **I band** contains mainly thin filaments attached to both sides of the Z line, and the dark-staining anisotropic **A band** contains mainly thick filaments.
- **Thick filaments** primarily consist of **myosin II molecules**; **thin filaments** are composed of **actin** and two major regulatory proteins (**tropomyosin** and **troponin**).
- **Z lines** located between sarcomeres contain an actin-binding protein (**α-actinin**) and Z matrix proteins.
- The **actomyosin cross-bridge cycle** represents a series of coupled biochemical and mechanical events between myosin heads and actin molecules that lead to muscle contraction. There are five recognizable stages of the cycle: **attachment**, **release**, **bending**, **force generation**, and **reattachment**.
- Regulation of muscle contraction involves Ca^{2+}, sarcoplasmic reticulum, and the transverse tubular system.
- The **sarcoplasmic reticulum** forms enlarged **terminal cisternae** that serve as reservoirs for Ca^{2+}. Their plasma membrane contains an abundance of **gated Ca^{2+}-release channels (ryanodine receptors [RyR1])**.
- **Transverse tubules (T tubules)** are formed by invaginations of the sarcoplasm that penetrate the muscle fiber between the adjacent terminal cisternae. They have an abundance of **voltage-sensor proteins (dihydropyridine-sensitive receptors [DHSRs])**.
- The T tubule and the two adjacent terminal cisternae are called a **triad**. Triads are located at the junction between A and I bands (two per each sarcomere).
- The depolarization of the **T-tubule** membrane triggers the release of Ca^{2+} from the terminal cisternae to initiate muscle contraction by binding to the troponin–tropomyosin complex.
- **Muscle relaxation** results from a decrease in cytosolic-free Ca^{2+} concentration.
- The **neuromuscular junction** (motor end plate) is the contact area of the axon endings with muscle fiber. The axon terminal contains the neurotransmitter **acetylcholine (ACh)**.
- Release of ACh into the synaptic cleft of the neuromuscular junction initiates depolarization of the plasma membrane, which leads to muscle contraction.
- Encapsulated **muscle spindles** and **Golgi tendon organs** are sensory (proprioceptive) stretch receptors in muscles and tendons.

CARDIAC MUSCLE

- **Cardiac muscle** is striated and has the same type and arrangement of contractile filaments as skeletal muscle.
- **Cardiac muscle cells** (cardiac myocytes) are short cylindrical cells with a centrally positioned single nucleus. They are attached to each other by intercalated discs to form a cardiac muscle fiber.
- The **intercalated discs** represent highly specialized cell-to-cell adhesion junctions containing **fascia adherens, gap junctions**, and **maculae adherentes** (desmosomes).
- **Terminal cisternae** are much smaller than in skeletal muscle and with the T tubules form **diads** that are located at the level of the Z line (one per sarcomere).
- Passage of Ca^{2+} from the lumen of the T tubule to the sarcoplasm of a cardiac myocyte is essential to initiate the contraction cycle.
- Specialized **cardiac-conducting muscle cells (Purkinje fibers)** exhibit a spontaneous rhythmic contraction. They generate and rapidly transmit action potentials to various parts of the myocardium.
- The **autonomic nervous system** regulates the rate of cardiac muscle contraction.

SMOOTH MUSCLE

- **Smooth muscle** generally occurs as bundles or sheets of small, elongated fusiform cells (called **fibers**) with finely tapered ends. They are specialized for slow, prolonged contractions.
- **Smooth muscle cells** possess a contractile apparatus of thin and thick filaments and a cytoskeleton of desmin and vimentin intermediate filaments. Smooth muscle myosin assembles into **side-polar myosin thick filament.**
- They do not form sarcomeres and do not exhibit striations.
- **Thin filaments** contain actin, tropomyosin (a smooth muscle isoform), caldesmon, and calponin. **No troponin** is associated with smooth muscle tropomyosin.
- Thin filaments are attached to cytoplasmic densities or **dense bodies**, which contain **α-actinin** and are located throughout the sarcoplasm and close to the sarcolemma.
- **Contraction** of smooth muscle is triggered by a variety of impulses, including mechanical (passive stretching), electrical (depolarization at nerve endings), and chemical (hormones acting by a second messenger) stimuli.
- Because smooth muscle cells lack T tubules, Ca^{2+} is delivered by **caveolae** and cytoplasmic vesicles.
- Contraction of smooth muscle is initiated by activation of **myosin light-chain kinase (MLCK)** by the **Ca^{2+}–calmodulin complex.**

DEVELOPMENT, REPAIR, HEALING, AND RENEWAL

- **Myoblasts** are derived from multipotential myogenic stem cells that originate in the mesoderm. Early in development, these cells express **MyoD transcription factor**, which plays a key role in activation of muscle-specific gene expressions and differentiation of all skeletal muscle lineages.
- Repair of skeletal muscle and its regeneration can occur from multipotential myogenic stem cells called **satellite cells.** These cells are left over from fetal development and express **Pax7 transcription factor.**
- After muscle tissue injury, satellite cells are activated. They coexpress Pax7 with MyoD to become myogenic precursors of skeletal muscle cells.
- Injury to **cardiac muscle** tissue results in death of cardiac myocytes. Cardiac muscle is repaired with fibrous connective tissue.
- **Smooth muscle** cells are capable of dividing to maintain or increase their number and size.

PLATE 11.1 ■ SKELETAL MUSCLE I

Muscle tissue is classified on the basis of the appearance of its contractile cells. Two major types are recognized: striated muscle, in which the cells exhibit a cross-striation pattern when observed at the light microscope level, and smooth muscle, in which the cells lack striations. Striated muscle is further subclassified based on location, namely, skeletal muscle, visceral striated muscle, and cardiac muscle. Skeletal muscle is attached to bone and is responsible for movement of the axial and appendicular skeleton and for maintenance of body position and posture. Visceral striated muscle is morphologically identical but is restricted to soft tissues, including the tongue, pharynx, upper part of the esophagus, and diaphragm. Cardiac muscle is a type of striated muscle found in the heart and at the base of the large veins that empty into the heart.

The cross-striations in striated muscle are due to the organization of the contractile elements that occur in the muscle cell, namely, thin filaments composed largely of the protein actin and thick filaments composed of the protein myosin II. The two types of myofilaments occupy the bulk of the cytoplasm. The skeletal and visceral striated muscle cells, more commonly called *fibers*, are a multinucleated syncytium formed during development by the fusion of individual small muscle cells called *myoblasts*.

Surrounding each fiber is a delicate mesh of collagen fibrils referred to as *endomysium*. In turn, bundles of muscle fibers that form functional units within a muscle are surrounded by a thicker connective tissue layer. This connective tissue is referred to as *perimysium*. Lastly, a sheath of dense connective tissue that surrounds the muscle is referred to as *epimysium*. The force generated by individual muscle fibers is transferred to the collagenous elements of each of these connective tissue elements to end in a tendon.

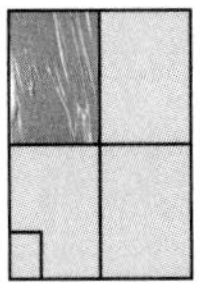

Skeletal muscle, human, hematoxylin and eosin (H&E) ×33.

This low-power micrograph shows a longitudinal section of striated muscle. The muscle tissue within the muscle is arranged in a series of **fascicles** (*F*). The individual muscle fibers within a fascicle are in close proximity to one another, but are not individually discernible. However, the small, blue dot-like structures are the nuclei of the fibers. Between the fascicles, although difficult to see at this magnification, is connective tissue, the **perimysium** (*P*). A nerve (*Nv*) is also evident in the micrograph.

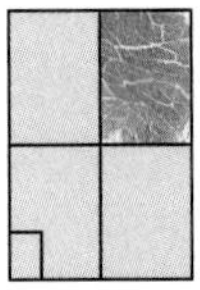

Skeletal muscle, human, H&E ×33.

This micrograph reveals part of a muscle that has been cut in cross section. Again, individual bundles of muscle fibers or **fascicles** (*F*) can be readily identified. In contrast to the previous micrograph, even at this low magnification, upon careful examination, individual **muscle fibers** (*MF*) can be identified in many of the fascicles. Each is bounded by connective tissue, which constitutes the **perimysium** (*P*). Also identifiable in this micrograph is a dense connective tissue surrounding the muscle, namely, **epimysium** (*E*).

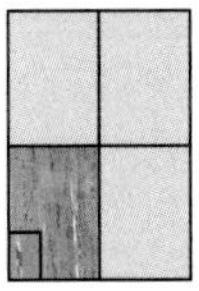

Skeletal muscle, human, H&E ×256; inset ×700.

This higher magnification of a longitudinal section of a muscle reveals two **muscle fascicles** (*F*). At this magnification, the cross-banding pattern is just perceptible. With few exceptions, the nuclei (*N*), which tend to run in linear arrays, belong to individual muscle fibers. Also evident in this micrograph is a small blood vessel (*BV*). The *inset*, taken from a glutaraldehyde-fixed, plastic-embedded specimen, is a much higher magnification of a portion of two muscle fibers. The major bands are readily identifiable at this magnification and degree of specimen preservation. The thick, dark-stained band is the A band. Between A bands is a lightly stained area, the I band, which is bisected by the Z line. The two elongated nuclei (*N*) belong to the muscle fibers. Below them are a capillary (*C*) and a portion of an endothelial cell nucleus (*End*). At this higher magnification, the endothelial nuclei, as well as the nuclei of the fibroblasts, can be distinguished from the muscle cell nuclei by their smaller size and heterochromatin, giving them a dark stain. The muscle cell nuclei (*N*) exhibit more euchromatin with a speckling of heterochromatin, thus giving them a lighter staining appearance.

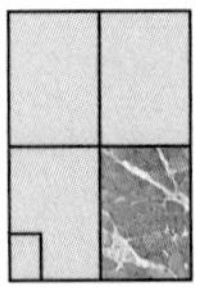

Skeletal muscle, human, H&E ×256.

In this cross section, individual **muscle fibers** (*MF*) are more readily discernible than individual muscle fibers in longitudinal sections. For example, if one imagines a cut crossing a number of cells (see *dashed line*), the close proximity of the muscle cells can mask the boundary between individual cells within a fascicle when observed in the opposite or longitudinal plane. The **connective tissue** (*CT*) that is readily apparent here belongs to the perimysium, which separates fascicles. The nuclei of the individual fibers are located at the periphery of the cell. At this magnification, it is difficult to distinguish between occasional fibroblasts that belong to the endomysium from the nuclei of the muscle cells.

BV, blood vessel
C, capillary
CT, connective tissue
E, epimysium
End, endothelial cell nucleus
F, fascicle
MF, muscle fibers
N, nuclei
Nv, nerve
P, perimysium

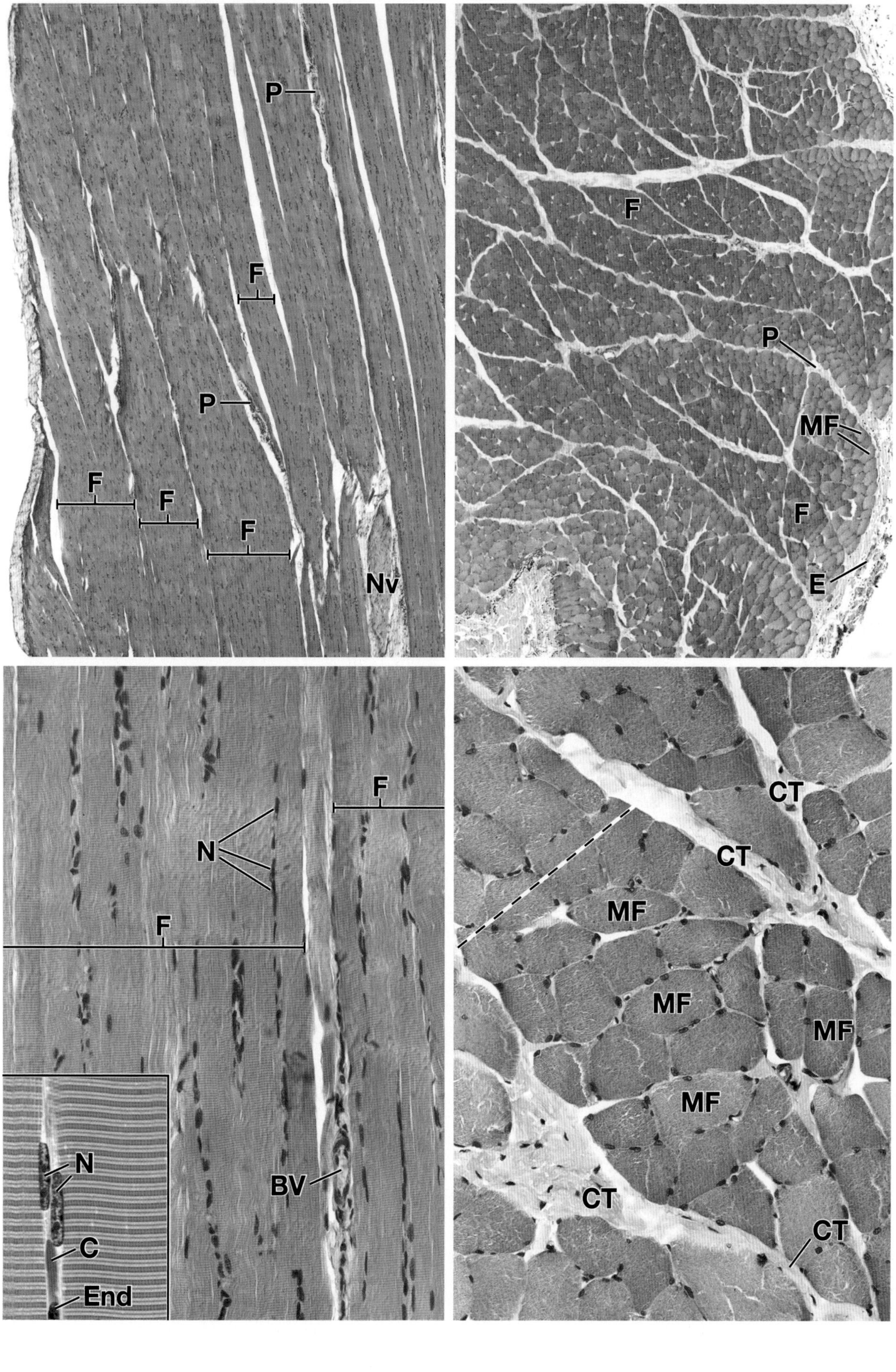
P
F
P
F
F
F
Nv
F
P
MF
F
E
F
N
F
N
C
End
BV
CT
CT
MF
MF
MF
MF
CT
CT

PLATE 11.2 ■ SKELETAL MUSCLE II AND ELECTRON MICROSCOPY

The **myofibril** is the structural and functional subunit of a muscle fiber containing **sarcomeres**. Myofibrils are best seen at higher magnification in the light microscope in a cross section of the cell where they appear as dot-like structures. The overall effect is a stippled appearance of the cytoplasm. Each myofibril is composed of two types of myofilaments arranged in sarcomeres: (1) the myosin II thick filament and (2) actin and its associated proteins that make up the thin filaments. It is the arrangement of the thick and thin filaments that produce density differences that, in turn, create the cross-striations of the myofibril when viewed in longitudinal section. The site of overlap of thin and thick filaments produces the dark A band. The light-appearing I band contains thin filaments. Careful examination of the A band in the light microscope reveals a light-staining area in the middle of the A band. This is referred to as the *H band*, which is occupied by thick filaments and is devoid of thin filaments. At the middle of each I band is the thin, dense Z line to which the thin filaments are attached.

The distance between Z lines is referred to as a *sarcomere*. When a muscle contracts, the sarcomere and I band shorten. The filaments, however, maintain a constant length. In this way, muscle contraction is produced by an increase in the overlap between the two filament types.

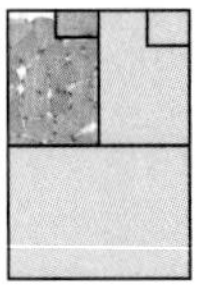

Skeletal muscle, human, hematoxylin and eosin (H&E) ×512; inset ×985.

This micrograph reveals a cross section of a muscle fascicle. The individual **muscle fibers** (*MF*) exhibit a polygonal shape but vary only slightly in width. Of the many nuclei that can be observed in this plane of section, only some belong to the muscle fibers. The muscle fiber nuclei (*MFN*) appear to be embedded within the extreme periphery of the fiber. In contrast, fibroblast nuclei (*FN*) that belong to the endomysium lie clearly outside the muscle fiber, are typically smaller, and exhibit a greater density than the nuclei of the muscle fibers. Also present between the muscle fibers are capillaries (*C*). The endothelial cell nuclei (*ECN*) are also relatively dense. Other nuclei that may be present but are very difficult to identify belong to satellite cells. The *inset*, which shows the *boxed area*, reveals several nuclei, two of which belong to the muscle fibers (*MF*). The small, very dense nucleus (*FN*) probably belongs to a fibroblast of the endomysium. Also clearly evident here is a cross-sectioned capillary (*C*). The more striking feature at this magnification is the appearance of the muscle cells' myofibrils, which appear as punctate or dot-like structures.

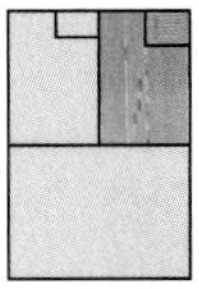

Skeletal muscle, human, H&E ×512; inset ×985.

This micrograph, a longitudinal section of a glutaraldehyde-fixed, plastic-embedded specimen reveals four **muscle fibers** (*MF*). Although they appear to be markedly different in width, the difference is due mainly to the plane of section through each of the fibers. Because the nuclei of the muscle fibers are located at the periphery of the cell, their location is variable when observed in a longitudinal section. For example, three nuclei (*N*) are seen in what appears to be a central location of a fiber. This is due to the section grazing the periphery of this fiber. The clear space at either end of two of these nuclei represents the cytoplasmic portion of the cell that contains organelles and is devoid of myofibrils. Other muscle fiber nuclei (*MFN*) can be seen at the periphery of the fibers. Note that they exhibit a similar chromatin pattern as the three nuclei previously described. Also present in this micrograph is a **capillary** (*C*) coursing along the *center* of the micrograph. In this plane of section, it is difficult to clearly distinguish between the endothelial cell nuclei and the nuclei of fibroblasts in the endomysium. Perhaps, the most significant feature of a longitudinal section of a muscle fiber is the striations that they exhibit. The *inset* shows the banding pattern of the muscle fiber at higher magnification. The dark-staining lines represent the A band. The light-staining area is the I band, which is bisected by the dark-staining Z line.

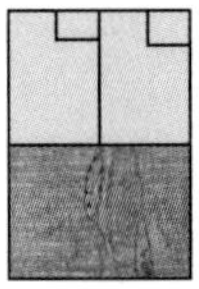

Skeletal muscle, human, electron micrograph ×5,000.

The low-power electron micrograph shown here should be compared to the previous *inset* of the longitudinally sectioned muscle fibers. It reveals portions of three **muscle fibers** (*MF*), two of which exhibit a nucleus (*N*). Between cells, various amounts of collagenous fibers are present, representing the **endomysium** (*E*). The micrograph illustrates the banding pattern of the **myofibrils** (*My*) to advantage. In contrast to the longitudinally sectioned muscle in the previous *inset*, individual myofibrils (*My*) can be identified in this electron micrograph. They correspond to the dot-like structures seen in the previous *inset* of the cross-sectioned muscle fibers. Note that adjacent myofibrils are aligned with one another with respect to their banding pattern and also that they exhibit different widths. Each muscle fibril is essentially a cylindrical structure much like a dowel; thus, when sectioned in a longitudinal plane, the width of each myofibril will vary depending on what portion of the cylindrical structure has been cut.

C, capillaries
E, endomysium
ECN, endothelial cell nuclei
FN, fibroblast nuclei
MF, muscle fiber
MFN, muscle fiber nuclei
My, myofibril
N, nucleus

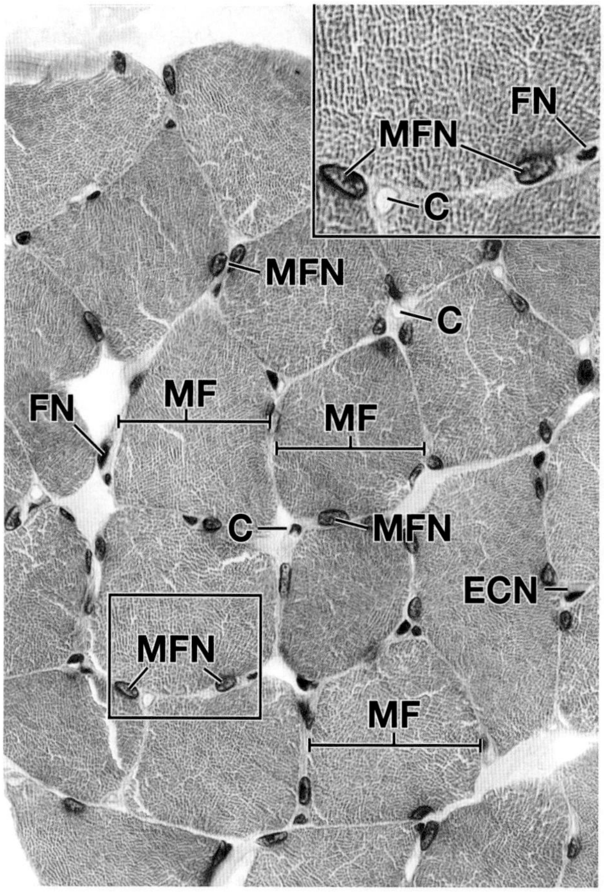
FN
MFN
C
MFN
C
FN
MF
MF
C
MFN
ECN
MFN
MF

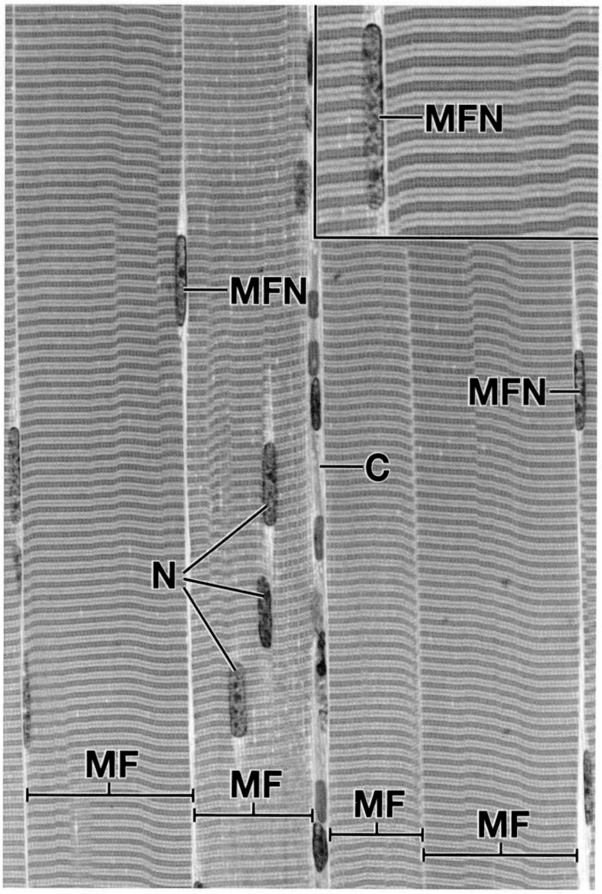
MFN
MFN
MFN
C
N
MF
MF
MF
MF

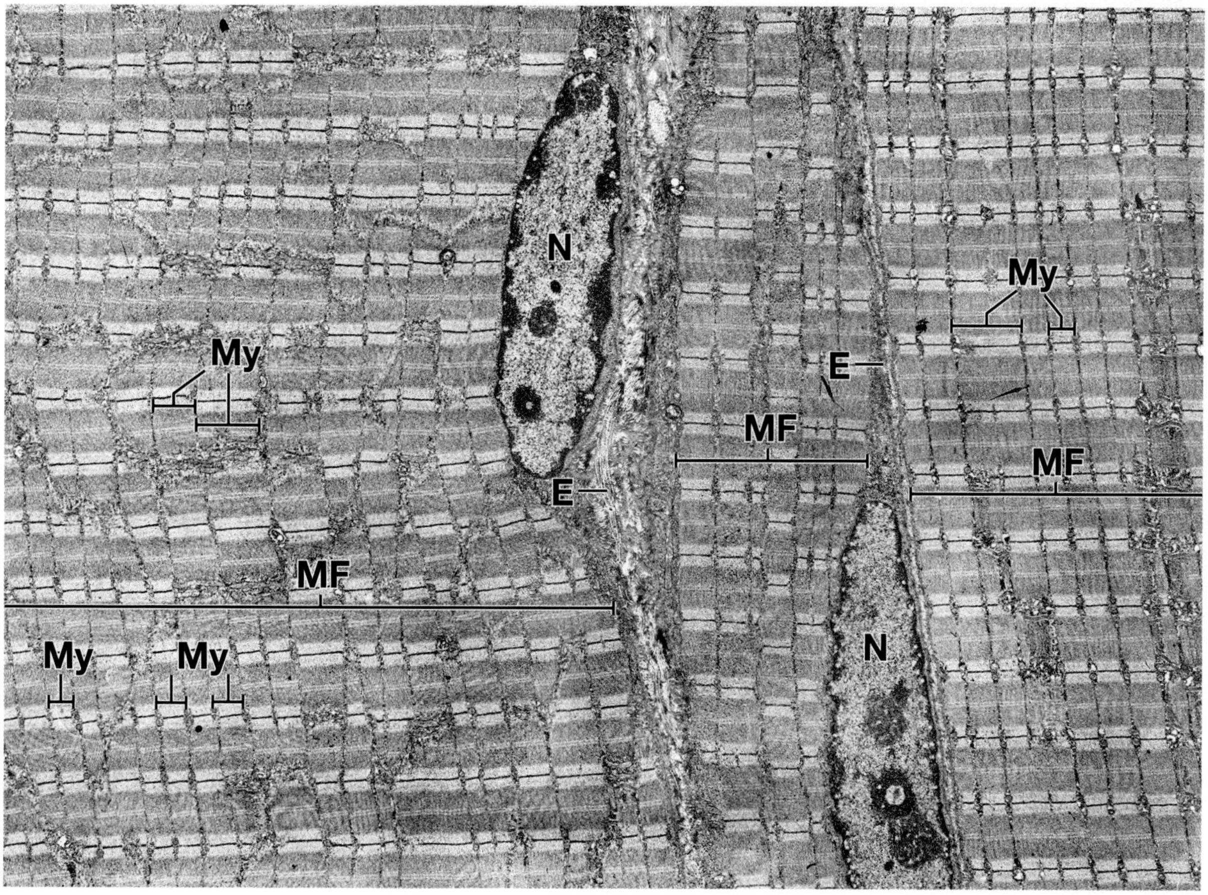
N
My
My
E
MF
E
MF
MF
My
My
N

PLATE 11.3 ■ MYOTENDINOUS JUNCTION

The force generated by skeletal muscle to allow body movement is transmitted through tendons to which the muscle fibers are attached. The site of attachment between a muscle fiber and the collagen of the tendon is referred to as the **myotendinous junction.** The muscle fibers at the junction site end in numerous finger-like cytoplasmic projections to increase the contact area of muscle and tendon. At the ends of each projection and between these projections, the collagen fibrils of the tendon attach to the cell at its basal lamina (see Electron Micrograph on this plate). In the light microscope, these finger-like projections appear to merge into the tendon. The detailed relationship is seen at the electron microscope level. The last sarcomeres in the muscle fiber end where the finger-like projections begin. At this point, the ending sarcomere lacks its Z line and the actin filaments from the A band continue into the cytoplasmic fingers ending at the sarcolemma.

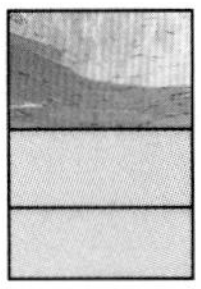

Myotendinous junction, monkey, hematoxylin and eosin (H&E) ×365.

This light micrograph reveals a **tendon** (*T*) and adjacent to it are several **muscle fibers** (*MF*). The tendon contains dispersed tendinocytes whose nuclei (*N*) are compressed between the collagenous bundles of the tendon. Several of the muscle fibers (*MF′*) are seen at the point where they terminate and are attached to the tendon fibers. The area in the *rectangle* is seen in higher magnification in the micrograph that follows.

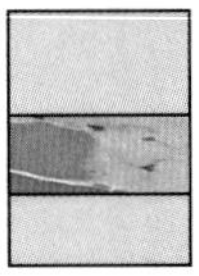

Myotendinous junction, monkey, H&E ×1,560.

The **muscle fiber** (*MF*) in this micrograph is seen at the point where it ends. Note the banding pattern of the muscle fiber. At this magnification, the finger-like projections (*arrows*) at the end of the muscle fiber are clearly seen. Between the finger-like structures are the collagen fibers of the tendon. The nuclei of the tendinocytes (*Tc*) are seen in the tendon where it continues from the muscle fiber.

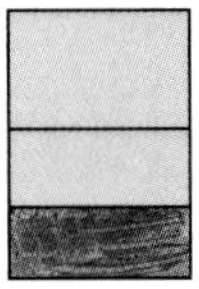

Myotendinous junction, monkey, electron micrograph ×24,000.

This electron micrograph shows the end of part of a muscle. Note that the last **sarcomere** (*S*) lacks a Z line. The actin filaments appear to extend from the A band and continue along the length of the finger projections and seemingly attach to the sarcolemma. Between the finger projections are the **collagen fibrils** (*arrows*) that make up the tendon. (Courtesy of Dr. Douglas Kelly.)

MF, muscle fibers **MF′,** terminating muscle fibers	**N,** nuclei **S,** sarcomere	**T,** tendon **Tc,** tendinocytes

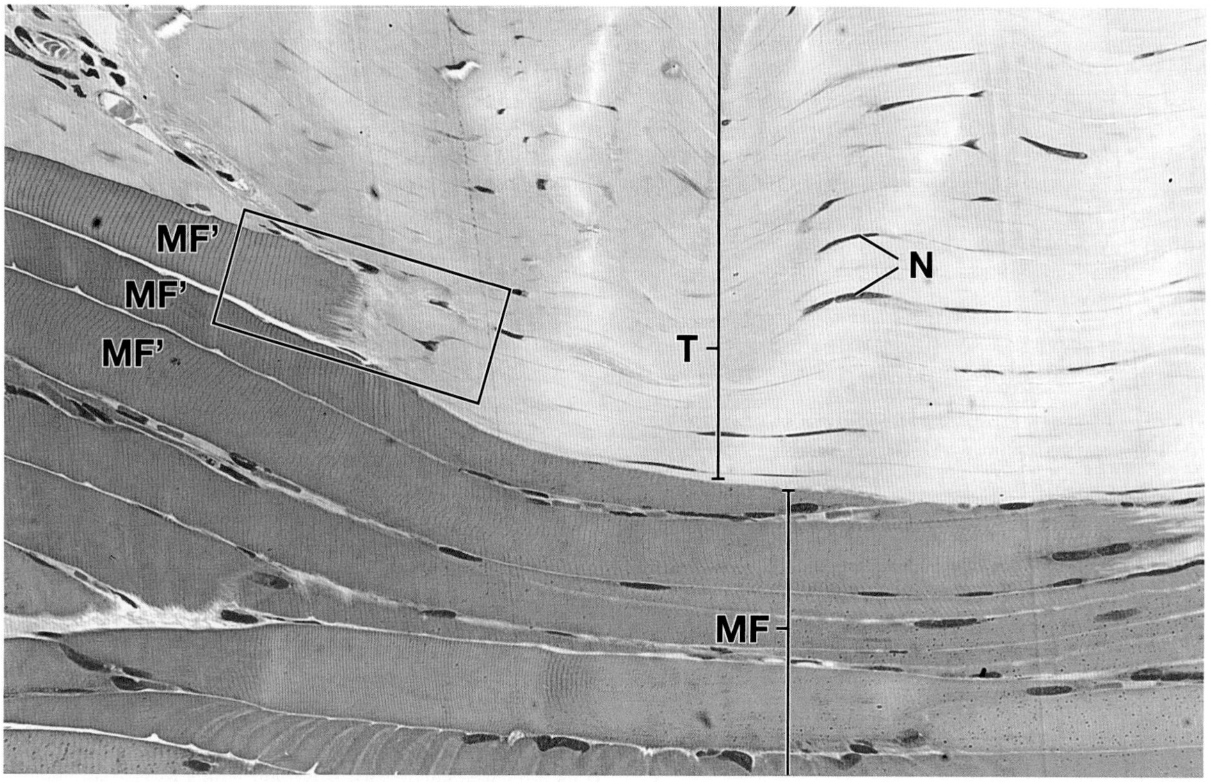
MF'
MF'
MF'
N
T
MF

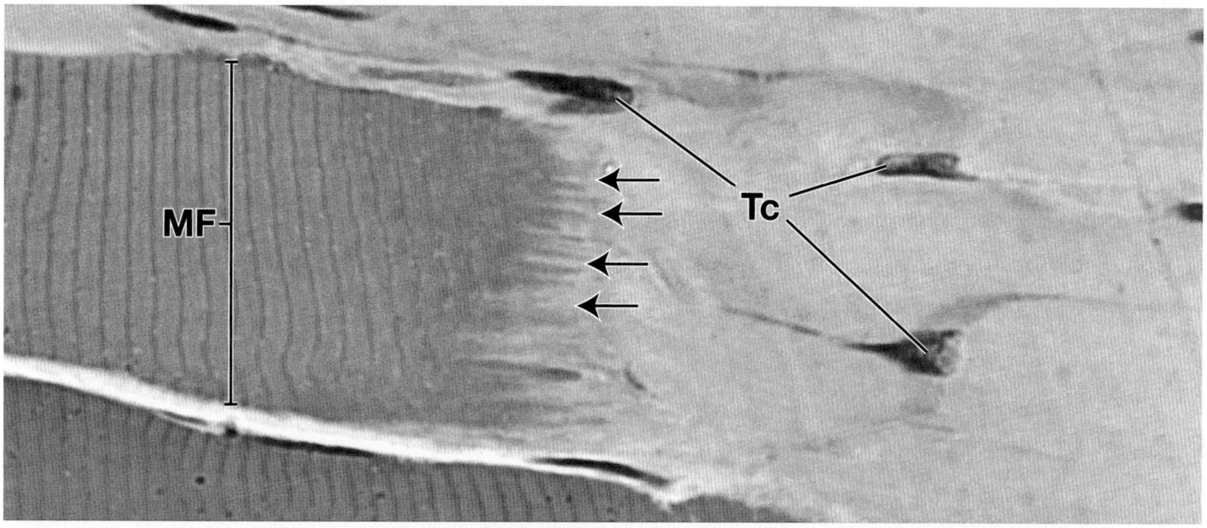
MF
Tc

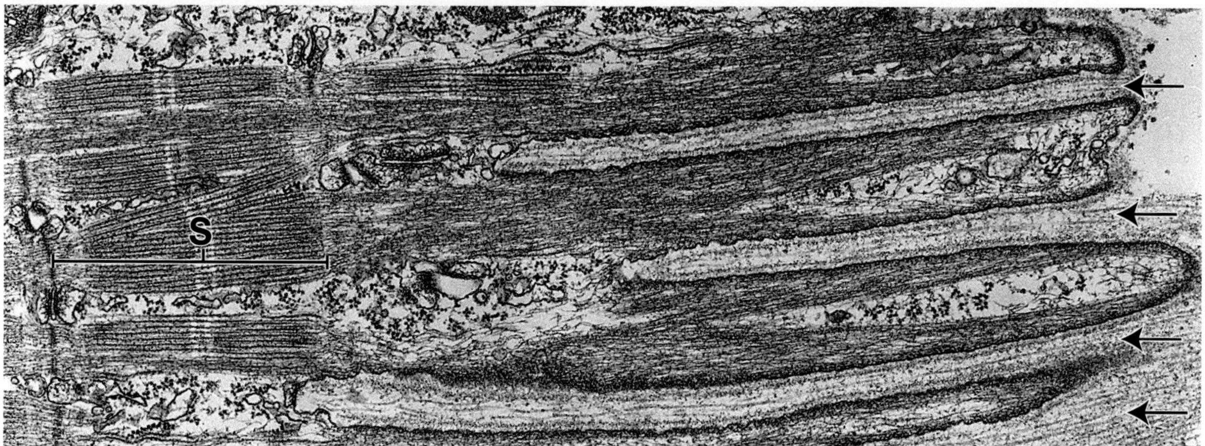
S

PLATE 11.4 ■ CARDIAC MUSCLE

Cardiac muscle consists of fibers that possess the same arrangement of contractile filaments and thus the same cross-banding patterns that are present in striated skeletal and visceral muscles. Although cardiac muscle is striated, it differs in many significant respects from skeletal and striated visceral muscles. Cardiac muscle consists of individual cells that are joined by complex cell-to-cell junctions to form a functional unit (fiber). The histologically obvious differences between cardiac and the other striated muscle fibers are the presence in cardiac muscle of **intercalated discs** (the light microscopic representations of the cell-to-cell junctions), the location of cardiac muscle cell nuclei in the center of the fiber, and the branching of the cardiac muscle fibers. All of these characteristics are evident in a well-prepared longitudinal section of the muscle.

Cardiac muscle, heart, human, hematoxylin and eosin (H&E) ×160.

This figure shows a longitudinal section of cardiac muscle. The muscle fibers are disposed horizontally in the illustration and show cross-striations. In addition to the regular cross-striations (those of greater frequency), however, there is another group of very pronounced cross-bands, namely, the **intercalated discs** (*ID*). Intercalated discs most often appear as a straight band, but sometimes, they are arranged in a stepwise manner (see also figure on the *right*). These discs are not always displayed in routine H&E sections; therefore, one may not be able to depend on these structures for identifying cardiac muscle. Intercalated discs are opposing cell-to-cell contacts. Thus, cardiac muscle fibers differ in a very fundamental respect from fibers of skeletal muscle. The cardiac muscle fiber consists of an end-to-end alignment of individual cells (cardiac myocyte); in contrast, the skeletal muscle fiber is a single multinucleated protoplasmic unit. In examining a longitudinal section of cardiac muscle, it is useful to scan specific fibers along their long axes. By doing so, one can find places where the fibers obviously branch. Two such branchings are indicated by the *arrows* in this figure. Cardiac muscle fibers are surrounded by endomysium, a thin layer of connective tissue (*CT*), which is represented in this figure by elongated nuclei of fibroblasts.

Cardiac muscle, heart, human, H&E ×400.

Like skeletal muscle, the cardiac muscle is composed of linear contractile units, the **myofibrils**. These are evident in this figure as the longitudinally disposed linear structures that extend through the length of the cell. The myofibrils separate to bypass the nuclei, and in doing so, they delineate a perinuclear region of cytoplasm that is free of myofibrils and their cross-striations. These perinuclear cytoplasmic areas (*asterisks*) contain the cytoplasmic organelles that are not directly involved in the contractile process. Many cardiac muscle cells are binucleate; both nuclei typically occupy the myofibril-free region of cytoplasm, as shown in the cell marked by the *asterisks*. The third nucleus in this region appears to belong to the connective tissue either above or below the "in-focus" plane of section. Often, the staining of muscle cell nuclei in a specific specimen is very characteristic, especially when seen in face view as here. Note, in the nucleus between the *asterisks*, the well-stained nucleolus and the delicate pattern of the remainder of the nucleus. Once such features have been characterized for a particular specimen, it becomes easy to identify nuclei with similar staining characteristics throughout the specimen. For example, survey the field in figure on the *left* for nuclei with similar features. Having done this, it is substantially easier to identify nuclei of connective tissue cells (*CT*), which display different staining properties and are not positioned in the same relationship to the muscle cells. In addition, several **intercalated discs** (ID) are well visualized in this figure. They often appear as straight bands, but they also can be seen arranged in a stepwise manner.

Cardiac muscle, heart, human, H&E ×160.

This figure shows cross-sectioned cardiac muscle fibers. Many have rounded or smooth-contoured polygonal profiles. Some fibers, however, are generally more irregular and elongated in profile. These probably reflect a profile of both a fiber and a branch of the fiber. The more lightly stained region in the center of many fibers represents the myofibril-free region of the cell already referred in the previous figure and indicated by the *asterisks* in the *top right* figure. Delicate connective tissue surrounds the individual muscle fibers. This contains capillaries and sometimes larger vessels, such as the venule (*V*) in the center of the bundle of muscle fibers. Larger amounts of connective tissue (*CT*) surround bundles of fibers, and this tissue contains larger blood vessels, such as the arteriole (*A*) marked in the figure.

Cardiac muscle, heart, human, H&E ×400.

At higher magnification, it is possible to see the cut ends of the myofibrils. These appear as the numerous *red* areas that give the cut face of the muscle cell a stippled appearance. The nuclei (*N*) occupy a central position surrounded by myofibrils. Recall that the nuclei of skeletal muscle fibers are located at the periphery of the cell. Note, also, that as mentioned, the nucleus-free central area of the cell, devoid of myofibrils, shows areas of perinuclear cytoplasm (*asterisks*) similar to that marked in the previous figure. Note that connective tissue surrounding the individual muscle fibers containing capillaries (*C*) and sometimes larger vessels, such as the venule (*V*), is well visualized at this higher magnification.

A, arteriole
C, capillaries
CT, connective tissue
ID, intercalated discs
N, nuclei of cardiac muscle cells
V, venule
arrows, sites where fibers branch
asterisks, perinuclear cytoplasmic areas

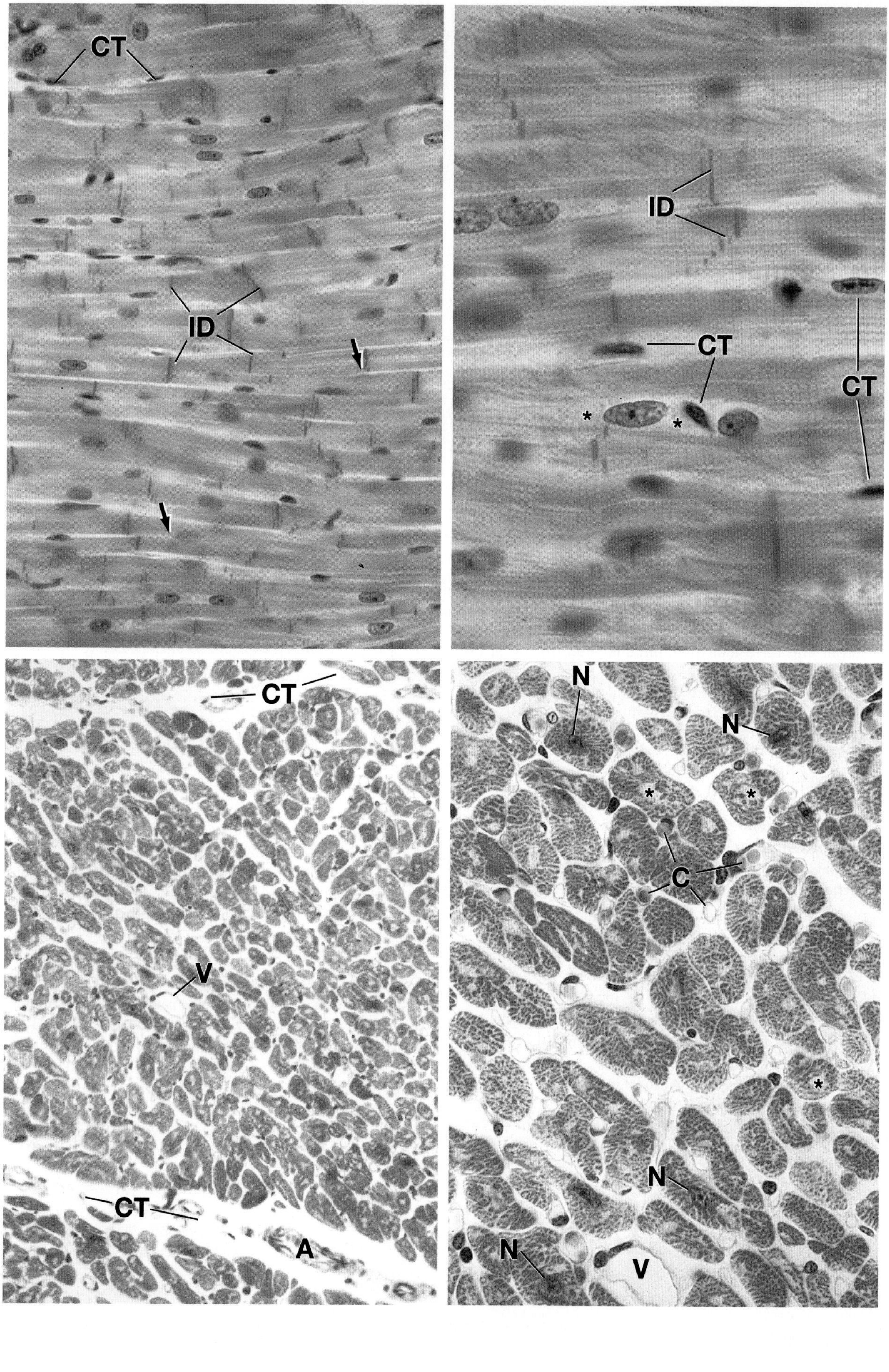
CT
ID
ID
CT
CT
*
*
CT
V
CT
A
N
N
*
*
C
*
N
N
V

PLATE 11.5 ■ CARDIAC MUSCLE, PURKINJE FIBERS

Cardiac muscle cells possess the ability for spontaneous rhythmic contractions. The contraction or beat of the heart is regulated and coordinated by specialized and modified cardiac muscle cells that are found in nodes and muscle bundles. The beat of the heart is initiated at the **sinoatrial (SA) node**, which consists of a group of specialized cardiac muscle cells located at the junction of the superior vena cava in the right atrium. The impulse spreads from this node along the cardiac muscle fibers of the atria. The impulse is then received at the **atrioventricular (AV) node**, which is located on the inner or medial wall of the right ventricle adjacent to the tricuspid valve. Specialized cardiac muscle cells then conduct impulses from the AV node along the ventricular septum and into the ventricular walls. Within the ventricular septum, the specialized cells are grouped into a bundle, the **AV bundle** (of His). This bundle then divides into two main branches, a left and right bundle branch, the former going to the left ventricle and the latter to the right ventricle. The specialized conducting fibers carry the impulse at a rate that is ~4 times faster than the cardiac muscle fibers. They are responsible for the final distribution of the electrical stimulus to the myocardium. Although the SA node on its own exhibits a constant or inherent rhythm, it is modulated by the autonomic nervous system. Thus, the rate of the heartbeat can be decreased by parasympathetic fibers from the vagus nerve or increased by fibers from sympathetic ganglia. The specialized conducting cells within the ventricles are referred to as **Purkinje fibers**. The cells that make up the Purkinje fibers differ from cardiac muscle cells in that they are larger and have their myofibrils located mostly at the periphery of the cell. Their nuclei are also larger. The cytoplasm between the nucleus and the peripherally located myofibrils stains poorly, a reflection, in part, of the large amount of glycogen present in this part of the cell.

ORIENTATION MICROGRAPH: The specimen shown here is a sagittal section revealing part of the atrial wall (*A*) and the ventricular wall (*V*). Between these two portions of the heart is the atrioventricular septum (*AS*). The clear space is the interior of the atrium.

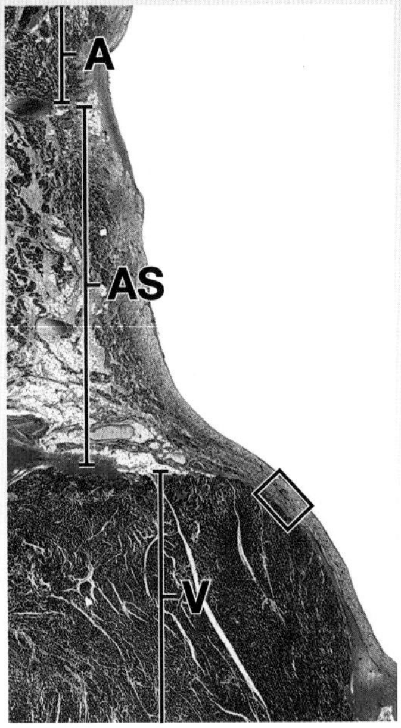

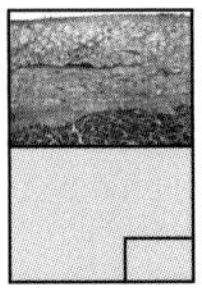

Purkinje fibers, heart, human, Masson ×180.

This micrograph shows the area in the *rectangle* of the orientation micrograph. At this site, the **endocardium** (*Ec*) occupies the upper three-quarters of the micrograph. It consists of the **endothelium** (*Et*) that lines the ventricle but is barely detectable at this magnification. Beneath the endothelium is the **subendothelial layer of dense connective tissue** (*SELCT*), in which elastic fibers are present as well as some smooth muscle cells. The deeper layer is called the **subendocardial layer of the endocardium** (*SELE*); it contains bundles of **Purkinje fibers** (bundle of His) (*PF*) coursing along the ventricle wall. The deeper part of subendocardial layer (*SELE*) consists of more irregularly arranged connective tissue (*DICT*) with blood vessels and occasional adipocytes separating the Purkinje fibers from the **myocardium** (*My*) at the *bottom* of the micrograph. Note how darkly stained the cardiac muscle fibers are compared with those of the Purkinje fibers.

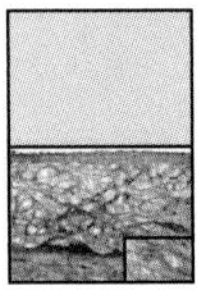

Purkinje fibers, heart, human, Masson ×365; inset ×600.

This higher magnification is the *boxed area* in the previous photomicrograph. It reveals endothelial cells (*EtC*) of the endocardium and underlying containing smooth muscle cells (*SM*). The remaining part of this micrograph below the **subendothelial layer of connective tissue** (*SELCT*) is occupied by the **subendocardial layer of the endocardium** (*SELE*), where the Purkinje fibers are cut in different profiles. Cross-sectioned and obliquely sectioned fibers are near the *top* of the micrograph, and longitudinally sectioned fibers are at the *bottom*. In cross-sectioned fibers, the myofibrils (*M*) are seen at the periphery of the cell. The cytoplasm in the inner portion of the cell appears unstained. Where the nuclei are included in the section of the cell, they are surrounded by the clear cytoplasm. In the *lower portion* of the figure, several longitudinally sectioned Purkinje fibers can be seen. Note the **intercalated discs** (*ID*) in the longitudinally sectioned fibers. The *inset* reveals the intercalated discs and the myofibrils with their cross-banding. Note the clear area or unstained cytoplasm surrounding the nuclei.

A, atrial wall
AS, atrioventricular septum
DICT, dense irregular connective tissue
Ec, endocardium
Et, endothelium
EtC, endothelial cells
ID, intercalated discs
M, myofibrils
My, myocardium
PF, Purkinje fibers
SELCT, subendothelial layer of connective tissue
SELE, subendocardial layer of endocardium
SM, smooth muscle cells
V, ventricular wall

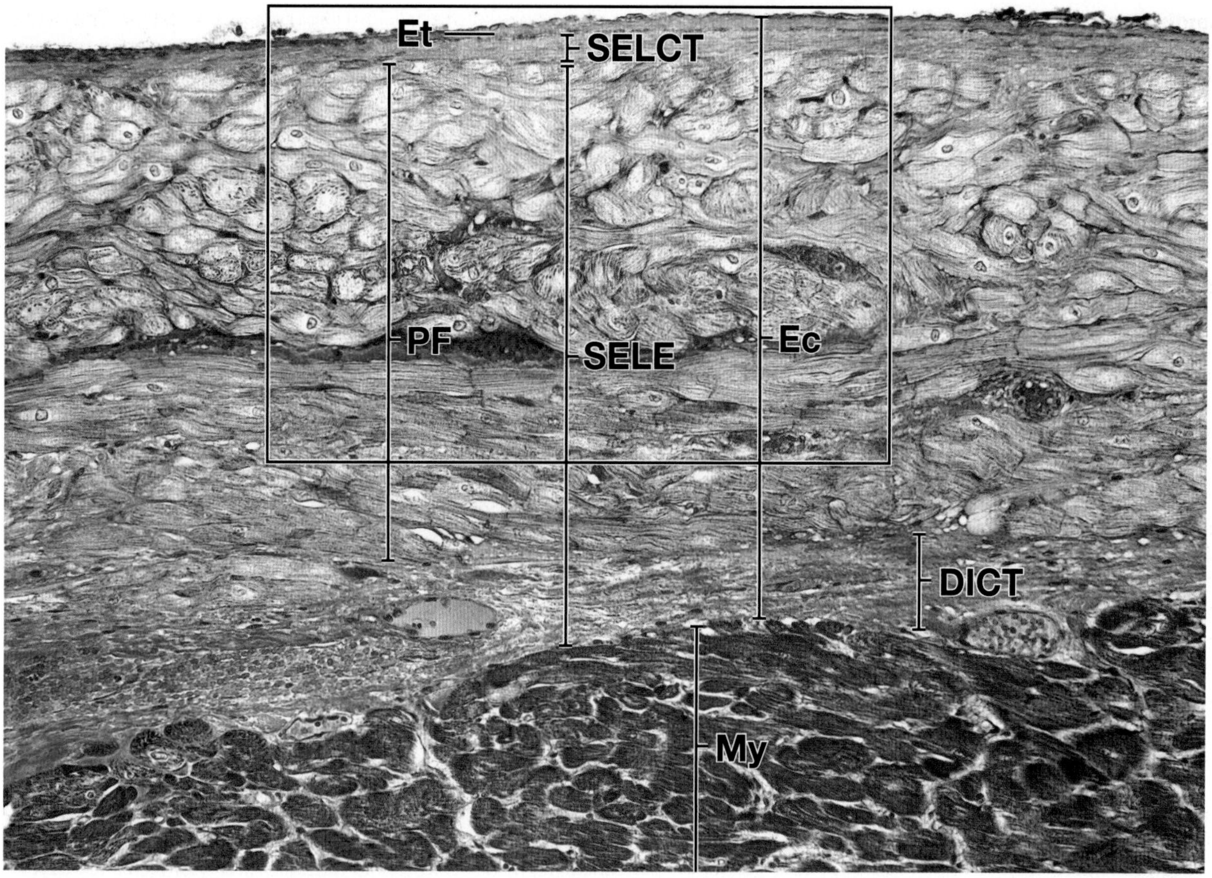
Et
SELCT
PF
SELE
Ec
DICT
My

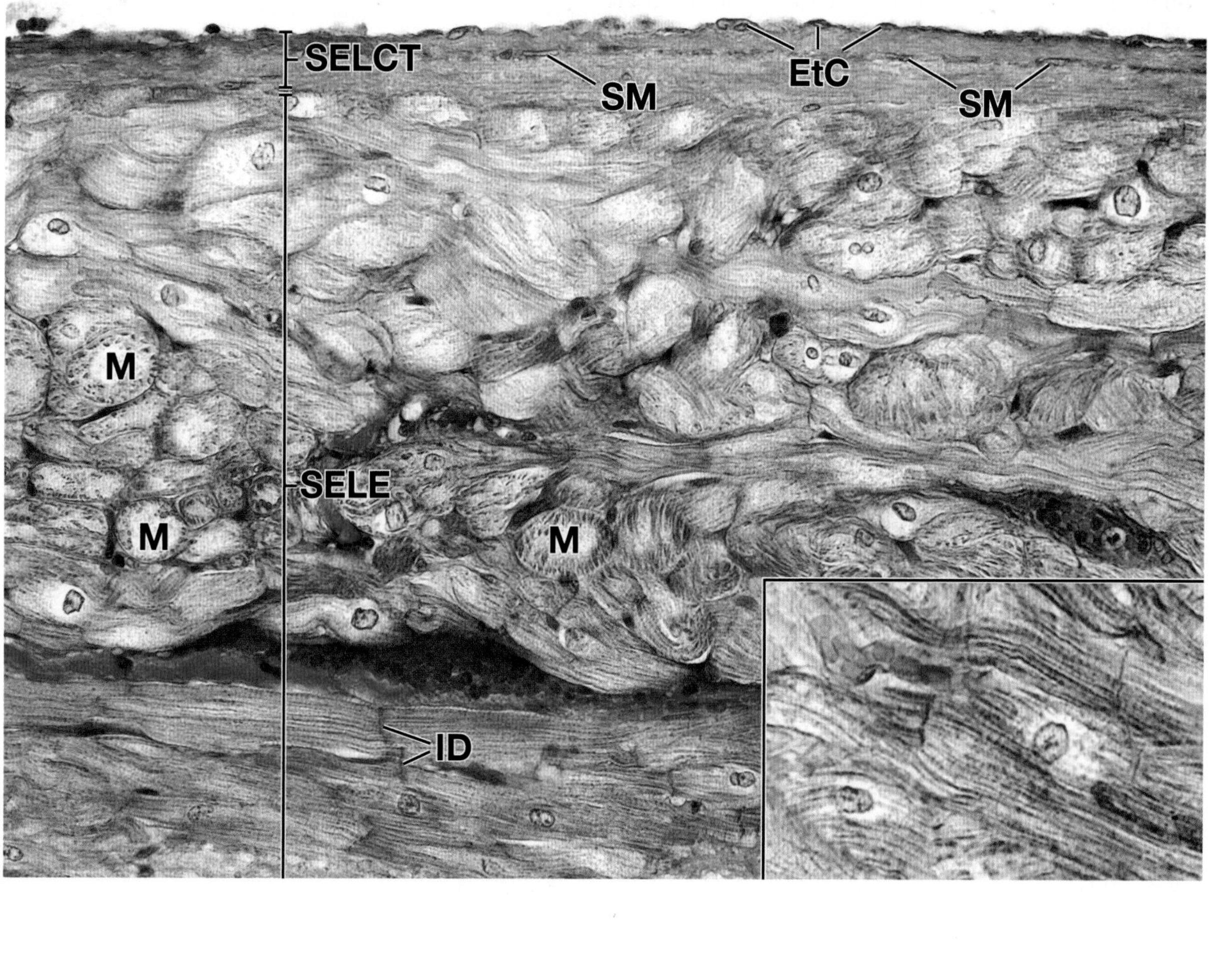
SELCT
SM
EtC
SM
M
SELE
M
M
ID

PLATE 11.6 ■ SMOOTH MUSCLE

Smooth muscle is the intrinsic muscle of the alimentary canal, blood vessels, the genitourinary and respiratory tracts, and other hollow and tubular organs. It is also a component of the nipple, scrotum, skin (arrector pili muscle), and parts of the eye (iris). In most locations, smooth muscle consists of bundles or layers of elongated fusiform cells. They lack the striated banding pattern found in skeletal and cardiac muscle cells. Smooth muscle cells may range in length from 20 μm in the walls of small blood vessels to about 200 μm in the intestinal wall. In the case of the uterus, they may become as long as 500 μm during pregnancy. Smooth muscle cells are joined by **gap junctions** that allow small molecules or ions to pass from cell to cell and allow regulation of contraction of the entire bundle or sheet of smooth muscle. The cytoplasm of smooth muscle cells stains uniformly with eosin in routine hematoxylin and eosin (H&E) preparations because of the concentration of actin and myosin that these cells contain. The nucleus of the cell is located in its center and is elongated with tapering ends, matching the shape of the cell. When the cell is maximally contracted, the nucleus displays a corkscrew shape. During lesser degrees of contraction, the nucleus may appear to have a slight spiral shape. Often in H&E preparations, smooth muscle stains much the same as dense connective tissue. A distinguishing feature relative to smooth muscle is that nuclei are considerably more numerous and they tend to look the same, appearing as elongated profiles when smooth muscle is longitudinally sectioned and as circular profiles when smooth muscle is cross-sectioned. In contrast, the nuclei of dense connective tissue, although fewer in number per unit area, may appear in varying profiles in a given section.

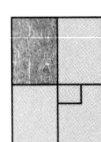

Smooth muscle, small intestine, human, H&E ×256.

This low-power micrograph reveals part of the wall of the small intestine, the **muscularis externa**. The *left side* of the micrograph shows two bundles in longitudinal section (*LS*), whereas on the *right side*, smooth muscle bundles are seen in cross section (*CS*). Note that the nuclei of the smooth muscle cells in the longitudinally sectioned bundles are all elongated; in contrast, the nuclei in the cross-sectioned smooth muscle bundles appear as circular profiles. Intermixed between the bundles is dense irregular connective tissue (*DICT*). Although both the smooth muscle cells and the dense connective tissue stain with eosin, the dense connective tissue exhibits a paucity of nuclei compared to the smooth muscle cell bundles.

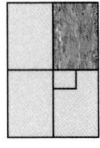

Smooth muscle, small intestine, human, H&E ×512.

This higher magnification photomicrograph shows a bundle of **smooth muscle cells** (*SMC*). Note how the nuclei exhibit an undulating or wavy form indicating that the cells are partially contracted. In contrast, the nuclei seen in the dense irregular connective tissue (*DICT*) show a variety of shapes. In this micrograph, as in the previous micrograph, the collagen fibers have *brighter red* coloration than the cytoplasm of the smooth muscle cells, which provides further distinction between the two types of tissue. However, this is not always the case, and the two may appear similarly stained.

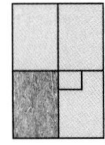

Smooth muscle, small intestine, human, H&E ×256.

This micrograph shows at low magnification several cross-sectioned bundles of smooth muscle (*SMB*). Again, note how the smooth muscle bundles are separated from one another by **dense irregular connective tissue** (*DICT*) and the numerous circular profiles of the smooth muscle cell nuclei.

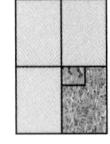

Smooth muscle, small intestine, human, H&E ×512; inset ×1,185.

At this higher magnification, the smooth muscle is again seen in cross section. As is typically the case, the distribution of the smooth muscle cell nuclei is not uniform; thus, in some areas, there appears to be a crowding of nuclei (*lower box*), whereas in other areas, there appears to be a paucity of nuclei (*upper box*). This is a reflection of the side-by-side orientation of the smooth muscle cells; thus, in this area, the cells are aligned in a manner that the nucleus has not been included in the thickness of the section. The *inset* is a higher magnification of this area and shows the cross-sectioned smooth muscle cells as circular profiles of varying size. Where the nuclei appear more numerous, the cells simply are aligned where the section has included the nucleus.

CS, cross-sectioned bundles
DICT, dense irregular connective tissue
LS, longitudinally sectioned bundles
SMB, smooth muscle bundle
SMC, smooth muscle cells

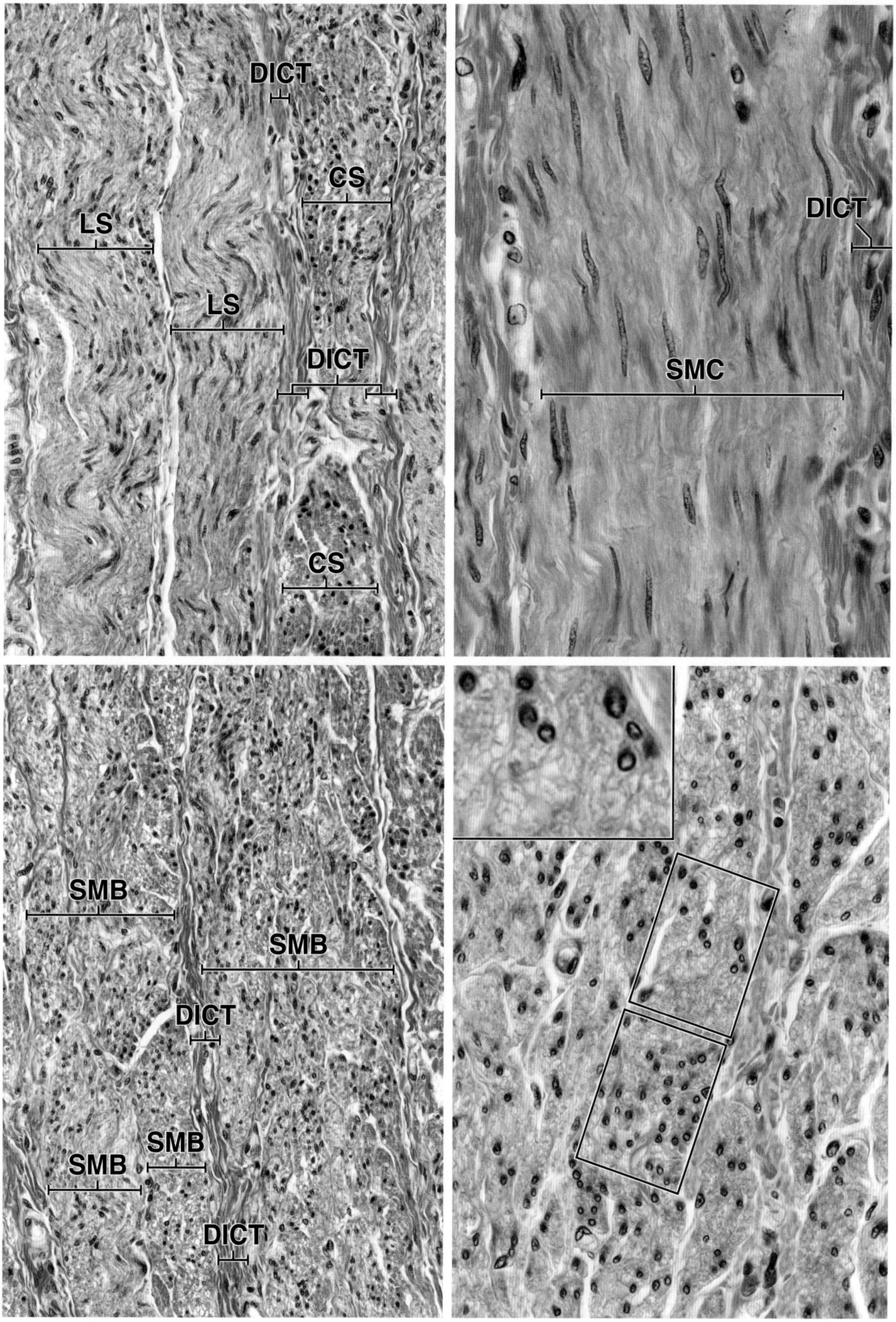
DICT
CS
LS
LS
DICT
CS
DICT
SMC
SMB
SMB
DICT
SMB
SMB
DICT

12 NERVE TISSUE

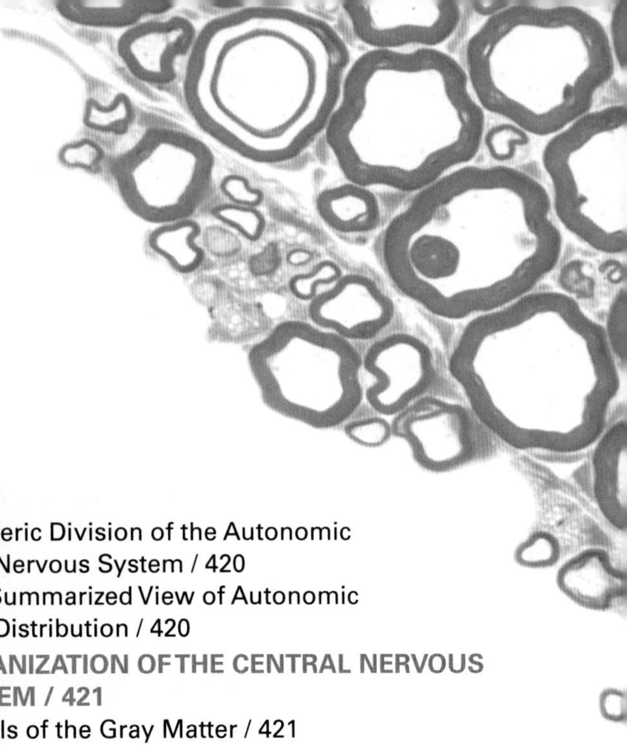

■ OVERVIEW OF THE NERVOUS SYSTEM

The **nervous system** enables the body to respond to continuous changes in its external and internal environment. It controls and integrates the functional activities of organs and organ systems. Anatomically, the nervous system is divided into the following:

- The **central nervous system (CNS)** consists of the brain and the spinal cord, which are located in the cranial cavity and spinal canal, respectively.
- The **peripheral nervous system (PNS)** consists of cranial, spinal, and peripheral **nerves** that conduct impulses from (efferent or motor nerves) and to (the afferent or sensory nerves of) the CNS; collections of nerve cell bodies outside the CNS called **ganglia**; and specialized nerve endings (both motor and sensory). Interactions between sensory (afferent) nerves that receive stimuli, the CNS that interprets them, and motor (efferent) nerves that initiate responses create **neural pathways**. These pathways mediate reflex actions called **reflex arcs.** In humans, most sensory neurons do not pass directly into the brain but instead communicate by specialized terminals (synapses) with motor neurons in the spinal cord.

Functionally, the nervous system is divided into the following:

- The **somatic nervous system (SNS)** consists of somatic *[Gr. soma, body]* parts of the CNS and PNS. The SNS controls functions that are under conscious voluntary control, with the exception of reflex arcs. It provides sensory and motor innervation to all parts of the body except viscera, smooth and cardiac muscle, and glands.

- The **autonomic nervous system (ANS)** consists of autonomic parts of the CNS and PNS. The ANS provides efferent involuntary motor innervation to smooth muscle, the conducting system of the heart, and glands. It also provides afferent sensory innervation from the viscera (pain and autonomic reflexes). The ANS is further subdivided into a **sympathetic division** and a **parasympathetic division**. A third division of ANS, the **enteric division**, serves the alimentary canal. It communicates with the CNS through the parasympathetic and sympathetic nerve fibers; however, it can also function independently of the other two divisions of the ANS (see page 418).

■ COMPOSITION OF NERVE TISSUE

Nerve tissue consists of two principal types of cells: neurons and supporting cells.

The **neuron** or **nerve cell** is the functional unit of the nervous system. It consists of a cell body, containing the nucleus, and several processes of varying length. Nerve cells are specialized to receive stimuli from other cells and to conduct electrical impulses to other parts of the system via their processes. Several neurons are typically involved in sending impulses from one part of the system to another. These neurons are arranged in a chain-like manner as an integrated communications network. Specialized contacts between neurons that provide for transmission of information from one neuron to the next are called **synapses**.

Supporting cells are nonconducting cells that are located close to the neurons. They are referred to as **neuroglial cells** or simply **glia**. The CNS contains four types of glial cells: oligodendrocytes, astrocytes, microglia, and ependymal cells (see page 409). Collectively, these cells are called the **central neuroglia**. In the PNS, supporting cells are called **peripheral neuroglia** and include Schwann cells, satellite cells, and a variety of other cells associated with specific structures. Schwann cells surround the processes of nerve cells and isolate them from adjacent cells and extracellular matrix. Within the ganglia of the PNS, peripheral neuroglial cells are called **satellite cells**. They surround the nerve cell bodies, the part of the cell that contains the nucleus, and are analogous to nonmyelinating Remak Schwann cells. The supporting cells of the ganglia in the wall of the alimentary canal are called **enteric neuroglial cells**. They are morphologically and functionally similar to central neuroglia (see page 409).

Functions of the various neuroglial cell types include the following:

- Physical support (protection) for neurons
- Insulation for nerve cell bodies and processes, which facilitates rapid transmission of nerve impulses
- Repair of neuronal injury
- Regulation of the internal fluid environment of the CNS
- Clearance of neurotransmitters from synaptic clefts
- Metabolic exchange between the vascular system and the neurons of the nervous system

In addition to neurons and supporting cells, an extensive vasculature is present in both the CNS and the PNS. The **blood vessels** are separated from the nerve tissue by the basal laminae and variable amounts of connective tissue, depending on vessel size. The boundary between blood vessels and nerve tissue in the CNS excludes many substances that normally leave blood vessels to enter other tissues. This selective restriction of blood-borne substances in the CNS is called the **blood–brain barrier**, which is discussed on page 424.

The nervous system allows rapid response to external stimuli.

The nervous system evolved from the simple neuroeffector system of invertebrate animals. In primitive nervous systems, only simple receptor–effector reflex loops exist to respond to external stimuli. In higher level animals and humans, the SNS retains the ability to respond to stimuli from the external environment through the action of effector cells (such as skeletal muscle), but the neuronal responses are infinitely more varied. They range from simple reflexes that require only the spinal cord to complex operations of the brain, including memory and learning.

The autonomic part of the nervous system regulates the function of internal organs.

The specific effectors in the internal organs that respond to the information carried by autonomic neurons include the following:

- **Smooth muscle**. Contraction of smooth muscle modifies the diameter or shape of tubular or hollow viscera, such as the blood vessels, gut, gallbladder, and urinary bladder.
- **Cardiac-conducting cells (Purkinje fibers)**. These cells are located within the conductive system of the heart. The inherent frequency of Purkinje fiber depolarization regulates the rate of cardiac muscle contraction and can be modified by autonomic impulses.
- **Glandular epithelium**. The ANS regulates the synthesis, composition, and release of secretions.

The regulation of the function of internal organs involves close cooperation between the nervous system and the endocrine system. Neurons in several parts of the brain and other sites behave as secretory cells and are referred to as **neuroendocrine tissue**. The varied roles of neurosecretions in regulating the functions of the endocrine, digestive, respiratory, urinary, and reproductive systems are described in subsequent chapters.

■ THE NEURON

The neuron is the structural and functional unit of the nervous system.

The human nervous system contains more than 10 billion neurons. Although neurons show the greatest variation in size and shape of any group of cells in the body, they can be grouped into three general categories.

- **Sensory neurons** convey impulses from receptors to the CNS. Processes of these neurons are included in somatic afferent and visceral afferent nerve fibers. **Somatic afferent fibers** convey sensations of pain, temperature, touch, and pressure from the body surface. In addition, these fibers convey pain and proprioception (nonconscious sensation) from organs within the body (e.g., muscles, tendons, and joints) to provide the brain with information related to the orientation of the body and limbs. **Visceral afferent fibers** transmit pain impulses and other sensations from internal organs, mucous membranes, glands, and blood vessels.

- **Motor neurons** convey impulses from the CNS or ganglia to effector cells. Processes of these neurons are included in somatic efferent and visceral efferent nerve fibers. **Somatic efferent neurons** send voluntary impulses to skeletal muscles. **Visceral efferent neurons** transmit involuntary impulses to smooth muscle, cardiac-conducting cells (Purkinje fibers), and glands (Fig. 12.1).
- **Interneurons**, also called **intercalated neurons**, form a communicating and integrative network between the sensory and motor neurons. It is estimated that more than 99.9% of all neurons belong to this integrative network.

The functional components of a neuron include the cell body, axon, dendrites, and synaptic junctions.

The **cell body (perikaryon)** of a neuron contains the nucleus and the organelles that maintain the cell. The processes extending from the cell body constitute the single common structural characteristic of all neurons. Most neurons have only one **axon**, usually the longest process extending from the cell, which transmits impulses away from the cell body to a specialized terminal (synapse). The synapse makes contact with another neuron or an effector cell (e.g., a muscle cell or glandular epithelial cell). A neuron usually has many **dendrites**, shorter processes that transmit impulses from the periphery (i.e., other neurons) toward the cell body.

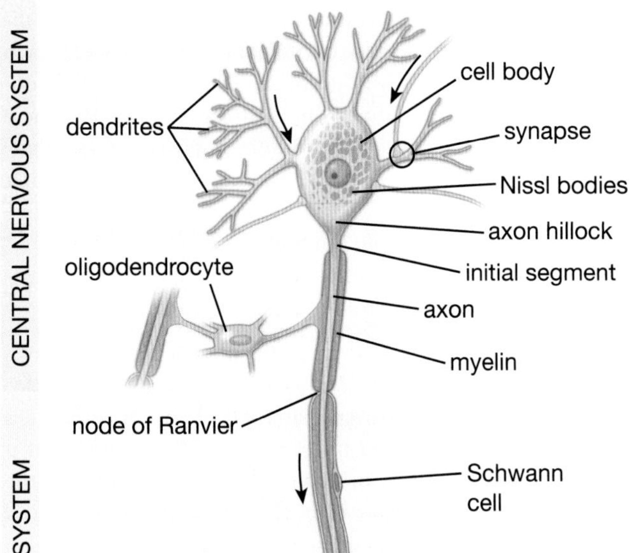

FIGURE 12.1. Diagram of a motor neuron. The nerve cell body, dendrites, and proximal part of the axon are within the central nervous system (CNS). The axon leaves the CNS and, while in the peripheral nervous system (PNS), is part of a nerve (not shown) as it courses to its effectors (striated muscle). In the CNS, the myelin for the axon is produced by, and is part of, an oligodendrocyte; in the PNS, the myelin is produced by, and is part of, a Schwann cell.

Neurons are classified on the basis of the number of processes extending from the cell body.

Most neurons can be anatomically characterized as the following:

- **Multipolar** neurons have one axon and two or more dendrites (Fig. 12.2). The direction of impulses is from dendrite to cell body to axon or from cell body to axon. Functionally, the dendrites and cell body of multipolar neurons are the receptor portions of the cell, and their plasma membrane is specialized for impulse generation. The axon is the conducting portion of the cell, and its plasma membrane is specialized for impulse conduction. The terminal portion of the axon, the synaptic ending, contains various neurotransmitters—that is, small molecules released at the synapse that affect other neurons as well as muscle cells and glandular epithelium. **Motor neurons** and **interneurons** constitute most of the multipolar neurons in the nervous system.
- **Bipolar** neurons have one axon and one dendrite (see Fig. 12.2). Bipolar neurons are rare. They are most often associated with the receptors for the **special senses** (taste, smell, hearing, sight, and equilibrium). They are generally found within the retina of the eye and the ganglia of the vestibulocochlear nerve (cranial nerve VIII) of the ear. Some neurons in this group do not fit the abovementioned generalizations. For example, amacrine cells of the retina have no axons, and olfactory receptors resemble neurons of primitive neural systems in that they retain a surface location and regenerate at a much slower rate than other neurons.
- **Pseudounipolar** (unipolar) neurons have one process, the axon that divides close to the cell body into two long axonal branches. One branch extends to the periphery (**peripheral dendritic branch**), and the other extends to the CNS (**central axonal branch**; see Fig. 12.2). The two axonal branches are the conducting units. Impulses are generated in the peripheral arborizations (branches) of the neuron that are the receptor portions of the cell. Each pseudounipolar neuron develops from a bipolar neuron as its axon and dendrite migrate around the cell body and fuse into a single process. The majority of pseudounipolar neurons are **sensory neurons** located close to the CNS (Fig. 12.3). Cell bodies of sensory neurons are situated in the **dorsal root ganglia** and **cranial nerve ganglia**.

Cell Body

The cell body of a neuron has characteristics of a protein-producing cell.

The **cell body** is the dilated region of the neuron that contains a large, euchromatic **nucleus** with a prominent nucleolus and surrounding **perinuclear cytoplasm** (Fig.12.4a and Plate 12.1, page 432). The perinuclear cytoplasm reveals abundant rough-surfaced endoplasmic reticulum (rER) and free ribosomes when observed with the transmission electron microscope (TEM), a feature consistent with its protein

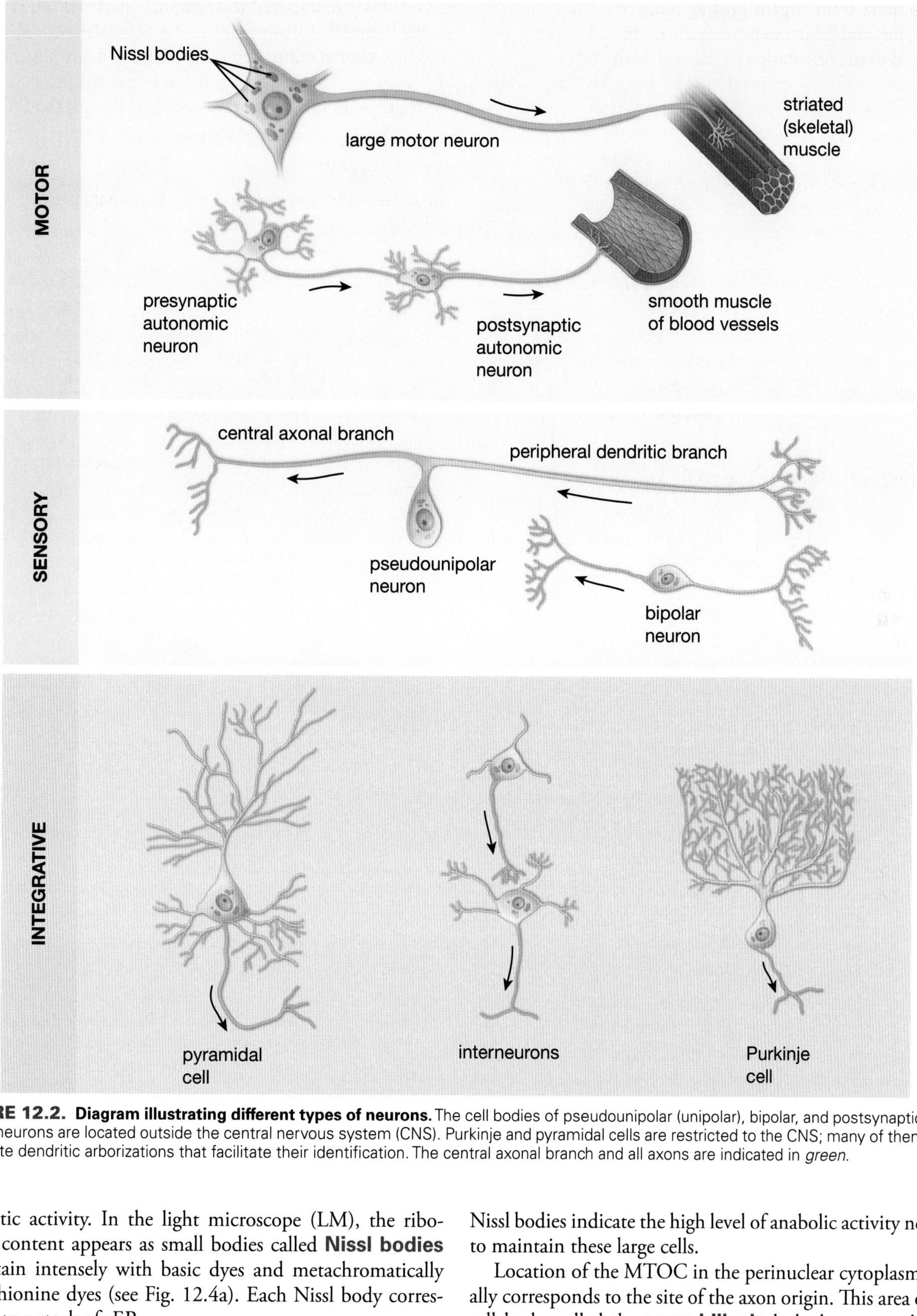

FIGURE 12.2. Diagram illustrating different types of neurons. The cell bodies of pseudounipolar (unipolar), bipolar, and postsynaptic autonomic neurons are located outside the central nervous system (CNS). Purkinje and pyramidal cells are restricted to the CNS; many of them have elaborate dendritic arborizations that facilitate their identification. The central axonal branch and all axons are indicated in *green*.

synthetic activity. In the light microscope (LM), the ribosomal content appears as small bodies called **Nissl bodies** that stain intensely with basic dyes and metachromatically with thionine dyes (see Fig. 12.4a). Each Nissl body corresponds to a stack of rER.

The perinuclear cytoplasm also contains numerous mitochondria, a large perinuclear Golgi apparatus, lysosomes, microtubules, microtubule-organizing center (MTOC) (centrosome), neurofilaments (intermediate filaments), transport vesicles, and inclusions (Fig. 12.4b). Nissl bodies, free ribosomes, and, occasionally, the Golgi apparatus extend into the dendrites, but not into the axon. The euchromatic nucleus, large nucleolus, prominent Golgi apparatus, and Nissl bodies indicate the high level of anabolic activity needed to maintain these large cells.

Location of the MTOC in the perinuclear cytoplasm usually corresponds to the site of the axon origin. This area of the cell body, called the **axon hillock**, lacks large cytoplasmic organelles and serves as a landmark to distinguish between axons and dendrites in both LM and TEM preparations.

Neurons do not divide; however, in some areas of the brain, neural stem cells are present and are able to differentiate and replace damaged nerve cells.

Although neurons do not replicate, the subcellular components of the neurons are regularly renewed and have

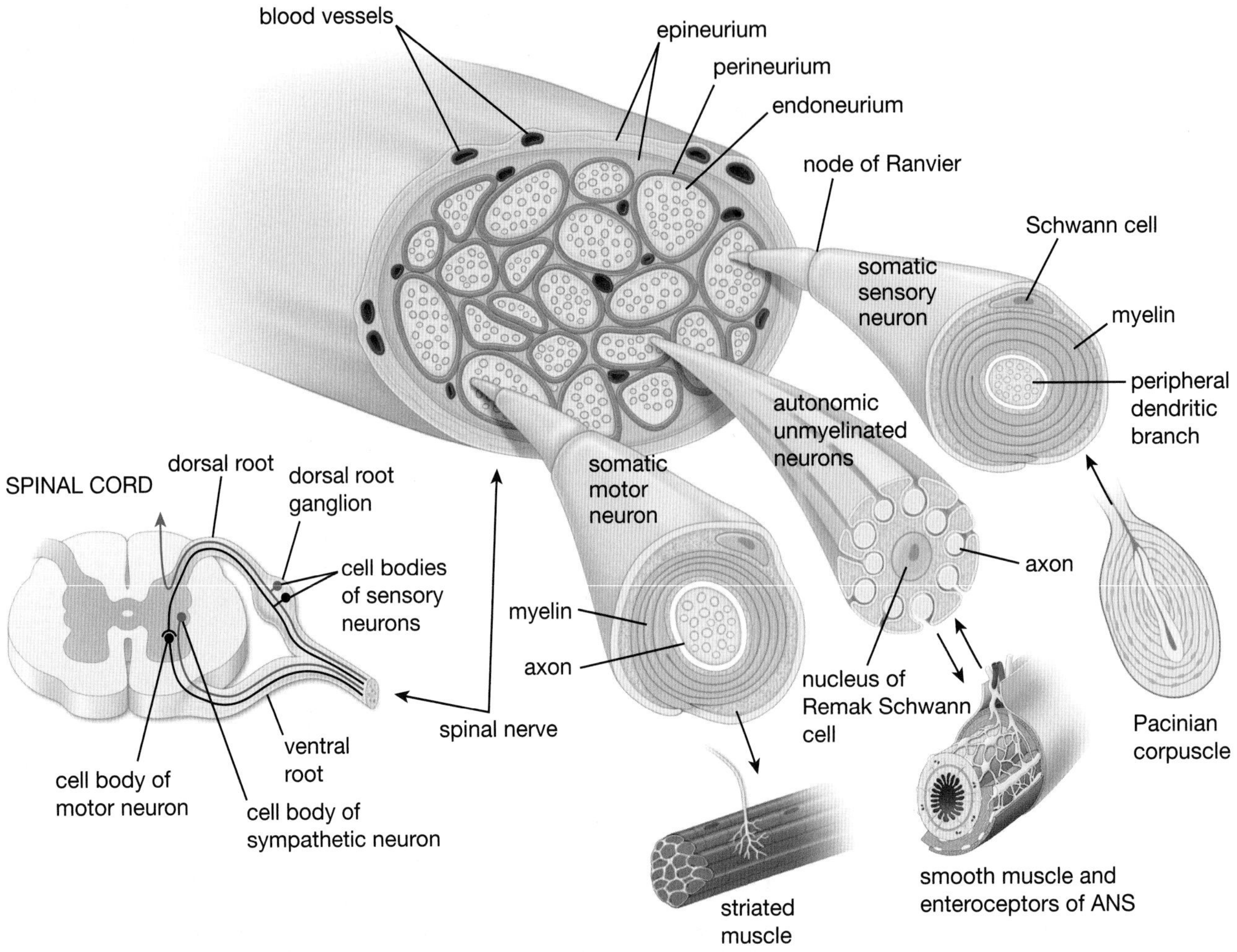

FIGURE 12.3. Schematic diagram showing arrangement of motor and sensory neurons. The cell body of a motor neuron is located in the ventral (anterior) horn of the gray matter of the spinal cord. Its axon, surrounded by myelin, leaves the spinal cord via a ventral (anterior) root and becomes part of a spinal nerve that carries it to its destination on striated (skeletal) muscle fibers. The sensory neuron originates in the skin within a receptor (here, a Pacinian corpuscle) and continues as a component of a spinal nerve, entering the spinal cord via the dorsal (posterior) root. Note the location of its cell body in the dorsal root ganglion (sensory ganglion). A segment of the spinal nerve is enlarged to show the relationship of the nerve fibers to the surrounding connective tissue (endoneurium, perineurium, and epineurium). In addition, segments of the sensory, motor, and autonomic unmyelinated neurons have been enlarged to show the relationship of the axons to the Schwann cells. *ANS*, autonomic nervous system.

life spans measured in hours, days, and weeks. The constant need to replace enzymes, neurotransmitter substances, membrane components, and other complex molecules is consistent with the morphologic features characteristic of a high level of synthetic activity. Newly synthesized protein molecules are transported to distant locations within a neuron in a process referred to as **neuronal transport** (pages 396-397).

It is generally accepted that nerve cells do not divide. However, recently, it has been shown that the adult brain retains some cells that exhibit the potential to regenerate. In certain regions of the brain, such as the olfactory bulb and dentate gyrus of the hippocampus, these **neural stem cells** are able to divide and generate new neurons. They are characterized by continuous expression of a 240-kDa intermediate filament protein **nestin**, which is used to identify these cells by histochemical methods. **Neural stem cells** are also able to migrate to the sites of injury and differentiate into new nerve cells. Research studies on animal models demonstrate that newly generated cells mature into functional neurons in the adult mammalian brain. These findings may lead to therapeutic strategies that use neural cells to replace nerve cells lost or damaged by neurodegenerative disorders, such as Alzheimer and Parkinson diseases.

Dendrites and Axons

As mentioned earlier, neurons extend two distinct types of nerve processes: dendrites and axons, which contain different types of proteins and organelles and thus differ in both structure and function.

Dendrites are receptor processes that receive stimuli from other neurons or the external environment.

The main function of **dendrites** is to receive information from other neurons or the external environment and carry that information to the cell body. Generally, dendrites are located in the vicinity of the cell body. They have a greater diameter than axons and are usually unmyelinated and tapered. Dendrites form extensive arborizations called **dendritic trees**. Dendritic trees significantly increase the receptor surface area of a neuron. Many neuron types are characterized by the extent and shape of their dendritic trees (see Fig. 12.2). In most of the excitatory neurons, they possess **dendritic spines**.

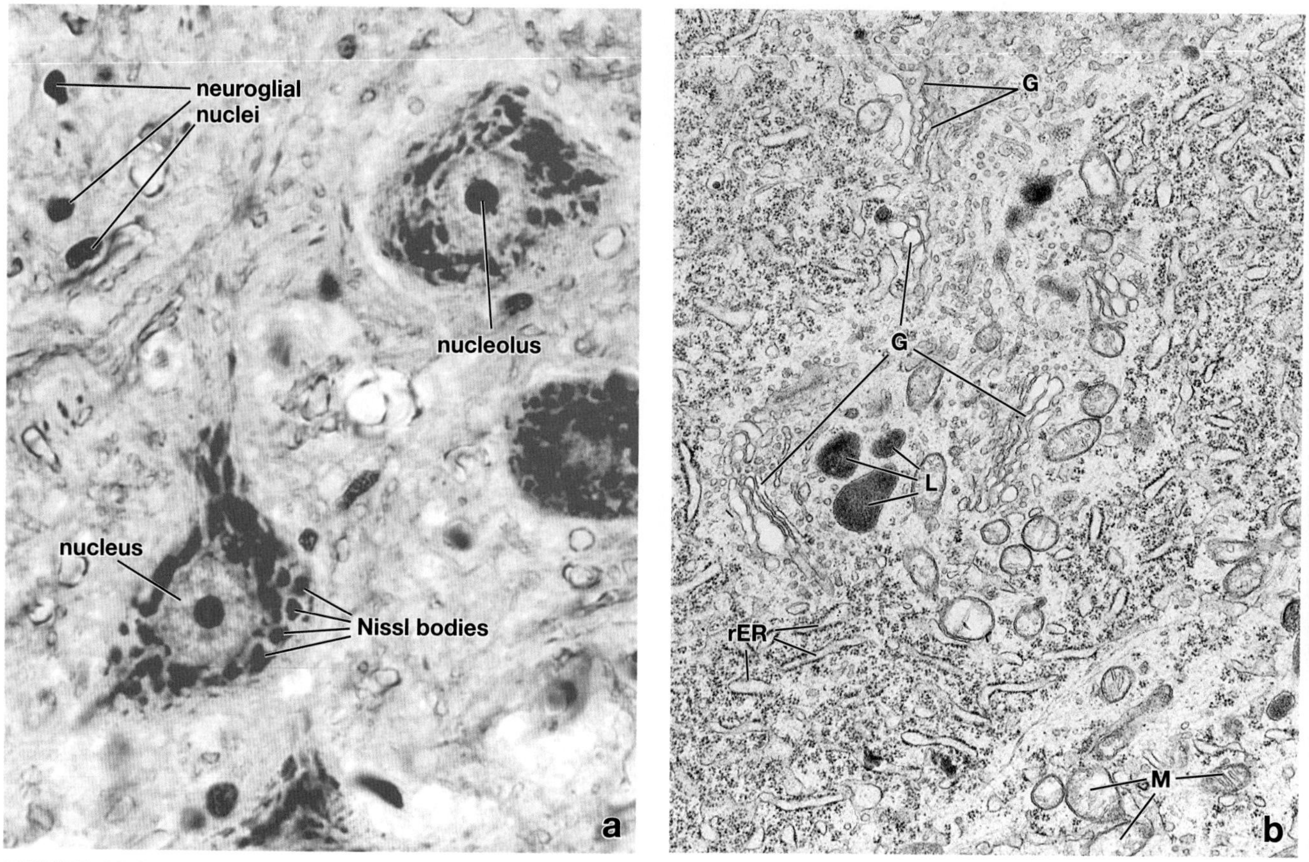

FIGURE 12.4. Nerve cell bodies. a. This photomicrograph shows a region of the ventral (anterior) horn of a human spinal cord stained with toluidine blue. Typical features of the nerve cell bodies visible in this image include large, spherical, pale-stained nuclei with a single prominent nucleolus and abundant Nissl bodies within the cytoplasm of the nerve cell body. Most of the small nuclei belong to neuroglial cells. The remainder of the field consists of nerve fibers and cytoplasm of central neuroglial cells. ×640. **b.** Electron micrograph of a nerve cell body. The cytoplasm is occupied by aggregates of free ribosomes and profiles of rough-surfaced endoplasmic reticulum (*rER*) that constitute the Nissl bodies of light microscopy. The Golgi apparatus (*G*) appears as isolated areas containing profiles of flattened sacs and vesicles. Other characteristic organelles include mitochondria (*M*) and lysosomes (*L*). The neurofilaments and neurotubules are difficult to discern at this relatively low magnification. ×15,000.

In general, the contents of the perinuclear cytoplasm of the cell body and cytoplasm of dendrites are quite similar. Other organelles characteristic of the cell body, including **ribosomes** and **rER**, are found in the dendrites, especially in the base of the dendrites. In addition, small **Golgi outposts**, which are discrete functional Golgi structures not connected with the Golgi apparatus in the cell body, are present in the cytoplasm of dendrites and may serve as nucleation centers for microtubules.

Dendrites are characterized by the presence of dendritic spines that are involved in synaptic plasticity, learning, and memory formation.

Many neurons in the CNS have dendrites that can be identified by the presence of **dendritic spines** (Fig. 12.5). They represent small protrusions of the dendritic plasma membrane containing actin filaments and postsynaptic density. Their shape varies considerably from short projections, resembling thin filopodia–like structures to mushroom-shaped structures. The mushroom-shaped spines are regarded as mature spines and account for the majority (~70%–80%) of spines found on dendrites.

Electron micrographs of mature dendritic spines reveal the presence of a **postsynaptic density** that contains clusters of neurotransmitter receptors as well as voltage-gated Na^+ and K^+ channels similar to those found in nerve synapses. The spines also appear to have a well-developed actin cytoskeleton associated with a variety of actin-binding proteins, occasional microtubules, and vesicles with elongated profiles of endoplasmic reticulum. The postsynaptic density is apposed by a plasma membrane of the neighboring axon containing an active zone with round synaptic vesicles (Fig. 12.6) that forms a fully functional synapse. Most of the synapses formed between dendritic spines and axons contain the neurotransmitter **glutamate (GLU)**, which mediates fast **excitatory synaptic transmission** in the CNS (see pages 401-403).

Dendritic spines are dynamic and can quickly be formed and dismantled; however, some remain stable and persist for months and years. In experimental animal models, acquisition of new memories is associated with increased spine density in pyramidal cells in the CNS. The learning process induces the formation of stable spines that are able to persist for months after training. These experimental findings provide evidence that dendritic spines are involved in **synaptic plasticity and learning** and mediate the long-term encoding for **memory** in the brain cortex.

Axons are effector processes that transmit stimuli to other neurons or effector cells.

The main function of the **axon** is to convey information away from the cell body to another neuron or to an effector cell, such as a muscle cell. *Each neuron has only one axon*, and

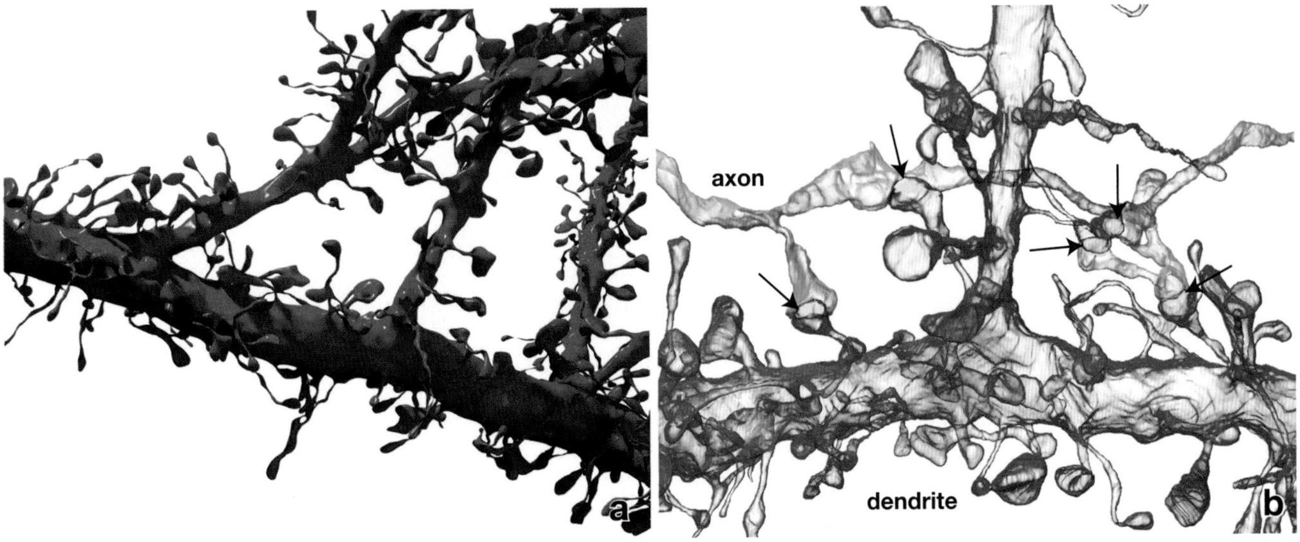

FIGURE 12.5. Three-dimensional (3D) computer reconstructions of nerve cell processes from the mouse somatosensory cerebral cortex. These images represent computer-generated 3D renderings of nerve cells and their processes extracted from a high-resolution stack of 1,850 scanning electron microscope (SEM) images of serially sectioned brain tissue. The automated tape-collecting ultramicrotome (ATUM) was used to cut 29-nm-thick sections that were stained with osmium and carbon coated for imaging with the SEM at sufficient resolution to detect individual synaptic vesicles. A multiscale digital volume image set was then processed for automated annotation and segmentation of nerve cell processes and organelles. Segmented structures were manually painted with a computer-assisted program and combined in a 3D data set. **a.** This image shows the 3D rendering of a single dendrite containing spines. Note the branching pattern of the dendrite. **b.** Semitransparent rendering of synaptic interactions between dendrite (*red*) and axon (*green*). In this image, dendritic spines form five synapses (*arrows*) with the same axon; the postsynaptic densities are indicated in *yellow*. ×13,000. (Courtesy of Drs. Daniel Berger and Jeff W. Lichtman, Harvard University, Cambridge, MA.)

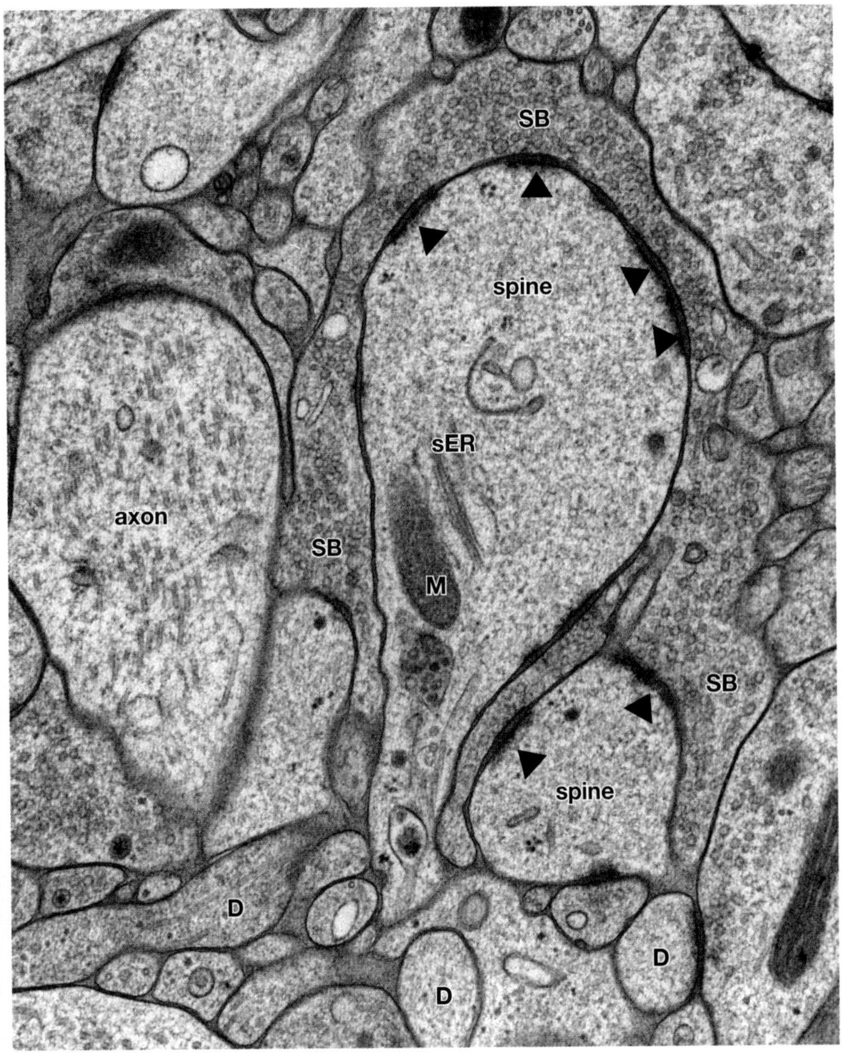

FIGURE 12.6. Electron micrograph of dendritic spines in proximal dendrites of pyramidal nerve cells in the mouse hippocampus. Thin slices (300 μm) of brain tissue were cultured for a period of 1–2 weeks, allowing for damaged tissue to recover and reorganize in vitro by removing cell debris from the tissue slices. After incubation, slices were prepared for electron microscopy (EM) using high-pressure freezing followed by cryosubstitution of tissue water with acetone, stained with osmium, and embedded in an EM-suitable medium. This preparation provides exceptional quality of EM images by avoiding that distortion of the tissue by protein denaturation that occurs in conventional fixation in aldehydes. Note that dendritic spines are surrounded by a large synaptic button (*SB*) containing synaptic vesicles. *Arrowheads* indicate postsynaptic densities. In these areas, synaptic clefts are visible separating active zones of presynaptic elements from postsynaptic densities. Spine cytoplasm contains an actin cytoskeleton with occasional profiles of smooth-surfaced endoplasmic reticulum (*sER*) and transport vesicles visible in the narrow part of the spine. Note an electron-dense organelle, which most likely represents mitochondrion (*M*). Several profiles of dendrites (*D*) are also visible. The large profile on the *left* most likely represents an oblique section of the unmyelinated axon with visible profiles of microtubules. ×95,000. (Courtesy of Prof. Michael Frotscher, Institute for Structural Neurobiology, Center for Molecular Neurobiology Hamburg, Germany.)

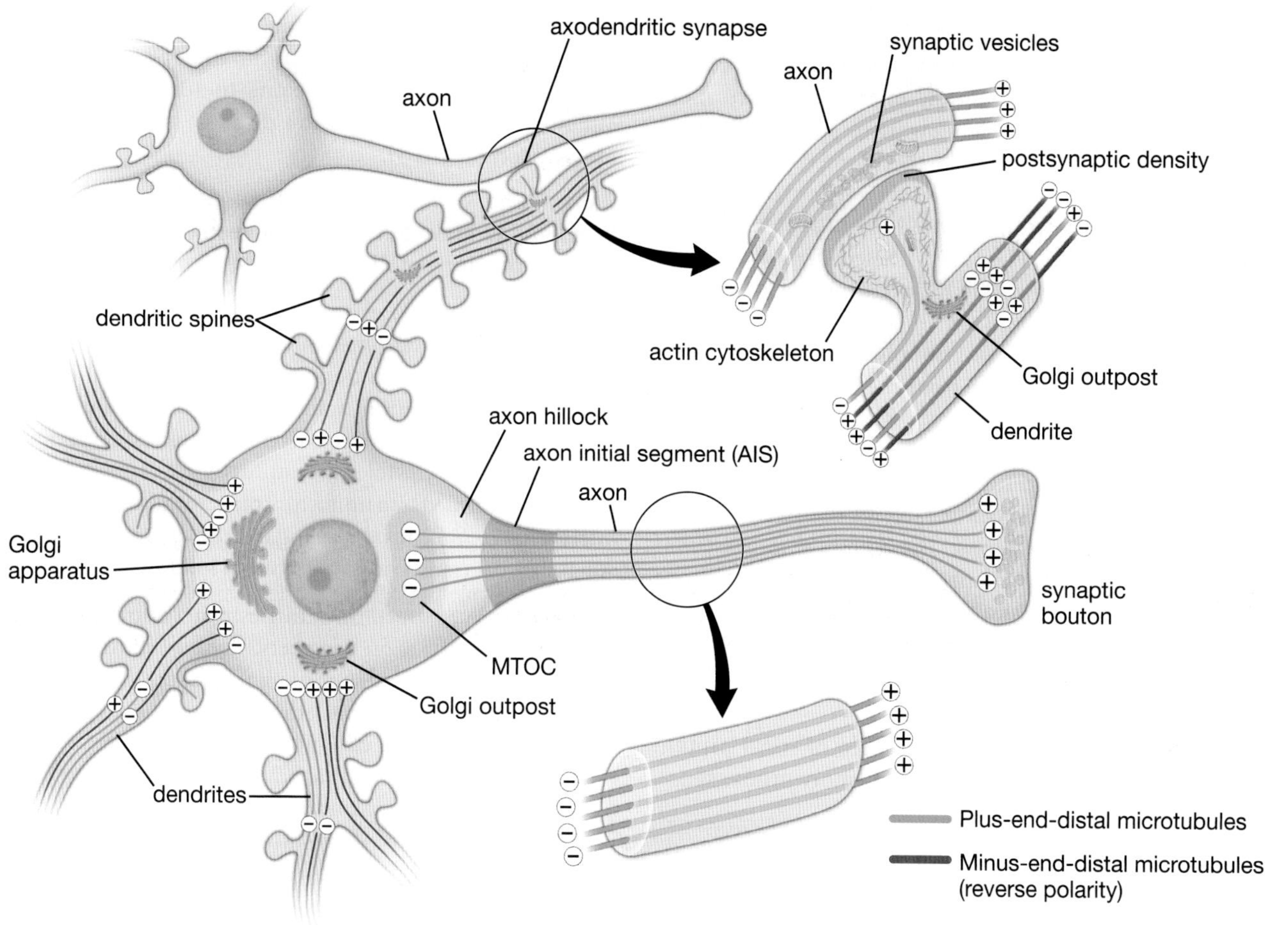

FIGURE 12.7. Organization of microtubules in axons and dendrites. Organization of the microtubule network in the neuron differs between dendrites and axons. All microtubules in axons originate from the microtubule-organizing center (*MTOC*), and they are uniformly oriented with their plus (+) ends directed distally. In contrast, microtubules in dendrites display a mixed polar orientation. The majority of microtubules in dendrites have reversed polarity with their minus (−) ends directed distally away from the cell body. Microtubules of normal polarity (with plus [+] ends directed distally) in dendrites are in the minority. In the central nervous system (CNS), some of them terminate in the cytoplasm of dendritic spines. Note the location of the axon hillock, an area where cargo materials destined for axonal transport are loaded on microtubule-associated motor proteins known as *kinesins*. Also, the axon initial segment (*AIS*) separates proteins and lipids of the axonal plasma membrane from the plasma membrane of the rest of the axon. Note also that dendritic spines form axodendritic synapses with neighboring presynaptic axons. A Golgi apparatus is positioned within the nerve cell body; however, a more characteristic feature of dendrites is the inclusion of small Golgi outposts. These are functional Golgi structures not connected with the main Golgi apparatus that can be found within dendrites and at their junctions with the nerve cell body. Reversed polarity microtubules are not anchored in the *MTOC*, and the Golgi outpost may serve as their nucleation centers.

it may be extremely long. Axons that originate from neurons in the motor nuclei of the CNS **(Golgi type I neurons)** may travel more than a meter to reach their effector targets, skeletal muscle. In contrast, interneurons of the CNS **(Golgi type II neurons)** have very short axons. Although an axon may give rise to a recurrent branch near the cell body (i.e., one that turns back toward the cell body) and to other collateral branches, the branching of the axon is most extensive in the vicinity of its targets.

The axon originates from the **axon hillock**. The axon hillock usually lacks large cytoplasmic organelles, such as Nissl bodies and Golgi cisternae. Microtubules, neurofilaments, mitochondria, and vesicles, however, pass through the axon hillock into the axon (Fig. 12.7). The surface region of the axon between the apex of the axon hillock and the beginning of the myelin sheath (see later in this chapter) is called the **axon initial segment (AIS)**. The molecular composition of the plasma membrane of the AIS acts as a diffusion barrier or "picket fence" to exclude passage of proteins and lipids that do not belong to the axonal plasma membrane. The underlying actin cytoskeleton also acts as a selective filter for organelles and transport vesicles that attempt to enter the axonal cytoplasm. This function can be likened to that of a border crossing checkpoint, where travelers are inspected for proper authorization required to enter the country.

The AIS is the site at which an **action potential** is generated in the axon. The action potential (described in more detail later) is stimulated by impulses carried to the axon hillock on the membrane of the cell body after other impulses are received on the dendrites or the cell body itself.

Organization of microtubules and their arrangement in axons and dendrites are unique and critical to the functional polarity of neurons.

Microtubules are important regulators of cell polarity. As discussed in Chapter 2, Cell Cytoplasm (pages 65-69), microtubules are part of the cell's cytoskeleton. They are composed of tubulin heterodimers and consist of two distinct ends: a plus (+) end and a minus (−) end. At the plus (+) end, microtubules elongate via tubulin polymerization and extend into the cell's periphery. The minus ends are often anchored to an MTOC.

The microtubule network within neurons has certain unique characteristics. In general, microtubules are more stable in axons than in dendrites owing to post-translational modification of tubulin and the protective role of microtubule-associated proteins (MAPs). **Microtubules in axons** are uniformly **oriented with their plus (+) ends directed distally** (see Fig 12.7). These microtubules originate from the area of the MTOC located in the perinuclear cytoplasm. In contrast, **microtubules in dendrites** display a **mixed polar orientation**: Both plus (+) and minus (−) ends are directed distally away from the cell body, although microtubules with reverse polarity (those with their minus [−] ends directed distally) comprise most of the microtubules within dendrites (see Fig. 12.7). These microtubules are generally more stable and are comparable to the plus (+) end–oriented microtubules in axons. These findings suggest that microtubules of reverse polarity are not anchored in the MTOC and that their nucleation occurs independently from the MTOC in the cytoplasm of dendrites. This arrangement is a critical regulator of cell polarity and thus has implications for dendritic transport.

Some large axon terminals are capable of local protein synthesis, which may be involved in memory processes.

Almost all of the structural and functional protein molecules are synthesized in the nerve cell body. These molecules are distributed to the axons and dendrites via **neuronal transport systems** (described on pages 396-397). However, contrary to the common view that the nerve cell body is the only site of protein synthesis, recent studies indicate that limited local synthesis of axonal proteins takes place in some large nerve terminals. Some vertebral axon terminals (i.e., from the retina) contain polyribosomes with complete translational machinery for protein synthesis. These discrete areas within the axon terminals, called **periaxoplasmic plaques**, possess biochemical and molecular characteristics of active protein synthesis. Protein synthesis within the periaxoplasmic plaques is modulated by neuronal activity. These proteins may be involved in the processes of **neuronal cell memory**.

Neuronal Transport Systems

Substances needed in the axons and dendrites are synthesized in the cell body and require transport to those sites.

Because the synthetic activity of the neuron is concentrated in the nerve cell body, microtubule-based **neuronal transport** is required to convey newly synthesized material to the correct neuronal compartment. Transport often takes place over long distances from the site of synthesis to its target destination in the axons or dendrites. Neuronal transport serves as a mode of intracellular communication, carrying molecules and information along the microtubules. Neuronal transport is bidirectional and occurs in both neurons and axons. Neurons are especially vulnerable to defects in neuronal transport because of the extreme length of the neuronal processes. Mutations in α- or β-tubulin and microtubule-based molecular motors have been directly linked to several neurologic disorders in both the CNS and the PNS. Disruption of neuronal transport is most likely responsible for abnormal accumulations of cytoskeletal proteins and organelles in axons in **Alzheimer disease**, **Parkinson disease**, **Huntington disease**, and **amyotrophic lateral sclerosis (ALS)**.

Kinesin and dynein motors drive axonal transport by directing the movement of cargo vesicles and organelles between the nerve cell body and the axon terminal.

Axonal transport is essential for supplying the distal part of the axon and its terminal with newly synthesized proteins, lipids, and neurotransmitters required to maintain synaptic transmission. In addition, aging proteins and organelles from the distal axon are transported for degradation and recycling to the nerve cell body. Molecular motors drive axonal transport along tracks formed by a uniform arrangement of microtubules with their plus (+) ends extending distally toward the axon terminal. Axonal transport is described as follows:

- **Anterograde transport** carries material from the nerve cell body to the axon periphery. Because all microtubules in axons are polarized in the same directions with their plus (+) ends directed toward the axon terminal, **kinesins**, microtubule-associated motor proteins, are involved in anterograde transport. Kinesins move the transport vesicles destined for axons along the microtubules toward their plus (+) ends. They utilize energy from adenosine triphosphate (ATP) hydrolysis to power their movement.
- **Retrograde transport** carries material from the axon terminal to the nerve cell body. This transport is mediated by the microtubule-associated motor proteins called **dyneins** that travel along the microtubules toward their minus (−) ends (see page 69).

The **motor properties** of both **kinesin** and **dynein** are regulated by external signals to allow transported cargo vesicles to slow down or speed up their movement. This is most likely achieved by alternate use of active and inactive conformations of these motor proteins that are attached to the same cargo vesicle. The presence of several motor proteins on the same cargo vesicle allows them to step around obstacles to resolve "road blocks" or "traffic jams" by switching to different microtubule tracks without exchanging the motors attached to the cargo vesicle.

Transport systems may also be distinguished by the rate at which substances are transported.

- A **slow anterograde transport system** conveys substances from the cell body to the axon terminal at the speed of 0.2–4 mm/d. Structural elements, such as tubulin molecules (microtubule precursors), actin molecules, and the proteins that form neurofilaments, are carried from the nerve cell body by this transport system. Cytoplasmic matrix proteins such as actin, calmodulin, and various metabolic enzymes are also transported this way.
- A **fast transport system** conveys substances in both directions at a rate of 20–400 mm/d. Thus, it is both an anterograde and a retrograde system. The **fast anterograde** transport system carries different membrane-limited organelles, such as smooth-surfaced endoplasmic reticulum (sER) components, synaptic vesicles, and mitochondria,

and low-molecular-weight materials, such as sugars, amino acids, nucleotides, some neurotransmitters, and calcium to the axon terminal. The **fast retrograde** transport system carries many of the same materials as well as proteins and other molecules endocytosed at the axon terminal to the nerve cell body. Fast transport in either direction requires ATP, which is used by microtubule-associated motor proteins, and depends on the microtubule arrangement that extends from the nerve cell body to the termination of the axon. Retrograde transport is the pathway followed by toxins and viruses that enter the CNS at nerve endings. Retrograde transport of exogenous enzymes, such as horseradish peroxidase, and radiolabeled or immunolabeled tracer materials is now used to trace neuronal pathways and to identify the nerve cell bodies related to specific nerve endings.

Dynein molecular motors are preferentially involved in dendritic transport, which is more complex than axonal transport owing to the antiparallel organization of microtubules.

Dendritic transport progresses along bundles of **mixed polarity microtubules**, which contain both "normal" microtubules' plus (+) ends and "reversed" microtubules' minus (−) ends oriented away from the nerve cell body. Therefore, a single unidirectional type of motor protein carrying transport vesicle could mediate bidirectional (anterograde and retrograde) transport by switching between normal and reverse polarity microtubule tracts. Recent studies indicate that **dyneins** play an important role in the initial sorting of vesicles that are destined for dendritic transport. Dyneins, which travel along the microtubules toward their minus (−) ends, are also **exclusively involved in anterograde transport** of cargo vesicles into dendrites utilizing microtubules with reversed polarity. Dyneins are also responsible for retrograde transport of vesicles from the dendritic processes into the body of the neuron. Kinesins play only a supporting role and providing assistance in dendritic transport once the transport vesicle is inside the dendrite.

Synapses

Neurons communicate with other neurons and effector cells by synapses.

Synapses are specialized junctions between neurons that facilitate the transmission of impulses from one (presynaptic) neuron to another (postsynaptic) neuron. Synapses also occur between axons and effector (target) cells, such as muscle and gland cells. Synapses between neurons may be classified morphologically as follows:

- **Axodendritic.** These synapses occur between axons and dendrites. In the CNS, some axodendritic synapses are found between axons and dendritic spines (Fig. 12.8).
- **Axosomatic.** These synapses occur between axons and the cell body.
- **Axoaxonic.** These synapses occur between axons and axons (see Fig. 12.8).

Synapses are not resolvable in routine hematoxylin and eosin (H&E) preparations. However, silver precipitation staining methods (e.g., Golgi method) not only demonstrate the overall shape of some neurons but also show synapses as oval bodies on the surface of the receptor neuron. Typically, a presynaptic axon makes several of these button-like contacts with the receptor portion of the postsynaptic neuron. Often, the axon of the presynaptic neuron travels along the surface of the postsynaptic neuron, making several synaptic contacts along the way that are called **boutons en passant** *[Fr. buttons in passing]*. The axon then continues, ending finally as a terminal branch with an enlarged tip, a **bouton terminal** *[Fr. terminal button]*, or end bulb. The number of synapses on a neuron or its processes vary from a few to tens of thousands per neuron (Fig. 12.9); this number appears to be directly related to the number of impulses that a neuron is receiving and processing.

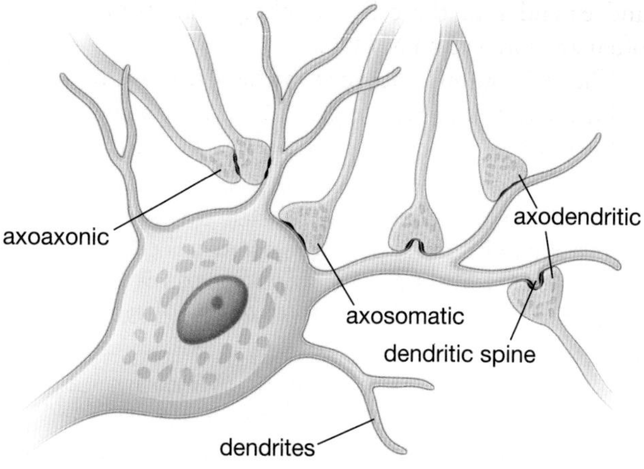

FIGURE 12.8. Schematic diagram of different types of synapses. Axodendritic synapses represent the most common type of connection between the presynaptic axon terminal and the dendrites of the postsynaptic neuron. Note that some axodendritic synapses possess dendritic spines, which are linked to learning and memory. Axosomatic synapses are formed between a presynaptic axon terminal and the postsynaptic nerve cell body; axoaxonic synapses are formed between the axon terminal of a presynaptic neuron and the axon of a postsynaptic neuron. The axoaxonic synapse may enhance or inhibit axodendritic (or axosomatic) synaptic transmission.

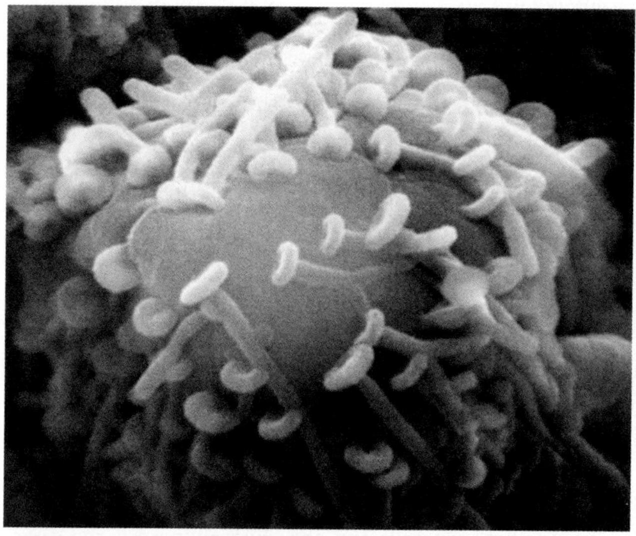

FIGURE 12.9. Scanning electron micrograph of the nerve cell body. This micrograph shows the cell body of a neuron. Axon endings forming axosomatic synapses are visible, as are numerous oval bodies with tail-like appendages. Each oval body represents a presynaptic axon terminal from different neurons making contact with the large postsynaptic nerve cell body. ×76,000. (Courtesy of Dr. George Johnson.)

FOLDER 12.1

CLINICAL CORRELATION: PARKINSON DISEASE

Parkinson disease is a slowly progressive neurologic disorder caused by the loss of dopamine (DA)-secreting cells in the substantia nigra and basal ganglia of the brain. DA is a neurotransmitter responsible for synaptic transmission in the nerve pathways coordinating smooth and focused activity of skeletal muscles. Loss of DA-secreting cells is associated with a classic pattern of symptoms, including the following:

- Resting tremor in the limb, especially of the hand when in a relaxed position; tremor usually increases during stress and is often more severe on one side of the body
- Rigidity or increased tone (stiffness) in all muscles
- Slowness of movement (bradykinesia) and inability to initiate movement (akinesia)
- Lack of spontaneous movements
- Loss of postural reflexes, which leads to poor balance and abnormal walking (festinating gait)
- Slurred speech, slowness of thought, and small, cramped handwriting

The cause of **idiopathic Parkinson disease**, in which DA-secreting neurons in the substantia nigra are damaged and lost by degeneration or apoptosis, is not known. However, some evidence suggests a hereditary predisposition; about 20% of Parkinson patients have a family member with similar symptoms.

Symptoms that resemble idiopathic Parkinson disease may also result from infections (e.g., encephalitis), toxins (e.g., MPTP), drugs used in the treatment of neurologic disorders (e.g., neuroleptics used to treat schizophrenia), and repetitive trauma. Symptoms with these causes are called **secondary parkinsonism**.

On the microscopic level, degeneration of neurons in the substantia nigra is very evident. This region loses its typical pigmentation, and an increase in the number of glial cells is noticeable (**gliosis**). In addition, nerve cells in this region display characteristic intracellular inclusions called **Lewy bodies**, which represent accumulation of intermediate neurofilaments in association with proteins α-synuclein and ubiquitin.

Treatment of Parkinson disease is primarily symptomatic and must strike a balance between relieving symptoms and minimizing psychotic side effects. L-Dopa is a precursor of DA that can cross the blood–brain barrier and is then converted to DA. It is often the primary agent used to treat Parkinson disease. Other drugs that are used include a group of cholinergic receptor blockers and amantadine, a drug that stimulates the release of DA from neurons.

Some patients may benefit from a therapeutic approach called *deep brain stimulation*. In this procedure, electrodes attached to a pulse-generating electrical stimulator are implanted into the subthalamic nucleus of the brain. The electrical pulses act on neurons to modulate nerve impulses. This therapy has been shown to reduce tremor, slowness of movement, and rigidity associated with Parkinson disease. It also reduces the need for L-Dopa to control signs and symptoms, which helps mitigate the debilitating side effects of this medication.

Synapses are classified as chemical or electrical.

Classification of synapses depends on the mechanism of conduction of the nerve impulses and the way the action potential is generated in the target cells. Thus, synapses may also be classified as follows:

- **Chemical synapses.** Conduction of impulses is achieved by the release of chemical substances (neurotransmitters) from the presynaptic neuron. Neurotransmitters then diffuse across the narrow intercellular space that separates the presynaptic neuron from the postsynaptic neuron or target cell. A specialized type of chemical synapse called a **ribbon synapse** is found in the receptor hair cells of the internal ear and photoreceptor cells of the retina (see Chapter 25, Ear, pages 1028-1029).
- **Electrical synapses.** Common in invertebrates, these synapses contain gap junctions that permit the movement of ions between cells and consequently permit the direct spread of electrical current from one cell to another. These synapses do not require neurotransmitters for their function. Mammalian equivalents of electrical synapses include **gap junctions** in smooth muscle and cardiac muscle cells.

A typical chemical synapse contains a presynaptic element, synaptic cleft, and postsynaptic membrane.

Components of a typical chemical synapse include the following:

- A **presynaptic element** (presynaptic knob, presynaptic component, or synaptic bouton) is the end of the neuronal process from which neurotransmitters are released. The presynaptic element is characterized by the presence of **synaptic vesicles**, membrane-bound structures that range from 30 to 100 nm in diameter and contain neurotransmitters (Fig. 12.10). The binding and fusion of synaptic vesicles to the presynaptic plasma membrane are mediated by a family of transmembrane proteins called **SNAREs** (which stands for "**S**oluble **N**SF **A**ttachment **RE**ceptors"; see pages 42-43). The specific SNARE proteins involved in this activity include **synaptobrevin**, a vesicle-bound v-SNARE, and **syntaxin** and **SNAP-25**, which are target membrane-bound t-SNARE proteins found in specialized areas of the presynaptic membrane. Another vesicle-bound protein called **synaptotagmin 1** then displaces the SNARE complex, which is subsequently dismantled and recycled by NSF/SNAP25 protein

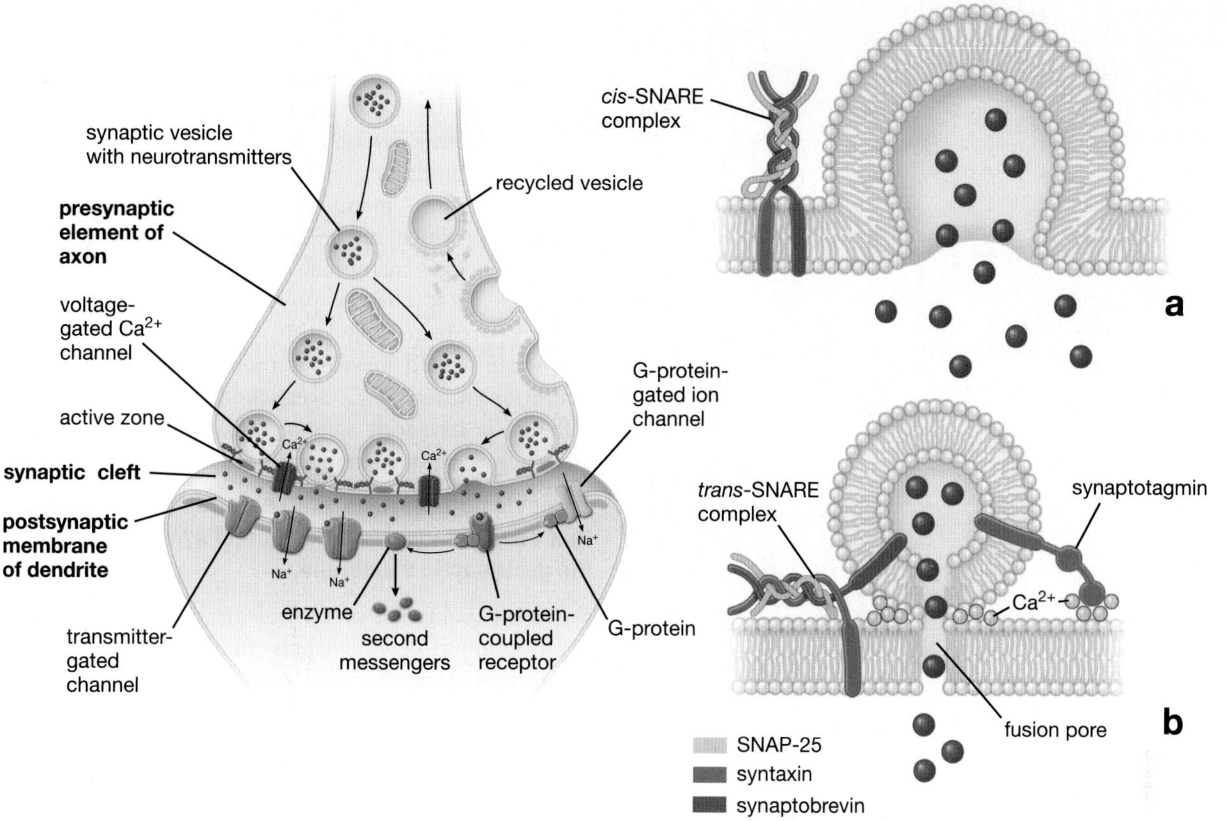

FIGURE 12.10. Diagram of a chemical axodendritic synapse. This diagram illustrates three components of a typical synapse. The presynaptic knob is located at the distal end of the axon from which neurotransmitters are released. The presynaptic element of the axon is characterized by the presence of numerous neurotransmitter-containing synaptic vesicles. The plasma membrane of the presynaptic knob is recycled by the formation of clathrin-coated endocytotic vesicles. The synaptic cleft separates the presynaptic knob of the axon from the postsynaptic membrane of the dendrite. The postsynaptic membrane of the dendrite is frequently characterized by a postsynaptic density and contains receptors with an affinity for the neurotransmitters. Note two types of receptors: *Green*-colored molecules represent transmitter-gated channels, and the *purple*-colored structure represents a G-protein–coupled receptor that, when bound to a neurotransmitter, may act on G-protein–gated ion channels or on enzymes producing a second messenger. **a.** Diagram showing neurotransmitter release from a presynaptic knob by fusion of the synaptic vesicles with the presynaptic membrane. The fusion mechanism that involves SNARE proteins is described in Chapter 2, Cell Cytoplasm (pages 42-44). Note the *cis*-SNARE complex, which is formed after the vesicle fuses to the presynaptic membrane. **b.** Diagram showing a proposed model of neurotransmitter release via porocytosis. In this model, the synaptic vesicle is anchored and juxtaposed to calcium-selective channels in the presynaptic membrane. In the presence of Ca^{2+}, the bilayers of the vesicle and presynaptic membranes are reorganized to create a 1-nm transient fusion pore connecting the lumen of the vesicle, with the synaptic cleft allowing the release of a neurotransmitter. Note the presence of the *trans*-SNARE complex and the synaptotagmin that anchor the vesicle to the active zones within the plasma membrane of the presynaptic element.

complexes. Dense accumulations of proteins are present on the cytoplasmic side of the presynaptic plasma membrane. These presynaptic densities represent specialized areas called **active zones** where synaptic vesicles are docked and where neurotransmitters are released. Active zones are rich in **Rab-GTPase docking complexes** (see pages 42-43), **t-SNAREs**, and **synaptotagmin-binding proteins**. The vesicle membrane that is added to the presynaptic membrane is retrieved by endocytosis and reprocessed into synaptic vesicles by the sER located in the nerve ending. Numerous small mitochondria are also present in the presynaptic element.

- The **synaptic cleft** is the 20- to 30-nm space that separates the presynaptic neuron from the postsynaptic neuron or target cell, which the neurotransmitter must cross.
- The **postsynaptic membrane** (postsynaptic component) contains receptor sites with which the neurotransmitter interacts. This component is formed from a portion of the plasma membrane of the postsynaptic neuron (Fig. 12.11) and is characterized by an underlying layer of dense material. This **postsynaptic density** represents an elaborate complex of interlinked proteins that serve numerous functions, such as translation of the neurotransmitter–receptor interaction into an intracellular signal, anchoring of and trafficking neurotransmitter receptors to the plasma membrane, and anchoring various proteins that modulate receptor activity.

Synaptic Transmission

Voltage-gated Ca^{2+} channels in the presynaptic membrane regulate transmitter release.

When a nerve impulse reaches the synaptic bouton, the voltage reversal across the membrane produced by the impulse (called **depolarization**) causes **voltage-gated Ca^{2+} channels** to open in the plasma membrane of the bouton. The influx of Ca^{2+} from the extracellular space causes the synaptic vesicles to migrate, anchor, and fuse with the presynaptic membrane, thereby releasing the neurotransmitter into the synaptic cleft by exocytosis. Vesicle docking and fusion are mainly driven by the actions of SNARE and synaptotagmin proteins. An alternative process that releases neurotransmitter following vesicle

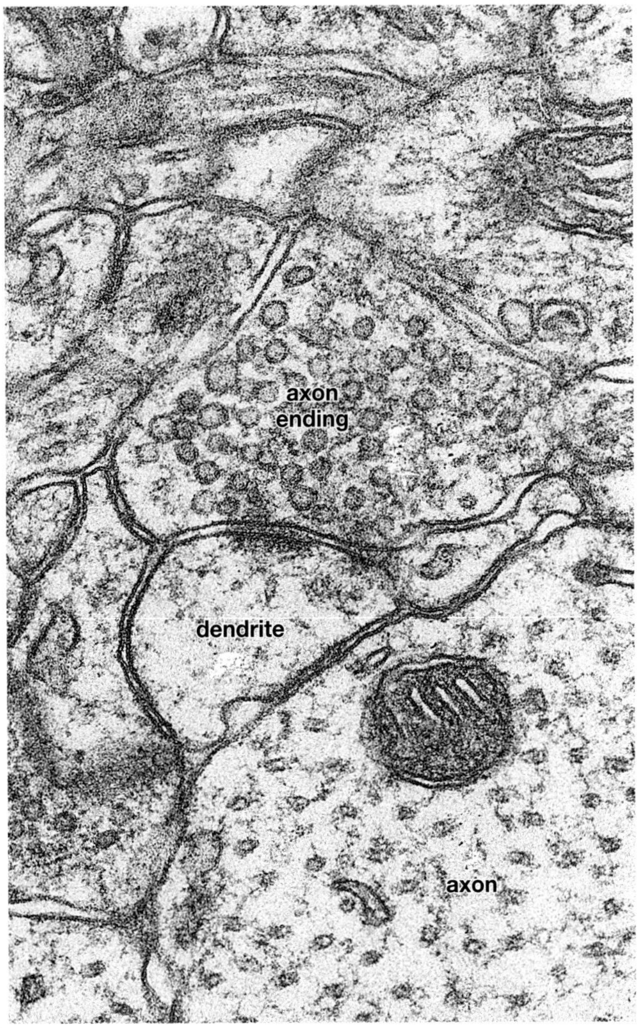

FIGURE 12.11. Electron micrograph of nerve processes in the cerebral cortex. A synapse can be seen in the *center* of the micrograph, where an axon ending is in apposition to a dendrite. The ending of the axon exhibits numerous neurotransmitter-containing synaptic vesicles that appear as circular profiles. The postsynaptic membrane of the dendrite shows a postsynaptic density. A substance of similar density is also present in the synaptic cleft (intercellular space) at the synapse. ×76,000. (Courtesy of Drs. George D. Pappas and Virginia Kriho.)

fusion is called **porocytosis**, in which vesicles anchored at the active zones release neurotransmitters through a transient fusion pore connecting the lumen of the vesicle with the synaptic cleft. At the same time, the presynaptic membrane of the synaptic bouton that released the neurotransmitter quickly forms endocytotic vesicles that return to the endosomal compartment of the bouton for recycling or reloading with neurotransmitter.

The neurotransmitter binds to either transmitter-gated channels or G-protein–coupled receptors on the postsynaptic membrane.

The released neurotransmitter molecules bind to the extracellular part of postsynaptic membrane receptors called **transmitter-gated channels**. Binding of neurotransmitter induces a conformational change in these channel proteins that causes their pores to open. The response that is ultimately generated depends on the identity of the ion that enters the cell. For instance, influx of Na^+ causes local depolarization in the postsynaptic membrane, which, under favorable conditions (sufficient amount and duration of neurotransmitter release), prompts the opening of **voltage-gated Na^+ channels**, thereby generating a nerve impulse.

Some amino acid and amine neurotransmitters may bind to **G-protein–coupled receptors** to produce longer lasting and more diverse postsynaptic responses. The neurotransmitter binds to a transmembrane receptor protein on the postsynaptic membrane. Receptor binding activates G-proteins, which move along the intracellular surface of the postsynaptic membrane and eventually activate effector proteins. These effector proteins may include transmembrane **G-protein–gated ion channels** or **enzymes** that synthesize second messenger molecules (page 401). Several neurotransmitters (e.g., acetylcholine [ACh]) can generate different postsynaptic actions, depending on which receptor system they act (see later in this chapter).

Porocytosis describes the secretion of neurotransmitter that does not involve the fusion of synaptic vesicles with the presynaptic membrane.

Based on evaluation of physiologic data and the structural organization of nerve synapses, an alternate model of neurotransmitter secretion called **porocytosis** has recently been proposed to explain the regulated release of neurotransmitters. In this model, secretion from the vesicles occurs without the fusion of the vesicle membrane with the presynaptic membrane. Instead, the synaptic vesicle is anchored to the presynaptic membrane next to Ca^{2+}-selective channels by SNARE and synaptotagmin proteins. In the presence of Ca^{2+}, the vesicle and presynaptic membranes are reorganized to create a 1-nm transient **fusion pore** that connects the lumen of the vesicle with the synaptic cleft. Neurotransmitters can then be released in a controlled manner through these transient membrane pores (see Fig. 12.10).

The chemical nature of the neurotransmitter determines the type of response at that synapse in the generation of neuronal impulses.

The release of neurotransmitter by the presynaptic component can cause either **excitation** or **inhibition** at the postsynaptic membrane.

- In **excitatory synapses**, the release of neurotransmitters such as **acetylcholine**, **glutamine**, or **serotonin** opens **transmitter-gated Na^+ channels** (or other cation channels), prompting an influx of Na^+ that causes local reversal of voltage of the postsynaptic membrane to a threshold level (depolarization). This leads to initiation of an action potential and generation of a nerve impulse.
- In **inhibitory synapses**, the release of neurotransmitters such as **γ-aminobutyric acid (GABA)** or **glycine** opens **transmitter-gated Cl^- channels** (or other anion channels), causing Cl^- to enter the cell and hyperpolarize the postsynaptic membrane, making it even more negative. In these synapses, the generation of an action potential then becomes more difficult.

The ultimate generation of a nerve impulse in a postsynaptic neuron (firing) depends on the summation of excitatory and inhibitory impulses reaching that neuron. This allows precise regulation of the reaction of a postsynaptic neuron (or muscle fiber or gland cell). The function of synapses is not simply to transmit impulses in an unchanged manner from one neuron to another. Rather, synapses allow for the processing of neuronal input. Typically, the impulse passing from the presynaptic to the postsynaptic neuron is modified at the synapse by other neurons that, although not in the direct pathway, nevertheless have access to the synapse (see Fig. 12.8). These other neurons may influence the membrane of the presynaptic neuron or the postsynaptic neuron and facilitate or inhibit the transmission of impulses. The firing of impulses in the postsynaptic neuron is caused by the summation of the actions of hundreds of synapses.

Neurotransmitters

Many molecules that serve as **neurotransmitters** have been identified in various parts of the nervous system. A neurotransmitter that is released from the presynaptic element diffuses through the synaptic cleft to the postsynaptic membrane, where it interacts with a specific receptor. Action of the neurotransmitter depends on its chemical nature and the characteristics of the receptor present on the postsynaptic plate of the effector cell.

Neurotransmitters act on either ionotropic receptors to open membrane ion channels or metabotropic receptors to activate G-protein signaling cascade.

Almost all known neurotransmitters act on multiple receptors, which are integral membrane proteins. These receptors can be divided into two major classes: ionotropic and metabotropic receptors. **Ionotropic receptors** contain integral transmembrane ion channels, also referred to as **transmitter-gated channels** or **ligand-gated channels**. Binding of neurotransmitter to ionotropic receptors triggers a conformational change of the receptor proteins that leads to the opening of the channel and subsequent movement of selective ions into or out of the cell. This generates an action potential in the effector cell. In general, signaling using ionotropic channels is very rapid and occurs in the major neuronal pathways of the brain and somatic motor pathways in the PNS. **Metabotropic channels** are responsible not only for binding a specific neurotransmitter but also for interacting with **G-protein** at their intracellular domain. G-protein is an important protein that is involved in intracellular signaling. It conveys signals from the outside to the inside of the cell by altering the activities of enzymes involved in the synthesis of a second messenger. Activation of metabotropic receptors is mostly involved in the modulation of neuronal activity.

The most common neurotransmitters are described as follows. A summary of selected neurotransmitters and their characteristics in both the PNS and the CNS is provided in Table 12.1.

- **Acetylcholine (ACh)**. ACh is the neurotransmitter between axons and striated muscle at the neuromuscular junction (see page 357) and serves as a neurotransmitter in the ANS. ACh is released by the presynaptic sympathetic and parasympathetic neurons and their effectors. ACh is also secreted by postsynaptic parasympathetic neurons as well as by a specific type of postsynaptic sympathetic neuron that innervates sweat glands. Neurons that use ACh as their neurotransmitter are called **cholinergic neurons**. The receptors for ACh in the postsynaptic membrane are known as **cholinergic receptors** and are divided into two classes. Metabotropic receptors interact with muscarine, a substance isolated from poisonous mushrooms **(muscarinic ACh receptors)**, and ionotropic receptors interact with nicotine isolated from tobacco plants **(nicotinic ACh receptors)**. The muscarinic ACh receptor in the heart is an example of a G-protein–coupled receptor that is linked to K^+ channels. Parasympathetic stimulation of the heart releases ACh, which, in turn, opens K^+ channels, causing hyperpolarization of cardiac muscle fibers. This hyperpolarization slows rhythmic contraction of the heart. In contrast, the nicotinic ACh receptor in skeletal muscles is an ionotropic ligand–gated Na^+ channel. Opening of this channel causes rapid depolarization of skeletal muscle fibers and initiation of contraction. Various drugs affect the release of ACh into the synaptic cleft as well as its binding to its receptors. For instance, **curare**, the South American arrow-tip poison, binds to nicotinic ACh receptors, blocking their integral Na^+ channels and causing muscle paralysis. **Atropine**, an alkaloid extracted from the belladonna plant *(Atropa belladonna)*, blocks the action of muscarinic ACh receptors.
- **Catecholamines** such as **norepinephrine (NE)**, **epinephrine (EPI, adrenaline)**, and **dopamine (DA)**. These neurotransmitters are synthesized in a series of enzymatic reactions from the amino acid tyrosine. Neurons that use catecholamines as their neurotransmitter are called **catecholaminergic neurons**. Catecholamines are secreted by cells in the CNS that are involved in the regulation of movement, mood, and attention. Neurons that utilize EPI (adrenaline) as their neurotransmitter are called **adrenergic neurons**. They all contain an enzyme that converts NE to adrenaline (EPI), which serves as a transmitter between postsynaptic sympathetic axons and effectors in the ANS. EPI is also released into the bloodstream by the endocrine cells (chromaffin cells) of the adrenal medulla during the **fight-or-flight response**.
- **Serotonin** or **5-hydroxytryptamine (5-HT)**. Serotonin is formed by the hydroxylation and decarboxylation of tryptophan. It functions as a neurotransmitter in the neurons of the CNS and enteric nervous system. Neurons that use serotonin as their neurotransmitter are called **serotonergic**. After the release of serotonin, a portion is recycled by reuptake into presynaptic serotonergic neurons. Serotonin has been found to be an important molecule that helps establish **asymmetrical right–left development** in embryos.
- **Amino acids** such as GABA, GLU, aspartate (ASP), and glycine (GLY) act as neurotransmitters, mainly in the CNS.
- **Nitric oxide (NO)**, a simple gas with free radical properties, also has been identified as a neurotransmitter. At low concentrations, NO carries nerve impulses from one neuron to another. Unlike other neurotransmitters, which are synthesized in the nerve cell body and stored in synaptic vesicles, NO is synthesized within the synapse and used immediately. It is postulated that excitatory neurotransmitter GLU induces a chain reaction in which **NO synthase** is activated to produce NO, which, in turn, diffuses from the presynaptic knob via the synaptic cleft and postsynaptic membrane to the adjacent cell. Biological actions of NO are due to the activation of guanylyl cyclase,

TABLE 12.1 Characterizations of the Most Common Neurotransmitters

Class of Molecule	Neurotransmitter	Receptor Type and Action: Ionotropic	Receptor Type and Action: Metabotropic	Physiologic Role
Ester	ACh	Nicotinic ACh receptors (nAChR); activates Na^+ channels	Muscarinic ACh receptor (mAChR); acts via G-protein	Fast excitatory synaptic transmission at the neuromuscular junction (acting on nAChR); also present in PNS (e.g., sympathetic ganglia, adrenal medulla) and CNS; both excitatory and inhibitory action (acting on mAChR) (e.g., decreases heart rate, smooth muscle relaxation of gastrointestinal tract)
Monoamine	Epinephrine, norepinephrine	NA	α- and β-adrenergic receptors; acts via G-protein	Slow synaptic transmission in CNS and in smooth muscles
	Dopamine	NA	D_1 and D_2 dopamine receptors; acts via G-protein	Slow synaptic transmission in CNS
	Serotonin	5-HT_3 ligand–gated Na^+/K^+ channel; activates ion channels	5-$HT_{1,2,4–7}$ receptors	Fast excitatory synaptic transmission (acting on 5-HT_3); both excitatory and inhibitory depending on receptor; acts in CNS and PNS (enteric system)
Amino acids	Glutamate	NMDA, kainite, and AMPA; activates Na^+, K^+, and Ca^{2+} channels	mGluR receptor; acts via G-protein	Fast excitatory synaptic transmission in CNS
	GABA	$GABA_A$ receptor; activates Cl^- channels	$GABA_B$ receptor; acts via G-protein	Both fast and slow inhibitory synaptic transmission in CNS
	Glycine	Glycine receptor (GlyR); activates Cl^- channels	NA	Fast inhibitory synaptic transmission in CNS
Small peptides	Substance P	NA	Neurokinin-1 (NK1) receptor; acts via G-protein	Slow excitation of smooth muscles and sensory neurons in CNS, especially when conveying pain sensation
	Enkephalins	NA	δ (DOP) and μ (MOP) opioid receptors; acts via G-protein	Reduces synaptic excitability (slow synaptic signaling); relaxes smooth muscles in gastrointestinal tract; causes analgesia
	β-Endorphin	NA	κ Opioid (KOP) receptor; acts via G-protein	Slow synaptic signaling in brain and spinal cord; causes analgesia
Free radical	NO	NO does not act on receptors; it activates guanylyl cyclase and then via cGMP signaling increases G-protein synthesis in target cells		Influences neurotransmitter release in CNS and PNS; acts as potent vasodilator, relaxes smooth muscles in gastrointestinal tract

5-HT, 5-hydroxytryptamine; *ACh*, acetylcholine; *AMPA*, α-amino-3-hydroxy-5-methyl-4-isoxazolepropionic acid; *cGMP*, cyclic guanosine monophosphate; *CNS*, central nervous system; *GABA*, γ-aminobutyric acid; *mGluR*, metabotropic glutamate receptor; *NA*, not applicable; *NMDA*, *N*-methyl D-aspartate receptor; *NO*, nitric oxide; *PNS*, peripheral nervous system.

which then produces cyclic guanosine monophosphate (cGMP) in target cells. cGMP, in turn, acts on G-protein synthesis, ultimately resulting in generation/modulation of neuronal action potentials.

- **Small peptides** have been shown to act as synaptic transmitters. Among these are **substance P** (so named because it was originally found in a powder of acetone extracts of brain and intestinal tissue), **hypothalamic-releasing hormones**, **endogenous opioid peptides** (e.g., **β-endorphin**, **enkephalins**, **dynorphins**), **vasoactive intestinal peptide (VIP)**, **cholecystokinin (CCK)**, and **neurotensin**. Many of these same substances are synthesized and released by **enteroendocrine cells** of the intestinal tract. They may act immediately on neighboring cells (paracrine secretion) or be carried in the bloodstream as hormones to act on distant target cells (endocrine secretion). They are also synthesized and released by endocrine organs and the neurosecretory neurons of the hypothalamus.

Neurotransmitters released into the synaptic cleft may be degraded or recaptured.

The degradation or recapture of neurotransmitters is necessary to limit the duration of stimulation or inhibition of the postsynaptic membrane. The most common process of neurotransmitter removal after its release into the synaptic cleft is called **high-affinity reuptake**. About 80% of released neurotransmitters are removed by this mechanism, in which they are bound into **specific neurotransmitter transport proteins** located in the presynaptic membrane. Neurotransmitters that were transported into the cytoplasm of the presynaptic bouton are either enzymatically destroyed or reloaded into empty synaptic vesicles. For example, the action of **catecholamines** on postsynaptic receptors is terminated by the reuptake of neurotransmitters into the presynaptic bouton utilizing **Na^+-dependent transporters**. The efficiency of this uptake can be regulated by several pharmacologic agents such as amphetamine and cocaine, which block catecholamine reuptake and prolong the actions of neurotransmitters on the postsynaptic neurons. Once inside the presynaptic bouton, catecholamines are reloaded into synaptic vesicles for future use. The excess of catecholamines is inactivated by the enzyme **catechol *O*-methyltransferase (COMT)** or is destroyed by another enzyme found on the outer mitochondrial membrane, **monoamine oxidase (MAO)**. Therapeutic substances that inhibit the action of MAO are frequently used in the treatment of **clinical depression**; selective COMT inhibitors have been also developed.

Enzymes associated with the postsynaptic membrane degrade the remaining 20% of neurotransmitters. For example, **acetylcholinesterase (AChE)**, which is secreted by the muscle cell into the synaptic cleft, rapidly degrades ACh into acetic acid and choline. Choline is then taken up by the cholinergic presynaptic bouton and reused for ACh synthesis. The **AChE action** at the **neuromuscular junction** can be inhibited by various pharmacologic compounds, nerve agents, and pesticides, resulting in prolonged muscle contraction. Clinically, **AChE inhibitors** have been used in the treatment of **myasthenia gravis** (see Folder 11.3 in Chapter 11, Muscle Tissue, page 358), an autoimmune neuromuscular disorder, and **glaucoma**. AChE inhibitors also improve many of the symptoms of **Alzheimer disease** and are considered the first-line therapeutic agents for these patients.

■ SUPPORTING CELLS OF THE NERVOUS SYSTEM: THE NEUROGLIA

In the PNS, supporting cells are called **peripheral neuroglia**; in the CNS, they are called **central neuroglia**.

Peripheral Neuroglia

Peripheral neuroglia include **Schwann cells**, **satellite cells**, and a variety of other cells associated with specific organs or tissues. Examples of the latter include **terminal neuroglia (terminal Schwann cells, teloglia)**, which are associated with the motor end plate; **enteric neuroglia** associated with the ganglia located in the wall of the alimentary canal; and **Müller cells** in the retina.

Schwann Cell Development and Synthesis of Myelin Sheath

In mature peripheral nerves, **Schwann cells** adopt one of the three distinct phenotypes: (1) a **myelinating phenotype** that is responsible for myelinating large-diameter axons in the PNS; (2) a **nonmyelinating phenotype** (also known as a **Remak Schwann cell)**, which is characterized by the enclosure of multiple small-diameter axons within grooves of the plasma membrane that invaginate deep into the cell cytoplasm; and (3) a **repair cell** phenotype that plays a major role during nerve injury, repair, and regeneration. Although Remak Schwann cells do not produce myelin, they are essential for the proper development and function of the peripheral nerves. During nerve injury, both myelinating Schwann cells and Remak Schwann cells undergo reprogramming and dedifferentiation into repair cells. For the purpose of this discussion, the term "Schwann cell" is used to describe myelin-producing cells, and "Remak Schwann cells" refers to the nonmyelin-producing cells that provide support for unmyelinated nerve fibers in the PNS.

- **Myelinating Schwann cells** are the major glial cell type in PNS. They produce the myelin that surrounds all large-diameter peripheral nerve processes and play essential roles in the development, maintenance, function, and regeneration of peripheral nerves. A detailed description of Schwann cell development, structure, and function is explained.

  Nonmyelinating Remak Schwann cells are the second major phenotype of Schwann cells. In the PNS, Remak Schwann cells do not produce myelin; instead, they envelope multiple small-diameter axons to form **unmyelinated fibers** called *Remak bundles.* Most unmyelinated fibers are composed of postsynaptic sympathetic and parasympathetic axons. Some nonmyelinating Schwann cells migrate toward the neuromuscular junction and cover the axon terminals, where they become **perisynaptic/terminal Schwann cells (teloglia)**. These cells are found at the distal ends of motor nerve terminals at neuromuscular junctions (see Fig. 11.14).
- **Repair Schwann cells** are the third phenotype of Schwan cells and are specialized to promote the repair of injured nerves in the PNS. Repair Schwann cells are derived from the conversion of myelinating Schwann cells and nonmyelinating Remak Schwann cells in response to nerve injury (Fig 12.12). This injury-induced conversion of Schwann and Remak Schwann cells is driven by the dedifferentiation of mature cells and cell reprogramming that involves the downregulation of myelin genes combined with activation of specific features used in nerve repair. These features include upregulation of trophic factors, increased synthesis of cytokines (i.e., for macrophage recruitment), activation of myelin autophagy (myelin clearance), and the formation of **regeneration tracks** called **bands of Büngner** that direct growing axonal sprouts to their targets. A detailed description of nerve regeneration is found in the section on response of neurons to injury (see pages 426-429).

Schwann cell precursors originate from neural crest cells and further differentiate into myelinating Schwann cells or nonmyelinating Remak Schwan cells according to axon-derived signals.

During nerve development in the PNS, some **neural crest cells** give rise to **Schwann cell precursors** under the influence of transcription factor SOX10 (see Fig 12.12). Schwann cell precursors migrate along developing axons to their final destination. Once this migration is complete, the Schwann cell precursors transition into **immature Schwann cells** and perform **radial sorting**, which sorts the axons based on their diameter. This process determines the final phenotype

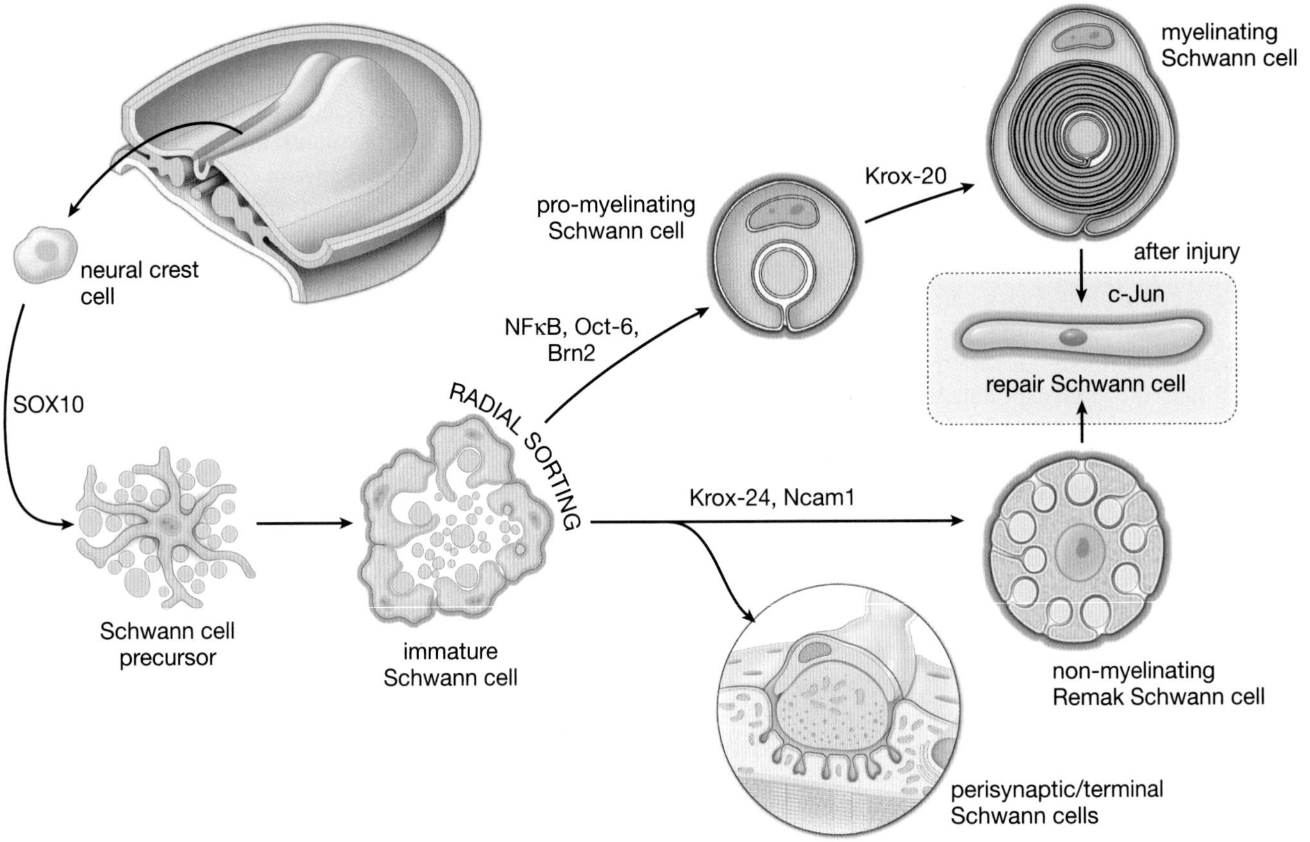

FIGURE 12.12. Schwann cell development and transformation after peripheral nerve injury. Schwann cell precursors originate from neural crest cells under the influence of transcription factor Sox-10. They further transition into immature Schwann cells and perform radial sorting of the axons based on their diameter. Immature Schwann cells, which have a one-to-one relationship with large-diameter axons, under influence of NF-κB, Oct-6, and Brn2 transcription factors, become promyelinating Schwan cells. Under further influence of Krox-20 transcription factor, these cells develop into myelinating Schwann cells. The remaining small-diameter fibers are engulfed in the cytoplasm of the remaining immature Schwan cells and eventually, under the influence of Krox-24 and Ncam1, differentiate into nonmyelinated Remak Schwann cells. Some immature Schwann cells near the neuromuscular junctions develop into perisynaptic/terminal Schwann cells, which also do not produce myelin. Radial sorting determines the final phenotype of the Schwann cell and the designation of the nerve fiber as myelinated or unmyelinated. Following peripheral nerve injury, c-Jun transcription factor is rapidly upregulated, downregulating the expression of Krox-20 and causing dedifferentiation of Schwann cells into repair Schwann cells. Similar processes occur in the Remak Schwan cells, leading to their differentiation during nerve injury.

of the Schwann cell and the designation of the nerve fiber as myelinated or unmyelinated.

Radial sorting begins by secluding a cohort of axons of mixed diameters into small bundles. These bundles are surrounded by three to eight immature Schwann cells that organize a common external lamina around them. Next, the immature Schwan cells extend their cytoplasmic processes between axons to progressively choose, segregate, and reposition larger axons (>6–7 μm in diameter) toward their own cell body at the periphery of the bundle. As immature Schwann cells continue to proliferate, large-diameter axons are sorted into a one-to-one relationship with immature Schwann cells. This close interaction with a single large axon allows immature Schwann cells to receive axonal signals from a transmembrane protein expressed on the axolemma of the axon called **neuregulin-1 (Nrg1)**. The Nrg1 signal upregulates the expression of **promyelinating transcription factors**, including nuclear factor κB (NF-κB), octamer-binding transcription factor 6 (Oct-6), and brain 2 class III POU-domain protein (Brn2) (see Fig 12.12). These transcription factors promote promyelination, in which **promyelinating Schwann cells** express early myelin markers. Further upregulation of KROX20 is required for maturation to **myelinated Schwann cells**, which express myelin-specific proteins and produce myelin sheaths.

As myelinating Schwann cell development progresses, large axons are pooled out from the initial axonal bundles. The bundles become smaller and smaller until they contain only the remaining small-diameter axons (<1 μm in diameter). They are subsequently engulfed by the cytoplasm of the remaining immature Schwan cells and eventually differentiate into **nonmyelinated Remak Schwann cells** (see Fig 12.12).

In the PNS, myelinating Schwann cells produce the myelin sheath.

The main function of Schwann cells is to support myelinated and unmyelinated nerve cell fibers. In the PNS, **Schwann cells** produce a lipid-rich layer called the **myelin sheath** that surrounds the axons (Fig. 12.13). The myelin sheath isolates the axon from the surrounding extracellular compartment of endoneurium. Its presence ensures the rapid conduction of nerve impulses. The axon hillock and the terminal arborizations where the axon synapses with its target cells are not covered by myelin. Unmyelinated fibers are also enveloped and nurtured by Remak Schwann cell's cytoplasm. In addition, Schwann cells aid in removing PNS debris and guide the regrowth of PNS axons (see pages 426-429).

Myelination begins when a Schwann cell surrounds the axon and its cell membrane becomes polarized.

During formation of the myelin sheath (also called **myelination**), the axon initially lies in a groove on the surface of the Schwann cell (Fig. 12.14a). A 0.08- to 0.1-mm segment of the axon then becomes enclosed within each Schwann cell that lies along the axon. The Schwann cell surface becomes polarized

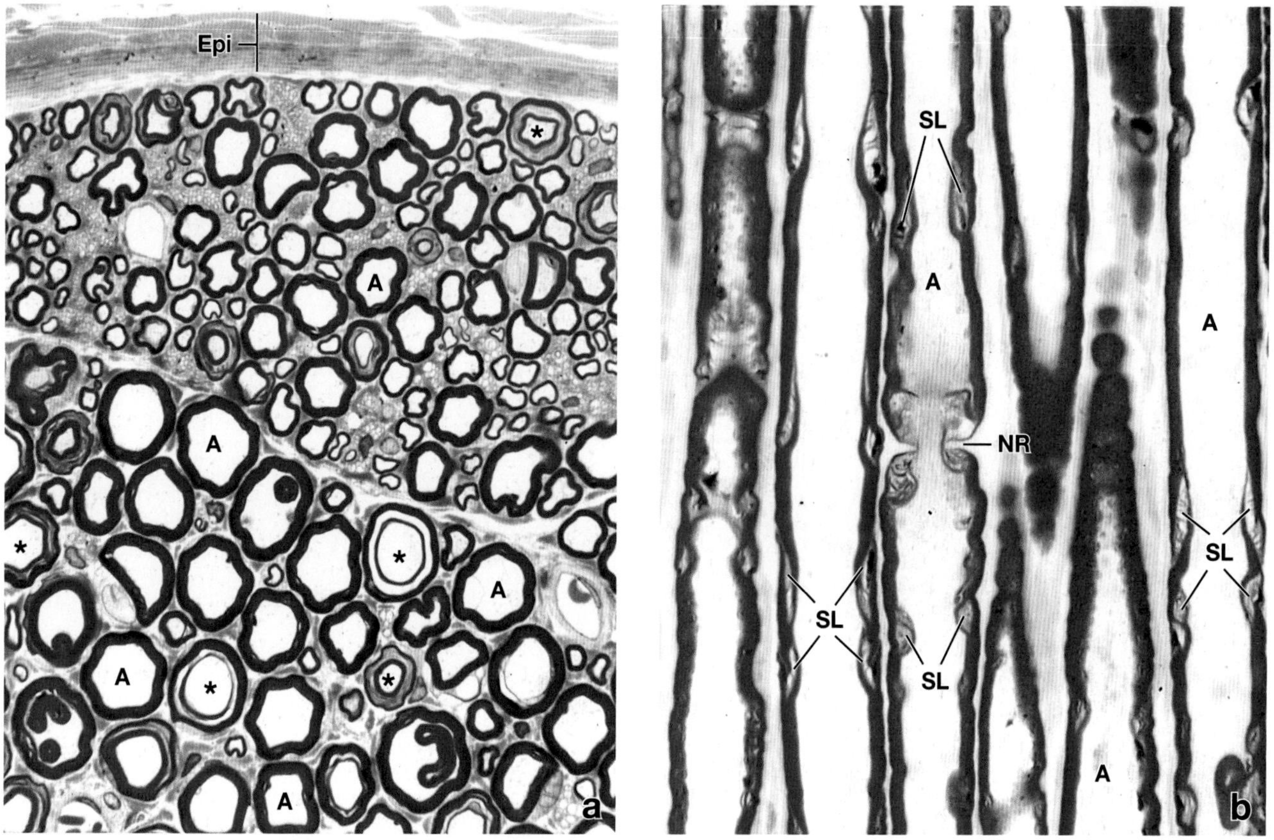

FIGURE 12.13. Photomicrographs of a peripheral nerve in cross and longitudinal sections. a. Photomicrograph of an osmium-fixed, toluidine blue–stained peripheral nerve cut in cross section. The axons (*A*) appear clear. The myelin is represented by the *dark ring* surrounding the *A*. Note the variation in diameter of the individual *A*. In some of the nerves, the myelin appears to consist of two separate rings (*asterisks*). This is caused by the section passing through a Schmidt–Lanterman cleft. *Epi*, epineurium. ×640. **b.** Photomicrograph showing longitudinally sectioned myelinated nerve *A* in the same preparation as earlier. A node of Ranvier (*NR*) is seen *near the center* of the micrograph. In the same *A*, a Schmidt–Lanterman cleft (*SL*) is seen on each side of the node. In addition, a number of *SL* clefts can be seen in the adjacent *A*. The perinodal cytoplasm of the Schwann cell at the *NR* and the Schwann cell cytoplasm at the *SL* cleft appear virtually unstained. ×640.

into two functionally distinct membrane domains. The part of the Schwann cell membrane that is exposed to the external environment or endoneurium, the **abaxonal plasma membrane**, represents one domain. The other domain is represented by the **adaxonal** or **periaxonal plasma membrane**, which is in direct contact with the axon. When the axon is completely enclosed by the Schwann cell membrane, a third domain, the **mesaxon**, is created (Fig. 12.14b). This third domain is a double membrane that connects the abaxonal and adaxonal membranes and encloses the narrow extracellular space.

The myelin sheath develops from compacted layers of Schwann cell mesaxon wrapped concentrically around the axon.

Myelin sheath formation is initiated when the Schwann cell mesaxon surrounds the axon. A sheet-like extension of the mesaxon then wraps around the axon in a spiraling motion. The first few layers or **lamellae** of the spiral are not compactly arranged—that is, some cytoplasm is left in the first few concentric layers (Fig. 12.14c). The TEM reveals the presence of a 12- to 14-nm gap between the outer (extracellular) leaflets and the Schwann cell's cytoplasm that separates the inner (cytoplasmic) leaflets. As the wrapping progresses, cytoplasm is squeezed out from between the membrane of the concentric layers of the Schwann cell.

External to, and contiguous with, the developing myelin sheath is a thin **outer collar of perinuclear cytoplasm** called the **sheath of Schwann**. This part of the cell is enclosed by an abaxonal plasma membrane and contains the nucleus and most of the organelles of the Schwann cell. Surrounding the Schwann cell is a basal or external lamina. The apposition of the mesaxon of the last layer to itself as it closes the ring of the spiral produces the **outer mesaxon**, the narrow intercellular space adjacent to the external lamina. Internal to the concentric layers of the developing myelin sheath is a narrow **inner collar of Schwann cell cytoplasm** surrounded by the adaxonal plasma membrane. The narrow intercellular space between mesaxon membranes communicates with the adaxonal plasma membrane to produce the **inner mesaxon** (Fig. 12.14d).

Once the mesaxon spirals on itself, the 12- to 14-nm gaps disappear and the membranes form the compact **myelin sheath**. Compaction of the sheath corresponds with the expression of transmembrane **myelin-specific proteins**, such as **protein 0 (P0)**, a **peripheral myelin protein of 22 kDa (PMP22)**, and **myelin basic protein (MBP)**. The inner (cytoplasmic) leaflets of the plasma membrane come close together as a result of the positively charged cytoplasmic domains of P0 and MBP. With the TEM, these closely aligned inner leaflets are electron opaque, appearing as the **major dense lines** in the TEM image of myelin (see Fig. 12.14d). The concentric dense lamellae alternate with the slightly less dense **intraperiod lines** that are formed by closely apposed, but not fused, outer (extracellular) membrane leaflets. The narrow 2.5-nm gap corresponds to the remaining extracellular space containing the extracellular domains of P0 protein (see Fig. 12.14d). P0 is a 30-kDa cell adhesion molecule expressed within the mesoaxial plasma membrane during myelination. This transmembrane glycoprotein mediates strong adhesions between the two opposite

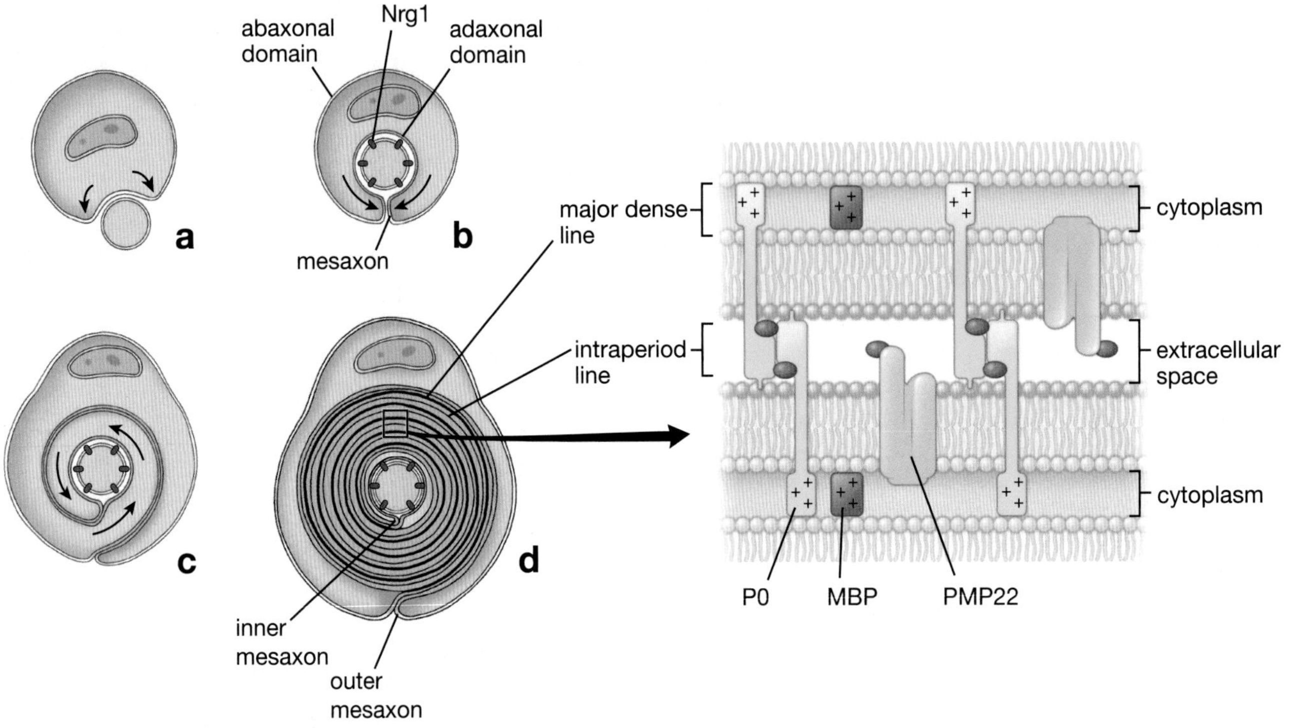

FIGURE 12.14. Diagram showing successive stages in the formation of myelin sheath by a Schwann cell. a. The axon initially lies in a groove on the surface of the immature Schwann cell. **b.** The axon is surrounded by a promyelinating Schwann cell. Note the two domains of the Schwann cell, the adaxonal plasma membrane domain and abaxonal plasma membrane domain. The mesaxon plasma membrane links these domains. The mesaxon membrane initiates myelination by surrounding the embedded axon. **c.** A sheet-like extension of the mesaxon membrane then wraps around the axon, forming multiple membrane layers. **d.** During the wrapping process, the cytoplasm is extruded from between the two apposing plasma membranes of the Schwann cell, which then become compacted to form myelin. The outer mesaxon represents the invaginated plasma membrane extending from the abaxonal surface of the Schwann cell to the myelin sheath. The inner mesaxon extends from the adaxonal surface of the Schwann cell (the part facing the axon) to the innermost layer of the myelin sheath. The *inset* shows the major proteins responsible for compaction of the myelin sheath. *MBP*, myelin basic protein; *Nrg1*, neuregulin; *P0*, protein 0; *PMP22*, peripheral myelin protein of 22 kDa.

membrane layers and represents a key structural component of peripheral nerve myelin. Structural and genetic studies indicate that mutations in human genes encoding P0 produce unstable myelin and may contribute to the development of **demyelinating diseases** (see Folder 12.2).

The thickness of the myelin sheath at myelination is determined by axon diameter and not by the Schwann cell.

Myelination is an example of cell-to-cell communication in which the axon interacts with the Schwann cell. Experimental studies show that the number of layers of myelin is

FOLDER 12.2

CLINICAL CORRELATION: DEMYELINATING DISEASES

In general, **demyelinating diseases** are characterized by preferential damage to the myelin sheath. Clinical symptoms of these diseases are related to decreased or lost ability to transmit electrical impulses along nerve fibers. Several immune-mediated diseases affect the myelin sheath.

Guillain–Barré syndrome, also known as **acute inflammatory demyelinating polyradiculoneuropathy**, is one of the most common life-threatening diseases of the peripheral nervous system (PNS). Microscopic examination of nerve fibers obtained from patients affected by this disease shows a large accumulation of lymphocytes, macrophages, and plasma cells around nerve fibers within nerve fascicles. Large segments of the myelin sheath are damaged, leaving the axons exposed to the extracellular matrix. These findings are consistent with a T-cell–mediated immune response directed against myelin, which causes its destruction and slows or blocks nerve conduction. Patients exhibit symptoms of ascending muscle paralysis, loss of muscle coordination, and loss of cutaneous sensation.

Multiple sclerosis (MS) is a disease that attacks myelin in the central nervous system (CNS). MS is also characterized by immune-mediated damage to myelin, which becomes detached from the axon and is eventually destroyed. In addition, destruction of oligodendroglia, the cells responsible for the synthesis and maintenance of myelin, occurs. Myelin basic protein appears to be the major autoimmune target in this disease. Chemical changes in the lipid and protein constituents of myelin produce irregular, multiple **plaques** throughout the white matter of the brain. Symptoms of MS depend on the area in the CNS in which myelin is damaged. MS is usually characterized by distinct episodes of neurologic deficits, such as unilateral vision impairment, loss of cutaneous sensation, lack of muscle coordination and movement, and loss of bladder and bowel control.

Treatment of both diseases is related to diminishing the causative immune response by immunomodulatory therapy with interferon and monoclonal antibodies directed against specific molecular targets on immune cells. For more severe, progressive forms, immunosuppressive drugs may be used.

determined by the axon and not by the Schwann cell. Myelin sheath thickness is regulated by a glial growth factor (GGF) called **neuregulin (Ngr1)** that induces growth, differentiation, and migration of Schwann cells throughout their development. Ngr1 is a transmembrane protein expressed on the axolemma (cell membrane) of the axon.

The node of Ranvier represents the junction between two adjacent Schwann cells.

The myelin sheath is segmented because it is formed by numerous Schwann cells arrayed sequentially along the axon. The junction where two adjacent Schwann cells meet is devoid of myelin. This site is called the **node of Ranvier**. Therefore, the myelin between two sequential nodes of Ranvier is called an **internodal segment** (Plate 12.2, page 434). The node of Ranvier constitutes a region where the electrical impulse is regenerated for high-speed propagation down the axon. The highest density of voltage-gated Na^+ channels in the nervous system occurs at the node of Ranvier; their expression is regulated by interactions with the perinodal cytoplasm of Schwann cells.

Myelin is composed of about 80% lipids because, as the Schwann cell membrane winds around the axon, the cytoplasm of the Schwann cell, as noted, is extruded from between the opposing layers of the plasma membranes. Electron micrographs, however, typically show small amounts of cytoplasm in several locations (Figs. 12.15 and 12.16): the inner collar of Schwann cell cytoplasm, between the axon and the myelin; the **Schmidt–Lanterman clefts**, small islands within successive lamellae of the myelin; **perinodal cytoplasm**, at the node of Ranvier; and the outer collar of perinuclear cytoplasm, around the myelin (Fig. 12.17). These areas of cytoplasm are what light microscopists identified as the Schwann sheath.

However, if one conceptually unrolls the Schwann cell process, as shown in Fig. 12.18, its full extent can be appreciated, and the inner collar of Schwann cell cytoplasm can be seen to be continuous with the body of the Schwann cell through the Schmidt–Lanterman clefts and the perinodal cytoplasm. Cytoplasm of the clefts contains lysosomes and occasional mitochondria and microtubules, as well as cytoplasmic inclusions, or dense bodies. The number of Schmidt–Lanterman clefts correlates with the diameter of the axon; larger axons have more clefts.

Unmyelinated axons in the peripheral nervous system are enveloped by nonmyelinating Remak Schwan cells and their external lamina.

The nerves in the PNS described as **unmyelinated** are nevertheless enveloped by **nonmyelinating Remak Schwann cell's** cytoplasm, as shown in Fig. 12.19, and can accommodate multiple small-diameter axons. The Remak Schwann cells are elongated in parallel to the long axis of the axons, and the axons fit into grooves on the cell surface. The lips of the groove may be open, exposing a portion of the axolemma of the axon to the adjacent external lamina of the Remak Schwann cell, or the lips may be closed, forming a mesaxon.

A single axon or a group of axons may be enclosed in a single invagination of the Remak Schwann cell surface. Large Remak Schwann cells in the PNS may have 20 or more grooves, each containing either one completely isolated axon (in the distal part of the nerve) or multiple axons (in the proximal part of the nerve close to ganglia). In the ANS, it is common for bundles of unmyelinated axons to occupy a single groove. Because they form bundles within the Remak Schwann cell's cytoplasm, unmyelinated nerves are often called **Remak bundles**. An interesting feature of unmyelinated nerve fibers has been observed in which axons may switch their position between neighboring Remak bundles along the nerve.

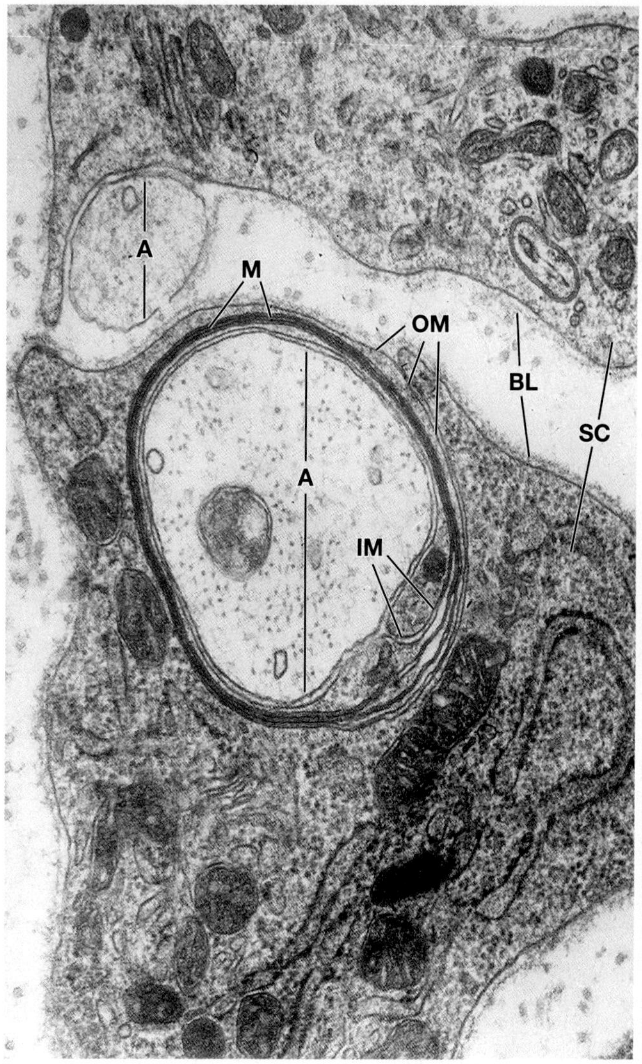

FIGURE 12.15. Electron micrograph of an axon in the process of myelination. At this stage of development, the myelin (*M*) sheath consists of about six membrane layers. The inner mesaxon (*IM*) and outer mesaxon (*OM*) of the Schwann cell (*SC*) represent parts of the mesaxon membrane. Another axon (see *upper left A*) is present that has not yet been embedded within an *SC* mesaxon. Other notable features include the *SC* basal (external) lamina (*BL*) and the considerable amount of Schwann cell cytoplasm associated with the myelination process. ×50,000. (Courtesy of Dr. Stephen G. Waxman.)

Satellite Cells

The neuronal cell bodies of ganglia are surrounded by a layer of small cuboidal cells called **satellite cells**. Although they form a complete layer around the cell body, only their nuclei are typically visible in routine H&E preparations (Fig. 12.20a and b). In paravertebral and peripheral ganglia, neural cell processes must penetrate between the satellite cells to establish a synapse (there are no synapses in sensory ganglia). They help to establish and maintain a controlled microenvironment around the neuronal body in the ganglion, providing electrical insulation as well as a pathway for metabolic exchanges. Thus, the functional role of the satellite cell is analogous to that of the Schwann cell, except that it does not make myelin.

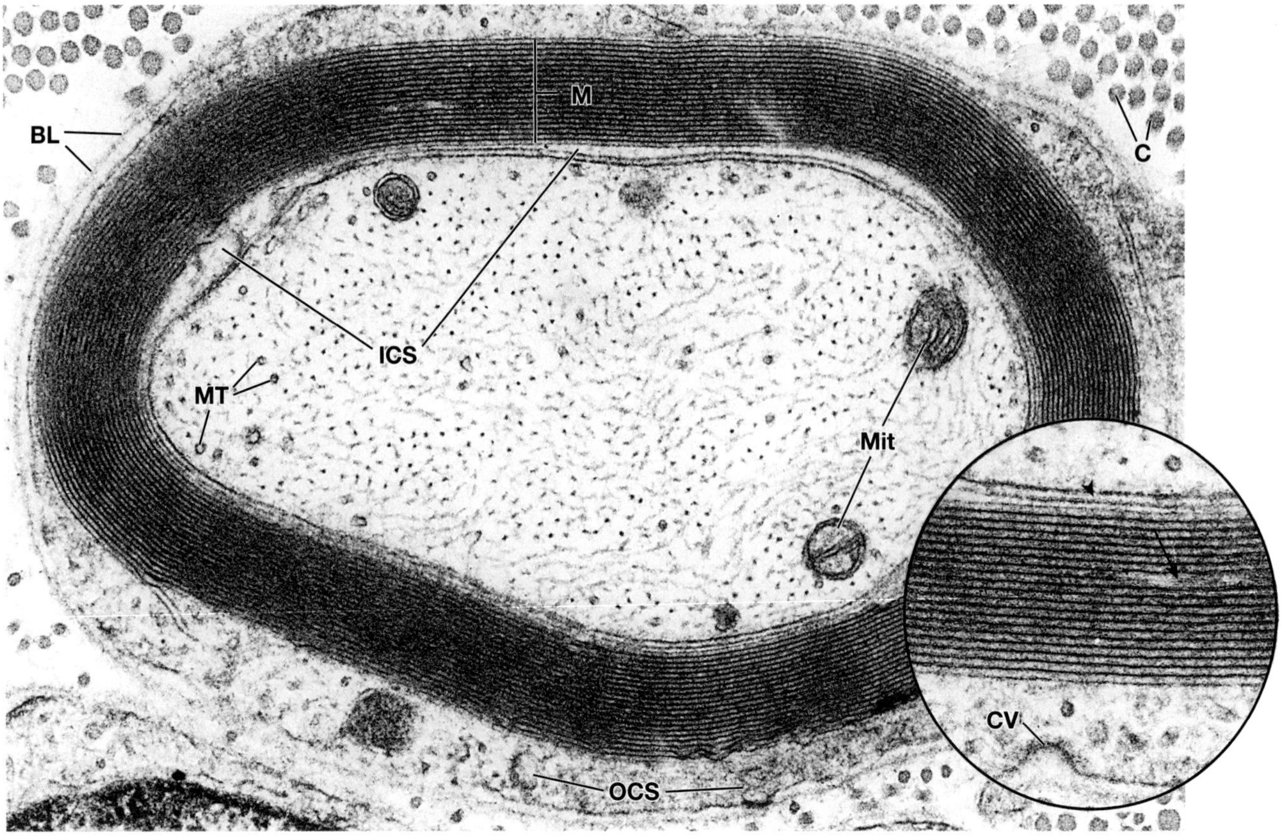

FIGURE 12.16. Electron micrograph of a mature myelinated axon. The myelin sheath (*M*) shown here consists of 19 paired layers of Schwann cell membrane. The pairing of membranes in each layer is caused by the extrusion of the Schwann cell's cytoplasm. The axon displays an abundance of neurofilaments, most of which have been cross-sectioned, giving the axon a stippled appearance. Also evident in the axon are microtubules (*MT*) and several mitochondria (*Mit*). The outer collar of Schwann cell's cytoplasm (*OCS*) is relatively abundant compared with the inner collar of Schwann cell's cytoplasm (*ICS*). The collagen fibrils (*C*) constitute the fibrillar component of the endoneurium. *BL*, basal (external) lamina. ×70,000. **Inset.** Higher magnification of the myelin. The *arrow* points to cytoplasm within the myelin that would contribute to the appearance of the Schmidt–Lanterman cleft as seen in the light microscope. It appears as an isolated region here because of the thinness of the section. The intercellular space between the axon and Schwann cell is indicated by the *arrowhead*. A coated vesicle (*CV*) in an early stage of formation appears in the outer collar of the Schwann cell cytoplasm. ×130,000. (Courtesy of Dr. George D. Pappas.)

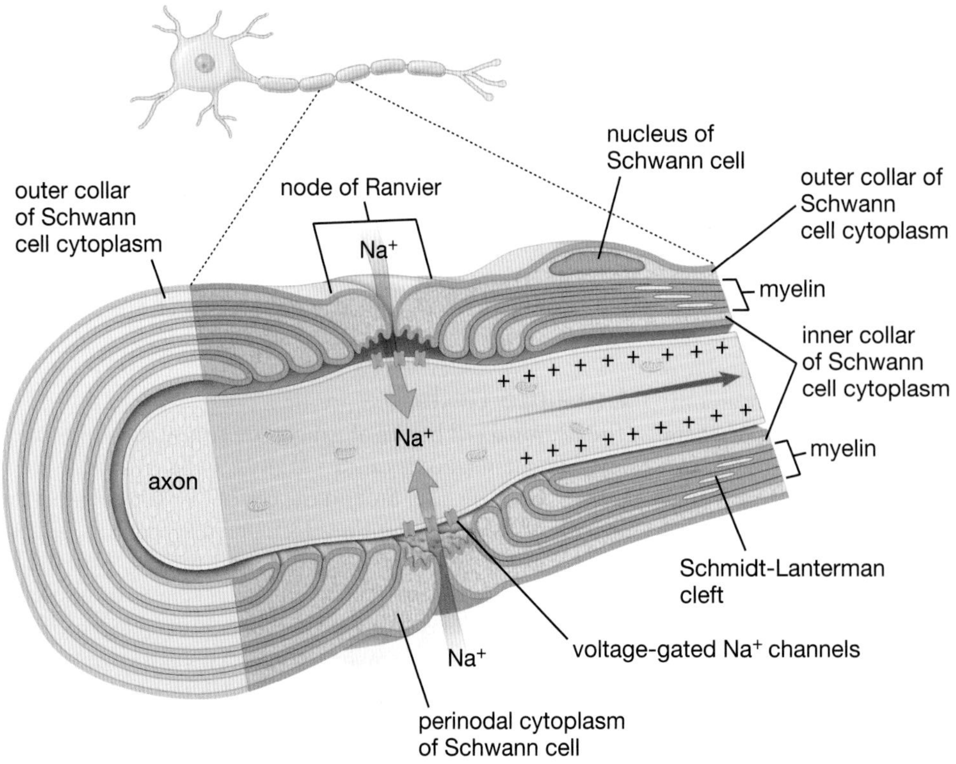

FIGURE 12.17. Diagram of the node of Ranvier and associated Schwann cells. This diagram shows a longitudinal section of the axon and its relationships to the myelin, cytoplasm of the Schwann cell, and node of Ranvier. Schwann cell's cytoplasm is present at four locations: the inner and the outer cytoplasmic collar of the Schwann cell, the nodes of Ranvier, and the Schmidt–Lanterman clefts. Note that the cytoplasm throughout the Schwann cell is continuous (see Fig. 12.18); it is not a series of cytoplasmic islands as it appears on the longitudinal section of the myelin sheath. The node of Ranvier is the site at which successive Schwann cells meet. The adjacent plasma membranes of the Schwann cells are not tightly apposed at the node, and extracellular fluid has free access to the neuronal plasma membrane. The node of Ranvier is also the site of depolarization of the neuronal plasma membrane during nerve impulse transmission and contains clusters of high-density, voltage-gated Na^+ channels.

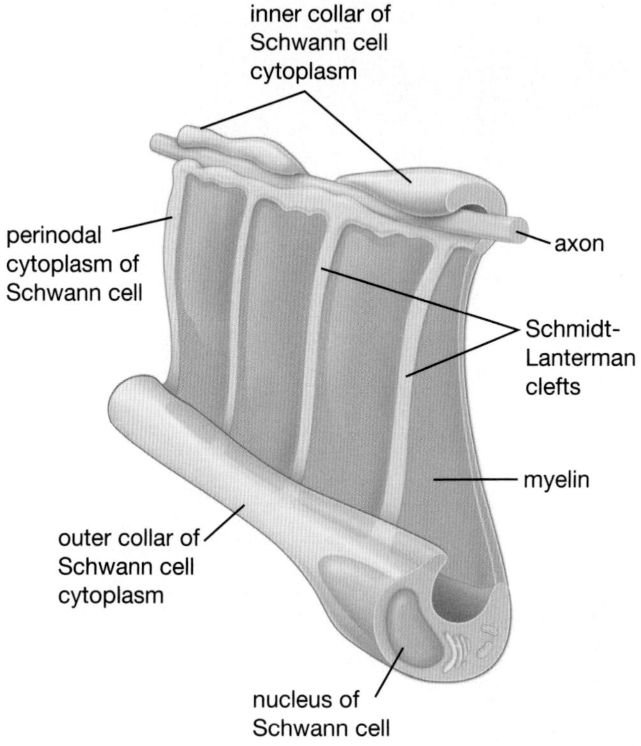

FIGURE 12.18. Three-dimensional diagram conceptualizing the relationship of myelin and cytoplasm of a Schwann cell. This diagram shows a hypothetically uncoiled Schwann cell. Note how the inner collar of the Schwann cell's cytoplasm is continuous with the outer collar of Schwann cell's cytoplasm via Schmidt–Lanterman clefts.

Enteric Neuroglial Cells

Neurons and their processes located within ganglia of the enteric division of the ANS are associated with **enteric neuroglial cells**. These cells are morphologically and functionally similar to **astrocytes** in the CNS (see later). Enteric neuroglial cells share common functions with astrocytes, such as structural, metabolic, and protective support of neurons. However, recent studies indicate that enteric glial cells may also participate in enteric neurotransmission and help coordinate activities of the nervous and immune systems of the gut.

Central Neuroglia

There are four types of central neuroglia:

- **Astrocytes** are morphologically heterogeneous cells that provide physical and metabolic support for neurons of the CNS.
- **Oligodendrocytes** are small cells that are active in the formation and maintenance of myelin in the CNS.
- **Microglia** are inconspicuous cells with small, dark, elongated nuclei that possess phagocytotic properties.
- **Ependymal cells** are columnar cells that line the ventricles of the brain and the central canal of the spinal cord.

Only the nuclei of glial cells are seen in routine histologic preparations of the CNS. Heavy metal staining or immunocytochemical methods are necessary to demonstrate the shape of the entire glial cell.

Although **glial cells** have long been described as supporting cells of nerve tissue in the purely physical sense, current concepts emphasize the **functional interdependence** of neuroglial cells and **neurons**. The most obvious example of physical support occurs during development. The brain and spinal cord develop from the **embryonic neural tube**. In the head region, the neural tube undergoes remarkable thickening and folding, leading ultimately to the final structure, the brain. During the early stages of the process, embryonic glial cells extend through the entire thickness of

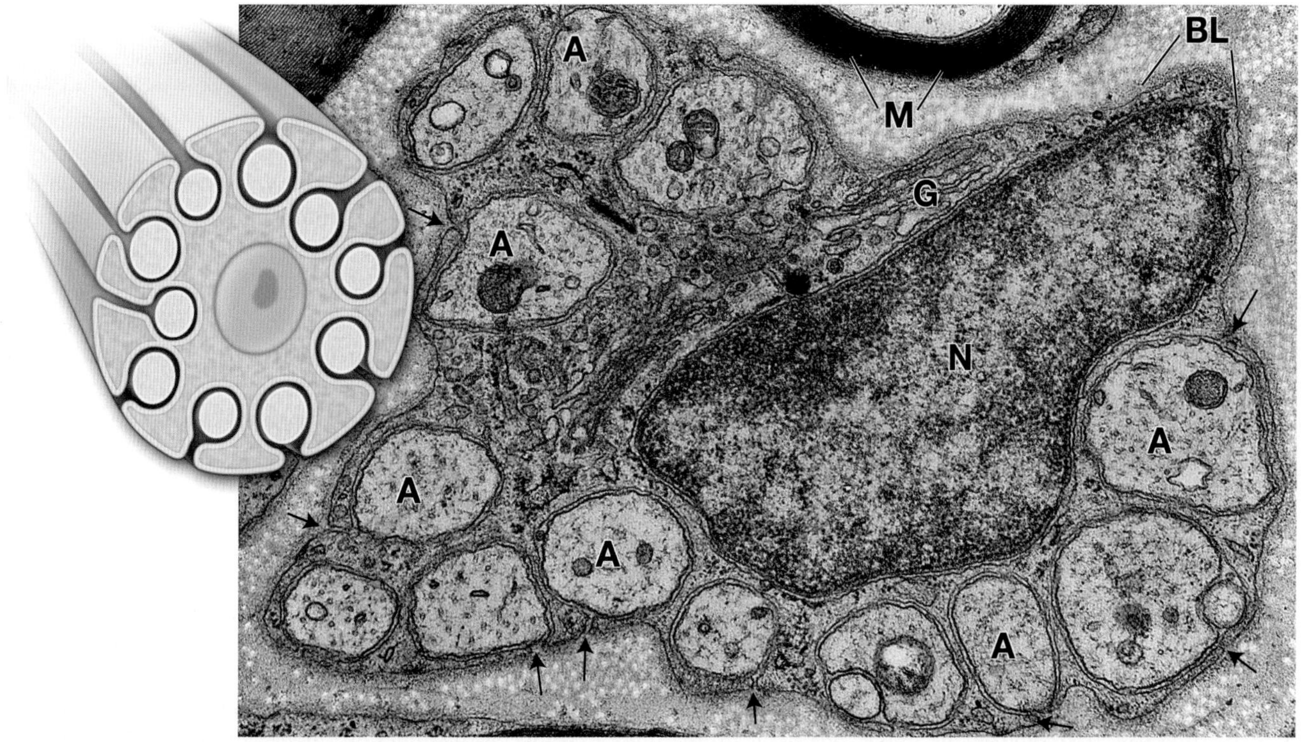

FIGURE 12.19. Electron micrograph of unmyelinated nerve fibers. The individual fibers or axons (*A*) are engulfed by the cytoplasm of a nonmyelinating Remak Schwann cell. The *arrows* indicate the site of mesaxons. In effect, each *A* is enclosed by the Remak Schwann cell's cytoplasm, except for the intercellular space of the mesaxon. Other features evident in the Remak Schwann cell are its nucleus (*N*), the Golgi apparatus (*G*), and the surrounding basal (external) lamina (*BL*). In the *upper part* of the micrograph, myelin (*M*) of two myelinated nerves is also evident. ×27,000. **Inset.** Schematic diagram showing the relationship of *A* engulfed by the Remak Schwann cell.

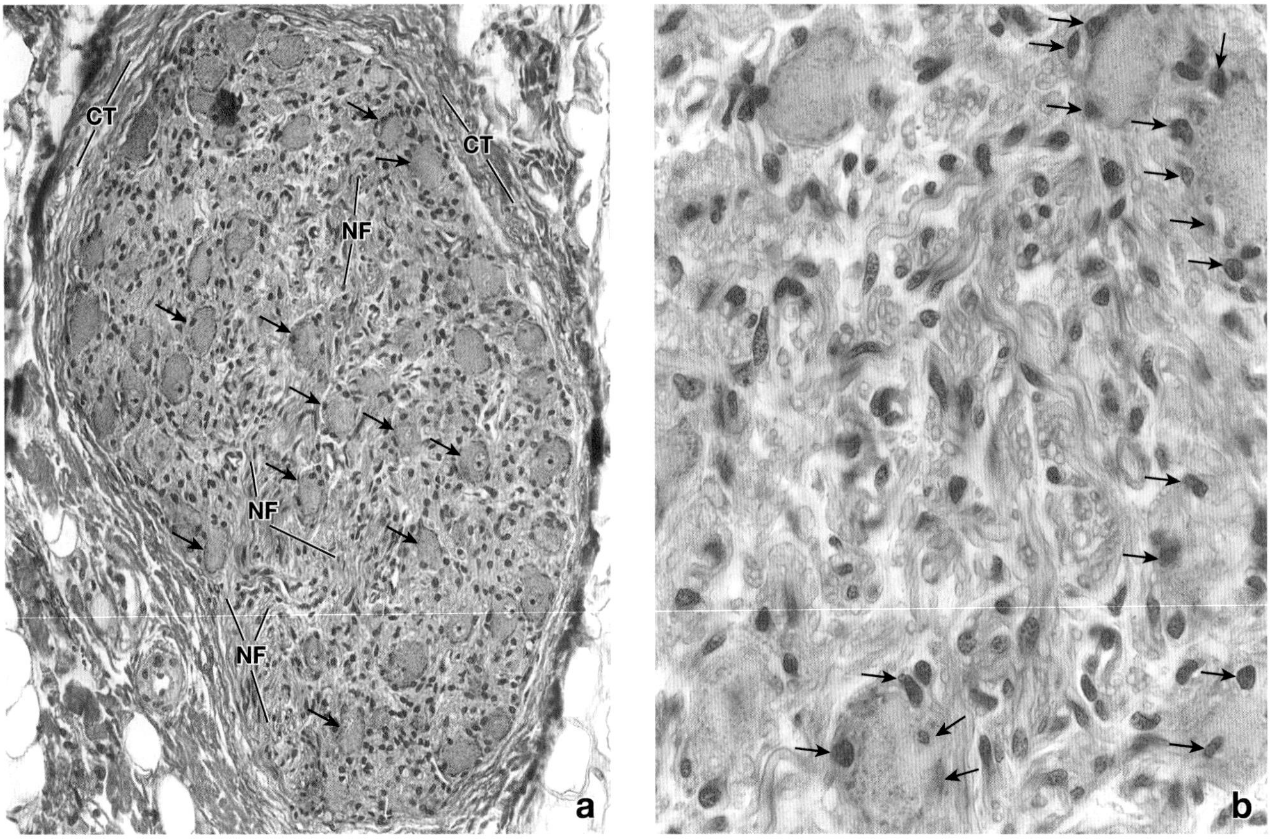

FIGURE 12.20. Photomicrograph of a nerve ganglion. a. Photomicrograph showing a ganglion stained by the Mallory–Azan method. Note the large nerve cell bodies (*arrows*) and nerve fibers (*NF*) in the ganglion. Satellite cells are represented by the very small nuclei at the periphery of the neuronal cell bodies. The ganglion is surrounded by a dense irregular connective tissue capsule (*CT*) that is comparable to, and continuous with, the epineurium of the nerve. ×200. **b.** Higher magnification of the ganglion showing individual axons and a few neuronal cell bodies with their satellite cells (*arrows*). The nuclei in the region of the axons are mostly Schwann cell's nuclei. ×640.

the neural tube in a radial manner. These **radial glial** cells serve as the physical scaffolding that directs the migration of neurons to their appropriate position in the brain.

Astrocytes are closely associated with neurons to support and modulate their activities.

Astrocytes are the largest of the neuroglial cells. They form a network of cells within the CNS and communicate with neurons to support and modulate many of their activities. Some astrocytes span the entire thickness of the brain, providing a scaffold for migrating neurons during brain development. Other astrocytes stretch their processes from blood vessels to neurons. The ends of the processes expand, forming end-feet that cover large areas of the outer surface of the vessel or axolemma. Recently, it has been shown that **reactive astrocytes** possess **phagocytic ability** and are involved in eliminating parts of live neurons such as synapses, nerve cell processes, as well as neuronal debris in the developing and injured brain. During brain development, neurons generate excess synapses. Astrocytic phagocytosis selectively eliminates these unnecessary synapses to achieve precise neural connectivity. Although astrocytes do not form myelin, they provide a compensatory mechanism to clear myelin debris after nerve cell injury if microglia (the primary phagocytic cells in the brain) are unable to execute phagocytosis (see page 413).

Two kinds of astrocytes are identified:

- **Protoplasmic astrocytes** are more prevalent in the outermost covering of the brain called *gray matter*. These astrocytes have numerous short, branching cytoplasmic processes (Fig. 12.21). Fine processes of a single protoplasmic astrocyte form an extensive network interacting with up to two million synapses in humans, allowing the gray matter to relay information at neuronal synapses. They also contribute to neurotransmitter, ion, and energy homeostasis.
- **Fibrous astrocytes** are more common in the inner core of the brain called *white matter*. These astrocytes have fewer, longer, relatively straight, and less branched processes (Fig. 12.22). In the white matter, electrical impulses are mainly propagated along the axons (most often myelinated), with little information processing. The processes of fibrous astrocytes run along axons throughout the white matter and make contact with axons only at the node of Ranvier.

Both types of astrocytes contain prominent bundles of intermediate filaments composed of **glial fibrillary acidic protein (GFAP)**. The filaments are much more numerous in the fibrous astrocytes, however, hence the name. Antibodies to GFAP are used as specific stains to identify astrocytes in sections and tissue cultures (see Fig. 12.22b). Tumors arising from fibrous astrocytes, **fibrous astrocytomas**, account for about 80% of adult primary brain tumors. They can be identified microscopically and by their **GFAP specificity**.

Astrocytes play important roles in the movement of metabolites and wastes to and from neurons. They help maintain the tight junctions of the capillaries that form the **blood–brain barrier** (see pages 424-425). In addition, astrocytes provide a covering for the "bare areas" of myelinated axons—for example, at the nodes of Ranvier and synapses. They may confine neurotransmitters to the synaptic cleft and remove excess neurotransmitters by pinocytosis. **Protoplasmic astrocytes** on the brain and spinal cord surfaces extend

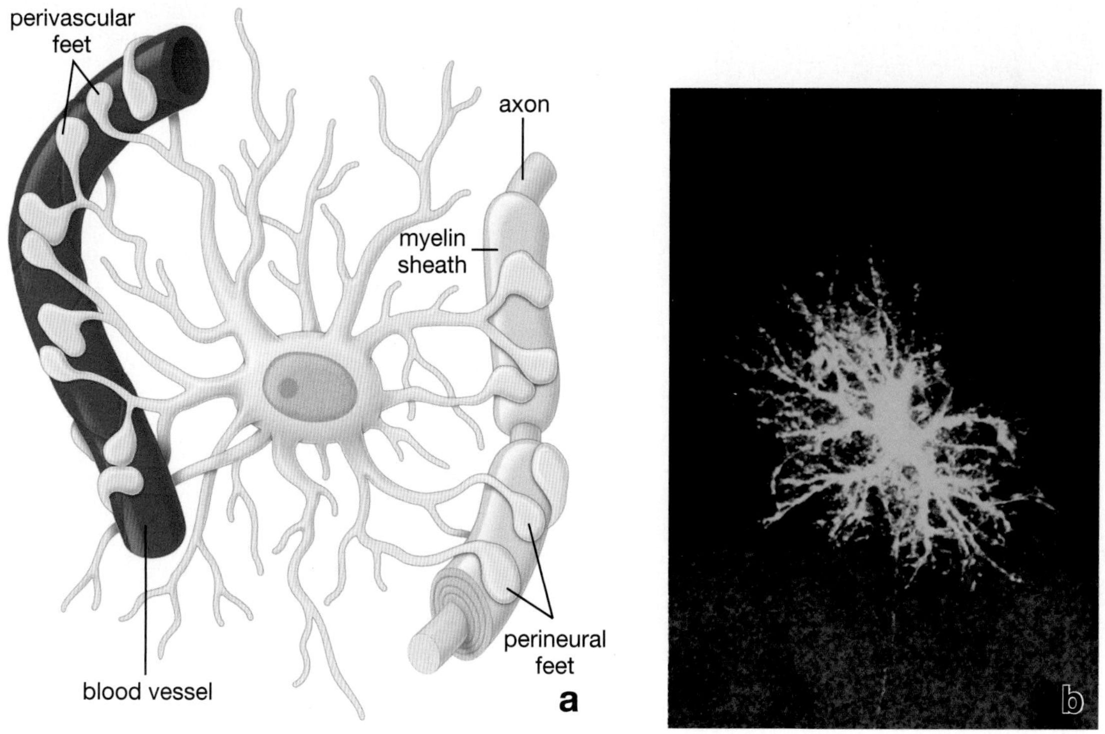

FIGURE 12.21. Protoplasmic astrocyte in the gray matter of the brain. a. This schematic drawing shows the foot processes of a protoplasmic astrocyte terminating on a blood vessel and the axonal process of a nerve cell. The foot processes terminating on the blood vessel contribute to the blood–brain barrier. The bare regions of the vessel as shown in the drawing would be covered by processes of neighboring astrocytes, thus forming the overall barrier. **b.** This laser scanning confocal image of a protoplasmic astrocyte in the gray matter of the dentate gyrus was visualized by intracellular labeling method. In lightly fixed tissue slices, selected astrocytes were impaled and iontophoretically injected with fluorescent dye (Alexa Fluor 568) using pulses of negative current. Note the density and spatial distribution of cell processes. ×480. (Reprinted with permission from Bushong EA, Martone ME, Ellisman MH. Examination of the relationship between astrocyte morphology and laminar boundaries in the molecular layer of adult dentate gyrus. *J Comp Neurol.* 2003;462:241–251.)

their processes (subpial feet) to the basal lamina of the pia mater to form the **glia limitans**, a relatively impermeable barrier surrounding the CNS (Fig. 12.23).

Astrocytes modulate neuronal activities by buffering the K^+ concentration in the extracellular space of the brain.

It is now generally accepted that astrocytes **regulate K^+ concentrations** in the brain's extracellular compartment, thus maintaining the microenvironment and modulating the activities of the neurons. The astrocyte plasma membrane contains an abundance of K^+ pumps and K^+ channels that mediate the transfer of K^+ ions from areas of high to low concentration. Accumulation of large amounts of intracellular K^+ in astrocytes decreases local extracellular K^+ gradients. The astrocyte membrane becomes depolarized, and the charge is dissipated over a large area by the extensive network of

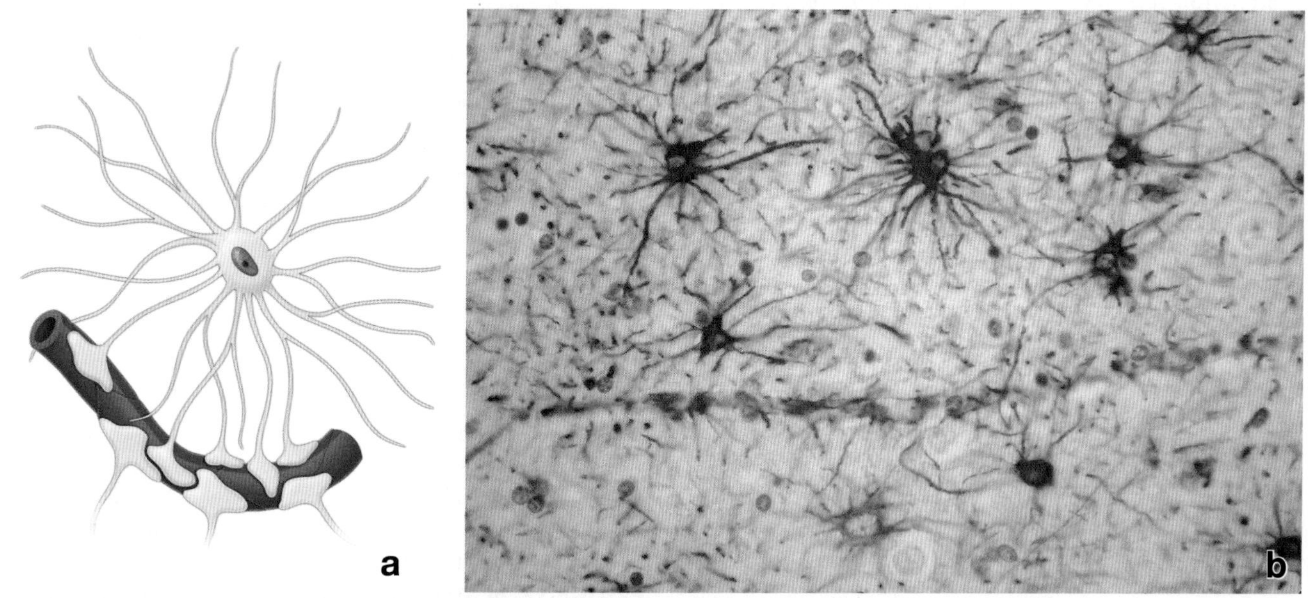

FIGURE 12.22. Fibrous astrocytes in the white matter of the brain. a. Schematic drawing of a fibrous astrocyte in the white mater of the brain. **b.** Photomicrograph of the white matter of the brain showing the extensive radiating cytoplasmic processes for which astrocytes are named. They are best visualized, as shown here, with immunostaining methods that use antibodies against glial fibrillary acidic protein (GFAP). ×220. (Reprinted with permission from Fuller GN, Burger PC. Central nervous system. In: Sternberg SS, ed. *Histology for Pathologists*. Lippincott-Raven; 1997.)

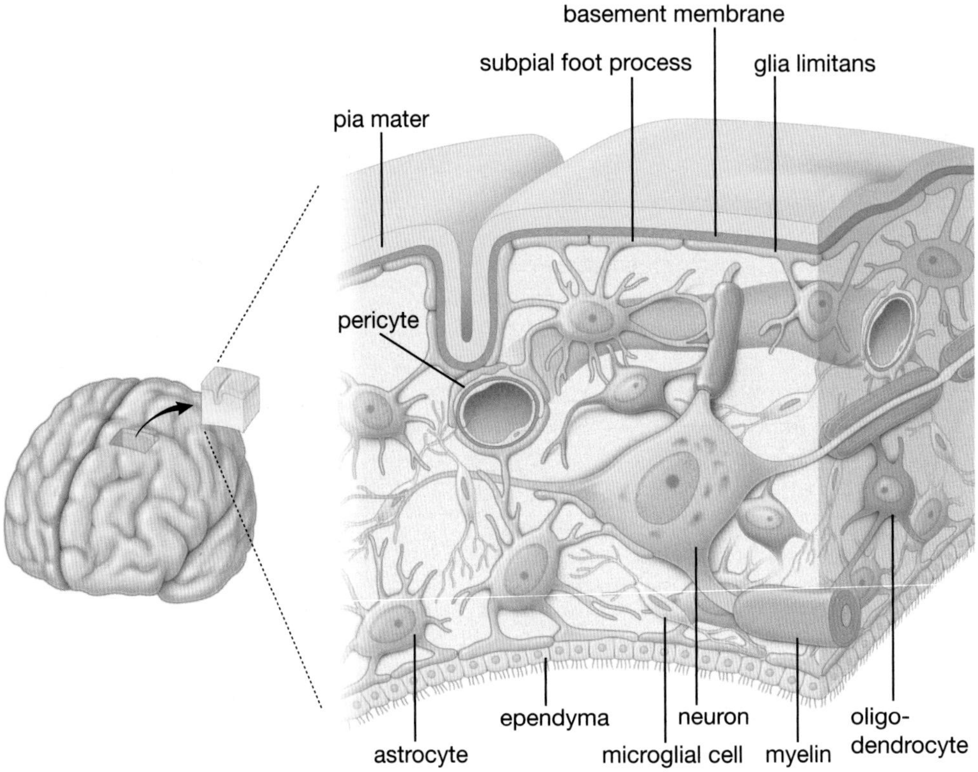

FIGURE 12.23. Distribution of glial cells in the brain. This diagram shows the four types of glial cells—astrocytes, oligodendrocytes, microglial cells, and ependymal cells—interacting with several structures and cells found in the brain tissue. Note that the astrocytes and their processes interact with the blood vessels as well as with axons and dendrites. Astrocytes also send their processes toward the brain surface, where they contact the basement membrane of the pia mater, forming the glia limitans. In addition, processes of astrocytes extend toward the fluid-filled spaces in the central nervous system (CNS), where they contact the ependymal lining cells. Oligodendrocytes are involved in myelination of the nerve fibers in the CNS. Microglia exhibit phagocytotic functions.

astrocyte processes. The maintenance of the K^+ concentration in the brain's extracellular space by astrocytes is called **potassium spatial buffering**.

Oligodendrocytes produce and maintain the myelin sheath in the CNS.

The **oligodendrocyte** is the cell responsible for producing CNS myelin. The myelin sheath in the CNS is formed by concentric layers of oligodendrocyte plasma membrane. The formation of the sheath in the CNS is more complex, however, than the simple wrapping of Schwann cell's mesaxon membranes that occurs in the PNS (pages 405-407).

Oligodendrocytes appear in specially stained LM preparations as small cells with relatively few processes compared with astrocytes. They are often aligned in rows between the axons. Each oligodendrocyte gives off several tongue-like processes that make contact with nearby axons. Each process wraps itself around a portion of an axon, forming an **internodal segment of myelin**. The multiple processes of a single oligodendrocyte may myelinate one axon or several nearby axons (Fig. 12.24). The nucleus-containing region of the oligodendrocyte may be at some distance from the axons it myelinates.

Because a single oligodendrocyte may myelinate several nearby axons simultaneously, the cell cannot embed multiple axons in its cytoplasm and allow the mesaxon membrane to spiral around each axon. Instead, each tongue-like process appears to spiral around the axon, always staying in proximity to it, until the myelin sheath is formed.

The myelin sheath in the CNS differs from that in the PNS.

There are several other important differences between the myelin sheaths in the CNS and those in the PNS. Oligodendrocytes in the CNS express different myelin-specific proteins during myelination than those expressed by Schwann cells in the PNS. Instead of P0 and PMP22, which are expressed only in myelin of the PNS, other proteins, including **proteolipid protein (PLP)**, **myelin oligodendrocyte glycoprotein (MOG)**, and **oligodendrocyte myelin glycoprotein (OMgp)**, perform similar functions in CNS myelin.

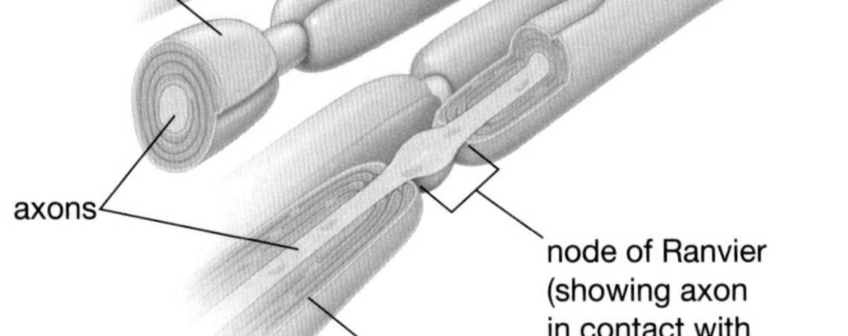

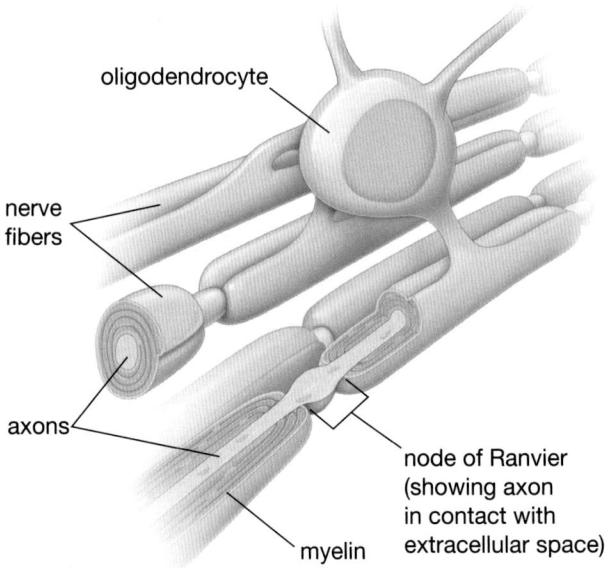

FIGURE 12.24. Three-dimensional view of an oligodendrocyte as it relates to several axons. Cytoplasmic processes from the oligodendrocyte cell body form flattened cytoplasmic sheaths that wrap around each of the axons. The relationship of cytoplasm and myelin is essentially the same as that of Schwann cells.

Deficiencies in the expression of these proteins appear to be important in the pathogenesis of several autoimmune **demyelinating diseases** of the CNS.

On the microscopic level, myelin in the CNS exhibits fewer Schmidt–Lanterman clefts because the astrocytes provide metabolic support for CNS neurons. Unlike Schwann cells of the PNS, oligodendrocytes do not have an external lamina. Furthermore, because of the manner in which oligodendrocytes form CNS myelin, little or no cytoplasm may be present in the outermost layer of the myelin sheath, and with the absence of external lamina, the myelin of adjacent axons may come into contact. Thus, where myelin sheaths of adjacent axons touch, they may share an intraperiod line. Finally, the nodes of Ranvier in the CNS are larger than those in the PNS. The larger areas of exposed axolemma thus make **saltatory conduction** (see later) even more efficient in the CNS.

Another difference between the CNS and the PNS in regard to the relationships between supporting cells and neurons is that unmyelinated neurons in the CNS are often found to be bare—that is, they are not embedded in glial cell processes. The lack of supporting cells around unmyelinated axons as well as the absence of basal lamina material and connective tissue within the substance of the CNS helps to distinguish the CNS from the PNS in histologic sections and TEM specimens.

Microglia possess phagocytotic properties.

Microglia are phagocytotic cells. They normally account for about 5% of all glial cells in the adult CNS but proliferate and become actively phagocytotic (**reactive microglial cells**) in regions of injury and disease. Microglial cells are considered part of the mononuclear phagocyte system (see Folder 6.4, page 203) and originate from erythro-myeloid progenitor cells in the yolk sac. Microglia precursor cells migrate to developing CNS during the embryonic and perinatal stages of development (see page 415). In the past, microglia have been regarded as the primary phagocytic cells in the brain. However, recent evidence shows that astrocytic phagocytosis provides a compensatory mechanism for microglial dysfunction. Similar to astrocytes, microglial cells are involved in synaptic pruning, a process that forms the cellular basis for learning and memory, especially during brain development and brain injury (see page 410). Recent evidence suggests that microglia play a critical role in **defense against invading microorganisms** and neoplastic cells. They remove bacteria, injured cells, and the debris of cells that undergo apoptosis. They also mediate neuroimmune reactions, such as those occurring in chronic pain conditions.

Microglia are the smallest of the neuroglial cells and have relatively small, elongated nuclei (Fig. 12.25). When stained with heavy metals, microglia exhibit short, twisted processes. Both the processes and the cell body are covered with numerous spikes. The spikes may be the equivalent of the ruffled border seen on other phagocytotic cells. The TEM reveals numerous lysosomes, inclusions, and vesicles. However, microglia contain little rER and few microtubules or actin filaments.

Ependymal cells form the epithelial-like lining of the ventricles of the brain and spinal canal.

Ependymal cells form the epithelium-like lining of the fluid-filled cavities of the CNS. They form a single layer of cuboidal-to-columnar cells that have the morphologic and physiologic characteristics of fluid-transporting cells (Fig. 12.26). They are tightly bound by junctional complexes located at the apical surfaces. Unlike a typical epithelium, ependymal cells lack an external lamina. At the TEM level, the basal cell surface exhibits numerous infoldings that interdigitate with adjacent astrocyte processes. The apical surface of the cell possesses cilia and microvilli. The latter are involved in absorbing cerebrospinal fluid (CSF).

Tanycytes are specialized types of ependymal cells. They are most numerous in the floor of the third ventricle. The free surface of tanycytes is in direct contact with CSF, but in contrast to the ependymal cells, they do not possess cilia. The cell body of tanycytes gives rise to a long process that projects into the brain parenchyma. Their role remains unclear; however, they are involved in the transport of substances from the CSF to the blood within the portal circulation of the hypothalamus. Tanycytes are sensitive to glucose concentration; therefore, they may be involved in detecting and responding to changes in energy balance as well as in monitoring other circulating metabolites in the CSF.

Within the **system of brain ventricles**, the epithelium-like lining is further modified to produce the CSF by transport and secretion of materials derived from adjacent capillary loops. The modified ependymal cells and associated capillaries are called the **choroid plexus**.

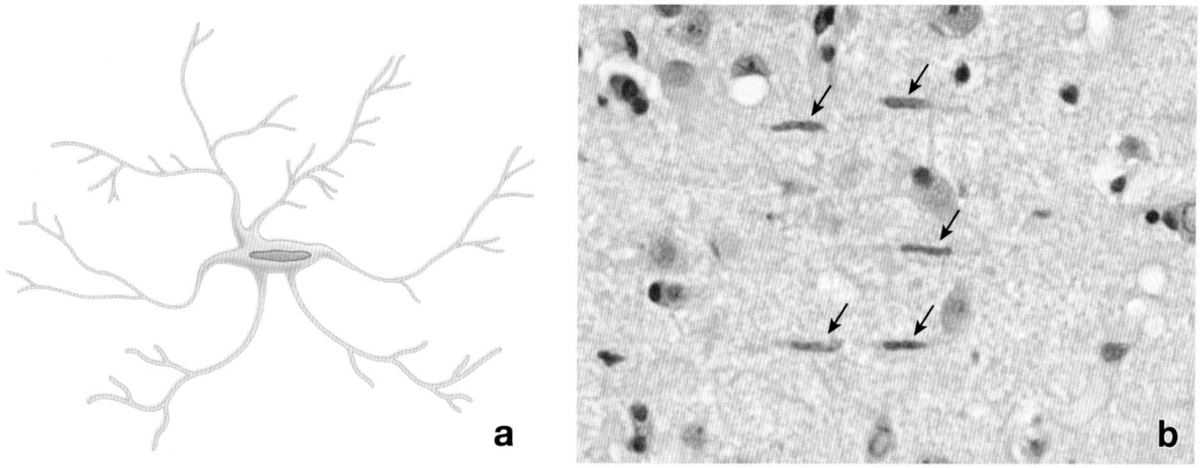

FIGURE 12.25. Microglial cell in the gray matter of the brain. a. This diagram shows the shape and characteristics of a microglial cell. Note the elongated nucleus and relatively few processes emanating from the body. **b.** Photomicrograph of microglial cells (*arrows*) showing their characteristic elongated nuclei. The specimen was obtained from an individual with diffuse microgliosis. In this condition, the microglial cells are present in large numbers and are readily visible in a routine hematoxylin and eosin (H&E) preparation. ×420. (Reprinted with permission from Fuller GN, Burger PC. Central nervous system. In: Sternberg SS, ed. *Histology for Pathologists*. Lippincott-Raven; 1997.)

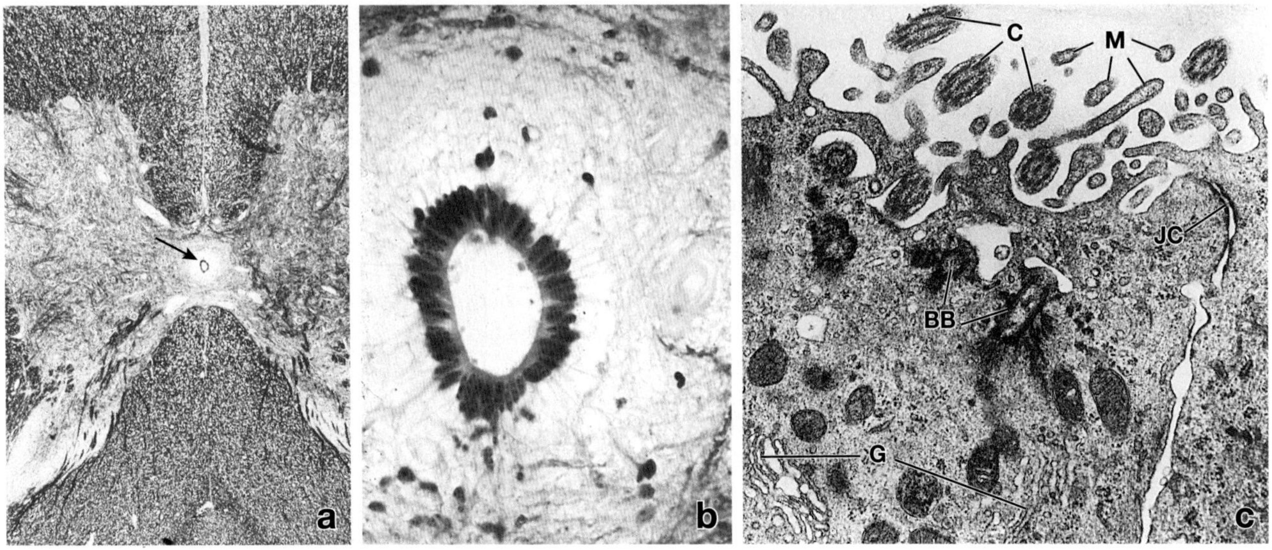

FIGURE 12.26. Ependymal lining of the spinal canal. a. Photomicrograph of the central region of the spinal cord stained with toluidine blue. The *arrow* points to the central canal. ×20. **b.** At higher magnification, ependymal cells, which line the central canal, can be seen to consist of a single layer of columnar cells. ×340. (Courtesy of Dr. George D. Pappas.) **c.** Transmission electron micrograph showing a portion of the apical region of two columnar ependymal cells. They are joined by a junctional complex (*JC*) that separates the lumen of the canal from the lateral intercellular space. The apical surface of the ependymal cells has both cilia (*C*) and microvilli (*M*). Basal bodies (*BB*) and a Golgi apparatus (*G*) within the apical cytoplasm are also visible. ×20,000. (Courtesy of Dr. Paul Reier.)

Impulse Conduction

An action potential is an electrochemical process triggered by impulses carried to the axon hillock after other impulses are received on the dendrites or the cell body itself.

A **nerve impulse** is conducted along an axon much as a flame travels along the fuse of a firecracker. This electrochemical process involves the generation of an **action potential**, a wave of membrane depolarization that is initiated at the initial segment of the axon hillock. Its membrane contains a large number of **voltage-gated Na^+ and K^+ channels**. In response to a stimulus, voltage-gated Na^+ channels in the initial segment of the axon membrane open, causing an influx of Na^+ into the axoplasm. This influx of Na^+ briefly reverses (depolarizes) the negative membrane potential of the resting membrane (−70 mV) to positive (+30 mV). After depolarization, the voltage-gated Na^+ channels close and voltage-gated K^+ channels open. K^+ rapidly exits the axon, returning the membrane to its resting potential. Depolarization of one part of the membrane sends electrical current to neighboring portions of unstimulated membrane, which is still positively charged. This local current stimulates adjacent portions of the axon's membrane and repeats depolarization along the membrane. The entire process takes less than 1,000th of a second. After a very brief (refractory) period, the neuron can repeat the process of generating an action potential once again.

Rapid conduction of the action potential is attributable to the nodes of Ranvier.

Myelinated axons conduct impulses more rapidly than unmyelinated axons. Physiologists describe the nerve impulse as "jumping" from node to node along the myelinated axon. This process is called **saltatory** *[L. saltus, to jump]* or **discontinuous conduction**. In myelinated nerves, the myelin sheath around the nerve does not conduct an electric current and forms an insulating layer around the axon. However, the voltage reversal can *only* occur at the nodes of Ranvier, where the axolemma lacks a myelin sheath. Here, the axolemma is exposed to extracellular fluids and possesses a high concentration of voltage-gated Na^+ and K^+ channels (see Figs. 12.17 and 12.24). Thus, the voltage reversal (and thus the impulse) jumps as current flows from one node of Ranvier to the next. The speed of saltatory conduction is related not only to the thickness of the myelin but also to the diameter of the axon. Conduction is more rapid along axons of greater diameter.

In **unmyelinated axons**, Na^+ and K^+ channels are distributed uniformly along the length of the fiber. The nerve impulse is conducted more slowly and moves as a continuous wave of voltage reversal along the axon.

■ ORIGIN OF NERVE TISSUE CELLS

CNS neurons and central glia, except microglial cells, are derived from neuroectodermal cells of the neural tube.

Neurons, oligodendrocytes, astrocytes, and ependymal cells are derived from cells of the **neural tube**. After developing neurons have migrated to their predestined locations in the neural tube and have differentiated into mature neurons, they no longer divide. However, in the adult mammalian brain, a very small number of **neural stem cells** retain the ability to divide. These cells migrate into the sites of injury and differentiate into fully functional nerve cells.

Oligodendrocyte precursors are highly migratory cells. They appear to share a developmental lineage with motor neurons migrating from their site of origin to developing axonal projections (tracts) in the white matter of the brain or spinal cord. The precursors then proliferate in response to the local expression of mitogenic signals. The matching of oligodendrocytes to axons is accomplished through a combination of local regulation of cell proliferation, differentiation, and apoptosis.

Astrocytes are also derived from cells of the neural tube. During the embryonic and early postnatal stages, immature astrocytes migrate into the cortex, where they differentiate and become mature astrocytes. **Ependymal cells** are derived from the proliferation of neuroepithelial cells that immediately surround the canal of the developing neural tube.

In contrast to other central neuroglia, **microglia cells** are derived from mesodermal macrophage precursors, specifically from **erythro-myeloid progenitor cells** in the yolk sac. They infiltrate the neural tube in the early stages of its development and under the influence of growth factors such as colony-stimulating factor 1 (CSF-1) produced by developing neural cells as they undergo proliferation and differentiation into motile amoeboid cells. These motile cells are commonly observed in the developing brain. As the only glial cells of mesenchymal origin, microglia possess the **vimentin class of intermediate filaments**, which can be useful in identifying these cells with immunocytochemical methods.

PNS ganglion cells and peripheral glia are derived from the neural crest.

The development of the **ganglion cells** of the PNS involves the proliferation and migration of ganglion precursor cells from the **neural crest** to their future ganglionic sites, where they undergo further proliferation. Here, the cells develop processes that reach the cells' target tissues (e.g., glandular tissue or smooth muscle cells) and sensory territories. Initially, more cells are produced than are needed. Those that do not make functional contact with a target tissue undergo apoptosis.

Schwann cells also arise from migrating neural crest cells that become associated with the axons of early embryonic nerves. Several genes have been implicated in Schwann cell development. Sex-determining region Y (SRY) box 10 (*Sox10*) is required for the generation of all peripheral glia from neural crest cells. Axon-derived neuregulin-1 (*Nrg-1*) sustains the **Schwann cell precursors** that undergo differentiation and divide along the growing nerve processes. The fate of all immature Schwann cells is determined by the nerve processes with which they have immediate contact. Immature Schwann cells that associate with large-diameter axons mature into myelinating Schwann cells, whereas those that associate with small-diameter axons mature into nonmyelinating cells.

■ ORGANIZATION OF THE PERIPHERAL NERVOUS SYSTEM

The **peripheral nervous system (PNS)** consists of peripheral nerves with specialized nerve endings and ganglia-containing nerve cell bodies that reside outside the CNS.

Peripheral Nerves

A peripheral nerve is a bundle of nerve fibers held together by connective tissue.

The nerves of the PNS are made up of many nerve fibers that carry sensory and motor (effector) information between the organs and tissues of the body and between the brain and spinal cord. The term **nerve fiber** is used in different ways that can be confusing. It can connote the axon with all of its coverings (myelin and Schwann cell), as used earlier, or it can connote the axon alone. It is also used to refer to any process of a nerve cell, either dendrite or axon, especially if insufficient information is available to identify the process as either an axon or a dendrite.

The cell bodies of peripheral nerves may be located either within the CNS or outside the CNS in **peripheral ganglia**. Ganglia contain clusters of neuronal cell bodies and the nerve fibers leading to and from them (see Fig. 12.20). The cell bodies in the dorsal root ganglia as well as ganglia of cranial nerves belong to sensory neurons (**somatic afferents** and **visceral afferents** that belong to the ANS discussed earlier), whose distribution is restricted to specific locations (Table 12.2 and Fig. 12.3). The cell bodies in the paravertebral,

TABLE 12.2 Peripheral Ganglia[a]

Ganglia that contain cell bodies of sensory neurons; these are not synaptic stations

- **Dorsal root ganglia of all spinal nerves**
- **Sensory ganglia of cranial nerves**
  - Trigeminal (semilunar, Gasserian) ganglion of the trigeminal (V) nerve
  - Geniculate ganglion of the facial (VII) nerve
  - Spiral ganglion (contains bipolar neurons) of the cochlear division of the vestibulocochlear (VIII) nerve
  - Vestibular ganglion (contains bipolar neurons) of the vestibular division of the vestibulocochlear (VIII) nerve
  - Superior and inferior ganglia of the glossopharyngeal (IX) nerve
  - Superior and inferior ganglia of the vagus (X) nerve

Ganglia that contain cell bodies of autonomic (postsynaptic) neurons; these are synaptic stations

- **Sympathetic ganglia**
  - Sympathetic trunk (paravertebral) ganglia (the highest of these is the superior cervical ganglion)
  - Prevertebral ganglia (adjacent to origins of large unpaired branches of abdominal aorta), including celiac, superior mesenteric, inferior mesenteric, and aorticorenal ganglia
  - Adrenal medulla, which may be considered a modified sympathetic ganglion (each of the secretory cells of the medulla, as well as the recognizable ganglion cells, is innervated by cholinergic presynaptic sympathetic nerve fibers)
- **Parasympathetic ganglia**
  - Head ganglia
    - Ciliary ganglion associated with the oculomotor (III) nerve
    - Submandibular ganglion associated with the facial (VII) nerve
    - Pterygopalatine (sphenopalatine) ganglion of the facial (VII) nerve
    - Otic ganglion associated with the glossopharyngeal (IX) nerve
  - Terminal ganglia (near or in wall of organs), including ganglia of the submucosal (Meissner) and myenteric (Auerbach) plexuses of the gastrointestinal tract (these are also ganglia of the enteric division of the ANS) and isolated ganglion cells in a variety of organs

[a]Practical note: Neuron cell bodies seen in tissue sections such as tongue, pancreas, urinary bladder, and heart are invariably terminal ganglia or "ganglion cells" of the parasympathetic nervous system.

prevertebral, and terminal ganglia belong to postsynaptic "motor" neurons (**visceral efferents**) of the ANS (see Table 12.1 and Fig. 12.20).

To understand the PNS, it is also necessary to describe some parts of the CNS.

Motor neuron cell bodies of the PNS lie in the CNS.

The cell bodies of motor neurons that innervate skeletal muscle (**somatic efferents**) are located in the brain, brainstem, and spinal cord. The axons leave the CNS and travel in peripheral nerves to the skeletal muscles that they innervate. A single neuron conveys impulses from the CNS to the effector organ.

Sensory neuron cell bodies are located in ganglia outside, but close to, the CNS.

In the sensory system (both the **somatic afferent** and the **visceral afferent** components), a single neuron connects the receptor, through a sensory ganglion, to the spinal cord or brainstem. **Sensory ganglia** are located in the dorsal roots of the spinal nerves and in association with sensory components of cranial nerves V, VII, VIII, IX, and X (see Table 12.2).

Connective Tissue Components of a Peripheral Nerve

The bulk of a **peripheral nerve** consists of nerve fibers and their supporting Schwann cells. The individual nerve fibers and their associated Schwann cells are held together by connective tissue organized into three distinctive components, each with specific morphologic and functional characteristics (Fig. 12.27; see also Fig. 12.3).

- The **endoneurium** includes loose connective tissue surrounding each individual nerve fiber.

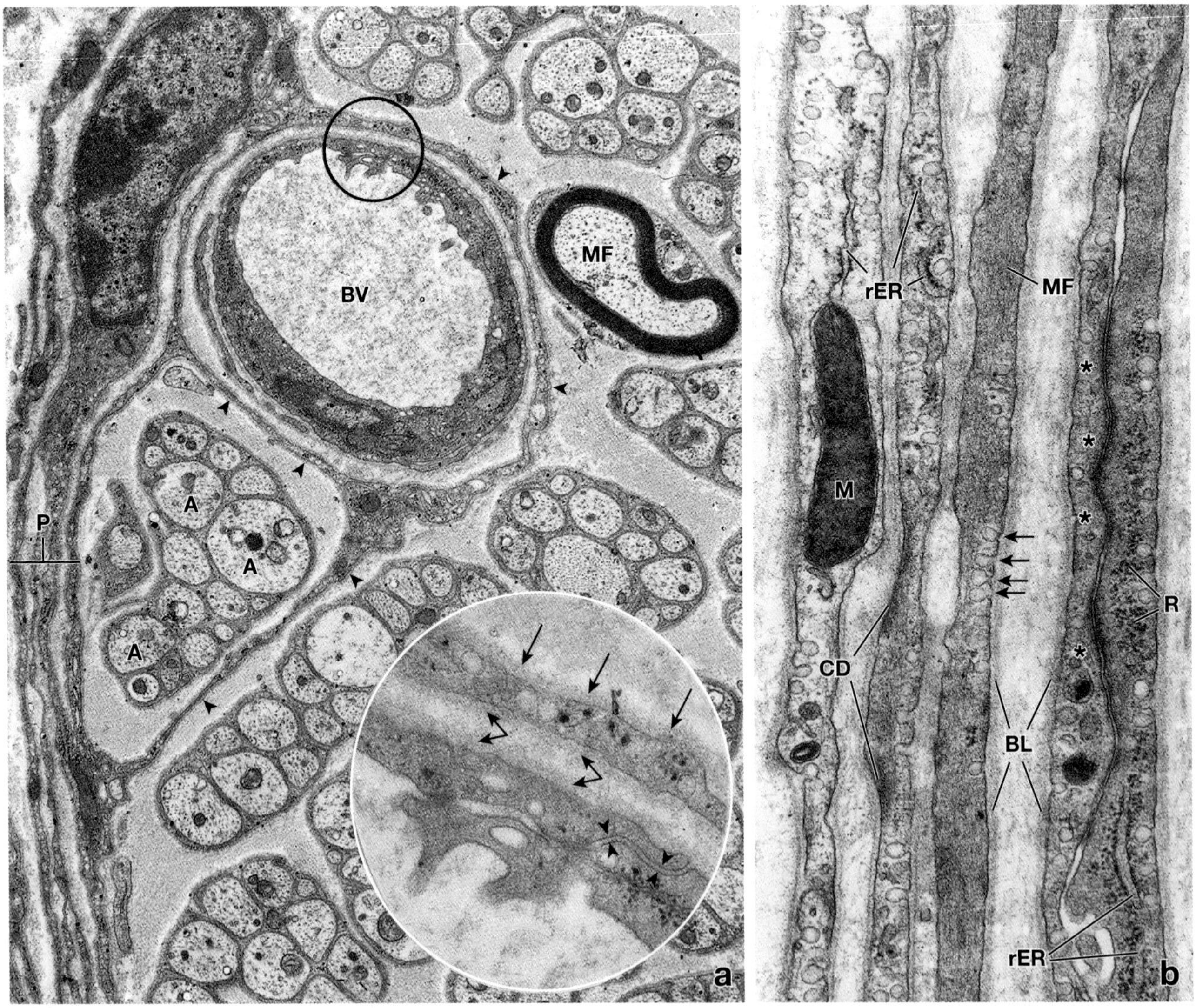

FIGURE 12.27. Electron micrograph of a peripheral nerve and its surrounding perineurium. a. Electron micrograph of unmyelinated nerve fibers and a single myelinated fiber (*MF*). The perineurium (*P*), consisting of several cell layers, is seen on the *left* of the micrograph. Perineurial cell processes (*arrowheads*) have also extended into the nerve to surround a group of axons (*A*) and their Remak Schwann cell as well as a small blood vessel (*BV*). The enclosure of this group of *A* represents the root of a small nerve branch that is joining or leaving the larger fascicle. ×10,000. The area within the *circle* encompassing the endothelium of the vessel and the adjacent perineurial cytoplasm is shown in the *inset* at higher magnification. Note the basal (external) laminae of the vessel and the perineurial cell (*arrows*). The junction between endothelial cells of the blood vessel is also apparent (*arrowheads*). ×46,000. **b.** Electron micrograph showing the perineurium of a nerve. Four cellular layers of the perineurium are present. Each layer has a basal (external) lamina (*BL*) associated with it on both surfaces. Other features of the perineurial cell include an extensive population of actin microfilaments (*MF*), pinocytotic vesicles (*arrows*), and cytoplasmic densities (*CD*). These features are characteristic of smooth muscle cells. The innermost perineurial cell layer (*right*) exhibits tight junctions (*asterisks*) where one cell is overlapping a second cell in forming the sheath. Other features seen in the cytoplasm are mitochondria (*M*), rough-surfaced endoplasmic reticulum (*rER*), and free ribosomes (*R*). ×27,000.

- The **perineurium** includes specialized connective tissue surrounding each nerve fascicle.
- The **epineurium** includes dense irregular connective tissue that surrounds a peripheral nerve and fills the spaces between nerve fascicles.

Endoneurium constitutes the loose connective tissue associated with individual nerve fibers.

The **endoneurium** is not conspicuous in routine LM preparations, but special connective tissue stains permit its demonstration. At the electron microscope level, collagen fibrils that constitute the endoneurium are readily apparent (see Figs. 12.15 and 12.16). The fibrils run both parallel to and around the nerve fibers, binding them together into a fascicle or bundle. Because **fibroblasts** are relatively sparse in the interstices of the nerve fibers, it is likely that most of the collagen fibrils are secreted by the Schwann cells. This conclusion is supported by tissue culture studies in which collagen fibrils are formed in pure cultures of Schwann cells and dorsal root neurons.

Other than occasional fibroblasts, the only other connective tissue cells normally found within the endoneurium are **mast cells** and **macrophages**. Macrophages mediate immunologic surveillance and also participate in nerve tissue repair. Following nerve injury, they proliferate and actively phagocytose myelin debris. In general, most of the nuclei (90%) found in cross sections of peripheral nerves belong to Schwann cells; the remaining 10% is equally distributed between the occasional fibroblasts and other cells, such as **endothelial cells** of capillaries, macrophages, and mast cells.

Perineurium is the specialized connective tissue surrounding a nerve fascicle that contributes to the formation of the blood–nerve barrier.

Surrounding the nerve bundle is a sheath of unique connective tissue cells that constitutes the **perineurium**. The perineurium serves as a metabolically active diffusion barrier that contributes to the formation of a **blood–nerve barrier**. This barrier maintains the ionic milieu of the ensheathed nerve fibers. In a manner similar to the properties exhibited by the endothelial cells of brain capillaries forming the blood–brain barrier (see pages 424-425), **perineurial cells** possess receptors, transporters, and enzymes that provide for the active transport of substances.

The perineurium may be one or more cell layers thick, depending on the nerve diameter. The cells that compose this layer are squamous; each layer exhibits an external (basal) lamina on both surfaces (Fig. 12.27b and Plate 12.1, page 432). The cells are contractile and contain an appreciable number of actin filaments, a characteristic of smooth muscle cells and other contractile cells. Moreover, when there are two or more perineurial cell layers (as many as five or six layers may be present in larger nerves), collagen fibrils are present between the perineurial cell layers, but fibroblasts are absent. **Tight junctions** provide the basis for the **blood–nerve barrier** and are present between the cells located within the same layer of the perineurium. In effect, the arrangement of these cells as a barrier—the presence of tight junctions and external (basal) lamina material—likens them to an epithelioid tissue. On the other hand, their contractile nature and their apparent ability to produce collagen fibrils also liken them to smooth muscle cells and fibroblasts.

The limited number of connective tissue cell types within the endoneurium (page 416) undoubtedly reflects the protective role that the perineurium plays. Typical immune system cells (i.e., lymphocytes, plasma cells) are not found within the endoneurial and perineurial compartments. This absence of immune cells (other than the mast cells and macrophages) is accounted for by the protective barrier created by the perineurial cells. Typically, only fibroblasts, a small number of resident macrophages, and occasional mast cells are present within the nerve compartment.

Epineurium consists of dense irregular connective tissue that surrounds and binds nerve fascicles into a common bundle.

The **epineurium** forms the outermost tissue of the peripheral nerve. It is a typical **dense irregular connective tissue** that surrounds the fascicles formed by the perineurium (Plate 12.2, page 434). Adipose tissue is often associated with the epineurium in larger nerves.

The blood vessels that supply the nerves travel in the epineurium, and their branches penetrate into the nerve and travel within the perineurium. Tissue at the level of the endoneurium is poorly vascularized; metabolic exchange of substrates and wastes in this tissue depends on diffusion from and to the blood vessels through the perineurial sheath (see Fig. 12.27).

Afferent (Sensory) Receptors

Afferent receptors are specialized structures located at the distal tips of the peripheral processes of sensory neurons.

Although **receptors** may have many different structures, they have one basic characteristic in common: They can initiate a nerve impulse in response to a stimulus. Receptors may be classified as follows:

- **Exteroceptors** react to stimuli from the external environment—for example, temperature, touch, smell, sound, and vision.
- **Enteroceptors** react to stimuli from within the body—for example, the degree of filling or stretch of the alimentary canal, bladder, and blood vessels.
- **Proprioceptors**, which also react to stimuli from within the body, provide sensation of body position and muscle tone and movement.

The simplest receptor is a bare axon called a **nonencapsulated (free) nerve ending**. This ending is found in epithelia, connective tissue, and in close association with hair follicles.

Most sensory nerve endings acquire connective tissue capsules or sheaths of varying complexity.

Sensory nerve endings with connective tissue sheaths are called **encapsulated endings**. Many encapsulated endings are mechanoreceptors located in the skin and joint capsules (Krause end bulb, Ruffini corpuscles, Meissner corpuscles, and Pacinian corpuscles) and are described in Chapter 15, Integumentary System (pages 555-559). **Muscle spindles** are encapsulated sensory endings located in skeletal muscle; they are described in Chapter 11, Muscle Tissue (pages 359-360). Functionally, related Golgi tendon organs are encapsulated tension receptors found at musculotendinous junctions.

■ ORGANIZATION OF THE AUTONOMIC NERVOUS SYSTEM

Although the ANS was introduced early in this chapter (see page 389), it is useful here to describe some of the salient features of its organization and distribution. The ANS is classified into three divisions:

- **Sympathetic division**
- **Parasympathetic division**
- **Enteric division**

The ANS controls and regulates the body's internal environment.

The **ANS** is the portion of the PNS that conducts involuntary impulses to smooth muscle, cardiac muscle, and glandular epithelium. These effectors are the functional units in the organs that respond to regulation by nerve tissue. The term *visceral* is sometimes used to characterize the ANS and its neurons, which are referred to as **visceral motor (efferent) neurons**. However, visceral motor neurons are frequently accompanied by **visceral sensory (afferent) neurons** that transmit pain and reflexes from visceral effectors (i.e., blood vessels, mucous membrane, and glands) to the CNS. These pseudounipolar neurons have the same arrangement as other sensory neurons—that is, their cell bodies are located in sensory ganglia, and they possess long peripheral and central axons, as described earlier.

The main organizational difference between the efferent flow of impulses to skeletal muscle (somatic effectors) and the efferent flow to smooth muscle, cardiac muscle, and glandular epithelium (visceral effectors) is that one neuron conveys the impulses from the CNS to the somatic effector, whereas a chain of two neurons conveys the impulses from the CNS to the visceral effectors (Fig. 12.28). Thus, there is a synaptic station in an autonomic ganglion outside the CNS where a presynaptic neuron makes contact with postsynaptic neurons. Each presynaptic neuron synapses with several postsynaptic neurons.

Sympathetic and Parasympathetic Divisions of the Autonomic Nervous System

The presynaptic neurons of the sympathetic division are located in the thoracic and upper lumbar portions of the spinal cord.

The **presynaptic neurons** send axons from the thoracic and upper lumbar spinal cord to the vertebral and paravertebral ganglia. The **paravertebral ganglia** in the **sympathetic trunk**

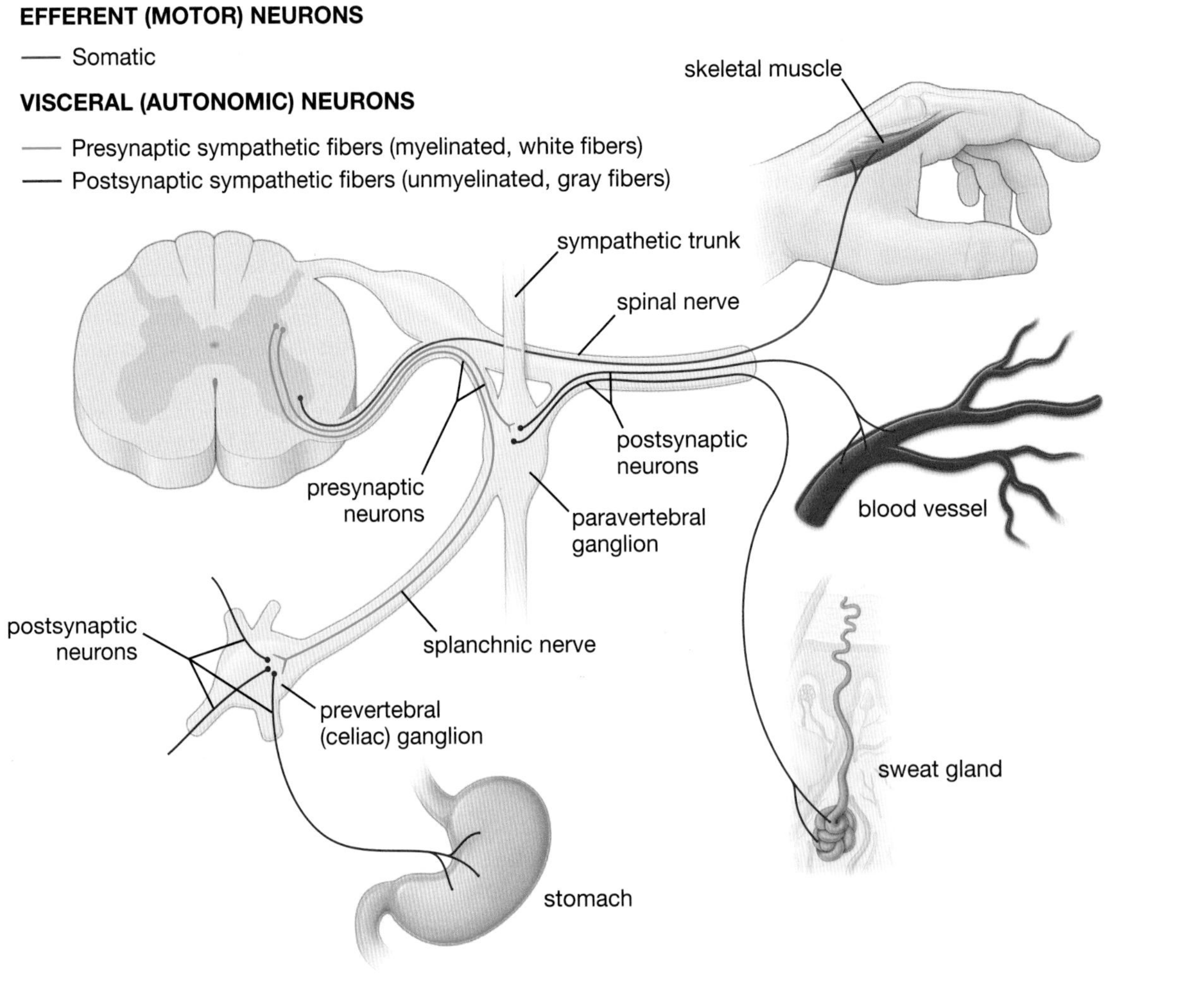

FIGURE 12.28. Schematic diagram of somatic efferent and visceral efferent neurons. In the somatic efferent (motor) system, one neuron conducts the impulses from the central nervous system (CNS) to the effector (skeletal muscle). In the visceral (autonomic) efferent system (represented in this drawing by the sympathetic division of the autonomic nervous system [ANS]), a chain of two neurons conducts the impulses: a presynaptic neuron located within the CNS and a postsynaptic neuron located in the paravertebral or prevertebral ganglia. Moreover, each presynaptic neuron makes synaptic contact with more than one postsynaptic neuron. Postsynaptic sympathetic fibers supply smooth muscles (as in blood vessels) or glandular epithelium (as in sweat glands). Neurons of the ANS that supply organs of the abdomen reach these organs by way of the splanchnic nerves. In this example, the splanchnic nerve joins with the celiac ganglion, where most of the synapses of the two-neuron chain occur.

contain the cell bodies of the postsynaptic effector neurons of the **sympathetic division** (see Figs. 12.28 and 12.29).

The presynaptic neurons of the parasympathetic division are located in the brainstem and sacral spinal cord.

The **presynaptic parasympathetic neurons** send axons from the brainstem—that is, the midbrain, pons, medulla, and the sacral segments of the spinal cord (S2–S4)—to **visceral ganglia.** The ganglia in or near the wall of abdominal and pelvic organs and the visceral motor ganglia of cranial nerves III, VII, IX, and X contain cell bodies of the postsynaptic effector neurons of the **parasympathetic division** (see Figs. 12.28 and 12.29).

The sympathetic and parasympathetic divisions of the ANS often supply the same organs. In these cases, the actions of the two are usually antagonistic. For example, sympathetic

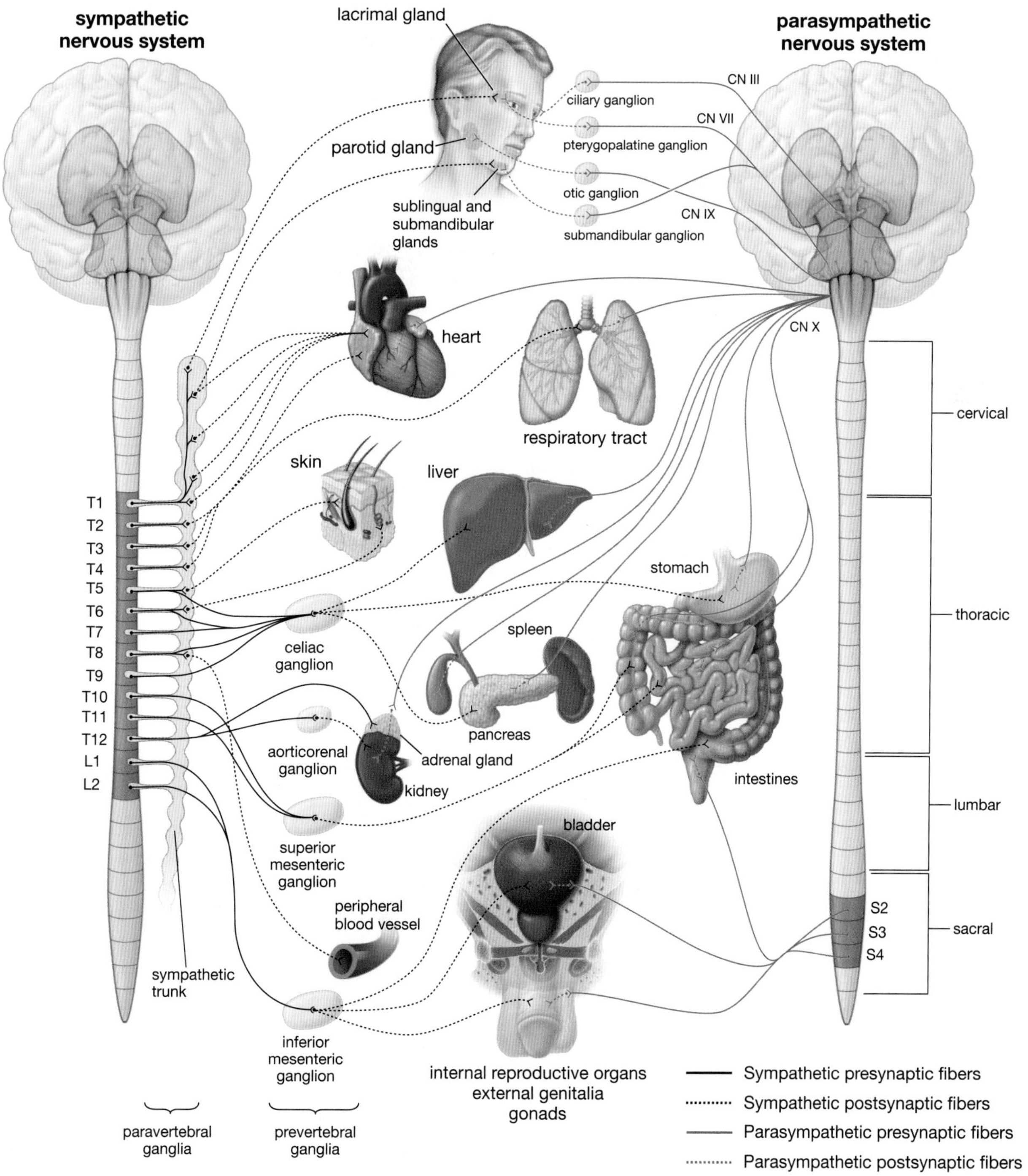

FIGURE 12.29. Schematic diagram showing the general arrangement of sympathetic and parasympathetic neurons of the autonomic nervous system (ANS). The sympathetic outflow is shown on the *left*, the parasympathetic on the *right*. The sympathetic (thoracolumbar) outflow leaves the central nervous system (CNS) from the thoracic and upper lumbar segments (T1–L2) of the spinal cord. These presynaptic fibers communicate with postsynaptic neurons in two locations: the paravertebral and prevertebral ganglia. Paravertebral ganglia are linked together and form two sympathetic trunks on each side of the vertebral column (*drawn as a single column on the side of the spinal cord*). Prevertebral ganglia are associated with the main branches of the abdominal aorta (*yellow ovals*). Note the distribution of postsynaptic sympathetic nerve fibers to the viscera. The parasympathetic (craniosacral) outflow leaves the CNS from the gray matter of the brainstem within cranial nerve (CN) III, CN VII, CN IX, and CN X and the gray matter of sacral segments (S2–S4) of the spinal cord and is distributed to the viscera. The presynaptic fibers traveling with CN III, CN VII, and CN IX communicate with postsynaptic neurons in various ganglia located in the head and neck region (*yellow ovals in front of the head*). The presynaptic fibers traveling with CN X and those from sacral segments (S2–S4) have their synapses with postsynaptic neurons in the wall of visceral organs (terminal ganglia). The viscera thus contains both sympathetic and parasympathetic innervation. Note that a two-neuron chain carries impulses to all viscera, except the adrenal medulla.

stimulation increases the rate of cardiac muscle contractions, whereas parasympathetic stimulation reduces the rate.

Many functions of the SNS are similar to those of the adrenal medulla, an endocrine gland. This functional similarity is partly explained by the developmental relationships between the cells of the adrenal medulla and the postsynaptic sympathetic neurons. Both are derived from the neural crest, are innervated by presynaptic sympathetic neurons, and produce closely related physiologically active agents, EPI and NE. A major difference is that the sympathetic neurons deliver the agent directly to the effector, whereas the cells of the adrenal medulla deliver the agent indirectly through the bloodstream. The innervation of the adrenal medulla may constitute an exception to the rule that autonomic innervation consists of a two-neuron chain from the CNS to an effector unless the adrenal medullary cell is considered the functional equivalent of the second neuron (in effect, a neurosecretory neuron).

Enteric Division of the Autonomic Nervous System

The enteric division of the ANS consists of the ganglia and their processes that innervate the alimentary canal.

The **enteric division of the ANS** represents a collection of neurons and their processes within the walls of the alimentary canal. It controls motility (contractions of the gut wall), exocrine and endocrine secretions, and blood flow through the gastrointestinal tract; it also regulates immunologic and inflammatory processes.

The enteric nervous system can function independently from the CNS and is regarded as the "**brain of the gut**." However, digestion requires communication between enteric neurons and the CNS, which is provided by parasympathetic and sympathetic nerve fibers. Enteroceptors located in the alimentary tract provide sensory information to the CNS regarding the state of digestive functions. The CNS then coordinates sympathetic stimulation, which inhibits gastrointestinal secretion, motor activity, and contraction of gastrointestinal sphincters and blood vessels as well as parasympathetic stimuli that produce opposite actions. **Interneurons** integrate information from sensory neurons and relay this information to enteric motor neurons in the form of reflexes. For instance, the gastrocolic reflex is elicited when distention of the stomach stimulates contraction of musculature of the colon, triggering defecation.

Ganglia and postsynaptic neurons of the enteric division are located in the lamina propria, muscularis mucosae, submucosa, muscularis externa, and subserosa of the alimentary canal from the esophagus to the anus (Fig. 12.30). Because the enteric division does not require presynaptic input from the vagus nerve and sacral outflow, the intestine will continue peristaltic movements, even after the vagus nerve or pelvic splanchnic nerves are severed.

Neurons of the enteric division are not supported by Schwann or satellite cells; instead, they are supported by **enteric neuroglial cells** that resemble astrocytes (see pages 410-411). Cells of the **enteric division** are also affected by the same pathologic changes that can occur in neurons of the brain. Lewy bodies associated with **Parkinson disease** (see Folder 12.1) as well as amyloid plaques and neurofibrillary tangles associated with **Alzheimer disease** have been found in the walls of the large intestine. This finding may lead to the development of routine gastrointestinal biopsies for early diagnosis of these conditions rather than the more complex and risk-associated biopsy of the brain for Alzheimer disease and postmortem identification of Parkinson disease.

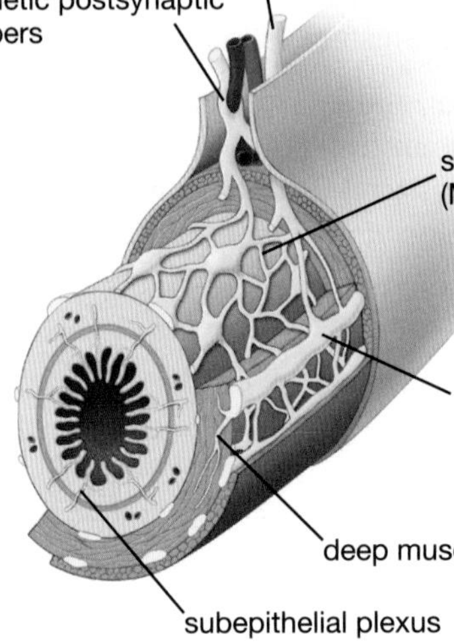

FIGURE 12.30. Enteric nervous system. This diagram shows the organization of the enteric system in the wall of the small intestine. Note the location of two nerve plexuses containing ganglion cells. The more superficial plexus, the myenteric plexus (Auerbach plexus), lies between two muscle layers. Deeper in the region of the submucosa is a network of unmyelinated nerve fibers and ganglion cells, forming the submucosal plexus (Meissner plexus). Parasympathetic fibers originating from the vagus nerve enter the mesentery of the small intestine and synapse with the ganglion cells of both plexuses. Postsynaptic sympathetic nerve fibers also contribute to the enteric nervous system.

A Summarized View of Autonomic Distribution

Figures 12.28 and 12.29 summarize the origins and distribution of the ANS. Refer to these figures as you read the descriptive sections. Note that the diagrams indicate both the paired innervation (parasympathetic and sympathetic) common to the ANS and the important exceptions to this general characteristic.

Head

- **Parasympathetic presynaptic outflow** to the head leaves the brain with the cranial nerves, as indicated in Figure 12.29, but the routes are quite complex. Cell bodies may also be found in structures other than head ganglia listed in Table 12.1 and Figure 12.28 (e.g., in the tongue). These are "terminal ganglia" that contain nerve cell bodies of the parasympathetic system.
- **Sympathetic presynaptic outflow** to the head comes from the thoracic region of the spinal cord. The *postsynaptic neurons* have their cell bodies in the superior cervical ganglion; the axons leave the ganglion in a nerve network that hugs the wall of the internal and external carotid arteries to form the periarterial plexus of nerves. The internal carotid plexus and external carotid plexus follow the branches of the carotid arteries to reach their destination.

Thorax

- **Parasympathetic presynaptic outflow** to the thoracic viscera is via the vagus nerve (X). The *postsynaptic neurons* have their cell bodies in the walls or in the parenchyma of the organs of the thorax.

- **Sympathetic presynaptic outflow** to the thoracic organs is from the upper thoracic segments of the spinal cord. *Sympathetic postsynaptic neurons* for the heart are mostly in the cervical ganglia; their axons make up the cardiac nerves. *Postsynaptic neurons* for the other thoracic viscera are in ganglia of the thoracic part of the sympathetic trunk. The axons travel via small splanchnic nerves from the sympathetic trunk to organs within the thorax and form the pulmonary and esophageal plexuses.

Abdomen and pelvis

- **Parasympathetic presynaptic outflow** to the abdominal viscera is via the vagus (X) and pelvic splanchnic nerves. *Postsynaptic neurons* of the parasympathetic system to abdominopelvic organs are in terminal ganglia that generally are in the walls of the organs, such as the ganglia of the submucosal (Meissner) plexus and the myenteric (Auerbach) plexus in the alimentary canal. These ganglia are part of the enteric division of the ANS.
- **Sympathetic presynaptic outflow** to the abdominopelvic organs is from the lower thoracic and upper lumbar segments of the spinal cord. These fibers travel to the prevertebral ganglia through abdominopelvic splanchnic nerves consisting of the greater, lesser, and least thoracic splanchnic and lumbar splanchnic nerves. *Postsynaptic neurons* have their cell bodies mostly in the prevertebral ganglia (see Fig. 12.28). Only presynaptic fibers terminating on cells in the medulla of the suprarenal (adrenal) gland originate from paravertebral ganglia of the sympathetic trunk. The adrenal medullary cells function as a special type of postsynaptic neuron that releases neurotransmitter directly into the bloodstream instead of into the synaptic cleft.

Extremities and body wall

There is no parasympathetic outflow to the body wall and extremities. Anatomically, the autonomic innervation in the body wall is only sympathetic (see Fig. 12.28). Each spinal nerve contains postsynaptic sympathetic fibers—that is, unmyelinated visceral efferents of neurons whose cell bodies are in paravertebral ganglia of the sympathetic trunk. For sweat glands, the neurotransmitter released by the "sympathetic" neurons is ACh instead of NE.

■ ORGANIZATION OF THE CENTRAL NERVOUS SYSTEM

The **central nervous system** consists of the **brain** located in the cranial cavity and the **spinal cord** located in the vertebral canal. The CNS is protected by the skull and vertebrae and is surrounded by three connective tissue membranes called **meninges**. The brain and spinal cord essentially float in the CSF that occupies the space between the two inner meningeal layers. The brain is further subdivided into the **cerebrum**, **cerebellum**, and **brainstem**, which connects with the spinal cord.

In the brain, the gray matter forms an outer covering or cortex; the white matter forms an inner core or medulla.

The **cerebral cortex** that forms the outermost layer of the brain contains nerve cell bodies, axons, dendrites, and central glial cells, and it is the site of synapses. In a freshly dissected brain, the cerebral cortex has a gray color, hence the name **gray matter**. In addition to the cortex, islands of gray matter called **nuclei** are found in the deep portions of the cerebrum and cerebellum.

The **white matter** contains only axons of nerve cells plus the associated glial cells and blood vessels (axons in fresh preparations appear white). These axons travel from one part of the nervous system to another. Whereas many of the axons going to, or coming from, a specific location are grouped into functionally related bundles called **tracts**, the tracts themselves do not stand out as delineated bundles. The demonstration of a tract in the white matter of the CNS requires a special procedure, such as the destruction of cell bodies that contribute fibers to the tract. The damaged fibers can be displayed by the use of appropriate staining or labeling methods and then traced. Even in the spinal cord, where the grouping of tracts is most pronounced, there are no sharp boundaries between adjacent tracts.

Cells of the Gray Matter

The types of cell bodies found in the gray matter vary according to which part of the brain or spinal cord is being examined.

Each functional region of the gray matter has a characteristic variety of cell bodies associated with a meshwork of axonal, dendritic, and glial processes.

The meshwork of axonal, dendritic, and glial processes associated with the gray matter is called the **neuropil**. The organization of the neuropil is not demonstrable in H&E-stained sections. It is necessary to use methods other than H&E histology to decipher the cytoarchitecture of the gray matter (Plate 12.3, page 436).

Although general histology programs usually do not deal with the actual arrangements of the neurons in the CNS, the presentation of two examples will add to the appreciation of H&E sections that students usually examine. These examples present a region of the cerebral cortex (Fig. 12.31 and Plate 12.3, page 436) and the cerebellar cortex (Fig. 12.32 and Plate 12.4, page 438).

Notable in the cerebellar cortex (see Fig. 12.32) is the Purkinje cell layer. Individuals infected by **rabies virus (RABV)** have characteristic inclusions in the cytoplasm of affected neurons called **Negri bodies**. These eosinophilic, sharply outlined, 2–10 µm in diameter inclusions visible in LM represent intracellular **viral replication compartments** formed during viral infection. They are easily observed in the cytoplasm of the Purkinje cells and pyramidal cells of the hippocampus. Negri bodies have been used for decades as primary histologic proof of RABV infection. The current approach for postmortem diagnosis of human and animal rabies is based on the direct fluorescent antibody (DFA) test. Recently, an LN34 pan-lyssavirus real-time reverse transcription-polymerase chain reaction (RT-PCR) assay has been introduced and has improved rabies diagnostics and surveillance.

The **brainstem** is not clearly separated into regions of gray matter and white matter. The nuclei of the cranial nerves located in the brainstem, however, appear as islands surrounded by more or less distinct tracts of white matter. The nuclei contain the cell bodies of the motor neurons of the cranial nerves and are both the morphologic and functional counterparts of the anterior horns of the spinal cord. In other sites in the brainstem, as in the **reticular formation**, the distinction between white matter and gray matter is even less evident.

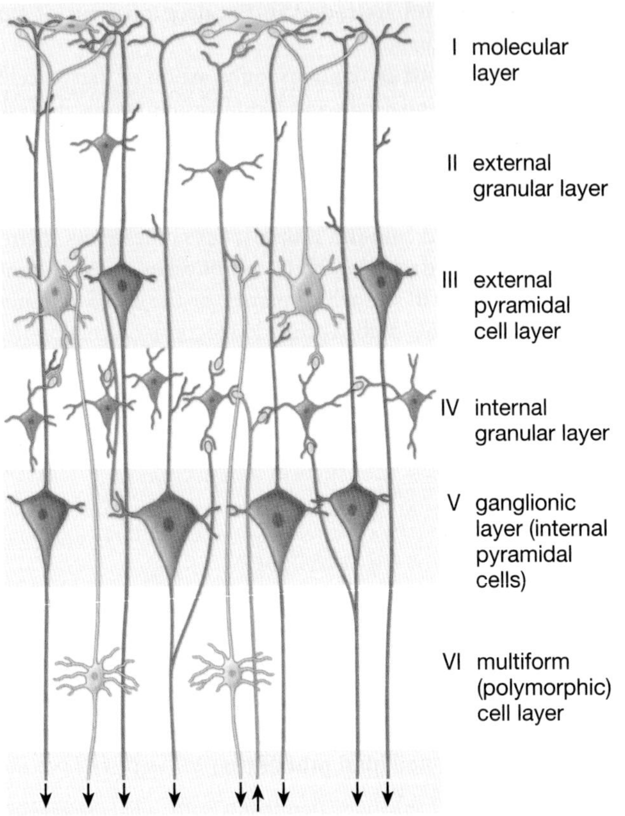

FIGURE 12.31. Nerve cells in intracortical cerebral circuits. This simplified diagram shows the organization and connections between cells in different layers of the cortex contributing to cortical afferent fibers (*arrows pointing up*) and cortical efferent fibers (*arrows pointing down*). The small interneurons are indicated in *yellow*.

Organization of the Spinal Cord

The **spinal cord** is a flattened cylindrical structure that is directly continuous with the brainstem. It is divided into 31 segments (8 cervical, 12 thoracic, 5 lumbar, 5 sacral, and 1 coccygeal), and each segment is connected to a pair of **spinal nerves.** Each spinal nerve is joined to its segment of the cord by a number of rootlets grouped as dorsal (posterior) or ventral (anterior) roots (Fig. 12.33; see also Fig. 12.3).

In cross section, the spinal cord exhibits a butterfly-shaped grayish-tan inner substance surrounding the **central canal**, the **gray matter**, and a whitish peripheral substance, the **white matter** (Fig. 12.34). White matter (see Fig. 12.3) contains only tracks of myelinated and unmyelinated axons traveling to and from other parts of the spinal cord and to and from the brain.

Gray matter contains neuronal cell bodies and their dendrites, along with axons and central neuroglia (Plate 12.5, page 440). Functionally related groups of nerve cell bodies in the gray matter are called **nuclei.** In this context, the term *nucleus* means a cluster or group of neuronal cell bodies plus fibers and neuroglia. Nuclei of the CNS are the morphologic and functional equivalents of the ganglia of the PNS. Synapses occur only in the gray matter.

The cell bodies of motor neurons that innervate striated muscle are located in the ventral (anterior) horn of the gray matter.

Ventral motor neurons, also called **anterior horn cells**, are large basophilic cells easily recognized in routine histologic preparations (see Fig. 12.34 and Plate 12.5, page 440). Because the motor neuron conducts impulses away from the CNS, it is an efferent neuron.

The axon of a motor neuron leaves the spinal cord, passes through the ventral (anterior) root, becomes a component of the spinal nerve of that segment, and, as such, is conveyed to the muscle. The axon is myelinated, except at its origin and termination. Near the muscle cell, the axon divides into numerous terminal branches that form neuromuscular junctions with the muscle cell (see page 357).

The cell bodies of sensory neurons are located in ganglia that lie on the dorsal root of the spinal nerve.

Sensory neurons in the dorsal root ganglia are pseudounipolar (Plate 12.1, page 432). They have a single process that divides

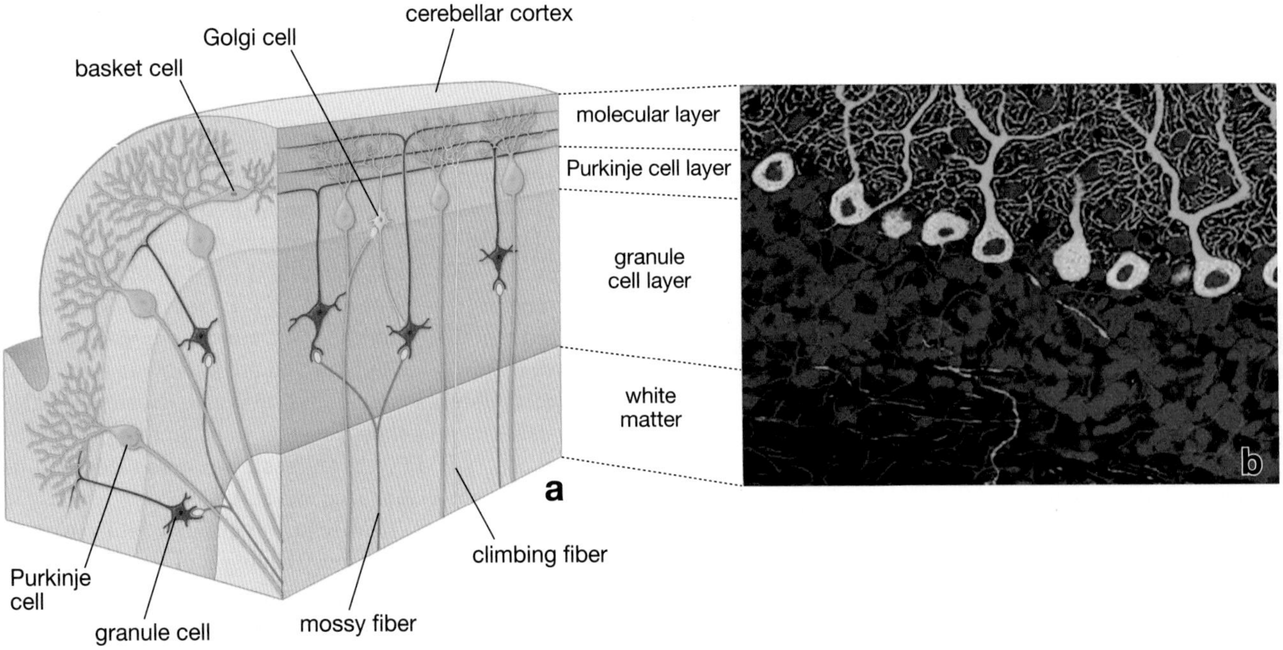

FIGURE 12.32. Cytoarchitecture of the cerebellar cortex. a. This diagram shows a section of the folium, a narrow, leaf-like gyrus of the cerebellar cortex. The longer cut edge is parallel to the folium. Note that the cerebellar cortex contains white matter and gray matter. Three distinct layers of gray matter are identified on this diagram: the superficially located molecular layer, the middle Purkinje cell layer, and the granule cell layer adjacent to the white matter. Mossy fibers and ascending fibers are major afferent fibers of the cerebellum. **b.** Purkinje cell layer from rat cerebellum visualized using double-fluorescent–labeling methods. Red DNA staining indicates the nuclei of cells in molecular and granule cell layer thin section. Note that each Purkinje cell exhibits an abundance of dendrites. ×380. (Courtesy of Thomas J. Deerinck.)

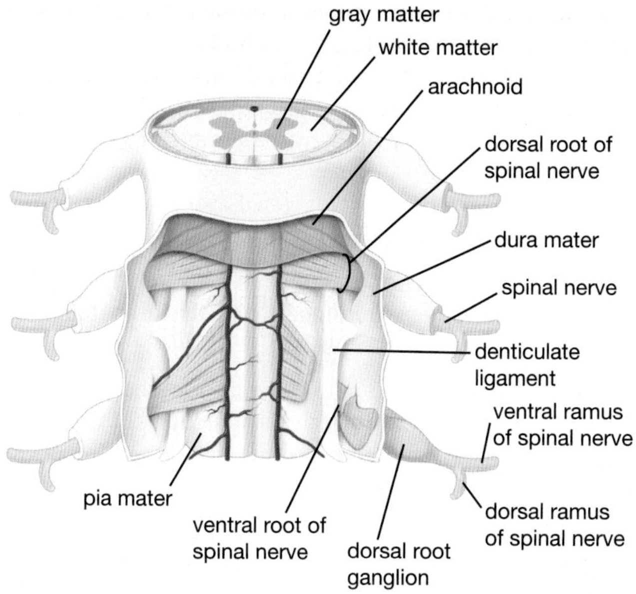

FIGURE 12.33. Posterior view of the spinal cord with surrounding meninges. Each spinal nerve arises from the spinal cord by rootlets, which merge to form dorsal (posterior) and ventral (anterior) nerve roots. These roots unite to form a spinal nerve that, after a short course, divides into larger ventral (anterior) and smaller dorsal (posterior) primary rami. Note the dura mater (the outer layer of the meninges) that surrounds the spinal cord and emerging spinal nerves. The denticulate ligament of the pia mater that anchors the spinal cord to the wall of the spinal canal is also visible.

into a peripheral segment that brings information from the periphery to the cell body and a central segment that carries information from the cell body into the gray matter of the spinal cord. Because the sensory neuron conducts impulses to the CNS, it is an *afferent neuron*. Impulses are generated in the terminal receptor arborization of the peripheral segment.

Connective Tissue of the Central Nervous System

Three sequential connective tissue membranes, the **meninges**, cover the brain and spinal cord.

- The **dura mater** is the outermost layer.
- The **arachnoid** layer lies beneath the dura.
- The **pia mater** is a delicate layer resting directly on the surface of the brain and spinal cord.

Meninges develop from a single layer of mesenchyme surrounding the developing brain. This layer, called the **primary meninx**, is the primordium for the developing meninges, bones of the skull, and dermal layer of the skin. The primary meninx further differentiates into an outer dense layer (that gives rise to the dermal layer of the skin and bones of the skull) and an inner reticular layer, which is considered the **meningeal mesenchyme**. This layer is separated into the **pachymeninx** (which develops into the dura mater) and **leptomeninx** (which develops into the arachnoid and pia mater). The pachymeninx contains longitudinally arranged fibroblasts that produce collagen fibers, whereas the leptomeninx represents a meshwork of loosely organized leptomeningeal cells. The cavitation of the leptomeninx generates arachnoid trabeculae and the subarachnoid space. In adults, the pia mater represents the visceral portion, and the arachnoid represents the parietal portion of the leptomeninx. The common origin of both meninges is evident in adults in which numerous delicate arachnoid trabeculae composed of leptomeningeal cells and fine collagen bundles pass between the pia mater and the arachnoid.

The dura mater is a relatively thick sheet of dense irregular connective tissue.

In the cranial cavity, the thick layer of connective tissue that attaches to the inner surface of the skull forms the **dura mater** *[L. tough mother]*. It consists of two layers:

- The **periosteal (outer) layer** that serves as the periosteum of the internal surface of the skull bones
- The **meningeal (inner) layer** that is fused to the periosteal layer in most regions

These two layers are separated only at the sites of **venous (dural) sinuses**, which are lined by endothelium. Venous (dural) sinuses serve as the principal channels for blood returning from the brain; they receive blood from the cerebral veins and carry it to the internal jugular veins.

Sheet-like extensions of the inner (meningeal) layer of the dura mater are called **dural reflections**. They form partitions between parts of the brain, supporting those parts within the cranial cavity and carrying the arachnoid to deeper parts of the brain. For example, the **falx cerebri** separates the two cerebral hemispheres along the midline, and the **tentorium cerebelli** separates the cerebral hemispheres posteriorly from the cerebellum.

In the spinal canal, the periosteal layer becomes the periosteum of the vertebrae and is separated from the inner meningeal layer by the epidural space, which contains adipose tissue and venous plexuses. The meningeal layer of the dura mater forms a separate tube surrounding the spinal cord (see Fig. 12.33).

The arachnoid is a delicate sheet of connective tissue adjacent to the inner surface of the dura.

The **arachnoid** forms a water-proof layer that abuts the inner surface of the dura and extends delicate **arachnoid trabeculae**

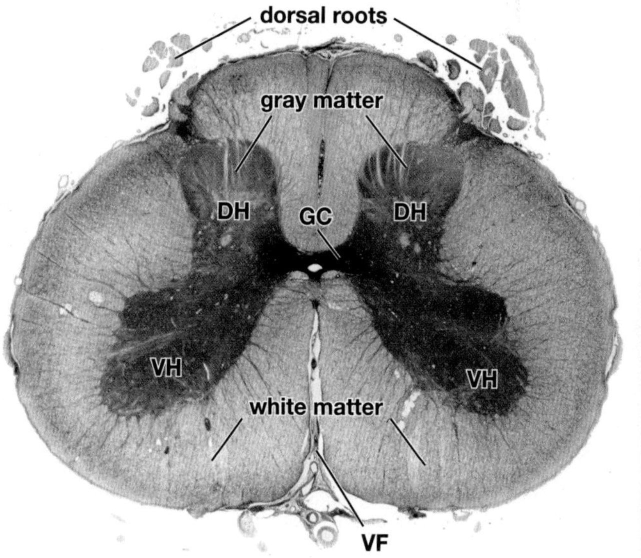

FIGURE 12.34. Cross section of the human spinal cord. This photomicrograph shows a cross section through the lower lumbar (most likely L4–L5) level of the spinal cord stained by the Bielschowsky silver method. The spinal cord is organized into an outer part, the white matter, and an inner part, the gray matter, which contains nerve cell bodies and associated nerve fibers. The gray matter of the spinal cord appears roughly in the form of a butterfly. The anterior and posterior prongs are referred to as *ventral horns* (*VH*) and *dorsal horns* (*DH*), respectively. They are connected by the gray commissure (*GC*). The white matter contains nerve fibers that form ascending and descending tracts. The outer surface of the spinal cord is surrounded by the pia mater. Blood vessels of the pia mater, the ventral fissure (*VF*), and some dorsal roots of the spinal nerves are visible in the section. ×5.

to the pia mater on the surface of the brain and spinal cord. The web-like trabeculae of the arachnoid give this tissue its name *[Gr. arachne—resembling a spider's web]*. Trabeculae are composed of loose connective tissue fibers containing elongated fibroblasts. The space bridged by these trabeculae is the **subarachnoid space**; it contains the **cerebrospinal fluid** (Fig. 12.35). In some areas, the arachnoid mater protrudes through the meningeal layer of the dura mater into the dural venous sinuses. These areas, called **arachnoid granulations**, are involved in the transport of CSF from the subarachnoid space into the venous sinuses (see Fig. 12.35).

The pia mater lies directly on the surface of the brain and spinal cord.

The **pia mater** *[L. tender mother]* is also a delicate connective tissue layer. It lies directly on the surface of the brain and spinal cord and is continuous with the perivascular connective tissue sheath of the blood vessels of the brain and spinal cord. Both surfaces of the arachnoid, the inner surface of the pia mater, and the trabeculae are covered with a thin squamous epithelial layer. Both the arachnoid and the pia mater fuse around the opening for the cranial and spinal nerves as they exit the dura mater.

Blood–Brain Barrier

The blood–brain barrier protects the CNS from fluctuating levels of electrolytes, hormones, and tissue metabolites circulating in the blood vessels.

The observation more than 100 years ago that vital dyes injected into the bloodstream can penetrate and stain nearly all organs, except the brain, provided the first description of the **blood–brain barrier**. More recently, advances in microscopy and molecular biology techniques have revealed the precise

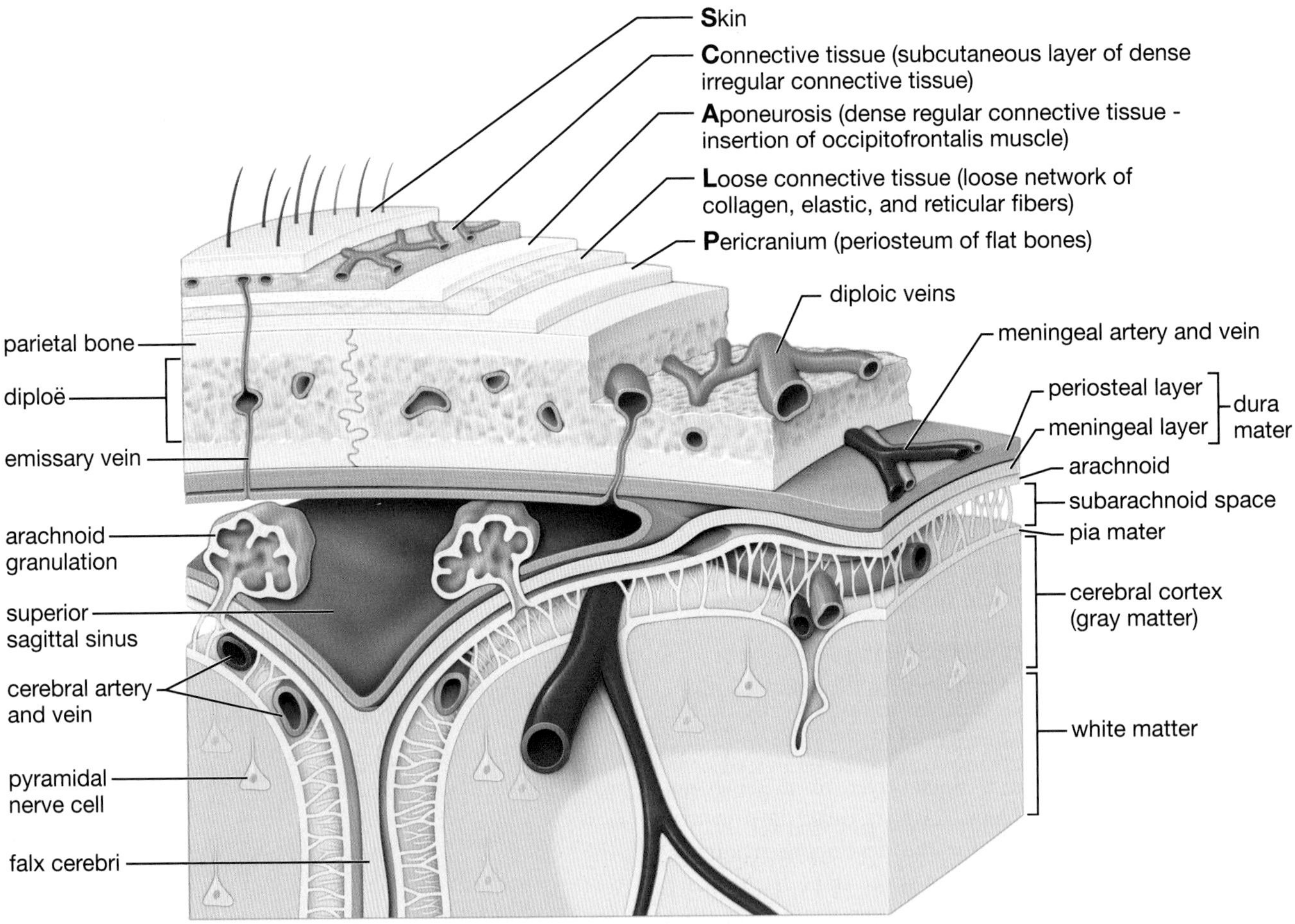

FIGURE 12.35. Schematic diagram of the layers of the scalp and cerebral meninges. This diagram of the frontal section of the top of the head shows the layers of the scalp, organization of the parietal bones of the skull, and arrangement of meninges and blood vessels within the cranial cavity. The five layers of the scalp can be remembered with the mnemonic SCALP: (1) Skin; (2) Connective tissue (dense irregular) located below the skin with an embedded subcutaneous layer of the vascular network; (3) Aponeurosis, which represents a flat tendon (dense regular connective tissue) for the attachment of occipital and frontalis muscles; (4) Loose connective tissue network of collagen, elastic, and reticular fibers; and (5) Pericranium, which represents the periosteum on the outer surface of the bone. Below the scalp, the section through the parietal bone reveals a middle spongy bone layer called *diploë* located between the inner and outer plates of compact bone. Diploic veins in the diploë connect dural sinuses with the extracranial venous systems through emissary veins. Within the cranial cavity, the superficial, outer layer of the dura mater, called the *periosteal layer*, is firmly attached to bone and serves as a periosteum (darker color). Note the branches of meningeal arteries with accompanying veins located between the periosteal layer of the dura mater and bone. The deeper, inner layer of the dura mater is called the *meningeal layer* (*lighter color*). In most regions of the cranial cavity, both layers of dura mater are fused, except at the sites of venous (dural) sinuses; here, the layers are separated from each other by a vascular space lined by endothelium. In a few regions of the cranial cavity, fused meningeal layers of the dura mater project away from the bone to form dural infoldings (reflections) that separate the different regions of the brain. Note the falx cerebri, the largest dural infolding that separates the right and left cerebral hemispheres. Deep to the dura mater is the arachnoid. It is adjacent, but not attached, to the dura mater. The arachnoid sends numerous web-like arachnoid trabeculae to the pia mater that adheres to the brain surface and follows all its contours. The subarachnoid space is located between the arachnoid and the pia mater; it contains cerebrospinal fluid. The space also contains the larger blood vessels (cerebral arteries and veins) that send branches into and receive tributaries from the brain. Note that in some areas called *arachnoid granulations*, the arachnoid mater protrudes through the meningeal layer of the dura mater into the dural venous sinuses. Arachnoid granulations are involved in the transport of cerebrospinal fluid from the subarachnoid space into venous sinuses.

location of this unique barrier and the role of brain endothelial cells in transporting essential substances to the brain tissue.

The blood–brain barrier maintains the optimal microenvironment in the CNS for proper brain function. In essence, it separates the brain tissue from circulating blood. The major functions of the blood–brain barrier are to:

- protect the brain from potential blood-borne toxins,
- meet the metabolic demands of the brain tissue, and
- regulate the homeostatic microenvironment in the CNS.

The blood–brain barrier resides in the single layer of uninterrupted vascular endothelial cells lining continuous capillaries in the CNS.

The blood–brain barrier develops early in the embryo through an interaction between glial astrocytes and capillary endothelial cells. The barrier is created largely by the elaborate **tight junctions** between the **endothelial cells**, which form continuous-type capillaries. Studies with the TEM using electron-opaque tracers show complex tight junctions between the endothelial cells. Morphologically, these junctions more closely resemble epithelial tight junctions than tight junctions present between other endothelial cells. In addition, TEM studies reveal a close association of astrocytes and their end-foot processes with the **endothelial basal lamina** (Fig. 12.36). The tight junctions eliminate gaps between endothelial cells and prevent simple diffusion of solutes and fluid into the neural tissue. Evidence suggests that the integrity of blood–brain barrier tight junctions depends on the normal functioning of the associated **astrocytes;** however, the astrocytes themselves and their end-foot processes do not significantly contribute to the physical barrier. Several brain diseases are characterized by a breakdown in the **blood–brain barrier**. Examination of brain tissue in these conditions with the TEM reveals loss of tight junctions as well as alterations in the morphology of astrocytes. Other experimental evidence has revealed that astrocytes release soluble factors that increase barrier properties and tight junction protein content.

The blood–brain barrier restricts passage of certain ions and substances from the bloodstream to tissues of the CNS.

The presence of only a few small vesicles indicates that pinocytosis across the brain endothelial cells is severely restricted. Substances with a molecular weight **greater than 500 Da** generally cannot cross the blood–brain barrier. However, some molecules leave and enter the blood capillaries through endothelial cells. For instance, O_2, CO_2, and certain lipid-soluble molecules (e.g., ethanol and steroid hormones) easily penetrate the endothelial cells and pass freely between the blood and extracellular fluid of the CNS. Owing to the high K^+ permeability of the neuronal membrane, neurons are particularly sensitive to changes in the concentration of extracellular K^+. As previously discussed, astrocytes are responsible for buffering the concentration of K^+ in the brain extracellular fluid (see pages 411-412). They are assisted by endothelial cells of the blood–brain barrier that effectively limit the movement of K^+ into the extracellular fluid of the CNS.

Substances that do cross the brain capillary wall are actively transported by influx and efflux transporters.

Many molecules that are required for neuronal integrity leave and enter the blood capillaries through endothelial cells. Brain endothelial cells use highly polarized transmembrane transporters to regulate the influx of nutrients and efflux of metabolic waste and toxins between the blood and the extracellular fluid of the CNS. The major class of known **efflux transporters** is the **ATP-binding cassette (ABC)** transporters. These efflux transporters utilize ATP to transport molecules into the blood against their concentration gradients. Brain endothelial cells also express specialized **influx transporters** that facilitate the transport of nutrients such as glucose (which neurons depend on almost exclusively for energy), ions, amino acids, nucleotides, vitamins, and proteins from the blood to the extracellular fluid of the CNS. Many of these transporters belong to the superfamily **solute carrier proteins (SLCs)**, which include glucose transporters (GLUT1) and cationic amino acid transporters (SLC7A1). The permeability of the blood–brain barrier to these macromolecules is attributable to the level of expression of specific transporters on the brain endothelial cell surface.

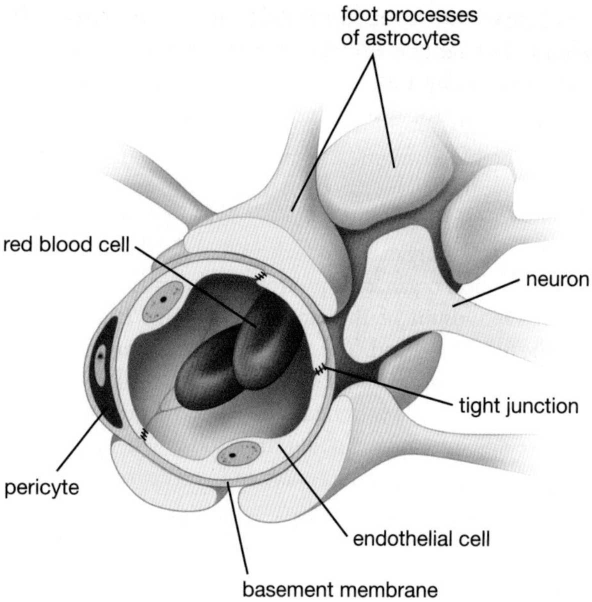

FIGURE 12.36. Schematic drawing of the blood–brain barrier. This drawing shows the blood–brain barrier, which consists of endothelial cells joined together by elaborate, complex tight junctions, endothelial basal lamina, and the end-foot processes of astrocytes.

Several other proteins that reside within the plasma membrane of endothelial cells protect the brain by metabolizing certain molecules, such as drugs and foreign proteins, thus preventing them from crossing the barrier. The restrictive nature of the blood–brain barrier hinders the delivery of therapeutics for many neurologic disorders. For example, **L-dopa (levodopa)**, the precursor of the neuromediators dopamine and noradrenaline, easily crosses the blood–brain barrier. However, the **dopamine** formed from the decarboxylation of L-dopa in endothelial cells cannot cross the barrier and is restricted from the CNS. In this case, the blood–brain barrier regulates the concentration of L-dopa in the brain. Clinically, this restriction explains why L-dopa is administered for the treatment of **dopamine deficiency** (e.g., Parkinson disease) rather than dopamine.

Recent studies indicate that the end-feet of astrocytes also play an important role in maintaining **water homeostasis** in brain tissue. **Water channels** (aquaporin AQP4) are found in end-foot processes in which water crosses the blood–brain barrier. In pathologic conditions, such as brain edema, these channels play a key role in reestablishing osmotic equilibrium in the brain.

The midline structures bordering the third and fourth ventricles are unique areas of the brain that are outside the blood–brain barrier.

Some parts of the CNS, however, are not isolated from substances carried in the bloodstream. The barrier is ineffective or absent in the sites located along the third and fourth ventricles of the brain, which are collectively called **circumventricular organs**. Circumventricular organs include the pineal gland, median eminence, subfornical organ, area postrema, subcommissural organ, organum vasculosum of the lamina terminalis, and posterior lobe of the pituitary gland. These barrier-deficient areas are most likely involved in the sampling of materials circulating in the blood that are normally excluded by the blood–brain barrier and then conveying information about these substances to the CNS. Circumventricular organs are important in regulating body fluid homeostasis and controlling neurosecretory activity of the nervous system. Some researchers describe them as "windows of the brain" within the central neurohumoral system.

■ RESPONSE OF NEURONS TO INJURY

Neuronal injury induces a complex sequence of events termed **axonal degeneration** and **neural regeneration**. Neurons, Schwann cells, oligodendrocytes, macrophages, and microglia are involved in these responses. In contrast to the PNS, in which injured axons rapidly regenerate, axons severed in the CNS usually cannot regenerate. This striking difference is most likely related to the inability of oligodendrocytes and microglia cells to phagocytose myelin debris quickly and the restriction of large numbers of migrating macrophages by the blood–brain barrier. Because myelin debris contains several inhibitors of axon regeneration, its removal is essential to the regeneration progress.

Degeneration

The portion of a nerve fiber distal to a site of injury degenerates because of interrupted axonal transport.

Degeneration of an axon distal to a site of injury is called **anterograde (Wallerian) degeneration** (Fig. 12.37a and b). The first sign of injury, which occurs 8–24 hours after the axon is damaged, is axonal swelling. The axon then disintegrates, and the components of the cytoskeleton, including microtubules and neurofilaments, are disassembled, resulting in fragmentation of the axon. Myelin is also destroyed. This process is known as **granular disintegration of the axonal cytoskeleton**. In the PNS, loss of axon contact induces several changes in myelinating Schwann cells. After injury, Schwann cells lose their characteristic gene expression pattern and undergo dedifferentiation and reprogramming into **repair Schwann cells**. This reprogramming involves the activation of a set of repair-related transcription factors and reexpression of molecules characteristic of immature Schwann cells during their early stages of development. Schwann cells undergoing reprogramming downregulate promyelin transcription factors and

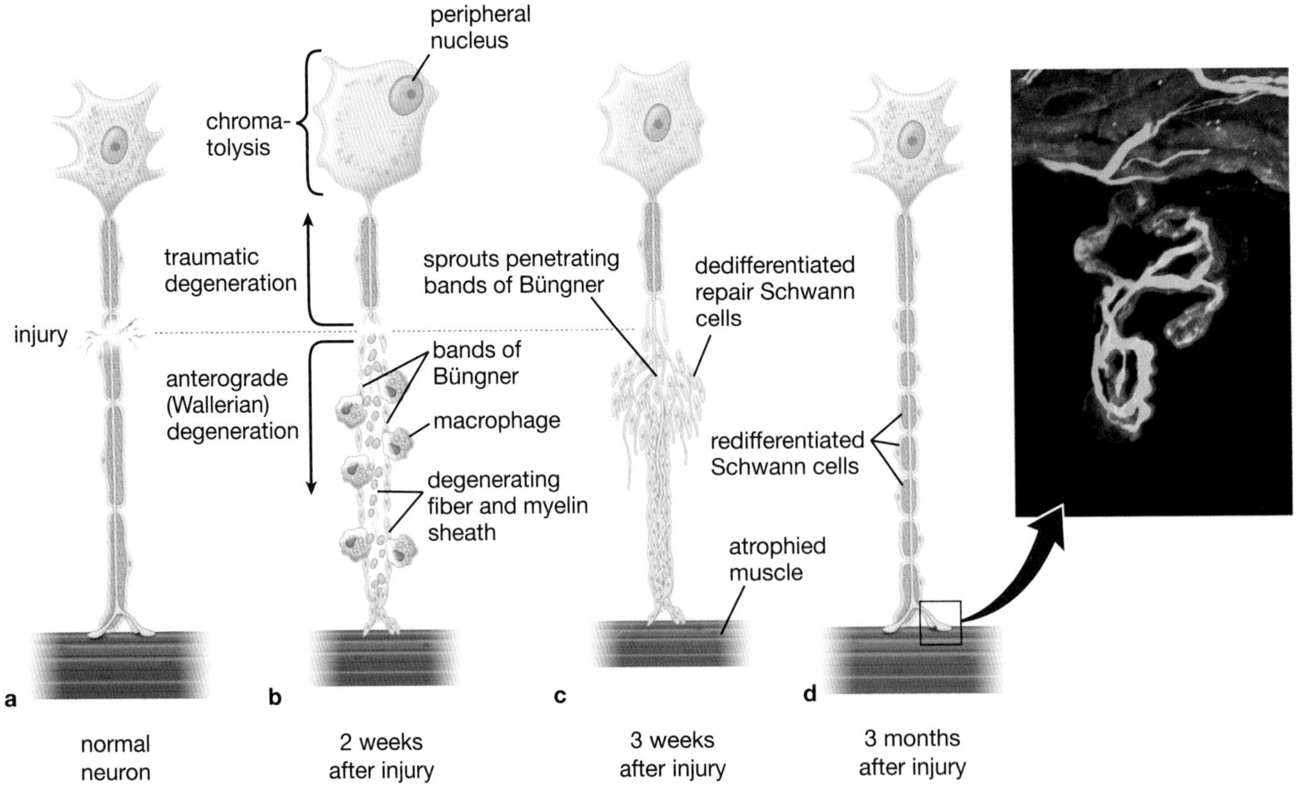

FIGURE 12.37. Response of a nerve fiber to injury. a. A normal nerve fiber at the time of injury, with its nerve cell body and the effector cell (striated skeletal muscle). Note the position of the neuron nucleus and the number and distribution of Nissl bodies. **b.** When the fiber is injured, the neuronal nucleus moves to the cell periphery, and the number of Nissl bodies is greatly reduced. The nerve fiber distal to the injury degenerates along with its myelin sheath. Schwann cells dedifferentiate into repair Schwann cell; myelin debris is phagocytosed by macrophages. **c.** Proliferating repair Schwann cells form cellular bands (of Büngner) that are penetrated by the growing axonal sprout. The axon grows at a rate of 0.5–3 mm/d. Note that the muscle fibers show a pronounced atrophy. **d.** If the growing axonal sprout reaches the muscle fiber, the regeneration is successful and new neuromuscular junctions are developed; thus, the function of skeletal muscle is restored. **Inset.** A confocal immunofluorescent image showing reinnervated skeletal muscle of the mouse. Regenerating motor axons are stained *green* for neurofilaments; reestablished connections with two neuromuscular junctions are visualized in *pink*, which reflects specific staining for postsynaptic acetylcholine receptors; repair Schwann cells are stained *blue* for S100, which represents a Schwann cell–specific calcium-binding protein. Regenerating axons have extended along repair Schwann cells, which has led them to the original synaptic sites of the muscle fibers. ×640. (Courtesy of Dr. Young-Jin Son.)

expression of myelin-specific proteins (see pages 405-407). Genes associated with epithelial-to-mesenchymal transition (EMT) are upregulated, triggering myelin autophagy that breaks down the myelin sheath enclosing the axon. At the same time, transformed repair Schwann cells upregulate and secrete several **glial growth factors (GGFs)**, members of a family of axon-associated neuregulins and potent stimulators of axonal proliferation. Increased secretion of cytokines allows repair Schwann cells to interact with immune cells and recruit **macrophages** to the site of nerve injury. Under the influence of GGFs, repair Schwann cells divide and arrange themselves in a line along their external laminae. Because axonal processes distal to the site of injury have been removed by phagocytosis, the linear arrangement of the repair Schwann cells' external laminae resembles a long tube with an empty lumen (Fig. 12.37b). In the CNS, oligodendrocyte survival is dependent on signals from axons. In contrast to Schwann cells, if oligodendrocytes lose contact with axons, they respond by initiating apoptotic programmed cell death.

The most important cells in clearing myelin debris from the site of nerve injury are monocyte-derived macrophages.

In the PNS, even before the arrival of phagocytotic cells at the site of nerve injury, **repair Schwann cells** initiate the removal of myelin debris. It is estimated that during the first 5–7 days after nerve injury, about 50% of the myelin is degraded by repair Schwann cells. The rest of myelin clearance is performed by macrophages, which migrate to the site of injury and phagocytose myelin debris. Several cytokines, such as interleukin-6 (IL-6), leukemia inhibitory factor (LIF), and monocyte chemotactic protein 1 (MCP-1), are secreted by repair Schwann cells. These cytokines activate **resident macrophages** (normally present in small numbers in the peripheral nerves) to migrate to the site of nerve injury, proliferate, and then phagocytize remaining myelin debris.

The efficient clearance of myelin debris in the PNS is attributed to the massive recruitment of **monocyte-derived macrophages** that migrate from blood vessels and infiltrate the vicinity of the nerve injury (Fig. 12.38). When an axon

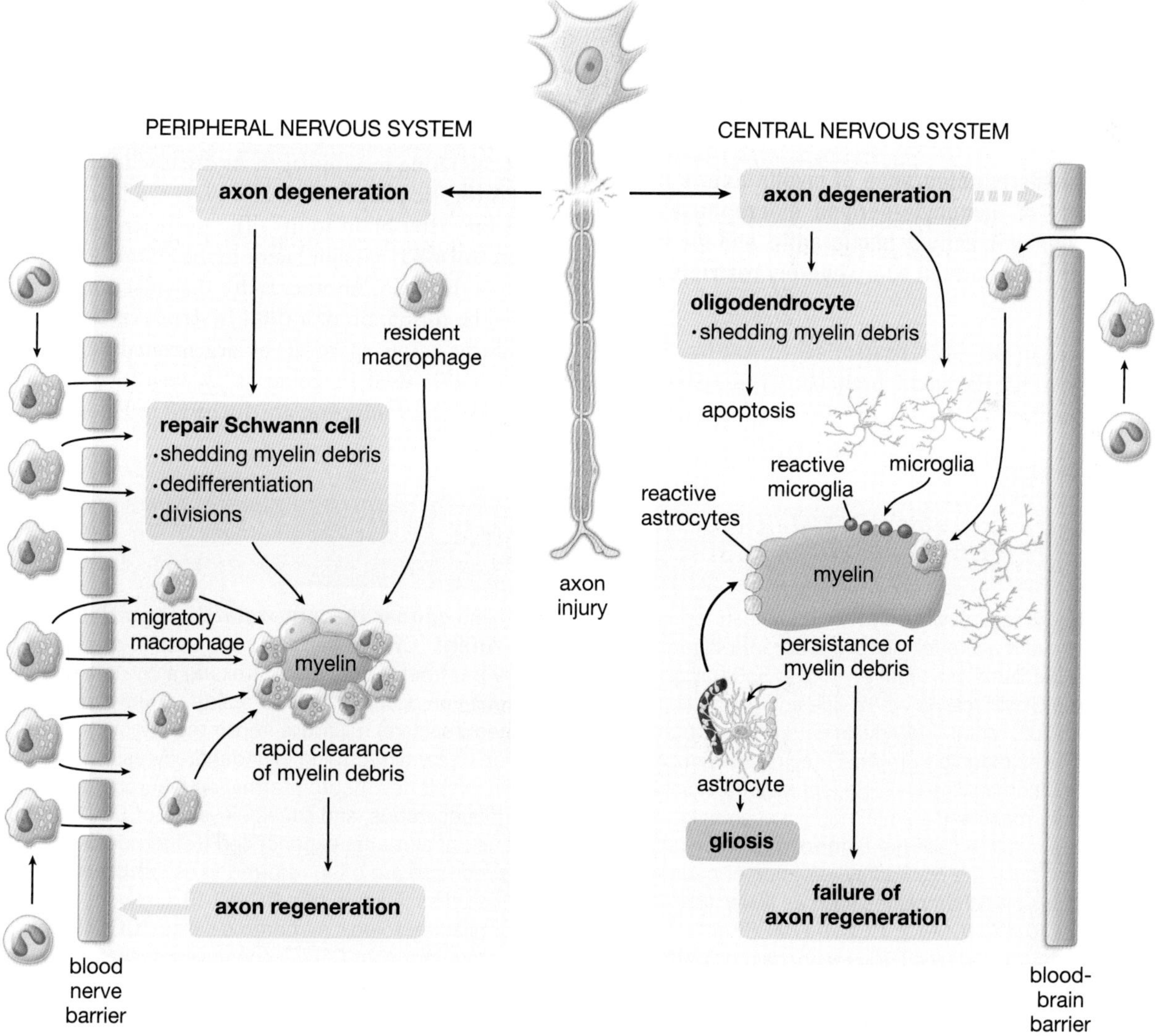

FIGURE 12.38. Schematic diagram of response to neuronal injury within peripheral and central nervous systems. Injuries of nerve processes (axons and dendrites) in both the peripheral nervous system (PNS) and the central nervous system (CNS) induce axonal degeneration and neural regeneration. These processes involve not only neurons but also supportive cells such as Schwann cells and oligodendrocytes as well as phagocytic cells such as macrophages and microglia. Injuries to axons in the PNS lead to their degeneration, which triggers the reprogramming and dedifferentiation of Schwann cells into repair Schwan cells and disruption of the blood–nerve barrier along the entire length of the injured axon. Repair Schwann cells play a major part in the initial phase of myelin degradation and clearance. About 50% of the myelin is degraded during this phase. Dismantling of the blood–nerve barrier allows massive infiltration of monocyte-derived macrophages, which phagocytose myelin debris. Rapid clearance of myelin debris allows for axon regeneration and subsequent restoration of the blood–nerve barrier. In the CNS, limited disruption of the blood–brain barrier restricts infiltration of monocyte-derived macrophages, dramatically slowing the process of myelin removal. Myelin is primarily removed by reactive microglia and secondarily by reactive astrocytes. In addition, apoptosis of oligodendrocytes, inefficient phagocytic activity of microglia, and the formation of an astrocyte-derived scar lead to failure of nerve regeneration in the CNS.

FOLDER 12.3

CLINICAL CORRELATION: REACTIVE GLIOSIS: SCAR FORMATION IN THE CENTRAL NERVOUS SYSTEM

When a region of the central nervous system (CNS) is injured, astrocytes near the lesion become activated. They divide and undergo marked hypertrophy with a visible increase in the number of their cytoplasmic processes. In time, the processes become densely packed with **glial fibrillary acidic protein (GFAP) intermediate filaments**. Eventually, scar tissue is formed. This process is referred to as **reactive gliosis**, whereas the resulting permanent scar is most often called a **plaque**. Reactive gliosis varies widely in duration, degree of hyperplasia, and time course of expression of GFAP immunostaining.

Several biological mechanisms for induction and maintenance of reactive gliosis have been proposed. The type of glial cell that responds during reactive gliosis depends on the brain structure that is damaged. In addition, activation of the microglial cell population occurs almost immediately after any kind of injury to the CNS. These reactive microglial cells migrate toward the site of injury and exhibit marked phagocytic activity. However, their phagocytic activity and ability to remove myelin debris are much less than that of monocyte-derived macrophages. Gliosis is a prominent feature of many diseases of the CNS, including stroke, neurotoxic damage, genetic diseases, inflammatory demyelination, and neurodegenerative disorders, such as multiple sclerosis. Much of the research in CNS regeneration is focused on preventing or inhibiting glial scar formation.

is injured, the blood–nerve barrier (see pages 424-425) is disrupted along the entire length of the injured axon, which allows for the influx of these cells into the site of injury. The presence of large numbers of monocyte-derived macrophages speeds up the process of myelin removal, which, in peripheral nerves, is usually completed within 2 weeks.

In the CNS, inefficient clearance of myelin debris due to limited access of monocyte-derived macrophages, the inefficient phagocytic activity of microglia, and the formation of an astrocyte-derived scar severely restricts nerve regeneration.

A key difference in the **CNS response to axonal injury** relates to the fact that the blood–brain barrier (see pages 424-425) is disrupted only at the site of injury and not along the entire length of the injured axon (see Fig. 12.38). This limits infiltration of monocyte-derived macrophages to the CNS and dramatically slows the process of myelin removal, which can take months or even years. Although the number of microglial cells increases at the sites of CNS injury, these **reactive microglia cells** do not possess the full phagocytotic capabilities of migrating macrophages. As discussed earlier (see page 410), astrocytic phagocytosis also plays a role in nerve tissue remodeling after brain injury. The inefficient **clearance of myelin debris** is a major factor in the failure of nerve regeneration in the CNS. Another factor that affects nerve regeneration is the formation of a **glial (astrocyte-derived) scar** that fills the empty space left by degenerated axons. Scar formation is discussed in Folder 12.3; cognitive impairments after COVID-19 infection are discussed in Folder 12.4.

FOLDER 12.4

CLINICAL CORRELATION: COGNITIVE IMPAIRMENTS AFTER COVID-19 INFECTIONS

The **COVID-19** (coronavirus disease 2019) pandemic caused by severe acute respiratory syndrome coronavirus 2 (SARS-CoV-2) has resulted in over 550 million documented COVID cases worldwide and 6.3 million deaths (mid-2022 data). Individuals with COVID-19 experience symptoms ranging from mild respiratory symptoms to severe multiorgan illnesses. Recent studies indicate that in both humans and animal models, even mild COVID infection can result in detrimental **neuroinflammatory responses**. These are marked by elevation of neurotoxic cytokines and chemokines such as IFN-γ, IL6, TNF-α, CXCL10, CCL7, CCL2, CCL11, GMCSF, BAFF, and others that characteristically react against **white matter microglial cells**. In a mouse model of mild respiratory COVID-19 infection, researchers discovered hippocampal changes that included a decreased number of oligodendrocytes with subsequent myelin loss. These changes were accompanied by elevated levels of cerebrospinal fluid (CSF) chemokines, including **CCL11** (also known as *eosinophil chemotactic protein* or *eotaxin-1*), which is associated with the cognitive impairments seen in aging. Similarly, individuals that recovered from COVID-19 experience persistent neurologic symptoms resembling **cancer therapy–related cognitive impairment (CRCI).** Certain drugs used in chemotherapy treatment (e.g., methotrexate) activate a distinct subpopulation of microglia that reside in white matter. Activated (reactive) microglia impair the ongoing differentiation of myelin-forming oligodendrocytes (loss of myelin), inhibit new neuron formation (neurogenesis) in the hippocampus, and cause elevation of CCL11. The cognitive impairments experienced by individuals with CRCI syndrome are often referred to as "**chemo fog.**" Recent studies indicate that COVID-19 survivors experience similar neurologic symptoms called "**COVID fog**," which represent post-COVID cognitive impairments. These include **impaired attention, decreased concentration, slowed information processing speed, memory problems,** as well as other impairments of executive function. As a result of these impairments, individuals who recovered from COVID-19 may present in the clinic with increased rates of **anxiety, depression, disordered sleep**, and **fatigue**. These symptoms of post–COVID-19 cognitive impairments represent a major public health crisis preventing people from returning to their previous level of occupational activity.

Traumatic degeneration occurs in the proximal part of the injured nerve.

Some retrograde degeneration also occurs in the proximal axon and is called **traumatic degeneration**. This process appears to be histologically similar to anterograde (Wallerian) degeneration. The extent of traumatic degeneration depends on the severity of the injury and usually extends to only one or a few internodal segments. Sometimes, traumatic degeneration extends more proximally than one or a few nodes of Ranvier and may result in death of the cell body. When a motor fiber is cut, the muscle innervated by that fiber undergoes atrophy (Fig. 12.37c).

Retrograde signaling to the cell body of an injured nerve causes a change in gene expression that initiates reorganization of the perinuclear cytoplasm.

Axonal injury also initiates retrograde signaling to the nerve cell body, leading to the upregulation of a gene called **c-jun.** C-jun transcription factor is involved in the early as well as later stages of nerve regeneration. Reorganization of the perinuclear cytoplasm and organelles starts within a few days. The cell body of the injured nerve swells, and its nucleus moves peripherally. Initially, Nissl bodies disappear from the center of the neuron and move to the periphery of the neuron in a process called **chromatolysis.** Chromatolysis is first observed within 1–2 days after injury and reaches a peak at about 2 weeks (see Fig. 12.37b). The changes in the cell body are proportional to the amount of axoplasm destroyed by the injury; extensive loss of axoplasm can lead to the death of the cell.

Before the development of modern dyes and radioisotope tracer techniques, Wallerian degeneration and chromatolysis were used as research tools. These tools allowed researchers to trace the pathways and destination of axons and the localization of the cell bodies of experimentally injured nerves.

Regeneration

In the PNS, repair Schwann cells divide and develop cellular bands that bridge a newly formed scar and direct growth of new nerve processes.

As mentioned previously, at the site of the injury, cells are reprogrammed to generate specialized **repair Schwann cells** to promote tissue repair. Division of repair Schwann cells is the first step in the regeneration of a severed or crushed peripheral nerve. Initially, these cells arrange themselves in a series of cylinders called **endoneurial tubes**. Removal of myelin and axonal debris inside the tubes eventually causes them to collapse. Proliferating repair Schwann cells elongate, extending long, parallel processes, and organize themselves into cellular bands resembling longitudinal columns called regeneration tracks or **bands of Büngner** (Fig. 12.39). These cellular bands guide the growth of new nerve processes (**neurites** or **sprouts**) of regenerating axons. Once the bands are in place, large numbers of sprouts begin to grow from the proximal stump (see Fig. 12.37c). A **growth cone** develops in the distal portion of each sprout that consists of filopodia rich in actin filaments. The tips of the filopodia establish a direction for the advancement of the growth cone. They preferentially interact with proteins of the extracellular matrix such as fibronectin and laminin found within the external lamina

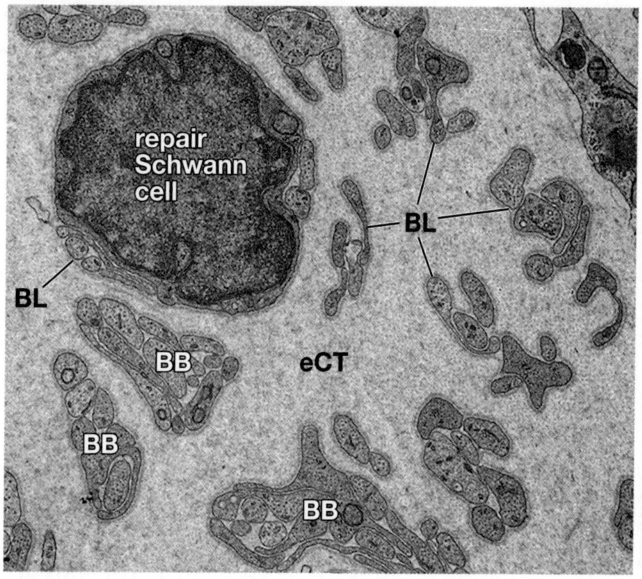

FIGURE 12.39. Electron micrograph of a distal stump of regenerating nerve. This image shows a cross section through the distal stump of the mouse tibial nerve 4 weeks after transection. A repair Schwan cell with a large nucleus and a thin rim of cytoplasm is enclosed by the basal (external) lamina (*BL*). Several cross sections of Büngner bands (*BB*) are embedded in the endoneurial connective tissue (*eCT*). They contain elongated parts of repair Schwann cells and their parallel processes. Note that every band and their components are also surrounded by the basal laminae. The cell in the *right upper corner* represents connective tissue cell (lack of basal lamina), and it may represent part of fibroblast or macrophage. × 65,000. (Courtesy of Dr. Kristjan R. Jessen, University College London, London, UK).

of the repair Schwann cell. Thus, if a sprout associates itself with a band of Büngner, it regenerates between the layers of external lamina of the repair Schwann cell. This sprout will grow along the band at a rate of about **3 mm/day**. Although many new sprouts do not make contact with cellular bands and degenerate, their large number increases the probability of reestablishing sensory and motor connections. After crossing the site of injury, sprouts enter the surviving cellular bands in the distal stump. These bands then guide the neurites to their destination as well as provide a suitable microenvironment for continued growth (Fig. 12.37d). Axonal regeneration leads to Schwann cell redifferentiation, which occurs in a proximal-to-distal direction. In addition, redifferentiated Schwann cells upregulate genes for myelin-specific proteins and downregulate **c-Jun transcription factor**, which is central to the reprogramming of myelinating and nonmyelinating Remak Schwann cells to repair Schwann cells after injury.

If physical contact is reestablished between a motor neuron and its muscle, function is usually reestablished.

Microsurgical techniques that rapidly reestablish intimate apposition of severed nerve and vessel ends have made reattachment of severed limbs and digits, with subsequent reestablishment of function, a relatively common procedure. If the axonal sprouts do not reestablish contact with the appropriate Schwann cells, then the sprouts grow in a disorganized manner, resulting in a mass of tangled axonal processes known as a **traumatic neuroma** or **amputation neuroma.** Clinically, a traumatic neuroma usually appears as a freely movable nodule at the site of nerve injury and is characterized by pain, particularly on palpation. Formation of a traumatic neuroma of the injured motor nerve prevents reinnervation of the affected muscle.

101 HISTOLOGY NOTEBOOK

NERVE TISSUE

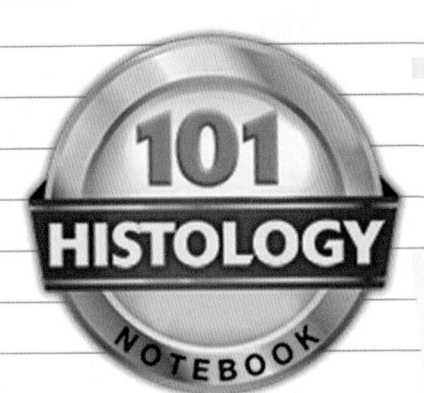

OVERVIEW OF THE NERVOUS SYSTEM

- The **nervous system** enables the body to respond to changes in its external environment and controls the functions of internal organs and systems.
- Anatomically, the nervous system is divided into the **central nervous system** (CNS; (brain and spinal cord) and the **peripheral nervous system** (PNS; peripheral and cranial nerves and ganglia).
- Functionally, the nervous system is divided into the **somatic nervous system** (SNS; under conscious voluntary control) and the **autonomic nervous system** (ANS; under involuntary control).
- The ANS is further subdivided into **sympathetic**, **parasympathetic**, and **enteric divisions**. The enteric division serves the alimentary canal and regulates the function of internal organs by innervating smooth and cardiac muscle cells as well as glandular epithelium.

SUPPORTING CELLS OF THE NERVOUS SYSTEM: NEUROGLIA

- **Peripheral neuroglia** includes Schwann cells and satellite cells.
- In **myelinated** nerves, **Schwann cells** produce the **myelin sheath** from compacted layers of their own cell membranes that are wrapped concentrically around the nerve cell process.
- The junction between two adjacent Schwann cells, the **node of Ranvier**, is the site where the electrical impulse is regenerated for high-speed propagation along the axon.
- In **unmyelinated** nerves, nerve processes are enveloped in the cytoplasm of **Remak Schwann cells.**
- **Satellite cells** maintain a controlled microenvironment around the nerve cell bodies in ganglia of the PNS.
- There are four types of **central neuroglia: astrocytes** (provide physical and metabolic support for neurons of the CNS), **oligodendrocytes** (produce and maintain the myelin sheath in the CNS), **microglia** (possess phagocytotic properties and mediate neuroimmune reactions), and **ependymal cells** (form the epithelial-like lining of the ventricles of the brain and spinal canal).

NEURONS

- **Nerve tissue** consists of two principal types of cells: **neurons** (specialized cells that conduct impulses) and **supporting cells** (nonconducting cells in close proximity to nerve cells and their processes).
- The neuron is the structural and functional unit of the nervous system.
- **Neurons** do not divide; however, in certain regions of the brain, **neural stem cells** may divide and differentiate into new neurons.
- Neurons are grouped into three categories: **sensory neurons** (carry impulses from receptors to the CNS), **motor neurons** (carry impulses from the CNS or ganglia to effector cells), and **interneurons** (communicate between sensory and motor neurons).
- Each neuron consists of a **cell body** or **perikaryon** (contains the nucleus, Nissl bodies, and other organelles), an **axon** (usually the longest process of the cell body; transmits impulses away from the cell body), and several **dendrites** (shorter processes that transmit impulses toward the cell body).
- Neurons communicate with other neurons and with effector cells by specialized junctions called **synapses.**
- **Chemical synapses** are the most common type of synapse. Each has a **presynaptic element** containing vesicles filled with neurotransmitter, a **synaptic cleft** into which neurotransmitter is released from the presynaptic vesicles, and a **postsynaptic membrane** containing receptors to which the neurotransmitter binds.
- **Electrical synapses** are less common and are represented by **gap junctions.**
- The chemical structure of a **neurotransmitter** determines either an **excitatory** (e.g., acetylcholine, glutamine) or **inhibitory** (e.g., GABA, glycine) response from the postsynaptic membrane.

ORIGIN OF NERVE TISSUE CELLS

- CNS neurons and central glia (except microglial cells) are derived from neuroectodermal cells of the **neural tube**. Microglial cells represent population of resident macrophages derived from erythromyeloid progenitor cells in the **yolk sac.**
- PNS ganglion cells and peripheral glia are derived from the **neural crest**.

ORGANIZATION OF THE PERIPHERAL NERVOUS SYSTEM

- The PNS consists of **peripheral nerves** with specialized nerve endings (synapses) and **ganglia**-containing nerve cell bodies.
- **Motor neuron cell bodies** of the PNS lie in the CNS, and **sensory neuron cell bodies** are located in the dorsal root ganglia.
- Individual nerve fibers are held together by connective tissue organized into **endoneurium** (surrounds each individual nerve fiber and associated Schwann cell), **perineurium** (surrounds each nerve fascicle), and **epineurium** (surrounds a peripheral nerve and fills the spaces between nerve fascicles).
- **Perineurial cells** are connected by tight junctions and contribute to the formation of the **blood–nerve barrier.**

ORGANIZATION OF THE CENTRAL NERVOUS SYSTEM

- The CNS consists of the **brain** and **spinal cord**. It is protected by the skull and vertebrae and is surrounded by three connective tissue membranes called **meninges** (**dura matter**, **arachnoid**, and **pia matter**).
- The **cerebrospinal fluid (CSF)** produced by the choroid plexus in the brain ventricles occupies the **subarachnoid space** located between arachnoid and pia matter. CSF surrounds and protects the CNS within the cranial cavity and the vertebral column.
- In the brain, the **gray matter** forms an outer layer of the cerebral cortex, whereas the **white matter** forms the inner core that is composed of axons, associated glial cells, and blood vessels.
- In the **spinal cord**, gray matter exhibits a butterfly-shaped inner substance, whereas the white matter occupies the periphery.
- The **cerebral cortex** contains nerve cell bodies, axons, dendrites, and central glial cells.
- The **blood–brain barrier** protects the CNS from fluctuating levels of electrolytes, hormones, and tissue metabolites circulating in the blood.

ORGANIZATION OF THE AUTONOMIC NERVOUS SYSTEM

- The **ANS** controls and regulates the body's internal environment. Its neural pathways are organized in a chain of two neurons (**presynaptic** and **postsynaptic neurons**) that convey impulses from the CNS to the visceral effectors.
- The ANS is subdivided into sympathetic, parasympathetic, and enteric divisions.
- **Presynaptic neurons** of the **sympathetic division** are located in the thoracolumbar portion of the spinal cord, whereas the **presynaptic neurons** of the **parasympathetic division** are located in the brainstem and sacral spinal cord.
- The **enteric division** of the ANS consists of ganglia and their processes that innervate the alimentary canal.

RESPONSE OF NEURONS TO INJURY

- Injured axons in the PNS usually regenerate, whereas axons severed in the CNS do not regenerate. This difference is related to the inability of microglial cells and astrocytes to efficiently phagocytose myelin debris.
- In the PNS, neuronal injury initially induces complete degeneration of an axon distal to the site of injury (**Wallerian degeneration**).
- **Traumatic degeneration** occurs in the proximal part of the injured nerve, followed by **neural regeneration**, in which repair Schwann cells divide and develop cellular bands that guide the growing axonal sprouts to the effector site.

PLATE 12.1 ■ SYMPATHETIC AND DORSAL ROOT GANGLIA

Ganglia are clusters of neuronal cell bodies located outside the *central nervous system* (CNS); nerve fibers lead to and from them. Sensory ganglia lie just outside the CNS and contain the cell bodies of sensory nerves that carry impulses into the CNS. Autonomic ganglia are peripheral motor ganglia of the *autonomic nervous system* (ANS) and contain the cell bodies of postsynaptic neurons that conduct nerve impulses to smooth muscle, cardiac muscle, and glands. Synapses between presynaptic neurons (all of which have their cell bodies in the CNS) and postsynaptic neurons occur in autonomic ganglia. *Sympathetic ganglia* constitute a major subclass of autonomic ganglia; *parasympathetic ganglia* and *enteric ganglia* constitute the other subclasses.

Sympathetic ganglia are located in the sympathetic chain (**paravertebral ganglia**) and on the anterior surface of the aorta (**prevertebral ganglia**). They send long postsynaptic axons to the viscera. **Parasympathetic ganglia (terminal ganglia)** are located in, or close to, the organs innervated by their postsynaptic neurons. The **enteric ganglia** are located in the *submucosal plexus* and the *myenteric plexus* of the alimentary canal. They receive parasympathetic presynaptic input as well as intrinsic input from other enteric ganglia and innervate smooth muscle of the gut wall.

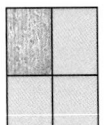

Sympathetic ganglion, human, silver and hematoxylin and eosin (H&E) stains ×160.

This micrograph shows a sympathetic ganglion stained with silver and counterstained with H&E is illustrated here. Shown to advantage are several discrete bundles of nerve fibers (*NF*) and numerous large circular structures, namely, the cell bodies (*CB*) of the postsynaptic neurons. Random patterns of nerve fibers are also seen. Moreover, careful examination of the cell bodies shows that some display several processes joined to them. Thus, these are multipolar neurons (one contained within the *rectangle* is shown at higher magnification). Generally, the connective tissue is not conspicuous in a silver preparation, although it can be identified by virtue of its location around the larger blood vessels (*BV*), particularly in the *upper part* of this figure.

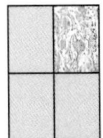

Sympathetic ganglion, human, silver and H&E stains ×500.

The cell bodies of the sympathetic ganglion are typically large, and the one labeled here shows several processes (*P*). In addition, the cell body contains a large, pale-staining spherical nucleus (*N*); this, in turn, contains a spherical, intensely staining nucleolus (*NL*). These features, namely, a large pale-staining nucleus (indicating much-extended chromatin) and a large nucleolus, reflect a cell active in protein synthesis. Also shown in the cell body are accumulations of lipofuscin (*L*), a yellow pigment that is darkened by silver. Because of the large size of the cell body, the nucleus is not always included in the section; in that case, the cell body appears as a rounded cytoplasmic mass.

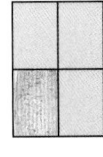

Dorsal root ganglion, cat, H&E ×160.

Dorsal root ganglia differ from autonomic ganglia in a number of ways. Whereas the latter contain multipolar neurons and have synaptic connections, dorsal root ganglia contain pseudounipolar sensory neurons and have no synaptic connections in the ganglion.

Part of a dorsal root ganglion stained with H&E is shown in this figure. The specimen includes the edge of the ganglion, where it is covered with connective tissue (*CT*). The dorsal root ganglion contains large cell bodies (*CB*) that are typically arranged as closely packed clusters. Also, between and around the cell clusters, there are bundles of nerve fibers (*NF*). Most of the fiber bundles indicated by the label have been sectioned longitudinally.

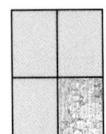

Dorsal root ganglion, cat, H&E ×350.

At higher magnification of the same ganglion, the constituents of the nerve fiber show their characteristic structure, namely, a centrally located axon (*A*) surrounded by an empty space after myelin was washed out during slide preparation (not labeled), which, in turn, is bounded on its outer border by the thin cytoplasmic strand of the neurilemma (*arrowheads*).

The cell bodies of the sensory neurons display large, pale-staining spherical nuclei (*N*) and intensely staining nucleoli (*NL*). Also seen in this H&E preparation are the nuclei of satellite cells (*Sat C*) that completely surround the cell body and are continuous with the Schwann cells that invest the axon. Note how much smaller these cells are compared with the neurons. Clusters of cells (*asterisks*) within the ganglion that have an epithelioid appearance are en-face views of satellite cells where the section tangentially includes the satellite cells but barely grazes the adjacent cell body.

A, axon
BV, blood vessels
CB, cell body of neuron
CT, connective tissue
L, lipofuscin
N, nucleus of nerve cell
NF, nerve fibers
NL, nucleolus
P, processes of nerve cell body
Sat C, satellite cells
arrowheads, neurilemma
asterisks, clusters of satellite cells

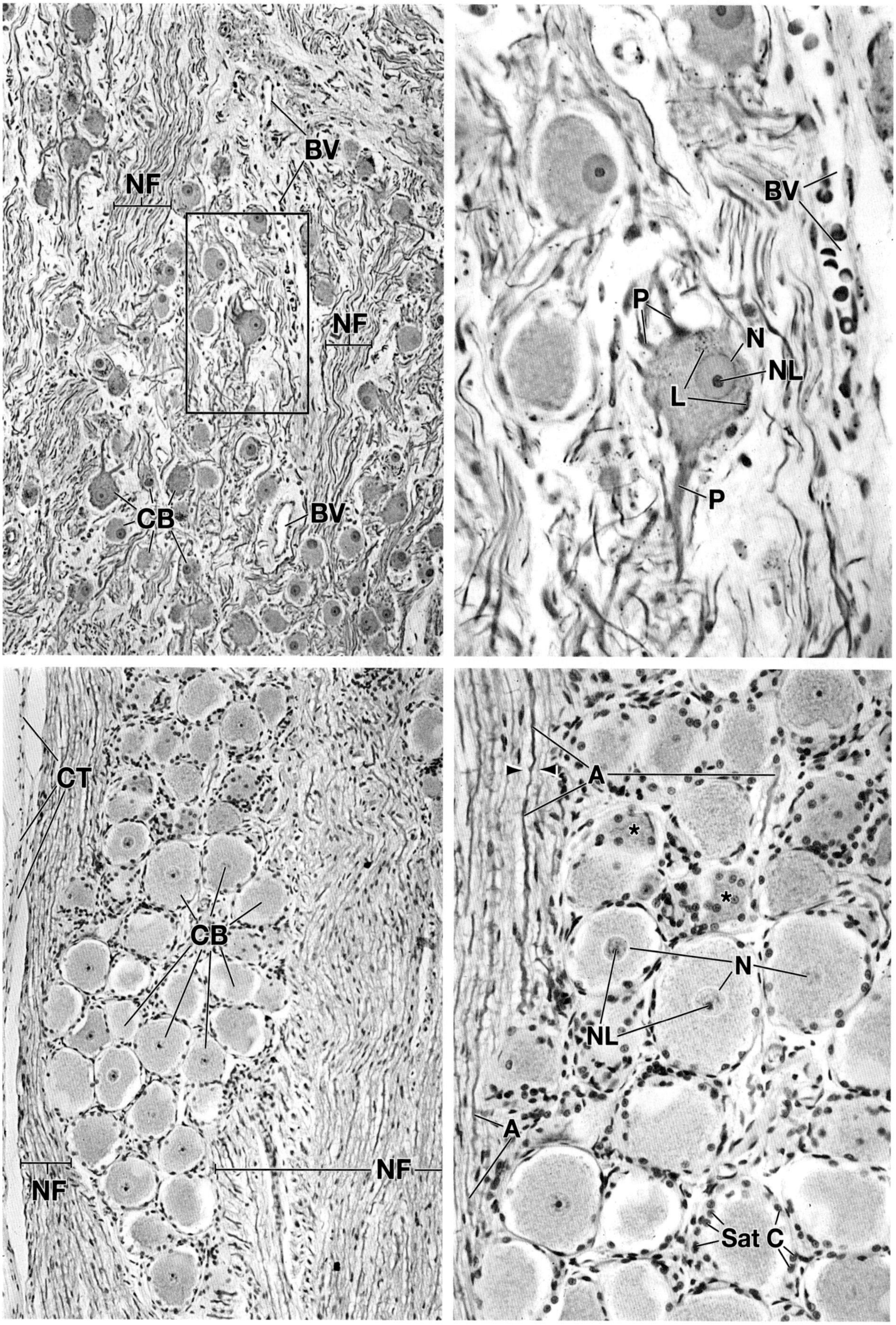
BV
NF
NF
CB
BV
P
N
NL
L
P
BV
CT
CB
NF
NF
A
*
*
N
NL
A
Sat C

PLATE 12.2 ■ PERIPHERAL NERVE

Peripheral nerves are composed of bundles of nerve fibers held together by connective tissue and a specialized layer (or layers) of cells, the **perineurium.** The connective tissue consists of an outer layer, the **epineurium**, surrounding the whole nerve; the perineurium, surrounding bundles of nerve fibers; and the **endoneurium**, associated with individual nerve fibers. Each nerve fiber consists of an axon that is surrounded by a cellular investment called the **neurilemma** or the sheath of Schwann. The fiber may be myelinated or unmyelinated. The myelin, if present, is immediately around the axon and is formed by the concentric wrapping of the Schwann cell around the axon. This, in turn, is surrounded by the major portion of the cytoplasm of the Schwann cell, forming the neurilemma. Unmyelinated axons rest in grooves in the Remak Schwann cell.

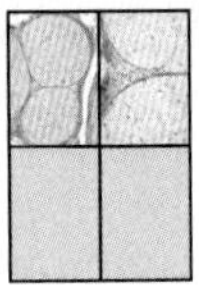

Peripheral nerve, cross section, femoral nerve, hematoxylin and eosin (H&E) ×200 and ×640.

This cross section shows several bundles of nerve fibers (*BNF*). The external cover for the entire nerve is the **epineurium** (*Epn*), the layer of dense connective tissue that one touches when a nerve has been exposed during a dissection. The epineurium may also serve as part of the outermost cover of individual bundles. It contains blood vessels (*BV*) and may contain some fat cells. Typically, adipose tissue (*AT*) surrounds the nerve.

The figure on the *right* shows, at higher magnification, the perineurial septum (marked with *arrows* on the *left* image, which is now rotated and vertically disposed).

The layer beneath the epineurium that directly surrounds the bundle of nerve fibers is the **perineurium** (*Pn*). As seen in the cross section through the nerve, the nuclei of the perineurial cells appear flat and elongated; they are actually being viewed on edge and belong to flat cells that are also being viewed on edge. Again, as noted by the distribution of nuclei, it can be ascertained that the perineurium is only a few cells thick. The perineurium is a specialized layer of cells and extracellular material whose arrangement is not evident in H&E sections. The perineurium (*Pn*) and epineurium (*Epn*) are readily distinguished in the *triangular area* formed by the diverging perineurium of the two adjacent nerve bundles.

The nerve fibers included in the figure on the *right* are mostly myelinated, and because the nerve is cross-sectioned, the nerve fibers are also seen in this plane. They have a characteristic cross-sectional profile. Each nerve fiber shows a centrally placed axon (*A*); this is surrounded by a myelin space (*M*) in which some radially disposed precipitate may be retained, as in this specimen. External to the myelin space is a thin cytoplasmic rim representing the **neurilemma**. On occasion, a Schwann cell's nucleus (*SS*) appears to be perched on the neurilemma. The *upper* edge of the nuclear crescent appears to occupy the same plane as that occupied by the neurilemma (*NI*). These features enable one to identify the nucleus as belonging to a Schwann (neurilemma) cell. Other nuclei are not related to the neurilemma but, rather, appear to be located between the nerve fibers. Such nuclei belong to the rare fibroblasts (*F*) of the endoneurium. The latter is the delicate connective tissue between the individual nerve fibers; it is extremely sparse and contains the capillaries (*C*) of the nerve bundle.

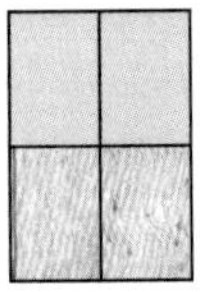

Peripheral nerve, longitudinal section, femoral nerve, H&E ×200 and ×640.

The edge of a longitudinally sectioned nerve bundle is shown on the *left*; a portion of the same nerve bundle is shown at higher magnification on the *right*. The boundary between the epineurium (*Epn*) and perineurium is ill-defined. Within the nerve bundle, the nerve fibers show a characteristic wavy pattern. Included among the wavy nerve fibers are nuclei belonging to **Schwann cells** and cells within the endoneurium. Higher magnification allows one to identify certain specific components of the nerve. Note that the nerve fibers (*NF*) are now shown in longitudinal profile. Moreover, each myelinated nerve fiber shows a centrally positioned axon (*A*) surrounded by a myelin space (*M*), which, in turn, is bordered on its outer edge by the thin cytoplasmic band of the neurilemma (*NI*). Another diagnostic feature of myelinated nerve fibers is also seen in longitudinal section, namely, the **node of Ranvier** (*NR*). This is the site at which the ends of the two Schwann cells meet. Histologically, the node appears as a constriction of the neurilemma, and sometimes, the constriction is marked by a cross-band, as in the figure on the *right*. It is difficult to determine whether the nuclei (*N*) shown here belong to Schwann cells or endoneurial fibroblasts.

A, axon
AT, adipose tissue
BNF, bundle of nerve fibers
BV, blood vessels
C, capillary
Epn, epineurium
F, fibroblast
M, myelin
N, nucleus of Schwann cell
NF, nerve fiber
NI, neurilemma
NR, node of Ranvier
Pn, perineurium
SS, Schwann cell nucleus
arrows, septum formed by perineurium

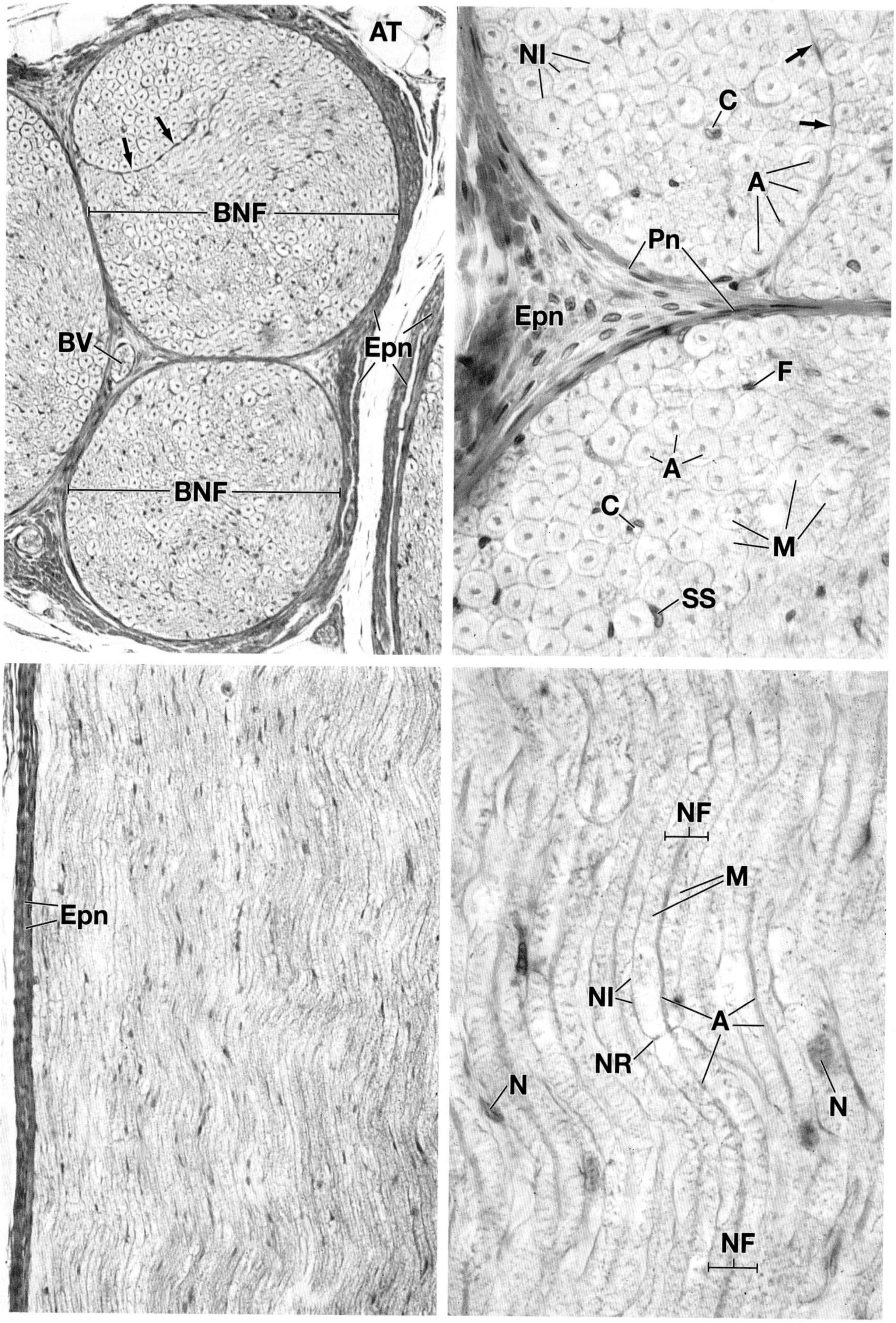
AT
BNF
BV
Epn
BNF
NI
C
A
Pn
Epn
F
A
C
M
SS
Epn
NF
M
NI
A
NR
N
N
NF

PLATE 12.3 ■ CEREBRUM

The cerebrum is the principal portion of the brain and contains the cell bodies of nerves that receive and store sensory information, nerves that control voluntary motor activity, and nerves that integrate and coordinate the activity of other nerves as well as the nerves and neural pathways that constitute memory.

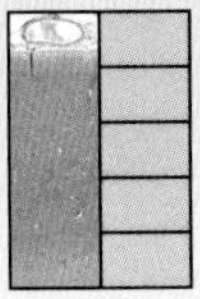

Cerebral cortex, brain, human, Luxol fast blue—(Periodic acid–Schiff) PAS ×65.

This micrograph shows a low-magnification view of the cerebral cortex (*CC*). It includes the full thickness of the gray matter and a small amount of white matter at the bottom of the micrograph (*WM*). The white matter contains considerably fewer cells per unit area; these are neuroglial cells rather than nerve cell bodies that are present in the cortex. Covering the cortex is the pia mater (*PM*). A vein (*V*) can be seen enclosed by the pia mater. Also, a smaller blood vessel (*BV*) can be seen entering the substance of the cortex. The six layers of the cortex are marked by *dashed lines*, which represent only an approximation of the boundaries. Each layer is distinguished on the basis of predominant cell types and fiber (axon and dendrite) arrangement. Unless the fibers are specifically stained, they cannot be utilized to further aid in the identification of the layers. Rather, the delineation of the layers, as they are identified here, is based on cell types and more specifically, the shape and appearance of the cells.

The six layers of the cortex are named and described as follows:

I. The **plexiform layer** (or molecular layer) consists largely of fibers, most of which travel parallel to the surface, and relatively few cells, mostly neuroglial cells and occasional horizontal cells of Cajal.

II. The **small pyramidal cell layer** (or outer granular layer) consists mainly of small pyramidal cells and granule cells, also called *stellate cells*.

III. The **layer of medium pyramidal cells** (or layer of outer pyramidal cells) is not sharply demarcated from layer II. However, the pyramidal cells are somewhat larger and possess a typical pyramidal shape.

IV. The **granular layer** (or inner granular layer) is characterized by the presence of many small granule cells (stellate cells).

V. The **layer of large pyramidal cells** (or inner layer of pyramidal cells) contains pyramidal cells that, in many parts of the cerebrum, are smaller than the pyramidal cells of layer III but, in the motor area, are extremely large and are called *Betz cells*.

VI. The **layer of polymorphic cells** contains cells with diverse shapes, many of which have a spindle of fusiform shape. These cells are called *fusiform cells*.

In addition to pyramidal cells, granule cells, and fusiform cells, two other cell types are also present in the cerebral cortex but are not recognizable in this preparation: the horizontal cells of Cajal, which are present only in layer I and send their processes laterally, and the cells of Martinotti, which send their axons toward the surface (opposite to that of pyramidal cells).

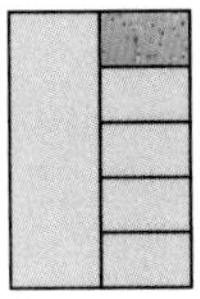

Layer I of cerebral cortex, brain, human, Luxol fast blue—PAS ×350.

This higher power micrograph shows layer I, the **plexiform layer**. It consists of nerve fibers, numerous neuroglial cells (*NN*), and occasional horizontal cells of Cajal. The neuroglial cells appear as naked nuclei, with the cytoplasm being indistinguishable from the nerve fibers that make up the bulk of this layer. Also present is a small capillary (*Cap*). The *pink* outline of the vessel is due to the PAS-staining reaction of its basement membrane.

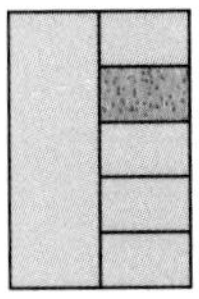

Layer II of cerebral cortex, brain, human, Luxol fast blue—PAS ×350.

This micrograph shows layer II, the **small pyramidal cell layer**. Many small pyramidal cells (*PC*) are present. Granule cells (*GC*) are also numerous, although difficult to identify here.

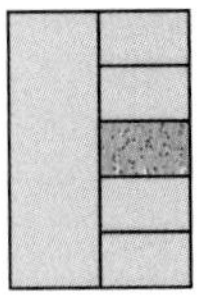

Layer IV of cerebral cortex, brain, human, Luxol fast blue—PAS ×350.

This micrograph shows layer IV, the **granular layer**. Many of the cells here are granule cells, but neuroglial cells are also prominent. The micrograph also reveals a number of capillaries. Note how they travel in various directions.

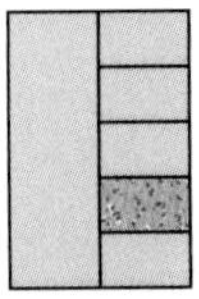

Layer VI of cerebral cortex, brain, human, Luxol fast blue—PAS ×350.

This micrograph shows layer VI, the **layer of polymorphic cells**, so named because of the diverse shape of the cells in this region. Pyramidal cells (*PC*) are readily recognized. Other cell types present include fusiform cells (*FC*), granule cells, and Martinotti cells.

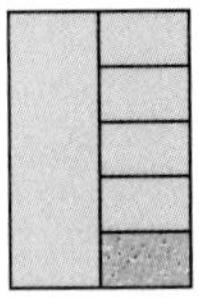

White matter, brain, human, Luxol fast blue—PAS ×350.

This micrograph shows the outer portion of the **white matter**. The small round nuclei (*NN*) belong to neuroglial cells. As in the cortex, the cytoplasm of the cell is not distinguishable. Thus, they appear as naked nuclei in the bed of nerve processes. The neuropil is essentially a densely packed aggregation of nerve fibers and neuroglial cells.

BV, blood vessel
Cap, capillary
CC, cerebral cortex
FC, fusiform cells
GC, granule cells
NN, neuroglial nuclei
PC, pyramidal cells
PM, pia mater
V, vein
WM, white matter

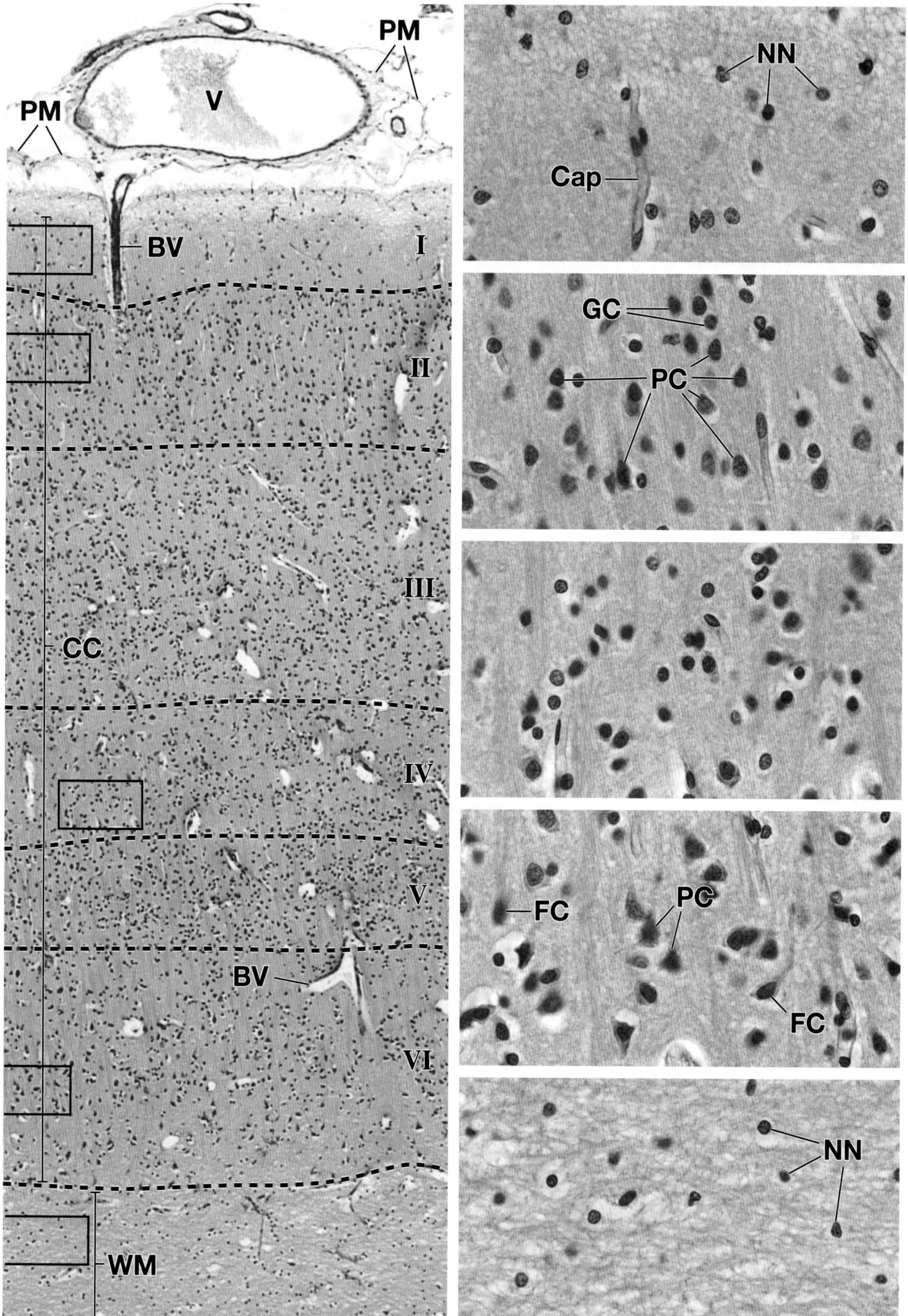
PM
V
PM
BV
I
II
III
CC
IV
V
BV
VI
WM
NN
Cap
GC
PC
FC
PC
FC
NN

PLATE 12.4 ■ CEREBELLUM

The cerebellum is a portion of the brain lying behind and below the cerebrum; it serves to coordinate both voluntary movements and muscle function in the maintenance of normal posture.

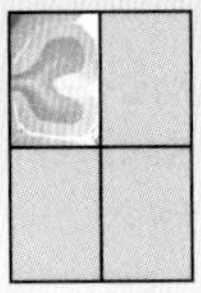

Cerebellum, brain, human, hematoxylin and eosin (H&E) ×40.

The **cerebellar cortex** has the same appearance regardless of which region is examined. In this low-magnification view of the cerebellum, the outermost layer, the **molecular layer** (*Mol*), is lightly stained with eosin. Beneath this layer is the **granule cell layer** (*Gr*), which stains intensely with hematoxylin. Together, these two layers constitute the cortex of the cerebellum. Deep in the granule cell layer is another region that stains lightly with H&E and, except for location, shows no distinctive histologic features. This is the white matter (*WM*). As in the cerebrum, it contains nerve fibers, supporting neuroglial cells, and small blood vessels but no neuronal cell bodies. The fibrous cover on the cerebellar surface is the pia mater (*Pia*). Cerebellar blood vessels (*BV*) travel in this layer. (Shrinkage artifact has separated the pia mater from the cerebellar surface.) The *rectangular area* is shown at higher magnification in the figure on the *right*.

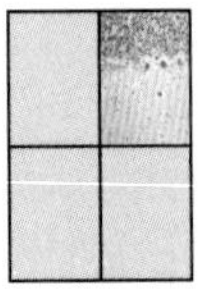

Cerebellum, brain, human, H&E ×400.

At the junction between the molecular and granule cell layers are the extremely large flask-shaped cell bodies of the **Purkinje cells** (*Pkj*). These cells are characteristic of the cerebellum. Each possesses numerous dendrites (*D*) that arborize in the molecular layer. The Purkinje cell has a single axon that is not usually evident in H&E sections. This nerve fiber represents the beginning of the outflow from the cerebellum.

The figure shows relatively few neuron cell bodies, those of the basket cells (*BC*), in the molecular layer; they are widely removed from each other and, at best, show only a small amount of cytoplasm surrounding the nucleus. In contrast, the granule cell layer presents an overall spotted-blue appearance due to the staining of numerous small nuclei with hematoxylin. These small neurons, called **granule cells**, receive incoming impulses from other parts of the CNS and send axons into the molecular layer, where they branch in the form of a T, so that the axons contact the dendrites of several Purkinje cells and basket cells. Incoming (mossy) fibers contact granule cells in the lightly stained areas called *glomeruli* (*arrows*). Careful examination of the granule cell layer where it meets the molecular layer will reveal a group of nuclei (*G*) that are larger than the nuclei of granule cells. These belong to Golgi type II cells.

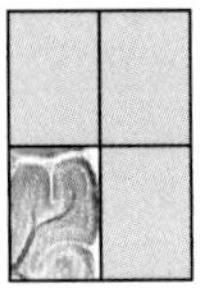

Cerebellum, brain, human, silver stain ×40.

The specimen in this figure has been stained with a silver procedure. Such procedures do not always color the specimen evenly, as does H&E. Note that the part of the molecular layer on the *right* is much darker than that on the *left*. A *rectangular area* on the *left* has been selected for examination at higher magnification in the *lower right* figure. Even at the relatively low magnification shown here, however, the Purkinje cells can be recognized in the silver preparation because of their large size, characteristic shape, and location between an outer molecular layer (*Mol*) and an inner granule cell layer (*Gr*). The main advantage of this silver preparation is that the **white matter** (*WM*) can be recognized as being composed of fibers; they have been blackened by the silver-staining procedure. The pia mater (*Pia*) and cerebellar blood vessels (*BV*) are also evident in the preparation.

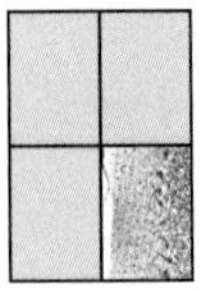

Cerebellum, brain, human, silver stain ×400.

At higher magnification, the **Purkinje cell** bodies (*Pkj*) stand out as the most distinctive and conspicuous neuronal cell type of the cerebellum, and numerous dendritic branches (*D*) can be seen. Note, also, the blackened fibers within the granule cell layer (*Gr*), about the Purkinje cell bodies, and in the molecular layer (*Mol*) disposed in a horizontal direction (relative to the cerebellar surface). Basket cells (*BC*) are the most common neurons that are visible in the molecular layer. The *arrow* indicates a T-turn characteristic of the turn made by axons of granule cells. As these axonal branches travel horizontally, they make synaptic contact with numerous Purkinje cells.

BC, basket cells
BV, blood vessels
D, dendrites
G, Golgi type II cells
Gr, granule cell layer
Mol, molecular layer
Pia, pia mater
Pkj, Purkinje cells
WM, white matter
arrows, upper right figure, glomeruli; lower right figure, T branching of axon in molecular layer
rectangular area, areas shown at higher magnification

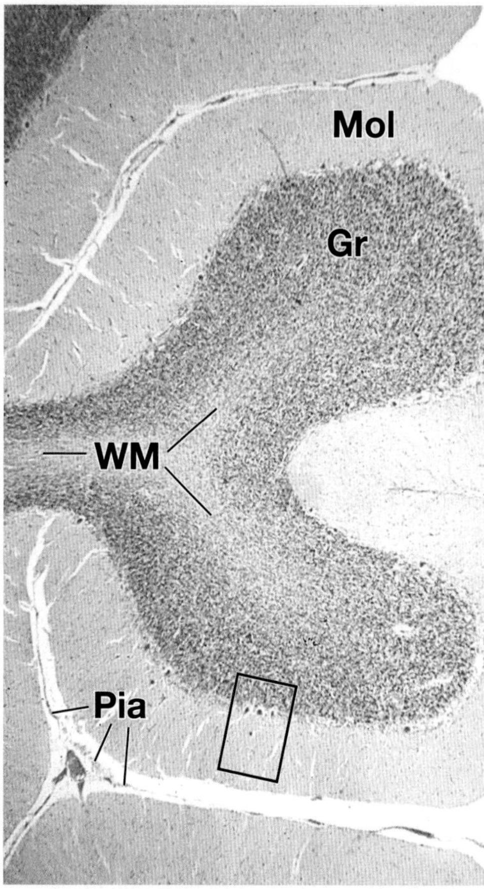
Mol
Gr
WM
Pia
BV

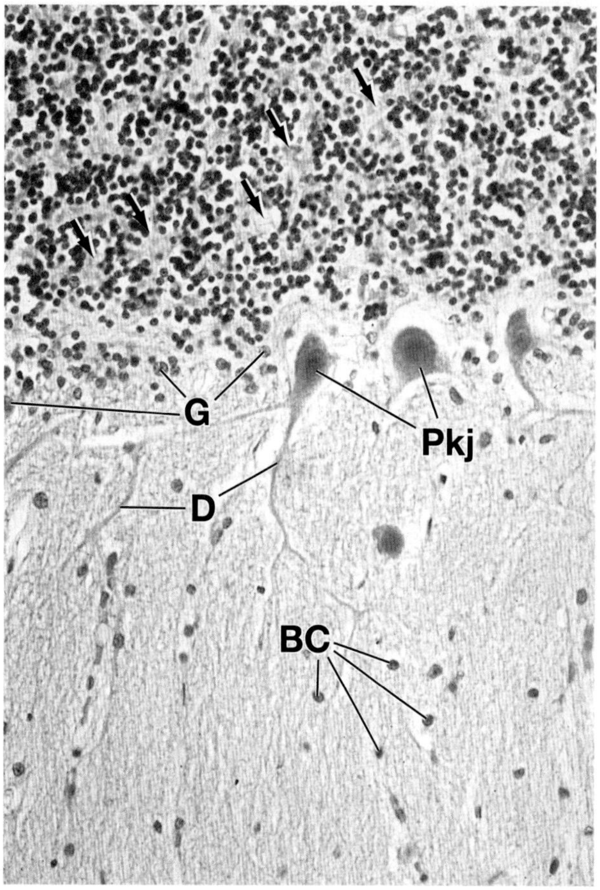
G
Pkj
D
BC

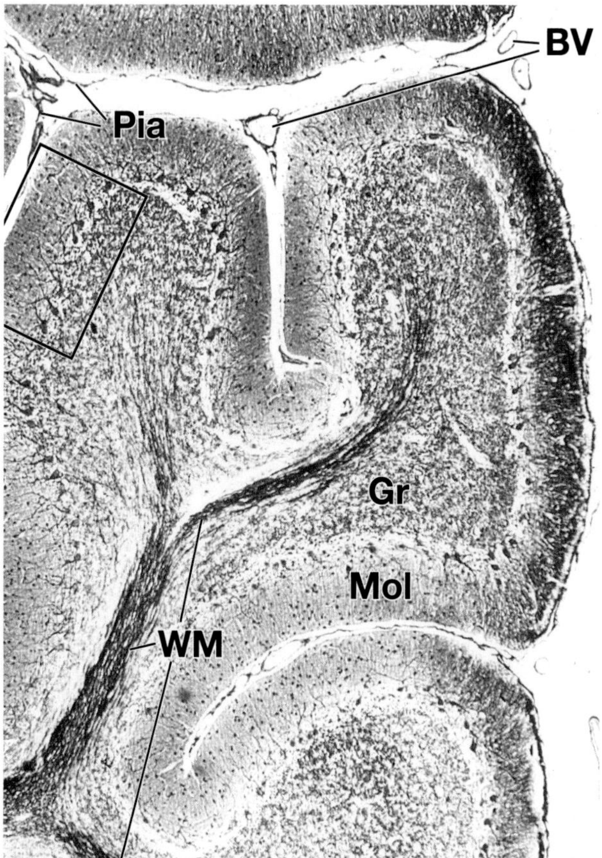
BV
Pia
Gr
Mol
WM

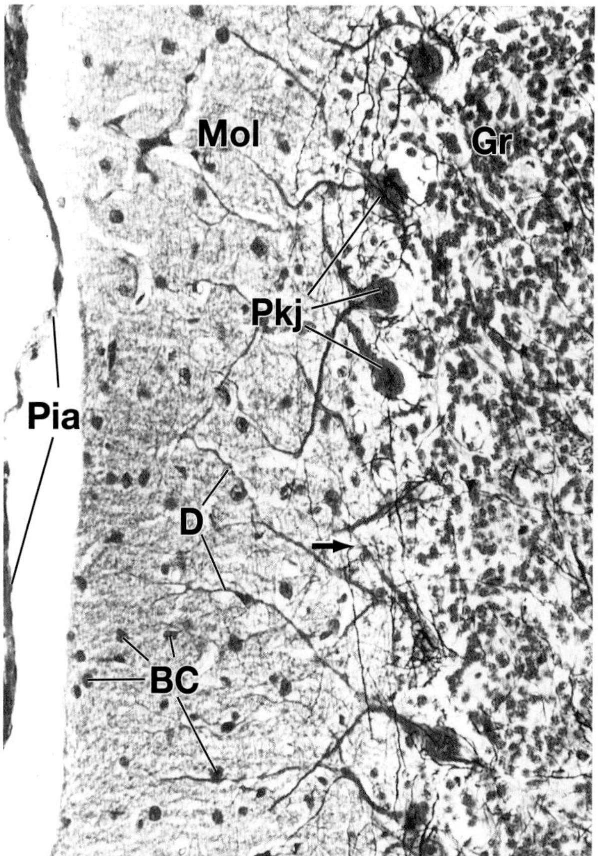
Mol
Gr
Pkj
Pia
D
BC

The spinal cord is organized into two discrete parts. The outer part, called the **white matter** of the cord because of its appearance in unfixed specimens, contains ascending and descending nerve fibers. Some of the fibers go to and from the brain, whereas others connect different levels of the spinal cord. The inner part of the spinal cord, called the **gray matter** because of its appearance in unfixed specimens, contains the cell bodies of neurons as well as nerve fibers. The gray matter forms an H- or butterfly-shaped pattern surrounding the central canal. The gray matter is described as having **dorsal (posterior) horns** and **ventral (anterior) horns.** The ventral horns contain the large cell bodies of ventral motor neurons, whereas the dorsal horns contain neurons that receive, process, and retransmit information from the sensory neurons whose cell bodies are located in the dorsal root ganglia. The size of the gray matter (and, therefore, the size of the spinal cord) is different at different levels. Where the gray matter contains many large motor nerve cells that control the movement of the upper and lower limbs, the gray matter and the spinal cord are considerably larger than where the gray matter contains only the motor neurons for the muscle of the torso.

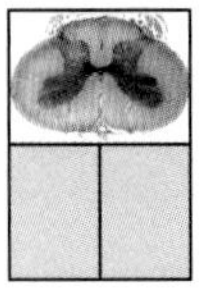

Spinal cord, human, silver stain ×16.

A cross section through the lower lumbar region of the spinal cord is shown here. The preparation is designed to stain the gray matter that is surrounded by the ascending and descending nerve fibers. Although the fibers that have common origins and destinations in the physiologic sense are arranged in tracts, these tracts cannot be distinguished unless they have been marked by special techniques, such as causing injury to the cell bodies from which they arise or by using special dyes or radioisotopes to label the axons.

The **gray matter** of the spinal cord appears roughly in the form of a butterfly. The anterior and posterior prongs are referred to as *ventral horns* (*VH*) and *dorsal horns* (*DH*), respectively. The connecting bar is called the *gray commissure* (*GC*). The neuron cell bodies that are within the ventral horns (ventral horn cells) are so large that they can be seen even at this extremely low magnification (*arrows*). The pale-staining fibrous material that surrounds the spinal cord is the **pia mater** (*Pia*). It follows the surface of the spinal cord intimately and dips into the large ventral fissure (*VF*) and the shallower sulci. Blood vessels (*BV*) are present in the pia mater. Some dorsal roots (*DR*) of the spinal nerves are included in the section.

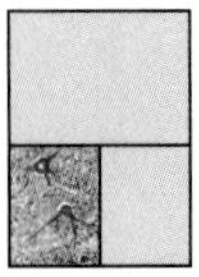

Ventral horn, spinal cord, human, silver stain ×640.

This preparation shows a region of a ventral horn. The nucleus (*N*) of the **ventral horn cell** (ventral motor neuron) is the large, spherical, pale-staining structure within the cell body. The ventral horn cell has many obvious processes. A number of other nuclei belong to neuroglial cells. The cytoplasm of these cells is not evident. The remainder of the field consists of nerve fibers and neuroglial cells whose organization is hard to interpret. This is called the neuropil (*Np*).

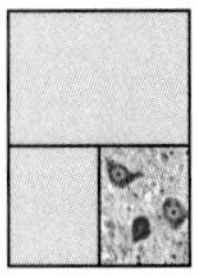

Ventral horn, spinal cord, human, toluidine blue ×640.

This preparation of the spinal cord is from an area comparable to the *left* image. Three ventral horn cells (ventral motor neurons) are visible. Owing to the plane of section, only two of them exhibit large pale-staining nuclei (*N*) with dark-staining nucleoli in the center. The toluidine blue reveals the **Nissl bodies** (*NB*) that appear as the large, dark-staining bodies in the cytoplasm. Nissl bodies do not extend into the axon hillock. The axon leaves the cell body at the axon hillock. The nuclei of neuroglial cells (*NN*) are also evident here.

BV, blood vessels
DH, dorsal horn
DR, dorsal root
GC, gray commissure
N, nucleus of ventral horn cell
NB, Nissl bodies
NN, nucleus of neuroglial cell
Np, neuropil
Pia, pia mater
VF, ventral fissure
VH, ventral horn
arrows, cell bodies of ventral horn cell

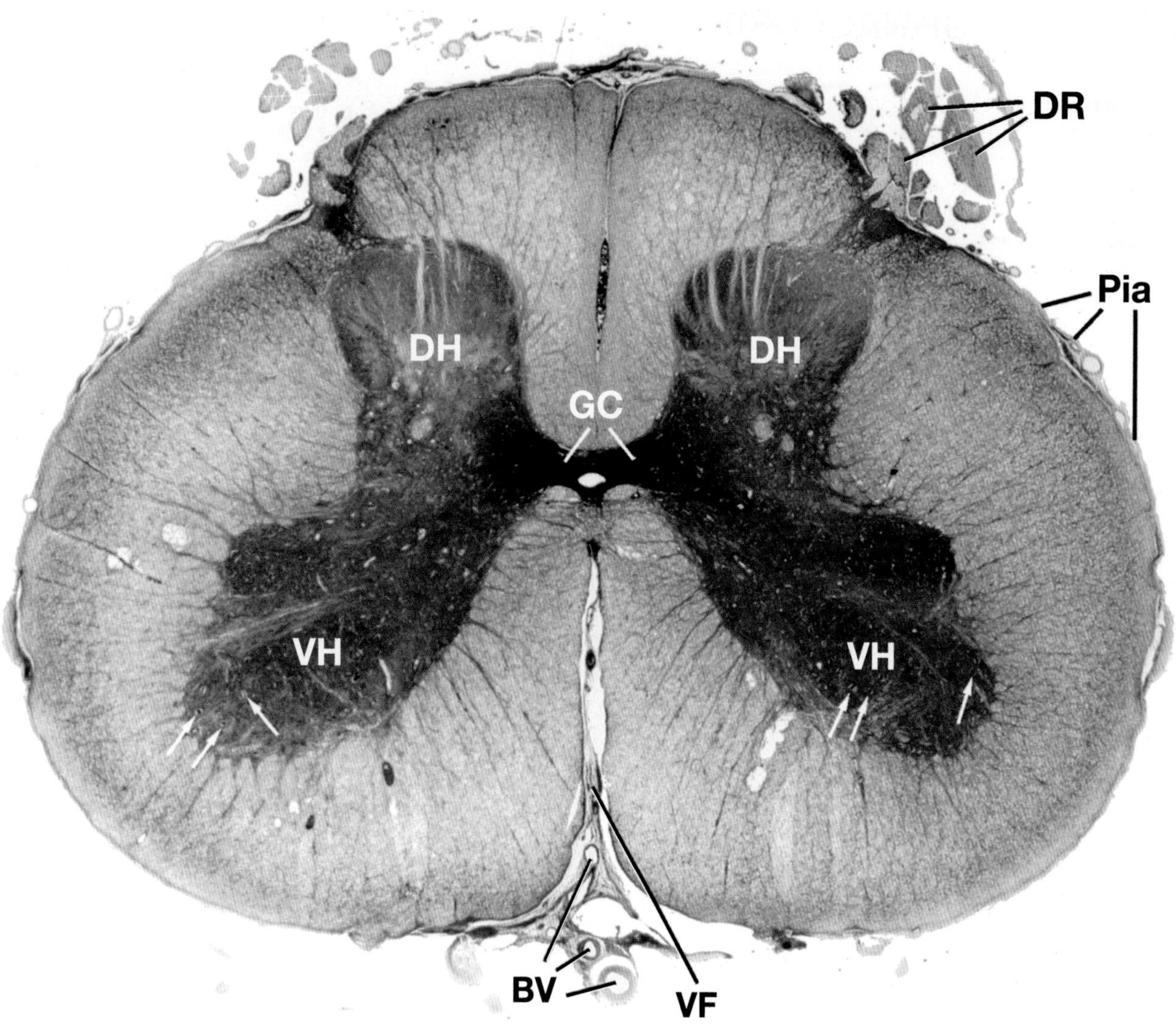
DR
Pia
DH
DH
GC
VH
VH
BV
VF

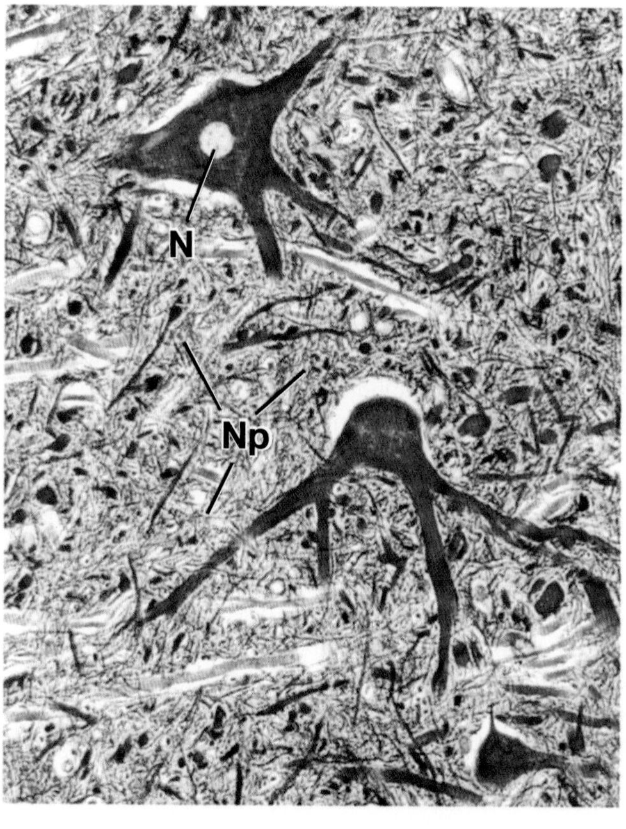
N
Np

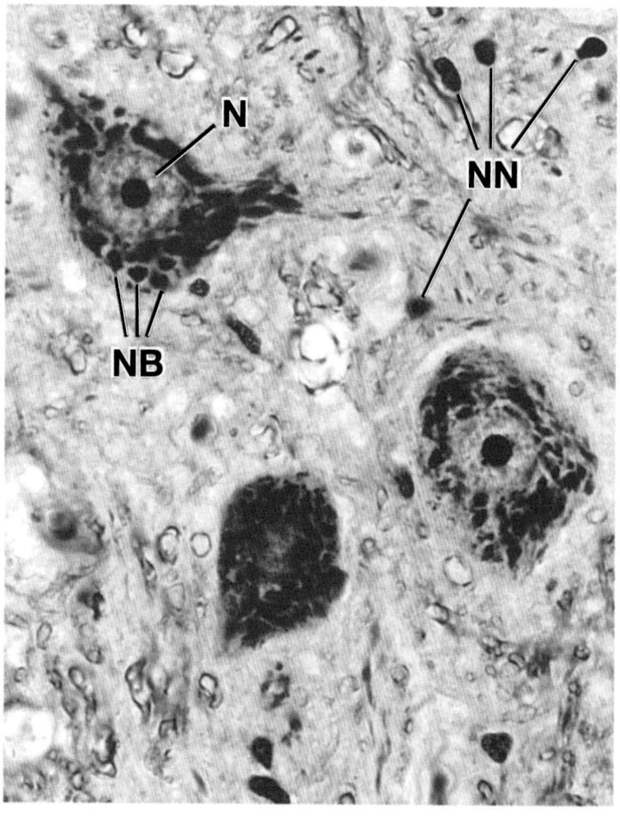
N
NN
NB

13 CARDIOVASCULAR SYSTEM

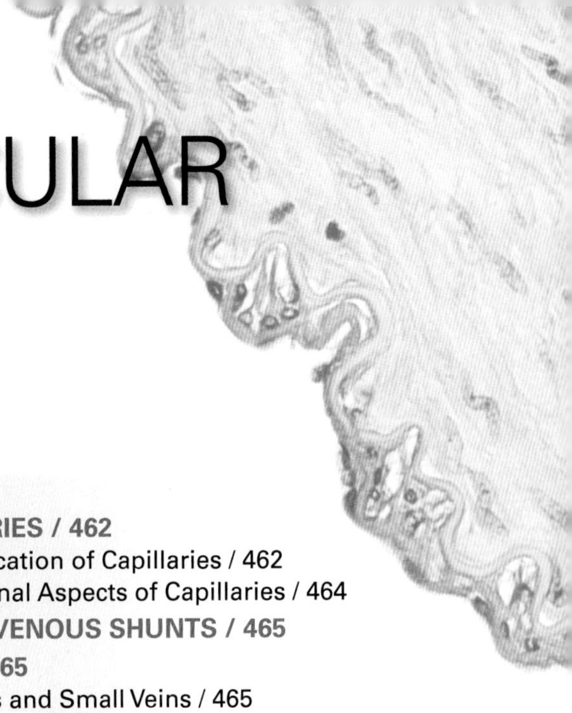

■ OVERVIEW OF THE CARDIOVASCULAR SYSTEM

The cardiovascular system is a transport system that carries blood and lymph to and from the tissues of the body. The constitutive elements of these fluids include cells, nutrients, waste products, hormones, and antibodies.

The cardiovascular system includes the heart, blood vessels, and lymphatic vessels.

The **cardiovascular system** consists of a pump, represented by the heart, and the blood vessels, which provide the route by which blood circulates to and from all parts of the body (Fig. 13.1). The **heart** pumps the blood through the arterial system under significant pressure; blood is returned to the heart under low pressure with the assistance of negative pressure in the thoracic cavity during inspiration and compression of the veins by skeletal muscle. The **blood vessels** are arranged so that blood delivered from the heart quickly reaches a network of narrow, thin-walled vessels—the blood **capillaries**—within or in proximity to the tissues in every part of the body.

In the capillaries, a two-directional exchange of fluid occurs between the blood and tissues. The liquid extracellular material of the blood, called **plasma**, carries oxygen and metabolites and passes through the capillary wall. In the tissues, these molecules are exchanged for carbon dioxide and waste products. Most of the fluid reenters the distal or venous end of the blood capillaries. The remaining fluid enters lymphatic capillaries as lymph and is ultimately returned to the bloodstream through a system of **lymphatic vessels** that join the blood system at the junction of the internal jugular veins with the subclavian veins. Normally, many of the white blood cells conveyed in the blood leave the blood vessels to enter the tissues. This occurs at the level of the **postcapillary venules**. When pathologic changes occur in the body, such as an inflammatory reaction, large numbers of white blood cells emigrate from these venules.

Arteries are the vessels that deliver blood to the capillaries. The smallest arteries, called **arterioles**, are functionally associated with networks of capillaries into which they deliver blood. The arterioles regulate the amount of blood that enters these capillary networks. Together, the arterioles, associated capillary network, and postcapillary venules form a functional unit called the **microcirculatory** or **microvascular bed** of that tissue. **Veins**, beginning with the postcapillary venule, collect blood from the microvascular bed and carry it away.

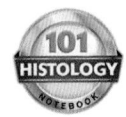

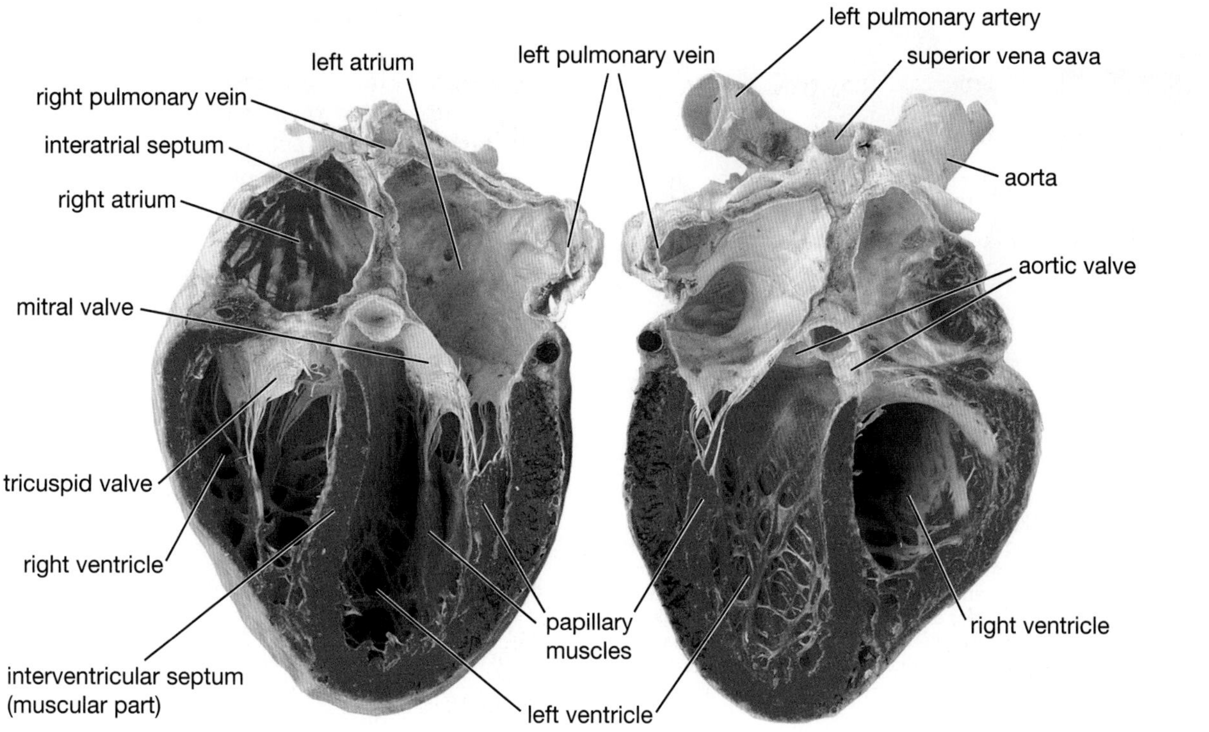

FIGURE 13.1. Photograph of the human heart. This specimen was sectioned in the oblique plane to visualize all of the chambers of the heart. The posterior part of the heart is on the *left*; the anterior part has been removed and is shown on the *right*. Note the thickness of the ventricular walls and the interventricular septum. The interatrial septum, which separates the atria, is also visible.

Two circuits distribute blood in the body: the systemic and pulmonary circulations.

Two pathways of circulation are formed by the blood vessels and the heart:

- **Pulmonary circulation** conveys blood from the heart to the lungs and from the lungs to the heart (Fig. 13.2).
- **Systemic circulation** conveys blood from the heart to other tissues of the body and from other tissues of the body to the heart.

Although the general arrangement of blood vessels in both circulations is from arteries to capillaries to veins, in some parts of the systemic circulation, it is modified so that a vein or an arteriole is interposed between two capillary networks; these vessels constitute a **portal system**. Venous portal systems occur in vessels carrying blood to the liver, namely, the **hepatic portal system (portal vein)**, and in vessels leading to the pituitary, the **hypothalamic–hypophyseal portal system**.

■ HEART

The **heart** lies obliquely, about two-thirds into the left side of the thoracic cavity, in the **middle mediastinum**—the space enclosed by the sternum, vertebral column, diaphragm, and lungs. It is surrounded by a tough fibrous sac, the **pericardium**, from which the great vessels enter and leave the heart. Through the pericardium, the heart is attached to the diaphragm and neighboring organs that lie in the thoracic cavity.

The heart is a muscular pump that maintains unidirectional flow of blood.

The heart contains four chambers—the right and left atria and the right and left ventricles—through which blood is pumped (see Fig. 13.1). Valves guard the exits of the chambers, preventing the backflow of blood. An **interatrial septum** and an **interventricular septum** separate the right and left sides of the heart.

The right side of the heart pumps blood through the pulmonary circulation. The **right atrium** receives deoxygenated

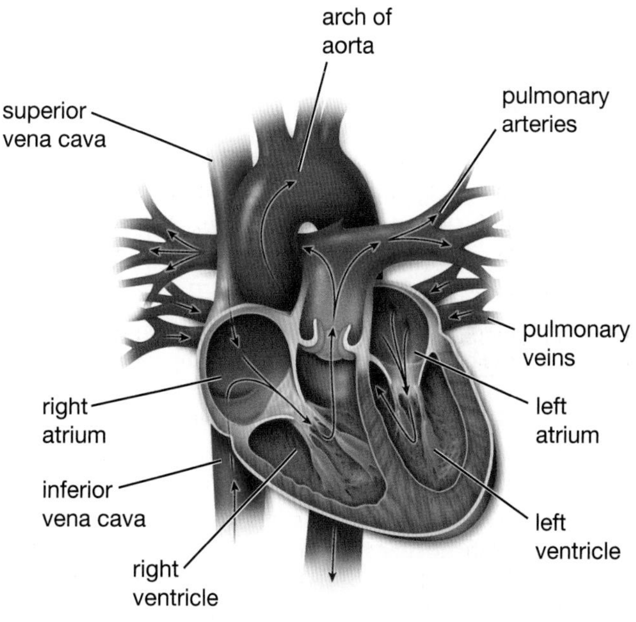

FIGURE 13.2. Diagram depicting circulation of blood through the heart. Blood returns from the tissues of the body via the superior vena cava and inferior vena cava. These two major venous vessels carry the blood to the right atrium. Blood then passes into the right ventricle and is pumped into the pulmonary trunk before flowing into the pulmonary arteries, which convey the blood to the lungs. The blood is oxygenated in the lungs and is then returned to the left atrium via the pulmonary veins. Blood then passes to the left ventricle and is pumped into the aorta, which conveys the blood to the tissues of the body. From the heart to the lungs and from the lungs to the heart constitutes the *pulmonary circulation*; from the heart to the tissues and from the tissues to the heart constitutes the *systemic circulation*.

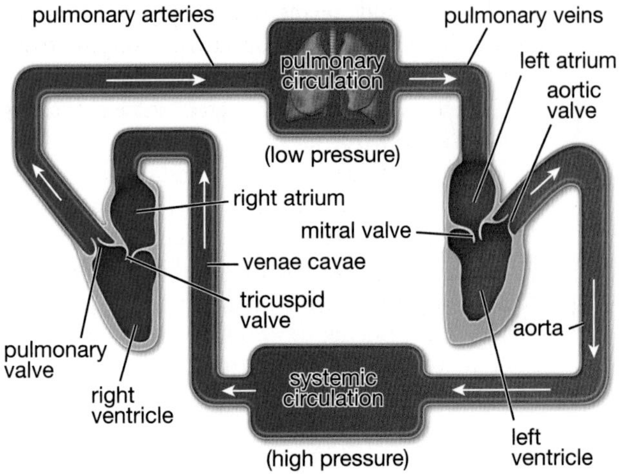

FIGURE 13.3. Diagram of the blood circulation. This diagram shows the right and left sides of the heart artificially separated. The right side of the heart pumps blood through the low-pressure pulmonary circulation. The right atrium receives deoxygenated blood returning from the body via the inferior and superior venae cavae. The right ventricle receives blood from the right atrium and pumps it to the lungs for oxygenation via the pulmonary arteries. The left side of the heart pumps blood through the high-pressure systemic circulation. The left atrium receives the oxygenated blood returning from the lungs via the four pulmonary veins. The left ventricle receives blood from the left atrium and pumps it into the aorta for systemic distribution.

blood returning from the body via the inferior and superior venae cavae, the two largest veins of the body (Fig. 13.3). The **right ventricle** receives blood from the right atrium and pumps it to the lungs for oxygenation via the pulmonary arteries. The left side of the heart pumps blood through the systemic circulation. The **left atrium** receives the oxygenated blood returning from the lungs via the four pulmonary veins. The **left ventricle** receives blood from the left atrium and pumps it into the aorta for distribution to the body.

The heart contains the following:

- A musculature of **cardiac muscle** for contraction to propel the blood
- A **fibrous skeleton** that consists of four fibrous rings surrounding the valve orifices, two fibrous trigones connecting the rings, and the membranous part of the interventricular and interatrial septa. The **fibrous rings** are composed of dense irregular connective tissue. They encircle the base of the two arteries, leaving the heart (aorta and pulmonary trunk) and the openings between the atria and the ventricles (right and left atrioventricular [AV] orifices) (Fig. 13.4). These rings provide the attachment site for the leaflets of all four valves of the heart that allow blood flow in only one direction through the openings. The **membranous part of the interventricular septum** is devoid of cardiac muscle; it consists of dense connective tissue that contains a short length of the AV bundle of the conducting system of the heart. The fibrous skeleton provides independent attachments for the atrial and ventricular myocardium. It also acts as an electrical insulator by preventing the free flow of electrical impulses between the atria and the ventricles.
- A **conducting system** for initiation and propagation of rhythmic depolarizations, which results in rhythmic cardiac muscle contractions (Fig. 13.5). This system is formed by **modified cardiac muscle cells (Purkinje fibers)**, which generate and conduct electrical impulses rapidly through the heart. In **cardiac arrest**, the sudden cessation of normal heart rhythm leads to abrupt cessation of blood circulation, and the conducting system of the heart fails to produce or conduct electrical impulses that cause the heart to contract and supply blood to the body. Sudden cardiac arrest is a medical emergency; first-aid treatment such as **cardiopulmonary resuscitation (CPR)** and defibrillation (delivering a therapeutic dose of electrical energy to the heart) can improve the chances of survival. If not treated, cardiac arrest leads to **sudden cardiac death**. Heart rhythm pathologies associated with cardiac arrest include tachycardia (accelerated heart rhythm), fibrillation (rapid, irregular, and ineffective contractions), bradycardia (decelerated heart rhythm), and asystole (total absence of heart rhythm).
- A **coronary vasculature** that consists of two coronary arteries and cardiac veins. The right and left **coronary arteries** provide the arterial blood supply to the heart. They originate from the initial part of the ascending aorta near the aortic valves and circle the base of the heart, with branches converging toward the apex of the heart. Venous drainage of the heart occurs via several **cardiac veins**, most of which drain into the coronary sinus located on the posterior surface of the heart. The coronary sinus drains into the right atrium.

Wall of the Heart

The wall of the heart is composed of three layers: epicardium, myocardium, and endocardium.

The structural organization of the wall of the heart is continuous within the atria and ventricles. The wall of the heart

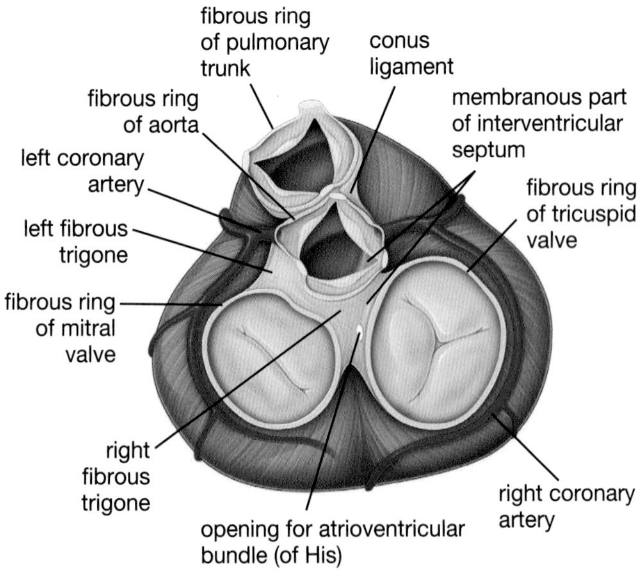

FIGURE 13.4. Fibrous skeleton of the heart as seen with the two atria removed. This fibrous network (indicated in *light blue*) serves for the attachment of cardiac muscle; it also serves for the attachment of the cuspid valves between the atria and the ventricles and for the semilunar valves of the aorta and the pulmonary artery. The atrioventricular bundle passes from the right atrium to the ventricular septum via the membranous septum of the fibrous skeleton.

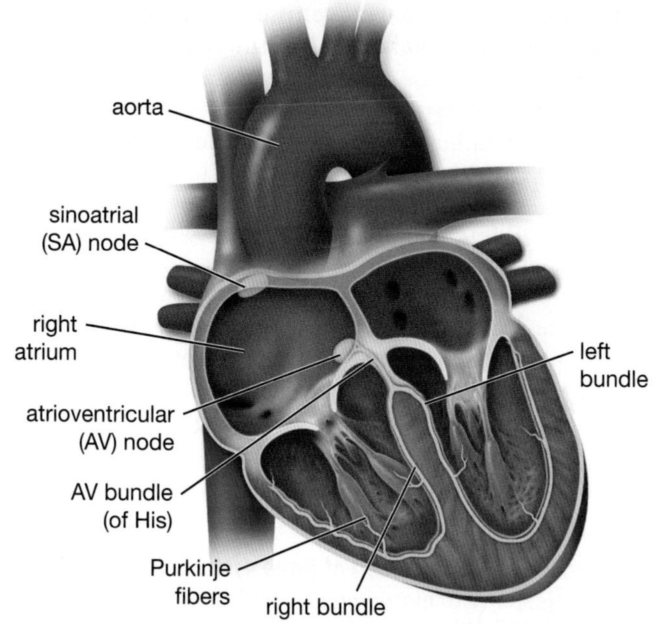

FIGURE 13.5. Chambers of the heart and the impulse-conducting system. The heart has been cut open in the coronal plane to expose its interior and the main parts of its impulse-conducting system (indicated in *yellow*). Impulses are generated in the sinoatrial (*SA*) node, transmitted through the atrial wall to the atrioventricular (*AV*) node, and then sent along the *AV* bundle to the Purkinje fibers.

is composed of three layers. From the outside to the inside, they are as follows:

- The **epicardium**, also known as the **visceral layer of serous pericardium**, adheres to the outer surface of the heart (Fig. 13.6). It consists of a single layer of mesothelial cells and underlying connective and adipose tissue. The blood vessels and nerves that supply the heart lie in the epicardium and are surrounded by adipose tissue that cushions the heart in the pericardial cavity. The epicardium is reflected back at the great vessels entering and leaving the heart as the **parietal layer of serous pericardium**, which lines the inner surface of the pericardium that surrounds the heart and roots of great vessels. Thus, there is a potential space containing a minimal amount (15–50 mL) of serous (pericardial) fluid between the visceral and parietal layers of the serous pericardium. This space is known as the **pericardial cavity**; its lining consists of mesothelial cells (see Fig. 13.6).
- **Cardiac tamponade** is a condition in which excess fluid (blood or pericardial effusion) rapidly accumulates in the pericardial cavity. It is commonly caused by both blunt and penetrating chest injuries and by myocardial rupture or pericarditis (inflammation of pericardium). This condition is potentially life-threatening because the accumulating fluid may compress the heart and prevent the heart's chambers from filling properly with blood. Relieving the pressure is usually accomplished with **pericardiocentesis** (a procedure to drain the fluid from the pericardial cavity).
- The **myocardium**, consisting of cardiac muscle, is the principal component of the heart. The detailed histologic structure and function of cardiac muscle is discussed in Chapter 11, Muscle Tissue (pages 361-366). The myocardium of the atria is substantially thinner than that of the ventricles. The atria receive blood from the large veins and deliver it to adjacent ventricles, a process that requires relatively low pressure. The myocardium of the ventricles is substantially thicker because of the higher pressure required

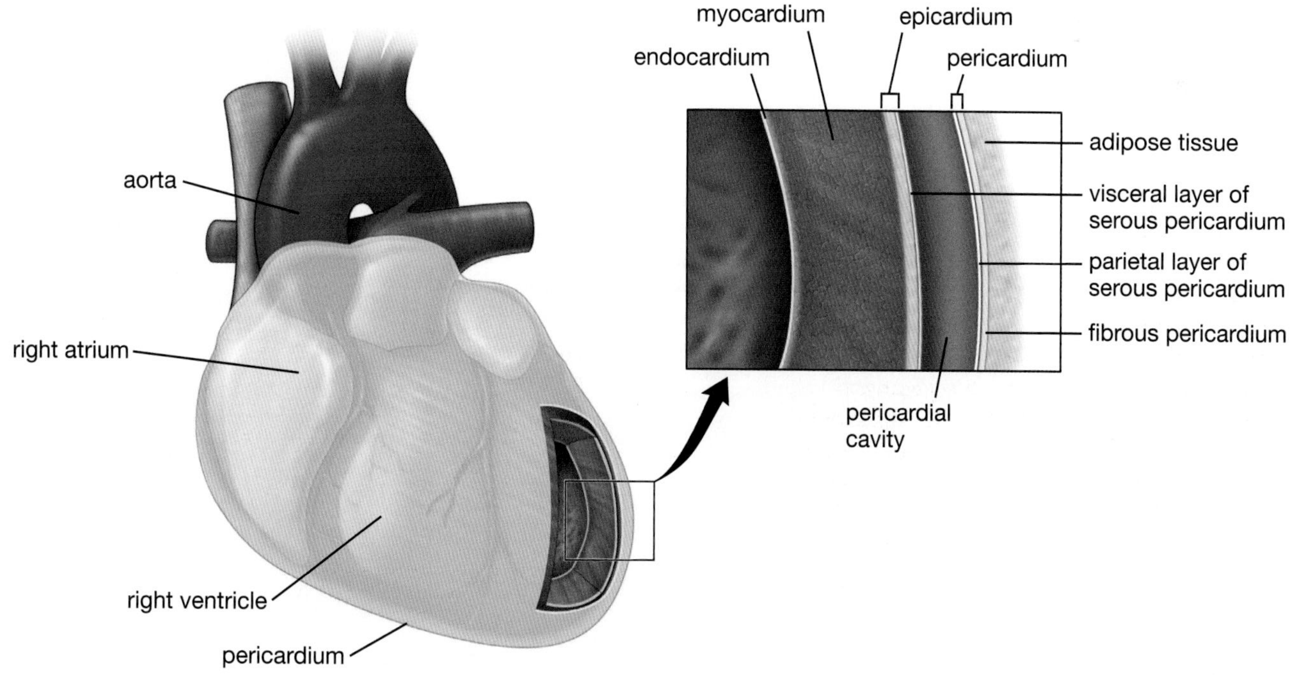

FIGURE 13.6. Layers of the heart and pericardium. This schematic diagram shows the anatomic relationship between the layers of the heart. In the middle mediastinum, the heart and roots of the great vessels are surrounded by the pericardium, which is often covered by highly variable amounts of adipose tissue. The pericardium has two layers: a tough external fibrous layer called the *fibrous pericardium* and a parietal layer of serous pericardium that lines its inner surface. The parietal layer of the serous pericardium is reflected back at the great vessels entering and leaving the heart as the visceral layer of the serous pericardium or epicardium. The epicardium lines the outer surface of the heart. The pericardial cavity is a space between the visceral and parietal layers of the serous pericardium, and it is lined by the mesothelial cells. Deep to the epicardium is the myocardium, which consists of cardiac muscle. Note the small amount of adipose tissue in the epicardium, which contains the coronary arteries and cardiac veins. The inner layer of the myocardium is called the *endocardium*, which is lined by the mesothelium with an underlying thin layer of connective tissue.

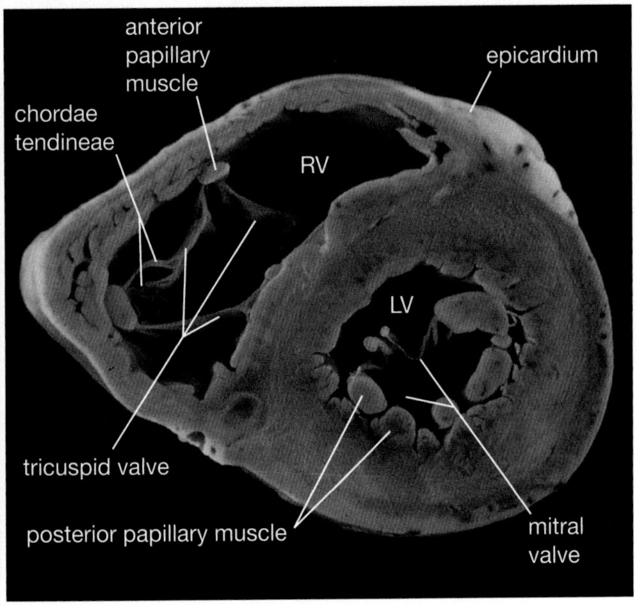

FIGURE 13.7. Horizontal section through the ventricles of the heart. This photograph shows a cross section of the human heart at the level of the ventricles. Cusps of both the tricuspid valve in the right ventricle and the mitral valve in the left ventricle are visible with their attachments to the chordae tendineae. Cross sections of the papillary muscles in both the ventricles are visible. Note the differences in the thickness between the wall of the right and left ventricles. Adipose tissue of the epicardium contains branches of the coronary arteries and tributaries of the cardiac veins. *RV*, right ventricle; *LV*, left ventricle. (Courtesy of Dr. William D. Edwards.)

to pump the blood through the pulmonary and systemic circulations (Fig. 13.7).

- The **endocardium** consists of an inner layer of endothelium and subendothelial connective tissue, a middle layer of connective tissue and smooth muscle cells, and a deeper layer of connective tissue, which is also called the **subendocardial layer**. The latter is continuous with the connective tissue of the myocardium. The conducting system of the heart is located in the subendocardial layer of the endocardium (see the section on intrinsic regulation of heart rate).

The **interventricular septum** is the wall between the right and left ventricles. It contains cardiac muscle in all but the membranous portion. Endocardium lines each surface of the interventricular septum. The **interatrial septum** is much thinner than the interventricular septum. Except in certain localized areas that contain fibrous tissue, it has a center layer of cardiac muscle and a lining of endocardium facing each chamber.

Heart Valves

Heart valves are composed of three distinct layers of connective tissue with overlying endocardium.

The heart valves attach to the complex framework of dense irregular connective tissue that forms the fibrous rings of the heart and surrounds the orifices containing the valves (Fig. 13.8). Each valve is composed of three distinct layers: **fibrosa**, **spongiosa**, and either **ventricularis** (on the ventricular surface of the aortic and pulmonary semilunar valves) or **atrialis** (on the atrial surface of the mitral and tricuspid AV valves):

- The **fibrosa** is situated on the ventricular surface of AV valves and the arterial surface (facing the aorta or pulmonary trunk) of semilunar valves. This layer is derived from the dense irregular connective tissue of the skeletal

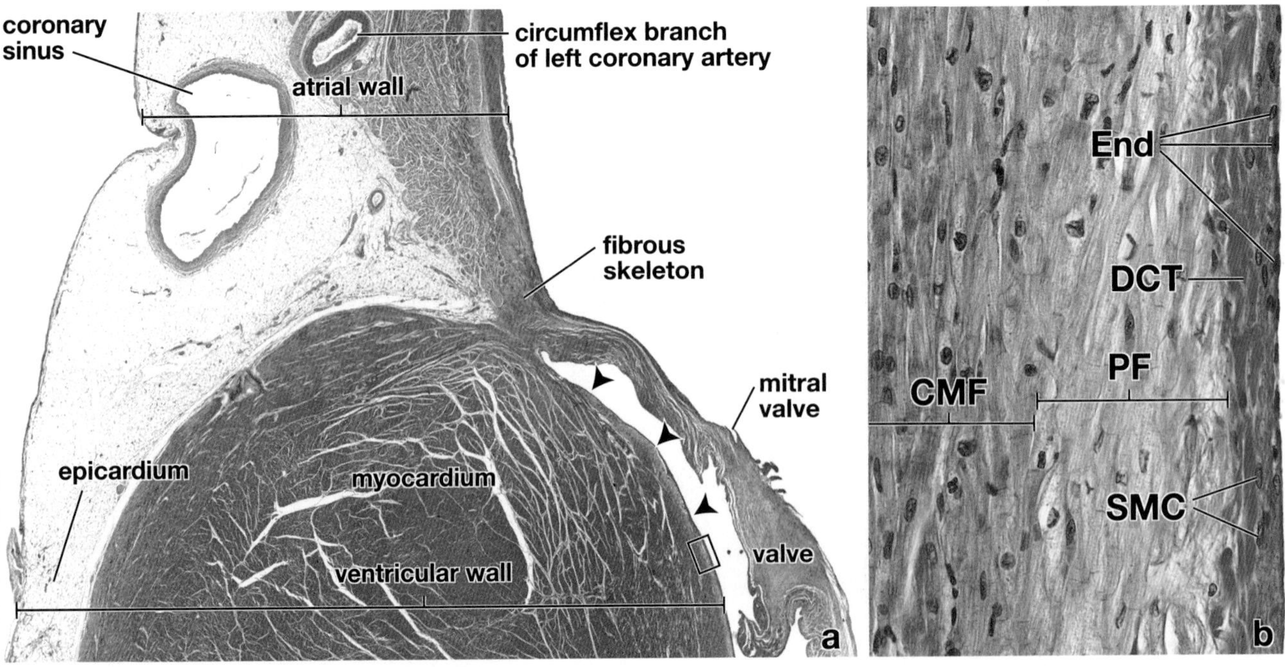

FIGURE 13.8. Photomicrograph of the left atrial and left ventricular walls. a. This photomicrograph shows a sagittal section of the posterior wall of the left atrium and left ventricle. The line of section crosses the coronary (*AV*) groove containing the coronary sinus and circumflex branch of the left coronary artery. Note that the section has cut through the fibrous *AV* ring of the mitral valve, which provides the attachment site for the muscle of the left atrium and the left ventricle and the cusp of the mitral valve. The ventricular wall consists of three layers: (1) endocardium (*arrowheads*), (2) myocardium, and (3) epicardium. The visible blood vessels lie in the epicardium and are surrounded by adipose tissue. The layers of the mitral valve are shown at higher magnification in Figure 13.9b. ×35. **b.** This high magnification of the area indicated by the *rectangle* shows the characteristic features of the inner surface of the heart. Note that the endocardium consists of a squamous inner layer of endothelium (*End*), a middle layer of subendothelial dense connective tissue (*DCT*) containing smooth muscle cells (*SMC*), and a deeper subendocardial layer containing Purkinje fibers (*PF*). The myocardium contains cardiac muscle fibers (*CMF*) and is seen on the *left*. ×120.

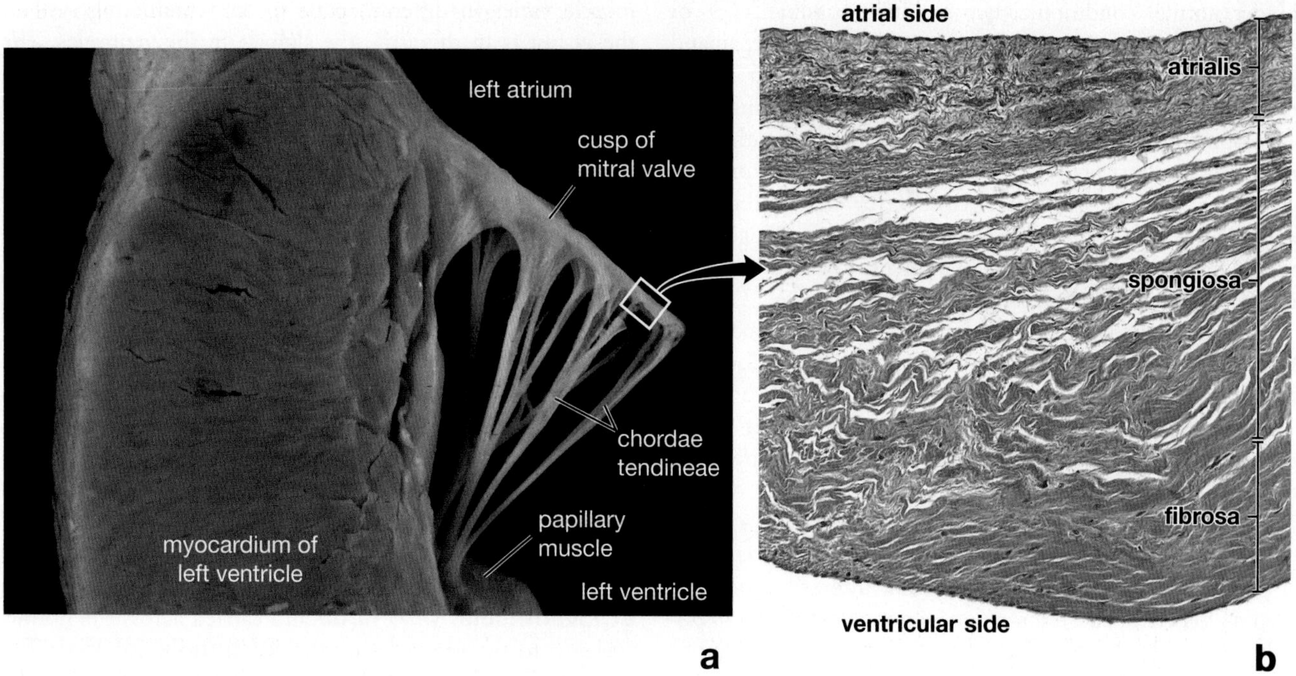

FIGURE 13.9. Mitral valve in the human heart. a. This photograph shows a sagittal section of the posterior wall of the left ventricle and the posterior cusp of the mitral valve. The chordae tendineae extend from the papillary muscle to the ventricular side of the mitral valve cusp. Note the thickness of the myocardium in the left ventricle. The glistening inner surface of the heart represents the endocardium; the outer surface of the myocardium is covered by the epicardium. ×2. (Courtesy of Dr. William D. Edwards.) **b.** Photomicrograph of a mitral valve. This photomicrograph shows a section through one of the two cusps of the mitral valve. Both sides of the cusp are covered by the endothelium. Note that the valve exhibits a layered architecture. Beginning at the atrial side (*top*), the first layer underlying the endothelium is the atrialis composed of densely packed collagen and elastic fibers. The second (middle) layer is the spongiosa, which forms the majority of the core of the valve and contains loosely arranged collagen fibers embedded in ground substance rich in proteoglycans and glycosaminoglycans. This layer gets thinner toward the attachment of the mitral valve to the annulus fibrosus and becomes more prominent toward the leaflet-free edge. The third layer, the fibrosa, is formed by dense connective tissue containing layers of elastic lamellae and collagen fibers. At this magnification, nuclei of valvular interstitial cells that resemble fibroblasts are difficult to identify. ×125.

rings of the heart. It is predominantly composed of densely packed type I (74%) and type III (24%) collagen fibers and elastic fibers that are arranged parallel to the leaflet-free edge. On the ventricular/arterial surface, the fibrosa is covered by a layer of endothelial cells. The fibrosa provides tensile stiffness to the leaflet. In AV valves, the fibrosa continues into the **chordae tendineae**, which are fibrous, thread-like cords also covered with endothelium (Fig. 13.9). At the sites of chordae tendineae insertion, the fibrosa changes from a flat layer to a cylindrical chord that enables the gradual transition of forces between the chordae and leaflet without its deformation. Chordae tendineae extend from the ventricular surfaces of the mitral and tricuspid valves into muscular projections from the wall of the ventricles, which are called **papillary muscles**.

- The **spongiosa** comprises the middle layer of the valve leaflet. It is composed of loosely arranged collagen and elastic fibers infiltrated by large amounts of **ground substance** containing **proteoglycans** and **glycosaminoglycans**. The spongiosa acts as a shock absorber to dampen vibrations associated with the closing of the valve. It also confers flexibility and plasticity to the valve cusps. Spongiosa is thin at the base of the leaflet but becomes very prominent toward the leaflet's free edge, where it contributes to the correct apposition of leaflets during valve closure that helps prevent valve leakage (regurgitation).
- The **ventricularis/atrialis** layer is immediately adjacent to the ventricular or atrial surface of each valve and is covered with endothelium. It represents a dense connective tissue layer with well-organized **collagen fibers** containing a large number of **elastic fibers** and **elastic lamellae**. The atrialis/ventricularis layer facilitates valve movement by allowing extension and recoil of the valve leaflet during the cardiac contraction cycle. In AV valves, this layer also contains cardiac muscle cells derived from atria (not ventricles) and small bundles of smooth muscle cells that may modulate leaflet stiffness and deformation during valve closure.

Although heart valves share a basic structural pattern and common functional requirements, each valve is structurally different, and emerging evidence suggests that molecular variations maintain distinct structural and biomechanical characteristics of individual valves.

Valve cusps are avascular and contain unique valvular interstitial cells that maintain the valve's internal structure throughout life.

Valve cusps are normally avascular. Small blood and lymphatic vessels, nerves, and smooth muscle can be found only at the base of the mitral and tricuspid valves. The surfaces of the valve are exposed to blood, and the cusps are thin enough to allow nutrients and oxygen to diffuse from the blood.

The leaflets of valves are populated by **valvular interstitial cells** that have unique features and sustain valve homeostasis throughout life. These cells originate from endocardial endothelial cells, but in a microscopic examination, they **resemble fibroblasts**. They are positive for vimentin and chondromodulin 1, which inhibit blood vessel formation.

Under normal conditions, they maintain baseline levels of extracellular matrix gene expression necessary for the repair and synthesis of connective tissue fibers and extracellular matrix proteins. However, in activated conditions (e.g., during valve development or heart valve diseases), valvular interstitial cells transition into activated **myofibroblast-like cells** expressing genes that encode proteins necessary for the synthesis of collagens, elastin, smooth muscle α-actin, proteoglycans, matrix metalloproteinases, and inflammatory cytokines, which rapidly remodel the extracellular matrix of the valve.

Several diseases affect the valves of the heart, causing their degeneration and resulting in heart malfunction because of insufficiency or stenosis of valvular orifices. These conditions, known collectively as **heart valve diseases**, include myxomatous mitral valve disease, rheumatic heart disease, vegetative endocarditis, degenerative calcific aortic valve stenosis, and mitral annular calcification. At the cellular level, heart valve diseases are characterized by activation of **valvular interstitial cells** as well as by increased expression of genes encoding extracellular matrix proteins and remodeling enzymes. Pathologic changes to the valves can be divided into three categories based on the type of valvular damage. The first category includes **degeneration of extracellular matrix** by accumulation of pathologic proteoglycans, collagen degradation, and elastic fiber fragmentation. These changes are characteristic of **myxomatous mitral valve disease** and result in a "floppy" valve that is prone to prolapse and regurgitation. The second category includes **fibrosis**, which is characterized by accumulation of collagen, degradation of proteoglycans, and elastic fiber fragmentation. These changes occur in **rheumatic heart disease** and result in a thick, rigid, and inflexible valve that is prone to restricted movement and stenosis. The fibrosis is initiated by inflammation of the valves (**valvulitis**) that occurs during the bacterial infection known as rheumatic fever. Inflammation induces angiogenesis in the valve and vascularization in the normally avascular layers of the valve. These changes most commonly affect the mitral valve (65%–70%) and aortic valve (20%–25%). Inflammation can lead to progressive replacement of elastic tissue by irregular masses of collagen fibers, causing the valve to thicken. The third category includes **nodular calcification** that begins within valvular interstitial cells. Such changes occur in **degenerative calcific aortic valve stenosis** that is characterized by thickening of the valve leaflets and formation of calcium nodules. Valvular calcification is also a common late finding in chronic kidney disease and in the older patient.

Intrinsic Regulation of Heart Rate

Contraction of the heart is synchronized by specialized cardiac-conducting cells.

Cardiac muscle can contract in a rhythmic manner without any direct stimulus from the nervous system. For the heart to be an effective pump, it is necessary for the atria and ventricles to contract in a coordinated rhythmic manner. The electrical activity (impulses) that results in the rhythmic pulsations of the heart is initiated and propagated by the **conducting system of the heart**. The rate of depolarization of cardiac muscle varies in different parts of the conducting system; the fastest is in the atria, the slowest in the ventricles. The contraction cycle of the heart is initiated in the atria, forcing blood into the ventricles. A wave of contraction in the ventricles then begins at the apex of the heart, forcing blood from the heart into the aorta and pulmonary trunk.

The **conducting system of the heart** consists of two nodes—the sinoatrial (or sinu-atrial) (SA) node and the AV node—and a series of conduction fibers or bundles (tracts). Electrical impulses are generated at the **sinoatrial (SA) node**, a group of specialized nodal cardiac muscle cells located near the junction of the superior vena cava and the right atrium (see Fig. 13.5). Because the SA node has the fastest rate of depolarizations, it is referred to as the dominant **pacemaker of the heart**. The pacemaker rate of the SA node is about 60–100 beats/min. The SA node initiates an impulse that spreads along the cardiac muscle fibers of the atria and over internodal tracts composed of modified cardiac muscle fibers. The impulse is then picked up at the **atrioventricular (AV) node** and carried across the fibrous skeleton to the ventricles by the **AV bundle (of His)**. The bundle divides into smaller right and left bundle branches and then into subendothelial branches, commonly called **Purkinje fibers**. The components of the conducting system convey impulses at a rate approximately 4 times faster than the cardiac muscle fibers and are the only elements that can convey impulses across the fibrous skeleton.

If the SA node fails to function (e.g., because of insufficient blood supply), then the area with the next fastest intrinsic rate of depolarization will take over. In this situation, the AV node will drive the heart contractions at a rate of about 50 beats/min. In **complete heart block**, in which the conduction of electric impulses to the ventricles is interrupted, the ventricles will beat at their own rate of about 30–40 beats/min, driven by depolarization of Purkinje fibers. Purkinje fibers have the slowest rate of intrinsic depolarization of the entire conducting system. The spread of electrical impulses through the myocardium can be monitored and recorded by an **electrocardiogram (ECG)**. The ECG is obtained by placing electrodes at different points on the skin at specific distances from the heart. Electrodes record the electrical activity of the heart by measuring voltage differences between different points. The coordinated spread of the electrical activity through the heart is responsible for the shape of the ECG waveform, careful analysis of which can provide information about heart rate, cardiac rhythm, conduction times through various parts of the heart, effects of electrolyte concentration, effects of cardiac medication, and location of pathologic (ischemic) damages in the heart.

The **nodal cardiac muscle cells** in both the SA and AV nodes are modified cardiac muscle fibers that are smaller than the surrounding atrial cardiac muscle cells. They contain fewer myofibrils and lack typical intercalated discs. The AV bundle, the bundle branches, and the Purkinje fibers are also composed of modified cardiac muscle cells, but they are larger than the surrounding ventricular muscle cells (Fig. 13.10 and Plate 13.1, page 474). Electrophysiologic studies of the cells in the SA node reveal the existence of two different functional groups of cells. These include the **pacemaker cells (P cells)**

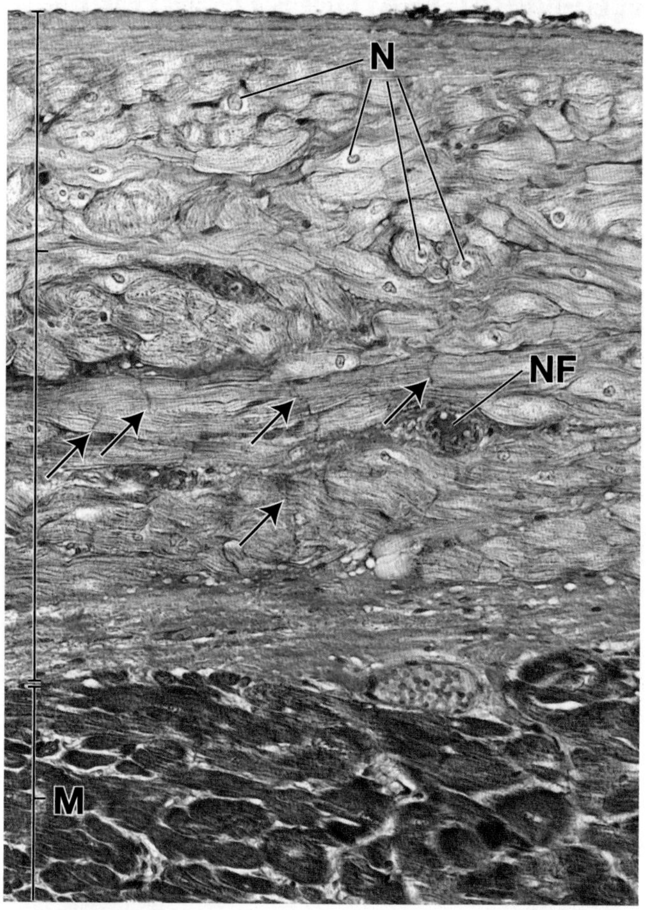

FIGURE 13.10. Photomicrograph of the ventricular wall containing the conducting system. This photomicrograph shows a Mallory–Azan-stained section of the ventricular wall of a human heart. The *upper two-thirds* of the micrograph is occupied by the endocardium (*E*) containing a thick layer of Purkinje fibers. The free luminal surface of the ventricle (*top*) is covered by endothelium and an underlying layer of subendothelial connective tissue (stained *blue*). The deep layer of endocardium contains the Purkinje fibers. Note the intercalated discs in the fibers (*arrows*). The Purkinje fibers contain large amounts of glycogen, which appear as homogeneous, pale-staining regions that occupy the center portion of the cell surrounded by the myofibrils. The nuclei (*N*) are round and larger than the nuclei of the cardiac muscle cells in the myocardium (*M*). They are frequently surrounded by the lighter stained cytoplasm, which represents the juxtanuclear region of the cell. Because of the considerable size of the Purkinje cells, the nuclei are often not included in the section. Among the Purkinje fibers are course nerves (*NF*) that belong to the autonomic nervous system. ×320.

with intrinsic spontaneous pacemaker function that generate impulses and **transitional cells (T cells)**, which are responsible for propagating impulses into the right atrium. P cells are grouped in elongated clusters in the middle of the SA node.

Dysfunction of the nodal cardiac muscle cells, known as a **sick sinus syndrome (SSS)**, is primarily a disease of the older adult and is the most common indication for the implantation of an electronic pacemaker worldwide. It results from age-related degeneration of nodal cardiac muscle cells in the SA node that affects its ability to generate and transmit impulses to the atrial musculature. SSS is characterized by abnormal, irregular heart rhythm disturbances (arrhythmia), which include a slow abnormal heart rate (**bradyarrhythmia**) alternating with a fast abnormal heart rate (**tachyarrhythmia**). Failure of pacemaker cells is manifested by a sinus pause or arrest of up to 3 seconds or more without generating impulses. Failure of transitional cells results in SA block, in which the cells are unable to transmit generated impulses into the atrial musculature. Symptoms of SSS include **palpitations** (irregular heartbeat) and tissue hypoperfusion leading to **fatigue, presyncope** (lightheadedness, muscular weakness, blurred vision, and feeling faint), and **syncope** (fainting). Recent genetic studies of patients with SSS have identified several gene mutations associated with familial and congenital forms of SSS. The main treatment of SSS is permanent placement of an electronic pacemaker.

The terminal ramifications of the conducting system consist of Purkinje fibers.

Cardiac-conducting cells that make up the bundle of His originate at the AV node, pass through the fibrous skeleton of the heart, course along both sides of the interventricular septum (see Fig. 13.5), and terminate as Purkinje fibers in the myocardium of the ventricles. The cells that form the **Purkinje fibers** are larger than ventricular muscle cells. Their myofibrils are located at the periphery of the cell. The nuclei are round and larger than the nuclei of the cardiac muscle cells in the myocardium. Because of the considerable size of the cells, the nuclei are often not included in the section. Intercalated discs are present in Purkinje fibers, but they are variable in appearance and number depending on their location. They are positive for periodic acid–Schiff (PAS) staining because of the large amount of glycogen they contain. With hematoxylin and eosin (H&E) and most other stains, the glycogen-rich center portion of the cell appears homogeneous and stains pale (see Fig. 13.10). Because of the stored glycogen, Purkinje fiber cells are more resistant to hypoxia than are ventricular muscle cells.

Systemic Regulation of Heart Function

As mentioned earlier, the **heart beats independently** of any nervous stimulation. This spontaneous rhythm of the heart can be altered by nerve impulses from both sympathetic and parasympathetic divisions of the autonomic nervous system. The **autonomic nerves** do not initiate contraction of the cardiac muscle but rather regulate the heart rate (**a chronotropic effect**) according to the body's immediate needs.

Stimulation of the parasympathetic nerves decreases the heart rate.

The **parasympathetic nerve supply** to the heart originates in the vagus nerve (cranial nerve X). Presynaptic parasympathetic fibers synapse with postsynaptic neurons within the heart. Their short postsynaptic fibers not only terminate chiefly at the SA and AV nodes but also extend into the coronary arteries that supply the heart. The release of the neurotransmitter **acetylcholine** from the terminals of these fibers slows the resting heart rate below 60 beats per minute (an effect known as **bradycardia**), reduces the force of the heartbeat, and constricts the coronary arteries of the heart.

Stimulation of the sympathetic nerves increases the heart rate.

The **sympathetic presynaptic fibers** that supply the heart originate in the lateral horns at the level of the T1–T6 segments of the spinal cord. They conduct electrical signals to the cell bodies of postsynaptic neurons located in the cervical and thoracic paravertebral ganglia of sympathetic trunks (see Fig. 12.28, page 418). The **postsynaptic fibers** terminate at the SA and AV nodes, extend into the myocardium, and also pass through the epicardium to reach the coronary arteries. The autonomic fibers secrete **norepinephrine** that regulates the rate of impulses emanating from the SA node. The sympathetic component causes the rate of contraction to increase (an effect known as **tachycardia**) and increases the force of muscle contraction. Sympathetic stimulation produces dilation of the coronary arteries by inhibiting their constriction.

The heart rate and the force of contraction can be regulated by circulating hormones and other substances.

Changes in the force and rate of cardiac muscle contractions are regulated by hormones secreted from the adrenal medulla. These hormones include **epinephrine** and **norepinephrine** that reach the heart muscle cells via the coronary circulation. Activation of adrenergic receptors (mainly β_1 type) by epinephrine and less efficiently by norepinephrine increases the force of contraction (a **positive inotropic effect**) and the heart rate (a **positive chronotropic effect**). Other substances that have positive inotropic and chronotropic effects on the heart include Ca^{2+}, thyroid hormones, caffeine, theophylline, and cardiac glycoside digoxin. These substances all increase intracellular Ca^{2+} levels in cardiac myocytes. Substances that have **negative inotropic and chronotropic actions** on the heart muscle include adrenergic receptor antagonists, such as propranolol or Ca^{2+} channel blockers. These substances decrease the heart rate and the force of cardiac muscle contraction.

The central nervous system monitors arterial pressure and heart function through specialized receptors located within the cardiovascular system.

The activity of the cardiovascular system is monitored by specialized centers in the central nervous system (CNS). Specialized sensory nerve receptors that supply afferent information about blood pressure are located in the walls of large blood vessels near the heart and within the heart itself. The information received from all types of **cardiovascular receptors** initiates the appropriate physiologic reflexes. The receptors function as follows:

- **Baroreceptors** (high-pressure receptors) sense arterial blood pressure. These receptors are located in the carotid sinus and aortic arch.
- **Volume receptors** (low-pressure receptors) located within the walls of the atria and ventricles sense central venous pressure and provide the CNS with information about cardiac distention.
- **Chemoreceptors** detect alterations in oxygen, carbon dioxide tension, and pH. These receptors are the **carotid** and **aortic bodies** located at the bifurcation of the common carotid arteries and in the aortic arch, respectively.

The carotid bodies consist of cords and irregular groups of epithelioid cells. A rich supply of nerve fibers is associated with these cells. The neural elements are both afferent and efferent. The structure of the aortic bodies is essentially similar to that of the carotid bodies. Both receptors function in neural reflexes that adjust cardiac output and respiratory rate.

■ GENERAL FEATURES OF ARTERIES AND VEINS

Layers of Vascular Wall

The walls of arteries and veins are composed of three layers called *tunics*.

The three layers of the vascular wall, from the lumen outward (Fig. 13.11 and Plate 13.2, page 476), are as follows:

- The **tunica intima**, the innermost layer of the vessel, consists of three components: (1) a single layer of squamous epithelial cells, the **endothelium**; (2) the **basal lamina** of the endothelial cells (a thin extracellular layer composed chiefly of collagen, proteoglycans, and glycoproteins); and (3) the **subendothelial layer**, consisting of loose connective tissue. Occasional smooth muscle cells are found in the loose connective tissue. The subendothelial layer of the intima in arteries and arterioles contains a sheet-like layer or lamella of fenestrated elastic material called the **internal elastic membrane**. Fenestrations enable substances to diffuse readily through the layer and reach cells deep within the wall of the vessel.

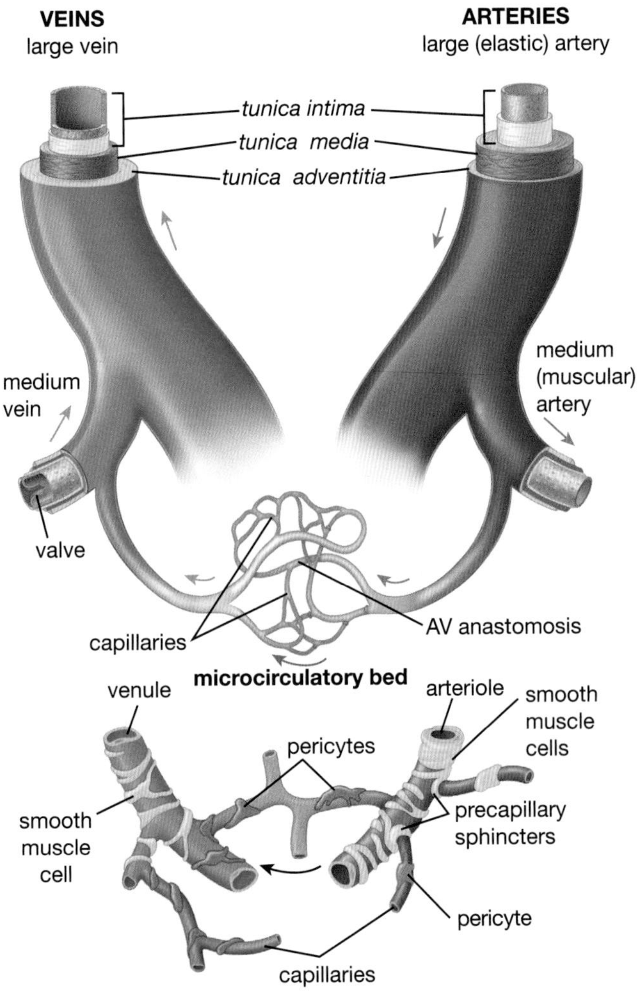

FIGURE 13.11. Schematic diagram of the major structural features of blood vessels. The layers or tunics of the blood vessel walls are labeled in the *upper two panels*. The arrangement of the microcirculatory bed in certain parts of the body is shown in the *lowest panel*. Note the location of pericytes and their relationship to the basal lamina. Also, an arteriovenous (*AV*) anastomosis is shown within the microcirculatory bed.

- The **tunica media**, or middle layer, consists primarily of circumferentially arranged layers of vascular smooth muscle cells. In arteries, this layer is relatively thick and extends from the internal elastic membrane to the **external elastic membrane.** The external elastic membrane is a layer of elastin that separates the tunica media from the tunica adventitia. Variable amounts of elastin, reticular fibers, and proteoglycans are interposed between the smooth muscle cells of the tunica media. The sheets or lamellae of elastin are fenestrated and arranged in circular concentric layers. All of the extracellular components of the tunica media are produced by the vascular smooth muscle cells.
- The **tunica adventitia**, or outermost connective tissue layer, is composed primarily of longitudinally arranged collagenous tissue and a few elastic fibers. These connective tissue elements gradually merge with the loose connective tissue surrounding the vessels. The tunica adventitia ranges from relatively thin in most of the arterial system to quite thick in the venules and veins, where it is the major component of the vessel wall. In addition, the tunica adventitia of large arteries and veins contains a system of vessels called the **vasa vasorum** that supplies blood to the vascular walls themselves as well as a network of autonomic nerves called **nervi vasorum (vascularis)** that controls contraction of the smooth muscle in the vessel walls.

Histologically, the various types of arteries and veins are distinguished from each other by the thickness of the vascular wall and differences in the composition of the layers. Table 13.1 summarizes the features of the various types of blood vessels.

TABLE 13.1 Characteristics of Blood Vessels

Vessel	Diameter	Tunica Intima (Inner Layer)	Tunica Media (Middle Layer)	Tunica Adventitia (Outer Layer)
Arteries				
Large artery (elastic artery)	>10 mm	Endothelium Connective tissue Smooth muscle	Smooth muscle Elastic lamellae	Thinner than tunica media Connective tissue Elastic fibers
Medium artery (muscular artery)	2–10 mm	Endothelium Connective tissue Smooth muscle Prominent internal elastic membrane	Smooth muscle Collagen fibers Relatively little elastic tissue	Thinner than tunica media Connective tissue Some elastic fibers
Small artery	0.1–2 mm	Endothelium Connective tissue Smooth muscle Internal elastic membrane	Smooth muscle (8–10 cell layers) Collagen fibers	Thinner than tunica media Connective tissue Some elastic fibers
Arteriole	10–100 μm	Endothelium Connective tissue Smooth muscle	Smooth muscle (one or two cell layers)	Thin, ill-defined sheath of connective tissue
Capillary	4–10 μm	Endothelium	None	None
Veins				
Vessel	**Diameter**	**Tunica Intima (Inner Layer)**	**Tunica Media (Middle Layer)**	**Tunica Adventitia (Outer Layer)**
Postcapillary venule	10–50 μm	Endothelium Pericytes	None	None
Muscular venule	50–100 μm	Endothelium	Smooth muscle (one or two cell layers)	Thicker than tunica media Connective tissue Some elastic fibers
Small vein	0.1–1 mm	Endothelium Connective tissue Smooth muscle (two or three layers)	Smooth muscle (two or three layers continuous with tunica intima)	Thicker than tunica media Connective tissue Some elastic fibers
Medium vein	1–10 mm	Endothelium Connective tissue Smooth muscle Internal elastic membrane in some cases	Smooth muscle Collagen fibers	Thicker than tunica media Connective tissue Some elastic fibers
Large vein	>10 mm	Endothelium Connective tissue Smooth muscle	Smooth muscle (2–15 layers) Collagen fibers	Much thicker than tunica media Connective tissue Some elastic fibers, longitudinal smooth muscles Cardiac muscle extensions (myocardial sleeves) into great veins near the heart

Vascular Endothelium

In the adult human body, the circulatory system consists of about 60,000 miles of different-sized vessels that are lined by a simple squamous epithelium called **endothelium**. The endothelium is formed by a continuous layer of flattened, elongated, and polygonally shaped **endothelial cells** that are aligned with their long axes in the direction of the blood flow. At the luminal surface, they express a variety of **surface adhesion molecules** and **receptors** (i.e., low-density lipoprotein [LDL], insulin, and histamine receptors). Endothelial cells play an important role in blood homeostasis. The functional properties of these cells change in response to various stimuli. This process, known as **endothelial activation**, is also responsible for the pathogenesis of many vascular diseases (e.g., atherosclerosis; Folder 13.1). Inducers of endothelial activation include bacterial and viral antigens, cytotoxins, complement products, lipid products, and hypoxia. Activated endothelial cells exhibit new surface adhesion molecules and produce different classes of cytokines, lymphokines, growth factors, and vasoconstrictor and vasodilator molecules as well as molecules that control blood coagulation.

FOLDER 13.1

CLINICAL CORRELATION: ATHEROSCLEROSIS

Atherosclerotic lesions are the most common acquired abnormality of blood vessels. More than one half of the annual deaths in the United States are related to complications of atherosclerotic disease, which includes **coronary heart disease** (see Folder 13.3), myocardial infarction, stroke, and **peripheral artery disease**. Lesions develop primarily in the tunica intima of large elastic arteries following endothelial injury, which leads to **endothelial dysfunction**. Factors that predispose to endothelial injuries include high levels of low-density lipoprotein (LDL) cholesterol, hyperlipidemia, hyperglycemia (in diabetes), hypertension, increased toxin levels associated with cigarette smoking, and certain viral and bacterial infections caused by cytomegalovirus (CMV) or *Chlamydia pneumoniae*, respectively. Altered function of vascular endothelium leads to increased expression of surface adhesion molecules (e.g., ICAM-1), increased permeability to LDL cholesterol, and increased adherence of white blood cells (mostly monocytes) to the endothelium. Endothelial injury also increases the production of reactive oxygen species such as O_2^-, H_2O_2, OH^-, and $ONOO^-$, which, in turn, oxidize LDL in the tunica intima of the artery.

In response to this injury, **monocytes** from the bloodstream enter the tunica intima and differentiate into macrophages. Macrophages phagocytize oxidized LDL, slowly transforming into **foam cells** as their cytoplasm fills with lipid-containing vesicles, which gives these cells their characteristic spongy appearance. Foam cells and infiltrated T lymphocytes form the initial atherosclerotic lesion or **fatty streak**. In this early lesion, vascular smooth muscle cells from the tunica media proliferate and migrate toward the fatty streak in response to platelet-derived growth factor (PDGF) produced by endothelial cells. At later stages, this lesion undergoes further remodeling and growth into a **fibrofatty plaque** as smooth muscle cells migrate from the media and synthesize collagen to form a protective capsule of connective tissue that encloses the growing lipid core (Fig. F13.1.1). A thick layer of fibrous

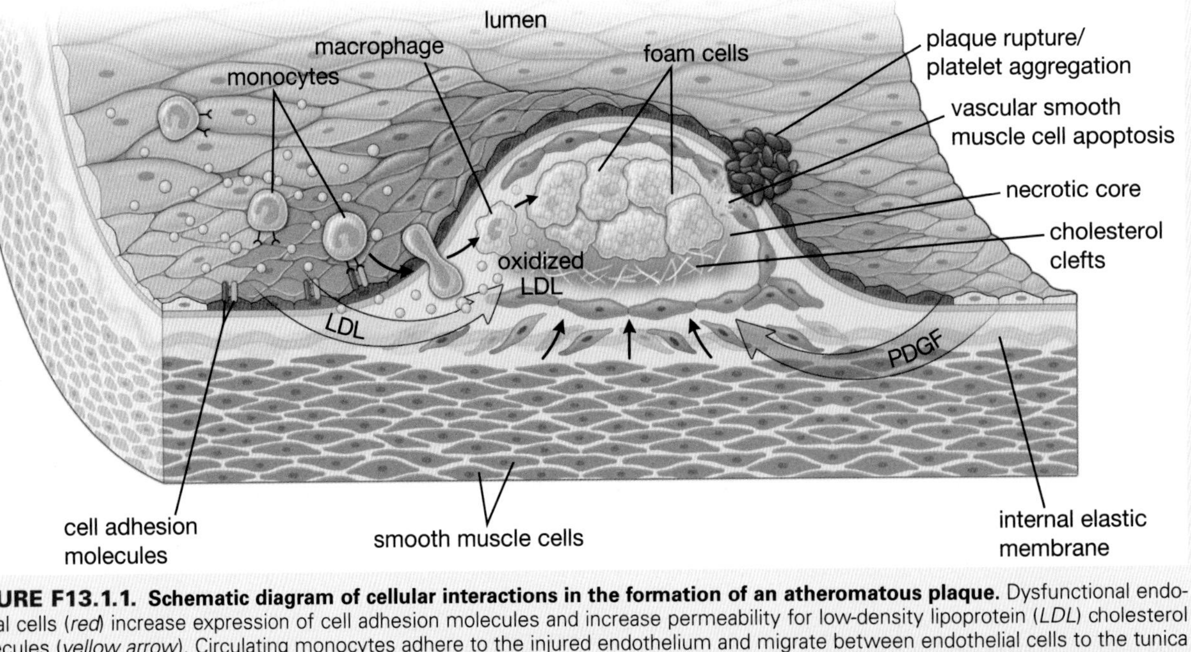

FIGURE F13.1.1. Schematic diagram of cellular interactions in the formation of an atheromatous plaque. Dysfunctional endothelial cells (*red*) increase expression of cell adhesion molecules and increase permeability for low-density lipoprotein (*LDL*) cholesterol molecules (*yellow arrow*). Circulating monocytes adhere to the injured endothelium and migrate between endothelial cells to the tunica intima, where they differentiate into macrophages. Free radicals produced by the endothelial cells oxidize *LDLs*, which are subsequently phagocytosed by macrophages. Platelet-derived growth factor (*PDGF*) and other growth factors (*blue arrow*) released from endothelial cells stimulate migration of the smooth muscle cells from the tunica media to the tunica intima. Foam cells derived from macrophages (and also from vascular smooth muscle cells) accumulate intracellular *LDLs*, whereas cholesterol is deposited in crystals within the necrotic core. In the tunica intima, smooth muscle cells produce large amounts of extracellular matrix (proteoglycans, collagen) that further increases the thickness of the tunica intima.

CLINICAL CORRELATION: ATHEROSCLEROSIS (*continued*)

connective tissue containing scattered smooth muscle cells, macrophages, foam cells, T lymphocytes, cholesterol crystals, and cell debris is known as an **atheromatous plaque**. Progression of the plaque is marked by accumulation of lipids and increased activity of matrix-degrading enzymes with accumulation of necrotic tissue. Gradual loss of the vascular smooth muscle cells by apoptosis and loss of integrity of the endothelium lead to plaque rupture with subsequent platelet attachment and clotting (thrombosis). In advanced lesions, blood stasis and clotting may lead to occlusion of the vessel. Other changes seen in advanced lesions include thinning of the tunica media, calcification of accumulated extracellular lipids, and accumulation of cholesterol crystals visible on histologic sections as open, needle-like spaces called *cholesterol clefts* (Fig. F13.1.2a,b). Progression from simple to complicated lesions can be found in some people as early as their 20s and in most individuals by age 50 or 60 years.

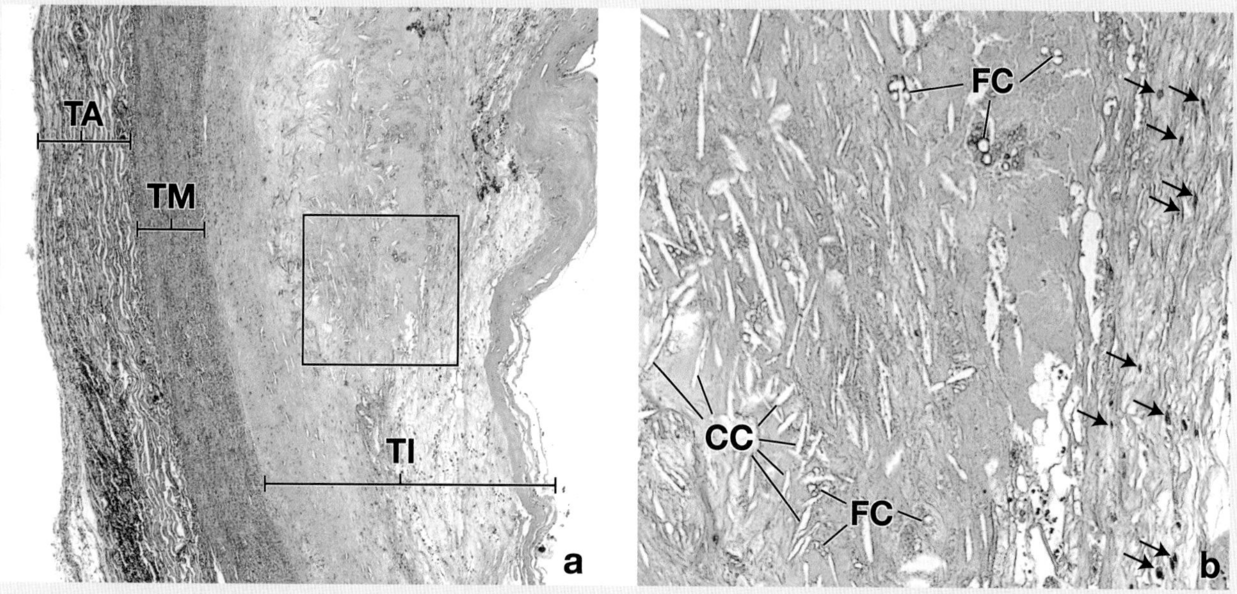

FIGURE F13.1.2. Photomicrographs of an atheromatous lesion. a. This specimen is from a human aorta stained by the Masson trichrome method. The lesion, referred to as a *fibrous plaque*, consists of connective tissue fibers, smooth muscle cells, fat-containing macrophages (foam cells), and a necrotic material. It occupies the site of the tunica intima (*TI*), which is greatly expanded in thickness. *TA*, tunica adventitia; *TM*, tunica media. ×40. **b.** A higher power magnification of the area in the *rectangle* in **a.** On the *right*, some of the fibrous connective tissue of the plaque is evident. The *arrows* point to smooth muscle cell nuclei that have produced the collagen fibers of the fibrous plaque. Also evident are foam cells (*FC*) and characteristic cholesterol clefts (*CC*). The latter are spaces occupied previously by cholesterol crystals that have been dissolved during specimen preparation. The remainder of the plaque consists of necrotic material and lipid. ×240.

Endothelial cells contribute to the structural and functional integrity of the vascular wall.

Endothelial cells are active participants in a variety of interactions between the blood and the underlying connective tissue and are responsible for many properties of the vessels (Table 13.2). These properties include the following:

- **Maintenance of a selective permeability barrier** allows selective movement of small and large molecules from the blood to the tissues and from the tissues to the blood. The barrier is mediated by endothelial cell–cell adhesion complexes, including tight junctions, zonula adherens junctions, and a variety of other adhesion molecules that are connected to the actin cytoskeleton. This movement across the endothelium is related to the size and charge of the molecules. The endothelium is permeable to small hydrophobic (lipid-soluble) molecules (e.g., oxygen, carbon dioxide) that readily pass through the lipid bilayer of the endothelial cell membrane (a process called **simple diffusion**). However, water and hydrophilic (water-soluble) molecules (e.g., glucose, amino acids, electrolytes) cannot diffuse across the endothelial cell membrane. These molecules and solutes must be either actively transported across the plasma membrane and released into the extracellular space (**transcellular pathways**) or transported across the zonula occludens between two epithelial cells (**paracellular pathway**; see Chapter 5, Epithelial Tissue, pages 141-145). The transcellular pathway utilizes **micropinocytotic** and **macropinocytotic vesicles** (a clathrin-independent form of endocytosis) to transport bulk material from the blood into the cell. In addition, some specific molecules (e.g., LDL, cholesterol, transferrin) are transported via **receptor-mediated endocytosis** (a clathrin-dependent process), which uses endothelial-specific surface receptors. In some blood vessels, larger molecules are transported through fenestrations within the endothelial cells visible in transmission electron microscope (TEM) preparations.
- **Maintenance of a nonthrombogenic barrier** between blood platelets and subendothelial tissue results from the production of **anticoagulants** (agents that prevent coagulation such as thrombomodulin and others) and **antithrombogenic** substances (agents that prevent or interfere with platelet aggregation and release of factors that cause the formation of clots, or **thrombi**, such as prostacyclin [PGI_2] and tissue plasminogen activator). In addition, the endothelial cell surface is rich in

heparin-like sulfated glycosaminoglycans that bind and activate circulating antithrombogenic substances. Normal endothelium does not support the adherence of platelets or the formation of thrombi on its surface. Damage to endothelial cells causes them to release **prothrombogenic agents** (agents that promote thrombi formation), such as von Willebrand factor or plasminogen-activator inhibitor.

- **Modulation of blood flow and vascular resistance** is achieved by the secretion of **vasoconstrictors** (endothelins, angiotensin-converting enzyme [ACE], prostaglandin H_2, thromboxane A_2) and **vasodilators** (nitric oxide [NO], prostacyclin). This subject is discussed in more depth in the next section.
- **Regulation and modulation of immune responses** occur through the interaction of lymphocytes with the endothelial surface, which is mainly achieved through the expression of adhesion molecules and their receptors on the endothelial-free surface as well as by secretion of three classes of interleukins (IL-1, IL-6, and IL-8).
- **Hormonal synthesis and other metabolic activities** occur through the synthesis and secretion of various **growth factors**—for example, hemopoietic colony-stimulating factors (CSFs), such as granulocyte–macrophage CSF (GM-CSF), granulocyte CSF (G-CSF), and macrophage CSF (M-CSF); fibroblast growth factor (FGF); and platelet-derived growth factor (PDGF). Endothelial cells also synthesize growth inhibitors, such as heparin and transforming growth factor β (TGF-β). Endothelial cells function in the conversion of angiotensin I to angiotensin II in the renin–angiotensin system that controls blood pressure as well as in the inactivation or conversion of several compounds conveyed in the blood (norepinephrine, thrombin, prostaglandins, bradykinin, and serotonin) to inactive forms.
- **Modification of the lipoproteins** occurs by oxidation. Lipoproteins, mainly LDLs with a high cholesterol content and very low-density lipoproteins (VLDLs), are oxidized by free radicals produced by endothelial cells. Modified LDLs, in turn, are rapidly endocytosed by macrophages to form **foam cells** (see Fig. F13.1.1). Foam cells are a characteristic feature in the formation of atheromatous plaques.

Endothelium of blood vessels controls contraction and relaxation of vascular smooth muscle cells in the tunica media, influencing local blood flow and pressure.

Endothelial-derived relaxing factor (EDRF) was historically one of the early compounds discovered in endothelial cells that cause relaxation of blood vessels. For years, researchers had difficulty characterizing EDRF chemically. It is now known that most of the vascular effects of EDRF can be attributed to **nitric oxide (NO)** and its related compounds, which are released by endothelial cells in arteries, blood capillaries, and even lymphatic capillaries. As a chemical compound, NO is a gas with a very short physiologic half-life measured in seconds, hence the difficulty with its discovery.

Shear stress produced during the interaction of blood flow with vascular endothelial cells initiates nitric oxide (NO)-derived relaxation of blood vessels.

Vasodilation (the relaxation of vascular smooth muscle cells) increases the luminal diameter of the vessels, decreasing vascular resistance and systemic blood pressure. Endothelium-derived **nitric oxide (NO)** is one of several critical regulators of cardiovascular homeostasis. It regulates the blood vessel diameter, inhibits monocyte adhesion to dysfunctional endothelial cells, and maintains an antiproliferative and antiapoptotic environment in the vessel wall.

NO is an endogenous vasodilatory gas continuously synthesized in endothelial cells by **endothelial nitric oxide synthase (eNOS)**. This Ca^{2+}-dependent enzyme catalyzes oxidation of L-arginine and acts through the G-protein signaling cascade. Endothelial cells are constantly subjected to **shear stress**, the dragging force generated by the blood flow. Shear stress increases synthesis of a potent eNOS stimulator and vascular endothelial growth factor (VEGF) and triggers a variety of other molecular and physical changes in the structure and function of endothelial cell. Once NO is produced by endothelial cells, it diffuses out through the cell and basement membrane to the underlying tunica media and binds to guanylate cyclase in smooth muscle cytoplasm. This enzyme increases the production of cyclic guanosine monophosphate (cGMP), which activates smooth muscle protein kinase G (PKG). Activation of PKG has a negative effect on intracellular concentration of Ca^{2+}, causing smooth muscle relaxation (Fig. 13.12). NO is a signaling molecule in many pathologic and physiologic processes. It acts as an anti-inflammatory agent under normal physiologic conditions, although its overproduction induces inflammation. NO is also involved in immune reactions (it stimulates macrophages to release high concentrations of NO), is a potent neurotransmitter in the nervous system, and contributes to the regulation of apoptosis. The pathogenesis of inflammatory disorders of the joint, gut, and lungs is linked to local overproduction of NO. Researchers are studying the pharmaceutical applications of NO inhibitors to treat a variety of disorders, including inflammatory diseases, migraines, and traumatic brain injury.

Metabolic stress in endothelial cells also contributes to smooth muscle relaxation. EDRFs include **prostacyclin (PGI_2)**, which, in addition to relaxing smooth muscles, is a potent inhibitor of platelet aggregation. PGI_2 binds to receptors on the smooth muscles; stimulates cyclic adenosine monophosphate (cAMP)-activated PKA, which, in turn, phosphorylates myosin light-chain kinase (MLCK); and prevents activation of the calcium–calmodulin complex. This type of relaxation occurs without changing the intracellular Ca^{2+} concentration. **Endothelium-derived hyperpolarizing factor (EDHF)** represents another EDRF that acts on Ca^{2+}-dependent potassium channels, causing hyperpolarization of vascular smooth muscle cells and their relaxation (see Fig. 13.12).

Endothelins produced by vascular endothelial cells play an important role in both physiologic and pathologic mechanisms of the circulatory system.

Vasoconstriction (contraction of smooth muscle) in the tunica media of small arteries and arterioles reduces the luminal diameter of these vessels and increases **vascular resistance**. Vasoconstriction increases systemic blood pressure. In the past, vasoconstriction was thought to be mainly induced by nerve impulses or circulating hormones. It is now known that endothelium-derived factors play

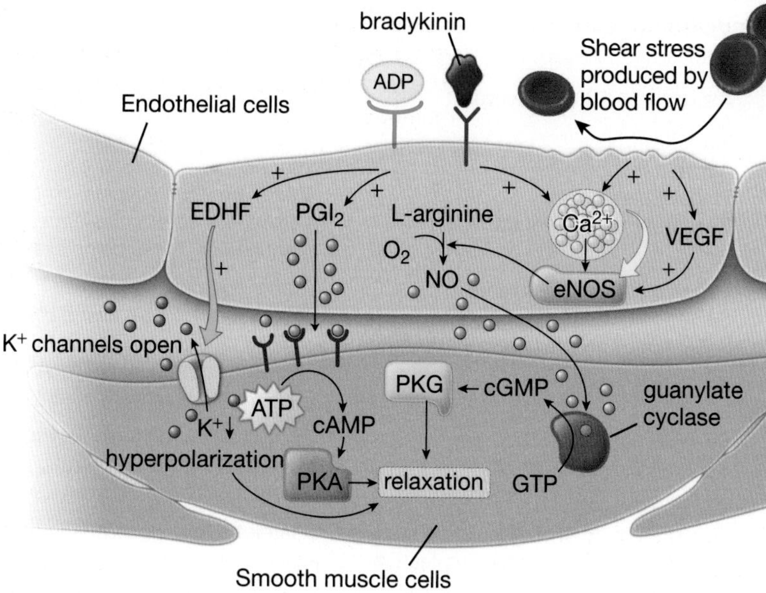

FIGURE 13.12. Molecular mechanism of blood vessel vasodilation. Relaxation of smooth muscle cells in the wall of the blood vessel causes an increase in its diameter and decreases in vascular resistance and systemic blood pressure. Nitric oxide (*NO*) produced by endothelial nitric oxide synthase (*eNOS*) in endothelial cells is an important molecule regulating relaxation of vascular smooth muscles. Other molecules include adenosine diphosphate (*ADP*), vascular endothelial growth factor (*VEGF*), bradykinin, prostacyclin (*PGI_2*), and endothelium-derived hyperpolarizing factor (*EDHF*). Shear stress produced between erythrocytes and endothelial cells as well as VEGF activates eNOS, increasing the production of NO. Once NO is produced, it diffuses into the underlying smooth muscles and activates guanylate cyclase production of cGMP, which, in turn, activates cGMP-dependent protein kinase G (PKG) metabolic pathways, causing smooth muscle relaxation. Metabolic stress of endothelial cells caused by increased levels of ADP or PGI_2 stimulates cAMP-activated protein kinase A (PKA) metabolic pathways in smooth muscles, causing their relaxation. In addition, EDHF opens potassium channels, causing hyperpolarization of smooth muscle cell membranes, further leading to their relaxation. *ATP*, adenosine triphosphate; *cAMP*, cyclic adenosine monophosphate; *cGMP*, cyclic guanosine monophosphate; *GTP*, guanosine triphosphate. (Based on Noble A, Johnson R, Thomas A, et al. *The Cardiovascular System*. Churchill Livingstone; 2005.)

an important role in both physiologic and pathologic mechanisms of the circulatory system. Members of the **endothelin family** of 21-amino-acid peptides produced by vascular endothelial cells are the most potent vasoconstrictors. The family consists of three members: **endothelin-1 (ET-1)**, **endothelin-2 (ET-2)**, and **endothelin-3 (ET-3)**. Endothelins act mainly as paracrine and autocrine agents and bind to their own receptors on the epithelial cells and vascular smooth muscles (Fig. 13.13). ET-1 is the most potent naturally occurring vasoconstricting agent that interacts with its ETA receptor on vascular smooth muscles. High levels of ET-1 gene expression are associated with many diseases

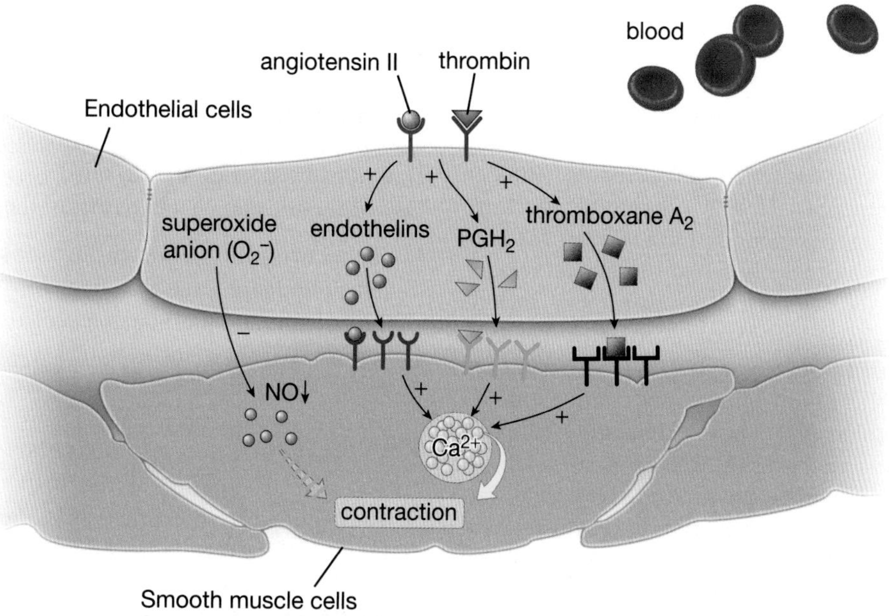

FIGURE 13.13. Molecular mechanism of blood vessel vasoconstriction. Contraction of vascular smooth muscle in a blood vessel (vasoconstriction) decreases its diameter and increases vascular resistance, leading to increased systemic blood pressure. Binding of angiotensin II and thrombin to vascular endothelial cells stimulates synthesis of endothelium-derived factors that regulate smooth muscle contraction. These include endothelins (the most potent family of vasoconstrictors), prostaglandin H_2 (PGH_2), and its derivative thromboxane A_2. They bind to their own receptors on the smooth muscle cell membrane, causing an influx of Ca^{2+} and an increase in the release of intracellular-stored Ca^{2+} from the sarcoplasmic reticulum. The reduced rate of nitric oxide (*NO*) production, which is a potent vasodilator, or inactivation of NO by the superoxide anion (*O_2^-*) has a stimulating effect on smooth muscle contraction. (Based on Noble A, Johnson R, Thomas A, et al. *The Cardiovascular System*. Churchill Livingstone; 2005.)

TABLE 13.2 Summary of Endothelial Cell Properties and Functions

Major Properties	Associated Functions	Active Molecules Involved
Maintenance of selective permeability barrier	Simple diffusion Active transport Pinocytosis Receptor-mediated endocytosis	Oxygen, carbon dioxide Glucose, amino acids, electrolytes Water, small molecules, soluble proteins LDL, cholesterol, transferrin, growth factors, antibodies, MHC complexes
Maintenance of nonthrombogenic barrier	Secretion of anticoagulants Secretion of antithrombogenic agents Secretion of prothrombogenic agents	Thrombomodulin Prostacyclin (PGI_2), tissue plasminogen activator (TPA), antithrombin III, heparin Tissue thromboplastin, von Willebrand factor, plasminogen-activator inhibitor
Modulation of blood flow and vascular resistance	Secretion of vasoconstrictors Secretion of vasodilators	Endothelin, angiotensin-converting enzyme (ACE) Endothelial-derived relaxation factor (EDRF)/nitric oxide (NO), prostacyclin
Regulation of cell growth	Secretion of growth-stimulating factors Secretion of growth-inhibiting factors	Platelet-derived growth factor (PDGF), hemopoietic colony-stimulating factors (GM-CSF, G-CSF, M-CSF) Heparin, transforming growth factor β (TGF-β)
Regulation of immune responses	Regulation of leukocyte migration by expression of adhesion molecules Regulation of immune functions	Selectins, integrins, CD marker molecules Interleukin molecules (IL-1, IL-6, IL-8), MHC molecules
Maintenance of extracellular matrix	Synthesis of basal lamina Synthesis of glycocalyx	Type IV collagen, laminin Proteoglycans
Involvement in lipoprotein, cholesterol, metabolism	Production of free radicals Oxidation of LDL	Reactive oxygen species (ROS), LDL, VLDL

CD, cluster of differentiation; *G-CSF*, granulocyte colony-stimulating factor; *GM-CSF*, granulocyte–macrophage colony-stimulating factor; *LDL*, low-density lipoprotein; *M-CSF*, macrophage colony-stimulating factor; *MHC*, major histocompatibility complex; *VLDL*, very low-density lipoprotein. Modified from Cotran S, Kumar V, Collins T, et al. eds. *Robbins Pathologic Basis of Disease*. Saunders; 1999.

that are caused in part by sustained endothelium-induced vasoconstriction. These include **systemic hypertension** (see Folder 13.2), pulmonary hypertension, atherosclerosis, congestive heart failure, idiopathic cardiomyopathy, and renal failure. It is interesting to note that snake venom from the Israeli burrowing asp (*Atractaspis engaddensis*) contains **sarafotoxin**, a highly toxic protein that exhibits a high degree of sequence homology with ET-1. After it enters the circulation, the toxin binds to ETA receptors and causes life-threatening, intense coronary vasoconstriction. This is remarkable because endothelin is a natural compound of the human vascular system, whereas sarafotoxin is a toxin in snake venom. The other endothelium-derived vasoconstrictors include **thromboxane A_2** and **prostaglandin H_2**. Thromboxane A_2 is synthesized from prostaglandin H_2. In addition, decreased rate of NO production or inactivation of NO by the superoxide anion (O_2^-) has a stimulating effect on smooth muscle contraction (see Fig. 13.13).

In summary, under normal physiologic conditions, vascular endothelial cells become activated by environmental factors, such as mechanical stimuli (pressure and shear stress) and chemical compounds (hormones and locally secreted vasoactive substances). In response to these stimuli, the endothelium releases factors that regulate vasomotor function, inflammatory processes, cell growth, and hemostasis. However, **endothelial dysfunction**, a term that comprises multiple potential defects of the endothelial cells, may shift the actions of the endothelium toward reduced vasodilation and various proliferative, prothrombotic, and pro-inflammatory conditions. Endothelial dysfunction is an important early event that may lead to many pathologic conditions, such as progressive **atherosclerotic disease** (see Folder 13.1).

■ ARTERIES

Traditionally, arteries are classified into three types on the basis of the size and characteristics of the tunica media:

- **Large arteries** or **elastic arteries**, such as the aorta and pulmonary arteries, convey blood from the heart to the systemic and pulmonary circulations, respectively (see Fig. 13.2). Their main branches—the brachiocephalic trunk, common carotid, subclavian, and common iliac arteries—are also classified as elastic arteries.
- **Medium arteries** or **muscular arteries** (most of the "named" arteries of the body) cannot be sharply distinguished from elastic arteries. Some of these arteries are difficult to classify because they have features that are intermediate between the two types.
- **Small arteries** and **arterioles** are distinguished from one another by the number of smooth muscle layers in the tunica media. By definition, arterioles have only one or two layers, and small arteries may have as many as eight layers of smooth muscle in their tunica media.

Large Arteries (Elastic Arteries)

The walls of elastic arteries contain multiple sheets of elastic lamellae.

From a functional standpoint, **elastic arteries** serve primarily as conduction tubes; however, they also facilitate the continuous and uniform movement of blood along the tube. Blood flow occurs as follows: The ventricles of the heart pump blood into the elastic arteries during **systole** (the contraction phase of the cardiac cycle). The pressure generated by contraction of the ventricles moves the blood through the elastic arteries and along the arterial tree. Simultaneously, it also causes the wall of the large elastic arteries to distend. The distension is limited by the network of collagenous fibers in the tunica media and tunica adventitia (Fig. 13.14). During **diastole** (the relaxation phase of the cardiac cycle), when no pressure is generated by the heart, the recoil of the distended elastic arteries serves to maintain arterial blood pressure and the flow of blood within the vessels. Initial elastic recoil forces blood both away from and back toward the heart. The flow of blood toward the heart causes the aortic and pulmonary valves to close. Continued elastic recoil then maintains a continuous flow of blood away from the heart.

The tunica intima of the elastic artery consists of endothelium, subendothelial connective tissue, and an inconspicuous internal elastic membrane.

The **tunica intima of elastic arteries** is relatively thick and consists of the following:

- An **endothelial lining** with its **basal lamina**, in which the cells are typically flat and elongated, with their long axes oriented parallel to the direction of blood flow in the artery (Fig. 13.15). In forming the epithelial sheet, the cells are joined by tight junctions (zonulae occludentes) and gap junctions. Endothelial cells possess rod-like inclusions called **Weibel–Palade bodies** that are present in the cytoplasm. These specific endothelial organelles are electron-dense structures and contain **von Willebrand factor** and **P-selectin.** Von Willebrand factor is a glycoprotein synthesized by arterial endothelial cells. When secreted into the blood, it binds **coagulating factor VIII** and plays an important role in platelets' adhesion to the site of endothelial injury. The antibody to von Willebrand factor is commonly used as an immunohistochemical marker for the identification of endothelium-derived tumors. P-selectin is a cell adhesion molecule involved in the mechanism of

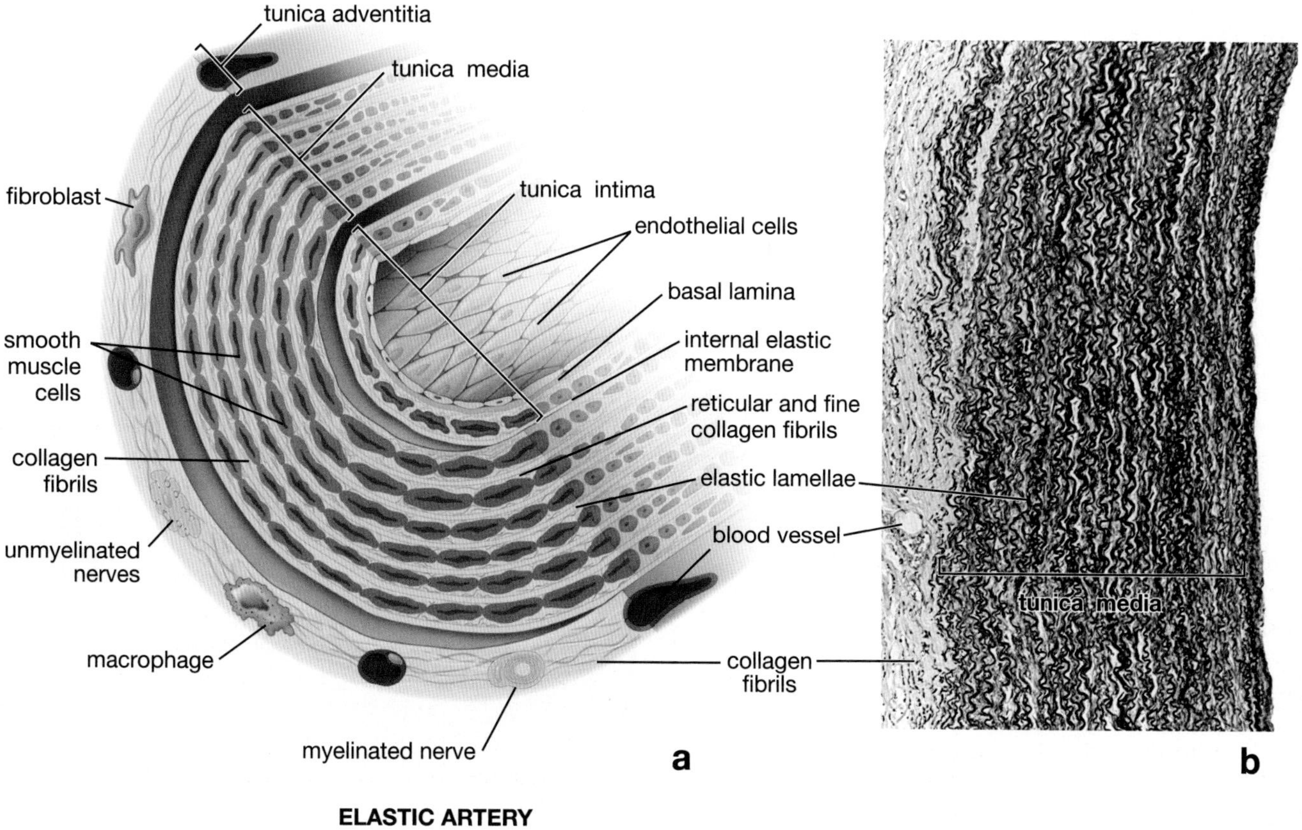

FIGURE 13.14. Diagram and photomicrograph of an elastic artery. a. This schematic diagram of a typical elastic artery shows its cellular and extracellular components. Note the organization of smooth muscle cells in the tunica media and the distribution of elastic lamellae. The internal elastic membrane is not well defined and is represented by the innermost elastic lamellae of the arterial wall. **b.** This low-magnification photomicrograph shows the section of the wall of the human aorta stained with Weigert resorcin-fuchsin elastic stain to visualize elastic lamellae interspersed with the smooth muscle cells of the tunica media. Only the tunica media, which is the thickest of the three layers of the elastic arteries, is labeled on this image. Note that elastic lamellae, collagen fibrils, and blood vessels are present in the tunica adventitia. ×48.

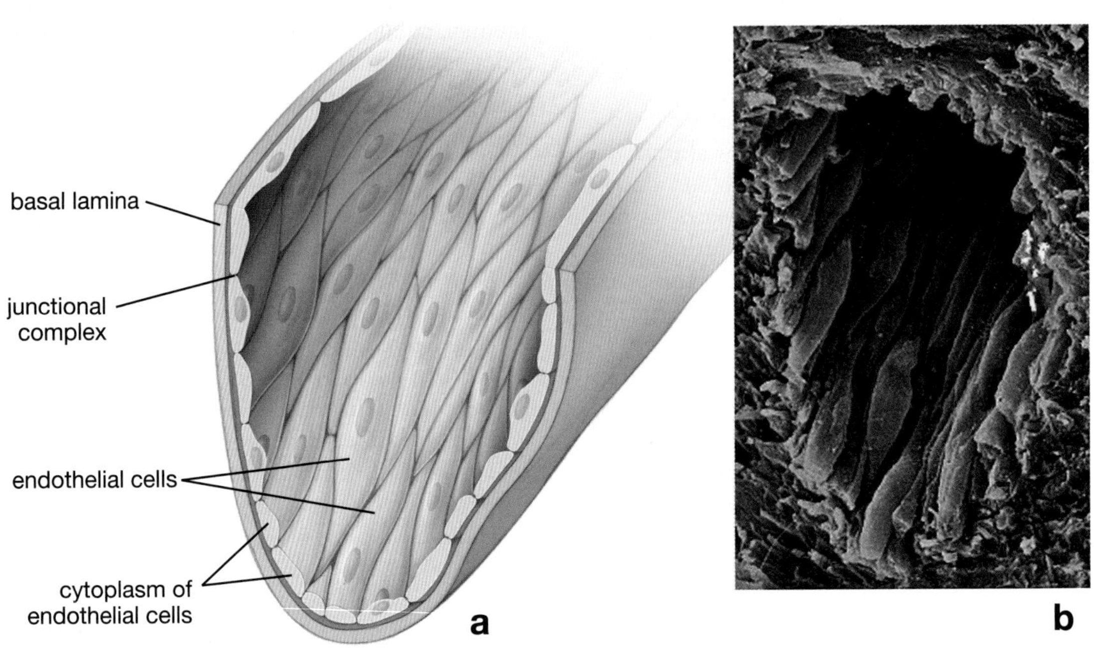

FIGURE 13.15. Diagram and scanning electron micrograph of the endothelium. a. This schematic drawing shows the luminal surface of the endothelium. The cells are elongated with their long axis parallel to the direction of blood flow. Nuclei of endothelial cells are also elongated in the direction of blood flow. **b.** Scanning electron micrograph of a small vein showing the cells of the endothelial lining. Note the spindle shape with the long axis of the cells running parallel to the vessel. ×1,100.

neutrophil–endothelial cell recognition. It initiates neutrophil migration from the blood to the site of action in the connective tissue (see pages 306-308).

- The **subendothelial layer** of connective tissue in larger elastic arteries consists of connective tissue with both collagen and elastic fibers. The main cell type in this layer is the smooth muscle cell. It is contractile and secretes extracellular ground substance as well as collagen and elastic fibers. Occasional macrophages may also be present.

FOLDER 13.2

CLINICAL CORRELATION: HYPERTENSION

Hypertension, or high blood pressure, occurs in about 25% of the population and is defined by a sustained diastolic pressure >80 mm Hg or a sustained systolic pressure >130 mm Hg. Hypertension is often associated with atherosclerotic vascular disease and with an increased risk of cardiovascular disorders, such as stroke and angina pectoris. In most cases of hypertension, the luminal diameter of small muscular arteries and arterioles is reduced, which leads to increased vascular resistance. Restriction in the luminal size may also result from active contraction of smooth muscle in the vessel wall, an increase in the amount of smooth muscle in the wall, or both.

In individuals with hypertension, smooth muscle cells multiply. The additional smooth muscle then adds to the thickness of the tunica media. Concomitantly, some of the smooth muscle cells accumulate lipid. This is one reason why hypertension is a major risk factor for atherosclerosis. In fat-fed animals, hypertension accelerates the rate of lipid accumulation in vessel walls. In the absence of a fatty diet, hypertension increases the rate of intimal thickening that occurs naturally with age.

Cardiac muscle is also affected by chronic hypertension that leads to pressure overload, resulting in compensatory left ventricular hypertrophy. Ventricular hypertrophy in this condition is caused by an increased diameter (not length) of cardiac muscle cells with characteristic enlarged and rectangular nuclei. Left ventricular hypertrophy is a common manifestation of **hypertensive heart disease**. Ventricular hypertrophy makes the wall of the left ventricle uniformly much thicker and less elastic, and the heart must then work harder to pump blood (Fig. F13.2.1). Untreated hypertensive heart disease may lead to cardiac failure. Studies have shown that prolonged reduction of blood pressure in patients with ventricular hypertrophy as a result of chronic hypertension can reduce the degree of hypertrophy.

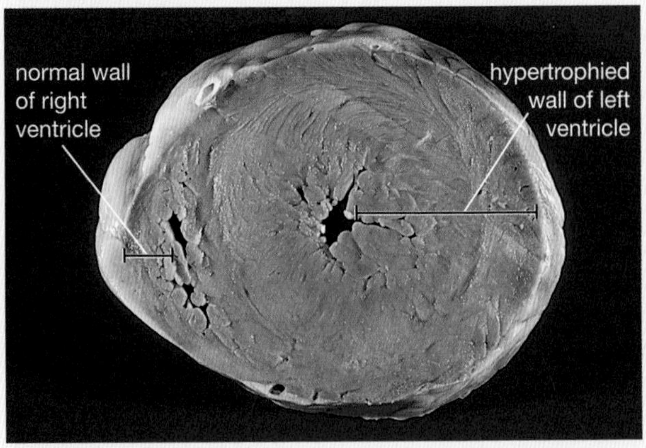

FIGURE F13.2.1. Horizontal section of the heart with left ventricular hypertrophy. This photograph shows a cross section of the ventricles of the heart of a patient with chronic hypertension. The walls of the left ventricle are concentrically thickened, resulting in decreases in the cavity diameter. Note the wall of the right ventricle, which has normal dimensions. (Reprinted with permission from Rubin R, Strayer DS, Rubin E, et al. *Rubin's Pathology: Clinicopathologic Foundations of Medicine*, 5th ed. Lippincott Williams & Wilkins; 2008.)

- The **internal elastic membrane** in elastic arteries is not conspicuous because it is one of many elastic layers in the wall of the vessel. It is usually identified only because it is the innermost elastic layer of the arterial wall.

Endothelial cells participate in the structural and functional integrity of the vascular wall.

Endothelial cells not only provide a physical barrier between the circulating blood and the subendothelial tissues but also produce **vasoactive agents** that cause constriction and relaxation of underlying vascular smooth muscles. Multiple roles and functions of the endothelium lining of blood vessels are described in detail at the beginning of this chapter (see pages 452-456).

The tunica media of elastic arteries consists of multiple layers of vascular smooth muscle cells separated by elastic lamellae.

The **tunica media** is the thickest of the three layers of elastic arteries and consists of the following:

- **Elastin** is in the form of fenestrated sheets or lamellae between the muscle cell layers. These lamellae are arranged in concentric layers (see Figs. 13.14 and 13.16a and Plate 13.2, page 476). As noted, fenestrations in the lamellae facilitate the diffusion of substances within the arterial wall. The number and thickness of these lamellae are related to blood pressure and age. At birth, the aorta is almost devoid of lamellae; in adult, the aorta has 40–70 lamellae. In individuals with hypertension, both the number and thickness of the lamellae are increased.
- **Vascular smooth muscle cells** are arranged in layers. The smooth muscle cells are arranged in a low-pitch spiral relative to the long axis of the vessel; thus, in cross sections of the artery, they appear in a circular array. The smooth muscle cells are spindle shaped with an elongated nucleus. They are invested with an external (basal) lamina, except where they are joined by gap junctions. **Fibroblasts are not present in the tunica media**. Vascular smooth muscle cells synthesize collagen, elastin, and other molecules of the extracellular matrix. In addition, in response to growth factors (i.e., PDGF, FGF) produced by endothelial cells, smooth muscle cells may proliferate and migrate to the adjacent intima. This characteristic is important in normal repair of the vascular wall and in pathologic processes similar to those occurring in **atherosclerosis**.
- **Collagen fiber** and **ground substance** (proteoglycans) are synthesized and secreted by vascular smooth muscle cells.

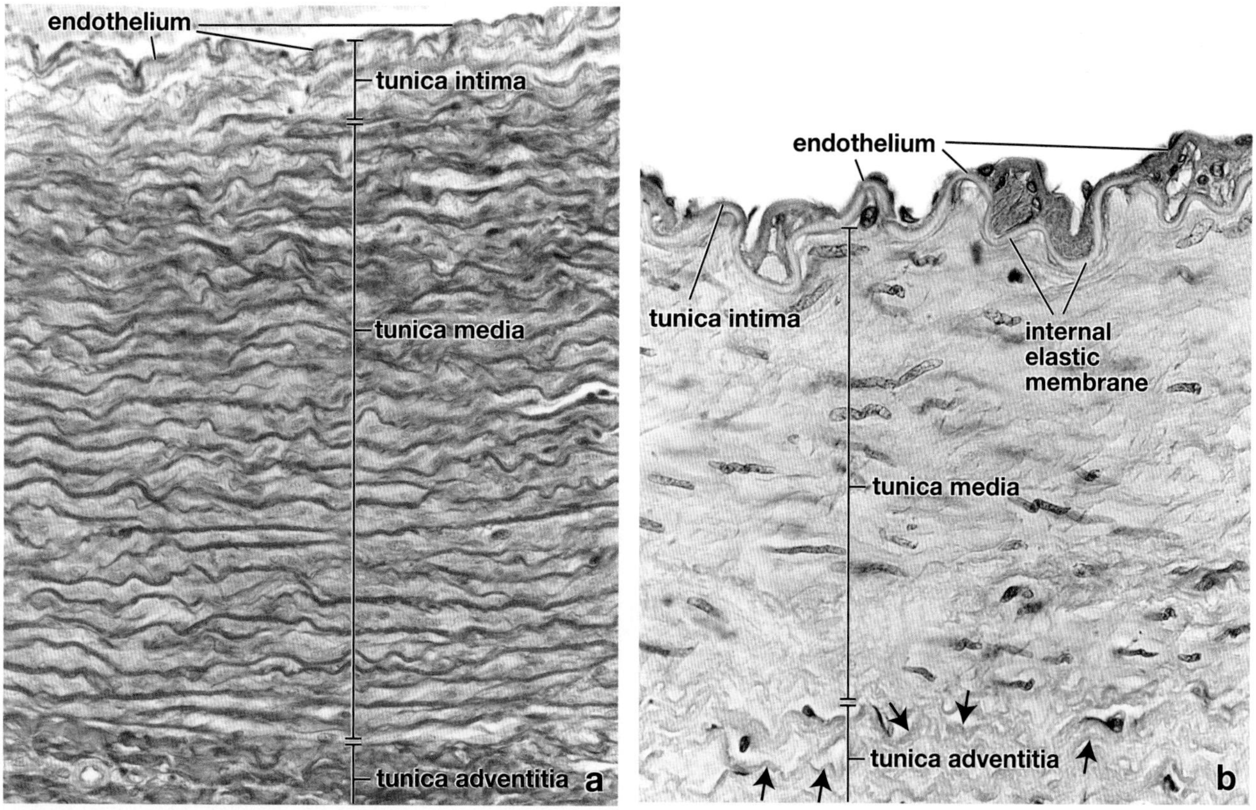

FIGURE 13.16. Photomicrographs of the wall of elastic and muscular types of arteries. a. This photomicrograph shows a cross section of the human aorta stained with resorcin-fuchsin to demonstrate elastic material. Three layers can be recognized: the tunica intima, the tunica media, and the tunica adventitia. The tunica intima consists of a lining of endothelial cells that rest on a thin layer of connective tissue containing smooth muscle cells, occasional macrophages, and collagen and elastic fibers. The boundary between it and the tunica media is not sharply defined. The tunica media contains an abundance of smooth muscle cells (note the *blue*-staining nuclei) and numerous elastic fenestrated membranes (the *red, wavy* lamellae). The tunica adventitia, the outermost part, lacks elastic laminae, consists mainly of connective tissue, and contains the blood vessels and nerves that supply the aortic wall. ×300. **b.** Photomicrograph of a cross section through a muscular artery in a routine hematoxylin and eosin (H&E) preparation shows that the wall of the muscular artery is also divided into the same three layers as in the elastic artery. The tunica intima consists of an endothelial lining, a small amount of connective tissue, and the internal elastic membrane. This structure has a scalloped appearance when the vessel is constricted and is highly refractile. Constriction also causes the endothelial cell nuclei to appear rounded. The tunica media consists mainly of circularly arranged smooth muscle cells and collagen and elastic fibers. The nuclei of the smooth muscle cells, when contracted, have a corkscrew appearance. The tunica adventitia consists mostly of connective tissue. A well-defined external elastic membrane is not apparent in this vessel, but profiles of elastic material (*arrows*) are present. ×360.

The tunica adventitia in the elastic artery is a relatively thin connective tissue layer.

In elastic arteries, the tunica adventitia is usually less than half the thickness of the tunica media. It consists of the following:

- **Collagen fibers** and **elastic fibers**, which form a loose network of elastic fibers (not lamellae) that are less organized than those in the tunica media. The collagen fibers help prevent the expansion of the arterial wall beyond physiologic limits during systole of the cardiac cycle.
- **Fibroblasts** and **macrophages**, which are the principal cells of the tunica adventitia
- **Vasa vasorum** (blood vessels), which includes small arterial branches, their capillary network, and corresponding veins similar to the vasculature in general
- **Nervi vasorum (vascularis)**, also called *vasoconstrictor nerves*, which represent unmyelinated postsynaptic sympathetic nerve fibers. These neurons release norepinephrine (NE) as their synaptic neurotransmitter, resulting in the narrowing of the lumen of the affected blood vessel (vasoconstriction).

The functions of the vasa vasorum are to deliver nutrients and oxygen into the vascular wall and to remove waste products.

In larger vessels, the transport of oxygen, nutrients, and waste products to and from the lumen is supplemented by diffusion from the network of small blood vessels called **vasa vasorum**. It consists of small arteries that enter the vascular wall from outside the vessel and then divide into a network of arterioles and capillaries supplying the outer part of the wall. Small veins emerging from the vasa vasorum network drain the capillaries and venules into larger veins that accompany the arteries. The inner part of the vascular wall is supplied by diffusion of nutrients from the lumen. In humans, vessels with a lumen of less than 0.5 mm in diameter usually do not have a vasa vasorum. In this type of vessel, the tunica media is usually thinner than a 30-cell layer. The function of the vasa vasorum is to deliver nutrients and oxygen to the vascular wall and to remove waste products produced by cells residing in the wall or diffused from the lumen of the vessel. There is a strong association between the higher density of vasa vasorum in an arterial wall and the severity of atheromatous plaque formation. The hemodynamic impact (i.e., increased blood pressure, low oxygen tension, and increased delivery or impaired removal of LDL cholesterol) on the function of the vasa vasorum may play a role in the pathogenesis of **atheromatous plaques**.

Medium Arteries (Muscular Arteries)

Muscular arteries have more smooth muscle and less elastin in the tunica media than do elastic arteries.

Generally, in the region of transition between elastic arteries and large muscular arteries, the amount of elastic material decreases, and smooth muscle cells become the predominant constituent of the tunica media (Fig. 13.17 and Plate 13.3, page 478). Also, a prominent **internal elastic membrane**

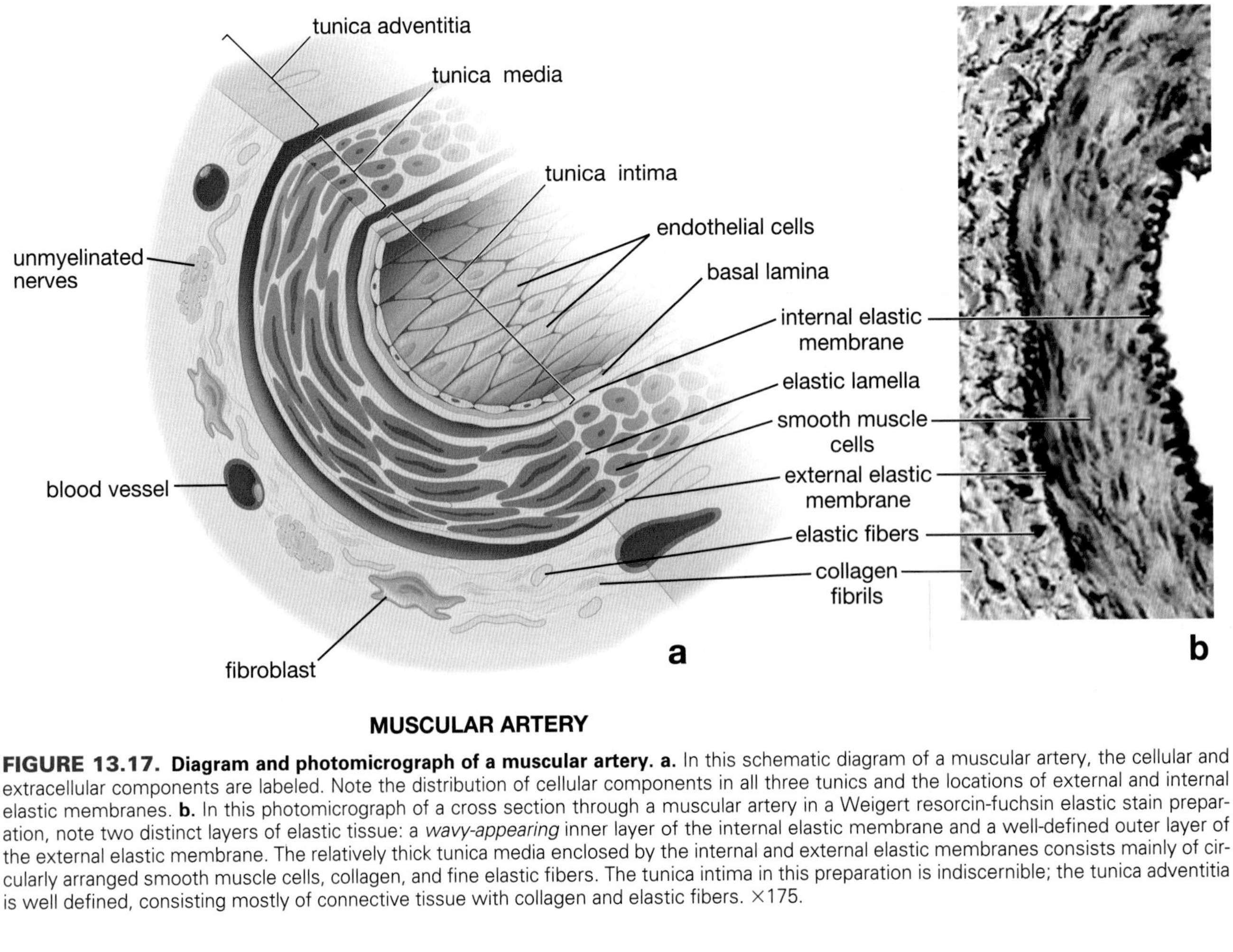

FIGURE 13.17. Diagram and photomicrograph of a muscular artery. a. In this schematic diagram of a muscular artery, the cellular and extracellular components are labeled. Note the distribution of cellular components in all three tunics and the locations of external and internal elastic membranes. **b.** In this photomicrograph of a cross section through a muscular artery in a Weigert resorcin-fuchsin elastic stain preparation, note two distinct layers of elastic tissue: a *wavy-appearing* inner layer of the internal elastic membrane and a well-defined outer layer of the external elastic membrane. The relatively thick tunica media enclosed by the internal and external elastic membranes consists mainly of circularly arranged smooth muscle cells, collagen, and fine elastic fibers. The tunica intima in this preparation is indiscernible; the tunica adventitia is well defined, consisting mostly of connective tissue with collagen and elastic fibers. ×175.

becomes apparent, helping to distinguish muscular arteries from elastic arteries. In many instances, a recognizable **external elastic membrane** is also evident.

The tunica intima is thinner in muscular arteries and contains a prominent internal elastic membrane.

The **tunica intima** is relatively thinner in muscular arteries than in elastic arteries and consists of an endothelial lining with its basal lamina, a sparse subendothelial layer of connective tissue, and a prominent **internal elastic membrane**. In some muscular arteries, the subendothelial layer is so scanty that the basal lamina of the endothelium appears to make contact with the internal elastic membrane. In histologic sections, the internal elastic membrane usually appears as a well-defined, undulating, or wavy structure because of the contraction of the smooth muscle (Fig. 13.16b).

The thickness of the tunica intima varies with age and other factors. In young children, it is very thin. In the muscular arteries of young adults, the tunica intima accounts for about one-sixth of the total wall thickness. In older adults, the tunica intima may be expanded by lipid deposits, often in the form of irregular "fatty streaks."

The tunica media of muscular arteries is composed almost entirely of vascular smooth muscle, with little elastic material.

The **tunica media** of muscular arteries consists of vascular smooth muscle cells amid collagen fibers and relatively little elastic material. The smooth muscle cells are arranged in a spiral manner in the arterial wall. Their contraction helps maintain blood pressure. As in elastic arteries, there are **no fibroblasts** in this layer. The smooth muscle cells possess an external (basal) lamina, except at the sites of gap junctions, and produce extracellular collagen, elastin, and ground substance.

The tunica adventitia of muscular arteries is relatively thick and often separated from the tunica media by a recognizable external elastic membrane.

The **tunica adventitia** of muscular arteries consists of fibroblasts, collagen fibers, elastic fibers, and, in some vessels, scattered adipose cells. Compared with elastic arteries, the tunica adventitia of muscular arteries is relatively thick—about the same thickness as the tunica media. Collagen fibers are the principal extracellular component. However, a concentration of elastic material immediately adjacent to the tunica media is often present and, as such, constitutes the **external elastic membrane.** Nerves and small vessels travel in the adventitia and give off branches that penetrate into the tunica media in the large muscular arteries as the vasa vasorum.

Small Arteries and Arterioles

Small arteries and arterioles are distinguished from one another by the number of smooth muscle cell layers in the tunica media.

As mentioned previously, **arterioles** have only one or two layers, and a small artery may have as many as eight layers of smooth muscle in the tunica media (Fig. 13.18 and Plate 13.4, page 480). Typically, the tunica intima of a small artery has an internal elastic membrane, whereas this layer may or may not

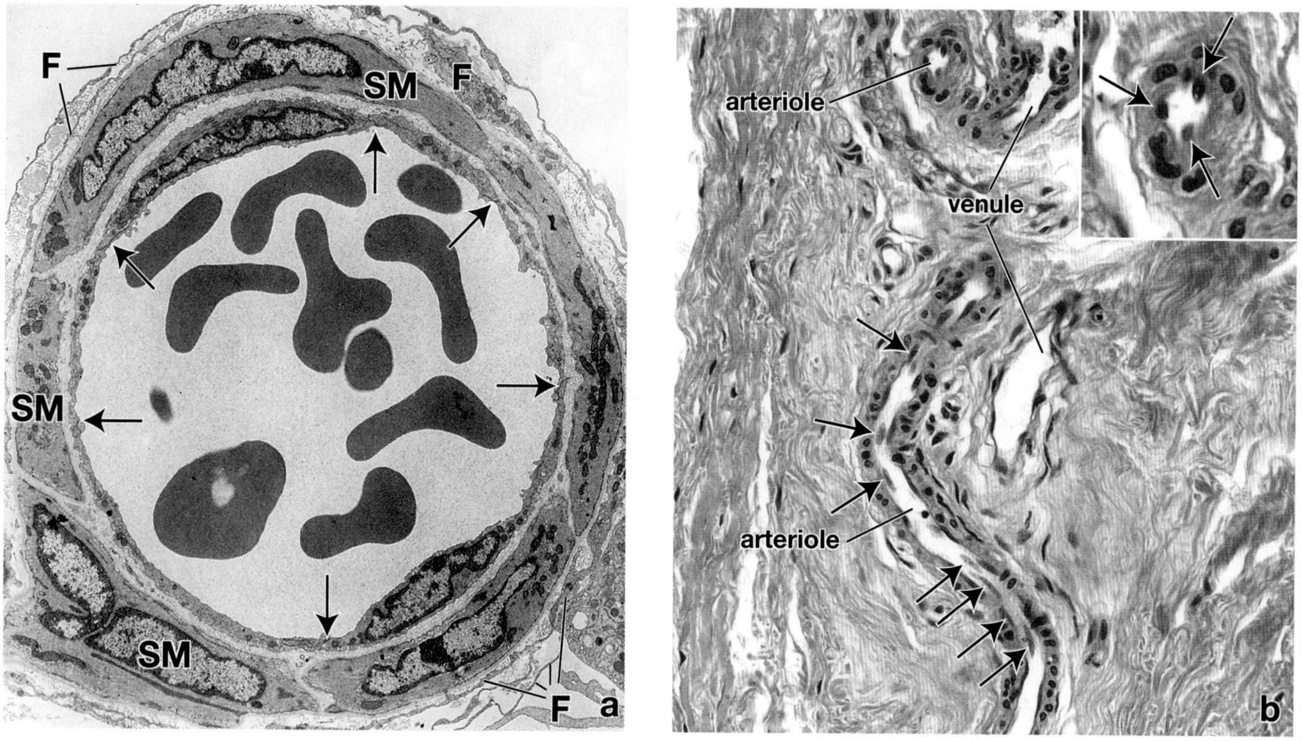

FIGURE 13.18. Electron micrograph and photomicrograph of arterioles. a. This electron micrograph shows a cross section of an arteriole. The tunica intima of the vessel is composed of an endothelium and a very thin layer of subendothelial connective tissue (collagen fibrils and ground substance). The *arrows* indicate the site of junction between adjoining endothelial cells. The tunica media consists of a single layer of smooth muscle cells (*SM*). The tunica adventitia is composed of collagen fibrils and several layers of fibroblasts (*F*) with extremely attenuated processes. Red blood cells are visible in the lumen. ×6,000. **b.** Photomicrograph of arteriole and venule in the dermis. One arteriole is seen in longitudinal section, and another is seen in cross section. The round and ovoid nuclei in the wall of the longitudinally sectioned arteriole belong to the smooth muscle cells of the tunica media. Their round to ovoid shape indicates that these cells have been cut in cross section. The elongated nuclei (*arrows*) belong to endothelial cells. ×320. **Inset.** The cross-sectioned arteriole is shown here at higher magnification and reveals the endothelial cell nuclei bulging into the lumen (*arrows*). They reflect a cross-sectional cut. The nuclei of the smooth muscle cells in the tunica media appear as elongate profiles reflecting their circular pattern around the vessel. ×600.

be present in the arteriole. The endothelium in both is essentially similar to endothelium in other arteries, except that at the electron microscope level, gap junctions may be found between endothelial cells and the smooth muscle cells of the tunica media. Lastly, the tunica adventitia is a thin, ill-defined sheath of connective tissue that blends with the connective tissue in which these vessels travel.

Arterioles control blood flow to capillary networks by contraction of the smooth muscle cells.

Arterioles serve as flow regulators for the capillary beds. In the normal relationship between an arteriole and a capillary network, contraction of the smooth muscle in the wall of an arteriole increases the **vascular resistance**, reducing or shutting off the blood going to the capillaries. The slight thickening of the smooth muscle at the origin of a capillary bed from an arteriole is called the **precapillary sphincter**. Most arterioles can dilate 60%–100% from their resting diameter and can maintain as much as 40% constriction for a long time. Precapillary sphincters also undergo rhythmic contractions and relaxations, a phenomenon called **vasomotion**, which regulates arteriolar diameter over time. A large decrease or increase in vascular resistance has a direct effect on the distribution of blood flow and systemic arterial pressure. Contractions and relaxation of arterioles direct blood to where it may be most needed. For instance, during strenuous physical exertion such as running, blood flow to skeletal muscle is increased by dilation of arterioles, and blood flow to the intestine is reduced by arteriolar constriction. After ingestion of a large meal, however, the reverse is true.

■ CAPILLARIES

Capillaries are the smallest diameter blood vessels, often smaller than the diameter of an erythrocyte.

Capillaries form blood vascular networks that allow fluid-containing gases, metabolites, and waste products to move through their thin walls. The human body contains approximately 50,000 miles of capillaries. Each consists of a single layer of **endothelial cells** and their **basal lamina**. The endothelial cells form a tube just large enough to allow the passage of red blood cells one at a time. In many capillaries, the lumen is so narrow that the red cells literally fold on themselves to pass through the vessel (Fig. 13.19). The passing red blood cells fill virtually the entire capillary lumen, minimizing the diffusion path for gases and nutrients between the capillary and the extravascular tissue. In cross sections and with the TEM, the tube appears to be formed by only one cell or portions of several cells. Because of their thin walls and close physical association with metabolically active cells and tissues, capillaries are particularly well suited for the exchange of gases and metabolites between cells and the bloodstream. The ratios of capillary volume to endothelial surface area and thickness also favor movement of substances across the vessel wall.

Classification of Capillaries

There are three different types of capillaries: continuous, fenestrated, and discontinuous (or sinusoidal).

Capillary structure varies in different tissues and organs. On the basis of their morphology, capillaries are divided into three types: continuous, fenestrated, and discontinuous.

Continuous capillaries are typically found in connective tissue; cardiac, skeletal, and smooth muscles; skin; lungs; and the CNS. They are characterized by an **uninterrupted vascular endothelium** that rests on a **continuous basal lamina** (Fig. 13.20a). Endothelial cells contain the usual organelles, a few short microvilli on their luminal surfaces, a variable number of electron-dense membrane-bound vesicles, and numerous pinocytotic vesicles that underlie both the luminal and basal plasma membrane surfaces. The vesicles are approximately 70 nm in diameter and function in **transcytosis**, a process that transports larger molecules between the lumen and the connective tissue and vice versa. With the TEM, continuous capillaries appear in cross sections as two plasma membranes enclosing a ribbon of cytoplasm that may include the nucleus (Fig. 13.21). Individual endothelial cells are joined by tight (occluding) junctions that can be seen in the typical cross section of a continuous capillary. The tight junctions restrict the passage of molecules between adjacent endothelial cells, only allowing the passage of relatively small molecules (<10 kDa).

Fenestrated capillaries are typically found in endocrine glands and sites of fluid or metabolite absorption, such as the gallbladder, kidney, pancreas, and intestinal tract. Their endothelial cells are characterized by the presence of numerous circular openings known as **fenestrations** (70–80 nm in diameter) that provide channels across the capillary wall (see Fig. 13.20b). The **continuous basal lamina** is found across the fenestrations on the basal plasma membrane surfaces. Endothelial cells in fenestrated capillaries also have numerous pinocytotic vesicles. Fenestrations are most

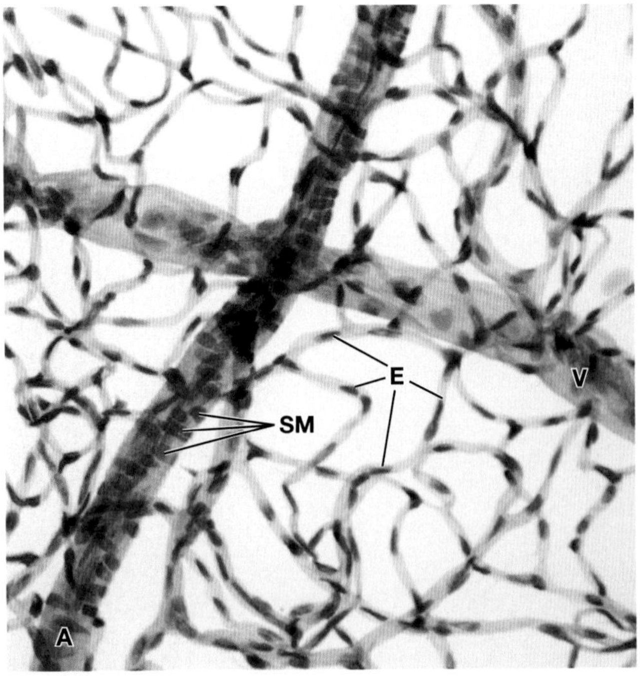

FIGURE 13.19. Photomicrograph of the capillary network in the retina. This is a whole-mount preparation of retinal capillaries. After mild enzymatic digestion, the retina was spread on a glass slide, stained with the periodic acid–Schiff (PAS) procedure, and counterstained with hematoxylin. Vertically crossing the image is an arteriole (*A*) with a clearly visible layer of circularly arranged smooth muscle cells (*SM*). This arteriole is crossed perpendicularly by a venule (*V*). Note the extensive network of capillaries connecting both vessels. Nuclei of endothelial cells (*E*) are clearly visible within capillaries. At this magnification, pericytes are difficult to discern. ×560. (Courtesy of Mr. Denifield W. Player.)

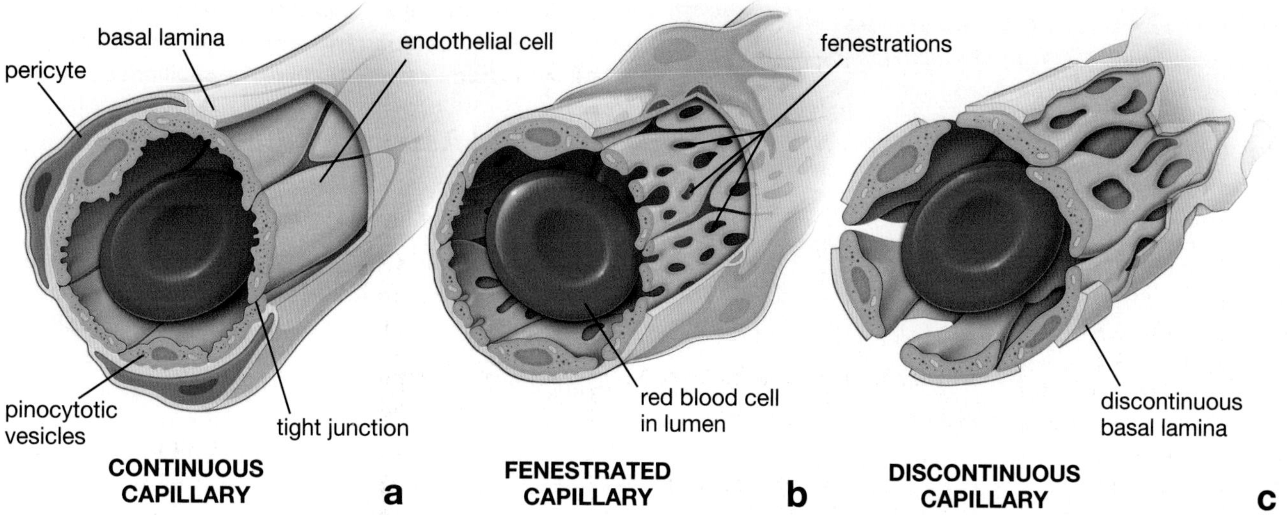

FIGURE 13.20. Diagram of the three types of capillaries. a. Continuous capillaries are characterized by an uninterrupted vascular endothelium that rests on a continuous basal lamina. Individual endothelial cells are joined by tight junctions that restrict the passage of molecules from the lumen into underlying tissue. **b.** Fenestrated capillaries have endothelial cells that are characterized by the presence of numerous fenestrations. The continuous basal lamina surrounds this type of capillary. In some organs, fenestrations may have a thin, nonmembranous diaphragm across their openings. **c.** Discontinuous capillaries (sinusoidal capillaries, sinusoids) have large openings in their endothelial cells and are separated by wide irregular intercellular gaps. Also, endothelial cells rest on a discontinuous basal lamina, which, in some organs, is rudimental and may be absent.

likely formed when a developing pinocytotic vesicle spans the narrow cytoplasmic layer and simultaneously opens on the opposite surface (Fig. 13.22). A fenestration may have a thin, nonmembranous **diaphragm** across its opening. When viewed from the luminal surface, this diaphragm has a cartwheel-like shape with a central thickening and 14 wedge-shaped gaps. It is derived from the glycocalyx formerly enclosed within the pinocytotic vesicle from which the fenestration may have formed. These fenestrations, also referred to as **filtration pores**, constitute specific transport sites within endothelial cells, but they do not allow passage of plasma like the gaps between endothelial cells in sinusoidal capillaries (see Fig. 13.20b).

Fenestrated capillaries in the gastrointestinal tract and gallbladder have fewer fenestrations and a thicker wall when no absorption is occurring. When absorption takes place, the walls are thin, and the number of pinocytotic vesicles and fenestrations increases rapidly. The ionic changes in the perivascular connective tissue, caused by the absorbed solutes, stimulate pinocytosis. These observations support the suggested mode of fenestration formation described earlier.

Discontinuous capillaries (also called **sinusoidal capillaries** or **sinusoids**) are typically found in the liver, spleen, and bone marrow. They are larger in diameter and more irregularly shaped than other capillaries. Vascular endothelial cells lining these capillaries have large openings in their cytoplasm, and they are separated by wide, irregular, intercellular gaps that allow for the passage of blood plasma proteins (see Fig. 13.20c). The endothelial cells rest on a **discontinuous basal lamina**. Structural features of these capillaries vary from organ to organ and include specialized cells. **Kupffer cells** (stellate sinusoidal macrophages) and vitamin A–storing **Ito cells** (hepatic stellate cells) in the liver occur in association with the endothelial cells of hepatic sinusoids. In the spleen, endothelial cells exhibit a unique spindle shape with gaps between the neighboring cells; the basal lamina underlying the endothelium is rudimentary and may be partially or even completely absent.

Pericytes represent a population of undifferentiated mesenchymal stem cells that are associated with capillaries.

Capillaries and some postcapillary venules are associated with perivascular cells exhibiting cellular processes that wrap around vascular endothelial cells. **Pericytes** (historically known as *Rouget cells*) are examples of perivascular cells that are associated with the endothelium (see Figs. 13.21

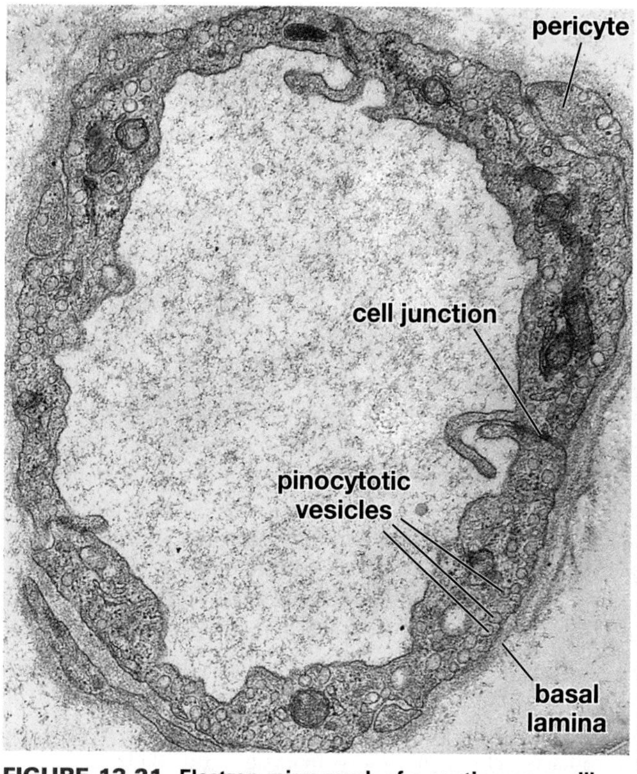

FIGURE 13.21. Electron micrograph of a continuous capillary. The endothelial cells that make up the wall of a continuous capillary contain numerous pinocytotic vesicles. The cell junctions are frequently marked by cytoplasmic (marginal) folds that protrude into the lumen. The endothelial cell nuclei are not included within the plane of section in the micrograph. Similarly, the electron micrograph shows only a small amount of pericyte cytoplasm. Note that the pericyte cytoplasm is enclosed by basal lamina. ×30,000.

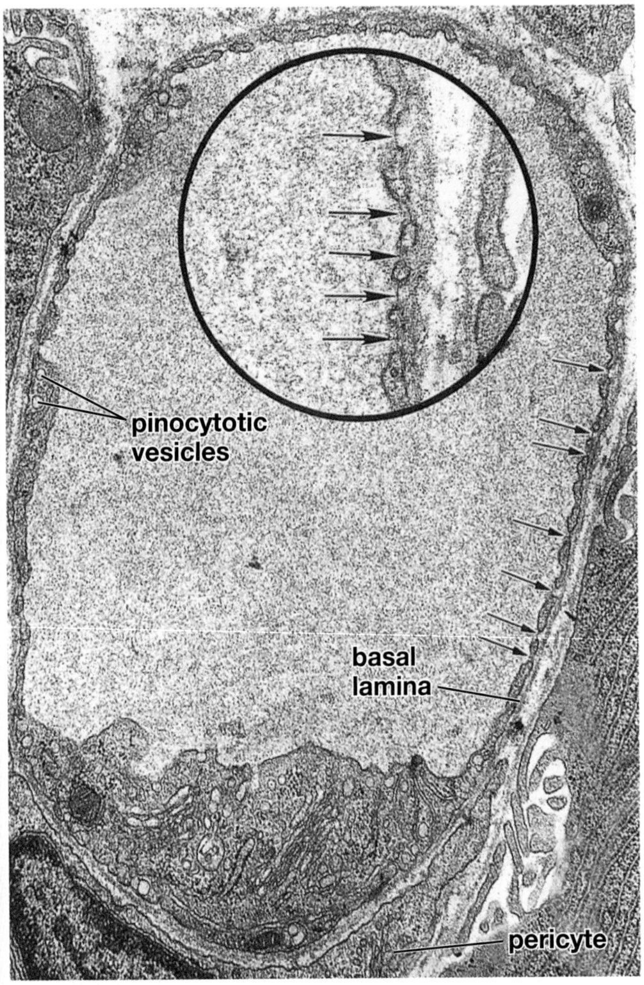

FIGURE 13.22. Electron micrograph of a fenestrated capillary. The cytoplasm of the endothelial cells contains numerous fenestrations (*small arrows*). In some of the thicker regions of the endothelial cells where the fenestrations are absent, pinocytotic vesicles are present. Part of a pericyte is seen on the *bottom* of the electron micrograph, including its nucleus in the *lower left* corner of the micrograph. ×21,500. The *inset* shows to advantage the fenestrations and the diaphragm that spans the openings (*large arrows*). ×55,000.

and 13.22). They intimately surround the capillary with branching cytoplasmic processes and are enclosed by a basal lamina that is continuous with that of the endothelium. Pericytes are contractile and are controlled by NO produced by endothelial cells. There is some evidence to suggest that pericytes can modulate capillary blood flow in specific capillary beds (e.g., brain).

Pericytes provide vascular support and promote the stability of capillaries and postcapillary venules through complex, bidirectional physical and chemical communication with vascular endothelial cells. Histologically, pericytes display features of **undifferentiated mesenchymal stem cells** with large nuclei rich in heterochromatin. Experiments have shown that environmental signals can stimulate proliferation, migratory capability, and differentiation of pericytes into a variety of cell types, including adipocytes, fibroblasts, chondrocytes, osteocytes, and skeletal muscle cells. During **embryonic development** or **angiogenesis** (e.g., wound healing), pericytes give rise to both endothelial cells and smooth muscle cells. Pericytes are directly involved in the pathogenesis of vascular-driven diseases (e.g., diabetic retinopathy and tumor angiogenesis). In addition, uncontrolled divisions of pericytes give rise to **hemangiopericytoma**, a rare vascular tumor that can originate in the body anywhere there are capillaries.

Functional Aspects of Capillaries

In the capillaries, a two-directional exchange of fluid occurs between the blood and the tissues.

Blood pressure causes the plasma, which carries oxygen, nutrients, and other constituents, to pass through the capillary wall from the proximal or **arterial end** of the **capillary network** into the tissue. In the tissues, these molecules are exchanged for carbon dioxide, waste products, and other metabolites. Approximately 90% of the extravasated fluids are reabsorbed at the distal or **venous end** of the capillary network. The remaining 10% is returned to the blood vascular system via the lymphatic vasculature (see page 469). The extravasated fluid initially enters blind-ended **lymphatic capillaries**, which connect with larger collecting lymphatic vessels, and the lymph is ultimately returned to the bloodstream through a system of large **lymphatic vessels**, such as the thoracic duct and right lymphatic trunk.

To understand capillary network function, two important points—**vasomotion** (i.e., intermittent capillary blood flow) and the extent or **density of the capillary network**—should be considered.

- **Vasomotion** represents the phenomenon of **intermittent blood flow** through the capillary network due to rhythmical contraction and relaxation of the **precapillary sphincters**. Blood flow through capillaries is not continuous; instead, it turns on and off every few seconds. Vasomotion regulates fluid and nutrient exchange between the vascular system and peripheral tissue. For instance, blood flow into the capillary network of skeletal muscle during exercise requires more oxygen and nutrients. When oxygen concentrations are reduced during increased oxygen utilization by the muscle, the intervals of blood flow through the capillary network occur more often and last longer. As a result, the muscle receives more oxygen and other nutrients. The intermittent contraction of arterioles and resulting vasomotion are regulated by oxygen, reactive oxygen intermediates (ROIs), NO, and waste products of tissue metabolism.
- The **density of the capillary network** determines the total surface area available for exchange between the blood and tissue. It is related to the metabolic activity of the tissue. The liver, kidney, cardiac muscle, and skeletal muscle have rich capillary networks. Dense connective tissue is less metabolically active and has less extensive capillary networks. Blood flow is controlled through local and systemic signals.

In response to vasodilating agents (e.g., NO, low O_2 tension), the smooth muscle in the walls of the arterioles relaxes, resulting in vasodilation and increased blood flow through the capillary system. Pressure within the capillaries increases, and much of the plasma fluid is driven into the tissue. This process occurs in **peripheral edema**. Local endothelial-derived factors, systemic signals carried by the autonomic nervous system, and norepinephrine released by the adrenal gland cause the smooth muscle of the arterioles to contract (vasoconstriction), resulting in decreased blood flow through the capillary bed. In this condition, capillary pressure decreases and greatly increases the absorption of tissue fluid. This situation occurs during a loss of blood volume and can add a considerable amount of fluid to the blood, preventing hypovolemic shock.

ARTERIOVENOUS SHUNTS

Arteriovenous shunts allow blood to bypass capillaries by providing direct routes between the arteries and the veins.

Generally, in a **microvascular bed**, arteries convey blood to the capillaries, and veins convey blood away from the capillaries. However, all the blood does not necessarily pass from arteries to capillaries and then to veins. In many tissues, there are direct routes between the arteries and the veins that divert blood from the capillaries. These routes are called **arteriovenous (AV) anastomoses** or **AV shunts** (see Fig. 13.11). AV shunts are commonly found in the skin of the fingertips, nose, and lips and in the erectile tissue of the penis and clitoris. The arteriole of AV shunts is often coiled, has a relatively thick smooth muscle layer, is enclosed in a connective tissue capsule, and is richly innervated. Contrary to the ordinary precapillary sphincter, contraction of the arteriole smooth muscle of the AV shunt sends blood to a capillary bed; relaxation of the smooth muscle sends blood to a venule, bypassing the capillary bed. AV shunts serve in **thermoregulation** at the body surface. Closing an AV shunt in the skin causes blood to flow through the capillary bed, enhancing heat loss. Opening an AV shunt in the skin reduces the blood flow to the skin capillaries, conserving body heat. In erectile tissue such as the penis, closing the AV shunt directs blood flow into the corpora cavernosa, initiating the erectile response.

Preferential thoroughfares, whose proximal segment is called a **metarteriole** (Fig. 13.23), also allow some blood to pass more directly from artery to vein. Capillaries arise from both arterioles and metarterioles. Although capillaries themselves have no smooth muscle in their walls, a sphincter of smooth muscle called the **precapillary sphincter** is located at their origin from either an arteriole or a metarteriole. These sphincters control the amount of blood passing through the capillary bed.

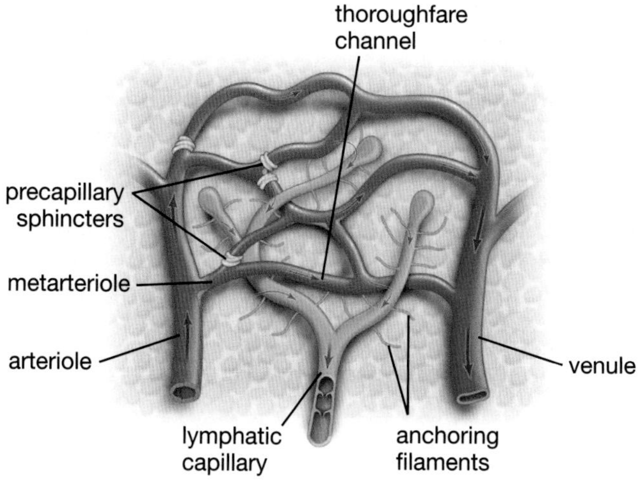

FIGURE 13.23. Diagram of microcirculation. This schematic diagram shows a metarteriole (initial segment of a thoroughfare channel) giving rise to capillaries. The precapillary sphincters of the arteriole and metarteriole control the entry of blood into the capillaries. The distal segment of the thoroughfare channel receives capillaries from the microcirculatory bed, but no sphincters are present where the afferent capillaries enter the thoroughfare channels. Blind-ended lymphatic vessels are shown in association with the capillary bed. Note the presence of anchoring filaments and the valve system within the lymphatic capillaries.

VEINS

The tunics of veins are not as distinct or well defined as the tunics of arteries. Traditionally, veins are divided into four types based on size:

- **Venules** are further subclassified as **postcapillary** and **muscular venules**. They receive blood from capillaries and have a diameter as small as 0.1 mm.
- **Small veins** are less than 1 mm in diameter and are continuous with muscular venules.
- **Medium veins** represent most of the named veins in this category. They are usually accompanied by arteries and have a diameter of as much as 10 mm.
- **Large veins** usually have a diameter greater than 10 mm. Examples include the superior and inferior venae cavae and hepatic portal vein.

Although large and medium veins have three layers—also designated tunica intima, tunica media, and tunica adventitia—these layers are not as distinct as they are in arteries. Large- and medium-sized veins usually travel with large- and medium-sized arteries; arterioles and muscular venules also sometimes travel together, thus allowing comparison in histologic sections. Typically, veins have thinner walls than their accompanying arteries, and the lumen of the vein is larger than that of the artery. The arteriole lumen is usually patent; that of the vein is often collapsed. Many veins, especially those that convey blood against gravity, such as those of the limbs, contain valves that allow blood to flow in only one direction, back toward the heart. The valves are semilunar flaps consisting of a thin connective tissue core covered by endothelial cells.

Venules and Small Veins

Postcapillary venules collect blood from the capillary network and are characterized by the presence of pericytes.

Postcapillary venules possess an endothelial lining with its basal lamina and pericytes (Plate 13.4, page 480). The **endothelium** of postcapillary venules is the principal site of action of vasoactive agents, such as histamine and serotonin. Response to these agents results in extravasation of fluid and migration of white blood cells from the vessel during inflammatory and allergic reactions. Postcapillary venules of lymph nodes are specialized in the transmural migration of lymphocytes from the vascular lumen into the lymphatic tissue. Because they are lined by cuboidal or columnar endothelial cells, they are often referred to as **high endothelial venules (HEVs)**. For a detailed description and function of HEVs, see Chapter 14, Immune System and Lymphatic Tissues and Organs (pages 509-510). **Pericytes** represent undifferentiated mesenchymal stem cells that form umbrella-like connections with the endothelial cells. The relationship between endothelial cells and pericytes promotes their mutual proliferation and survival.

Both synthesize and share a basal lamina (see Fig. 13.21), synthesize growth factors, and communicate with each other through tight and gap junctions. Pericyte coverage is more extensive in the postcapillary venules than in the capillaries.

High endothelial venules are specialized postcapillary venules found in lymphoid tissues that support high levels of lymphocyte migration from the blood.

The postcapillary venules in the lymphatic system are also called **high endothelial venules (HEVs)** because of the prominent cuboidal appearance of their endothelial cells and ovoid nuclei. They are found in all secondary (peripheral) lymphatic organs (with the exception of the spleen) such as lymph nodes, tonsils, and in solitary as well as aggregated lymph nodules. The endothelium of HEVs is able to recruit a large number of lymphocytes; they can be often seen migrating through the wall of the venule. When observed with an electron microscope, endothelial cells of HEVs exhibit a prominent Golgi apparatus, abundant polyribosomes, and an extensive network of rough-surfaced endothelium reticulum (rER). These features are typical for cells with a secretory function, which is reflected by the presence of secretory vesicles in their cytoplasm. They also contain multivesicular bodies, transport vesicles, and Weibel–Palade bodies.

Muscular venules are distinguished from postcapillary venules by the presence of a tunica media.

Muscular venules are located distal to the postcapillary venules in the returning venous network and have a diameter of as much as 0.1 mm. Whereas postcapillary venules have no true tunica media, the muscular venules have one or two layers of vascular smooth muscle that constitute a tunica media. These vessels also have a thin tunica adventitia. Pericytes are usually not found in muscular venules.

Small veins are a continuation of muscular venules.

Small veins are a continuation of muscular venules and their diameters vary from 0.1 to 1 mm. All three tunics are present and recognizable in a routine slide preparation. Tunica media usually constitutes two or three layers of vascular smooth muscle. These vessels also have thicker tunica adventitia.

Medium Veins

Medium veins have a diameter of as much as 10 mm. Most deep veins that accompany arteries are in this category (e.g., radial vein, tibial vein, popliteal vein). Valves are a characteristic feature of these vessels and are most numerous in the inferior portion of the body, particularly the lower limbs, to prevent retrograde movement of blood because of gravity. Often, deep veins of the lower limbs are the site of thrombus (blood clot) formation, a condition known as **deep venous thrombosis (DVT)**. DVT is associated with immobilization of the lower limbs and may occur as a result of prolonged bed rest (after surgery or hospitalization), orthopedic casts, or restricted movement (such as during long airline flights). DVT may cause a blood clot originating from deep veins breaks off and becomes lodged in a pulmonary artery, a condition called **pulmonary embolism**.

The three tunics of the venous wall are most evident in medium-sized veins (Fig. 13.24).

- The **tunica intima** consists of an endothelium with its basal lamina; a thin subendothelial layer with occasional

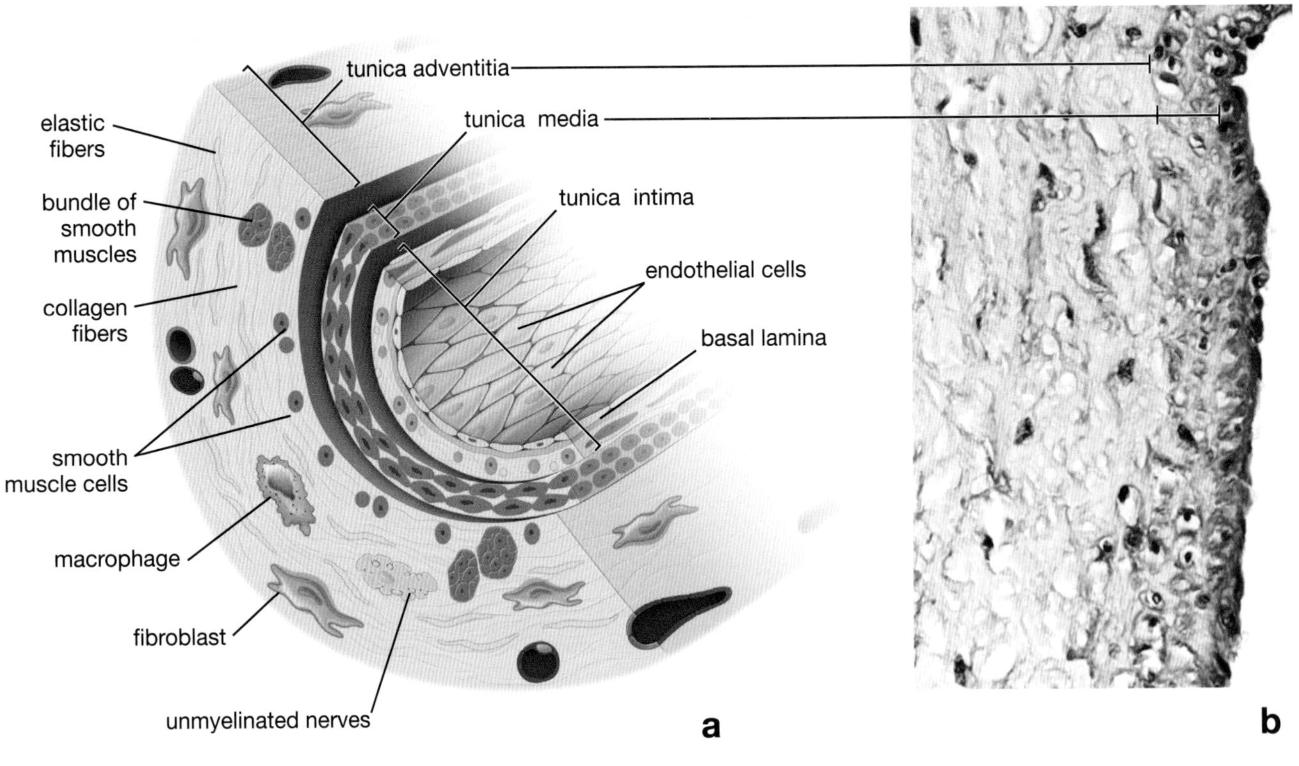

FIGURE 13.24. Schematic diagram and photomicrograph of a medium-sized vein. a. The cellular and extracellular components are labeled. Note that the tunica media contains a few layers of circularly arranged smooth muscle cells with interspersed collagen and elastic fibers. Also, longitudinally arranged smooth muscle cells are present at the junction with the tunica adventitia. **b.** This photomicrograph shows a section through the wall of a medium-sized vein in routine hematoxylin and eosin (H&E) preparation. The tunica intima consists of endothelium and a very thin subendothelial layer of connective tissue containing some smooth muscle cells. The tunica media contains a few layers of circularly and spirally arranged smooth muscle cells with collagen and elastic fibers. Note that the thickest layer is the tunica adventitia, which contains an abundance of collagen and some elastic fibers. The few nuclei seen in this layer belong to fibroblasts. ×360.

smooth muscle cells scattered in the connective tissue elements; and, in some cases, a thin, often discontinuous internal elastic membrane.

- The **tunica media** of medium-sized veins is much thinner than the same layer in medium-sized arteries. It contains several layers of circularly arranged smooth muscle cells with interspersed collagen and elastic fibers. In addition, longitudinally arranged smooth muscle cells may be present just beneath the tunica adventitia.
- The **tunica adventitia** is typically thicker than the tunica media and consists of collagen fibers and networks of elastic fibers (Fig. 13.24b).

Large Veins

In large veins, the tunica media is relatively thin, and the tunica adventitia is relatively thick.

Veins with a diameter greater than 10 mm are classified as large veins.

- The **tunica intima** of these veins (Fig. 13.25 and Plate 13.3, page 478) consists of an endothelial lining with its basal lamina, a small amount of subendothelial connective tissue, and some smooth muscle cells. Often, the boundary between the tunica intima and the tunica media is not clear, and it is not always easy to decide whether the smooth muscle cells close to the intimal endothelium belong to the tunica intima or the tunica media.
- The **tunica media** is relatively thin and contains circumferentially arranged smooth muscle cells, collagen fibers, and some fibroblasts.
- The **tunica adventitia** of large veins (e.g., the subclavian veins, portal vein, and venae cavae) is the thickest layer of the vessel wall. Along with the usual collagen and elastic fibers and fibroblasts, the tunica adventitia also contains longitudinally disposed smooth muscle cells (Fig. 13.26). Atrial myocardial extensions known as **myocardial sleeves** are present in the adventitia of both superior and inferior venae cavae as well as the pulmonary trunk. The arrangement, length, orientation, and thickness of myocardial sleeves may vary in different individuals. The presence of a myocardial extension containing cardiac muscle cells into the adventitia of large veins may lead to **atrial fibrillation**, the most common abnormal heart rhythm disorder that contributes to cardiac morbidity and mortality. Postmortem examinations of pulmonary veins from patients with atrial fibrillation frequently reveal the presence of **myocardial sleeves** containing altered cardiac muscle cells.

■ ATYPICAL BLOOD VESSELS

In several locations in the body, blood vessels—both arteries and veins—with an atypical structure are present, following:

- **Coronary arteries**, considered to be medium-sized muscular arteries, originate from the proximal part of the

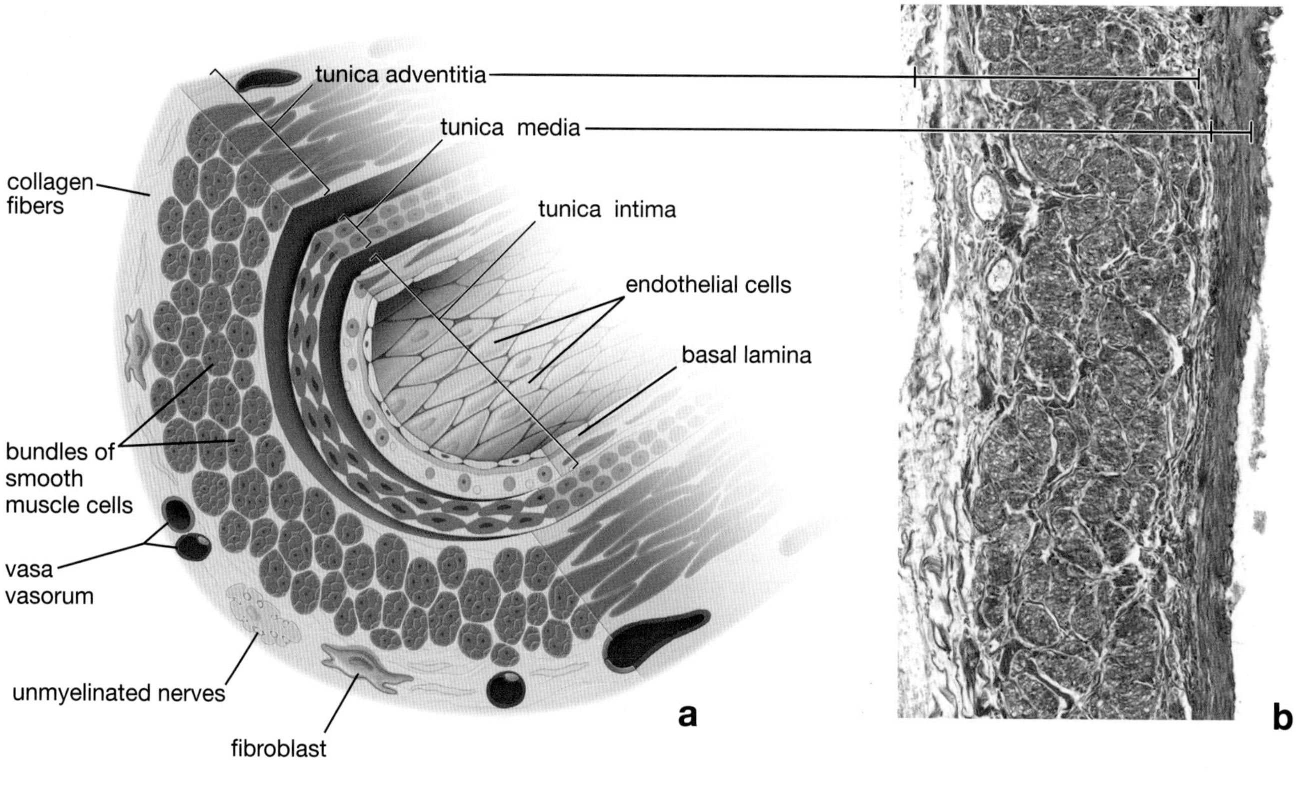

FIGURE 13.25. Schematic diagram and photomicrograph of a large vein. a. The cellular and extracellular components are labeled. Note a thin layer of circumferentially arranged smooth muscles of tunica media and the tunica adventitia with a large amount of longitudinally arranged smooth muscle bundles. **b.** This photomicrograph shows a section through the wall of a human portal vein in a routine hematoxylin and eosin (H&E) preparation. The tunica intima is indiscernible at this magnification. The tunica media contains a layer of circumferentially arranged smooth muscle cells with collagen and elastic fibers. Note the thickest layer of this wall is the tunica adventitia. In addition to an extensive collagen and elastic fiber network, the tunica adventitia contains a broad layer of smooth muscle cells arranged in longitudinal bundles. These bundles are variable in size and separated from each other by connective tissue fibers. ×125. (Courtesy of Dr. Donald J. Lowrie Jr., University of Cincinnati College of Medicine.)

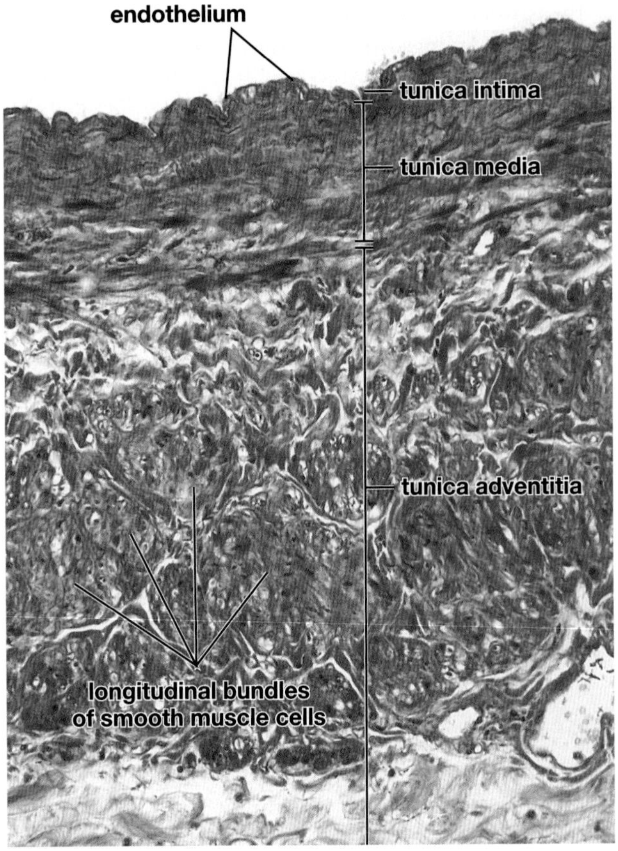

FIGURE 13.26. Photomicrograph of a large vein. This photomicrograph shows the three tunics in a section through the wall of the portal vein stained with hematoxylin and eosin (H&E). The tunica intima consists of endothelium and a thin subendothelial layer of connective tissue containing a few smooth muscle cells. The tunica media contains a relatively thin layer of circularly arranged smooth muscle cells. Tunica adventitia is the thickest layer of this vessel. It contains a thick layer of longitudinally arranged smooth muscle bundles (seen here in cross section) separated by collagen and elastic fibers. Note a layer of connective tissue containing coarse collagen and elastic fibers that separates longitudinal bundles of smooth muscle in the tunica adventitia from a layer of smooth muscles of the tunica media. ×240. (Courtesy of Dr. Donald J. Lowrie Jr., University of Cincinnati College of Medicine.)

ascending aorta and lie on the surface of the heart in the epicardium surrounded by adipose tissue. The walls of coronary arteries are usually thicker than those of comparable arteries in the upper or lower limb because of the large amounts of circular smooth muscle layers in the tunica media. In routine H&E preparation, the subendothelial layer of the tunica intima of younger people is inconspicuous, but it progressively thickens as increasing amounts of smooth muscle cell and fibroelastic tissue are added with aging (Fig. 13.27). The internal elastic membrane is well developed, although it may be fragmented, duplicated, or focally lost in older individuals. The relatively "loose" consistency of the tunica adventitia is reinforced by the longitudinal bundles of collagen fibers that allow for continuous changes of the vascular diameter. Atherosclerotic changes in coronary arteries that restrict blood flow and oxygen supply to cardiac muscle lead to **coronary heart disease** (see Folder 13.3).

- **Dural venous sinuses** represent venous channels in the cranial cavity. They are essentially broad spaces within the dura mater that are lined with endothelial cells and devoid of smooth muscles.
- The **great saphenous vein** represents a long subcutaneous vein of the lower limb that originates in the foot and drains into the femoral vein just below the inguinal ligament. This vein is often described as a **muscular vein** because of the presence of an unusual amount of smooth muscle (Fig. 13.28). In addition to the thick circular arrangement of smooth muscle in its tunica media, the great saphenous vein possesses numerous longitudinal smooth muscle bundles in the intima and in the well-developed adventitia. A thin, poorly developed internal elastic membrane separates the tunica intima from the media. The great saphenous vein is frequently harvested from the lower limb and used for autotransplantation in **coronary artery bypass graft (CABG)** surgery when arterial grafts (usually taken from the internal thoracic artery) are not available or many grafts are required for multiple bypass anastomoses. CABG is the most common type of open-heart surgery performed in the United States.
- The **central adrenomedullary vein** that passes through the adrenal medulla and its tributaries has an unusual tunica media. It contains several longitudinally oriented bundles of smooth muscle cells that vary in size and appearance (Fig. 13.29). These irregularly arranged smooth muscle bundles (also called **muscle cushions**) extend into larger tributaries of the central adrenomedullary vein. This unique eccentric arrangement of smooth muscle bundles results in irregularity of the thickness of the vascular wall. In areas where muscle bundles are absent, cells of the adrenal medulla or sometimes adrenal cortex are separated from the lumen of the vein by only a thin layer of the tunica intima (see Fig. 13.29). Contraction of the longitudinally arranged smooth muscles in the tunica media enhances the efflux of hormones from the adrenal medulla into the circulation.

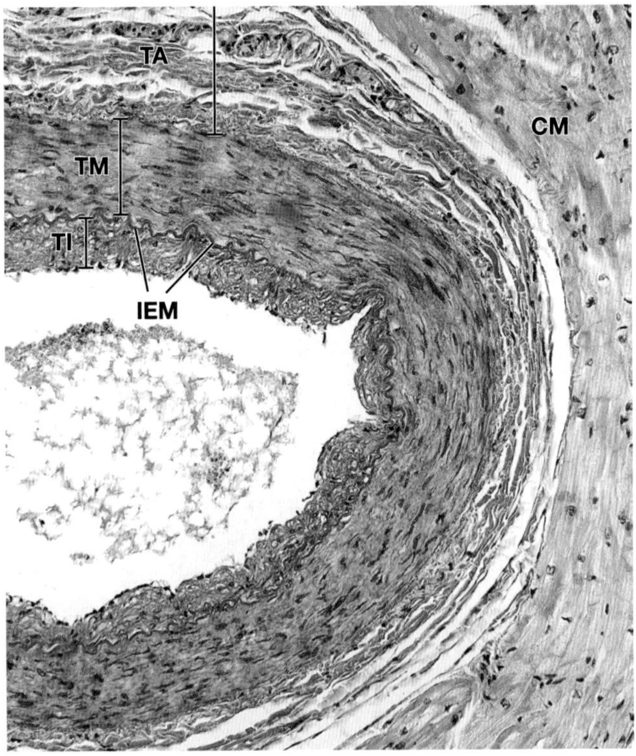

FIGURE 13.27. Photomicrograph of the coronary artery. This photomicrograph of a cross section of the coronary artery obtained from an adult human shows all three vascular tunics similar to those in muscular arteries. The subendothelial layer of the tunica intima (*TI*) is considerably thicker because of the aging process than a comparable muscular artery. The internal elastic membrane (*IEM*) is visible at the border with the tunica media (*TM*), which is also thicker than in other muscular-type arteries. Connective tissue of the tunica adventitia (*TA*) is loosely arranged and contains peripherally positioned longitudinal bundles of collagen fibers. There is an artificial separation between cardiac muscle (*CM*) and tunica adventitia. ×175.

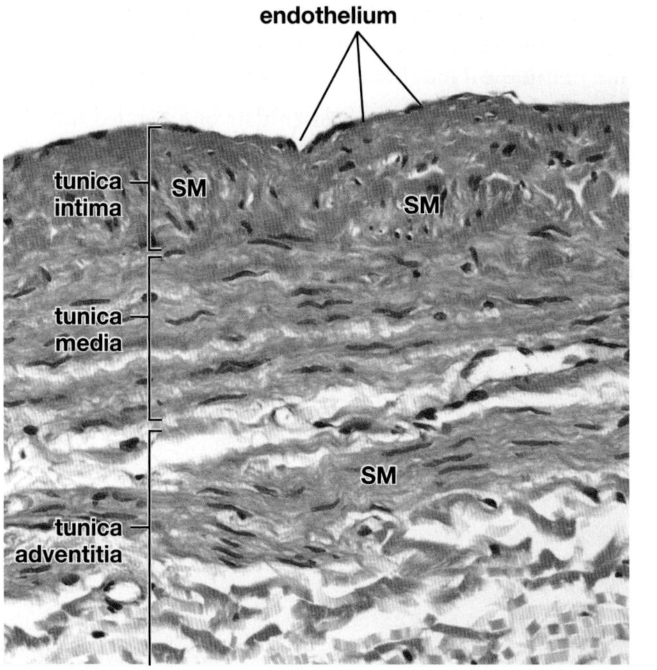

FIGURE 13.28. Photomicrograph of the great saphenous vein. This photomicrograph shows a section through the wall of the great saphenous vein. The tunica intima is usually thicker than in the other medium-sized veins and is characterized by the presence of numerous longitudinal smooth muscle bundles (*SM*) separated by connective tissue fibers. The tunica media contains a relatively thick layer of circularly arranged smooth muscles. The tunica adventitia is well developed and contains additional layers of smooth muscle fibers arranged in spiral, oblique, and longitudinal bundles. ×380. (Courtesy of Dr. Joseph J. Maleszewski.)

Veins in certain other locations (e.g., retina, placenta, trabeculae of the spleen) also have atypical walls and are discussed in the chapters that describe these organs.

■ LYMPHATIC VESSELS

Lymphatic vessels convey fluids from the tissues to the bloodstream and are important in the immunologic surveillance.

In addition to blood vessels, another set of vessels circulates fluid called **lymph** through most parts of the body. These lymph-carrying vessels serve as adjuncts to the blood vessels. Unlike the blood vessels, which convey blood to and from tissues, the **lymphatic vessels** are unidirectional, conveying fluid only from tissues. As mentioned earlier, approximately 90% of the extravasated fluid is reabsorbed at the venous side of the capillary network. Lymphatic vessels return the remaining 10% to the blood vascular system. In healthy adult individuals, the lymphatic system returns as much as 8 L of interstitial fluid with 20–30 g of protein per L to the blood circulation each day. In addition to this fluid **homeostasis function**, the lymphatic vessels are involved in the **immunologic surveillance** transporting antigens and antigen-presenting cells from the periphery to lymph nodes. In the gastrointestinal tract, lymphatics (lacteals) are crucial for **absorption of dietary fats** in the form of chylomicrons (an assembly of triglycerides, cholesterol, cholesteryl esters, phospholipids with apolipoprotein B). These processes all depend on the organized movement of fluid, solutes, and cells across the wall of the lymphatic vessel.

Defects affecting lymphatic vessels can lead to **lymphedema**, a clinical condition that is characterized by a localized accumulation of interstitial fluid and tissue swelling. The most common presentations involve swelling of upper and lower limbs, tissue fibrosis, susceptibility to infections, and accumulation of adipose tissue. **Primary lymphedema** has origin from genetic defects that affect the development of the lymphatic vessels, whereas **secondary lymphedema** is most likely caused by surgery, radiation therapy, infection, or trauma.

The smallest lymphatic vessels are called **lymphatic capillaries.** They are especially numerous in the loose connective tissues under the epithelium of the skin and mucous membranes. The lymphatic capillaries begin as "blind-ended" tubes in the microcapillary beds (see Fig. 13.23). Lymphatic capillaries converge into increasingly larger **collecting vessels** called **lymphatic vessels**, and they connect with chains of **lymph nodes** where lymph is filtrated. They ultimately unite to form two large lymphatic vessels that empty into the blood vascular system by draining into the large veins in the base of the neck. Lymph enters the vascular system at the junctions of the internal jugular and subclavian veins. The largest lymphatic vessel, draining most of the body and emptying into the veins on the left side, is the **thoracic duct**. The other main channel is the **right lymphatic trunk**.

Lymphatic capillaries are more permeable than blood capillaries and collect excess protein-rich tissue fluid.

Lymphatic capillaries are a unique part of the circulatory system, forming a network of small vessels within the tissues.

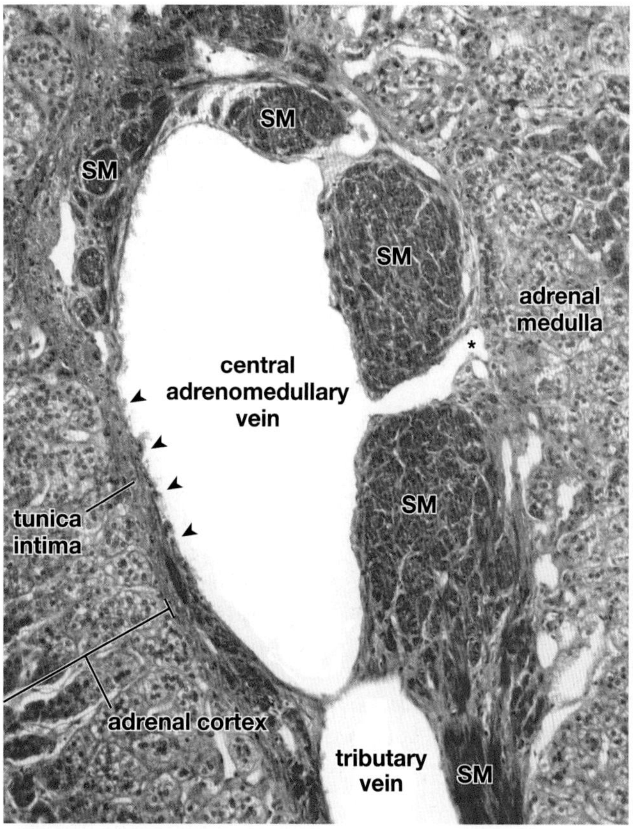

FIGURE 13.29. Photomicrograph of the central adrenomedullary vein. This photomicrograph of the human adrenal gland shows a large central adrenomedullary vein with its tributary stained with hematoxylin and eosin (H&E). The wall of the vein is highly irregular, containing several longitudinally oriented bundles of smooth muscles (*SM*) that extend into the wall of a tributary. This unique eccentric arrangement of smooth muscles, sometimes called *muscle cushions*, results in the irregularity of the thickness of the vascular wall. Note that in the cleft between two smooth muscle bundles (*asterisk*), the lumen of the vein is separated from the chromaffin cells of the adrenal medulla only by the tunica intima. On the opposite side of the wall, muscle bundles are absent (*arrowheads*) and the cells of the adrenal cortex are in direct contact with the tunica intima. ×120. (Courtesy of Dr. Donald J. Lowrie Jr., University of Cincinnati College of Medicine.)

Because of their greater permeability, lymphatic capillaries are more effective than blood capillaries in removing protein-rich fluid from the intercellular spaces. They are also specialized in the uptake of inflammatory molecules, dietary lipids, and immune cells. Once the collected fluid enters the lymphatic vessel, it is called **lymph**. Lymphatic vessels also serve to convey proteins and lipids that are too large to cross the fenestrations of the absorptive capillaries in the small intestine.

Before lymph is returned to the blood, it passes through **lymph nodes**, where it is exposed to the cells of the immune system. Thus, the lymphatic vessels serve not only as an adjunct to the blood vascular system but also as an integral component of the immune system.

Lymphatic capillaries have unique oak leaf–shaped endothelial cells with discontinuous basal lamina and button-like cell-to-cell junctions.

Lymphatic capillaries are essentially blind-ended tubes of endothelium that are approximately 30–80 μm in diameter. Unlike typical blood capillaries, they are not surrounded by pericytes or smooth muscle cells and **lack a continuous basal lamina** (Fig. 13.30). Lymphatic endothelial cells in lymphatic capillaries have a distinctive oak leaf shape. The overlapping flaps of adjacent endothelial cells interdigitate with one another (see Fig 13.30, inset). Lymphatic endothelial cells have characteristic **discontinuous** or **button-like**

FOLDER 13.3

CLINICAL CORRELATION: CORONARY HEART DISEASE

Coronary heart disease (CHD) is caused by an imbalance between the supply and demand of the heart for oxygenated blood. CHD is the most common type of heart disease in the United States and affects ~6% of the population. The most common cause of CHD is **atherosclerosis**, also called "hardening of the arteries." The risk of developing atherosclerosis increases with age, family history, hypertension, cigarette smoking, hypercholesterolemia, and diabetes. In atherosclerosis, the lumina of the coronary arteries progressively narrows because of the accumulation of lipids, extracellular matrix, and cells, leading to the development of **atheromatous plaques** (Fig. F13.3.1). Plaques are formed by intracellular and extracellular lipid deposition, smooth muscle

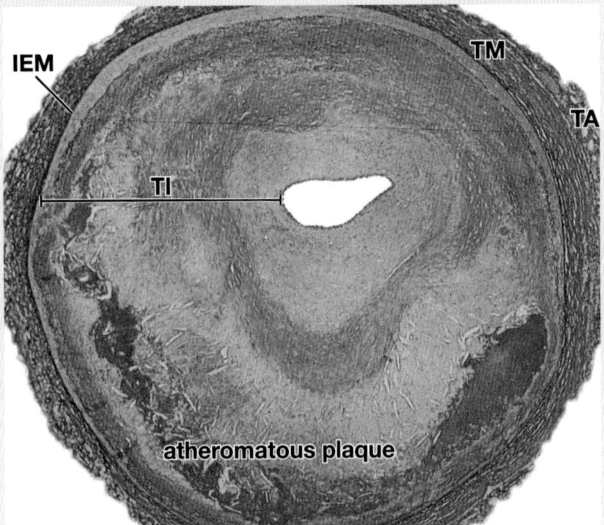

FIGURE F13.3.1. Photomicrograph of an atheromatous plaque in the coronary artery. This low-magnification photomicrograph shows a cross section of the human coronary artery with chronic coronary heart disease. The specimen is stained with the Verhoeff van Gieson technique for elastic and connective tissue fibers. The *black strands* represent elastic lamellae; a distinct intact internal elastic membrane (*IEM*) is present between the *dark red*–stained tunica media (*TM*) containing smooth muscle cells and the pathologically changed tunica intima (*TI*). Variable shades of *pink* material represent collagen fibers deposited in a thick tunica intima, which contains an advanced atheromatous plaque with visible calcifications (*dark pink-orange*) and accumulation of extracellular lipids (cholesterol clefts). The *light pink* color surrounding the lumen of the vessel represents the most recent deposition of the pathologic material. Note that the lumen of the vessel is occluded almost 90%, which leads to inadequate coronary blood flow. Tunica adventitia (*TA*) represents the outermost layer of the vessel. ×34. (Courtesy of Dr. William D. Edwards.)

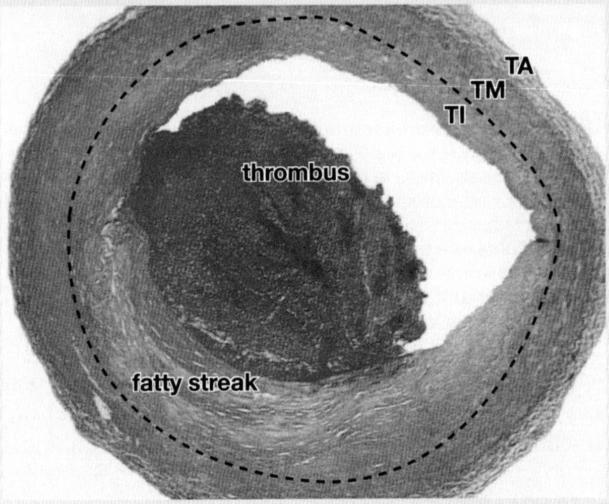

FIGURE F13.3.2. Photomicrograph of the coronary artery with a mural thrombus. This photomicrograph shows a cross section of the coronary artery in a less advanced stage of atherosclerotic disease. The fibrofatty plaque is visible in the tunica intima (*TI*) and a thrombus is superimposed on a plaque, partially obstructing the arterial lumen. The *dashed line* indicates the border between the tunica intima and the tunica media (*TM*). The tunica adventitia (*TA*) forms the outermost layer of the vessel. ×40. (Courtesy of Dr. William D. Edwards.)

proliferation, and increased synthesis of proteoglycans and collagen within the intima of the vessel wall. Blood flow becomes critical when it is reduced by ≥90%. Sudden occlusion of the narrowed lumen by a thrombus (blood clot) released from the surface of an atheromatous plaque precipitates an acute ischemic event. Ischemic events are characterized by **anginal pain** associated with loss of oxygenated blood flow to the region of the heart supplied by the affected coronary vessel. **Coronary artery thrombosis** usually precedes and precipitates a **myocardial infarction**—that is, a sudden insufficiency of blood supply that results in an area of muscle cell death. A mural thrombus may develop and is usually associated with dysfunctional or ruptured endothelium overlying atheromatous plaque (Fig. F13.3.2). With time, the area of the heart affected by the myocardial infarction heals. A scar forms and replaces the damaged tissue, but the area of infarction loses contractile function. Multiple infarctions over time can produce sufficient loss of cardiac function to cause death. Infarction also commonly occurs in the brain, spleen, kidney, lung, intestine, testes, and tumors (especially of the ovaries and uterus).

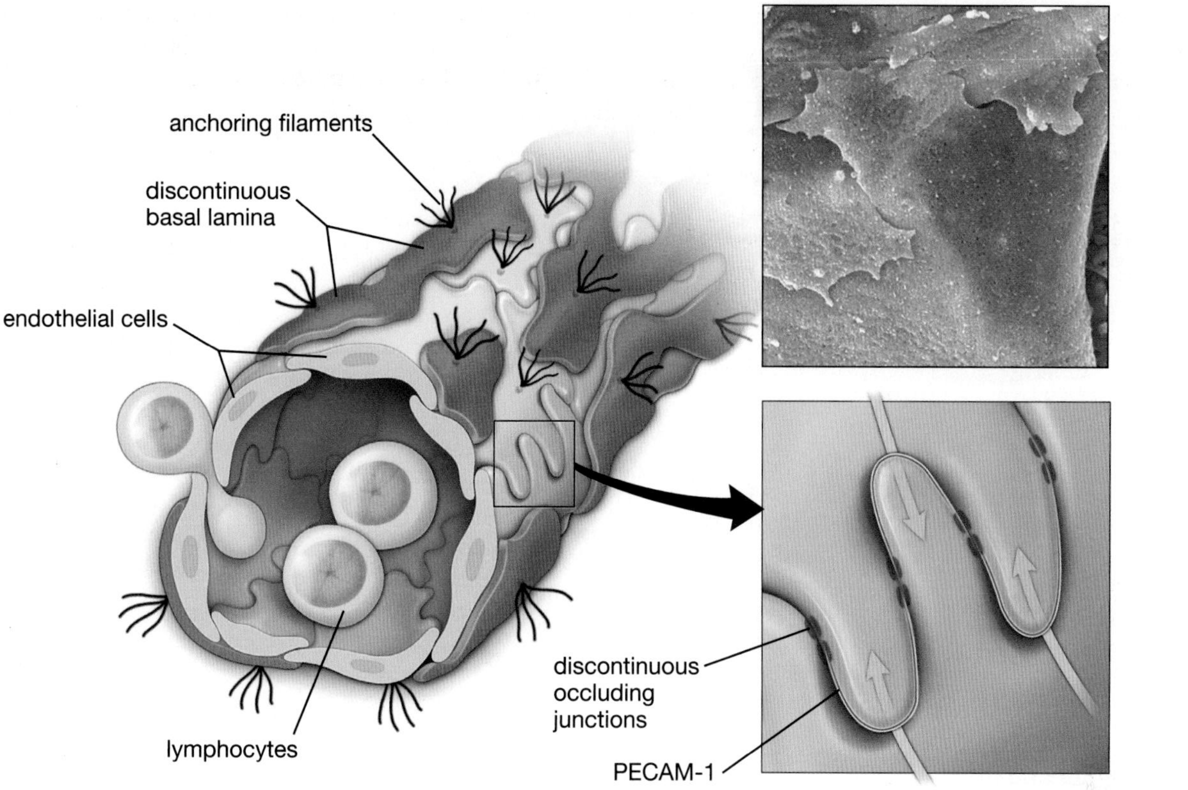

FIGURE 13.30. Diagrams and scanning electron microscope of a lymphatic capillary. Lymphatic capillaries are characterized by a discontinuous basal lamina and anchoring filaments that extend from endothelial cells to the extracellular matrix. Anchoring filaments consist of fibrillin microfibrils similar to those found in the elastic fibers. In the large figure on the *left*, note the overlapping flaps of adjacent endothelial cells that interdigitate with one another. The *lower inset* is an enlarged view of the basal domain of lymphatic endothelial cells containing discontinuous occluding junctions (button-like cell-to-cell adhesions). These junctions are concentrated at the overlapping edges of the cells. The gaps between tight junctions at the tip of the flaps express platelet and endothelial cell adhesion molecule-1 (PECAM-1). Interactions between leukocyte PECAM-1 and endothelial PECAM-1 are required for the migration of lymphocytes into the lymphatic capillary in the direction shown by the *yellow arrows*. The *upper inset* is a scanning electron micrograph showing the loosely apposed overlapping borders of lymphatic endothelial cells as they are visible from the basal domain of lymphatic endothelial cells following the removal of surrounding connective tissue. ×32,000. (Reprinted with permission from Baluk P, McDonald DM. Buttons and zippers: endothelial junctions in lymphatic vessels. *Cold Spring Harb Perspect Med.* 2022,12:a041178.)

cell-to-cell junctions concentrated at the scalloped edges of the cells. These junctions are similar to **occluding (tight) junctions** in vascular epithelial cells composed of occludins, claudins, zonula occludens-1 (ZO-1), and junctional adhesion molecules (JAMs). They also contain **vascular endothelial cadherin** (VE-cadherin), which is found in the anchoring junctions. The gaps between tight junctions at the tip of the flaps express **platelet and endothelial cell adhesion molecule-1 (PECAM-1**; also known as CD31). Homophilic interactions between leukocyte PECAM-1 and endothelial PECAM-1 are required for the migration of lymphocytes into the lymphatic capillary. Therefore, these areas provide the entry point for leukocytes, dendritic cells, and interstitial fluid into the vessels. The incomplete basal lamina and discontinuous cell-to-cell junctions are correlated with their high permeability, which enables optimal uptake of lymph components.

The lymphatic capillaries are connected to the surrounding extracellular matrix by **anchoring filaments** that extend between endothelial cells and their incomplete basal lamina and the perivascular collagen (see Fig. 13.30). They consist of **fibrillin microfibrils** composed of **fibrillin-1** molecules and microfibril-associated protein **emilin-1**, which are similar to those found in elastic fibers of connective tissue. Anchoring filaments maintain the patency of the vessels during times of increased tissue pressure, such as in inflammation. Deficiency in emilin-1 synthesis in animals is related to structural and functional defects of lymphatic capillaries.

The lymphatic endothelial cells are terminally differentiated cells distinct from blood vascular endothelial cells. In the early embryo, under the influence of prospero-related homeobox transcription factor (**Prox-1**) or vascular endothelial growth factor C (**VEGF-C**), lymphatic endothelial cells bud from cardinal veins, giving rise to primitive lymph sacs. Lymphatic vessels subsequently sprout from lymphatic sacs, forming a separate vascular network with lymphatic vascular–specific molecules expressed on the surface of lymphatic endothelial cells. Markers used for identifying lymphatic vessels in tissues include **Prox-1**, the transmembrane glycoprotein **podoplanin (PDPN)**, vascular endothelial growth factor receptor-3 (**VEGFR-3**), and lymphatic vessel hyaluronan receptor-1 (**LYVE-1**). Clinically, podoplanin is widely utilized as a marker for lymphatic differentiation in the evaluation of vascular tumors.

In contrast to lymphatic capillaries, the lumens of **lymphatic vessels** exhibit features to prevent leakage of lymph. These include **continuous (zipper-like) tight junctions** between the endothelial cells and a continuous basal lamina that is surrounded by smooth muscle cells. As lymphatic vessels become larger, their walls thicken as more connective tissue and bundles of smooth muscle are added. Lymphatic vessels possess bileaflet **valves** that prevent backflow of the lymph, thus aiding unidirectional flow (Plate 13.4, page 480). There is no central pump in the lymphatic system. Lymph moves sluggishly, driven primarily by compression of the lymphatic vessels by adjacent skeletal muscles. In addition, contraction of the smooth muscle layer surrounding lymphatic vessels may help propel the lymph.

HISTOLOGY 101 NOTEBOOK

CARDIOVASCULAR SYSTEM

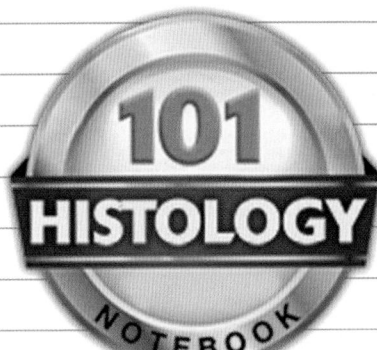

OVERVIEW OF THE CARDIOVASCULAR SYSTEM

- The **cardiovascular system** includes the heart, blood vessels, and lymphatic vessels. It carries blood and lymph to and from tissues of the body.
- The cardiovascular system consists of the **pulmonary circulation** (conveys arterial blood from the heart to the lungs and returns venous blood back to the heart) and **systemic circulation** (conveys arterial blood from the heart to all other tissues and returns venous blood back to the heart).

HEART

- The **heart** is a four-chambered muscular pump (two atria and two ventricles). It contains **cardiac muscle** (for contraction to propel blood), a **fibrous skeleton** (for attachment of valves and separation of atrial and ventricular musculature), a **conducting system** (for initiation and propagation of rhythmic contractions), and **coronary vasculature** (coronary arteries and cardiac veins).
- The wall of the heart is composed of three layers: epicardium, myocardium, and endocardium.
- **Epicardium** (visceral layer of serous pericardium) is the outer layer of the heart and consists of mesothelium with underlying connective and adipose tissue. It contains coronary vasculature.
- **Myocardium** is the middle layer and consists of cardiac muscle.
- **Endocardium** is the inner layer and consists of endothelium, subendothelial connective tissue, and a subendocardial layer containing cells of the conducting system of the heart.
- **Heart valves** are composed of three layers: **fibrosa**, **spongiosa**, and either **ventricularis** (in semilunar valves) or **atrialis** (in atrioventricular valves).
- Contraction of the heart is initiated and synchronized by the **conducting system**, which consists of modified cardiac myocytes forming the **sinoatrial (or sinu-atrial) (SA) node, atrioventricular (AV) node, AV bundle (of His),** and **Purkinje fibers.**
- The heart rate is regulated by the sympathetic nerves (increase rate) and parasympathetic nerves (decrease rate) as well as by circulating hormones (**epinephrine** and **norepinephrine**) and other substances (Ca^{2+}, thyroid hormones, caffeine, etc.).

GENERAL FEATURES OF ARTERIES AND VEINS

- The walls of arteries and veins are composed of three layers called *tunics*.
- **Tunica intima**, the innermost layer of the vessel, consists of **endothelium**, a **subendothelial layer** of connective tissue, and an **internal elastic membrane.**
- **Tunica media**, the middle layer, consists of circumferentially arranged layers of vascular smooth muscle cells with elastic lamellae interposed between them. In arteries, tunica media is relatively thick and extends between the internal and external elastic membranes.
- **Tunica adventitia**, the outermost connective tissue layer, is composed primarily of collagen with few dispersed elastic fibers. It contains **vasa vasorum** and a network of autonomic nerves called **nervi vasorum (vascularis).**
- **Endothelial cells** actively interact with underlying vascular smooth muscle cells and connective tissue. In addition to maintaining a selective permeability barrier between blood and connective tissue, the endothelial cells prevent blood clotting (by secretion of anticoagulants and antithrombogenic agents), modulate vascular resistance (by secretion of vasoconstrictors and vasodilators), and regulate immune responses.

ARTERIES

- **Arteries** are classified into three types based on the size and thickness of their tunica media: large arteries (elastic arteries), medium arteries (muscular arteries), and small arteries (including arterioles).
- **Elastic arteries** have a tunica media that consists of multiple layers of vascular smooth muscle cells separated by elastic lamellae. Fibroblasts are not present in the tunica media.
- **Muscular arteries** have a tunica media with more smooth muscle and less elastic lamellae than the elastic arteries. They also have a prominent internal elastic membrane in the tunica intima.
- **Small arteries** and arterioles are distinguished from one another by the number of smooth muscle cell layers in the tunica media.
- **Arterioles** have one to two layers of smooth muscles and regulate **vascular resistance,** thus controlling blood flow to capillary networks.
- **Arteriovenous shunts** allow blood to bypass capillaries by providing direct routes between the arteries and the veins. This pathway is regulated by contraction of precapillary sphincters on the **metarterioles.**

CAPILLARIES

- **Capillaries** are the smallest diameter blood vessels and are classified into three different types: **continuous** (characterized by uninterrupted vascular endothelium), **fenestrated** (characterized by numerous openings in the capillary wall and the continuous basal lamina), and **discontinuous** or **sinusoidal** capillaries (larger in diameter with large openings, intercellular gaps, and a **discontinuous basal lamina**).
- **Pericytes** associated with capillaries represent a population of undifferentiated mesenchymal stem cells.

VEINS

- **Veins** are divided into four types based on their size (diameter): **venules** (<0.1 mm), **small veins** (<1 mm), **medium veins** (<10 mm), and **large veins** (>10 mm).
- **Postcapillary venules** collect blood from the capillary network and are characterized by the presence of pericytes. In lymphoid tissues, they are lined by cuboidal endothelium (**high endothelial venules**), which facilitates extensive lymphocyte migration from the blood.
- **Small, medium,** and **large veins** have a relatively thin layer of tunica media and a more pronounced tunica adventitia.
- Veins, especially of limbs, may contain **valves** preventing the backflow of blood.
- **Large veins** near the heart may contain **myocardial sleeves** in the tunica adventitia.

LYMPHATIC VESSELS

- **Lymphatic vessels** convey interstitial fluids from tissues to the bloodstream.
- The smallest and most permeable lymphatic vessels are called **lymphatic capillaries.** They drain lymph into larger collecting lymphatic vessels and then into the thoracic duct or right lymphatic trunk before emptying it into the venous system.
- All collecting lymphatic vessels possess valves that prevent the backflow of lymph.

PLATE 13.1 ■ HEART

The **cardiovascular system** is a transport system that carries blood and lymph to and from the tissues of the body. The cardiovascular system includes the heart, blood vessels, and lymphatic vessels. Blood vessels provide the route by which blood circulates to and from all parts of the body. The heart pumps the blood. Lymphatic vessels carry tissue-derived fluid, called *lymph*, back to the blood vascular system.

The **heart** is a four-chambered organ consisting of a right and left atrium and a right and left ventricle. Blood from the body is returned to the right atrium from which it enters the right ventricle. Blood is pumped from the right ventricle to the lungs for oxygenation and returns to the left atrium. Blood from the left atrium enters the left ventricle from which it is pumped to the rest of the body, that is, the systemic circulation.

The heart, which forms from a straight vascular tube in the embryo, has the same basic three-layered structure in its wall as do the blood vessels above the level of capillaries and postcapillary venules. In the blood vessels, the three layers are called the **tunica intima**, including the vascular endothelium and its underlying connective tissue; the **tunica media**, a muscular layer that varies in thickness in arteries and veins; and the **tunica adventitia**, the outermost layer of relatively dense connective tissue. In the heart, these layers are called the *endocardium*, the *myocardium*, and the *epicardium*, respectively.

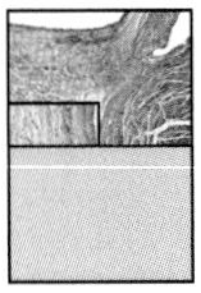

Atrioventricular septum, heart, human, hematoxylin and eosin (H&E) ×45; inset ×125.

This micrograph of the field shows portions of the atrial (*A*) and ventricular (*V*) walls at the level of the **atrioventricular septum** and the root of the mitral valve (*MV*). Both chambers and the valve are lined with squamous endothelium of the endocardium (*En*). **Purkinje fibers** (*PF*) of the cardiac conduction system are seen in the atrial wall between the relatively thin subendocardial connective tissue (*CT*) and the underlying modified **cardiac muscle cells** (*CM*) of the atrioventricular node (*AVN*). Dense fibrous connective tissue (*DCT*) that is continuous with that of the septum and the subendocardial layers of the atrium and ventricle extends from the root of the valve into the leaflet. Thin cardiac muscle fibers can also be seen extending from the wall of the atrium into the upper portion of the valve. **Inset.** This higher magnification view of the area outlined by the *rectangle* (turned ~90°) shows more clearly the endothelial layer of the **endocardium** (*En*) and the dense fibrous connective tissue of the endocardium (*DCT*) and subendocardial layer. A thin layer of smooth muscle (*SM*) appears between the more densely packed fibrous tissue immediately subjacent to the endothelium and the more loosely packed dense fibrous tissue of the subendocardium. Particularly evident are the longitudinally sectioned Purkinje fibers (*PF*) of the cardiac conduction system. These modified cardiac muscle cells contain the same fibrillar contractile system as their smaller counterparts in the myocardium, but the fibrils are fewer, more loosely packed, and often surround what appear to be vacuolated areas. **Intercalated discs** (*ID*), typical of cardiac muscle cell organization, are evident in some areas.

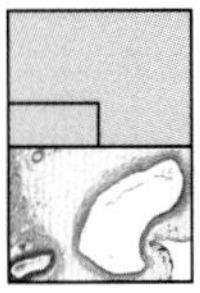

Coronary artery and cardiac vein, heart, human, H&E ×30.

This micrograph shows cross sections of a coronary artery and cardiac vein in the coronary sulcus. The surrounding adipose tissue (*AT*) serves to cushion the blood vessels that run in the coronary sulcus. The **coronary artery** (*CA*) in the *lower left* of this micrograph is surrounded by small bundles of small cardiac muscle cells (*CM*) that are part of the atrioventricular node (*AVN*). A small lymph node (*LN*) and a loop of the conduction bundle (*CB*) containing **Purkinje fibers** are evident next to the artery. The darkly stained tunica intima (*TI*) is delimited by an internal elastic membrane (*IEM*) that is easily distinguished even at this relatively low magnification. The thick muscular tunica media (*TM*) is also easily distinguished from the thinner, fibrous tunica adventitia (*TA*). A smaller arterial vessel (*A′*) is visible in the *upper left* of the micrograph. The larger vessel, the cardiac vein (*CV*), has a large lumen and thin wall relative to its size, a feature typical of veins compared to arteries. The tunica intima (*TI*) of this vein again appears as a darker layer. At this magnification, it is not possible to distinguish the tunica media from the adventitia. Partial aggregates of blood (*B*) cellular elements are present in the lumens of the vessels.

A, atrium
A′, small artery
AT, adipose tissue
AVN, atrioventricular node
B, blood
CA, coronary artery
CB, conduction bundle
CM, cardiac muscle
CT, connective tissue
CV, cardiac vein
DCT, dense connective tissue
En, endothelium
ID, intercalated disc
IEM, internal elastic membrane
LN, lymph node
MV, mitral valve
PF, Purkinje fibers
SM, smooth muscle
TA, tunica adventitia
TI, tunica intima
TM, tunica media
V, ventricle

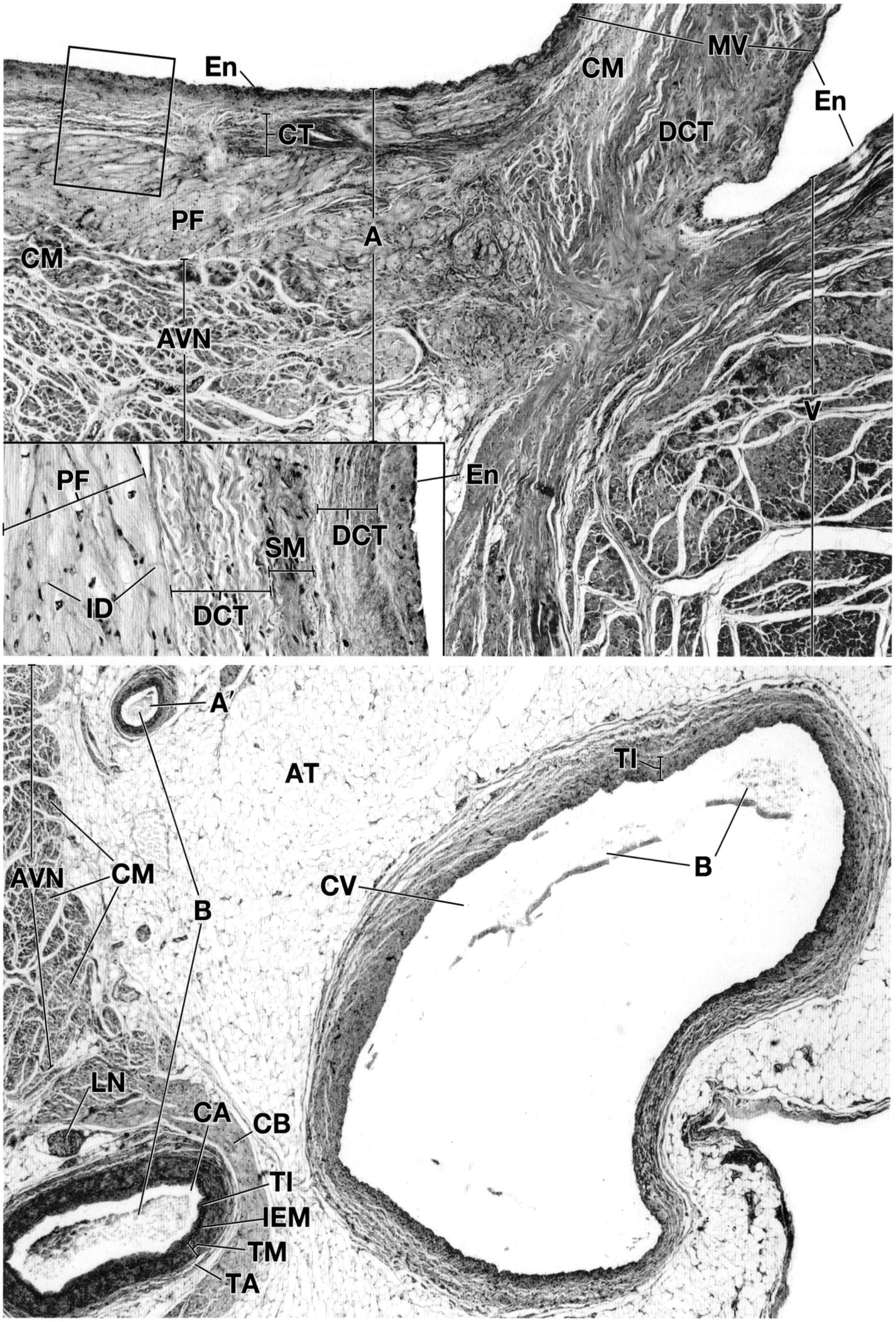

En
MV
CM
En
CT
DCT
A
PF
CM
AVN
V
PF
En
DCT
SM
ID
DCT
A
AT
TI
B
AVN
CM
CV
B
LN
CA
CB
TI
IEM
TM
TA

PLATE 13.2 ■ AORTA

The **aorta**, the main systemic artery of the body, is an elastic artery. The presence of numerous fenestrated elastic lamellae allows it to resist the pressure variations caused by a rhythmic contraction of the left ventricle. The **intima** is comparatively much thicker than that seen in muscular arteries. The subendothelial layer of the intima consists of connective tissue with both collagen and elastic fibers. The cellular component consists of smooth muscle cells and fibroblasts. The external border of the intima is bounded by an internal elastic membrane that represents the first layer of the many concentric fenestrated laminae in the media of the vessel. The **media** constitutes the bulk of the wall. Between the elastic laminae are collagen fibers and smooth muscle cells. The latter are responsible for the synthesis of collagen and elastic fibers. With increasing age, the number and thickness of elastic laminae in the wall increase. By the age 35 years, as many as 60 laminae are found in the thoracic aorta. At ~50 years of age, individual laminae begin to show signs of degeneration and gradually become replaced by collagen, leading to a gradual loss of elasticity of the aortic wall.

The **adventitia** consists of irregular dense connective tissue with intermixed elastic fibers that tend to be organized in a circumferential pattern. It also contains small blood vessels that supply the outer portion of the media. They are the vasa vasorum of the aorta. Also present in the adventitia are lymphatic capillaries.

ORIENTATION MICROGRAPHS: The *upper micrograph* shows a cross section of a hematoxylin and eosin (H&E)-stained human aorta from a child. The intima (*I*) stains considerably lighter than the adjacent media (*M*). The adventitia (*A*) contains an abundance of collagenous fibers and stains more densely than that of either the media or the intima. The *lower micrograph* is from an adult and has been stained to reveal the elastic component of the vessel wall. The intima (*I*) is very lightly stained, in this case, owing to the paucity of elastic material. The media (*M*) is heavily stained owing to the presence of large amounts of elastic laminae. The adventitia (*A*) contains, in addition to the dense connective tissue, a moderate amount of elastic fibers.

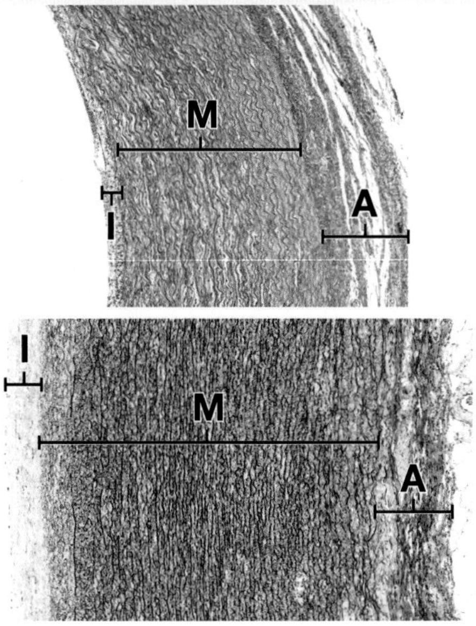

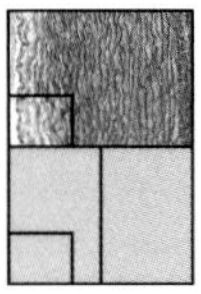

Aorta, human, H&E ×365; inset ×700.

This micrograph shows the layers of the aortic wall. The intima consists of an endothelium (*En*) overlying loose connective tissue (*LCT*). The thickest portion of the vessel wall is the media (*M*). The wavy eosinophilic material is the collagenous fibers. The eosin stain does not reveal the elastic laminae. The nuclei are those of smooth muscle cells. Fibroblasts are absent. The outer layer of the vessel wall is the adventitia (*A*). The eosinophilic material here consists of dense connective tissue. The nuclei that are evident belong to fibroblasts. Also note the small blood vessel (*BV*) in the adventitia. The *inset* shows the intima at higher magnification and includes part of the media. Note the endothelium (*En*). The eosinophilic material in the intima consists of collagenous fibers (*CF*). The main cell type here is the smooth muscle cell (*SMC*).

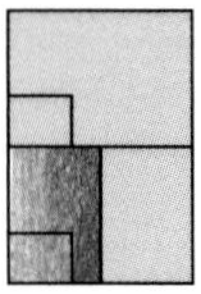

Aorta, human, iron hematoxylin and aniline blue ×255; inset ×350.

The specimen shown here has been stained to distinguish collagen from elastic material. The intima (*I*) consists mostly of collagenous fibers. The endothelium (*En*) represented by several nuclei is just barely evident. The media (*M*) contains numerous elastic lamellae that appear as the *black wavy lines*. The intervening *blue*-stained material consists of collagen fibers. Careful examination of the media reveals nuclei of smooth muscle cells dispersed between the elastic lamellae. The *inset* shows the intima at higher magnification. Note the nuclei of the endothelial cells (*EnC*) at the luminal surface. The remainder of the intima consists mostly of collagenous fibers (stained *blue*) with occasional elastic fibers (*EF*) identified by their *darker coloration*. The nuclei of the fibroblasts and occasional smooth muscle cells (*SMC*) appear randomly arranged.

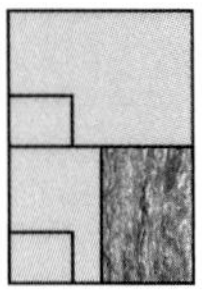

Aorta, human, iron hematoxylin and aniline blue ×255.

This micrograph shows the outer portion of the media (*M*) with its elastic lamellae. The major portion of the micrograph is the adventitia (*A*). Here, the thick collagenous fibers (*CF*) are readily recognized. The outer portion of the adventitia contains numerous elastic fibers that appear as *black*, *dot-like* structures. These elastic fibers are arranged in a circumferential pattern, thus when sectioned, they appear as *black*, *dot-like* structures.

A, adventitia
BV, blood vessel
CF, collagenous fibers
EF, elastic fibers
En, endothelium
EnC, endothelial cells
I, intima
LCT, loose connective tissue
M, media
SMC, smooth muscle cells

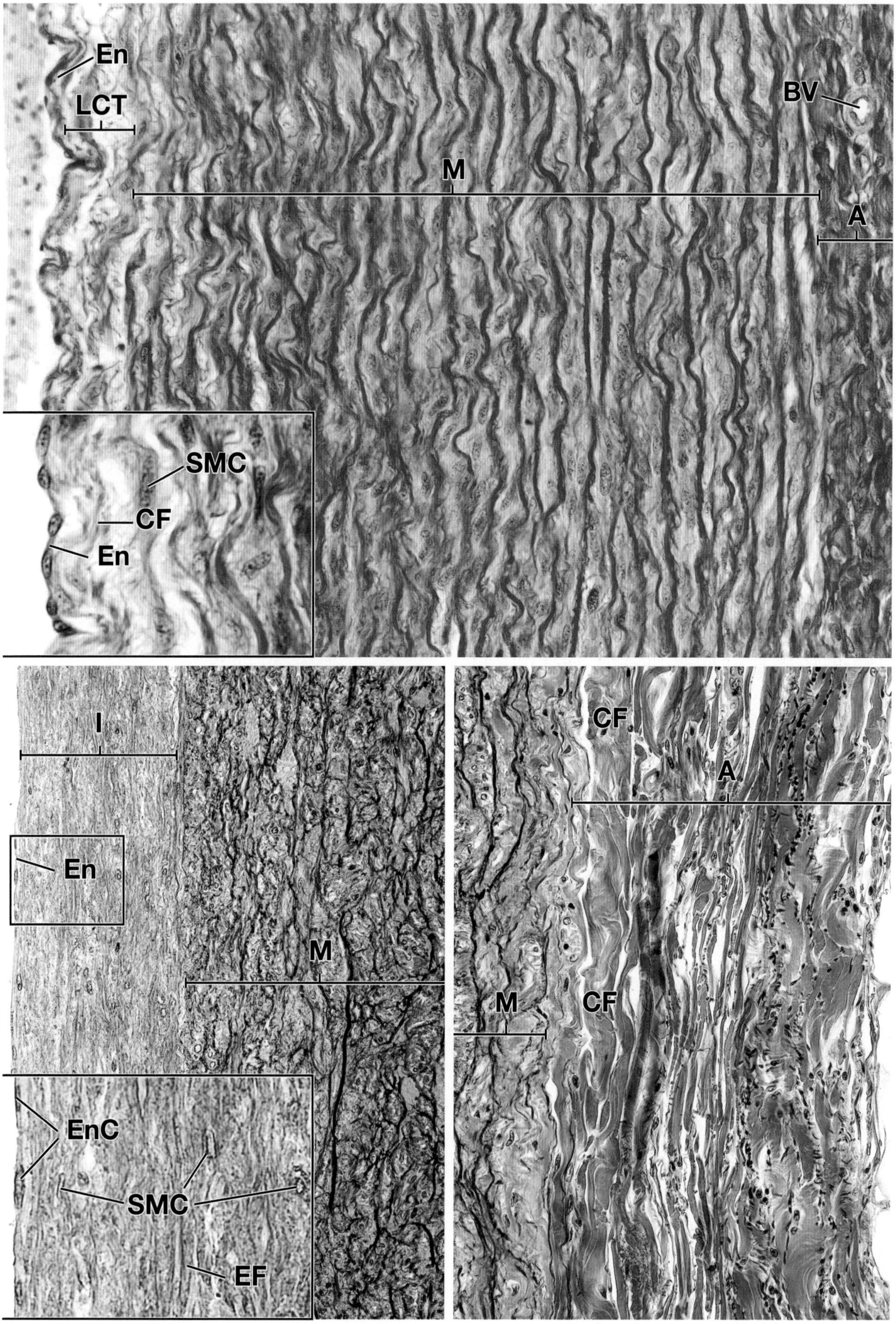
En
LCT
BV
M
A
SMC
CF
En
I
En
M
EnC
SMC
EF
CF
A
M
CF

PLATE 13.3 ■ MUSCULAR ARTERIES AND MEDIUM VEINS

Muscular arteries have more smooth muscle and less elastin in the tunica media than do elastic arteries. Thus, as the arterial tree is traced further from the heart, the elastic tissue is considerably reduced, and smooth muscle becomes the predominant component of the tunica media. The muscular arteries are characterized, however, by a refractile **internal elastic membrane** separating the tunica intima from the tunica media and usually by an **external elastic membrane** separating the tunica media from the tunica adventitia. Muscular arteries, or arteries of medium caliber, constitute the majority of the named arteries in the body. Veins usually accompany arteries as they travel in the loose connective tissue. The veins have the same three layers in their walls, but the tunica media is thinner than in the accompanying artery, and the tunica adventitia is the predominant layer in the wall. The veins usually have the same name as the artery they accompany.

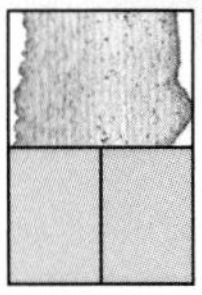

Muscular artery and medium vein, monkey, hematoxylin and eosin (H&E) ×365.

In this photomicrograph, the lumen of the artery is at the *left* and the lumen of the vein is at the *right*. Both vessels are joined by their outermost layers of tunica adventitia in the *middle* of this image. The arterial endothelium (*AEn*) is clearly seen on the corrugated surface of the tunica intima, whereas the venous endothelium (*VEn*) is somewhat harder to distinguish. The internal elastic membrane (*IEM*) of the artery is seen as a corrugated thin clear ribbon immediately beneath the endothelial layer, separating the tunica intima from the underlying smooth muscle (*SM*) layer of the tunica media (*TM*). The external elastic membrane containing elastic fibers (*EF*) separates the tunica media (TM) from the tunica adventitia of the artery (*TA′*). It is evident here that the tunica media is almost twice as thick as the tunica adventitia (TA′). The tunica media of the vein at the *right* is thin and difficult to detect. It contains a layer of small smooth muscles (*SSm*) that is adjacent to thick tunica adventitia (*TA*), which is about twice as thick as the tunica media in the vein. Tunica adventitia represents the outermost connective tissue layer containing bundles of collagen fibers with visible nuclei (*N*) of fibroblasts.

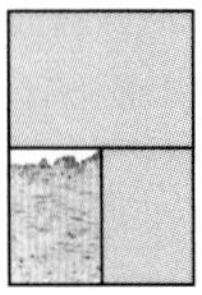

Muscular artery, monkey, H&E ×545.

This is a higher magnification micrograph of the portion of the previous figure outlined by the *rectangle* turned 90 degree. At this magnification, it is evident that the flattened endothelial cells (*EN*) follow the contours of the refractile, corrugated internal elastic membrane (*IEM*), which rests directly on the most luminal layer of smooth muscle cells (*SM*) of the thick tunica media (*TM*). The *lower portion* of the micrograph is occupied by the tunica adventitia (*TA′*), which is ~3 times thinner than that of the tunica media. Nuclei (*N*) of fibroblasts are visible among bundles of collagen fibers (*C*) and elastic fibers (*EF*) at the intersection between the tunica media (*TM*) and the tunica adventitia (*TA′*) of the artery.

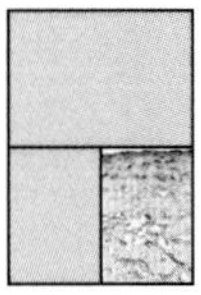

Medium vein, monkey, H&E ×600.

In this higher magnification view of a portion of the wall of the vein in the previous figure, the endothelial cells (*EN*) are more easily recognized and are seen to be plumper than those of the arterial endothelium. The margin between the tunica intima (*TI*) and the thin tunica media (*TM*) is difficult to discern, but the smooth muscle cells (*SM*) in the thin media are more easily recognized than in the previous figure because of the shape of their nuclei and the slight basophilia of their cytoplasm. The tunica adventitia (*TA*) is about twice as thick as the tunica media and appears to contain only bundles of collagen fibers and fibroblasts, with the latter recognizable by their nuclei (*N*). The collagen bundles of the loose connective tissue beneath the tunica adventitia are larger than those of the adventitia, and there are fewer cells in this portion of the specimen.

AEn, arterial endothelium
C, collagen bundles
EF, elastic fibers
EN, endothelial cells
IEM, internal elastic membrane
N, nuclei
SM, smooth muscle
SSm, small smooth muscle
TA, tunica adventitia of accompanying vein
TA′, tunica adventitia of artery
TI, tunica intima
TM, tunica media
VEn, venous endothelium

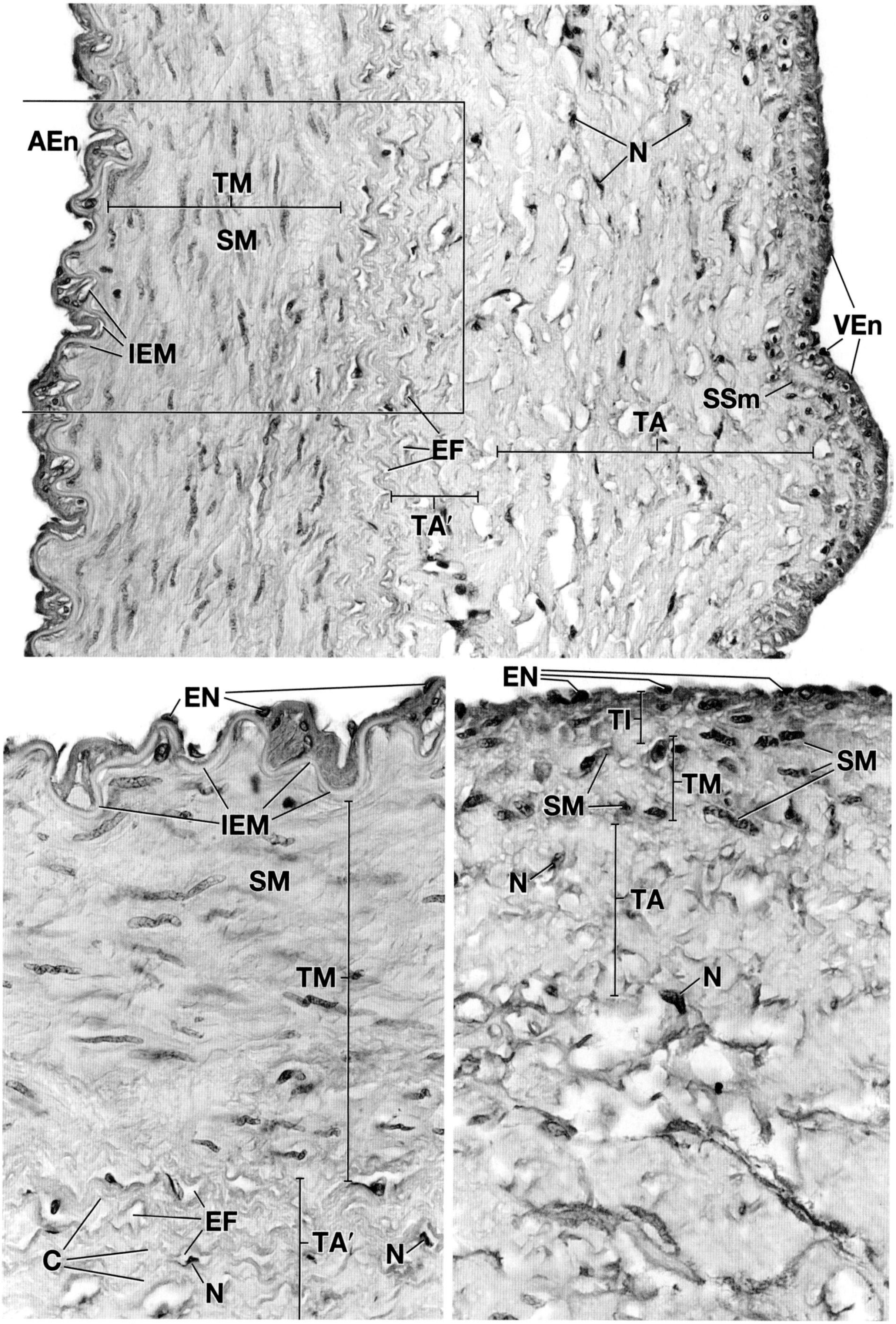
AEn
TM
SM
IEM
N
VEn
SSm
TA
EF
TA′
EN
IEM
SM
TM
EF
C
N
TA′
N
EN
TI
SM
TM
SM
N
TA
N

PLATE 13.4 ■ ARTERIOLES, VENULES, AND LYMPHATIC VESSELS

The terminal components of the arterial tree just before a capillary bed or an arteriovenous shunt are the **arterioles.** Arterioles have an endothelial lining and smooth muscle in the wall, but the smooth muscle is limited in thickness to one or two cells. There may or may not be an internal elastic membrane, according to the size of the vessel. Arterioles control blood flow into capillary networks. In the normal relationship between an arteriole and a capillary network, contraction of the smooth muscle of the arteriole wall reduces or shuts off the blood going to the capillaries. A **precapillary sphincter** is formed by a slight thickening of the smooth muscle at the origin of a capillary bed from an arteriole. Nerve impulses and hormonal stimulation can cause the muscle cells to contract, directing blood into capillary beds where it is most needed.

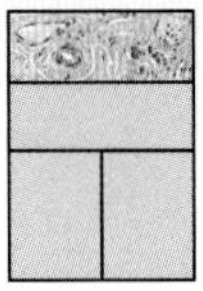

Arteriole, venule, and small nerve, fingertip, human, hematoxylin and eosin (H&E) ×600.

This micrograph shows two cross-sectioned arterioles (*A*) and a venule (*V*). The **arteriole** on the *left* is identified as a large arteriole, based on the presence of two discrete layers of smooth muscle cells that form the tunica media of the vessel. The nuclei of the muscle cells appear in longitudinal profile as a result of the circumferential arrangement of the cells. The endothelial cell nuclei of the vessel appear as small round profiles surrounding the lumen. These cells are elongated and oriented with their long axis in the direction of flow. Thus, their nuclei are seen here as cross-sectioned profiles. The arteriole on the *right* is a very small arteriole, having only a single layer of smooth muscle. Again, the muscle cell nuclei are seen in longitudinal profile. The endothelial cell nuclei appear as *small round* profiles at the luminal surface. A venule is seen in proximity to the larger arteriole, and a cross section of peripheral nerve (*N*) is seen in proximity to the smaller arteriole. Compare the wall of the **venule**, consisting only of endothelium and a thin layer of connective tissue, with the arterioles. Also, note the relatively large lumen of the venule.

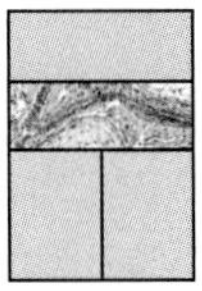

Arteriole, fingertip, human, H&E ×350.

This micrograph shows a longitudinal section of an **arteriole.** Because of its twisting path through the section, its wall has been cut such that the single layer of muscle cells of the tunica media is seen in different planes along its length. In segment numbered *1*, at the *left*, the vessel wall has been cut tangentially. Thus, the vessel lumen is not included in the plane of section, but the smooth muscle cell nuclei of the tunica media are seen in longitudinal profile. After the arteriole makes an acute turn (segment numbered *2*), the vessel wall is cut to reveal the lumen. Here, the smooth muscle nuclei appear as round profiles, and the nuclei of the endothelial cells lining the lumen appear in longitudinal profile. In segment numbered *3*, the vessel wall is again only grazed. In segment numbered *4*, the cut is deeper, again showing the lumen and some of the endothelial cells in face view (*arrowheads*). The washed-out area above segment numbered *4* represents adipose tissue (*AT*). The area below the vessel is occupied by dense irregular connective tissue (*DCT*) and contains an encapsulated nerve ending known as a Pacinian corpuscle (*P*) that detects pressure and vibration applied to the skin surface.

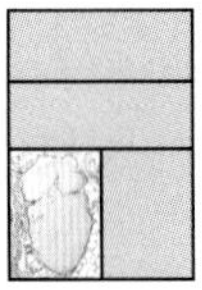

Lymphatic vessel, fingertip, human, H&E ×175.

The **lymphatic vessel** shown in this figure shows a region where the vessel is making a U-shaped turn in the plane of the section, thus disappearing at the *top* and *bottom* of the micrograph. The wall of the vessel consists of an endothelial lining and a small amount of connective tissue, with one being indistinguishable from the other. A **valve** (*Val*), which is characteristic of lymphatic vessels, is seen within the vessel. It is formed from a minuscule layer of connective tissue that is covered on both sides by endothelium. The *arrows* indicate nuclei that are just barely visible at this magnification; most of them belong to endothelial cells. Typically, the lumen contains precipitated lymph material (*L*); sometimes, lymphocytes may be present. Adjacent to the vessel, on the *right*, is adipose tissue (*AT*), and on the *upper left* is dense irregular connective tissue (*DCT*).

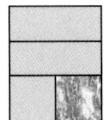

Lymphatic vessel, fingertip, human, Mallory trichrome ×375.

The **lymphatic vessel** shown here is contained within dense irregular connective tissue (*DCT*). The lumen is irregular, appearing relatively narrow below the valve (*Val*). A few endothelial cell nuclei are evident (*arrows*). A thin layer of connective tissue that is present outside the endothelium blends with the dense connective tissue beyond the wall of the vessel. A venule (*V*) and arteriole (*A*) are also present; they can readily be distinguished from the lymphatic vessel by thicker walls and by the presence of red blood cells in the lumen. Also at the *bottom left*, note a single adipocyte (*Ad*) from which a lipid droplet has been removed during slide preparation. In contrast to the lumen of the lymphatic vessel, which contains precipitated lymph material (*L*), the space occupied by the lipid droplet is borderless and clear.

A, arteriole
Ad, adipocyte
AT, adipose tissue
DCT, dense irregular connective tissue
L, lymph material
N, nerve
P, Pacinian corpuscle
V, venule
Val, valve
arrowheads, endothelial cells
arrows, endothelial cell nuclei

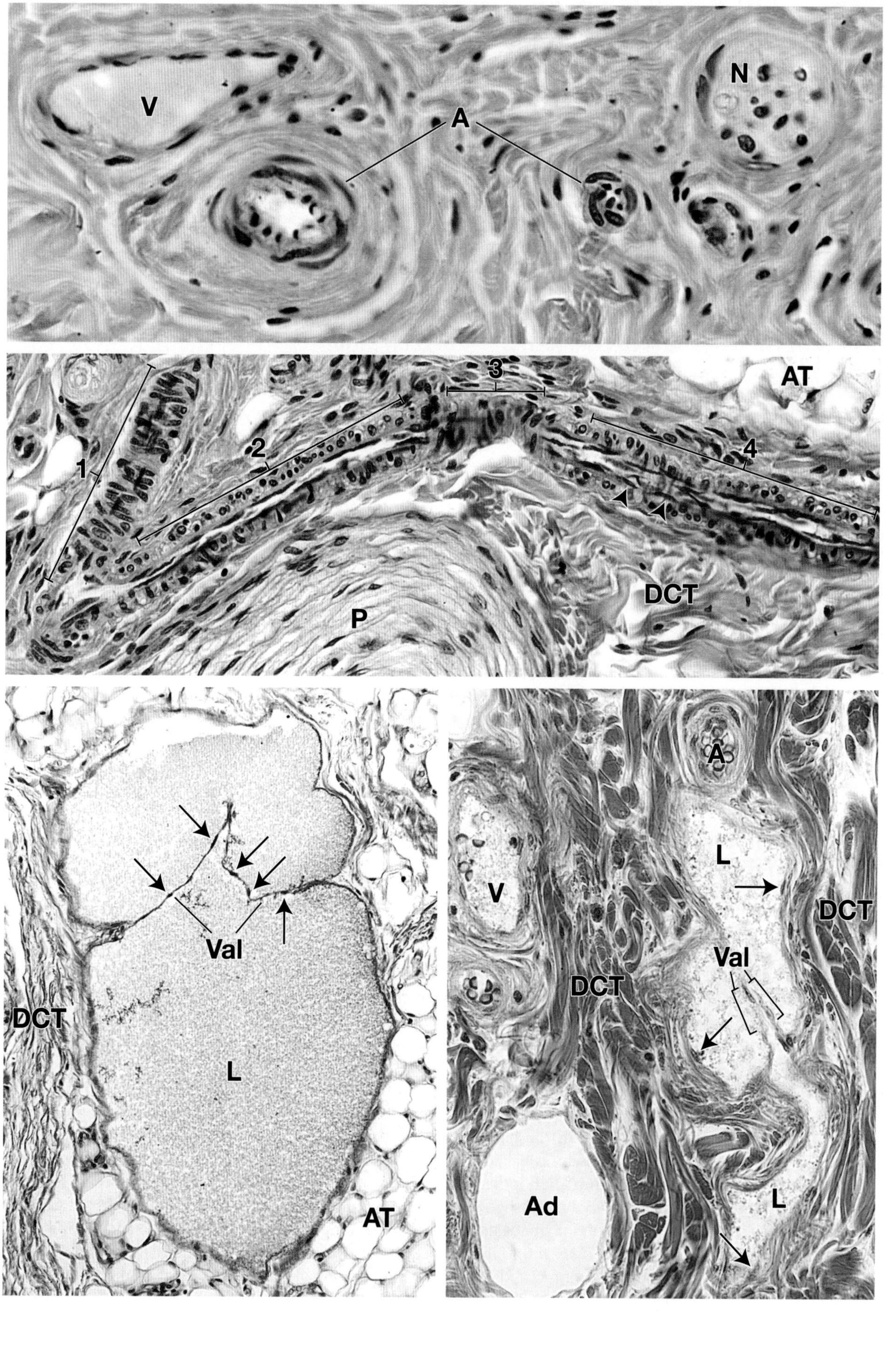
V
A
N
1
2
3
4
AT
P
DCT
Val
DCT
L
AT
A
L
V
DCT
Val
DCT
Ad
L

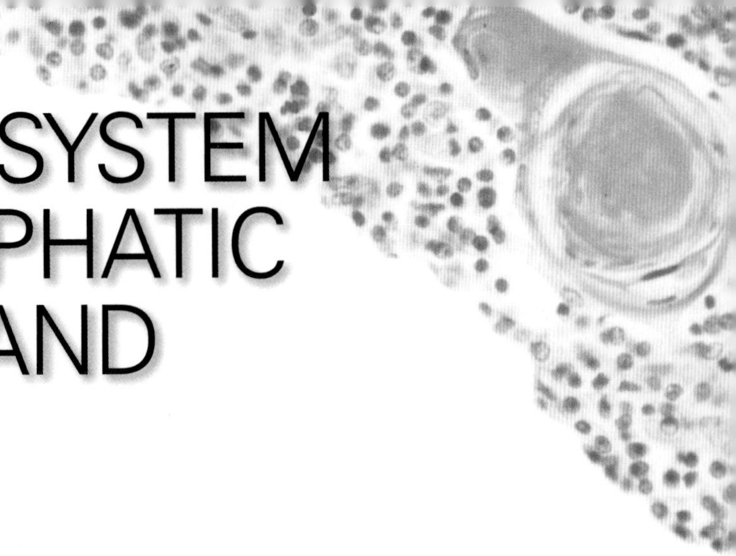

14 IMMUNE SYSTEM AND LYMPHATIC TISSUES AND ORGANS

■ OVERVIEW OF THE IMMUNE AND LYMPHATIC SYSTEMS

The physiologic role of the **immune system** is to defend the body against infectious microorganisms and pathogenic agents as well as noninfectious foreign substances and transformed cells and their products. The **lymphatic system** is a morphologic counterpart of the immune system and consists of groups of cells, tissues, and organs that monitor body surfaces and internal fluid compartments (Fig. 14.1). Thus, the term *immune system* reflects the physiologic role (i.e., defense mechanisms) of the lymphatic system. Included in the lymphatic system are primary and secondary lymphatic organs connected by lymphatic vessels that terminate in the blood vascular system. The two systems are so closely associated that they are virtually indistinguishable from each other. Throughout history, it has been noted that individuals who recover from certain diseases such as chickenpox, measles, and mumps become resistant or immune *[Lat., immūnis, free, exempt]* to the same disease. Another long-standing observation is that immunity is specific—that is, immunity to chickenpox does not prevent infection with measles. It is also recognized that the immune system can react against the body's own tissues, causing autoimmune diseases such as lupus erythematosus, autoimmune hemolytic anemia, some forms of diabetes mellitus, and autoimmune thyroiditis (Hashimoto thyroiditis).

Almost all **cells of the immune system** are derived from **hemopoietic stem cells (HSCs)** in the bone marrow. Based on their progenitor stem cells (see pages 321-323), immune cells are derived from either the myeloid linage (monocytes, macrophages, granulocytes, and dendritic cells) or lymphoid lineage (all lymphocytes). **Lymphocytes** are the definitive cell type of the immune system and the effector cells in the response of the immune system to harmful substances. Lymphatic tissues serve as primary sites where lymphocytes proliferate, differentiate, and mature. The **thymus** and **bone marrow** are the **primary lymphatic organs** in mammals (see Fig. 14.1) where lymphocytes are "born and educated" and equipped with diverse antigen receptors to recognize and destroy specific antigens. After undergoing maturation and a careful selection process in the primary lymphatic organs, lymphocytes migrate to the **secondary lymphatic organs** and tissues, including the spleen, lymph nodes, appendix, lymphatic nodules, and

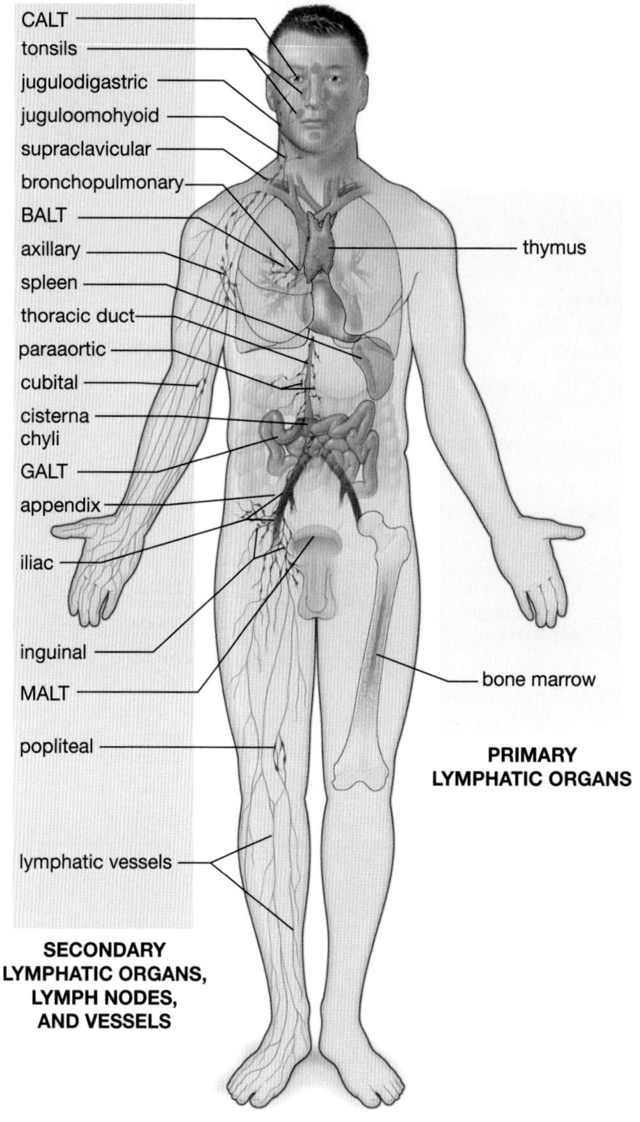

FIGURE 14.1. Overview of the structures constituting the lymphatic system. The lymphatic system consists of a group of cells, tissues, and organs that are responsible for monitoring body surfaces and internal compartments in order to combat foreign microorganisms, transformed cells, and other harmful substances. Lymphocytes are the most important cells of the lymphatic system. They differentiate and mature in the primary lymphatic organs, which for B lymphocytes is the bone marrow and for T lymphocytes is the thymus. Lymphocytes then enter into the blood or lymphatic vessels to colonize secondary lymphatic organs and tissues, where they undergo the final stages of antigen-dependent activation. Secondary lymphatic tissues consist of the spleen; various groups of lymph nodes and aggregations of lymphatic nodules, such as tonsils; conjunctiva-associated lymphatic tissue (*CALT*) in eyelids; bronchus-associated lymphatic tissue (*BALT*) in lungs; gut-associated lymphatic tissues (*GALT*) in the gastrointestinal tract; and mucosa-associated lymphatic tissue (*MALT*) throughout the genitourinary system (i.e., shown here is the mucosa of the bladder). Lymph is the fluid that is removed from the extracellular spaces of the connective tissues. It flows in lymphatic vessels into the lymph nodes, which are interspersed along the superficial lymphatic vessels (associated with the skin and superficial fascia) and deep lymphatic vessels (associated with main arteries). Ultimately, the lymphatic vessels empty into the bloodstream by joining the large veins at the base of the neck. The thoracic duct is the largest lymphatic vessel.

diffuse lymphatic tissues (see Fig. 14.1). Within these secondary lymphatic tissues in the presence of antigen, lymphocytes interact with each other and with nonlymphoid cells to become activated, such as **immunocompetent effector T and B cells**. These cells are able to distinguish between "self" (molecules normally present within an organism) and "nonself" (foreign molecules—i.e., those not normally present) and initiate an appropriate immune response.

An antigen is any substance that can induce a specific immune response.

The body is constantly exposed to pathogenic (disease-causing) organisms and hazardous substances from the external environment (infectious microorganisms, toxins, and foreign cells). In addition, changes may occur in cells (such as transformation of normal cells into cancerous cells) that give them characteristics of foreign cells. An immune response is generated against a specific **antigen**, which can be a soluble substance (e.g., a foreign protein, polysaccharide, or toxin) or an infectious organism, foreign tissue, or transformed (e.g., virus-infected or malignant) tissue. It is important to note that the term "antigen" refers to a molecule that can be recognized by the cells of the immune system and does not necessarily imply pathogenic origin. Most antigens must be "processed" by cells of the immune system before other cells can mount the immune response.

Historically, the term **antigen** has been used to refer to any substance that is able to induce the **specific (adaptive) immune response** culminating with the production of **antibodies** to which the antigen is capable of binding. However, it is now known that some antigens are too small (typically under 20 kDa) or too difficult to be detected by cells of immune system, and they are thus unable to trigger an immune response. For this reason, the term **immunogen** was introduced to describe a specific type of antigen that is always able to elicit an immune response. Therefore, all immunogens are antigens, but not all antigens are necessarily immunogens. The terms *antigen* and *immunogen* are often used interchangeably. In this chapter, because the difference between an immunogen and an antigen is not relevant, the term "antigen" is used exclusively.

The immune responses can be divided into nonspecific (innate) and specific (adaptive) defenses.

The body has two lines of immune defenses against foreign invaders and transformed cells: nonspecific immunity and specific immunity.

- **Nonspecific (innate) immunity**, comprising preexisting, nonspecific defenses, represents the first line of defense against microbial invasion. It consists of (1) **physical barriers** (e.g., the skin and mucous membranes) that prevent foreign organisms from invading the tissues; (2) **chemical defenses** (e.g., low pH in the stomach and vagina) that destroy many invading microorganisms; (3) various **secretory substances** (e.g., thiocyanate in saliva, lysozymes, interferons, fibronectin, and complement in serum) that neutralize foreign microorganisms; and (4) **cells** of the innate immune system, including phagocytic cells (e.g., **neutrophils**, **monocytes**, and **macrophages**), natural killer (NK) cells, mast cells, basophils, eosinophils, and dendritic cells (Fig. 14.2). In addition, a specific **type of gamma/delta (γ/δ) T lymphocytes** that reside in various epithelial tissues (e.g., the skin, oral mucosa, respiratory mucosa, intestines, and vagina) can be considered a part of these first-line defense mechanisms. For example, **neutrophils** can recognize invading bacteria via **pattern recognition receptors (PRRs)** such as **toll-like receptors (TLRs)**. These receptors recognize various pathogen-associated molecules commonly expressed on the bacterial surface (but not on the surface of its own cells), triggering an immune response (see page 309). PRRs are a key element of the innate immune system. In the case of **viral infection**, infected cells produce a pathogen-nonspecific antiviral agent, **interferon**, that

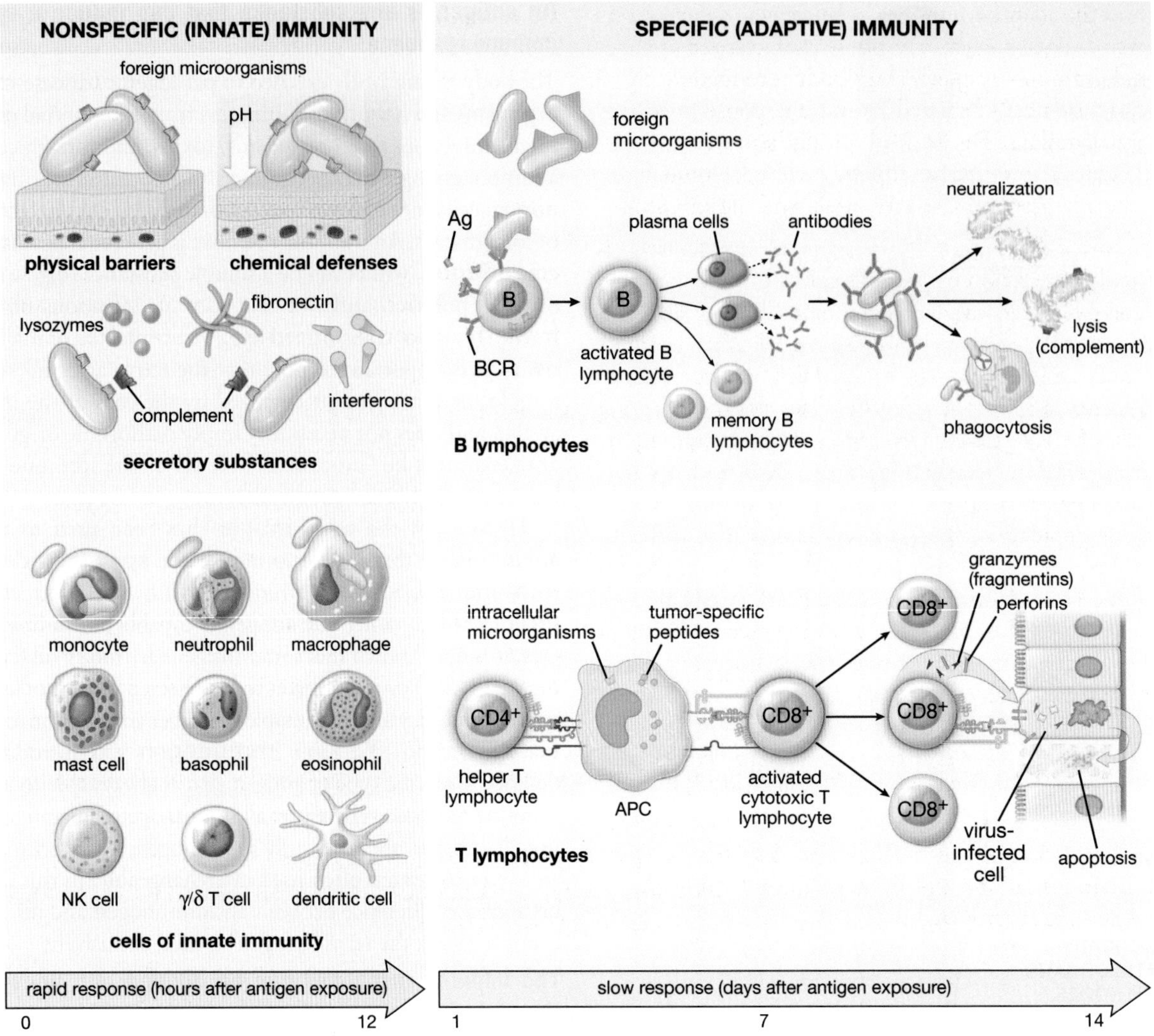

FIGURE 14.2. Nonspecific (innate) and specific (adaptive) immunity. The body has two lines of immune defenses against foreign invaders and transformed cells. Nonspecific (innate) immunity represents the first line of defense against microorganisms (microbial invasion). It consists of physical barriers, chemical defenses, various secretory substances, and a variety of cells that support the innate immune system. Specific (adaptive) immunity provides defenses that can precisely target antigens specific to invaders. Initial contact with foreign microorganisms activates specialized antigen-presenting cells (*APCs*) and initiates a chain of events involving effector cells. During an adaptive immune response, specific B and T lymphocytes become activated in secondary lymphatic organs and tissues to destroy invading organisms. *Ag*, antigen; *NK*, natural killer.

inhibits the replication of viruses in neighboring cells by decreasing protein synthesis.

- **Specific (adaptive) immunity**, activated when nonspecific defenses fail, precisely targets antigens specific to the invader. **B lymphocytes** and **T lymphocytes** provide both the **specificity** and **immune memory** characteristics of the adaptive immune response (see Fig. 14.2). Initial contact with an antigen or foreign agent activates specialized antigen-presenting cells and initiates a chain of reactions that involve effector cells of the immune system and may eventually lead to a state of immune memory. Adaptive immunity is possible due to **acquired resistance** against microbial aggression through random somatic rearrangements of genes that encode membrane-bound forms of immunoglobulin on B lymphocytes (i.e., B-cell receptors or BCRs) and specific receptors on T lymphocytes (i.e., T-cell receptors or TCRs). This rearrangement occurs in the thymus for T cells and bone marrow for B cells. During an adaptive immune response, specific **B and T lymphocytes** become activated in secondary lymphatic organs and tissues to destroy invading organisms.

Both nonspecific (innate) and specific (adaptive) immunity systems are interconnected and overlapping. In most cases, innate immunity is activated first. Shortly after invasion by a pathogenic agent, the innate immune system activates an **inflammatory response** to destroy infectious agents. **Neutrophils** are the main cell types that are recruited in the initial phases of the inflammatory response. As discussed earlier, neutrophils possess PRRs and complement receptors that trigger phagocytosis and destruction of invading pathogenic agents. The influx of neutrophils is followed by the influx of **monocytes** that differentiate into **macrophages**. Both macrophages and neutrophils are, therefore, also known as *inflammatory cells*. Because the inflammation site is drained by lymphatic vessels, the pathogenic agents (and antigens) flow with the lymph to neighboring lymph nodes, resulting in the activation of T and B lymphocytes. They generate a specific (adaptive) immune response that may produce long-term memory against pathogens.

Specific (adaptive) immunity can be divided into humoral and cell-mediated immunity.

Adaptive immunity is induced by innate immunity and is generally activated if innate immunity (i.e., the inflammatory response) fails. Adaptive immunity is activated by the presence of antigen. The longer the innate system takes to clear a pathogen, the more antigens are accumulated and the more robust the adaptive response is. In general, an encounter with a given antigen triggers a response characterized as either a humoral immune response (antibody production by B lymphocytes) or a cell-mediated immune response (mediated by T lymphocytes) (see Fig. 14.2). Typically, however, both cellular and humoral immune systems are involved, although one system generally predominates, depending on the stimulus.

- The **humoral response (humoral immunity)** is mediated by secretion of proteins called **antibodies** that coat and neutralize invaders (e.g., toxins, viruses, and bacteria) and mark them for destruction by other immune cells. **B lymphocytes** are the primary effector cells in this system. A B lymphocyte recognizes a pathogen using its surface BCR, which is specific to a single corresponding (cognate) antigen. Interaction of the BCR with its cognate antigen induces the proliferation of the B cell. Different populations of the B-cell clones then differentiate into **memory B cells** and **plasma cells**. Plasma cells can secrete soluble forms of the BCR as **antibodies** (see Fig. 14.2). Humoral immunity represents the major defense mechanism against pathogenic microorganisms and their toxins located outside cells (e.g., on cell surfaces and within the lumens of the gastrointestinal [GI], respiratory, and urogenital tracts) and within extracellular fluids (e.g., blood, lymph, and other body secretions). Humoral immunity promotes their elimination by macrophages and by activation of complement system, which consists of circulating small proteins that enhance the function of antibodies and macrophages. In some diseases (e.g., **tetanus, rabies, COVID-19**), antibodies are so critical and effective that a nonimmune person can be rendered "immune" by receiving an injection of antibody purified from the blood of an immune person (or animal). The effectiveness of this passive transfer proves that it is the antibody that is responsible for the protection.
- **Cell-mediated response (cellular immunity)** is mediated by **T lymphocytes** and their products (e.g., cytokines) that target cancer-transformed and virus-infected cells for destruction by specific "killer" cells. Cytotoxic $CD8^+$ lymphocytes are involved in direct killing of infected cells. Cellular immunity also promotes the destruction of infectious microorganisms inside phagocytic cells as well as foreign (transplanted) cells. T lymphocytes do not produce antibodies but possess specialized **antigen receptors** that recognize peptide-derived antigens (see Fig. 14.2). Unlike B lymphocytes, T lymphocytes cannot recognize antigen on their own. T lymphocytes require antigen to be presented to them on major histocompatibility complex (MHC) molecules (see pages 492-493) that are expressed on the surface of other antigen-presenting cells (APCs). Cell-mediated immunity is important in the defense against viral, fungal, and mycobacterial infections as well as tumor cells. Cell-mediated immunity is also responsible for transplant rejection.

■ CELLS OF THE IMMUNE SYSTEM

Overview

Cells of the immune system include lymphocytes and various supporting cells.

Lymphocytes and various supporting cells comprise the cells of the immune system. Three major types of **lymphocytes** are recognized: B cells, T cells, and NK cells. Supporting cells interact with lymphocytes and play important roles in the presentation of antigen to lymphocytes and the regulation of immune responses. These cells include **monocytes, macrophages, neutrophils, basophils, mast cells, eosinophils, reticular cells, dendritic cells, follicular dendritic cells, Langerhans cells,** and **epithelioreticular cells**. In addition, a series of specialized epithelial and stromal cells provide the environment for many immune reactions to occur by secreting specific substances that regulate growth, migration, and the activation of effector and supporting cells.

Supporting cells in the lymphatic organs are organized into loose meshworks.

In lymph nodules, lymph nodes, and the spleen, **reticular cells** and the **reticular fibers** produced by these cells form elaborate meshworks. Lymphocytes, macrophages, dendritic cells, follicular dendritic cells, and other cells of the immune system reside in these meshworks and in the loose connective tissue of the body; Langerhans cells are found only in the middle layers of the epidermis. At these sites, they carry out their mission of surveillance and defense. In the thymus, **epithelioreticular cells** form the structural meshwork within the tissue. Despite their name, these cells neither produce nor are related to reticular fibers.

Different types of cells in lymphatic tissue are identified by a specific cluster of differentiation (CD) molecules on their surfaces.

Different lymphatic and hematopoietic tissue cells possess unique cell surface molecules. Until the early 1980s, the various names of these surface molecules used in the scientific literature were inconsistent and confusing. The First International Workshop on Human Leucocyte Differentiation Antigens held in Paris in 1982 proposed a new nomenclature system that linked different antibodies with clusters of corresponding molecules. The specific markers, now called **cluster of differentiation (CD) molecules**, became designated by numbers that related them to antigens expressed at different stages of cell differentiation. For example, CD4 is a protein complex specific to T lymphocytes, whereas the CD4 antibody is the monoclonal antibody reacting to the CD4 molecule. CD molecules can be visualized by immunohistochemical or immunofluorescent methods using monoclonal antibodies and are useful in identifying specific subtypes of lymphatic or hematopoietic cells. Some CD markers are expressed by cells throughout their entire life span; others are expressed only during one phase of differentiation or cell activation. To date, there are more than 400 identified CD markers. **CD markers** are useful in the diagnosis and treatment of many hematopoietic tissue disorders. For instance, the absence (or presence in large quantities) of one particular CD marker in lymphocytes in a biopsy sample may indicate that the patient has a disorder related to the production and differentiation of a specific lymphocyte expressing this marker. CD markers are also useful in distinguishing between T-cell and B-cell leukemia (cancer of white blood cell–forming tissues) and other hematopoietic tissue disorders. Table 14.1 lists the most clinically useful markers.

TABLE 14.1 Most Common Cluster of Differentiation Markers Used in Clinical Practice

Marker	Main Cellular Expression	Function/Identity	Molecular Weight (kDa)
CD1	T cells in the midstage of development, Langerhans cells, dendritic cells	Presentation of lipid antigen to T cells MHC I–like molecules associated with β_2 microglobulin Developmental markers for T cells and Langerhans cells of the skin	49
CD2	T cells, NK cells	Adhesion molecules Used as clinical markers for T-cell activation	50
CD3	T cells	Form complex with T-cell receptor (TCR)	25–28
CD4	Helper T cells, monocytes, macrophages	Members of Ig superfamily Interact with MHC II molecules Bind viral protein gp120 of HIV-1 and HIV-2	56
CD5	T cells, some B cells	Costimulatory molecules that appear on mature T and B cells Required for Th2 and Th17 cells differentiation High levels in chronic lymphocytic leukemia	67
CD7	T cells, pluripotential hematopoietic cells	Members of Ig superfamily Bind the PI-3 kinase Useful clinical markers for T-cell acute lymphocytic leukemia and stem cell leukemia	40
CD8	Cytotoxic T cells	Members of Ig superfamily Interact with MHC I molecules	34
CD9	B cells, T cells, monocytes, eosinophils, basophils, platelets, endothelial cells, exosomes	Facilitate aggregation of platelets, cell adhesion, and cell migration. General exosome marker	24
CD10	Pre–B cells, pre–T cells, monocytes, eosinophils	Zinc metalloprotease Common markers for acute lymphoblastic leukemia	100
CD16a	NK cells also mast cells, macrophages	Clinical markers for NK cells Function as F_c receptors for aggregated IgG Mediate phagocytosis and antibody-dependent cell–mediated cytotoxicity	50–70
CD16b	Neutrophils	Function as F_c receptors for aggregated IgG Mediate neutrophil activation (degranulation, phagocytosis oxidative burst reaction)	50–70
CD19	B cells, dendritic cells	Co-receptors with CD21 and CD81 Clinical markers for all stages of B-cell development	95
CD20	B cells	Form Ca^{2+} channels Role in B-cell activation and plasma cell development Markers for late stage of B-cell development Monoclonal antibodies to CD20 are used to achieve B cell depletion in chronic lymphocytic leukemia	35–37
CD21	B cells, follicular dendritic cells	Receptors for C3d complement protein and for Epstein–Barr virus	145
CD22	B cells	B-lymphocyte cell adhesion molecules Mediate B-cell to T-cell adhesion	130–140
CD23	B cells, monocytes, macrophages, eosinophils, platelets, dendritic cells	Low-affinity receptor for the F_c portion of IgE that mediates IgE-dependent cytotoxicity and phagocytosis by macrophages and eosinophils	45
CD24	B cells, granulocytes, epithelial cells	Sialoglycoprotein at the cell surface Expressed in late stage of B-cell differentiation	41
CD25	Activated T cells and B cells	Binds to IL-2 (IL-2 receptor α-chain)	55
CD28	T cells (all $CD4^+$ and >50% of $CD8^+$ in humans)	T-cell costimulatory molecule interacts with CD80 (B7-1) and CD86 (B7-2); the costimulatory signal induces T-cell activation and IL-2 production.	44
CD31	Lymphatic endothelial cells, platelets, macrophages, leukocytes, megakaryocytes	Also known as platelet and endothelial cell adhesion molecule-1 (PECAM-1A) involved in leukocyte migration into lymphatic capillaries	130
CD34	Hemopoietic stem cells (HSCs)	Clinical markers for HSCs and ligand for CD62L Mediate attachment of stem cells to bone marrow extracellular matrix	105–120
CD35	T cells, B cells, monocytes, dendritic cells, granulocytes, erythrocytes	Complement receptor 1 Promote phagocytosis of complement-coated particles Bind C3b and C4b complement proteins	250
CD38	Early B and T cells, activated T cells	NAD glycohydrolase Used as markers for T-cell activation and proliferation	45

Marker	Main Cellular Expression	Function/Identity	Molecular Weight (kDa)
CD40	B cells, macrophages, follicular dendritic cells, dendritic cells, activated monocytes, endothelial and vascular smooth muscle cells	Active in proliferating B cells Costimulatory molecules for CD40L (CD154) Facilitate cytokine production in macrophages and dendritic cells	48
CD40L	Activated $CD4^+$ T cells; known as CD154	Facilitate interaction between T and B cells Regulate B-cell function Costimulatory molecules for CD40	39
CD45	All human leukocytes	Tyrosine phosphatase Leukocyte common antigen Required for T- and B-cell receptor signal transduction	220
CD45RO, CD45RA	Memory T cells (CD45RO), naïve T cells (CD45RA), some B cells, monocytes, macrophages	Tyrosine phosphatase Isoforms of CD45 Regulate T- and B-cell activation	180
CD49a	Tissue resident memory $CD8^+$ cells (Trm)	$\alpha1$ subunit of $\alpha1\beta1$ integrin, a receptor associated with adhesion of lymphocytes to collagen IV	200
CD56	NK cells	Clinical markers for NK cells Isoforms of neural adhesion molecules (N-CAM)	135–220
CD62E	Endothelial cells (only)	Represent ELAM-1 Binds to Sialyl-Lewis^x (s-Le^x) carbohydrates on leukocytes	140
CD62L	Leukocytes	Bind CD34 Represent L-selectins, a leukocyte adhesion molecules that allow lymphocytes to roll along the endothelial surface	150
CD63	All cells, activated platelets, exosomes	LAMP-3 protein associated with lysosomes and membranes of intracellular vesicles General exosome marker	30–60
CD69	Tissue resident memory $CD8^+$ cells (Trm), γ/δ T cells	Represent a membrane-bound, type II C-lectin receptor Considered as marker of lymphocyte tissue retention	28–32
CD80	B cells, macrophages, dendritic cells, monocytes; known as B7-1 receptor	APC costimulatory molecule interacts with CD28 and CTLA-4	60
CD86	Activated B cells, macrophages, monocytes, dendritic cells, endothelial cells; known as B7-2 receptor	APC costimulatory molecule interacts with CD28 and CTLA-4	80
CD94	NK cells	Regulate function of NK cells Clinical markers for NK cells	43
CD103	Tissue resident memory $CD8^+$ cells (Trm) in skin, lungs, and GI tract	Represent $\alpha4\beta7$ integrin and directs lymphocytes to its ligand E-cadherin Considered as marker of lymphocyte tissue retention	175

APC, antigen-presenting cell; *CTLA-4*, cytotoxic T-lymphocyte–associated protein 4; *ELAM-1*, endothelial–leukocyte adhesion molecule 1; *GI*, gastrointestinal; *HIV-1*, human immunodeficiency virus-1; *Ig*, immunoglobulin; *LAMP*, lysosome-associated membrane protein, *MHC*, major histocompatibility complex; *NAD*, nicotinamide adenine dinucleotide; *N-CAM*, neural cell adhesion molecule; *NK*, natural killer; *PECAM-1A*, platelet and endothelial cell adhesion molecule-1A; *PI-3 kinase*, phosphatidylinositol-3 kinase.

Lymphocytes

Circulating lymphocytes are the chief cellular constituents of lymphatic tissue.

To understand the function of **lymphocytes**, it is important to recognize that most lymphocytes (~70%) in blood or lymph represent a **circulating pool** of immunocompetent cells. These cells participate in a cycle during which they exit the systemic circulation to enter the lymphatic tissue. While there, they are responsible for **immunologic surveillance** of surrounding tissues. The cells then return to the systemic circulation. This population of cells is represented mainly by long-lived, mature lymphocytes (mainly T cells) that have developed the capacity to recognize and respond to foreign antigens and are in transit from one lymphatic tissue site to another.

The remaining 30% of lymphocytes in the blood vessels do not circulate between the lymphatic tissues and the systemic circulation. This population comprises mainly short-lived, immature cells or activated cells destined for a specific tissue. These cells leave the capillaries and migrate directly to the tissues, especially into the connective tissue that underlies the lining epithelium of the respiratory, GI, and urogenital tracts as well as into the intercellular spaces of these epithelia. Functionally, three major types of lymphocytes are present in the body: **T lymphocytes**, **B lymphocytes**, and **NK cells.** The functional classification of lymphocytes is independent of their morphologic (size) characteristics.

T lymphocytes differentiate in the thymus and account for the majority of circulating lymphocytes.

T lymphocytes (T cells) are named for the thymus, where they differentiate. They have a long life span and are involved in **cell-mediated immunity**. They account for 60%–80% of circulating lymphocytes. T cells express CD2, CD3, CD5, and CD7 markers and TCRs; however, they are subclassified according to the presence or absence of two other important surface markers: CD4 and CD8. It is essential to mention here that both CD4 and CD8 proteins are not only passive cell markers but also active co-receptors that recognize peptide antigens bound to MHC molecules (see pages 492-493).

- **Helper $CD4^+$ T lymphocytes** are T cells that express CD4 markers. These cells are further subdivided into three major subsets by their ability to secrete cytokines (see page 498); however, more subsets are actively being discovered. The first subset incudes helper T cells that synthesize primary interferon-γ (IFN-γ) and other cytokines (e.g., interleukin-2 [IL-2] and tumor necrosis factor [TNF]); these cells are called **Th1 cells.** Th1 cells activate **macrophages** that destroy intracellular pathogens, such as bacteria and other microorganisms. The second subset of helper T cells synthesizes IL-4, IL-5, IL-10, and IL-13 and is called **Th2 cells.** Th2 cells activate **eosinophils**, **mast cells**, and **B cells** (for IgE production). Th2 cells initiate antibody E (IgE)-, mast cell- and eosinophil-mediated immune responses that destroy extracellular parasites (helminths) and mediate allergic reactions. The third subset of helper T cells synthesizes IL-17 and IL-22 and is called **Th17 cells.** Their principal function is to destroy extracellular bacteria and fungi by recruiting neutrophils to the site of inflammation. In addition, IL-22 produced by Th17 cells increases the production of antimicrobial peptides (e.g., defensins) and supports epithelial barrier function. Defective Th17 function is associated with **Job syndrome (hyper-IgE syndrome)**, which is characterized by frequent and recurrent fungal and bacterial infections of the skin.
- **Cytotoxic $CD8^+$ T lymphocytes (CTLs)** are T cells that express CD8 markers. Following recognition of the antigen and subsequent activation, these cells kill target cells–expressing antigen by delivery of cytotoxic proteins that induce apoptosis. The major cytotoxic proteins found in cytoplasmic granules in cytotoxic T cells are the same as those in NK cells, including granzymes, perforin, and granulysin. Cytotoxic T cells kill target cells, such as virus-infected cells, cancer-transformed cells, cells infected with intracellular microorganisms, and parasites, and play a critical role in the acute rejection of transplanted cells and organs.
- **Regulatory (suppressor) T lymphocytes** represent a phenotypically diverse population of T lymphocytes that can functionally suppress an immune response to foreign and self-antigens by influencing the activity of other cells in the immune system. For example, T lymphocytes with $CD4^+CD25^+FOXP3^+$ markers are regulatory cells that can diminish the ability of T lymphocytes to initiate immune responses. The FOXP3 marker indicates an expression of the forkhead family of transcription factors that are characteristic of many T cells. Another tumor-associated T lymphocyte with $CD8^+CD45RO^+$ markers is able to suppress T-cell activation. Other suppressor T cells may also function in suppressing B-cell differentiation and in regulating erythroid cell maturation in the bone marrow.
- **Gamma/delta (γ/δ) T lymphocytes** represent a small population of T cells (<5%) that possess a distinct TCR on their surface composed of one γ-chain and one δ-chain. Most other TCRs are composed of two glycoprotein chains: α-chain and β-TCR chain. These cells develop in the thymus and **migrate to various epithelial tissues** (e.g., the skin, oral mucosa, respiratory mucosa, intestines, and vagina). Once they colonize an epithelial tissue, they do not recirculate between blood and lymphatic organs. Gamma/delta (γ/δ) T cells are strategically positioned at the interfaces of the external and internal environments and function as the first line of defense against invading organisms. They encounter antigen on the surface of the epithelial cells even before it enters the body.
- **Mucosa-associated invariant T (MAIT) lymphocytes** represent a subset of T cells that express receptors composed of two invariant α- and β-TCR chains. These cells recognize **metabolites of riboflavin** (vitamin B_2) synthesis pathway that occurs in fungi and bacteria. These metabolites must be presented to MAIT lymphocytes by other cells expressing MHC I–like complexes called **MHC I–related proteins (MR1)**. After activation, MAIT cells secrete inflammatory cytokines, such as IFN-γ and TNF-α, and are capable of destroying infected cells. MAIT cells account for about 50% of all T lymphocytes found in the liver. A functional impairment of MAIT cells was found in chronic hepatitis B virus (HBV) and human immunodeficiency virus (HIV) infections. They most likely represent a second defense mechanism against microorganisms that cross the mucosal epithelial barrier of the gastrointestinal tract and enter the portal circulation.
- **Resident memory T lymphocytes (Trm)** represent a new T-lymphocyte lineage of nonrecirculating memory T cells. They are generated after exposure to antigen in peripheral tissues and provide immunologic memory at the site of initial exposure. Trm cells express specific markers of residency CD69, CD103, and CD49a but lack molecules enabling them to leave the peripheral tissues and migrate to lymph nodes. Trm cells are distributed throughout the epithelial barrier tissues, including the GI tract, lung, skin, and reproductive tract. They are more potent effector cells compared with other circulating T cells. Resident Trm cells maintain immune surveillance of the specific tissue, and they are crucial for initiating rapid robust immune responses at times of infection.

B lymphocytes differentiate in the bursa-equivalent organ and participate in humoral immunity.

B lymphocytes (B cells) are so named because they were first recognized as a separate population in the bursa of Fabricius in birds (page 315) or bursa-equivalent organ such as bone marrow in mammals (see Folder 14.1). They have variable life spans and are involved in the production and secretion of the various circulating **antibodies**, also called **immunoglobulins (Ig)**, the immune proteins associated with **humoral immunity** (Fig. 14.3 and Table 14.2). B cells account for 20%–30% of the circulating lymphocytes. In addition to secreting circulating Igs, B cells express membrane-bound forms of Ig called **B-cell receptors (BCRs)** that serve as the antigen-specific binding site. During differentiation, the BCR isotope switches from a single immunoglobulin M (IgM) in immature B cells to a mixture of **IgD** and M **(IgM)** in **mature B cells**. The recognition of antigens by BCRs activates these lymphocytes and initiates the humoral response. B cells also express **major histocompatibility complex II (MHC II) molecules** on the cell surface for antigen presentation to T cells. Their CD markers are CD9, CD19, and CD20. Mature B cells equipped with membrane-bound forms of IgM and IgD enter the blood circulation and migrate to the periphery where they colonize the spleen and the other secondary lymphatic organs.

Natural killer lymphocytes (NK cells) are neither T nor B cells and are specialized to kill certain types of target cells.

Natural killer (NK) cells are part of nonspecific (innate) immunity but share similarities with cells of the adaptive immune system, including T and B cells. NK cells are named for their ability to kill certain target cells. They develop from the common lymphoid progenitor (CLP) cell in the bone marrow, similar to B and T cells. NK cells constitute about 5%–15% of circulating lymphocytes. Because NK cells are larger than T and B cells and possess cytoplasmic granules, they are sometimes called large granular lymphocytes (LGLs). They do not mature in the thymus and, therefore, do not express TCRs. However, during their development, they are genetically programmed to recognize transformed cells by expressing **natural cytotoxicity receptors (NCRs)** on their surface. These germline-encoded activating receptors can bind directly to stress-induced or pathogen-derived antigens on tumor- and virus-infected cells. NK cells kill these target cells in a similar manner to that of cytotoxic $CD8^+$ T lymphocytes. After recognition of the target cell, NK cells directly eliminate these cells by releasing **perforins** (pore-forming proteins) and **granzymes** (necessary for triggering **apoptosis** of target cells). The specific markers expressed on NK cells are CD16a, CD56, and CD94.

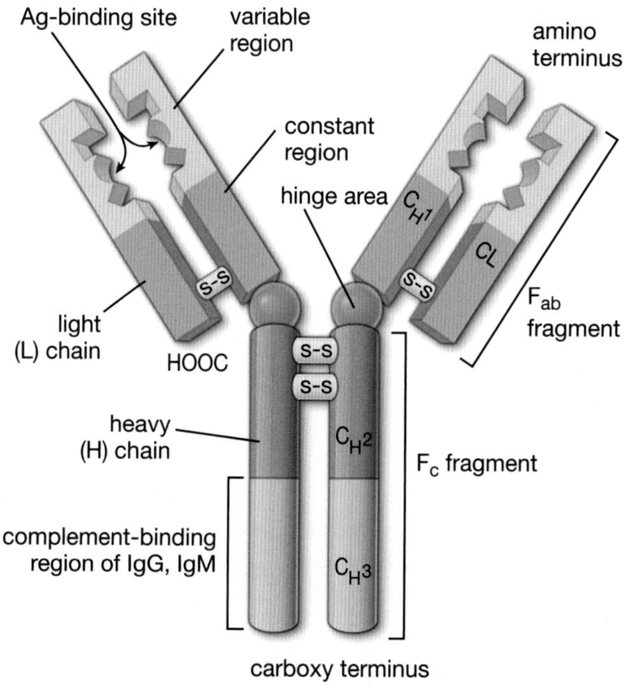

FIGURE 14.3. Schematic diagram of an antibody molecule. Antibodies are Y-shaped molecules produced by plasma cells. They consist of two heavy (*H*) and two light (*L*) polypeptide chains connected by disulfide bonds (S–S). Both *H* and *L* chains are composed of domains of amino acids that are constant (at the carboxy-terminus) or variable (at the amino-terminus) in their sequence. The five different immunoglobulin (*Ig*) isotypes are determined by the type of heavy chain present. An antibody molecule binds an antigen (*Ag*) at the two sites of the amino-terminus, where the heavy and light chains are associated with each other. Digestion of an antibody molecule by the proteolytic enzyme papain cleaves the antibody into two F_{ab} fragments and one crystallizable F_c fragment. The F_{ab} fragments bind to specific antigens, whereas the F_c fragment, which is composed of two carboxy-terminus heavy-chain segments (C_H2 and C_H3), fulfills the effector functions (e.g., in complement activation). Many cells express F_c receptors on their surfaces, which anchor antibodies at the F_c fragment.

In addition to directly triggering apoptosis in target cells, NK cells employ additional mechanisms to kill cells. NK cells kill target cells indirectly by secretion of pro-inflammatory cytokines that lead to inflammatory responses and cell lysis. They kill antibody-coated target cells using the **antibody-dependent cell–mediated cytotoxicity (ADCC)** immune response (see pages 495-496). **CD16a** ($F_c\gamma$RIIIa) is an **F_c receptor for IgG** antibodies. Interaction between the CD16a receptor on NK cells and IgG antibodies coating a microorganism triggers the ADCC mechanism. Through this mechanism, the antigen specificity of the adaptive immune system (represented by IgG antibodies secreted from plasma cells) is paired with the toxicity of NK cells to provide antigen-specific killing. Thus, the engagement of CD16a on NK cells acts as a strong proapoptotic signal and induces NK cell–mediated killing.

Natural killer (NK) cells are activated to kill target cells by recognizing an imbalance between activating and inhibitory signals derived from their surface receptors.

The function of NK cells is determined by the integration of numerous signals generated by activating and inhibitory receptors on their surfaces (Fig. 14.4). Under physiologic conditions, circulating NK cells are mostly inactive. They become activated through various signaling pathways that cause them to migrate and infiltrate certain tumor- or virus-infected tissues. In general, among other receptors, NK cells express two classes of regulatory receptors on their surface:

- **Activating receptors** known as **natural cytotoxicity receptors (NCRs)**, such as NKp46, NKp44, and NKp30, that recognize ligands expressed by tumor- and virus-infected cells and send activating signals, and
- **Inhibitory receptors**, such as killer cell immunoglobulin-like receptors (KIRs), NKG2A, KLRG1, and TIGIT, that react with MHC I molecules that inhibit the action of NK cells.

NK cell activation is controlled by a **dynamic imbalance** between **activating** and **inhibitory pathways** initiated by respective receptors during interaction with potential target cells. All normal healthy cells express sufficient MHC I molecules that act as ligands for inhibitory receptors on NK cells. The balance between inhibitory and activating pathways keeps NK cells inactive (in the no-killing mode), sparing healthy normal cells from NK cell attack (see Fig. 14.4). However, during viral infection, MHC I molecules are usually

TABLE 14.2 Characteristics of Human Immunoglobulins

Isotype	Molecular Weight (kDa)	Serum Level (mg/mL)	Percentage of All Ig in Adult Blood	Cells to Which Bind via F_c Region	Major Functions
IgG	145	12.0	85	Macrophages, B cells, NK cells, neutrophils, eosinophils	Principal Ig in secondary immune response Longest half-life (23 days) of all five Igs Activates complement Stimulates chemotaxis Crosses placenta, providing newborn with passive immunity
IgM	190 (950)[a]	1.5	5–10	B cells	Principal Ig produced during primary immune response Most efficient Ig in fixing complement Activates macrophages Serves as Ag receptor of B lymphocytes
IgA	160 (385)[b]	2.0	5–15	B cells	Ig present in body secretions, including tears, colostrum, saliva, and vaginal fluid, and in secretions of nasal cavity, bronchi, intestine, and prostate Provides protection against proliferation of microorganisms in these fluids and aids in defense against microbes and foreign molecules penetrating body via cell linings of these cavities
IgD	185	0.03	<1	B cells	Acts as an antigen receptor (together with IgM) on surface of mature B lymphocytes (only traces in serum)
IgE	190	3×10^{-5}	<1	Mast cells, basophils	Stimulates mast cells to release histamine, heparin, leukotrienes, and eosinophil chemotactic factor of anaphylaxis Responsible for anaphylactic hypersensitivity reactions Increased levels in parasitic infections

[a]IgM found in serum as a pentameric molecule.
[b]IgA found in serum as dimeric molecule.
Ag, antigen; *Ig*, immunoglobulin; *NK*, natural killer.

downregulated or sometimes lost, which decreases the signaling to the NK inhibitory pathways and creates an imbalance between inhibitory and activating signals. A similar imbalance is also created when tumor-transformed cells overexpress activating ligands on their surface, which is recognized by increased signaling from NK-activating receptors. NK cells are thus regulated by the integration of activating and inhibitory signals via surface receptors that recognize the appropriate ligand. Any imbalance between these signals activates natural killer cells into the killing mode (see Fig. 14.4).

FOLDER 14.1

FUNCTIONAL CONSIDERATIONS: ORIGIN OF THE NAMES *T LYMPHOCYTE* AND *B LYMPHOCYTE*

In the early 1960s, investigators using chicken embryos demonstrated that the bursa of Fabricius, a mass of lymphatic tissue associated with the cloaca of birds, was one of the anatomic sites of lymphocyte differentiation. When this tissue was destroyed in the chicken embryos (by either surgical removal or administration of high doses of testosterone), the adult chickens were unable to produce antibodies, leading to impaired humoral immunity. The chickens also demonstrated a marked reduction in the number of lymphocytes found in specific bursa-dependent areas of the spleen and lymph nodes. These affected lymphocytes were, therefore, named **B lymphocytes** or **B cells**. The bursa-equivalent organ in mammals (including humans) is the **bone marrow**, where B lymphocytes differentiate into immunocompetent cells. Thus, the "B" refers to the **bursa of Fabricius** in birds or the **bursa-equivalent organ** in mammals.

Investigators studying newborn mice found that removal of the thymus results in profound deficiencies in cell-mediated immune responses. The rejection of transplanted skin from a heterologous donor is an example of a cell-mediated immune response. Thymectomized mice demonstrate a marked reduction in the number of lymphocytes found in specific regions of the spleen and the lymph nodes (thymus-dependent areas). The areas of depletion differ from those identified after removal of the bursa of Fabricius in the chicken. These affected lymphocytes were, therefore, named **T lymphocytes** or **T cells**; thus, the "T" refers to **thymus**.

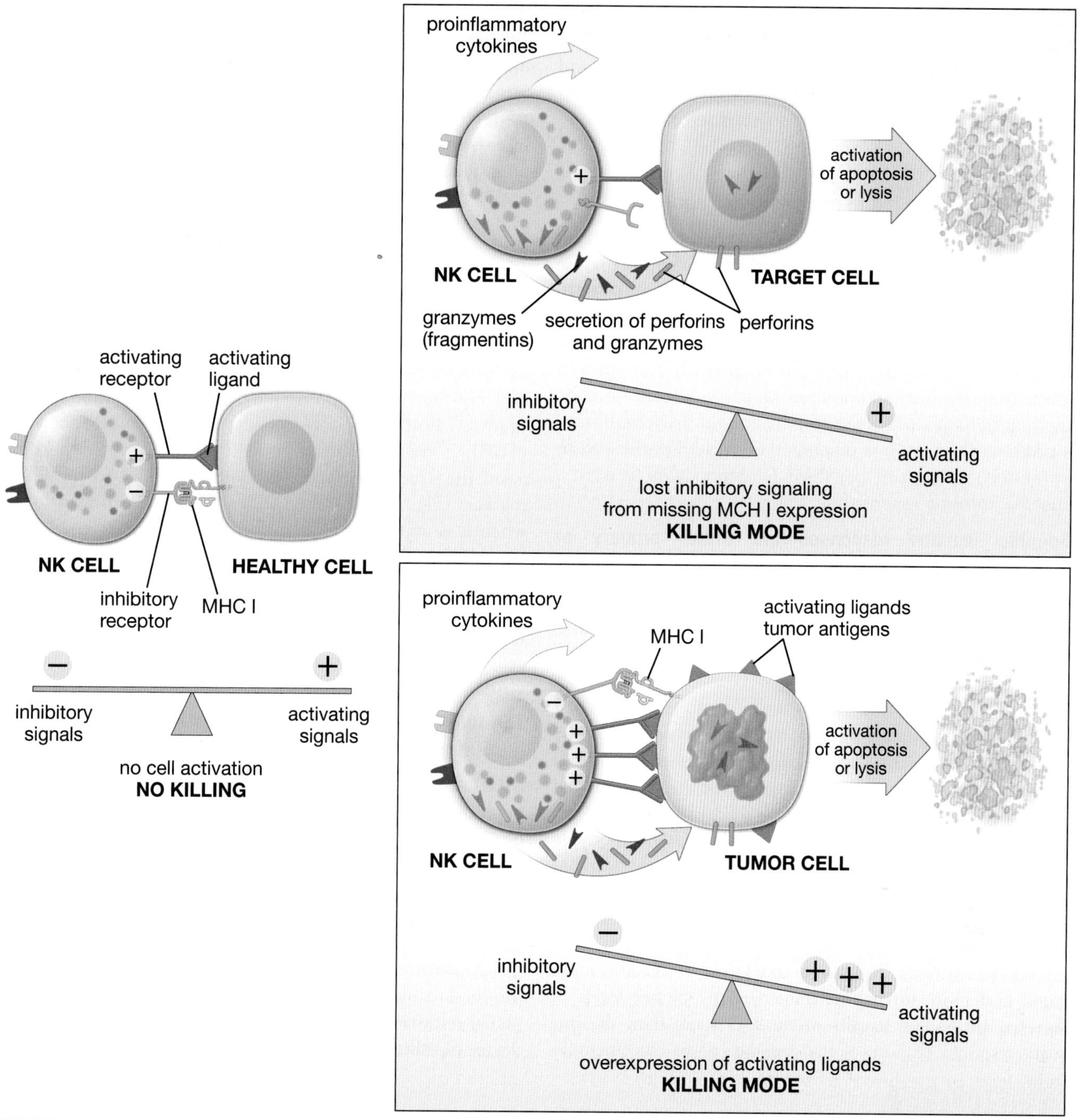

FIGURE 14.4. Activation of NK cells. Natural killer (*NK*) cells are activated to kill target cells by recognizing the imbalance between activating and inhibitory signals derived from their surface receptors. Note that under normal conditions (*left panel*), activating receptors (i.e., NKp46, NKp44, or NKp30) recognize ligands expressed on most "healthy" cells by sending activating signals to *NK* cells. These signals are neutralized by inhibitory signals derived from inhibitory receptors (i.e., KIR, NKG2A, KLRG1, or TIGIT), which interact with major histocompatibility complex class I (*MHC I*) molecules. *NK* cells are inactive when both inhibitory and signals are present and appropriately balanced. Under pathologic conditions, such as viral infection, *MHC I* molecules are downregulated or lost, lowering *NK* inhibitory signaling (*upper right panel*). In addition, tumor-transformed cells often overexpress activating ligands on their surface, which are recognized by activating receptors on NK cells (*lower right panel*). It is the imbalance between activating and inhibitory signals that causes *NK* cells to become activated and enter killing mode.

Lymphocyte development and differentiation

Lymphocytes undergo antigen-independent differentiation in the primary lymphatic organs.

In humans and other mammals, the **bone marrow** (called the **bursa-equivalent organ**) and the **thymus** have been identified as **primary (central) lymphatic organs**. Lymphocytes differentiate into immunocompetent cells in these organs. Initially, lymphocytes are genetically programmed to recognize a single antigen out of virtually an infinite number of possible antigens, a process called **antigen-independent proliferation and differentiation**. These immunocompetent naïve cells then enter the blood or lymph and are transported throughout the body, where a large number of them are dispersed in the secondary lymphatic organs.

Lymphocytes undergo antigen-dependent activation in the secondary lymphatic organs.

Immunocompetent lymphocytes (together with plasma cells derived from B lymphocytes and with macrophages) organize around reticular cells and their reticular fibers to form the adult effector lymphatic tissues and organs (i.e., lymphatic nodules, lymph nodes, tonsils, and spleen). Within these **secondary (peripheral) lymphatic organs**, naïve T and B lymphocytes undergo **antigen-dependent activation into effector lymphocytes and memory cells.**

Immune responses to antigens

Inflammation is the initial response to an antigen.

The initial reaction of the body to invasion by an antigen, either a foreign molecule or a pathogenic organism, is the nonspecific defense known as the **inflammatory response.** The inflammatory response may either sequester the antigen, physically digest it with enzymes secreted by neutrophils, or phagocytose and degrade the antigen in the cytoplasm of macrophages. Degradation of antigens by macrophages may lead to subsequent presentation of a portion of the antigen displayed on MHC II molecules to immunocompetent helper $CD4^+$ T lymphocytes to elicit a specific immune response.

Specific immune responses are either primary or secondary.

When immunocompetent cells encounter a foreign antigen (e.g., antigen associated with pathogenic microorganisms, tissue transplants, or toxins), a **specific immune response** to the antigen is generated.

A **primary immune response** refers to the body's first encounter with an antigen. This response is characterized by a lag period of several days before antibodies (mostly IgM) or specific lymphocytes directed against the invading antigen can be detected in the blood. The initial response to an antigen is initiated by only one or a few B lymphocytes that have been genetically programmed to respond to that specific antigen. After this initial immune response, a few antigen-specific **B lymphocytes** remain in circulation as **memory cells**.

The **secondary immune response** is usually more rapid and more intense (characterized by higher levels of secreted antibodies, usually of the IgG class) than the primary response because of the presence of specific memory B lymphocytes already programmed to respond to that specific antigen. The secondary response is the basis of most **immunizations** for common bacterial and viral diseases. Some antigens, such as penicillin and insect venoms, may trigger intense secondary immune responses that produce **hypersensitivity reactions** such as type I, also known as **anaphylactic hypersensitivity** (see Folder 14.2). However, antibodies themselves do not kill or destroy invading antigens; they simply neutralize them and mark them for destruction by cells of the immune system.

Helper T and cytotoxic T lymphocytes recognize and bind to antigens that are bound to MHC molecules.

Helper and cytotoxic T lymphocytes play central roles in initiating **specific immune responses** (humoral and cell-mediated responses) by acting as immune system "patrols." Both kinds of lymphocytes have a **T-cell receptor (TCR)**, a transmembrane protein whose exposed portion is on the T-cell membrane in close proximity to the CD3 marker (Fig. 14.5). The TCR recognizes antigen only when it is attached to "identification molecules," the **MHC molecules.** In addition, helper T lymphocytes can only recognize an antigen when it is "presented" to them by cells called **antigen-presenting cells (APCs).** Cytotoxic T lymphocytes can only react to "foreign" antigen exposed on cells, such as those transformed by cancer or infected with a virus.

The two classes of MHC molecules display peptides on the surface of cells.

MHC molecules serve as peptide display molecules for recognition by T lymphocytes. They display short fragments of digested "foreign" and "self" proteins on the cell surface. These proteins bind to MHC molecules inside the cell and are then transported to the cell surface. MHC I and MHC II molecules are products of a "supergene" located on chromosome 6 in humans known as the **major histocompatibility gene complex.** The expression of this gene complex produces molecules that are specific not only to the individual cell that produces them but also to the tissue type and degree of cellular differentiation.

FOLDER 14.2

CLINICAL CORRELATION: HYPERSENSITIVITY REACTIONS

When an individual has been immunologically sensitized by exposure to an **antigen**, subsequent exposure may lead not only to a secondary immune response but also to undesirable tissue-damaging reactions called **hypersensitivity reactions**. Such reactions are observed in sensitized humans after insect bites or injections of penicillin. There are several types of hypersensitivity reactions; however, the most common type is the **allergic reaction (type I, immediate, or anaphylactic hypersensitivity)**. The reaction usually develops ~15–30 minutes from the time of exposure to the **antigen (allergen)** and may cause a variety of symptoms involving the skin (urticaria and eczema), eyes (conjunctivitis), nasal cavities (rhinorrhea, rhinitis), lungs (airway constriction), and alimentary tract (gastritis). Allergic reactions are mediated by **IgE antibodies** that are responsible for the antibody-induced discharge of **mast cell** or **basophil** granules. These granules contain preformed mediators (i.e., histamine, serine proteases, eosinophil chemotactic factor) and newly synthesized mediators (i.e., leukotrienes, interleukins), which account for the distressing features of hypersensitivity reactions. **Eosinophils** are attracted by eosinophil chemotactic factor to the site of mast cell degranulation, where they neutralize the effects of mediators released by mast cells and basophils. Thus, eosinophils are frequently seen in connective tissue at allergic or other hypersensitivity reaction sites. The allergic reactions are amplified by platelet activation factor (PAF), which causes platelet aggregation and additional release of histamine, heparin, and vasoactive substances. Treatment of symptoms is achieved with **antihistamine medications** that block histamine receptors.

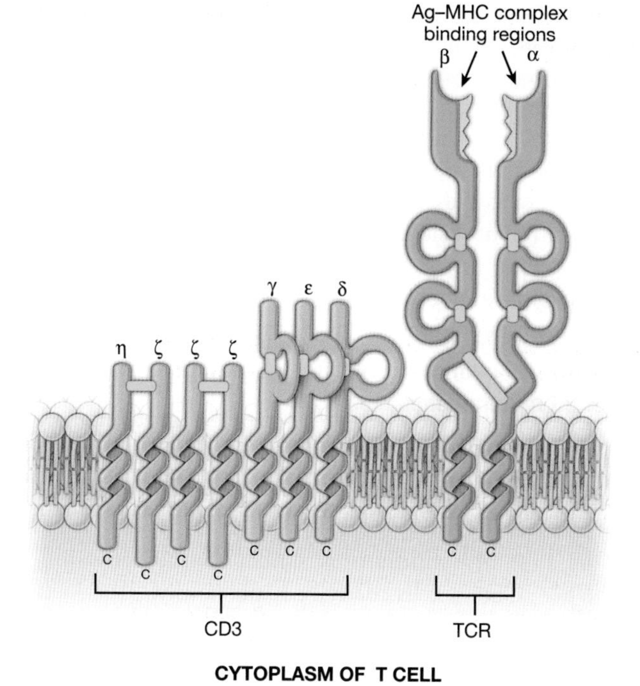

FIGURE 14.5. Schematic diagram of the molecular structure of the CD3–TCR complex. The CD3 molecule consists of five different polypeptide chains with molecular weights ranging from 16 to 28 kDa. This molecule is closely associated with the T-cell receptor (*TCR*), which has two polypeptide chains (α and β). The T cell may be activated after the interaction of the *TCR* with antigen (*Ag*) displayed on the surface of a major histocompatibility complex (*MHC*) molecule. This interaction transmits the signals to the interior of the cell through the CD3 molecule. This signal stimulates the T cell to secrete interleukins, which, in turn, stimulate T cells to divide and differentiate.

MHC I is expressed on the surface of all nucleated cells and platelets. The MHC I molecules present fragments of peptides derived from **cytosolic** proteins to **cytotoxic CD8$^+$ T lymphocytes.** MHC I molecules perform this function by displaying on their surface short fragments of all peptides (8–10 amino acids in length) that are actively synthesized by the cell. MHC I molecules act as a target to allow the elimination of abnormal host cells (e.g., virus-infected or cancer-transformed cells). Therefore, all endogenous "self" peptides are displayed on the surface of every cell in the body, but viral or cancer-specific peptides are displayed only on the surface of infected or transformed cells (Fig. 14.6).

MHC II is limited in its distribution (see Fig. 14.6). It is expressed on the surface of all APCs (e.g., macrophages, dendritic cells, and lymphocytes B) and is critical in immune interactions. The MHC II molecules present partially digested, endocytosed foreign peptides (18–20 amino acids in length) acquired by APCs through phagocytosis to **helper CD4$^+$ T lymphocytes.**

Tissue distribution of MHC molecules uniquely restricts T-cell responses.

It is important to recognize that the tissue distribution of MHC I and MHC II molecules uniquely restricts T-cell responses. Because all nucleated cells contain the cellular machinery for the replication and reproduction of viruses, they must be equipped with **MHC I** molecules that allow them to communicate with **cytotoxic CD8$^+$ T lymphocytes** if they become infected or transformed. In this way, MHC I molecules present intracellular antigens to cytotoxic CD8$^+$ T lymphocytes. In the absence of infection or transformation, MHC I molecules present endogenous antigen peptides to cytotoxic CD8$^+$ T lymphocytes. Because self-reactive T cells are selected and eliminated in the thymus, the presentation of self-antigen allows for constant surveillance by the cytotoxic CD8$^+$ T lymphocytes, which react only to cells expressing aberrant, nonself antigens. Through this mechanism, infected and transformed cells are eliminated.

In contrast, **MHC II** molecules are only expressed on the surface of professional APCs, which obtain antigen peptides by sampling the extracellular environment through phagocytosis. Presentation of antigen to helper CD4$^+$ T lymphocytes leads to the **coordination of an immune response** and recruitment of innate immune cells and cytotoxic CD8$^+$ T lymphocytes to the site of infection. The subset of helper CD4$^+$ T lymphocytes produced after antigen presentation depends on the cytokines secreted by the APC. Different cytokines are secreted in response to the activation of different PRRs and their downstream transcription factors.

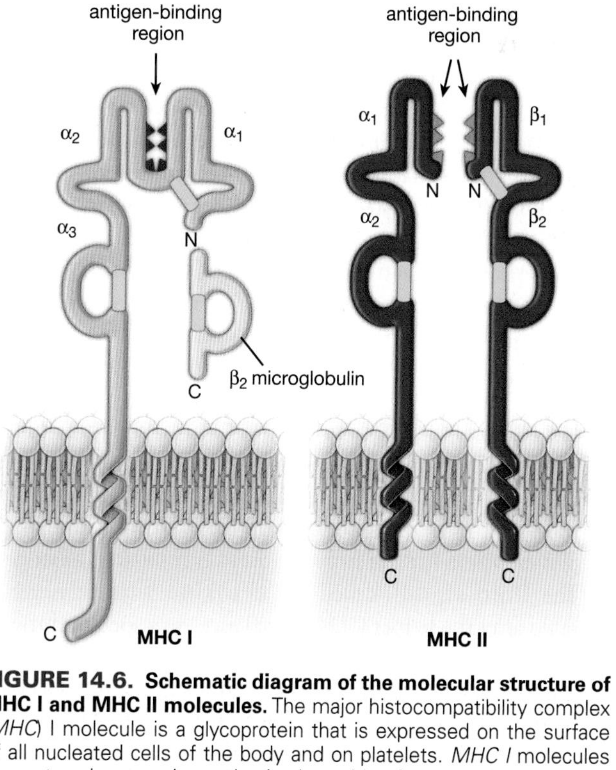

FIGURE 14.6. Schematic diagram of the molecular structure of MHC I and MHC II molecules. The major histocompatibility complex (*MHC*) I molecule is a glycoprotein that is expressed on the surface of all nucleated cells of the body and on platelets. *MHC I* molecules present endogenously synthesized peptides for recognition by cytotoxic CD8$^+$ T lymphocytes. Therefore, the *MHC I* molecule acts as the target for the elimination of abnormal host cells producing abnormal proteins (e.g., cells infected by an intracellular agent such as a virus or cells that have been transformed such as cancer cells). *MHC I* consists of an α heavy chain (45 kDa) and a smaller, noncovalently attached β_2 microglobulin polypeptide (12 kDa). The β_2 microglobulin promotes maturation of T cells and acts as a chemotactic factor. The *MHC II* molecule is also a glycoprotein but is expressed only on a restricted population of cells known as *antigen-presenting cells* (*APCs*). *MHC II* molecules present exogenous (foreign) peptides to helper CD4$^+$ T lymphocytes. They consist of two chains—an α-chain (33 kDa) and a β-chain (29 kDa)—each of which possesses oligosaccharide groups. Note that the antigen-binding region on the *MHC I* molecule is narrower than that on *MHC II*; therefore, the size of the displayed peptides varies from 8 to 10 amino acids in *MHC I* and 18 to 20 amino acids in *MHC II*.

Activation of T and B Cells

Activation of helper CD4$^+$ T cell requires the presence of three stimulatory signals.

Helper CD4$^+$ T cells require **three stimulatory signals** to become fully activated and subsequently differentiate and proliferate.

- The **first signal**, called the **antigen signal**, is generated by the interaction of the **TCR** with the **antigen–MHC** complex. This binding triggers the initial activation of the naïve helper T cell. Subsequent binding of the **CD4 molecule** to the TCR–antigen–MHC complex helps to stabilize this interaction. This process usually takes place in the secondary lymphatic organs.
- The **second signal**, called the **costimulatory signal**, is delivered by the interaction of membrane molecules on T cells and molecules on the APC. The most well-characterized interactions are between the **CD28** molecule expressed on the T-cell membrane and **B7** molecules, either B7-1 (CD80) or B7-2 (CD86) expressed on the APC membrane. Another pair of costimulatory signals is generated by the interaction of **CD40** (on APCs) with **CD40L** (CD154) on T cells. T cells also possess high-affinity inhibitory receptors known as *cytotoxic T lymphocyte–associated protein 4* (**CTLA-4**), which competes for binding with B7 (CD80 and CD86) protein. Thus, CTLA-4 is a competitive inhibitor of B7-CD28 interaction and inhibits the immune response, which is important for maintaining tolerance (nonresponsiveness) to self-antigens. Interaction of the TCR with antigen–MHC complex in the absence of costimulatory signal shuts down the activation process of the T cells, so they do not respond inappropriately. Recently, a new therapeutic **CTLA-4-Ig** fusion protein has been developed to inhibit the immune response by blocking the B7-CD28 costimulatory signal. This protein, which consists of the extracellular domain of the CTLA-4 receptor fused with the F_c fragment of human IgG, binds to and blocks B7 molecules. CTLA-4-Ig (abatacept) is used to treat rheumatoid and juvenile idiopathic arthritis and is in clinical trials for the prevention of transplant rejection.
- The **third signal,** called the **cytokine signal**, is generated after the helper CD4$^+$ T cell receives a specific antigen signal (first signal) and a costimulatory (second) signal. The third signal consists of instructions for future development in the form of **cytokines** secreted by an APC. These different cytokines activate specific transcription factors that determine the pathway for helper T-cell differentiation. Cytokines trigger further differentiation of helper CD4$^+$ T cells into a specific subset (Th1, Th2, or Th17). Each of these cells performs a different role in furthering the immune response. For example, IFN-γ and IL-12 lead to activation of the T-box transcription factor TBX21, also called *T-bet* (T-box expressed in T cells), which induces differentiation of the helper CD4$^+$ **Th1 cell** phenotype. In contrast, IL-4 activates the transcription factor GATA-3, leading to a differentiation of **Th2 cell** phenotype, and IL-6 and IL-23 lead to activation of RORγT transcription factor, leading to helper CD4$^+$ **Th17 cell** differentiation. The selection of which cytokines to be secreted by the APC when it presents antigen to the helperT cell depends on pattern recognition receptors (PRRs) activated by the pathogen-associated molecules expressed on invading microorganisms. For example, the specific PRR called toll-like receptor-9 (TLR9) detects viral and bacterial DNA within the endosomal compartment, leading to the secretion of interferon (IFN-γ). INF-γ not only inhibits protein synthesis in neighboring cells to prevent viral or bacterial spread but also induces helper Th1 phenotype differentiation to promote intracellular killing of endosomal contents within macrophages.

Activation of cytotoxic CD8$^+$ T cell is achieved through two different mechanisms.

Cytotoxic CD8$^+$ T lymphocytes (CTLs) can be activated by interacting with **antigen-presenting cells** (i.e., macrophage, dendritic cells) through two different mechanisms.

- The **first mechanism** is similar to the activation of helper CD4$^+$ cells described previously. The activation process of naïve cytotoxic T cells is initiated by the interaction of its TCR with the antigen–MHC complex. In contrast to helper T cells, cytotoxic T cells can only recognize the processed antigen displayed on MHC I molecules. This binding triggers the initial activation of the naïve cytotoxic T cell, and the TCR–MHC I complex is subsequently stabilized by the CD8 molecule. A required costimulatory signal is generated from interactions between the CD28 molecule expressed on the T-cell membrane and B7 molecules expressed on APC. If the initial binding stimulus is strong enough, the APC provides a strong enough costimulatory signal to induce IL-2 secretion by cytotoxic CD8$^+$ cells. IL-2 then acts in an autocrine manner to induce and advance the differentiation of cytotoxic CD8$^+$ cells into fully activated immunocompetent effector cells.
- The **second mechanism** of cytotoxic CD8$^+$ T-cell activation **requires help from CD4$^+$ T helper cells**, which recognize the same processed antigen on the same APC as the naïve cytotoxic T cell. Recall that APCs express both MHC I and MHC II molecules so they can display the same antigen peptide to both cytotoxic CD8$^+$ and helper CD4$^+$ T cells simultaneously on different MHCs. TCRs of helper CD4$^+$ and cytotoxic CD8$^+$ cells bind to the respective MHCs. In this mechanism, the B7 molecule on the APC activates the expression of CD40L molecules and secretion of IL-2 cytokine by the effector helper CD4$^+$ cell. Interaction between CD40L on helper CD4$^+$ cells and CD40 on the APC increases expression of costimulatory molecules on the APCs, which, in turn, enhances the activation process of the naïve cytotoxic CD8$^+$ cells. Given the highly toxic nature of cytotoxic CD8$^+$ cells, this activation mechanism ensures that only those cytotoxic CD8$^+$ cells targeting relevant antigens are activated.

When a fully activated **cytotoxic CD8$^+$ T lymphocyte** recognizes an antigen–MHC I complex, the TCR attaches to it. Interaction of the cytotoxic CD8$^+$ TCR with the MHC I molecule–presenting antigen peptide on the target cell results in secretion of perforin and granzyme B, which induces the intrinsic pathway of apoptosis in target cells by activating the enzymatic cascade of caspases.

Cytotoxic CD8⁺ T lymphocytes are MHC I restricted, and helper CD4⁺ T lymphocytes are MHC II restricted.

As mentioned earlier, MHC molecules are recognized by helper $CD4^+$ T lymphocytes or cytotoxic $CD8^+$ T lymphocytes, depending on the class of the MHC molecule engaged. *This restricted presentation of foreign antigens by MHC molecules to either cytotoxic or helper T lymphocytes is a key component of immune surveillance.*

The MHC I molecule with the peptide antigen displayed on its surface interacts only with the TCR and CD8 molecule expressed on cytotoxic **$CD8^+$ T lymphocytes**; these cells are, therefore, described as **MHC I restricted**. This interaction allows cytotoxic T lymphocytes to recognize infected or transformed target cells (Fig. 14.7a).

In contrast, the MHC II molecule with the peptide antigen displayed on its surface interacts only with the TCR and CD4 molecule expressed on helper **$CD4^+$ T lymphocytes** (Fig. 14.7b); these cells are, therefore, described as **MHC II restricted**. MHC II molecules are found on APCs, such as macrophages, whose main function is to present antigen to T lymphocytes.

For B cells to become activated and differentiate into plasma cells, they require interactions with helper T lymphocytes.

Each **B lymphocyte** reacts only with a single antigen or type of antigenic site that it has been genetically programmed to recognize. Activation of B cells requires **two signals**. The first signal is derived from interaction between **BCRs** and **antigen**. The bound antigen molecules are engulfed into B cells by receptor-mediated endocytosis, and fragments of the antigen are then displayed at the cell surface with the help of MHC II molecules. Helper T cells with complementary TCRs bind B cells and provide the second **costimulatory signal**. The binding usually involves a reaction between **CD40** molecules on a B-cell surface with their ligands (**CD40L** or CD154) residing at the surface of a helper T cell. These interactions complete the activation process of a B lymphocyte and induce an involved T cell to secrete specific cytokines that stimulate divisions and differentiation of B cells. Details of B-cell activation are illustrated in Figure 14.8. Activated B lymphocytes differentiate into plasma cells and memory B cells.

- **Plasma cells** synthesize and secrete a specific antibody. During this process, activated B cells switch from synthesizing their BCRs as integral membrane proteins to forming a soluble version, which are called **antibodies**.
- **Memory B cells** respond more quickly to the next encounter with the same antigen. Memory B cells express high levels of Bcl-2 proteins, which, on lymphocytes, act as antiapoptotic agents contributing to their long life span. In humans, a marker for memory B cells is CD27.

The specific antibody produced by the plasma cell binds to the stimulating antigen, forming an **antigen–antibody complex**. These complexes are eliminated in a variety of ways, including destruction by NK cells and phagocytosis by macrophages and eosinophils.

In antibody-dependent cell–mediated cytotoxicity (ADCC), the specificity of IgG molecules directs NK cells to their targets.

The membranes of several cells, including NK cells, macrophages, neutrophils, and eosinophils, possess **immunoglobulin F_c receptors** and can kill certain target cells. The target cells are usually coated with IgG antibodies. NK cells express CD16a ($F_c\gamma$RIIIa) receptor on their surface to recognize the F_c region of antibodies and preferentially attack and destroy these target cells (Fig. 14.9). The recognition and subsequent destruction of antibody-coated target cells by NK cells is called **antibody-dependent cell–mediated cytotoxicity (ADCC)**. The antibodies in

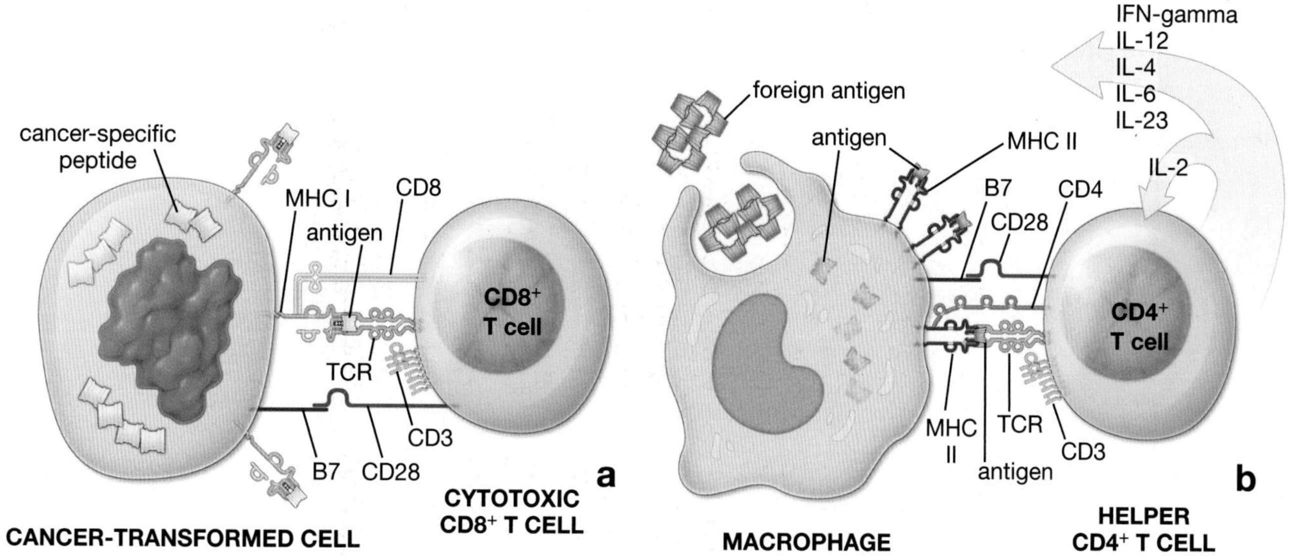

FIGURE 14.7. Schematic diagram of the molecular interactions that occur during antigen presentation. To become activated, both cytotoxic and helper T lymphocytes need to identify presented antigens as "nonself" as well as recognize the appropriate class of major histocompatibility complex (MHC) molecules. Note that each interaction between an antigen–MHC complex with its specific T-cell receptor (*TCR*) requires a costimulatory signal from the interaction of CD28 with B7 molecules. Without a costimulatory signal, the T cell cannot be fully activated. **a.** In all nucleated cells of the body, viral antigen or cancer (tumor-specific) proteins are displayed in the context of *MHC I* molecules to interact with cytotoxic $CD8^+$ T lymphocytes. **b.** On antigen-presenting cells (e.g., macrophages), the foreign antigen is displayed in the context of *MHC II* molecules to interact with a helper $CD4^+$ T lymphocyte.

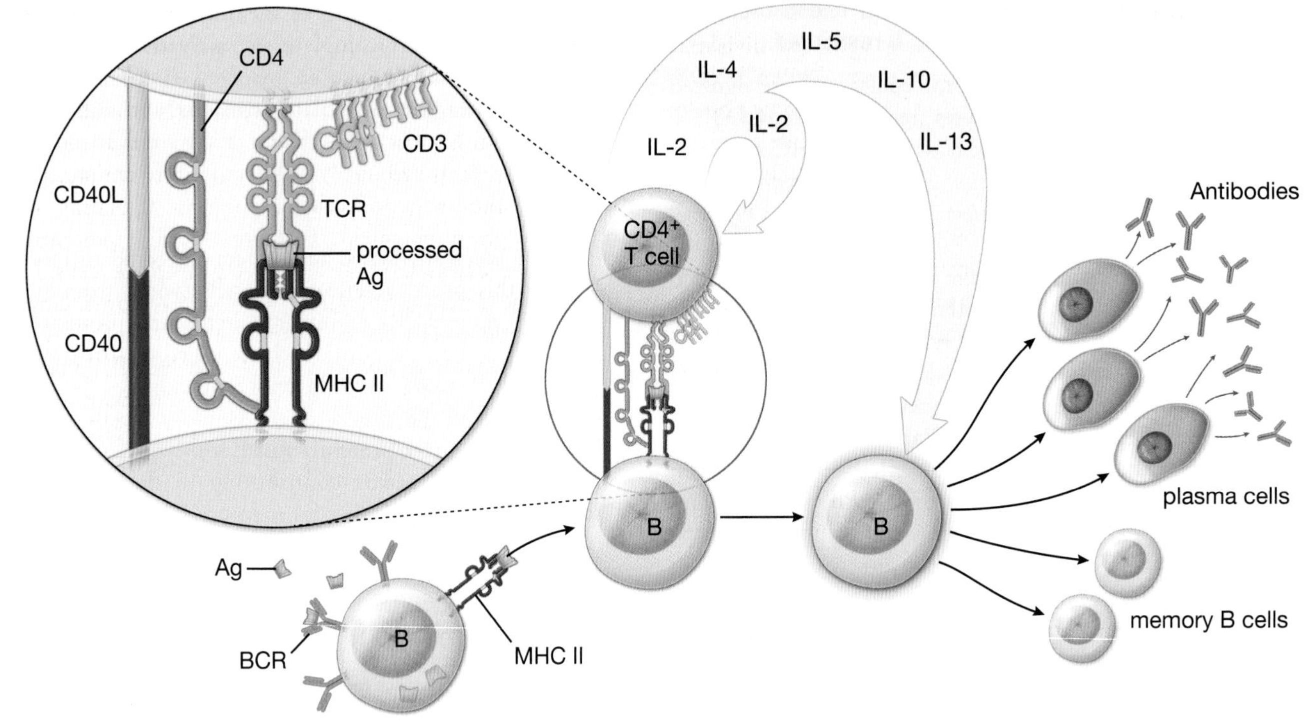

FIGURE 14.8. Schematic diagram of B lymphocyte activation leading to plasma cell and B memory cell formation. B cells are activated by the binding of antigen (*Ag*) to B-cell receptors (*BCRs*; membrane-bound antibodies) expressed on their surface. As an antigen-presenting cell, a B cell internalizes the *BCR*–antigen complex, partially digests the antigen, and then displays parts of it on the surface of its own major histocompatibility complex (*MHC*) II molecules. The T-cell receptor (*TCR*) on a helper CD4$^+$ T lymphocyte (Th2 cell) recognizes both the antigen and the MHC II molecule, activating the helper CD4$^+$ T lymphocyte. The activated helper CD4$^+$ T lymphocyte releases interleukins, including IL-2, IL-4, IL-5, IL-10, and IL-13, which promote division and differentiation of the B lymphocyte into plasma cells and memory B cells. Note the presence of a costimulatory molecule complex between the B and T cells.

ADCC that coat the target cells often include tumor-specific antibodies. As mentioned earlier (see page 489), through this mechanism, the antigen specificity of IgG antibodies, representing the adaptive immune system, is paired with the toxicity of NK cells to provide antigen-specific killing. This binding (through the F_c region) results in the apoptosis and lysis of the target cell.

If the antigen is a bacterium, the antigen–antibody complex may also activate a system of plasma proteins called the **complement system** and cause one of its components, usually C3, to bind to the bacterium and act as a ligand for its phagocytosis by macrophages. Complement-bound foreign cells are also the targets of ADCC.

In the cell-mediated immune response, cytotoxic CD8$^+$ T lymphocytes (CTLs) target and destroy transformed and virus-infected cells.

When the TCR of a cytotoxic T cell recognizes and binds to an antigen–MHC I complex on the surface of a transformed or virus-infected cell, the activation process is triggered.

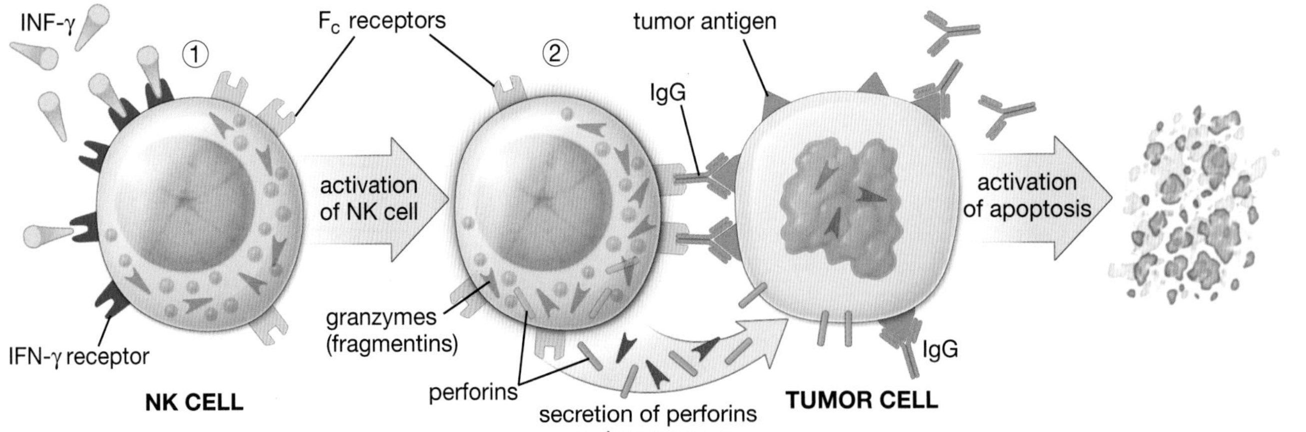

FIGURE 14.9. Schematic diagram of activation of natural killer cells leading to destruction of a transformed tumor cell by antibody-dependent cell–mediated cytotoxicity (ADCC). The *ADCC* reaction involves **(1)** activation of natural killer (*NK*) cells by the binding of interferon-γ (*IFN-γ*), the powerful *NK* cell activator, to its cell surface receptor (*IFN-γ receptor*) and **(2)** the binding of an antibody- or an antibody- and complement-coated target cell to an *NK* cell–bearing F_c receptors. These reactions induce apoptosis, or lysis, of the target cell, usually through the action of tumor-specific antibodies or the action of perforins and granzymes (fragmentins) secreted by activated *NK* cells. *IgG*, immunoglobulin G.

First, cytotoxic T cells undergo "**clonal expansion**" by entering the cell cycle and proceeding with cell divisions, followed by differentiation into effector ("killer") cells. During differentiation, a large number of secretory vesicles are formed containing specific proteins that include perforins and granzymes (fragmentins). Cytotoxic T cells secrete these proteins as a result of their interaction with antigen. **Perforins** are pore-forming proteins that attach to the target cell and form ring-like transmembrane channels in the target cell membranes. These channels cause an increase in the permeability of the membrane that contributes to cell death. **Granzymes** are exogenous serine proteinases that are released from cytoplasmic granules and pass into the target cells through the pores created by perforins. Once inside the cell, granzymes activate caspases that induce the cell to undergo apoptosis (Fig. 14.10). After killing the target cell, the majority of activated cytotoxic T cells will die (apoptosis), but some of them that interacted with helper T cells will become memory cells.

$CD4^+$ $CD25^+$ $FOXP3^+$ regulatory (suppressor) T lymphocytes represent a subset of helper $CD4^+$ cells that suppress the immune responses of other lymphocytes.

Once the immune reactions are initiated by contact with antigen, the immune system is capable of controlling the magnitude of this response and terminating it over time. As discussed earlier, this process is regulated by **CTLA-4 receptors** expressed on activated T cells that inhibit B7-CD28 costimulatory signals (see page 494). In addition, certain T lymphocytes called **regulatory (suppressor) T cells** diminish or suppress responses of other lymphocytes to antigen. They play an important role in regulating and maintaining immunologic **self-tolerance**, thus preventing autoimmune diseases. Characterization of these cells has proved to be difficult, but recent studies have convincingly shown that these cells belong to the population of $CD4^+$ T lymphocytes that coexpress the CD25 and $FOXP3^+$ marker proteins. **$CD4^+$ $CD25^+$ $FOXP3^+$ T cells** originate in the thymus and account for about 5% of the total population of T cells. They secrete cytokines such as IL-10 and transforming growth factor β (TGF-β), the latter a potent suppressor of proliferation of specific classes of T and B effector cells.

Regulatory (suppressor) T cells diminish or suppress antibody formation by B cells as well as mitigate the ability of cytotoxic T cells to provide a cell-mediated immune response. They play important roles in **delayed hypersensitivity reactions (type IV hypersensitivity reactions)** by downregulating responses to antigen that enter the body through the skin or mucosa. The classic example of the delayed hypersensitivity reactions is the **tuberculin**

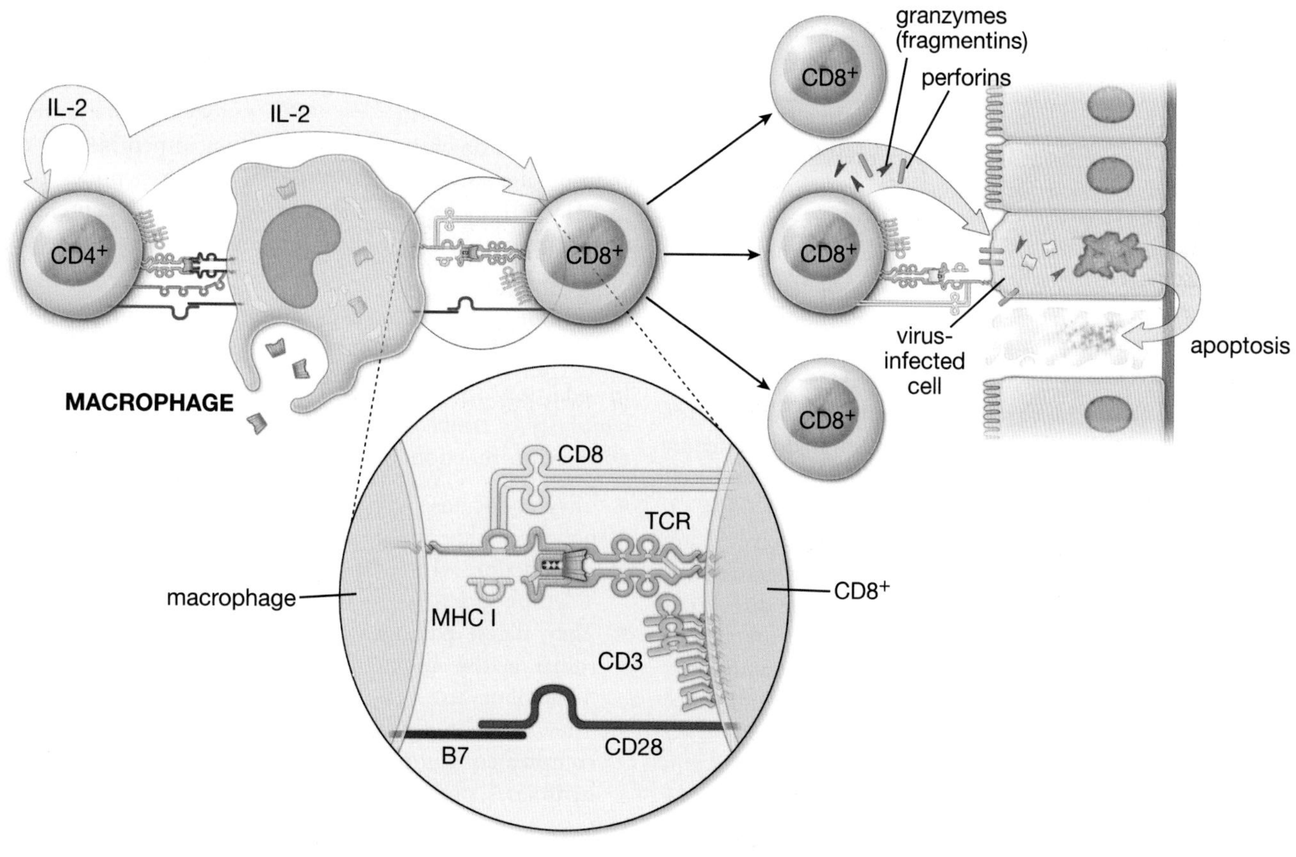

FIGURE 14.10. Schematic diagram of T-cell activation leading to elimination of a virus-infected host cell. The T-cell receptor (*TCR*)–CD3 complex on a helper $CD4^+$ T lymphocyte recognizes foreign antigen displayed on a major histocompatibility complex (*MHC*) II molecule on the surface of a macrophage. This recognition triggers a rapid response from B lymphocytes and the release of interleukin-2 (*IL-2*). The same macrophage also expresses *MHC I* molecules (like every other cell in the body) that interact with the appropriate *TCR* on the surface of a cytotoxic $CD8^+$ T lymphocyte. The cytotoxic $CD8^+$ T lymphocyte also possesses IL-2 receptors. IL-2 binding to these receptors stimulates the cell to divide and differentiate. The newly formed cytotoxic $CD8^+$ T lymphocytes migrate to the site of viral infection. There, the *TCRs* recognize the viral antigens displayed on the surface of *MHC I* molecules of infected cells. After successfully recognizing these "nonself" proteins, the cytotoxic $CD8^+$ T lymphocytes secrete perforins and granzymes, killing the infected cells. Note that interaction of cytotoxic $CD8^+$ T lymphocytes with an infected cell does not require costimulatory signals.

screening (Mantoux) test, in which tuberculin (an extract of *Mycobacterium tuberculosis*) is injected between the layers of dermis causing skin induration (hardening) and erythema (redness) in individuals exposed to tuberculosis. The Mantoux reaction peaks 48 hours after the injection of tuberculin.

Regulatory (suppressor) T cells are involved in the pathogenesis of many autoimmune and infectious diseases and also play an important role in the prevention of **graft rejection**. Suppressor T lymphocytes may also function in the regulation of erythroid cell maturation in the bone marrow.

Activated T lymphocytes synthesize a variety of cytokines.

Cytokines are soluble polypeptide substances that modulate the immune responses. They are synthesized mainly by activated T lymphocytes, which affect the function of immune system effector cells (T, B, and NK cells), monocytes, macrophages, and other APCs. In general, cytokines and growth factors are similar in nature; the distinction between them is related to their effects on their target cell populations. **Cytokines** are defined as substances that are involved in immune defense mechanisms and **act on lymphocytes**, whereas growth factors act on other somatic cells. Included among these substances are chemotactic and mitogenic agents, migration inhibitory factors, interferon, and interleukins.

Cytokines serve as **chemical messengers** between cells of the immune system and act locally on the same cell that secreted them (autocrine control) or on neighboring cells (paracrine control). In a way similar to hormones, they may also communicate the state of the immune system to cells in other systems (e.g., central nervous system, endocrine system, and hemopoietic system). Cytokines function through specific receptors. Therefore, cells regulated by cytokines possess cytokine receptors.

Interleukins are synthesized by helper $CD4^+$ T lymphocytes, monocytes, macrophages, and endothelial cells. Interleukins promote growth and differentiation of T, B, NK, and hematopoietic cells. Signaling transduction pathways downstream of cytokine receptors result in activation of specific transcription factors, which affect many different processes including differentiation, proliferation, and cell metabolism. Through interleukin secretion, helper $CD4^+$ T cells can coordinate an immune response that involves many different cell types. Currently, more than 38 interleukins have been identified. IL-2 was the first cytokine to be discovered and characterized. It is also the most important cytokine that induces proliferation of T cells. Several **immunosuppressive agents** (e.g., cyclosporine A, tacrolimus, rapamycin) are widely used to prevent transplant rejection. They block T-cell proliferation by inhibiting expression of the **gene encoding IL-2**, an important growth factor for T lymphocytes. Rapamycin also inhibits T-cell proliferation by arresting them in the G_1 phase of the cell cycle and promoting apoptosis.

Mutations in the genes encoding several cytokine receptors have been identified in several immunodeficiency disorders, bacterial sepsis, certain lymphoid cancers, and autoimmune diseases. For instance, individuals with a mutation in the **IL-12 receptor gene** cannot mount an effective immune response against mycobacterial (fungal) infections. In addition, cytokines are being used to reverse cellular deficiencies after chemotherapy and radiation therapy and treat certain cancers. The major functions of selected interleukins are summarized in Table 14.3.

Antigen-Presenting Cells

APCs interact with helper $CD4^+$ T lymphocytes to facilitate immune responses.

The interaction between most antigens and antibodies is insufficient to stimulate immune responses. The antigen must be broken into small peptides and presented in conjunction with MHC II molecules by specialized APCs to the appropriate helper $CD4^+$ T lymphocytes. Antigen can also be processed as a part of the B-cell activation pathway (see Fig. 14.8). Most APCs belong to the mononuclear phagocyte system (MPS; described in Chapter 6, Connective Tissue, Folder 6.4, page 203). Examples of APCs include **macrophages**, **sinusoidal macrophages (Kupffer cells)** of the liver, **Langerhans cells** in the epidermis, **dermal macrophages** in the dermis, and **dendritic cells** of the spleen, thymus, lymph nodes, and skin. Two APCs that do not belong to the MPS are **B lymphocytes** and type II and type III **epithelioreticular cells** of the thymus.

To present an antigen to a helper T cell, the APC first processes the antigen intracellularly and then displays antigen peptides on its surface using MHC II molecules. Antigen processing begins when the APC endocytoses the antigen and breaks it down into 18–20 amino acid peptides. In the endosomal compartment of the APC, the peptides bind to MHC II molecules. The antigen–MHC II complex is then translocated to the plasma membrane of the APC and displayed on the cell surface (Fig. 14.11).

In addition to acting as APCs, macrophages perform other crucial functions in the immune response.

In addition to presenting antigens to both T and B lymphocytes, **macrophages** have other important, although nonspecific, functions in the immune response:

- They endocytose and partially degrade both protein and polysaccharide antigens before they present them in conjunction with MHC II molecules to helper $CD4^+$ T lymphocytes.
- They digest pathogenic microorganisms through lysosomal action in combination with the helper $CD4^+$ T lymphocytes.
- They secrete multiple cytokines, including lymphokines, complement components, and interleukins as well as acid hydrolases, proteases, and lipases.

Activated macrophages destroy phagocytosed bacteria and foreign antigens.

After contact with an antigen, activated helper $CD4^+$ T lymphocytes trigger the macrophage activation process. Macrophages undergo one of two activation processes characterized by multiple functional and morphologic

TABLE 14.3 **Characteristics of Interleukins**

Name	Symbol	Source	Major Functions
Interleukin-1	IL-1	Neutrophils, monocytes, macrophages, endothelial cells	Stimulates various cells in inflammatory response; induces fever; facilitates proliferation and differentiation of $CD4^+$ T (Th17) cells and B cells
Interleukin-2	IL-2	T cells	Induces proliferation and differentiation of $CD4^+$ T cells and, to a lesser degree, $CD8^+$ T cells, B cells, and NK cells; stimulus for Ig synthesis
Interleukin-3	IL-3	$CD4^+$ T cells, epithelioreticular cells of thymus, stromal cells	Induces early proliferation of hematopoietic stem cells
Interleukin-4	IL-4	$CD4^+$ T (Th2) cells, γ/δ T cells, mast cells, basophiles	Induces proliferation and differentiation of B cells and Th2 subset of $CD4^+$ T cells; activates macrophages; promotes synthesis of IgE and IgG
Interleukin-5	IL-5	$CD4^+$ T (Th2) cells, γ/δ T cells, NK cells, mast cells, eosinophils	Induces proliferation and differentiation of eosinophils; stimulates B cells to secrete IgA
Interleukin-6	IL-6	Endothelial cells, neutrophils, macrophages, T cells, osteoblasts, smooth muscle cells	Stimulates differentiation of hematopoietic cells; induces growth of activated B cells, differentiation of Th17 subset of $CD4^+$ T cells
Interleukin-7	IL-7	Adventitial cells of bone marrow, endothelial cells	Stimulates growth and differentiation of progenitor B and T cells
Interleukin-8	IL-8	Macrophages, monocytes, endothelial cells	Acts as chemotactic factor on T lymphocytes, NK cells, and neutrophils
Interleukin-9	IL-9	$CD4^+$ T (Th2, Th17) cells	Facilitates growth and activation of mast cells; stimulates growth of Th2 subset of $CD4^+$ T cell and hematopoietic cells
Interleukin-10	IL-10	Macrophages, dendritic cells, T cells, B cells	Immunosuppressive effect through APCs; acts on T cells as cytokine synthesis inhibitory factor; inhibits macrophage functions
Interleukin-11	IL-11	Bone marrow stromal cells (fibroblasts)	Facilitates growth of hematopoietic cells, mainly megakaryocytes
Interleukin-12	IL-12	Macrophages, monocytes, dendritic cells	Stimulates growth of NK cells, differentiation of Th1 subset of $CD4^+$ T cells and $CD8^+$ T cells
Interleukin-13	IL-13	T cells, mast cells, basophils	Modulates B-cell responses; promotes IgE synthesis; stimulates alternative activation of M2 macrophages; stimulates MHC II expression on B cells
Interleukin-14	IL-14	T cells, follicular dendritic cells, malignant B cells	Induces proliferation of both normal and malignant B cells
Interleukin-15	IL-15	$CD4^+$ T cells, macrophages, monocytes, other cell types	Induces proliferation and differentiation of $CD8^+$ T cells; stimulates activation of NK cells
Interleukin-16	IL-16	T cells, mast cells, eosinophils	Activates migration of $CD8^+$ and $CD4^+$ T cells, monocytes, and eosinophils
Interleukin-17	IL-17	Th17 subset of $CD4^+$ T cells, $CD8^+$ T cells, NK cells, γ/δ T cells, neutrophils	Stimulates epithelial, endothelial cells and fibroblasts to secrete cytokines, chemokines, and metalloproteases
Interleukin-18	IL-18	Activated macrophages dendritic cells, keratinocytes, and Kupffer cells	Indices differentiation of Th1 subset of $CD4^+$ T cells; induces synthesis of IFN-γ by T cells and NK cells
Interleukin-19	IL-19	Monocytes	Activates monocytes
Interleukin-20	IL-20	Th1 subset of $CD4^+$ T cells, monocytes, epithelial cells	Promotes differentiation of Th2 subset of $CD4^+$ T cell; stimulates keratinocytes proliferation

APC, antigen-presenting cell; *IFN-γ*, interferon-γ; *Ig*, immunoglobulin; *NK*, natural killer.

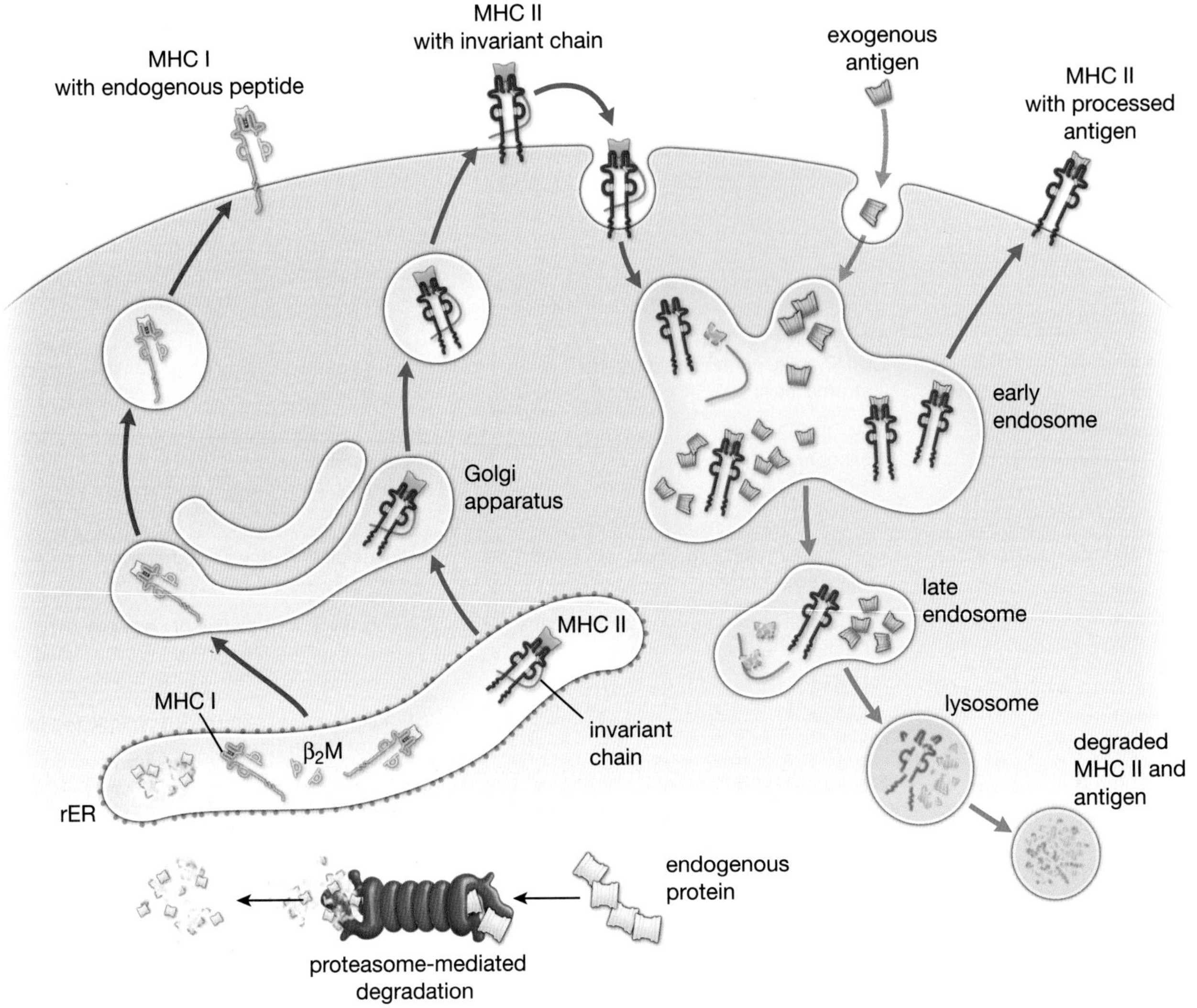

FIGURE 14.11. Schematic diagram of processing pathways for MHC I and MHC II synthesis and antigen presentation. During the processing and presentation of cytoplasmic antigen (*Ag*) for major histocompatibility complex (*MHC*) I molecules (*red pathway*), cytoplasmic protein antigens undergo proteasome-mediated degradation into 8–10 amino acid fragments that then enter the rough-surfaced endoplasmic reticulum (*rER*). In the *rER*, newly synthesized α-chains of *MHC I* molecules interact with both the processed antigen (*yellow*) and β_2 microglobulin (β_2M) and form a stable complex. This complex leaves the *rER* via the typical secretory pathway through the Golgi apparatus. The antigen–*MHC I* complex is displayed on the cell surface, where it is available for recognition by cytotoxic $CD8^+$ T lymphocytes. *MHC II* molecules are assembled in the *rER* and then bind to an invariant chain, which blocks the antigen-binding site. At this point, the *MHC II* molecule and the invariant chain are secreted to the cell surface (*blue pathway*). After a brief stay on the cell surface, the *MHC II* molecule and invariant chain are endocytosed, and in an early endosome, the invariant chain is degraded. The foreign (exogenous) antigen (*orange*) is endocytosed and partially digested by proteolytic degradation in endosomes (*grey pathway*). The *MHC II* molecule can now bind the processed foreign antigen and return with it to the cell surface. On the cell surface, the antigen–MHC II complex is recognized by helper $CD4^+$ T lymphocytes, which initiates the immune response. If the MHC II molecule fails to capture the antigen, it will be degraded in the lysosomal compartment (*green pathway*).

changes. When **Th1 lymphocytes** are stimulated by antigen, the cells express CD40L markers on their surface and secrete IFN-γ. Macrophages that are activated by IFN-γ and costimulated by interaction of CD40L and CD40 (at the surface of macrophage) are called **classically activated macrophages (M1 macrophages)**. They increase in size, as do the number of lysosomes and cytoplasmic vacuoles (Fig. 14.12). M1 macrophages become avidly phagocytotic with a greater ability to lyse ingested pathogenic microorganisms and foreign antigens. They promote inflammation, the destruction of extracellular matrix, and apoptosis. In contrast, macrophages that are activated by interleukins produced by **Th2 lymphocytes** are called **alternatively activated macrophages (M2 macrophages)**. They downregulate inflammation; promote rebuilding of extracellular matrix, fibroblast proliferation, and collagen synthesis; and stimulate angiogenesis. Cytokines produced by Th2 cells also suppress classically activated macrophages (M1 macrophages). A detailed description of both types of macrophages, their activation pathways, and their functions is provided in Chapter 6, Connective Tissue (page 200).

Macrophages also play a vital role in sequestering and removing foreign materials and organisms that either do not provoke an immune response or are ingested but not digested. These include both organic and inorganic particulate materials (e.g., carbon particles), pigment (e.g., from tattoos), cellulose, and asbestos as well as tuberculosis and leprosy bacilli and the organisms that cause malaria and other diseases. In these instances, macrophages often fuse to form multinucleate giant cells called **Langhans giant cells** that isolate these pathogens from the body.

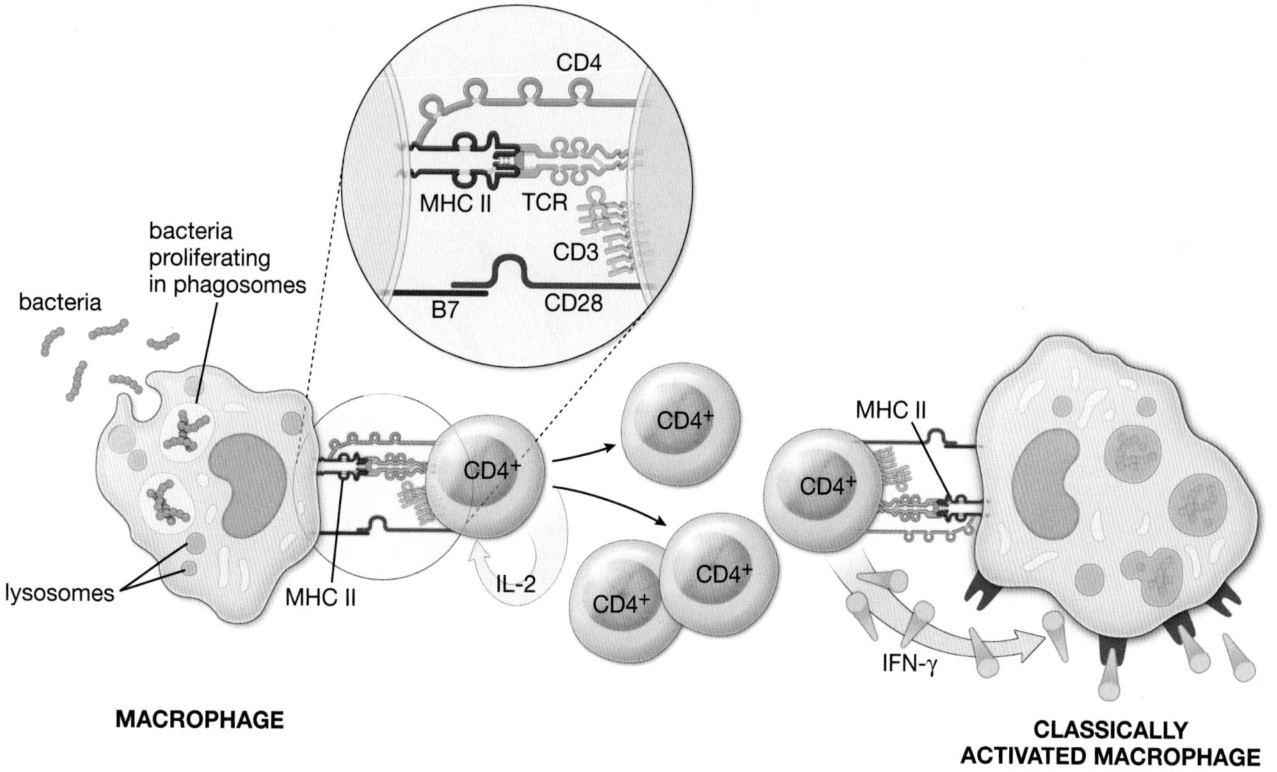

FIGURE 14.12. Classic activation process of the macrophage by a helper CD4⁺ T cell. Helper CD4⁺ T lymphocytes recognize the bacterial antigen expressed in the context of major histocompatibility complex (*MHC*) II molecules on the surface of a macrophage that has phagocytosed the bacteria. The recognition of *MHC II* molecules activates the T cell, which, in turn, secretes IL-2. IL-2 acts as an autocrine hormone to stimulate T-cell division and differentiation. Newly formed helper CD4⁺ T lymphocytes also interact with *MHC II* molecules and release interferon-γ (*IFN-γ*). This cytokine stimulates the macrophage to transform into classically activated (M1) macrophage to destroy the bacteria inside its phagosomes. CD4 molecules on the surface of the T cell also potentiate antibacterial reactions. *TCR*, T-cell receptor.

■ LYMPHATIC TISSUES AND ORGANS

Lymphatic Vessels

Lymphatic vessels are the route by which cells and large molecules pass from the tissue spaces back to the blood.

Lymphatic vessels begin as networks of blind capillaries in loose connective tissue. They are most numerous beneath the epithelium of skin and mucous membranes. These vessels remove substances and fluid from the extracellular spaces of the connective tissues, thus producing lymph. Because the walls of the lymphatic capillaries are more permeable than the walls of blood capillaries, large molecules, including antigens and cells, gain entry more readily into the lymphatic capillaries than into blood capillaries.

As lymph circulates through the lymphatic vessels, it passes through lymph nodes. Within the lymph nodes, foreign substances (antigens) conveyed in the lymph are trapped by follicular dendritic cells. The antigen exposed on the surface of follicular dendritic cells can be processed by antigen-presenting cells which reside within the lymph node.

Lymphocytes circulate through both lymphatic and blood vessels.

The circulation of lymphocytes through the lymphatic vessels and the bloodstream enables them to move from one part of the lymphatic system to another at different stages in their development and to reach sites within the body where they are needed. Lymphocytes conveyed in the lymph enter lymph nodes via **afferent lymphatic vessels**, whereas lymphocytes conveyed in the blood enter the node through the walls of **postcapillary venules** (**high endothelial venules [HEVs]**; Fig. 14.13). B and T cells that enter lymph node migrate to and populate distinct regions within the lymph node. Activated lymphocytes pass through the substance of the node and leave via the **efferent lymphatic vessels**, which lead to the right lymphatic trunk or to the thoracic duct. In turn, both of these channels empty into the blood circulation at the junctions of the internal jugular and subclavian veins at the base of the neck. The lymphocytes are conveyed to and from the various lymphatic tissues via the blood vessels.

■ DIFFUSE LYMPHATIC TISSUE AND LYMPHATIC NODULES

Diffuse lymphatic tissue and lymphatic nodules guard the body against pathogenic substances and are the site of the initial immune response.

The alimentary canal, respiratory passages, and genitourinary tract are guarded by accumulations of lymphatic tissue that is not enclosed by a capsule. Lymphocytes and other free cells of this tissue are found in the **lamina propria** (subepithelial tissue) of these tracts. This form of lymphatic tissue is called **diffuse lymphatic tissue** or **mucosa-associated lymphatic tissue (MALT)** because of its association with

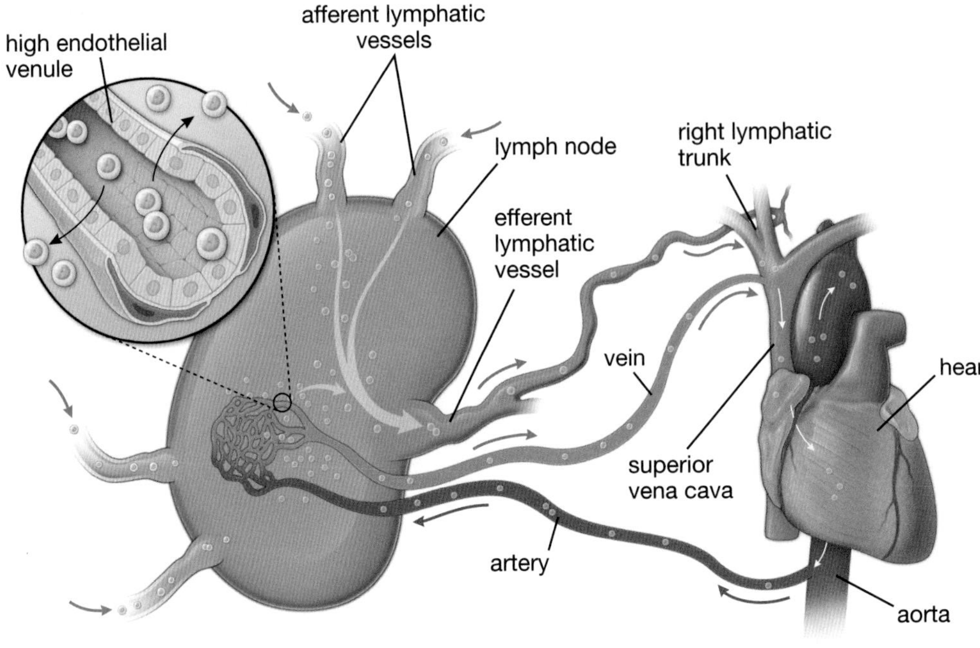

FIGURE 14.13. Diagram depicting circulation of lymphocytes in the body. Lymphocytes enter lymph nodes by two routes: afferent lymphatic vessels and through the wall of high endothelial venules (*HEVs*) in the deep cortex. *Inset* shows details of the *HEV*, which include cuboidal endothelium, continuous basement membrane, and occasional pericytes (*purple*). Some lymphocytes move to the T and B domains of the lymph node; others pass through the parenchyma of the node and leave via an efferent lymphatic vessel. Ultimately, the lymphocytes enter a major lymphatic vessel—in this case, the right lymphatic trunk—that opens into the junction of the right internal jugular and right subclavian vein. The lymphocytes continue to the arterial side of the circulation and, via the arteries, to the lymphatic tissues of the body or to tissues where they participate in immune reactions. From the lymphatic tissues, lymphocytes again return to the lymph nodes to gain entry via the *HEV*.

mucous membranes (Fig. 14.14). These cells are strategically located to intercept antigens and initiate an immune response. After contact with antigen, they travel to regional lymph nodes, where they undergo proliferation and differentiation. Progeny of these cells then returns to the lamina propria as effector B and T lymphocytes.

The importance of **diffuse lymphatic tissue** in protecting the body from antigens is indicated by two factors:

- The regular presence of large numbers of plasma cells, especially in the lamina propria of the GI tract, a morphologic indication of local antibody secretion
- The presence of large numbers of eosinophils, also frequently observed in the lamina propria of the intestinal and respiratory tracts, an indication of chronic inflammation and hypersensitivity reactions

Lymphatic nodules are discrete concentrations of lymphocytes contained in a meshwork of reticular cells.

In addition to diffuse lymphatic tissue, localized concentrations of lymphocytes are commonly found in the walls of the alimentary canal, respiratory passages, and genitourinary tract. These concentrations, called **lymphatic nodules** or **lymphatic follicles**, are sharply defined, but not encapsulated (Fig. 14.15). A lymphatic nodule consisting chiefly of small lymphocytes is called a **primary nodule**. However, most nodules are **secondary lymphatic nodules** and have distinctive features that include the following:

- A **germinal center** is located in the central region of the nodule (Fig. 14.16) and appears lightly stained in

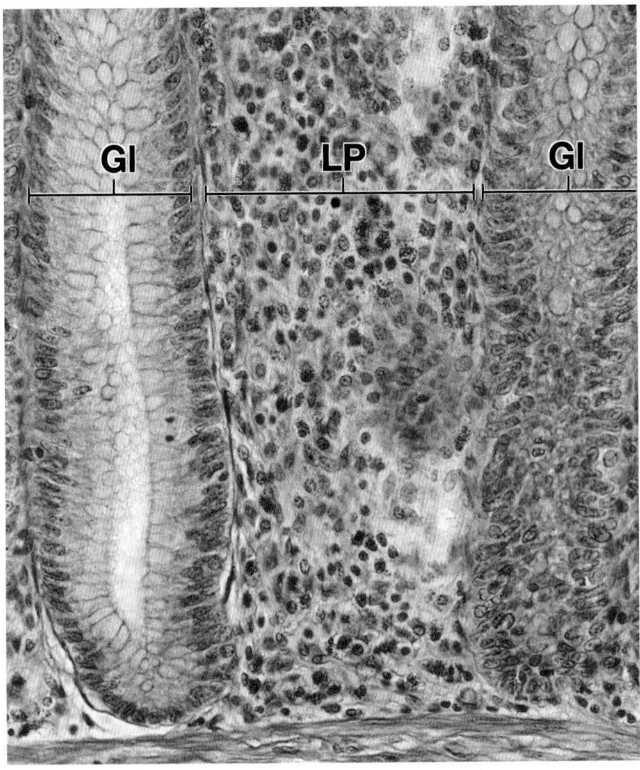

FIGURE 14.14. Photomicrograph of diffuse lymphatic tissue. This photomicrograph shows the diffuse lymphatic tissue in the lamina propria (*LP*) of the large intestine. The lower portion of two intestinal glands (*GI*) is also evident. The highly cellular, diffuse lymphatic tissue includes fibroblasts, plasma cells, and eosinophils. However, the most abundant cell component, whose presence characterizes diffuse lymphatic tissue, is the lymphocyte, which can be identified by its small, round, dark-staining nucleus. ×320.

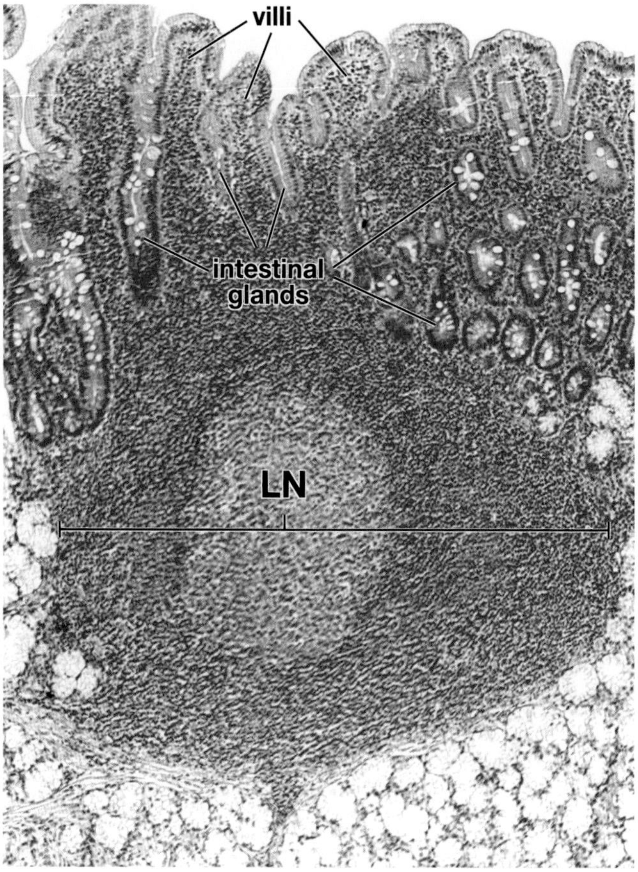

FIGURE 14.15. Photomicrograph of a lymphatic nodule. This photomicrograph shows a section of the wall of the small intestine (duodenum). Short villi and intestinal glands are present in the *upper part* of the micrograph. A lymphatic nodule (*LN*) occupies most of the remainder of the micrograph. The lighter central region of the nodule is the germinal center. The lymphocytes in the germinal center are larger than those in the denser region of the nodule. They have more cytoplasm, so their nuclei are more dispersed, giving the appearance of a less compact cellular mass. ×120.

histologic sections. The germinal center develops when a B lymphocyte that has recognized an antigen undergoes extensive division and proliferation. The lighter staining is attributable to the presence of the large lymphocytes (**lymphoblasts**) and migratory B cells committed to secreting antibodies called **plasmablasts**. These cells have large amounts of dispersed euchromatin in their nuclei rather than the dense heterochromatin of small lymphocytes. **Follicular dendritic cells (FDCs)**, **follicular helper CD4$^+$ lymphocytes (T_{FH})**, and resident **macrophages** are also present in germinal centers interspersed between populations of B lymphocytes. The germinal center is a morphologic indication of lymphatic tissue response to antigen. The presence of a germinal center represents a cascade of events (often called the **germinal center reaction**) that includes helper T cell–dependent activation, proliferation, and genetic diversification of B lymphocytes; generation of memory B cells; differentiation of plasma cells; and antibody production. Mitotic figures are frequently observed in the germinal center, reflecting the proliferation of new lymphocytes at this site. The number of follicular dendritic cells and macrophages in the germinal center often increases dramatically after a period of intense response to an antigen.

- A **mantle zone** or **corona** is present that represents an outer ring of small lymphocytes that encircles the germinal center. These lymphocytes represent **naïve B lymphocytes** that have not been previously stimulated by antigen.

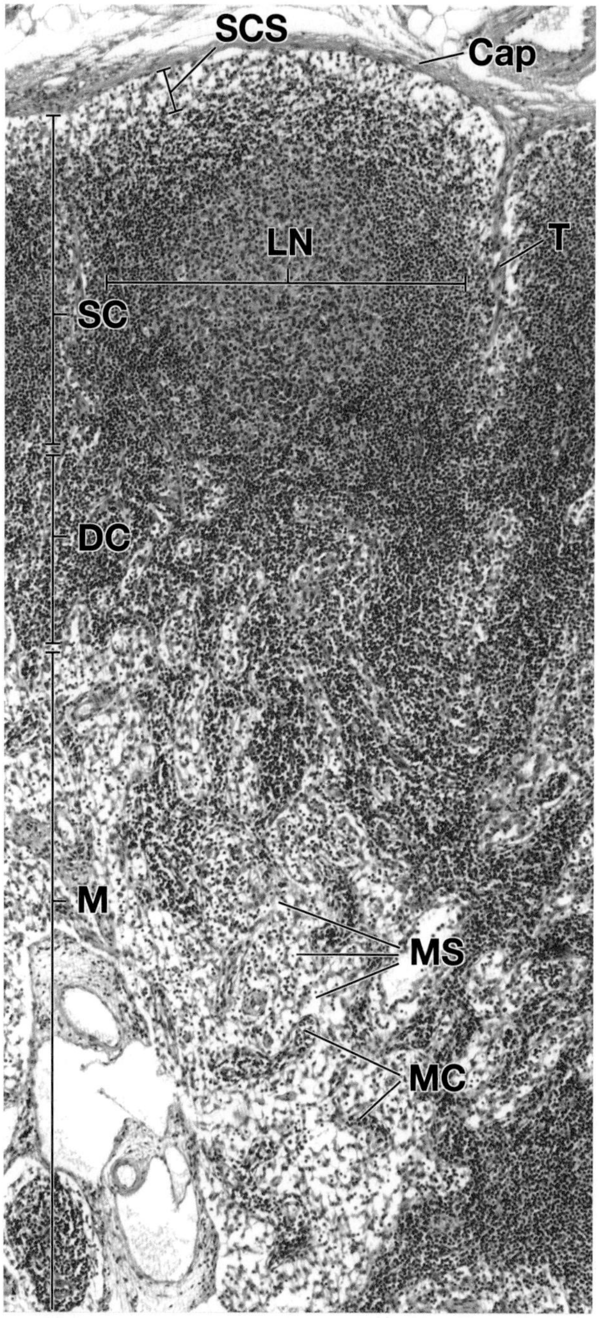

FIGURE 14.16. Photomicrograph of a lymph node. This photomicrograph shows the superficial cortex (*SC*), deep cortex (*DC*), and medulla (*M*) of the lymph node in a routine hematoxylin and eosin (H&E) preparation. The capsule (*Cap*) is composed of dense connective tissue from which trabeculae (*T*) penetrate into the organ. Below the capsule is the subcapsular sinus (*SCS*). It receives lymph from afferent lymphatic vessels that penetrate the capsule. The subcapsular sinus is continuous with the trabecular sinuses that course along the trabeculae. The superficial cortex contains the lymphatic nodules (*LN*). The deep cortex is nodule free. It consists of densely packed lymphocytes and contains the unique high endothelial venules (not visible at this magnification). The medulla consists of narrow strands of anastomosing lymphatic tissue called *medullary cords* (*MC*), which are separated by light-appearing spaces, the medullary sinuses (*MS*). The medullary sinuses receive lymph from the trabecular sinuses as well as lymph that has filtered through the cortical tissue. ×140.

FOLDER 14.3

CLINICAL CORRELATION: HUMAN IMMUNODEFICIENCY VIRUS (HIV) AND ACQUIRED IMMUNODEFICIENCY SYNDROME (AIDS)

Human immunodeficiency virus (HIV) is an RNA retrovirus; it contains an enzyme called *reverse* transcriptase. HIV is the virus that causes **acquired immunodeficiency syndrome (AIDS)**. It has an incubation period that may be as long as 11 years before symptoms of clinical AIDS occur. The great majority of HIV-infected individuals eventually develop AIDS. HIV gains entry to helper T cells by binding to CD4 molecules. The virus then injects its own genetic information into the cell cytoplasm (Fig. F14.3.1). This injected genetic information consists of single-stranded RNA. The viral RNA is incorporated into the infected host T-cell genome through reverse transcription of the RNA into DNA. The T cell then makes copies of the virus, which are extruded from the T cell through exocytosis. These HIV particles then infect other helper T cells. The immune system responds to this condition by generating cytotoxic $CD8^{+}$ T cells and antibodies directed against the virus particles. Cytotoxic $CD8^{+}$ T cells kill HIV-infected helper $CD4^{+}$ T cells, reducing the number of helper T cells (the helper T-cell count is actually used as a clinical indicator of the progress of HIV infection). As the helper $CD4^{+}$ T-cell population becomes depleted, infected individuals eventually become incapable of generating an immune response against bacterial or viral infections. They usually die of secondary infections caused by opportunistic microorganisms or cancer.

Anti-HIV treatment is the major strategy against HIV infection and AIDS. Azidothymidine (AZT), an inhibitor of reverse transcriptase, was the first promising drug used to treat HIV infection. Currently, the most effective treatment is **multidrug antiretroviral therapy (ART)**, which uses a combination of several chemotherapeutic agents. Regimens generally include nucleoside reverse transcriptase inhibitors (NRTIs) plus either a non-nucleoside reverse transcriptase inhibitor, protease inhibitor (which blocks viral protease), or integrase strand transfer inhibitor (which prevents integration of the virus into the host cell). ART offers several advantages over monotherapy, such as synergistic dosage effects and reduced side effects as well as reduced drug resistance.

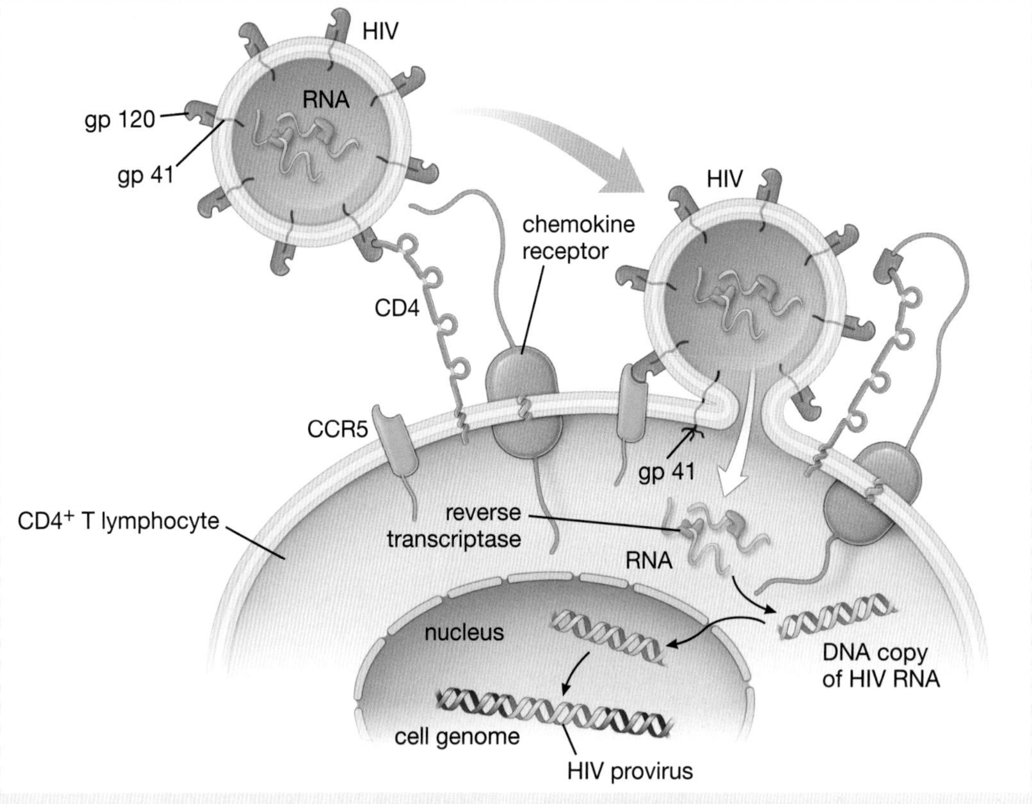

FIGURE F14.3.1. Schematic diagram of the interaction between HIV and the helper $CD4^{+}$ T cell. Human immunodeficiency virus (*HIV*) is an RNA virus that possesses the enzyme reverse transcriptase. The envelope of the HIV virus contains a high concentration of glycoproteins called *gp120,* which bind to the CD4 molecules on helper T cells. This results in the formation of the CD4-gp120 complex, which pulls the gp120 away from the viral envelope, allowing for another glycoprotein, gp41, to be exposed on the viral surface. The unveiled gp41 interacts with the helper T cell by anchoring the virus into the lymphocyte's cell membrane. In addition, gp120 interacts with C-C chemokine receptor type 5 (CCR5), which is a major coreceptor for this binding. Other chemokine receptors may also interact with gp120 proteins. Next, the viral envelope fuses with the T-cell membrane, thus allowing the virus to inject its genetic information (viral RNA with reverse transcriptase) into the T-cell cytoplasm. The reverse transcriptase produces a double-stranded DNA copy of a single-stranded viral RNA. The newly synthetized viral DNA is then transported into the T-cell nucleus. With the help of another viral enzyme integrase, this viral DNA is incorporated into the cell genome, at which point it is referred to as a "provirus." Simultaneously, the viral RNA in the T-cell cytoplasm is translated using protein-making machinery, resulting in the synthesis of new viral proteins.

Lymphatic nodules are usually found in structures associated with the alimentary canal, such as the tonsils, ileum, and vermiform appendix.

Generally, nodules are dispersed singly in a random manner. In the alimentary canal, however, **aggregations of nodules** are found in specific locations, including:

- **Tonsils** form a ring of lymphatic tissue at the entrance of the oropharynx. The **pharyngeal tonsils** (**adenoids**, located in the roof of the pharynx), the **palatine tonsils** (or simply the tonsils, located on either side of the pharynx and between the palatopharyngeal and palatoglossal arches), and the **lingual tonsils** at the base of the tongue all contain aggregates of lymphatic nodules. The palatine tonsils consist of dense accumulations of lymphatic tissue located in the mucous membrane. The squamous epithelium that forms the surface of the tonsil dips into the underlying connective tissue in numerous places, forming **tonsillar crypts** (Fig. 14.17 and Plate 14.1, page 526). The walls of these crypts usually possess numerous lymphatic nodules. Like other aggregations of lymph nodules, tonsils do not possess afferent lymphatic vessels; however, lymph drains from the lymphatic tissue of the tonsil via efferent lymphatic vessels.
- **Peyer patches** are located in the **ileum** (distal portion of the small intestine) and consist of numerous aggregations of lymphatic nodules containing T and B lymphocytes (Fig. 14.18). In addition, numerous isolated **single (solitary) lymph nodules** are located along both the large and small intestines.
- The **vermiform appendix** arises from the cecum. The lamina propria is heavily infiltrated with lymphocytes and contains numerous lymphatic nodules. Although the appendix is often described as a *vestigial organ*, the abundant lymphatic tissue that it contains during early life suggests that it is functionally associated with immune reactions. With age, the amount of lymphatic tissue within the organ regresses and is difficult to recognize.

As noted, diffuse lymphatic tissue and lymphatic nodules are named according to the region or organ in which they appear. In the alimentary canal, they are collectively referred to as **gut-associated lymphatic tissue (GALT)**; in the bronchial tree, they are known as **bronchus-associated lymphatic tissue (BALT)**; and in the eyelids, they are referred as **conjunctiva-associated lymphatic tissue (CALT)**. The term **mucosa-associated lymphatic tissue (MALT)** includes GALT, CALT, and BALT. Diffuse lymphatic tissue and lymphatic nodules of MALT are present in many other regions of the body (e.g., female reproductive tract) where the mucosa is exposed to the external environment. All lymphatic nodules become enlarged as a consequence of encounters with antigen.

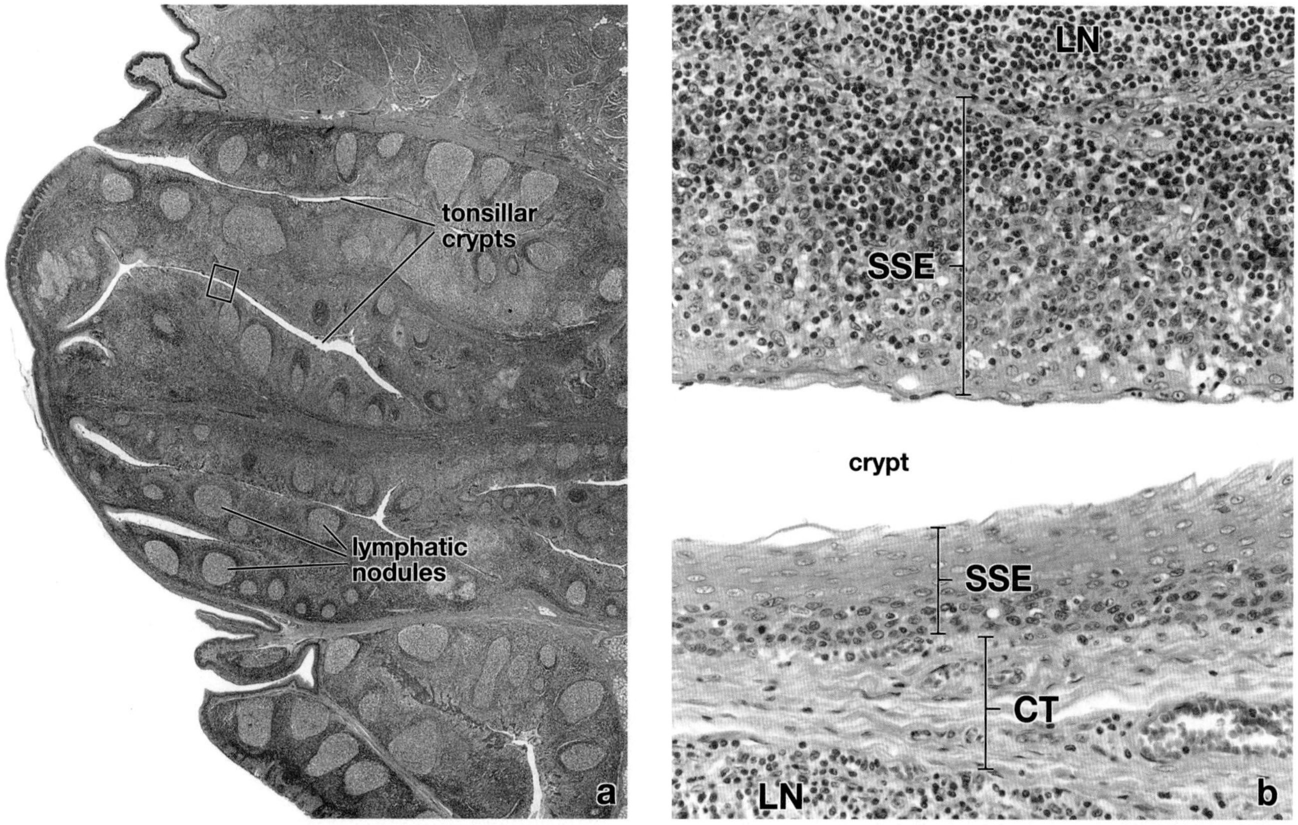

FIGURE 14.17. Photomicrograph of a palatine tonsil. a. This low-magnification photomicrograph shows a hematoxylin and eosin (H&E)-stained palatine tonsil. The stratified squamous epithelium that forms the surface of the tonsil dips into the underlying connective tissue in numerous places, forming tonsillar crypts. ×25. **b.** This higher magnification photomicrograph of the *rectangular area* in **a** shows the stratified squamous epithelium (*SSE*) lining the tonsillar crypt. In the portion of the photomicrograph below the lumen of the crypt, *SSE* is well defined and separated by a connective tissue layer (*CT*) from the lymphatic nodule (*LN*). In the *upper portion* of the photomicrograph, the *SSE* is just barely recognized because of the heavy infiltration of lymphocytes; the epithelial cells are present, however, although they are difficult to identify. In effect, the lymphatic nodule has literally grown into the epithelium, distorting it and resulting in the disappearance of the more typical, well-defined epithelial–connective tissue boundary. ×450.

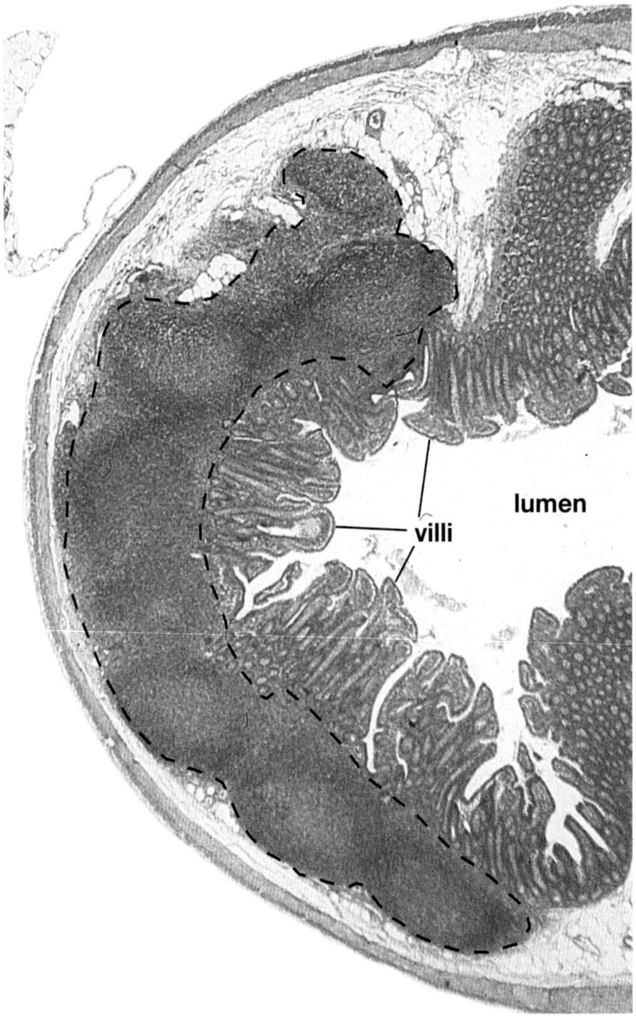

FIGURE 14.18. Photomicrograph of aggregated nodules in the wall of the ileum. This low-magnification photomicrograph provides an example of aggregated nodules. The multiple lymphatic nodules (indicated by a *dashed line*) with visible germinal centers are typically found in the ileum. This accumulation of lymphatic tissue is known as a *Peyer patch*. The nodules originate in the lamina propria and extend into the submucosa of the ileum. ×5.

■ LYMPH NODES

Lymph nodes filter lymph along the pathway of lymphatic vessels and initiate adaptive immune responses to antigens.

Lymph nodes are small, bean-shaped, encapsulated lymphatic organs. They range in size from about 1 mm (barely visible with the unaided eye) to about 1–2 cm in their longest dimension. Lymph nodes are interposed along lymphatic vessels (Fig. 14.19) and serve as filters through which **lymph** percolates on its way to the blood vascular system. Because of their location, lymph nodes have access to the antigens that enter the organism through the epithelia or originate in tissues drained by lymphatic vessels. As **antigens** enter the lymph node, they **activate antigen-specific lymphocytes** that undergo proliferation and differentiation into effectors cells. These cells then leave the lymph node and travel to the tissue where they will act. Although widely distributed throughout the body, lymph nodes are concentrated in certain regions, such as the axilla, groin, neck, and mesenteries.

Two types of lymphatic vessels serve the lymph node:

- **Afferent lymphatic vessels** convey lymph toward the node and enter it at various points on the convex surface of the capsule.
- **Efferent lymphatic vessels** convey lymph away from the node and leave at the hilum, a depression on the concave surface of the node that also serves as the entrance and exit for blood vessels and nerves.

The supporting elements of the **lymph node** are as follows:

- **Capsule**, composed of dense connective tissue that surrounds the node
- **Trabeculae**, also composed of dense connective tissue, which extend from the capsule into the substance of the node, forming a gross framework
- **Reticular tissue**, composed of reticular cells and reticular fibers that form a fine supporting meshwork throughout the remainder of the organ (Fig. 14.20). The reticular meshwork of lymphatic tissues and organs (except the thymus) consists of cells of mesenchymal origin and reticular fibers and ground substance produced by those cells.

Cells of the Reticular Meshwork

The reticular meshwork of the lymph node contains several types of cells that perform different functions in generating immune responses.

The **cells of the reticular meshwork** appear as stellate or elongated cells with an oval euchromatic nucleus and a small amount of acidophilic cytoplasm. These cells can take up dyes and colloidal materials. Using immunocytochemistry and transmission electron microscopy (TEM), several populations of cells have been identified:

- **Reticular cells** are indistinguishable from typical fibroblasts. These cells synthesize and secrete type III collagen (reticular fibers) and the associated ground substance that forms the stroma observed with the light microscope (Plate 14.3, page 530). Elongated cytoplasmic processes of these cells wrap around the bundles of reticular fibers, effectively isolating these structural components from the parenchyma of the lymphatic tissue and organs (Fig. 14.21). Besides their supporting role, they express surface molecules and produce substances (chemokines) that attract lymphocytes and dendritic cells.
- **Dendritic cells (DCs)** are unique bone marrow–derived antigen-presenting cells. Dendritic cells monitor the local environment for foreign substances that they then process and present to antigen-specific T cells. They are much more efficient in antigen presentation than other antigen-presenting cells and can present virtually any form of protein antigen on both MHC I and MHC II molecules. They express an exceptionally high level of MHC II and costimulatory molecules necessary for **activation of T cells**. In the lymph node, dendritic cells are usually localized in T lymphocyte–rich areas.
- **Macrophages** are both phagocytic cells and antigen-presenting cells that express MHC I, MHC II, and

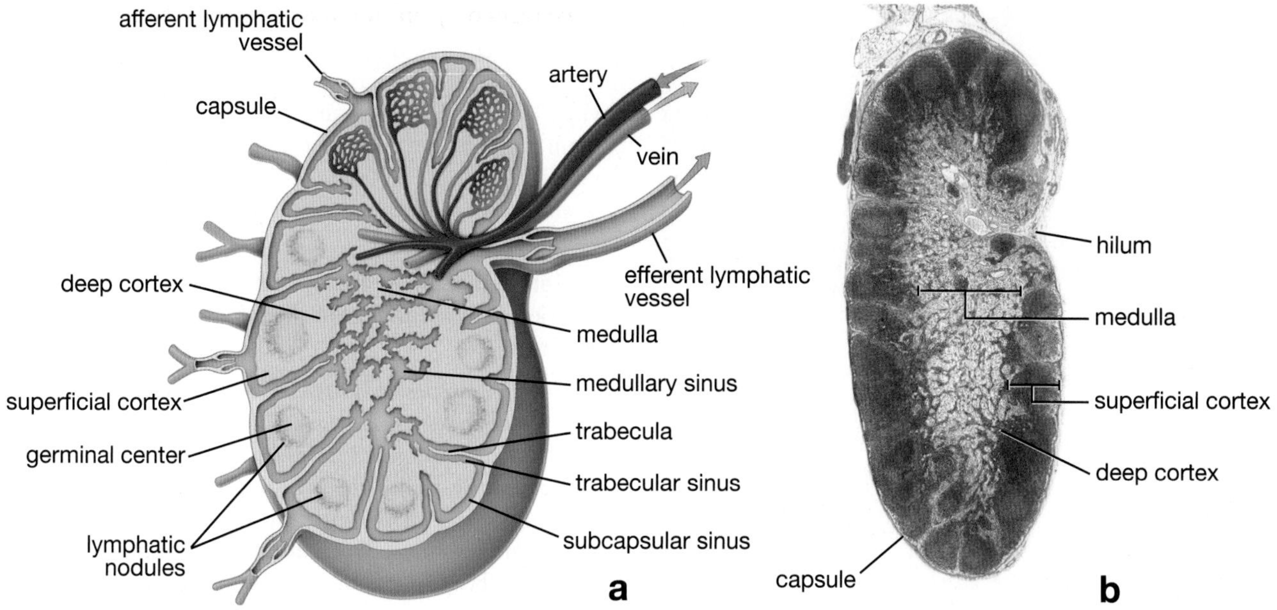

FIGURE 14.19. Structure of a lymph node. a. This diagram depicts the general features of a lymph node as seen in a section. The substance of the lymph node is divided into a cortex, including a deep cortex, and a medulla. The cortex, the outermost portion, contains spherical or oval aggregates of lymphocytes called *lymphatic nodules*. In an active lymph node, nodules contain a lighter center called the *germinal center*. The medulla, the innermost region of the lymph node, consists of lymphatic tissue that appears as irregular cords separated by lymphatic medullary sinuses. The dense population of lymphocytes between the superficial cortex and the medulla constitutes the deep cortex. It contains the high endothelial venules. Surrounding the lymph node is a capsule of dense connective tissue from which trabeculae extend into the substance of the node. Under the capsule and adjacent to the trabeculae are, respectively, the subcapsular sinus and the trabecular lymphatic sinuses. Afferent lymphatic vessels (*arrows*) penetrate the capsule and empty into the subcapsular sinus. The subcapsular sinus and trabecular sinuses communicate with the medullary sinuses. The *upper portion* of the lymph node shows an artery and a vein and the location of high endothelial venules of the lymph node. **b.** Photomicrograph of a lymph node in a routine hematoxylin and eosin (H&E) preparation. The *dense outer portion* of the lymph node is the cortex. It consists of aggregations of lymphocytes organized as nodules and a nodule-free deep cortex. The *innermost portion* of the lymph node, the medulla, extends to the surface at the hilum, where blood vessels enter or leave and where efferent lymphatic vessels leave the node. Surrounding the lymph node is the capsule, and immediately beneath it is the subcapsular sinus. ×18.

costimulatory molecules. However, the expression levels of MHC II and costimulatory molecules are much lower than those of the dendritic cells, making them less efficient APCs. Instead, they have an immense capacity for endocytosis and digestion of internalized materials. The structure, microscopic characteristics, and functions of macrophages are described in Chapter 6, Connective Tissue (pages 199-200).

- **Follicular dendritic cells (FDCs)** have multiple, thin, hair-like branching cytoplasmic processes that interdigitate between **B lymphocytes** in the germinal centers (Fig. 14.22). Antigen–antibody complexes adhere to the dendritic cytoplasmic processes by means of the antibody's F_c receptors, and the cell can retain antigen on its surface for weeks, months, or years. Although this mechanism is similar to the adhesion of antigen–antibody complexes to macrophages, the antigen is not generally endocytosed, as it is by the macrophage. Follicular dendritic cells are thus not antigen-presenting cells because they lack MHC II molecules.

General architecture of the lymph node

The **parenchyma** of the lymph node is divided into a cortex and medulla (Fig. 14.23). The **cortex** forms the outer portion of the node, except at the hilum. It consists of a dense mass of lymphatic tissue (reticular framework, dendritic cells, follicular dendritic cells, lymphocytes, macrophages, and plasma cells) and lymphatic sinuses, the lymph channels. The **medulla** is the inner part of the lymph node.

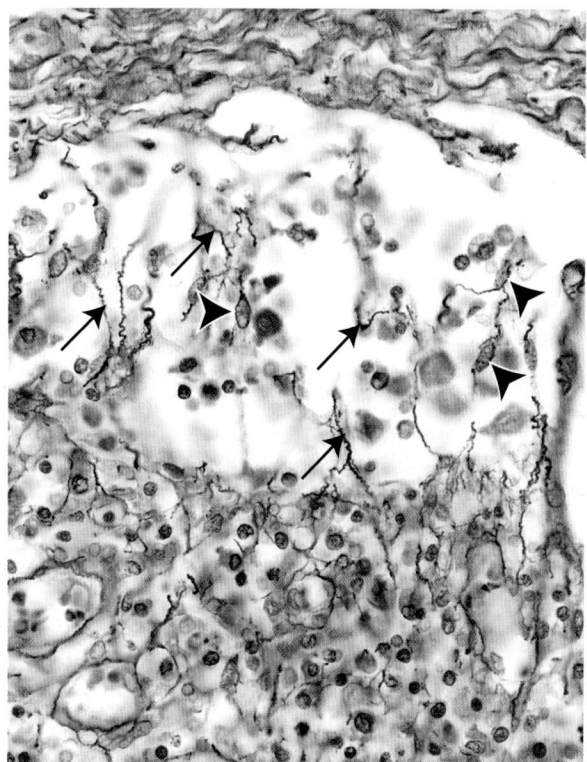

FIGURE 14.20. Photomicrograph of a lymph node. This silver preparation shows the connective tissue capsule (*top*), subcapsular sinus, and the superficial cortex of the lymph node (*bottom*). The reticular fibers (*arrows*) form an irregular anastomosing network throughout the stroma of the lymph node. Note elongated oval nuclei of reticular cells (*arrowheads*), which are in intimate contact with reticular fibers in the sinus. ×640.

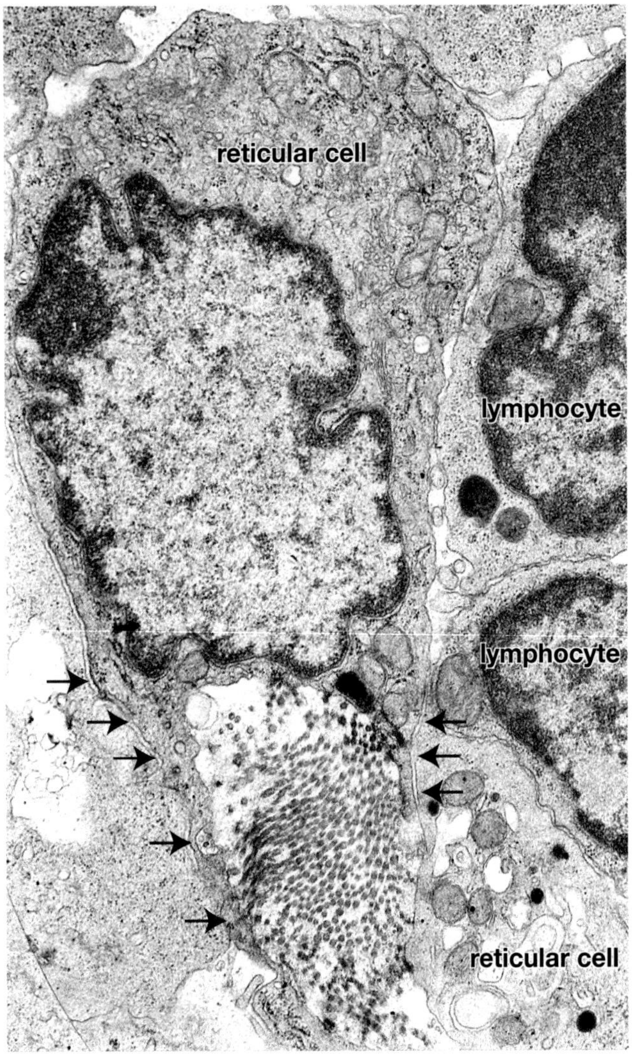

FIGURE 14.21. Electron micrograph of a reticular cell. The body of a reticular cell and its processes (*arrows*) are evident. The arrangement of the reticular cells contains and isolates the collagen fibrils from exposure to the lymphocytes. Note the adjacent lymphocytes on the *right*. In the light microscope and using a silver-staining method, these collagen fibrils are recognized as a reticular fiber. ×12,600.

Lymphocytes in the superficial cortex are organized into nodules.

Similar to other lymphatic tissues, the lymphatic nodules of the cortex of lymph node are designated primary nodules if they consist chiefly of small lymphocytes or secondary nodules if they possess a germinal center. Lymphatic nodules are found in the outer part of the cortex, called the **superficial (nodular) cortex** (Plate 14.2, page 528). The portion of the cortex between the medulla and the superficial cortex is free of nodules; it is called the **deep cortex (paracortex)**. This region contains most of the T cells in the lymph node (Fig. 14.24a). Because of its dependence on the thymus, perinatal thymectomy in animals results in a poorly developed deep cortex. On the basis of this observation, the deep cortex is also called the **thymus-dependent cortex**.

The medulla of the lymph node consists of the medullary cords and medullary sinuses.

The **medulla**, the inner part of the lymph node, consists of cords of lymphatic tissue separated by lymphatic sinuses called **medullary sinuses**. As described earlier, a network of reticular cells and fibers traverses the medullary cords and medullary sinuses and serves as the framework of the parenchyma. In addition to reticular cells, the **medullary cords** contain lymphocytes (mostly B lymphocytes), macrophages, dendritic cells, and plasma cells (Fig. 14.24b). The medullary sinuses converge near the hilum, where they drain into efferent lymphatic vessels.

Filtration of lymph in the lymph node occurs within a network of interconnected lymphatic channels called *sinuses*.

There are three types of **lymphatic channels** called *sinuses* in the lymph node. Just beneath the capsule of the lymph node is a sinus interposed between the capsule and the cortical lymphocytes called the **subcapsular (cortical) sinus** (Plate 14.3, page 530). Afferent lymphatic vessels drain lymph into this sinus. **Trabecular sinuses** that originate from the subcapsular sinuses extend through the cortex along the trabeculae and drain into **medullary sinuses**. Lymphocytes and macrophages or their processes readily pass back and forth between the lymphatic sinuses and the parenchyma of the node. The sinuses have a lining of endothelium that is continuous where it is directly adjacent to the connective tissue of the capsule or trabeculae but discontinuous where it faces the lymphatic parenchyma. Although a macrophage may reside in the lymphatic parenchyma, it often sends pseudopods (long cytoplasmic processes) into the sinus through these endothelial discontinuities. These pseudopods monitor the lymph as it percolates through the sinus.

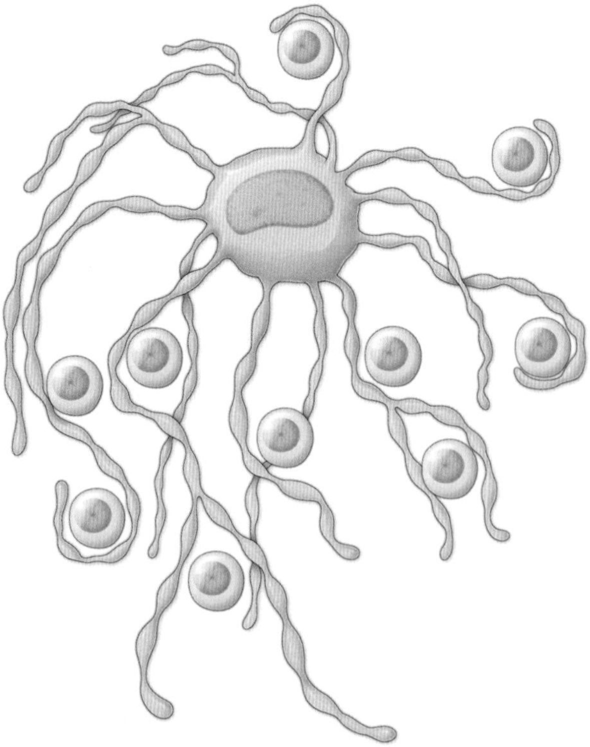

FIGURE 14.22. Diagram of a follicular dendritic cell. This cell, usually found in germinal centers, has multiple, thin, hair-like cytoplasmic processes that interdigitate between B lymphocytes. Antigen–antibody complexes adhere to the dendritic cytoplasmic processes by means of F_c receptors. Follicular dendritic cells are not antigen-presenting cells because they lack MHC II molecules.

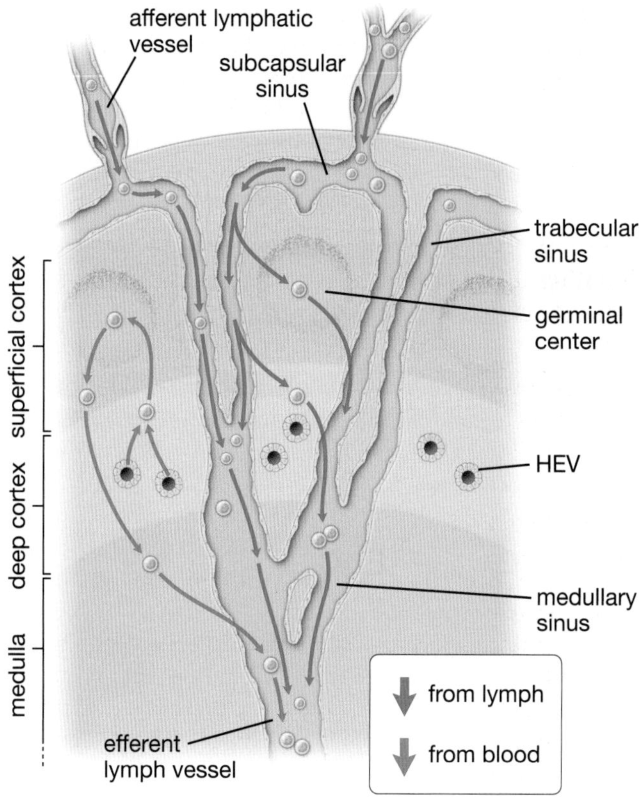

FIGURE 14.23. Schematic diagram of lymphocyte circulation within a lymph node. The *green arrows* indicate the circulation pathway of lymphocytes that enter the lymph node with the flow of lymph. Afferent lymphatic vessels carry lymph from the surrounding tissues and neighboring lymph nodes into the elaborate network of lymphatic sinuses. The wall of the sinuses allows lymph to percolate freely into the superficial and deep cortex, allowing lymphocytes to engage in immunosurveillance. The lymphocytes that enter the tissue next migrate back to the sinuses and leave the lymph node with the flow of the lymph. Lymphocytes that migrate to the lymph node from the blood (*blue arrows*) enter the deep cortex via high endothelial venules (*HEVs*) and also migrate to the superficial cortex. Here, lymphocytes perform the same functions as lymphocytes that enter via lymphatic vessels. They also leave the lymph node by the efferent lymph vessels.

Lymphatic sinuses are not open spaces, as are blood sinuses. Particularly in the medulla, macrophage processes, along with the reticular fibers surrounded by reticular cell processes, span the lumen of the sinus and form a crisscrossing meshwork that retards the free flow of lymph and enhances its filtration. Antigenic material and transformed cells of malignant tumors are trapped by this mechanical filter and then phagocytosed by macrophages. In metastatic cancer, the system can be overwhelmed by an excessive number of cancer cells flowing through the lymphatic sinuses; as a result, the cells may establish a new metastatic site in the lymph node.

Specialized high endothelial venules (HEVs) are the site of entrance for circulating lymphocytes into the lymph node and fluid absorption.

In addition to lymph, **lymphocytes** also circulate through the lymph nodes. Although some lymphocytes enter nodes through afferent lymphatic vessels as components of lymph, most (about 90%) enter the node through the walls of postcapillary venules located in the deep cortex (see Fig. 14.23 and Plate 14.3, page 530). Because the postcapillary venules are lined by cuboidal or columnar endothelial cells, they are referred to as **high endothelial venules (HEVs)**. In histologic sections, the wall of the venule is often infiltrated by a number of lymphocytes in various stages of migration (Fig. 14.25). HEVs are also present in other parts of the lymphatic system, such as diffuse lymphatic tissue and lymph nodules in Peyer patches of the ileum.

Endothelial cells of HEVs play an important role in attracting T and B lymphocytes to migrate to underlying lymphatic tissues by expressing specific adhesion molecules and secretion of specific chemokines. Endothelial cells are also involved in circulating and concentrating lymph by transporting approximately 35% of the fluid and electrolytes entering via afferent lymph vessels directly into the bloodstream. The cells of HEVs express a high concentration of water channels (aquaporin-1 [AQP1] molecules). The rapid resorption of the interstitial fluid via water channels into the bloodstream causes lymph entering through the afferent lymph vessels to be drawn into the deep cortex by solvent drag.

Migration of naïve T and B lymphocytes through the high endothelial venules (HEVs) into the lymph node is mediated by specific adhesion molecules and chemokines.

Naïve circulating T and B cells are mature lymphocytes that have not been previously stimulated by antigen. These cells

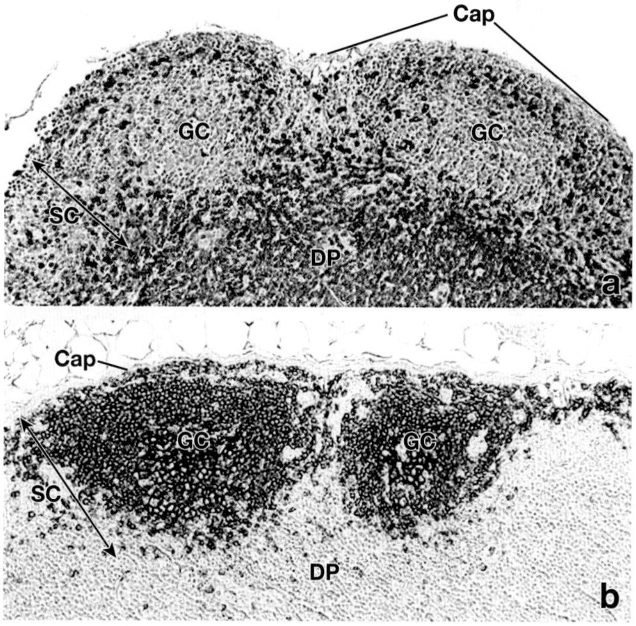

FIGURE 14.24. Distribution of T and B lymphocytes in the superficial cortex of the lymph node. a. Distribution of T lymphocytes in the lymph node of a marmoset monkey was visualized using an immunocytochemical method employing antibodies against CD3 protein, a specific marker for T lymphocytes. Tissue sections were initially treated with primary rabbit antihuman antibodies against a CD3 marker and later exposed to biotinylated secondary swine antirabbit antibodies. After incubation with avidin-biotin-peroxidase complex, the positive response was then visualized with diaminobenzidine (DAB) solution (*brown-colored reaction*). Cell nuclei were counterstained with hematoxylin. Note that the majority of T cells are distributed within the deep cortex (*DP*); a small number of T cells are present in the superficial cortex (*SC*), mainly around germinal centers (*GC*). **b.** Using the same immunoperoxidase DAB reaction described in **a**, B cells were localized using primary monoclonal antibodies against human CD20 protein (specific marker for B lymphocytes). Subsequently, secondary rabbit antimouse antibodies were used to visualize location of B cells, the accumulations of which are found within germinal centers (*GC*) of the superficial cortex (*SC*). *Cap*, capsule. ×200. (Courtesy of Dr. Douglas F. Paulsen.)

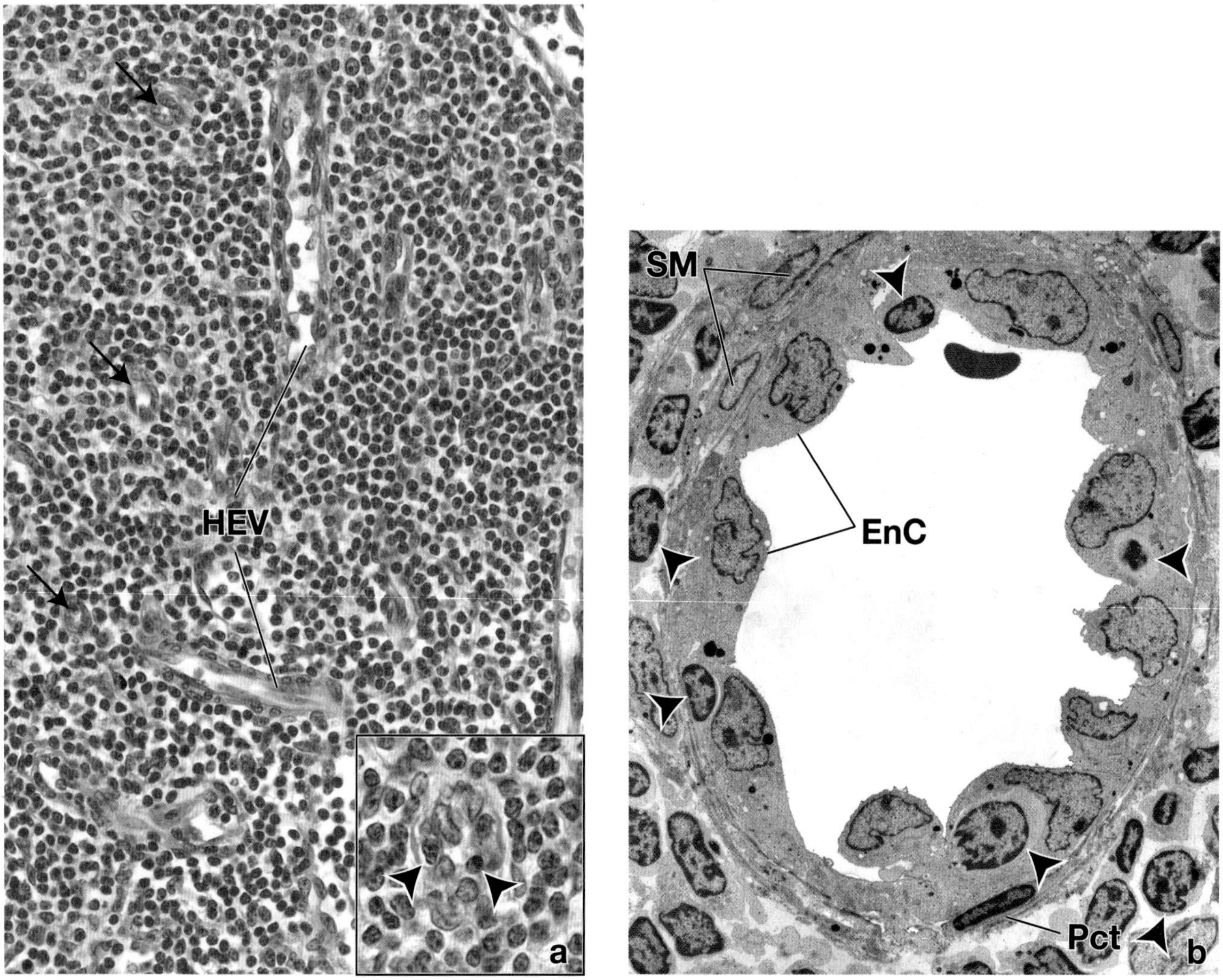

FIGURE 14.25. The deep cortex of a lymph node containing high endothelial venules. a. This photomicrograph shows several longitudinally sectioned high endothelial venules (*HEVs*) as well as several that are seen in cross section (*arrows*). These vessels are lined by cuboidal endothelial cells. In some preparations, the walls of an *HEV* may be infiltrated with migrating lymphocytes, making it difficult to recognize. ×400. **Inset.** The cross section of an *HEV* shown here at higher magnification reveals several lymphocytes (*arrowheads*) in the process of migrating from the *HEV* into the parenchyma of the lymph node. ×640. **b.** This relatively low-magnification electron micrograph shows a cross section of a high endothelial venule from the deep cortex of a lymph node lined by cuboidal endothelial cells (*EnC*). Cells are resting on a fenestrated basal lamina and are surrounded by occasional smooth muscle (*SM*) cells and pericytes (*Pct*). Note several lymphocytes (*arrowheads*) in various stages of migration between the lumen of the vessels and the parenchyma of the lymph node. ×5,000. (Copyright © 2010. Regents of the University of Michigan. Reprinted with permission.)

recirculate between the blood and lymphatic organs. The endothelial cells of specialized HEVs possess specific adhesion molecules that interact with **L-selectin** and **integrins** expressed on migrating lymphocytes. Both B and T cells leave the bloodstream crossing the endothelium by diapedesis—that is, by migrating between the endothelial cells in a manner similar to that described for neutrophils (see Fig. 10.9, page 308). The cytokines that determine and regulate migration of lymphocytes through the HEVs in lymph node are called **chemokines**, and they bind to chemokine receptors on the lymphocytes. Chemokines signal lymphocytes to leave the circulation and migrate into the lymph node. T cells express CCR7 receptors that interact with the chemokines CCL19 and CCL21 produced by the HEV's endothelial cells. In a similar manner, B cells express different CXCR5 receptors that bind to another chemokine called CXCL13. Interactions of these chemokines with their receptors on respective T and B lymphocytes allow them to enter the lymph node.

Chemokines also determine the regional distribution of T and B cells within the lymph node. **T cells** remain in the thymus-dependent **deep cortex** attracted by CCL19 and CCL21 chemokines that are produced by reticular and other stromal cells in this region. In contrast, **B cells** migrate to the **superficial cortex** following secretion of CXCL13 chemokine that is produced by follicular dendritic cells residing in lymph nodules and germinal centers of the superficial cortex (see Fig. 14.24). After B cells have been exposed to antigen, a subset of T cells differentiates into **follicular helper $CD4^{+}$ lymphocytes (TFH)**, which also express CXCR5 receptors (the same as those on B cells). These cells are essential in the formation and function of germinal centers, especially formation of memory B cells.

The lymph node is an important site for phagocytosis and initiation of immune responses.

Phagocytosis of particulate material by macrophages and APCs within the lymph nodes is an important step in initiating an immune response. Antigens conveyed to the lymph percolate through the sinuses and penetrate the lymph nodules to initiate an immune response. Some antigens become trapped on the surface of follicular dendritic cells, whereas others are processed by macrophages, dendritic cells, and B cells, leading to activation of both T and B lymphocytes. **Activated B cells** differentiate into plasma cells, memory B cells, and plasmablasts. These cells represent the population of migratory B cells committed to secreting antibody.

Plasma cells migrate to the medullary cords where they synthesize and release specific antibodies into the lymph flowing through the sinuses. Plasma cells account for 1%–3% of the cells in resting lymph nodules. Their number increases dramatically during an immune response, thereby increasing the amount of circulating Igs. **Plasmablasts** leave the lymph node and migrate into the bone marrow where they further differentiate into plasma cells that secrete antibodies for a long period of time. **Memory B cells** may leave the lymph nodes and circulate to various regions throughout the body, where they can proliferate in response to subsequent exposure to their specific antigen. The presence of memory cells in various sites throughout the body ensures a more rapid secondary response to an antigen.

Lymph nodes in which lymphocytes are responding to antigens often enlarge, reflecting the formation of germinal centers and proliferation of lymphocytes. This phenomenon is often seen in the lymph nodes of the neck in response to nasal or oropharyngeal infection and in axillary and inguinal regions because of infection in extremities. **Lymphadenitis**, a reactive (inflammatory) lymph node enlargement, is a common complication of microbial infections. These enlarged lymph nodes are commonly referred to as **swollen glands** (see Folder 14.4).

Exit of T and B lymphocytes from the lymph node is regulated by chemotactic lipid sphingosine-1-phosphate (S1P) and expression of its receptors on the lymphocyte cell surface.

Most lymphocytes leave the lymph node by entering lymphatic sinuses from which they flow to an efferent lymphatic vessel. Their exit from the lymph node is regulated by **S1P exit pathway**, which depends on expression of **sphingosine-1-phosphate receptor 1 (S1PR1) molecules** on the surface of lymphocytes and their interactions with **sphingosine-1-phosphate (S1P)**. S1P, which has signaling properties similar to those of chemokines, is a blood-borne lipid that is present at higher concentrations in lymph and blood than in other tissues. Naïve T cells entering the lymph node express small amounts of S1PR1. If they fail to recognize antigen for several hours, their expression of S1PR1 increases and the T cells are allowed to leave the lymph node via efferent lymphatic vessels. If a naïve T cell is activated by antigen, its expression of S1PR1 is suppressed for several days and the ability of the cell to leave the lymph node is delayed. This process allows activated T cells to remain in the lymph node and undergo division and differentiation into effector and memory T cells that will eventually return to the blood circulation using the same S1P exit pathway.

Naïve B cells that are not activated by antigen leave the lymph node in a manner similar to that of naïve T cells. Activated B cells that differentiate into memory B cells and plasmablasts also leave the lymph node and enter the circulation via the S1P pathway.

The regulation of the exit of lymphocytes from lymph nodes and other secondary lymphatic organs is the basis of development of new immunomodulating drugs. For instance, a fungus-derived metabolite called fingolimod (FTY720) is used in the treatment of **multiple sclerosis (MS)**. When introduced into the body, it becomes phosphorylated and mimics activity of S1P molecule. After binding to the S1PR1 receptor on lymphocytes, the S1PRI–receptor complex is internalized, which inhibits the body's immune response and prevents fully immunocompetent effector cells from exiting the lymph nodes. Lymphocytes then become sequestered in secondary lymphatic organs, causing peripheral lymphopenia (abnormally low level of lymphocytes in the blood).

Specific features of lymph nodes in comparison with other major lymphatic organs are summarized in Table 14.4.

■ THYMUS

The thymus is a lymphoepithelial organ located in the superior mediastinum.

The **thymus** is a bilobed lymphoepithelial organ located in the superior mediastinum, anterior to the heart and great vessels. It develops bilaterally from the third (and sometimes also the fourth) branchial (oropharyngeal) pouch. During development, the epithelium invaginates, and the thymic rudiment grows caudally as a tubular projection of the endodermal epithelium into the mediastinum of the chest. The advancing tip proliferates and ultimately becomes disconnected from the branchial epithelium. **Common lymphoid progenitor (CLP) cells** from the bone marrow that are destined to develop into immunocompetent T cells invade the epithelial rudiment and occupy spaces between the epithelial cells.

The thymus is fully formed and functional at birth. It persists as a large organ until about the time of puberty, when T-cell differentiation and maturation are reduced and most of the lymphatic tissue is replaced by adipose tissue (involution). However, some maturation of T cells may continue throughout adult life in the involuted thymus. The organ function can be restimulated under specific conditions that require a high demand for new mature T cells, such as in adult recipients of bone marrow transplants.

General Architecture of the Thymus

Connective tissue surrounds the thymus and subdivides it into thymic lobules.

The thymus possesses a thin connective tissue **capsule** from which **trabeculae** extend into the parenchyma of the organ. The capsule and trabeculae contain blood vessels, efferent (but not afferent) lymphatic vessels, and nerves. In addition to collagen fibers and fibroblasts, the connective tissue of the thymus contains variable numbers of plasma cells, granulocytes, lymphocytes, mast cells, adipose cells, and macrophages.

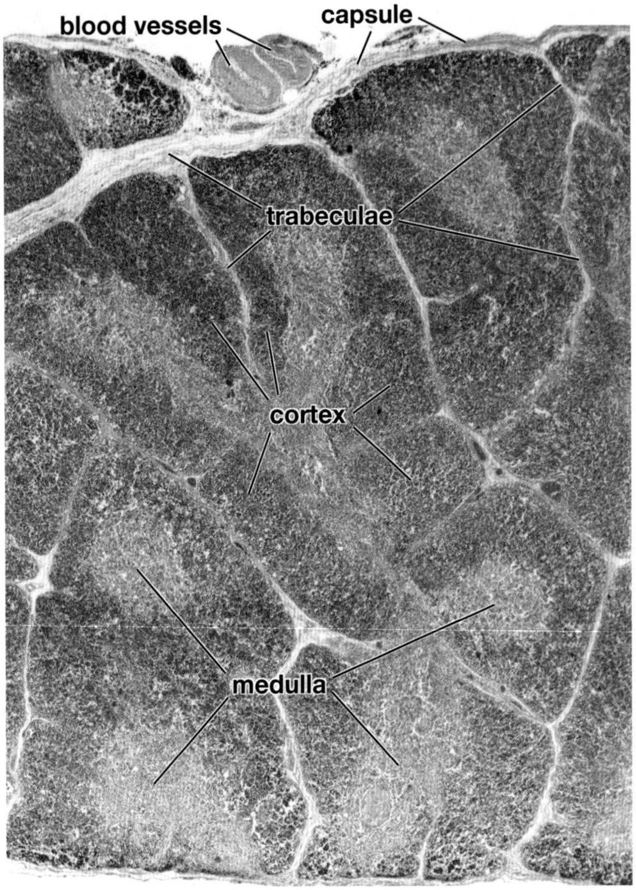

FIGURE 14.26. Photomicrograph of an infant human thymus. This hematoxylin and eosin (H&E) preparation reveals multiple lobules separated by connective tissue trabeculae that extend into the organ from the surrounding capsule. Each lobule is composed of a dark-staining basophilic cortex and a lighter staining and relatively eosinophilic medulla. The medulla is actually a continuous branching mass surrounded by the cortex. The cortex contains numerous densely packed lymphocytes, whereas the medulla contains fewer lymphocytes. Note that in some instances, the medulla may bear a resemblance to germinal centers of lymphatic nodules (*upper right* and *center left*). Such isolated medullary profiles are continuous with the overall medullary tissue, but this continuity may not be seen within the plane of section. ×25.

The trabeculae establish domains in the thymus called **thymic lobules**. They are not true lobules but cortical caps over portions of the highly convoluted but continuous inner medullary tissue (Fig. 14.26 and Plate 14.6, page 536). In some planes of section, the "lobular" arrangement of the cortical cap and medullary tissue superficially resembles a lymphatic nodule with a germinal center, which often confuses students. Other morphologic characteristics (described later in this chapter) allow positive identification of the thymus in histologic sections.

The thymic parenchyma contains developing T cells in an extensive meshwork formed by epithelioreticular cells.

The outer portion of the parenchyma, the **thymic cortex**, is markedly basophilic in hematoxylin and eosin (H&E) preparations because of the closely packed developing T lymphocytes with their intensely staining nuclei. These developing T lymphocytes, also called **thymocytes**, occupy spaces within an extensive meshwork of **epithelioreticular cells** (Fig. 14.27). **Macrophages** and **dendritic cells** are also dispersed among the cortical cells. The developing T cells arise from CLPs, which originate in the bone marrow. As development proceeds in the thymus, the cells derived from CLPs pass through a series of developmental stages that are reflected by their expression of different CD molecules.

As their name implies, epithelioreticular cells have features of both epithelial and reticular cells. They provide a framework for the developing T cells; thus, they correspond to the reticular cells and their associated reticular fibers in other lymphatic tissues and organs. Reticular connective tissue cells and their fibers, however, are not present in the thymic parenchyma. Epithelioreticular cells exhibit certain features characteristic of epithelium, such as intercellular junctions and intermediate filaments.

Six types of epithelioreticular cells are recognized on the basis of function: three types in the cortex and three types in the medulla. Each type is designated by roman numerals. In the cortex, the following cell types are recognized:

- **Type I epithelioreticular cells** are located at the boundary of the cortex and the connective tissue capsule as well as between the cortical parenchyma and the trabeculae. They also surround the adventitia of the cortical blood vessels. In essence, type I epithelioreticular cells serve to separate the thymic parenchyma from the connective tissue of the organ. The occluding junctions between these cells reflect their function as a barrier that isolates developing T cells from the connective tissue of the organ—that is, capsule, trabeculae, and perivascular connective tissue.
- **Type II epithelioreticular cells** are located within the cortex. The TEM reveals maculae adherents (desmosomes) that join long cytoplasmic processes of adjacent cells. The cell body and cytoplasmic processes contain abundant intermediate filaments. Because of their processes, these cells are stellate. They have a large nucleus that stains lightly with H&E because of its abundant euchromatin. This nuclear feature allows the cell to be easily identified in the light microscope. Type II cells compartmentalize the cortex into isolated areas for developing T cells. Unlike type I cells, type II cells express MHC I and MHC II molecules, which are involved in thymic cell education.
- **Type III epithelioreticular** cells are located at the boundary of the cortex and medulla. The TEM reveals occluding junctions between sheet-like cytoplasmic processes of adjacent cells. Like type I cells, type III epithelioreticular cells create a functional barrier—in this case, between the cortex and the medulla. Like type II cells, they possess MHC I and MHC II molecules.
- **Macrophages** and **dendritic cells** reside within the thymic cortex and are responsible for phagocytosis of T cells that do not fulfill thymic education requirements. These T cells are programmed to die before leaving the cortex. Approximately 98% of the T cells undergo this apoptosis and are then phagocytosed by the macrophages. The macrophages in the cortex are difficult to identify in H&E preparations. However, the periodic acid–Schiff (PAS) reaction readily defines them because of the staining of their numerous large lysosomes. Accordingly, these macrophages are called **PAS cells**. Dendritic cells within the thymus regulate the expression of FOXP3 markers on the regulatory (suppressor) $CD4^{+}$ T lymphocytes (see pages 497 and 498).

Although the epithelioreticular cells of the thymic cortex play an important role in the development of immunocompetent mature T cells, experimental evidence shows

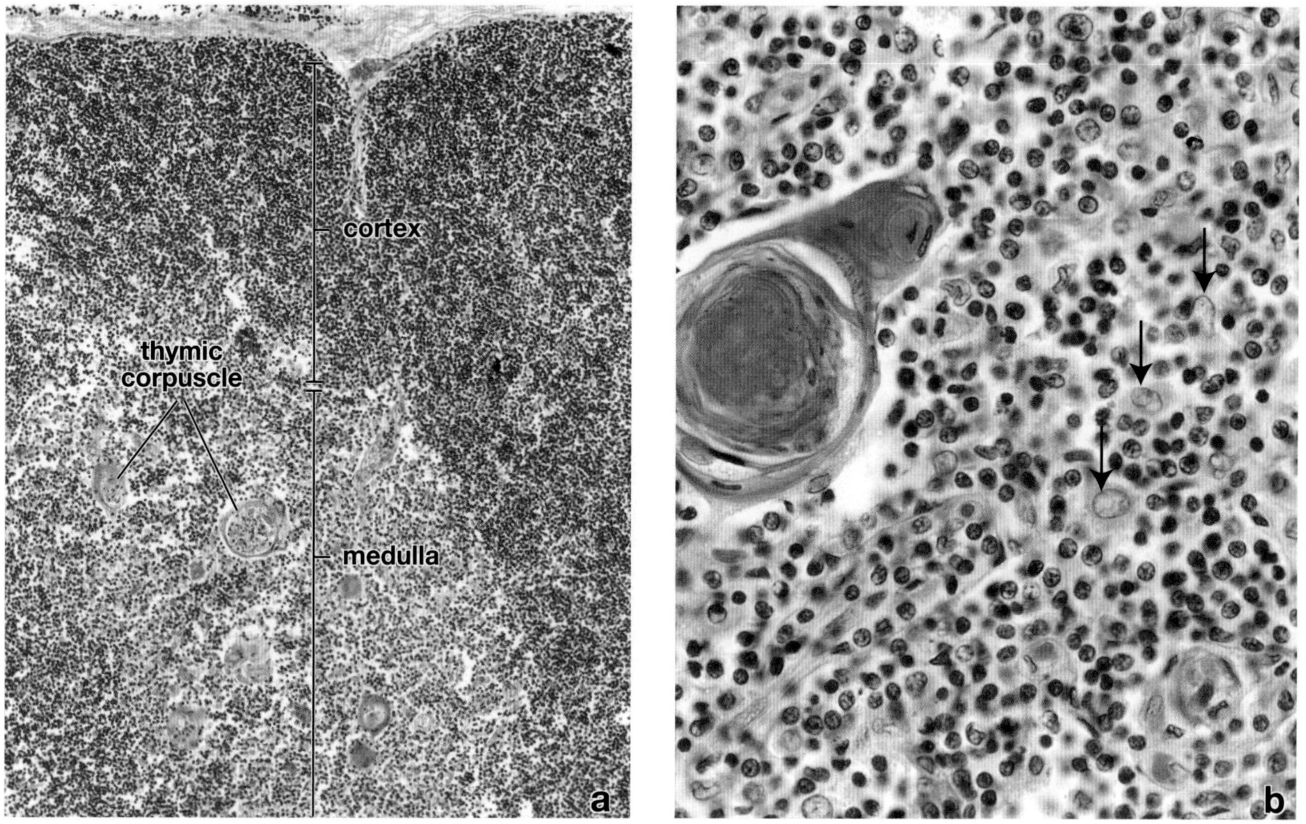

FIGURE 14.27. Photomicrograph of a human thymus. a. The cortex contains a dense population of small, maturing T cells that create the dark staining of this region of the thymus. The medulla, in contrast, appears lighter. The medulla also contains the thymic corpuscles that stain with eosin and give it a further distinction. ×120. **b.** This higher magnification photomicrograph shows the medulla with a thymic corpuscle (*left*) and surrounding cells. Thymic corpuscles are isolated masses of closely packed, concentrically arranged type VI epithelioreticular cells; these cells exhibit flattened nuclei. The more central mass of the corpuscle contains fully keratinized cells. In addition to numerous lymphocytes, the micrograph also shows type V epithelioreticular cells (*arrows*), with their eosinophilic cytoplasm and large, pale-staining nuclei. ×600.

that T cells at different stages of differentiation control the microarchitecture of the thymic epithelioreticular cells, a phenomenon called **cross-talk**. The developing lymphocytes and epithelioreticular cells thus influence each other during T-cell development.

Thymic or Hassall corpuscles (derived from type VI epithelioreticular cells) are a distinguishing feature of the thymic medulla.

The **thymic medulla**, the inner portion of the parenchyma, contains a large number of epithelioreticular cells and loosely packed T cells (see Fig. 14.27). The medulla stains less intensely than the cortex because it contains mostly large lymphocytes. These lymphocytes have pale-staining nuclei and quantitatively more cytoplasm than small lymphocytes. Like the cortex, the medulla also contains three types of epithelioreticular cells:

- **Type IV epithelioreticular cells** are located between the cortex and the medulla close to type III cells. They possess sheet-like processes with occluding junctions between adjacent cells as well as between them and type III cells. In cooperation with type III cells, they create the barrier at the corticomedullary junction.
- **Type V epithelioreticular cells** are located throughout the medulla. Like the type II cells located in the cortex, processes of adjacent cells are joined by desmosomes to provide the cellular framework of the medulla and to compartmentalize groups of lymphocytes. These nuclei contrast markedly with the densely staining lymphocyte nuclei.
- **Type VI epithelioreticular cells** form the most characteristic feature of the thymic medulla, the **thymic (Hassall) corpuscles** (Fig. 14.28 and Plate 14.5, page 534). Thymic corpuscles are isolated masses of closely packed, concentrically arranged type VI epithelioreticular cells that exhibit flattened nuclei. TEM studies of these cells reveal **keratohyalin granules**, bundles of cytoplasmic intermediate filaments, and lipid droplets. The cells are joined by desmosomes. The center of a thymic corpuscle may display evidence of keratinization, not a surprising feature for cells developed from oropharyngeal epithelium. Thymic corpuscles are unique, antigenically distinct, and functionally active multicellular components of the medulla. Although the function of thymic corpuscles is not fully understood, it is thought that thymic corpuscles produce interleukins (IL-4 and IL-7) that function in thymic differentiation and education of T lymphocytes.

Blood vessels pass from the trabeculae to enter the parenchyma of the thymus. Typically, the blood vessels enter the medulla from the deeper parts of the trabeculae and carry a sheath of connective tissue along with them. This perivascular connective tissue sheath varies in thickness. It is thicker around larger vessels and gradually becomes thinner around smaller vessels. Where it is thick, it contains reticular fibers, fibroblasts, macrophages, plasma cells, and other cells found in loose connective tissue; where it is thin, it may contain only reticular fibers and occasional fibroblasts. Specific features of the thymus in comparison to other major lymphatic organs are summarized in Table 14.4.

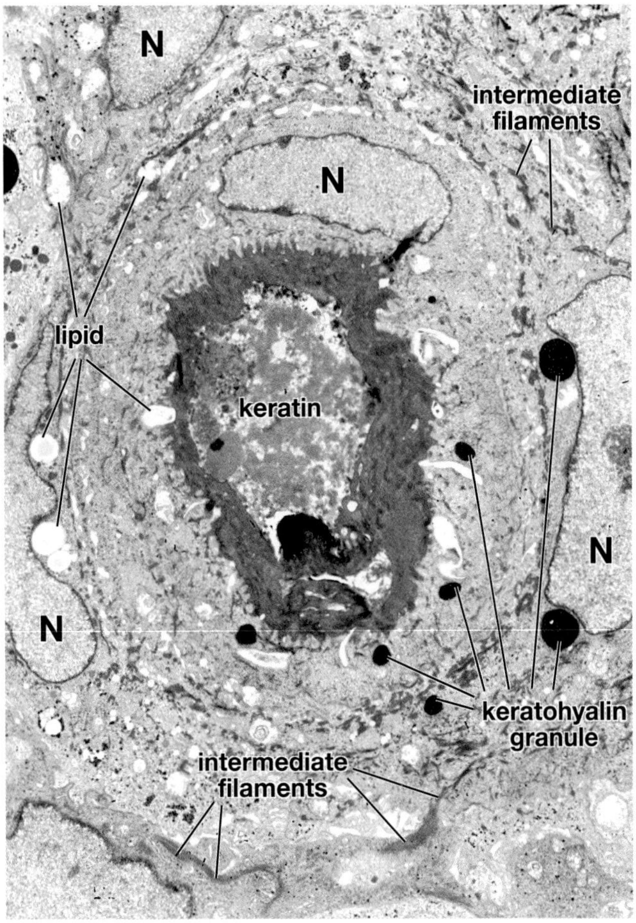

FIGURE 14.28. Electron micrograph of a thymic (Hassall) corpuscle. This relatively low-magnification electron micrograph shows some of the nuclei (*N*) and cytoplasm of the concentrically arranged epithelioreticular cells of a thymic (Hassall) corpuscle. Bundles of intermediate filaments, keratohyalin granules, and lipid droplets are also evident within the cytoplasm of the epithelioreticular cells. Fully keratinized cells (*black layer*) are present in the center of the thymic corpuscle. ×5,000. (Courtesy of Dr. Johannes A. G. Rhodin.)

Blood–Thymus Barrier and Thymic Cell Education

The blood–thymus barrier protects developing lymphocytes in the thymus from exposure to antigens.

Lymphocytes reaching the thymic cortex are prevented from contact with antigen by a physical barrier called the **blood–thymus barrier** (Fig. 14.29). The following components constitute the blood–thymus barrier between the T cells and the lumen of cortical blood vessels, from the lumen outward:

- The **endothelium** lining the capillary wall is of the continuous type with occluding junctions. It is highly impermeable to macromolecules and is considered a major structural component of the barrier within the cortical parenchyma. The underlying **basal lamina** of endothelial cells and occasional **pericytes** are also part of the capillary wall.
- **Macrophages** residing in the surrounding perivascular connective tissue may phagocytose antigenic molecules that escape from the capillary lumen into the cortical parenchyma.
- **Type I epithelioreticular cells** with their occluding junctions provide further protection to the developing T cells. The epithelioreticular cells surround the capillary wall in the cortex; with their basal lamina, they represent another major structural component of the blood–thymus barrier.

The thymus is the site of intense T-cell education where thymocytes must pass two sequential life-and-death tests to survive.

During fetal life, the thymus is populated by multipotential lymphoid stem cells that originate from the bone marrow and are destined to develop into immunocompetent, mature T cells. Stem cell maturation is also called **thymic cell education** (Fig. 14.30) and is driven by a precise order in which TCR genes are rearranged. This process is characterized by expression or deletion of specific surface CD molecules. These surface changes reflect the state of functional maturation of T cells, and expressed CD proteins are used as markers for T-cell differentiation.

The expression of CD2 and CD7 molecules on the T-cell surface indicates an **early stage of differentiation (double-negative stage)**. The term *double-negative* refers to the absence of both CD4 and CD8 molecules. This early stage is followed by the expression of the CD1 molecule, which indicates the **middle stage of T-cell differentiation**. As maturation progresses, the T cells express CD3 and both CD4 and CD8 molecules. This is the **double-positive stage** of T-cell differentiation. The double-positive T cells, which have developed without any antigenic stimulation from outside, begin to express TCRs.

At this stage, the cells then undergo **positive selection** to make sure they have functional TCRs. Double-positive T cells encounter types II and III epithelioreticular cells that display a variety of self-peptides bound to MHC I and MHC II

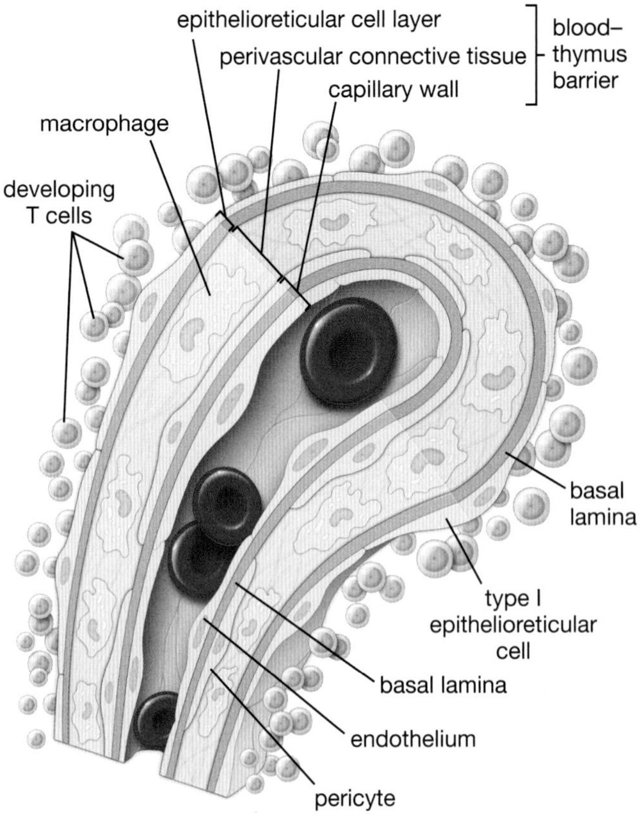

FIGURE 14.29. Schematic diagram of the blood–thymus barrier. The blood–thymus barrier consists of three major elements: (1) capillary endothelium and its basal lamina, (2) perivascular connective tissue space occupied by macrophages, and (3) type I epithelioreticular cells with their basal lamina. The perivascular connective tissue is enclosed between the basal lamina of the epithelioreticular cells and the endothelial cell basal lamina. These layers provide the necessary protection to the developing immature T cells and separate them from mature immunocompetent lymphocytes circulating in the bloodstream.

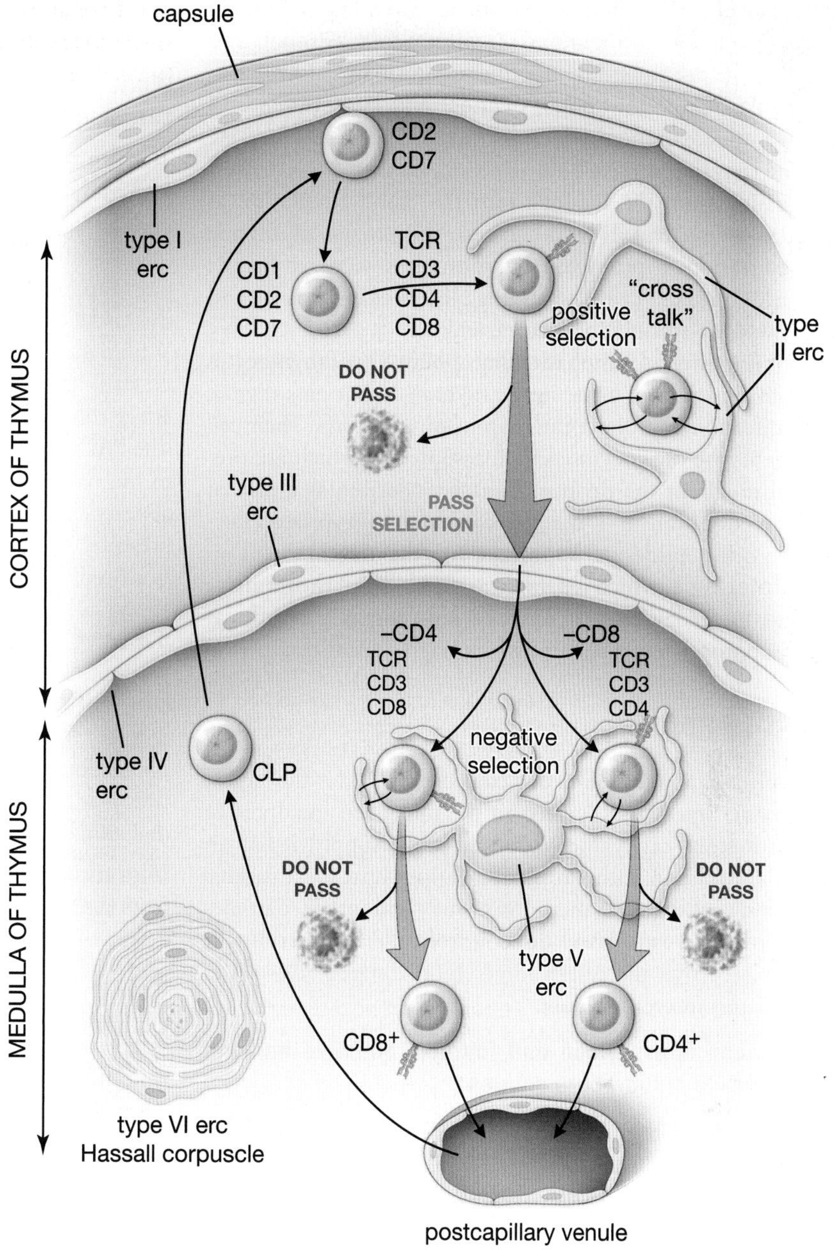

FIGURE 14.30. Schematic drawing of the major steps in thymic education. The process of common lymphoid progenitor (*CLP*) cell maturation and differentiation into immunocompetent T cells is accomplished by the expression and deletion of specific surface CD antigens. The *CLP* stem cells enter the medulla of the thymus via a postcapillary venule and then migrate to the periphery of the thymic lobule. The presence of CD2 and CD7 molecules on the cell surface indicates an early stage of differentiation. This is followed by expression of the CD1 molecule, indicating the middle stage of T-cell differentiation. As maturation progresses, the cells express TCRs, CD3, CD4, and CD8 molecules. These cells are then presented with self-antigens and foreign antigens by types II and III epithelioreticular (*erc*) cells. If the lymphocyte recognizes self-MHC and self-antigen, it will survive the selection (positive selection); if not, death of the cell will occur. Cells that pass the positive selection test leave the cortex and enter the medulla. Here, they undergo another selection process in which cells that react too strongly to self-antigen displayed by self-MHC are eliminated (negative selection). Cells that survive negative selection then become mature cytotoxic $CD8^+$ T lymphocytes or helper $CD4^+$ T lymphocytes. These cells are now mature (but naïve) T lymphocytes; they leave the thymus from the medulla and enter the blood circulation. Hormonal substances secreted by type VI epithelioreticular cells within the thymic (Hassall) corpuscle promote the process of thymic cell education. Note the distribution of all six types of epithelioreticular cells. *MHC*, major histocompatibility complex; *TCR*, T-cell receptor.

molecules. If the lymphocyte recognizes self-MHC molecules and displayed self-peptides with enough affinity to generate survival signals, it will survive this positive selection test. If the lymphocyte's TCR does not recognize self-MHC molecules, this nonreacting cell is eliminated by a process called **death by neglect** (a default pathway of apoptosis). During the positive selection process, T cells with TCRs that recognize self-MHC I molecules become cytotoxic $CD8^+$ T lymphocytes (by losing CD4 and retaining CD8), and cells with TCRs that recognize self-MHC II molecules become helper $CD4^+$ T lymphocytes (by losing CD8 and retaining CD4). This stage is called the **single-positive stage** of T-cell differentiation.

Cells that pass the positive selection test leave the cortex and enter the medulla. Here, they undergo another test called **negative selection** that checks whether their TCRs respond too enthusiastically to self-antigens. This process is performed by the epithelioreticular cells (types IV–VI), which display many tissue-specific self-antigens on their MHCs. A specific transcription factor known as the **autoimmune regulator (AIRE) protein** expressed by epithelioreticular cells promotes the promiscuous expression of upregulated **tissue-specific self-antigens** from every tissue and organ that are not normally required for the direct function of epithelioreticular cells. These antigens are specifically generated for the negative selection test and are presented to developing T cells as the antigenic mirror of self. The negative selection process eliminates cells that recognize self-antigens with high avidity by apoptosis. Any excessive stimulation of these immature T cells by self-antigens at this stage is unwanted and is the basis for their elimination.

The negative selection of T cells in the thymus regulated by AIRE is necessary to maintain self-tolerance. Mutations in the gene encoding AIRE protein cause abnormal negative selection (due to incomplete expression of tissue-specific self-antigens) and a breakdown in self-tolerance that allows self-reactive T cells to escape their death by apoptosis in the thymus. These lymphocytes are released into the blood circulation and colonize peripheral tissue and organs, leading to multiorgan autoimmune diseases. An example is **autoimmune polyendocrinopathy-candidiasis-ectodermal dystrophy (APECED) syndrome.** This syndrome is characterized by the presence of autoantibodies directed toward multiple endocrine (e.g., parathyroid, adrenal, and thyroid glands) and nonendocrine organs (e.g., skin, gastrointestinal tract, liver, lungs, ovaries) and susceptibility to chronic mucocutaneous fungal infection with *Candida*.

The cells that survive both selection tests leave the thymus by passing from the medulla into the blood circulation as mature (but naïve) T lymphocytes. The process of thymic cell education is promoted by substances secreted by the epithelioreticular cells, including interleukins (IL-4 and IL-7), colony-stimulating factors, and IFN-γ.

It is important to emphasize that about 98% of thymocytes that divide and proliferate in the thymus do not pass thymic cell education and die in the thymus by apoptosis. Their cell fragments are phagocytosed by macrophages, which are present throughout the thymus. Negative selection as a part of intense education of T cells to learn and appropriately recognize self-peptides is important for the development of **self-tolerance**, which is defined as the ability of the immune system to recognize self-produced antigens as a nonthreat while appropriately responding to foreign substances.

■ SPLEEN

The spleen is about the size of a clenched fist and is the largest lymphatic organ. It is located in the upper left quadrant of the abdominal cavity and has a rich blood supply. It has no direct connection with lymph circulation; instead, it gathers antigens, pathogenic microorganisms, and other particles (e.g., immune complexes) directly from the bloodstream. It is estimated that the spleen filters approximately 5% of the cardiac output every minute.

The spleen filters blood and initiates adaptive immune responses to blood-borne antigens.

The **spleen** has both morphologic and immunologic filtering functions. In addition to large numbers of lymphocytes, it contains specialized vascular spaces or channels, a meshwork of reticular cells and reticular fibers, and a rich supply of macrophages and dendritic cells. These contents allow the spleen to monitor the blood immunologically, much as the macrophages and dendritic cells of the lymph nodes monitor the lymph.

The spleen is enclosed by a dense connective tissue **capsule** from which **trabeculae** extend into the parenchyma of the organ (Fig. 14.31). The connective tissue of the capsule and trabeculae contains **myofibroblasts**. These contractile cells also produce extracellular connective tissue fibers. In many mammals, the spleen holds large volumes of red blood cells in reserve. In these species, contraction in the capsule and trabeculae helps discharge stored red blood cells into the systemic circulation. The human spleen normally retains relatively little blood, but it has the capacity for contraction by means of the contractile cells in its capsule and trabeculae.

The **hilum**, located on the medial surface of the spleen, is the site for the passage of the splenic artery and vein, nerves, and lymphatic vessels. The lymphatic vessels originate in the white pulp near the trabeculae and constitute a route for lymphocytes, leaving the spleen.

Most of the spleen consists of splenic pulp. Splenic pulp, in turn, is divided into two functionally and morphologically different regions: **white pulp** and **red pulp**, based on the color of fresh sections. White pulp appears as circular or elongated whitish gray areas surrounded by red pulp.

White pulp consists of a thick accumulation of lymphocytes surrounding an artery.

The **white pulp** consists of lymphatic tissue, mostly densely packed **lymphocytes**, which give the impression of white nodules against the background of red blood cells occupying splenic sinuses and splenic cords. In H&E-stained sections, white pulp appears basophilic because of the dense heterochromatin in the nuclei of the numerous lymphocytes (Plate 14.4, page 532). Within the white pulp, the branch of the splenic artery is called the **central artery**. Lymphocytes that aggregate around the central artery constitute the **periarterial lymphatic sheath (PALS)**. The PALS has a roughly cylindrical configuration that conforms to the course of the central artery. In cross sections, the PALS appears circular and may resemble a **lymphatic nodule**. The presence of the central artery, however, distinguishes the PALS from typical lymphatic nodules found in other sites. Nodules appear as localized expansions of the PALS and displace the central artery so that it occupies an eccentric rather than a central position. The architecture of white pulp is analogous to organization of a lymph node in which T and B cells are separated into different zones. In addition to lymphocytes, white pulp contains populations of specialized dendritic cells and macrophages. They later play an important role in phagocytosis of apoptotic B cells that arise during the germinal center reaction.

Migration of T and B lymphocytes into the spleen differs from that observed in lymph node.

Naïve T and B cells released from the thymus and bone marrow, respectively, enter the spleen through the open circulation. In contrast to lymph nodes, there are no HEVs in the spleen; thus, entry of lymphocytes is unregulated, and there is no need for adhesion molecules (i.e., selectin, integrins) or chemokines to be involved in the entry process.

T and B cells are then attracted to the external surface of small arteries and arterioles, forming the white pulp. The lymphatic nodules in the white pulp are the territory of B lymphocytes; other lymphocytes of the PALS are chiefly T lymphocytes that surround the nodules. Thus, the PALS may be considered a thymus-dependent zone similar to the deep cortex of a lymph node. The distribution of B and T lymphocytes is dependent on the production of different chemokines by the stromal cells and expression of specific receptors on B cells (CXCR5) and T cells (CCR7) in a process similar to that found in the lymph node (see pages 509-510). The nodules usually contain germinal centers, which, as in other lymphatic tissues, develop as B cells proliferate after their activation by antigen. Exit of lymphocytes from the white pulp to the red pulp is regulated and uses an S1P pathway similar to that found in lymph nodes (see page 511).

The lymphocytes pass through the spleen at very high rate; almost 50% of all circulating lymphocytes circulate through the spleen every 24 hours. In humans, germinal centers develop within 24 hours after antigen exposure and may become extremely large and visible with the naked eye. These enlarged nodules are called **splenic nodules** or Malpighian corpuscles (not to be confused with the renal corpuscles that have the same name).

Red pulp contains large numbers of red blood cells that it filters and degrades.

Red pulp has a red appearance in the fresh state as well as in histologic sections because it contains large numbers of

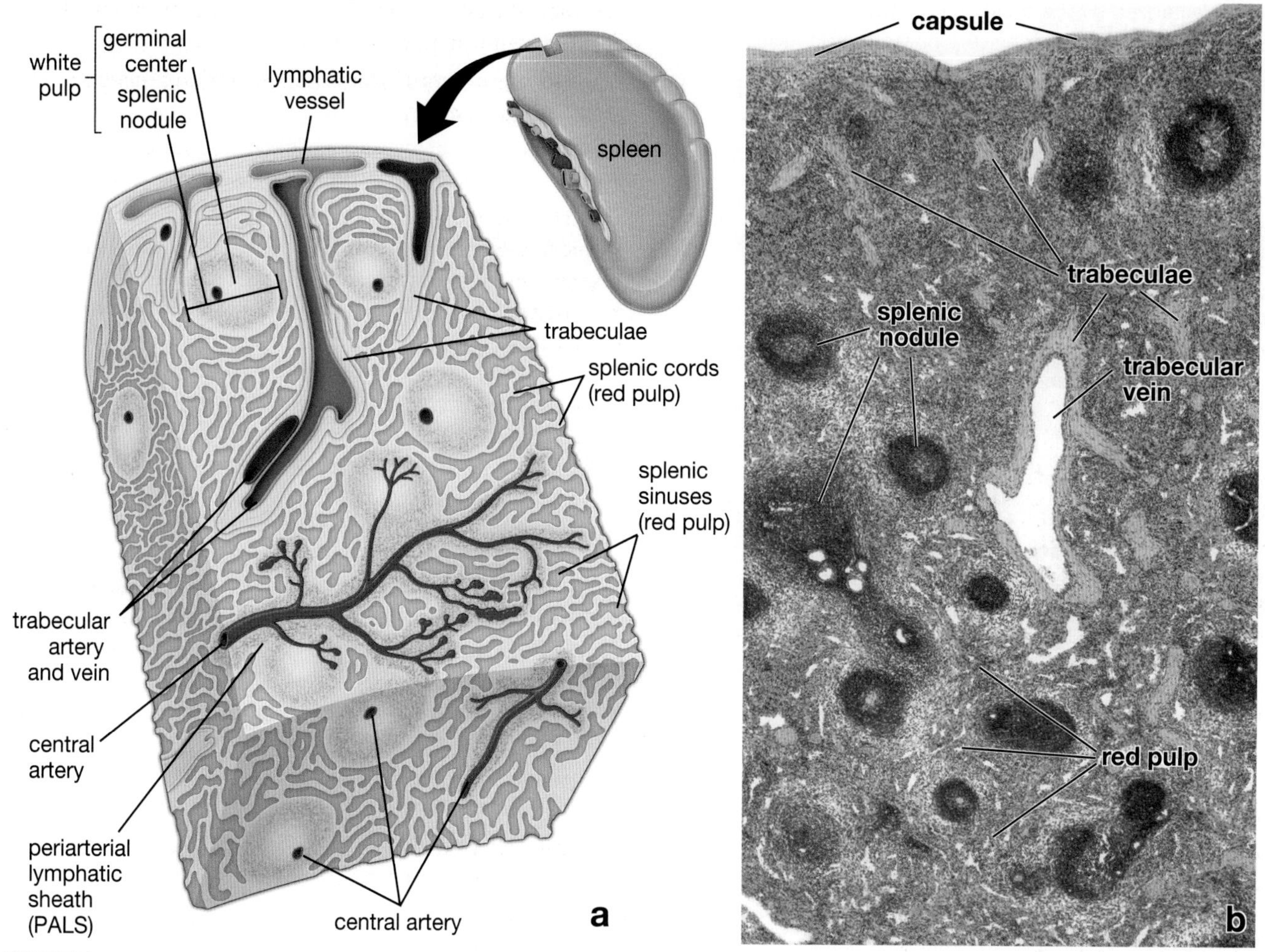

FIGURE 14.31. Schematic diagram and photomicrograph of splenic structure. a. The substance of the spleen is divided into white pulp and red pulp. White pulp consists of a cylindrical mass of lymphocytes arranged around a central artery that constitutes the periarterial lymphatic sheath (*PALS*). Splenic nodules occur along the length of the *PALS*. When observed in cross section through part of the sheath that contains a nodule, the central artery appears eccentrically located with respect to the lymphatic mass. The red pulp consists of splenic sinuses surrounded by splenic cords (cords of Billroth). A capsule surrounds the spleen; trabeculae project from it into the substance of the spleen. Both capsule and trabeculae give the appearance of dense connective tissue infiltrated by numerous myofibroblasts. Blood vessels traverse the capsule and trabeculae before and after passage within the substance of the spleen. Lymphatic vessels originate in the white pulp near the trabeculae. **b.** This low-magnification photomicrograph of the spleen reveals the same components shown in the previous drawing. Note the capsule with several trabeculae projecting into the substance of the spleen. In the *center*, there is a trabecula containing a trabecular vein through which blood leaves the organ. The red pulp constitutes the greater bulk of the splenic tissue. The white pulp contains lymphatic tissue that follows and ensheathes the central artery. Expansion of the white pulp creates the splenic nodules. ×45.

red blood cells (Plate 14.5, page 534). Essentially, red pulp consists of **splenic sinuses** separated by **splenic cords** (cords of Billroth). Splenic cords consist of the now-familiar loose meshwork of reticular cells and reticular fibers that contain type III and type V collagen molecules. Large numbers of erythrocytes, platelets, macrophages, monocytes, lymphocytes, dendritic cells, plasma cells, and granulocytes reside within the reticular meshwork of splenic cords. **Red pulp macrophages** differ from macrophages associated with white pulp; they primarily phagocytose damaged red blood cells and other materials that need to be removed from the blood. The iron from destroyed red blood cells is either released from the macrophage or stored by the cell as ferritin or its aggregate hemosiderin, which is an insoluble complex of partially degraded ferritin. Inclusions of ferritin can easily be observed in red pulp macrophages. Red pulp macrophages are essential to initiating the process of hemoglobin breakdown and iron reclamation, which is critical in the formation of new red blood cells.

The red pulp is also a large reservoir of monocytes that are clustered in splenic red cords. This pool of monocytes is larger than the pool of circulating monocytes in the blood and can be rapidly mobilized to be released from the spleen (e.g., as a response to infection). Megakaryocytes are also present in certain species, such as rodents and the cat, but not in humans, except during fetal life. Specific features of the spleen in comparison to other major lymphatic organs are summarized in Table 14.4.

The splenic or venous sinuses are special sinusoidal vessels lined by rod-shaped endothelial cells.

The **endothelial cells** that line the **splenic sinuses** are extremely long. Their longitudinal axis runs parallel to the direction of the vessel (Fig. 14.32). There are few contact points between adjacent cells, thus producing prominent intercellular spaces. These spaces allow blood cells to pass readily into and out of the sinuses. TEM images clearly demonstrate that human erythrocytes reenter the circulation from the splenic cords by squeezing through intracellular spaces between the sinus endothelial cells (Fig. 14.33). Endothelial cells contain actin filaments (stress fibers) arranged longitudinally just underneath the plasma membrane. Stress fibers are most prominent at the neighboring edges of adjacent cells. The presence of actin, myosin-like filaments, and α-actinin in stress fibers indicates their contractile properties and possible role in regulating the

FOLDER 14.4
CLINICAL CORRELATION: REACTIVE (INFLAMMATORY) LYMPHADENITIS

Reactive (inflammatory) lymphadenitis refers to enlargement of the lymph nodes that is often secondary to bacterial and other microbial infections. Lymph nodes enlarge because of edema and hyperplasia of lymphatic nodules and their cellular components (Fig. F14.4.1). These include B lymphocytes, T lymphocytes, macrophages, and other antigen-presenting cells. In addition, infiltration of lymphatic sinuses by neutrophils is also prominent. In severe bacterial infections, lymphadenitis may be accompanied by lymphangitis, an inflammation of afferent lymphatic vessels that carry infected lymph into regional lymph nodes. Inflamed lymph vessels may be visible as red streaks under the skin in the affected area of lymphatic drainage.

Common symptoms of acute lymphadenitis are swollen lymph nodes that are tender to palpation, fever, chills, loss of appetite, tachycardia, and general weakness. Lymph nodes are usually palpable and tender, with red discoloration on the overlying skin. In severe cases of suppurative necrosis (necrosis with pus formation), a fistula (false opening) may develop that allows pus to drain from the enlarged lymph node to the surface.

The most common microbial organisms that cause lymphadenitis are streptococcal and staphylococcal bacteria. Other less common organisms are viruses (as in mononucleosis or rubella), protozoa, rickettsiae, fungi, and the tuberculosis bacillus. Tonsillitis, infections originating from teeth, and bacterial pharyngitis (sore throats) are the most common causes of lymphadenitis in the neck area. Generalized lymphadenopathy is typical for rheumatoid arthritis and is detected as an early sign of HIV infection. In chronic lymphadenitis, lymph nodes are enlarged, but they are usually not tender.

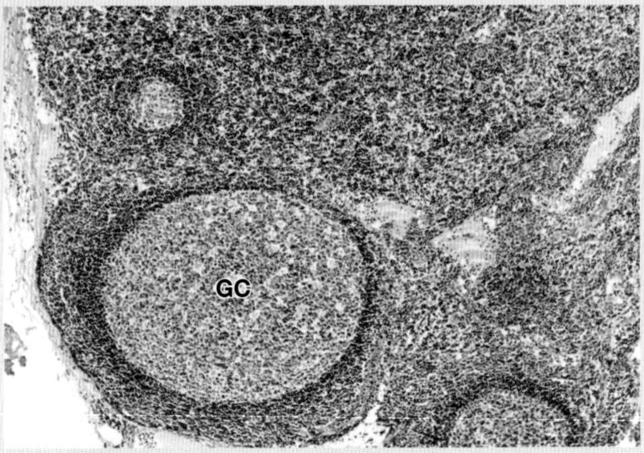

FIGURE F14.4.1. Photomicrograph of a lymph node with reactive lymphadenitis. Section through a superficial cortex of the lymph node shows a hyperplastic germinal center (*GC*) projecting toward the connective tissue capsule. The majority of pale-staining cells within the germinal center are represented by B lymphocytes and macrophages; accumulation of T lymphocytes forms a distinct mantle zone that encircles the germinal center. ×120. (Reproduced from Schwarting R, McKenzie S, Rubin R. Hematopathology. In: Rubin R, Strayer DS, eds. *Rubin's Pathology: Clinicopathologic Foundations of Medicine*. 5th ed. Lippincott Williams & Wilkins; 2008.)

size of intercellular spaces, which could, in turn, control the passage of blood cells from the splenic cords into the sinuses.

The sinuses do not possess a continuous basal lamina. **Strands of basal lamina** containing collagen IV and laminin loop around the outside of the sinus much like the hoops that loop around the staves of a barrel. These strands are at right angles to the long axes of the endothelial cells. This material stains with silver-containing reagents or with the PAS reaction (Plate 14.5, page 534). Neither smooth muscle nor pericytes are present in the wall of splenic sinuses. Reticular cell processes extend to the basal side of the endothelial cells and are associated with the **reticular fibers** that appear to merge with the perisinusoidal loops of basal lamina. Blood fills both the sinuses and cords of the red pulp, often obscuring the underlying structures and making it difficult to distinguish between the cords and the sinuses in histologic sections.

Blood Circulation in Spleen

Circulation within red pulp allows macrophages to screen antigens in the blood.

Blood entering the spleen through the **splenic artery** is distributed through the branches of **trabecular arteries** that enter the white pulp. They branch throughout the spleen to reach a terminating vessel called the **central artery,** which is surrounded by lymphatic cells. The central artery in some animals (not humans) sends branches to the white pulp itself and to the sinuses at the perimeter of the white pulp called *marginal sinuses* (see Fig. 14.31). In contrast to other animals (i.e., mice and rats), humans do not exhibit marginal sinuses. The central artery continues into the red pulp, where it branches into several relatively straight arterioles called **penicillar arterioles**. The penicillar arterioles then continue as **arterial capillaries**. Some arterial capillaries are surrounded by aggregations of macrophages and are thus called **sheathed capillaries**. Sheathed capillaries have an open trumpet- or funnel-shaped ends, allowing blood to empty directly into the reticular meshwork of the splenic cords rather than connecting to the endothelium-lined splenic sinuses. Blood entering the red pulp in this manner percolates through the cords and is exposed to the macrophages of the cords before returning to the circulation by squeezing through the narrow (1–3-μm wide) interendothelial slits in the wall of splenic sinuses. These slits are the smallest openings for erythrocyte passage in the body, which makes the spleen the largest filter of erythrocytes. In addition, the processes of macrophages extend between the endothelial cells and into the lumen of the sinuses to monitor the passing blood for foreign antigens (Figs. 14.33 and 14.34).

This type of circulation is referred to as **open circulation**, and it is the only route by which blood returns to the venous circulation in humans. It is important to underline that all research data and three-dimensional (3D) imaging support the notion that splenic circulation forms an **entirely open system in humans**. In other species such as the rat and dog, some of the blood from the sheathed capillaries passes directly to the splenic sinuses of the red pulp. This type of circulation is referred to as **closed circulation**.

Open circulation exposes the blood more efficiently to the macrophages of the red pulp. Both TEM and scanning electron micrograph often show blood cells in transit across the

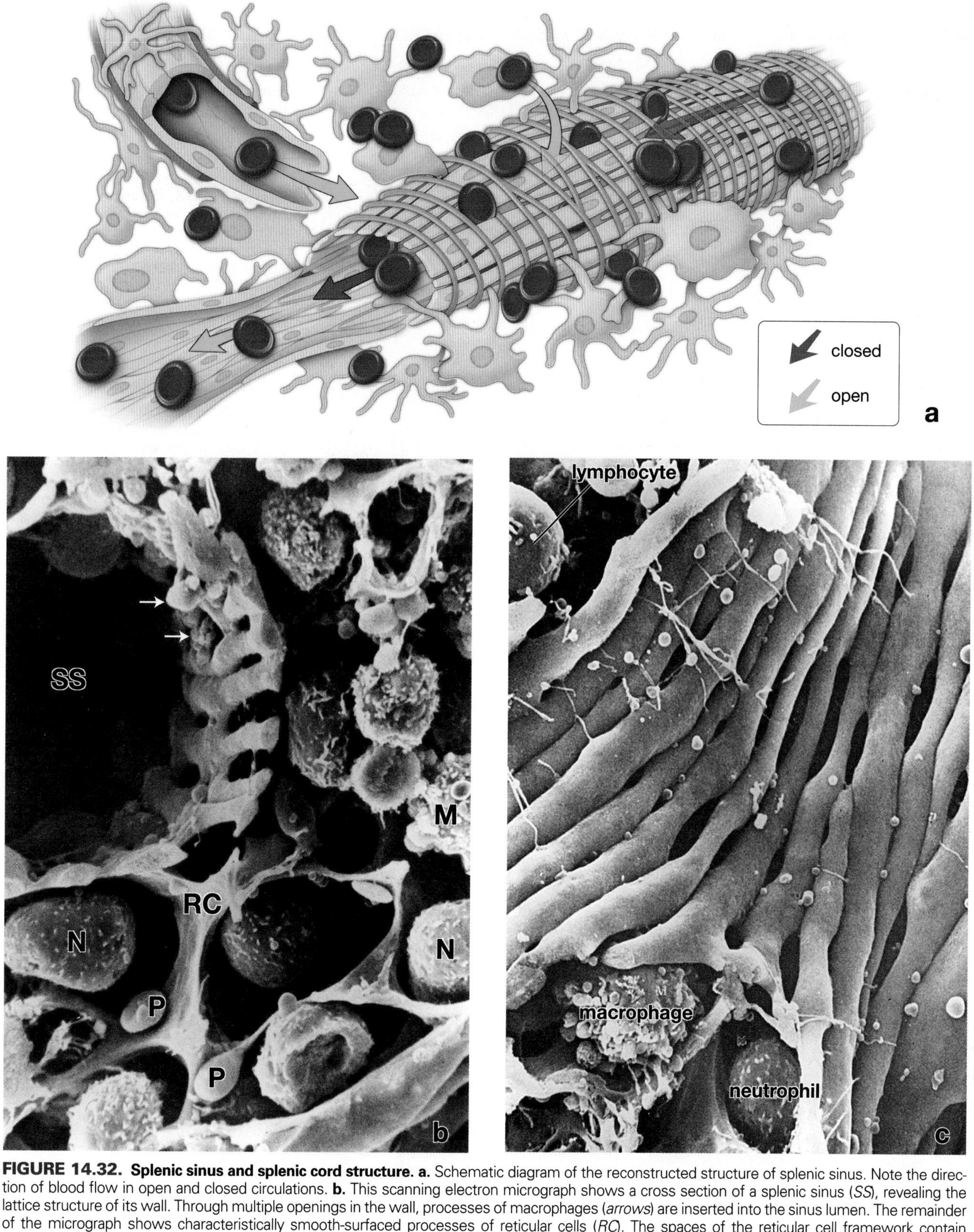

FIGURE 14.32. Splenic sinus and splenic cord structure. a. Schematic diagram of the reconstructed structure of splenic sinus. Note the direction of blood flow in open and closed circulations. **b.** This scanning electron micrograph shows a cross section of a splenic sinus (*SS*), revealing the lattice structure of its wall. Through multiple openings in the wall, processes of macrophages (*arrows*) are inserted into the sinus lumen. The remainder of the micrograph shows characteristically smooth-surfaced processes of reticular cells (*RC*). The spaces of the reticular cell framework contain neutrophils (*N*), macrophages (*M*), and blood platelets (*P*). ×4,400. **c.** Scanning electron micrograph of the splenic sinus showing the architecture of the sinus wall as seen from its luminal side. Rod-like endothelial cells run in parallel and are intermittently connected to each other by side processes. A nuclear swelling is shown at *lower right*. The tapered ends of a few of the rod cells are seen. The macrophage, neutrophil, and lymphocyte are outside the sinus. ×5,300. (Reprinted with permission from Fujita T, Tanaka K, Tokunga J. *SEM Atlas of Cells and Tissues*. Igaku-Shoin; 1981.)

endothelium of the sinus, presumably reentering the vascular system from the red pulp cords (see Fig. 14.33). The blood collected in the sinuses drains to tributaries of the trabecular veins that converge into larger veins and eventually leaves the spleen by the splenic vein. The splenic vein, in turn, joins the drainage from the intestine in the hepatic portal vein.

The spleen initiates adaptive immune responses and performs hemopoietic functions.

Because the spleen filters blood as the lymph nodes filter lymph, it functions in both the immune and the hemopoietic systems. The spleen is the largest secondary lymphatic organ in an adult human.

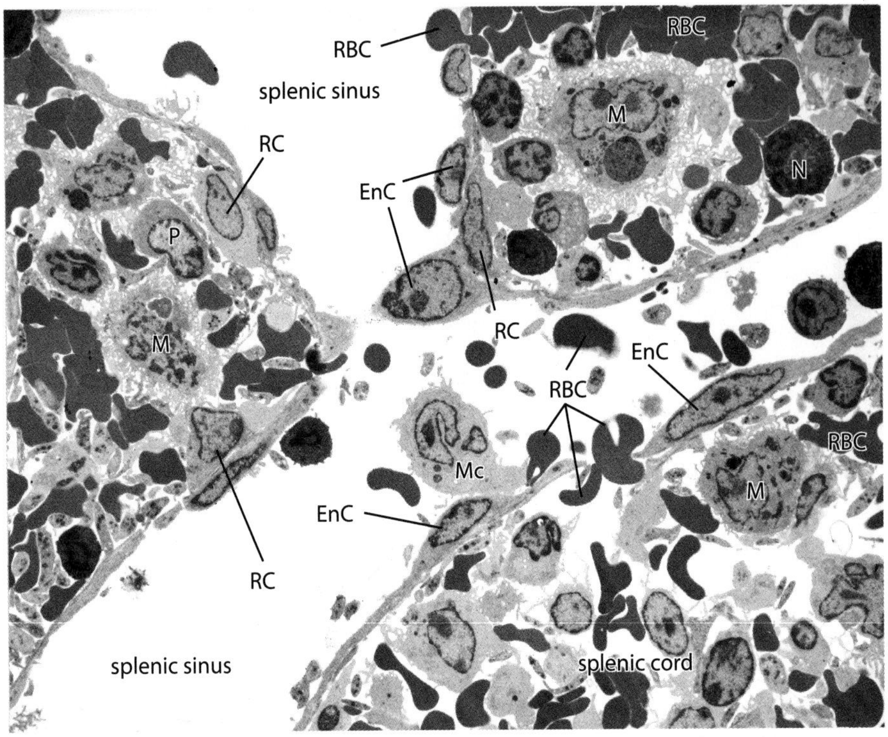

FIGURE 14.33. Electron micrograph of the red pulp of the spleen. This low-magnification electron micrograph shows a section of the red pulp of the spleen. The junction of two splenic sinuses is visible in the *center*; the sinuses are surrounded by the stromal cells of the red pulp. Elongated nuclei belong to the rod-like endothelial (*EnC*) cells lining the sinuses. Note many profiles of red blood cells in the red pulp and in the splenic sinuses (*RBC*); several of them are in the process of passing through intercellular spaces between endothelial cells. Reticular cells (*RC*) are adjacent to the wall of the sinus. Many red pulp macrophages (*M*) are visible outside the wall of the sinus. *Mc*, monocyte; *N*, neutrophil; *P*, plasma. ×2,800. (Copyright © 2010. Regents of the University of Michigan. Reprinted with permission.)

Immune system functions of the spleen include the following:

- Antigen presentation by antigen-presenting cells (mostly dendritic cells and macrophages) and initiation of immune response to blood-borne antigens
- Antigen activation and proliferation of B and T lymphocytes
- Production of antibodies against antigen present in circulating blood
- Removal of macromolecular antigens and opsonized microorganisms from the blood

Activation and proliferation of T cells and differentiation of B cells and plasma cells, as well as secretion of antibodies, occur in the white pulp of the spleen; in this regard, the white pulp is the equivalent of other lymphatic organs.

Hemopoietic functions of the spleen include the following:

- Removal and destruction of senescent, damaged, and abnormal erythrocytes and platelets
- Retrieval of iron from erythrocyte hemoglobin
- Formation of erythrocytes during early fetal life (10th–25th week of gestation)
- Storage of blood, especially red blood cells and platelets, in some species

The role of the red pulp is primarily **blood filtration** (i.e., removal of particulate material; macromolecular antigens; and

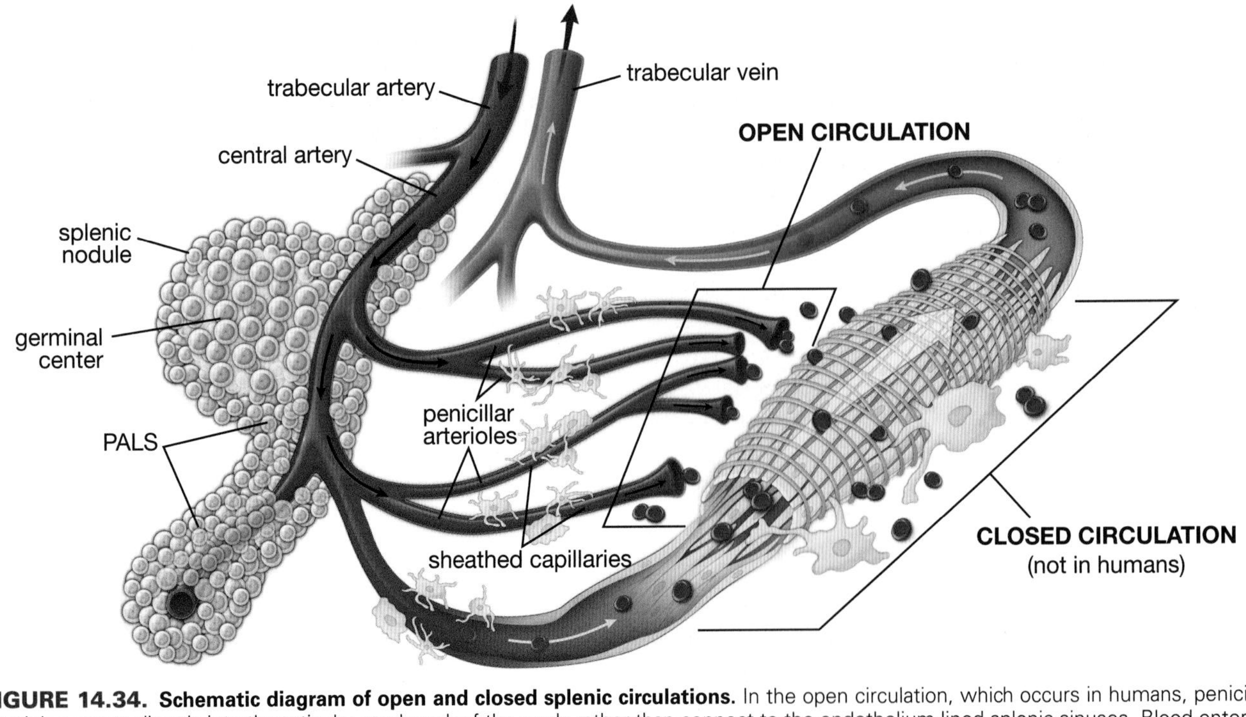

FIGURE 14.34. Schematic diagram of open and closed splenic circulations. In the open circulation, which occurs in humans, penicillar arterioles empty directly into the reticular meshwork of the cords rather than connect to the endothelium-lined splenic sinuses. Blood entering the red pulp then percolates through the cords and is exposed to the macrophages residing there. In the closed circulation, which occurs in other species, the penicillar arterioles empty directly into the splenic sinuses of the red pulp. *PALS*, periarterial lymphatic sheath.

TABLE 14.4 Comparisons of the Major Lymphatic Organs

Features	Lymphatic Nodules (CALT, BALT, GALT, MALT)	Lymph Nodes	Thymus	Spleen
	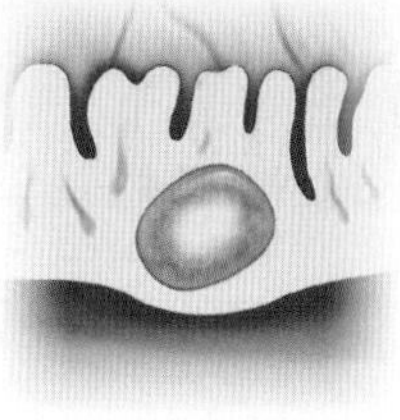	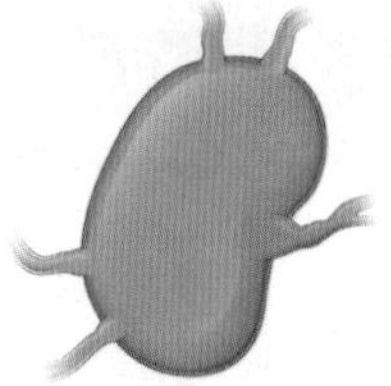	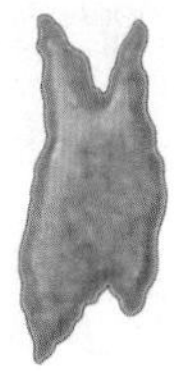	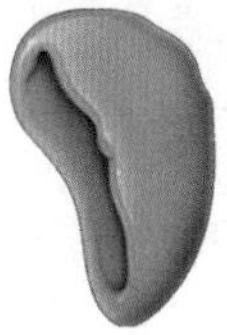
Major function	Immune surveillance of mucosal membranes	Filter lymph Generate immune responses to antigens in the lymph	Develops immunocompetent T lymphocytes	Filters blood Eliminates senescent erythrocytes Generates immune responses to circulating antigens
Connective tissue capsule	No	Yes	Yes	Yes; contains myofibroblasts
Cortex	No	Yes	Yes	No
Medulla	No	Yes	Yes	No
Lymph nodules	Yes	Yes; in the superficial cortex only	No	Yes; in white pulp only
Afferent lymphatic vessels	No	Yes; passing through the capsule	No	No
Efferent lymphatic vessels	Yes	Yes; leaving the node at the hilum	Yes (few); originate in connective tissue septa and capsule	Yes; inconspicuous, originate in white pulp near trabeculae
High endothelial venules (HEVs)	Yes; in well-established lymph nodules (i.e., tonsils, appendix, Peyer patches)	Yes; associated with deep cortex	No	No
Characteristic features	Diffuse lymphatic tissue with randomly distributed lymphatic nodules underlying epithelial surface	Presence of lymphatic sinuses (subcapsular, trabecular, and medullary) Reticular meshwork	Thymic lobules Meshwork of epithelioreticular cells Hassall corpuscles in medulla only	White pulp with PALS splenic nodules containing central artery Red pulp containing splenic sinuses, penicillar arteries, sheathed capillaries, and splenic cords

BALT, bronchus-associated lymphatic tissue; *CALT*, conjunctiva-associated lymphatic tissue; *GALT*, gut-associated lymphatic tissue; *HEV*, high endothelial venule; *MALT*, mucosa-associated lymphatic tissue; *PALS*, periarterial lymphatic sheath.

aged, abnormal, or damaged blood cells and platelets from the circulating blood). These functions are accomplished by the macrophages embedded in the reticular meshwork of the red pulp, especially those that are situated directly beneath the endothelium of splenic sinuses. The open circulation in the spleen ensures that all materials circulating in the blood have direct access to red pulp macrophages. Senescent, damaged, or abnormal red cells are broken down by the lysosomes of the red pulp macrophages, and iron from the hemoglobin is retrieved and stored as ferritin or hemosiderin for future recycling. The heme portion of the molecule is broken down to bilirubin, which is transported to the liver via the portal system and there conjugated to glucuronic acid. Conjugated bilirubin is secreted into the bile, giving it a characteristic color.

Red pulp macrophages recognize senescent or abnormal blood cells by several different mechanisms:

- **Nonspecific mechanisms** involve morphologic and biochemical changes that occur in aged erythrocytes; they become more rigid and are thus more easily trapped in the mesh of the red pulp.
- **Specific mechanisms** include opsonization of the cell membrane with antiband 3 IgG antibodies, which trigger F_c receptor–dependent phagocytosis of erythrocytes. In addition, specific changes in glycosylation of glycophorins (see page 302) in aging erythrocytes act as a recognition signal that triggers the elimination of senescent erythrocytes by macrophages.

Despite these important functions, the spleen is not essential for human life. It can be removed surgically (**splenectomy**), which may be performed after trauma that causes intractable bleeding from the spleen. The removal and destruction of aging red blood cells then occur in the bone marrow and liver. The crucial role of the spleen in protection against blood-borne pathogens is demonstrated by studies of splenectomized patients, who cannot generate immune responses to several types of encapsulated bacteria such as **meningococci, pneumococci**, and ***Haemophilus influenzae* type b**. Polysaccharide capsules surrounding these microorganisms enable them to evade adaptive and specific immune defense mechanisms. Several studies have shown that antibody responses to polysaccharides occur more readily in the spleen than in other lymphatic tissues. In addition, specialized splenic macrophages are crucial for removing antibody-coated encapsulated organisms from the blood. People who have undergone splenectomy have an increased risk of infections caused by encapsulated bacteria (i.e., pneumococcal pneumonia).

HISTOLOGY 101 NOTEBOOK

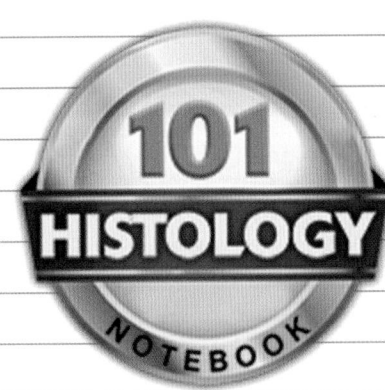

IMMUNE SYSTEM AND LYMPHATIC TISSUES AND ORGANS

OVERVIEW OF THE IMMUNE SYSTEM

- The **immune system** is the body's defense system that generates immune responses against their own transformed cells and foreign invaders. The **lymphatic system** is practically indistinguishable from the immune system; it consists of groups of cells, tissues, and organs involved in immune responses.
- **Lymphocytes** are the definitive cells of the immune system and the effector cells in immune responses.
- Tissues and organs of the lymphatic system include diffuse lymphatic tissues, lymphatic nodules, lymph nodes, spleen, tonsils, bone marrow, and thymus.
- Immune responses can be divided into **nonspecific (innate) immunity** (represents the first line of defense against microbial aggression) and **specific (adaptive) immunity** (gradually acquired and based on contact with antigen and its presentation to various types of lymphocytes).
- Two types of responses are characteristic of specific immunity: the **humoral response** (production of antibodies against invaded foreign antigen) and the **cellular immune response** (targets transformed and virus-infected cells for destruction by specific "killer" cells).

CELLS OF THE IMMUNE SYSTEM

- Three major types of **lymphocytes** are present in the body: T lymphocytes, B lymphocytes, and NK cells.
- **T lymphocytes (T cells)** differentiate and mature in the thymus and are characterized by the presence of TCRs. They account for 60%–80% of the circulating lymphocytes and are subclassified based on the presence of different surface marker proteins named by the **cluster of differentiation (CD)** numbering system.
- **B lymphocytes (B cells)** differentiate and mature in the bone marrow and are characterized by the presence of BCRs (IgM and IgD bound to cell membranes). They participate in humoral immunity and differentiate into antibody-producing plasma cells.
- **Natural killer lymphocytes (NK cells)** are specialized in killing target cells by releasing perforins and granzymes.
- Lymphocytes undergo antigen-independent differentiation in the **primary lymphatic organs** (**thymus** and **bone marrow**). They undergo antigen-dependent activation in the **secondary lymphatic organs and tissues.**

TYPES OF IMMUNE RESPONSES

- **Primary immune response** refers to the body's first encounter with an antigen; it is delayed by several days and generates mainly IgM antibodies.
- **Secondary immune response** is more rapid and intense than the primary response; it generates IgG antibodies.
- **Humoral (antibody-mediated) immunity** is mediated by antibodies produced by B cells and plasma cells.
- **Cell-mediated immunity** is mediated by specific T cells.
- In **antibody-dependent cell–mediated cytotoxicity (ADCC)**, IgG antibodies direct NK cells to their target.

ACTIVATION OF T AND B CELLS

- To initiate an immune response, helper and cytotoxic T cells must recognize and bind to an antigen (polypeptide) that is displayed on the **major histocompatibility complex (MHC) molecules.**
- Two classes of MHC molecules are found on cells: **MHC I** is expressed on the surface of all nucleated cells and platelets; **MHC II** has limited distribution and is expressed only on the surface of the **antigen-presenting cells (APCs).**
- **Cytotoxic CD8$^+$ T cells** are MHC I restricted, and **helper CD4$^+$ T cells** are MHC II restricted.
- Activation of T cells requires three signals.
  1. **First (antigen) signal:** The TCR and the CD4 or CD8 molecules interact with the antigen displayed on the MHC molecule.
  2. **Second (costimulatory) signal:** Interaction between the different CD molecules expressed on T cells and the antigen-presenting cells.
  3. **Third (cytokine) signal** derives from the secretion of cytokines for differentiation of a specific subset of T cells.
- **Activated helper T cells** release cytokines (interleukins) that stimulate other T, B, and NK cells to differentiate and proliferate. **Activated cytotoxic T cells** also release cytokines that stimulate cells to proliferate and destroy the abnormal host cells.
- **Activation of B cells** requires interaction with helper T cells to produce specific cytokines and to differentiate into plasma cells and memory B cells.
- **Regulatory (suppressor) T cells** suppress the immune responses of other activated lymphocytes, thereby preventing autoimmune diseases.

LYMPHATIC TISSUES AND ORGANS

- **Diffuse lymphatic tissues** in the GI tract (GALT), respiratory system (BALT), eyelids (CALT), and genitourinary tract (MALT) guard the body against pathogenic substances.
- Diffuse lymphatic tissue is a site for the **initial immune response** that is characterized by clonal proliferation of B cells and subsequent development of **lymphatic nodules** (or **follicles**).
- A **germinal center** is located in the center of the lymph nodule; it contains **activated B lymphocytes, plasmablasts,** antigen-presenting **follicular dendritic cells (FDCs)**, and a subset of **follicular helper T (TFH) cells.**
- **Lymphatic nodules** are found in the GALT (tonsils, Peyer patches, solitary lymph nodules, and vermiform appendix), BALT (bronchial tree), CALT (eyelids), and MALT (mucosa of urogenital system).
- **Lymphatic vessels** begin as networks of blind capillaries in loose connective tissue that collect **lymph** composed of extracellular fluid, large molecules (antigens), and cells (mainly lymphocytes). Many lymphatic vessels originate in the diffuse lymphatic tissues.

LYMPH NODES

- As lymph circulates through the lymphatic vessels, it passes through **lymph nodes**, which are small, encapsulated organs in which antigens are trapped by follicular dendritic cells and exposed to lymphocytes for their activation.
- **Afferent lymphatic vessels** pass the capsule and enter the cortex of a lymph node. Lymph is then filtrated within a network of interconnected **lymphatic sinuses** (subcapsular, trabecular, and medullary) and leaves the lymph node by an **efferent lymphatic vessel.**
- The **reticular meshwork** of the lymph node contains reticular cells, dendritic cells, follicular dendritic cells, and macrophages. They all interact with T and B cells that are dispersed throughout the **superficial cortex**, **deep cortex**, and the **medulla** of the lymph node.
- Lymphocytes from blood vessels enter the lymph node via specialized **high endothelial venules (HEVs)** located in the **deep cortex**, which contains most of the **T cells.**
- Most of the **B cells** are located in the lymph nodules within the **superficial cortex.**

THYMUS

- The **thymus** is a lymphoepithelial organ located in the superior mediastinum that contains developing **T cells** within an extensive meshwork of interconnected **epithelioreticular cells**. The thymus is fully formed at birth and persists until puberty.
- **Epithelioreticular cells** form compartments (cortex and medulla), secrete cytokines, surround blood vessels in the blood–thymus barrier, and, as APCs, are involved in **cross-talk** with developing T cells.
- The most characteristic microscopic feature of the **thymic medulla** is the presence of **thymic (Hassall) corpuscles** formed by type VI epithelioreticular cells.
- During **thymic cell education** (characterized by synthesis of TCRs and expression and deletion of specific surface CD molecules), T cells undergo differentiation and a **two-stage selection process** (**positive** and **negative selection**) that leads to the development of immune tolerance by eliminating all T cells directed against the body's own tissues.

SPLEEN

- The **spleen** is the largest lymphatic organ and is located in the abdominal cavity. The spleen filters blood and reacts immunologically to blood-borne antigens. It removes senescent and defective erythrocytes and recycles iron from degraded hemoglobin.
- The spleen has two functionally and morphologically different regions: **white pulp** and **red pulp**.
- **White pulp** consists of lymphatic tissue associated with branches of the central artery. T cells that surround the central artery constitute the **periarterial lymphatic sheath (PALS)**.
- **Red pulp** consists of **splenic sinuses** separated by **splenic cords**, which contain large numbers of erythrocytes, macrophages, and other immune cells.
- The **splenic sinuses** are lined by rod-shaped endothelial cells with strands of incomplete basal lamina looping around the outside.
- Blood entering the spleen flows via **open circulation**, where capillaries open directly into the splenic cords (outside the circulatory system), or **closed circulation**, where blood circulates without leaving the vascular network. In humans, open circulation is the only route by which blood returns to the venous circulation.

PLATE 14.1 ■ PALATINE TONSIL

The **palatine tonsils** are paired structures consisting of masses of lymphatic tissue located on either side of the pharynx. They, along with the pharyngeal tonsils (adenoids) and lingual tonsils, form a ring at the entrance to the oropharynx (Waldeyer ring). Structurally, the tonsils contain numerous lymphatic nodules located in the mucosa. The stratified squamous epithelium that covers the surface of the palatine tonsil (and pharyngeal) dips into the underlying connective tissue forming many crypts, the **tonsillar crypts**. The walls of these crypts contain lymphatic nodules. The epithelial lining of the crypts is typically infiltrated with lymphocytes and often to such a degree that the epithelium may be difficult to discern. While the nodules principally occupy the connective tissue, the infiltration of lymphocytes into the epithelium tends to mask the epithelial connective tissue boundary. The tonsils guard the opening of the pharynx, the common entry to the respiratory and digestive tracts. The palatine and pharyngeal tonsils can become enflamed due to repeated infection in the oropharynx and nasopharynx and can harbor bacteria that cause repeated infections if they are overwhelmed. When this occurs, the enflamed tonsils are removed surgically (tonsillectomy and adenoidectomy). Tonsils, like other aggregations of lymphatic nodules, do not possess afferent lymphatic vessels. Lymph, however, does drain from the tonsillar lymphatic tissue through efferent lymphatic vessels.

ORIENTATION MICROGRAPH: This low-magnification micrograph is a section through a palatine tonsil. The hematoxylin-staining areas represent the lymphatic tissue (*L*). The tonsil is surfaced by stratified squamous epithelium (*SSE*), which dips into the underlying connective tissue forming the tonsillar crypts (*TC*). At the base of one of the crypts are a number of mucus-secreting glands (*MG*).

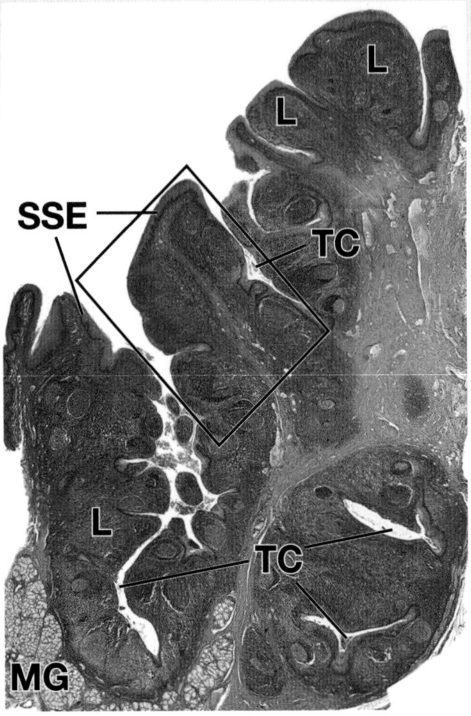

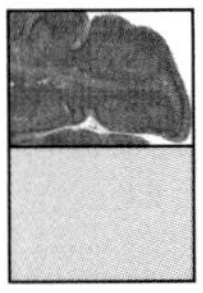

Tonsil, human, hematoxylin and eosin (H&E) ×47.

This micrograph is from the area in the *rectangle* of the orientation micrograph. At this higher magnification, part of the surface epithelium (*SE*) of the tonsil can be readily identified. In other sites, the lymphocytes (*Ly*) have infiltrated the epithelium to such an extent that the epithelium is difficult to identify. The body of the nodules (*N*) lies within the mucosa, and because of their close proximity, they tend to merge. Several of the nodules have been cut in a plane that includes their germinal center (*GC*). Note the eosinophilic staining in these areas. Beneath the nodules is the submucosa (*S*) consisting of dense connective tissue, which is continuous with the dense connective tissue beyond the tonsillar tissue.

Tonsil, human, H&E ×365.

At the higher magnification of this micrograph, the characteristic invasiveness of the lymphocytes into the overlying epithelium is readily evident. Note on the *lower left side* of the micrograph a clear boundary between the epithelium and the underlying lamina propria. The basal cells (*BC*) of the stratified squamous epithelium can be recognized. The underlying lamina propria is occupied by numerous lymphocytes; only a few have entered the epithelial compartment. Also note the thin band of collagen fibers (*CF*) that can be seen at the boundary between the epithelium and the lamina propria. In contrast, the *lower right side* of the micrograph displays numerous lymphocytes that have invaded the epithelium. More striking is the presence of what appear as isolated islands of epithelial cells (*Ep*) within the periphery. The thin band of collagen (*C*) lying at the interface of the epithelium is so disrupted in this area that it appears as small fragments. In effect, the small portion of the nodule seen on the *right side* of the micrograph has literally grown into the epithelium with the consequent disappearance of the well-defined epithelial–connective tissue boundary.

BC, basal cells
C, collagen
CF, collagen fibers
Ep, islands of epithelial cells
GC, germinal center
L, lymphatic tissue
Ly, lymphocytes
MG, mucus-secreting glands
N, nodule
S, submucosa
SE, surface epithelium
SSE, stratified squamous epithelium
TC, tonsillar crypts

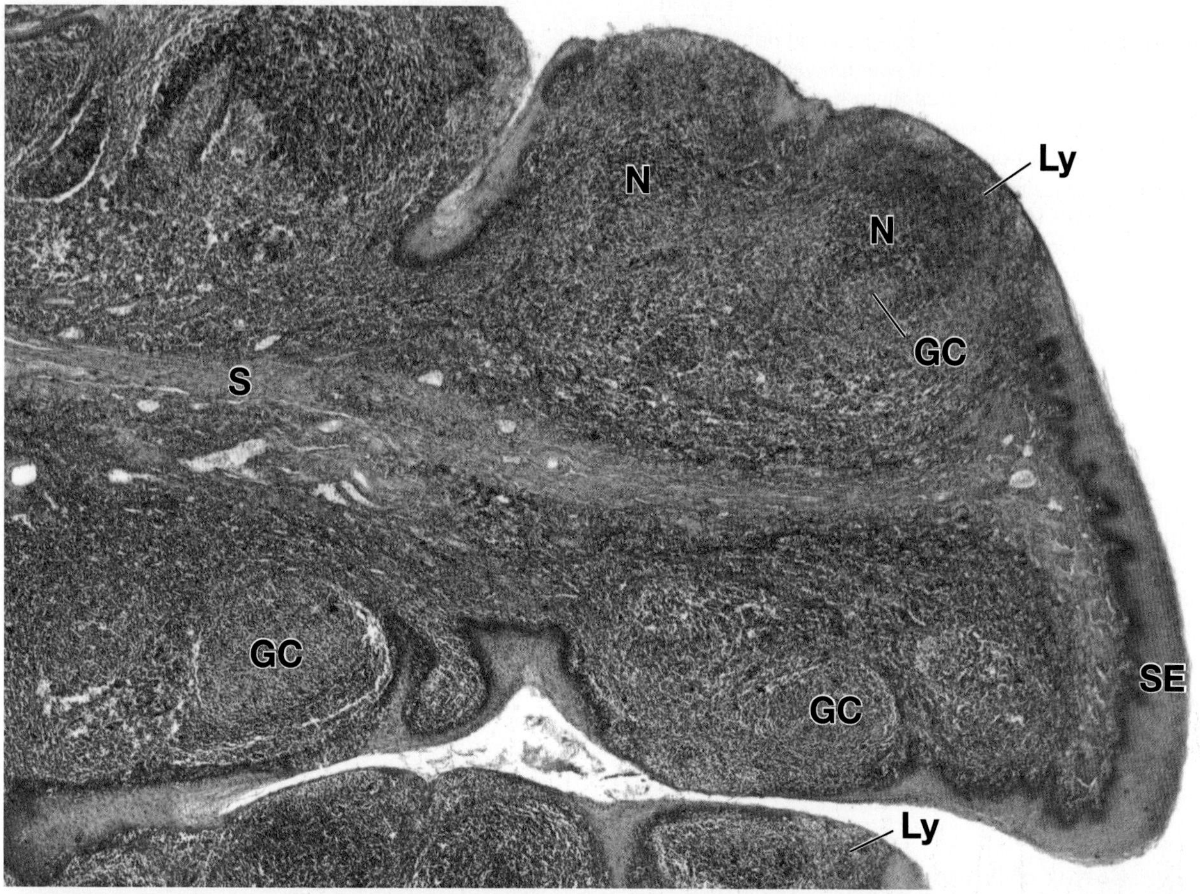
N
N
Ly
GC
S
GC
GC
SE
Ly

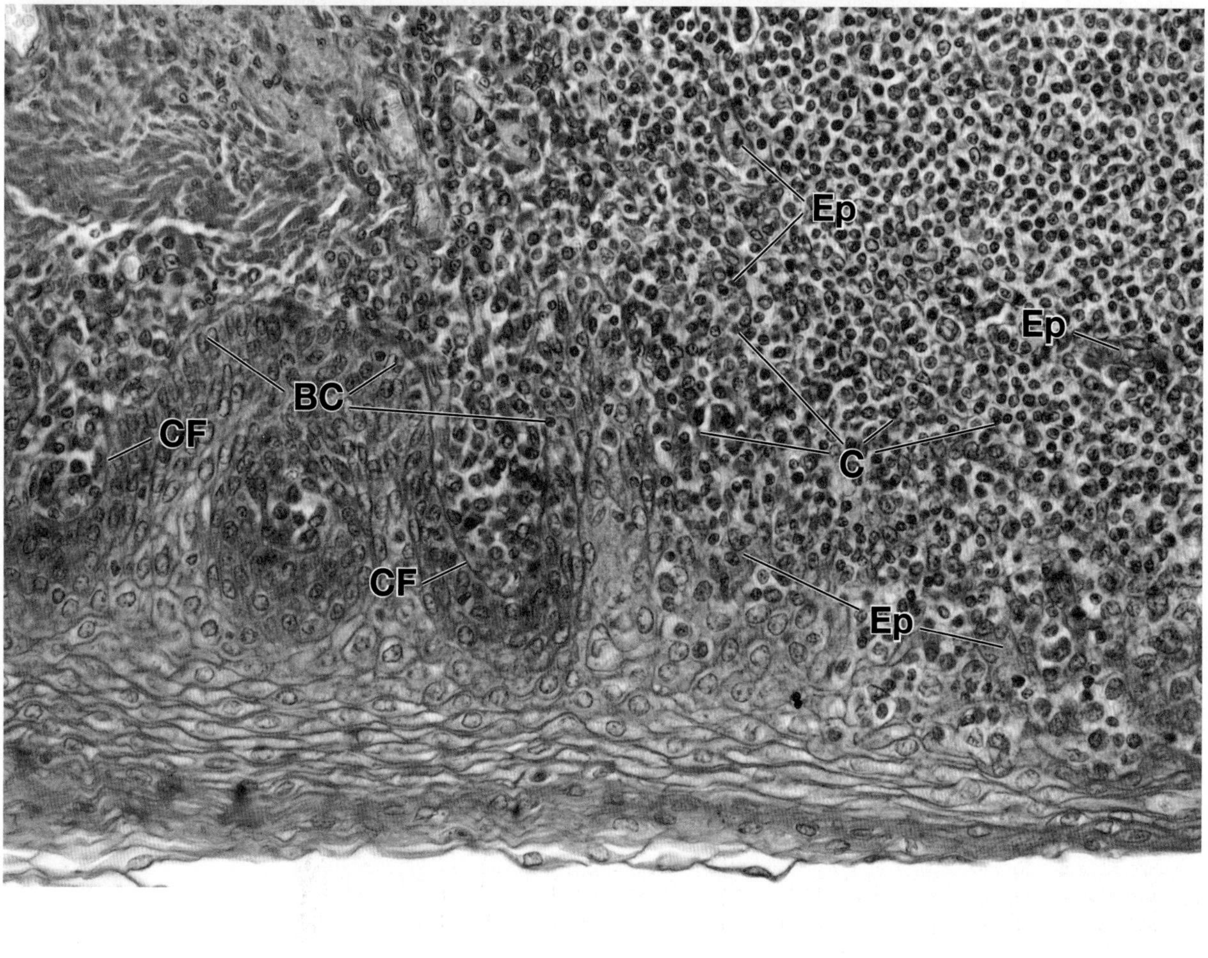
Ep
Ep
BC
CF
C
CF
Ep

PLATE 14.2 ■ LYMPH NODE I

Lymph nodes are small, encapsulated lymphatic organs that are located in the path of the lymph vessels. They serve as filters of the lymph and as the principal site in which T and B lymphocytes undergo *antigen-dependent* proliferation and differentiation into *effector lymphocytes* (plasma cells and T cells) and *memory B cells* and *T cells.* A low-magnification (×14) micrograph of a section through a human lymph node is shown on this page for orientation. The **capsule** appears as a thin connective tissue covering.

The parenchyma of the node is composed of a mass of lymphatic tissue, arranged as a **cortex** (*C*) that surrounds a less dense area, the **medulla** (*M*). The cortex is interrupted at the **hilum** of the organ (*H*), where there is a recognizable concavity. It is at this site that blood vessels enter and leave the lymph node; the efferent lymphatic vessels also leave the node at the hilum.

Afferent lymphatic vessels penetrate the capsule at multiple sites to empty into an endothelium-lined space, the *cortical* or *subcapsular sinus.* This sinus drains into the trabecular sinuses that extend through the cortex alongside the trabeculae and then supply the *medullary sinuses.* These, in turn, drain to the *efferent lymphatic vessels* that leave the node at the hilum.

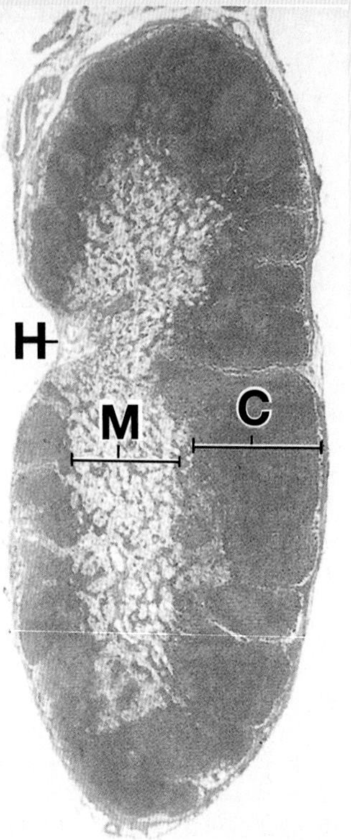

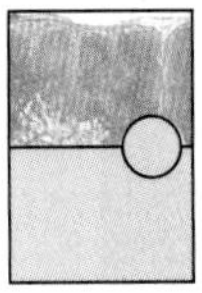

Cortex of lymph node, human, hematoxylin and eosin (H&E) ×120.

An area from the **cortex** is shown here at higher magnification. The **capsule** (*Cap*) is composed of dense connective tissue from which **trabeculae** (*T*) penetrate into the organ. Immediately below the capsule is the cortical or **subcapsular sinus** (*CS*), which receives lymph from the afferent lymphatic vessels after they penetrate the capsule. The cortical sinus is continuous with the trabecular sinuses (*TS*) that course along the trabeculae.

The cortex contains the lymphatic nodules (*LN*) and a deeper component that lacks nodules, known as the *deep cortex.* Whereas lymph nodules and their lighter staining germinal centers characterize the outer cortex, a more dense mass of lymphocytes, which imparts a distinct basophilia, characterizes the deep cortex. In contrast to these areas, the medulla is characterized by narrow strands of anastomosing lymphatic tissue containing numerous lymphocytes, the medullary cords (*MC*), separated by light-appearing areas known as the *medullary sinuses* (*MS*). The medullary sinuses receive lymph from the trabecular sinuses and lymph filtered through the cortical tissue.

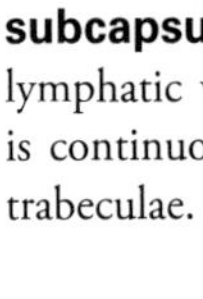

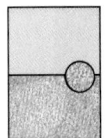

Lymphatic nodule, lymph node, human, H&E ×400; inset ×640.

This higher magnification micrograph of a **lymphatic nodule** from the previous figure illustrates the **germinal center** (*GC*) containing medium and large lymphocytes (majority of activated B cells). Germinal centers also contain plasma cells. Dividing lymphocytes are shown at slightly higher magnification in the *inset* (*arrows*), which corresponds to the area in the *circle* in this figure. The *inset* also reveals nuclei of the **reticular cells** (*RC*) that form the connective tissue stroma throughout the organ. The ovoid reticular cell has a large pale-staining nucleus, and its cytoplasm forms long processes that surround the reticular fibers. In H&E preparations, the reticular fibers and the surrounding cytoplasm are difficult to identify. Reticular cells are best seen in the sinuses, where they extend across the lymphatic space and are relatively unobscured by other cells.

A unique vessel, the **high endothelial venule** (*HEV*), is found in relation to the lymphatic nodules, particularly in the deep cortex. These vessels have an endothelium composed of tall cells between which lymphocytes migrate from the vessel lumen into the parenchyma.

C, cortex
Cap, capsule
CS, cortical or subcapsular sinus
GC, germinal center
H, hilum
HEV, high endothelial venule
LN, lymphatic nodule
M, medulla
MC, medullary cords
MS, medullary sinus
RC, reticular cells
T, trabecular
TS, trabecular sinus
arrows, dividing lymphocytes

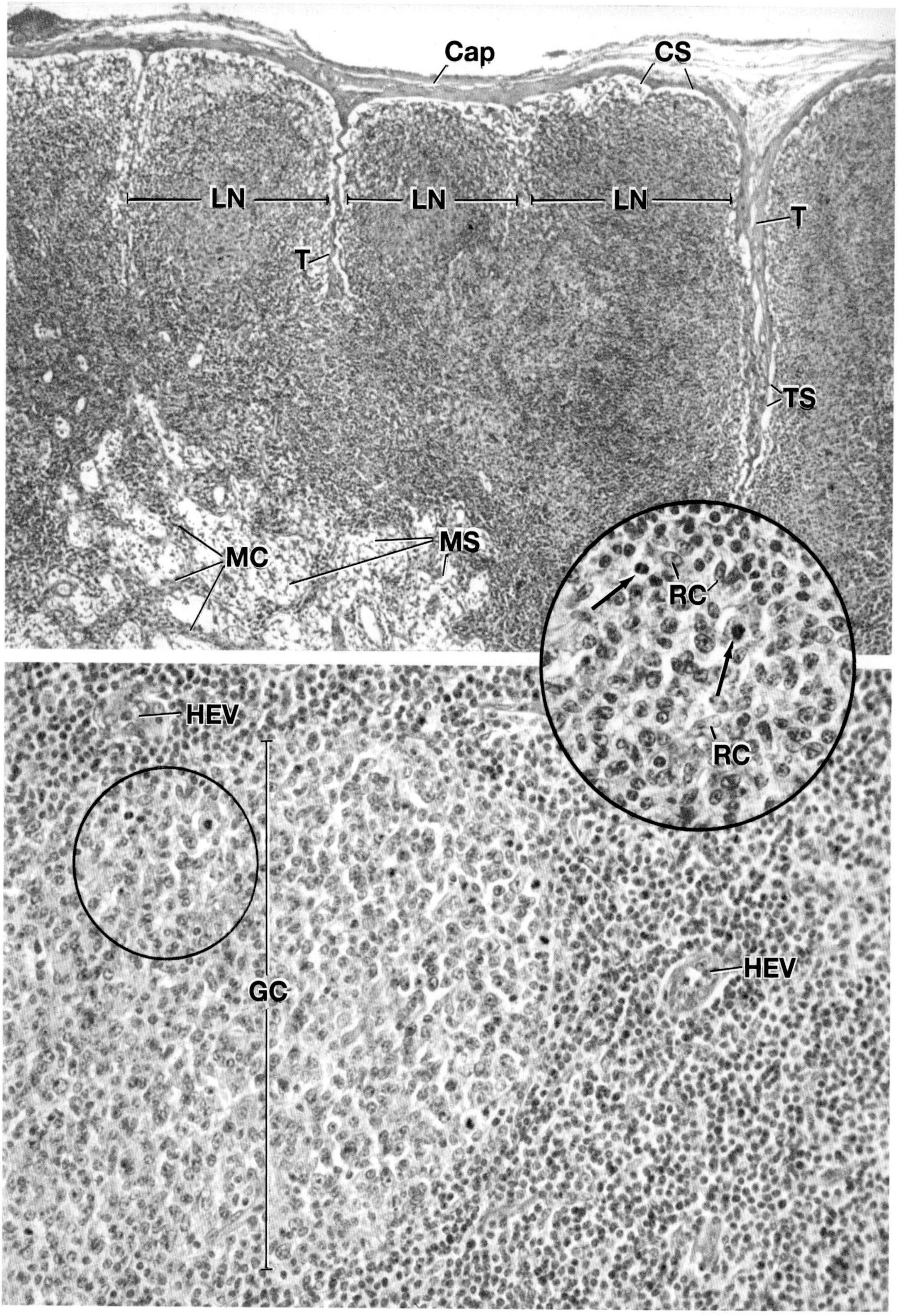
Cap
CS
LN
LN
LN
T
T
TS
MC
MS
RC
RC
HEV
GC
HEV

PLATE 14.3 ■ LYMPH NODE II

Immunocompetent B cells that have been exposed to an antigen that they can recognize and bind migrate to a lymph node, where they undergo activation and begin a series of mitotic divisions that produce large numbers of immature lymphocytes. They proliferate further in **superficial cortex** into a clone of lymphocytes that differentiate into antibody-secreting plasma cells and memory cells. B-cell proliferation and differentiation take place in **germinal centers** in the superficial cortex of the lymph node. T-cell activation and differentiation take place in the **deep cortex**. Newly differentiated plasma cells migrate to the medulla, where they release antibodies into the lymph leaving the node. They may also leave the node, enter the blood vascular system at the thoracic duct, and travel to localized sites in the connective tissue where they may continue to produce antibodies.

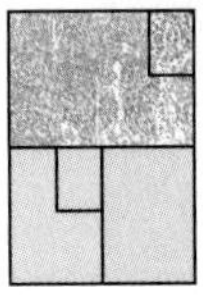

Deep cortex, lymph node, human, hematoxylin and eosin (H&E) ×365.

This micrograph shows the lymph node **deep cortex**. As noted in the previous plate, it lies below the region containing the lymph nodules and consists of closely packed lymphocytes. A number of blood vessels can be seen in this region. Whereas typical small blood vessels such as capillaries (*Cap*) and venules are present, the more unusual postcapillary venule called **high endothelial venule** (*HEV*) is also found in this region. A small vessel that can be identified as a venule (*Ven*), based on lumen size and wall thickness, is seen at a point of transition to become a high endothelial venule (*arrowheads*). The endothelial cell nuclei at this point of juncture have become cuboidal. The high endothelial venule is identified by its endothelium, which is composed of cells that are cuboidal. A cross-sectioned profile of a postcapillary venule is shown in the *inset* at higher magnification (×700). The endothelial cell's nuclei are round and lightly stained, in contrast to the nuclei of the surrounding lymphocytes, which are of similar size and shape but are densely stained. This vessel also shows three lymphocytes (*arrows*) that are in the process of migrating through the wall of the vessel. The *lower right* corner of this figure reveals a region where there is a considerably lesser concentration of lymphocytes. This area, part of the medulla, contains spaces that represent medullary sinuses (*MS*).

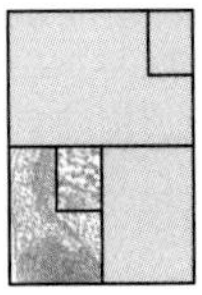

Hilar region, lymph node, human, H&E ×250.

The areas shown here, near the hilar region of the node, are part of a **lymph nodule** (*LN*), the **cortical sinus** (*CS*) just below the capsule (*Caps*), and some of the medullary sinus (*MS*). Both the cortical sinus and the medullary sinus are spanned by **reticular cells** (*RC*). These cells wrap around the collagen bundles that form the supporting trabecular framework of the node. The *inset* reveals the *boxed area* at higher magnification (×530). The nuclei of the reticular cells (*RC*) are larger and less densely staining than the lymphocyte nuclei, which are round and densely stained. In H&E preparations, these characteristics allow for the distinction between the reticular cell and the lymphocyte.

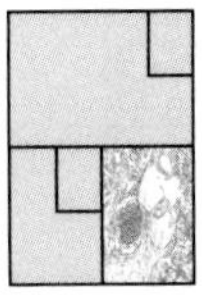

Hilar region, lymph node, monkey, H&E ×530.

This micrograph shows an area in the region of the hilum of the node. Two of the vessels here are **efferent lymphatics**; both contain a valve (*Val*). The upper lymphatic vessel exhibits what appears to be an incomplete wall. The openings in the vessel wall (*arrows*) are sites in which the medullary sinuses are emptying their contents into the lymphatic vessel. Also present are a small artery (*A*) and a vein (*V*).

A, artery
Cap, capillary
Caps, capsule
CS, cortical sinus
HEV, high endothelial venule
LN, lymph nodule
MS, medullary sinus
RC, reticular cells
V, vein
Val, valve
Ven, venule
arrowheads, endothelial cells of postcapillary venule
arrows, top image endothelial cells of HEV; bottom image opening of medullary sinus to lymph vessel

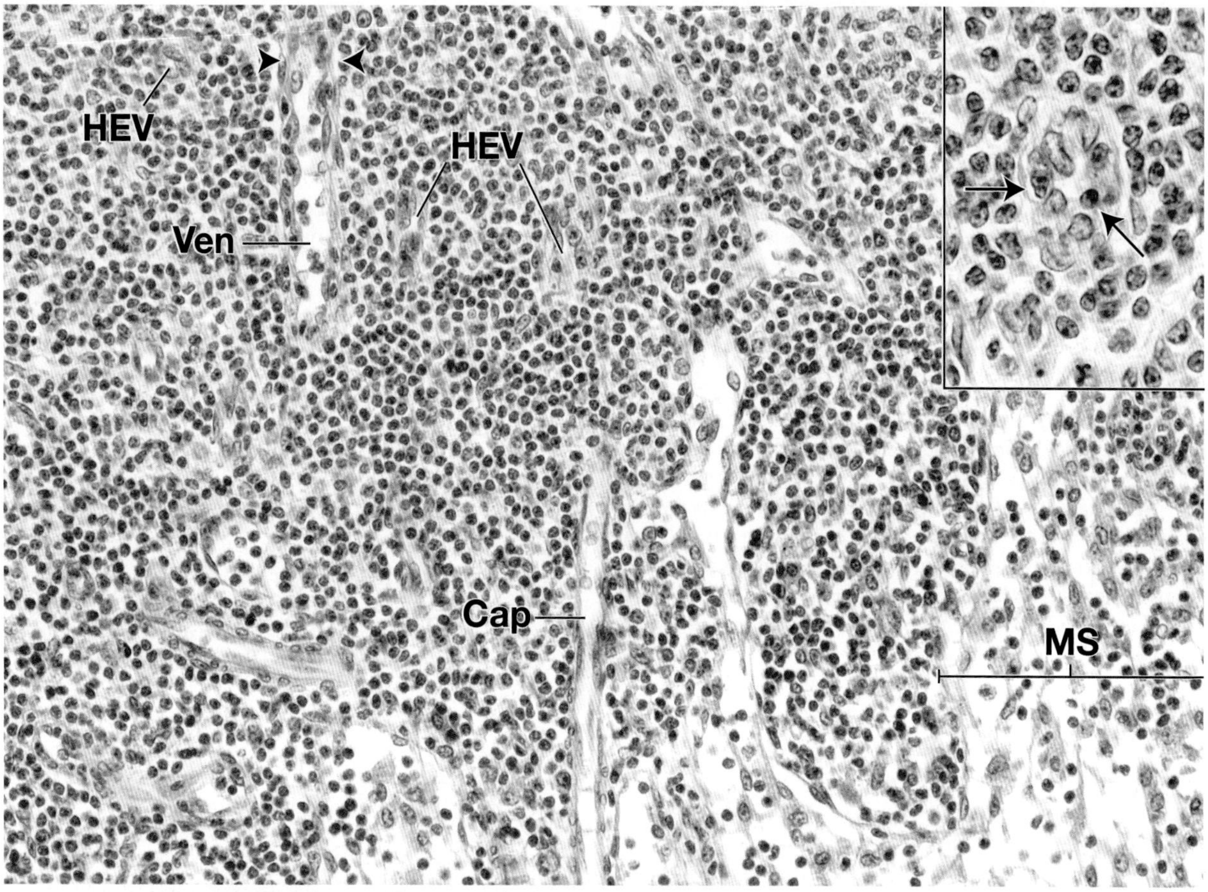
HEV
HEV
Ven
Cap
MS

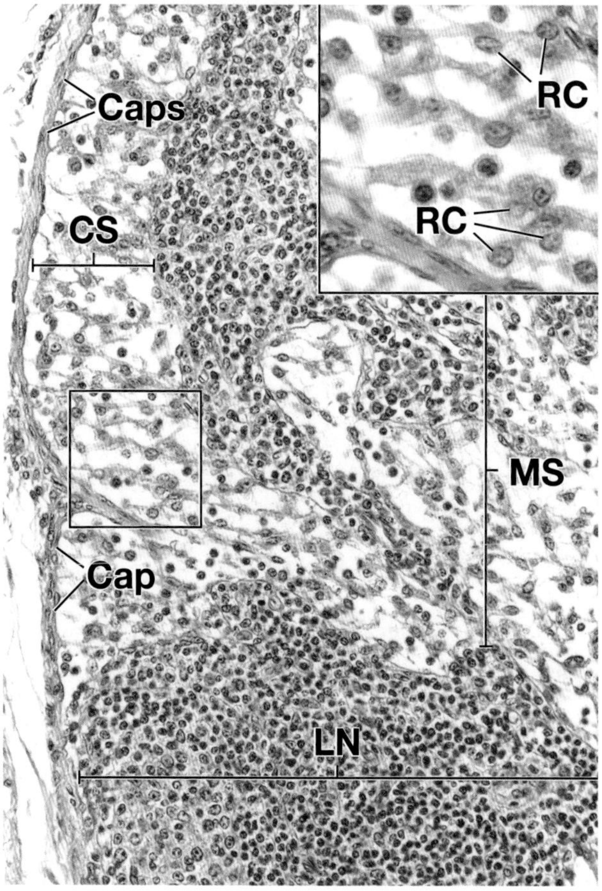
Caps
CS
RC
RC
MS
Cap
LN

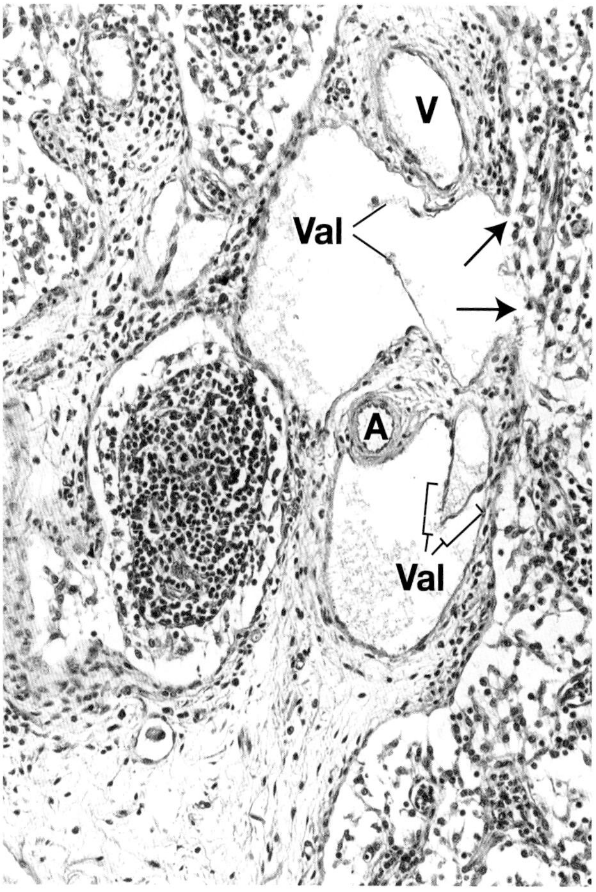
V
Val
A
Val

PLATE 14.4 ■ SPLEEN I

The **spleen** is the largest lymphatic organ; it is surrounded by a capsule and located in the path of the bloodstream (splenic artery and vein). The spleen filters the blood and reacts immunologically to blood-borne antigens. It has both morphologic and immunologic filtering functions. The substance of the spleen, the splenic pulp, consists of **red pulp** and **white pulp**, so named because of their appearance in fresh tissue. The white pulp is rich in lymphocytes that form a **periarterial lymphatic sheath (PALS)** around branches of the splenic artery that penetrate the white pulp. The red pulp contains large numbers of red blood cells that it filters and degrades. Aged, damaged, or abnormal red blood cells are trapped by macrophages associated with unusual vascular sinuses in the red pulp. These macrophages break down the red cells, begin the metabolic breakdown of hemoglobin, and retrieve and store the iron from the heme for reutilization in the formation of new red blood cells in the bone marrow.

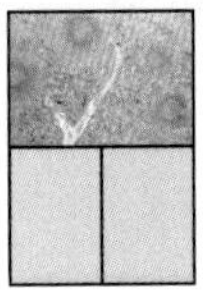

Spleen, human, hematoxylin and eosin (H&E) ×65.

This low-magnification micrograph of the spleen reveals its two major components, the **red pulp** (*RP*) and **white pulp** (*WP*). In the *center* of the figure, there is a trabecula containing a blood vessel, a trabecular vein (*TV*) through which blood leaves the organ. The red pulp constitutes the greater bulk of the splenic tissue. In life, the red pulp has pulp-like texture; it is red as a result of the natural coloration of the numerous red blood cells present, hence its name.

The white pulp, on the other hand, is so named because its content of lymphocytes appears in life as whitish areas. In tissue sections, however, the nuclei of the closely packed lymphocytes impart an overall blue-staining response. The lymphatic tissue that constitutes the white pulp differs from nodules seen elsewhere in that it follows and ensheathes a blood vessel, the central artery. The lymphatic tissue surrounding the artery exhibits periodic expansion, thus forming the nodules. When this occurs, the **central artery** (*CA*) is displaced peripherally within the nodule.

In those regions where the lymphatic tissue is not in nodular form, it is present as a thin cuff around the central artery and is referred to as the *periarterial lymphatic sheath*. If the plane of section does not include the artery, the sheath may appear only as a localized and irregular aggregation of lymphocytes.

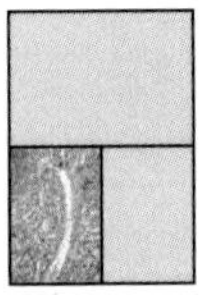

Red pulp, spleen, human, H&E ×160.

This figure reveals, at a higher magnification, the **red pulp** and a portion of the trabecular vein from the area enclosed in the *uppermost rectangle* in the *top* figure. The red pulp is composed of two elements: **venous sinuses** (*VS*) and the **splenic cords** (of Billroth), the tissue that lies between the sinuses. In this specimen, the venous sinuses can be seen to have advantages because the red blood cells in the sinuses have lysed and appear as unstained "ghosts"; only the nuclei of the white cells are readily seen. (This is better seen in Plate 14.5, page 534.) The paler, unstained areas thus represent the sinus lumina.

Near the *top* of the micrograph, two venous sinuses (*arrows*) empty into the trabecular vein (*TV*), thus showing the continuity between venous sinuses and the trabecular veins. The wall of the vein is thin, but the trabecula (*T*) containing the vessel gives the appearance of being part of the vessel wall. In humans as well as in other mammals, the capsule and the trabeculae that extend from the capsule contain myofibroblasts. Under conditions of increasing physical stress, contraction of these cells will occur and cause rapid expulsion of blood from the venous sinuses into the trabecular veins and thus into the general circulation. Note the small area of white pulp in the *upper right* portion of this image with labeled marginal zone (*MZ*) that separates white pulp and red pulp. This zone is not well defined in humans.

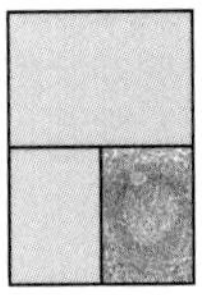

White pulp, spleen, human, H&E ×240.

This figure reveals, at higher magnification, the **splenic nodule** in the *rectangle* in the *right* portion of the previous figure. Present are a **germinal center** (*GC*) and a cross section through the thick-walled **central artery** (*CA*). As noted earlier, the central artery is eccentrically placed in the nodule. The marginal zone (*MZ*) is not well defined in humans, but it is assumed to be in the area that separates white pulp and red pulp (*RP*). Small arterial vessels and capillaries, branches of the central artery, supply the white pulp, and some pass into the reticular network terminating in a funnel-shaped orifice. The details of the vascular supply are, at best, difficult to resolve in typical H&E preparations. The penicillar arterioles, the terminal branches of the central artery, supply the red pulp but are likewise difficult to resolve.

CA, central artery
GC, germinal center
MZ, marginal zone
RP, red pulp
T, trabecular
TV, trabecular vein
VS, venous sinus
WP, white pulp
arrows, venous sinuses emptying into the trabecular vein

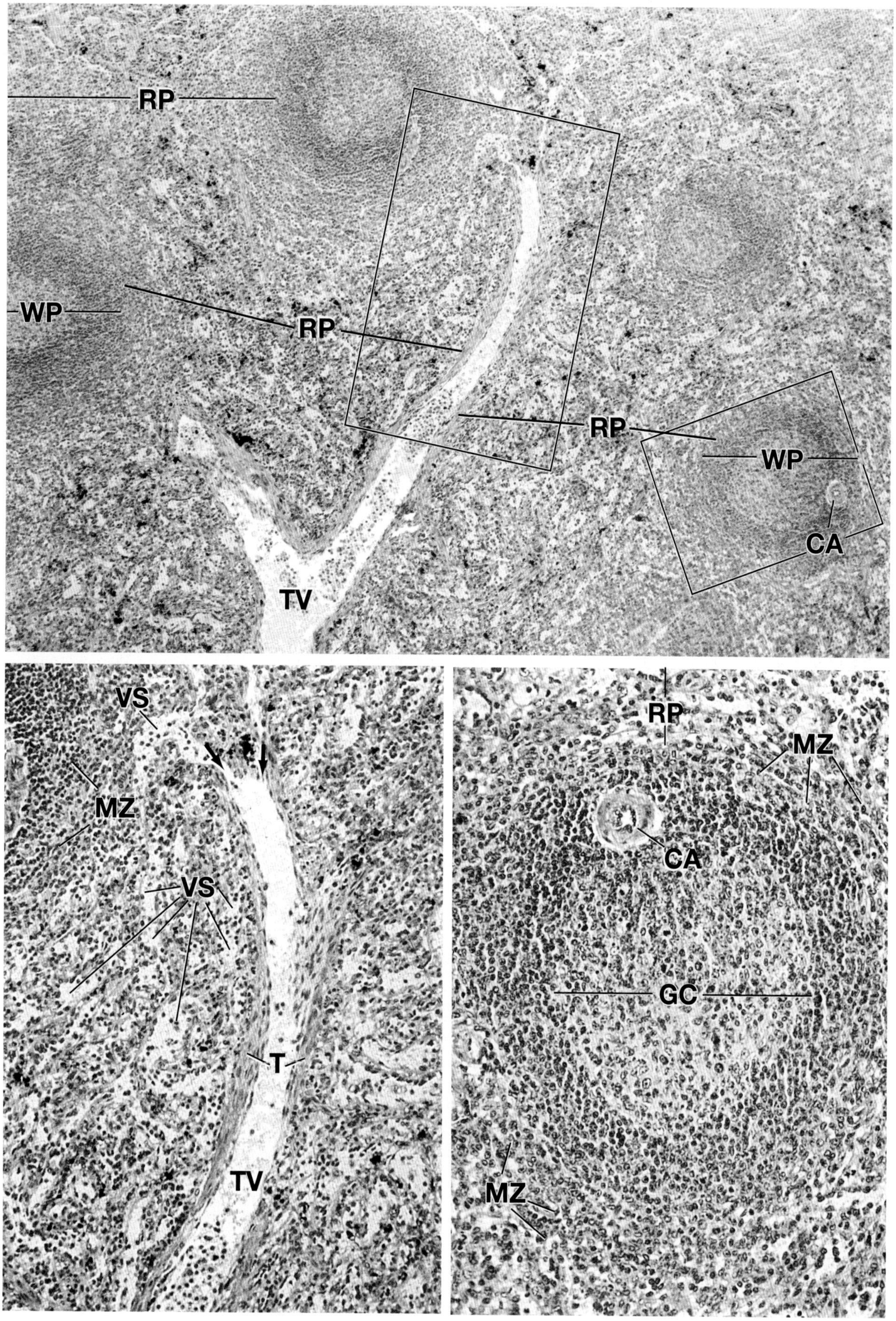
RP
WP
RP
RP
WP
CA
TV
VS
MZ
VS
T
TV
RP
MZ
CA
GC
MZ

PLATE 14.5 ■ SPLEEN II

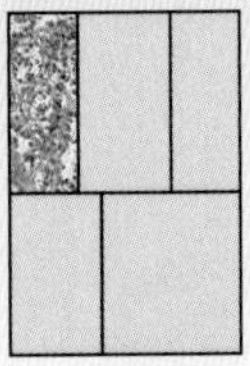

Red pulp, spleen, human, hematoxylin and eosin (H&E) ×360.

As previously noted, the **red pulp** consists of the **venous sinuses** (*VS*) and the area between the venous sinuses, the **splenic cords** (of Billroth) (*SC*). In this specimen, the red blood cells have been lysed, leaving only a clear outline of the individual cells. Thus, the relatively clear spaces with scattered nuclei represent the lumen of the venous sinus; the nuclei are those of white blood cells. When the wall of a venous sinus is tangentially sectioned (*VW*), as in this figure, the endothelial cells, which are rod like in shape, appear as a series of thin, linear bodies.

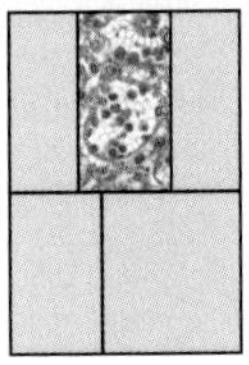

Red pulp, spleen, human, H&E ×1,200.

This micrograph is a high magnification of the area in the *rectangle* of the previous micrograph. The **venous sinus** in the *center* of the micrograph has been cut in cross section. Other than the lysed red blood cells, which appear as empty circular profiles, a number of lymphocytes (*Ly*) are present in the lumen. The wall of the sinus as seen here consists of rod-like endothelial cells (*EC*) that have been cut in cross section. A narrow but clearly visible intercellular space is present between adjacent cells. These spaces allow blood cells to pass readily into and out of the sinuses. Also, processes of macrophages located outside the sinuses in the splenic cords extend between the endothelial cells and into the lumen of the sinuses to monitor the passing blood for foreign antigens. The endothelial cell nuclei (*ECN*) project into the lumen of the vessel and appear to be sitting on top of the cell. A macrophage (*M*), identified by residual bodies in its cytoplasm, is seen just outside the sinus.

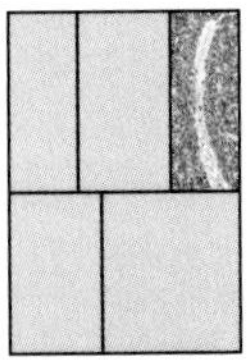

Spleen, human, H&E ×160.

This figure shows a **trabecular vein** (*TV*) and surrounding red pulp. At the *top* of the micrograph, two venous sinuses (*arrows*) can be seen emptying into the trabecular vein. These small trabecular veins converge into larger veins, which eventually unite giving rise to the splenic vein.

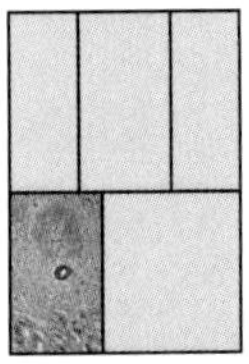

Spleen, human, silver preparation ×128.

This micrograph shows a **splenic nodule** (*SN*) occupying the *upper portion* of the micrograph and below red pulp (*RP*). The components that can be identified are a germinal center (*GC*), a central artery (*CA*), and venous sinuses (*VS*) in the red pulp. The structural elements that are stained by the silver in the nodule consist of reticular fibers. Note their paucity within the germinal center. The fine, thread-like stained material that encircles the venous sinuses is a usual modification of basement membrane.

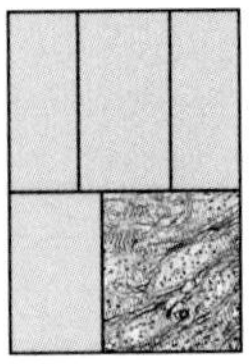

Venous sinuses, spleen, human, silver preparation ×515.

This micrograph reveals several **venous sinuses** (*VS*). Where the vessel wall has been tangentially sectioned, the **basement membrane** appears as a ladder-like structure (*BM*). Where the vessel has been cut deeper along its long axis, the basement membrane appears as dot-like structures (*arrowheads*). A three-dimensional reconstruction of the basement membrane would reveal it as a series of ring-like structures.

BM, basement membrane
CA, central artery
EC, rod-like endothelial cells
ECN, endothelial cell nuclei
GC, germinal center
Ly, lymphocytes
M, macrophage
RP, red pulp
SC, splenic cords
SN, splenic nodule
TV, trabecular vein
VS, venous sinuses
VW, venous sinus wall

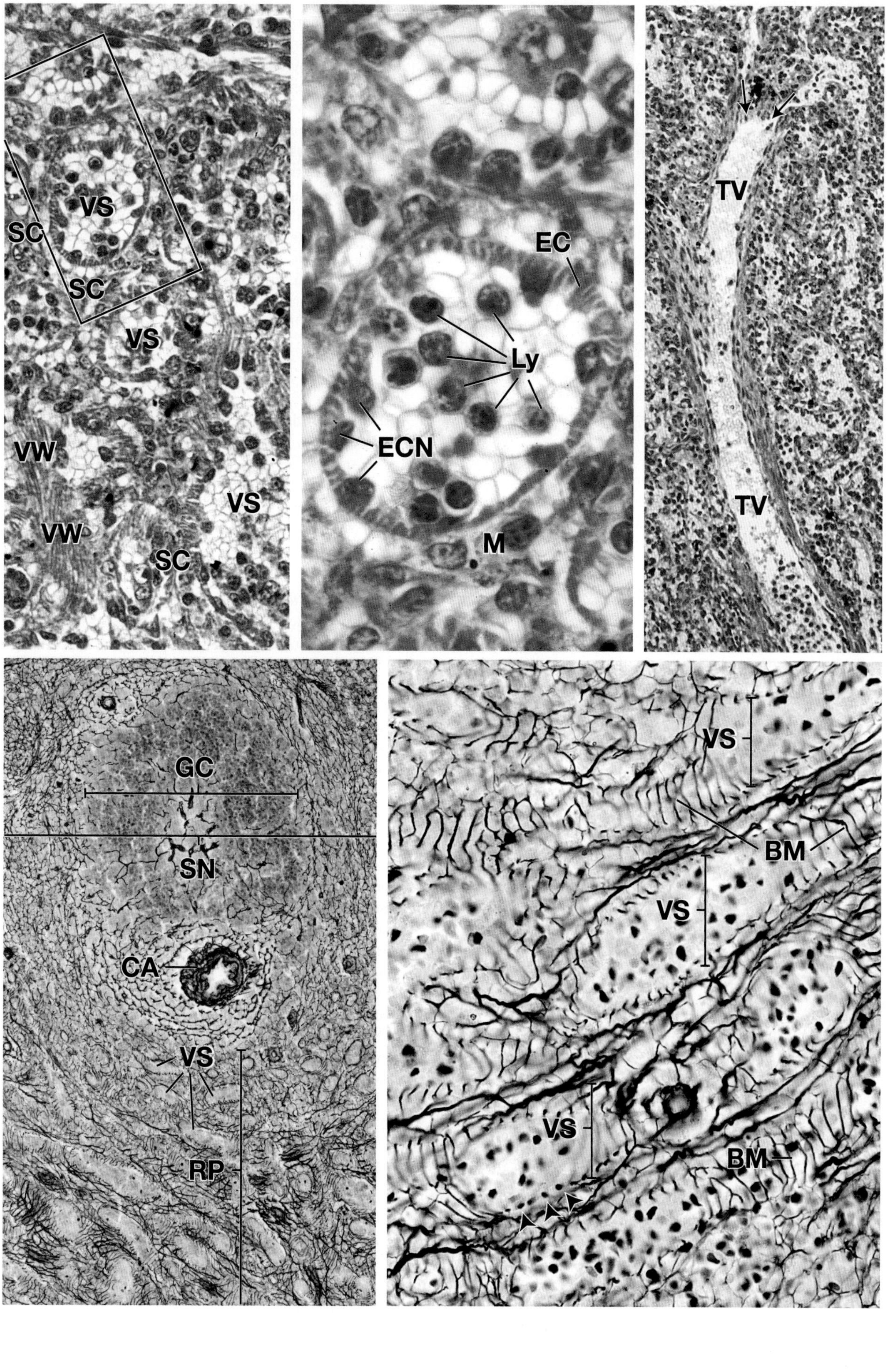
VS
SC
SC
VS
VW
VW
VS
SC
EC
Ly
ECN
M
TV
TV
GC
SN
CA
VS
RP
VS
BM
VS
VS
BM

PLATE 14.6 ■ THYMUS

The **thymus** is a lymphatic organ that exhibits certain unique structural features. The supporting **reticular stroma** arises from endodermal epithelium and produces a cellular reticulum. There are no reticular fibers associated with these cells; instead, the cells, designated **epithelioreticular cells**, serve as the stroma. Lymphocytes come to lie in the interstices of the cellular reticulum, and these two cellular elements, the lymphocytes and the epithelioreticular cells, comprise the bulk of the organ. The stem lymphocytes that migrate into the endodermal rudiment in the embryo derive from the yolk sac and later from the red bone marrow. These lymphocytes proliferate and become immunologically competent in the thymus, differentiating into the **thymus-dependent lymphocytes** (i.e., T lymphocytes). Some of these lymphocytes migrate to other tissues to populate the thymus-dependent portions of lymph nodes and spleen as well as to reside in the loose connective tissue. Many lymphocytes die or are destroyed in the thymus because in the random process by which they acquire the ability to recognize and react to antigens, they become programmed against "self" antigens. Numerous macrophages are present to phagocytize these destroyed lymphocytes. A **blood–thymus barrier** is formed by the sheathing of the perivascular connective tissue of the thymus by the epithelioreticular cells. In addition, there are no afferent lymphatic vessels to the thymus. Thus, it cannot react to circulating antigens. The thymus involutes during adolescence and is often difficult to recognize in the adult.

A connective tissue **capsule** (*Cap*) surrounds each lobe of the two lobes of the thymus and sends trabeculae (*T*) into the parenchyma to form lobules. The lobules are not completely separate units; rather, they interconnect because of the discontinuous nature of the trabeculae.

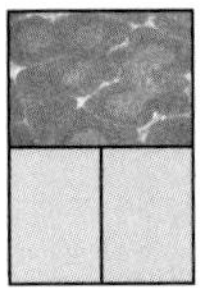

Thymus, human, hematoxylin and eosin (H&E) ×40.

Examination of the thymus at low magnification reveals the lobules (*L*) composed of a dark-staining basophilic **cortex** (*C*) and a lighter staining and relatively eosinophilic **medulla** (*M*). The cortex contains numerous densely packed lymphocytes, whereas the medulla contains fewer lymphocytes and is consequently less densely packed. A connective tissue capsule of the thymus sends trabeculae (*T*) into the parenchyma of the gland to form lobules. However, trabeculae do not completely separate lobules owing to their discontinuous nature.

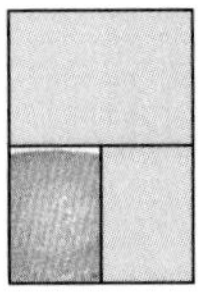

Thymus, human, H&E ×140.

It is the relative difference in the lymphocyte population (per unit area) and, in particular, the staining of their nuclei with hematoxylin that creates the difference in appearance between **cortex** (*C*) and **medulla** (*M*). Note that some of the medullary areas bear a resemblance to germinal centers of other lymphatic organs because of the medulla appearing as isolated circular areas (*upper left of top figure*). The medullary component, however, is actually a continuous branching mass surrounded by cortical tissue. Thus, the "isolated" medullary profiles are actually united with one another, although not within the plane of section. A suggestion of such continuity can be seen on the *right in the top figure* where the medulla appears to extend across several lobules.

The main cellular constituents of the thymus are lymphocytes (thymocytes), with characteristic small, round, dark-staining nuclei, and epithelioreticular supporting cells, with large pale-staining nuclei. Both of the cell types can be distinguished in the figure on the *right*, which provides a high-magnification view of the medulla. Because there are fewer lymphocytes in the medulla, it is the area of choice to examine the epithelioreticular cells. The thymus also contains macrophages; however, they are difficult to distinguish from the epithelioreticular cells.

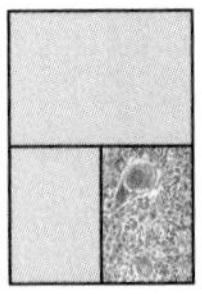

Medulla, thymus, human, H&E ×600.

The medulla usually possesses varying numbers of circular bodies called **Hassall corpuscles**, or **thymic, corpuscles** (*HC*). In addition to type IV and type V of **epithelioreticular cells** (*Ep*) that serve as a reticular stroma of the medulla, the Hassall corpuscles contain large concentric layers of flattened type VI **epithelioreticular cells** (*arrowheads*). They stain readily with eosin and can be distinguished easily with low magnification, as in the *top figure* and *lower left* (*arrows*). The center of a corpuscle, particularly a large one, may show evidence of keratinization and appear somewhat amorphous. Note a blood vessel (*BV*) in the medulla that is surrounded by lymphocytes.

The thymus gland remains as a large structure until the time of puberty. At that time, regressive changes occur that result in a significant reduction in the amount of thymic tissue. The young thymus is highly cellular and contains a minimum of adipose tissue. On the other hand, in the older thymus, much adipose tissue is present between the lobules. With continued involution, adipose cells are found even within the thymic tissue itself. Occasional plasma cells may be present in the periphery of the thymic cortex of the involuting thymus gland.

BV, blood vessels
C, cortex
Cap, capsule
Ep, epithelioreticular cells
HC, Hassall corpuscles
L, lobule
M, medulla
T, trabeculae
arrowheads, nuclei of type VI epithelioreticular cells of Hassall corpuscles
arrows, Hassall corpuscles

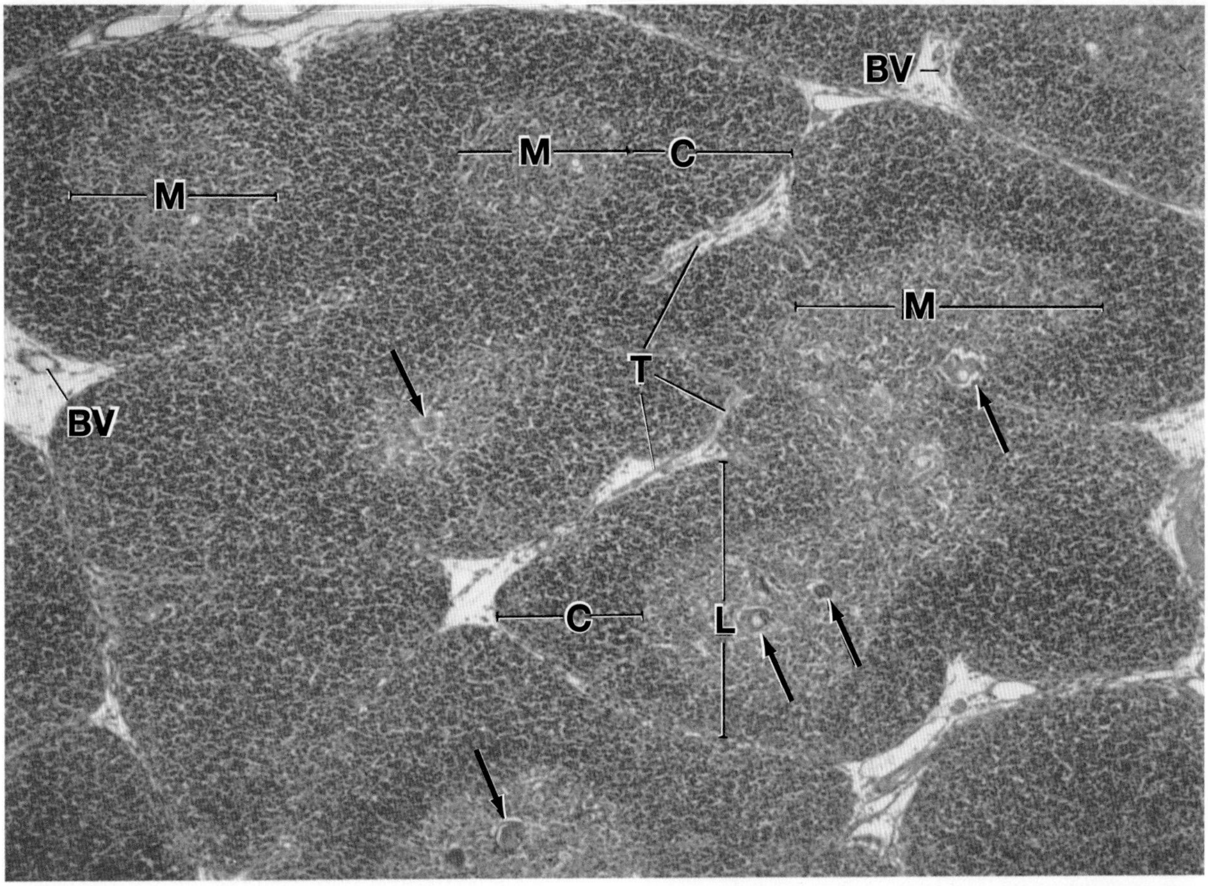
BV
M
C
M
M
T
BV
C
L

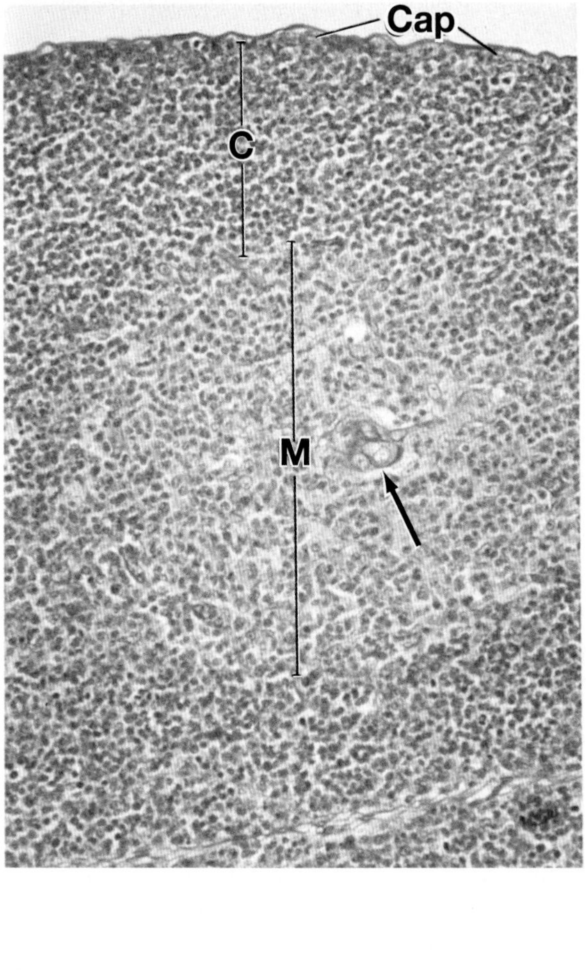
Cap
C
M

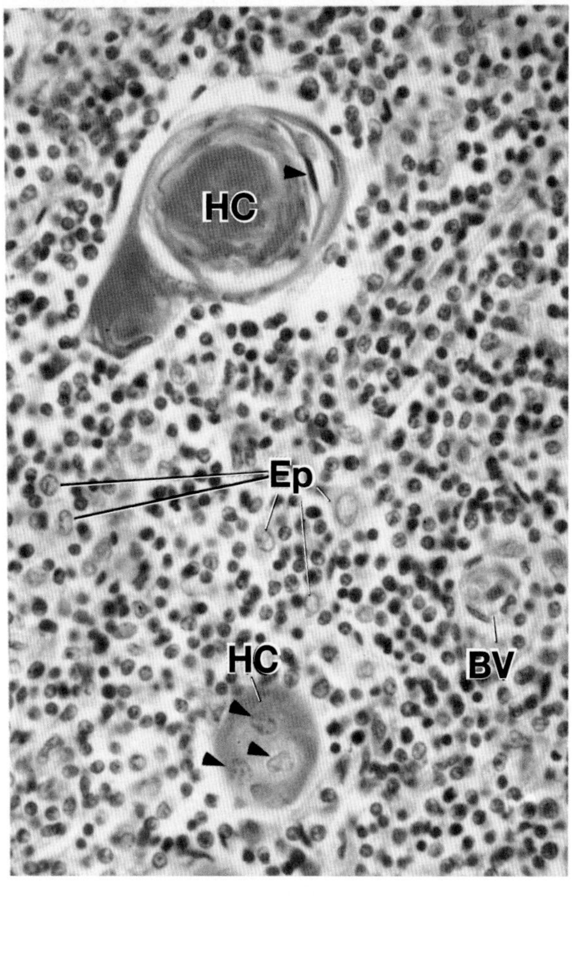
HC
Ep
HC
BV

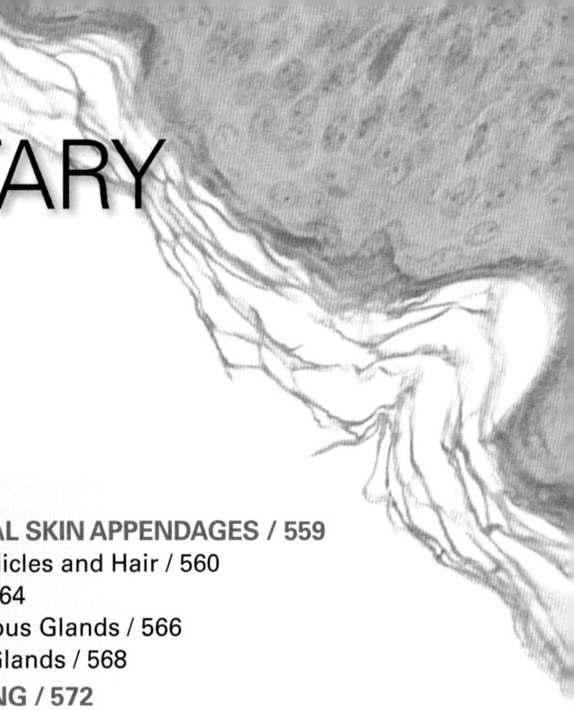

15 INTEGUMENTARY SYSTEM

■ OVERVIEW OF THE INTEGUMENTARY SYSTEM

The **skin (cutis, integument)** and its derivatives constitute the **integumentary system**. The skin forms the external covering of the body with an extensive surface area of approximately 1.8 m^2. It is also the largest organ of the body, constituting 15%–20% of its total body mass. The skin consists of two main layers:

- The **epidermis** is composed of a keratinized stratified squamous epithelium that grows continuously but maintains its normal thickness through desquamation. Epidermis is derived from ectoderm.
- The **dermis** is composed of a dense irregular connective tissue that imparts mechanical support, strength, and thickness to the skin. Dermis is derived from mesoderm.

The **hypodermis** contains variable amounts of adipose tissue arranged into lobules separated by connective tissue septa. It lies deep to the dermis and is equivalent to the **subcutaneous fascia** described in gross anatomy. The adipose tissue can be quite thick in well-nourished individuals and those living in cold climates.

The **epidermal derivatives of the skin** (epithelial skin appendages) include the following structures and integumentary products:

- **Hair follicles** and **hair**
- **Nails**
- **Sweat (sudoriferous) glands**
- **Sebaceous glands**
- **Mammary glands**

The integumentary system performs essential functions related to its external surface location.

Skin and its derivatives constitute a complex organ composed of many different cell types. The diversity of these cells and their ability to work together provide many functions that allow the individual to cope with the external environment. Major functions of the skin include the following:

- It acts as a **barrier** that protects against physical, chemical, and biologic agents in the external environment (i.e., mechanical barrier, permeability barrier, ultraviolet [UV] barrier).
- It provides **immunologic information** obtained during antigen processing to the appropriate effector cells in the lymphatic tissue.
- It participates in **homeostasis** by regulating body temperature and water loss.
- It conveys **sensory information** about the external environment to the nervous system.
- It performs **endocrine functions** by secreting hormones, cytokines, and growth factors and converting precursor molecules into hormonally active molecules (vitamin D_3).
- It functions in **excretion** through the exocrine secretion of sweat, sebaceous, and apocrine glands.

In addition, certain lipid-soluble substances may be absorbed through the skin. Although not a function of skin, this property is frequently used to deliver therapeutic agents. For example, nicotine, steroid hormones, and seasickness medications are frequently delivered through the skin in the form of patches, sprays, creams, or gels. To reduce **nicotine withdrawal symptoms** during smoking cessation, nicotine patches are often used to provide a small, constant dose of nicotine without the dangerous effects of tobacco smoke.

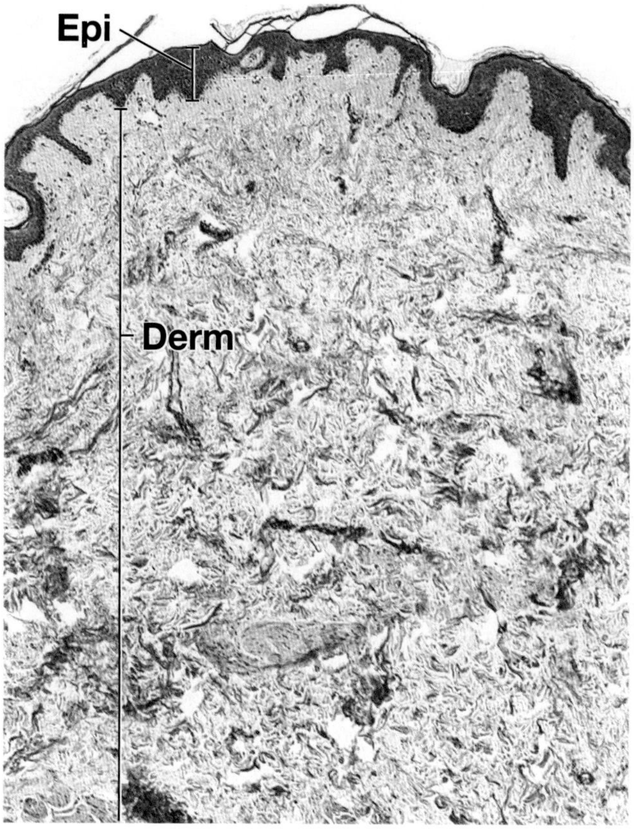

FIGURE 15.1. Photomicrograph showing the layers of thin skin. This hematoxylin and eosin (H&E)-stained specimen from human skin shows the two chief layers of the skin—the epidermis (*Epi*) and dermis (*Derm*). The epidermis forms the surface; it consists of stratified squamous epithelium that is keratinized. The dermis consists of two layers: the papillary layer, which is the most superficial layer and is adjacent to the epidermis, and the more deeply positioned reticular layer. The boundary between these two layers is not conspicuous; the papillary layer is, however, more cellular than the reticular layer. In addition, the collagen fibers of the reticular layer are thick (clearly visible in the *lower part* of the figure); those of the papillary layer are thin. ×45.

■ SKIN

Skin is categorized as thick or thin, reflecting its thickness and location.

The thickness of the skin varies over the surface of the body, from less than 1 mm to more than 5 mm. However, the skin is grossly and histologically different at two locations: the palms of the hands and the soles of the feet. These areas are subject to the most abrasion, are hairless, and have a much thicker epidermal layer than skin in any other location. This hairless skin is referred to as **thick skin**. Elsewhere, the skin possesses a much thinner epidermis and is called **thin skin**. It contains hair follicles in all but a few locations.

The histologic terms thick skin and thin skin are misnomers and refer only to **the thickness of the epidermal layer**. Anatomically, the thickest skin is found on the upper back, where the dermis is exceedingly thick. However, the epidermis of the upper back is comparable to that of thin skin found elsewhere on the body. In contrast, in certain other sites, such as the eyelid, the skin is extremely thin.

■ EPIDERMIS

Layers of the Epidermis

The **epidermis** is composed of stratified squamous epithelium in which four distinct layers can be identified. In the case of thick skin, a fifth layer is observed (Figs. 15.1 and 15.2). Beginning with the deepest layer, these layers are as follows:

- **Stratum basale**, also called the **stratum germinativum** because of the presence of mitotically active cells, the stem cells of the epidermis
- **Stratum spinosum**, also called the **spinous layer** or **prickle cell layer** because of the characteristic light microscopic appearance of short processes extending from cell to cell
- **Stratum granulosum**, which contains numerous intensely staining granules
- **Stratum lucidum**, which is limited to thick skin and considered a subdivision of the stratum corneum
- **Stratum corneum**, which is composed of keratinized cells

Differentiation of epithelial cells constitutes a specialized form of apoptosis.

Terminal differentiation of the epidermal cells, which begins with the cell divisions in the stratum basale, is considered a specialized form of apoptosis. Cells in the stratum granulosum exhibit typical apoptotic nuclear morphology, including fragmentation of their DNA. However, the cellular fragmentation associated with normal apoptosis does not occur; instead, the cells become filled with filaments of the intracellular protein **keratin** and are later sloughed from the skin surface.

The stratum basale provides for epidermal cell renewal.

The **stratum basale** is represented by a single layer of cells that rests on the basal lamina (Plate 15.1, page 576). It contains the **stem cells** from which new cells, called

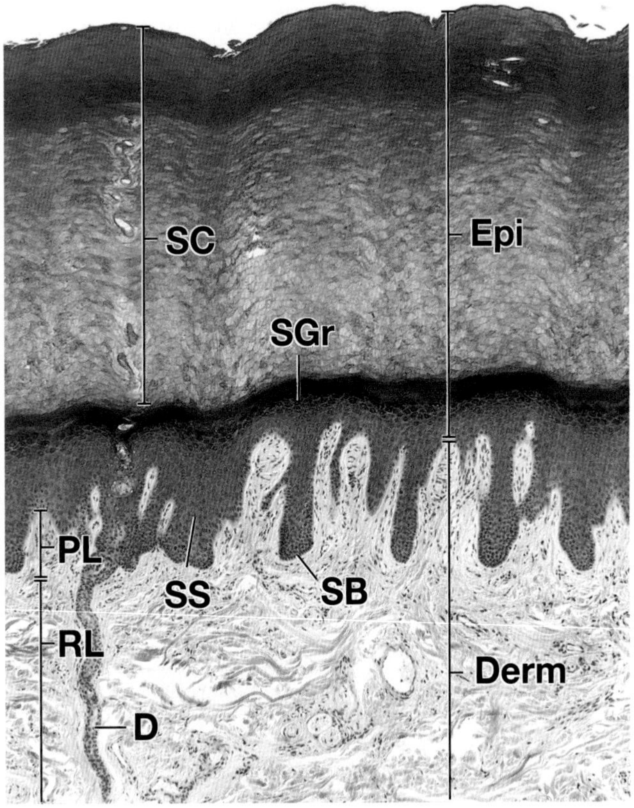

FIGURE 15.2. Photomicrograph showing the layers of thick skin. This specimen obtained from the skin of the sole of the foot (human) shows epidermis (*Epi*) containing the extremely thick stratum corneum (*SC*). Remaining layers of the epidermis (except for the stratum lucidum, which is not present on this slide)—the stratum basale (*SB*), the stratum spinosum (*SS*), and the stratum granulosum (*SGr*)—are clearly visible in this routine hematoxylin and eosin (H&E) preparation. The duct of a sweat gland (*D*) can be seen on the *left* as it traverses the dermis (*Derm*) and further spirals through the epidermis. At the sites where the ducts of the sweat gland enter the epidermis, note the epidermal downgrowths known as *interpapillary pegs.* The dermis contains papillae, protrusions of connective tissue that lie between the interpapillary pegs. Note also the greater cellularity of the papillary layer (*PL*) and that the collagen fibers of the reticular layer (*RL*) are thicker than those of the papillary layer. ×65.

keratinocytes, arise by mitotic division. For this reason, the stratum basale is also called the **stratum germinativum**. The cells are small and cuboidal to low columnar. They have less cytoplasm than the cells in the layer above; consequently, their nuclei are more closely spaced. The closely spaced nuclei, in combination with the basophilic cytoplasm of these cells, impart a noticeable basophilia to the stratum basale. Basal cells also contain various amounts of **melanin** (described later) in their cytoplasm that is transferred from neighboring melanocytes interspersed in this layer. Basal cells exhibit extensive cell junctions; they are connected to each other and to keratinocytes by desmosomes and to the underlying basal lamina by hemidesmosomes. As new keratinocytes arise in this layer by mitotic division, they move into the next layer, thus beginning their process of upward migration. This process terminates when the cell becomes a mature keratinized cell, which is eventually sloughed off at the skin surface.

The cells of the stratum spinosum characteristically exhibit spinous processes.

The **stratum spinosum** is at least several cells thick. **Keratinocytes** in this layer are larger than those of the stratum basale. They exhibit numerous **cytoplasmic processes** or spines, which gives this layer its name (Fig. 15.3 and Plate 15.1, page 576). The processes are attached to similar processes of adjacent cells by **desmosomes**. In the light microscope, the site of the desmosome appears as a slight thickening called the node of Bizzozero. The processes are usually conspicuous, in part because the cells shrink during preparation and a resultant expanded intercellular space develops between the spines. Because of their appearance, the cells that constitute this layer are often referred to as **prickle cells**. As the cells mature and move to the surface, they increase in size and become flattened in a plane parallel to the surface. This arrangement is particularly notable in the most superficial spinous cells, where the nuclei also become elongate instead of ovoid, matching the acquired squamous shape of the cells.

The cells of the stratum granulosum contain conspicuous keratohyalin granules.

The **stratum granulosum** is the most superficial layer of the nonkeratinized portion of the epidermis. This layer varies from one to three cells thick. **Keratinocytes** in this layer contain numerous **keratohyalin granules**, hence the name of the layer. These granules contain cystine-rich and histidine-rich proteins, which are the precursors of the protein **filaggrin**

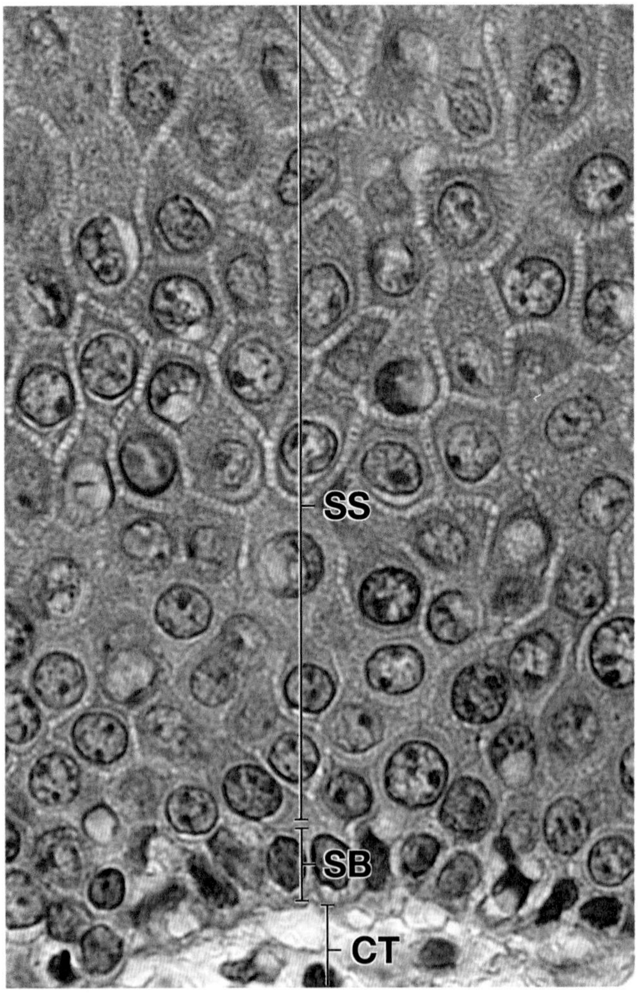

FIGURE 15.3. Photomicrograph of the stratum spinosum and stratum basale. The epidermis of thin skin is shown here at higher magnification. The one-cell-deep layer at the base of the epidermis just above the connective tissue (*CT*) of the dermis is the stratum basale (*SB*). The cells of this layer rest on the basement membrane. The *stratum spinosum* (*SS*) is located just above the stratum basale. It consists of cells with spinous processes on their surfaces. These processes are attached to spinous processes of neighboring cells by desmosomes and together appear as intercellular bridges. ×640.

(keratin **fil**ament **aggr**egating prote**in**), which aggregates the **keratin filaments** present within the cornified cells of the stratum corneum. Keratohyalin granules are irregular in shape and variable in size. Because of their intense basophilic staining, they are readily seen in routine histologic sections.

The stratum corneum consists of anucleate squamous cells largely filled with keratin filaments.

Usually, an abrupt transition occurs between the nucleated cells of the stratum granulosum and the flattened, desiccated, anucleate cells of the **stratum corneum**. The cells in the stratum corneum are the most differentiated cells in the skin. They lose their nucleus and cytoplasmic organelles and become filled almost entirely with keratin filaments. The thick plasma membrane of these cornified, keratinized cells is coated from the outside, in the deeper portion of this layer, with an extracellular layer of lipids that form the major constituent of the **water barrier** in the epidermis.

The stratum corneum is the layer that varies most in thickness, being thickest in thick skin. The thickness of this layer constitutes the principal difference between the epidermis of thick and thin skin. This cornified layer will become even thicker at sites subjected to unusual amounts of friction, as in the formation of calluses on the palms of the hands and the fingertips.

The **stratum lucidum**, considered a subdivision of the stratum corneum by some histologists, is normally only well seen in thick skin. In the light microscope, it often has a refractile appearance and may stain poorly. This highly refractile layer contains eosinophilic cells in which the process of keratinization is well advanced. The nucleus and cytoplasmic organelles become disrupted and disappear as the cell gradually fills with keratin.

■ CELLS OF THE EPIDERMIS

There are four different types of cells in the epidermis:

- **Keratinocytes** are highly specialized epithelial cells designed to perform a specific function: separating the organism from its external environment. They account for 85% of the cells in the epidermis.
- **Melanocytes** are the pigment-producing cells of the epidermis. They account for approximately 5% of the cells in the epidermis.
- **Langerhans cells** are antigen-presenting cells involved in signaling in the immune system. They account for approximately 2%–5% of the cells in the epidermis.
- **Merkel cells** are the sensitive mechanoreceptor cells associated with sensory nerve endings. They account for approximately 6%–10% of the cells in the epidermis.

Keratinocytes

The **keratinocyte** is the predominant cell type of the epidermis. These cells originate in the stratum basale of the epidermis. On leaving this layer, keratinocytes perform two essential activities:

- They produce **keratins (cytokeratins)**, major heteropolymeric structural proteins of the epidermis (see Table 2.3, page 74). Keratins form intermediate filaments; they constitute almost 85% of fully differentiated keratinocytes.
- They participate in the formation of the **epidermal water barrier**.

The keratinocytes in the basal layer contain numerous free ribosomes, scattered 7- to 9-nm intermediate (keratin) filaments, a small Golgi apparatus, mitochondria, and rough endoplasmic reticulum (rER). The cytoplasm of immature keratinocytes appears basophilic in histologic sections because of the large number of free ribosomes, most of which are engaged in synthesizing keratins, which will later be assembled into **keratin filaments**. These filaments are classified as intermediate filaments, although they are more commonly called **tonofilaments**.

As the cells enter and are moved through the stratum spinosum, the synthesis of keratin filaments continues, and the filaments become grouped into bundles sufficiently thick to be visualized in the light microscope. These bundles are called **tonofibrils**. The cytoplasm becomes eosinophilic because of the staining reaction of the tonofibrils that fill more and more of the cytoplasm.

Keratohyalin granules contain intermediate filament–associated proteins that aid in the aggregation of keratin filaments.

In the upper part of the stratum spinosum (Fig. 15.4), the free ribosomes within the keratinocytes begin synthesizing **keratohyalin granules** that become the distinctive feature of the cells in the stratum granulosum (Plate 15.1, page 576). Keratohyalin granules contain the two major intermediate filament–associated proteins: **filaggrin** and **trichohyalin**. The appearance of the granules and expression of filaggrin in keratinocytes are often used as a clinical marker for the initiation of the final stage of apoptosis. As the number of granules increases, their contents are released into the keratinocyte cytoplasm. Filaggrin and trichohyalin function as promoters in the aggregation of keratin filaments into tonofibrils, thus initiating the conversion of granular cells into cornified cells. This process is called **keratinization** and occurs in 2–6 hours, the time it takes for the cells to leave the stratum granulosum and enter the stratum corneum. The keratin fibril formed in this process is called **soft keratin** in contrast to the **hard keratin** of hair and nails (see later).

The transformation of a granular cell into a keratinized cell also involves breakdown of the nucleus and other organelles and thickening of the plasma membrane. This is accompanied by a change in pH, which decreases from approximately neutral (pH 7.17) in the stratum granulosum to acidic at the surface of the stratum corneum, ranging between pH 4.5 and 6.0.

Desquamation of surface keratinocytes from the stratum corneum is regulated by proteolytic degradation of the cells' desmosomes.

Cells are regularly exfoliated or desquamated from the surface of the stratum corneum. The **continuous exfoliation** of surface keratinocytes is a regulated proteolytic process that involves the degradation of the cells' desmosomes. The human **kallikrein-related serine peptidases**, such as **KLK5**, **KLK7**, and **KLK14**, cause cleavage of desmosomes in a pH-dependent manner. A physiologic serine protease inhibitor, **lymphoepithelial Kazal-type inhibitor (LEKTI)**, through its interactions with KLKs in neutral pH, prevents desmosomal cleavage. However, as pH decreases in more superficial portions of the stratum corneum as described, LEKTI progressively releases KLKs at the lower pH, thus allowing KLKs to degrade the desmosomes and cause keratinocyte release

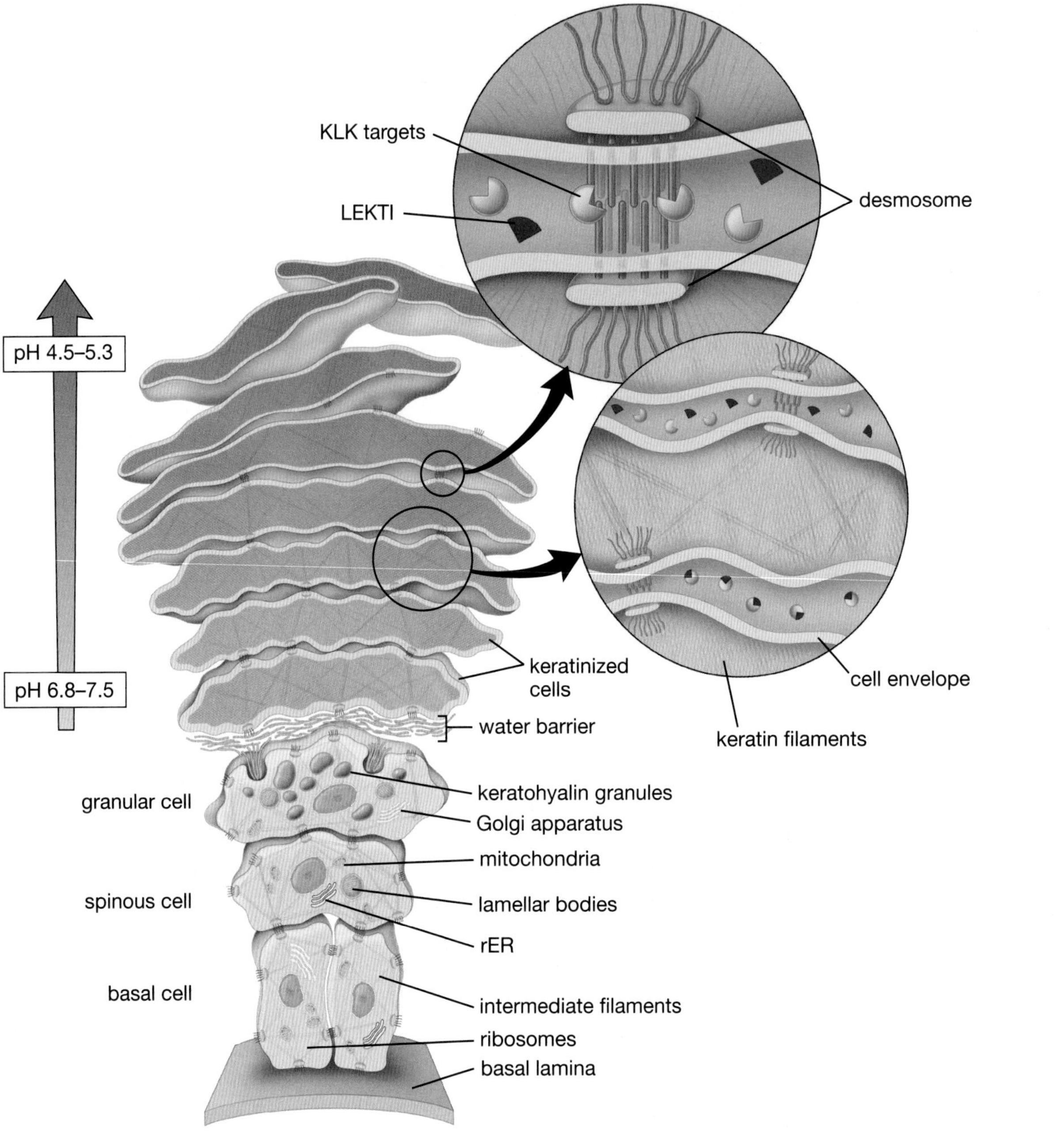

FIGURE 15.4. Schematic diagram of keratinocytes in the epidermis. The keratinocytes in this figure reflect different stages in the life cycle of the cell as it passes from the basal layer to the skin surface, where it becomes desquamated. The basal cell begins to synthesize intermediate (keratin) filaments; these are grouped into bundles and are seen in the light microscope as tonofibrils. The cell enters the spinous layer, where the synthesis of intermediate filaments continues. In the upper part of the spinous layer, the cells begin to produce keratohyalin granules containing intermediate filament–associated proteins and glycolipid-containing lamellar bodies. Within the granular layer, the cell discharges lamellar bodies that contribute to formation of the water barrier of the epidermis; the remainder of the cell cytoplasm contains numerous keratohyalin granules that, in close association with tonofilaments, form the cell envelope. The surface cells are keratinized; they contain a thick cell envelope and bundles of tonofilaments in a specialized matrix. Desquamation of keratinized cells is regulated by the activity of KLK and its interaction with LEKTI in desmosomes, which in turn is dependent on pH. Keratinocytes positioned near the granular layer exhibit neutral pH, which maintains desmosomal interactions and allows a strong interaction in the extracellular matrix between LEKTI and its KLK targets. As the pH acidifies toward the skin surface, LEKTI and KLK dissociate, releasing KLKs into the extracellular space. In the most superficial layers of keratinocytes, the pH is low enough for active KLK molecules to digest desmosomal proteins. In concert with other proteinase activities, this action leads to a complete degradation of desmosomal junctions, resulting in the detachment of the most superficial layer of keratinocytes. *rER*, rough-surfaced endoplasmic reticulum; *LEKTI*, lymphoepithelial Kazal-type inhibitor; *KLK*, kallikrein-related serine peptidase.

(see Fig. 15.4). Under normal conditions, the process allows a controlled renewal of the epidermis by means of its pH gradient. There are known pathogenic mutations in the gene called **serine protease inhibitor Kazal-type 5 (SPINK5)**, which encodes LEKTI. **Netherton syndrome**, a rare genetic disorder, is associated with a mutation in the SPINK5 gene. This syndrome is characterized by decreased skin barrier function, generalized redness of the skin (erythroderma), and scaling.

Lamellar bodies contribute to the formation of the intercellular epidermal water barrier.

An **epidermal water barrier** is essential for mammalian "dry" epithelia and is responsible for **maintaining body homeostasis.** The barrier is established primarily by two factors in terminally differentiating keratinocytes: (1) deposition of insoluble proteins on the inner surface of the plasma membrane and (2) a lipid layer that is attached to the outer surface of the plasma membrane.

As the keratinocytes in the stratum spinosum begin to produce keratohyalin granules, they also produce membrane-bounded **lamellar bodies (membrane-coating granules)**. They are tubular or ovoid-shaped membrane-bound organelles that are unique to the mammalian epidermis (Fig. 15.5). Spinous and granular cells synthesize a heterogeneous mixture of **probarrier lipids** and their respective **lipid-processing enzymes**, such as glycosphingolipids, phospholipids, ceramides, acid sphingomyelinase, and secretory phospholipase A2; this mixture is assembled into lamellar bodies in the Golgi apparatus (Fig. 15.6). In addition, lamellar bodies contain **proteases** (i.e., stratum corneum chymotryptic enzyme, cathepsin D, acid phosphatase, glycosidases, and protease inhibitors). The contents of the granules are then secreted by exocytosis into the intercellular spaces between the stratum granulosum and stratum corneum. The organization of these **intercellular lipid lamellae** is responsible for the formation of the **epidermal water barrier** (see Fig. 15.6). In addition to their major role in the formation of barrier homeostasis, lamellar bodies are also involved in the formation of the cornified envelope, desquamation of cornified cells, and antimicrobial defenses in the skin.

The **epidermal water barrier** thus consists of two structural elements:

- The **cell envelope (CE)** is a 15-nm-thick layer of insoluble proteins deposited on the inner surface of the plasma membrane that contributes to the strong mechanical properties of the barrier. The thickness of the CE increases in epithelia that are subject to considerable mechanical stress (e.g., lip, palm of the hand, sole of the foot). The CE is formed by cross-linking **small proline-rich (SPR) proteins** and larger structural proteins. The structural proteins include **cystatin, desmosomal proteins (desmoplakin), elafin, envoplakin, filaggrin, involucrin**, five different **keratin** chains, and **loricrin**. Loricrin is the major structural protein and accounts for almost 80% of the total CE protein mass. This 26-kDa insoluble protein has the highest glycine content of any known protein in the body.
- The **lipid envelope** is a 5-nm-thick layer of lipids attached to the cell surface by ester bonds. The major lipid components of the lipid envelope are **ceramides**, which belong to the class of sphingolipids, **cholesterol**, and **free fatty acids**. However, the most important component is the monomolecular layer of **acylglucosylceramide**, which provides a "Teflon-like" coating on the cell surface. Ceramides also play

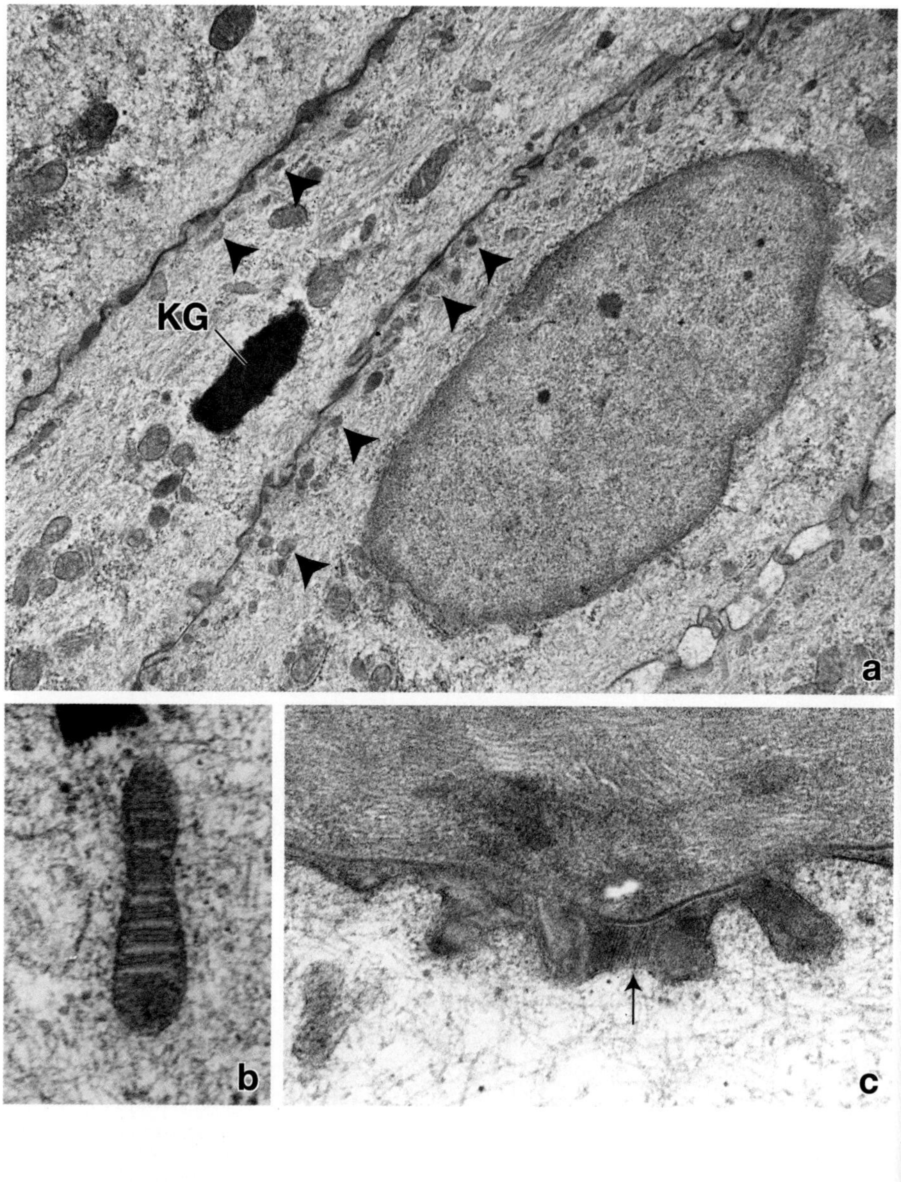

FIGURE 15.5. Electron micrographs of keratinocytes. a. Much of the keratinocyte cytoplasm is filled with tonofilaments. One keratinocyte exhibits a keratohyalin granule (*KG*). Near the plasma membrane closest to the surface (*upper left*), two keratinocytes display lamellar bodies (*arrowheads*). ×8,500. **b.** A lamellar body at higher magnification. ×135,000. **c.** Part of a keratinized cell and the underlying keratinocyte. Located between the cells are the contents of the lamellar bodies, which have been discharged into the intercellular space (*arrow*) to form the lipid envelope. ×90,000. (Courtesy of Dr. Albert I. Farbman.)

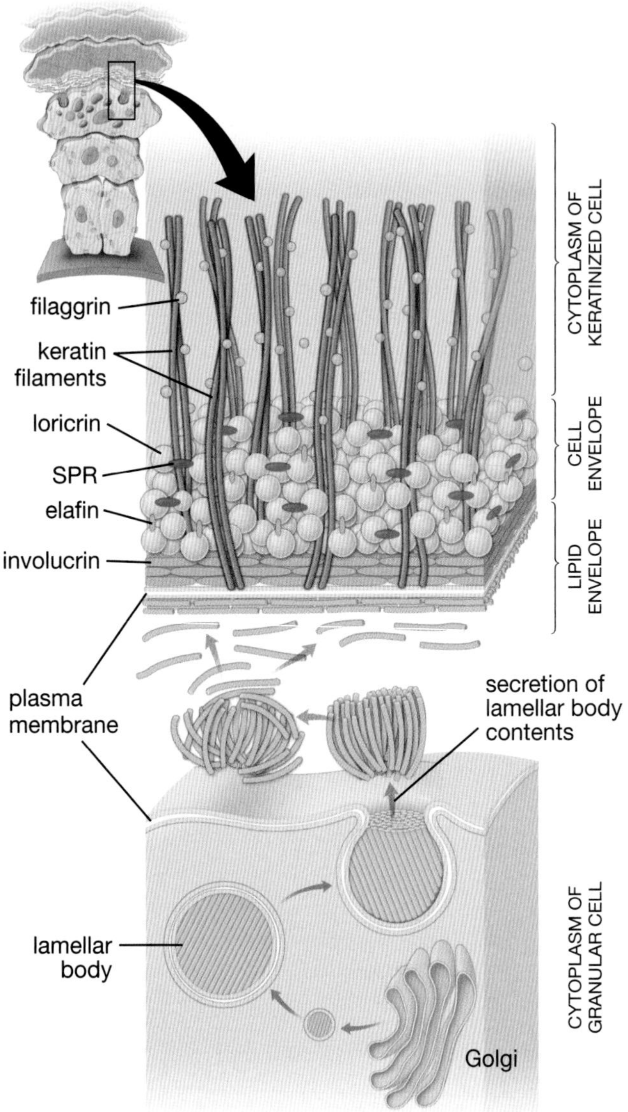

FIGURE 15.6. Schematic diagram of the epidermal water barrier. The heterogeneous mixture of glycosphingolipids, phospholipids, and ceramides makes up the lamellae of the lamellar bodies. The lamellar bodies, produced within the Golgi apparatus, are secreted by exocytosis into the intercellular spaces between the stratum granulosum and stratum corneum, where they form the lipid envelope. The lamellar arrangement of lipid molecules is depicted in the intercellular space just below the thickened plasma membrane and forms the cell envelope of the keratinized keratinocyte. The innermost part of the cell envelope consists primarily of loricrin molecules (*pink spheres*) that are cross-linked by small proline-rich (*SPR*) proteins and elafin. The layer adjacent to the cytoplasmic surface of the plasma membrane consists of the two tightly packed proteins involucrin and cystatin α. Keratin filaments (tonofilaments) bound by filaggrin are anchored into the cell envelope.

an important role in cell signaling and are partially responsible for inducing cell differentiation, triggering apoptosis, and reducing cell proliferation. As the cells continue to move toward the free surface, the barrier is constantly maintained by keratinocytes entering the process of terminal differentiation. Lamellae may remain as recognizable discs in the intercellular space or may fuse into broad sheets or layers.

Experiments have shown that the epidermis of animals with induced **essential fatty acid deficiency (EFAD)** is more permeable than normal to water. The membrane-coating granules also have fewer lamellae than normal. Destruction of the epidermal water barrier over large areas, as in **severe burns**, can lead to life-threatening loss of fluid from the body.

The epidermis is in a state of dynamic equilibrium in which exfoliated keratinized cells are constantly replaced by a steady flow of terminally differentiated cells.

Epidermal cell replacement is maintained by the following processes:

- Division of basal cells in the stratum basale
- Differentiation and programmed cell death as the cells move upward to the stratum corneum
- Cell loss by exfoliation from the skin surface

To maintain this equilibrium, each cell in the epidermis has a predetermined amount of time to perform specific functions. Several scientific experiments and empirical calculations have concluded that the turnover time for the keratinocyte compartment (stratum spinosum and granulosum) is about 31 days, with an additional 14 days for the stratum corneum (average thickness in humans, 16–20 cell layers). Adding 1–2 days for mitotic divisions in the stratum basale, total **epidermal turnover** takes approximately **47 days** (Fig. 15.7). One cell layer in the stratum corneum has been found to produce and exfoliate every 22.4 hours. In hyperproliferative diseases, such as **psoriasis**, the epidermal turnover time is accelerated and takes approximately 8–10 days. In this disorder, epidermal thickness increases, and the rate of cell death is reduced. Clinically, psoriasis appears as elevated, reddish patches of itchy skin, often covered by silvery-white scales. Patches vary in size and typically appear on knees, elbows, lower back, and scalp.

Melanocytes

Neural crest–derived melanocytes are scattered among the basal cells of the stratum basale.

During embryonic life, **melanocyte precursor cells** migrate from the neural crest and enter the developing epidermis. A specific functional association is then established—the **epidermal–melanin unit**—in which one melanocyte maintains an association with a given number of keratinocytes. In humans, each epidermal–melanin unit is estimated to contain one melanocyte associated with approximately 36 keratinocytes. The ratio of melanocytes to keratinocytes or their precursors in the stratum basale may vary from 1:4 to 1:40 or even higher, depending on the area of the body. This ratio is constant in all individuals but is influenced by age and environmental factors, such as exposure to sunlight.

In adults, a pool of undifferentiated melanocyte stem cells resides in the area of the hair follicle called the **follicular bulge**. Differentiation of the melanocyte stem cell is regulated by the expression of the **Pax3 gene** that belongs to the paired box (PAX) family of transcription factors. Pax3 activates the expression of the **microphthalmia-associated transcription factor (MITF)**, which is critical for the development and differentiation of melanocytes (melanogenesis). Melanocytes maintain the capacity to replicate throughout their life, although at a much slower rate than keratinocytes, thus maintaining cell ratio in the epidermal–melanin unit.

The epidermal **melanocyte** is a dendritic cell scattered among the basal cells of the stratum basale (Fig. 15.8). They are called dendritic cells because the rounded cell body resides in the basal layer and extends long processes between the keratinocytes of the stratum spinosum. Neither the processes nor the cell body forms desmosomal attachments

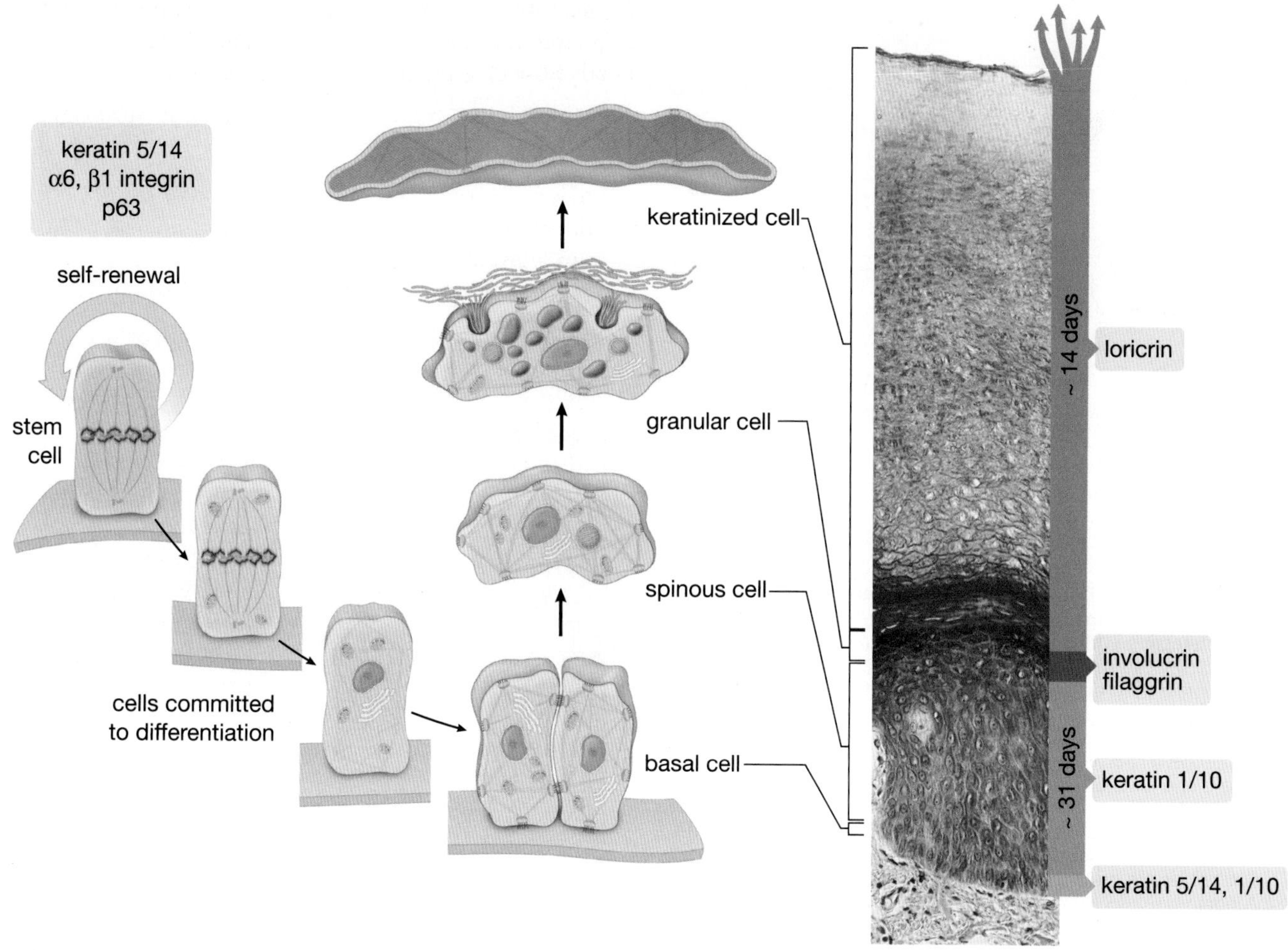

FIGURE 15.7. Schematic diagram of epidermal cell differentiation and replacement. Epidermal cell replacement is initiated by the division of stem cells in the stratum basale. Newly formed cells undergo additional divisions in the stratum basale and move upward as they differentiate into keratinized cells, which eventually are lost by exfoliation on the skin surface. To maintain this equilibrium between cell division and cell loss at the skin surface, each cell has a predetermined time to travel through specific compartments of the epidermis and to perform specific functions. Mitotic divisions in the stratum basale take about 1–2 days; after that, it takes an average of 31 days for keratinocytes to move through the stratum spinosum (spinous cells) and differentiate into granular cells in the stratum granulosum. It takes an additional 14 days for the keratinized cell to cross the stratum corneum (assuming an average thickness of 16–20 cells in humans). Therefore, the total epidermal turnover time is approximately 47 days. At each stage of differentiation, cells express different molecular markers (see *yellow boxes*), which can be useful in identifying specific cells using immunocytochemical methods. *Inset* on the *left* shows full-thickness section of the epidermis from a human fingertip stained with Mallory trichrome. ×260.

with neighboring keratinocytes. However, melanocytes that reside close to the basal lamina have structures that resemble hemidesmosomes. In routine hematoxylin and eosin (H&E) preparations, melanocytes are seen in the stratum basale with elongated nuclei surrounded by a clear cytoplasm. With the transmission electron microscope (TEM), however, they are readily identified by the presence of developing and mature melanin granules in the cytoplasm (see Fig. 15.8).

Melanocytes produce two forms of melanin pigment, a brownish-black eumelanin and a reddish-yellow pheomelanin.

Epidermal **melanocytes** produce and secrete two forms of **melanin** pigment, a brownish-black pigment called **eumelanin** and a reddish-yellow pigment called **pheomelanin**. The relative amounts of these two pigments are responsible for hair and skin color. The most important function of melanin is to protect the organism against the damaging effects of nonionizing UV irradiation. Individuals who produce more eumelanin than pheomelanin have brown or black hair and darker skin that is protected from damage caused by UV radiation in sunlight. In contrast, individuals who produce more pheomelanin than eumelanin have red or blond hair and lighter skin that is poorly protected from UV radiation. These individuals are at increased risk of skin damage caused by UV radiation.

Melanocytes produce melanin in membrane-bounded organelles called melanosomes.

Melanin production occurs in membrane-bounded, lysosome-related organelles called **melanosomes**, which are derived from the Golgi apparatus (Fig. 15.9). Melanin is produced by hydroxylation of the amino acid **L-tyrosine** to **L-3,4-dihydroxyphenylalanine (L-DOPA)** by the enzyme **tyrosinase**. The subsequent oxidation of L-DOPA produces the melanin precursor known as **L-DOPAquinone**. This compound undergoes further modification via two different pathways depending on the availability of the amino acid **cysteine**. With cysteine present in sufficient amounts, the L-DOPAquinone is gradually transformed into **pheomelanin** pigment. When cysteine is insufficient, L-DOPAquinone is spontaneously converted to **eumelanin** pigment. This conversion pathway requires the presence of tyrosinase-related protein 1 (TRP1) and tyrosinase-related protein 2 (TRP2), which are enzyme regulators in this process.

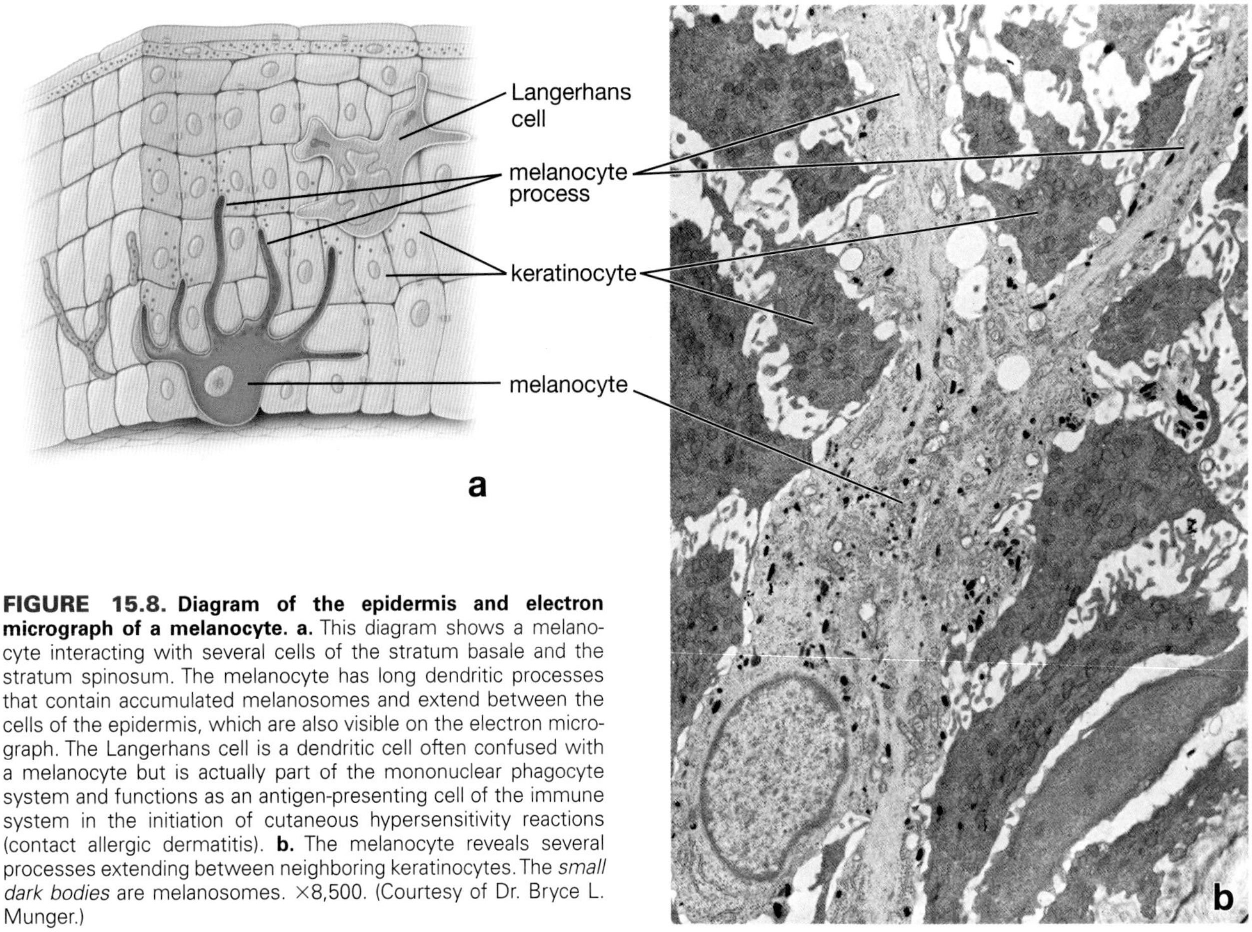

FIGURE 15.8. Diagram of the epidermis and electron micrograph of a melanocyte. a. This diagram shows a melanocyte interacting with several cells of the stratum basale and the stratum spinosum. The melanocyte has long dendritic processes that contain accumulated melanosomes and extend between the cells of the epidermis, which are also visible on the electron micrograph. The Langerhans cell is a dendritic cell often confused with a melanocyte but is actually part of the mononuclear phagocyte system and functions as an antigen-presenting cell of the immune system in the initiation of cutaneous hypersensitivity reactions (contact allergic dermatitis). **b.** The melanocyte reveals several processes extending between neighboring keratinocytes. The *small dark bodies* are melanosomes. ×8,500. (Courtesy of Dr. Bryce L. Munger.)

Melanosomes are formed through a series of well-defined stages.

There are four stages (I–IV) of melanosome development, starting with the premelanosome and ending with the mature melanosome. With each stage, their location within the cell shifts as more melanin accumulates. **Premelanosomes (stage I)** and **early melanosomes (stage II)** are concentrated near the Golgi apparatus and interact with the rER, smooth ER (sER), and mitochondria. **Nearly mature melanosomes (stage III)** are relocated using microtubule-dependent transport to the bases of the melanocyte processes. **Mature melanosomes (stage IV)** travel further toward the ends of the melanocyte processes (see Fig. 15.9).

- In **eumelanin**-producing melanocytes, the lumen of **premelanosomes (stage I)** lacks pigment. With the TEM, premelanosomes exhibit a finely ordered internal structure composed of proteinaceous fibrils. These fibrils are composed primarily of **premelanosome protein (PMEL17)** and become the core for melanin deposition within the melanosome. The assembly of this internal structure is usually completed in the **early melanosome (stage II)**, which confers an ellipsoid shape to the premelanosomes.
- In **pheomelanin-producing** melanocytes, PMEL17 expression is downregulated, which might explain why melanosomes in these cells lack internal fibrils and have spherical-shaped nucleosomes.

Production of the electron-opaque melanin granules begins when they acquire an elliptical shape at the end of stage II, and the process continues throughout **stages III and IV**. During the last two stages, the internal structure of melanosomes becomes obscured. The mature organelles **(stage IV)** filled with melanin granules are transported to the tips of the melanocyte processes for transfer into keratinocytes.

During development, melanosomes share several features with lysosomes, such as a **lower pH** necessary for melanin synthesis and the presence of lysosomal membrane proteins and lysosomal hydrolases. **Melanosomal pH** is an important factor in the regulation of skin pigmentation. Melanosomes derived from melanocytes in light skin are more acidic and have lower tyrosinase activity than melanosomes in dark skin, which have a more neutral pH and higher tyrosinase activity. Therefore, **tyrosinase activity** is increased in dark skin without upregulation of tyrosinase gene expression.

Melanocytes distribute melanin to keratinocytes in the process of pigment donation.

The melanin transfer mechanism called **pigment donation** between pigment-producing melanocytes and pigment-recipient keratinocytes is critical in determining skin color. Its molecular mechanism remains unclear; however, the classical description of pigment donation based on **phagocytosis of the tips of the melanocyte processes** by keratinocytes is the most accepted. This model has been confirmed by TEM observation of cells cultured in vitro. In this model, a keratinocyte engulfs the tip of a melanocyte process, pinching it off to form a melanosome-filled cytoplasmic vesicle. A small amount of cytoplasm surrounding the melanosome is also phagocytosed, which characterizes this process as a type of **cytocrine secretion**. Other recent models of pigment donation include: direct membrane fusion between melanocytes and keratinocytes with melanosome transfer; phagocytosis of membrane-bound vesicles by keratinocytes containing melanosomes originating from the melanocyte cytoplasmic blebs; and exocytosis of melanin pigment by melanocytes and subsequent endocytosis by keratinocytes.

After pigment transfer, most melanosomes in light skin reside in keratinocytes near the basal layer of the epidermis (60%–80% of total melanosomes); however, in dark skin, distribution of melanosomes is equal throughout all layers of the epidermis. Melanosomes in keratinocytes are generally positioned around and above the nucleus, forming an umbrella-like structure called the "**dark umbrella**" or **melanosome microparasol**, which protects nuclear DNA against harmful UV radiation (Fig. 15.10).

Melanin production is genetically determined and highly regulated by many factors.

More than 125 genes regulate melanocyte differentiation, survival, synthesis, and function. In humans, approximately 15 genes have been associated with variations in skin pigmentation. Variations in the **melanocortin 1 receptor (MC1R) gene**, the key gene in human pigmentation, appear to be associated with normal differences in skin and hair color.

The critical enzymes in melanin synthesis are **tyrosinase**, **TRP1**, and **TRP2**, which dramatically affect the quality and quantity of melanin produced. Melanin synthesis is also regulated by **melanocyte-stimulating hormone (MSH)** produced by the anterior lobe of the pituitary gland. MSH binds to the **melanocortin 1 receptor (MC1R)** on melanocytes and affects tyrosinase activity through the G-protein signaling cascade. Stimulation of MC1R receptors

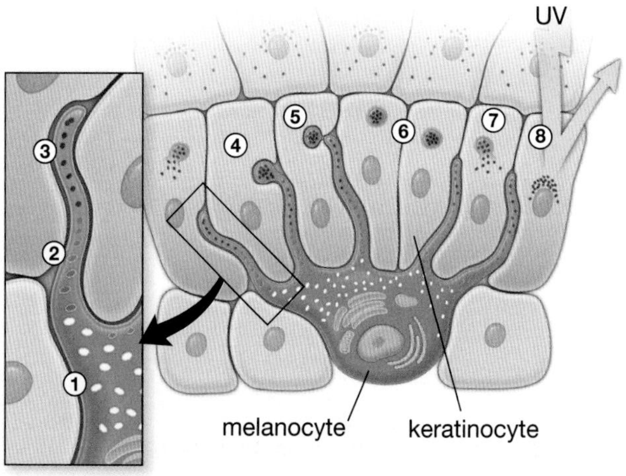

FIGURE 15.9. Formation of melanin and mechanism of pigment donation. Melanocytes produce lysosome-related membrane-bound structures that originate from the Golgi apparatus as premelanosomes **(1)** that are involved in melanin synthesis. Melanin is produced from tyrosine by a series of enzymatic reactions and its accumulation is visible in the melanosomes **(2)**. As maturation progresses, melanosomes travel toward the ends of the melanocyte processes. Mature melanosomes **(3)** have a high concentration of melanin and accumulate at the ends of melanocyte processes that invaginate into the keratinocyte's cell membrane **(4)**. Keratinocytes phagocytose the tips of the melanocyte processes containing the melanosomes **(5)**. In the process described as pigment donation, melanin is transferred to neighboring keratinocytes in vesicles containing melanosomes with a small amount of melanocyte cytoplasm **(6)**. Once inside the keratinocytes, melanosomes are released into the cytoplasm **(7)**. Melanosomes are distributed within the keratinocytes but are most numerous in areas over and around the nuclei, creating "dark umbrellas"—so-called melanosome microparasol **(8)**—that protect the nuclear DNA from the sun's harmful ultraviolet (*UV*) radiation.

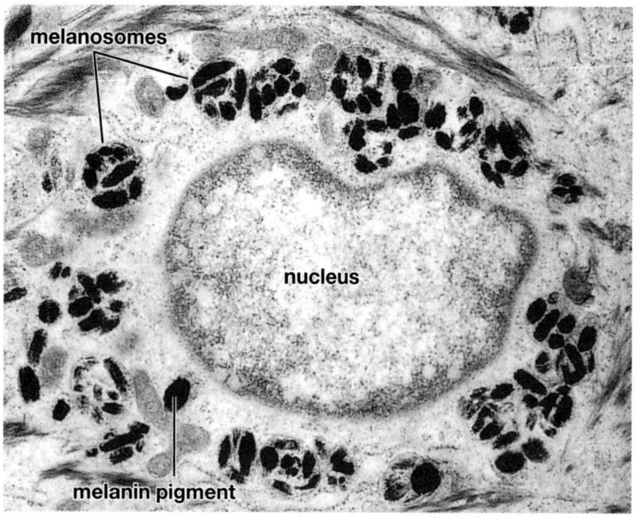

FIGURE 15.10. Electron micrograph of a keratinocyte. This high-magnification electron micrograph shows the nucleus of the keratinocyte surrounded by melanosomes containing melanin pigment. This arrangement is often described as the "dark umbrella," or melanosome microparasol, which protects nuclear DNA against harmful sun ultraviolet radiation. During pigment donation, the tips of the melanocyte process containing melanosomes are pinched off by a keratinocyte, and the resulting cytoplasmic vesicle fuses with a lysosome to produce phagolysosome. Note that a few melanin pigments are not surrounded by the cytoplasmic membrane, which was most likely dissolved in the phagolysosomes of the keratinocyte. ×19,200. (Reprinted with permission from Kanik A. Skin. In: Mills SM, ed. *Histology for Pathologists.* Wolters Kluwer; 2020:3–30.)

by MSH and **adrenocorticotropic hormone (ACTH)** leads to increased tyrosinase activity, resulting in eumelanin synthesis. The opposite effect is achieved by the **Agouti signaling protein (ASIP)**, which decreases tyrosinase activity and results in pheomelanin production. In this way, the MC1R signaling regulates the balance between eumelanin and pheomelanin synthesis within melanocytes, leading to diversity in skin pigmentation.

Steroid hormones do not act on MC1R receptors. However, recent studies show that sex steroids such as **estrogen (17β-estradiol)** and **progesterone** may indirectly regulate melanin synthesis. This finding may explain **pregnancy-associated hyperpigmentation** of specific areas of the skin (i.e., face, external genitalia, linea alba of the abdomen, and areolae surrounding the nipples). Researchers suggest that the newly discovered, nonclassical membrane-bound G-protein-coupled sex hormone receptors **GPER** and **PAQR7** are involved in melanocyte signaling (see pages 817-818 for membrane-initiated steroid signaling). Activation of these receptors is sufficient to change skin pigmentation. Estrogen increases melanin synthesis, whereas progesterone counterbalances the effect of estrogen by decreasing melanin production. Some individuals who use hormonal contraceptives containing estrogen and progesterone might develop darkening or discoloration of the skin called **melasma.** Therapeutic use of inhibitors or stimulators of GPER or PAQR7 receptors could potentially modulate melanin pigment production and alter skin color.

In addition to regulating melanin synthesis in melanocytes, recent research shows that **paracrine regulators** of melanocyte microenvironment (i.e., growth factors and cytokines) can result in skin pigmentation changes. Skin also responds to sun exposure (see Folder 15.3, page 580). Epidermal keratinocytes have been shown to release exosomes that may also be responsible for stimulation of pigmentation after UV exposure.

The number of melanocytes in normal skin is constant in all individuals.

Despite variations in skin color among different individuals, the number of melanocytes remains constant, with a similar ratio of melanocytes to keratinocytes. This ratio oscillates in the range of one melanocyte for every 4–40 basal keratinocytes. Changes in the melanocyte-to-keratinocyte ratio are diagnostically useful in identifying certain pigmented skin lesions. For instance, **vitiligo** (acquired loss of skin pigmentation) is characterized by selective loss of melanocytes. In contrast, skin from individuals with **albinism** (a disorder resulting in the partial or complete absence of skin color) has a normal melanocyte-to-keratinocyte ratio; however, the melanin synthesis pathway is defective (see page 547). The number of melanocytes also decreases with age, diminishing the number of melanosomes in keratinocytes. The skin becomes lighter in color, and the incidence of skin cancer increases. The increased number of melanocytes is observed in **lentigo** (pigmented skin lesions) and **melanocytic neoplasms**.

Skin color is mainly determined by the number and size of melanosomes, not by the number of melanocytes.

Dark skin has the largest number of more prominent melanosomes with larger pigment cores, and these melanosomes are distributed throughout the cytoplasm of keratinocytes. **Light skin** has fewer, less prominent melanosomes with smaller pigment cores; these melanosomes are aggregated in clusters. In addition, in light skin, keratinocytes do not have detectable melanin content in the upper layers of the epidermis; in contrast, in dark skin, keratinocytes maintain the melanin pigment throughout the entire thickness of the epidermis (Fig. 15.11).

Melanosomes and their contents are degraded in the process of **macroautophagy** at various rates in different individuals. In individuals with dark skin, melanin is degraded slowly, and melanosomes remain discrete; in those with light skin, melanin is degraded more rapidly (see Fig. 15.11). Degradation efficacy is attributed to the higher expression of hydrolytic enzymes, particularly **cathepsin L2** in light skin, and the higher autophagic activity of keratinocytes in light skin compared with dark skin.

Because of the complexity of melanin biogenesis, protein trafficking, organelle movement, and cell-to-cell interactions within the epidermal–melanin unit, even minor changes in the cellular environment can affect melanosome structure and the pigment donation process. Numerous intrinsic and extrinsic factors are also responsible for **skin pigmentation**, including age, ethnicity, and sex differences; variable hormone levels and affinities of their receptors; genetic defects; UV radiation; climate and season changes; and chemical exposure to toxins and pollutants.

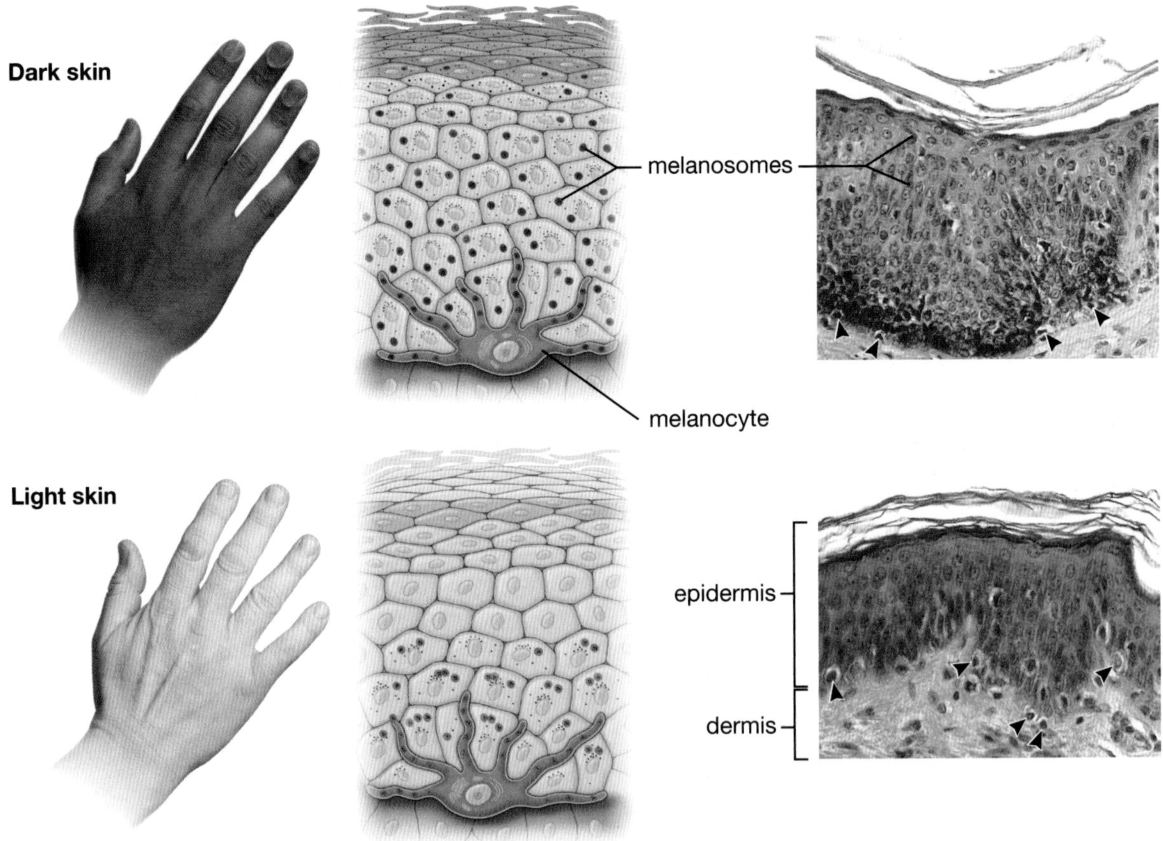

FIGURE 15.11. Melanosome number and size differences in light and dark skin. The first column shows photographs of the dorsum of the hand from a dark- and light-skinned individual. These correspond to the diagrams in the middle column showing the distribution of melanosomes in dark and light skin. Note that the melanosomes and melanin pigments accumulate around and above the nuclei, forming the melanosome micoparasol that protects nuclear DNA against harmful sun ultraviolet radiation. Dark skin has numerous prominent melanosomes with larger pigment cores that are equally distributed throughout the keratinocyte cytoplasm. Keratinocytes in dark skin maintain melanin pigment throughout the entire thickness of the epidermis. In contrast, light skin has fewer, less prominent melanosomes with smaller pigment cores aggregated in clusters in the keratinocyte cytoplasm. In addition, most of the melanosomes reside in keratinocytes near the basal layer of the epidermis. The corresponding photomicrograph in the last column shows that the number of melanocytes (*arrowheads*) is similar. Note the differences in the distribution of melanosomes. Note also that the keratinocytes in light skin do not have detectable melanin content in the upper layers of the epidermis.

Langerhans Cells

Langerhans cells represent the population of antigen-presenting resident macrophages in the epidermis.

Langerhans cells are dendritic-appearing, antigen-presenting resident macrophages in the epidermis. They are derived from **erythro-myeloid progenitor cells** originating from the **yolk sac.** Yolk sac–derived resident macrophages (i.e., Langerhans cells in the epidermis and dermal macrophages in the dermis) are self-sustaining and represent a resident self-renewing phagocyte population in the tissues (see page 203). Langerhans cells in the epidermis are long-lived and cannot be replenished by bone marrow–derived monocytes. In early development, their precursors migrate through the bloodstream and ultimately enter the epidermis, where they differentiate into immunocompetent cells. Langerhans cells provide immunosurveillance of the epidermis by processing antigens on the skin.

Langerhans cells are specialized at "sensing" the microenvironment of the epidermis by extending their processes through intercellular tight junctions to sample the outermost layers of the skin (stratum corneum). Once the antigen is phagocytized, processed, and displayed on the surface of the Langerhans cell, the cell presents antigen to T cells within the epidermis to initiate a local immune response. They also can migrate from the epidermis to a regional lymph node. Within the lymph node, the interaction of Langerhans cells with T lymphocytes initiates instruction of the adaptive immune system toward either immune tolerance or immune activation and response to the antigen. Exposure to UV radiation depletes Langerhans cells and decreases their ability to present antigen to T cells. Several experimental studies have determined that the ratio of Langerhans cells to other cells in the epidermis of normal human skin is constant at 1:53.

Langerhans cells cannot be distinguished with certainty in routine H&E-stained paraffin sections. Like melanocytes, Langerhans cells do not form desmosomes with neighboring keratinocytes. The nucleus stains heavily with hematoxylin, and the cytoplasm is clear. With special techniques, such as gold chloride impregnation or immunostaining with antibody against **CD1a molecules**, Langerhans cells can be readily seen in the stratum spinosum (Fig. 15.12). CD1a is a clinically useful marker expressed on the human Langerhans cell (see later) and is structurally related to the MHC I molecule. Langerhans cells possess dendritic processes resembling those of melanocytes. However, the TEM reveals several distinctive

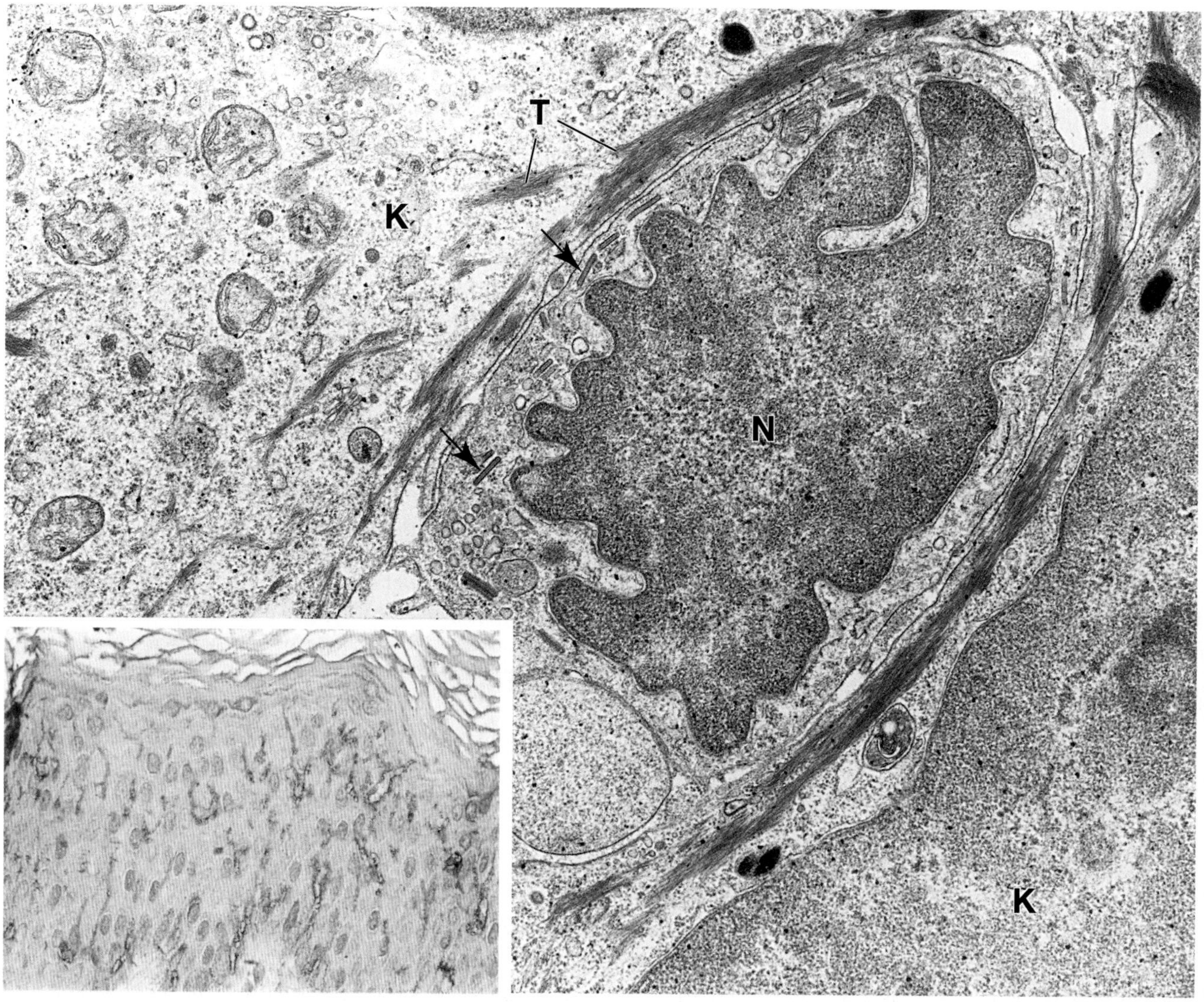

FIGURE 15.12. Electron micrograph of a Langerhans cell. The nucleus (*N*) of a Langerhans cell is characteristically indented in many places, and the cytoplasm contains distinctive rod-shaped bodies (*arrows*). Note the presence of tonofilaments (*T*) in adjacent keratinocytes (*K*) but the absence of these filaments in the Langerhans cell. ×19,000. **Inset.** Photomicrograph of the epidermis shows the distribution and dendritic nature of the Langerhans cells that were stained via immunostaining techniques with antibodies against CD1a surface antigen. ×300. (Reprinted with permission from Urmacher CD. Normal skin. In: Sternberg SS, ed. *Histology for Pathologists*. Lippincott-Raven; 1997:25–45.)

features of the Langerhans cell (see Fig. 15.12). Its nucleus is characteristically indented in many places, so the nuclear profile is uneven. Also, it possesses characteristic tennis racket–shaped **Birbeck granules**. These small vesicles appear as rods with a bulbous expansion at their end. For many years, Birbeck granules remained enigmatic until the **langerin (CD207) molecule**, a C-type lectin receptor, was finally identified as the main molecular component of these granules.

Birbeck granules play a role in the immune response against certain pathogens, including *Human immunodeficiency virus (HIV-1), Mycobacterium leprae,* and *Candida albicans.* These pathogens express carbohydrates in the form of complex *N*-glycan residues that protect them from antibodies. **Langerin** expressed on the surface of Langerhans cells recognizes and binds to *N*-glycan residues. After the pathogen binds to langerin, the entire complex is internalized and degraded in the Birbeck granule. Skin biopsy specimens from individuals with **acquired immunodeficiency syndrome (AIDS)** or AIDS-related diseases reveal that Langerhans cells contain *HIV* in their cytoplasm. Langerhans cells appear to be more resistant than T cells to the deadly effects of *HIVs* and may thus serve as a reservoir for the virus while waiting for degradation.

Like macrophages, Langerhans cells express both **MHC I** and **MHC II** molecules, which are essential for presenting antigen to cytotoxic $CD8^+$ and helper $CD4^+$ lymphocytes, respectively. They also express **F_c receptors (FcγRs)** for immunoglobulin G (IgG), **complement C3b receptors**, and fluctuating quantities of **CD1a** molecules, which are used as a specific clinical marker for Langerhans cells. As an antigen-presenting cell, the **Langerhans cell** is involved in **delayed-type hypersensitivity reactions** (e.g., contact allergic dermatitis and other cell-mediated immune responses in the skin) through their recognition of antigens in the skin and their transport to the lymph nodes.

In addition, a malignant transformation of Langerhans cells is responsible for **histiocytosis X** (Langerhans cell histiocytosis), a group of immune diseases that are characterized by an abnormal increase and accumulation of Langerhans cells, which may form tumors affecting various parts of the body, including the bones, lungs, skull, and other areas and organs.

Merkel Cells

Merkel cells are epidermal cells that function in cutaneous sensation.

Merkel cells are dendritic cells located in the stratum basale. The origin of Merkel cells is unknown; they possess antigenic markers of both epidermal and neural types. They are most abundant in skin where sensory perception is acute, such as the fingertips and lips. Merkel cells are bound to adjoining keratinocytes by desmosomes and contain intermediate (keratin) filaments in their cytoplasm. The nucleus is lobed, and the cytoplasm is somewhat denser than that of melanocytes and Langerhans cells. They may contain some melanosomes in their cytoplasm, but they are best characterized by the presence of **80-nm dense-core neurosecretory granules** that resemble those found in the adrenal medulla and carotid body (Fig. 15.13). Merkel cells are closely associated with the expanded terminal bulb of afferent myelinated nerve fibers. The neuron terminal loses its

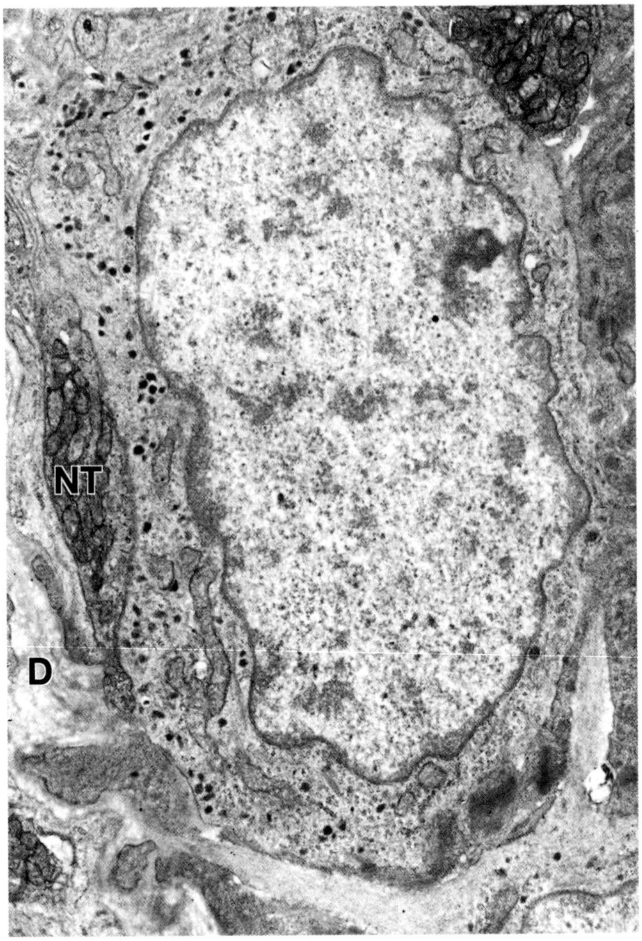

FIGURE 15.13. Electron micrograph of a Merkel cell. The cell has small neurosecretory granules in the cytoplasm and makes contact with a peripheral nerve terminal (*NT*) of a sensory neuron. The dermis (*D*) is in the *lower part* of the micrograph. ×14,450. (Courtesy of Dr. Bryce L. Munger.)

Schwann cell covering and immediately penetrates the basal lamina, where it expands into a plate-like ending called a *disc receptor* that lies in close apposition to the base of the Merkel cell. The combination of the neuron and epidermal cell, called a **Merkel corpuscle**, is a sensitive **mechanoreceptor**.

Merkel cell carcinoma (MCC) is a rare but highly aggressive type of skin cancer that develops when Merkel cells undergo uncontrolled proliferation. It most often starts in areas of skin exposed to the sun, such as the head, neck, and upper and lower limbs. MCC tends to grow quickly and metastasizes via lymph vessels at an early stage.

■ DERMIS

The attachment of the epidermis to the dermis is enhanced by an increased interface between the two tissues.

The junction between the epidermis and dermis (**epidermal–dermal junction**) is seen in the light microscope as an uneven boundary except in the thinnest skin. Sections of skin cut perpendicular to the surface reveal numerous finger-like connective tissue protrusions, **dermal papillae**, that project into the undersurface of the epidermis (see Fig. 15.2). The papillae are complemented by what appear to be similar epidermal protrusions, called **epidermal ridges** or **rete ridges**, that project into the dermis. If the plane of section is parallel to the surface of the epidermis and passes at a level that includes the dermal papillae, however, the epidermal tissue appears as a continuous sheet of epithelium, containing circular islands of connective tissue within it. The islands are cross sections of true finger-like dermal papillae that project into the epidermis. At sites where increased **mechanical stress** is placed on the skin, the epidermal ridges are much deeper (the epithelium is thicker), and the dermal papillae are much longer and more closely spaced, creating a more extensive interface between the dermis and epidermis. This phenomenon is particularly well demonstrated in histologic sections that show both palmar and dorsal surfaces of the hand, as in a section of a finger.

Friction ridge skin contains a genetically unique pattern of dermal ridges located on the palmar surface of the hand and plantar surface of the foot.

The thick skin on the palmar surface of the hands and the plantar surface of the feet is specialized. It is called **friction ridge skin** because it has a corrugated surface with elevated **dermal ridges** broken up by lower **furrows (grooves)** (Fig. 15.14). Friction ridge skin assists in gripping objects and surfaces. Eccrine sweat gland openings occur at regular intervals along the tops of the dermal ridges. The furrows are involved in a moisture-regulating mechanism (i.e., channel excess fluid), which provides optimal hydration to the keratinized cells in the epidermis that maximizes friction and reduces the possibility of slip. With the development of touchscreen devices and artificial hands for robotic and prosthetic applications, there is a renewed interest in the study of the structure and function of friction ridge skin.

The interface between the epidermis and dermis is also uneven. The pattern of dermal ridges and furrows on the skin surface correlates with a complementary pattern of **epidermal ridges** and **dermal papillae** (see Fig 15.14). The epidermal ridges and dermal papillae are most prominent in the friction ridge skin. Here, the basal surface of the epidermis greatly exceeds its free surface. The germinal layer is thus spread over a large area; assuming a near-constant rate of mitosis in the stratum germinativum, more cells per unit of time enter the stratum corneum in thick skin than in thin skin. These additional cells are thought to account for the greater thickness of the cornified layer in thick skin.

Dermal ridges tend to have a parallel arrangement, with the dermal papillae located between them (see Fig. 15.14a). These ridges form a distinctive pattern that is genetically unique to each individual and is reflected in the appearance of furrows (grooves) and dermal ridges on the skin surface. An impression of the friction ridges of all or any part of the finger is called a fingerprint. The patterns of friction ridges are the basis of the science of fingerprint and footprint identification, which is called **dermatoglyphics** or **dactyloscopy**.

Hemidesmosomes strengthen the attachment of the epidermis to the underlying connective tissue.

When studied with the TEM, the basal surface of the basal epidermal cells exhibits a pattern of irregular cytoplasmic protrusions that increase the attachment surface between the epithelial cell and its subjacent basal lamina. A series of **hemidesmosomes** links the intermediate filaments of the cytoskeleton into the basal lamina. In addition, **focal adhesions** that anchor actin filaments into the basal lamina are also present. These specialized anchoring junctions are discussed on pages 145-150.

Layers of the Dermis

The dermis is composed of two layers: the papillary layer and the reticular layer.

Examination of the full thickness of the dermis in the light microscope level reveals two structurally distinct layers:

- The **papillary layer**, the more superficial layer, consists of loose connective tissue immediately beneath the epidermis (Plate 15.2, page 578). The collagen fibers located in this part of the dermis are not as thick as those in the deeper portion. This delicate collagen network contains predominately type I and type III collagen molecules. The number and diameter of collagen fibers decreases with age and the ratio of type III to type I collagen increases. Similarly, the elastic fibers are thread-like and form an irregular network. The papillary layer is relatively thin and includes the substance of the dermal papillae and dermal ridges. It contains blood vessels that serve but do not enter the epidermis. It also contains nerve processes that either

FOLDER 15.1

CLINICAL CORRELATION: CANCERS OF EPIDERMAL ORIGIN

Three major types of **skin cancer** originate from cells in the epidermis. In general, skin cancer is caused by unprotected, long-term exposure to the sun's ultraviolet radiation. The most common type is **basal cell carcinoma**, which microscopically, as its name implies, resembles cells from the stratum basale of the epidermis. Basal cell carcinoma is a slow-growing tumor that usually does not metastasize. Typically, the cancer cells arise from the follicular bulge of the external root sheath of the hair follicle. In almost all cases of basal cell carcinoma, the recommended treatment is Mohs micrographic surgical removal of the tumor. Histologic monitoring of the excised tumor during the surgical procedure for the presence of malignant cells ensures that margins of excised tissue are cancer free (for details about Mohs micrographic surgery, see Folder 15.2).

The second most common skin cancer is **squamous cell carcinoma**, with more than 200,000 cases each year. Individuals with this form of cancer usually develop a small painless nodule or patch surrounded by an area of inflammation. Squamous cell carcinoma is characterized by highly atypical cells at all levels of the epidermis (carcinoma in situ). Disruption of the basement membrane results in spread (metastasis) of tumor cells to the lymph nodes. Squamous cell carcinoma is known for variable differentiation patterns ranging from polygonal squamous cells arranged in orderly lobules and zones of keratinization to rounded cells with foci of necrosis and occasional single keratinized cells. Treatment for squamous cell carcinoma depends on histologic type, size, and location. It may include surgical excision, curettage and electrodesiccation, cryotherapy

(continued)

FOLDER 15.1

CLINICAL CORRELATION: CANCERS OF EPIDERMAL ORIGIN (*continued*)

(freezing with liquid nitrogen), or chemotherapy or radiotherapy.

Malignant melanoma is the most serious form of skin cancer if not recognized at an early stage and surgically removed. Individual melanoma cells, which originate from melanocytes, contain large nuclei with irregular contours and prominent eosinophilic nucleoli. These cells either aggregate in nests or are scattered through the entire thickness of the epidermis (Fig. F15.1.1). They may reside only in the epidermis (melanoma in situ) or extend into the underlying papillary layer of the dermis. With time, the melanoma undergoes a **radial growth phase**. The melanocytes grow in all directions, upward in the epidermis, downward into the dermis, and peripherally in the epidermis. At this early stage, the melanoma tends not to metastasize. On the skin surface, it presents as an irregularly pigmented multicolor lesion, appearing black with parts brown to light brown, and a mixture of pink to red or shades of blue (Fig. F15.1.2). In time (approximately 1 or 2 years), melanocytes exhibit mitotic activity and form round nodules growing perpendicularly to the surface of the skin. In this **vertical growth phase**, the melanocytes display little or no pigment and usually metastasize into regional lymph nodes.

The **ABCD rule** is helpful for remembering the signs and symptoms of melanoma (see Fig. F15.1.2):

- **A**symmetrical shape of skin lesion
- **B**order of the lesion is irregular.
- **C**olor variations; melanomas usually have multiple colors.
- **D**iameter of skin lesion; moles greater than 6 mm are more likely to be suspicious.

Surgery is the treatment of choice for localized malignant melanoma of the skin. A multidisciplinary approach is used for advanced malignant melanoma, including surgery combined with chemotherapy or immunotherapy with adjuvant treatment.

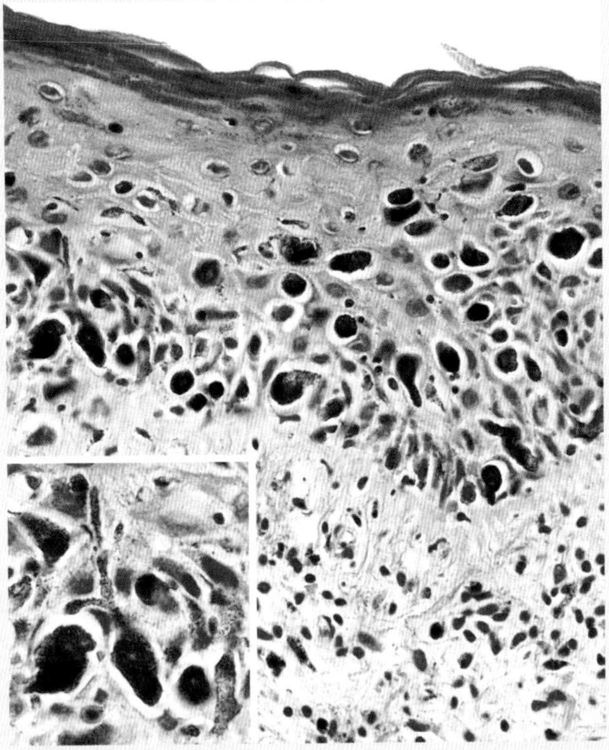

FIGURE F15.1.1. Photomicrograph of a malignant melanoma lesion early in the radial growth phase. This section of the skin shows a layer of the epidermis containing atypical (hyperplasic) cells loaded with dark brown pigment granules containing melanin. These cells represent atypical melanocytes that normally should reside in the stratum basale of the epidermis. At this stage of disease, these abnormal melanocytes migrate to the upper layers of the epidermis (melanocytic hyperplasia). There are scattered small nests of atypical cells in the dermis. Note the accumulation of lymphocytes in the superficial dermis. ×320. *Inset* shows an enlarged nest containing melanocytes with clearly visible processes containing melanin granules. ×640.

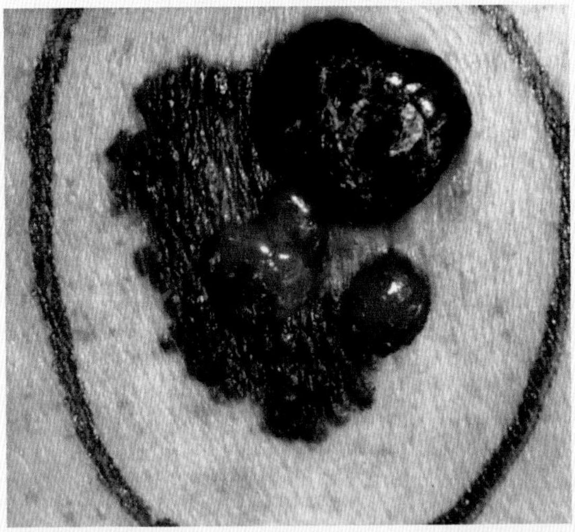

FIGURE F15.1.2. Photograph of the skin with malignant melanoma during the radial growth phase. In this individual, malignant melanoma is represented by the relatively flat, irregularly pigmented multicolor lesion. The largest nodule appears *ebony black*. It is adjacent to a slightly elevated region that is colored in shades from *dark brown* to *light brown* with two *reddish* smaller nodules. At this early stage, melanocytes grow in all directions, upward in the epidermis, downward into the dermis, and peripherally in the epidermis. (Reproduced from Storm CA, Elder DE. The skin. In: Rubin R, Strayer DS, eds. *Rubin's Pathology: Clinicopathologic Foundations of Medicine*, 5th ed. Lippincott Williams & Wilkins; 2008.)

terminate in the dermis or penetrate the basal lamina to enter the epithelial compartment. Because the blood vessels and sensory nerve endings are concentrated in this layer, they are particularly apparent in the dermal papillae.

- The **reticular layer** lies deep to the papillary layer. Although its thickness varies in different parts of the body, it is always considerably thicker and less cellular than the papillary layer. It is characterized by thick, irregular bundles of mostly type I collagen and coarser elastic fibers. Collagen fibers provide the skin with tensile strength and tissue integrity, whereas elastic fibers provide elasticity and resiliency. The collagen and elastic fibers are not randomly oriented but form regular lines of tension in the skin called **Langer lines**, also known as **cleavage lines**. Skin incisions made parallel to Langer lines heal with the least scarring.

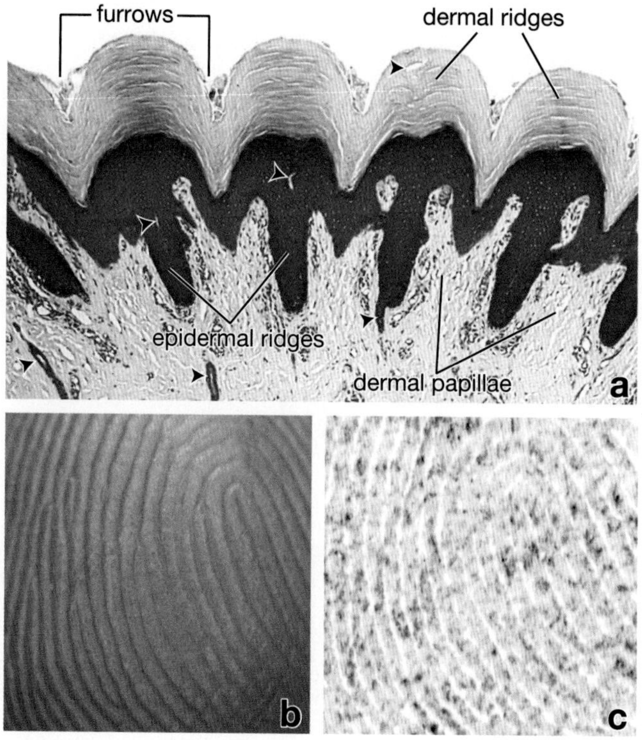

FIGURE 15.14. Friction ridge skin in a histologic section, surface photograph, and fingerprint image. a. This low-magnification hematoxylin and eosin (H&E)-stained photomicrograph shows a section of friction ridge skin from the human fingertip. The epidermis is at the top of this image. Note that the upper layer of the epidermis is keratinized, forming dome-shaped surface projections. These represent cross sections through the dermal ridges separated by the furrows. The interface between the epidermis and dermis (on the bottom) is well demarcated by the corrugated pattern of epidermal ridges and dermal papillae. The secretory segments of eccrine sweat glands are deeper in the dermis and are not visible on this image; however, their ducts pierce the epidermis to open at the top of the dermal ridges. Note eccrine sweat ducts (*arrowheads*) traversing through both the dermis and epidermis. The surface features of friction ridge skin produce the characteristic fingerprints of an individual. ×45. **b.** This enlarged photograph of friction ridge skin from the fingertip shows the unique pattern of dermal ridges and furrows. At this magnification, the openings of the eccrine sweat ducts on the top of the dermal ridges are barely visible. ×10. **c.** An impression of the unique arrangement of dermal ridges on the friction ridge skin is called a fingerprint. This image was obtained using an inkless fingerprinting technique in which a towelette moistened with a colorless, nontoxic solution is used to wipe the friction ridge skin of the finger, which is then imprinted on chemically treated paper. ×10.

■ CELLS OF THE DERMIS

Dermal fibroblasts and a diverse population of cells belonging to the mononuclear phagocyte system are found in the dermis.

The papillary and reticular layers of the dermis have a typical resident cell population embedded in the extracellular matrix of the dense irregular connective tissue. The dermis is rich in blood vessels, lymphatic vessels, and nerves. The network of lymphatic vessels in the dermis facilitates the migration of dermis-resident immune cells toward the lymph nodes. A few cells, such as **dermal fibroblasts**, deserve a closer look because of their unique function within the skin. Immune cell populations in the dermis are predominantly comprised of **dermal dendritic cells** and **resident dermal macrophages**. These cells belong to the mononuclear phagocyte system (see page 203). In addition, a transient population of other connective tissue cells, including **mast cells** and **several types of lymphocytes**, such as $CD4^+$ and $CD8^+$ lymphocytes, gamma/delta (γ/δ) T lymphocytes, regulatory $CD4^+$ $CD25^+$ $FOXP3^+$ T lymphocytes, NK cells, and skin resident memory T lymphocytes (T_{rm}), are present in the dermis. Under normal skin conditions, neutrophils are usually absent. However, if the skin is injured or after exposure to sunlight, neutrophils infiltrate the dermis and contribute to the inflammatory reaction (i.e., sunburn).

Dermal Fibroblasts

Dermal fibroblasts are the structural cells of the dermis. Their primary function is to secrete extracellular matrix molecules (i.e., procollagen I, III, V, VII, proteoglycans, glycosaminoglycans, and multiadhesive glycoproteins). They control the self-assembly and arrangement of collagen and elastic fibers in the dermis. In addition to maintaining connective tissue integrity, dermal fibroblasts are involved in immune defense mechanisms. They express a full range of **toll-like receptors (TLRs)** that play an important role in pathogen pattern recognition. When triggered, these receptors lead to the production of inflammatory cytokines that initiate an immune response.

Dermal Dendritic Cells

Like the Langerhans cells in the epidermis, **dermal dendritic cells** also originate from yolk sac–derived erythro-myeloid progenitor cells. They are abundant in the papillary layer of the dermis. Dendritic cells sample the microenvironment and either present antigen to the T cells in the dermis or migrate through the lymphatics to the lymph node to initiate an immune response. They all express MHC II molecules and do not possess markers defining T cells, B cells, or NK cells. There are several subsets of dendritic cells characterized by the expression of different cell markers such as **CD1c, CD14,** and **CD141**. Dermal dendritic cells have increased expression of costimulatory receptors and are strong stimulators of T-cell proliferation.

Resident Dermal Macrophages

Resident dermal macrophages also originate from yolk sac–derived erythro-myeloid progenitor cells. They are long-lived, self-renewing cells with a slow turnover. They can be replenished by macrophages derived from circulating monocytes. Resident dermal macrophages are antigen-presenting cells that reside deep in the dermis; they respond to foreign substances (i.e., tattoo ink), tissue damage, and pathogens and initiate an appropriate immune response. Resident dermal macrophages maintain tissue homeostasis through anti-inflammatory mechanisms and contribute to wound healing. **CD163** has been proposed as a specific marker for resident dermal macrophages, as its expression distinguishes them from other monocyte-derived macrophages that migrated more recently into the skin.

Dermal macrophages are responsible for phagocytosis of the ink pigment injected into the skin during the tattoo procedure.

A **tattoo** involves inserting a needle through the epidermis and delivering ink into the underlying dermis (Fig. 15.15). The injection of the ink pigment, an insoluble foreign body resistant to enzymatic degradation, damages the skin and triggers the immune system to respond to the injury. Newly tattooed skin becomes inflamed and infiltrated by immune cells. Although **resident dermal macrophages** phagocytize the ink, their

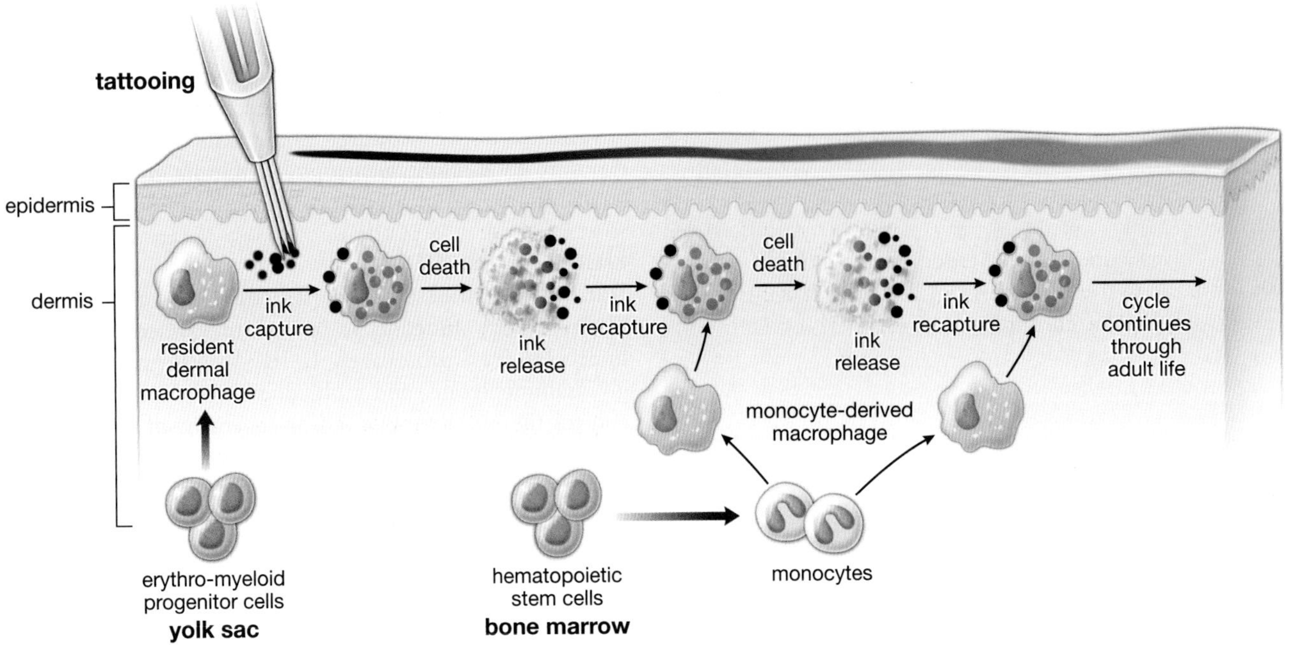

FIGURE 15.15. Diagram of the role of dermal macrophages in the ink capture–release–recapture cycle in tattooed skin. The tattoo machine operates like a sewing machine, moving a set of needles up and down to deliver ink deep into the dermis. Resident dermal macrophages, which colonized the skin in early development from the erythro-myeloid progenitor cells of the yolk sac, phagocytize the ink, capturing it within cytoplasmic vacuoles throughout the life of the cell. The resident dermal macrophages are long-lived cells; however, these ink-laden cells sometimes die during adult life. The phagocytosed ink particles are then released into the extracellular matrix, where they are once again phagocytized by newly arrived monocyte-derived macrophages. When these macrophages die, the cycle of ink capture–release–recapture continues in the tattooed skin. Note that over time and with multiple cycles, ink is passed from one macrophage to another, and the edges of the tattoo become less sharp and washed out.

lysosomal enzymes cannot break it down, and the ink remains in the cytoplasmic vacuoles throughout the life of the macrophage (Fig. 15.16). As a result, most injected ink is trapped in macrophages in the skin region where the ink was originally injected (see Fig. 15.15). Most macrophages loaded with ink stay in the tissue, whereas others migrate to the perivascular spaces (see Fig. 15.16). In addition, small ink particles are removed from the injection site via blood and lymph vessels and could be observed in local lymph nodes.

In the past, it was thought that ink responsible for the visible part of the tattoo resides mainly in dermal fibroblasts, perivascular macrophages, and the connective tissue between the collagen fibers (free ink particles). More recent studies have found that resident dermal macrophages are the only cells to take

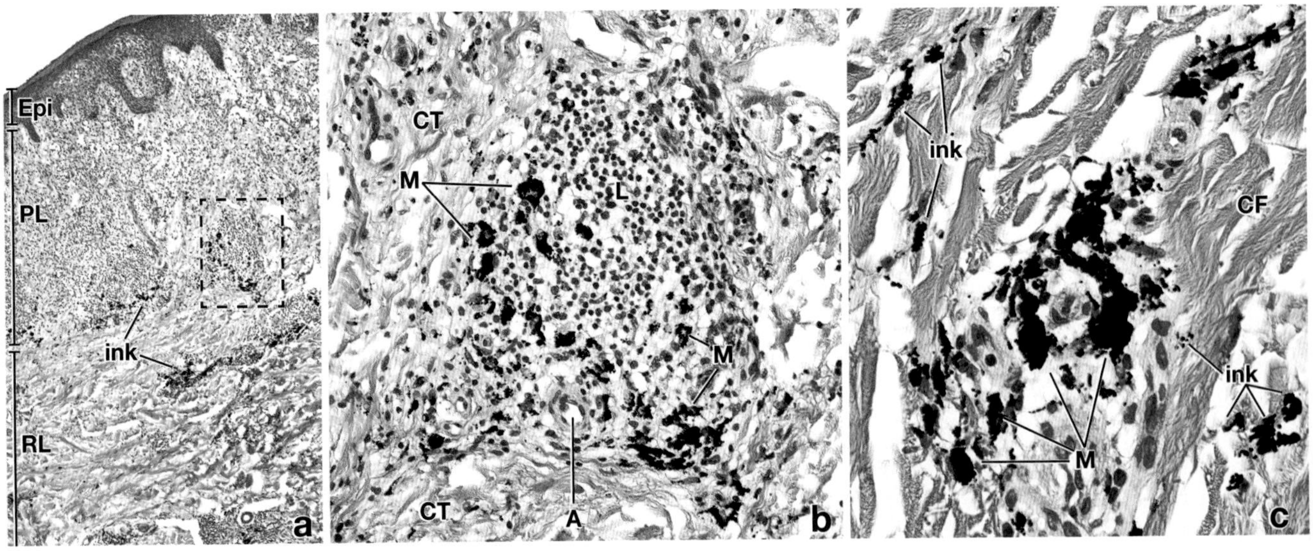

FIGURE 15.16. Photomicrograph of a biopsy specimen from tattooed skin. a. This low-magnification hematoxylin and eosin (H&E)-stained photomicrograph shows skin with injected black ink particles. They are visible below the epidermis (*Epi*) in the reticular layer (*RL*) of the dermis and near the interface with the papillary layer (*PL*). Note the presence of lymphocytes in the papillary layer of the dermis and areas around visible ink particles, representing a chronic immune response with lymphocyte infiltration. These changes are characteristic of an inflammatory reaction as this patient was allergic to the specific tattoo ink. ×40. **b.** This photomicrograph shows an enlargement of the area marked by the *rectangle* in panel a. Most of the ink is phagocytosed by dermal macrophages (*M*), which are surrounded by lymphocytes and other immune system cells. Some of the macrophages have visible nuclei. Dermal macrophages are aggregated near the perivascular spaces near a small artery (*A*). The pattern of irregular connective tissue (*CT*) of the dermis is visible. ×240. **c.** This high-magnification photomicrograph shows a nest of ink-laden macrophages in which the ink obscures their nuclei. Note that a few small pigment particles appear to be dispersed between collagen fibers (*CF*). These small particles could be in the process of removal from the tissue by lymphatic vessels or have not been recaptured yet by newly arrived macrophages during the continuous ink "capture–release–recapture" cycle. ×480. (Specimen courtesy of Dr. Kevin Christensen, Winona Health.)

up pigment in the same way they engulf invading pathogens. As discussed earlier, resident dermal macrophages are long-lived cells; however, after a certain time, these ink-laden dermal macrophages die and the ink particles are released into the extracellular matrix. These particles are once again phagocytized by newly arrived monocyte-derived macrophages (see Fig. 15.15). Therefore, the **cycle of ink capture, ink release,** and **ink recapture** occurs continuously in tattooed skin. This cycle is the basis of "tattoo aging," where the tattoo loses its sharpness over time (see Fig. 15.15). The aging process is also aggravated by chronic sun exposure. The **tattoo** does not remain histologically inert during one's lifetime. The ink pigment causes **chronic nonspecific macrophage activation** and generates **mild inflammatory** changes. They can be observed in the tissue biopsy as moderate fibrosis of the papillary layer of the dermis, reactive capillary proliferation, and nonspecific lymphocytic infiltration (see Fig. 15.16).

The ink capture–release–recapture cycle makes **tattoo removal** difficult. Removal can only be successful if the treatment (surgery, laser, dermabrasion) extends to the dermis. Although **laser therapy** breaks down the ink and kills the ink-laden macrophages, new monocyte-derived macrophages are recruited to the damaged tissue and recapture much of the released pigment. Combining laser surgery with the **transient ablation of the macrophages** could improve the procedure. In this combined treatment, the fragmented ink particles released to the dermis after laser treatment are not immediately phagocytized by macrophages, which increases their likelihood of being drained away via the lymphatic vessels.

Dermal T-Resident Memory Cells

Dermal T-resident memory (T_{rm}) cells. These recently discovered cells are **noncirculating memory T cells** present in the skin. Dermal T_{rm} cells are generated after exposure to antigen and provide memory at the site of initial exposure. They are more potent effector cells compared with other circulating T cells. Dermal T_{rm} cells maintain immune surveillance of the skin and are crucial for initiating rapid, robust immune responses during infection. They lack molecules enabling them to leave the skin and migrate to lymph nodes. They express specific markers of residency (**CD69, CD103, CD49a**).

■ HYPODERMIS

Layers of adipose tissue, smooth muscle, and, in some sites, striated muscle may be found just beneath the reticular layer.

Deep to the reticular layer is a **layer of adipose tissue**, the **panniculus adiposus**, which varies in thickness. This layer serves as a major energy storage site and also provides insulation. It is particularly thick in individuals who live in cold climates. This layer and its associated loose connective tissue constitute the **hypodermis** or **subcutaneous fascia**.

In the skin of the areolae, penis, scrotum, and perineum, **smooth muscle** cells form a loose plexus in the reticular layer. This arrangement accounts for the puckering or wrinkled appearance of the skin at these sites, particularly in the scrotum (see pages 890-893).

Individual smooth muscle cells or small bundles of smooth muscle cells that originate in this layer form the **arrector pili muscles** that connect the deep part of hair follicles to the more superficial dermis. Contraction of these muscles in humans produces the erection of hairs and puckering of skin called "goose flesh." In other animals, the erection of hairs serves in both thermal regulation and fright reactions.

A thin layer of striated muscle, the **panniculus carnosus**, lies deep to the subcutaneous fascia in many animals. Although largely vestigial in humans, it remains well defined in the skin of the neck, face, and scalp, where it constitutes the **platysma** muscle and the other **muscles of facial expression**.

■ SENSORY NERVE RECEPTORS OF THE SKIN

The skin is endowed with sensory receptors of various types that are peripheral terminals of sensory nerves (Fig. 15.17). It is also well supplied with motor nerve endings to the blood vessels, arrector pili muscles, and sweat glands.

Free nerve endings are the most numerous neuronal receptors in the epidermis.

Free nerve endings in the epidermis terminate in the stratum granulosum. The endings are "free" in that they lack a connective tissue or Schwann cell investment. Such neuronal endings subserve multiple sensory modalities including fine touch, heat, cold, and pain without apparent morphologic distinction. Networks of free dermal endings surround most hair follicles and attach to their external root sheath (Figs. 15.18 and 15.19). In this position, they are particularly sensitive to hair movement and serve as mechanoreceptors. This relationship imparts a sophisticated degree of specialization in the receptors that surround tactile hairs (vibrissae), such as the whiskers of a cat or rodent, in which each vibrissa has a specific representation in the cerebral cortex.

Other nerve endings in the skin are enclosed in a connective tissue capsule. **Encapsulated nerve endings** include the following:

- **Pacinian corpuscles** detect pressure changes and vibrations applied on the skin surface.
- **Meissner corpuscles** are responsible for sensitivity to light touch.
- **Ruffini corpuscles** are sensitive to skin stretch and torque.

Pacinian corpuscles are deep pressure receptors for mechanical and vibratory pressure.

Pacinian corpuscles are large ovoid structures found in the deeper dermis and hypodermis (especially in the fingertips), in connective tissue in general, and in association with joints, periosteum, and internal organs. Pacinian corpuscles usually have macroscopic dimensions, measuring more than 1 mm along their long axis. They are composed of a myelinated nerve ending surrounded by a capsule structure (see Figs. 15.17 and 15.18a). The nerve enters the capsule at one pole with its myelin sheath intact. The myelin is retained for one or two nodes and is then lost. The unmyelinated portion of the axon extends toward the opposite pole from which it entered. Its length is covered by a series of tightly packed, flattened Schwann cell lamellae that form the inner core of the corpuscle. The remainder of the capsule, the outer core, is formed by a series of concentric lamellae; each lamella is separated from its neighbor by a narrow space containing lymph-like fluid (Plate 15.5, page 584). The appearance of

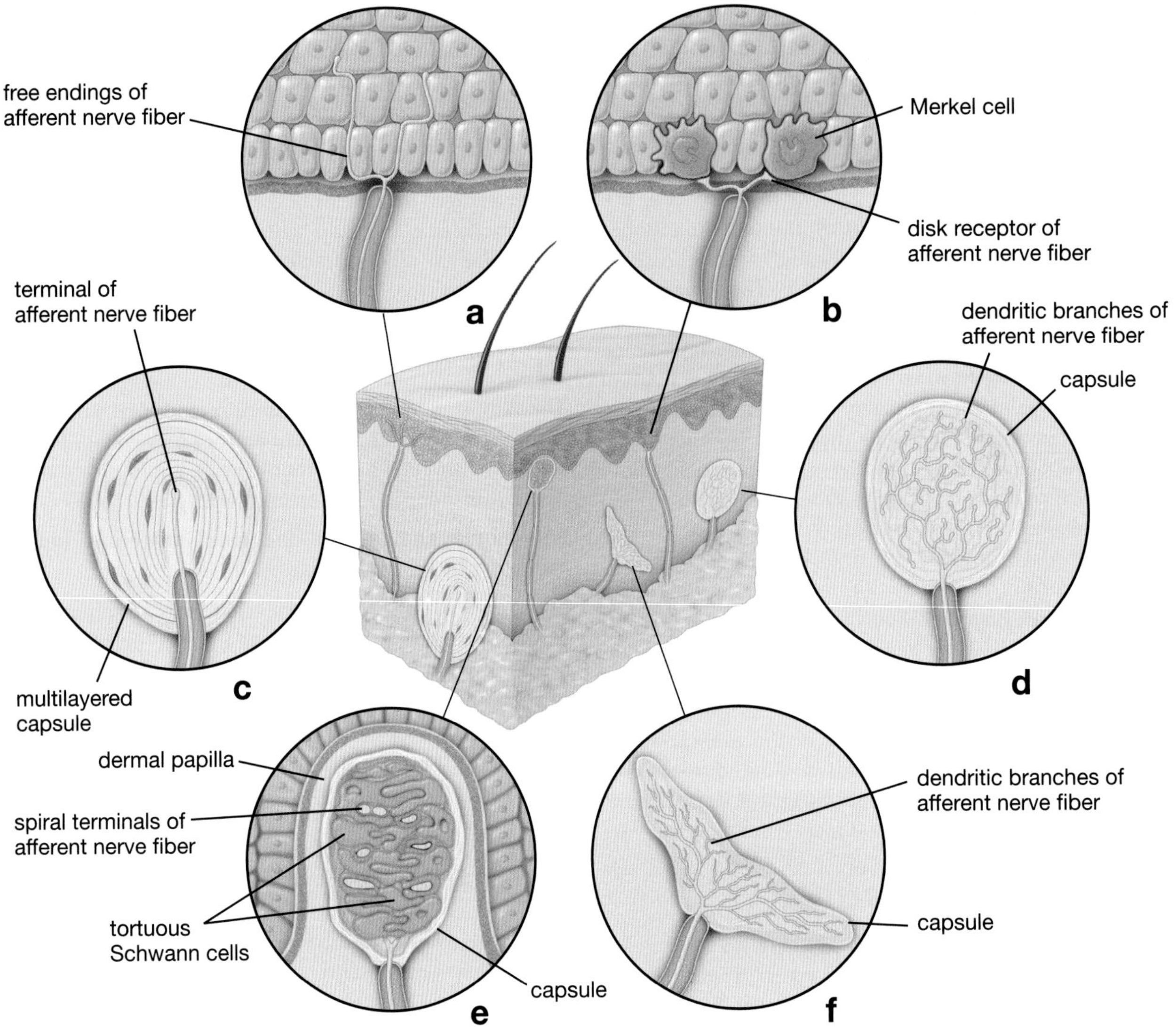

FIGURE 15.17. Diagram of the sensory receptors in skin. a. Epidermal free endings. **b.** Merkel corpuscles containing Merkel cells and disc receptors of afferent myelinated nerve fiber. **c.** Pacinian corpuscle located in the deep layer of deep dermis and hypodermis. **d.** Krause end bulb serves as cold receptor. **e.** Meissner corpuscle in dermal papilla. **f.** Ruffini corpuscle in deep layers of the dermis. Note that sensory nerve fibers in receptors shown in **c** to **f** are encapsulated.

FOLDER 15.2

CLINICAL CORRELATION: MOHS MICROGRAPHIC SURGERY

Mohs micrographic surgery (MMS), also referred to as **Mohs surgery**, is a specialized microscopically guided surgical technique for removing certain types of skin cancers. This technique, developed by Dr. Frederic E. Mohs in the 1930s and refined over the following decades, utilizes uniquely prepared frozen sections of excised skin to guide the surgeon in excision of the entire lesion.

The surgical specimen, usually excised in the shape of a disc, is placed on a glass slide so that the surgical margin is pressed outward and toward the surface of the slide. It is important that the surgical margins be pulled into the same plane as the remainder of the specimen. To achieve this, a shallow, circumferential relaxing incision is made parallel to the resection edge of the skin. Four radial incisions are often necessary to produce a flat surgical margin (Figs. F15.2.1 and F15.2.2a). The edges of the specimen are marked with color ink for orientation. A frozen tissue embedding medium (commonly called optimal cutting temperature [OCT]) is poured on both the specimen and the metal stub. Next, the specimen (still a flattened surgical surface attached to the glass slide) is flipped so that it is attached surgical side up on the metal stub. Liquid nitrogen is applied to the metal stub to snap-freeze the specimen. The glass slide is then removed to expose the OCT-embedded surgical surface, and the frozen specimen is transferred to a cryostat (a microtome placed in a freezer compartment) for sectioning. The sections taken are very thin horizontal ("en face") slices cut from the bottom-most layers of the resected specimen. These slices are mounted on a glass slide, stained with hematoxylin and eosin (H&E), and examined with a microscope by the surgeon (see Fig. F15.2.1).

Flattening of the specimen as described earlier ensures that 100% of the true surgical margin is visible on the first cryostat cut. Such preparation of excised skin tumors allows for complete examination of the entire peripheral and deep margins of the specimen in one single focal plane (see Fig F15.2.2a). It differs from the conventional

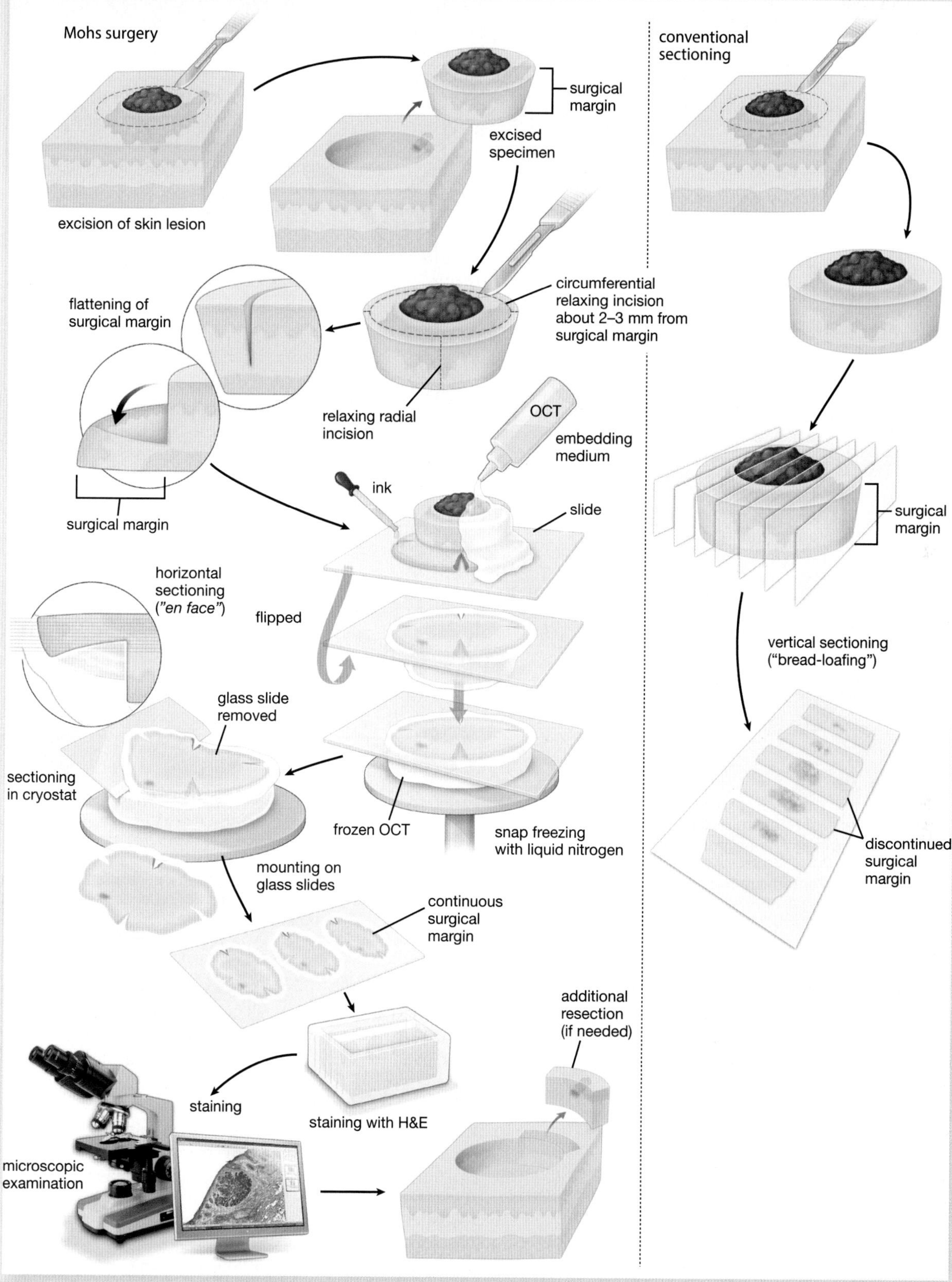

FIGURE F15.2.1. Diagram illustrating steps in Mohs micrographic surgery in comparison with conventional surgical slide preparation. Mohs surgical technique allows unique histologic processing of excised tissue that is examined by the surgeon during the tumor removal procedure. In this preparation, 100% of the continuous peripheral surgical margin is displayed on the same focal plane as the deep margin. Frozen sections are cut horizontally ("en face") from the bottom-most layers of the resected specimen. If tumor cells are found in the surgical margin during microscopic examination, the surgeon is able to remove additional tissue within the specific area indicated by color ink markings on the slide that correspond to the patient skin incision. In conventional surgical slide preparation, the specimen is cut vertically in a "bread-loafing" fashion, and individual sections show only discontinuous peripheral and deep surgical margins. Cancer cells may be lost with the discarded tissue between sections. Also, it is difficult to orient the location of the tumor to the specific region on the patient's skin. *OCT*, optimal cutting temperature.

(*continued*)

FOLDER 15.2

CLINICAL CORRELATION: MOHS MICROGRAPHIC SURGERY (*continued*)

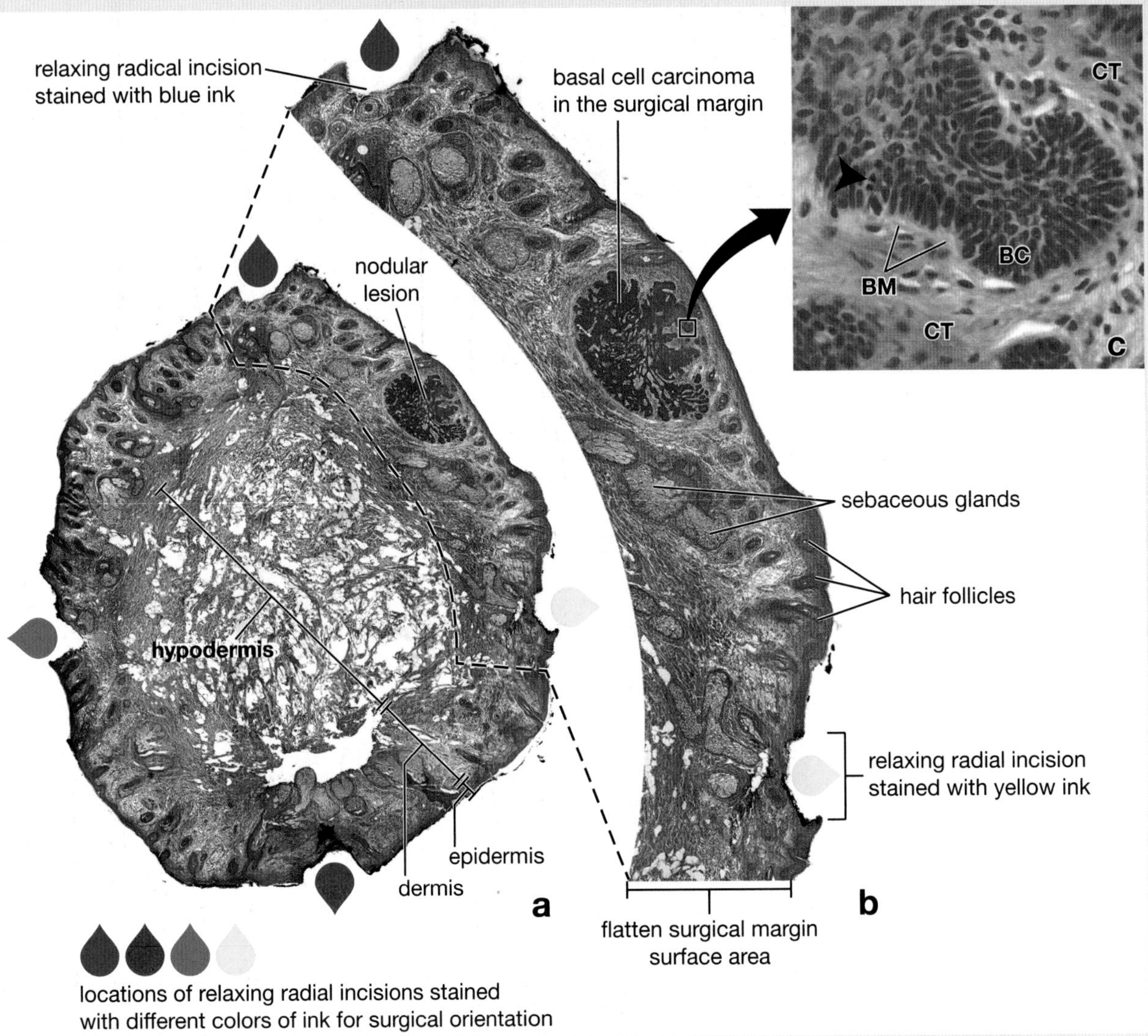

FIGURE F15.2.2. Photomicrograph of a specimen removed from the skin of the upper lip during Mohs micrographic surgery. A small, round (0.5 cm in diameter) specimen from the skin has been excised from the patient diagnosed with basal cell carcinoma and processed according to the tissue preparation procedure for Mohs frozen sections. **a.** This image shows the entire specimen with its clearly visible flattened surgical margin surface and underlying hypodermis in one focal plane. Note that 100% of the margin surface is visible. Four radial incisions are visible and stained with four different colors of ink for orientation. At this low magnification, a darker stained nodule indicates the presence of cancer cells in the surgical margin of the incision. ×8. **b.** This higher magnification image of a flattened surgical margin shows features of the skin containing epidermis, dermis with hair follicles, and sebaceous glands. The structure of the nodule can be clearly visible. It contains well-outlined multiple cords and islands consisting of deeply stained basophilic epithelial cells. This nodular lesion is characteristic of basal cell carcinoma that grows downward into the dermis and has no connection with upper layers of the epidermis. ×20. **c.** Higher magnification shows an island of cancer cells surrounded by connective tissue (*CT*) of the dermis. The island is composed of organized layers of cells resembling columnar cells of the stratum basale, hence their name basaloid cells (*BC*). In the periphery, basaloid cells are organized into parallel (palisade) arrangement with their long axis being perpendicular to the underlying basement membrane (*BM*). Their elongated nuclei are deeply basophilic and surrounded by a small rim of cytoplasm; occasional mitoses are also visible (*arrowhead*). Cells in the center of the island are spindle-shaped and more irregular. ×280. (Specimen courtesy of Dr. Kevin Christensen, Winona Health.)

vertical ("bread-loafing") sectioning of the specimen that does not allow the surgeon to see the continuous surgical edge of excised tissue (see Fig. F15.2.1).

Because the edges of the specimen are marked with color ink that is visible under the microscope, the surgeon is able to identify the precise location of any remaining cancer cells. The surgeon is able then to remove the corresponding area on the patient, allowing superior tissue conservation compared with standard blind excision. This makes the technique ideal for removing skin tumors from certain areas of the body including the face, hands, feet, and genitalia.

MMS only works for contiguously growing tumors, as multifocal lesions could potentially appear to have a negative margin. Fortunately, most primary skin cancers, including basal and squamous cell carcinomas, as well as melanomas, grow contiguously and are amenable to this technique. In MMS, the surgeon also acts as the pathologist, both excising the tissue and progressively examining the processed slides. This allows for direct clinical pathologic correlation and precise mapping of the tumor. Once the tumor is completely removed, reconstruction of the defect can occur in the same day under local anesthesia in the outpatient setting.

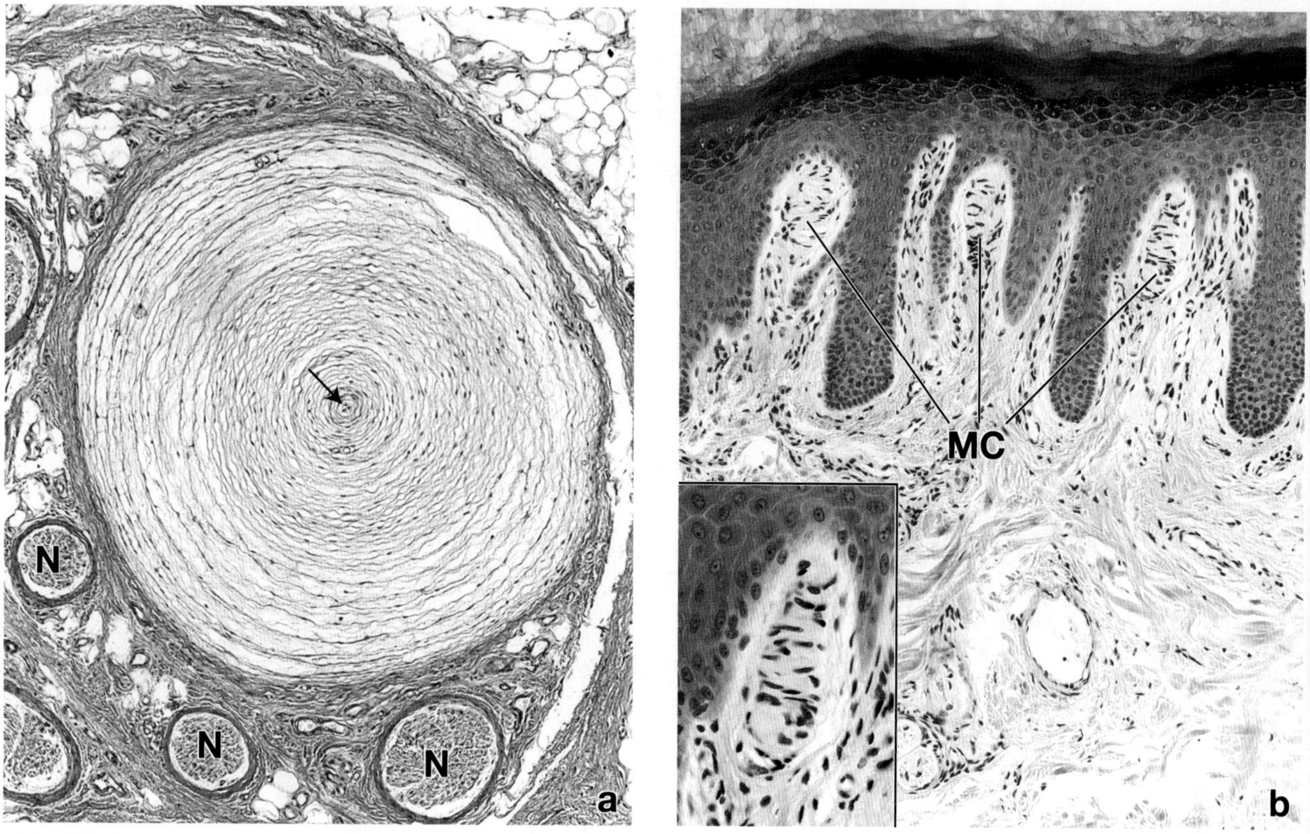

FIGURE 15.18. Pacinian and Meissner corpuscles in hematoxylin and eosin (H&E) preparations. a. In this photomicrograph, the concentric cellular lamellae of the Pacinian corpuscle are visible because of flat, fibroblast-like supportive cells. Although not evident within the tissue section, these cells are continuous with the endoneurium of the nerve fiber. The spaces between lamellae contain mostly fluid. The neural portion of the Pacinian corpuscle travels longitudinally through the center of the structure (*arrow*). Several nerves (*N*) are present adjacent to the corpuscle. ×85. **b.** Three Meissner corpuscles (*MC*) are shown residing within the dermal papillae. Note the direct proximity of the corpuscle to the undersurface of the epidermis. ×150. **Inset.** A higher magnification of a Meissner corpuscle. The nerve fiber terminates at the superficial pole of the corpuscle. Note that supporting cells are oriented approximately at right angles to the long axis of the corpuscle. ×320.

the concentric lamellae as observed in the light microscope is reminiscent of the cut surface of a hemisected onion. Each lamella is composed of flattened cells that correspond to the cells of the endoneurium outside the capsule. In addition to fluid between the lamellae, collagen fibrils are present, although sparse, as are occasional capillaries.

Pacinian corpuscles respond to **pressure** and **vibration** by displacing the capsule lamellae. This displacement effectively causes depolarization of the axon.

Meissner corpuscles are localized within dermal papillae and serve as touch receptors.

Meissner corpuscles (see Figs. 15.17 and 15.18b) are touch receptors that are particularly responsive to **low-frequency stimuli** in the papillary layer of hairless skin (e.g., the lips and the palmar and volar surfaces, particularly those of the fingers and toes). Generally, they are tapered cylinders that measure about 150 μm along their long axis and are oriented perpendicular to the skin surface. Meissner corpuscles are present in the dermal papillae just beneath the epidermal basal lamina (Plate 15.5, page 584). Within these receptors, one or two unmyelinated endings of myelinated nerve fibers follow spiral paths in the corpuscle. The cellular component consists of flattened Schwann cells that form several irregular lamellae through which the axons course to the pole of the corpuscle. In H&E-stained slides of sagittal sections, this structure resembles a loose, twisted skein of wool. It is the Schwann cells that give this impression.

Ruffini corpuscles respond to mechanical displacement of adjacent collagen fibers.

Ruffini corpuscles are the simplest encapsulated mechanoreceptors. They have an elongated fusiform shape and measure 1–2 μm in length (see Fig. 15.17f). Structurally, they consist of a thin connective tissue capsule that encloses a fluid-filled space. Collagen fibers from the surrounding connective tissue pass through the capsule. The neural element consists of a single myelinated fiber that enters the capsule, where it loses its myelin sheath and branches to form a dense arborization of fine axonal endings, each terminating in a small knob-like bulb. The axonal endings are dispersed and intertwined inside the capsule. The axonal endings respond to displacement of the collagen fibers induced by sustained or continuous mechanical stress; thus, they respond to **stretch** and **torque**. Ruffini corpuscles functionally belong to the family of rapidly adapting receptors (phasic receptors) that generate short action potentials at the beginning and end of a stimulus.

■ EPIDERMAL SKIN APPENDAGES

Skin appendages are derived from downgrowths of epidermal epithelium during development. They include the following:

- **Hair follicles** and their product, **hair**
- **Nail beds** and their product **nails**
- **Sebaceous glands** and their product, **sebum**

- **Eccrine sweat glands** and their product, **sweat**
- **Apocrine sweat glands** and their mixed product containing a form of sweat with a high concentration of carbohydrates, lipids, and proteins

Both hairs and sweat glands play specific roles in the regulation of body temperature. Sebaceous glands secrete an oily substance that may have protective functions. Apocrine glands produce a serous secretion containing pheromones that act as a sex attractant in other animals and possibly in humans. The epithelium of the skin appendages (especially hair follicles) can serve as a source of new epithelial stem cells for skin wound repair.

Hair Follicles and Hair

Each hair follicle represents an invagination of the epidermis in which a hair is formed.

Hair follicles and **hairs** are present over almost the entire body; they are absent only from the sides and palmar surfaces of the hands, sides, and plantar surfaces of the feet, the lips, and the region around the urogenital orifices. Hair distribution is influenced to a considerable degree by sex hormones; these include, in the male, the thick, pigmented facial hairs that begin to grow at puberty and the pubic and axillary hair that develops at puberty in both sexes. In the male, the hairline tends to recede with age; in both sexes, the scalp hair thins with age because of reduced secretion of estrogen and estrogen-like hormones.

The **hair follicle** is responsible for the production and growth of a hair. Coloration of the hair is attributable to the content and type of melanin that the hair contains. The follicle's histologic appearance varies depending on whether it is in a growing or resting phase. The growing follicle shows the most elaborate structure; thus, it is described here.

The hair follicle is divided into four regions:

- The **infundibulum** extends from the surface opening of the follicle to the level of the opening of its sebaceous gland. The infundibulum is a part of the **pilosebaceous canal**, which is used to discharge the oily substance **sebum**.

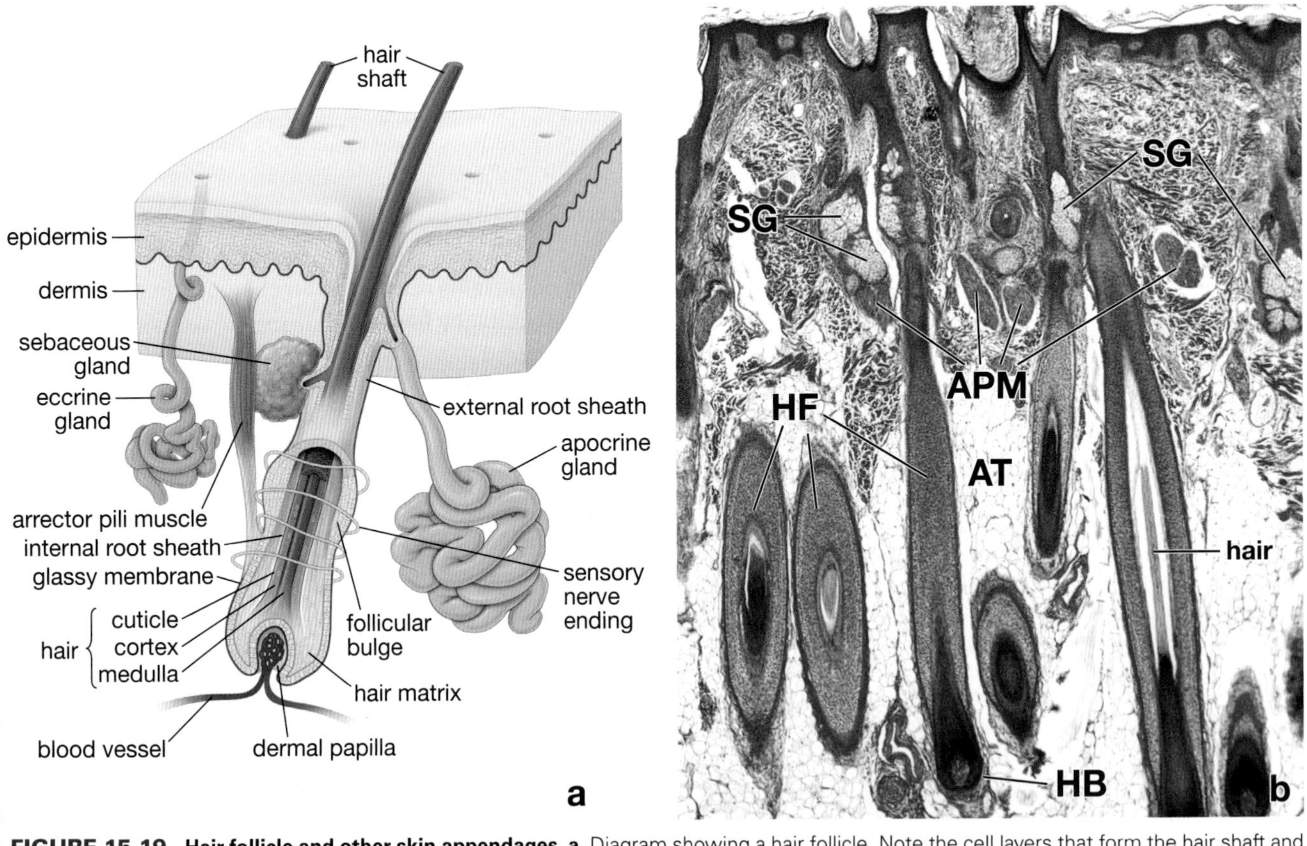

FIGURE 15.19. Hair follicle and other skin appendages. a. Diagram showing a hair follicle. Note the cell layers that form the hair shaft and the surrounding external and internal root sheaths. The sebaceous gland consists of the secretory portion and a short duct that empties into the infundibulum, the upper part of the hair follicle. The arrector pili muscle accompanies the sebaceous gland; contraction of this smooth muscle assists in gland secretion and discharges the sebum into the infundibulum of the hair follicle. Projection of the external root sheath near insertion of the arrector pili muscle forms the follicular bulge that contains epidermal stem cells. Nerve endings (*yellow*) surround the follicular bulge with nearby insertion of arrector pili muscle. The apocrine sweat gland also empties into the infundibulum. Note that eccrine sweat glands are independent structures and are not associated directly with the hair follicle. **b.** Photomicrograph of hematoxylin and eosin (H&E)-stained section of thin skin from human scalp. The growing end of a hair follicle consists of an expanded hair bulb (*HB*) of epithelial cells that is invaginated by a connective tissue dermal papilla. Hair matrix that fills the bulb consists of cells that differentiate into the hair shaft and the internal root sheath of the hair follicle (*HF*). Note that several oblique and longitudinal sections of the hair follicles are embedded in the adipose tissue (*AT*) of the hypodermis. Some of them reveal a section of the hair. Sebaceous glands (*SG*) are visible in conjunction with the infundibulum of the hair follicle. ×60. *APM*, arrector pili muscle.

FOLDER 15.3

FUNCTIONAL CONSIDERATIONS: SKIN COLOR

The **color of an individual's skin** is determined by several factors, including genetic makeup, hormonal and environmental influences, such as exposure to ultraviolet radiation. The most significant are **melanosome number** and **melanin content**. Although the number of melanocytes is essentially the same in all individuals, the fate of the melanin produced by melanocytes differs. For example, because of the lysosomal activity of keratinocytes, melanin is degraded more rapidly in individuals with light skin than in individuals with dark skin. In the former, melanosomes are concentrated in the keratinocytes nearest the basal layer and are relatively sparse in the midregion of the stratum granulosum. In contrast, dark skin may exhibit melanosomes throughout the epidermis, including the stratum corneum.

In addition, melanin pigment comprises two chemically distinct forms. One form, **eumelanin**, is a brownish-black pigment. The other form, **pheomelanin**, is a reddish-yellow pigment. Each is genetically determined. Coloration is most apparent in hair because of the concentration of melanin pigment granules, but it is also reflected in skin coloration.

Exposure to **ultraviolet radiation**, particularly the sun's rays, is called **sun tanning**. It increases the number of melanocytes and accelerates the rate of melanin production, thus protecting against further radiation effects. Response to ultraviolet radiation is genetically determined, and the skin is more protected in individuals with dark skin color.

On the molecular level, exposure to UV radiation causes keratinocytes in the upper layers of the epidermis to activate the **p53 signaling cascade**, leading to the secretion of a variety of growth factors such as fibroblast growth factor 2 (FGF2), epithelial growth factor kit ligand (KITL), endothelin 1 (EDN1), and α-melanocyte-stimulating hormone (α-MSH). These signaling molecules bind to their respective melanocyte receptors to activate their growth and differentiation by increasing the synthesis of the **paired box 3 (PAX3) protein** and **microphthalmia-associated transcription factor (MITF)**. MITF is a main transcriptional activator of genes involved in pigment synthesis and melanosome formation and trafficking. Under MITF expression, melanocytes increase melanosome production, develop a more robust dendritic structure, and increase the rate of pigment donation to keratinocytes, which causes the skin to darken. In the absence of sunlight and UV exposure, keratinocytes secrete transforming growth factor β (TGF-β) to keep the melanocytes in a quiescent state. Recently, keratinocytes have been shown to release **exosomes** that may also be responsible for stimulation of melanin synthesis after UV exposure.

Increased pigmentation of the skin may also result from hormonal factors, for example, in Addison disease. Lack of pigmentation occurs in a condition known as **albinism**. In this hereditary condition, premelanosomes are produced by melanocytes, but because of the absence of tyrosinase, the transformation of L-tyrosine to L-3,4-dihydroxyphenylalanine (L-DOPA) and the subsequent transformation of L-DOPA into melanin fail to occur. Thus, there is no pigmentation in the skin or hair of these individuals.

Two genes encoding **Bcl2 apoptosis regulator** and **microphthalmia-associated transcription factor (MITF)** appear to be responsible for the **process of graying**. The expression of Bcl2 in melanocyte stem cells is essential to maintaining their population within the niche of the follicular bulge. **Deficiency in Bcl2 expression** causes apoptosis of melanocyte stem cells and a consequent decrease in the number of melanocytes. Melanocyte depletion occurs with age, resulting in a decreased rate of pigment donation to keratinocytes. Therefore, the skin becomes lighter with increased age, and the incidence of skin cancer also increases. Melanocyte depletion caused by defective self-maintenance of melanocyte stem cells is also linked to hair graying, the most obvious sign of aging in humans. Individuals with a mutation in the **Bcl2 gene** may become prematurely gray.

Other normal factors that affect skin coloration include the presence of **oxyhemoglobin** in the dermal vascular bed, which imparts a red hue; the presence of carotenes, an exogenous orange pigment taken up from foods and concentrated in tissues containing fat; and the presence of certain endogenous pigments. The latter include degradation products of hemoglobin, iron-containing **hemosiderin**, and iron-free bilirubin, all of which impart color to the skin. Hemosiderin is a golden-brown pigment, whereas bilirubin is a yellowish-brown pigment. **Bilirubin** is normally removed from the bloodstream by the liver and eliminated via the bile. A yellowish skin color as a result of abnormal accumulation of bilirubin reflects liver dysfunction and is evidenced as **jaundice**.

- The **isthmus** extends from the infundibulum to the level of insertion of the arrector pili muscle.
- The **follicular bulge** protrudes from the hair follicle near the insertion of the arrector pili muscle and contains **epidermal stem (ES) cells** (Fig. 15.19).
- The **inferior segment** in the growing follicle (see Fig. 15.19) is of nearly uniform diameter except at its base, where it expands to form the **bulb**. The base of the bulb is invaginated by a tuft of vascularized loose connective tissue called, not surprisingly, a **dermal papilla** (Plate 15.6, page 586).

Other cells forming the bulb, including those surrounding the connective tissue dermal papilla, are collectively referred to as the **hair matrix**, which consists simply of **matrix cells**. Matrix cells immediately adjacent to the dermal papilla represent the population of rapidly dividing and

FOLDER 15.4

CLINICAL CORRELATION: CLINICAL SIGNIFICANCE OF SKIN COLOR VARIATION

Skin color and skin type are important concepts in dermatology and oncology. **Skin color** can affect the appearance of malignant and nonmalignant lesions, which may lead to missed or incorrect diagnoses. **Skin type**—how the skin reacts to various insults and events—can be useful in both the diagnosis and management of skin conditions. Clinicians and researchers recognize two types of skin color: **constitutive skin color**, which refers to the genetically determined distribution of melanin in the epidermis, and **facultative skin color**, which refers to the increases in melanin content that occur as a result of environmental factors, such as ultraviolet (UV) radiation exposure or hormonal influences.

Skin Classification Systems

There have been many attempts to classify skin color. In older systems, such as the **Classifications of Human Varieties** created by Swedish physician and taxonomist Carl Linnaeus in 1758, skin color, other physical characteristics, and geographic location were used to categorize people into four different races. It is now recognized that racial classifications based on skin color and other physical features are subjective and arbitrary and that race is a social rather than a biologic construct. In current medical practice, race is no longer used as a demographic variable similar to socioeconomic status or educational level.

Another classification system was created in the late 18th century by Austrian physician and anthropologist Felix von Luschan. The **von Luschan Chromatic Scale** classified human skin colors into 36 tones using glass tiles of varying colors. The obvious limitation of this chromatic scale is that it could not be reliably reproduced, as researchers would assign different tones to the same individual.

Classification systems based only on the subjective assessment of skin color and appearance were eventually replaced by systems that classify how the skin responds to UV radiation (called phototypic systems), esthetic procedures, and the effects of aging. The most widely accepted phototyping classification in clinical practice is the **Fitzpatrick Phototyping Scale**, developed by Harvard dermatologist Thomas B. Fitzpatrick in 1975. The Fitzpatrick phototypes, graded from I to VI, are based on the self-reported tendency to sunburn or tan as a result of sun exposure. Individuals are asked to answer questions about hair color, eye color, freckling, and their skin's reaction to sunlight exposure without sunblock after 1 day of sun exposure (Table F15.4.1). The Fitzpatrick phototypes are shown in Table F15.4.2.

TABLE F15.4.1 Fitzpatrick Skin Type Classification Questionnaire

Question	Score 0	1	2	3	4	Score/ Question
What is the natural color of your hair (before aging)?	Sandy red	Blonde	Chestnut or dark blonde	Dark brown	Black	
What is the color of your eyes?	Light blue, gray, or green	Blue, gray, or green	Dark blue, green, or light brown (hazel)	Dark brown	Brownish-black	
What is the color of your sun unexposed skin areas?	Pink or reddish	Very pale	Pale with beige tint	Light brown	Dark brown	
Do you have freckles on unexposed areas?	Many	Several	Few	Incidental	None	
What happens to your skin if you stay in the sun for an extended period of time without sunblock?	Severe burns, painful, redness, blistering, followed by peeling	Moderate burns, blistering, followed by peeling	Burns sometimes followed by peeling	Rarely burns	No burns, never had a problem	
How well do you turn brown after sun exposure?	Hardly or not at all	Light color tan	Reasonable tan	Tan very easily	Turn dark very quickly	
Do you turn brown within a day of sun exposure?	Never	Seldom	Sometimes	Often	Always	
Is your face sensitive to the sun?	Very sensitive	Sensitive	Normal	Resistant	Very resistant, never had a problem	
When did you last expose your skin to the sun or artificial sun treatments (tanning beds)?	>3 months	In the last 2–3 months	In the last 1–2 months	<1 month	<2 weeks	
How often do you tan?	Never	Hardly ever	Sometimes	Often	Always	
Skin type (total score)						

Questionnaire score: Skin type I = 0–7 points; Skin type II = 8–16 points; Skin type III = 17–25 points; Skin type VI = 25–30 points; Skin type V and VI = 30–40 points

FOLDER 15.4

CLINICAL CORRELATION: CLINICAL SIGNIFICANCE OF SKIN COLOR VARIATION (*continued*)

TABLE F15.4.2 Fitzpatrick Skin Type Classification

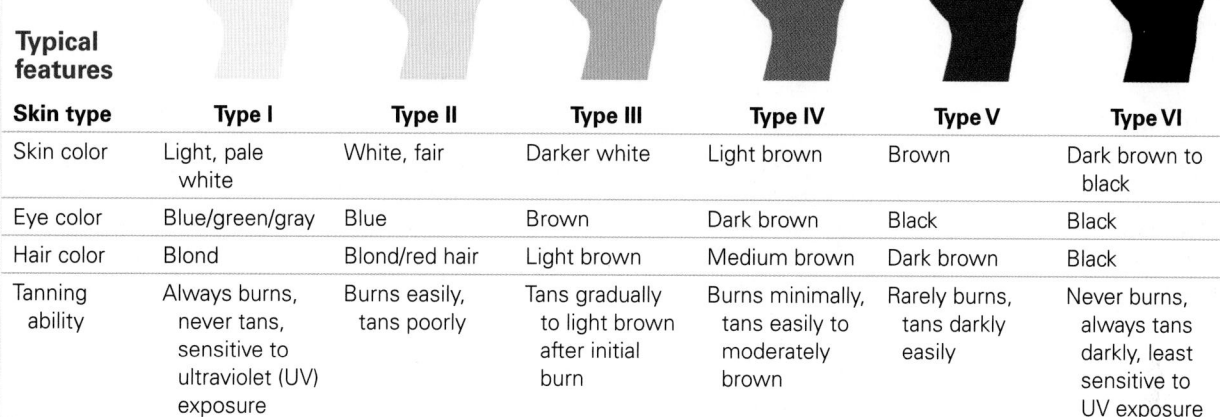

Typical features

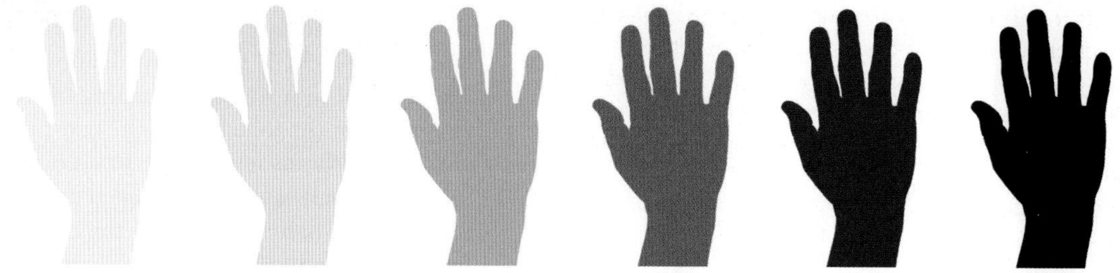

Skin type	**Type I**	**Type II**	**Type III**	**Type IV**	**Type V**	**Type VI**
Skin color	Light, pale white	White, fair	Darker white	Light brown	Brown	Dark brown to black
Eye color	Blue/green/gray	Blue	Brown	Dark brown	Black	Black
Hair color	Blond	Blond/red hair	Light brown	Medium brown	Dark brown	Black
Tanning ability	Always burns, never tans, sensitive to ultraviolet (UV) exposure	Burns easily, tans poorly	Tans gradually to light brown after initial burn	Burns minimally, tans easily to moderately brown	Rarely burns, tans darkly easily	Never burns, always tans darkly, least sensitive to UV exposure

In recent years, the validity of the Fitzpatrick scale has been questioned because of its reliance on self-report and its use of skin color changes as a basis for the skin's reactivity to the sun. Darker skin may also be sensitive to the sun but may not visibly "burn" in response to sun exposure. Although the epidermis of a darker-skinned person contains a greater amount of melanin than that of a lighter-skinned person, melanin is not the only factor contributing to photoprotection. Research shows that additional mechanisms involving antioxidants, DNA repair, and cellular survival pathways also play important roles and are not determined by melanin content. Nevertheless, the Fitzpatrick scale remains the gold standard for skin classification systems.

Skin Color and Diagnosis of Skin Cancer

Clinicians and researchers in dermatology and oncology now acknowledge that the appearance of skin cancer can differ significantly according to skin color. Skin cancer can occur in people of any skin color, although the risk of skin cancer is decreased in those with darker skin. When skin cancer does occur in a person with darker skin, it tends to be diagnosed at a later stage, which correlates with a worse prognosis. Efforts are currently directed at educating everyone, regardless of skin color, about the risks of skin cancer and the need for photoprotection. In addition, medical educational materials, such as textbooks and websites, currently strive to include photos showing skin cancer and other dermatologic conditions in individuals with different skin colors.

differentiating cells that migrated from the follicular bulge containing ES cells (Fig. 15.20). Division and proliferation of these cells account for the growth of the hair. Scattered melanocytes are also present in this germinative layer. They contribute melanosomes to the developing hair cells in a manner analogous to that in the stratum basale of the epidermis. The dividing matrix cells differentiate into the keratin-producing cells of the hair and the internal root sheath.

The **internal root sheath** is a multilayered cellular covering that surrounds the deep part of the hair (Fig. 15.21). The internal root sheath has three layers:

- **Henle layer** consists of a single outer layer of cuboidal cells. These cells are in direct contact with the outermost part of the hair follicle, which represents a downgrowth of the epidermis and is designated the **external root sheath**.
- **Huxley layer** consists of a single or double layer of flattened cells that form the **middle plate of the internal root sheath**.
- The **internal root sheath cuticle** consists of squamous cells whose outer free surface faces the hair shaft.

The **external root sheath** encloses the inner root sheath and is continuous with the epidermis of the skin (see Fig. 15.21). A periodic acid–Schiff (PAS)-positive basement membrane separates the external root sheath from the connective tissue surrounding the hair follicle called the **dermal sheath**. The thickness of the external root sheath increases from the base of the hair follicle to its surface opening at the infundibulum. In the upper part of the hair follicle, the external root sheath is similar to the epidermis. It contains **basal cells**, **melanocytes**, **keratinocytes**, and other cells present in the epidermis. The stratum granulosum is visible near the skin surface. Near the follicular bulge, the

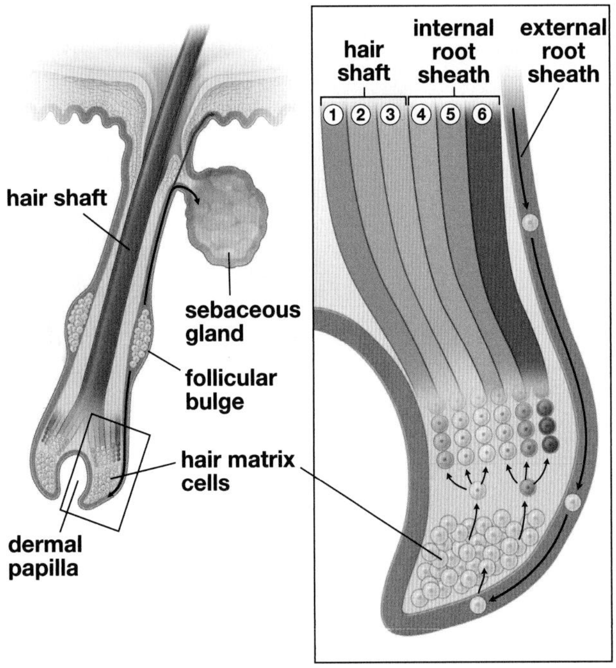

FIGURE 15.20. Hair follicle and pathways of epidermal stem cell migration. This diagram shows the location and migration pathways of epidermal stem cells that reside in the follicular bulge. Under normal conditions, epidermal stem cells migrate upward to the sebaceous gland and downward to reach the hair matrix in the bulb of the follicle (*black arrows*). Hair matrix is formed by differentiating cells that migrate along the external root sheath from the follicular bulge. As the differentiation progresses, cells leave the matrix; they form cell layers that differentiate into the hair shaft containing **(1)** medulla, **(2)** hair cortex, and **(3)** hair cuticle, and the internal root sheath containing **(4)** internal root sheath cuticle, **(5)** Huxley layer, and **(6)** Henle layer. During injury of the epidermis, the epidermal stem cells migrate from the follicular bulge toward the skin surface (*red arrow*) and participate in the initial resurfacing of damaged epidermis.

hair follicle contains a site for attachment of the arrector pili muscle (a smooth muscle that raises hair into a vertical position). Keratinocytes in the lower part of the external root sheath appear to have clear cytoplasm, which is attributed to the high glycogen content in their cytoplasm.

A niche of ES cells that resides within the follicular bulge of the external root sheath provides stem cells for hair growth and skin regeneration.

The progression of the external root sheath of the hair follicle upward toward the epidermal surface reveals the insertion site of the arrector pili muscle and the origin of the sebaceous duct and gland from the wall of the follicular canal (see Fig 15.19). Nerve endings surround the external root sheath at the level of arrector pili muscle insertion. In this general region resides an aggregate of relatively undifferentiated epithelial cells called the **follicular bulge**. Recent studies have identified the follicular bulge as a **niche of ES cells** (see Fig. 15.20). The ES cells can reside in this area indefinitely and undergo self-renewal or differentiation into specific cell lineages. Under normal conditions, ES cells are responsible for providing stem cells for the growth of hair follicles (the hair matrix, internal root sheath, cortex, and medulla) as well as sebaceous glands (see Fig. 15.20). The ES cells that normally reside in the follicular bulge do not contribute to the population of the basal stem cells of the epidermis. However, when the epidermis is injured or lost (such as in extensive skin burns and superficial skin wounds), the **ES cells** become reprogrammed, migrate toward the wound surface from their follicular niches, and participate in the initial resurfacing of the wound.

Hairs are composed of keratinized cells that develop from hair follicles.

Keratinization of the hair and internal root sheath occurs shortly after the cells leave the matrix in a region called the **keratogenous zone** in the lower third of the follicle. As the cortical cells pass through this zone, they differentiate, extrude their organelles, and become tightly packed with cross-linked keratin intermediate filaments. By the time the hair emerges from the follicle, it is entirely keratinized as **hard keratin**. The internal root sheath, consisting of soft keratin, does not emerge from the follicle with the hair but is broken down at about the isthmus level where sebaceous secretions enter the follicle. A thick basal lamina, called the **glassy membrane**, separates the hair follicle from the dermis. Surrounding the follicle is a dense irregular connective tissue. The **arrector pili muscle** is attached near the follicular bulge, which, as indicated earlier, serves as an ES cell niche.

Hairs are elongated filamentous structures that project from the hair follicles. They are composed of heavily cross-linked hard keratins and consist of three layers (see Fig. 15.19):

- The **medulla** forms the central part of the shaft and contains a column of large, loosely connected keratinized cells containing soft keratin. The medulla is present only in thick hairs.
- The **cortex** is the largest layer and accounts for approximately 80% of the total mass of each hair. It is located outside the medulla and is composed of cortical cells filled with hard keratin intermediate filaments. Each filament is surrounded by an amorphous space containing **keratin-associated proteins (KAPs)**. These high-sulfur KAPs are responsible for forming the rigid hair shaft by extensive cross-linking of keratin intermediate filaments by disulfide bonds. The cortex determines texture, elasticity, and the color of hair. Melanin pigment responsible for the color of hair is produced by melanocytes present in the germinative layer (hair matrix) of the hair bulb.
- The **cuticle of the hair shaft** is the outermost layer of the hair. It contains several layers of overlapping, semitransparent keratinized squamous cells. These cells resemble fish scales or roof tiles with their free edges lying away from the hair follicle. The cuticle protects the hair from physical and chemical damage and determines its porosity.

Hair structure in humans is determined by multiple genetic factors that include 17 keratin genes (11 genes for type I and 6 genes for type II keratins) and more than 85 KAP genes.

Nails

Nails are plates of keratinized cells containing hard keratin.

The **nails** are specialized skin appendages composed of keratinized, flattened epithelial cells derived from the germinative zones of the nail bed. The slightly arched fingernails and toenails, more properly referred to as **nail plates**, are strongly attached to underlying **nail beds**. The nail bed consists of epithelial cells that are continuous with the stratum basale and stratum spinosum of the epidermis (Fig. 15.22 and Plate 15.6, page 586).

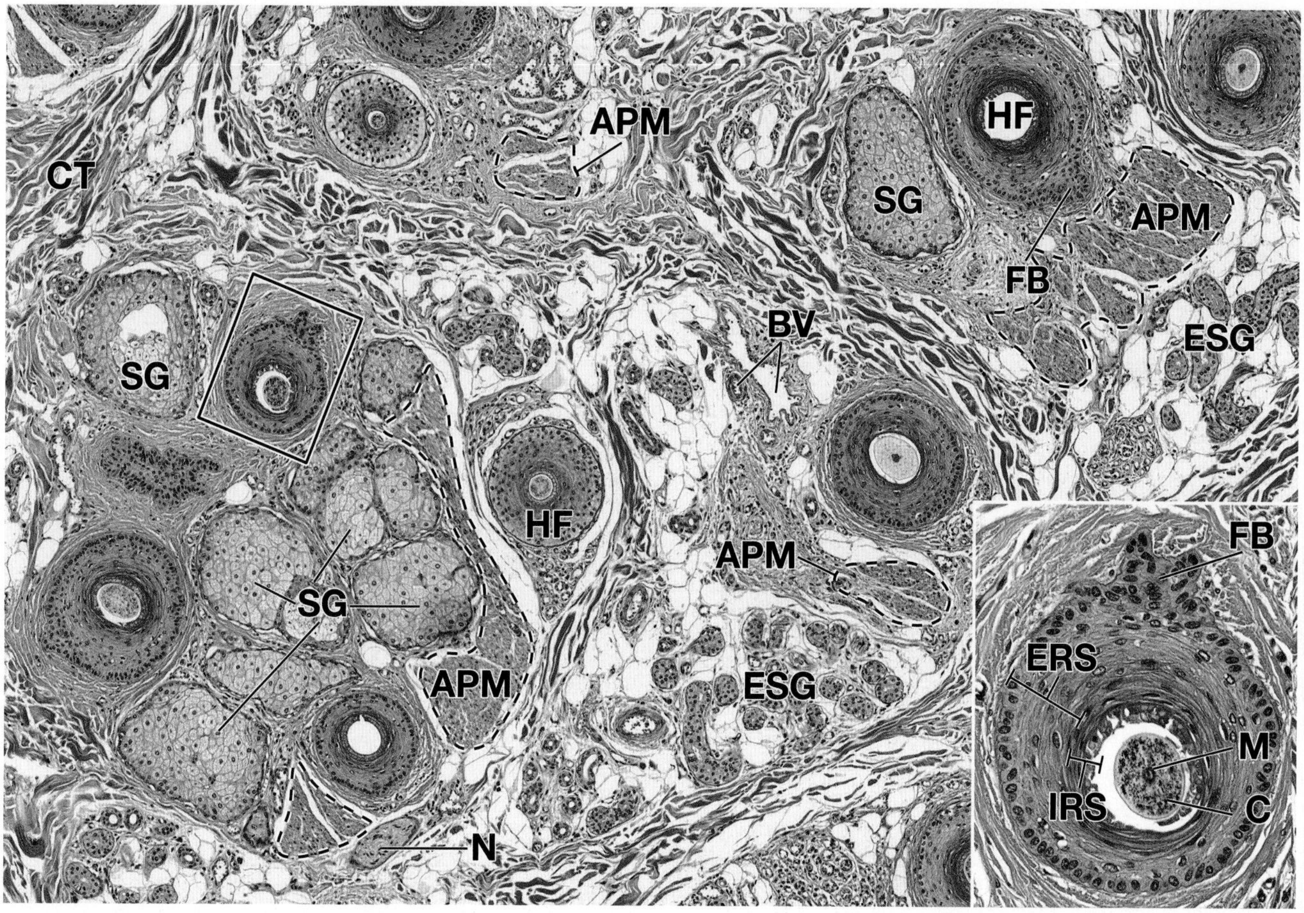

FIGURE 15.21. Photomicrograph showing a transverse section of hair follicles from the skin of the scalp. This hematoxylin and eosin (H&E)-stained specimen shows several cross-sectional profiles of hair follicles (*HF*) randomly distributed throughout the section. Some of the follicles are missing a hair shaft in the center that was lost during slide preparation. The sebaceous glands (*SG*) are visible in close association with hair follicles. Arrector pili muscles (*APM*) encircled by the *dashed line* comprise smooth muscle fibers accompanying the sebaceous gland; they attach to the hair follicle near the follicular bulge (*FB*). During contraction, they assist in gland secretion and discharge the sebum into the infundibulum of the hair follicles. Nerves (*N*) are frequently found near arrector pili muscles. Projection of the external root sheath near the insertion of the arrector pili muscle forms the follicular bulge (*FB*) visible in this cross section in two follicles. The hair follicle, hair shaft, arrector pili muscle, and sebaceous gland form the pilosebaceous unit. They are separated by dense irregular connective tissue (*CT*) and adipocytes containing blood vessels (*BV*). The secretory components and ducts of the eccrine sweat glands are found between groups of pilosebaceous units. ×120. *Inset* shows the hair follicle included in the *dashed rectangle* at higher magnification. The cross section of the hair follicle is at the level of the follicular bulge (*FB*), which is a protrusion of the external root sheath (*ERS*) containing a niche of the epidermal stem cells. An internal root sheath (*IRS*) and hair shaft in the center of the follicle are also visible. Note the melanin pigment transferred from the bulbar melanocytes residing in the hair matrix to the cortex (*C*) and the medulla (*M*) of the hair shaft. ×120. (Courtesy of Dr. Jamie Chapman, Tasmanian School of Medicine, University of Tasmania, Hobart, Australia.)

The proximal part of the nail, the **nail root**, is buried in a fold of epidermis and covers the cells of the **germinative zone** or **matrix**. The matrix contains a variety of cells, including stem cells, epithelial cells, melanocytes, Merkel cells, and Langerhans cells. The stem cells of the matrix regularly divide, migrate toward the root of the nail, and there differentiate and produce the keratin of the nail. Nail keratin is a **hard keratin**, like that of the hair cortex. Unlike the soft keratin of the epidermis, it does not desquamate. It consists of densely packed keratin filaments embedded in a matrix of amorphous keratin with a high sulfur content, which is responsible for the hardness of the nail. The process of hard keratin formation, as with the hair cortex, does not involve keratohyalin granules. In addition, a cornified CE contains proteins similar to those found in the epidermis.

The continuous addition and keratinization of new cells at the root account for nail growth. As the nail plate grows, it moves over the nail bed. The average growth rate for fingernails is estimated at 2 to 3 mm/month and for toenails about 1 mm/month; thus, complete replacement of nail requires 6 months for fingernails and 18 months for toenails. On the microscopic level, the nail plate resembles the modified stratum corneum of the skin. It contains closely packed, terminally differentiated interdigitating keratinocytes called **onychocytes** lacking nuclei and organelles. In contrast to the stratum corneum, the nail plate contains less fat and water, and surface onychocytes do not desquamate like keratinocytes on the skin surface.

The crescent-shaped white area near the root of the nail, the **lunula**, demarcates the distal portion of the germinative zone. Its color derives from the thick, opaque layer of partially keratinized matrix cells in this region. When the nail plate becomes fully keratinized, it is more transparent and takes on the coloring of the underlying vascular bed. The edge of the skin fold covering the root of the nail is the **eponychium** or **cuticle**. The cuticle is also composed of hard keratin; therefore, it does not desquamate. Because of its thinness, it tends to break off or, as with many individuals, it is trimmed and pushed back. A thickened epidermal layer, the hyponychium, secures the free edge of the nail plate at the fingertip.

FOLDER 15.5

FUNCTIONAL CONSIDERATIONS: HAIR GROWTH AND HAIR CHARACTERISTICS

Unlike the renewal of the surface epidermis, hair growth is not continuous but a cyclic process. A **period of growth (anagen)** in which a new hair develops is followed by a brief period in which **growth stops (catagen)**. Catagen is followed by a long (range 2–4 months) **rest period (telogen)** in which the follicle atrophies, and the hair is eventually lost. Epidermal stem cells found in the follicular bulge are capable of providing stem cells that give rise to mature anagen follicles. During the hair growth cycle, mature anagen hairs periodically undergo apoptosis and regress to the catagen stage. In this phase, cell division ceases, the hair matrix regresses, the dermal papilla retracts, capillary nourishment diminishes, and entire follicles retract toward the epidermal layer. As the base of the retracted follicle approximates the follicular bulge, the hair shaft is no longer supported by the nutrient-rich anagen bulb and eventually is ejected from the resting telogen follicle. This makes room for a new shaft that will grow during anagen regeneration.

Hairs in the anagen phase are susceptible to destruction by **laser hair removal (LHR)** procedures. Because of the cyclic nature of hair growth, repeated hair removal treatments are necessary to address new follicles entering the anagen phase. Professional and home-based laser and light devices are both currently available for removal of "unwanted hair" (the term used in describing facial and body hair but not scalp hair).

Out of a total of 100,000 hairs present in the normal scalp, more than 80% is in the anagen phase. In the catagen phase, the germinative zone is reduced to an epithelial strand still attached to a remnant of the dermal papilla. In the telogen phase, the atrophied follicle may contract to one-half or less of its original length. The hair may remain attached to the follicle for several months during this stage and is called a **club hair** because of the shape of its proximal end.

Hairs in humans grow to a specific length, which varies with the individual. Hairs vary in size from long, coarse **terminal hairs** that may reach a meter or more in length (scalp hair and beard hair in males) to short, fine **vellus hairs** that may be visible only with the aid of a magnifying lens (vellus hairs of the forehead and anterior surface of the forearm). Terminal hairs are produced by large-diameter, long follicles; vellus hairs are produced by relatively small follicles. Length of hair depends on genetic influences, location in the body, climate, age, nutrition, and hormonal status.

Hair length is determined by the rate and duration of anagen period. Terminal hair follicles may spend up to several years in anagen and only a few months in telogen. Average hair growth is estimated at 0.4 mm/day (1.2 cm/month), but with aging, the rate of hair growth declines and hair diminishes in thickness. Gray hair appears as the result of decreased melanin production within the hair matrix.

In the balding individual, large terminal follicles are gradually converted into small vellus follicles after several growth cycles. The ratio of vellus follicles to terminal follicles increases as baldness progresses. The "completely bald" scalp is not hairless but is populated by vellus follicles that produce fine hairs and remain in telogen for relatively long periods.

Sebaceous Glands

Most sebaceous glands are associated with hair follicles and form pilosebaceous units.

Sebaceous glands are usually found in association with hair follicles in most areas of the body surface except for the palms and soles. They form the **pilosebaceous units** comprising four structures: the hair follicle, hair shaft, arrector pili muscle, and sebaceous gland. The association between these structures is well demonstrated on a transverse section of hair follicles from the scalp (see Fig. 15.21). The highest density of sebaceous glands is found on the face. In some areas such as the eyelids (Meibomian and Zeis glands), areolae (pigmented regions surrounding the nipples of mammary glands), and vermilion border of the lips, sebaceous glands are not associated with a hair follicle and open directly onto the skin's surface.

Sebaceous glands develop early in fetal development as outgrowths of the external root sheath of the hair follicle in the epidermis. The glands can be either unilobular or multilobular (Fig. 15.23 and Plate 15.4, page 582). During the second trimester of fetal development, sebaceous glands are fully functional, and their secretion contributes to the **vernix caseosa**, a cheese-like white creamy substance that coats the skin of a newborn.

The development of sebaceous glands is highly regulated by several transcription factors such as Sox9, Blimp1, Wnt, BMP, and the hedgehog pathway. Proliferation, differentiation, and metabolism of these glands are regulated by sex hormones, particularly androgens. **Sebaceous gland activity** increases shortly after birth but then diminishes in the first few postnatal months. Increased androgen levels at puberty coincide with an increase in sebaceous

FOLDER 15.6

CLINICAL CORRELATION: SWEATING AND DISEASE

Although many neural and emotional factors can alter the **composition of sweat**, altered sweat composition can also be a sign of disease. For example, elevated sodium and chloride levels in sweat can serve as an indicator of **cystic fibrosis**. Individuals with cystic fibrosis have two to five times higher than normal amounts of sodium and chloride in their sweat.

In pronounced **uremia**, in which the kidneys are unable to rid the body of urea, the concentration of urea in sweat increases. In this condition, after the water evaporates, crystals may be discerned on the skin, especially on the upper lip. These include urea crystals and are called **urea frost**.

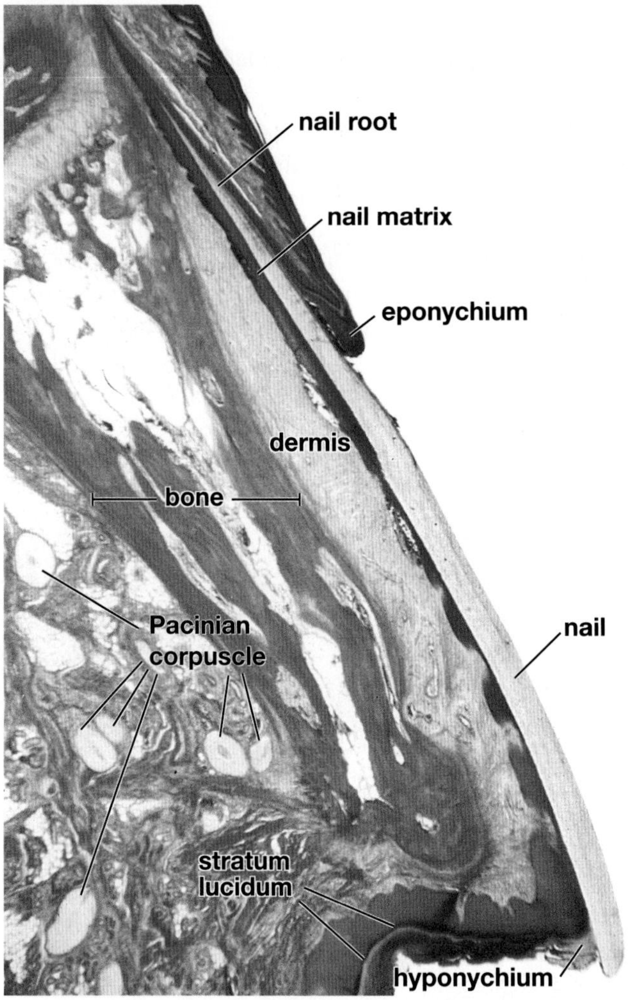

FIGURE 15.22. Photomicrograph of a sagittal section of distal phalanx with a nail. A nail is a keratinized plate located on the dorsal aspect of the distal phalanges. Beneath the free edge of the nail is a boundary layer, the hyponychium, which is continuous with the stratum corneum of the adjacent epidermis. The proximal end, the root of the nail, is overlapped by skin, the eponychium, which is also continuous with the stratum corneum of the adjacent epidermis. Deep to the nail is a layer of epithelium with underlying dermis. The proximal portion of this epithelium is referred to as the *nail matrix.* The bone in this section represents a distal phalanx. Numerous Pacinian corpuscles are present in the connective tissue of the palmar side of the finger. Note that even at this low magnification, the stratum lucidum is visible in the epidermis of the fingertip. ×10.

gland activity and sebum secretion. Sebum production decreases by about 23% per decade in males and 32% per decade in females.

Sebocytes are terminally differentiated epithelial cells that produce and accumulate sebum.

Sebocytes are the major cells within sebaceous glands that produce and accumulate lipids. The oily and waxy substance called **sebum** is produced by fully mature sebocytes in a process termed **holocrine secretion**. In this process, the entire cell produces and becomes filled with the fatty product while it simultaneously undergoes programmed cell death (apoptosis). Ultimately, both the secretory product and cellular debris are discharged from the gland as sebum into the infundibulum of a hair follicle, which forms the **pilosebaceous canal** with the short duct of the sebaceous gland. New sebocytes are produced by mitosis of the basal cells at the periphery of the gland, and the cells of the gland remain linked to one another by desmosomes and gap junctions regardless of their differentiation stage. The basal lamina of these cells is continuous with that of the epidermis and the hair follicle. The basal cells of the sebaceous gland contain sER, rER, free ribosomes, mitochondria, glycogen, and a well-developed Golgi apparatus. As the sebocytes move away from the basal layer and begin to produce their lipid secretory product, the amount of sER increases, reflecting the role of the sER in lipid synthesis and secretion. The sebocytes gradually become filled with numerous lipid droplets separated by thin strands of cytoplasm. The sebum production process takes about 8 days from the time of basal cell mitosis to the secretion of the sebum.

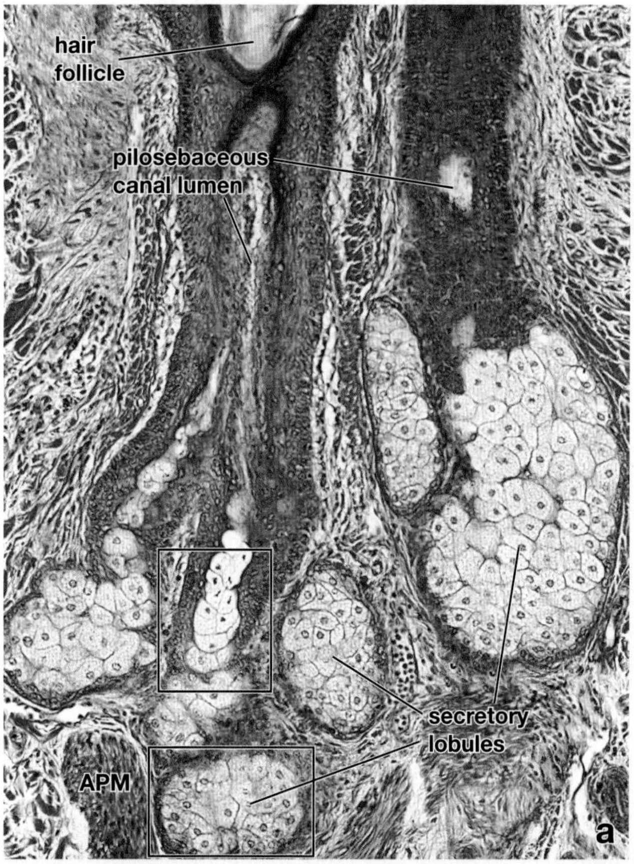

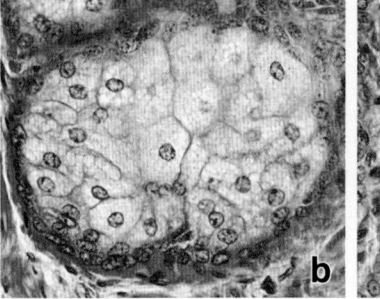

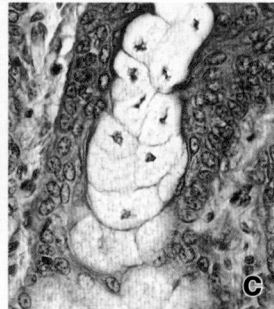

FIGURE 15.23. Photomicrograph of a sebaceous gland. a. This micrograph shows the secretory lobules and their pilosebaceous canal of two sebaceous glands. The canal of the gland on the *left* is about to enter the hair follicle seen at the *top* of the micrograph. The canal of the sebaceous gland on the *right* has been sectioned in a manner that shows mostly the wall of the canal. ×60. **b.** The secretory component of the lobule in the *lower box* of **a** is shown here at higher magnification. Note the light staining of the sebocytes because of the lack of staining of the sebum that they contain. These cells are actively producing sebum. The basal cells at the periphery of the lobule divide and replenish the population of new sebocytes. Also, the arrector pili muscle (*APM*) composed of smooth muscle fibers is visible in the periphery of the secretory lobule. ×120. **c.** The secretory component of the lobule in the upper box of **a** is shown here at higher magnification. The sebocytes are now within the canal. Note their pyknotic nuclei, signifying the death of the cell. ×120.

The complex mixture of oily substances in the sebum provides a personalized chemical signature unique for each individual.

Sebum represents a complex oily mixture that consists of triglycerides, diglycerides, and free fatty acids (57%); wax esters (26%); squalene (12%); cholesterol; and cholesterol esters (2%). Because of its complex composition, human sebum is remarkably specific as a result of individual genetic variations in enzyme concentrations, pH, and temperature. The secreted sebum provides each person with a highly individual and **unique chemical signature**. Animals with a highly developed sense of smell, such as dogs, may be able to identify individuals on the basis of this specific chemical signature. Besides contributing to the maintenance of a functional epidermal barrier and the well-defined function of the specialized sebaceous gland secretion from Meibomian glands in eyelids, the role of sebum in human skin remains elusive. Some theories suggest that it may play a role in protection against UV irradiation. Other studies suggest that it has both immune and communication functions because of the presence of antioxidants (especially vitamin E), anti-inflammatory and proinflammatory substances, antimicrobial peptides, and pheromones on the skin surface.

Differentiation, proliferation, and secretion of lipid substances from sebocytes are controlled by complex endocrine pathways. Androgens generally increase sebaceous gland function, whereas estrogens have an inhibitory effect on sebum production. In addition, histamine, substance P, corticotropin-releasing hormone (CRH), and dietary substances (e.g., free fatty acids, sugar, and fat) can induce sebum production. The increase in sebum secretion and alterations in its lipid composition during puberty in males and females may cause the chronic inflammatory disease of the pilosebaceous unit known as **acne vulgaris**. The three major events leading to acne development include (1) excessive sebum production (seborrhea), (2) abnormal follicular keratinization of the pilosebaceous canal, and (3) proliferation of *Propionibacterium acnes* bacteria within the pilosebaceous unit. On histologic examination, acne is characterized by the retention of sebum in the isthmus of the hair follicle with variable lymphocytic infiltration. In severe cases, dermal abscesses may form in association with inflamed hair follicles.

Sweat Glands

Humans have approximately 4 million **sweat glands** that are classified on the basis of their structure and the nature of their secretion. Two types of sweat glands are recognized:

- **Eccrine sweat glands** are distributed over the entire body surface except for the vermilion border of the lips, nail beds, and part of the external genitalia (glans penis, clitoris, and labia minora). The maximum density of sweat glands is found in the palms of the hands, soles of the feet, skin of axillae, forehead, and trunk.
- **Apocrine sweat glands** are limited to the axilla, areola and nipple of the mammary gland, skin around the anus, and the external genitalia. The **ceruminous glands** of the external acoustic meatus and the **apocrine glands of eyelashes (glands of Moll)** are also apocrine-type glands.

Eccrine Sweat Glands

Eccrine sweat glands are simple coiled glands that regulate body temperature.

Eccrine sweat glands are independent structures and are not associated with the hair follicle that arises as a downgrowth from the fetal epidermis. Each eccrine gland is arranged as a blind-ended, simple, coiled tubular structure. It consists of two segments: a **secretory segment** located deep in the dermis or in the upper part of the hypodermis and a directly continuous, less coiled **duct segment** that leads to the epidermal surface (Fig. 15.24 and Plate 15.3, page 580).

Eccrine sweat glands play a major role in **temperature regulation** through the cooling that results from the evaporation of water from sweat on the body surface. Eccrine sweat

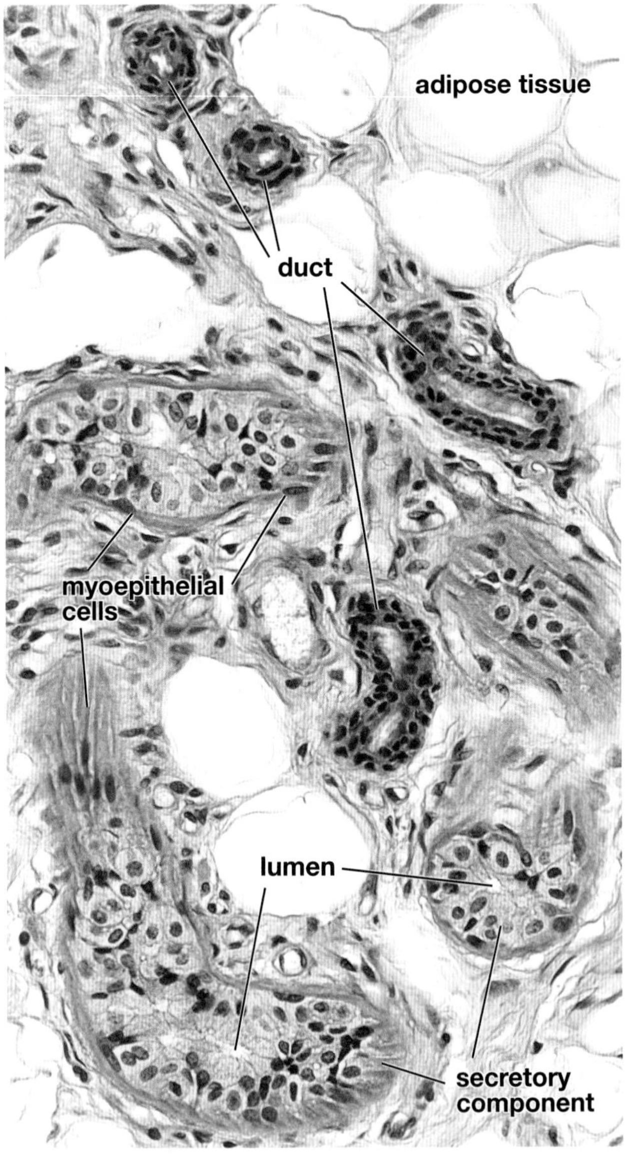

FIGURE 15.24. Photomicrograph of an eccrine sweat gland. This photomicrograph of a hematoxylin and eosin (H&E)-stained section of human skin shows profiles of both the secretory component and the duct of an eccrine sweat gland. The secretory component appears as a double layer of cuboidal epithelial cells and peripherally, within the basal lamina, a layer of myoepithelial cells. The duct portion of the gland has a narrower outside diameter and lumen than the secretory portion of the gland. It consists of a double layer of small cuboidal cells without the myoepithelial cells. ×320.

glands in the skin of the palm and soles increase gripping strength. The secretory portion of the glands produces a secretion similar in composition to an ultrafiltrate of blood. Resorption of some of the sodium and water in the duct results in the release of a hypotonic sweat at the skin surface. This hypotonic watery solution is low in protein and contains varying amounts of sodium chloride, urea, uric acid, and ammonia. Thus, the eccrine sweat gland also serves, in part, as an excretory organ.

Excessive sweating can lead to the loss of other electrolytes, such as potassium and magnesium as well as significant water loss. Normally, the body loses about 600 mL of water a day through evaporation from the lungs and skin. Under conditions of high ambient temperature, water loss can be increased in a regulated manner by an increased rate of sweating. This **thermoregulatory sweating** first occurs on the forehead and scalp, extends to the face and the rest of the body, and occurs last on the palms and soles. Under conditions of emotional stress, however, the palms, soles, and axillae are the first surfaces to sweat. Control of thermoregulatory sweating is cholinergic, whereas emotional sweating may be stimulated by adrenergic portions of the sympathetic division of the autonomic nervous system.

The secretory segment of the eccrine sweat gland contains three cell types.

Three cell types are present in the secretory segment of the gland: **clear cells** and **dark cells**, both of which are secretory epithelial cells, and **myoepithelial cells**, which are contractile epithelial cells (Fig. 15.25 and Plate 15.4, page 582). All of the cells rest on the basal lamina; their arrangement is that of a pseudostratified epithelium. These three cell types are described as follows:

- **Clear cells** are characterized by abundant glycogen. In the electron micrograph shown in Figure 15.25a, the glycogen is conspicuous; it would also stain intensely with the PAS method. In routine H&E preparations, the cytoplasm of clear cells stains poorly. Membranous organelles include numerous mitochondria, profiles of sER, and a relatively small Golgi apparatus. The plasma membrane is remarkably amplified at the lateral and apical surfaces by extensive cytoplasmic folds. In addition, the basal surface of the cell possesses infoldings, although they are considerably less complex than the cytoplasmic folds. The morphology of these cells indicates that they produce the watery component of sweat.
- **Dark cells** are characterized by abundant rER and secretory granules (see Fig. 15.25). The Golgi apparatus is relatively large, a feature consistent with the glycoprotein secretion of these cells. The apical cytoplasm contains mature secretory granules and occupies most of the luminal surface (see Fig. 15.25a). Clear cells have considerably less cytoplasmic exposure to the lumen; their secretion is largely via the lateral surfaces of the cell, which are in contact with intercellular canaliculi that allow the watery secretion to reach the lumen. Here it mixes with the proteinaceous secretion of the dark cells.
- **Myoepithelial cells** are limited to the basal aspect of the secretory segment. They lie between the secretory cells, with their processes oriented transversally to the tubule. The cytoplasm contains numerous contractile filaments (actin) that stain deeply with eosin, thus making them readily identifiable in routine H&E specimens. Contraction of these cells is responsible for rapid expression of sweat from the gland.

The duct segment of eccrine glands is lined by stratified cuboidal epithelium and lacks myoepithelial cells.

The **duct segment** of the gland continues from the secretory portion with coiling. In histologic sections, multiple duct profiles typically appear among the secretory profiles. As the duct passes upward through the dermis, it takes a gentle spiral course until it reaches the epidermis, where it then continues in a tighter spiral to the surface. When the duct enters the epidermis, however, the duct cells end, and the epidermal cells form the wall of the duct. Clinically, the dermal part of the eccrine duct is called **syrinx**, and the coiled intraepidermal part that opens onto the skin surface is called the **acrosyringium**. Benign tumors of the syrinx are termed **syringomas,** and tumors of the acrosyringium are **poromas**. The acrosyringium is also a place of origin for **eccrine porocarcinoma**, a rare type of skin cancer.

The dermal part of the duct is composed of **stratified cuboidal epithelium**, consisting of a basal cell layer and a luminal cell layer. The duct cells are smaller and appear darker than the cells of the secretory portion of the gland. Also, the duct has a smaller diameter than the secretory portion. In contrast to the secretory portion of the eccrine gland, the duct portion does not possess myoepithelial cells. These features are useful in distinguishing the duct from the secretory portion in a histologic section (see Fig. 15.24).

The basal or peripheral cells of the duct have a rounded or ovoid nucleus and contain a prominent nucleolus. The cytoplasm is filled with mitochondria and ribosomes. The apical or luminal cells are smaller than the basal cells, but their nuclei are similar in appearance. The most conspicuous feature of the luminal cells is the deeply stained, glassy (hyalinized) appearance of the apical cytoplasm. The glassy appearance is attributable to large numbers of aggregated tonofilaments in the apical cytoplasm.

Apocrine Sweat Glands

Apocrine glands are large-lumen tubular glands associated with hair follicles.

Apocrine sweat glands develop from the same downgrowths of epidermis that give rise to hair follicles. The connection to the follicle is retained, allowing the secretion of the gland to enter the follicle, typically at a level just above the entrance to the sebaceous duct. From here, the secretion makes its way to the surface.

Like eccrine glands, apocrine glands are coiled tubular glands, and they are sometimes branched. The secretory portion of the gland is located deep in the dermis or, more commonly, in the upper region of the hypodermis.

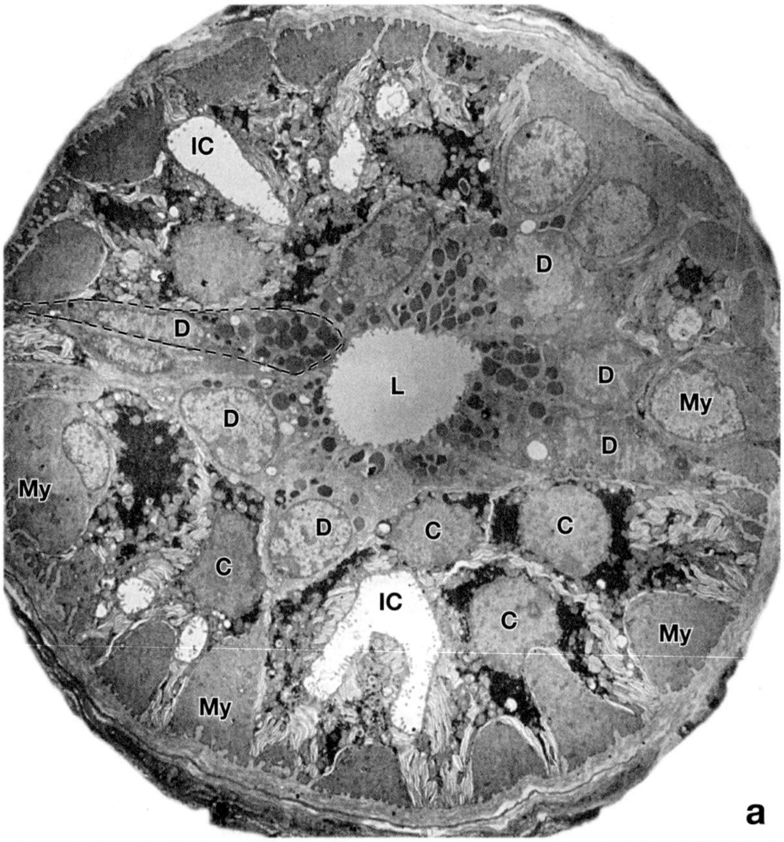

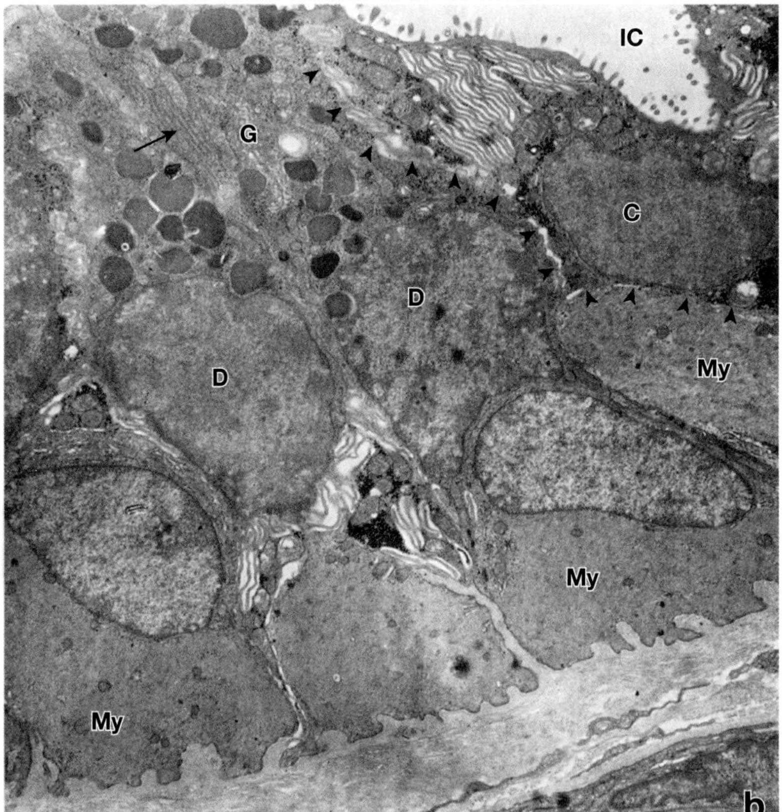

FIGURE 15.25. Electron micrographs of an eccrine sweat gland. a. This micrograph shows myoepithelial cells (*My*) and two distinctive gland cell types, dark cells (*D*) and clear cells (*C*). The apical portion of the dark cell is broad; it faces the lumen (*L*) of the gland and contains numerous secretory granules. The *dashed line* marks the boundary of one dark cell. The clear cell is more removed from the lumen of the gland. Its base rests on the myoepithelial cells or directly on the basal lamina. Most of the free surface of the clear cell faces an intercellular canaliculus (*IC*). Clear cells contain numerous mitochondria, extensive infoldings of the plasma membrane, and large numbers of electron-dense glycogen inclusions. ×5,600. **b.** At higher magnification, dark cells display rough-surfaced endoplasmic reticulum (rER) (*arrow*) and a Golgi apparatus (*G*) in addition to secretory granules. Clear cells show large amounts of folded membrane, mitochondria, and glycogen. The myoepithelial cells (*My*) contain large numbers of contractile actin filaments. *Arrowheads* (*upper right*) mark the boundary of a clear cell. ×17,500. (Courtesy of Dr. John A. Terzakis.)

The secretory portion of apocrine glands has a wider lumen than that of eccrine glands and is composed of a single cell type.

The secretory portion of apocrine glands differs in several respects from that of eccrine glands. The most obvious difference, readily noted in the light microscope, is its very wide lumen (Fig. 15.26 and Plate 15.3, page 580). Unlike eccrine glands, apocrine glands store their secretory product in the lumen. The secretory portion of the gland is composed of simple epithelium. Only one cell type is present, and the cytoplasm of the cell is eosinophilic. The apical part of the cell often exhibits a bleb-like protrusion. It was once thought that this part of the cell pinched off and was discharged into the lumen as an apocrine secretion, thus the name of the gland. However, TEM studies confirm that the secretion is a **merocrine type**. The apical cytoplasm contains numerous small granules, the secretory components within the cell, which are discharged by exocytosis. Other features of the cell include numerous lysosomes and lipofuscin pigment granules. The latter represent secondary and tertiary lysosomes. Mitochondria are also numerous. During the refractory phase, after expulsion of the secretion, the Golgi apparatus enlarges in preparation for a new secretory phase.

Myoepithelial cells are also present in the secretory portion of the gland and are situated between the secretory cells and the adjacent basal lamina. As in eccrine glands, contraction of the processes of myoid cells facilitates expulsion of the secretory product from the gland.

The duct portion of apocrine glands is lined by stratified cuboidal epithelium and lacks myoepithelial cells.

The **duct of the apocrine gland** is similar to that of the eccrine duct; it has a narrow lumen. However, it continues from the secretory portion of the gland in a relatively straight path to empty into the follicle canal. Because of its straight course, the probability of viewing both the duct and the secretory portion of an apocrine gland in the same histologic section is reduced. Also, in contrast to the eccrine duct, resorption does not occur in the apocrine duct. The secretory product is not altered in its passage through the duct.

The duct epithelium is stratified cuboidal, usually two but sometimes three cell layers thick. The apical cytoplasm of the luminal cells appears hyalinized, a consequence of the aggregated tonofilaments in the apical cytoplasm. In this aspect, they resemble the luminal cells of the eccrine duct.

Apocrine glands produce a protein-rich secretion containing pheromones.

Apocrine glands produce a secretion that contains protein, carbohydrates, ammonia, lipid, and certain organic compounds that may color the secretion. However, the secretions vary with the anatomic location. In the axilla, the secretion is milky and slightly viscous. When secreted, the fluid is odorless; through bacterial action on the skin surface, it develops an acrid odor.

Apocrine glands become functional at **puberty**; as with axillary and pubic hair, their development depends on sex hormones. In the female, axillary and areolar apocrine glands undergo morphologic and secretory changes that parallel the menstrual cycle.

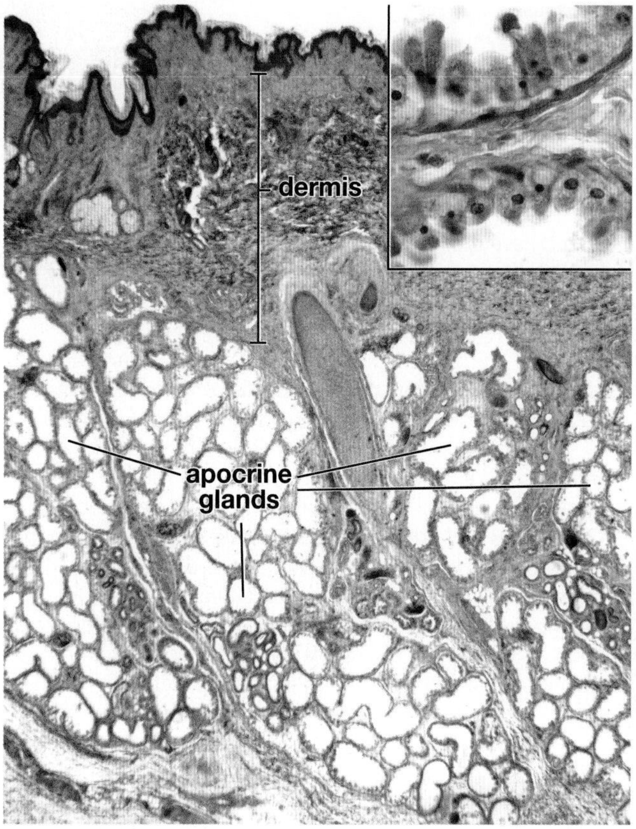

FIGURE 15.26. Photomicrograph of an apocrine sweat gland. This section of adult skin from the area around the anus shows several apocrine (anal) sweat glands, which are easily identified by the large lumen of their secretory components. This apocrine sweat gland is close to a hair follicle (*center* of photomicrograph) and deep to the dense, irregular connective tissue of the dermis. ×45. **Inset.** Higher magnification of secretory component shows the cell types of the apocrine gland. The gland consists of a simple epithelium whose cells are either cuboidal or columnar and myoepithelial cells located in the basal portion of the epithelial cell layer. ×230.

In many mammals, similar glands secrete **pheromones**, chemical signals used in marking territory, courtship behavior, and certain maternal and social behaviors. It is generally believed that apocrine secretions may function as pheromones in humans. Male pheromones (androstenol and androstenone) in the secretion of apocrine glands have been shown to influence the female menstrual cycle. Furthermore, female pheromones (copulins) influence male perception of females and may also induce hormonal changes in males.

The sympathetic portion of the autonomic nervous system innervates both eccrine and apocrine sweat glands.

The cholinergic neurotransmitter **acetylcholine** stimulates **eccrine sweat glands**; paradoxically, it is discharged from sympathetic nerve fibers, which typically use norepinephrine and not acetylcholine (acetylcholine serves as a neurotransmitter in the parasympathetic nerve fibers). Thus, eccrine sweat glands have a functional cholinergic innervation but are anatomically sympathetic. The adrenergic neurotransmitter **norepinephrine** stimulates the **apocrine glands.** As described earlier, eccrine glands respond to heat and stress. Sympathetic innervation to the sweat glands is mediated by the thermoregulatory center of the hypothalamus. Apocrine glands are involved in emotional sweating because of stress, fear, pain, and sexual stimulation but do not respond to heat.

FOLDER 15.7

CLINICAL CORRELATION: SKIN REPAIR

The process of wound healing of the skin is classically described as either a primary or secondary union. Healing by **primary union (first intention)** occurs after surgical incisions in which wounds that are usually clean and uninfected have their edges approximated by surgical sutures. Healing by **secondary union (secondary intention)** occurs in traumatic wounds with separated edges, which are characterized by more extensive loss of cells and tissues. Wound healing in such cases involves generating a large amount of **granulation tissue**, which represents a specialized type of tissue formed during the repair process.

The repair of an incision or laceration of the skin requires stimulated growth of both the dermis and the epidermis. Dermal repair involves (1) blood clot formation; (2) removal of damaged collagen fibers, primarily through the effort of macrophage activity that is associated with inflammation; (3) formation of granulation tissue; (4) reepithelialization of the exposed surface; (5) proliferation and migration of fibroblasts and differentiation of myofibroblasts involved in wound contraction; and (6) deposition and remodeling of the extracellular matrix of underlying connective tissue. Healing by primary union following application of sutures reduces the extent of the repair area through maximal closure of a wound, minimizing scar formation. Surgical incisions are typically made along cleavage lines; the cut tends to parallel the collagen fibers, thus minimizing the need for excess collagen production and the inherent scarring that may occur.

Repair of the epidermis involves the proliferation of the basal keratinocytes in the stratum basale in the undamaged site surrounding the wound (Fig. F15.7.1). Mitotic activity is markedly increased within the first 24 hours. In a short time, the wound site is covered by a **scab** that represents dehydrated blood clot. The proliferating basal cells of the stratum basale begin migrating beneath the scab and across the wound surface. The migration rate may be as much as 0.5 mm/day, starting within 8–18 hours after wounding. Further proliferation and differentiation occur behind the migration front, leading to restoration of the multilayered epidermis. As new cells ultimately keratinize and desquamate, the overlying scab is freed with the desquamating cells, which explains why a scab detaches from its periphery inward.

In cases in which the full thickness of the epidermal layer is removed either by trauma or in surgery, the parts of hair follicles, the follicular bulge that contains the niche of the epidermal stem cells, will produce cells that migrate over the exposed surface to reestablish a complete epithelial (epidermal) layer. Massive destruction of all of the epithelial structures of the skin, as in a third-degree burn or extensive full-thickness abrasion, prevents reepithelialization. Such wounds can be healed only by grafting the epidermis to cover the wounded area. In the absence of a graft, the wound would, at best, reepithelialize slowly and imperfectly by ingrowth of cells from the margins of the wound.

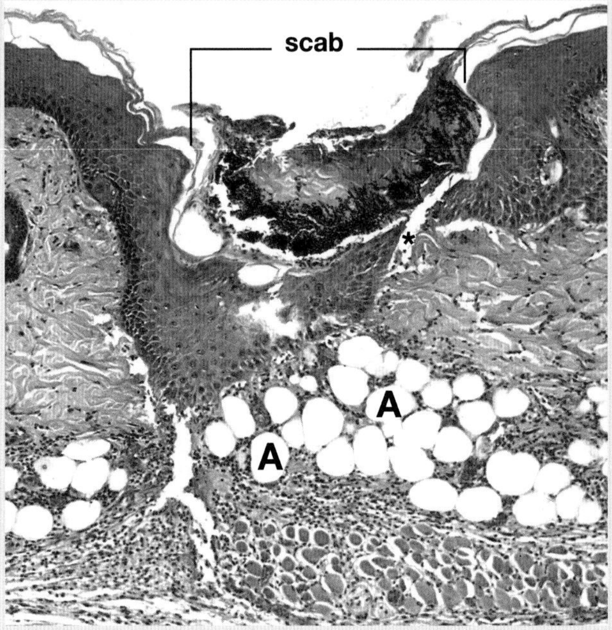

FIGURE F15.7.1. Photomicrograph showing a late stage in the epidermal repair of a skin wound. The initial injury was caused by an incision through the full thickness of the skin and partially into the hypodermis, which contains adipose cells (*A*). The epidermis has re-formed beneath the scab. The *asterisk* marks an artifact where epithelium separated during specimen preparation. The scab, which contains numerous dead neutrophils in its inferior aspect, is close to the point of release. The dermis at this stage shows little change during the repair process but will ultimately reestablish itself to form a continuous layer. ×110.

Hyperhidrosis is a pathologic disorder affecting 0.6%–5% of the population and is characterized by excessive sweat production above the quantity needed for thermoregulation. It can be idiopathic (primary hyperhidrosis) or be a result of another endocrine, neurologic, or infectious disorder. **Primary hyperhidrosis** is characterized by uncontrollable, excessive, and unpredictable sweating, which occurs at rest and is not related to temperature. The symptoms of hyperhidrosis can significantly affect quality of life and lead to social embarrassment, loneliness, anxiety, and depression. Treatment options include topical and oral anticholinergic medications, surgical procedures (i.e., endoscopic thoracic sympathectomy), laser therapy, or botulinum toxin injection.

■ SKIN AGING

Skin aging is influenced by several intrinsic and extrinsic factors, including genetics, environmental exposure, hormonal changes, and metabolic factors, all of which lead to a loss of structural integrity and physiologic function. The complex cellular and biochemical processes of the skin become altered with age and affect the balance between remodeling, regeneration, and repair. Additionally, the protective immune barrier of aged skin is less efficient. On the histologic level, several structural changes are noticeable in aged skin:

- **Keratinocyte atrophy**, which leads to decreased thickness of the epidermal layer of the skin. A thinner epidermis with a flattened interface between the epidermis and dermis makes aged skin less resistant to shearing forces and prone to injuries. In addition, keratinocyte atrophy affects the production of proteins and lipid components of the epidermal water barrier, increasing transepidermal water loss in elderly individuals that increases skin dryness.

- **Diminishment of mononuclear phagocyte system cell activity**, which affects the immunologic response to pathogens. Langerhans cells in the epidermis are reduced in number, and their capacity to migrate to lymph nodes is diminished. Dermal dendritic cells also show changes in the skin aging process. They exhibit impaired migration and phagocytic activity with decreased ability to interact with T cells. A possible decrease in the skin's T-resident memory (T_{rm}) cells may be related to the increased rate of infection seen in elderly individuals.
- **Reduction is the size and activity of dermal fibroblasts**, which adds to age-associated dermal thinning. Dermal fibroblasts from elderly individuals synthesize less procollagen and other structural extracellular matrix proteins. However, they have increased matrix metalloproteinase (MMP) expression that contributes to the remodeling/destruction of the extracellular matrix.
- **Collagen and elastic fibers fragmentation**, which is related to increased activity of MMPs. The total amount of collagen and elastin in the skin is reduced with age. Several MMPs (i.e., MMP-1, MMP-3, and MMP-9) specifically target elastin fibers and are responsible for their fragmentation. This results in reduced skin elasticity, causing wrinkling of aging skin.
- **Reduction in secretion of sweat and sebaceous glands**, which amplifies the effect of skin dryness. Both sweat and sebum contain antimicrobial peptides and lipids that control bacterial growth on the skin surface. Decreased secretion of these compounds affects the immunologic skin barrier in restricting the growth of pathogenic bacteria.
- **Subcutaneous adipose tissue reduction**, which occurs in the hypodermis and superficial fascia. Dermal adipose tissue chronically exposed to UV radiation reduces the number of adipocytes and is accompanied by a decrease in free fatty acids and triglycerides.

The process of skin aging is dependent to a degree on lifestyle choices, genetic factors, and environmental challenges, including UV exposure, tobacco smoking, and environmental pollution. Collectively, these changes render older individuals more susceptible to mechanical injury and infections. It is important to note that high levels of pigmentation in keratinocytes are protective with regard to the cumulative effects of sun UV exposure and skin damage.

INTEGUMENTARY SYSTEM

OVERVIEW OF THE INTEGUMENTARY SYSTEM

- The **integumentary system** consists of skin and its derivatives (epidermal skin appendages).
- The **skin** has two layers: the **epidermis**, a superficial layer that consists mainly of a stratified squamous keratinized epithelium, and the **dermis**, a deeper layer of dense irregular connective tissue.
- Deep to the skin is the **hypodermis**, which contains variable amounts of adipose tissue.

EPIDERMIS

- The **epidermis** is composed primarily of **keratinocytes** (85%) that undergo differentiation to form stratified squamous keratinized epithelium.
- Four distinct layers (strata) of epidermis can be distinguished.
- The **stratum basale** is a single layer of small, mitotically active basal cells that are attached by hemidesmosomes to underlying connective tissue and by desmosomes to each other.
- The **stratum spinosum** contains several layers of larger keratinocytes that are attached to each other by **desmosomes** located at the ends of their cytoplasmic processes containing intermediate filaments (keratin filaments).
- The **stratum granulosum** is a distinct layer of flattened keratinocytes filled with **keratohyalin granules** (contain precursors to **filaggrin**, which aggregates **keratin filaments**) and lamellar bodies containing lipids, which, when secreted, are responsible for the formation of the epidermal **water barrier**.
- The **stratum comeum** is the most superficial layer of terminally differentiated squamous cells (with no nuclei) that are entirely filled with keratin filaments. These cells are constantly desquamating from the skin surface.
- Total epidermal turnover time is approximately **47 days**.

SPECIALIZED CELLS OF THE EPIDERMIS

- **Melanocytes** (5% of cells in epidermis) reside in the stratum basale and have long processes that extend between keratinocytes into the stratum spinosum.
- Melanocytes synthesize **melanin** pigment in **melanosomes** that is then transferred (**pigment donation**) to adjacent keratinocytes. The transferred pigment accumulates above nuclei of keratinocytes to protect nuclear DNA from UV radiation and damage.
- Other cells in the epidermis include **Langerhans cells** (2%–5%), which are the antigen-presenting cells involved in signaling of the immune system, and **Merkel cells** (6%–10%), which are mechanoreceptor cells associated with sensory nerve endings.

DERMIS

- The **dermis** is composed of two layers.
- The **papillary layer** is superficial and consists of loose connective tissue (collagen I and III) that contains extensive plexus of blood, lymphatic vessels, and sensory nerve endings.
- The **reticular layer** is deeper and is composed of dense irregular connective tissue containing type I collagen, elastic fibers, and larger blood vessels.
- The **epidermal–dermal junction** has numerous finger-like connective tissue protrusions called **dermal papillae** that correspond to similar epidermal protrusions (**epidermal ridges**).
- **Dermal papillae** contain nerve endings and a network of blood and lymphatic capillaries.

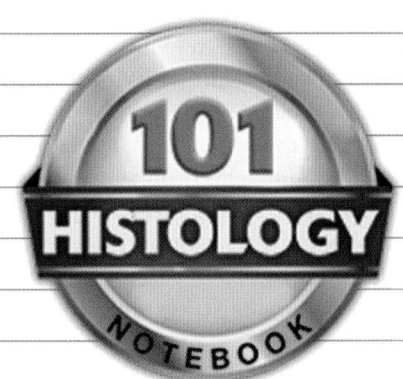

SPECIALIZED CELLS OF THE DERMIS

- **Dermal fibroblasts** have **toll-like receptors (TLRs)** for pathogen recognition; when they encounter pathogens, they produce inflammatory cytokines and initiate an immune response.
- **Dermal dendritic cells** present antigens to the T cells or migrate to the lymph node to initiate an immune response.
- **Resident dermal macrophages** are yolk sac–derived antigen-presenting cells in the dermis that initiate an immune response to foreign substances, tissue damage, and pathogens.
- **Dermal T-resident memory (T_{rm}) cells** are noncirculating memory T cells that provide immunologic memory to initiate a rapid, robust immune response.

SENSORY NERVE RECEPTORS OF THE SKIN

- The epidermis contains **free nerve endings**, which detect fine touch, heat, cold, and pain.
- In addition, **Merkel corpuscle** (Merkel cell with a nerve ending) is a sensitive mechanoreceptor.
- The dermis contains several encapsulated nerve endings, such as **Pacinian corpuscles** to detect pressure and vibrations, **Meissner corpuscles** to detect light touch, and **Ruffini corpuscles** to detect skin stretch and torque.

HAIRS AND NAILS

- **Hairs** and **hair follicles** are present over almost the entire body.
- The **hair follicle** contains a reservoir of epidermal stem cells (**follicular bulge**) that are responsible for differentiation into hair-forming matrix cells.
- **Hair** is formed by the differentiation of **matrix cells** in the **inferior segment** of the hair follicle (**bulb**) to form the medulla, cortex (80% of hair mass), and cuticle of a hair shaft.
- The **hair shaft** is surrounded by the internal and external root sheath. The **internal root sheath** has three layers of cells: **Henle layer, Huxley layer**, and the **internal root sheath cuticle**. The **external root sheath** is continuous with the epidermis.
- **Nails** are plates of keratinized cells resting on **nail beds** containing **hard keratin** that is formed in a nail root at the proximal part of the nail. Keratinocytes proliferate there and differentiate to form hard keratin.
- As the **nail plate** grows, it moves over the nail bed with edges covered by skin folds.

GLANDS OF THE SKIN

- **Sebaceous glands** produce **sebum** that coats the hair and skin surface. Sebum is produced by holocrine secretion by **sebocytes** and is discharged via the pilosebaceous canal into the hair follicle.
- **Apocrine sweat glands** secrete protein-rich sweat into the hair follicles, but they are restricted to specific regions of the body (axillae, perineum).
- Apocrine sweat glands are coiled tubular glands with a wide lumen. Their secretory parts contain **myoepithelial cells**, the contraction of which is responsible for expression of sweat.
- **Eccrine sweat glands** are not related to hair follicles. They produce sweat that is similar in composition to an ultrafiltrate of blood in the kidney.
- Eccrine sweat glands play a major role in **temperature regulation** through the cooling that results from the evaporation of water from sweat on the body surface. Their secretory parts also contain **myoepithelial cells.**

PLATE 15.1 ■ SKIN I

The **skin**, or integument, consists of two main layers: the **epidermis**, composed of stratified squamous epithelium that is keratinized, and the **dermis**, composed of connective tissue. Under the dermis is a layer of loose connective tissue called the **hypodermis**, which is also generally referred to as the **subcutaneous tissue** or, by gross anatomists, as the superficial fascia. Typically, the hypodermis contains large amounts of adipose tissue, particularly in an adequately nourished individual.

The epidermis gives rise to nails, hairs, sebaceous glands, and sweat glands. On the palms of the hands and soles of the feet, the epidermis has an outer keratinized layer that is substantially thicker than that over other parts of the body. Accordingly, the skin over the palms and soles is referred to as **thick skin**, in contrast to the skin over other parts of the body, which is referred to as **thin skin.**

There are no hairs in thick skin. In addition, the interface between the epidermis and the dermis is more complex in thick skin than in thin skin. The finger-like projections of the dermis into the base of the epidermis, the **dermal papillae**, are much longer and more closely spaced in thick skin. This provides greater resistance to frictional forces acting on this skin.

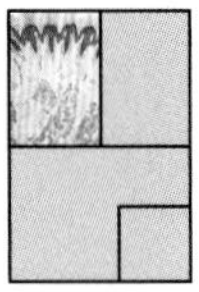

Thick skin, human, hematoxylin and eosin (H&E) ×45.

In this sample of thick skin, the **epidermis** (*Ep*) is at the top; the remainder of the field consists of dermis, in which a large number of **sweat glands** (*SW*) can be observed. Although the layers of the epidermis are examined more advantageously at higher magnification, it is easy to see, even at this relatively low magnification, that about half of the thickness of the epidermis consists of a distinctive surface layer that stains more lightly than the remainder of the epidermis. This is the keratinized layer. The dome-shaped surface contours represent a cross section through the minute dermal ridges on the surface of thick skin that produce the characteristic fingerprints of an individual.

In addition to sweat glands, the dermis displays blood vessels (*BV*) and adipose tissue (*AT*). The ducts of the sweat glands (*D*) extend from the glands to the epidermis. One of the ducts is shown as it enters the epidermis at the bottom of an epithelial ridge. It will pass through the epidermis in a spiral course to open onto the skin surface.

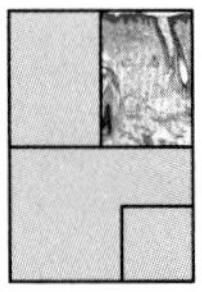

Thin skin, human, H&E ×60.

A sample of thin skin is shown here to compare with the thick skin in the above figure. Note a very thin keratinized layer of epidermis (*Ep*) in comparison to thick skin. In addition to sweat glands, thin skin contains hair follicles (*HF*) and their associated **sebaceous glands** (*SGl*). Each sebaceous gland opens into a hair follicle. Often, as in this tissue sample, the hair follicles and the glands, both sebaceous and sweat, extend beyond the dermis (*De*) and into the hypodermis. Note the blood vessels (*BV*) and adipose tissue (*AT*) in the hypodermis.

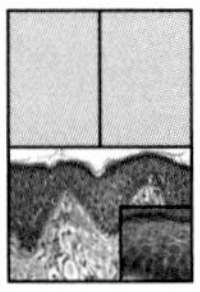

Epidermis, skin, human, H&E ×320; inset ×640.

The layers of the **epidermis of thin skin** are shown here at higher magnification. The cell layer that occupies the deepest location is the **stratum basale** (*SB*). This is one cell deep. Just above this is a layer several cells in thickness, the **stratum spinosum** (*SS*). It consists of cells that have spinous processes on their surface. These processes meet with spinous processes of neighboring cells and, together, appear as intercellular bridges (*arrows, inset*). The next layer is the **stratum granulosum** (*SGr*), whose cells contain keratohyalin granules (*arrowhead, inset*). On the surface is the **stratum corneum** (*SC*). This consists of keratinized cells, that is, cells that no longer possess nuclei. The keratinized cells are flat and generally adhere to other cells above and below without evidence of cell boundaries. In thick skin, a fifth layer, the **stratum lucidum**, is seen between the stratum granulosum and the stratum corneum. The pigment in the cells of the stratum basale is melanin; some of this pigment (*P*) is also present in connective tissue cells of the dermis. Note blood vessels (*BV*) extending into dermal papillae.

AT, adipose tissue
BV, blood vessels
D, duct of sweat glands
De, dermis
Ep, epidermis
HF, hair follicle
P, pigment
SB, stratum basale
SC, stratum corneum
SGl, sebaceous gland
SGr, stratum granulosum
SS, stratum spinosum
SW, sweat gland
arrowhead, granules in cell of stratum granulosum
arrows, intercellular bridges

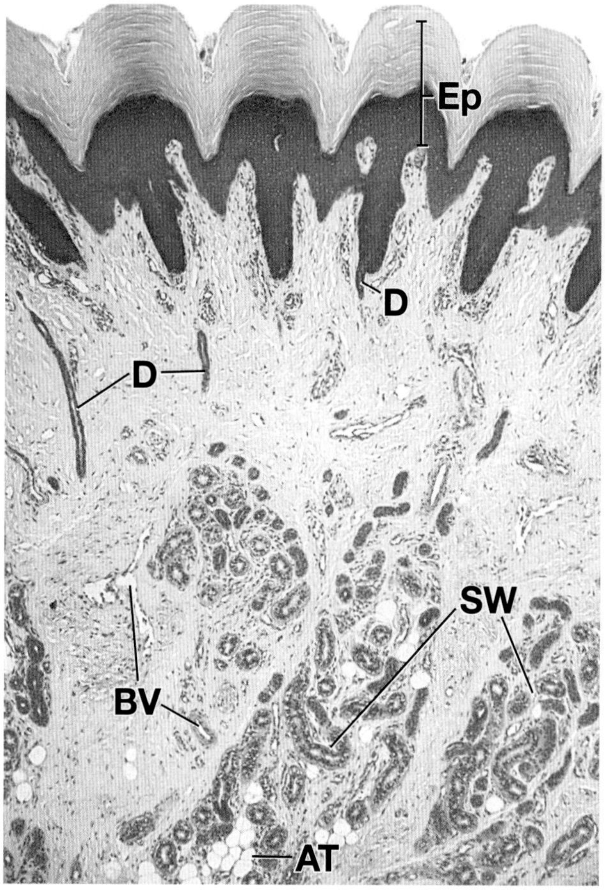
Ep
D
D
BV
SW
AT

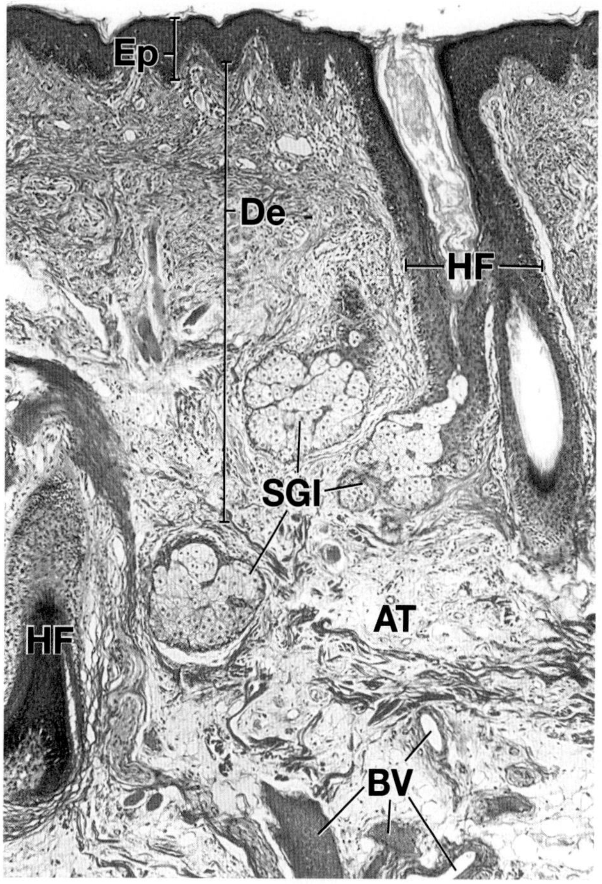
Ep
De
HF
SGl
HF
AT
BV

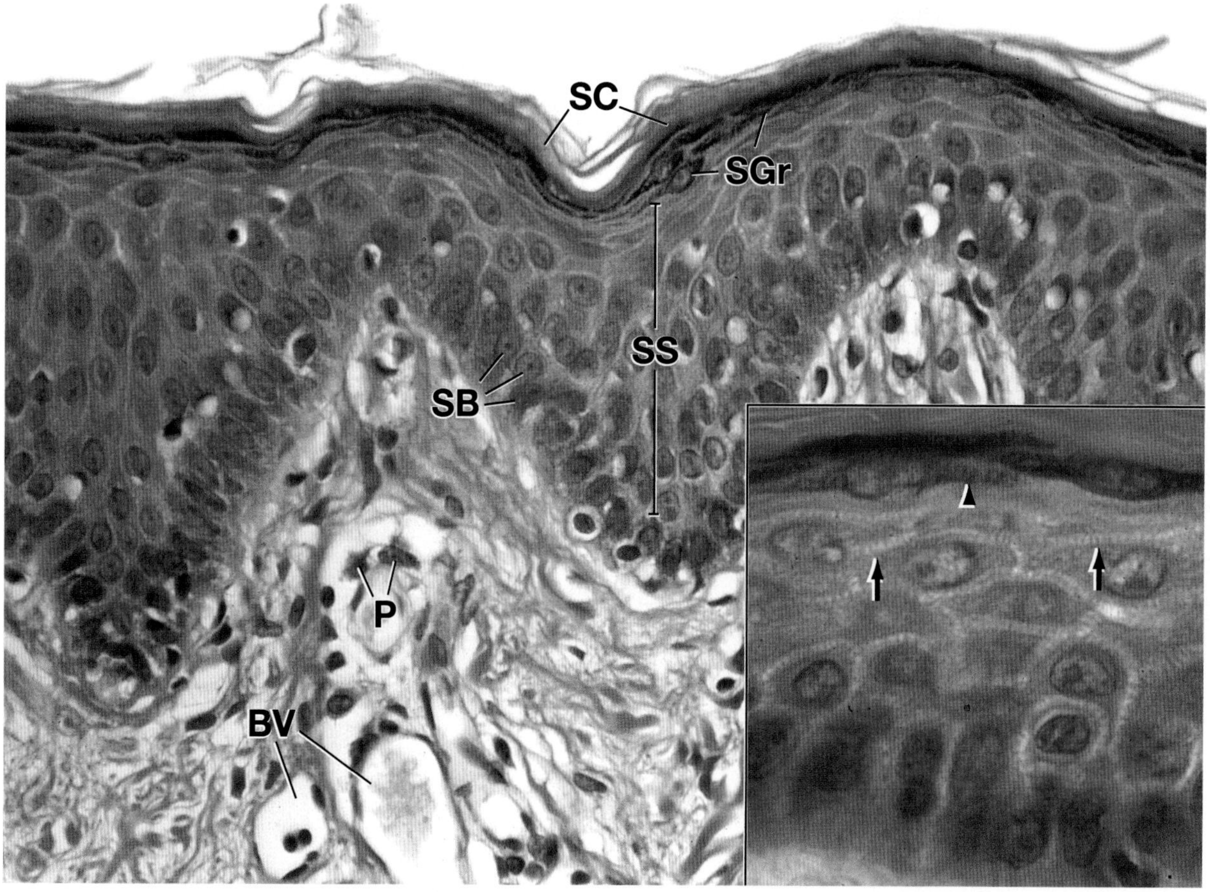
SC
SGr
SS
SB
P
BV

The **epidermis** contains four distinctive cell types: **keratinocytes, melanocytes, Langerhans cells,** and **Merkel cells**. Keratinocytes are the most numerous of these cells; they are generated in the **stratum basale** and move toward the surface. As they do so, they produce the intracellular protein **keratin** and the special extracellular lipid that serves as a water barrier in the upper layers of the epidermis. Histologically, the keratinocytes are the cells that show spinous processes in the **stratum spinosum**. The other three cell types are not readily identified in hematoxylin and eosin (H&E)-stained paraffin sections. The product of the melanocyte is, however, evident in H&E sections, and this is considered in the first two figures of this plate.

The skin contains a pigment, **melanin**, which protects the tissue against the harmful effects of ultraviolet light. It is formed by the melanocytes that then pass the pigment to the keratinocytes. More pigment is present in dark skin than in light skin; this can be seen by comparing light skin (*top figure*) and dark skin (*middle figure*). The epidermis and a small amount of the dermis are shown in each figure. Whereas the deep part of the dark skin contains considerable pigment, the amount of pigment in light skin is insufficient to be noticeable at this magnification. Cells for producing the pigment are present in both skin types and in approximately equal numbers. The difference is due to more rapid digestion of the pigment by lysosomes of keratinocytes in light skin. After prolonged exposure to sunlight, pigment is also produced in sufficient amounts to be seen in light skin.

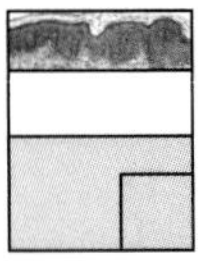

Light skin, human, H&E ×300.

In routine H&E-stained paraffin sections of light skin, such as this sample, the **melanocytes** are among the cells that appear as small, rounded, clear cells (*CC*) mixed with the other cells of the stratum basale. However, not all clear cells of the epidermis are melanocytes. For example, Langerhans cells may also appear as clear cells, but they are located more superficially in the stratum spinosum. Merkel cells may also appear as clear cells, thus making it difficult to identify these three cell types with certainty.

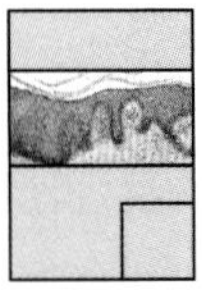

Dark skin, human, H&E ×300.

In dark skin, most of the pigment is in the basal portion of the epidermis, but it is also present in cells progressing toward the surface and within the nonnucleated cells of the keratinized layer. The *arrows* indicate the **melanin pigment** in keratinocytes of the stratum spinosum and in the stratum corneum. In light skin, the melanin is broken down before it leaves the upper part of the stratum spinosum. Thus, pigment is not seen in the upper layers of the epidermis.

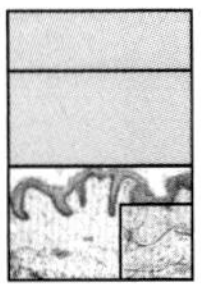

Dermis, skin, human, H&E and elastin stain ×200; inset ×450.

This figure is included because it shows certain features of the dermis, the connective tissue layer of the skin. The dermis is divided into two layers: the **papillary layer** (*PL*) of loose connective tissue and the reticular layer (*RL*) of denser connective tissue. The papillary layer is immediately under the epidermis. It includes the connective tissue papillae that project into the undersurface of the epidermis. The **reticular layer** is deep to the papillary layer. The boundary between these two layers is not demarcated by any specific structural feature except for the change in the histologic composition of the two layers.

This specimen was stained with H&E and also with a procedure to display elastic fibers (*EF*). They are relatively thick and conspicuous in the reticular layer (see also *inset*), where they appear as dark-blue profiles, some of which are elongate, whereas others are short. In the papillary layer, the elastic fibers are thinner and relatively sparse (*arrows*). The *inset* shows the typical eosinophilic staining of the thick collagenous fibers in the reticular layer. Although the collagenous fibers at the lower magnification of this figure are not as prominent, it is nevertheless possible to note that they are thicker in the reticular layer than in the papillary layer. The papillary layer is evidently more cellular than the reticular layer. Many of the small dark-blue profiles in the reticular layer represent oblique and cross sections through elastic fibers (see *inset*) and not nuclei of cells.

CC, clear cells
EF, elastic fibers
PL, papillary layer
RL, reticular layer
arrows, middle figure, pigment in different layers of epidermis; lower figure, delicate elastic fibers

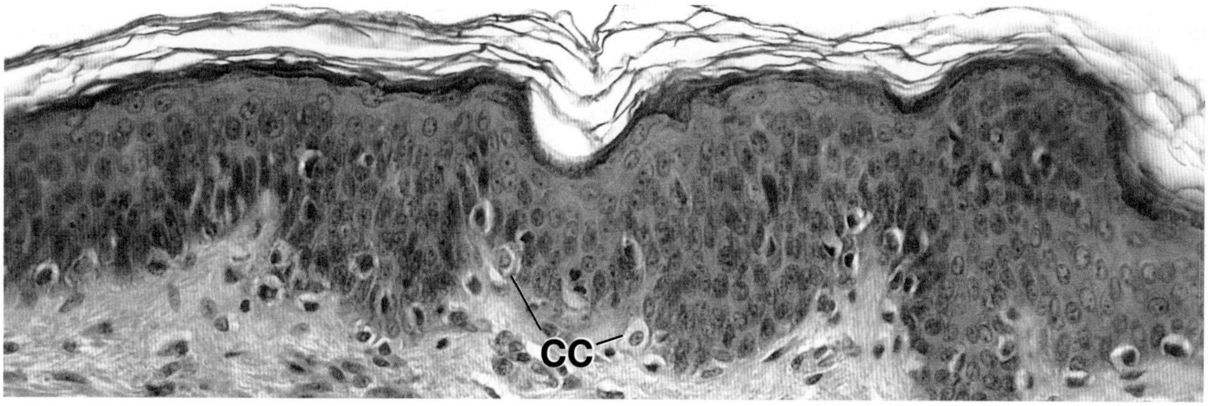
CC

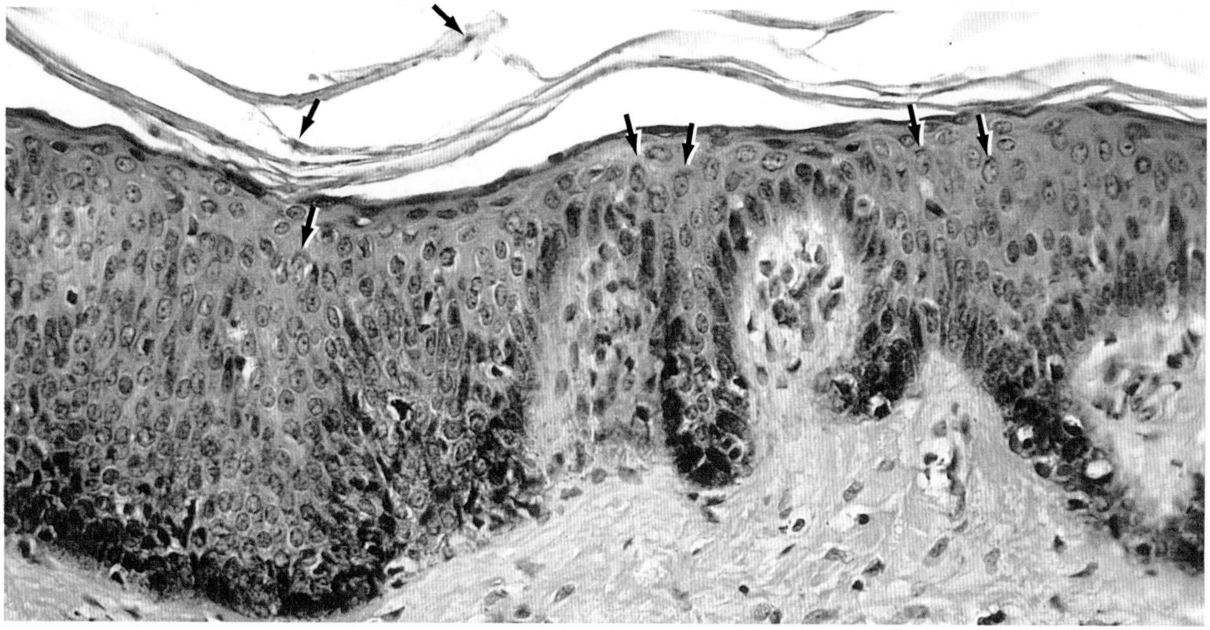

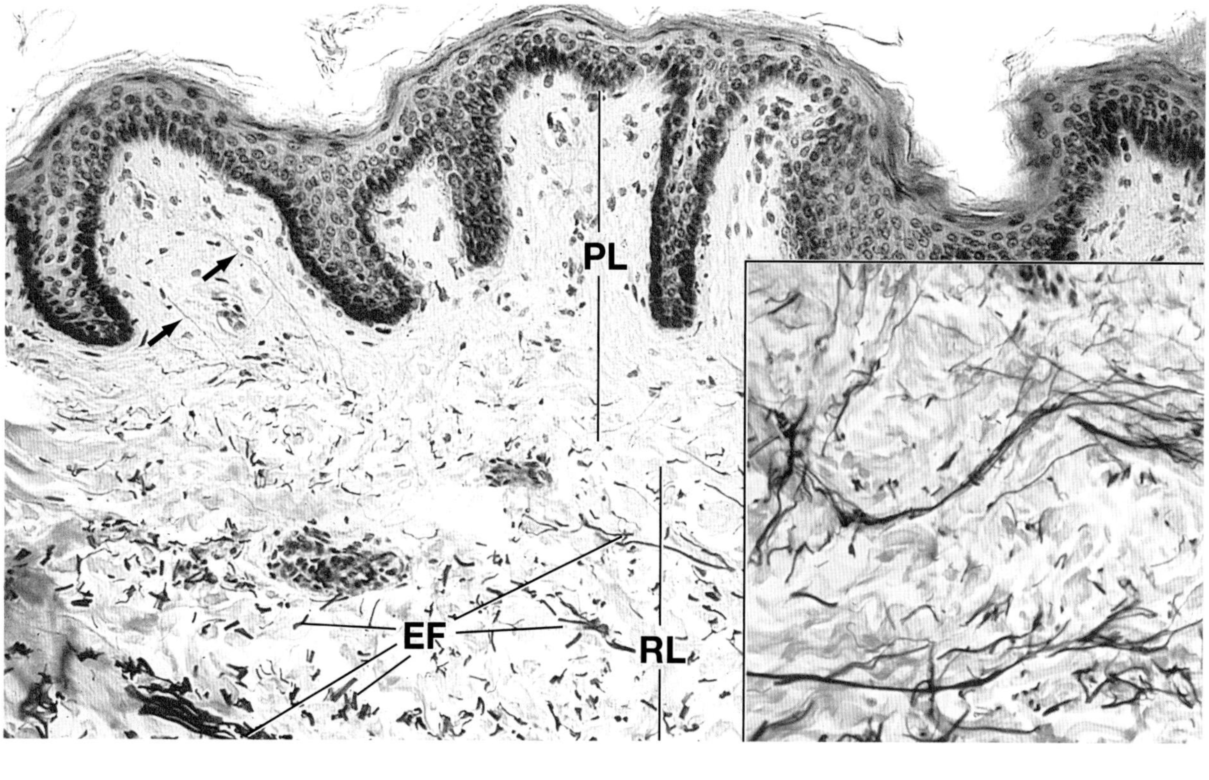
PL
EF
RL

PLATE 15.3 ■ APOCRINE AND ECCRINE SWEAT GLANDS

Skin possesses three types of glands: **eccrine**, **apocrine**, and **sebaceous**. Eccrine sweat glands are distributed over the entire body surface except for the lips, glans penis, prepuce, clitoris, and labia minora. They are especially numerous in the thick skin of the hands and feet. Evaporation of the secreted sweat on the skin surface cools the body.

Apocrine sweat glands are localized in the axilla, areolae, perineal and perianal area, prepuce, scrotum, mons pubis, and labia majora. Many of the epithelial cells in the secretory segment of these glands exhibit an apical bleb-like protrusion that was earlier thought to represent their mode of secretion (i.e., pinching off of the bleb as the secretory product, thus the name apocrine). It is now known that secretion occurs as a merocrine process. The secretion is a clear, viscous product that becomes odiferous through the action of resident microbes on the skin surface. In the human, its role is unclear, but it is generally believed that the secretion may act as a sex attractant (pheromone). Apocrine glands are present at birth but do not fully develop and become functional until puberty. In the female, these glands undergo changes that parallel the menstrual cycle.

ORIENTATION MICROGRAPH: The adjacent orientation micrograph of the skin of the axilla shows both the large, branched tubular apocrine glands (*A*) and the smaller, simple tubular eccrine glands (*E*) in the hypodermis (*H*). Also evident is a tangentially cut hair follicle (*HF*). The overlying dermis (*D*) consists of dense connective tissue and includes part of a sebaceous gland (*SG*).

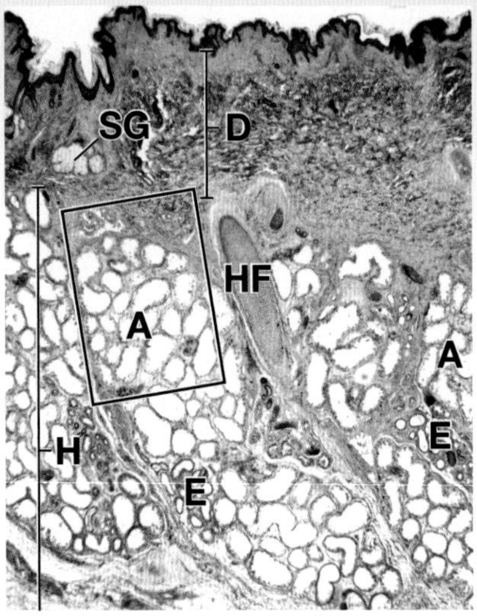

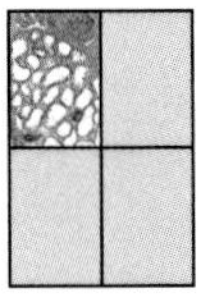

Apocrine sweat gland, skin, human, hematoxylin and eosin (H&E) ×33.

Low-power micrograph showing the secretory segment of an **apocrine sweat gland**. The sectioned profiles seen here represent several coiled branches of a single gland surrounded by dense connective tissue (*DCT*). In the *upper part* of this image are two **sweat glands** (*SwG*) also surrounded by dense connective tissue. Note the considerable difference in diameter and lumen size of the two types of glands.

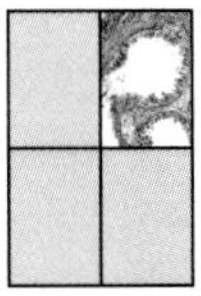

Apocrine sweat gland, skin, human, H&E ×256.

The epithelium (*Ep*) of the **apocrine sweat gland** from the *boxed area to the left* is simple columnar. The individual cells vary in height, and some show bleb-like protrusions (*B*). At the base of the epithelium are the spindle-shaped myoepithelial cells. In some regions of the tubule, these cells have been cut longitudinally and thus appear as a deeply stained eosin band (*EB*). At other sites, the cells have been sectioned tangentially and appear as a series of parallel linear profiles (*MyC*).

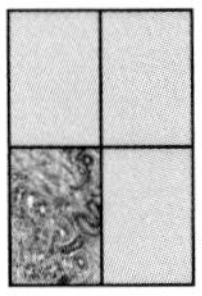

Eccrine sweat gland, skin, human, H&E ×256.

In this micrograph, the **eccrine sweat gland** from above is seen at higher magnification. Both secretory and duct segments are present. The **secretory segment** (*SS*) has a wider diameter and larger lumen than the duct segment (*DS*). The epithelium of the secretory segment is simple columnar; the **duct segment** is two cell layers thick, namely, stratified cuboidal. Also, the secretory segment possesses a myoepithelial component.

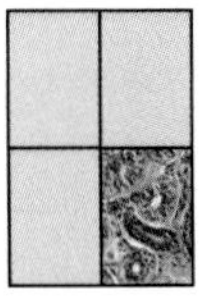

Eccrine sweat gland, skin, human, H&E ×512.

At this very high magnification, two cross-sectioned profiles of the secretory segment (*SS*) and one profile of the duct segment (*DS*) from the *boxed area to the left* are shown. When the tubule wall of the secretory segment is cut in a perpendicular plane, the simple columnar nature of the epithelium (*Ep*) is evident. Because the tubule is so tortuous, more often the epithelium appears to be multilayered. The **myoepithelial cells** of the secretory segment appear here both as a circumferential band (*CB*) and in a cross-sectioned array (*CA*) in which they resemble the teeth of a saw blade. Occasionally, myoepithelial cell nuclei (*MyN*) are present. Such profiles give the appearance of a pseudostratified epithelium. The duct segment (*DS*) lacks the myoepithelium and also differs in that it is stratified cuboidal. See next plate.

A, apocrine gland
B, bleb-like protrusions
CA, cross-sectioned array
CB, circumferential band
D, dermis
DCT, dense connective tissue
DS, duct segment
E, eccrine gland
EB, eosin band
Ep, epithelium
H, hypodermis
HF, hair follicle
MyC, linear profiles of myoepithelial cells
MyN, myoepithelial cell nuclei
SG, sebaceous gland
SS, secretory segment
SwG, sweat glands

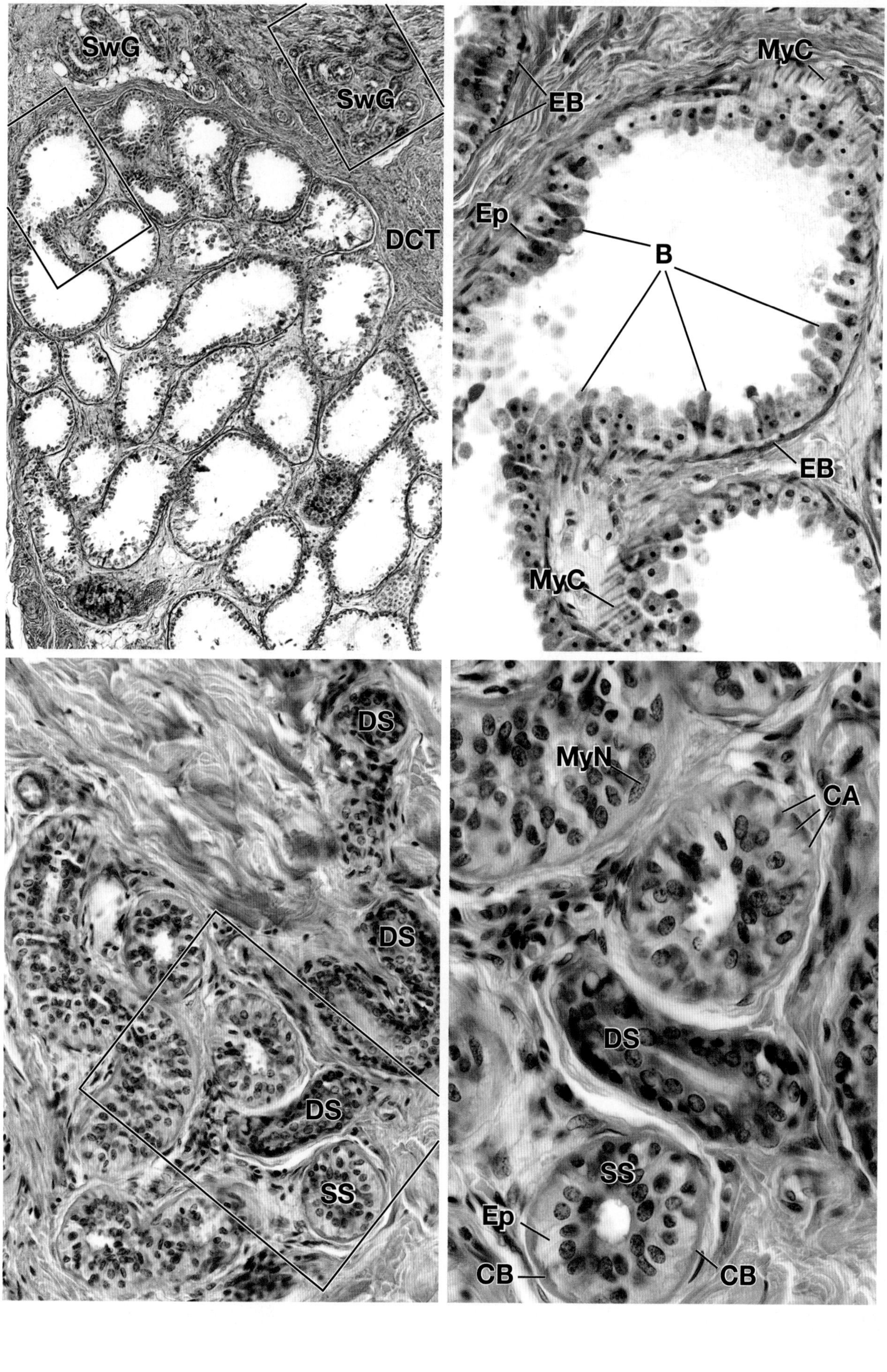
SwG
SwG
DCT
MyC
EB
Ep
B
EB
MyC
DS
DS
DS
SS
MyN
CA
DS
SS
Ep
CB
CB

PLATE 15.4 ■ SWEAT AND SEBACEOUS GLANDS

Normally, the body loses ~600 mL of water a day through evaporation from the lungs and skin. Under conditions of high ambient temperature, water loss is increased by an increased rate of sweating. This *thermoregulatory sweating* first occurs on the forehead and scalp, extends to the face and the rest of the body, and occurs last on the palms and soles. *Emotional sweating,* however, occurs first on the palms and soles and in the axillae. Sweating is under both nervous control through the autonomic nervous system and hormonal control.

Sebaceous glands secrete sebum, an oily substance that coats the hair and skin surface. Sebaceous secretion is a *holocrine* secretion; the entire cell produces, and becomes filled with, the fatty secretory product while it simultaneously undergoes progressive disruption, followed by apoptosis, as the product fills the cell. Both secretory product and cell debris are discharged into the **pilosebaceous canal**.

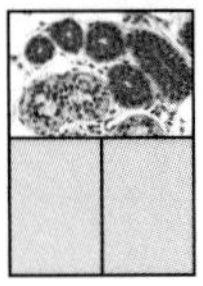

Sweat gland, skin, human, hematoxylin and eosin (H&E) ×1,000.

This section through a **sweat gland** shows five profiles of the ductal portion (*D*) and two profiles of the secretory portion (*SG*). The larger secretory segment is through a region either just below or above where a U turn was made; therefore, it shows two luminal profiles. The lumina of both the ductal and the secretory units are marked by *asterisks*.

The **glandular unit** of the eccrine sweat gland contains two epithelial cell types and myoepithelial cells (*M*). *Arrowheads* show small cross sections of myoepithelial cell cytoplasm; *large arrows* show where more elongate profiles of myoepithelial cytoplasm are evident. The epithelial cells are of two types, designated dark cells and clear cells. Unfortunately, the characteristic dark cytoplasmic staining of the dark cells is not evident unless special precautions are taken to preserve the secretory granules in their apical cytoplasm. Nevertheless, note that the dark cells are closer to the lumen, whereas the clear cells are closer to the base of the epithelial layer, making contact with either the basal lamina or, more frequently, the myoepithelial cells. In addition, the clear cells are in contact with intercellular canaliculi. Several such intercellular canaliculi are shown in the secretory units (*small arrows*). This figure also shows that the duct consists of two layers of small cuboidal cells.

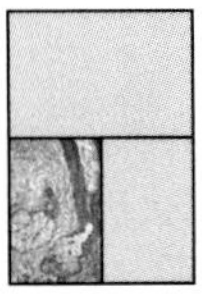

Sebaceous gland, skin, human, H&E ×160.

Sebaceous glands develop from the epithelial cells of the hair follicle and discharge their secretion into the follicle, from where it reaches the skin surface. The sebaceous secretion is rich in lipid, and this is reflected in the cells of the sebaceous gland. A section of a sebaceous gland and its related hair follicle is shown in this figure. At this level, the hair follicle consists of the external root sheath (*RS*) surrounding the hair shaft. The **sebaceous gland** (*Seb*) appears as a cluster of cells known as **sebocytes**, most of which display a washed-out or finely reticulated cytoplasm. This is because these cells contain numerous lipid droplets and the lipid is lost by dissolution in fat solvents during the routine preparation of the H&E-stained paraffin section. The opening of the sebaceous gland through the external root sheath (*eRS*) and into the hair follicle is shown in the *lower right*.

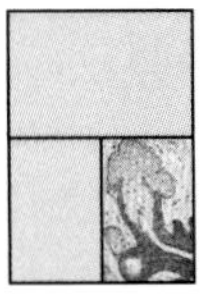

Sebaceous gland, skin, human, H&E ×280.

The **sebaceous gland** and **pilosebaceous canal** are shown here at higher magnification. *Numbers 1 to 4* show a series of sebocytes filled with an increasingly greater amount of lipid and progressively closer to the opening of the pilosebaceous canal (*PSC*) as it enters into the hair follicle. The sebaceous secretion includes the entire cell, and therefore, sebocytes need to be replaced constantly in the functional gland. Cells at the periphery of the gland are basal cells (*BC*). Dividing cells in the basal layer replace those that are lost with the secretion.

BC, basal cells
CT, connective tissue
D, duct of eccrine sweat gland
eRS, junction between sebaceous gland and external root sheath
M, myoepithelial cell
PSC, pilosebaceous canal
RS, external root sheath of hair follicle
Seb, sebaceous gland
SG, secretory component of eccrine sweat gland
arrowheads, myoepithelial cell cytoplasm (cross section)
asterisks, lumina of glands and ducts
large arrows, myoepithelial cell cytoplasm (longitudinal section)
numbers 1 to 4 (lower right image), see text
small arrows, intercellular canaliculi

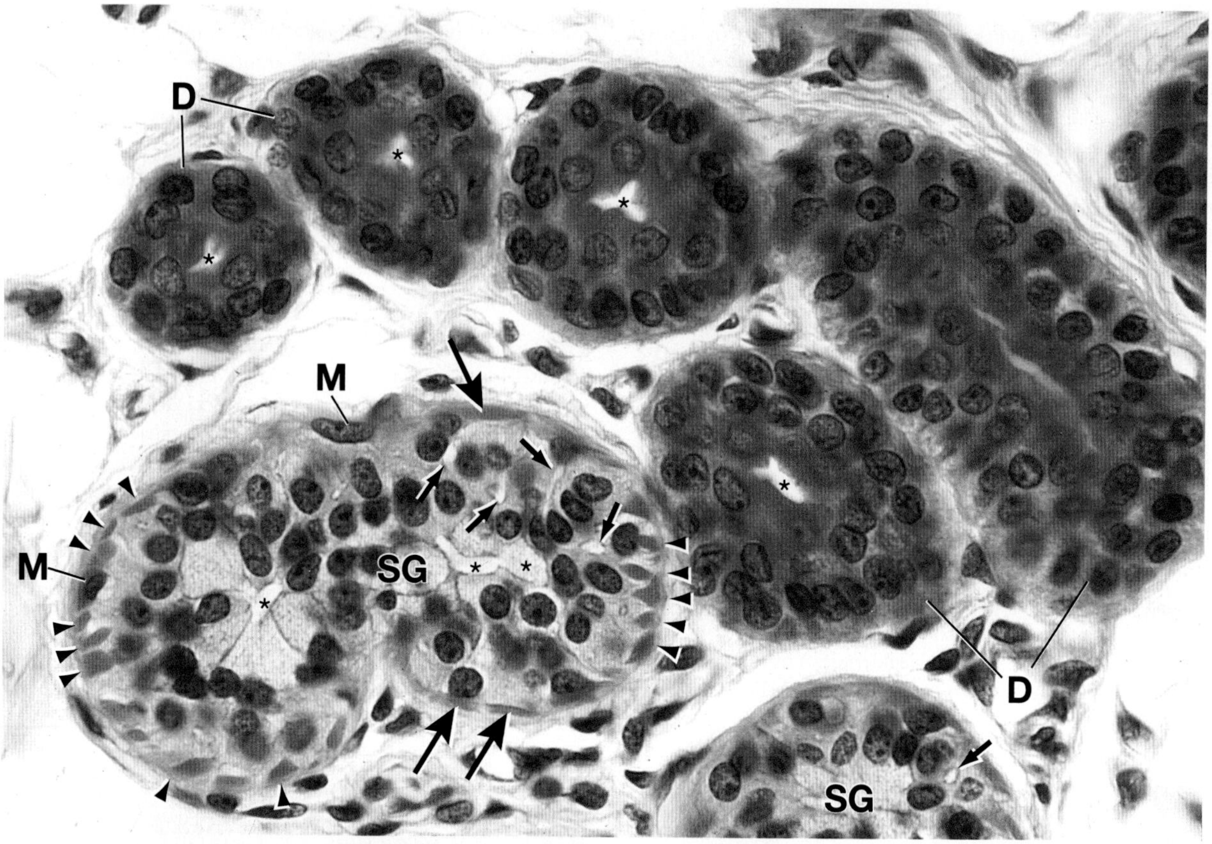
D
M
M
SG
D
SG

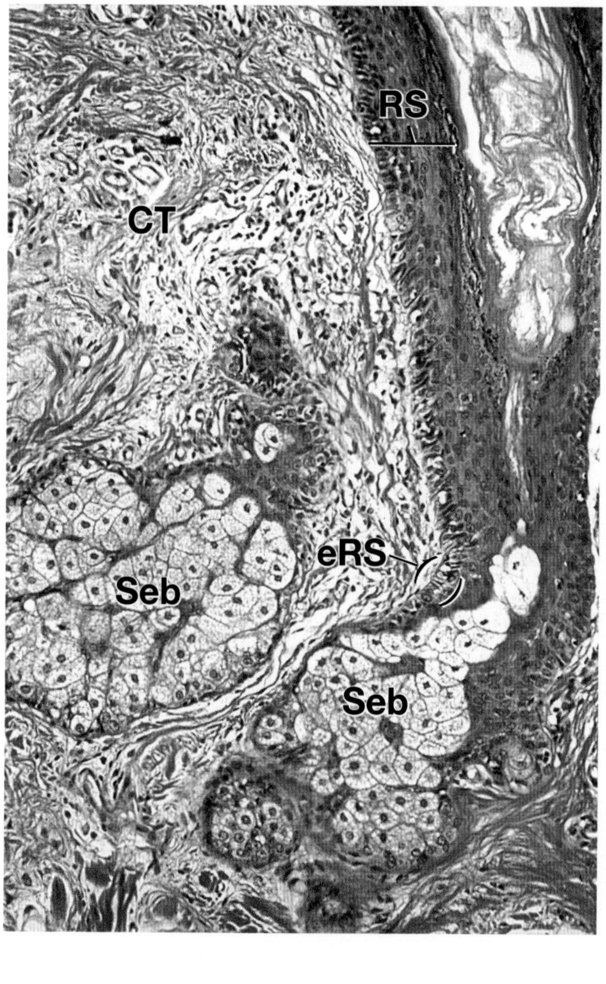
RS
CT
eRS
Seb
Seb

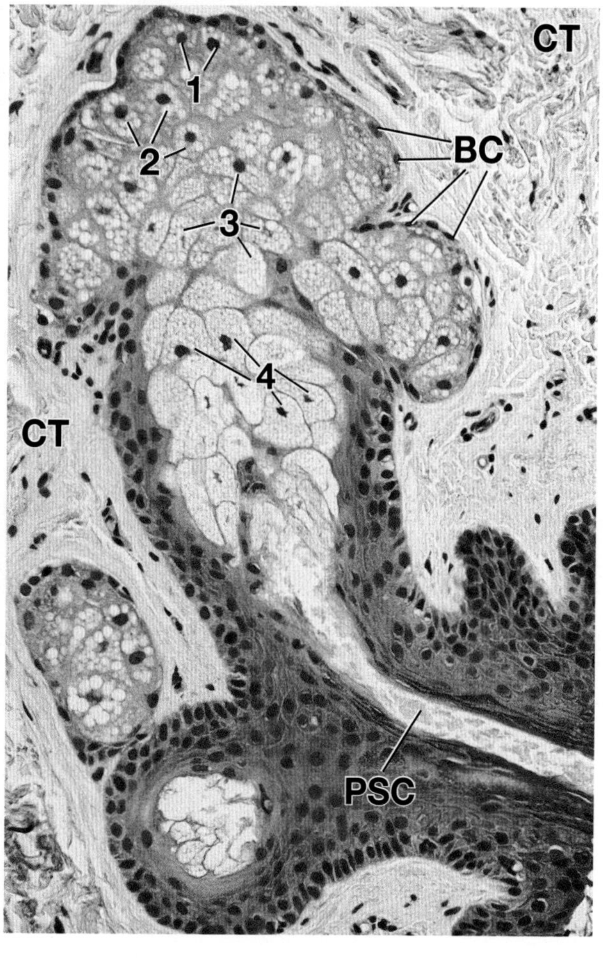
CT
1
2
BC
3
4
CT
PSC

PLATE 15.5 ■ INTEGUMENT AND SENSORY ORGANS

The **skin** is endowed with numerous **sensory receptors** of various types. These are the peripheral terminals of sensory nerves whose cell bodies are in the dorsal root ganglia. The receptors in the skin are described as **free nerve endings** and **encapsulated nerve endings**. Free nerve endings are the most numerous. They subserve fine touch, heat, and cold and are found in the basal layers of the epidermis and as a network around the root sheath of hair follicles. Encapsulated nerve endings include **Pacinian corpuscles** (deep pressure and vibration), **Meissner corpuscles** (touch, especially in the lips and thick skin of fingers and toes), and **Ruffini corpuscles** (sustained mechanical stress on the dermis).

Motor endings of the autonomic nervous system supply the blood vessels, the arrector pili muscles, and the apocrine and eccrine sweat glands.

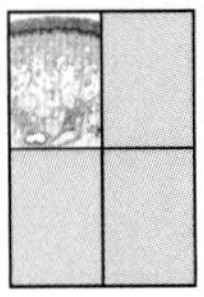

Skin, fingertip, human, hematoxylin and eosin (H&E) ×20.

This specimen is a section of thick skin from the fingertip, showing the **epidermis** (*Ep*) and the **dermis** (*De*) and, under the skin, a portion of the **hypodermis** (*Hy*). The thickness of the epidermis is largely due to the thickness of the stratum corneum. This layer is more lightly stained than the deeper portions of the epidermis. Note, even at this low magnification, the thick collagenous fibers in the reticular layer of the dermis. **Sweat glands** (*SG*) are present in the upper part of the hypodermis, and several sweat ducts (*D*) are seen passing through the epidermis. A feature of this specimen is that it depicts those sensory receptors that can be recognized in a routine low-power H&E-stained paraffin section. They are Meissner corpuscles and Pacinian corpuscles (*PC*). Several nerve bundles (*N*) are seen in proximity to the Pacinian corpuscles. Meissner corpuscles are in the upper part of the dermis, in the dermal papillae immediately under the epidermis. These corpuscles are small and difficult to identify at this low magnification; however, their location is characteristic. Knowing where they are located is a major step in finding Meissner corpuscles in a tissue section; they are shown at higher magnification in the figure below.

Pacinian corpuscles are seen in the lower part of the hypodermis. These corpuscles are large, slightly oval structures, and even at low magnification, a layered or lamellated pattern can be discerned.

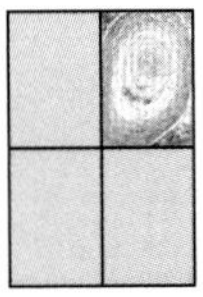

Pacinian corpuscle, skin, human, H&E ×320.

At this higher magnification, the concentric layers or lamellae of the **Pacinian corpuscle** can be seen to be due to flat cells. These are fibroblast-like cells, and although not evident within the tissue section, these cells are continuous with the perineurium of the nerve fiber. The space between the cellular lamellae contains mostly fluid. The neural portion of the Pacinian corpuscle travels longitudinally through the center of the corpuscle. In this specimen, the corpuscle has been cross-sectioned; an *arrowhead* points to the centrally located nerve fiber.

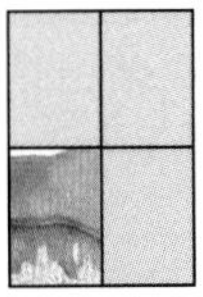

Meissner's corpuscle, skin, human, H&E ×190.

This high-magnification micrograph shows portions of the *upper left* field of the figure above in which two **Meissner corpuscles** (*MC*) are in direct proximity to the undersurface of the epidermis in adjacent dermal papillae. The section shows the long axis of the corpuscles. A Meissner corpuscle consists of an axon (sometimes two) taking a zigzag or flat spiral course from one pole of the corpuscle to the other. The nerve fiber terminates at the superficial pole of the corpuscle. Consequently, as seen here, the nerve fibers and supporting cells are oriented approximately at right angles to the long axis of the corpuscle. Meissner corpuscles are particularly numerous near the tips of the fingers and toes.

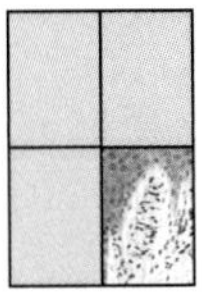

Meissner corpuscle, skin, human, H&E ×550.

At the even higher magnification of this figure, the close apposition of **Meissner corpuscle** to the undersurface of the epidermis is well demonstrated throughout the entire area of the dermal papilla. The flat spiral path of the nerve fiber (not seen) and its supporting cells is evident here, as is the fibrous capsule (*FC*) that surrounds the ending.

D, ducts of sweat glands
De, dermis
Ep, epidermis
FC, fibrous capsule
Hy, hypodermis
MC, Meissner corpuscles
N, nerve bundles
PC, Pacinian corpuscles
SG, sweat glands
arrowhead, nerve fiber in the center of Pacinian corpuscle

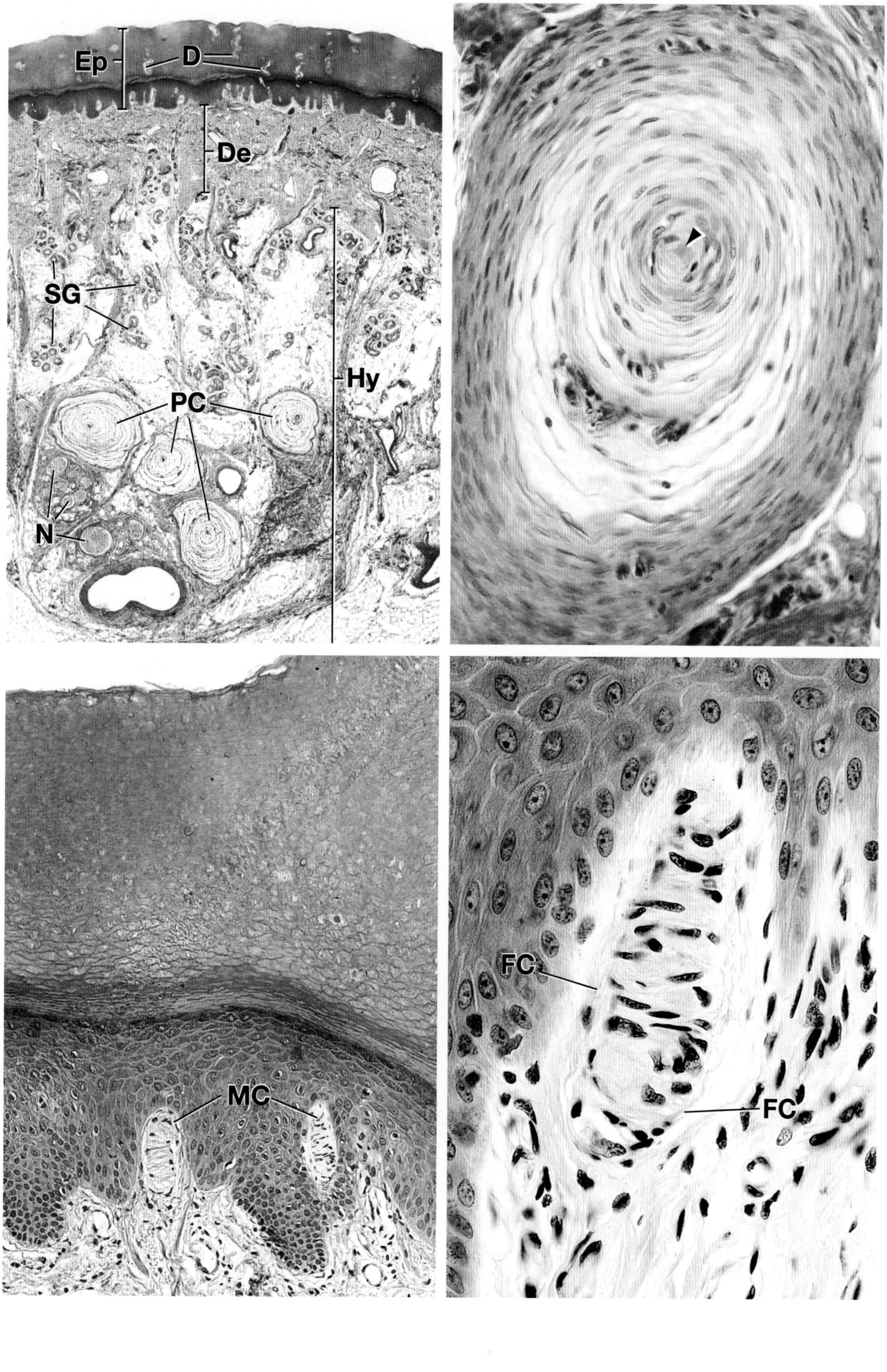
Ep
D
De
SG
Hy
PC
N
MC
FC
FC

PLATE 15.6 ■ HAIR FOLLICLE AND NAIL

Hairs are composed of keratinized cells that develop from hair follicles. Hairs are present over almost the entire body, being conspicuously absent only from the sides and palmar surfaces of the hands, from the sides and plantar surfaces of the feet, from the lips, and from the skin around the urogenital orifices. Coloration of the hair is due to the content and type of melanin that it contains. The follicle varies in appearance, depending on whether it is in a growing or a resting phase; the growing follicle is the more elaborate.

The **skin appendages** (adnexa), especially hair follicles and sweat glands, are particularly important in healing of skin wounds. They serve as the source of new epithelial cells when there is extensive loss of epidermis, as in deep abrasions and second-degree burns.

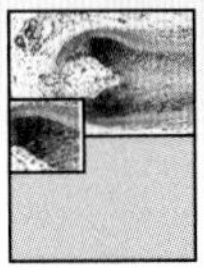

Hair follicle, skin, human, hematoxylin and eosin (H&E) ×300; inset ×440.

The growing end of a **hair follicle** consists of an expanded bulb of epithelial cells that is invaginated by a dermal papilla (*DP*) of connective tissue. The epithelial cells surrounding the papilla at the very tip of the follicle are not yet specialized; they constitute the **hair matrix** (*HM*), the region of the hair follicle where cell division occurs. As the cells leave the matrix, they form cell layers that will become the shaft of the hair and the internal and external root sheaths of the hair follicle.

The cells that will develop into the **shaft of the hair** are seen just to the right of the expanded bulb. They constitute the cortex (*C*), medulla (*M*), and cuticle (*asterisks*) of the hair. The cells of the cortex become keratinized. This layer will come to constitute most of the hair shaft as a thick cylinder. The medulla forms the centrally located axis of the hair shaft; it does not always extend through the entire length of the hair and is absent from some hairs. The cuticle consists of overlapping cells that ultimately lose their nuclei and become filled with keratin. The cuticle covers the hair shaft like a layer of overlapping shingles.

The **root sheath** (*RS*) has two parts: the external root sheath, which is continuous with the epidermis of the skin, and the internal root sheath, which extends only as far as the level at which sebaceous glands enter the hair follicle. The internal root sheath is further divided into three layers: Henle layer, Huxley layer, and the cuticle of the internal root sheath. These layers are seen in the growing hair follicle and are shown at higher magnification in the *inset* with *numbers 1 to 5*: *1*, cells of the external root sheath; *2*, Henle layer; *3*, Huxley layer; *4*, cuticle of the internal root sheath; and *5*, future cuticle of the hair.

Note that many of the cells in the hair matrix (*HM*) of the growing hair follicle contain melanin produced by melanocytes. The melanin, which is transferred to the cells forming cortex and medulla of the hair shaft, contributes to the color of the hair. Most of this pigment is inside the cell (*inset*); however, in very dark hair, some pigment is also extracellular.

The connective tissue surrounding the hair follicle forms a distinct layer referred to as the *sheath*, or *dermal sheath* (*DS*), of the hair follicle.

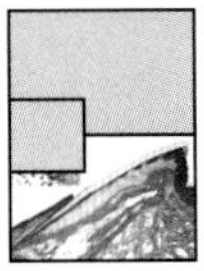

Nail, skin, human, H&E ×12.

A **nail** is a keratinized plate located on the dorsal aspect of the distal phalanges. A section through a nail plate is shown here. The **nail** itself (*N*) is difficult to stain. Under the free edge of the nail is a boundary layer, the **hyponychium** (*Hypon*), which is continuous with the stratum corneum of the adjacent epidermis. The proximal end of the nail is overlapped by skin; here, the junctional region is called the **eponychium** (*Epon*) and is also continuous with the stratum corneum of the adjacent epidermis. Under the nail is a layer of epithelium, the proximal portion of which is referred to as the **nail matrix** (*NM*). The cells of the nail matrix function in the growth of the nail. Together, the epithelium under the nail and the underlying dermis (*D*) constitute the nail bed. The proximal portion of the nail, covered by the fold of the skin, is the root of the nail (*NR*).

The relationship of the nail to other structures in the fingertip is also shown in this figure. The bone (*B*) in the specimen represents a distal phalanx. Note that in this bone, there is an epiphyseal growth plate (*EP*) at the proximal extremity of the bone but not at the distal extremity. Numerous Pacinian corpuscles (*PC*) are present in the connective tissue of the palmar side of the finger. Also seen to advantage in this section is the stratum lucidum (*SL*) in the epidermis of the thick skin of the fingertip.

B, bone
C, cortex
D, dermis
DP, dermal papilla of hair follicle
DS, dermal sheath
EP, epiphyseal plate
Epon, eponychium
HM, hair matrix
Hypon, hyponychium
M, medulla
N, nail or nail plate
NM, nail matrix
NR, nail root
PC, Pacinian corpuscles
RS, root sheath
SL, stratum lucidum
asterisks, cuticle of hair
numbers, *1*, external root sheath; *2*, Henle layer; *3*, Huxley layer; *4*, cuticle of internal root sheath; *5*, future cuticle of the hair

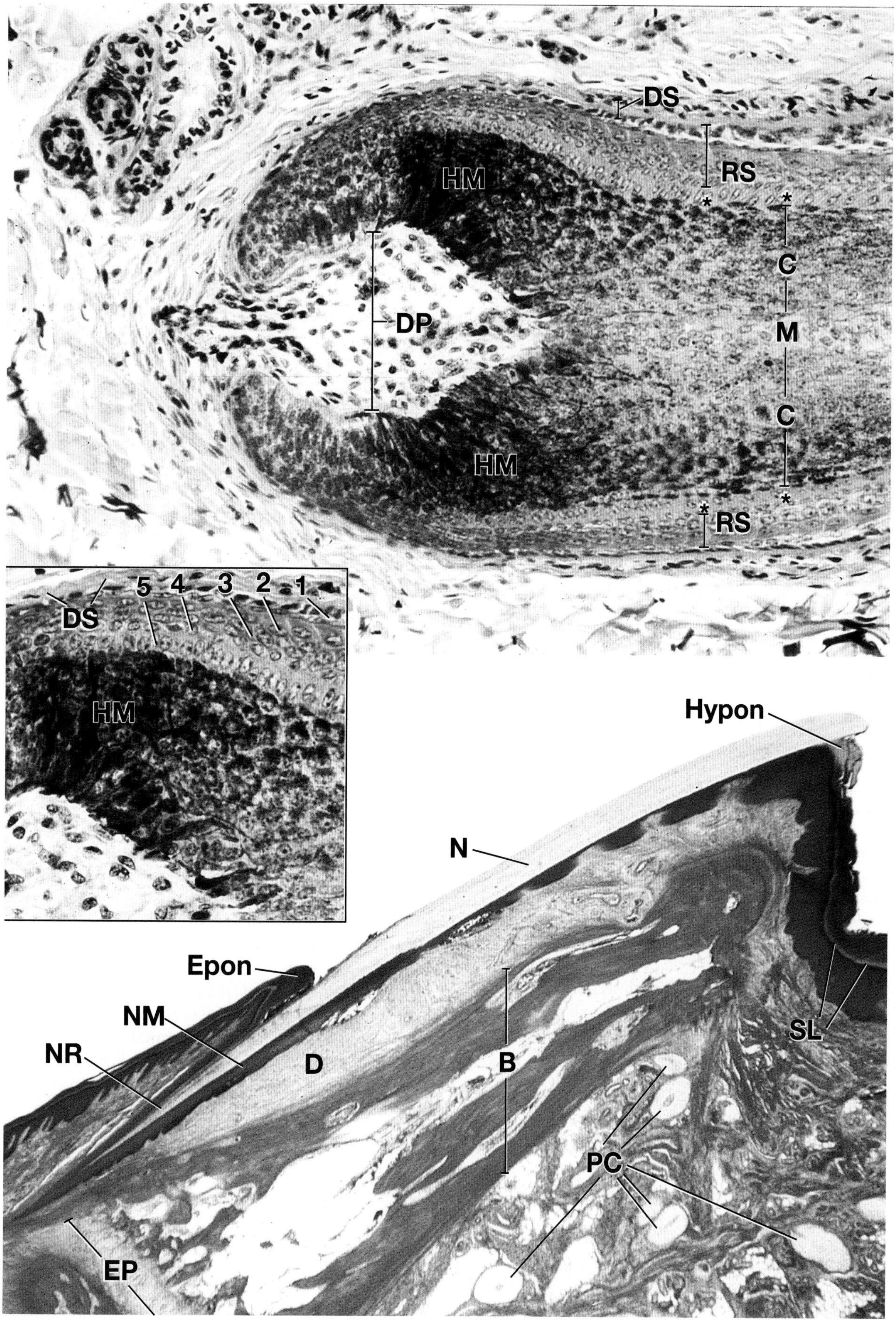
DS
RS
HM
C
DP
M
C
HM
RS
DS
5
4
3
2
1
HM
Hypon
N
Epon
NM
NR
D
B
SL
PC
EP

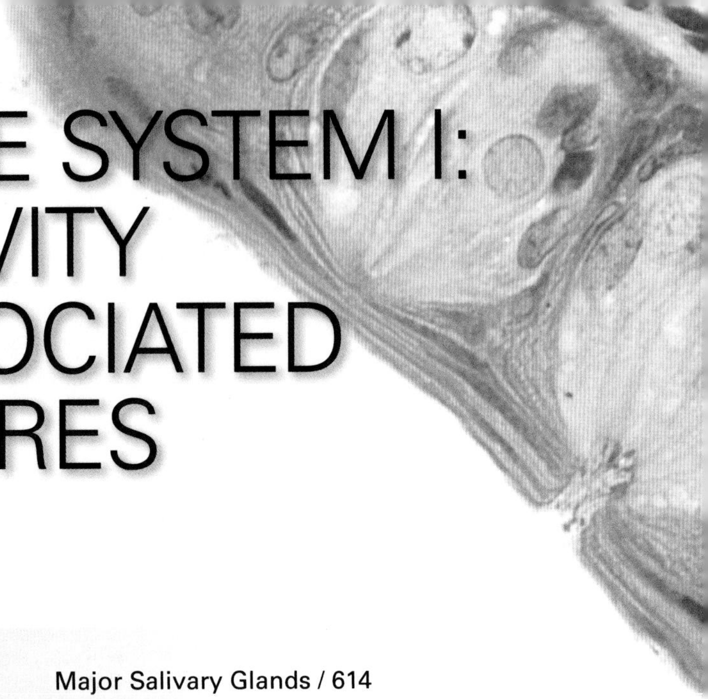

16 DIGESTIVE SYSTEM I: ORAL CAVITY AND ASSOCIATED STRUCTURES

■ OVERVIEW OF THE DIGESTIVE SYSTEM

The **digestive system** consists of the **alimentary canal** and its principal **associated organs**, namely, the tongue, teeth, salivary glands, pancreas, liver, and gallbladder. Major functions of the digestive system include transport of ingested water and food along the alimentary canal; secretion of fluids, electrolytes, and digestive enzymes; digestion and absorption of digested products; and excretion of indigestible remains.

The lumen of the alimentary canal is physically and functionally external to the body.

As it passes through the alimentary canal, food is broken down physically and chemically so that the degraded products can be absorbed into the body. The various segments of the **alimentary canal** are morphologically specialized for specific aspects of digestion and absorption.

Approximately 2 L of water and food are ingested into the body each day (Fig. 16.1). After preliminary maceration, moistening, and formation into a **bolus** by the actions of the structures of the oral cavity and by secretion of the salivary glands, food passes rapidly through the pharynx to the esophagus. The rapid passage of food through the pharynx ensures that only a brief interruption occurs in the airway for passage of air. The foodpasses more slowly through the **gastrointestinal tract**, aided by the secretion of digestive juices that may amount to 7 L or so per day. During food transit through the stomach and small intestine, the major alterations associated with digestion, solubilization, and absorption occur. Most of these fluids and nutrients are absorbed chiefly through the wall of the small intestine, but a small portion is absorbed in the large intestine (see Fig. 16.1). **Undigested food** and other substances within the alimentary canal, such as mucus, bacteria, desquamated cells, and bile pigments, are excreted as solids (**feces**).

The alimentary mucosa is the surface across which most substances enter the body.

The alimentary **mucosa** performs numerous functions in its role as an interface between the body and the environment. These functions include the following:

- **Secretion**. The lining of the alimentary canal secretes, at specific sites, digestive enzymes, hydrochloric acid, mucin, and antibodies.

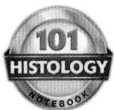

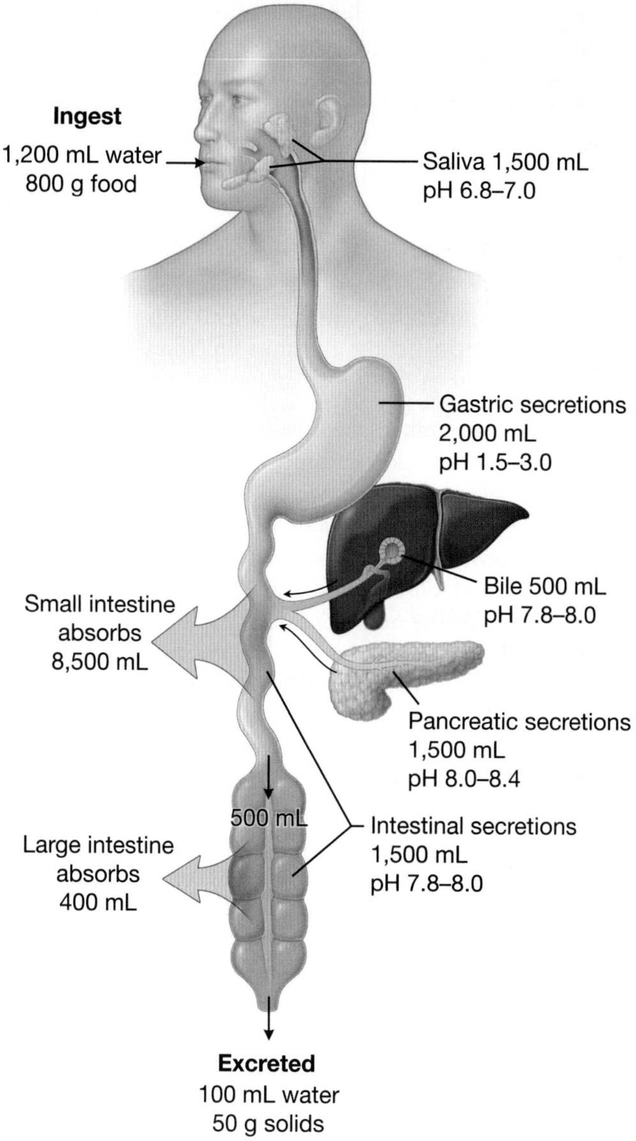

FIGURE 16.1. The alimentary canal and its function in secretion and absorption of fluids. This schematic diagram shows regions of the alimentary canal with associated exocrine glands that contribute to secretion of digestive juices. Almost all of the absorption of fluids, electrolytes, and nutrients occurs in the small intestine.

- **Absorption.** The epithelium of the mucosa absorbs metabolic substrates (e.g., the breakdown products of digestion) as well as vitamins, water, electrolytes, recyclable materials such as bile components and cholesterol, and other substances essential to the functions of the body.
- **Barrier.** The mucosa serves as a barrier to prevent the entry of noxious substances, antigens, and pathogenic organisms.
- **Immunologic protection.** Lymphatic tissue within the mucosa serves as the body's first line of immune defense.

The functions listed earlier are discussed at the beginning of the next chapter (see page 632). The digestive system is considered in three chapters that deal, respectively, with the oral cavity and pharynx (this chapter); the esophagus and gastrointestinal tract (see Chapter 17, Digestive System II: Esophagus and Gastrointestinal Tract, page 632); and the liver, gallbladder, and pancreas (see Chapter 18, Digestive System III: Liver, Gallbladder, and Pancreas, page 692).

■ ORAL CAVITY

The oral cavity consists of the mouth and its structures, which include the tongue, teeth, and their supporting structures (periodontium); major and minor salivary glands; and tonsils.

The **oral cavity** is divided into a vestibule and the oral cavity proper. The **vestibule** is the space between the lips, cheeks, and teeth. The **oral cavity proper** lies behind the teeth and is bounded by the hard and soft palates superiorly, the tongue and the floor of the mouth inferiorly, and the entrance to the oropharynx posteriorly.

The three **major salivary glands** are paired structures, including:

- **Parotid gland**, the largest of the three glands, located in the infratemporal region of the head. Its excretory duct, the parotid (Stensen) duct, opens at the parotid papilla, a small elevation on the mucosal surface of the cheek opposite the second upper molar tooth.
- **Submandibular gland**, located in the submandibular triangle of the neck. Its excretory duct, the submandibular (Wharton) duct, opens at a small fleshy prominence (the sublingual caruncle) on each side of the lingual frenulum on the floor of the oral cavity.
- **Sublingual gland**, lying inferior to the tongue within the sublingual folds at the floor of the oral cavity. It has a number of small excretory ducts; some enter the submandibular duct, and others enter individually into the oral cavity.

The parotid and submandibular glands have relatively long ducts that extend from the secretory portion of the gland to the oral cavity. The sublingual ducts are relatively short.

The **minor salivary glands** are located in the submucosa of the oral cavity. They empty directly into the cavity via short ducts and are named for their location (i.e., buccal, labial, lingual, and palatine).

The tonsils consist of aggregations of lymphatic nodules that are clustered around the posterior opening of the oral and nasal cavities.

Lymphatic tissue is organized into a **Waldeyer tonsillar ring** of immunologic protection located at the shared entrance to the digestive and respiratory tracts. This lymphatic tissue surrounds the posterior orifice of the oral and nasal cavities and contains aggregates of lymphatic nodules that include the following:

- **Palatine tonsils**, or simply the **tonsils**, which are located at either side of the entrance to the oropharynx between the palatopharyngeal and palatoglossal arches
- **Tubal tonsils**, which are located in the lateral walls of the nasopharynx posterior to the opening of the auditory tube
- **Pharyngeal tonsil**, or **adenoid**, which is located on the roof of the nasopharynx
- **Lingual tonsil**, which is located at the base of the tongue on its superior surface

The oral cavity is lined by the oral mucosa that consists of masticatory mucosa, lining mucosa, and specialized mucosa.

The **masticatory mucosa** is found on the gingiva (gums) and the hard palate (Fig. 16.2). It has a **keratinized** and, in some

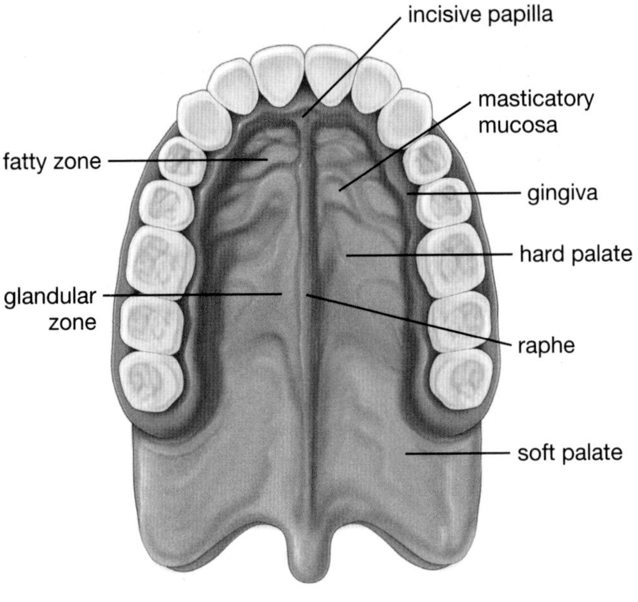

FIGURE 16.2. Roof of the oral cavity. The hard palate, which contains bone, is bisected into right and left halves by a raphe. Anteriorly, in the fatty zone, the submucosa of the hard palate contains adipose tissue; posteriorly, in the glandular zone, there are mucous glands within the submucosa. Neither the raphe nor the gingiva contains a submucosa; instead, the mucosa is attached directly to the bone. The soft palate has muscle instead of bone, and its glands are continuous with those of the hard palate in the submucosa.

areas, a **parakeratinized stratified squamous epithelium**. Parakeratinized epithelium is similar to keratinized epithelium, except that the superficial cells do not lose their nuclei and their cytoplasm does not stain intensely with eosin (Plate 16.1, page 620). The nuclei of the parakeratinized cells are pyknotic (highly condensed) and remain until the cell is exfoliated (Fig. 16.3). The keratinized epithelium of the masticatory mucosa resembles that of the skin but lacks a stratum lucidum. The underlying **lamina propria** consists of a thick papillary layer of loose connective tissue that contains blood vessels and nerves, some of which send bare axon endings into the epithelium as sensory receptors, and some of which end in Meissner corpuscles. Deep to the lamina propria is a reticular layer of denser connective tissue.

As in the skin, the depth and number of connective tissue papillae contribute to the relative immobility of the masticatory mucosa, thus protecting it from frictional and shearing stress. At the midline of the hard palate, in the **palatine raphe**, the mucosa adheres firmly to the underlying bone. The **reticular layer** of the lamina propria blends with the periosteum; thus, there is no submucosa. The same is true of the gingiva. Where there is a submucosa underlying the lamina propria on the hard palate (see Fig. 16.2), it contains adipose tissue anteriorly (fatty zone) and mucous glands posteriorly (glandular zone) that are continuous with those of the soft palate. In the submucosal regions, thick collagenous bands extend from the mucosa to the bone.

Lining mucosa is found on the lips, cheeks, alveolar mucosal surface, floor of the mouth, inferior surfaces of the tongue, and soft palate. At these sites, it covers striated muscle (lips, cheeks, and tongue), bone (alveolar mucosa), and glands (soft palate, cheeks, inferior surface of the tongue). The lining mucosa has fewer and shorter papillae so that it can adjust to the movement of its underlying muscles.

Generally, the epithelium of the lining mucosa is nonkeratinized, although, in some places, it may be parakeratinized (see Fig. 16.3). The epithelium of the vermilion border of the lip (the reddish portion between the moist inner surface and the facial skin) is keratinized. The nonkeratinized lining epithelium is thicker than keratinized epithelium. It consists of only three layers:

- **Stratum basale**, a single layer of cells resting on the basal lamina
- **Stratum spinosum**, which is several cells thick
- **Stratum superficiale**, the most superficial layer of cells, also referred to as the *surface layer of the mucosa*

The cells of the mucosal epithelium are similar to those of the epidermis of the skin and include keratinocytes, Langerhans cells, melanocytes, and Merkel cells.

The lamina propria contains blood vessels, nerves that send bare axon endings into the basal layers of the epithelium, and encapsulated sensory endings in some papillae. The sharp contrast between the numerous deep papillae of the alveolar mucosa and the shallow papillae in the rest of the lining mucosa allows easy identification of the two different regions in a histologic section.

Because it is highly vascularized, absorption of drugs through the **oral mucosa** is often used as an alternative method of systemic drug delivery. **Oral transmucosal delivery** offers several advantages because the absorbed substance directly enters the systemic circulation, bypassing the gastrointestinal tract and portal circulation, thus bypassing metabolism in the liver. Several cardiovascular drugs, such as nitroglycerin; analgesics; sedatives; antinausea drugs; drugs for erectile dysfunction; and hormonal drugs are available as oral transmucosal

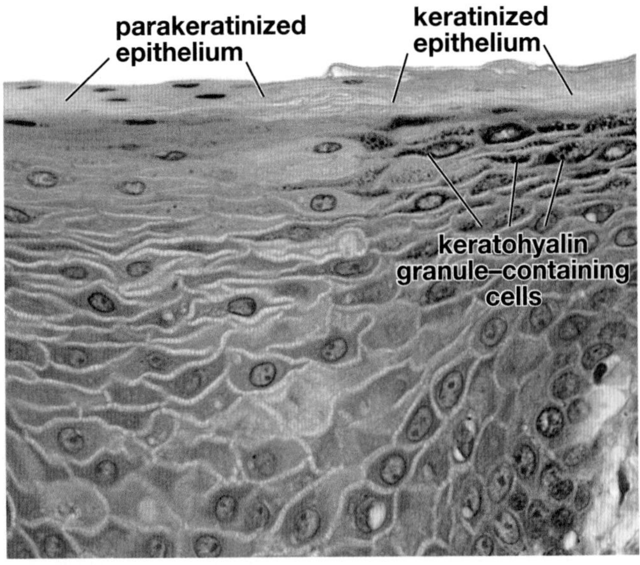

FIGURE 16.3. Stratified squamous epithelium at the mucocutaneous junction of the lip. This photomicrograph shows a transition in the oral mucosa from a stratified squamous epithelium (*on the right*) to a stratified squamous parakeratinized epithelium (*on the left*). The flattened surface cells of the keratinized epithelium are devoid of nuclei. The layer of keratohyalin granule–containing cells is clearly visible in this type of epithelium. The flattened surface cells of the parakeratinized epithelium display the same characteristics as the keratinized cells, except they retain their nuclei, that is, they are parakeratinized. In addition, note the paucity of keratohyalin granules present in the subsurface cells. ×380.

formulations. Some of these medications are administered by placement under the tongue (**sublingual administration**); other medications are administered by placement between the cheek and gum (**buccal administration**).

A distinct **submucosa** underlies the lining mucosa, except on the inferior surface of the tongue. This layer contains large bands of collagen and elastic fibers that bind the mucosa to the underlying muscle; it also contains the many minor salivary glands of the lips, tongue, and cheeks. Occasionally, **sebaceous glands** not associated with a hair follicle are found in the submucosa just lateral to the corner of the mouth and in the cheeks opposite the molar teeth. They are visible to the eye and are called **Fordyce spots**. The submucosa contains the larger blood vessels, nerves, and lymphatic vessels that supply the subepithelial neurovascular networks in the lamina propria throughout the oral cavity.

Specialized mucosa is associated with the sensation of taste and is restricted to the dorsal surface of the tongue. It contains papillae and **taste buds** responsible for generating the chemical sensation of taste.

Oral mucosa forms an important **protective barrier** between the external environment of the oral cavity and the internal environments of the surrounding tissues. It is resistant to the pathogenic organisms that enter the oral cavity and to indigenous microorganisms residing there as microbial flora. Epithelial cells, migratory neutrophils, and saliva all contribute to maintaining the health of the oral cavity and protecting the oral mucosa from bacterial, fungal, and viral infections. The protective mechanisms include several **salivary antimicrobial peptides**, β-defensins expressed in the epithelium, α-defensins expressed by neutrophils, and secretory immunoglobulin A (sIgA). However, in individuals with immunodeficiency or those undergoing antibiotic therapy, in which the balance between microorganisms and protective mechanisms is disrupted, oral infections are rather common.

■ TONGUE

The **tongue** is a muscular organ projecting into the oral cavity from its inferior surface. **Lingual muscles** (i.e., muscles of the tongue) are both extrinsic (having one attachment outside the tongue) and intrinsic (confined entirely to the tongue, without external attachment). The striated muscle of the tongue is arranged in bundles that generally run in three planes. They are divided into longitudinal, vertical, and transverse muscles, with each arranged at right angles to the other two. This arrangement of tongue muscles can be most clearly seen in the frontal section of the fetal head (Fig. 16.4a) and permits enormous flexibility and precision in the movements of the tongue, which are essential to human speech and its role in digestion and swallowing. This unique form of muscle organization is found only in the tongue, which allows easy identification of this tissue as lingual muscle. Variable amounts of adipose tissue are found among the muscle fiber groups (Fig. 16.4b).

Grossly, the **dorsal surface of the tongue** is divided into an anterior two-thirds and a posterior one-third by a V-shaped depression, the **sulcus terminalis** (Fig. 16.5). The apex of the V points posteriorly and is the location of the **foramen cecum**, the remnant of the site from which an evagination of the floor of the embryonic pharynx occurred to form the thyroid gland.

Papillae cover the dorsal surface of the tongue.

Numerous mucosal irregularities and elevations called **lingual papillae** cover the dorsal surface of the tongue anterior to the sulcus terminalis. The lingual papillae and their associated taste buds constitute the **specialized mucosa** of

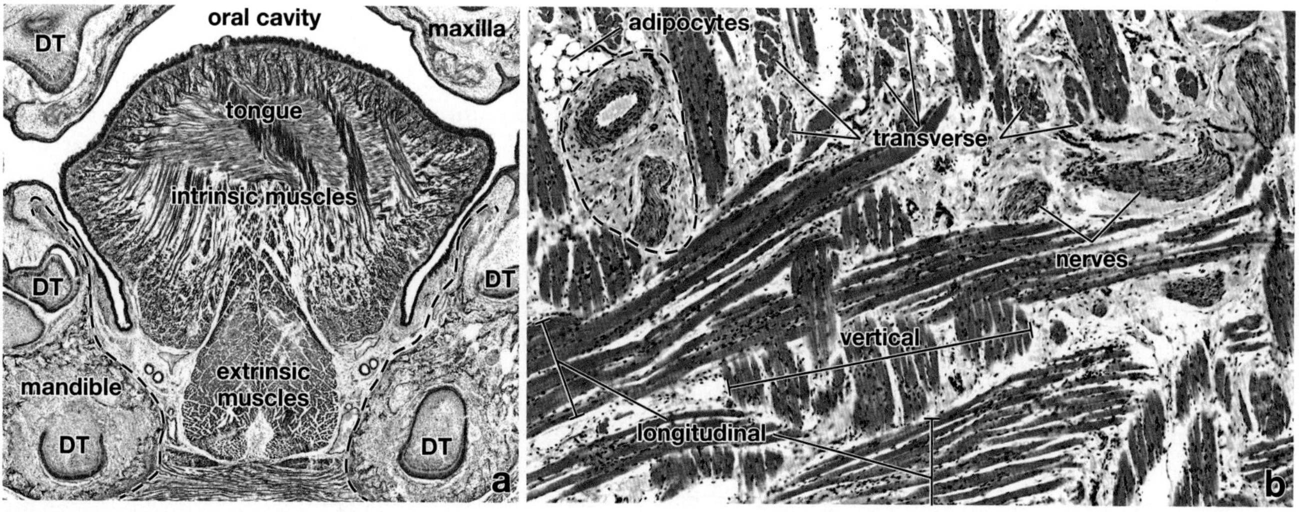

FIGURE 16.4. Muscle organization in the developing and adult human tongue. a. This photomicrograph of Mallory trichome–stained specimen shows the frontal section of the fetal head at the level of the developing oral cavity. The cross section of the tongue shows the organization of intrinsic muscles into longitudinal bundles (just deep to the surface of the tongue), transverse bundles (connecting lateral surfaces of the tongue), and vertical bundles (connecting superior [dorsal] surface with the base of the tongue). The extrinsic muscles attach the tongue into the floor of the mouth. Note the mandible on both sides of the tongue and the maxilla above with developing teeth (*DT*). ×40. **b.** This sagittal section of the hematoxylin and eosin (H&E)-stained tongue shows the unique arrangement of visceral striated muscle within the body of the tongue. All three directions of muscle fibers are visible, including cross-sectional profiles of transverse muscles and longitudinal profiles of both vertical and longitudinal muscles. In the *upper left corner,* note a small artery and nerve (*circled by dashed line*) next to accumulations of adipocytes. Nerve bundles are often visible between muscle fibers. ×380. (Courtesy Dr. Frank Daley, University of New England College of Osteopathic Medicine.)

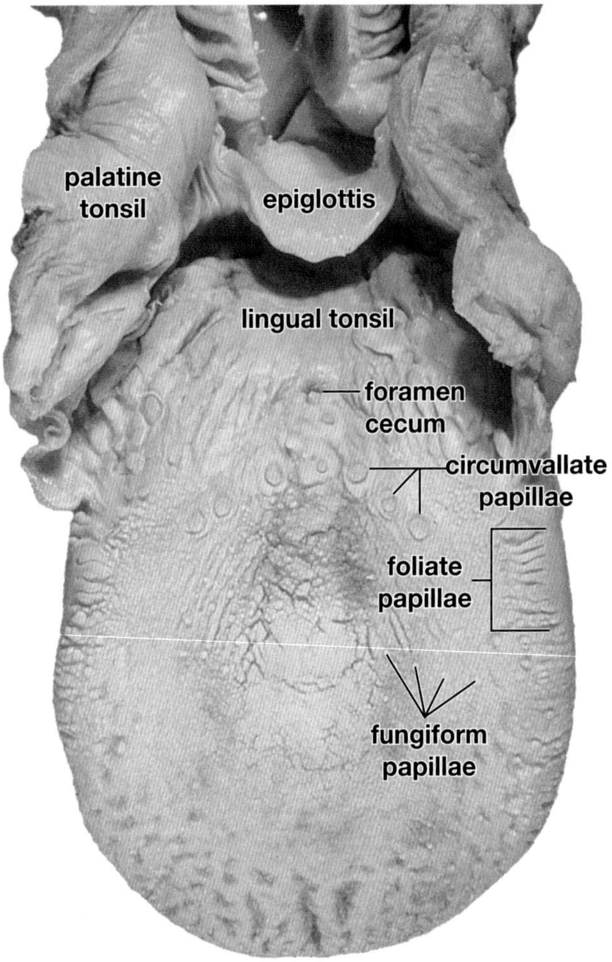

FIGURE 16.5. Human tongue. Circumvallate papillae are positioned in a V configuration, separating the anterior two-thirds of the tongue from the posterior third. Fungiform and filiform papillae are located on the anterior portion of the dorsal tongue surface. The uneven contour of the posterior tongue surface is attributable to the lingual tonsils. The palatine tonsil is at the junction between the oral cavity and the pharynx.

the oral cavity. Four types of papillae are described: filiform, fungiform, circumvallate, and foliate.

- **Filiform papillae** are the smallest and most numerous in humans. They are conical, elongated projections of connective tissue that are covered with highly keratinized stratified squamous epithelium (Fig. 16.6a and Plate 16.2, page 622). This epithelium does not contain taste buds. The papillae serve only a mechanical role. Filiform papillae are distributed over the entire anterior dorsal surface of the tongue, with their tips pointing backward. They appear to form rows that diverge to the left and right from the midline and that parallel the arms of the sulcus terminalis.
- **Fungiform papillae**, as the name implies, are mushroom-shaped projections located on the dorsal surface of the tongue (Fig. 16.6b). They project above the filiform papillae, among which they are scattered, and are just visible to the unaided eye as small spots (see Fig. 16.5 and Plate 16.2, page 622). They tend to be more numerous near the tip of the tongue. **Taste buds** are present in the stratified squamous epithelium on the dorsal surface of these papillae.
- **Circumvallate papillae** are large, dome-shaped structures that reside in the mucosa just anterior to the sulcus terminalis (see Fig. 16.5). The human tongue has 8–12 of these papillae. Each papilla is surrounded by a moat-like invagination lined with stratified squamous epithelium that contains numerous taste buds (Fig. 16.6d). Ducts of **lingual salivary (von Ebner) glands** empty their serous secretion into the base of the moats. This secretion presumably flushes material from the moat to enable the taste buds to respond rapidly to changing stimuli.
- **Foliate papillae** consist of parallel low ridges separated by deep mucosal clefts (see Fig. 16.6c and Plate 16.3, page 624), which are aligned at right angles to the long axis of the tongue. They occur on the lateral edge of the tongue. In older individuals, the foliate papillae may not be recognized; in younger individuals, they are easily found on the posterior lateral surface of the tongue and contain many taste buds in the epithelium of the facing walls of neighboring papillae (see Fig. 16.5). Small serous glands empty into the clefts. In some animals, such as the rabbit, foliate papillae constitute the principal site of aggregation of taste buds.

The dorsal surface of the base of the tongue exhibits smooth bulges that reflect the presence of the lingual tonsil in the lamina propria (see Fig. 16.5).

Taste buds are present on fungiform, foliate, and circumvallate papillae.

Humans have approximately 5,000–10,000 taste buds, of which about half are located on the sides of circumvallate papillae. In histologic sections, **taste buds** appear as oval, pale-staining bodies that extend through the thickness of the epithelium (Fig. 16.7). A small opening onto the epithelial surface at the apex of the taste bud is called the **taste pore**.

Three principal cell types are found in taste buds:

- **Neuroepithelial (sensory) cells** are the most numerous cells in the taste bud. These elongated cells extend from the basal lamina of the epithelium to the taste pore, through which the tapered apical surface of each cell extends microvilli (see Fig. 16.7). Near their apical surface, they are connected to neighboring neuroepithelial or supporting cells by tight junctions. At their base, they form a synapse with the processes of afferent sensory neurons of the **facial** (cranial nerve VII), **glossopharyngeal** (cranial nerve IX), or **vagus** (cranial nerve X) nerves. The turnover time of neuroepithelial cells is about 10–14 days.
- **Supporting cells** are less numerous. They are also elongated cells that extend from the basal lamina to the taste pore. Like neuroepithelial cells, they contain microvilli on their apical surface and possess tight junctions, but they do not synapse with the nerve cells. The turnover time of supporting cells is also about 10 days.
- **Basal cells** are small cells located in the basal portion of the taste bud, near the basal lamina. They are the stem cells for the two other cell types.

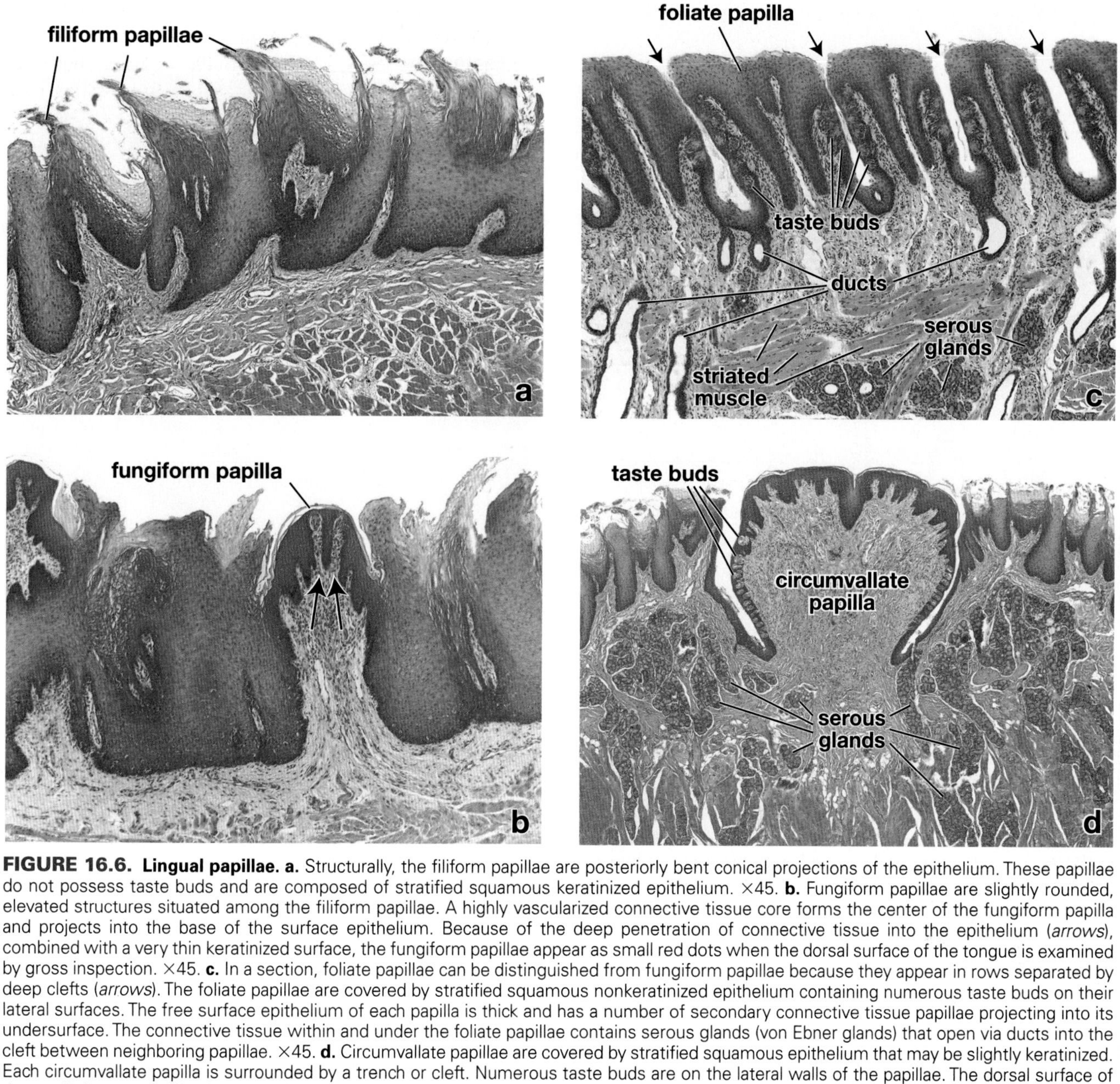

FIGURE 16.6. Lingual papillae. a. Structurally, the filiform papillae are posteriorly bent conical projections of the epithelium. These papillae do not possess taste buds and are composed of stratified squamous keratinized epithelium. ×45. **b.** Fungiform papillae are slightly rounded, elevated structures situated among the filiform papillae. A highly vascularized connective tissue core forms the center of the fungiform papilla and projects into the base of the surface epithelium. Because of the deep penetration of connective tissue into the epithelium (*arrows*), combined with a very thin keratinized surface, the fungiform papillae appear as small red dots when the dorsal surface of the tongue is examined by gross inspection. ×45. **c.** In a section, foliate papillae can be distinguished from fungiform papillae because they appear in rows separated by deep clefts (*arrows*). The foliate papillae are covered by stratified squamous nonkeratinized epithelium containing numerous taste buds on their lateral surfaces. The free surface epithelium of each papilla is thick and has a number of secondary connective tissue papillae projecting into its undersurface. The connective tissue within and under the foliate papillae contains serous glands (von Ebner glands) that open via ducts into the cleft between neighboring papillae. ×45. **d.** Circumvallate papillae are covered by stratified squamous epithelium that may be slightly keratinized. Each circumvallate papilla is surrounded by a trench or cleft. Numerous taste buds are on the lateral walls of the papillae. The dorsal surface of the papilla is smooth. The deep trench surrounding the circumvallate papillae and the presence of taste buds on the sides rather than on the free surface are features that distinguish circumvallate from fungiform papillae. The connective tissue near the circumvallate papillae also contains many serous-type glands that open via ducts into the bottom of the trench. ×25.

In addition to those associated with the papillae, taste buds are also present on the glossopalatine arch, the soft palate, the posterior surface of the epiglottis, and the posterior wall of the pharynx down to the level of the cricoid cartilage.

Taste is a chemical sensation in which various chemicals elicit stimuli from neuroepithelial cells of taste buds.

Taste is characterized as a chemical sensation in which various **tastants** (taste-stimulating substances) in food or beverages interact with taste receptors located at the apical surface of the neuroepithelial cells. There are three types of neuroepithelial cells that react to five basic stimuli: Type I reacts to **salty** taste; type II reacts to **sweet**, **bitter**, and **umami** *[Jap. delicious]* tastes; and type III detects **sour** taste. All taste buds have the same three neuroepithelial cell types; however, their ratios in different regions of the tongue vary. The molecular action of tastants can involve opening and passing through ion channels (i.e., salt and sour), closing ion channels (sour), or acting on a specific G-protein–coupled taste receptor (i.e., bitter, sweet, and umami).

Loss or changes in taste (ageusia or dysgeusia) are unique clinical symptoms reported by individuals infected by the **SARS-CoV-2 (COVID-19)** virus. These taste abnormalities frequently coexist with smell disorders (see Chapter 19, Respiratory System, page 735). Expression of **angiotensin-converting enzyme 2 (ACE2)** on the cell surface is responsible for the cellular entry of the SARS-CoV-2 virus. Once the viral spike protein binds to ACE2, more spike proteins are activated by **transmembrane protease serine 2 (TMPRSS2)**, thereby facilitating viral entry. In the

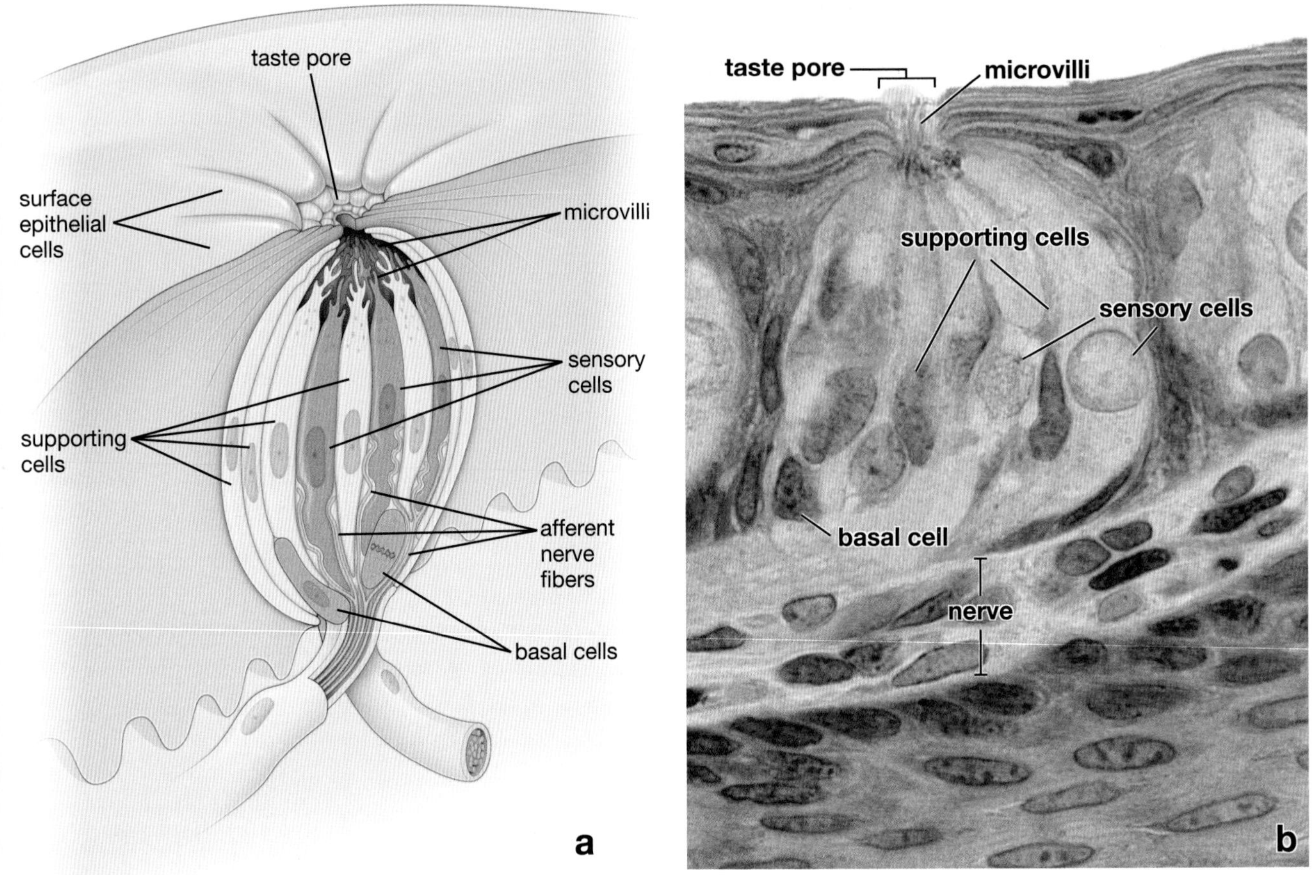

FIGURE 16.7. Diagram and photomicrograph of a taste bud. a. This diagram of a taste bud shows the neuroepithelial (sensory), supporting, and basal cells. One of the basal cells is shown in the process of dividing. Nerve fibers have synapses with the neuroepithelial cells. (Based on Warwick R, Williams PL, eds. *Gray's Anatomy.* 35th ed. Churchill Livingstone; 1973.) **b.** This high-magnification photomicrograph shows the organization of the cells within the taste bud. The sensory and supporting cells extend through the full length of the taste bud. The apical surface of these cells contains microvilli. The basal cells are located at the bottom of the taste bud. Note that the taste bud opens at the surface by means of a taste pore. ×1,100.

tongue, both ACE2 and TMPRSS2 proteins are coexpressed in the taste buds of lingual papillae. ACE2 expression has not been found in the neurons or ganglia of nerves innervating neuroepithelial cells. A recent study localized coexpression of ACE2 and TMPRSS2 proteins to **type II neuroepithelial cells,** which have **sweet, bitter,** and **umami** taste receptors. Taste receptor types I and II for salty and sour taste, respectively, are not involved in the replication of the SARS-CoV-2 virus. Direct injury to type II neuroepithelial cells may explain the high incidence of ageusia or dysgeusia in individuals with SARS-CoV-2 infection. Almost 90% of patients regain taste function in 4–15 days, which is compatible with the life span of the neuroepithelial cells.

Stimulation of bitter, sweet, and umami receptors activates G-protein–coupled taste receptors that belong to T1R and T2R chemosensory receptor families.

Bitter, sweet, and umami tastes in type II neuroepithelial cells are detected by a variety of receptor proteins encoded by two **taste receptor genes (T1R and T2R).** Their products are characterized as **G-protein–coupled taste receptors.**

- **Bitter taste** is detected by about 30 different types of **T2R chemosensory receptors.** Each receptor represents a single transmembrane protein coupled to its own **G-protein.** After receptor activation by the tastant, the G-protein stimulates the enzyme phospholipase C, leading to increased intracellular production of **inositol 1,4,5-trisphosphate (IP_3),** a second messenger molecule. IP_3, in turn, activates **taste-specific Na^+ channels** causing an influx of Na^+ ions, thus depolarizing the neuroepithelial cell. Depolarization of the plasma membrane causes **voltage-gated Ca^{2+} channels** in neuroepithelial cells to open. An increase in the concentration of intracellular Ca^{2+} levels, either by an influx of extracellular Ca^{2+} into the cell (the effect of depolarization) or by its release from intracellular stores (direct IP_3 stimulation), results in the release of neurotransmitter molecules, which generate nerve impulses along the gustatory afferent nerve fiber (Fig. 16.8a).
- **Sweet taste** receptors are also G-protein–coupled receptors. In contrast to bitter taste receptors, they have two protein subunits, **T1R2** and **T1R3.** The sweet tastants bound to these receptors activate the same second

messenger system cascade of reactions that the bitter receptors do (see Fig. 16.8a).

- **Umami taste** is linked to certain amino acids (e.g., L-glutamate, aspartate, and related compounds) and is common to asparagus, tomatoes, cheese, and meat. Umami taste receptors are very similar to sweet receptors; they are also composed of two subunits. One subunit, **T1R3**, is identical to that in the sweet receptor, but the second subunit formed by the **T1R1** protein is unique for umami receptors (see Fig. 16.8a). The transduction process is identical to that described previously for bitter taste pathways. Monosodium glutamate, added to many foods to enhance their taste (and the main ingredient of soy sauce), stimulates umami receptors.

The mechanism of transduction can be similar to several tastes (i.e., bitter or sweet); however, it is important to remember that neuroepithelial cells selectively express only one class of receptor proteins. Therefore, the messages about bitterness or sweetness from eating food are transferred to the central nervous system (CNS) along different nerve fibers.

Sodium ions and hydrogen protons, which are responsible for salty and sour taste, respectively, act directly on ion channels.

Signaling mechanisms, in the case of sour and salty tastes, are similar to other signaling mechanisms found in synapses and neuromuscular junctions.

- **Sour taste** in type III neuroepithelial cells is generated by H^+ protons that are formed by hydrolysis of acidic compounds. The H^+ proton primary blocks **K^+ channels** that are responsible for generating the cell membrane potential that causes depolarization of the cell membrane. In addition, H^+ protons enter the cell through **amiloride-sensitive Na^+ channels** and through specification channels, called *PKD1L3* and *PKD2L1*, found in neuroepithelial cells exclusively involved in sour taste transduction. The entry of H^+ into the receptor cell activates **voltage-sensitive Ca^{2+} channels.** Influx of Ca^{2+} triggers migration of synaptic vesicles, their fusion, and transmitter release, which results in generating action potentials in apposed sensory nerve fiber (Fig. 16.8b).

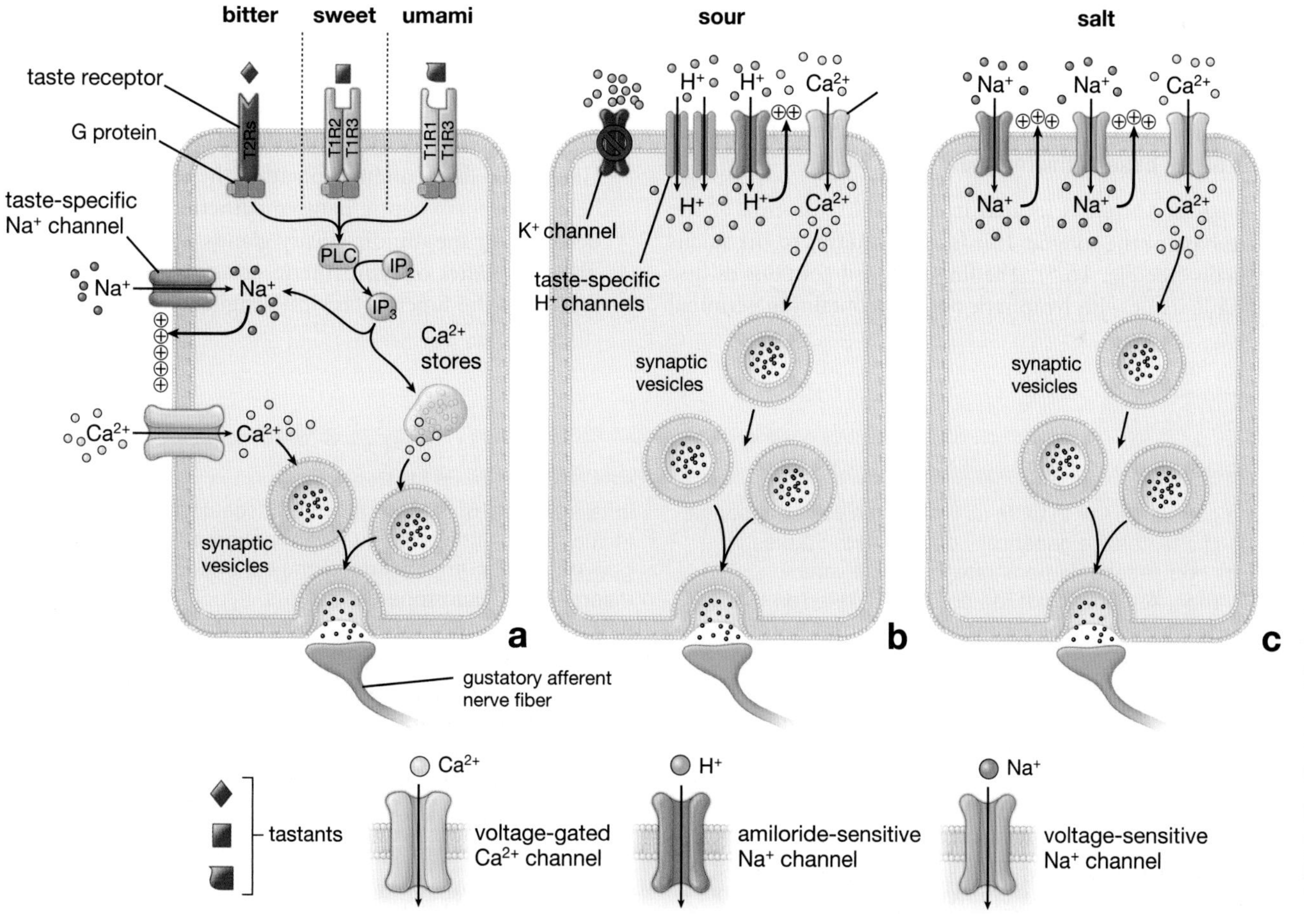

FIGURE 16.8. Diagram of taste receptors and their signaling mechanisms. a. This diagram shows the signaling mechanism of bitter, sweet, and umami receptors in the neuroepithelial cells. These cells selectively express only one class of receptor proteins; for simplicity, all three taste receptors are depicted in the apical cell membrane. See text for details. **b.** Signaling mechanism for the sour sensation is generated by H^+ protons that primarily block K^+ channels. The H^+ protons enter the cell via amiloride-sensitive Na^+ channels and through taste-specific H^+ channels (PKD1L3 and PKD2L1) exclusively expressed in cells involved in sour taste transduction. **c.** Salty sensation is generated from Na^+ ions that enter the neuroepithelial cells through amiloride-sensitive Na^+ channels. Intracellular Na^+ causes a depolarization of the membrane and activation of additional voltage-sensitive Na^+ and Ca^{2+} channels. Calcium-mediated release of neurotransmitters from synaptic vesicles results in the stimulation of gustatory nerve fibers. *IP_2*, inositol-1,4-diphosphate; *IP_3*, inositol 1,4,5-trisphosphate; *PLC*, phospholipase C.

- **Salty taste** that is stimulated by table salt (NaCl) is essentially derived from the taste of the sodium ions. The Na^+ enters the type I neuroepithelial cells through specific **amiloride-sensitive Na^+ channels** (the same that are involved in sour taste transmission). These channels are different from voltage-sensitive Na^+ channels that generate action potentials in nerve or muscle cells. The entry of Na^+ into a receptor cell causes depolarization of its membrane and activation of additional **voltage-sensitive Na^+ channels and voltage-sensitive Ca^{2+} channels.** As previously described, an influx of Ca^{2+} triggers migration and release of neurotransmitter from synaptic vesicles, which results in stimulating gustatory nerve fibers (Fig. 16.8c).

Some areas of the tongue are more responsive to certain tastes than others.

In general, taste buds at the tip of the tongue detect sweet stimuli, those immediately posterolateral to the tip detect salty stimuli, and those more posterolateral detect sour-tasting stimuli. Taste buds on the circumvallate papillae detect bitter and umami stimuli. However, studies with thermal stimulation of the tongue have shown that the classic taste maps as described earlier represent an oversimplified view of the distribution of taste receptors. Sensitivity to all tastes is distributed across the entire tongue, but some areas are more responsive to certain tastes than others.

The lingual tonsil consists of accumulations of lymphatic tissue at the base of the tongue.

The **lingual tonsil** is located in the lamina propria of the root or base of the tongue. It is found posterior to the sulcus terminalis (see Fig. 16.5). The lingual tonsil contains diffuse lymphatic tissue with lymphatic nodules containing germinal centers. These structures are discussed in Chapter 14, Immune System and Lymphatic Tissues and Organs (page 505).

Epithelial crypts usually invaginate into the lingual tonsil. However, the structure of the epithelium may be difficult to distinguish because of the extremely large number of lymphocytes that normally invade it. Between nodules, the lingual epithelium has the characteristics of lining epithelium. Mucous lingual salivary glands may be seen within the lingual tonsil and may extend into the muscle of the base of the tongue.

The complex nerve supply of the tongue is provided by cranial nerves and the autonomic nervous system.

- **General sensation** for the anterior two-thirds of the tongue (anterior to the sulcus terminalis) is carried in the **mandibular division of the trigeminal nerve** (cranial nerve V). General sensation for the posterior one-third of the tongue is carried in the **glossopharyngeal nerve** (cranial nerve IX) and the **vagus nerve** (cranial nerve X).
- **Taste sensation** is carried by the **chorda tympani**, a branch of the facial nerve (cranial nerve VII) anterior to the sulcus terminalis, and by the **glossopharyngeal nerve** (cranial nerve IX) and **vagus nerve** (cranial nerve X) posterior to the sulcus.
- **Motor innervation** for the musculature of the tongue is supplied by the **hypoglossal nerve** (cranial nerve XII).
- Vascular and glandular innervation is provided by the **sympathetic** and **parasympathetic nerves.** They supply blood vessels and small salivary glands of the tongue. Ganglion cells are often seen within the tongue. These cells belong to postsynaptic parasympathetic neurons and are destined for the minor salivary glands within the tongue. The cell bodies of sympathetic postsynaptic neurons are located in the superior cervical ganglion.

FOLDER 16.1

CLINICAL CORRELATION: THE GENETIC BASIS OF TASTE

The general ability to taste as well as the ability to sense specific tastes are genetically determined. Studies in large populations demonstrate that taste variation is common. About 25% of the population, referred to as "**supertasters**," have more than the normal number of lingual papillae and a high density of taste buds. Rare individuals in this group, such as wine, brandy, coffee, or tea tasters, have prodigious taste discrimination and taste memory. These individuals are characterized by their extreme sensitivity to the chemical phenylthiocarbamide (PTC) and its derivative 6-*N*-propylthiouracil (PROP); they typically report an intensely bitter taste after a drop of PTC/PROP solution is placed on the tip of their tongue. On the other side of the spectrum (about 25% of the population) are individuals known as "**nontasters**," with a smaller-than-normal number of lingual papillae and a lower density of taste buds. When tested with PTC/PROP solution, these individuals are unaware of its bitter taste.

Many clinical conditions can affect taste perception. They include lesions in the nerves that transmit the taste sensation to the central nervous system (i.e., facial nerve, chorda tympani, and lingual nerve); inflammations of the oral cavity; mucosal disorders, including radiation-induced inflammation of the lingual mucosa; nutritional deficiencies; endocrine disorders such as diabetes mellitus, hypogonadism, and pseudohypoparathyroidism; and hormonal fluctuations during menstruation and pregnancy. Some rare genetic disorders also affect taste sensation. **Type I familial dysautonomia (Riley–Day syndrome)** causes severe hypogeusia (decreased ability to detect taste) because of the developmental absence of taste buds and fungiform papillae. This sensory and autonomic neuropathy is an autosomal recessive disorder caused by a mutation in the DYS gene (also referred to as the IKBKAP gene) located on chromosome 9. In addition to hypogeusia, these individuals experience other symptoms related to developmental defects in the peripheral and autonomic nervous systems, including diminished lacrimation, defective thermoregulation, orthostatic hypotension, excessive sweating, loss of pain and temperature sensation, and absent reflexes. A test that detects the causative mutation in the DYS gene can be used to confirm the diagnosis of familial dysautonomia.

■ TEETH AND SUPPORTING TISSUES

Teeth are a major component of the oral cavity and are essential for initiating the digestive process. Teeth are embedded in and attached to the alveolar processes of the maxilla and mandible. Children have 10 **deciduous (primary, milk) teeth** in each jaw on each side:

- A **medial (central) incisor**, the first tooth to erupt (usually in the mandible) at approximately 6 months of age (in some infants, the first teeth may not erupt until 12 or 13 months of age)
- A **lateral incisor**, which erupts at approximately 8 months
- A **canine tooth**, which erupts at approximately 15 months
- Two **molar teeth**, the first of which erupts at 10–19 months and the second of which erupts at 20–31 months

During a period of years, usually beginning at about age 6 and ending at about age 12 or 13, deciduous teeth are gradually replaced by 16 **permanent (secondary) teeth** in each jaw (Folder 16.2). Each side of both the upper and lower jaws consists of the following:

- A **medial (central) incisor**, which erupts at age 7 or 8
- A **lateral incisor**, which erupts at age 8 or 9
- A **canine tooth**, which erupts at age 10 to 12
- Two **premolar teeth**, which erupt between ages 10 and 12
- Three **molar teeth**, which erupt at different times; the first molar usually erupts at age 6, the second molar in the early teens, and the third molar (**wisdom teeth**) during the late teens or early 20s

Incisors, canines, and premolars have one root each, except for the first premolar of the maxilla, which has two roots. Molars have either two roots (lower jaw) or three (upper jaw) and, on rare occasions, four roots. However, all teeth have the same basic structure.

Teeth consist of several layers of specialized tissues.

Teeth are made up of three specialized tissues:

- **Enamel**, a hard, thin, translucent layer of acellular mineralized tissue that covers the crown of the tooth
- **Dentin**, the most abundant dental tissue; it lies deep to the enamel in the crown and cementum in the root. Its unique tubular structure and biochemical composition support the more rigid enamel and cementum overlying the surface of the tooth.
- **Cementum**, a thin, pale yellowish layer of bone-like calcified tissue covering the dentin of the root of the teeth. Cementum is softer and more permeable than dentin and is easily removed by abrasion when the root surface is exposed to the oral environment.

FOLDER 16.2

CLINICAL CORRELATION: CLASSIFICATION OF PERMANENT (SECONDARY) AND DECIDUOUS (PRIMARY) DENTITION

Three systems (dental notations) are currently used to classify permanent and deciduous teeth (Fig. F16.2.1):

- ***Palmer system (military system)***, which is primarily used in the United Kingdom. In this system, uppercase letters are used for the deciduous teeth, and Arabic numerals are used for the permanent teeth. Each quadrant in this system is designated by angled line symbols (┘, └, ┐, ┌): ┘ for upper right (UR), └ for upper left (UL), ┐ for lower right (LR), and ┌ for lower left (LL). For example, permanent canines are called number 3 in each quadrant, and the quadrant is designated by its angled line. In the era of electronic medical records, Palmer notation symbols are encoded in the standard Unicode transformation format (UTF-16), which has been employed in modern operating systems and programming languages.
- ***International system (World Dental Federation [FDI] system or ISO 3950)***, which is the most commonly used notation worldwide, except the United States, which uses the American (universal) system, and the United Kingdom, where the Palmer notation is frequently used. The International system uses two Arabic numerals to designate the individual tooth. In this system, the first numeral indicates the location of the tooth in a specific quadrant. The permanent quadrants are designated UR = 1, UL = 2, LL = 3, and LR = 4; the deciduous quadrants are designated UR = 5, UL = 6, LL = 7, and LR = 8. The second numeral designates the individual tooth, which is numbered beginning from the dental midline. For example, in this system, the permanent canines are named 13, 23, 33, and 43, and the deciduous canines would be 53, 63, 73, and 83.
- ***American system (Universal system, UNS)***, which is the most commonly used notation in North America. In this system, the permanent dentition is designated by Arabic numerals, and the deciduous dentition is designated with uppercase letters. For permanent dentition, numbering begins in the UR quadrant, with the UR third molar designated number 1. Numbering continues across the maxillary arch to the UL third molar, designated tooth number 16. Tooth number 17 is the third molar located in the LL quadrant inferior and opposite tooth number 16. Then, the numbering progresses across the mandibular arch and terminates with tooth number 32, the LR third molar. *In this system, the sum of the numbers of opposing teeth adds up to 33.* For the deciduous dentition, the same pattern is followed, but the letters A–T are used to designate the individual teeth. Thus, in this system, the permanent canines are designated 6, 11, 22, and 27, and the deciduous canines C, H, M, and R.

(continued)

FOLDER 16.2

CLINICAL CORRELATION: CLASSIFICATION OF PERMANENT (SECONDARY) AND DECIDUOUS (PRIMARY) DENTITION (*continued*)

Also note that in Figure F16.2.1, the *red* color outline demonstrates the relationship of the deciduous and permanent dentitions. Examination of the table reveals that deciduous molars are replaced with permanent premolars after exfoliation and that the permanent molars have no deciduous precursors.

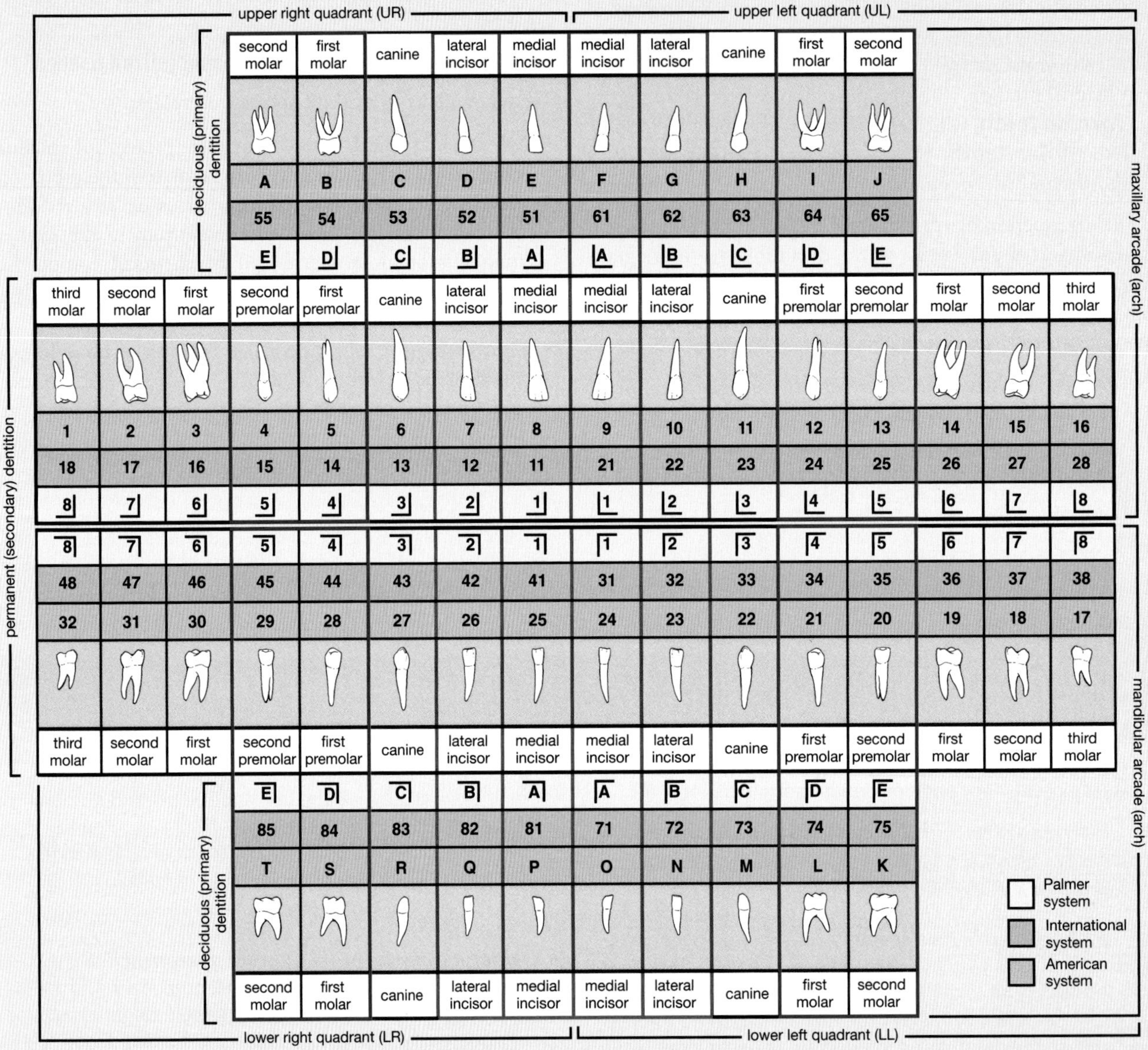

FIGURE F16.2.1. Classification of permanent and deciduous teeth. Three systems of tooth classification are used. The *central panel* of the diagram shows the permanent teeth, whereas the *upper and lower panels* show the deciduous teeth. Dentition is divided into four quadrants: upper left (UL), upper right (UR), lower left (LL), and lower right (LR). Each quadrant includes eight permanent teeth or five deciduous teeth. In the American (universal) system (*blue*), permanent teeth are designated with Arabic numerals. The numbering begins from the wisdom tooth in the upper right quadrant designated as tooth number 1 and continues along all the teeth in the maxilla to tooth number 16, which designates the third upper left molar. The numbering progresses to the mandible, beginning at the third left lower molar designated as number 17 to the third lower right molar designated as number 32. In the American system, deciduous teeth are marked with capital letters designated for each tooth. The pattern is the same as that for permanent teeth, so the numbering begins from the second upper right molar and finishes with the second lower right molar. In the International system (*red*), also referred to as the *two-digit system*, each tooth is designated with two numbers: The first number indicates the dentition quadrant, which is marked from 1 to 4 and from 5 to 8 in a clockwise direction beginning from the upper right quadrant for permanent and deciduous teeth, respectively. The second number specifies individual teeth in each quadrant beginning from the midline, where the medial incisors are designated as number 1 and third molars are designated as number 8. In the Palmer system (*yellow*), the dentition is divided into four quadrants with a right-angle bracket. The *vertical line* of the bracket divides the dentition into a right and a left side beginning at the midline. The *horizontal line* of the bracket divides the dentition into the upper and lower parts to designate teeth in the maxilla and mandible. In the Palmer system, permanent teeth are numbered with Arabic numerals beginning from the midline. The deciduous teeth are marked with capital letters, also starting from the midline. To mark a particular tooth with the Palmer system, two lines (vertical and horizontal) and the correct number or letter of the tooth are needed. (Table design courtesy of Dr. Wade T. Schultz.)

Enamel

Enamel is the hardest substance in the body; it consists of 96%–98% calcium hydroxyapatite.

Enamel is an acellular mineralized tissue that covers the crown of the tooth. Once formed, it cannot be replaced. Enamel is a unique tissue because, unlike bone, which is formed from connective tissue, it is a mineralized material derived from epithelium. Enamel is more highly mineralized and harder than any other mineralized tissue in the body; it consists of 96%–98% of calcium hydroxyapatite. The enamel that is exposed and visible above the gum line is called the **clinical crown**; the **anatomic crown** describes all of the tooth that is covered by enamel, some of which is below the gum line. Enamel varies in thickness over the crown and may be as thick as 2.5 mm on the **cusps** (biting and grinding surfaces) of some teeth. The enamel layer ends at the **neck**, or cervix, of the tooth at the **cementoenamel junction** (Fig. 16.9); the **root** of the tooth is then covered by **cementum**, a bone-like material.

Enamel is composed of enamel rods that span the entire thickness of the enamel layer.

The nonstoichiometric carbonated calcium hydroxyapatite enamel crystals that form the **enamel** are arranged as **rods** that measure 4 μm wide and 8 μm high. Each enamel rod spans the full thickness of the enamel layer from the dentinoenamel junction to the enamel surface. When examined in cross section at higher magnification, the rods reveal a keyhole shape (Fig. 16.10); the ballooned part, or head, is oriented superiorly, and the tail is directed inferiorly toward the root of the tooth. The **enamel crystals** are primarily oriented parallel to the long axis of the rod within the head, and in the tail, they are oriented more obliquely (Figs. 16.10 and 16.11). The limited spaces between the rods are also filled with enamel crystals. Striations observed on enamel rods (contour lines of Retzius) may represent evidence of rhythmic growth of the enamel in the developing tooth. A wider line of hypomineralization is observed in the enamel of the deciduous teeth. This line, called the *neonatal line*, marks the nutritional changes that take place between prenatal and postnatal life.

Although the enamel of an erupted tooth lacks cells and cell processes, it is not a static tissue. It is influenced by the secretion of the salivary glands, which are essential to its maintenance. The substances in saliva that affect teeth include digestive enzymes, secreted antibodies, and a variety of inorganic (mineral) components.

Mature enamel contains very little organic material. Despite its hardness, enamel can be decalcified by

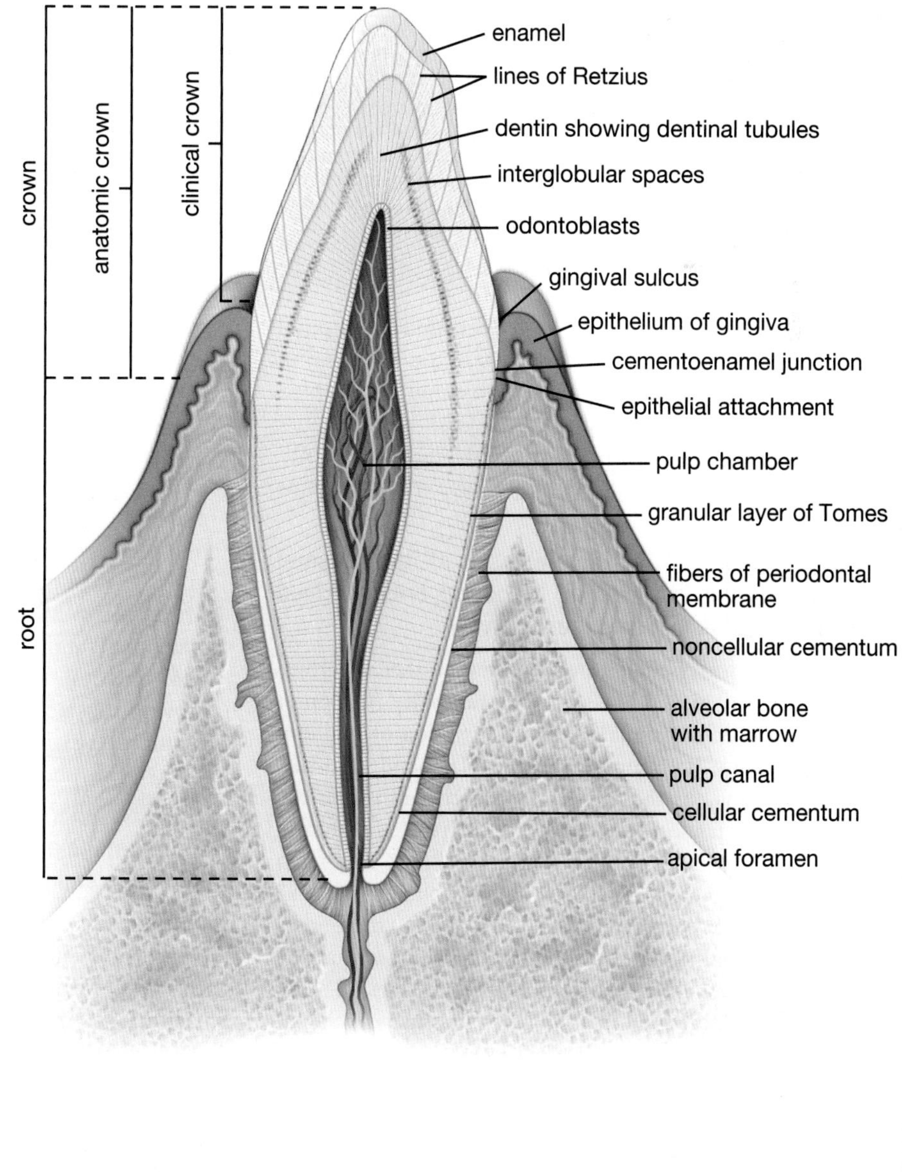

FIGURE 16.9. Diagram of a section of an incisor tooth and surrounding bony and mucosal structures. The three mineralized components of the tooth are dentin, enamel, and cementum. The central soft core of the tooth is the pulp. The periodontal ligament (membrane) contains bundles of collagenous fibers that bind the tooth to the surrounding alveolar bone. The clinical crown of the tooth is the portion that projects into the oral cavity. The anatomic crown is the entire portion of the tooth covered by enamel.

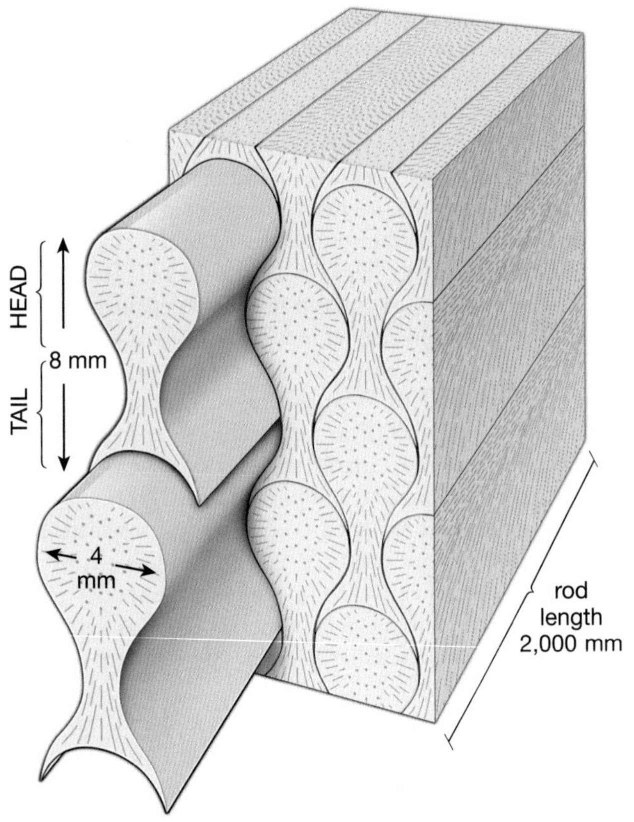

FIGURE 16.10. Diagram showing the basic organization and structure of enamel rods. The enamel rod is a thin structure extending from the dentinoenamel junction to the surface of the enamel. Where the enamel is thickest, at the tip of the crown, the rods are the longest, measuring up to 2,000 μm. On cross section, the rods reveal a keyhole shape. The upper, ballooned part of the rod, called the *head*, is oriented superiorly, and the lower part of the rod, called the *tail*, is directed inferiorly. Within the head, most of the enamel crystals are oriented parallel to the long axis of each rod. Within the tail, the crystals are oriented more obliquely.

acid-producing bacteria acting on food products trapped on the enamel surface. This is the basis of the initiation of dental caries. Fluoride added to the hydroxyapatite complex makes the enamel more resistant to acid demineralization. The widespread use of fluoride in drinking water, toothpaste, pediatric vitamin supplements, and mouthwashes significantly reduces the incidence of **dental caries**.

Enamel is produced by ameloblasts of the enamel organ, and dentin is produced by neural crest–derived odontoblasts of the adjacent mesenchyme.

The **enamel organ** is an epithelial formation that is derived from ectodermal epithelial cells of the oral cavity. The onset of tooth development is marked by proliferation of oral epithelium to form a horseshoe-shaped cellular band of tissue, the dental lamina, in the adjacent mesenchyme where the upper and lower jaws will develop. At the site of each future tooth, there is a further proliferation of cells that arise from the dental lamina, resulting in a rounded, cellular, bud-like outgrowth, one for each tooth, that projects into the underlying mesenchymal tissue. This outgrowth, referred to as the **bud stage**, represents the early enamel organ (Fig. 16.12a). Gradually, the rounded cell mass enlarges and then develops a concavity at the site opposite to which it arose from the dental lamina; this is referred to as the **cap stage** (Fig. 16.12b). Further growth and development of the enamel organ results in the **bell stage** (Fig. 16.12c and d). At this stage, the enamel organ consists of four recognizable cellular components:

- **Outer enamel epithelium**, made up of a cell layer that forms the convex surface
- **Inner enamel epithelium**, made up of a cell layer that forms the concave surface
- **Stratum intermedium**, a cell layer that develops internal to the inner enamel epithelium
- **Stellate reticulum**, made up of cells that have a stellate appearance and occupy the inner portion of the enamel organ

The neural crest–derived **preodontoblasts** lined up within the "bell" adjacent to the inner enamel epithelial cells become columnar and have an epithelial-type appearance. They will become **odontoblasts** and form the dentin of the tooth. The inner enamel epithelial cells of the enamel organ will become **ameloblasts.** Along with the cells of the stratum intermedium, they will be responsible for enamel production. At the early stage, just before dentinogenesis and amelogenesis, the dental lamina degenerates, leaving the developing tooth primordium detached from its site of origin.

Dental enamel is formed by a matrix-mediated biomineralization process known as **amelogenesis**. The major stages of amelogenesis are described as follows:

- **Matrix production** or **secretory stage**. In the formation of mineralized tissues of the tooth, dentin is produced first. Next, partially mineralized enamel matrix (Fig. 16.13) is deposited directly on the surface of the previously formed dentin. The cells producing this partially mineralized organic matrix are called **secretory-stage ameloblasts.** These cells produce an organic proteinaceous matrix by the activity of the rough endoplasmic reticulum (rER), Golgi apparatus, and secretory granules, similar to the process by which osteoblasts produce bone. The secretory-stage ameloblasts continue to produce enamel matrix until the full thickness of the future enamel is achieved.
- **Matrix maturation**. Maturation of the partially mineralized enamel matrix involves the removal of organic material as well as the continued influx of calcium and phosphate into the maturing enamel. Cells involved in this second stage of enamel formation are called **maturation-stage ameloblasts**. Maturation-stage ameloblasts differentiate from secretory-stage ameloblasts and function primarily as a transporting epithelium, moving substances into and out of the maturing enamel. Maturation-stage ameloblasts undergo cyclical alterations in their morphology that correspond to the cyclical entry of calcium into the enamel.

Secretory-stage ameloblasts are polarized columnar cells that produce enamel.

The **secretory-stage ameloblast** lies directly adjacent to the developing enamel. At the apical pole of each ameloblast is a process, **Tomes process**, which is surrounded by the developing enamel (Fig. 16.14). A cluster of mitochondria

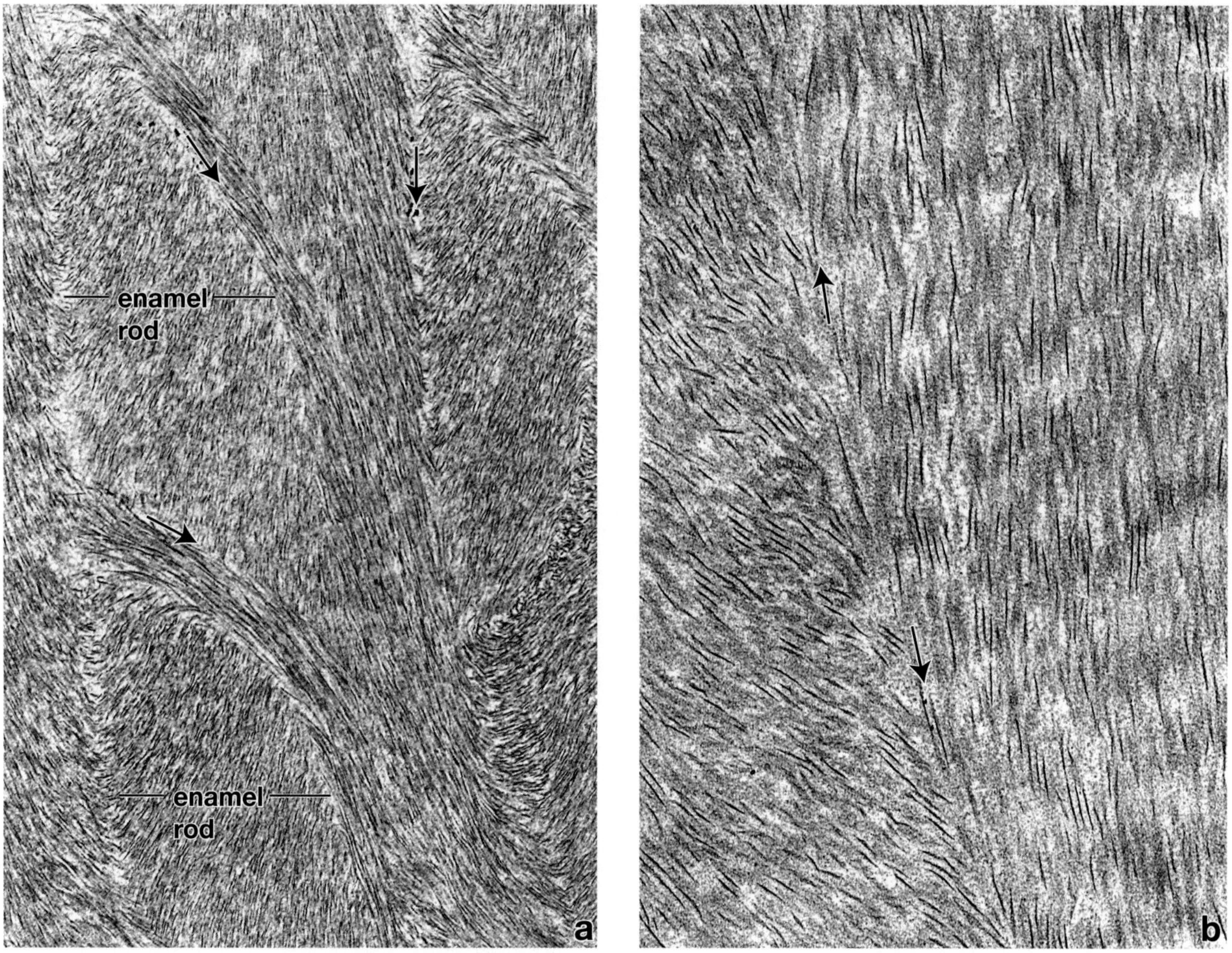

FIGURE 16.11. Structure of young enamel. a. This electron micrograph shows enamel rods cut obliquely. *Arrows* indicate the boundaries between adjacent rods. ×14,700. **b.** Parts of two adjacent rods are seen at higher magnification. *Arrows* mark the boundary between the two rods. The dark needle-like objects are young hydroxyapatite crystals; the substance between the hydroxyapatite crystals is the organic matrix of the developing enamel. As the enamel matures, the hydroxyapatite crystals grow, and the bulk of the organic matrix is removed. ×60,000.

and an accumulation of actin filaments in the proximal terminal web in the base of the cell account for the eosinophilic staining of this region in hematoxylin and eosin (H&E)-stained paraffin sections (Figs. 16.15 and 16.16a). Adjacent to the mitochondria is the nucleus; in the main column of cytoplasm are the rER, Golgi, secretory granules, and other cell elements. Junctional complexes are present at both the apical and basal parts of the cell. They maintain the integrity and orientation of the ameloblasts as they move away from the dentinoenamel junction. Actin filaments joined to these junctional complexes are involved in moving the secretory-stage ameloblast over the developing enamel. The rod produced by the ameloblast follows in the wake of the cell. Thus, in mature enamel, the direction of the enamel rod is a record of the path taken earlier by the secretory-stage ameloblast.

At their base, the secretory-stage ameloblasts are adjacent to a layer of enamel organ cells called the **stratum intermedium** (see Figs. 16.12b, c, and g and 16.13b). The plasma membrane of these cells, especially at the base of the ameloblasts, contains alkaline phosphatase, an enzyme active in calcification. Stellate enamel organ cells are external to the stratum intermedium and are separated from the adjacent blood vessels by a basal lamina.

Maturation-stage ameloblasts transport substances needed for enamel maturation.

The histologic feature that characterizes **maturation-stage ameloblasts** is the presence of a striated (or ruffled) border on their apical surface (Fig. 16.16b). At this stage, ameloblasts undergo **modulation**, a cyclic change in which the striated border appears, then disappears, and finally reappears. During the modulation, maturation-stage ameloblasts undergo extensive remodeling, which alternates between displaying a **striated border** or a **smooth border**. Maturation-stage ameloblasts with striated borders account for approximately 70% of all cells undergoing cyclic modulation. A well-developed striated border is responsible for secreting bicarbonate ions (CHO_3^-); it also contains plasma membrane Ca^{2+}-ATPases (PMCA) that extrude calcium ions (Ca^{2+}) into the maturing enamel. Maturation-stage ameloblasts with smooth-ended apical borders account for approximately 30% of this cell population. Although they have no detected

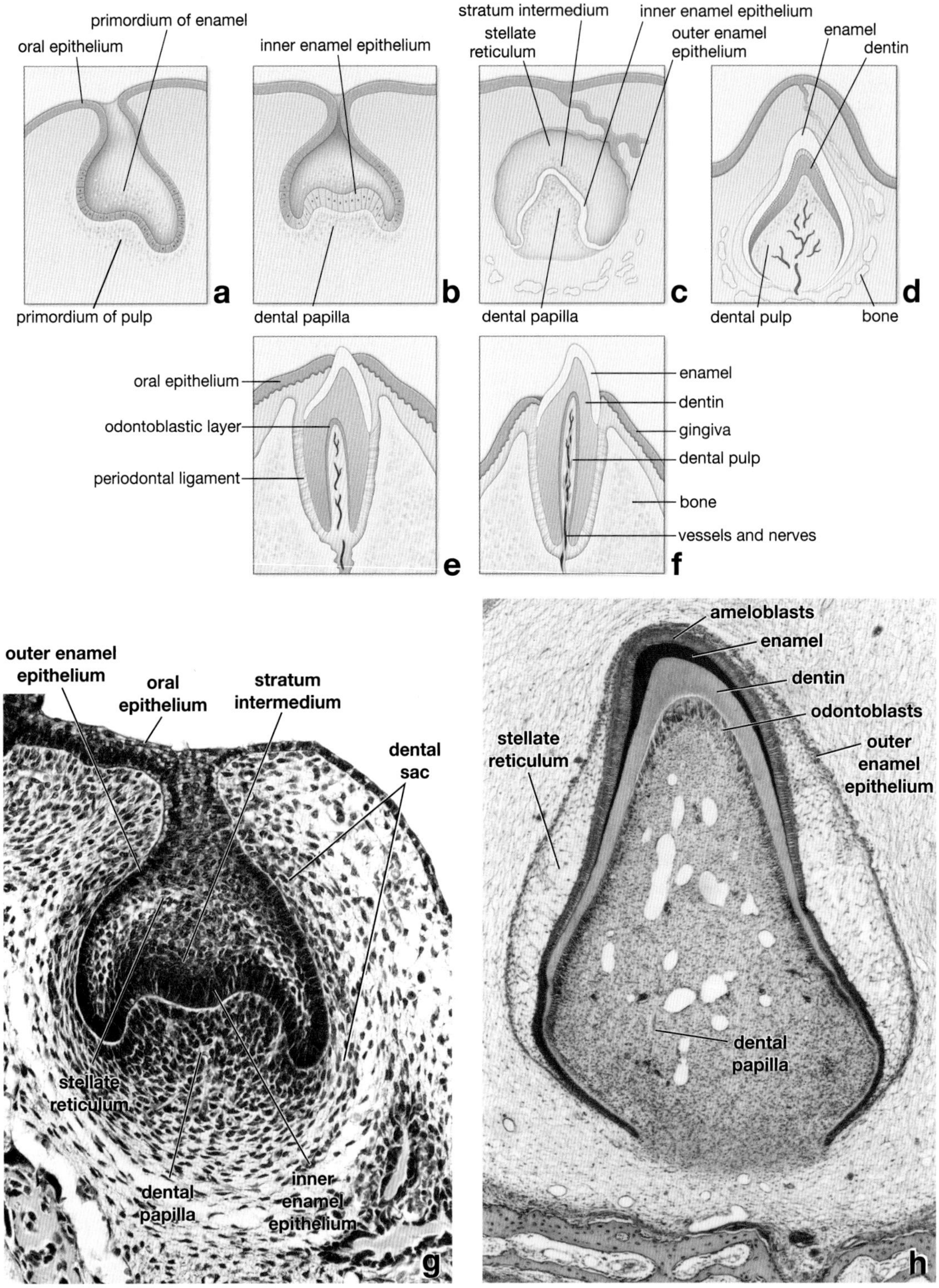

FIGURE 16.12. Diagrams and photomicrographs of a developing tooth. a. In the bud stage, the oral epithelium invaginates into the underlying mesenchyme, giving rise to the enamel organ (primordium of enamel). Mesenchymal cells adjacent to the tooth bud begin to differentiate, forming the dental papilla that protrudes into the tooth bud. **b.** Tooth bud in cap stage. In this stage, cells located in the concavity of the cap differentiate into tall, columnar cells (ameloblasts) forming the inner enamel epithelium. The condensed mesenchyme invaginates into the inner enamel epithelium, forming the dental papilla, which gives rise to the dentin and the pulp. **c.** In the bell stage, the connection with the oral epithelium is almost cut off. The enamel organ consists of a narrow line of outer enamel epithelium, an inner enamel epithelium formed by ameloblasts, several condensed layers of cells that form the stratum intermedium, and the widely spaced stellate reticulum. The dental papilla is deeply invaginated against the enamel organ. **d.** In this appositional dentin and enamel stage, the tooth bud is completely differentiated and independent from the oral epithelium. The relationship of the two mineralized tissues of the dental crown, enamel and dentin, is clearly visible. The surrounding mesenchyme has developed into bony tissue. **e.** In this stage of tooth eruption, the apex of the tooth emerges through the surface of the oral epithelium. The odontoblastic layer lines the pulp cavity. Note the developed periodontal ligaments that fasten the root of the tooth to the surrounding bone. The apex of the root is still open, but after eruption occurs, it becomes narrower. **f.** Functional tooth stage. Note the distribution of enamel and dentin. The tooth is embedded in the surrounding bone and gingiva. **g.** This photomicrograph of the developing tooth in the cap stage (comparable to **b**) shows its connection with the oral epithelium. The enamel organ consists of a single layer of cuboidal cells forming the outer enamel epithelium; the inner enamel epithelium has differentiated into columnar ameloblasts, and the layer of cells adjacent to the inner enamel epithelium has formed the stratum intermedium. The remainder of the structure is occupied by the stellate reticulum. The mesenchyme of the dental papilla has proliferated and pushed into the enamel organ. At this stage, the forming tooth is surrounded by condensed mesenchyme, called the *dental sac*, which gives rise to periodontal structures. ×300. **h.** This photomicrograph shows the developing crown of an incisor, which is surrounded by the outer enamel epithelium and remnants of the stellate reticulum. It is comparable to **d**. The underlying lighter stained layer of dentin is a product of the odontoblasts. These tall columnar odontoblasts have differentiated from cells of the dental papilla. The pulp cavity is filled with dental pulp, and blood vessels permeate the pulp tissue. ×40.

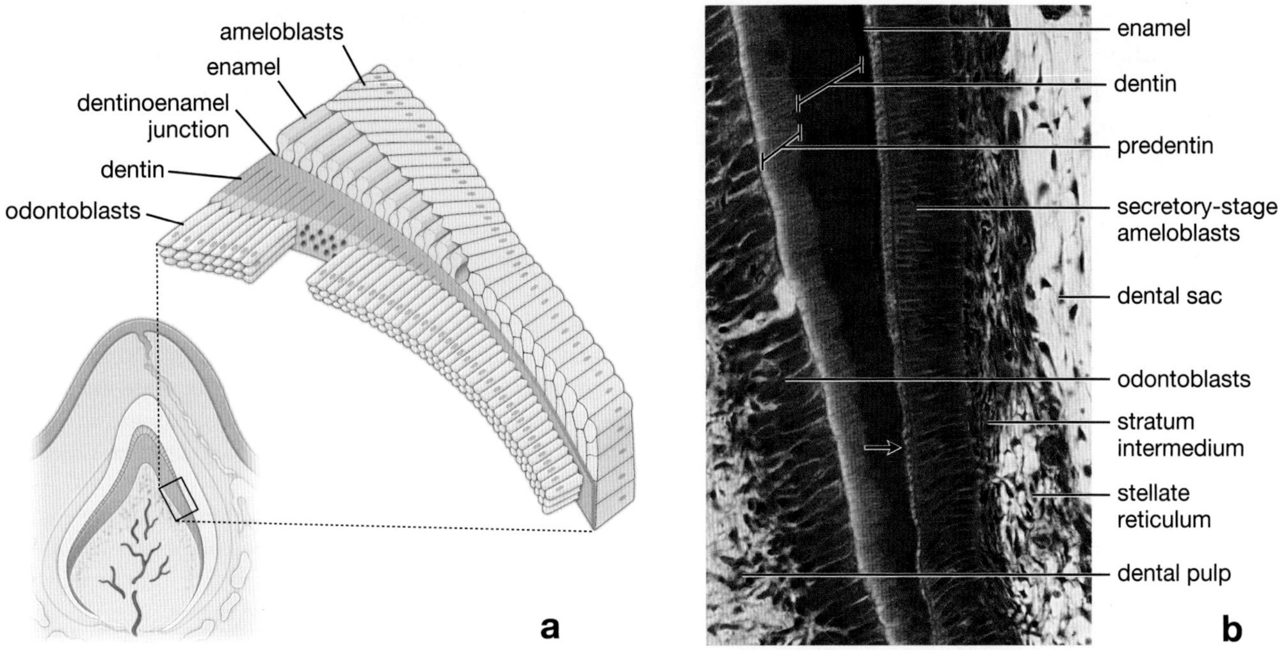

FIGURE 16.13. Diagram and photomicrograph showing the cellular relationships during enamel formation. a. In the initial secretory stage, dentin is produced first by odontoblasts. Enamel matrix is then deposited directly on the surface of the previously formed dentin by secretory-stage ameloblasts. The secretory-stage ameloblasts continue to produce enamel matrix until the full thickness of the future enamel is achieved. **b.** This photomicrograph of a hematoxylin and eosin (H&E)-stained section of a developing human tooth shows an early stage of enamel formation (amelogenesis). The secretory-stage ameloblasts lie directly adjacent to the developing enamel, which is being deposited on the layer of dentin. The beginning of enamel deposition is indicated by the *arrow*. As the first increment of enamel is formed, ameloblasts move away from the dentin surface. Basal domains of secretory-stage ameloblasts are adjacent to cells in the stratum intermedium (a part of the enamel organ). Dentin is secreted by odontoblasts. Note the *lightly stained layer* of the newly secreted organic matrix (predentin) is in close apposition to the apical surfaces of odontoblasts. Predentin further undergoes mineralization to mature dentin (*dark-stained layer*). The layer of odontoblasts separates enamel from the dental pulp. ×240. (Courtesy of Dr. Arthur R. Hand.)

Ca^{2+}-ATPase activity, they produce and secrete enzymes to degrade and reabsorb the extracellular matrix that is no longer necessary.

At this stage, there is no stratum intermedium in the enamel organ during enamel maturation. Cells from the underlying stratum intermedium, stellate reticulum, and outer dental epithelium collapse on each other and undergo reorganization, making it impossible to distinguish them as individual layers. Finally, the blood vessels invaginate into this newly reorganized layer to form the **papillary layer** containing stellate **papillary cells** that are adjacent to the maturation-stage ameloblasts.

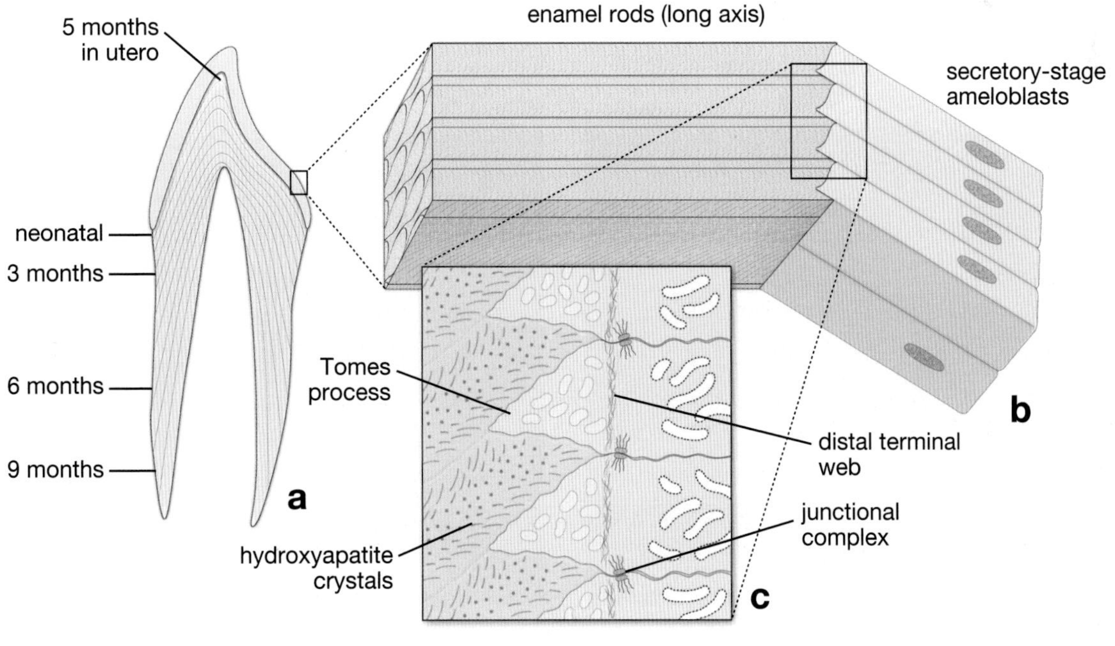

FIGURE 16.14. Schematic diagrams of a partially formed tooth showing details of amelogenesis. a. The enamel is drawn to show the enamel rods extending from the dentinoenamel junction to the surface of the tooth. Although the full thickness of the enamel is formed, the full thickness of the dentin has not yet been established. The contour lines within the dentin show the extent to which the dentin has developed at a particular time, as labeled in the illustration. Note that the pulp cavity in the center of the tooth becomes smaller as the dentin develops. (Based on Schour I, Massler M. The neonatal line in the enamel and dentin of the human deciduous teeth and first permanent molar. *J Am Dent Assoc.* 1936;23:1948.) **b.** During amelogenesis, enamel formation is influenced by the path of the ameloblasts. The rod produced by the ameloblast forms in the wake of the cell. Thus, in mature enamel, the direction of the enamel rod is a record of the path taken earlier by the secretory-stage ameloblast. **c.** At the apical pole of the secretory-stage ameloblasts are Tomes processes, surrounded by the developing enamel. Junctional complexes at the apical pole and distal terminal web are also shown. Note the numerous matrix-containing secretory vesicles in the cytoplasm of the processes.

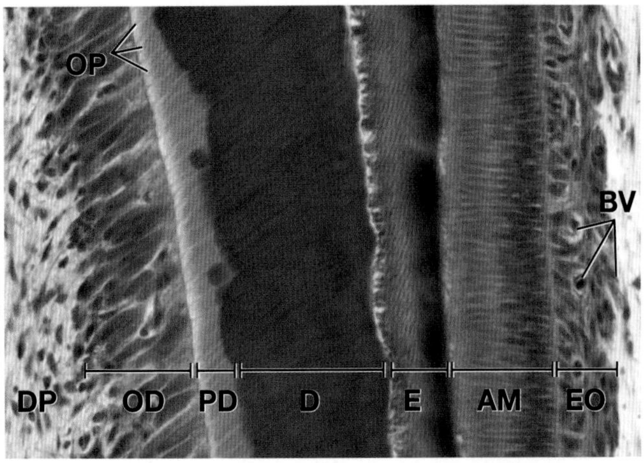

FIGURE 16.15. Enamel organ cells and odontoblasts in a developing tooth. This photomicrograph of a hematoxylin and eosin (H&E)-stained section of a developing human tooth shows ameloblasts and odontoblasts as they begin to produce enamel (*E*) and dentin (*D*), respectively. Enamel is deposited by the secretory-stage ameloblasts (*AM*) onto the previously formed dentin. The enamel appears *deep purple* in this image and is adjacent to the *reddish purple* layer of mature dentin (*D*). The blood vessels (*BV*) on the *right* belong to the enamel organ (*EO*), which is partially formed from the cells of the stratum intermedium. Basal domains of odontoblasts (*OD*) on the *left* are in contact with dental pulp (*DP*). The cytoplasm of odontoblasts is adjacent to predentin (*PD*). At this point, cytoplasmic processes of odontoblasts (*OP*) extend into dentinal tubules of predentin. ×280. (Courtesy of Dr. Arthur R. Hand.)

The maturation-stage ameloblasts and the adjacent papillary cells are characterized by numerous mitochondria. Their presence indicates cellular activity that requires large amounts of energy and reflects the function of maturation-stage ameloblasts and adjacent papillary cells as a transporting epithelium.

Recent advances in the molecular biology of ameloblast gene products have revealed the enamel matrix to be highly heterogeneous. It contains proteins encoded by a number of different genes. Listed as follows are the principal proteins in the extracellular matrix of the developing enamel:

- **Amelogenins**, important proteins in establishing and maintaining the spacing between enamel rods in the early stages of enamel development
- **Ameloblastins**, signaling proteins produced by ameloblasts from the early secretory to late maturation stages. Their function is not well understood; however, their developmental pattern suggests that ameloblastins play a much broader role in amelogenesis than the other proteins. Ameloblastins are believed to guide the enamel mineralization process by controlling elongation of the enamel crystals and to form junctional complexes between individual enamel crystals.
- **Enamelins**, proteins distributed throughout the enamel layer. These proteins undergo proteolytic cleavage as the enamel matures. Low-molecular-weight products of this cleavage are retained in the mature enamel, often localized on the surface of enamel crystals.
- **Tuftelins**, the earliest detected proteins located near the dentinoenamel junction. Their acidic and insoluble nature aids in the nucleation of enamel crystals. Tuftelins are present in **enamel tufts** and account for hypomineralization, that is, enamel tufts have a higher percentage of organic material than the remainder of the mature enamel.

The maturation of the developing enamel results in its continued mineralization so that it becomes the hardest substance in the body. Amelogenins and ameloblastins are removed during enamel maturation. Thus, mature enamel contains only enamelins and tuftelins. The ameloblasts degenerate after the enamel is fully formed, at about the time of tooth eruption through the gum.

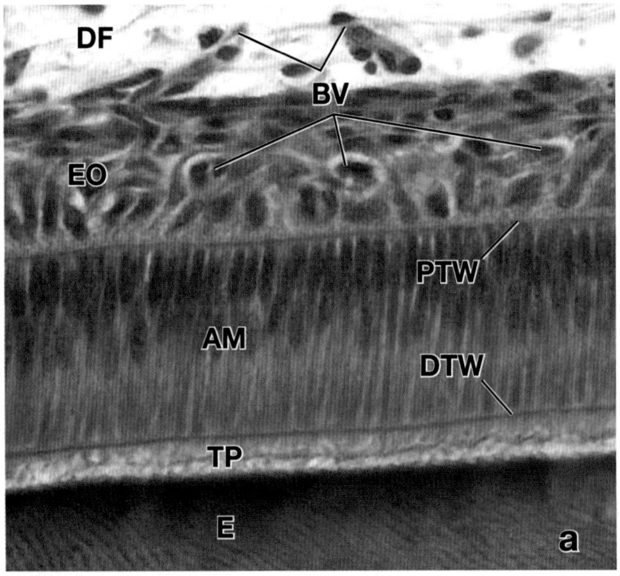

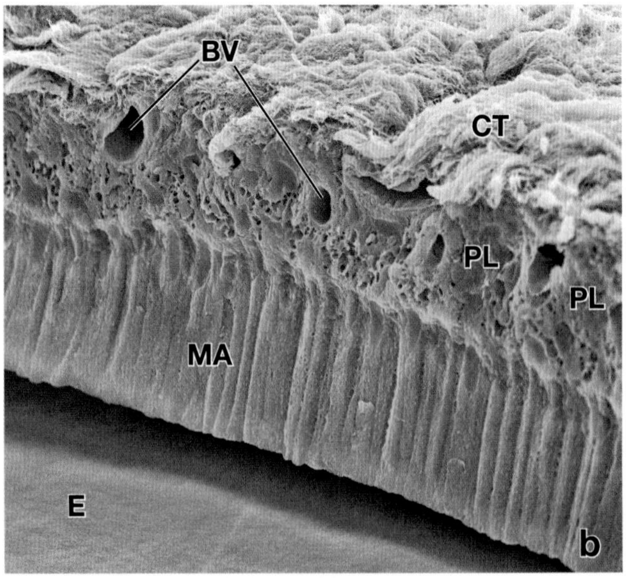

FIGURE 16.16. Ameloblasts in secretory and maturation stages. a. This high-magnification photomicrograph of a hematoxylin and eosin (H&E)-stained specimen shows the secretory-stage ameloblasts (*AM*). Note the lightly stained Tomes processes (*TP*) of the apical part of ameloblasts and the deeply stained enamel just below. The distinct *pink lines* are related to the accumulation of actin filaments in ameloblasts. The *first line* between Tomes processes and the cytoplasm of ameloblasts represents the distal terminal web (*DTW*), and the *second line* at the base of ameloblasts is the proximal terminal web (*PTW*). The enamel organ (*EO*) containing blood vessels (*BV*) is adjacent to the layer of ameloblasts. Stroma of dental follicles (*DF*) is visible at the top of this image. ×480. (Courtesy of Dr. Arthur R. Hand.) **b.** Colorized scanning electron micrograph of a freeze-fracture section of the tooth shows a layer of smooth-ended maturation-stage ameloblasts (*MA*, *green*) on the enamel surface (E, *orange*). At the basal pole of the ameloblasts are the cells of the papillary layer (*PL*) containing blood vessels (*BV*) and loose connective tissue (*CT*). A layer of stratum intermedium is no longer present during this stage of ameloblast maturation. During slide preparation, apical surfaces of ameloblasts were detached from the enamel. ×1,300. (Courtesy of SPL/Photo Researchers, Inc., with permission.)

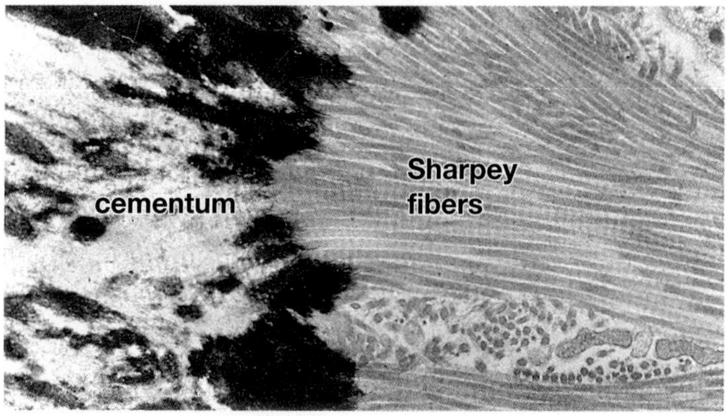

FIGURE 16.17. Electron micrograph of Sharpey fibers. Sharpey fibers extend from the periodontal ligament (*right*) into the cementum. They consist of collagen fibrils. Sharpey fibers within the cementum are mineralized; those within the periodontal ligament are not mineralized. ×13,000.

Cementum

Cementum covers the root of the tooth.

The **root** is the part of the tooth that fits into the **alveolus** or jaw socket in the maxilla or mandible. **Cementum** is a thin layer of bone-like material that covers the roots of the teeth beginning at the cervical portion of the tooth at the cementoenamel junction and continuing to the apex. Cementum is produced by **cementoblasts** (large cuboidal cells that resemble the osteoblasts of the surface of growing bone). Cementoblasts secrete an extracellular matrix called **cementoid** that undergoes mineralization. A layer of cementoblasts is present on the outer surface of the cementum, adjacent to the **periodontal ligament**. During cementogenesis, cementoblasts are incorporated into the cementum and become **cementocytes**, cells that closely resemble osteocytes in bone. Like bone, cementum is 65% mineral and contains the highest concentration of fluoride of any mineralized tissue. The lacunae and canaliculi in the cementum contain the cementocytes and their processes, respectively. They resemble structures in bone that contain osteocytes and osteocyte processes. Unlike bone, cementum is avascular. In addition, the lacunae are irregularly distributed throughout the cementum and their canaliculi do not form an interconnecting network.

Collagen fibers that project out of the matrix of the cementum and embed in the bony matrix of the socket wall form the bulk of the periodontal ligament. These fibers are another example of **Sharpey fibers** (Fig. 16.17). In addition, elastic fibers are also a component of the periodontal ligament. This mode of attachment of the tooth in its socket allows slight movement of the tooth to occur naturally. It also forms the basis of orthodontic procedures used to straighten teeth and reduce malocclusion of the biting and grinding surfaces of the maxillary and mandibular teeth. During corrective tooth movements, the alveolar bone of the socket is resorbed and resynthesized, but the cementum is not.

Dentin

Dentin is a calcified material that forms most of the tooth substance.

Dentin lies deep to the enamel and cementum. It contains less hydroxyapatite than enamel, about 70%, but more than is found in bone and cementum. Dentin is secreted by **odontoblasts** that form an epithelial layer over the inner surface of the dentin, that is, the surface that is in contact with the pulp (Fig. 16.18). Like ameloblasts, odontoblasts are columnar cells that contain a well-developed rER,

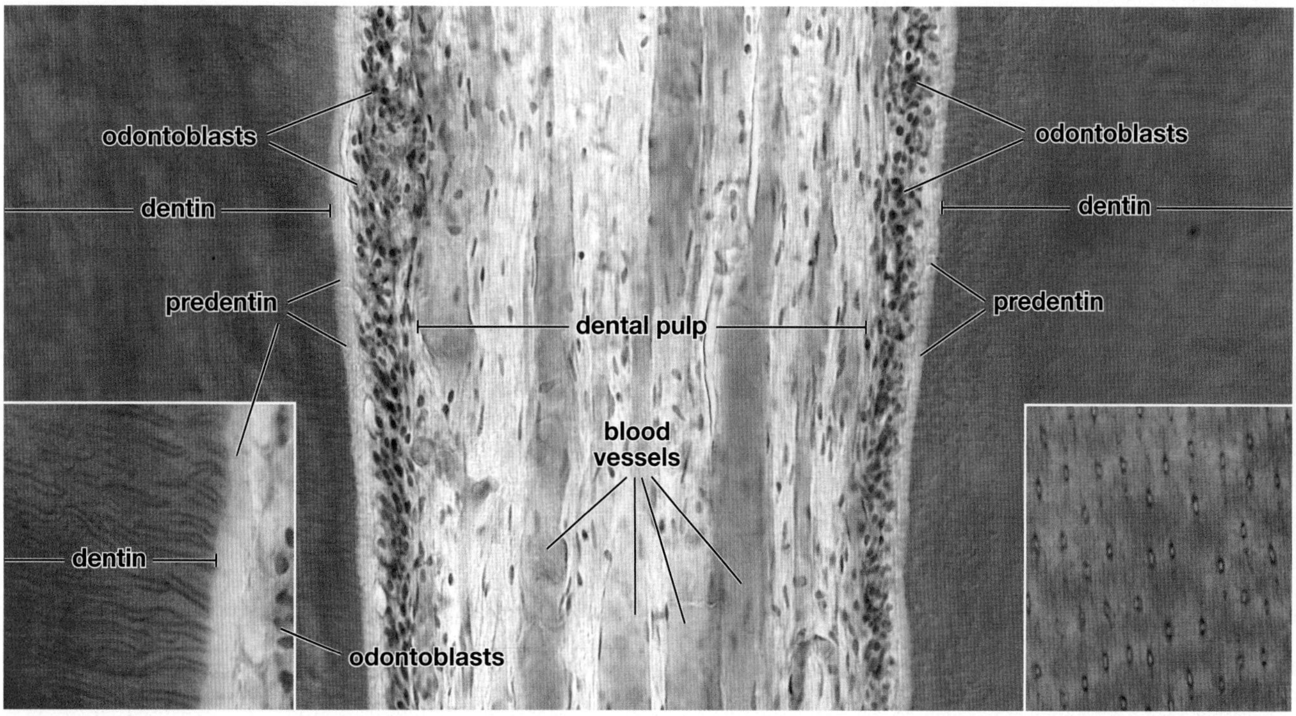

FIGURE 16.18. Dental pulp and structure of dentin. This photomicrograph of a decalcified tooth shows the centrally located dental pulp, surrounded by dentin on both sides. The dental pulp is a soft-tissue core of the tooth that resembles embryonic connective tissue, even in the adult. It contains blood vessels and nerves. Dentin contains the cytoplasmic processes of the odontoblasts within dentinal tubules. They extend into the dentinoenamel junction. The cell bodies of the odontoblasts are adjacent to the unmineralized dentin called the *predentin*. ×120. **Left inset.** Longitudinal profiles of the dentinal tubules. ×240. **Right inset.** Cross-sectional profiles of dentinal tubules. The dark outline of the dentinal tubules, as seen in both *insets*, represents the peritubular dentin, which is the more mineralized part of the dentin. ×240.

a large Golgi apparatus, and other organelles associated with the synthesis and secretion of large amounts of protein (Fig. 16.19). The apical surface of the odontoblast is in contact with the forming dentin; junctional complexes between the odontoblasts at that level separate the dentinal compartment from the pulp chamber.

The layer of odontoblasts retreats as the dentin is laid down, leaving odontoblast processes embedded in the dentin in narrow channels called **dentinal tubules** (see Fig. 16.18). The tubules and processes continue to elongate as the dentin continues to thicken by rhythmic growth. The rhythmic growth of dentin produces certain "growth lines" in the dentin (incremental lines of von Ebner and thicker lines of Owen) that mark significant developmental times such as birth (**neonatal line**) and when unusual substances such as lead are incorporated into the growing tooth. The study of growth lines has proved useful in forensic medicine.

Predentin is the newly secreted organic matrix, closest to the cell body of the odontoblast, which has yet to be mineralized. Although most of the proteins in the organic matrix are similar to those of bone, predentin contains two unique proteins:

- **Dentin phosphoprotein (DPP)**, a 45-kDa highly acidic phosphorylated protein, which is rich in aspartic acid and phosphoserine and binds large amounts of calcium. DPP is involved in the initiation of mineralization and the control of mineral size and shape.
- **Dentin sialoprotein (DSP)**, a 100-kDa proteoglycan that is rich in aspartic and glutamic acids, serine, glycine, and chondroitin 6-sulfate. DSP is also involved in the mineralization process.

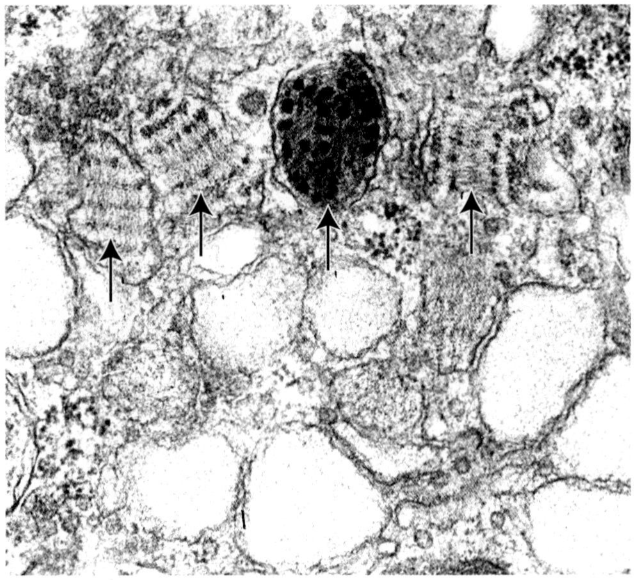

FIGURE 16.20. Golgi apparatus in an odontoblast. This electron micrograph shows a region of the Golgi apparatus containing numerous large vesicles. Note the abacus bodies (*arrows*) that contain parallel arrays of filaments studded with granules. ×52,000.

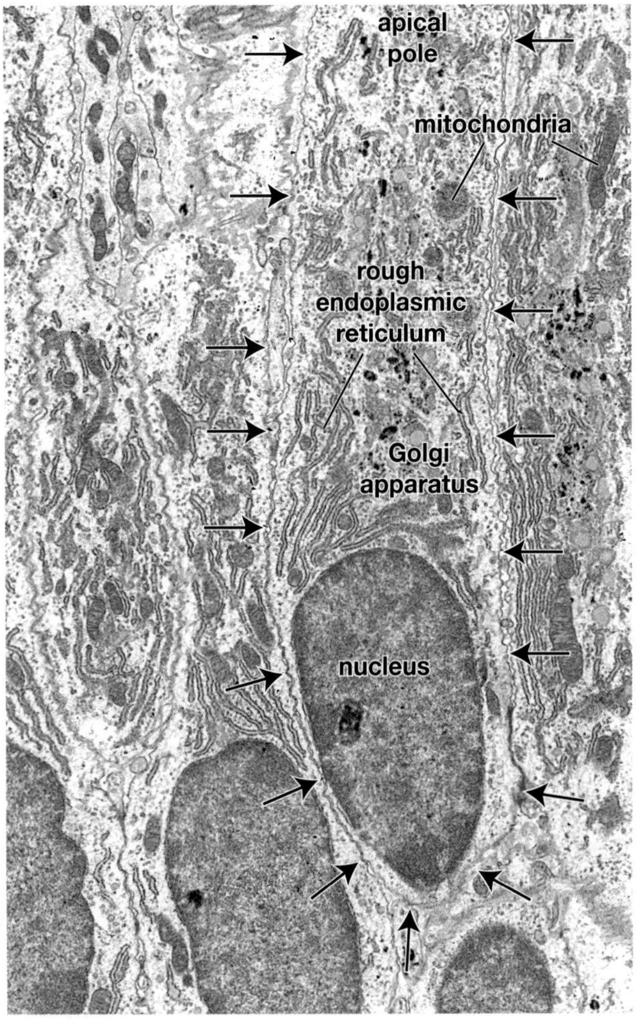

FIGURE 16.19. Electron micrograph of odontoblasts. The plasma membrane of one odontoblast has been marked with *arrows*. The cell contains a large amount of rough endoplasmic reticulum and a large Golgi apparatus. The odontoblast processes are not included in this image; one process would extend from the apical pole of each cell (*top*). The *black objects* in the Golgi region are abacus bodies. The tissue has been treated with pyroantimonate, which forms a black precipitate with calcium. ×12,000.

An unusual feature of the secretion of collagen and hydroxyapatite by odontoblasts is the presence, in Golgi vesicles, of arrays of a formed filamentous collagen precursor. Granules believed to contain calcium attach to these precursors, giving rise to structures called **abacus bodies** (Figs. 16.19 and 16.20). Abacus bodies become more condensed as they mature into secretory granules.

Dentin is produced by odontoblasts.

Dentin is the first mineralized component of the tooth to be deposited. The outermost dentin, which is referred to as **mantle dentin**, is formed by subodontoblastic cells that produce small bundles of collagen fibers (von Korff fibers). The **odontoblasts** differentiate from cells at the periphery of the dental papilla. The progenitor cells have the appearance of typical mesenchymal cells, that is, they contain little cytoplasm. During their differentiation into odontoblasts, the cytoplasmic volume and organelles characteristic of collagen-producing cells increase. The cells form a layer at the periphery of the dental papilla, and they secrete the organic matrix of dentin, or predentin, at their apical end (away from the dental papilla; Fig. 16.21). As the predentin thickens, the odontoblasts move or are displaced centrally (see Fig. 16.14). A **wave of mineralization** follows the receding odontoblasts; this mineralized product is dentin. As

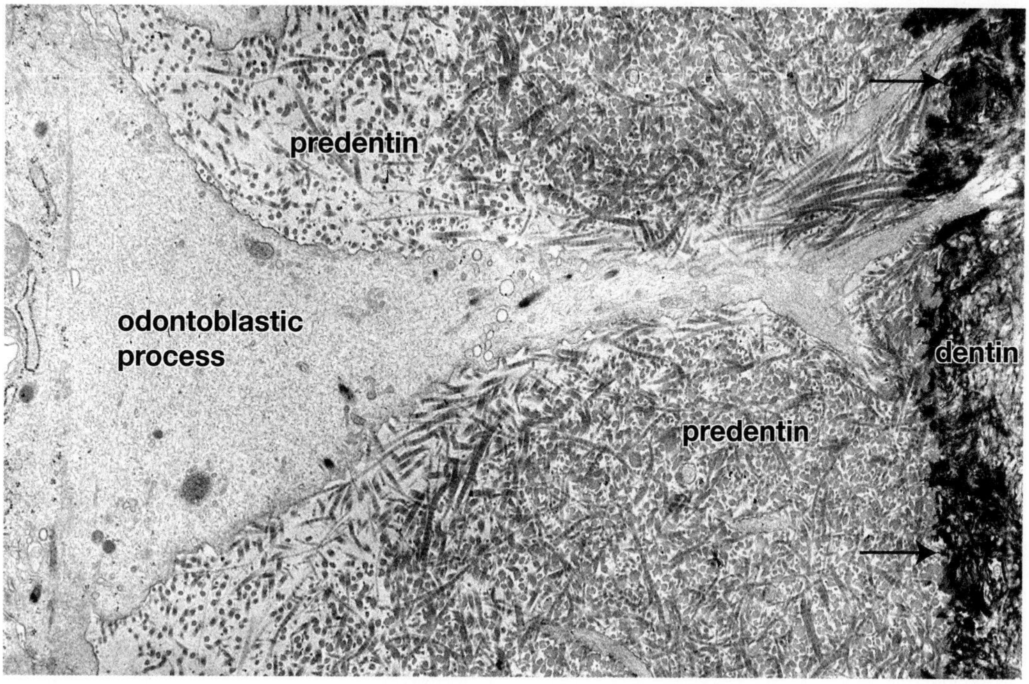

FIGURE 16.21. Odontoblast process of a young odontoblast. This electron micrograph shows a process of the odontoblast entering a dentinal tubule. The process extends into the predentin and, after passing the mineralization front (*arrows*), lies within the dentin. The collagen fibrils in the predentin are finer than the more mature, coarser fibrils of the mineralization front and beyond. ×34,000.

the cells move centrally, the odontoblastic processes elongate, the longest being surrounded by the mineralized dentin. In newly formed dentin, the wall of the dentinal tubule is simply the edge of the mineralized dentin. Over time, the dentin immediately surrounding the dentinal tubule becomes more highly mineralized; this more mineralized sheath of dentin is referred to as the **peritubular dentin**. The remainder of the dentin is called the **intertubular dentin**.

Dental Pulp and Central Pulp Cavity (Pulp Chamber)

The dental pulp cavity is a connective tissue compartment bounded by the tooth dentin.

The **central pulp cavity** is the space within a tooth that is occupied by **dental pulp**, a loose connective tissue that is richly vascularized and supplied by abundant nerves. The pulp cavity takes the general shape of the tooth. The blood vessels and nerves enter the pulp cavity at the tip (apex) of the root at a site called the **apical foramen**. (The designations *apex* and *apical* in this context refer only to the narrowed tip of the root of the tooth rather than to a luminal [apical] surface, as used in describing secretory and absorptive epithelia.)

The blood vessels and nerves extend to the crown of the tooth, where they form vascular and neural networks beneath and within the layer of odontoblasts. Some bare nerve fibers also enter the proximal portions of the dentinal tubules and contact with the odontoblast processes. The odontoblast processes are believed to serve a transducer function in transmitting stimuli from the tooth surface to the nerves in the dental pulp. In teeth with more than one cusp, **pulpal horns** extend into the cusps and contain large numbers of nerve fibers. More of these fibers extend into the dentinal tubules than at other sites. Because dentin continues to be secreted throughout life, the pulp cavity decreases in volume with age.

Supporting Tissues of the Teeth

Supporting tissues of the teeth include the alveolar bone of the alveolar processes of the maxilla and mandible, periodontal ligaments, and gingiva.

The alveolar processes of the maxilla and mandible contain the sockets or alveoli for the roots of the teeth.

The **alveolar bone proper**, a thin layer of compact bone, forms the wall of the alveolus (see Fig. 16.9) and is the bone to which the periodontal ligament is attached. The rest of the alveolar process consists of supporting bone.

The surface of the alveolar bone proper usually shows regions of bone resorption and bone deposition, particularly when a tooth is being moved (Fig. 16.22). **Periodontal disease** usually leads to loss of alveolar bone, as does the absence of functional occlusion of a tooth with its normal opposing tooth.

The **periodontal ligament** is the fibrous connective tissue joining the tooth to its surrounding bone. This ligament is also called the **periodontal membrane**, but neither term describes its structure and function adequately. The **periodontal ligament** provides for the following:

- Tooth attachment (fixation)
- Tooth support
- Bone remodeling (during movement of a tooth)
- Proprioception
- Tooth eruption

A histologic section of the periodontal ligament shows that it contains areas of both dense and loose connective tissues. The dense connective tissue contains collagen fibers and fibroblasts that are elongated parallel to the long axis of the collagen fibers. The fibroblasts are believed to move back and forth, leaving behind a trail of collagen fibers. Periodontal fibroblasts also contain internalized collagen fibrils

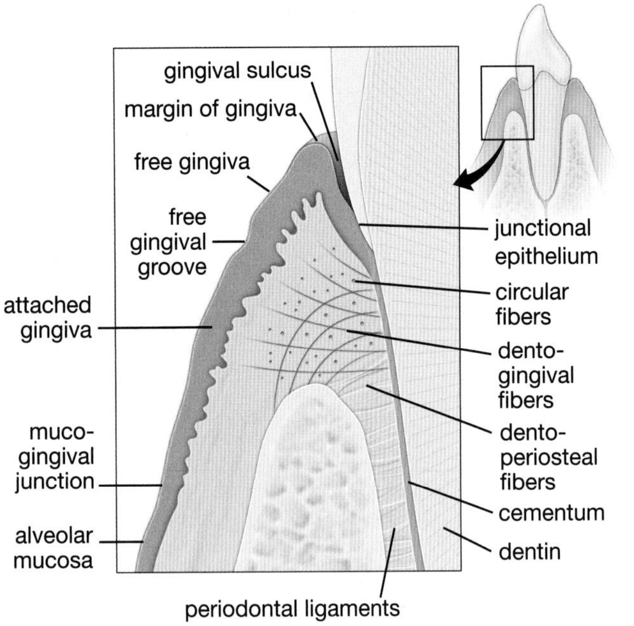

FIGURE 16.22. Schematic diagram of gingiva. This schematic diagram of gingiva corresponds to the *rectangular area* of the orientation diagram. The gingival epithelium is attached to the enamel of the tooth. Here, the junction between epithelium and connective tissue is smooth. Elsewhere, the gingival epithelium is deeply indented by connective tissue papillae, and the junction between the two is irregular. The *black lines* represent collagen fibers from the cementum of the tooth and from the crest of the alveolar bone that extend toward the gingival epithelium. Note the shallow papillae in the lining mucosa (alveolar mucosa) that contrast sharply with those of the gingiva.

that are digested by the hydrolytic enzymes of the cytoplasmic lysosomes. These observations indicate that the fibroblasts not only produce collagen fibrils but also resorb collagen fibrils, thereby adjusting continuously to the demands of tooth stress and movement.

The loose connective tissue in the periodontal ligament contains blood vessels and nerve endings. In addition to fibroblasts and thin collagenous fibers, the periodontal ligament also contains thin, longitudinally disposed **oxytalan fibers.** They are attached to bone or cementum at each end. Some appear to be associated with the adventitia of blood vessels.

The gingiva is the part of the mucous membrane commonly called the *gums*.

The **gingiva** is a specialized part of the oral mucosa located around the neck of the tooth. It is firmly attached to the teeth and underlying alveolar bony tissue. An idealized diagram of the gingiva is presented in Figure 16.22. The gingiva is composed of two parts:

- **Gingival mucosa**, which is synonymous with the masticatory mucosa described earlier
- **Junctional epithelium**, or **attachment epithelium**, which adheres firmly to the tooth. A basal lamina–like material is secreted by the junctional epithelium and adheres firmly to the tooth surface. The cells then attach to this material via hemidesmosomes. The basal lamina and the hemidesmosomes are together referred to as the **epithelial attachment.** In young individuals, this attachment is to the enamel; in older individuals, where passive tooth eruption and gingival recession expose the roots, the attachment is to the cementum.

Above the attachment of the epithelium to the tooth, a shallow crevice called the **gingival sulcus** is lined with **crevicular epithelium** that is continuous with the attachment epithelium.

The term **periodontium** refers to all the tissues involved in the attachment of a tooth to the mandible and maxilla. These include the crevicular and junctional epithelium, the cementum, the periodontal ligament, and the alveolar bone. **Periodontitis** is an inflammatory oral disease that leads to the destruction of periodontal tissue involved in the attachment of the tooth. Although conventional therapies are available to control the inflammatory process, they are unable to restore damaged periodontal structures. With the discovery of multipotent **periodontal ligament stem cells (PDLSCs)**, periodontal regenerative treatment that could restore the physiologic function of teeth by rebuilding damaged periodontal supporting tissues, including alveolar bone, gingiva, periodontal ligaments, and the cementum, may become possible. PDLSCs in humans can be obtained from healthy permanent and deciduous teeth. When isolated human PDLSCs are transplanted into laboratory animals, they differentiate into periodontal ligaments, alveolar bone, cementum, peripheral nerves, and blood vessels.

■ SALIVARY GLANDS

The major salivary glands are paired glands with long ducts that empty into the oral cavity.

The **major salivary glands**, as noted earlier, consist of the paired parotid, submandibular, and sublingual glands. The parotid and the submandibular glands are actually located outside the oral cavity; their secretions reach the cavity by ducts. The **parotid gland** is located subcutaneously, below and in front of the ear in the space between the ramus of the mandible and the styloid process of the temporal bone. The **submandibular gland** is located under the floor of the mouth, in the submandibular triangle of the neck. The **sublingual gland** is located on the floor of the mouth anterior to the submandibular gland.

The **minor salivary glands** are located in the submucosa of different parts of the oral cavity. They include the **lingual**, **labial**, **buccal**, **molar**, and **palatine glands**.

The embryologic development of the major salivary glands is a complex process requiring multidirectional signaling between invaginating epithelium and mesenchyme.

Each salivary gland arises from the developing oral cavity epithelium. The parotid glands develop first from invagination of the oral ectodermal lining the stomodeum (primitive oral cavity), whereas the submandibular and sublingual glands arise later from oral endoderm (near the junction between the ectoderm of the stomodeum and the endoderm of the gut tube). Initially, the gland forms a solid cord of cells that enters the mesenchyme. The invaginated epithelium interacts with the adjacent mesenchyme, and through multidirectional signaling networks, these interactions influence the growth and differentiation of the gland tissue. Under the influence of fibroblast growth factor-10 (FGF10), the proliferation of epithelial cells eventually produces highly branched epithelial cords with bulbous ends. Degeneration of the innermost cells of the cords and bulbous ends leads to their canalization. The cords become ducts, and the bulbous ends become **secretory acini**. Finally, the glands develop a dense irregular connective tissue capsule. In addition, both sympathetic and parasympathetic innervations are necessary for the proper development, growth, and maintenance of salivary gland tissue.

Any disruption in signaling networks between the developing glandular epithelium and mesenchyme, as well as disruption of autonomic nervous system innervation, may lead to **salivary gland aplasia** (lack of its development). Craniofacial abnormalities such as cleft palate, skeletal dysplasias, and branchial cleft anomalies are also associated with either unilateral or bilateral salivary gland aplasia and hypoplasia (arrested development).

Secretory Gland Acini

Secretory acini are organized into lobules.

The major salivary glands are surrounded by a capsule of moderately dense connective tissue from which septa divide the secretory portions of the gland into lobes and lobules. The septa contain the larger blood vessels and excretory ducts. The connective tissue associated with the groups of secretory acini blends imperceptibly into the surrounding loose connective tissue. The minor salivary glands do not have a capsule.

Numerous lymphocytes and plasma cells populate the connective tissue surrounding the acini in both the major and minor salivary glands. Their significance in the secretion of salivary antibodies is described later.

Acini are of three types: serous, mucous, or mixed.

The basic secretory unit of salivary glands, the **salivon**, consists of the acinus, intercalated duct, and excretory duct (Fig. 16.23). The **acinus** is a blind sac composed of secretory cells. The term *acinus [L, berry or grape]* refers to the secretory unit of the salivary glands. The acini of salivary glands contain **serous cells** (protein secreting), **mucous cells** (mucin secreting), or both. The relative frequencies of the three types of acini are the primary characteristic by which the major salivary glands are distinguished. Thus, three types of acini are described:

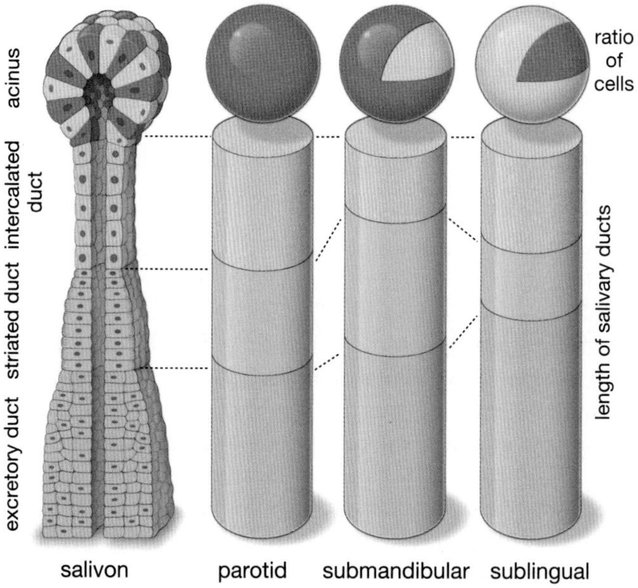

FIGURE 16.23. Diagram comparing the components of the salivon in the three major salivary glands. The four major parts of the salivon—the acinus, intercalated duct, striated duct, and excretory duct—are color coded. The three columns on the *right* of the salivon compare the length of the different ducts in the three salivary glands. The *red-colored* cells of the acinus represent serous-secreting cells, and the *yellow-colored* cells represent mucus-secreting cells. The ratio of serous-secreting cells to mucus-secreting cells is depicted in the acini of the various glands.

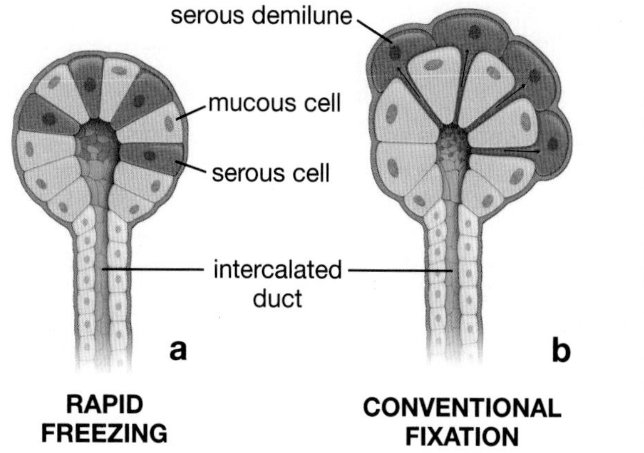

FIGURE 16.24. Relationship of serous-secreting cells and mucus-secreting cells in a mixed acinus. a. This drawing indicates the relationship of the mucous and serous cells as observed in the electron microscope after the rapid-freezing method. The serous cells extend from the basal lamina to the lumen of the acinus. **b.** In this drawing, serous cells are shown occupying the periphery of the acinus to form the so-called *serous demilune*. This feature is visible in routine preparations using immersion fixation. The swollen mucous cells have forced out the serous cells, leaving small remnants of the cytoplasm between the mucous cells.

- **Serous acini**, which contain only serous cells and are generally spherical
- **Mucous acini**, which contain only mucous cells and are usually more tubular
- **Mixed acini**, which contain both serous and mucous cells. In routine H&E preparations, mucous acini appear to have a cap of serous cells, in which the cytoplasm extends into the narrowed and highly convoluted intercellular space between the mucous cells. Because of their appearance in histologic sections, such caps are called **serous demilunes** *[Fr. half-moon]* and represent an artifact of fixation.

Serous demilunes are artifacts of the traditional fixation method.

As noted earlier, each mixed acinus, such as those found in the sublingual and submandibular glands, contains serous- and mucus-producing cells. In routine preparations for both light and electron microscopies, serous cells have traditionally been regarded as the structures that make up the **demilune**. Recent electron microscopic studies now challenge this classic interpretation of the demilune. Rapid freezing of the tissue in liquid nitrogen, followed by rapid-freeze substitution with osmium tetroxide in cold acetone, reveals that both mucous and serous cells are aligned in the same row to surround the lumen of the secretory acinus. No serous demilune is found (Fig. 16.24a). Sections prepared from the same specimen by conventional methods show swollen **mucous cells** with enlarged secretory granules. The serous cells have been squeezed out by swollen mucous cells to form typical demilunes. Most of the cell cytoplasm is relocated to the peripheral region of the

FOLDER 16.3

CLINICAL CORRELATION: DENTAL CARIES

Dental caries is an infectious microbial disease of teeth that results in the destruction of affected calcified tissues, that is, enamel, dentin, and cementum. Carious lesions generally occur under masses of bacterial colonies referred to as "dental plaque." The onset of dental caries is primarily associated with bacterial colonies of *Streptococcus mutans*, whereas lactobacilli are associated with an active progression of the disease. These bacterial colonies metabolize carbohydrates, producing an acidic environment that demineralizes the underlying tooth structure. Frequent sucrose ingestion is strongly associated with the development of these acidogenic bacterial colonies.

Trace amounts of **fluoride**, from sources such as water supplies (0.5–1.0 ppm is optimal), toothpaste, and even diet, can improve resistance to the effects of cariogenic bacteria. Fluoride improves the acid resistance of the tooth structure, acts as an antimicrobial agent, and promotes remineralization of small carious lesions. Resistance to acid breakdown of enamel is facilitated by the substitution of fluoride ion for the hydroxyl ion in the hydroxyapatite crystal. This decreases enamel crystal solubility in acid.

Treatment of cavitated lesions, or "tooth cavities" (Fig. F16.3.1), includes excavation of the infected tooth tissue and replacement with dental materials, such as amalgam, composite, and glass ionomer cements. Microbial invasion of tooth structure can reach the "pulp" of the tooth and elicit an inflammatory response. In this case, endodontic treatment, or a "root canal," is generally recommended, with subsequent placement of a crown to add strength to the compromised coronal tooth structure.

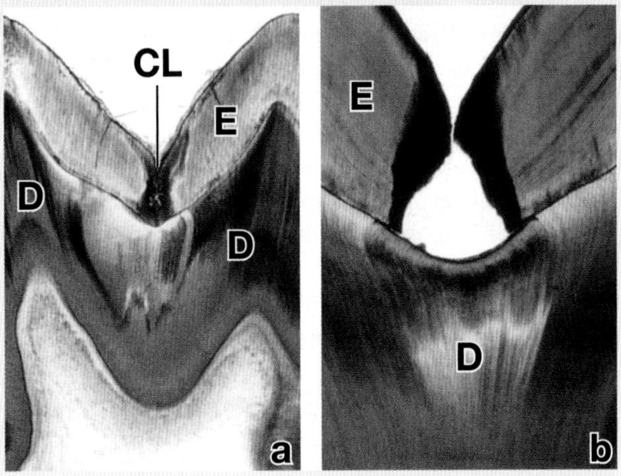

FIGURE F16.3.1. Photomicrographs of carious lesions. a. Photomicrograph of an unstained ground section of a tooth showing a carious lesion (*CL*) that has penetrated the entire thickness of the enamel (*E*) and spread laterally at the amelodentinal junction. *D*, dentin. **b.** The lesion here is more advanced. The enamel (*E*) has been undermined and weakened, causing fracture and a resulting cavity. At this point, bacteria can invade and penetrate into the exposed dental tubules, resulting in destructive liquefaction foci in the dentin (*D*) and, ultimately, exposure of the pulp. ×16. (From Eveson JW, Scully C. *Color Atlas of Oral Pathology*. Times Mirror International Publishers; 1995.)

acinus with slender cytoplasmic processes interposed between the mucous cells (Fig. 16.24b). These findings indicate that the demilune observed in light or electron microscopy is an **artifact of the routine fixation method** (see Fig. 16.24). The process of demilune formation can be explained by the expansion of mucinogen, a major component of secretory granules, during routine fixation. This expansion increases the volume of the mucous cells and displaces the serous cells from their original position, thus creating the demilune effect. A similar phenomenon is sometimes seen in the intestinal mucosa, in which swollen goblet cells displace adjacent absorptive cells.

Serous cells are protein-secreting cells.

Serous cells have a pyramidal shape, with a relatively wide basal surface facing the basal lamina and a small apical surface facing the lumen of the acinus. They contain large amounts of rER, free ribosomes, a prominent Golgi apparatus, and numerous spherical secretory granules (Fig. 16.25). As in most protein-secreting cells that store their secretions in **zymogen granules**, the granules are located in the apical cytoplasm. Most other organelles are located in the basal or perinuclear cytoplasm. In H&E sections, the basal cytoplasm of the serous cell stains with hematoxylin because of the presence of the rER and free ribosomes, whereas the apical region stains with eosin, in large part because of the presence of secretory granules.

When examined with the transmission electron microscope (TEM), the base of the serous cell may display infoldings of the plasma membrane and basolateral folds in the form of processes that interdigitate with similar processes of adjacent cells. The serous cells are joined near their apical surface by junctional complexes to neighboring cells of the acinus (see Fig. 16.25).

Mucous cells are mucin-secreting cells.

As in other mucus-secreting epithelia, the **mucous cells** of the mucous salivary acini undergo cyclic activity. During part of the cycle, mucus is synthesized and stored within the cell as **mucinogen granules**. When the product is discharged after hormonal or neural stimulation, the cell begins to resynthesize mucus. After discharge of most or all of the mucinogen granules, the cell is difficult to distinguish from an inactive serous cell. However, most mucous cells contain large numbers of mucinogen granules in their apical cytoplasm, and because the mucinogen is lost in H&E-stained paraffin sections, the apical portion of the cell usually appears empty. In TEM preparations, the rER, mitochondria, and other components are seen chiefly in the basal portion of the cell; this part of the cell also contains the nucleus, which is typically flattened against the base of the cell (Fig. 16.26). In rapid-freeze preparations (Fig. 16.27), cells are rounded and clearly isolated from each other. The nuclei are round and centrally located. The apical portion of the mucous cell

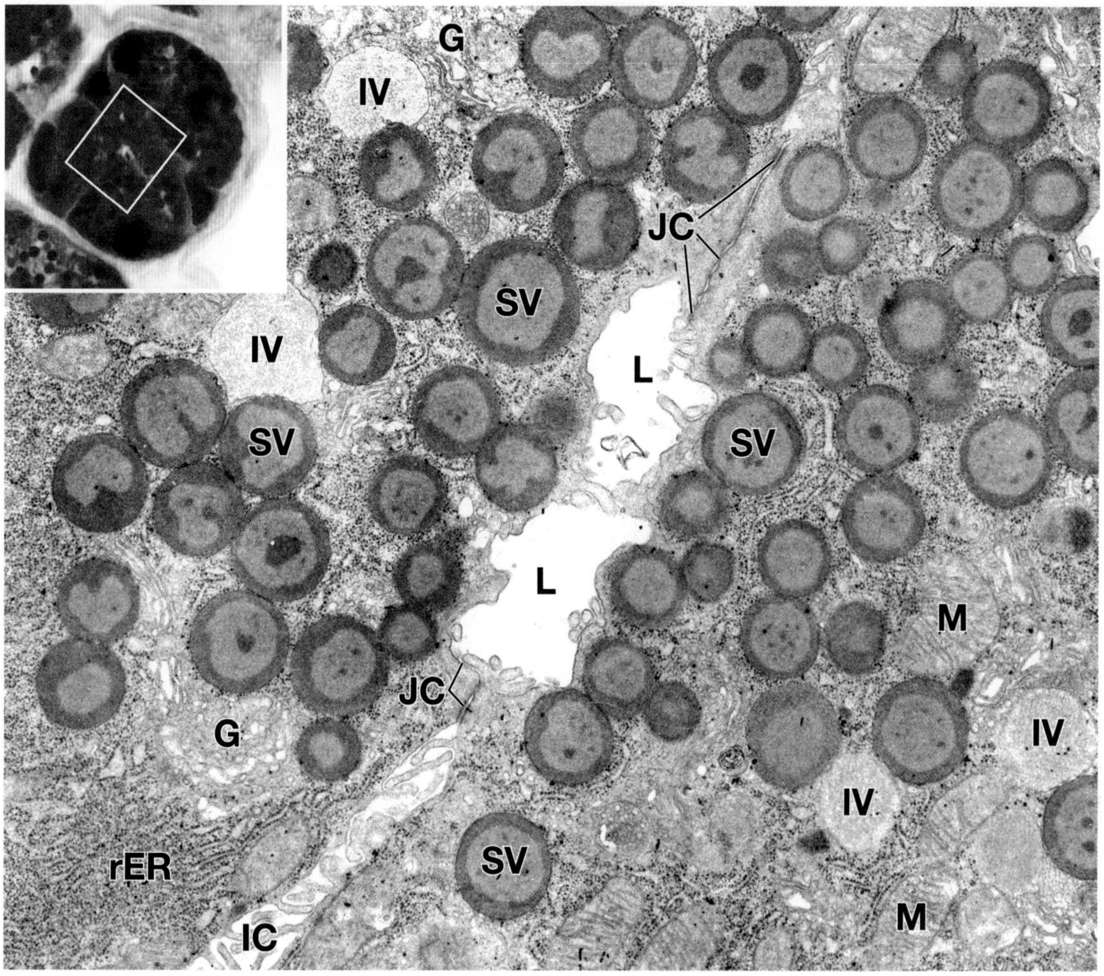

FIGURE 16.25. Electron micrograph of the apical portion of parotid gland serous cells. As indicated by the *box* in the orientation photomicrograph, only the apical portions of parotid gland serous acinus are shown in this electron micrograph. The cells are polarized, with their product packaged within the secretory vesicles (*SV*) near the lumen (*L*) of the acinus. The cells display rough endoplasmic reticulum (*rER*) and several profiles of the Golgi apparatus (*G*). Immature secretory vesicles (*IV*) are present close to the Golgi apparatus. At the apical pole of the cells are junctional complexes (*JC*). The intercellular space (*IC*) is dilated, and profiles of sectioned lateral plications are seen. *M*, mitochondria. ×15,000.

contains numerous mucinogen granules and a large Golgi apparatus, in which large amounts of carbohydrates are added to a protein base to synthesize the glycoprotein of the mucin. Mucous cells possess apical junctional complexes, the same as those seen between serous cells.

Secretion from salivary glands is largely dependent upon signals from the parasympathetic nerves. The protein content of the saliva is increased by sympathetic innervation and modified by neuropeptides (i.e., nerve growth factor [NGF], substance P).

Myoepithelial cells are contractile cells that embrace the base of the acinar secretory cells.

Myoepithelial cells are contractile cells with numerous processes. Owing to their shape and interwoven processes forming a basket around the acinus, they are commonly referred to as "basket cells." Other descriptions compare them to "an octopus sitting on a rock." They lie between the basal plasma membrane of the epithelial cells and the basal lamina of the epithelium (Fig. 16.28). They are not unique to the salivary gland and can be found in the secretory portion of most excretory glands, such as mammary, lacrimal, and sweat glands.

Myoepithelial cells also underlie the cells of the proximal portion of the duct system (intercalated and striated ducts), where they are oriented along the long axes of ducts. In both locations, the contraction of the myoepithelial cells is instrumental in reducing the acinus's luminal volume and shortening the length of the duct system (pumping effect) in moving secretory products toward the excretory duct.

Myoepithelial cells are sometimes difficult to identify in H&E sections. The nucleus of the cell is often seen as a small, round profile near the basement membrane. The contractile filaments stain with eosin and are sometimes recognized as a thin eosinophilic band adjacent to the basement membrane. On electron micrographs, cells exhibit electron density owing to the accumulation of contractile elements with visible cytoplasmic densities (dense bodies) similar to that found in muscle cells (Fig. 16.29). Myoepithelial cells produce and maintain a basement membrane; thus, their cytoplasm contains typical organelles, such as mitochondria, rER, Golgi apparatus, and occasional collections of glycogen particles. They secrete basement membrane–related proteins (type IV collagen and laminin) and other interstitial matrix proteins. The feature distinguishing them from smooth muscle cells is that myoepithelial cells are attached to acinar and ductal cells

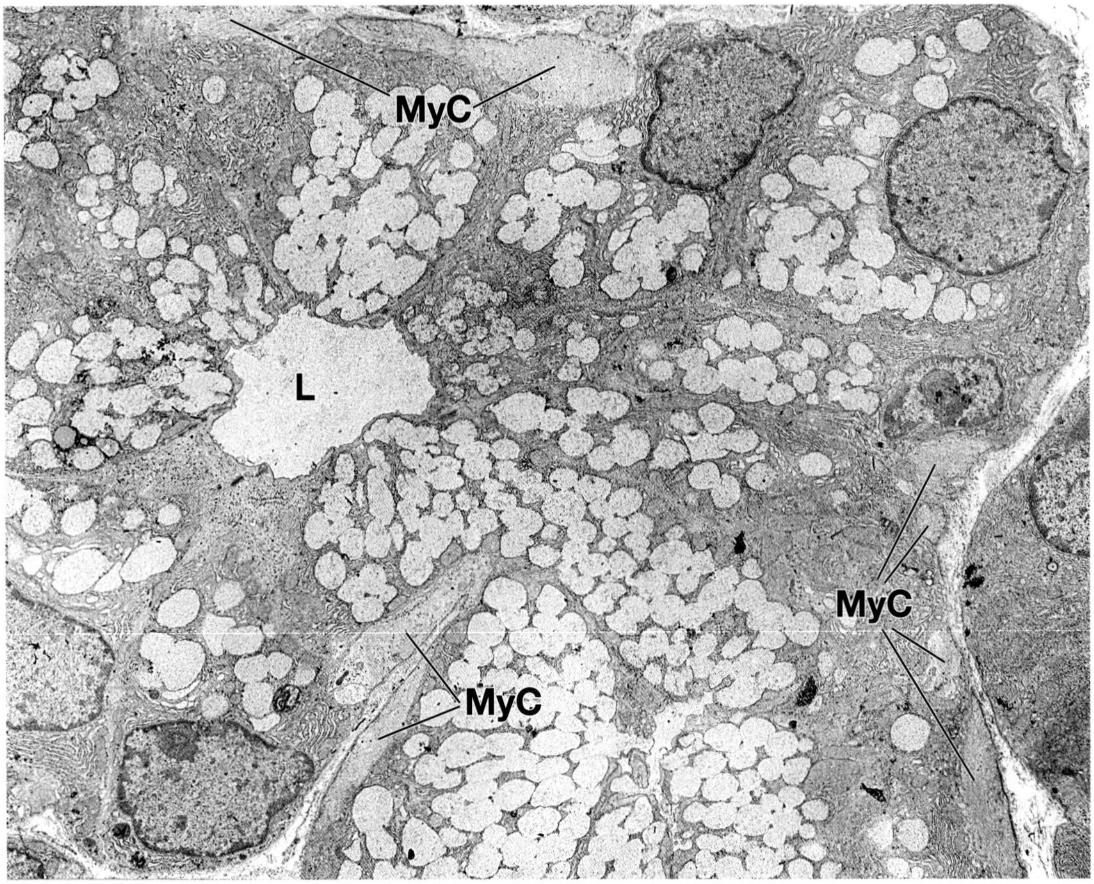

FIGURE 16.26. Low-magnification electron micrograph of a mucous acinus. The mucous cells contain numerous mucinogen granules. Many of the granules have coalesced to form larger irregular masses that will ultimately discharge into the lumen (*L*) of the acinus. Myoepithelial cell processes (*MyC*) are evident at the periphery of the acinus. ×5,000.

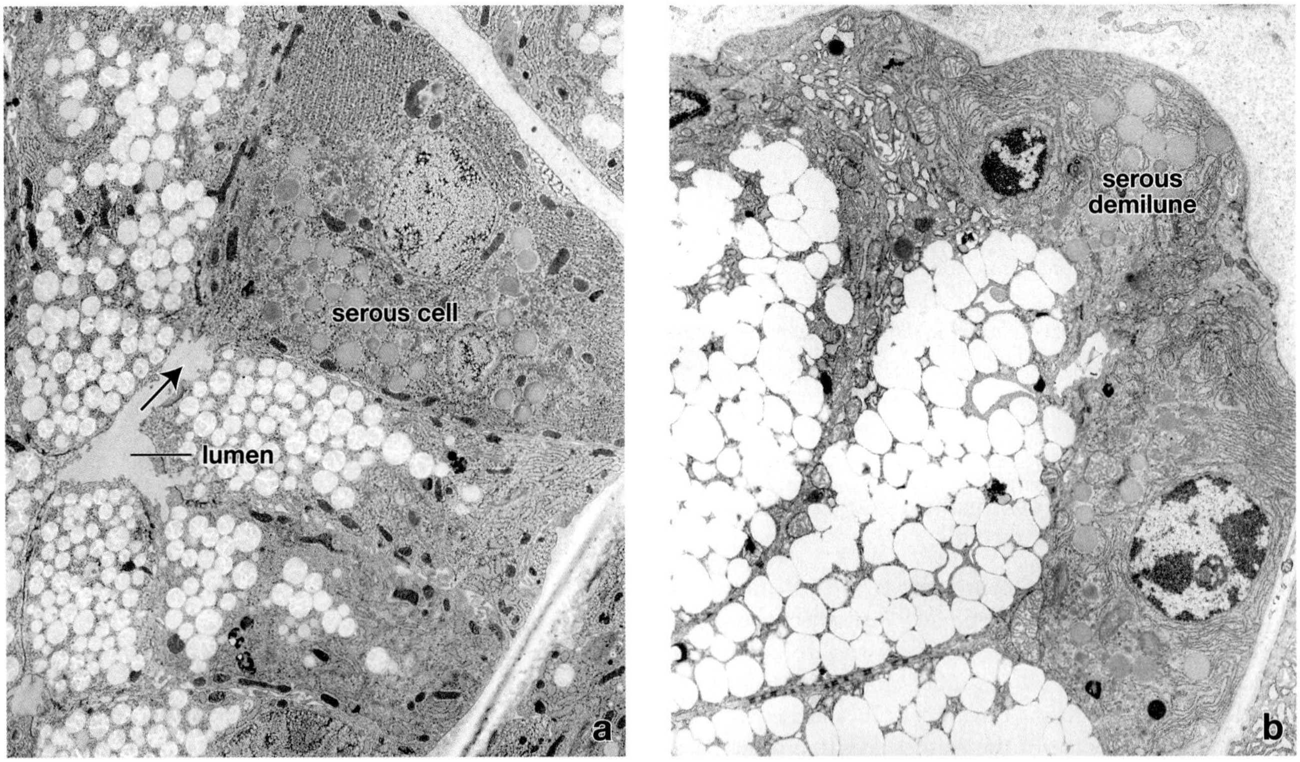

FIGURE 16.27. Electron micrographs of mixed acini. a. Low-magnification electron micrograph of the sublingual gland, prepared by the rapid-freezing and freeze-substitution method, shows the arrangement of the cells within a single acinus. The mucous cells have well-preserved round mucinogen granules. The mucous and serous cells are aligned to surround the acinus lumen. Serous demilunes are not evident. ×6,000. **b.** Electron micrograph of the sublingual gland prepared by traditional fixation in formaldehyde. Note the considerable expansion and coalescence of the mucinogen granules and the formation of a serous demilune. ×15,000. (Courtesy of Dr. Shohei Yamashina.)

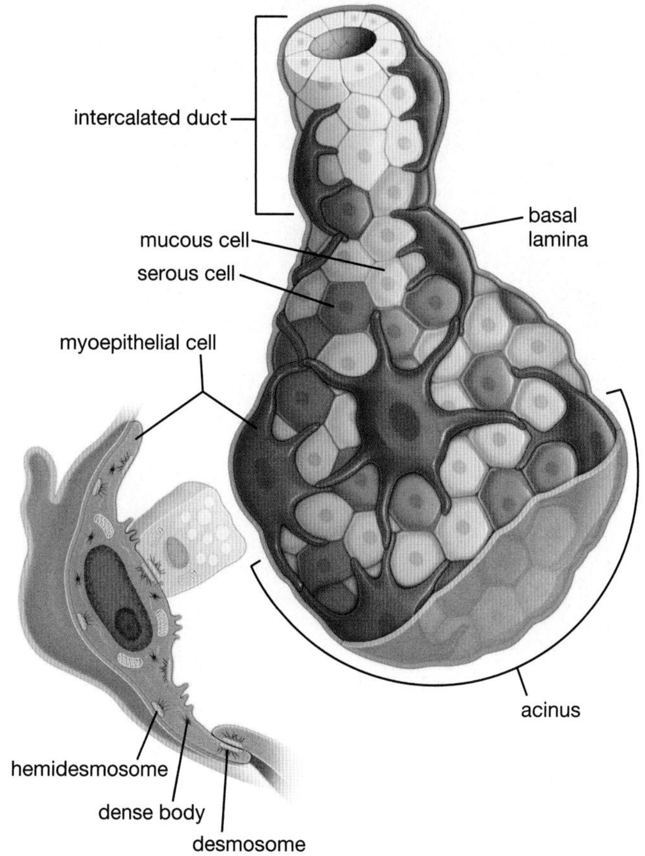

FIGURE 16.28. Schematic illustration of a mixed acinus of the salivary gland with its intercalated duct. The acinus of the salivary gland represents a blind sac composed of secretory acinar cells that are either serous (protein-secreting) or mucous (mucin-secreting) cells or both. Serous acini contain only serous cells, mucous acini contain only mucous cells, and mixed acini contain both serous and mucous cells. The illustration shows a mixed acinus with *yellow* mucous cells and *red* serous cells and its intercalated duct lined by *light pink* ductal cells. Note the myoepithelial cells that envelop the acinus (like an octopus sitting on a rock) extend onto the intercalated duct. This drawing clearly shows the basal lamina (*magenta*) as semitransparent sheath at the bottom of the acinus covering both acinar cells and overlying the myoepithelial cells. Basal lamina also extends over ductal cells and myoepithelial cells in the intercalated duct. Myoepithelial cells thus lie between the basal plasma membrane of the acinar and ductal cells and the basal lamina of the epithelium. The cytoplasm of myoepithelial cells possesses contractile elements (similar to that in smooth muscles), which can be seen in electron microscopies (EMs) as dense bodies. The myoepithelial cells and their overlapping processes are attached to each other and to acinar and ductal cells by desmosomes and gap junctions and to the basal lamina by hemidesmosomes. During contraction, myoepithelial cells compress the acinus to aid in the expulsion of saliva and its passage through the intercalated duct.

and to each other by desmosomes and gap junctions and to the basal lamina by hemidesmosomes.

Primary Sjögren syndrome is a systemic autoimmune inflammatory disease that involves salivary and lacrimal glands, resulting in dry mouth and dry eyes. A histologic section of the salivary gland from an affected individual shows focal **lymphocytic infiltration** of the gland with an increased number of macrophages and plasma cells. In advanced stages, normal secretory acini are replaced by lymphocytes. Recent studies also indicate the alteration of the **myoepithelial cells**. The amount of α-smooth muscle actin (α-SMA) that is responsible for contractile properties of myoepithelial cells in salivary glands is significantly reduced in patients with primary Sjögren syndrome when compared with healthy individuals. This may cause a loss of mechanical support for acini and the duct system and contribute to the reduction of salivary flow.

Salivary Ducts

The lumen of the salivary acinus is continuous with that of a **duct system** that may have as many as three sequential segments:

- **Intercalated duct**, which leads from the acinus
- **Striated duct**, so-called because of the presence of "striations," the infoldings of the basal plasma membrane of the columnar cells that form the duct
- **Excretory ducts**, which are the larger ducts that empty into the oral cavity

The degree of development of the intercalated ducts and striated ducts varies, depending on the nature of the acinar secretion (see Fig. 16.23). Serous glands have well-developed intercalated ducts and striated ducts that modify the serous secretion by both the absorption of specific components from the secretion and the secretion of additional components to form the final product. Mucous glands, in which the secretion is not modified, have very poorly developed intercalated ducts that may not be recognizable in H&E sections. Moreover, they do not display striated ducts.

Intercalated ducts are located between a secretory acinus and a larger duct.

Intercalated ducts are lined by low cuboidal epithelial cells that usually lack any distinctive feature to suggest a function other than that of a conduit. However, the cells of intercalated ducts possess carbonic anhydrase activity. In serous-secreting glands and mixed glands, they have been shown to

- **secrete HCO_3^-** into the acinar product and
- **absorb Cl^-** from the acinar product.

As noted earlier, intercalated ducts are most prominent in those salivary glands that produce a watery serous secretion. In mucus-secreting salivary glands, the intercalated ducts, when present, are short and difficult to identify.

Striated duct cells have numerous infoldings of the basal plasma membrane.

Striated ducts are lined by a simple cuboidal epithelium that gradually becomes columnar as it approaches the excretory duct. The infoldings of the basal plasma membrane are seen in histologic sections as "striations." Longitudinally oriented, elongated mitochondria are enclosed in the infoldings. Basal infoldings associated with elongated mitochondria are a morphologic specialization associated with reabsorption of fluid and electrolytes. The striated duct cells also have numerous basolateral folds that are interdigitated with those of adjacent cells. The nucleus typically occupies a central (rather than basal) location in the cell. Striated ducts are the sites of

- **reabsorption of Na^+** from the primary secretion and
- **secretion of K^+ and HCO_3^-** into the secretion.

More Na^+ is resorbed than K^+ is secreted, so the secretion becomes hypotonic. When the secretion is very rapid, more Na^+ and less K^+ appear in the final saliva because the reabsorption and secondary secretion systems cannot keep

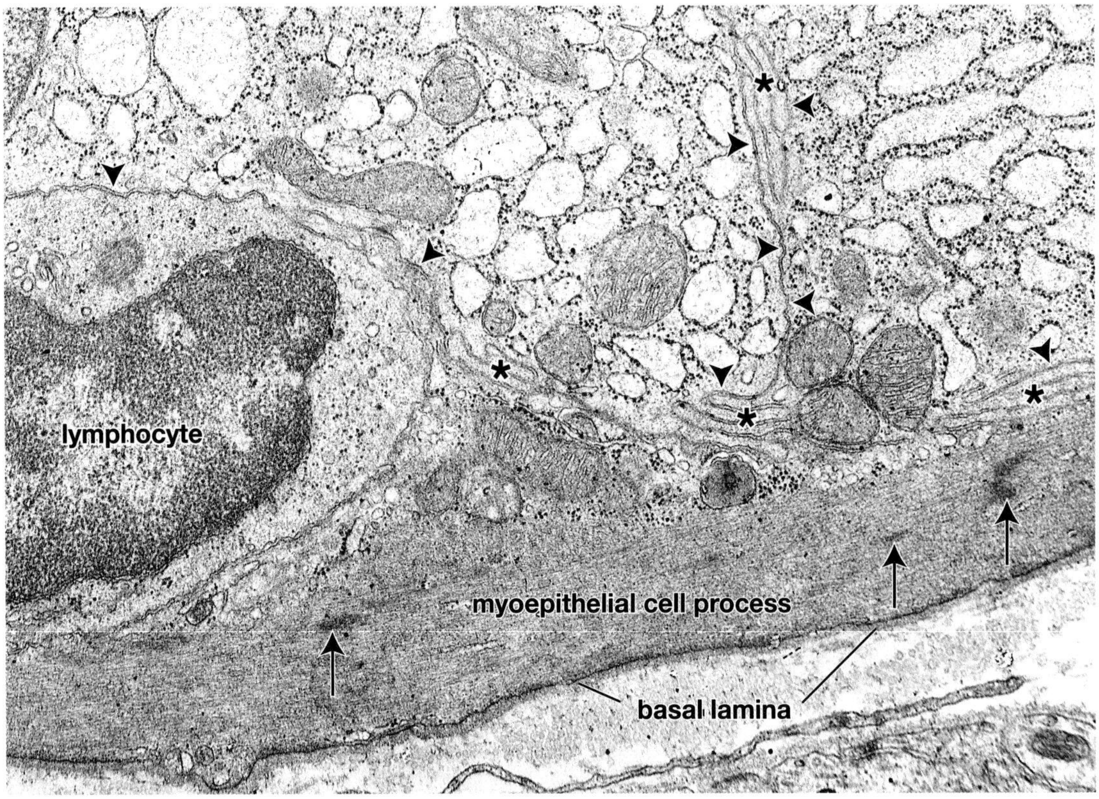

FIGURE 16.29. Electron micrograph of the basal portion of an acinus. This electron micrograph shows the basal portion of two secretory cells from a submandibular gland. A myoepithelial cell process is also evident. Note the location of the myoepithelial cell process on the epithelial side of the basal lamina. The cytoplasm of the myoepithelial cell contains contractile filaments and cytoplasmic densities or dense bodies (*arrows*) similar to those seen in smooth muscle cells. The cell on the *left* with the small nucleus is a lymphocyte. Having migrated through the basal lamina, it is also located within the epithelial compartment. *Arrowheads*, cell boundaries; *asterisks*, basolateral folds. ×15,000.

up with the rate of primary secretion. Thus, the saliva may become isotonic to hypertonic.

The diameter of striated ducts often exceeds that of the secretory acinus. Striated ducts are located in the parenchyma of the glands (they are **intralobular ducts**) but may be surrounded by small amounts of connective tissue in which blood vessels and nerves can be seen running in parallel with the duct.

Excretory ducts travel in the interlobular and interlobar connective tissue.

Excretory ducts constitute the principal ducts of each of the major glands. They ultimately connect to the oral cavity. The epithelium of small excretory ducts is a simple cuboidal. It gradually changes to pseudostratified columnar or stratified cuboidal. As the diameter of the duct increases, stratified columnar epithelium is often seen, and as the ducts approach the oral epithelium, stratified squamous epithelium may be present. The parotid duct (Stensen duct) and the submandibular duct (Wharton duct) travel in the connective tissue of the face and neck, respectively, for some distance from the gland before penetrating the oral mucosa.

Major Salivary Glands

Parotid gland

The parotid glands are composed of pure serous acini.

The paired serous **parotid glands** are the largest of the major salivary glands. The parotid duct travels from the gland, which is located below and in front of the ear, to enter the oral cavity opposite the second upper molar tooth. The secretory units in the parotid are serous and surround numerous, long, narrow intercalated ducts. Striated ducts are large and conspicuous (Fig. 16.30a).

Large amounts of adipose tissue often occur in the parotid gland; this is one of its distinguishing features (Plate 16.5, page 628). The **facial nerve** (cranial nerve VII) passes through the parotid gland; large cross sections of this nerve may be encountered in routine H&E sections of the gland and are useful in identifying the parotid. **Mumps**, a viral infection of the parotid gland, can damage the facial nerve.

Submandibular gland

The submandibular glands are mixed glands that are mostly serous in humans.

The large, paired, mixed **submandibular glands** are located under either side of the floor of the mouth, close to the mandible. A duct from each of the two glands runs forward and medially to a papilla located on the floor of the mouth just lateral to the frenulum of the tongue. Some mucous acini capped by serous demilunes are generally found among the predominant serous acini. Intercalated ducts are less extensive than in the parotid gland (Fig. 16.30b and Plate 16.4, page 626).

Sublingual gland

The small sublingual glands are mixed glands that are mostly mucus secreting in humans.

The **sublingual glands**, the smallest of the paired major salivary glands, are located on the floor of the mouth anterior

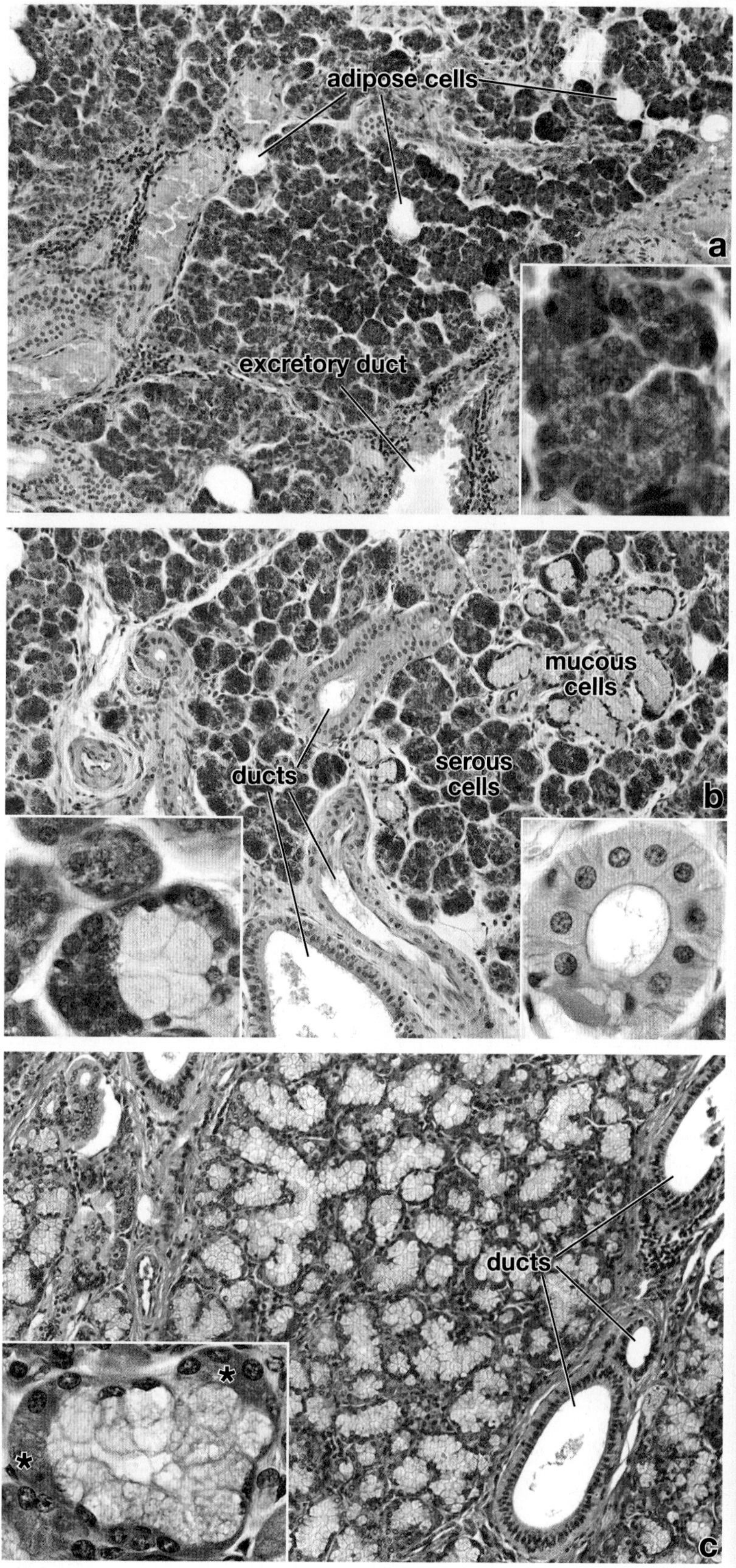

FIGURE 16.30. Photomicrographs of the three major salivary glands. a. The parotid gland in the human is composed entirely of serous acini and their ducts. Typically, adipose cells are also distributed throughout the gland. The *lower portion* of the figure reveals an excretory duct within a connective tissue septum. ×120. **Inset.** Higher magnification of the serous acinar cells. ×320. **b.** The submandibular glands contain both serous and mucous acini. In humans, the serous components predominate. The mucus-secreting acini are readily discernible at this low magnification because of their light staining. The remainder of the field is composed largely of serous acini. Various ducts—excretory, striated, and intercalated—are evident in the field. ×120. **Left inset.** Higher magnification of an acinus revealing a serous demilune surrounding mucus-secreting cells. ×360. **Right inset.** Higher magnification of a striated duct. These ducts have columnar epithelium with visible basal striations. ×320. **c.** The sublingual gland also contains both serous and mucous elements. Here, the mucous acini predominate. The mucous acini are conspicuous because of their light staining. Critical examination of the mucous acini at this relatively low magnification reveals that they are not spherical structures but, rather, elongated or tubular structures with branching outpockets. Thus, the acinus is rather large, and much of it is usually not seen within the plane of a single section. The ducts of the sublingual gland that are observed with the greatest frequency in a section are the interlobular ducts. ×120. **Inset.** The serous component of the gland is composed largely of demilunes (*asterisks*), artifacts of conventional fixation. ×320.

to the submandibular glands. Their multiple small sublingual ducts empty into the submandibular duct as well as directly onto the floor of the mouth. Some of the predominant mucous acini exhibit serous demilunes, but purely serous acini are rarely present (Fig. 16.30c and Plate 16.6, page 630). Intercalated ducts and striated ducts are short, difficult to locate, or sometimes absent. The mucous secretory units may be more tubular than purely acinar.

Saliva

Saliva includes the combined secretions of all the major and minor salivary glands.

Most **saliva** is produced by the salivary glands. The composition of saliva produced by each of the three major salivary glands is slightly different. The parotid glands produce the most serous fluid; the sublingual glands produce slightly more viscous fluid; and the submandibular glands produce the most viscous and mucinous saliva. A smaller amount of saliva is produced by general transudation from the epithelial lining of the oral cavity; minor salivary glands dispersed in the oral mucosa; and by the gingival sulcus and tonsillar crypts. One of the unique features of saliva is the large and variable volume produced. The volume (per weight of gland tissue) of saliva exceeds that of other digestive secretions by as much as 40 times. The large volume of saliva produced is undoubtedly related to its many functions, only some of which are concerned with digestion.

Saliva performs both protective and digestive functions.

The salivary glands produce about 1,500 mL of saliva a day. **Saliva** has numerous functions relating to metabolic and nonmetabolic activities:

- Moistening the oral mucosa, which helps controls water intake. Lack of saliva signals thirst.
- Moistening dry foods to aid chewing and swallowing

TABLE 16.1 Composition of Unstimulated Saliva

Organic Constituents	Mean (mg/mL)
Protein	220.0
Amylase	38.0
Mucin	2.7
Muramidase (lysozyme)	22.0
Lactoferrin	0.03
ABO group markers	0.005
EGF	3.4
sIgA	19.0
IgG	1.4
IgM	0.2
Glucose	1.0
Urea	20.0
Uric acid	1.5
Creatinine	0.1
Cholesterol	8.0
cAMP	7.0
Inorganic Constituents	
Sodium	15.0
Potassium	80.0
Thiocyanate	
Smokers	9.0
Nonsmokers	2.0
Calcium	5.8
Phosphate	16.8
Chloride	5.0
Fluoride	Traces (according to intake)

cAMP, cyclic adenosine monophosphate; *EGF*, epithelial growth factor; *Ig*, immunoglobulin; *sIgA*, secretory immunoglobulin A.

Modified from Jenkins GN. *The Physiology and Biochemistry of the Mouth.* 4th ed. Blackwell Scientific Publications; 1978.

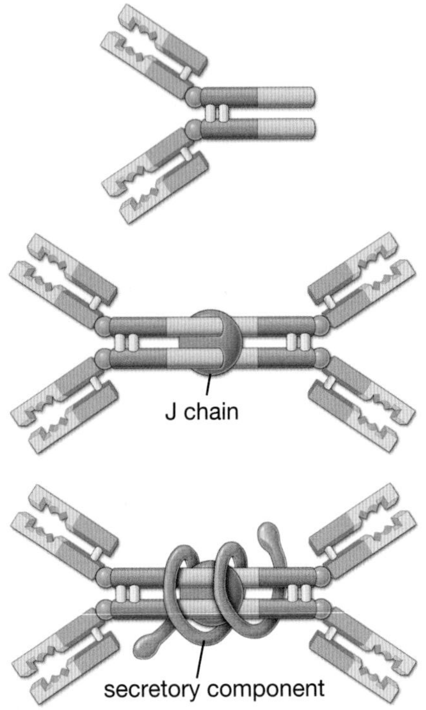

FIGURE 16.31. Diagram of different forms of immunoglobulin A (IgA). This drawing shows the monomer of IgA (*top*). The dimer of IgA is a product of the plasma cell and contains a J chain (*J*) connecting two monomers (*middle*). The secretory component (*SC*), a product of proteolytically cleaved pIgR, is added to the dimer to form secretory IgA (sIgA; *bottom*). *pIgR*, polymeric immunoglobulin receptor; *sIgA*, secretory immunoglobulin A.

- Providing a medium for dissolved and suspended food materials that chemically stimulate taste buds
- Buffering the contents of the oral cavity because of its high concentration of bicarbonate ions
- Digesting carbohydrates with the digestive enzyme α-amylase, which breaks 1,4 glycosidic bonds and continues to act in the esophagus and stomach
- Controlling the bacterial flora of the oral cavity by the use of lysozyme (muramidase), an enzyme that lyses the muramic acid in certain bacteria (e.g., staphylococci)

The unique composition of saliva is summarized in Table 16.1.

Saliva contains water, various proteins, and electrolytes.

Saliva contains chiefly water, proteins and glycoproteins (enzymes and antibodies), and electrolytes. It has a high potassium concentration that is approximately 7 times that of blood; a sodium concentration of approximately one-tenth that of blood; a bicarbonate concentration of approximately 3 times that of blood; and significant amounts of calcium, phosphorus, chloride, thiocyanate, and urea. Lysozyme and α-amylase are the principal enzymes present (see Table 16.1).

Saliva is a source of calcium and phosphate ions essential for normal tooth development and maintenance.

Calcium and phosphate in the saliva are essential for the mineralization of newly erupted teeth and the repair of precarious lesions of the enamel in erupted teeth. In addition, saliva serves several other roles in protecting the teeth. Proteins in saliva cover the teeth with a protective coat called

FOLDER 16.4

CLINICAL CORRELATION: SALIVARY GLAND TUMORS

Tumors of salivary glands usually occur in the major salivary glands (parotid, submandibular, and sublingual); however, a small percentage occurs in the minor glands located within the oral mucosa, palate, uvula, floor of the mouth, tongue, pharynx, larynx, and paranasal sinuses. Approximately 80% of salivary gland tumors are benign. Most originate in the parotid gland (Fig. F16.4.1a). The palate is the most common site of minor salivary gland tumors.

The most common benign tumor is the **pleomorphic adenoma**, which accounts for 65% of all salivary gland tumors. It is characterized by epithelial tissue containing ductal and myoepithelial cells intermingled with areas, resembling ground substance of connective tissues (e.g., in cartilage). These connective-like tissues are produced by myoepithelial cells (Fig. F16.4.1b).

Most individuals with benign tumors present with painless swelling of the involved gland. Because of nerve involvement, signs such as numbness or weakness of innervated muscle are also reported. For instance, paralysis of facial muscles or persistent facial pain may be present in some individuals with parotid tumors.

The most common treatment is surgical removal of the tumor. For parotid gland tumors, a total parotidectomy (excision of parotid gland) is often necessary. Postoperative radiation therapy is also used when the tumor is cancerous. Complications of surgical treatment of parotid gland tumors include facial nerve dysfunction and **Frey syndrome** (also known as *gustatory sweating*).

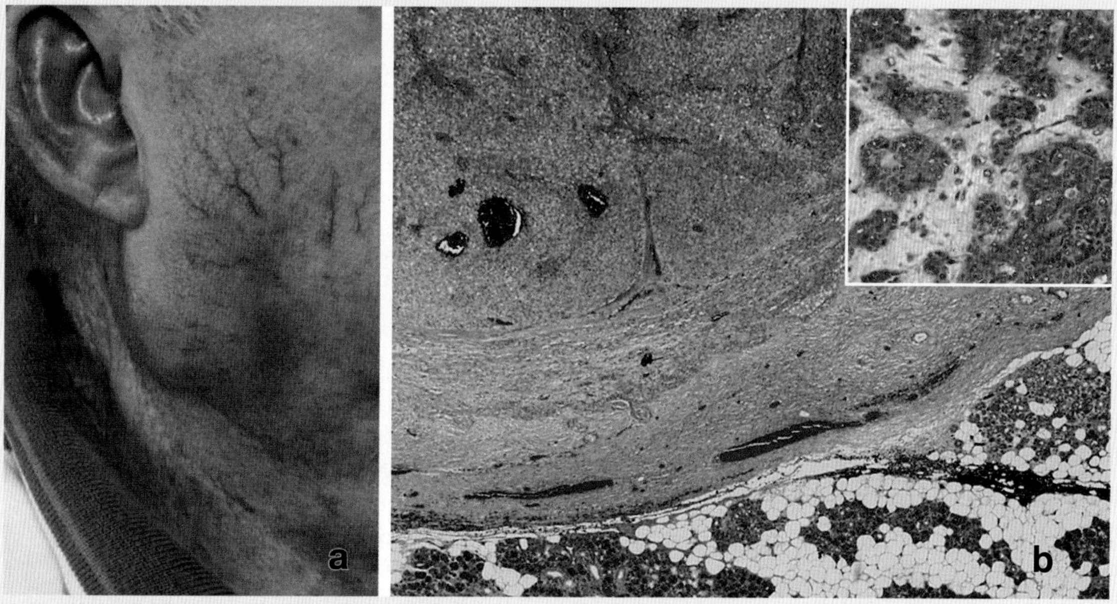

FIGURE F16.4.1. Pleomorphic adenoma of the parotid gland. a. This photograph shows an individual with a parotid mass located near the angle of the mandible. **b.** This low-magnification photomicrograph shows the features of a pleomorphic adenoma. (Courtesy of Dr. Kerry D. Olsen.) Note that normal parotid tissue (basophilic-stained areas in the *lower part*) is separated by the fibrous capsule of a nodule containing connective-like tissue that resembles the extracellular matrix of cartilage. ×40. Higher magnification *inset* shows a nest of cancer cells separated by lighter eosinophilic-stained stroma that resembles extracellular matrix of the hyaline cartilage. ×200. (Courtesy of Dr. Joaquín J. García.)

the **acquired pellicle**. Antibodies and other antibacterial agents retard bacterial action that would otherwise lead to tooth decay. Patients whose salivary glands are irradiated, as in the treatment of salivary gland tumors, fail to produce normal amounts of saliva; these patients typically develop numerous **dental caries**. Anticholinergic drugs used to treat some forms of heart disease also significantly reduce salivary secretion and induce the development of dental caries.

Saliva performs immunologic functions.

As noted, saliva contains antibodies, salivary **immunoglobulin A (IgA)**. IgA is synthesized by plasma cells in the connective tissue surrounding the secretory acini of the salivary glands, and both dimeric and monomeric forms are released into the connective tissue matrix (Fig. 16.31). A **polymeric immunoglobulin receptor (pIgR)** protein is synthesized by the salivary gland cells and inserted into the basal plasma membrane, where it serves as a receptor for dimeric IgA.

When dimeric IgA binds to the receptor, the **pIgR–dIgA complex** is internalized by receptor-mediated endocytosis and carried through the acinar cell to the apical plasma membrane. Here, pIgR is proteolytically cleaved and the extracellular part of the receptor that is bound to dIgA is released into the lumen as **secretory IgA (sIgA)**. This process of synthesis and secretion of IgA is essentially identical to that which occurs in the more distal parts of the gastrointestinal tract, where sIgA is transported across the absorptive columnar epithelium of the small intestine and colon (see page 658).

101 HISTOLOGY NOTEBOOK

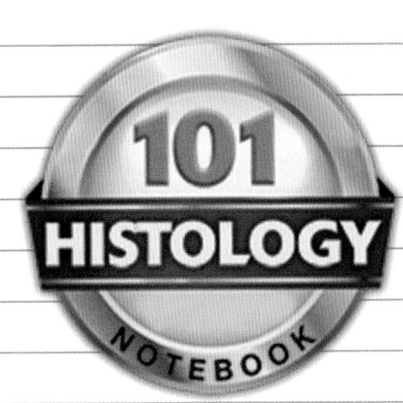

DIGESTIVE SYSTEM I: ORAL CAVITY AND ASSOCIATED STRUCTURES

OVERVIEW OF THE DIGESTIVE SYSTEM

- The **digestive system** consists of the **alimentary canal**, its associated organs (tongue and teeth), and exocrine glands (salivary glands, liver, pancreas).
- The major functions of the digestive system are transport of ingested water and food through the alimentary canal; secretion of fluids, electrolytes, and digestive enzymes; digestion and absorption of digested products; and excretion of undigested remains.
- Because the lumen of the alimentary canal is physically and functionally external to the body, the alimentary **mucosa** (lining of the digestive system) provides immunologic protection and acts as a barrier between the lumen and the internal body environment.

ORAL CAVITY

- The **oral cavity** consists of the mouth, which includes the tongue, teeth, and their supporting structures; major and minor salivary glands; and tonsils.
- **Oral mucosa** lines the oral cavity. Depending on its location, it is divided into **masticatory mucosa** (gingiva and hard palate), a stratified squamous keratinized or parakeratinized epithelium; **lining mucosa** (remaining parts of the oral cavity, except for the dorsum of the tongue), a stratified squamous nonkeratinized epithelium; and **specialized mucosa** (dorsal surface of the tongue), which contains lingual papillae.

TEETH

- Humans have 32 permanent **teeth**; each tooth has a root embedded in the alveolar bone and a **clinical crown** that projects into the oral cavity. The centrally located **pulp cavity** contains loose connective tissue, vessels, and nerves.
- The tooth has three specialized tissues: visible **enamel** covering its anatomic crown; **cementum**, found on the root for the attachment of periodontal ligaments; and **dentin**, which lies deep to enamel and cementum.
- **Enamel** is produced by **ameloblasts** (during **enamel organ** embryonic tooth development) and is composed of parallel **enamel rods**; enamel production is regulated by specific proteins (e.g., amelogenins, ameloblastins, enamelins).
- **Cementum** is a bone-like structure that covers the root of the tooth. Collagen fibers project from the cementum and form the **periodontal ligaments** connecting the tooth to the **alveolus** (socket).
- **Dentin** is initially deposited by odontoblasts as **predentin**, which, under the influence of **dentin phosphoprotein (DPP)** and **dentin sialoprotein (DSP)**, is mineralized to dentin. It has tubules containing elongated processes of odontoblasts.

TONGUE

- The specialized mucosa on the dorsal surface of the tongue has four types of projecting **lingual papillae: filiform** (made of stratified squamous keratinized epithelium), **foliate, fungiform**, and **circumvallate** (lined by stratified squamous nonkeratinized epithelium).
- The foliate, fungiform, and circumvallate papillae contain **taste buds** on their surface with neuroepithelial (sensory) cells for the detection of five basic tastes: sweet, salty, bitter, sour, and umami.
- **Sweet, bitter**, and **umami tastes** are detected by G-protein–coupled taste receptors, and **sour** and **sweet tastes** act on Na^+ and K^+ channels.
- The **lingual tonsil** represents aggregation of diffuse lymphatic tissue and lymphatic nodules at the base of the tongue.

SALIVARY GLANDS

- The **salivon** is the basic secretory unit of any salivary gland and consists of the acinus, intercalated duct, and excretory duct.
- The **acinus** is the secretory part of the salivon. Acini are spherical, containing **serous cells** (protein secreting); more tubular, containing **mucous cells** (mucin secreting); or mixed, with both types of cells. Mixed acini in routine preparation have **serous demilunes** (artifacts of fixation). Myoepithelial cells are present at the base of secretory cells.
- Secretion from the acinus is drained by the **intercalated duct** (lined by simple cuboidal epithelium), which merges into the **striated duct** (simple columnar epithelium with distinct basal striations) and finally into the **excretory duct** (stratified cuboidal or columnar epithelium), which is surrounded by connective tissue.
- Cells of striated ducts have numerous infoldings of the basal plasma membrane that contain mitochondria. The infoldings are specialized for reabsorption of electrolytes from the secretion.
- The **major salivary glands** are the paired parotid, submandibular, and sublingual glands.
- **Parotid glands** contain only serous acini with adipose tissue distributed throughout the gland.
- **Submandibular glands** contain predominantly serous but also mucous acini.
- **Sublingual glands** are also mixed but primarily contain elongated mucous acini. The serous component is visible as **demilunes.**
- **Saliva** is produced by salivary glands and has protective and digestive functions. It contains water, proteins and glycoproteins (enzymes and antibodies), and electrolytes.

PLATE 16.1 ■ LIP AND MUCOCUTANEOUS JUNCTION

The **lips** are the entry point of the alimentary canal. Here, the thin **keratinized epithelium** of the facial skin changes to the thick **parakeratinized epithelium** of the oral mucosa. At the mucocutaneous junction, the *red* portion of the lips is characterized by deep penetration of connective tissue papillae into the base of the **stratified squamous keratinized epithelium.** The blood vessels and nerve endings in these papillae are responsible for both the color and exquisite touch sensitivity of the lips.

ORIENTATION MICROGRAPH: A hematoxylin and eosin (H&E)-stained sagittal section through the upper lip in this low-power orientation photomicrograph to the *right* (×8) reveals the skin of the face, the red margin of the lip, and the transition to the oral mucosa (*OM*). The *marked rectangles* indicate representative areas of each of these sites, shown at higher magnifications in *upper, middle,* and *lower rows* of figures on the adjacent plate. Note the change in thickness of the epithelium from the exterior or facial portion of the lip (the *vertical surface on the left*) to the interior surface of the oral cavity (the surface beginning with *rectangle marked lower* and continuing upward along the right surface of the lip) in this micrograph.

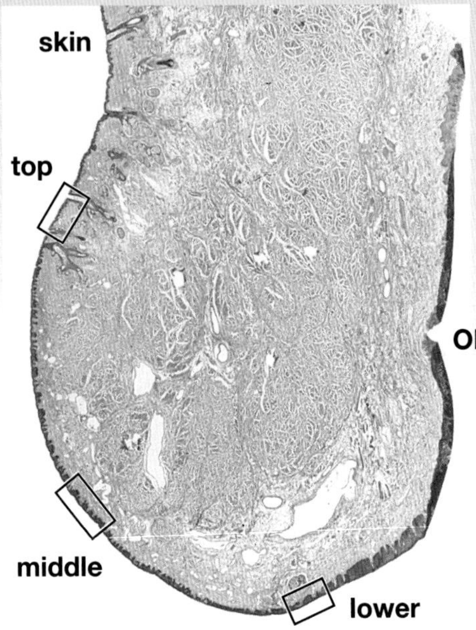

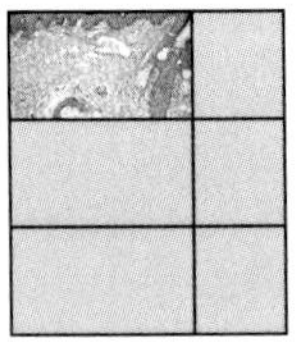

Keratinized epithelium, lip, human, H&E ×120.

The **keratinized epithelium** (*EP*) of the face is relatively thin and has the general features of thin skin found in other sites. Associated with it are hair follicles (*HF*), sebaceous glands (*SGl*), and blood vessels (*BV*).

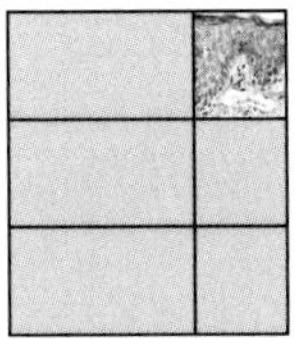

Keratinized epithelium, lip, human, H&E ×380.

The *circled area* in the figure on the *left* is shown at a higher magnification. The *reddish brown* material in the basal cells is the pigment melanin (*M*), and the *dark blue* near the surface is the stratum granulosum (*SG*) with its deep blue–stained keratohyalin granules.

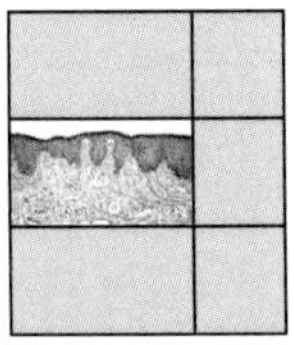

Red margin, lip, human, H&E ×120.

The epithelium of the **red margin** of the lip is much thicker than that of the face. The stratum granulosum is still present; thus, the epithelium is keratinized. The feature that accounts for the coloration of the red margin is the deep penetration of the connective tissue papillae into the epithelium (*arrowheads*). The thinness of the epithelium combined with the extensive vascularity of the underlying connective tissue, particularly the extensive venous blood vessels (*BV*), allows the color of the blood to show through.

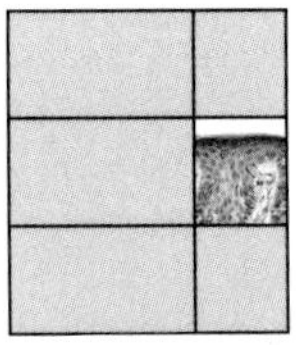

Red margin, lip, human, H&E ×380.

The sensitivity of the red margin to stimuli such as light touch is due to the presence of an increased number of sensory receptors. In fact, each of the two deep papillae seen in the figure on the *left* contains a Meissner corpuscle (*MC*), one of which is more clearly seen in this figure.

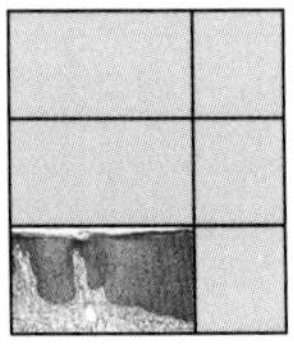

Mucocutaneous junction, lip, human, H&E ×120.

The transition from the keratinized red margin to the fairly thick stratified squamous parakeratinized epithelium of the oral mucosa is evident in this figure. Note how the stratum granulosum suddenly ends. This is more clearly shown at higher magnification in the figure on the *right*.

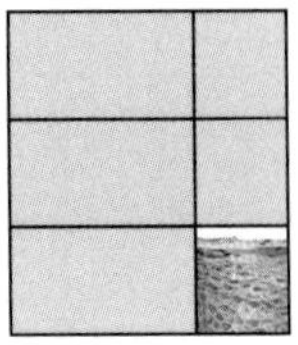

Mucocutaneous junction, lip, human, H&E ×380.

Beyond the site where the stratum granulosum cells disappear, nuclei are seen in the superficial cells up to the surface (*arrows*). The epithelium is also much thicker at this point and remains so throughout the oral cavity.

BV, venous blood vessels
EP, epithelium
HF, hair follicle
M, melanin pigment
MC, Meissner corpuscle
OM, oral mucosa
SG, stratum granulosum
SGl, sebaceous gland
arrowheads, connective tissue papillae
arrows, nuclei of superficial cells up to surface

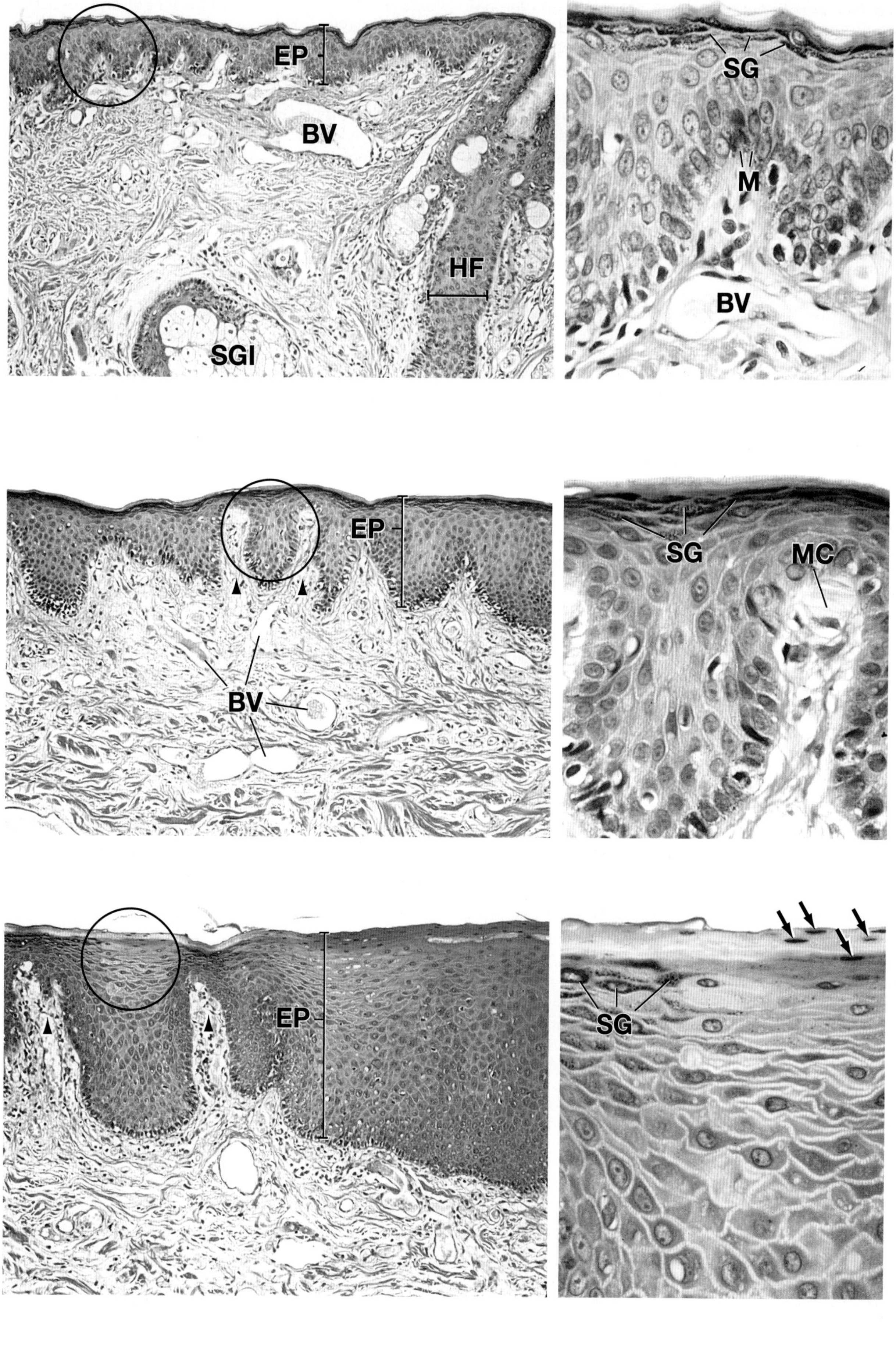
EP
BV
HF
SGl
SG
M
BV
EP
BV
SG
MC
EP
SG

PLATE 16.2 ■ TONGUE I

The tongue is a muscular organ projecting into the oral cavity from its inferior surface. It is covered with a mucous membrane that consists of **stratified squamous epithelium**, keratinized in parts, resting on loose connective tissue. The undersurface of the tongue is relatively uncomplicated. The mucosa of the dorsal surface, however, is modified to form three types of papillae: **filiform**, **fungiform**, and **circumvallate**. The circumvallate papillae form a V-shaped row that divides the tongue into a body and a root; the dorsal surface of the body, that is, the portion anterior to the circumvallate papillae, contains filiform and fungiform papillae. Parallel ridges bearing taste buds are found on the sides of the tongue and are particularly evident in infants. When sectioned at right angles to their long axis, they appear as papillae and, although not true papillae, are called **foliate papillae**.

The tongue contains both intrinsic and extrinsic voluntary striated muscles. The **striated muscles** of the tongue are arranged in three interweaving planes, with each arrayed at right angles to the other two. This arrangement is unique to the tongue. It provides enormous flexibility and precision in the movements of the tongue that are essential to human speech as well as to its role in digestion and swallowing. The arrangement also allows easy identification as lingual muscle.

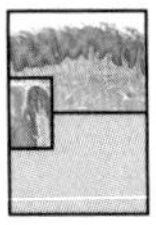

Dorsal surface, tongue, monkey, hematoxylin and eosin (H&E) ×65; inset ×130.

This figure shows the dorsal surface of the tongue with the **filiform papillae** (*Fil P*). They are the most numerous of the three types of papillae. Structurally, they are bent, conical projections of the epithelium, with the point of the projection directed posteriorly. These papillae do not possess taste buds and are composed of stratified squamous keratinized epithelium.

The **fungiform papillae** are scattered about as isolated, slightly rounded, elevated structures situated among the filiform papillae. A fungiform papilla is shown in the *inset*. A large connective tissue core (primary connective tissue papilla) forms the center of the fungiform papilla, and smaller connective tissue papillae (secondary connective tissue papillae) project into the base of the surface epithelium (*arrowhead*). The connective tissue of the papillae is highly vascularized. Because of the deep penetration of connective tissue into the epithelium, combined with a very thin keratinized surface, the fungiform papillae appear as small red dots when the dorsal surface of the tongue is examined by gross inspection.

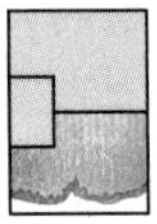

Ventral surface, tongue, monkey, H&E ×65.

The ventral surface of the tongue is shown in this figure. The smooth surface of the **stratified squamous epithelium** (*Ep*) contrasts with the irregular surface of the dorsum of the tongue. Moreover, the epithelial surface on the ventral surface of the tongue is usually not keratinized. The connective tissue (*CT*) is immediately deep to the epithelium; deeper still is the striated muscle (*M*). The numerous connective tissue papillae that project into the base of the epithelium of both ventral and dorsal surfaces give the epithelial–connective tissue junction an irregular profile. Often, these connective tissue papillae are cut obliquely and then appear as small islands of connective tissue within the epithelial layer (see the previous figure).

The connective tissue extends as far as the muscle without changing character, and no submucosa is recognized. The muscle (*M*) is striated and is unique in its organization, that is, the fibers travel in three planes. Therefore, most sections will show bundles of muscle fibers cut longitudinally, at right angles to each other, and in cross section. Nerves (*N*) that innervate the muscle are also frequently observed in the connective tissue septa between the muscle bundles.

The surface of the tongue behind the vallate papillae (the root of the tongue) contains lingual tonsils (not shown). These are similar in structure and appearance to the palatine tonsils illustrated in Plate 14.1 (page 526).

CT, connective tissue
Ep, epithelium
Fil P, filiform papillae
M, striated muscle bundles
N, nerves
arrowhead (inset), secondary connective tissue papilla

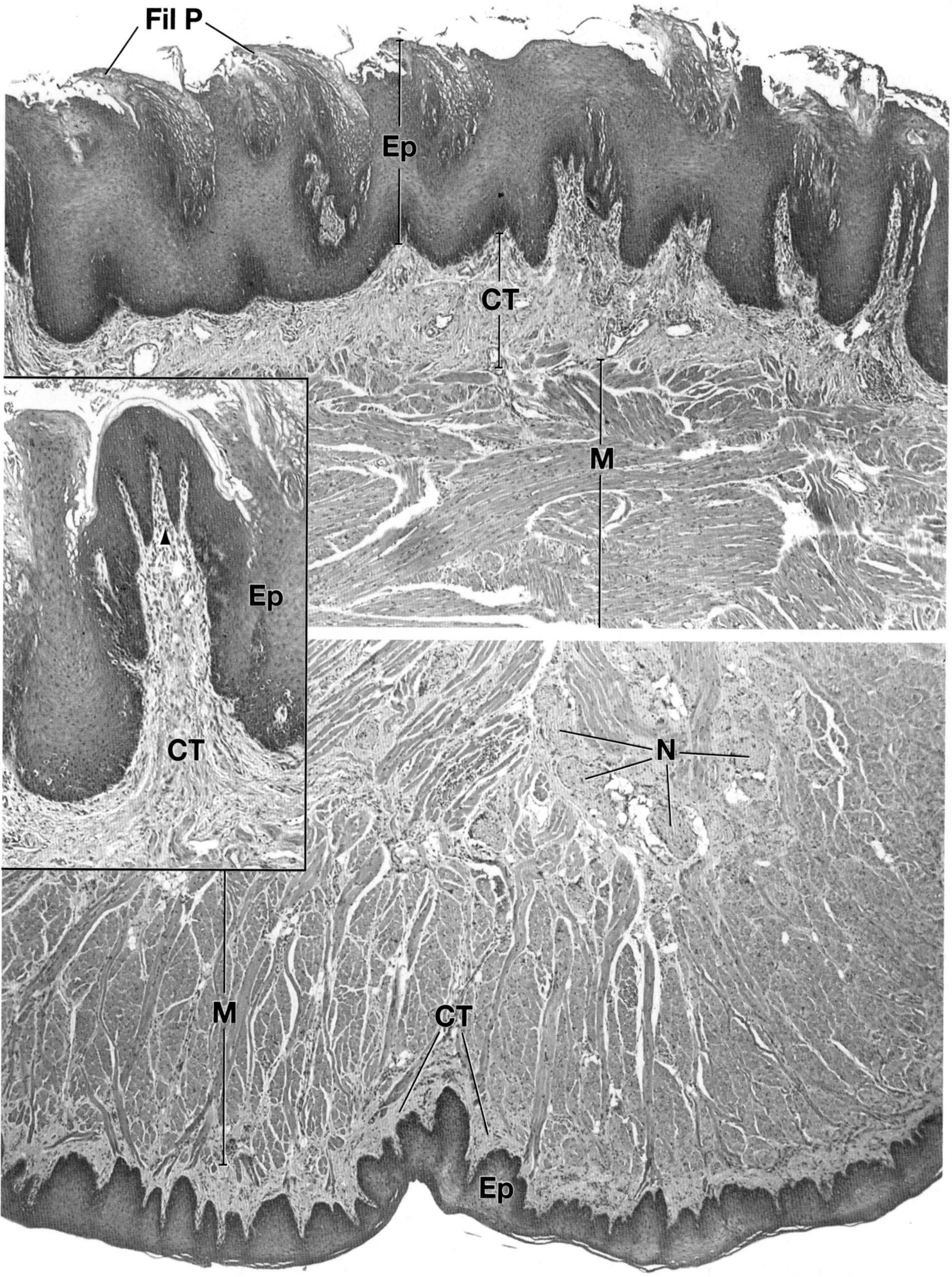
Fil P
Ep
CT
M
Ep
CT
N
M
CT
Ep

PLATE 16.3 ■ TONGUE II—FOLIATE PAPILLAE AND TASTE BUDS

The papillae and their associated **taste buds** constitute the specialized mucosa of the oral cavity. Although filiform papillae do not have taste buds, the other three types, namely, foliate, fungiform, and circumvallate, contain taste buds in their epithelium. The fungiform (i.e., mushroom-shaped) papillae (see *inset* on Plate 16.2, page 622) are most numerous near the tip of the tongue. Taste buds are present in the epithelium on their dorsal surface. The taste buds in the epithelium covering the circumvallate and foliate papillae are located in deep clefts that separate the papillae from adjacent mucosa or from each other, respectively. **Ducts of lingual salivary glands** (von Ebner glands; a component of the minor salivary glands) empty their serous secretions into the moat surrounding each circumvallate papilla. The secretions flush material from the moat to allow the taste buds to respond to new stimuli. Similarly, ducts of small serous glands empty into the clefts between foliate papillae. Taste buds in section appear as oval, pale-staining bodies that extend through the thickness of the epithelium. A small opening at the epithelial surface is called the **taste pore**. Taste buds react to only five stimuli: sweet, salty, bitter, sour, and umami. Sensitivity to all tastes is distributed across the entire tongue; however, taste receptors appear to be more concentrated in specific areas of the tongue; taste buds at the tip of the tongue detect sweet stimuli, those immediately posterolateral to the tip detect salty stimuli, and those on the circumvallate papillae detect bitter and umami stimuli.

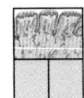

Foliate papillae, tongue, human, hematoxylin and eosin (H&E) ×50.

Foliate papillae consist of a series of parallel ridges that are separated by narrow, deep mucosal clefts (see Fig. 16.5, page 592). They are aligned at right angles to the long axis of the tongue on its posterior lateral edge. In younger individuals, they are readily observed by gross inspection. However, with age, foliate papillae may not be recognized. This micrograph shows three papillae; each is separated from its neighbor by a narrow cleft (*C*). The surface of these papillae is covered by a thick stratified nonkeratinized epithelium (*SE*). The basal surface of the epithelium is extremely uneven owing to the presence of deep, penetrating connective tissue papillae (*CTP*). In contrast, the epithelium lining the clefts (*Ep*) is relatively thin and uniform. It contains numerous taste buds. These are the light-staining objects seen in the cleft epithelium. Underlying the epithelium is a layer of loose connective tissue (*LCT*) and a central core of dense connective tissue. Within this core and between bundles of muscle fibers beneath the papillae are **lingual serous glands** (*LSG*). These glands, like the serous glands associated with the circumvallate papillae, have ducts (*D*) that empty into the base of the clefts between papillae.

Taste buds, tongue, human, H&E ×500.

This higher magnification micrograph shows the **taste buds** located within the cleft epithelium. The taste buds typically appear as oval, pale-staining structures that extend through much of the thickness of the epithelium. Beneath the taste bud are nerve fibers (*NF*) that are also lightly stained. At the apex of the taste bud, there is a small opening in the epithelium, which is the taste pore (*TP*).

Taste bud, tongue, human, H&E ×1,100.

This micrograph shows to advantage the **taste pore** (*TP*), the cells of the taste bud, and its associated nerve fibers (*NF*). The cells with large, round nuclei are **neuroepithelial sensory cells** (*NSC*). They are the most numerous cells of the taste bud. At their apical surface, they possess microvilli that extend into the taste pore. At their basal surface, they form a synapse with the afferent sensory fibers that make up the underlying nerve. Among the sensory cells are **supporting cells** (*SC*). These cells contain microvilli on their apical surface. Also present in the taste bud at its base are small cells simply referred to as **basal cells** (*BC*), one of which is identified here. They are the stem cells for the supporting and neuroepithelial cells, which have a turnover life of about 10 days.

BC, basal cells
C, cleft
CTP, connective tissue papillae
D, ducts
Ep, epithelium lining the clefts
LCT, loose connective tissue
LSG, lingual serous glands
NF, nerve fibers
NSC, neuroepithelial sensory cells
SC, supporting cells
SE, stratified nonkeratinized epithelium
TP, taste pore

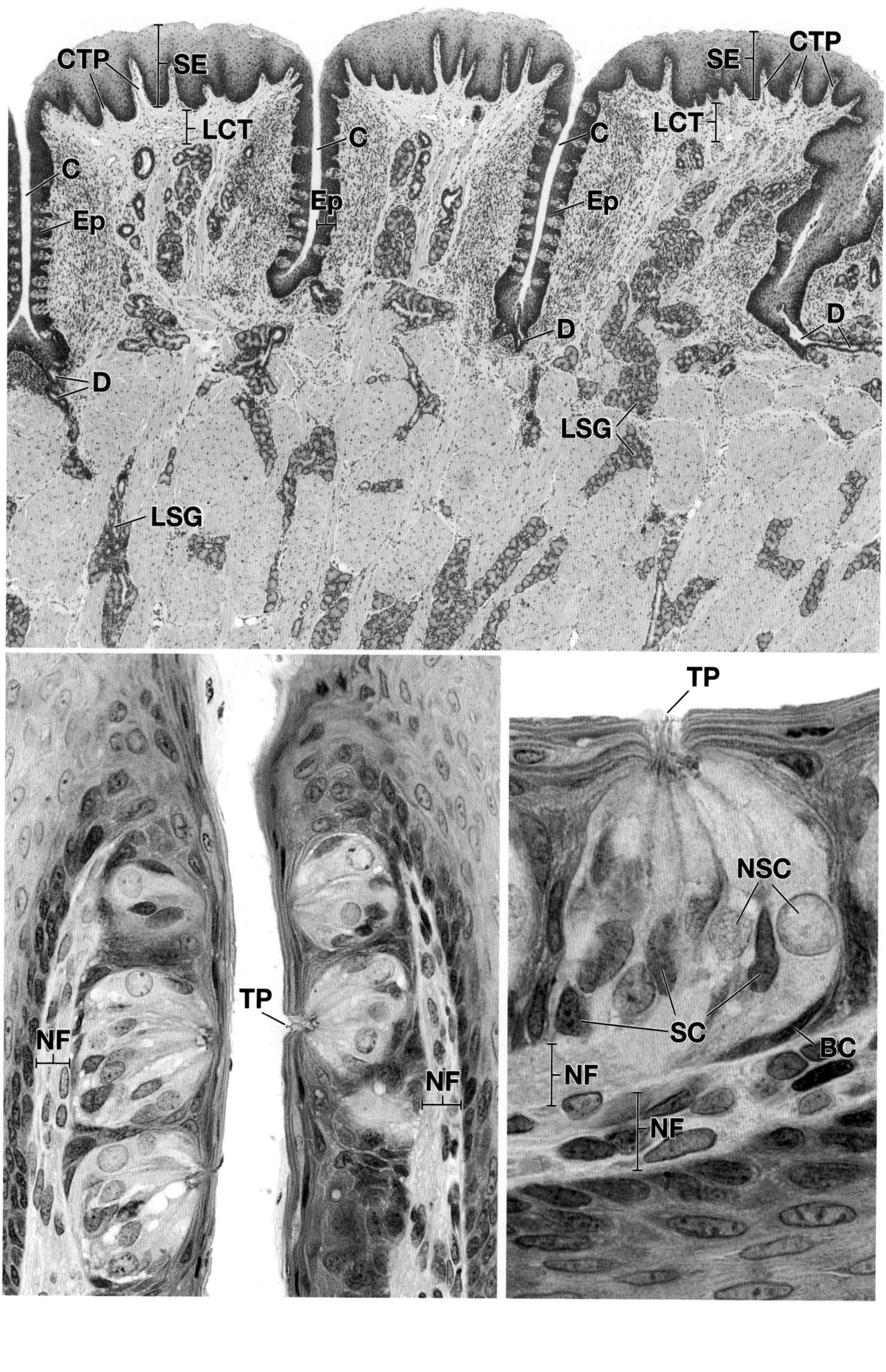
CTP
SE
LCT
C
Ep
D
LSG
C
Ep
D
SE
CTP
LCT
C
Ep
D
LSG
LSG
TP
NF
NF
TP
NSC
SC
BC
NF
NF

PLATE 16.4 ■ SUBMANDIBULAR GLAND

Like the parotid glands, the **submandibular glands** are located outside the oral cavity. They are located under either side of the floor of the mouth near the mandible. A duct runs forward and medially from each of the two glands to a papilla located on the floor of the mouth just lateral to the frenulum of the tongue. The secretory components of the submandibular glands are the acini, which are of three types: **serous acini**, which are protein secreting like those of the parotid gland; **mucous acini**, which secrete mucin; and acini containing both serous- and mucus-secreting cells. In the case of the **mixed acini**, the mucous cells are capped by serous cells, which are typically described as demilunes. Research suggests that the demilune is an artifact of tissue preparation and that all of the cells are aligned to secrete into the acinus lumen. Traditional fixation in formaldehyde appears to expand the mucous cells with the consequent squeezing of the serous cells to form their cap-like position.

ORIENTATION MICROGRAPH: This micrograph reveals a portion of the submandibular gland. A single well-defined lobe (*L*) is seen in the *upper part* of the micrograph. Within the central portion of the gland, there is a dense connective tissue core (*DCT*) containing the larger arteries (*A*), veins (*V*), and excretory ducts (*ED*) of the gland. The submandibular gland is a mixed gland; those regions containing serous acini (*SA*) are darkly stained, whereas regions containing mucous acini (*MA*) are lighter in appearance.

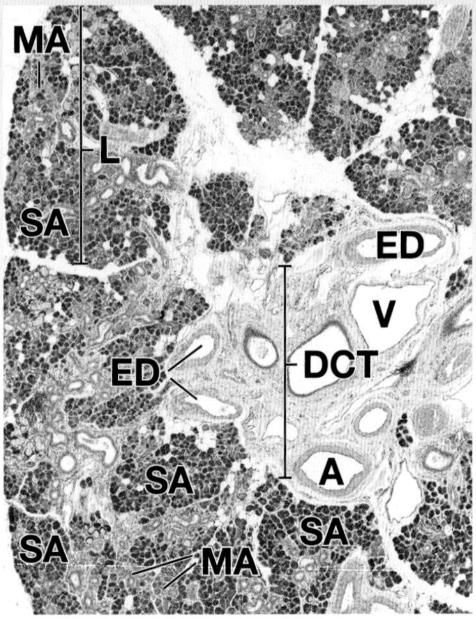

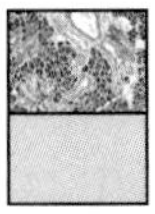

Submandibular gland, human, hematoxylin and eosin (H&E) ×175.

This micrograph reveals the various components of the submandibular gland. The **serous acini** (*SA*) are darkly stained in contrast to the lighter staining **mucous acini** (*MA*). Furthermore, the serous acini are generally spherical in shape. The mucous acini are more tubular or elongated and sometimes can be seen to branch. The secretion from the acini enters an intercalated duct. They are the smallest ducts and are of relatively short length. They reside within the lobule but are often difficult to find because of their shortness. These ducts, in turn, empty into the larger **striated duct** (*SD*). This type of duct is better demonstrated in the next micrograph. Their contents then empty into an **excretory duct** (*ED*), which is recognized by a stratified or pseudostratified epithelium. Other features of note in this micrograph are arteries (*A*) and veins (*V*), which are found coursing in the connective tissue with the larger ducts. Also evident in this micrograph is an area containing an accumulation of lymphocytes and plasma cells (*LP*).

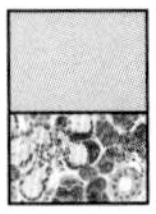

Submandibular gland, human, H&E ×725.

The *boxed area* in the previous micrograph is shown here at higher magnification. It includes several **mucous acini** (*MA*) on the *left side* of the micrograph, a number of **serous acini** (*SA*) on the *right side* of the micrograph, and in the *center*, two **mixed acini** (*MxA*) consisting of mucus- and serous-secreting cells. Characteristically, the mucus-secreting cells have a pale-staining cytoplasm with their nuclei flattened at the base of the cell. In contrast, the serous-secreting cells are deeply stained and exhibit round nuclei. In addition, the lumen (*Lu*) of the acini associated with the mucus-secreting cells is relatively wide; the lumen of the serous acini is relatively narrow and difficult to find. An additional point that should be made is that the serous cells of the mixed acini generally appear as a cap in relation to the mucous cells. These cells are referred to as *demilunes*. In evaluating some of those acini that appear to be serous in nature, it is possible that they simply represent a tangential section of a demilune. A **striated duct** (*SD*) is also included in the micrograph. It is so named because of the faint striations that can be seen in the basal cytoplasm. These ducts, as noted, receive secretion from the intercalated ducts and empty into the larger excretory ducts.

A, arteries
DCT, dense connective tissue core
ED, excretory ducts
L, lobe
LP, lymphocytes and plasma cells
Lu, lumen
MA, mucous acini
MxA, mixed acini
SA, serous acini
SD, striated duct
V, vein

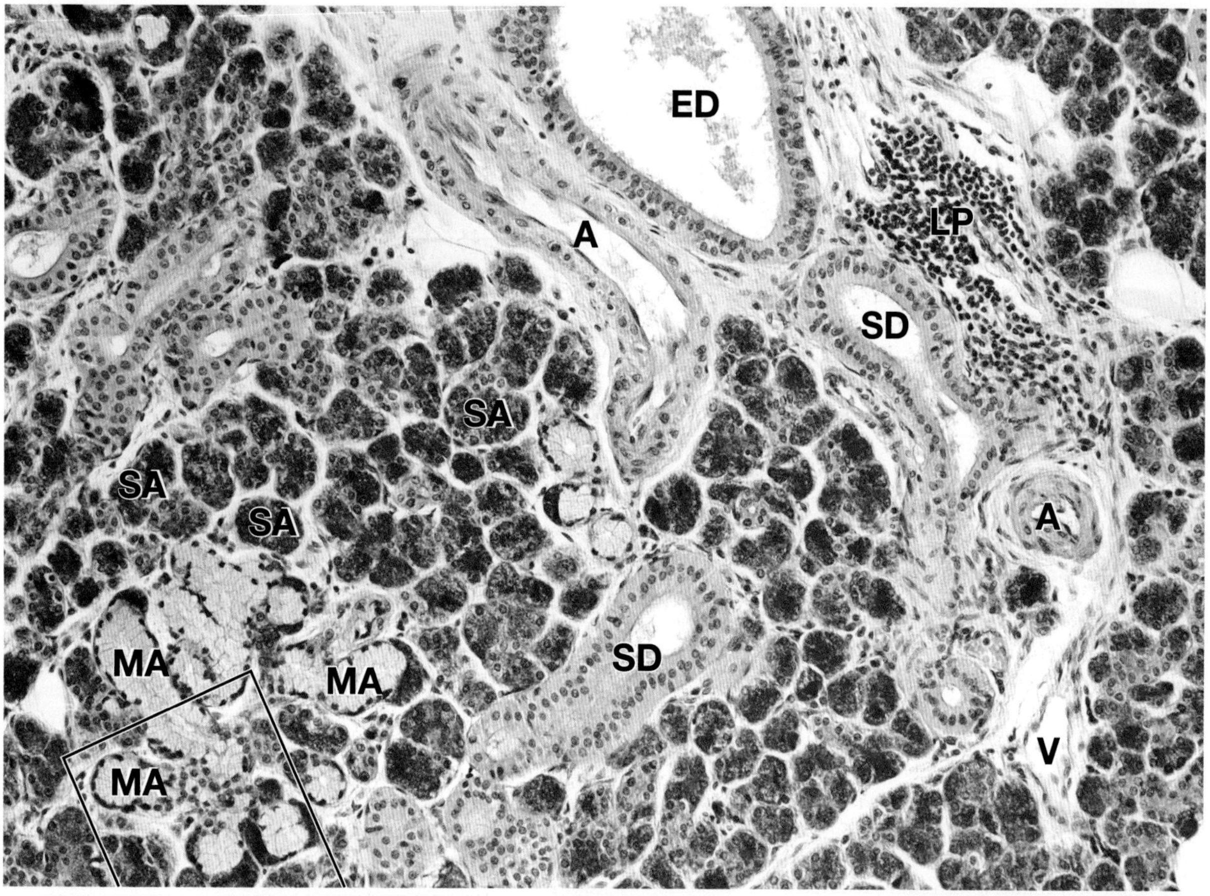
ED
A
LP
SD
SA
SA
SA
A
MA
MA
SD
MA
V

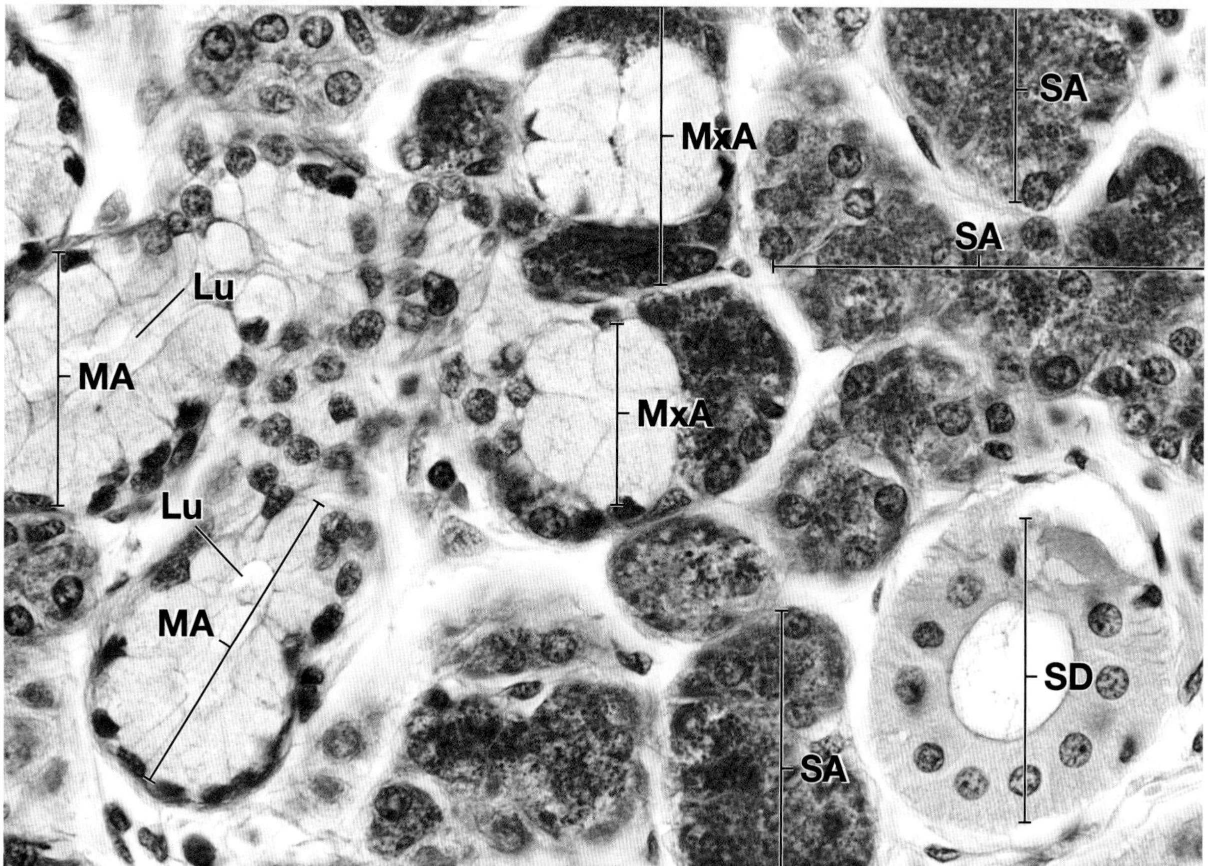
MxA
SA
SA
Lu
MA
MxA
Lu
MA
SA
SD

PLATE 16.5 ■ PAROTID GLAND

The **parotid glands** are the largest of the major salivary glands. They are composed of alveoli containing only serous secretory cells. Adipose tissue often occurs in the parotid gland and may be one of its distinguishing features. The facial nerve (cranial nerve VII) passes through the parotid gland; large cross sections of this nerve, often found in routine hematoxylin and eosin (H&E) sections of the gland, may also be of help in identifying the parotid. Mumps, a viral infection of the parotid gland, can damage the facial nerve.

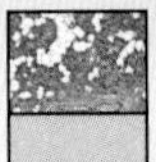

Parotid gland, human, H&E ×160.

The **parotid gland** in the human is composed entirely of **serous acini** (*A*) and their ducts. However, numerous **adipose cells** (*AC*) are usually distributed throughout the gland. Both the serous acini and their duct system in the parotid gland are comparable in structure and arrangement to the same components in the submandibular gland. Within the lobule, the striated ducts (*StD*) are readily observed. They exhibit a simple columnar epithelium. The intercalated ducts are smaller; at the low magnification of this figure, they are difficult to recognize. A few **intercalated ducts** (*ID*) are indicated. The *lower portion* of the figure reveals an **excretory duct** (*ED*) within a connective tissue septum (*CT*). The epithelium of this excretory duct exhibits two layers of nuclei and is either pseudostratified or, possibly, already true stratified epithelium.

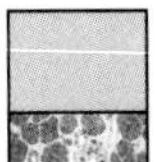

Parotid gland, monkey, glutaraldehyde-osmium tetroxide fixed, H&E ×640.

The **serous cells** are optimally preserved in this specimen and reveal their secretory (zymogen) granules. The granules appear as fine dot-like objects within the cytoplasm. The acinus in the *upper right* of the figure has been cut in cross section and reveals the acinar lumen (*AL*). The *small rectangle* drawn in the acinus represents an area comparable to the electron micrograph shown in Figure 16.25. The large acinar profile to the *left* of the striated duct (*StD*) shows that the acini are not simple spheres but, rather, irregular elongated structures. Because of the small size of the acinar lumen and the variability in sectioning an acinus, the lumen is seen infrequently.

A cross-sectional profile of an intercalated duct (*ID*) appears on the *left* of the micrograph; note its simple cuboidal epithelium. A single flattened nucleus is present at the top of the duct and may represent one of the myoepithelial cells that are associated with the beginning of the duct system as well as with the acini (*A*). The large duct occupying the *center* of the micrograph is a **striated duct** (*StD*). It is composed of columnar epithelium. The striations (*S*) that give the duct its name are evident. Also of significance is the presence of plasma cells (*PC*) within the connective tissue surrounding the duct. These cells produce the immunoglobulins taken up and resecreted by the acinar cells, particularly secretory IgA (sIgA).

A, acinus
AC, adipose cell
AL, acinar lumen
CT, connective tissue
ED, excretory duct
ID, intercalated duct
PC, plasma cells
S, striations of duct
StD, striated duct

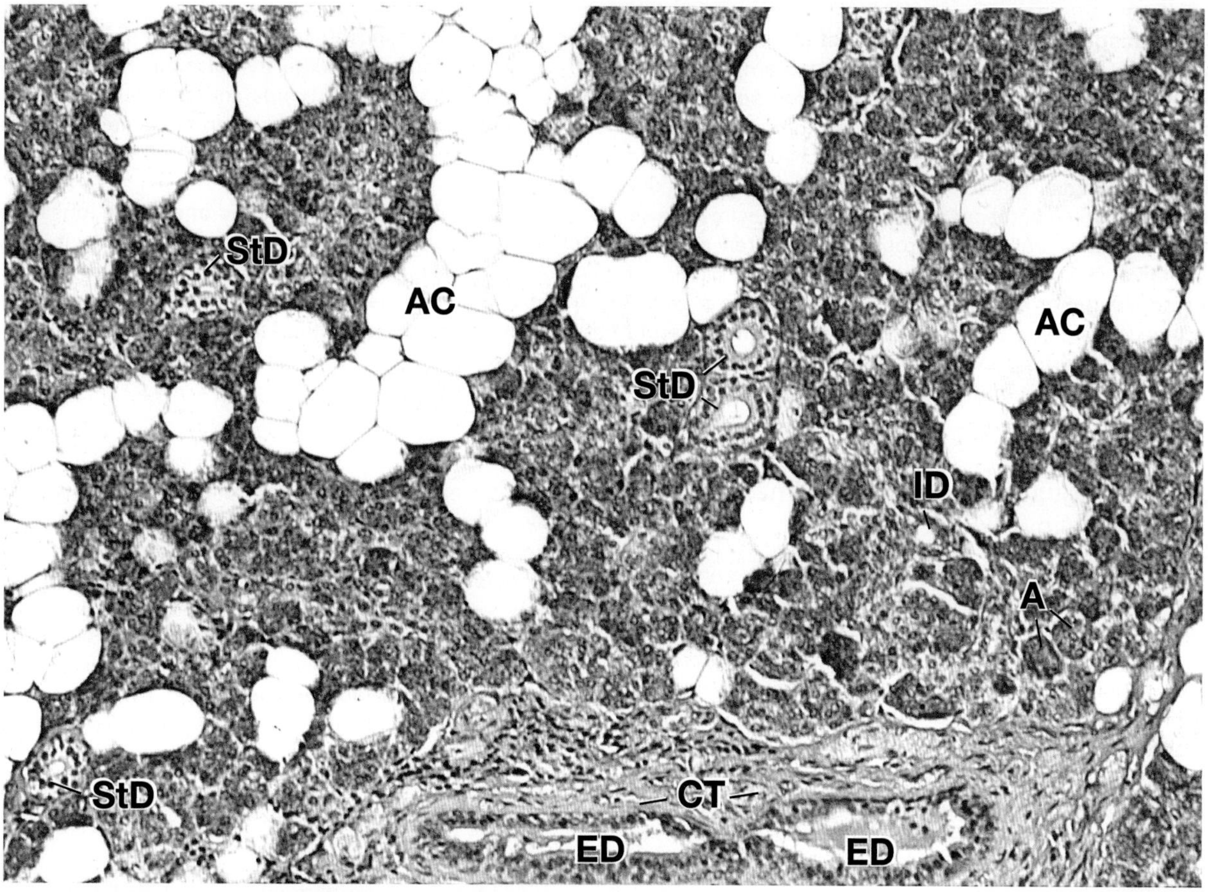
StD
AC
AC
StD
ID
A
StD
CT
ED
ED

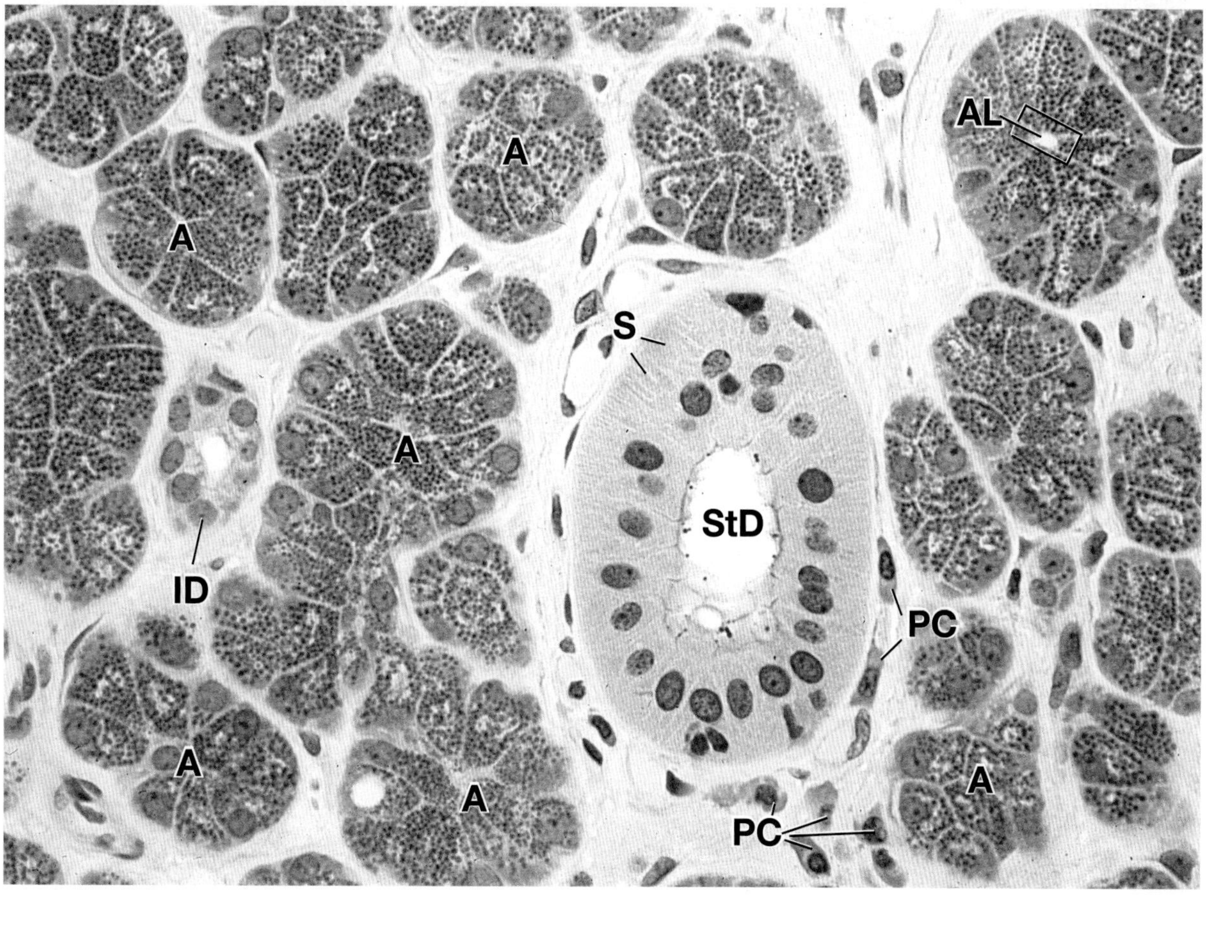
AL
A
A
S
A
StD
ID
PC
A
A
A
PC

PLATE 16.6 ■ SUBLINGUAL GLAND

The **sublingual glands** are the smallest of the paired major salivary glands. Their multiple small ducts empty into the submandibular ducts as well as directly onto the floor of the mouth. The sublingual gland resembles the submandibular gland in that it contains both serous and mucous elements. In the sublingual gland, however, the mucous acini predominate. Some of the predominant mucous acini have serous demilunes, but purely serous acini are rarely present.

Saliva includes the combined secretions of all the major and minor salivary glands. The functions of saliva include *moistening* dry foods to aid swallowing, *dissolving* and *suspending* food materials that chemically stimulate taste buds, *buffering* the contents of the oral cavity through its high concentration of bicarbonate ion, digestion of carbohydrates by the digestive enzyme α-amylase (which breaks the 1–4 glycoside bonds and continues to act in the esophagus and stomach), and *controlling* the bacterial *flora* of the oral cavity because of the presence of the antibacterial enzyme *lysozyme*.

Saliva is a source of calcium and phosphate ions essential for normal tooth development and maintenance. It also contains antibodies, notably salivary secretory immunoglobulin A (sIgA). Salivation is part of a reflex arc that is normally stimulated by the ingestion of food, although sight, smell, or even thoughts of food can also stimulate salivation.

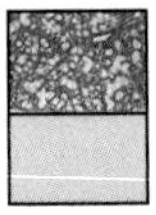

Sublingual gland, human, hematoxylin and eosin (H&E) ×160.

This figure shows a **sublingual gland** at low power. The mucous acini (*MA*) are conspicuous because of their light staining. Critical examination of the mucous acini at this relatively low magnification reveals that they are not spherical structures but, rather, elongated or tubular structures with branching outpockets. Thus, the acinus is rather large, and much of it is usually not seen within the plane of a single section.

The serous component of the gland is composed largely of **demilunes**, but occasional serous acini are present. As noted earlier, some of the serous demilunes may be sectioned in a plane that does not include the mucous component of the acinus, thus giving the appearance of a serous acinus.

The ducts of the sublingual gland that are observed most frequently in a section are the intralobular ducts. They are the equivalent of the striated duct of the submandibular and parotid glands but lack the extensive basal infoldings and mitochondrial array that creates the striations. One of the **intralobular ducts** (*InD*) is evident in this figure (*upper right*). The area within the *rectangle* includes part of this duct and is shown at higher magnification in the next figure.

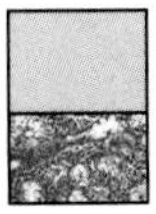

Sublingual gland, human, H&E ×400.

Note that through a fortuitous plane of section, the lumen of a **mucous acinus** (*MA*) (*upper right*) is seen joining an intercalated duct (*ID*). The juncture between the acinus and the beginning of the **intercalated duct** is marked by an *arrowhead*. The intercalated duct is composed of a flattened or low columnar epithelium similar to that seen in the other salivary glands. The intercalated ducts of the sublingual gland are extremely short, however, and thus are usually difficult to find. The intercalated duct seen in this micrograph joins with one or more other intercalated ducts to become the **intralobular duct** (*InD*), which is identified by its columnar epithelium and relatively large lumen. The point of transition from intercalated to intralobular duct is not recognizable in the micrograph, however, because the duct wall has only been grazed and the shape of the cells cannot be determined.

Examination of the acini at this higher magnification also reveals the serous demilunes (*SD*). Note how they form a cap-like addition to the mucous end pieces. The cytologic appearance of the mucous cells (*MC*) and serous cells is essentially the same as that described for the submandibular gland. The area selected for this higher magnification also reveals isolated cell clusters that bear some resemblance to serous acini. It is likely, however, that these cells are actually mucous cells that either have been cut in a plane parallel to their base and do not include the mucinogen-containing portions of the cell or are in a state of activity in which, after depletion of their granules, the production of new mucinogen granules does not yet suffice to give the characteristic "empty" mucous cell appearance.

An additional important feature of the connective tissue stroma is the presence of numerous lymphocytes and plasma cells. Some of the plasma cells are indicated by the *arrows*. The plasma cells are associated with the production of salivary IgA and are also present in the other salivary glands.

ID, intercalated duct
InD, intralobular duct
MA, mucous acinus
MC, mucous cells
SD, serous demilune
arrowhead, mucous acinus joining intercalated duct
arrows, plasma cells

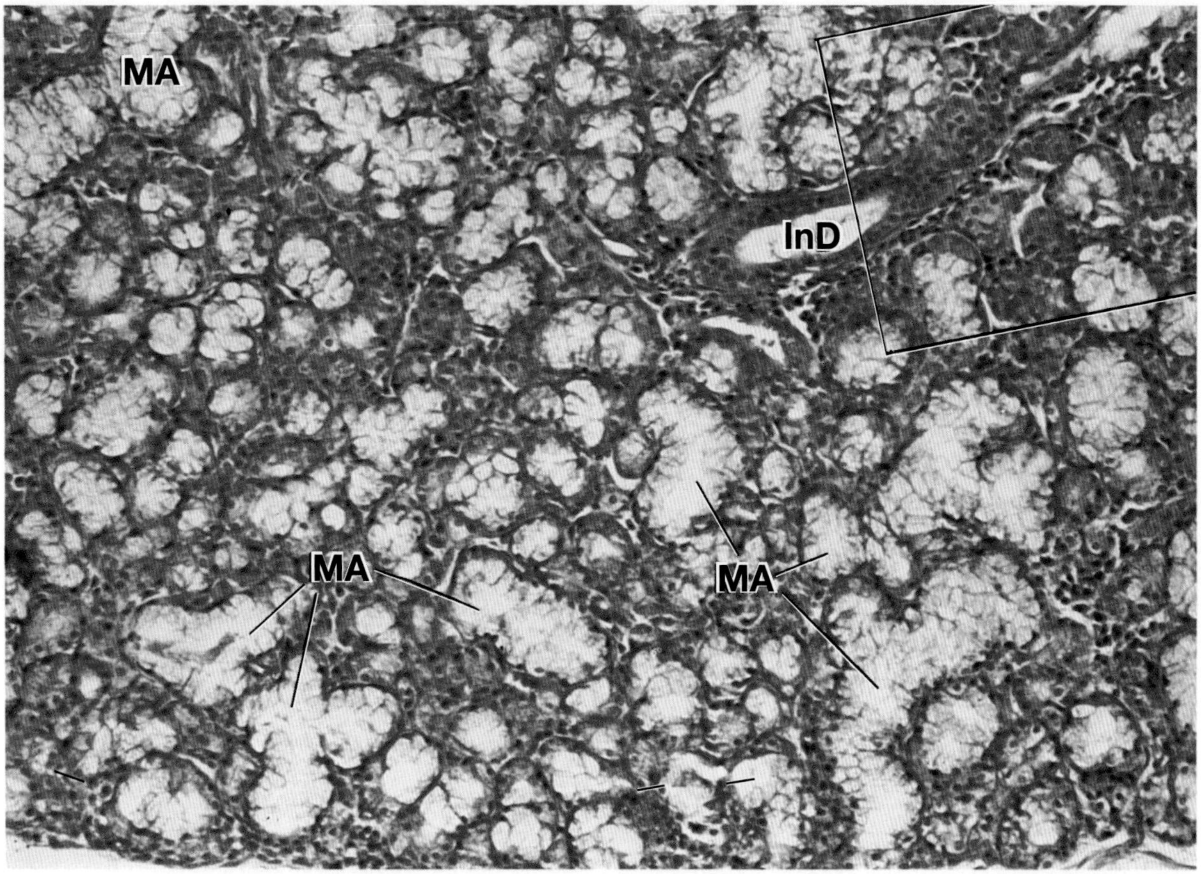
MA
InD
MA
MA

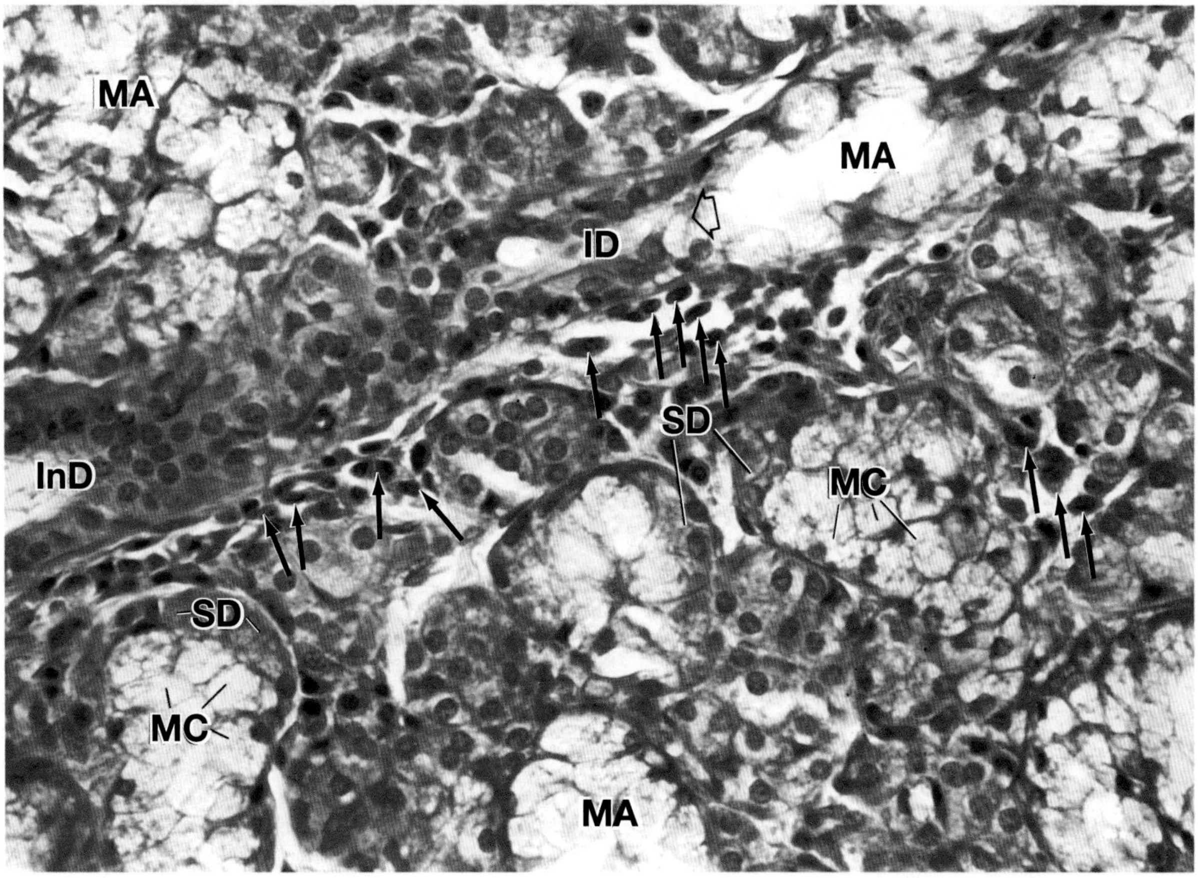
MA
MA
ID
InD
SD
MC
SD
MC
MA

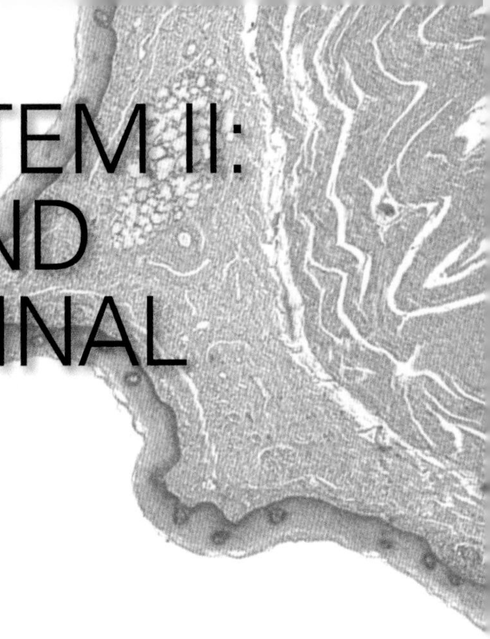

17 DIGESTIVE SYSTEM II: ESOPHAGUS AND GASTROINTESTINAL TRACT

OVERVIEW OF THE ESOPHAGUS AND GASTROINTESTINAL TRACT

The portion of the **alimentary canal** that extends from the proximal part of the esophagus to the distal part of the anal canal is a hollow tube of varying diameter. This tube has the same basic structural organization throughout its length. Its wall is formed by four distinctive layers. From the lumen outward (Fig. 17.1), they are as follows:

- **Mucosa**, consisting of a lining epithelium, an underlying connective tissue called the **lamina propria**, and the **muscularis mucosae**, composed of smooth muscle
- **Submucosa**, consisting of dense irregular connective tissue
- **Muscularis externa**, consisting, in most parts, of two layers of smooth muscle
- **Serosa**, a serous membrane consisting of a simple squamous epithelium, the mesothelium, and a small amount of underlying connective tissue. An **adventitia** consisting only of connective tissue is found where the wall of the tube is directly attached or fixed to adjoining structures (i.e., body wall and certain retroperitoneal organs).

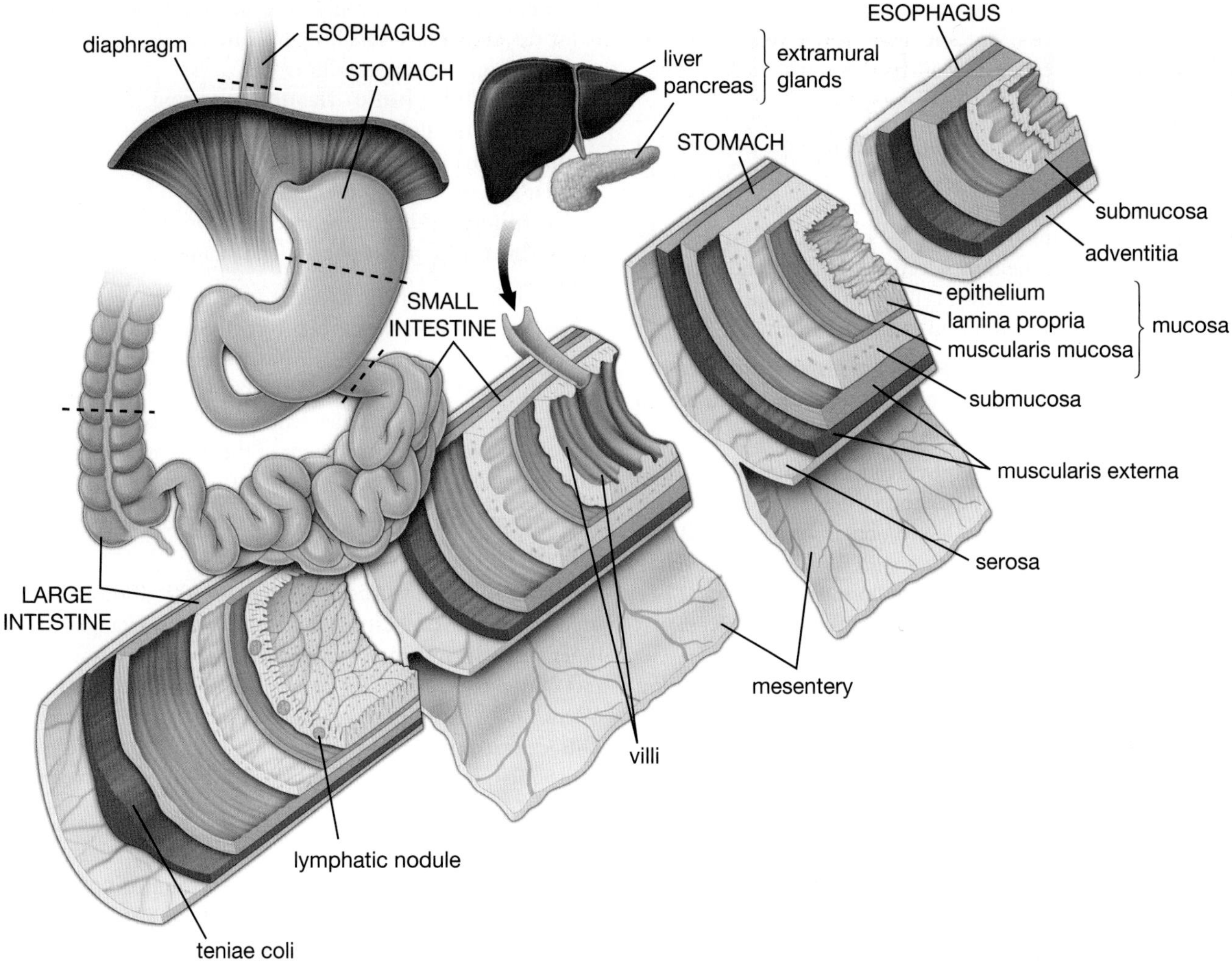

FIGURE 17.1. General organization of the alimentary canal. This composite diagram shows the wall structure of the alimentary canal in four representative organs: esophagus, stomach, small intestine, and large intestine. Note that villi, a characteristic feature of the small intestine, are not present in other parts of the alimentary canal. Mucosal glands are present throughout the length of the alimentary canal but sparingly in the esophagus and oral cavity. Submucosal glands are present in the esophagus and duodenum. The extramural glands (liver and pancreas) empty into the duodenum (first part of the small intestine). Diffuse lymphatic tissues and nodules are found in the lamina propria throughout the entire length of the alimentary canal (shown here only in the large intestine). Nerves, blood vessels, and lymphatic vessels reach the alimentary canal via the mesenteries or via adjacent connective tissue (tunica adventitia as in the retroperitoneal organs).

Mucosa

The structure of the **esophagus** and **gastrointestinal tract** varies considerably from region to region; most of the variation occurs within the mucosa. The epithelium differs throughout the alimentary canal and is adapted to the specific function of each part of the tube. The mucosa has three principal functions: **protection**, **absorption**, and **secretion**. The histologic characteristics of these layers and their functions are described later in this chapter in relation to specific regions of the digestive tube.

The epithelium of the mucosa serves as a barrier that separates the lumen of the alimentary canal from the rest of the organism.

The epithelial barrier separates the external luminal environment of the tube from the tissues and organs of the body. The barrier aids in the protection of the individual from the entry of antigens, pathogens, and other noxious substances. In the esophagus, a stratified squamous epithelium provides protection from physical abrasion by ingested food. In the gastrointestinal portion of the alimentary tract, tight junctions between the simple columnar epithelial cells of the mucosa serve as a selectively permeable barrier. Most epithelial cells transport products of digestion and other essential substances such as water through the cell and into the extracellular space beneath the tight junctions.

The absorptive function of the mucosa allows the movement of digested nutrients, water, and electrolytes into the blood and lymph vessels.

The **absorption** of digested nutrients, water, and electrolytes is possible because of projections of the mucosa and submucosa into the lumen of the digestive tract. These surface projections greatly increase the surface area available for absorption and vary in size and orientation. They consist of the following structural specializations (see Fig. 17.1):

- **Plicae circulares** are circumferentially oriented submucosal folds present along most of the length of the small intestine.
- **Villi** are mucosal projections that cover the entire surface of the small intestine, the principal site of absorption of the products of digestion.

- **Microvilli** are tightly packed, microscopic projections of the apical surface of intestinal absorptive cells. They further increase the surface available for absorption.

In addition, the **glycocalyx** consists of glycoproteins that project from the apical plasma membrane of epithelial absorptive cells. It provides an additional surface for adsorption and includes enzymes secreted by the absorptive cells that are essential for the final steps of digestion of proteins and sugars. The epithelium selectively absorbs the products of digestion both for its own cells and for transport into the vascular system for distribution to other tissues.

The secretory function of the mucosa provides lubrication and delivers digestive enzymes, hormones, and antibodies into the lumen of the alimentary tube.

Secretion is carried out largely by glands distributed throughout the length of the digestive tube. The various secretory products provide mucus for protective lubrication as well as buffering of the tract lining and substances that assist in digestion, including enzymes, hydrochloric acid, peptide hormones, and water (see Fig. 17.1). The mucosal epithelium also secretes antibodies that it receives from the underlying connective tissue.

The glands of the alimentary tract (see Fig. 17.1) develop from invaginations of the luminal epithelium and include the following:

- **Mucosal glands** that extend into the lamina propria
- **Submucosal glands** that deliver their secretions either directly to the lumen of mucosal glands or via ducts that pass through the mucosa to the luminal surface
- **Extramural glands** that lie outside the digestive tract and deliver their secretions via ducts that pass through the wall of the intestine to enter the lumen. The liver and pancreas are extramural digestive glands (see Chapter 18, Digestive System III: Liver, Gallbladder, and Pancreas, page 692) that greatly increase the secretory capacity of the digestive system. They deliver their secretions into the **duodenum**, the first part of the small intestine.

The lamina propria contains glands, vessels that transport absorbed substances, and components of the immune system.

As noted, the **mucosal glands** extend into the lamina propria throughout the length of the alimentary canal. In addition, in several parts of the alimentary canal (e.g., the esophagus and anal canal), the lamina propria contains aggregations of mucus-secreting glands. In general, they lubricate the epithelial surface to protect the mucosa from mechanical and chemical injury. These glands are described later in this chapter in relation to specific regions of the digestive tube.

In segments of the digestive tract in which absorption occurs, principally in the small and large intestines, the absorbed products of digestion diffuse into the **blood and lymphatic vessels** of the lamina propria for distribution. Typically, the blood capillaries are of the fenestrated type and collect most of the absorbed metabolites. In the small intestine, lymphatic capillaries are numerous and receive some absorbed lipids and proteins.

- The **lymphatic tissues** in the lamina propria function as an integrated immunologic barrier that protects against pathogens and other antigenic substances that could potentially enter through the mucosa from the lumen of the alimentary canal. Lymphatic tissues present in the lamina propria are as follows:
- **Diffuse lymphatic tissue** consisting of numerous lymphocytes and plasma cells located in the lamina propria and lymphocytes transiently residing in the intercellular spaces of the epithelium
- **Lymphatic nodules** with well-developed germinal centers
- **Eosinophils**, macrophages, and, sometimes, neutrophils

The diffuse lymphatic tissue and the lymphatic nodules are referred to as **gut-associated lymphatic tissue (GALT)**. In the distal small intestine, the **ileum**, extensive aggregates of nodules, called **Peyer patches**, occupy much of the lamina propria and submucosa. They tend to be located on the side of the tube opposite the attachment of the mesentery. Aggregated lymphatic nodules are also present in the appendix.

The muscularis mucosae forms the boundary between mucosa and submucosa.

The **muscularis mucosae**, the deepest portion of the mucosa, consists of **smooth muscle** cells arranged in an inner circular and outer longitudinal layer. Contraction of this muscle produces movement of the mucosa, forming ridges and valleys that facilitate absorption and secretion. This localized movement of the mucosa is independent of the peristaltic movement of the entire wall of the digestive tract.

Submucosa

The submucosa consists of a dense irregular connective tissue layer containing blood and lymphatic vessels, a nerve plexus, and occasional glands.

The **submucosa** contains the larger blood vessels that send branches to the mucosa, muscularis externa, and serosa. The submucosa also contains lymphatic vessels and a nerve plexus. The extensive nerve network in the submucosa contains visceral sensory fibers of mainly sympathetic origin, parasympathetic (terminal) ganglia, and preganglionic and postganglionic parasympathetic nerve fibers. The nerve cell bodies of parasympathetic ganglia and their postganglionic nerve fibers represent the **enteric nervous system**, the third division of the autonomic nervous system. This system is primarily responsible for innervating the smooth muscle layers of the alimentary canal and can function totally independently of the central nervous system. In the submucosa, the network of unmyelinated nerve fibers and ganglion cells constitute the **submucosal plexus** (also called **Meissner plexus**).

As noted, glands occur occasionally in the submucosa in certain locations. For example, they are present in the esophagus and the initial portion of the duodenum. In histologic sections, the presence of these glands often aids in identifying the specific segment or region of the tract.

Muscularis Externa

In most parts of the digestive tract, the **muscularis externa** consists of two concentric and relatively thick layers of smooth muscle. The cells in the inner layer form a tight spiral, described as a **circularly oriented layer**; those in the outer layer form a loose spiral, described as a **longitudinally oriented layer**. Located between the two muscle layers is a thin connective tissue layer. Within this connective tissue lies the **myenteric plexus** (also called the **Auerbach plexus**), containing nerve cell bodies (ganglion cells) of postganglionic parasympathetic neurons, neurons of the enteric nervous system, and satellite cells as well as blood vessels and lymphatic vessels.

Contractions of the muscularis externa mix and propel the contents of the digestive tract.

Contraction of the inner circular layer of the **muscularis externa** compresses and mixes the contents by constricting the lumen; contraction of the outer, longitudinal layer propels the contents by shortening the tube. The slow, rhythmic contraction of these muscle layers under the control of the enteric nervous system produces **peristalsis** (i.e., waves of contraction). Peristalsis is marked by constriction and shortening of the tube, which moves the contents through the intestinal tract.

A few sites along the digestive tube exhibit variations in the muscularis externa. For example, in the wall of the proximal portion of the esophagus (pharyngoesophageal sphincter) and around the anal canal (external anal sphincter), striated muscle forms part of the muscularis externa. In the stomach, a third, obliquely oriented layer of smooth muscle is present deep into the circular layer. Finally, in the large intestine, part of the **longitudinal smooth muscle layer** is thickened to form three distinct, equally spaced longitudinal bands called **teniae coli**. During contraction, the teniae facilitate shortening of the tube to move its contents.

The circular smooth muscle layer forms sphincters at specific locations along the digestive tract.

At several points along the digestive tract, the **circular muscle layer** is thickened to form **sphincters** or **valves**. From the oropharynx distally, these structures include the following:

- **Pharyngoesophageal sphincter**. Actually, the lowest part of the cricopharyngeus muscle is physiologically referred to as the **superior (upper) esophageal sphincter**. It prevents the entry of air into the esophagus.
- **Inferior (lower) esophageal sphincter**. As its name implies, this sphincter is located at the lower end of the esophagus; its action is reinforced by the diaphragm that surrounds this part of the esophagus as it passes into the abdominal cavity. It creates a pressure difference between the esophagus and the stomach that prevents reflux of gastric contents into the esophagus. Abnormal relaxation of this sphincter allows the acidic contents of the stomach to return (reflux) into the esophagus. If not treated, this condition may progress to **gastroesophageal reflux disease (GERD)**, characterized by inflammation of the esophageal mucosa (reflux esophagitis), strictures, and difficulty in swallowing (dysphagia) with accompanying chest pain.
- **Pyloric sphincter**. Located at the junction of the pylorus of the stomach and duodenum (gastroduodenal sphincter), this sphincter controls the release of **chyme**, the partially digested contents of the stomach, into the duodenum. Nitric oxide synthase (NOS), which **produces nitric oxide (NO)**, is responsible for physiologic relaxation of the pyloric sphincter. Deficiency in NOS causes smooth muscle spasm of the pyloric sphincter and subsequent **hypertrophic pyloric stenosis**. This condition occurs most commonly during the first 2–12 weeks of life and results in obstruction in flow of chyme into the duodenum, which causes projectile vomiting (without bile) after feeding. If untreated, it may lead to dehydration and hypochloremic, hypokalemic metabolic alkalosis. Hypertrophy of the pyloric muscle can be diagnosed by ultrasonography and is also easily palpable as an "olive" in the right upper quadrant of the abdomen. Laparoscopic pyloromyotomy that involves transection of pyloric muscle without disruption of underlying mucosa remains the primary surgical treatment.
- **Ileocecal valve**. Located at the junction of the small and large intestines, it prevents reflux of the contents of the colon with its high bacterial count into the distal ileum, which normally has a low bacterial count.
- **Internal anal sphincter**. This, the most distally located sphincter, surrounds the anal canal and prevents passage of the feces into the anal canal from the undistended rectum.

Serosa and Adventitia

Serosa or adventitia constitutes the outermost layer of the alimentary canal.

The **serosa** is a serous membrane consisting of a layer of simple squamous epithelium, called the **mesothelium**, and a small amount of underlying connective tissue. It is equivalent to the visceral peritoneum described in gross anatomy. The serosa is the most superficial layer of those parts of the digestive tract that are suspended in the peritoneal cavity. As such, the serosa is continuous with both the **mesentery** and lining of the abdominal cavity.

Large blood and lymphatic vessels and nerve trunks travel through the serosa (from and to the mesentery) to reach the wall of the digestive tract. Large amounts of adipose tissue can develop in the connective tissue of the serosa (and in the mesentery).

Parts of the digestive tract do not possess a serosa. These include the thoracic part of the esophagus and portions of structures in the abdominal and pelvic cavities that are fixed to the cavity wall—descending, horizontal, and ascending part of duodenum; ascending and descending colon; rectum; and anal canal. These structures are attached to the abdominal and pelvic walls by connective tissue, the **adventitia**, which blends with the connective tissue of the wall.

■ ESOPHAGUS

The esophagus is a fixed muscular tube that delivers food and liquid from the pharynx to the stomach.

The **esophagus** courses through the neck and mediastinum, where it is attached to adjacent structures by connective tissue. As it enters the abdominal cavity, it is free for a short distance, approximately 1–2 cm. The overall length of the esophagus is about 25 cm. On cross section (Fig. 17.2), the lumen in its normally collapsed state has a branched appearance because of longitudinal folds. When a bolus of food passes through the esophagus, the lumen expands without mucosal injury.

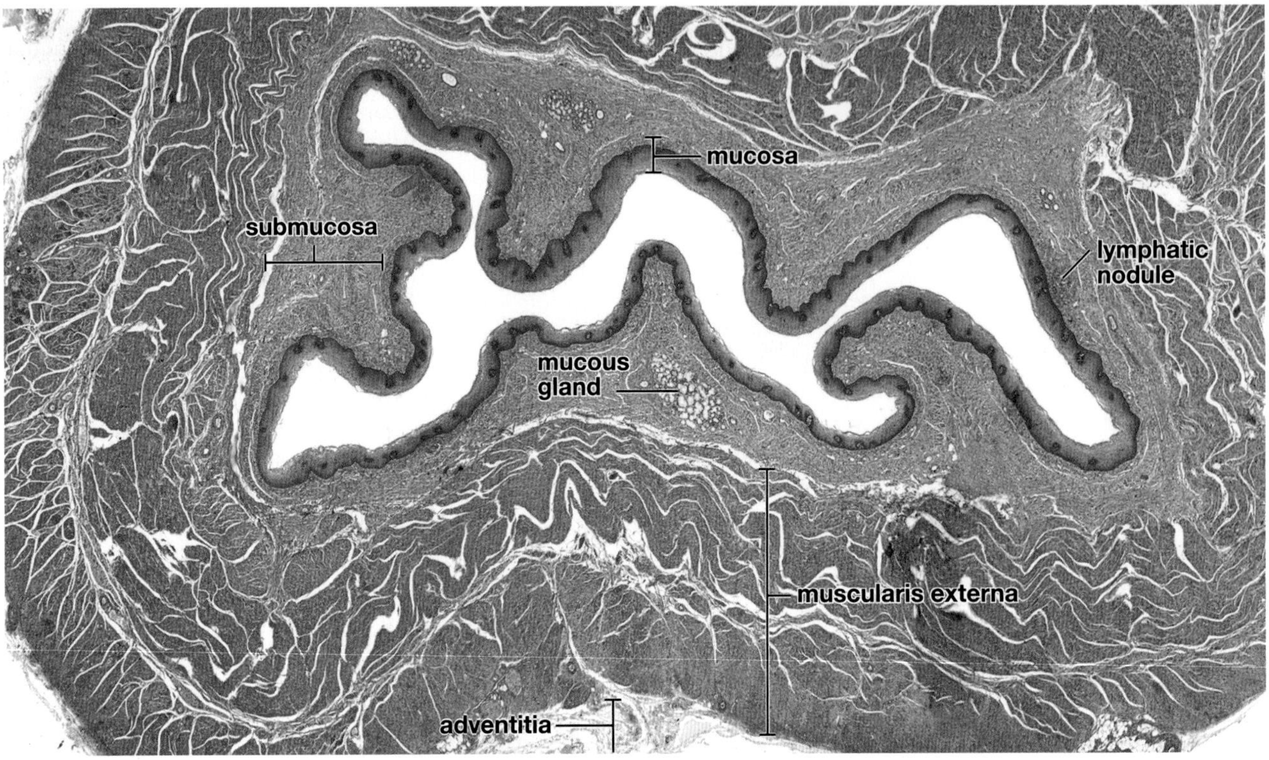

FIGURE 17.2. Photomicrograph of the esophagus. This low-magnification photomicrograph shows a hematoxylin and eosin (H&E)-stained section of the esophagus with its characteristically folded wall, giving the lumen an irregular appearance. The mucosa consists of a relatively thick stratified squamous epithelium, a thin layer of lamina propria containing occasional lymphatic nodules, and muscularis mucosae. Mucous glands are present in the submucosa; their ducts, which empty into the lumen of the esophagus, are not evident in this section. External to the submucosa in this part of the esophagus is a thick muscularis externa made up of an inner layer of circularly arranged smooth muscle and an outer layer of longitudinally arranged smooth muscle. The adventitia is seen just external to the muscularis externa. ×8.

The **mucosa** that lines the length of the esophagus has a nonkeratinized stratified squamous epithelium (Fig. 17.3 and Plate 17.1, page 670). In many animals, however, the epithelium is keratinized, reflecting a coarse food diet. In humans, the surface cells may exhibit some keratohyalin granules, but keratinization does not normally occur. The underlying lamina propria is similar to the lamina propria throughout the alimentary tract; diffuse lymphatic tissue is scattered throughout, and lymphatic nodules are present, often in proximity to ducts of the esophageal mucous glands (see page 638). The deep layer of the mucosa, the **muscularis mucosae**, is composed of longitudinally organized smooth muscle that begins near the level of the cricoid cartilage. It is unusually thick in the proximal portion of the esophagus and presumably functions as an aid in swallowing.

The **submucosa** consists of dense irregular connective tissue that contains the larger blood and lymphatic vessels, nerve fibers, and ganglion cells. The nerve fibers and ganglion cells make up the **submucosal plexus (Meissner plexus)**. Glands are also present (see page 634). In addition, diffuse lymphatic tissue and lymphatic nodules are present mostly in the upper and lower parts of the esophagus where submucosal glands are more prevalent.

The **muscularis externa** consists of two muscle layers, an inner circular layer and an outer longitudinal layer (Plate 17.1, page 670). It differs from the muscularis externa found in the rest of the digestive tract in that the upper one-third is striated muscle, a continuation of the muscle of the pharynx. Striated muscle and smooth muscle bundles are mixed and interwoven in the muscularis externa of the middle third of the esophagus; the muscularis externa of the distal third consists only of smooth muscle, as in the rest of the digestive tract. A nerve plexus, the **myenteric (Auerbach) plexus**, is present between the outer and inner muscle layers. As in the submucosal plexus (Meissner plexus), nerves and ganglion cells are present here. This plexus innervates the muscularis externa and produces peristaltic activity.

As noted, the esophagus is fixed to adjoining structures throughout most of its length; thus, its outer layer is composed of adventitia. After entering the abdominal cavity, the short remainder of the tube is covered by serosa, the visceral peritoneum.

Mucosal and submucosal glands of the esophagus secrete mucus to lubricate and protect the luminal wall.

Glands are present in the wall of the esophagus and are of two types. Both secrete mucus, but their locations differ.

- **Esophageal glands proper** lie in the submucosa. These glands are scattered along the length of the esophagus but are somewhat more concentrated in the upper half. They are small, compound, tubuloalveolar glands (Fig. 17.4). The excretory duct is composed of stratified squamous epithelium and is usually conspicuous when present in a section because of its dilated appearance.
- **Esophageal cardiac glands** are named for their similarity to the cardiac glands of the stomach and are found in the lamina propria of the mucosa. They are present in the terminal part of the esophagus and frequently, although not consistently, in the beginning portion of the esophagus.

The mucus produced by the esophageal glands proper is slightly acidic and serves to lubricate the luminal wall. Because the secretion is relatively viscous, transient cysts often occur in the ducts. The esophageal cardiac glands produce neutral mucus. Those glands near the stomach tend to protect the esophagus from regurgitated gastric contents. Under certain conditions, however, they are not fully effective, and excessive reflux results in **pyrosis**, a condition more commonly known as **heartburn**. This condition may progress to **gastroesophageal reflux disease (GERD)**.

The muscle of the esophageal wall is innervated by both autonomic and somatic nervous systems.

The **striated musculature** in the upper part of the esophagus is innervated by somatic motor neurons of the **vagus nerve**, cranial nerve X (from the nucleus ambiguus). The smooth muscle of the lower part of the esophagus is innervated by visceral motor neurons of the vagus nerve (from the dorsal motor nucleus). These motor neurons synapse with postsynaptic neurons whose cell bodies are located in the wall of the esophagus.

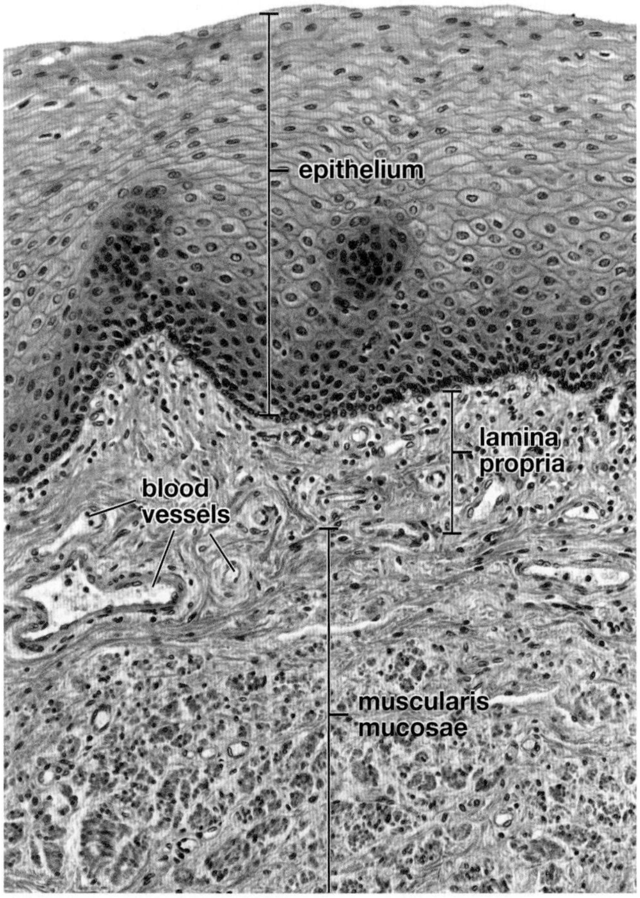

FIGURE 17.3. Photomicrograph of the esophageal mucosa. This higher magnification photomicrograph shows the mucosa of the wall of the esophagus in a hematoxylin and eosin (H&E) preparation. It consists of stratified squamous epithelium, lamina propria, and muscularis mucosae. The boundary between the epithelium and the lamina propria is distinct, although uneven, because of the connective tissue papillae. The basal layer of the epithelium stains intensely, appearing as a dark band because the basal cells are smaller and have a high nucleus-to-cytoplasm ratio. Note that the loose connective tissue of the lamina propria is very cellular, containing many lymphocytes. The deepest part of the mucosa is the muscularis mucosae, which is arranged in two layers (inner circular and outer longitudinal) similar in orientation to the muscularis externa. ×240.

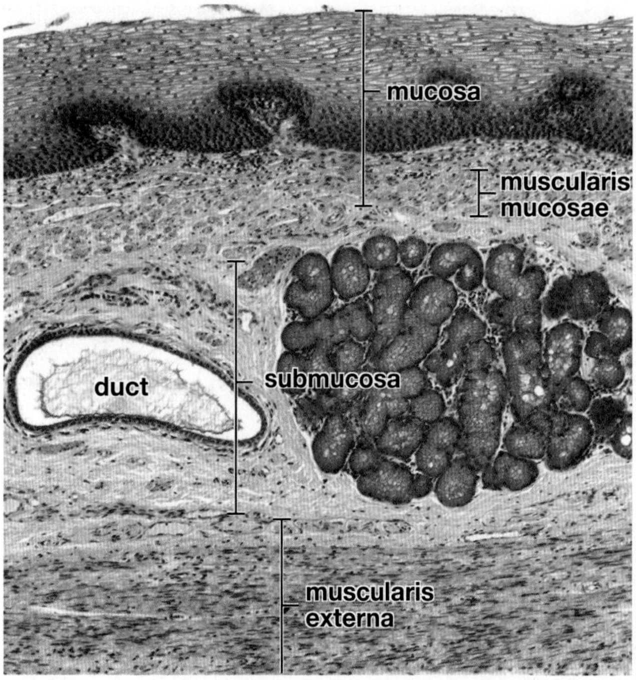

FIGURE 17.4. Photomicrograph of an esophageal submucosal gland. This photomicrograph shows a mucicarmine-stained section of the esophagus. An esophageal gland, deeply stained red by the carmine, and an adjacent excretory duct are seen in the submucosa. These small, compound, tubuloalveolar glands produce mucus that lubricates the epithelial surface of the esophagus. Note the stained mucus within the excretory duct. The remaining submucosa consists of dense irregular connective tissue. The inner layer of the muscularis externa (*bottom*) is composed of circularly arranged smooth muscle. ×110.

■ STOMACH

The **stomach** is an expanded part of the digestive tube that lies beneath the diaphragm. It receives the bolus of macerated food from the esophagus. Mixing and partial digestion of the food in the stomach by its gastric secretions produce a pulpy fluid mix called **chyme**. The chyme then passes into the duodenum, a critical step for further digestion and absorption in the small intestine. Regulation of the rate of gastric emptying is provided by feedback from the intestines via a variety of gastrointestinal hormones.

The stomach is divided histologically into three regions based on the type of gland that each contains.

Gross anatomists subdivide the **stomach** into four regions. The **cardia** surrounds the esophageal orifice; the **fundus** lies above the level of a horizontal line drawn through the esophageal (cardiac) orifice; the **body** lies below this line; and the **pyloric antrum** is the funnel-shaped region that leads into the **pylorus**, the distal, narrow sphincteric region between the stomach and duodenum. Histologists also subdivide the stomach but only into three regions (Fig. 17.5). These subdivisions are based not on location but on the types of glands that occur in the gastric mucosa. The histologic regions are as follows:

- **Cardiac region**, the part near the esophageal orifice, which contains the cardiac glands (Fig. 17.6 and Plate 17.2, page 672)
- **Pyloric region**, the part proximal to the pyloric sphincter, which contains the pyloric glands
- **Fundic region**, the largest part of the stomach, which is situated between the cardia and pylorus and contains the fundic or **gastric glands** (see Fig. 17.6)

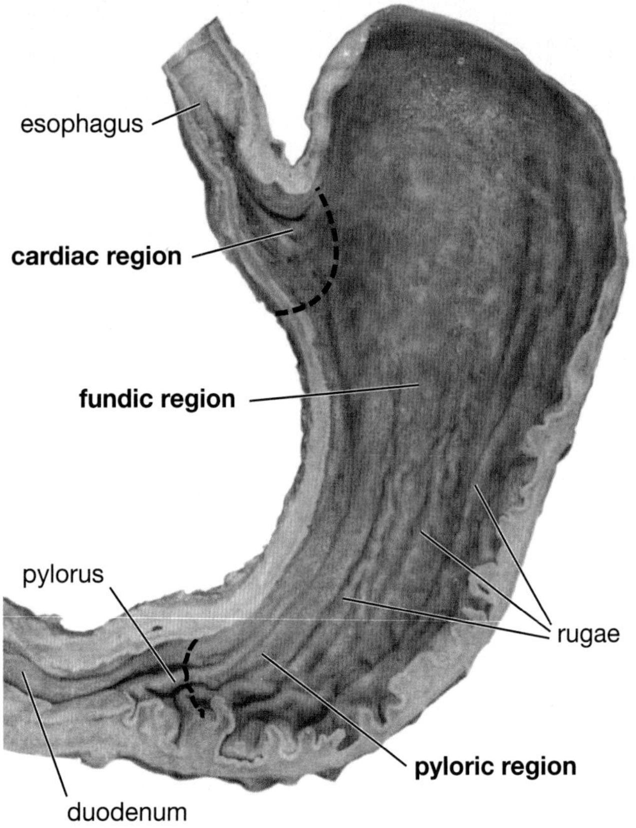

FIGURE 17.5. Photograph of a hemisected human stomach with its histologic divisions. This photograph shows the mucosal surface of the posterior wall of the stomach. Numerous longitudinal gastric folds are evident. These folds or rugae allow the stomach to distend as it fills. The histologic divisions of the stomach differ from the anatomic division. The former is based on the types of glands found in the mucosa. Histologically, the portion of the stomach adjacent to the entrance of the esophagus is the *cardiac region* in which cardiac glands are located. A *dashed line* approximates its boundary. A slightly larger region leading toward the pyloric sphincter, the *pyloric region*, contains the pyloric glands. Another *dashed line* approximates boundary of the pyloric sphincter. The remainder of the stomach, the *fundic region*, is located between the cardiac and pyloric regions and contains the fundic (gastric) glands.

Gastric Mucosa

Longitudinal submucosal folds, rugae, allow the stomach to distend when filled.

The **stomach** has the same general structural plan throughout, consisting of mucosa, submucosa, muscularis externa, and serosa. Examination of the **inner surface** of the empty stomach reveals a number of longitudinal folds or ridges called **rugae**. They are prominent in the narrower regions of the stomach but poorly developed in the upper portion (see Fig. 17.5). When the stomach is fully distended, the rugae, composed of the mucosa and underlying submucosa, virtually disappear. The rugae do not alter total surface area; rather, they serve to accommodate the expansion and filling of the stomach.

A view of the stomach's surface with a hand lens shows that smaller regions of the mucosa are formed by grooves or shallow trenches that divide the stomach surface into bulging irregular areas called **mamillated areas**. These grooves provide a slightly increased surface area for secretion.

At higher magnification, numerous openings can be observed in the mucosal surface. These are the **gastric pits** or **foveolae**. They can be readily demonstrated with the scanning electron microscope (Fig. 17.7). The gastric glands open into the bottom of the gastric pits.

Surface mucous cells line the inner surface of the stomach and the gastric pits.

The epithelium that lines the surface and gastric pits of the stomach is simple columnar. The columnar cells are designated **surface mucous cells**. Each cell possesses a large, apical cup of **mucinogen granules**, creating a glandular sheet of cells (Fig. 17.8). The mucous cup occupies most of the volume of the cell. It typically appears empty in routine hematoxylin and eosin (H&E) sections because the mucinogen is lost in fixation and dehydration. When the mucinogen is preserved by appropriate fixation, however, the granules stain intensely with toluidine blue and with the periodic acid–Schiff (PAS) procedure. The toluidine blue staining reflects the presence of many strongly anionic groups in the glycoprotein of the mucin, among which is bicarbonate.

The nucleus and Golgi apparatus of the surface mucous cells are located below the mucous cup. The basal part of the cell contains small amounts of rough endoplasmic reticulum

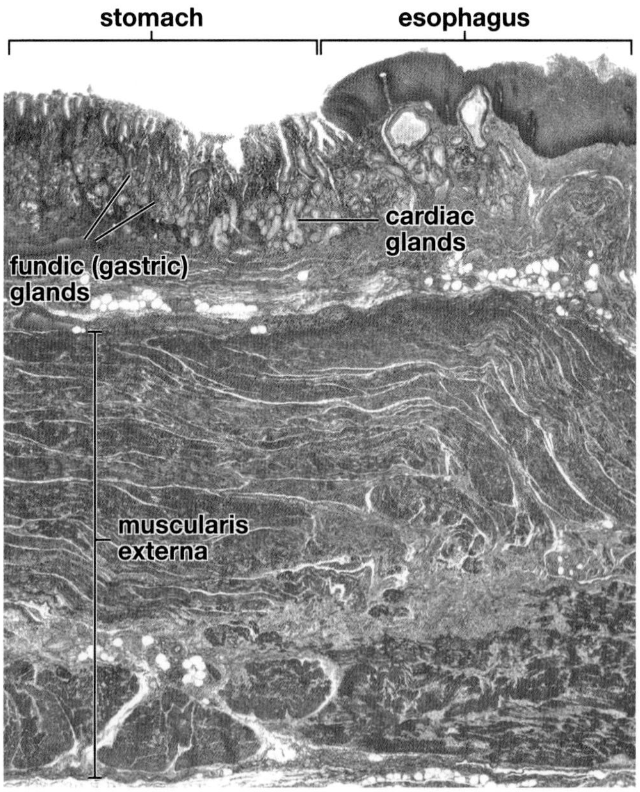

FIGURE 17.6. Photomicrograph of the esophagogastric junction. This low-magnification photomicrograph shows the junction between the esophagus and the stomach. At the esophagogastric junction, the stratified squamous epithelium of the esophagus ends abruptly, and the simple columnar epithelium of the stomach mucosa begins. The surface of the stomach contains numerous and relatively deep depressions called *gastric pits* that are formed by the surface epithelium. The glands in the vicinity of the esophagus, the cardiac glands, extend from the bottom of these pits. The fundic (gastric) glands similarly arise at the base of the gastric pits and are evident in the remaining part of the mucosa. Note the relatively thick muscularis externa. ×40.

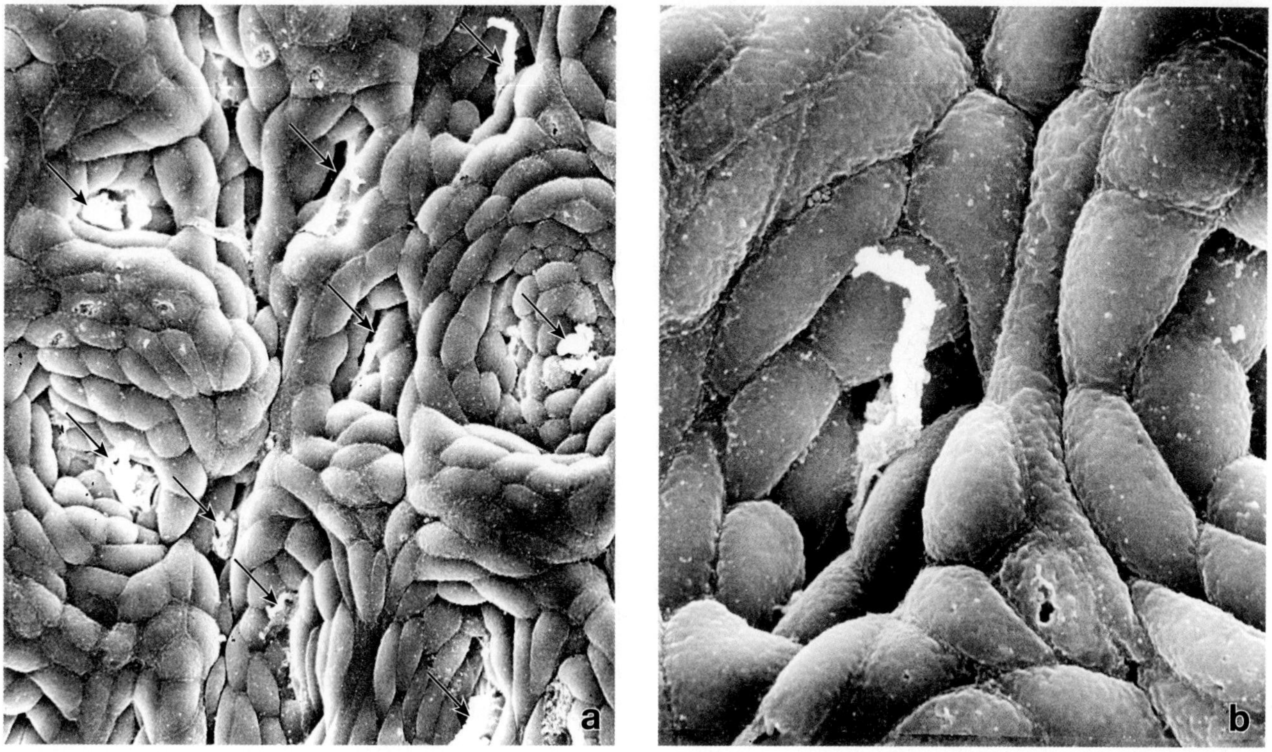

FIGURE 17.7. Mucosal surface of the stomach. a. Scanning electron micrograph showing the mucosal surface of the stomach. The gastric pits contain secretory material, mostly mucus (*arrows*). The surface mucus has been washed away to reveal the surface mucous cells. ×1,000. **b.** Higher magnification showing the apical surface of the surface mucous cells that line the stomach and gastric pits. Note the elongated polygonal shape of the cells. ×3,000.

(rER) that may impart a light basophilia to the cytoplasm when observed in well-preserved specimens.

Several mechanisms help protect the gastric mucosa from exogenous injury and contribute to recovery of its functional integrity after damage.

The first line of protection from injury of gastric mucosa is the mucous secretion from the surface mucous cells. It is described as **visible mucus** because of its cloudy appearance and forms a thick, viscous, gel-like coat that adheres to the epithelial surface. It protects against abrasion from rougher components of the chyme. In addition, its **high bicarbonate and potassium concentration** protects the epithelium from the acidic content of the gastric juice. The bicarbonate that makes the mucus alkaline is secreted by the surface cells but is prevented from mixing rapidly with the contents of the gastric lumen by its containment within the mucous coat.

The second line of protection is related to the regulation of the submucosal blood by a number of mediators, including prostaglandins (PGE_2), nitric oxide (NO), and sensory neuropeptides. **Prostaglandins (PGE_2)** and **nitric oxide (NO)** appear to play an important role in protecting the gastric mucosa. PGE_2 stimulate secretion of bicarbonates and increase the thickness of the mucous layer with accompanied vasodilatation in the lamina propria. NO released from vascular endothelium, sensory afferent nerves, and gastric epithelium **increases gastric mucosal blood flow**, thus improving the supply of nutrients to damaged areas of the gastric mucosa. This ability of the gastric mucosa to optimize conditions for tissue repair after injury (independently of the inhibition of acid secretion) is referred to as **gastric cytoprotection**.

The lining of the stomach does not function in an absorptive capacity. However, some water, salts, and lipid-soluble drugs may be absorbed. For instance, alcohol and certain drugs such as aspirin or nonsteroidal anti-inflammatory drugs (NSAIDs) enter the lamina propria by damaging the surface epithelium. Even small doses of aspirin suppress the production of protective prostaglandins by the gastric mucosa. In addition, aspirin's direct contact with the wall of the stomach interferes with the hydrophobic properties of the gastric mucosa.

Fundic glands of the gastric mucosa

The fundic glands produce the gastric juice of the stomach.

The **fundic glands**, also called **gastric glands**, are present throughout the entire gastric mucosa, except for the relatively small regions occupied by cardiac and pyloric glands. The fundic glands are simple, branched, tubular glands that extend from the bottom of the gastric pits to the muscularis mucosae (see Fig. 17.8). Located between the **gastric pit** and the gland below is a short segment known as the **isthmus**.

Typically, several glands open into a single gastric pit. Each gland has a narrow, relatively long **neck segment** and a shorter and wider base or **fundic segment**. The base of the gland usually divides into two and sometimes three branches that become slightly coiled near the muscularis mucosae. The cells of the gastric glands produce gastric juice (about 2 L/d), which contains a variety of substances. In addition

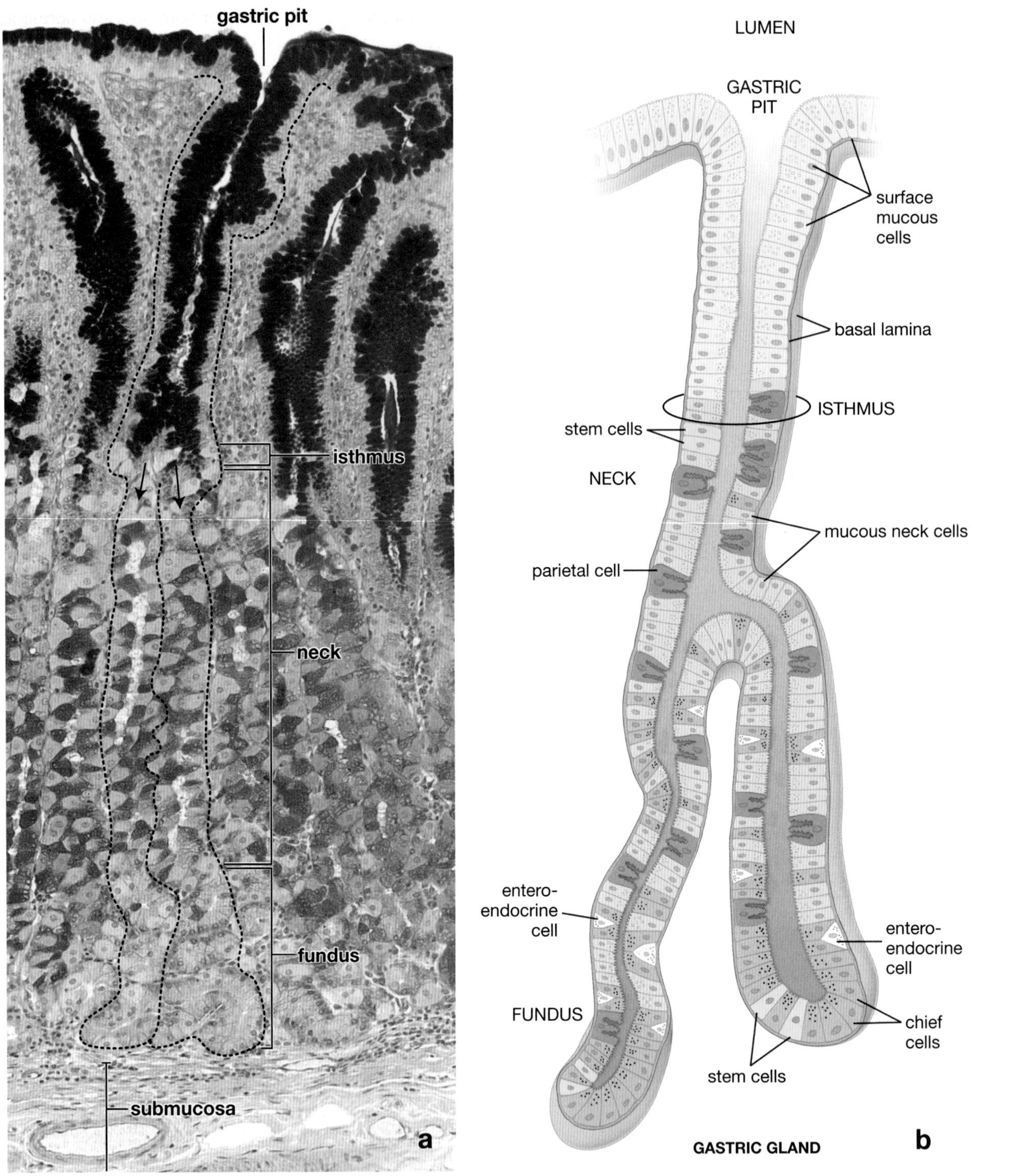

FIGURE 17.8. Gastric glands. a. This photomicrograph shows the fundic mucosa from an Alcian blue/periodic acid–Schiff (PAS) preparation to visualize mucus. Note that the surface epithelium invaginates to form gastric pits. The surface mucous cells and the cells lining the gastric pits are readily identified in this preparation because the neutral mucus within these cells is stained intensely. One of the gastric pits and its associated fundic gland are depicted by the *dashed lines*. This gland represents a simple branched tubular gland (*arrows* indicate the branching pattern). It extends from the bottom of the gastric pit to the muscularis mucosae. Note the segments of the gland: the short isthmus, the site of cell divisions; the relatively long neck; and a shorter and wider fundus. The mucous secretion of mucous neck cells is different from that produced by the surface mucous cells as evidenced by the *lighter magenta* staining in this region of the gland. ×320. **b.** Schematic diagram of a gastric gland illustrating the relationship of the gland to the gastric pit. Note that the isthmus region contains dividing cells and undifferentiated cells; the neck region contains mucous neck cells, parietal cells, and enteroendocrine cells, including amine precursor uptake and decarboxylation (APUD) cells. Parietal cells are large, pear-shaped acidophilic cells found throughout the gland. The fundus of the gland contains mainly chief cells, some parietal cells, and several types of enteroendocrine cells.

to water and electrolytes, gastric juice contains four major components:

- **Hydrochloric acid (HCl)** in a concentration ranging from 150 to 160 mmol/L, which gives the gastric juice a low pH (<1.0–2.0). It is produced by **parietal cells** and initiates the digestion of dietary protein (it promotes acid hydrolysis of substrates). It also converts inactive pepsinogen into the active enzyme pepsin. Because HCl is bacteriostatic, most of the bacteria entering the stomach with ingested food are destroyed. However, some bacteria can adapt to the low pH of the gastric contents. ***Helicobacter pylori*** contains large amounts of urease, the enzyme that hydrolyzes urea, in its cytoplasm and on its plasma membrane. This highly active enzyme creates a protective basic "ammonia cloud" around the bacterium, allowing it to survive in the acidic environment of the stomach (Folder 17.1).

- **Pepsin**, a potent proteolytic enzyme. It is formed from the conversion by HCl of **pepsinogen**, which is produced by the **chief cells**, when the pH is lower than 5. Pepsin hydrolyzes proteins into small peptides by splitting interior peptide bonds. Peptides are further digested into amino acids by enzymes in the small intestine.
- **Mucus**, an acid-protective coating for the stomach secreted by several types of mucus-producing cells. The mucus and bicarbonates trapped within the mucous layer maintain a neutral pH and contribute to the so-called **physiologic gastric mucosa barrier**. In addition, mucus serves as a physical barrier between the cells of the gastric mucosa and the ingested material in the lumen of the stomach.
- **Intrinsic factor**, a glycoprotein secreted by **parietal cells** that binds to vitamin B_{12}. It is essential for its absorption, which occurs in the distal part of the ileum. Lack of intrinsic factor leads to **pernicious anemia** and **vitamin B_{12} deficiency** (see Folder 17.1).

In addition, **gastrin** and other hormones and hormone-like secretions are produced by **enteroendocrine cells** in the fundic glands and secreted into the lamina propria, where they enter the circulation or act locally on other gastric epithelial cells.

Fundic glands are composed of four functionally different cell types.

The cells that constitute the fundic glands are of four functional types. Each has a distinctive appearance. In addition, undifferentiated cells that give rise to these cells are also present. The following are the various cells that constitute the gland:

- **Mucous neck cells**
- **Chief cells**
- **Parietal cells**, also called *oxyntic cells*
- **Enteroendocrine cells**
- **Stem cells**

Mucous neck cells are localized in the neck region of the gland and are interspersed with parietal cells.

As the name implies, the **mucous neck cells** are located in the neck region of the fundic gland. Parietal cells are usually interspersed between groups of these cells. The mucous neck cell is much shorter than the surface mucous cell and contains considerably less mucinogen in the apical cytoplasm. Consequently, these cells do not exhibit a prominent

FOLDER 17.1

CLINICAL CORRELATION: PERNICIOUS ANEMIA AND PEPTIC ULCER DISEASE

Achlorhydria is a chronic autoimmune disease characterized by the destruction of the gastric mucosa. Consequently, in the absence of parietal cells, the intrinsic factor is not secreted, thereby leading to **pernicious anemia**. Lack of **intrinsic factor** is the most common cause of **vitamin B_{12} deficiency**. However, other factors such as Gram-negative anaerobic bacterial overgrowth in the small intestine are associated with vitamin B_{12} deficiency. These bacteria bind to the vitamin B_{12}–intrinsic factor complex, preventing its absorption. Parasitic tapeworm infections also produce clinical symptoms of pernicious anemia. Because the liver has extensive reserve stores of vitamin B_{12}, the disease is often not recognized until long after significant changes in the gastric mucosa have taken place.

Another cause of reduced secretion of intrinsic factor and subsequent pernicious anemia is the loss of gastric epithelium in partial or total gastrectomy. Loss of functional gastric epithelium also occurs in chronic or recurrent **peptic ulcer disease (PUD)**. Often, even healed ulcerated regions produce insufficient intrinsic factor. Repeated loss of epithelium and consequent scarring of the gastric mucosa can significantly reduce the amount of functional mucosa.

Histamine H2 receptor–antagonist drugs such as ranitidine (Zantac) and cimetidine (Tagamet), which block the attachment of histamine to its receptors in the gastric mucosa, suppress both acid and intrinsic factor production and have been used extensively in the treatment of peptic ulcers and gastroesophageal reflux disease (GERD). These drugs prevent further mucosal erosion and promote healing of the previously eroded surface. However, long-term use can cause vitamin B_{12} deficiency. Recently, new proton-pump inhibitors (e.g., omeprazole and lansoprazole) have been designed that inhibit H^+/K^+-ATPase. They suppress acid production in the parietal cells and do not affect intrinsic factor secretion.

Although it was generally thought that the parietal cells are the direct target of the H_2 receptor–antagonist drugs, evidence from a combination of in situ hybridization histochemistry and antibody staining has unexpectedly revealed that the immunoglobulin A (IgA)-secreting plasma cells and some of the macrophages in the lamina propria display a positive reaction for gastrin receptor messenger RNA (mRNA), not the parietal cells. These findings indicate that the agents used to treat peptic ulcers may act directly on plasma cells or macrophages and that these cells then transmit their effects to the parietal cells to inhibit HCl secretion. The factor that mediates the interaction between the connective tissue cells and the epithelial cells has not been elucidated.

It is now recognized that most peptic ulcers (95%) are actually caused by a chronic infection of the gastric mucosa by the bacterium ***Helicobacter pylori***. Lipopolysaccharide antigens are expressed on its surface that mimics those on human gastric epithelial cells. The mimicry appears to cause an initial immunologic tolerance to the pathogen by the host immune system, thus helping to enhance the infection and ultimately causing the production of antibodies. These antibodies against *H. pylori* bind to the gastric mucosa and cause damage to the mucosal cells. Treatment includes antibiotic eradication of the bacteria. These treatments for ulcerative disease have made the common surgical interventions of the past infrequent.

mucous cup. Also, the nucleus tends to be spherical compared with the more prominent, elongated nucleus of the surface mucous cell.

The mucous neck cells secrete less alkaline **soluble mucus** compared with the high-alkaline **insoluble** or **cloudy mucus** produced by the surface mucous cell. Vagal stimulation induces the release of mucinogen granules; thus, secretion from these cells does not occur in the resting stomach. These mucous neck cells differentiate from stem cells, which reside in the neck region or the base of the fundic gland. Mucous neck cells are considered immature precursors of surface mucous cells.

Chief cells are located in the deeper part of the fundic glands.

Chief cells are typical protein-secreting cells (Fig. 17.9 and Plate 17.4, page 676). The abundant rER in the basal cytoplasm gives this part of the cell a basophilic appearance, whereas the apical cytoplasm is eosinophilic owing to the presence of the secretory vesicles, also called *zymogen granules* because they contain enzyme precursors. The basophilia, in particular, allows easy identification of these cells in H&E sections. The eosinophilia may be faint or absent when the secretory vesicles are not adequately preserved. Chief cells secrete **pepsinogen** and a weak lipase. On contact with the acid gastric juice, pepsinogen is converted to pepsin, a proteolytic enzyme.

Parietal cells secrete HCl and intrinsic factor.

Parietal (oxyntic) cells are found in the neck of the fundic glands, among the mucous neck cells, and in the deeper part of the gland. They tend to be most numerous in the upper and middle portions of the neck. They are large cells, sometimes binucleate, and appear somewhat triangular in sections, with the apex directed toward the lumen of the gland and the base resting on the basal lamina. The nucleus is spherical, and the cytoplasm stains with eosin and other acidic dyes. Their size and distinctive staining characteristics allow them to be easily distinguished from other cells in the fundic glands.

When examined with the transmission electron microscope (TEM), parietal cells (Fig. 17.10) are seen to have an extensive **intracellular canalicular system** that communicates with the lumen of the gland. Numerous microvilli project from the surface of the canaliculi, and

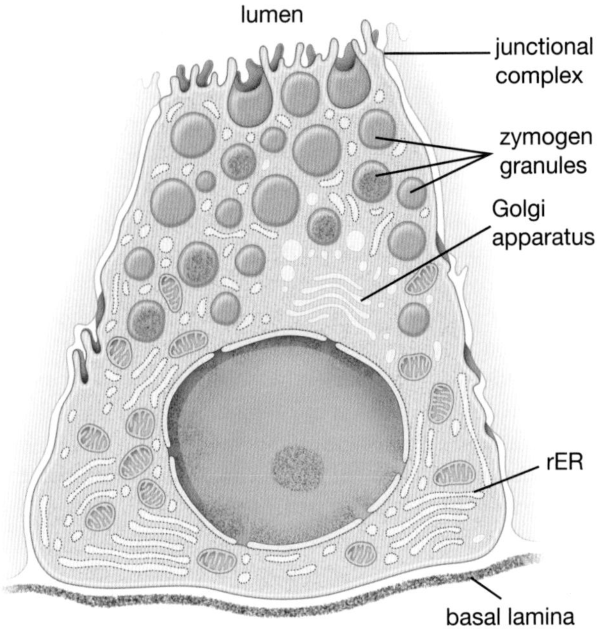

FIGURE 17.9. Diagram of a chief cell. The large amount of rough endoplasmic reticulum (*rER*) in the basal portion of the cell accounts for the intense basophilic staining seen in this region. Secretory vesicles (zymogen granules) containing pepsinogen and a weak lipase are not always adequately preserved, and thus, the staining in the apical region of the cell is somewhat variable. This cell produces and secretes the precursor enzyme of the gastric secretion.

an elaborate **tubulovesicular membrane system** is present in the cytoplasm adjacent to the canaliculi. In an actively secreting cell, the number of microvilli in the canaliculi increases, and the tubulovesicular system is reduced significantly or disappears. The membranes of the tubulovesicular system serve as a reservoir of plasma membrane containing active **proton pumps**. This membrane material can be inserted into the plasma membrane of the canaliculi to increase their surface area and the number of proton pumps available for acid production. Numerous mitochondria with complex cristae and many matrix granules supply the high levels of energy necessary for acid secretion.

FOLDER 17.2

CLINICAL CORRELATION: ZOLLINGER–ELLISON SYNDROME

Excessive secretion of **gastrin** is usually caused by a tumor of the gastrin-producing enteroendocrine cells located in the duodenum or the pancreatic islet. This condition, known as the **Zollinger–Ellison syndrome** or **gastrinomas**, is characterized by excessive secretion of hydrochloric acid (HCl) by continuously stimulated parietal cells. The excess acid cannot be adequately neutralized in the duodenum, thereby leading to gastric and duodenal ulcers. Gastric ulcers are present in 95% of patients with this syndrome and are 6 times more prevalent than duodenal ulcers. Patients with Zollinger–Ellison syndrome may experience intermittent abdominal pain, diarrhea, and steatorrhea (excretion of stool containing a large amount of fat). Patients without symptoms who have severe ulceration of the stomach and small intestine, especially if they fail to respond to conventional treatment, should be also suspected of having a tumor that is producing excess gastrin. Treatment of Zollinger–Ellison syndrome in the past involved blockage of the parietal cell membrane receptors that stimulate HCl production. Recently, proton-pump inhibitors have become the treatment of choice in managing HCl hypersecretion. In addition, surgical excision of the tumor, when possible, removes the source of gastrin production and alleviates symptoms.

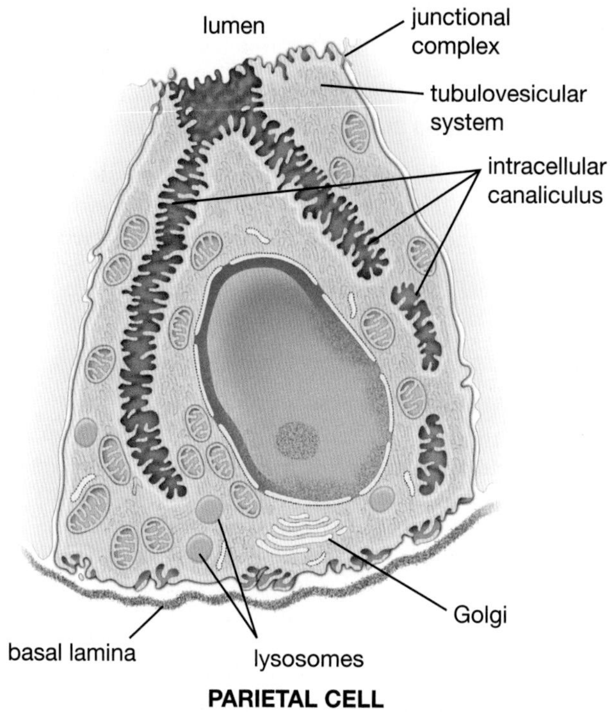

FIGURE 17.10. Diagram of a parietal cell. The cytoplasm of the parietal cell stains with eosin largely because of the extensive amount of membrane comprising the intracellular canaliculus, tubulovesicular system, mitochondria, and the relatively small number of ribosomes. This cell produces hydrochloric acid (HCl) and intrinsic factor.

HCl is produced in the lumen of the intracellular canaliculi.

Parietal cells have three different types of membrane receptors for substances that activate HCl secretion: **gastrin receptors, histamine H_2 receptors,** and **acetylcholine M_3 receptors**. Activation of gastrin receptors by **gastrin**, a gastrointestinal peptide hormone, is the major path for parietal cell stimulation (Folder 17.2). After stimulation, several steps occur in the production of HCl (Fig. 17.11):

- **Production of H^+ ions** in the parietal cell cytoplasm by the enzyme carbonic anhydrase. This enzyme catalyzes the combination of H_2O and CO_2 to form carbonic acid (H_2CO_3), which then rapidly dissociates into H^+ and HCO_3^-. Carbon dioxide (CO_2), necessary for synthesis of carbonic acid, diffuses across the basement membrane into the cell from the blood capillaries in the lamina propria.
- **Transport of H^+ ions** from the cytoplasm across the membrane to the lumen of the canaliculus by the H^+/K^+-ATPase proton pump. Simultaneously, K^+ from the canaliculus is transported into the cell cytoplasm in exchange for the H^+ ions.
- **Transport of K^+ and Cl^- ions** from the parietal cell cytoplasm into the lumen of the canaliculus through activation of K^+ and Cl^- channels (uniporters) in the plasma membrane
- **Formation of HCl** from the H^+ and Cl^- that were transported into the lumen of the canaliculus

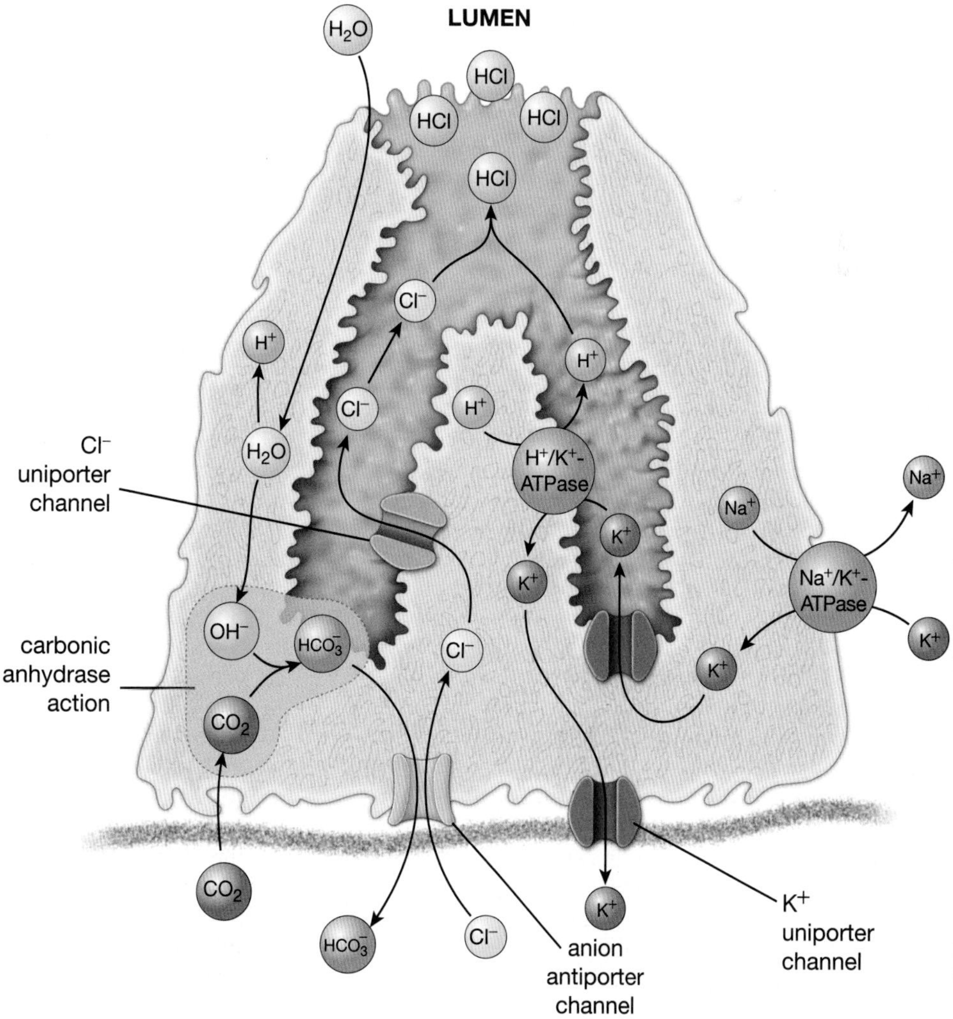

FIGURE 17.11. Diagram of parietal cell hydrochloric acid (HCl) synthesis. After parietal cell stimulation, several steps occur leading to the production of HCl. Carbon dioxide (CO_2) from the blood diffuses across the basement membrane into the cell to form H_2CO_3. The H_2CO_3 dissociates into H^+ and HCO_3^-. The reaction is catalyzed by carbonic anhydrase, which leads to the production of H^+ ions in the cytoplasm, which are then transported across the membrane to the lumen of the intracellular canaliculus by an H^+/K^+-ATPase proton pump. Simultaneously, K^+ within the canaliculus is transported into the cell in exchange for the H^+ ions. Cl^- ions are also transported from the cytoplasm of the parietal cell into the lumen of the canaliculus by Cl^- channels in the membrane. HCl is then formed from H^+ and Cl^-. The HCO_3^-/Cl^- anion channels maintain the normal concentration of both ions in the cell and Na^+/K^+-ATPase on the basolateral cell membrane.

In humans, **intrinsic factor** is secreted by the parietal cells (chief cells do so in some other species). Its secretion is stimulated by the same receptors that stimulate gastric acid secretion. **Intrinsic factor** is a 44-kDa glycoprotein that complexes with **vitamin B_{12}** in the stomach and duodenum, a step necessary for subsequent absorption of the vitamin in the ileum. Autoantibodies directed against intrinsic factor or parietal cells themselves lead to an intrinsic factor deficiency, resulting in malabsorption of vitamin B_{12} and **pernicious anemia** (see Folder 17.1).

Enteroendocrine cells secrete their products into either the lamina propria or the underlying blood vessels.

Enteroendocrine cells are found at every level of the fundic gland, although they tend to be somewhat more prevalent in the base (Folder 17.3). In general, **two types**

FOLDER 17.3

FUNCTIONAL CONSIDERATIONS: THE GASTROINTESTINAL ENDOCRINE SYSTEM

Enteroendocrine cells are specialized cells present in the mucosa of the digestive tract. They account for <1% of all epithelial cells in the gastrointestinal tract, but as a whole, they collectively constitute the largest endocrine "organ" in the body. Enteroendocrine cells are also found in the ducts of the pancreas, the liver, and the respiratory system, another endodermal derivative that originates by invagination of the epithelium of the embryonic foregut. Because enteroendocrine cells closely resemble neurosecretory cells of the central nervous system (CNS) that secrete many of the same hormones, signaling molecules, and regulatory agents, they are also called **neuroendocrine cells**. Most of these cells are not grouped as clusters in any specific part of the gastrointestinal tract. Rather, enteroendocrine cells are distributed singly throughout the gastrointestinal epithelium. For that reason, they are described as constituting part of a **diffuse neuroendocrine system (DNES)**. Figure 17.13 shows the parts of the gastrointestinal tract in which the gastrointestinal peptides are produced. One notable exception to this distribution pattern is found in the pancreas. Here, enteroendocrine cells, derived from pancreatic buds that also arise from the embryonic foregut, form specialized accumulations called **endocrine islets of Langerhans** (see pages 715-719).

In the current view, the DNES includes both neurons and endocrine cells that share common characteristics, including the expression of specific markers (e.g., neuropeptides, chromogranins, and neuropeptide-processing enzymes) and the presence of dense-core secretory granules. Secretory products of enteroendocrine cells derive from a variety of genes; they are expressed in different forms because of alternative splicing and differential processing. Secretion of enteroendocrine cells is regulated by G-protein–coupled receptors and tyrosine kinase activity. There is evidence that chromogranin A regulates biosynthesis of dense-core secretory granules, whereas chromogranin B controls sorting and packaging of produced peptides into secretory vesicles. Table 17.1 lists important gastrointestinal hormones, their sites of origin, and their major functions.

Neoplastic transformations of DNES cells are responsible for the development of **gastroenteropancreatic (GEP) neuroendocrine tumors**. These tumors represent rare neoplasms of the gastrointestinal tract and pancreas that often secrete hormonally active agents, causing distinct clinical syndromes. The appendix is the most common gastrointestinal site of origin for neuroendocrine tumors. The classic example is the **carcinoid syndrome** caused by the release of a variety of hormonally active substances by tumor cells. Symptoms include diarrhea (case by serotonin), episodic flushing, bronchoconstriction, and right-sided cardiac valve disease.

Some enteroendocrine cells may be classifiable functionally as **amine precursor uptake and decarboxylation (APUD) cells**. They should not, however, be confused with the APUD cells that are derived from the embryonic neural crest and migrate to other sites in the body. APUD cells secrete a variety of regulator substances in tissues and organs, including the respiratory epithelium, adrenal medulla, islets of Langerhans, thyroid gland (parafollicular cells), and pituitary gland. The enteroendocrine cells differentiate from the progeny of the same stem cells as all of the other epithelial cells of the digestive tract. The fact that two different cells may produce similar products should not imply that they have the same origin.

Enteroendocrine cells produce not only gastrointestinal hormones such as gastrin, ghrelin, secretin, cholecystokinin (CCK), gastric inhibitory peptide (GIP), and motilin but also **paracrine hormones**. A paracrine hormone differs from an endocrine hormone in that it diffuses locally to its target cell instead of being carried by the bloodstream to a target cell. A well-known substance that appears to act as a paracrine hormone within the gastrointestinal tract and pancreas is somatostatin, which inhibits other gastrointestinal and pancreatic islet endocrine cells.

In addition to the established gastrointestinal hormones, several gastrointestinal peptides have not been definitely classified as hormones or paracrine hormones. These peptides are designated **candidate** or **putative hormones**.

Other locally active agents isolated from the gastrointestinal mucosa are **neurotransmitters**. These agents are released from nerve endings close to the target cell, usually the smooth muscle of the muscularis mucosae, the muscularis externa, or the tunica media of a blood vessel. Enteroendocrine cells can also secrete neurotransmitters that activate afferent neurons, sending signals to the central nervous system (CNS) and enteric division of the autonomic nervous system. In addition to acetylcholine (not a peptide), peptides found in nerve fibers of the gastrointestinal tract are vasoactive intestinal peptide (VIP), bombesin, and enkephalins. Thus, a particular peptide may be produced by endocrine and paracrine cells and also be localized in nerve fibers.

of enteroendocrine cells can be distinguished throughout the gastrointestinal tract. Most represent small cells that rest on the basal lamina and do not always reach the lumen; they are known as **enteroendocrine "closed" cells** (Fig. 17.12a and b and Plate 17.4, page 676). Some cells, however, have a thin cytoplasmic extension bearing microvilli that are exposed to the gland lumen (Fig. 17.12c); these are referred to as **enteroendocrine "open" cells**. Open cells serve as **primary chemoreceptors** that sample the contents of the gland lumen and release hormones based on the information obtained from those samples. Taste receptors, similar to those found in taste buds of the specialized oral mucosa (pages 592-596), detect sweet, bitter, and umami sensations and are present on the free surface of open enteroendocrine cells. They belong to the T1R and T2R families of G-protein–coupled receptors described in Chapter 16, Digestive System I: Oral Cavity and Associated Structures (pages 594-595). Secretion from closed cells, however, is regulated by the luminal contents indirectly through neural and paracrine mechanisms.

Electron micrographs (EMs) reveal small membrane-bound secretory vesicles throughout the cytoplasm; however, these vesicles are typically lost in H&E preparations, and the cytoplasm appears clear because of the lack of sufficient stainable material. Although enteroendocrine cells are often difficult to identify because of their small size and lack of distinctive staining, their clear cytoplasm sometimes stands out in contrast to the adjacent chief or parietal cells, thus allowing their easy recognition.

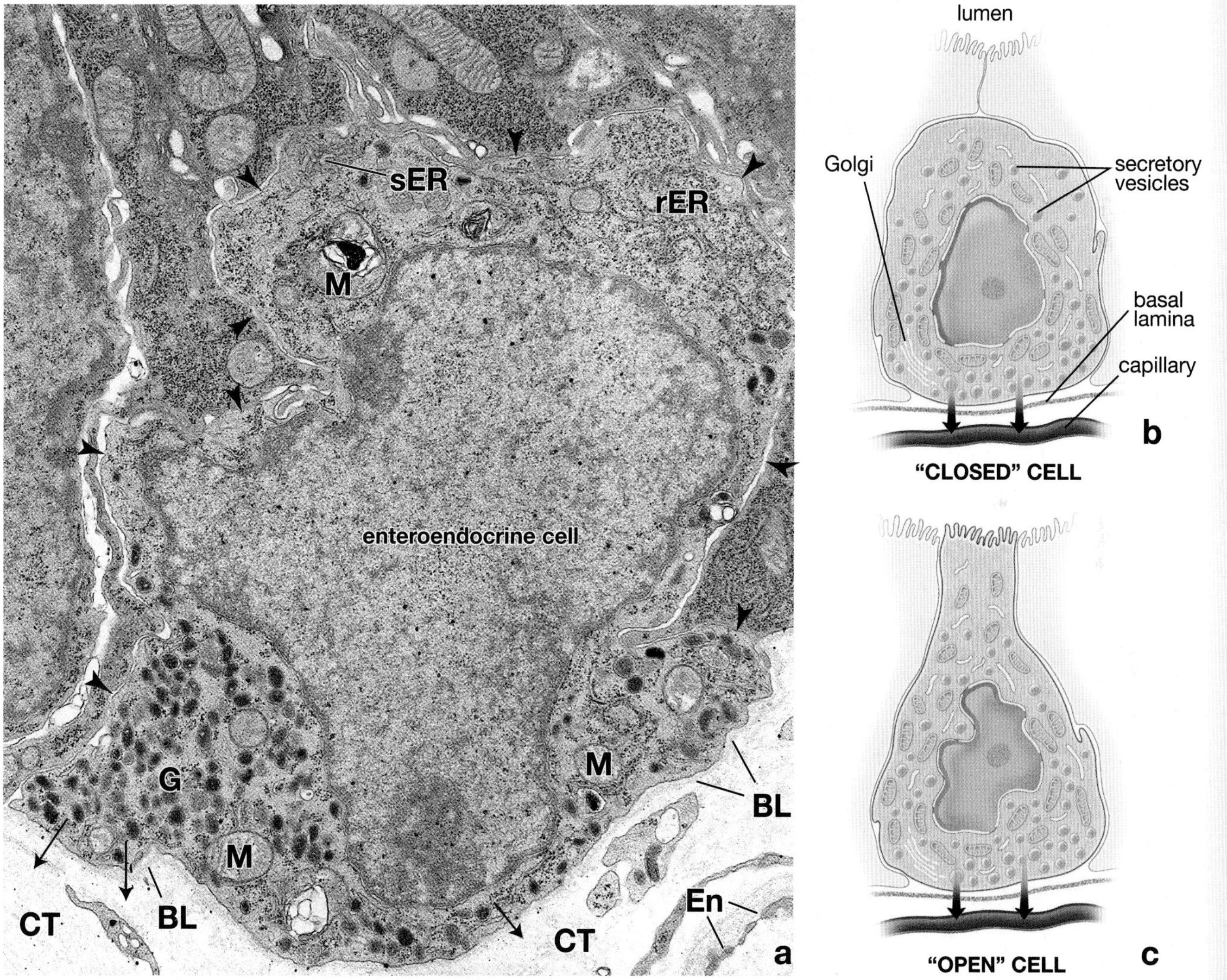

FIGURE 17.12. Electron micrograph and diagrams of enteroendocrine cells. a. This electron micrograph shows an example of a "closed" enteroendocrine cell. *Arrowheads* mark the boundary between the enteroendocrine cell and the adjacent epithelial cells. At its base, the enteroendocrine cell rests on the basal lamina (*BL*). This cell does not extend to the epithelial or luminal surface. Numerous secretory vesicles (*G*) in the base of the cell are secreted in the direction of the *arrows* across the *BL* and into the connective tissue (*CT*). **b.** This diagram of an enteroendocrine "closed" cell is drawn to show that it does not reach the epithelial surface. The secretory vesicles are regularly lost during routine preparation. Because of the absence of other distinctive organelles, the nucleus appears to be surrounded by a small amount of clear cytoplasm in hematoxylin and eosin (H&E)-stained sections. **c.** The enteroendocrine "open" cell extends to the epithelial surface. Microvilli on the apical surface of these cells possess taste receptors and are able to detect sweet, bitter, and umami sensations. These cells serve as chemoreceptor cells, which monitor the environment on the surface of the epithelium. They are involved in the regulation of gastrointestinal hormone secretion. *En*, endothelium of capillary; *M*, mitochondria; *rER*, rough endoplasmic reticulum; *sER*, smooth endoplasmic reticulum.

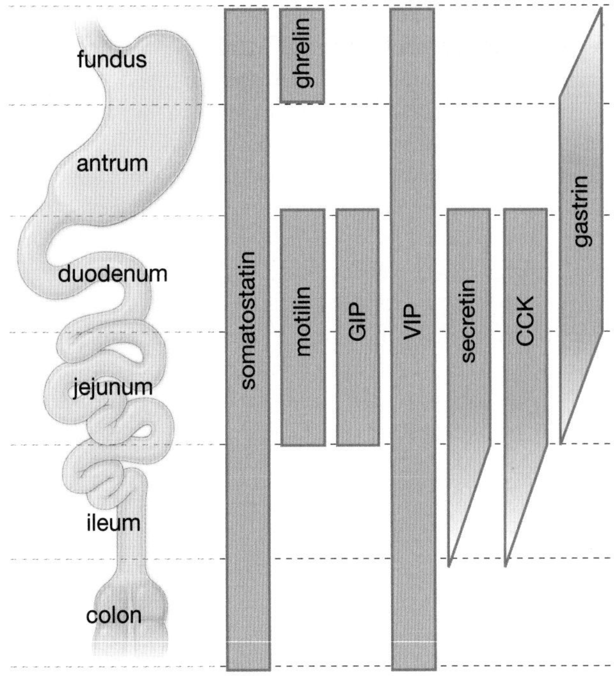

FIGURE 17.13. Gastrointestinal hormones. This schematic diagram shows the distribution of gastrointestinal peptide hormones produced by enteroendocrine cells in the alimentary canal. *CCK*, cholecystokinin; *GIP*, gastric inhibitory peptide; *VIP*, vasoactive intestinal peptide.

The names given to the enteroendocrine cells in the older literature were based on their staining with salts of silver and chromium (i.e., enterochromaffin cells, argentaffin cells, and argyrophil cells). Such cells are currently identified and characterized by immunochemical staining for the more than 20 peptide and polypeptide hormones and hormone-like regulating agents that they secrete (a list of many of these agents and their actions is given in Fig. 17.13 and Tables 17.1 and 17.2). With the aid of the TEM, at least 17 different types of enteroendocrine cells have been described on the basis of size, shape, and density of their secretory vesicles.

Cardiac glands of the gastric mucosa

Cardiac glands are composed of mucus-secreting cells.

Cardiac glands are limited to a narrow region of the stomach (the cardia) that surrounds the esophageal orifice. Their secretion, in combination with that of the esophageal cardiac glands, contributes to the gastric juice and helps protect the esophageal epithelium against gastric reflux. The glands are tubular, somewhat tortuous, and occasionally branched (Fig. 17.14 and Plate 17.3, page 674). They are composed mainly of mucus-secreting cells, with occasional interspersed enteroendocrine cells. The mucus-secreting cells are similar in appearance to the cells of the esophageal cardiac glands. They have a flattened basal nucleus, and the apical cytoplasm is typically filled with mucin granules. A short duct segment containing columnar cells with elongated nuclei is interposed between the secretory portion of the gland and the shallow pits into which the glands secrete. The duct segment is the site at which the surface mucous cells and the gland cells are produced.

Pyloric glands of the gastric mucosa

Pyloric gland cells are similar to surface mucous cells and help protect the pyloric mucosa.

Pyloric glands are located in the pyloric antrum (the part of the stomach between the fundus and the pylorus). They are branched, coiled, tubular glands (Plate 17.5, page 678). The lumen is relatively wide, and the secretory cells are similar in appearance to the surface mucous cells,

TABLE 17.1 Physiologic Actions of Gastrointestinal Hormones

		Major Action	
Hormone	**Site of Synthesis**	**Stimulates**	**Inhibits**
Gastrin	G cells in stomach	Gastric acid secretion	
Ghrelin	Gr cells in stomach	GH secretion Appetite and perception of hunger	Lipid metabolism Fat utilization in adipose tissue
Cholecystokinin (CCK)	I cells in duodenum and jejunum	Gallbladder contraction Pancreatic enzyme secretion Pancreatic bicarbonate ion secretion Pancreatic growth	Gastric emptying
Secretin	S cells in duodenum	Pancreatic enzyme secretion Pancreatic bicarbonate ion secretion Pancreatic growth	Gastric acid secretion
Gastric inhibitory peptide (GIP)	K cells in duodenum and jejunum	Insulin release	Gastric acid secretion
Motilin	Mo cells in duodenum and jejunum	Gastric motility Intestinal motility	

GH, growth hormone.

Modified from Johnson LR, ed. *Essential Medical Physiology*. Lippincott-Raven; 1998.

TABLE 17.2 Physiologic Actions of Additional Hormones in the Gastrointestinal Tract

Hormone	Site of Synthesis	Major Action: Stimulates	Major Action: Inhibits
Candidate hormones			
Pancreatic polypeptide	PP cells in pancreas	Gastric emptying and gut motility	Pancreatic enzyme secretion Pancreatic bicarbonate secretion
Peptide YY	L cells in ileum and colon	Electrolyte and water absorption in the colon	Gastric acid secretion Gastric emptying Food intake
Glucagon-like peptide-1 (GLP-1)	L cells in ileum and colon	Insulin release	Gastric acid secretion Gastric emptying
Paracrine hormones			
Somatostatin	D cells in mucosa throughout GI tract		Gastrin release Gastric acid secretion Release of other GI hormones
Histamine	Mucosa throughout GI tract	Gastric acid secretion	
Neurocrine hormones			
Bombesin	Stomach	Gastrin release	
Enkephalins	Mucosa and smooth muscle throughout GI tract	Smooth muscle contraction	Intestinal secretion
Vasoactive intestinal peptide (VIP)	Mucosa and smooth muscle throughout GI tract	Pancreatic enzyme secretion Intestinal secretion	Smooth muscle contraction Sphincter contraction

GI, gastrointestinal.

Modified from Johnson LR, ed. *Essential Medical Physiology*. 2nd ed. Lippincott-Raven; 1998.

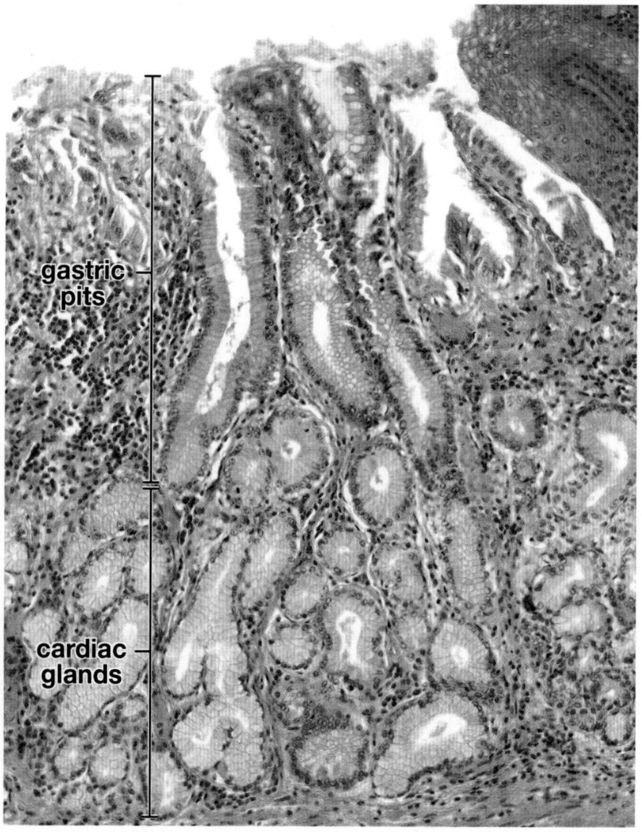

FIGURE 17.14. Photomicrograph of cardiac glands. This photomicrograph shows the esophagogastric junction. Note the presence of the stratified squamous epithelium of the esophagus in the *upper right corner* of the micrograph. The cardiac glands are tubular, somewhat tortuous, and occasionally branched. They are composed mainly of mucus-secreting cells similar in appearance to the cells of the esophageal glands. Mucous secretion reaches the lumen of the gastric pit via a short duct segment containing columnar cells. ×240.

suggesting a relatively viscous secretion. Enteroendocrine cells are found interspersed within the gland epithelium along with occasional parietal cells. The glands empty into deep gastric pits that occupy about half the thickness of the mucosa (Fig. 17.15).

Epithelial Cell Renewal in the Stomach

Gastric glands contain stem cell niches that are responsible for epithelial cell renewal.

Previous studies using nucleotide incorporation assays and EM showed that the **isthmus of the fundic gland** is a site of **stem cell location (stem cell niche)** in which stem cells replicate and differentiate. Cells destined to become mucous surface cells migrate upward in the gastric pits to the stomach surface. Other cells migrate downward, maintaining the population of the fundic gland epithelium. However, the differentiation of these stem cells and their migration routes has remained elusive.

Experimental studies using retrovirus-infected stem cells containing labeled transgenes (genes altered by genetic engineering) and in situ hybridization techniques (to trace the stem cells' progeny) show the location of these stem cells in two different regions of the gastric gland. These studies confirm the presence of an isthmus cell niche and identify a second stem cell location at the **base of the gastric glands**. These cells were also capable of self-renewing and differentiating into surface mucous cells, mucous neck cells, chief cells, parietal cells, and enteroendocrine cells. A similar distribution of stem cells is found in all regions of the stomach; however, in each region, stem cells express different molecular markers and play different roles in cell renewal. For instance, stem

FOLDER 17.4

FUNCTIONAL CONSIDERATIONS: DIGESTIVE AND ABSORPTIVE FUNCTIONS OF ENTEROCYTES

The plasma membrane of the microvilli of the enterocyte plays a role in digestion as well as absorption. Digestive enzymes are anchored in the plasma membrane, and their functional groups extend outward to become part of the glycocalyx. This arrangement brings the end products of digestion close to their site of absorption. Included among the enzymes are peptidases and disaccharidases. The plasma membrane of the apical microvilli also contains the enzyme **enteropeptidase (enterokinase)**, which is particularly important in the duodenum, where it converts trypsinogen into trypsin. Trypsin can then continue to convert additional trypsinogen into trypsin, and trypsin converts several other pancreatic zymogens into active enzymes (Fig. F17.4.1). A summary of digestion and absorption of the three major nutrients is outlined in the following paragraphs.

Carbohydrate final digestion is brought about by enzymes bound to the microvilli of the enterocytes (Fig. F17.4.2). Galactose, glucose, and fructose are absorbed directly into venous capillaries and conveyed to the liver by the vessels of the hepatic portal system. Some infants and a larger percentage of adults cannot tolerate milk and unfermented milk products because of the absence of lactase, the disaccharidase that splits lactose into galactose and glucose. These individuals are unable to break down milk or milk products, which leads to bloating caused by the buildup of gas from the bacterial digestion of the unprocessed lactose and diarrhea. The condition is completely alleviated if lactose (milk sugar) is eliminated from the diet. For some individuals, milk intolerance may be also partially or completely alleviated by using lactose-reduced milk products or tablets of lactase (enzyme that digests lactose), which are available as over-the-counter drugs.

Triglycerides are broken down into glycerol, monoglycerides, and long-, medium-, and short-chain fatty acids. These substances are emulsified by bile salts and pass into the apical portion of the enterocyte. Here, the glycerol and long-chain fatty acids are resynthesized into triglycerides. The resynthesized

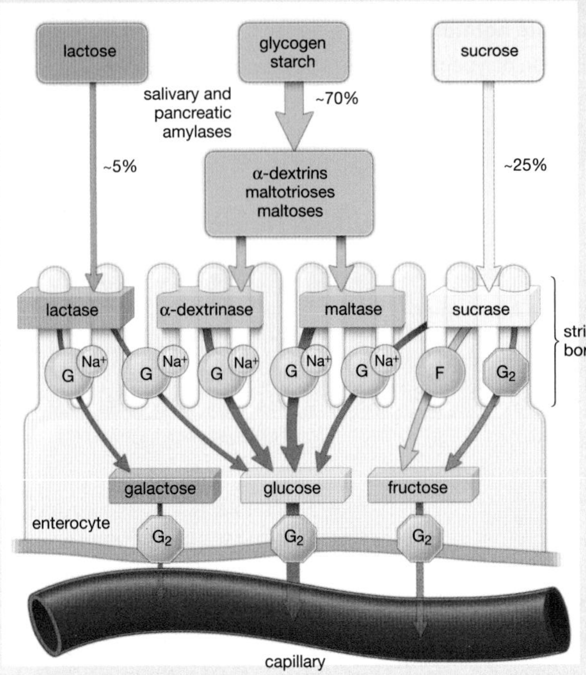

FIGURE F17.4.2. Diagram showing the digestion and absorption of carbohydrates by an enterocyte. Carbohydrates are delivered to the alimentary canal as monosaccharides (e.g., glucose, fructose, and galactose), disaccharides (e.g., sucrose, lactose, and maltose), and polysaccharides (e.g., glycogen and starch). Enzymes involved in the digestion of carbohydrates are classified as salivary and pancreatic amylases. Further digestion is performed at the striated border of the enterocytes by enzymes, breaking down oligosaccharides and polysaccharides into three basic monosaccharides (glucose, galactose, and fructose). Glucose and galactose are absorbed by the enterocyte via active transport using Na^+-dependent glucose transporters (SGLT1). These transporters are localized at the apical cell membrane (*circles with G and Na^+ labels*). Fructose enters the cell via facilitated Na^+-independent transport using GLUT5 (*gray circle with F label*) and GLUT2 glucose transporters (*orange octagons with G_2 label*). The three absorbed monosaccharides then pass through the basal membrane of the enterocyte, using GLUT2 glucose transporters, into the underlying capillaries of the portal circulation to reach their final destination in the liver.

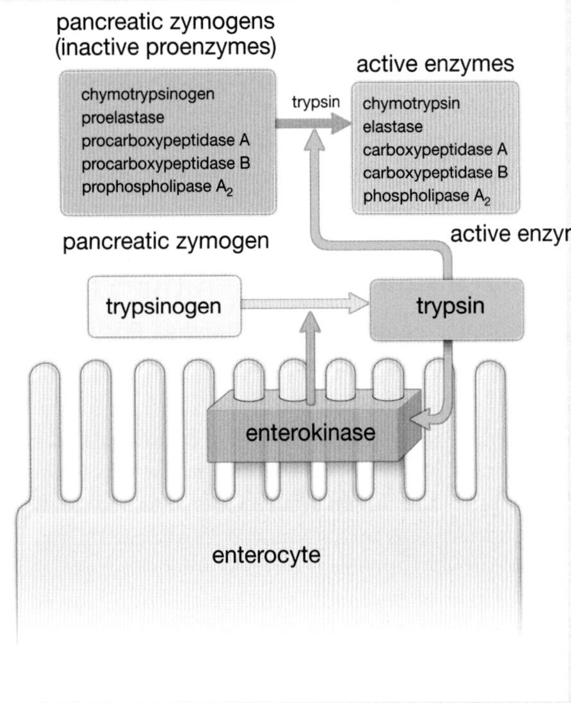

FIGURE F17.4.1. Diagram showing events in the activation of the proteolytic enzymes of the pancreas. The majority of pancreatic enzymes (proteases) are secreted as inactive proenzymes. Their activation is triggered by the arrival of chyme into the duodenum. This stimulates the mucosal cells to release and activate the enterokinase (*blue box*) within the glycocalyx. The enterokinase activates trypsinogen, converting it into its active form, trypsin (*green box*). In turn, trypsin activates other pancreatic proenzymes (*red box*) into their active forms (*purple box*). The active proteases hydrolyze peptide bonds of proteins or polypeptides and reduce them to small peptides and amino acids.

FOLDER 17.4

FUNCTIONAL CONSIDERATIONS: DIGESTIVE AND ABSORPTIVE FUNCTIONS OF ENTEROCYTES (*continued*)

triglycerides appear first in apical vesicles of the smooth endoplasmic reticulum (sER) (see Fig. 17.21), then in the Golgi (where they are converted into **chylomicrons**, small droplets of neutral fat), and finally in vesicles that discharge the chylomicrons into the intercellular space. Instead of being absorbed directly into venous capillaries, chylomicrons are conveyed away from the intestine via lymphatic vessels (lacteals) that penetrate into each villus. Chylomicron-rich lymph then drains into the thoracic duct, which flows into the venous blood system. When in the blood circulation, chylomicrons are rapidly disassembled, and their constituent lipids are utilized throughout the body. Short- and medium-chain fatty acids and glycerol cross the apical cell membrane and enter and leave the enterocyte exclusively via capillaries that lead to the portal vein and the liver.

Protein digestion and absorption are shown in Figure F17.4.3. The major end products of protein digestion are amino acids (about 30%) and oligopeptides (about 70%), which are absorbed by enterocytes. The mechanism of amino acid absorption is conceptually identical to that of carbohydrates. The apical plasma membrane of the enterocytes bears at least four Na^+-amino acid cotransporters. The dipeptides and tripeptides are transported across the apical membrane into the cell cytoplasm by the H^+-oligopeptide cotransporter (PepT1). Most of the dipeptides and tripeptides are then digested by cytoplasmic peptidases into free amino acids, which are subsequently transported through the basal membrane (without a need for cotransporter) into the underlying capillaries of the portal circulation. In one disorder of amino acid absorption (Hartnup disease), free amino acids appear in the blood when dipeptides are fed to patients, but not when free amino acids are fed. This supports the conclusion that dipeptides of certain amino acids are absorbed via the PepT1 cotransporter, which is involved in different pathways from those involved in absorption of free amino acids.

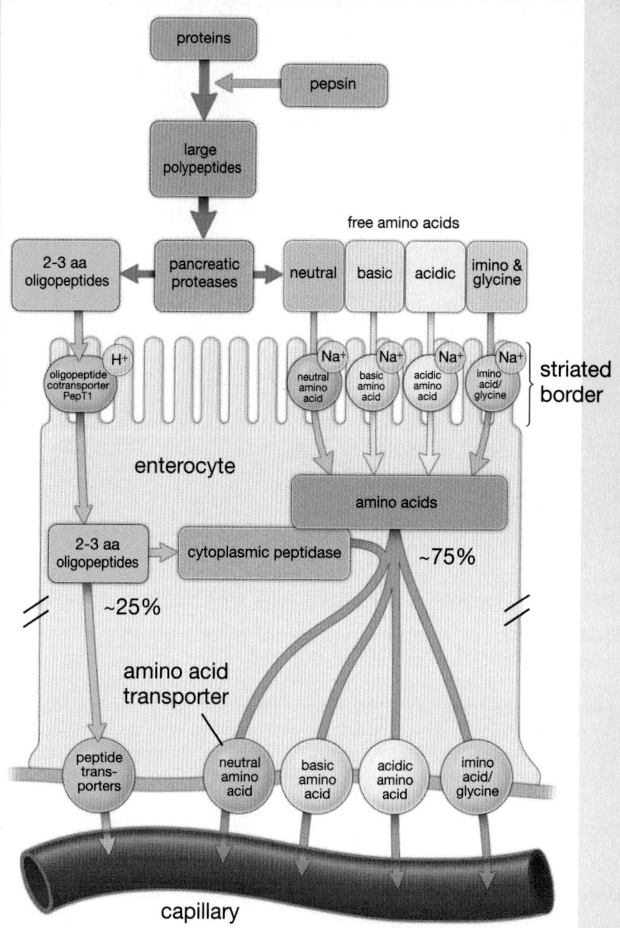

FIGURE F17.4.3. Diagram showing the digestion and absorption of protein by an enterocyte. Proteins entering the alimentary canal are completely digested into free amino acids (*aa*) and small dipeptide or tripeptide fragments. Protein digestion starts in the stomach with pepsin, which hydrolyzes proteins to large polypeptides. The next step occurs in the small intestine by the action of pancreatic proteolytic enzymes. The activation process is shown in Figure F17.4.1. Free amino acids are transported by four different amino acid Na^+ cotransporters. The dipeptides and tripeptides are transported across the apical membrane into the cell by H^+ oligopeptide cotransporters (PepT1). Most of the dipeptides and tripeptides are then broken down by cytoplasmic peptidases, and free amino acids are transported through the basal membrane into the underlying capillaries of the portal circulation.

cells located in the base of pyloric glands maintain epithelial cell renewal under normal homeostatic conditions, whereas in the fundic region, these cells remain quiescent under normal homeostatic conditions.

Surface mucous cells are renewed approximately every 3–5 days.

The relatively short life span of the **surface mucous cells**, 3–5 days, is accommodated by mitotic activity in the isthmus, the narrow segment that lies between the gastric pit and the fundic gland (Fig. 17.16). The isthmus of the fundic gland contains a reservoir of tissue stem cells that undergo mitotic activity, providing for continuous cell renewal. Most of the newly produced cells at this site become surface mucous cells. They migrate upward along the wall of the pit to the luminal surface of the stomach and are ultimately shed into the stomach lumen.

The cells of the fundic glands have a relatively long life span.

Other cells from the isthmus migrate down into the gastric glands to give rise to the parietal cells, chief cells, mucous gland cells, and enteroendocrine cells that constitute the gland epithelium. As mentioned previously, these cells also can differentiate from stem cells located at the base of the gland. These cells have a relatively long life span. **Parietal cells** have the longest life span, approximately 150–200 days. Although

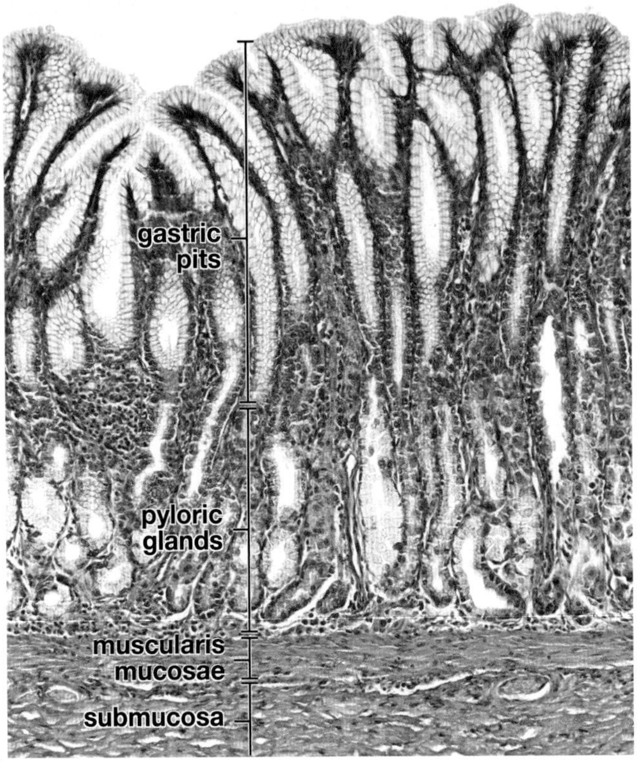

FIGURE 17.15. Photomicrograph of pyloric glands. This photomicrograph shows a section of the wall of the pylorus. The pyloric glands are relatively straight for most of their length but are slightly coiled near the muscularis mucosae. The lumen is relatively wide, and the secretory cells are similar in appearance to the surface mucous cells, suggesting a relatively viscous secretion. They are restricted to the mucosa and empty into the gastric pits. The boundary between the pits and glands is, however, hard to ascertain in routine hematoxylin and eosin (H&E) preparations. ×120.

parietal cells develop from the same undifferentiated stem cells, their life span is distinctly different. It has been hypothesized that parietal cells may have originated from a fungus called ***Neurospora crassa*** that previously existed in a symbiotic relationship with the cells of the human stomach. The basis for this hypothesis is that the human proton pump (H^+/K^+-ATPase) found in parietal cells bears a strong genetic resemblance to proton pumps found in this organism. The fungal DNA is thought to have been translocated and subsequently incorporated into the nucleus of the stem cells, probably with the help of a virus.

Chief and **enteroendocrine cells** are estimated to live for about 60–90 days before they are replaced by new cells migrating downward from the isthmus. **Mucous neck cells**, in contrast, have a much shorter life span, approximately 6 days.

Lamina Propria and Muscularis Mucosae

The **lamina propria** of the stomach is relatively scant and restricted to the limited spaces surrounding the gastric pits and glands. The stroma is composed largely of reticular fibers with associated fibroblasts and smooth muscle cells. Other components include cells of the immune system, namely, lymphocytes, plasma cells, macrophages, and some eosinophils. When inflammation occurs, as is often the case, neutrophils may also be prominent. Occasional lymphatic nodules are also present, usually intruding partially into the muscularis mucosae.

The **muscularis mucosae** is composed of two relatively thin layers, usually arranged as an inner circular and outer longitudinal layer. In some regions, a third layer may be present; its orientation tends to be in a circular pattern. Thin strands of smooth muscle cells extend toward the surface of the lamina propria from the inner layer of the muscularis mucosae. These smooth muscle cells in the lamina propria are thought to help outflow of the gastric gland secretions.

Gastric Submucosa

The **submucosa** is composed of a dense connective tissue containing variable amounts of adipose tissue and blood vessels as well as the nerve fibers and ganglion cells that compose the **submucosal (Meissner) plexus.** The latter innervates the vessels of the submucosa and the smooth muscle of the muscularis mucosae.

Gastric Muscularis Externa

The **muscularis externa** of the stomach is traditionally described as consisting of an outer longitudinal layer, a middle circular layer, and an inner oblique layer. This description is somewhat misleading, as distinct layers may be difficult to discern. As with other hollow, spheroidal organs (e.g., gallbladder, urinary bladder, and uterus), the smooth muscle of the muscularis externa of the stomach is somewhat more randomly oriented than the term *layer* implies. Moreover, the longitudinal layer is absent from much of the

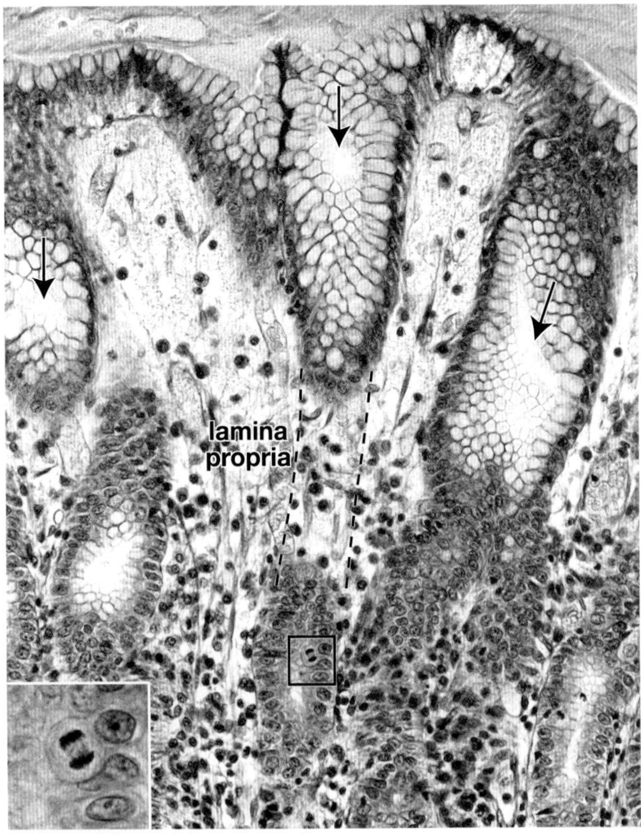

FIGURE 17.16. Photomicrograph of a dividing cell in the isthmus of a pyloric gland. The gastric pits in this photomicrograph were sectioned in a plane that is oblique to the axis of the pit. Note that in this section, gastric pits (*arrows*) can be recognized as invaginations of surface epithelium that are surrounded by lamina propria. The lamina propria is highly cellular because of the presence of large numbers of lymphocytes. ×240. **Inset.** This high magnification of the area indicated by the *square* shows a dividing cell in the isthmus. ×580.

anterior and posterior stomach surfaces, and the circular layer is poorly developed in the periesophageal region. The arrangement of the muscle layers is functionally important, as it relates to its role in mixing chyme during the digestive process as well as to its ability to force the partially digested contents into the small intestine. Groups of ganglion cells and bundles of unmyelinated nerve fibers are present between the muscle layers. Collectively, they represent the **myenteric (Auerbach) plexus**, which provides innervation of the muscle layers.

Gastric Serosa

The **serosa** of the stomach is, as described earlier, for the alimentary canal in general. It is continuous with the parietal peritoneum of the abdominal cavity via the greater omentum and with visceral peritoneum of the liver at the lesser omentum. Otherwise, it exhibits no special features.

■ SMALL INTESTINE

The small intestine is the longest component of the digestive tract, measuring over 6 m, and is divided into three anatomic portions:

- **Duodenum** (~25 cm long) is the first, shortest, and widest part of the small intestine. It begins at the pylorus of the stomach and ends at the duodenojejunal junction (Plate 17.6, page 680).
- **Jejunum** (~2.5 m long) begins at the **duodenojejunal junction** and constitutes the upper two-fifths of the small intestine. It gradually changes its morphologic characteristics to become the ileum (Plate 17.7, page 682).
- **Ileum** (~3.5 m long) is a continuation of the jejunum and constitutes the lower three-fifths of the small intestine. It ends at the **ileocecal junction**, the union of the distal ileum and cecum (Plate 17.8, page 684).

Mucosa

The small intestine is the principal site for the digestion of food and absorption of the products of digestion.

Chyme from the stomach enters the duodenum, where enzymes from the pancreas and bile from the liver are also delivered to continue the solubilization and digestion process. Enzymes, particularly disaccharidases and dipeptidases, are also located in the glycocalyx of the microvilli of the **enterocytes**, the **intestinal absorptive cells**. These enzymes contribute to the digestive process by completing the breakdown of most sugars and proteins to monosaccharides and amino acids, which are then absorbed (Folder 17.4). Water and electrolytes that reach the small intestine with the chyme and pancreatic and hepatic secretions are also reabsorbed in the small intestine, particularly in the distal portion.

Plicae circulares, villi, and microvilli increase the absorptive surface area of the small intestine.

The absorptive surface area of the small intestine is amplified by tissue and cell specializations of the submucosa and mucosa.

- **Plicae circulares (circular folds)**, also known as the *valves of Kerckring*, are permanent transverse folds that contain a core of submucosa. Each circular fold is circularly arranged and extends about one-half to two-thirds of the way around the circumference of the lumen (Fig. 17.17). The folds begin to appear about 5–6 cm beyond the pylorus. They are most numerous in the distal part of the duodenum and the beginning of the jejunum and become reduced in size and frequency in the middle of the ileum.
- **Villi** are unique, finger-like and leaf-like projections of the mucosa that extend from the theoretical mucosal surface for 0.5–1.5 mm into the lumen (Fig. 17.18). They completely cover the surface of the small intestine, giving it a velvety appearance when viewed with the unaided eye.
- **Microvilli** of the enterocytes provide the major amplification of the luminal surface. Each cell possesses several thousand closely packed microvilli. They are visible in the light microscope (LM) and give the apical region of the cell a striated appearance, the so-called **striated border**. Enterocytes and their microvilli are described later in this chapter (see pages 653-655).

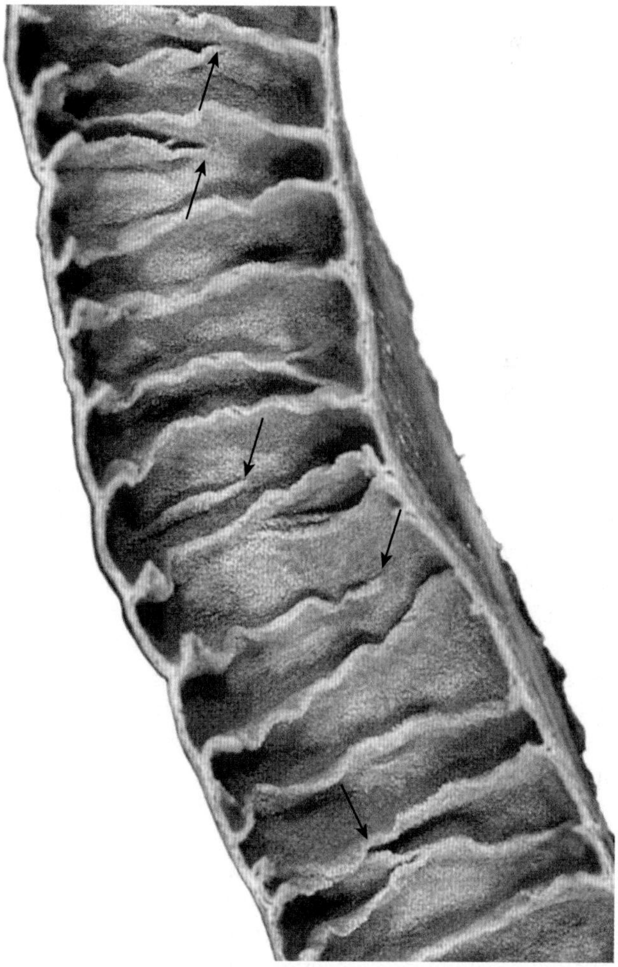

FIGURE 17.17. Photograph of the mucosal surface of the small intestine. This photograph of a segment of a human jejunum shows the mucosal surface. The circular folds (plicae circulares) appear as a series of transversely oriented ridges that extend partially around the lumen. Consequently, some of the circular folds appear to end (or begin) at various sites along the luminal surface (*arrows*). The entire mucosa has a velvety appearance because of the presence of villi.

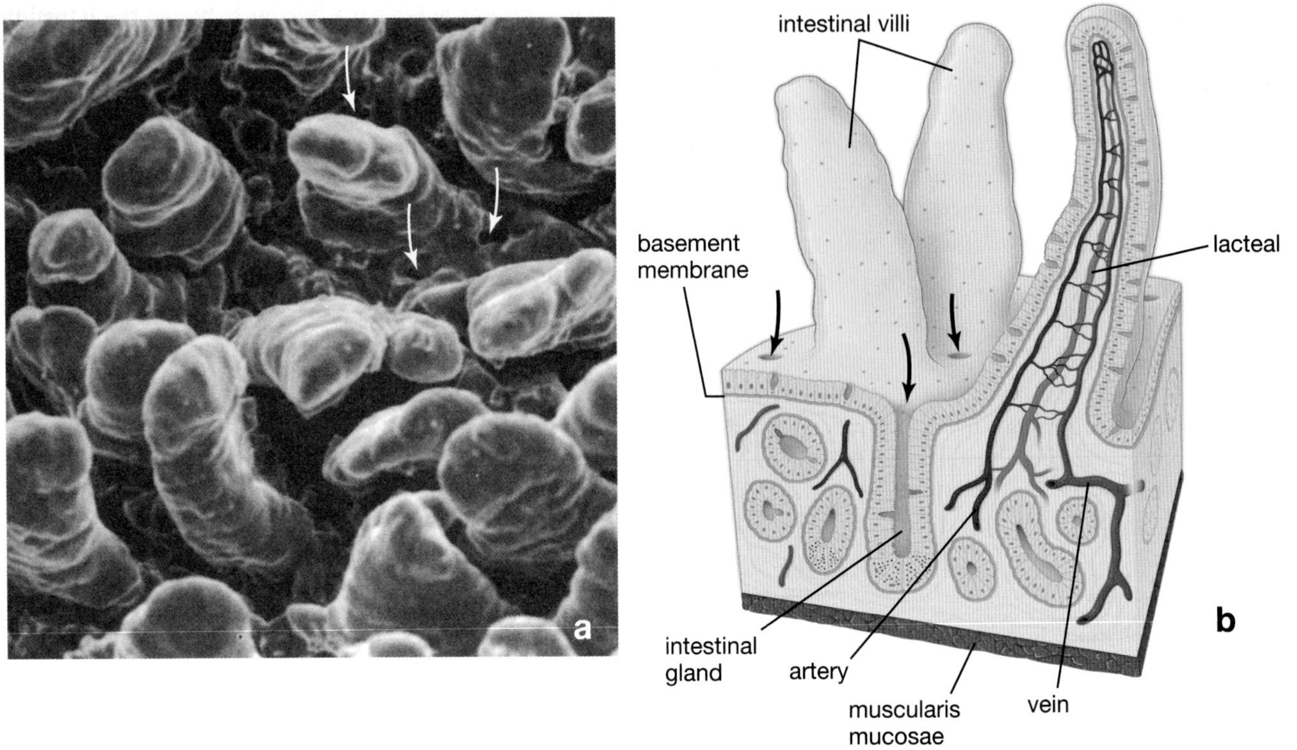

FIGURE 17.18. Intestinal villi in the small intestine. a. Scanning electron micrograph of the intestinal mucosa showing its villi. Note the openings (*arrows*) located between the bases of the villi that lead into the intestinal glands (crypts of Lieberkühn). ×800. **b.** This three-dimensional diagram of the intestinal villi shows the continuity of the epithelium covering the villi with the epithelium lining the intestinal glands. Note blood vessels and the blind-ending lymphatic capillary, called a *lacteal*, in the core of the villus. Between the bases of the villi, the openings of the intestinal glands can be seen (*arrows*). Also, the small openings on the surface of the villi indicate the location of discharged goblet cells.

The villi and intestinal glands, along with the lamina propria, associated GALT, and muscularis mucosae, constitute the essential features of the small intestinal mucosa.

Villi, as noted, are projections of the mucosa. They consist of a core of loose connective tissue covered by a simple columnar epithelium. The core of the villus is an extension of the lamina propria, which contains numerous fibroblasts, smooth muscle cells, lymphocytes, plasma cells, eosinophils, macrophages, and a network of fenestrated blood capillaries located just beneath the epithelial basal lamina. In addition, the lamina propria of the villus contains a central, blind-ending lymphatic capillary, the **lacteal** (Fig. 17.19 and Plate 17.7, page 682). Smooth muscle cells derived from the muscularis mucosae extend into the villus and accompany the lacteal. These smooth muscle cells may account for the observation that villi contract and shorten intermittently, an action that may force lymph from the lacteal into the lymphatic vessel network surrounding the muscularis mucosae.

The **intestinal glands**, or **crypts of Lieberkühn**, are simple tubular structures that extend from the muscularis mucosae through the thickness of the lamina propria, where they open onto the luminal surface of the intestine at the base of the villi (see Fig. 17.18). The glands are composed of a simple columnar epithelium that is continuous with the epithelium of the villi.

As in the stomach, the lamina propria surrounds the intestinal glands and contains numerous cells of the immune system (lymphocytes, plasma cells, mast cells, macrophages, and eosinophils), particularly in the villi. The **lamina propria** also contains numerous **nodules of lymphatic tissue** that represent a major component of the GALT. The nodules are particularly large and numerous in the ileum, where they are preferentially located on the side of the intestine opposite the mesenteric attachment (Fig. 17.20). These nodular aggregations are known as **aggregated nodules** or **Peyer patches**. In gross specimens, they appear as aggregates of white specks.

The **muscularis mucosae** consists of two thin layers of smooth muscle cells, an inner circular and an outer longitudinal layer. As noted earlier, strands of smooth muscle cells extend from the muscularis mucosae into the lamina propria of the villi.

At least five types of cells are found in the intestinal mucosal epithelium.

The mature cells of the intestinal epithelium are found both in the intestinal glands and on the surface of the villi. They include the following:

- **Enterocytes**, whose primary function is absorption
- **Goblet cells**, unicellular mucin-secreting glands
- **Paneth cells**, whose primary function is to maintain mucosal innate immunity by secreting antimicrobial substances
- **Enteroendocrine cells**, which produce various paracrine and endocrine hormones
- **M cells (microfold cells)**, specialized cells located in the epithelium that covers lymphatic nodules in the lamina propria

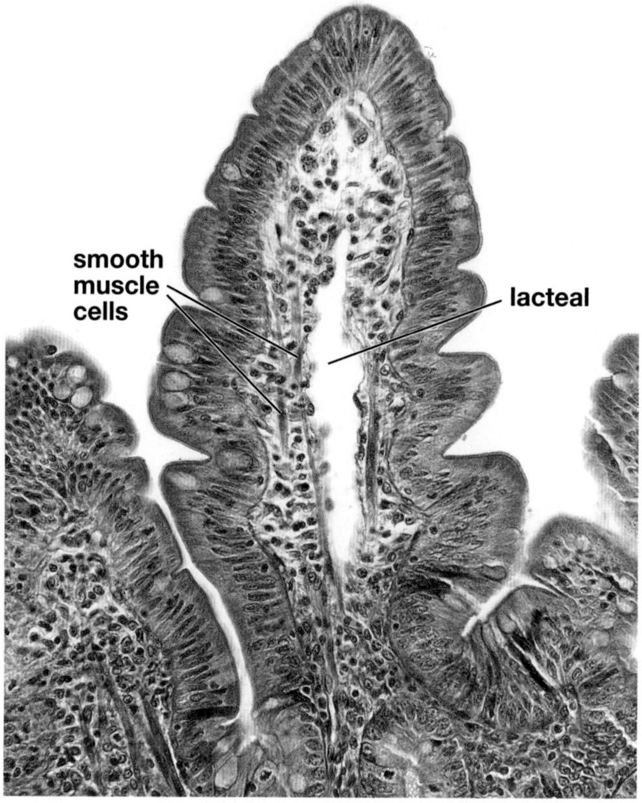

FIGURE 17.19. Photomicrograph of an intestinal villus. The surface of the villus consists of columnar epithelial cells, chiefly enterocytes with a striated border. Also evident are goblet cells that can be readily identified by the presence of the apical mucous cup. Located beneath the epithelium is the highly cellular loose connective tissue, the lamina propria. The lamina propria contains large numbers of round cells, mostly lymphocytes. In addition, smooth muscle cells can be identified. A lymphatic capillary called a *lacteal* occupies the center of the villus. When the lacteal is dilated, as it is in this specimen, it is easily identified. ×160.

Enterocytes are absorptive cells specialized for the transport of substances from the lumen of the intestine to the circulatory system.

Enterocytes are tall columnar cells with a basally positioned nucleus (see Figs. 17.18 and 17.21). Microvilli increase the apical surface area as much as 600 times; they are recognized in the LM as forming a **striated border** on the luminal surface.

Each microvillus has a core of vertically oriented actin microfilaments that are anchored to villin located in the tip of the microvillus and that also attach to the microvillus plasma membrane by myosin I molecules. The actin microfilaments extend into the apical cytoplasm and insert into the **terminal web**, a network of horizontally oriented contractile microfilaments that form a layer in the most apical cytoplasm and attach to the intracellular density associated with the zonula adherens. Contraction of the terminal web causes the microvilli to spread apart, thus increasing the space between them to allow more surface area exposure for absorption to take place. In addition, contraction of the terminal web may aid in "closing" the holes left in the epithelial sheet by exfoliation of aging cells. Enterocytes are bound to one another and to goblet, enteroendocrine, and other cells of the epithelium by junctional complexes.

Tight junctions establish a barrier between the intestinal lumen and the epithelial intercellular compartment.

The **tight junctions** between the intestinal lumen and the connective tissue compartment of the body allow selective retention of substances absorbed by the enterocytes. As noted in Chapter 5, Epithelial Tissue (pages 141-145), the "tightness" of these junctions can vary.

In relatively impermeable tight junctions, as in the ileum and colon, active transport is required to move solutes across the barrier. In simplest terms, active transport systems, for example, sodium pumps (Na^+/K^+-ATPase), located in the lateral plasma membrane, transiently reduce the cytoplasmic

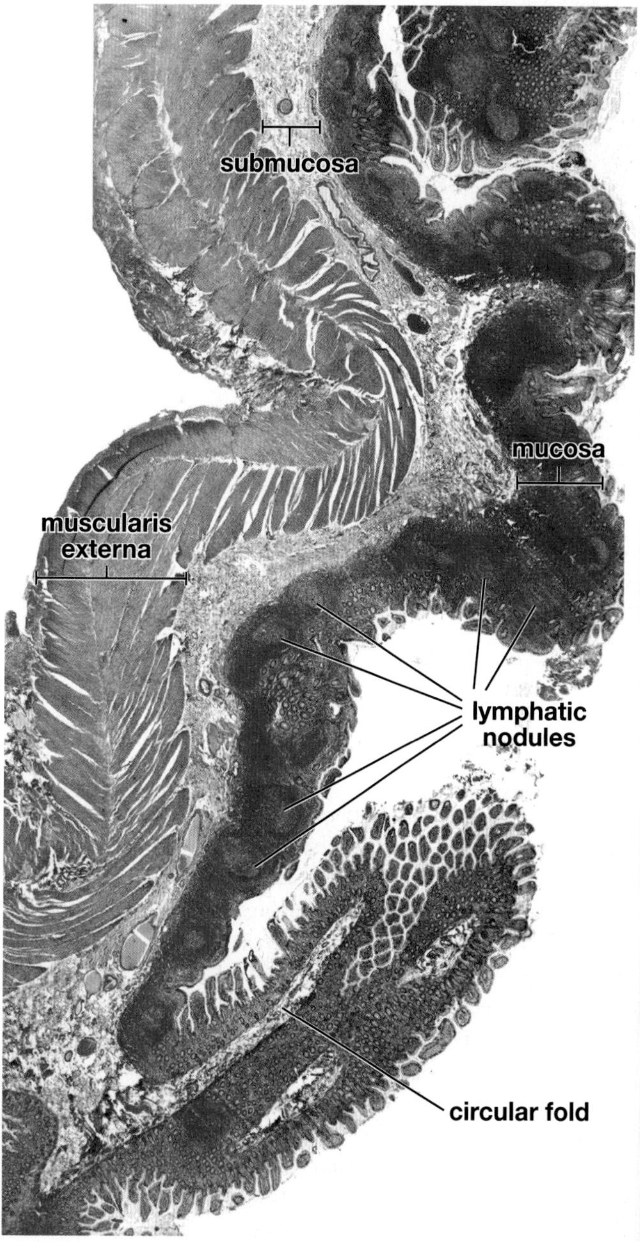

FIGURE 17.20. Photomicrograph of Peyer patches. This photomicrograph shows a longitudinal section through the wall of a human ileum. Note the extensive lymphatic nodules located in the mucosa and the section of a circular fold projecting into the lumen of the ileum. Lymphatic nodules within the Peyer patch are primarily located within the lamina propria, although many extend into the submucosa. They are covered by the intestinal epithelium, which contains enterocytes, occasional goblet cells, and specialized antigen-transporting M cells. ×40.

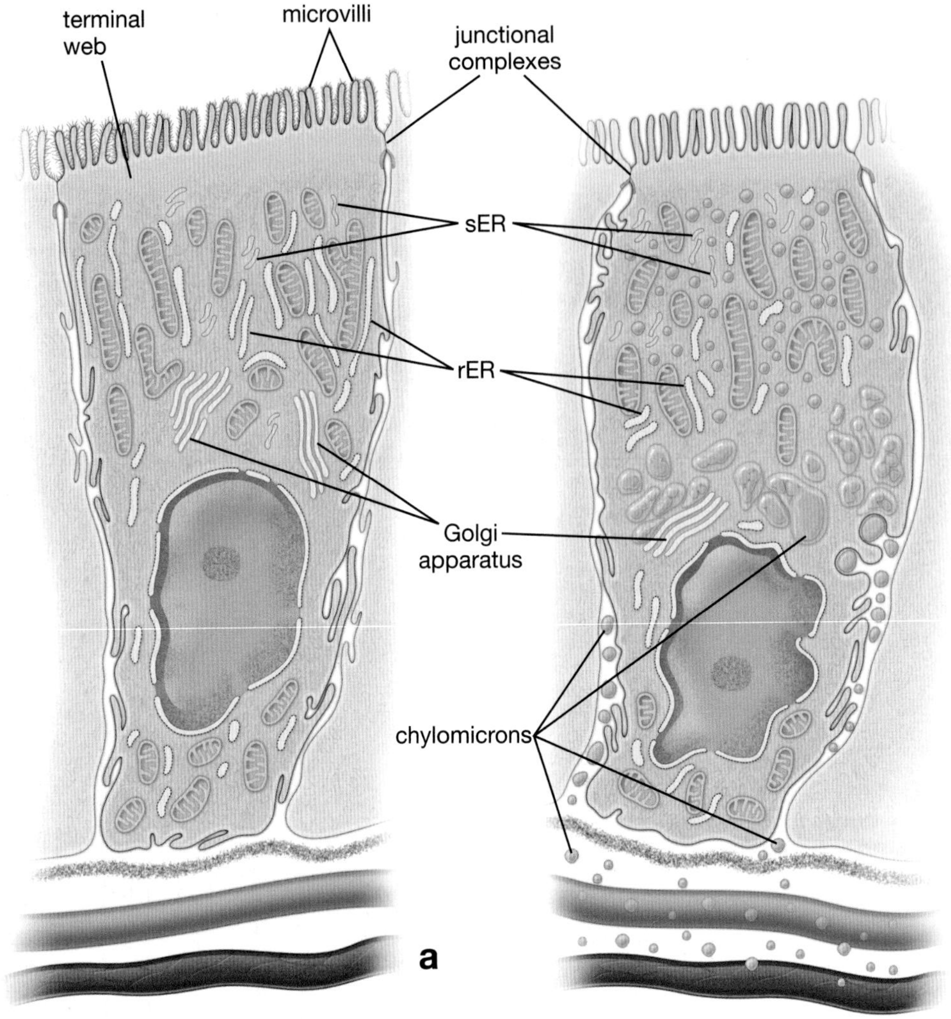

ABSORPTIVE CELLS

FIGURE 17.21. Diagrams of an enterocyte in different phases of absorption. a. This cell has a striated border on its apical surface and junctional complexes that seal the lumen of the intestine from the lateral intercellular space. The characteristic complement of major organelles is depicted in the diagram. **b.** This cell shows the distribution of lipid during fat absorption as seen with transmission electron microscopy (TEM). Initially, lipids are seen in association with the microvilli of the striated border. Lipids are internalized and seen in vesicles of the smooth endoplasmic reticulum (*sER*) in the apical portion of the cell. The membrane-bound lipid can be traced to the center of the cell, where many of the lipid-containing vesicles fuse. The lipid is then discharged into the intercellular space. The extracellular lipids, recognized as chylomicrons, pass beyond the basal lamina for further transport into lymphatic (*green*) and/or blood vessels (*red*). *rER*, rough endoplasmic reticulum.

concentration of Na^+ by transporting sodium ions across the lateral plasma membrane into the extracellular space below the tight junction. This transport of Na^+ creates a high intercellular Na^+ concentration, causing water from the cell to enter the intercellular space, reducing both the water and Na^+ concentrations in the cell. Consequently, water and Na^+ enter the cell at its apical surface, passing through the cell and exiting at the lateral plasma membrane as long as the sodium pump continues to function. Increased osmolarity in the intercellular space draws water into this space, establishing a hydrostatic pressure that drives Na^+ and water across the basal lamina into the connective tissue.

In epithelia with more permeable tight junctions, such as those in the duodenum and jejunum, a sodium pump also creates low intracellular Na^+ concentration. When the contents that pass into the duodenum and jejunum are hypotonic, however, considerable absorption of water, along with additional Na^+ and other small solutes, takes place directly across the tight junctions of the enterocytes into the intercellular spaces. This mechanism of absorption is referred to as **solvent drag**.

Other transport mechanisms also increase the concentrations of specific substances, such as sugars, amino acids, and other solutes in the intercellular space. These substances then diffuse or flow down their concentration gradients within the intercellular space to cross the epithelial basal lamina and enter the fenestrated capillaries in the lamina propria located immediately beneath the epithelium. Substances that are too large to enter the blood vessels, such as lipoprotein particles, enter the lymphatic lacteal.

The lateral cell surface of the enterocytes exhibits elaborate, flattened cytoplasmic processes (plicae) that interdigitate with those of adjacent cells (see Fig. 5.24). These folds increase the lateral surface area of the cell, thus increasing the amount of plasma membrane containing transport enzymes. During active absorption, especially of solutes, water, and lipids, these **lateral plications** separate, enlarging the intercellular compartment. The increased hydrostatic pressure from the accumulated solutes and solvents causes a directional flow through the basal lamina into the lamina propria (see Fig. 5.1).

In addition to the membrane specializations associated with absorption and transport, the enterocyte cytoplasm is also specialized for these functions. Elongated mitochondria that provide energy for transport are concentrated in the apical cytoplasm between the terminal web and the nucleus. Tubules and cisternae of the smooth endoplasmic reticulum (sER), which are involved in the absorption of fatty acids and glycerol and in the resynthesis of neutral fat, are found in the apical cytoplasm beneath the terminal web.

Enterocytes are also secretory cells, producing enzymes needed for terminal digestion and absorption as well as secretion of water and electrolytes.

The secretory function of **enterocytes**, primarily the synthesis of glycoprotein enzymes that will be inserted into the apical plasma membrane, is represented morphologically by aligned stacks of Golgi cisternae in the immediate supranuclear region and by the presence of free ribosomes and rER lateral to the Golgi apparatus (see Fig. 17.21). Small secretory vesicles containing glycoproteins destined for the cell surface are located in the apical cytoplasm, just below the terminal web, and along the lateral plasma membrane. Histochemical or autoradiographic methods are needed, however, to distinguish these secretory vesicles from endocytotic vesicles or small lysosomes.

The small intestine also secretes water and electrolytes. This activity occurs mainly in the cells within the intestinal glands. The secretion that occurs in these glands is thought to assist the process of digestion and absorption by maintaining an appropriate liquid state of the intestinal chyme. Under normal conditions, the absorption of fluid by the villus enterocyte is balanced by the secretion of fluid by the gland enterocyte.

Goblet cells represent unicellular glands that are interspersed among the other cells of the intestinal epithelium.

As in other epithelia, **goblet cells** produce mucus. In the small intestine, goblet cells increase in number from the duodenum to the terminal part of the ileum. Also, as in other epithelia, because water-soluble mucinogen is lost during preparation of routine H&E sections, the part of the cell that normally contains mucinogen granules appears empty. Examination with the TEM reveals a large accumulation of mucinogen granules in the apical cytoplasm that distends the apex of the cell and distorts the shape of neighboring cells (Fig. 17.22). With the apex of the cell

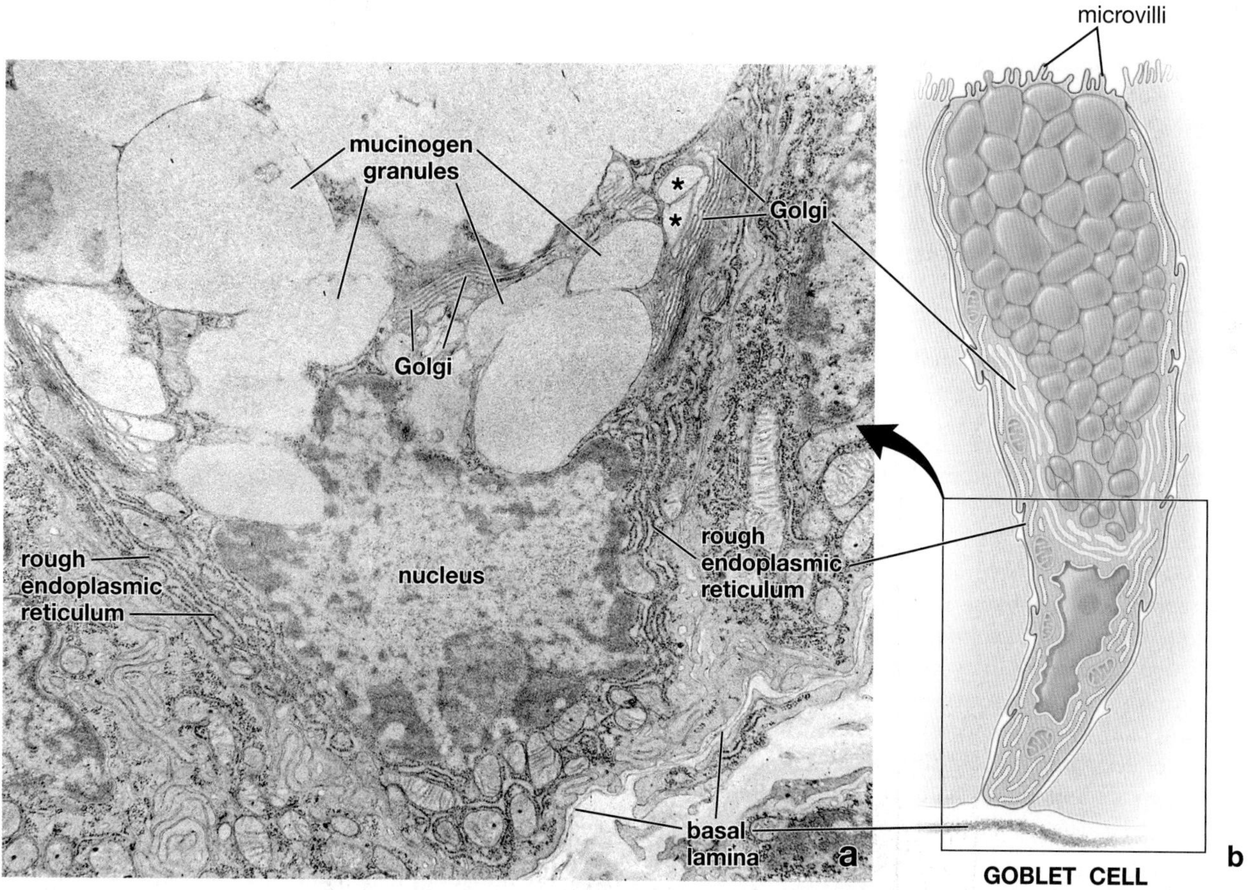

FIGURE 17.22. Electron micrograph and diagram of a goblet cell. a. This electron micrograph shows the basal portion of a goblet cell depicted on the adjacent diagram. The cell rests on the basal lamina. The basal portion of the cell contains the nucleus, rough endoplasmic reticulum, and mitochondria. Just apical to the nucleus are extensive profiles of the Golgi apparatus. As the mucous product accumulates in the Golgi cisternae, they become enlarged (*asterisks*). The large mucinogen granules fill most of the apical portion of the cell and collectively constitute the "mucous cup" seen in the light microscope. ×15,000. **b.** This diagram shows the entire goblet cell. The *boxed region* on this diagram represents an area from which the adjacent electron micrograph was most likely obtained. The nucleus is located at the basal portion of the cell. The major portion of the cell is filled with mucinogen granules forming the mucous cup that is evident in the light microscope. At the base and lower sides of the mucous cup are flattened saccules of the large Golgi apparatus. Other organelles are distributed throughout the remaining cytoplasm, especially in the perinuclear cytoplasm at the base of the cell.

containing a large accumulation of mucinogen granules, the basal portion of the cell resembles a narrow stem. This basal portion is intensely basophilic in histologic preparations because it is occupied by a heterochromatic nucleus, extensive rER, and free ribosomes. Mitochondria are also concentrated in the basal cytoplasm. The characteristic shape, with the apical accumulation of granules and the narrow basal stem, is responsible for the name of the cell, as in a glass "goblet." An extensive array of flattened Golgi cisternae forms a wide cup around the newly formed mucinogen granules adjacent to the basal part of the cell (see Fig. 17.22a). The microvilli of goblet cells are restricted to a thin rim of cytoplasm (the theca) that surrounds the apical–lateral portion of the mucinogen granules. Microvilli are more obvious on the immature goblet cells in the deep one-half of the intestinal gland.

Paneth cells play a role in the regulation of normal bacterial flora of the small intestine.

Paneth cells are found in the bases of the intestinal glands. (They are also occasionally found in the normal colon in small numbers; their number may increase in certain pathologic conditions.) They have a basophilic basal cytoplasm, a supranuclear Golgi apparatus, and large, intensely acidophilic, refractile apical secretory vesicles. These vesicles allow their easy identification in routine histologic sections (Fig. 17.23). The secretory vesicles contain the antibacterial enzyme lysozyme, α-defensins, other glycoproteins, an arginine-rich protein (probably responsible for the intense acidophilia), and zinc. **Lysozyme** digests the cell walls of certain groups of bacteria. **α-Defensins** are homologs of peptides that function as mediators in cytotoxic $CD8^+$ T lymphocytes. Their antibacterial action and ability to phagocytose certain bacteria and protozoa suggest that Paneth cells play a role in regulating the normal bacterial flora of the small intestine.

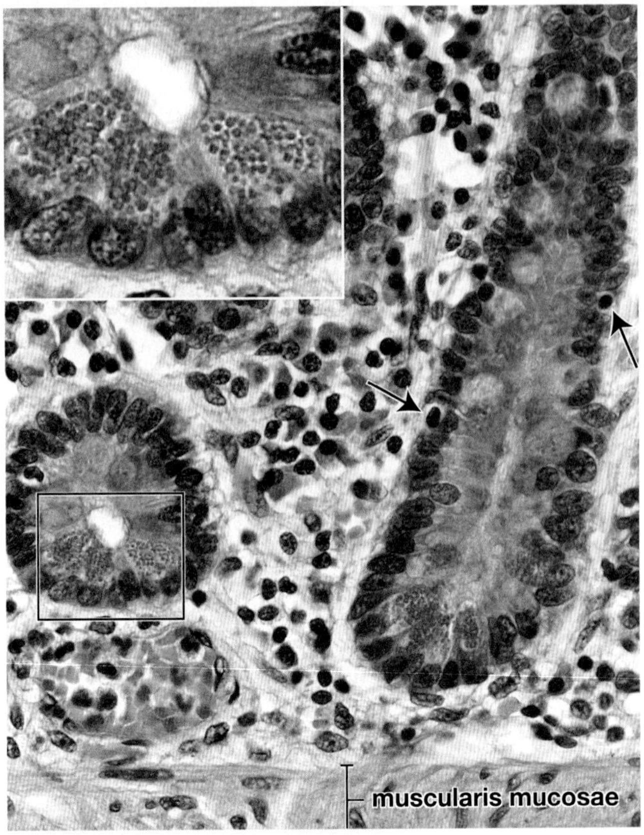

FIGURE 17.23. Photomicrograph of intestinal glands showing Paneth cells. This photomicrograph shows the base of intestinal (jejunal) glands in a hematoxylin and eosin (H&E) preparation. The gland on the *right* is sectioned longitudinally; the circular cross-sectional profile of another gland is seen on the *left*. Paneth cells are typically located in the base of the intestinal glands and are readily seen in the light microscope because of the intensive eosin staining of their vesicles. The lamina propria contains an abundance of plasma cells, lymphocytes, and other connective tissue cells. Note several lymphocytes in the epithelium of the gland (*arrows*). ×240. **Inset.** This high magnification of the area indicated by the *rectangle* shows the characteristic basophilic cytoplasm in the basal portion of the cell and large accumulations of intensely staining, eosinophilic, refractile secretory vesicles in the apical portion of the cell. An arginine-rich protein found in the vesicles is probably responsible for the intense eosinophilic reaction. ×680.

Enteroendocrine cells in the small intestine produce nearly all of the same peptide hormones as they do in the stomach.

Enteroendocrine cells in the small intestine resemble those that reside in the stomach (see Fig. 17.12). The "closed cells" are concentrated in the lower portion of the intestinal gland, whereas the "open cells" can be found at all levels of each villus. Activation of taste receptors found on the apical cell membrane of "open cells" activates the **G-protein signaling cascade**, resulting in the release of peptides that regulate a variety of gastrointestinal functions. These include pancreatic secretion, inducing digestion and absorption, and energy homeostasis by acting on neural pathways of the **brain–gut–adipose axis**. Nearly all of the same peptide hormones identified in this cell type in the stomach can be demonstrated in the enteroendocrine cells of the intestine (see Table 17.1). **Cholecystokinin (CCK)**, **secretin**, **gastric inhibitory polypeptide (GIP)**, and **motilin** are the most active regulators of gastrointestinal physiology that are released in this portion of the gut (see Fig. 17.13). CCK and secretin increase pancreatic and gallbladder activity and inhibit gastric secretory function and motility. GIP stimulates insulin release in the pancreas, and motilin initiates gastric and intestinal motility. Although other peptides produced by enteroendocrine cells have been isolated, they are not considered hormones and are, therefore, called **candidate hormones** (see Folder 17.3, page 644). Enteroendocrine cells also produce at least two hormones, somatostatin and histamine, which act as **paracrine hormones** (see Folder 17.3, page 644) (i.e., hormones that have a local effect and do not circulate in the bloodstream). In addition, several peptides are secreted by the nerve cells located in the submucosa and muscularis externa. These peptides, called **neurocrine hormones**, are represented by vasoactive intestinal peptide (VIP), bombesin, and enkephalins. The functions of these peptides are listed in Table 17.2 (page 647).

M cells convey microorganisms and other macromolecules from the intestinal lumen to Peyer patches.

M cells are epithelial cells that overlie **Peyer patches** and other large lymphatic nodules; they differ significantly from the surrounding intestinal epithelial cells (Folder 17.5). M cells have a characteristic shape because each cell develops a deep pocket–like recess connected to the extracellular space. Dendritic cells, macrophages, and T and B lymphocytes reside in this space. Owing to this unique shape, the basolateral cell

FOLDER 17.5

FUNCTIONAL CONSIDERATIONS: IMMUNE FUNCTIONS OF THE ALIMENTARY CANAL

Immunologists have shown that the gut-associated lymphatic tissue (GALT) not only responds to antigenic stimuli but also functions in a monitoring capacity. This function has been partially clarified for the lymphatic nodules of the intestinal tract. The **M cells** that are part of the epithelium that cover Peyer patches and lymphatic nodules have a distinctive surface that might be misinterpreted in sections as thick microvilli. The cells are readily identified with the scanning electron microscope because microfolds contrast sharply with the microvilli that constitute the striated border of the adjacent enterocytes.

It has been shown with **glycoprotein GP2** (molecular marker for M cells) that the M cells endocytose proteins and bacteria from the intestinal lumen, transport them in the vesicles through the cell, and discharge the contents by exocytosis into deep recesses that are continuous with the extracellular space (Fig. F17.5.1). Dendritic cells and lymphocytes within the deeply recessed extracellular space sample the luminal protein, including antigens, and thus have the opportunity to stimulate the development of specific antibodies against the antigens. The destination of these exposed lymphocytes has not yet been fully determined. Some remain within the local lymphatic tissue, but others may be destined for other sites in the body, such as the salivary and mammary glands. Recall that in the salivary glands, cells of the immune system (plasma cells) secrete immunoglobulin A (IgA), which the glandular epithelium then converts into secretory IgA (sIgA). Some experimental observations suggest that antigen contact necessary for the production of IgA by plasma cells occurs in the lymphatic nodules of the intestines. Recent findings using glycoprotein 2 (GP2)-deficient mice show that the interaction of GP2 with bacteria plays an important role in antigen-specific immune responses in Peyer patches. This discovery may lead to the development not only of new oral vaccines for infectious diseases but also of the innovative treatment of tumors and inflammatory bowel diseases.

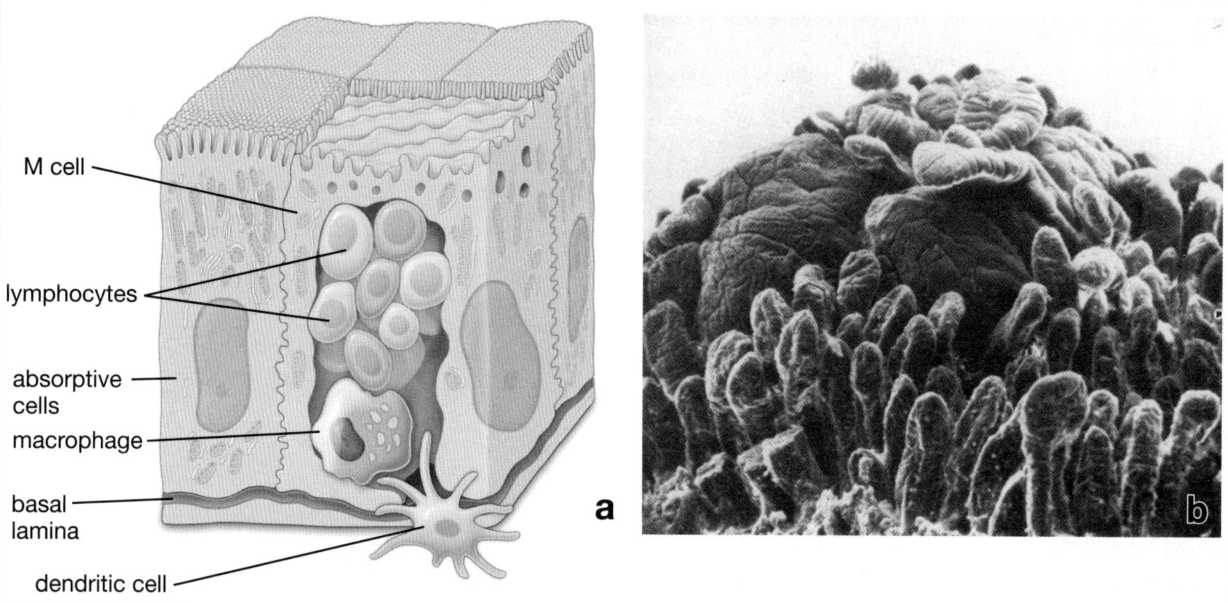

FIGURE F17.5.1. Diagram of M cells covering the lymphatic nodule of the intestine. a. This diagram shows the relationship of the M cells (microfold cells) and absorptive cells in the epithelium covering a lymphatic nodule. The M cell is an epithelial cell that displays microfolds rather than microvilli on its apical surface. It has deep recesses within which lymphocytes, macrophages, and processes of dendritic cells come close to the lumen of the small intestine. An intact antigen from the intestinal lumen is transferred across the thin layer of the M cell apical cytoplasm to lymphocytes and other antigen-presenting cells residing within the recesses. **b.** Scanning electron micrograph of a Peyer patch lymphatic nodule bulging into the lumen of the ileum. Note that the area of the follicle covered by M cells is surrounded by the finger-like projections of the intestinal villi. The surface of the M cells has a smooth appearance. The absence of absorptive cells and mucus-producing goblet cells in the area covered by M cells facilitates immunoreactions to antigens. ×80. (Reprinted with permission from Owen RL, Johns AL. Epithelial cell specialization within human Peyer's patches: an ultrastructural study of intestinal lymphoid follicles. *Gastroenterology.* 1974;66:189–203.)

surface of the M cell resides within a few microns of its apical surface, greatly reducing the distance that endocytic vesicles must travel to cross the epithelial barrier. On their apical surface, M cells have **microfolds** rather than microvilli and a thin layer of glycocalyx. The apical surface expresses an abundance of glycoprotein 2 (GP2) receptors that bind specific macromolecules and Gram-negative bacteria (e.g., *Escherichia coli*). The substances bound to GP2 receptors are internalized in endocytic vesicles and transported to the basolateral cell surface of the pocket-like recess. Within the recess, the released contents are immediately transferred to immune cells residing in this space. Thus, M cells function as highly specialized **antigen-transporting cells** that relocate intact antigens from the intestinal lumen across the epithelial barrier. Antigens that reach the immune cells in this manner stimulate a response in the GALT that is described later in this chapter.

Intermediate cells constitute the amplifying compartment of the intestinal stem cell niche.

Intermediate cells constitute most of the cells found within the intestinal stem cell niche that is located in the lower half of the intestinal gland. These cells constitute the amplifying compartment of the cells that are still capable of cell division and usually undergo one or two divisions before they become committed to differentiation into either absorptive or goblet cells. These cells have short, irregular microvilli with long core filaments extending deep into the apical cytoplasm and numerous macular (desmosomal) junctions with adjacent cells. Small mucin-like secretory granules form a column in the center of the supranuclear cytoplasm. Intermediate cells that are committed to becoming goblet cells develop a small, rounded collection of secretory granules just beneath the apical plasma membrane; those that are committed to becoming absorptive cells lose the secretory granules and begin to show concentrations of mitochondria, rER, and ribosomes in the apical cytoplasm.

GALT is prominent in the lamina propria of the small intestine.

As noted earlier, the **lamina propria** of the digestive tract is heavily populated with elements of the immune system; approximately one-fourth of the mucosa consists of a loosely organized layer of lymphatic nodules, lymphocytes, macrophages, plasma cells, and eosinophils in the lamina propria (Plate 17.2, page 672). Lymphocytes are also located between epithelial cells. The **GALT** serves as an immunologic barrier throughout the length of the gastrointestinal tract. In cooperation with the overlying epithelial cells, particularly M cells, the lymphatic tissue samples the antigens in the epithelial intercellular spaces. Lymphocytes, macrophages, and other antigen-presenting cells process the antigens and migrate to lymphatic nodules in the lamina propria where they undergo activation (see page 494), leading to antibody secretion by newly differentiated plasma cells.

The mucosal surface is protected by immunoglobulin-mediated responses.

The **mucosal surface** of the gut tube is constantly challenged by the presence of ingested microorganisms (i.e., viruses, bacteria, parasites) and toxins, which, after compromising the epithelial barrier, may cause infections or diseases. An example of a specific defense mechanism is the immunoglobulin-mediated response using immunoglobulin A (IgA), IgM, and IgE antibodies. Most of the plasma cells in the lamina propria of the intestine secrete **dimeric dIgA antibodies** rather than the more common IgG; other plasma cells produce **pentameric IgM** and IgE (see page 490). Diameric dIgA is composed of two monomeric IgA subunits and a polypeptide J chain (see Fig. 16.28). Secreted dIgA molecules bind to the **polymeric immunoglobulin receptor (pIgR)** located at the basal domain of the epithelial cells (Fig. 17.24). The pIgR is a transmembrane glycoprotein (75 kDa) synthesized by enterocytes and expressed on the basal plasma membrane. The pIgR–dIgA complex is then endocytosed and transported across the epithelium to the apical surface of the enterocyte (this type of transport refers to as *transcytosis*). After the pIgR–dIgA complex reaches the apical surface, pIgR is proteolytically cleaved and the extracellular part of the receptor that is bound to dIgA is released into the gut lumen (see Fig. 17.24). This cleaved

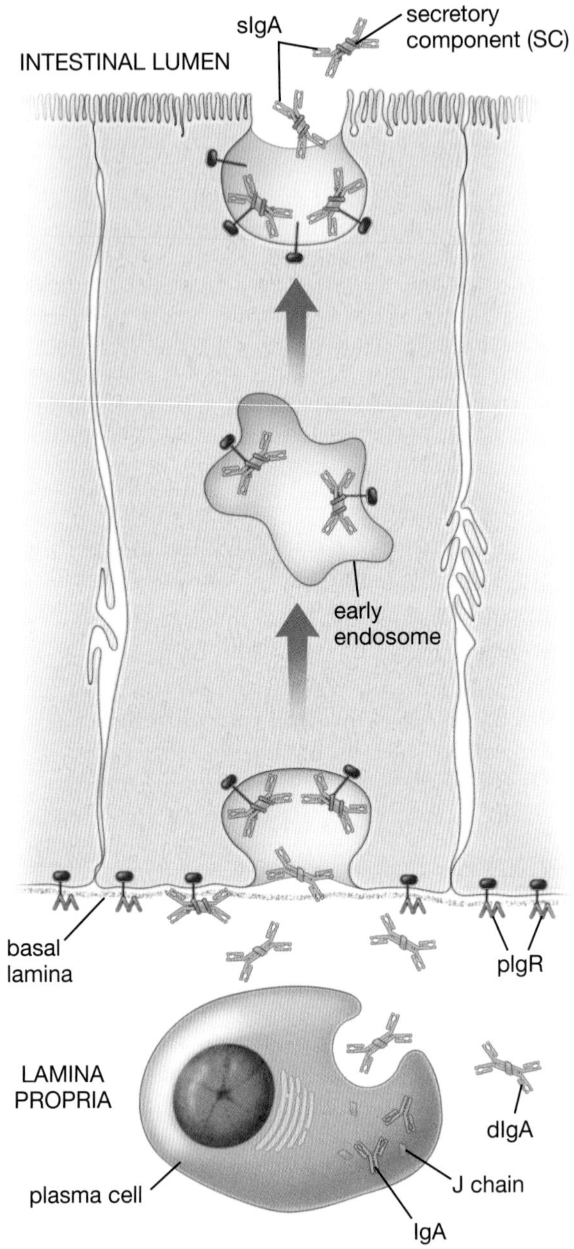

FIGURE 17.24. Diagram of immunoglobulin A (IgA) secretion and transport. A monomeric form of immunoglobulin A (*IgA*) is synthesized by the plasma cell. *IgAs* are secreted into the lamina propria in a dimeric form as *dIgA*. Dimeric *dIgA* is composed of two monomeric *IgA* subunits and a polypeptide J chain also produced by the plasma cell. In the lamina propria, *dIgA* binds to the polymeric immunoglobulin receptor (*pIgR*) on the basal cell membrane of the enterocyte. The *pIgR–IgA* complex enters the cell by endocytosis and is carried out within the endocytotic vesicles to the early endosomal compartment and then to the apical surface (a process called *transcytosis*). Endocytic vesicles fuse with the apical plasma membrane, the *pIgR* is proteolytically cleaved, and *dIgA* is released with the extracellular portion of the *pIgR*. This portion of the *pIgR* remains with the *IgA* dimer and becomes the secretory component (*SC*) of the secretory IgA (*sIgA*).

extracellular binding domain of the receptor is known as the **secretory component (SC)**; secreted dIgA in association with the SC is known as **secretory IgA (sIgA)**. The release of sIgA immunoglobulins is critical for proper **immunologic surveillance** by the mucosal immune system. In the lumen, sIgA binds to antigens, toxins, and microorganisms. Secretory IgA prevents the attachment and invasion of viruses and bacteria into the mucosa by either inhibiting their motility, causing microbial aggregation, or masking pathogen adhesion sites on the epithelial surface. For example, sIgA binds to a glycoprotein on the viral envelope of **HIV**, preventing its attachment, internalization, and subsequent replication in the cell.

Secretory IgA is the principal molecule of mucosal immunity. However, IgM molecules utilize similar pathways of receptor-mediated transcytosis to reach the mucosal surface. Some of the IgE binds to the plasma membranes of mast cells in the lamina propria (see pages 200-204), selectively sensitizing them to specific antigens derived from the lumen.

Epithelial Cell Renewal in the Small Intestine

Mature cells of the intestinal epithelium are derived from a single stem cell population.

Stem cells are located in the base of the intestinal gland. This **intestinal stem cell niche** (zone of cell replication) is restricted to the lower one-half of the gland and contains highly proliferative intermediate cells (as previously explained) and cells in various stages of differentiation. A cell destined to become a goblet cell or absorptive cell usually undergoes several additional divisions after it leaves the pool of stem cells. The epithelial cells migrate upward in the intestinal gland onto the villus where they undergo apoptosis and slough off into the lumen. Autoradiographic studies have shown that the renewal time for absorptive and **goblet cells** in the human small intestine is 4–6 days.

Enteroendocrine cells and Paneth cells are also derived from the stem cells at the base of the intestinal gland. Enteroendocrine cells appear to divide only once before differentiating. They migrate with the absorptive and goblet cells but at a slower rate. **Paneth cells** migrate downward and reside at the bottom of the intestinal gland. They live for approximately 4 weeks and are then replaced by differentiation of a nearby "committed" cell in the intestinal gland. Cells that are recognizable as Paneth cells no longer divide. As mentioned in Chapter 5, Epithelial Tissue (page 166), expression of **transcription factor Math1** appears to determine the fate of differentiating cells in the intestinal stem cell niche. The cells committed to the secretory lineage (i.e., they will differentiate into goblet, enteroendocrine, and Paneth cells) have increased expression of Math1. Inhibition of Math1 expression characterizes the default developmental pathway into absorptive intestinal cells (enterocytes).

Submucosa

A distinguishing characteristic of the duodenum is the presence of submucosal glands.

The **submucosa** consists of dense connective tissue and localized sites that contain aggregates of adipose cells. A conspicuous feature in the duodenum is the presence of **submucosal glands**, also called **Brunner glands**.

The branched, tubular submucosal glands of the duodenum have secretory cells with characteristics of both zymogen-secreting and mucus-secreting cells (Fig. 17.25).

The secretion of these glands has a pH of 8.1–9.3 and contains neutral and alkaline glycoproteins and bicarbonate ions. This highly alkaline secretion probably serves to protect the proximal small intestine by neutralizing the acid-containing chyme delivered to it. It also brings the intestinal contents close to the optimal pH for activation of pancreatic enzymes that are also delivered to the duodenum.

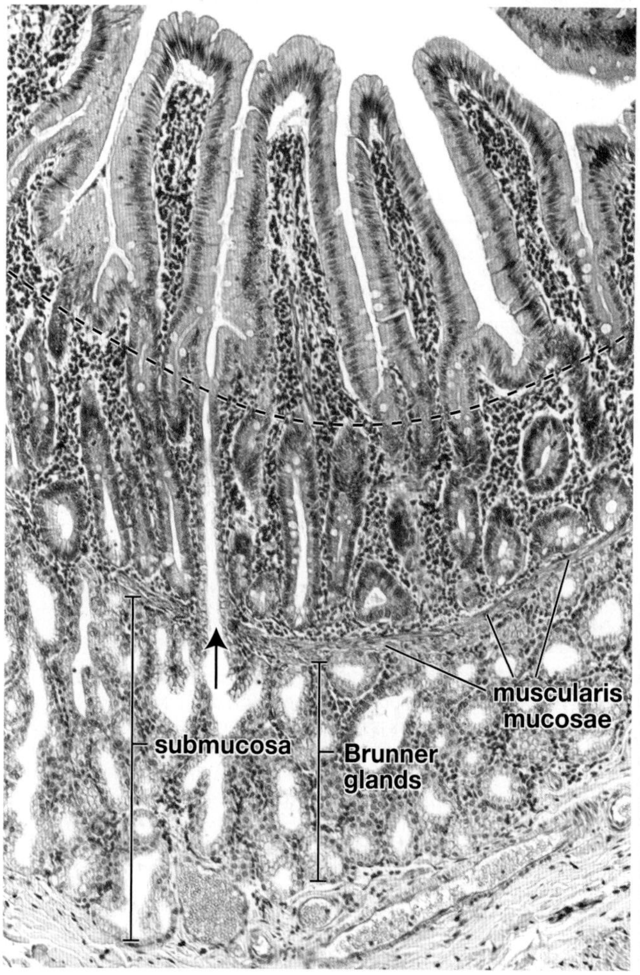

FIGURE 17.25. Photomicrograph of Brunner glands in the duodenum. This photomicrograph shows part of the duodenal wall in a hematoxylin and eosin (H&E) preparation. A distinctive feature of the duodenum is the presence of Brunner glands. The *dashed line* marks the boundary between the villi and the typical intestinal glands (crypts of Lieberkühn). The latter extend to the muscularis mucosae. Beneath the mucosa is the submucosa, which contains Brunner glands. These are branched tubular glands whose secretory component consists of columnar cells. The duct of Brunner gland opens into the lumen of the intestinal gland (*arrow*). ×120.

Muscularis Externa

The **muscularis externa** consists of an inner layer of circularly arranged smooth muscle cells and an outer layer of longitudinally arranged smooth muscle cells (Fig. 17.26). The main components of the **myenteric plexus (Auerbach plexus)** are located between these two muscle layers (see Fig. 17.26 for an LM image and 17.27 for an EM image). Two kinds of muscular contraction occur in the small intestine. Local contractions displace intestinal contents both proximally and distally; this type of contraction is called **segmentation**. These contractions primarily involve the circular muscle layer. They serve to circulate the chyme locally, mixing it with digestive juices and moving it into contact with the mucosa for absorption. **Peristalsis**, the second type of contraction, involves the coordinated action of both circular and longitudinal muscle layers and moves the intestinal contents distally.

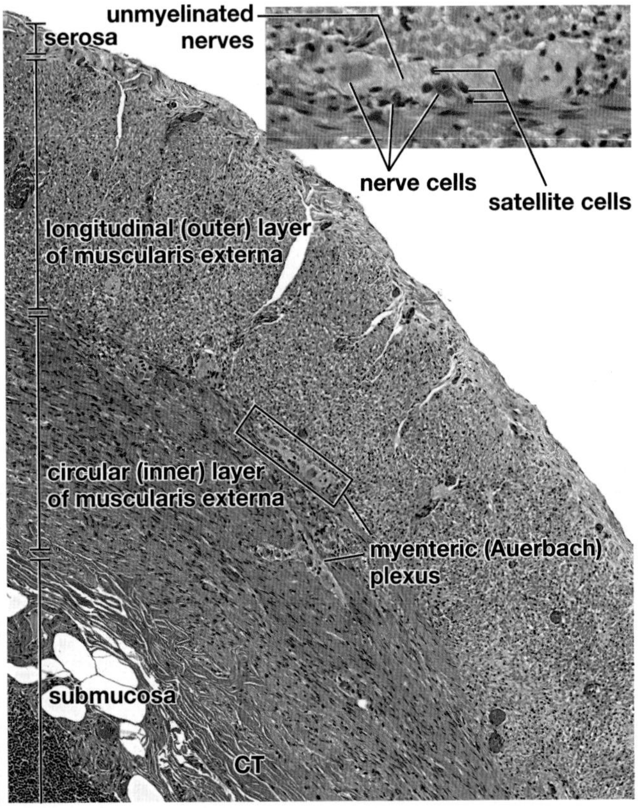

FIGURE 17.26. Photomicrograph of muscularis externa in the ileum. This photomicrograph of a hematoxylin and eosin (H&E)-stained specimen shows the cross section of the outer section of the intestinal wall. In this image, the most prominent structure is the muscularis externa, which consists of two layers of smooth muscle. The inner layer appears as circularly arranged smooth muscle cells distinguished in this section by the elongated profiles of their nuclei. In the outer layer, the smooth muscle cells are longitudinally arranged, and in this section, they display cross-sectional profiles with small round nuclei surrounded by cytoplasm. Owing to the plane of the section, many cytoplasmic profiles of smooth muscle cells in the outer layer do not have visible nuclei. The arrangement of smooth muscles in both layers can be seen at higher magnification in the *inset*. Located between these two muscle layers is the myenteric (Auerbach) plexus. In the section, the plexus exhibits lighter stained irregular profiles of tissue containing dispersed darker stained nerve cells. The main components of the myenteric plexus shown on the *inset* at higher magnification are nerve cell bodies of the postsynaptic parasympathetic neurons, satellite cells (peripheral neuroglia cells), and unmyelinated nerve fibers with nonmyelinating Remak Schwann cells. Nerve cells can be distinguished by their basophilic cytoplasm and prominent nucleus containing darker nucleolus. The free surface of the intestine is covered by the serosa, which consists of simple squamous epithelium (mesothelium) and a small amount of underlying connective tissue (*CT*). Deep into the muscularis externa toward the lumen of the intestine is a dense irregular connective tissue layer known as *submucosa*. Note collagen fibers, adipose cells, and accumulation of lymphocytes (*lower right corner*) in this layer. ×180; inset × 450.

Serosa

The **serosa** of the parts of the small intestine that are located intraperitoneally in the abdominal cavity corresponds to the general description at the beginning of the chapter. Parts of the duodenum that lie in the retroperitoneal space and have direct contact with structures and organs on the posterior abdominal wall have typical adventitia.

■ LARGE INTESTINE

The **large intestine** comprises the **cecum** with its projecting **vermiform appendix**, the **colon**, the **rectum**, and the **anal canal**. The colon is further subdivided on the basis of its anatomic locations into the ascending colon, transverse colon, descending colon, and sigmoid colon. The four layers characteristic of the alimentary canal are present throughout. However, several distinctive features exist at the gross level (Fig. 17.28):

- **Teniae coli** represent three narrowed, thickened, equally spaced bands of the outer longitudinal layer of the muscularis externa. They are primarily visible in the cecum and colon and are absent in the rectum, anal canal, and vermiform appendix.
- **Haustra coli** are visible sacculations between the teniae coli on the external surface of the cecum and colon.
- **Omental appendices** are small, fatty projections of the serosa, observed on the outer surface of the colon.

Mucosa

The **mucosa** of the large intestine has a "smooth" surface; neither plicae circulares nor villi are present. It contains numerous straight tubular intestinal glands (crypts of Lieberkühn) that extend through the full thickness of the mucosa (Fig. 17.29a). The glands consist of simple columnar epithelium, as does the intestinal surface from which they invaginate. Examination of the luminal surface of the large intestine at the microscopic level reveals the openings of the glands, which are arranged in an orderly pattern (Fig. 17.29b).

The principal functions of the large intestine are reabsorption of electrolytes and water and elimination of undigested food and waste.

The primary function of the **columnar absorptive cells** is reabsorption of water and electrolytes. The morphology of the absorptive cells of the large intestine is essentially identical to that of the enterocytes of the small intestine. Reabsorption is accomplished by the same Na^+/K^+-activated ATPase-driven transport system as described for the small intestine.

Elimination of semisolid to solid waste materials is facilitated by the large amounts of mucus secreted by the numerous **goblet cells** of the intestinal glands. Goblet cells are more numerous in the large intestine than in the small intestine (see Fig. 17.29a and Plate 17.9, page 686). They produce mucin that is secreted continuously to lubricate the bowel, facilitating the passage of increasingly solid contents.

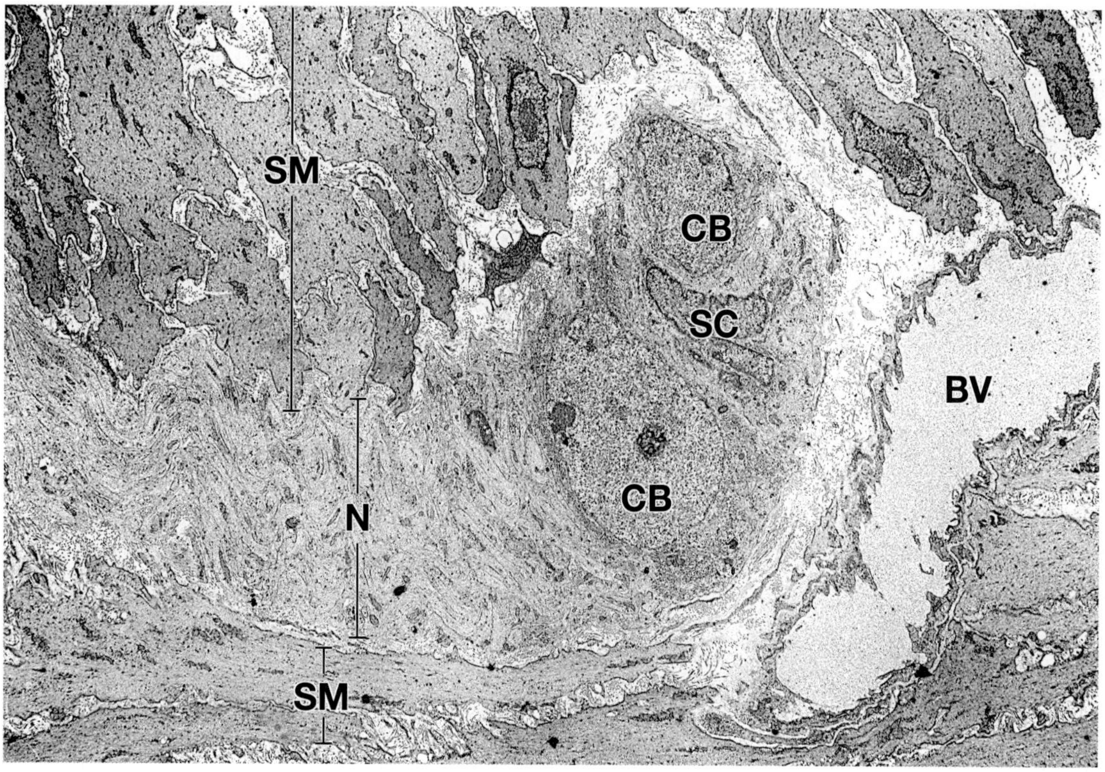

FIGURE 17.27. Electron micrograph of the myenteric (Auerbach) plexus. The plexus is located between the two smooth muscle (*SM*) layers of the muscularis externa. It consists of nerve cell bodies (*CB*) and an extensive network of nerve fibers (*N*). A satellite cell (*SC*), also referred to as an *enteric glial cell*, is seen in proximity to the neuron cell bodies. These cells have structural and chemical features in common with glial cells of the CNS. *BV*, blood vessel. ×3,800.

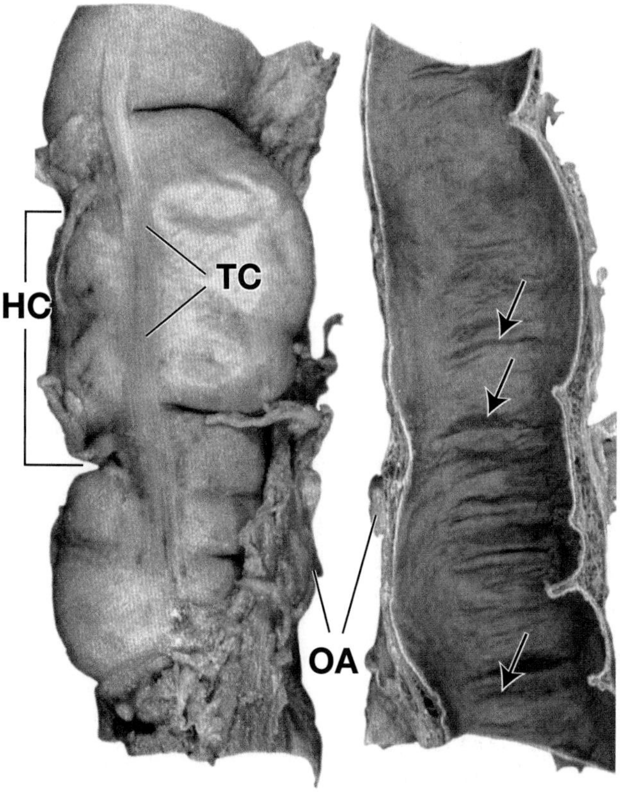

FIGURE 17.28. Photograph of the large intestine. This photograph shows the outer (serosal) surface (*left*) and internal (mucosal) surface (*right*) of the transverse colon. On the outer surface, note the characteristic features of the large intestine: a distinctive smooth muscle band representing one of the three teniae coli (*TC*); haustra coli (*HC*), the sacculations of the colon located between the teniae; and omental appendices (*OA*), small peritoneal projections filled with fat. The smooth mucosal surface shows semilunar folds (*arrows*) formed in response to contractions of the muscularis externa. Compare the mucosal surface as shown here with that of the small intestine (Fig. 17.17).

The mucosal epithelium of the large intestine contains the same cell types as the small intestine, except Paneth cells, which are normally absent in humans.

Columnar absorptive cells predominate (4:1) over goblet cells in most of the colon, although this is not always apparent in histologic sections (see Fig. 17.29a). The ratio decreases, however, approaching 1:1, near the rectum, where the number of goblet cells increases. Although the absorptive cells secrete glycocalyx at a rapid rate (turnover time is 16–24 hours in humans), this layer has not been shown to contain digestive enzymes in the colon. As in the small intestine, however, Na^+/K^+-ATPase is abundant and is localized in the lateral plasma membranes of the absorptive cells. The intercellular space is often dilated, indicating active transport of fluid.

Goblet cells may mature deep into the intestinal gland, even in the replicative zone (Fig. 17.30). They secrete mucus continuously, even to the point where they reach the luminal surface. Here, at the surface, the secretion rate exceeds the synthesis rate, and "exhausted" goblet cells appear in the epithelium. These cells are tall and thin and have a small number of mucinogen granules in the central apical cytoplasm. An infrequently observed cell type, the caveolated "tuft" cell, has also been described in the colonic epithelium; however, this cell may be a form of exhausted goblet cell.

Epithelial Cell Renewal in the Large Intestine

All intestinal epithelial cells in the large intestine derive from a single stem cell population.

As in the **small intestine**, all of the mucosal epithelial cells of the large intestine arise from stem cells located at

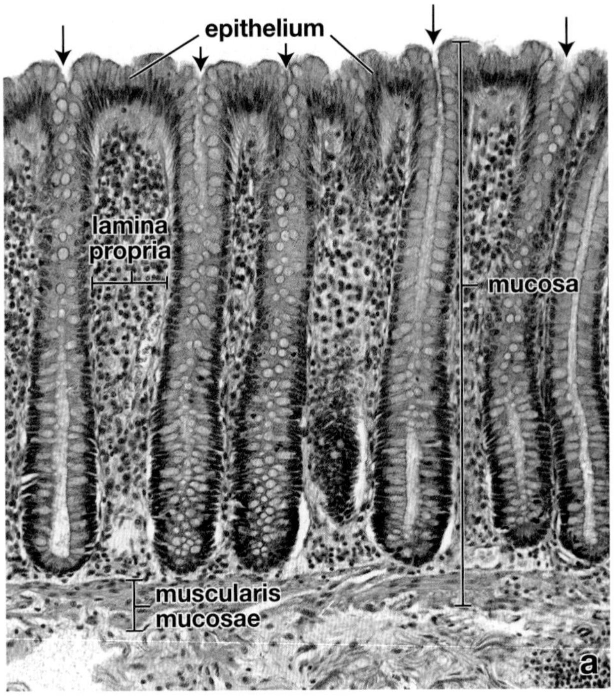

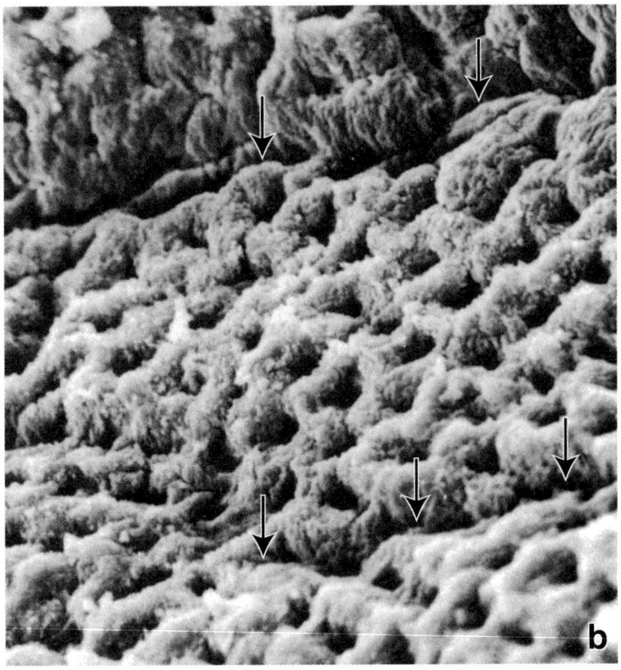

FIGURE 17.29. Mucosa of the large intestine. a. This photomicrograph of a hematoxylin and eosin (H&E) preparation shows the mucosa and part of the submucosa. The surface epithelium is continuous with the straight, unbranched, tubular intestinal glands (crypts of Lieberkühn). The openings of the glands at the intestinal surface are identified (*arrows*). The epithelial cells consist principally of absorptive and goblet cells. As the absorptive cells are followed into the glands, they become fewer in number, whereas the goblet cells increase in number. The highly cellular lamina propria contains numerous lymphocytes and other cells of the immune system. **b.** Scanning electron micrograph of the human mucosal surface of the large intestine. The surface is divided into territories by clefts (*arrows*). Each territory contains 25–100 gland openings. ×140. (Reprinted with permission from Fenoglio CM, Richart RM, Kaye GI. Comparative electron-microscopic features of normal, hyperplastic, and adenomatous human colonic epithelium. II. Variations in surface architecture found by scanning electron microscopy. *Gastroenterology*. 1975;69:100–109.)

the bottom of the intestinal gland. The lower third of the gland constitutes the intestinal stem cell niche, where newly generated cells undergo two to three more divisions as they begin their migration up to the luminal surface, where they are shed about 5 days later. The intermediate cell types found in the lower third of the intestinal gland are identical to those seen in the small intestine.

The turnover times of the epithelial cells of the large intestine are similar to those of the small intestine (i.e., about 6 days for absorptive cells and goblet cells and up to 4 weeks for enteroendocrine cells). Senile epithelial cells that reach the mucosal surface undergo apoptosis and are shed into the lumen at the midpoint between two adjacent intestinal glands.

Lamina Propria

Although the **lamina propria** of the large intestine contains the same basic components as the rest of the digestive tract, it demonstrates some additional structural features and greater development of some others, including:

- **Collagen table**, which represents a thick layer of collagen and proteoglycans that lies between the basal lamina of the epithelium and that of the fenestrated absorptive venous capillaries. This layer is as much as 5 μm thick in the normal human colon and can be up to 3 times that thickness in human hyperplastic colonic polyps. The collagen table participates in the regulation of water and electrolyte transport from the intercellular compartment of the epithelium to the vascular compartment.
- **Pericryptal fibroblast sheath**, which constitutes a well-developed fibroblast population of regularly replicating cells. They divide immediately beneath the base of the intestinal gland, adjacent to the stem cells found in the epithelium (in both the large and small intestines). The fibroblasts then differentiate and migrate upward in parallel and synchrony with the epithelial cells. Although the ultimate fate of the pericryptal fibroblast is unknown, most of these cells, after they reach the level of the luminal surface, take on the morphologic and histochemical characteristics of macrophages. Some evidence suggests that the macrophages of the core of the lamina propria in the large intestine may arise as a terminal differentiation of the pericryptal fibroblasts.
- **GALT**, which is continuous with that of the terminal ileum. In the large intestine, GALT is more extensively developed; large lymphatic nodules distort the regular spacing of the intestinal glands and extend into the submucosa. The extensive development of the immune system in the colon probably reflects the large number and variety of microorganisms and noxious end products of metabolism normally present in the lumen.

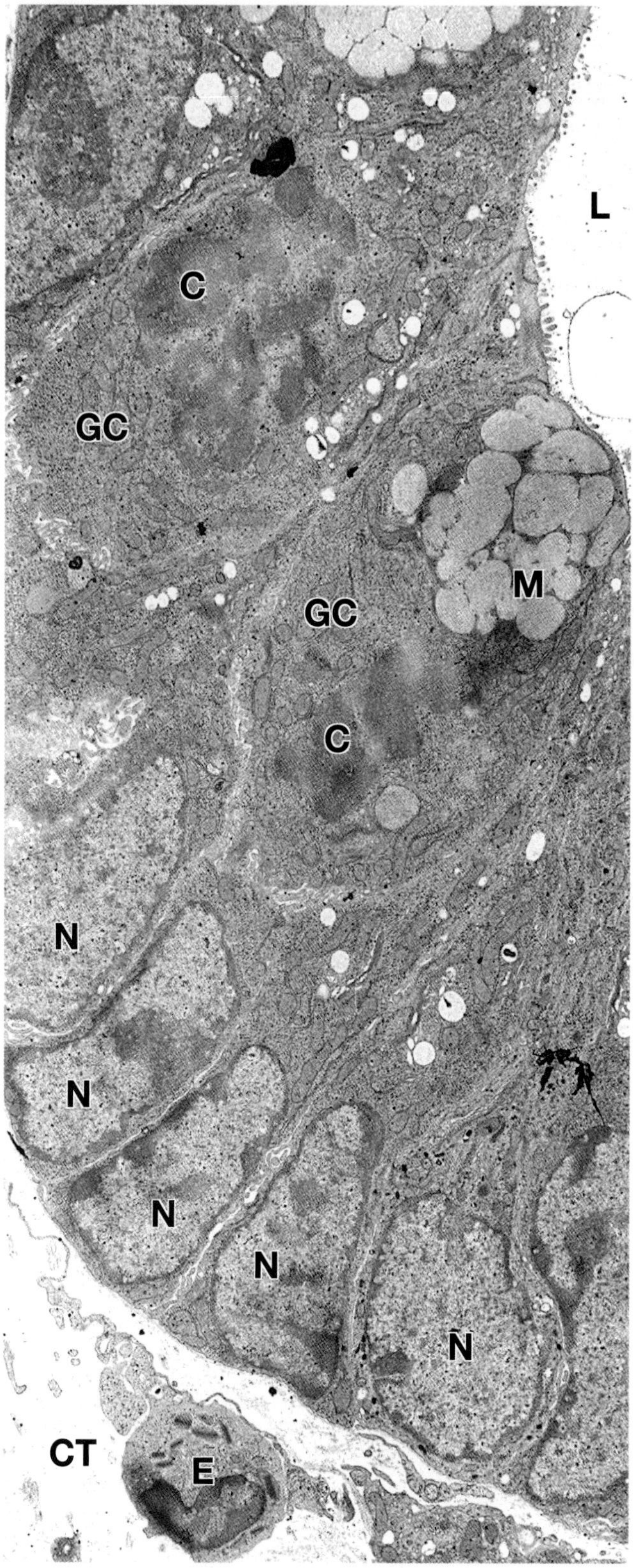

FIGURE 17.30. Electron micrograph of dividing goblet cells. This electron micrograph demonstrates that certain cells of the intestine continue to divide even after they have differentiated. Here, two goblet cells (*GC*) are shown dividing. Typically, dividing cells move away from the basal lamina toward the lumen. One of the goblet cells demonstrates mucinogen granules (*M*) in its apical cytoplasm. The chromosomes (*C*) of the dividing cells are not surrounded by a nuclear membrane. Compare with the nuclei (*N*) of the nondividing intestinal epithelial cells. The lumen of the gland (*L*) is on the *right*. *CT*, connective tissue; *E*, eosinophil. ×5,000.

- **Lymphatic vessels.** In general, lymphatic vessels are not present in the core of the lamina propria between the intestinal glands, and there are no vessels that extend toward the luminal surface of the large intestine. However, using a selective marker for lymphatic epithelium, researchers have found occasional small lymphatic vessels at the bases of the intestinal glands. These lymphatic vessels drain into the lymphatic network within the muscularis mucosae. The next step in lymph drainage occurs in the lymphatic plexuses in the submucosa and muscularis externa before lymph leaves the wall of the large intestine and drains into the regional lymph nodes. To understand the clinical significance of the lymphatic pattern in the large intestine, see Folder 17.6.

Muscularis Externa

As noted, in the cecum and colon (the ascending, transverse, descending, and sigmoid colons), the **outer layer of the muscularis externa** is, in part, condensed into prominent longitudinal bands of muscle, called **teniae coli**, which may be seen at the gross level (see Fig. 17.28). Between these bands, the longitudinal layer forms an extremely thin sheet. In the rectum, anal canal, and vermiform appendix, the outer longitudinal layer of smooth muscle is a uniformly thick layer, as in the small intestine.

Bundles of muscle from the teniae coli penetrate the **inner, circular layer of muscle** at irregular intervals along the length and circumference of the colon. These apparent discontinuities in the muscularis externa allow segments of the colon to contract independently, leading to the formation of **haustra coli**, sacculations of the colon wall.

The muscularis externa of the large intestine produces two major types of contraction: segmentation and peristalsis. Segmentation is local and does not result in the propulsion of contents. Peristalsis results in the distal mass movement of the colonic contents. Mass peristaltic movements occur infrequently; in healthy persons, they usually occur once a day to empty the distal colon.

Submucosa and Serosa

The **submucosa** of the large intestine corresponds to the general description already given. Where the large intestine is directly in contact with other structures (as on much of its posterior surface), its outer layer is an adventitia; elsewhere, the outer layer is a typical serosa.

Cecum and Appendix

The **cecum** forms a blind pouch just distal to the ileocecal valve; the appendix is a thin, finger-like extension of this pouch. The histology of the cecum closely resembles that of the rest of the colon; the **appendix** differs from it in having a uniform layer of longitudinal muscle in the muscularis externa (Fig. 17.31 and Plate 17.10, page 688). The most conspicuous feature of the appendix is the large number of lymphatic nodules that extend into THE submucosa. In many adults, the normal structure of the appendix is lost, and

FOLDER 17.6

CLINICAL CORRELATION: THE PATTERN OF LYMPH VESSEL DISTRIBUTION AND DISEASES OF THE LARGE INTESTINE

The normal **absence of lymphatic drainage** from the lamina propria of the large intestine was initially discovered using standard techniques of analyzing tissue samples obtained from biopsies with light and electron microscopy. A specific monoclonal antibody called *D2-40* is currently being used to study the distribution of lymphatic vessels within the lamina propria that may be associated with several disease processes. D2-40 reacts with a 40-kDa *O*-linked sialoglycoprotein expressed on the lymphatic endothelium. For instance, in the chronic superficial inflammation of the colon and rectum known as **ulcerative colitis**, the formation of granulation tissue is associated with proliferation of blood and lymphatic vessels within the lamina propria. Lymphangiogenesis (the growth of lymphatic vessels) in this disease is linked to the expression of vascular endothelial growth factors (VEGFs). The progress of treatment in ulcerative colitis can be monitored by biopsies, which show the disappearance of lymphatic vessels from the lamina propria. Conversely, an increased number of lymphatic vessels in the lamina propria signals the presence of active inflammation.

Discovery of the distribution of lymphatic vessels in the large intestine established the basis for the current management of **adenomas** (adenomatous polyps of the large intestine). These are intraepithelial neoplasms located on the mass of tissue that protrudes into the lumen of the large intestine (Fig. F17.6.1). The absence of lymphatic vessels from the lamina propria was important in understanding the slow rate of metastasis from certain colon cancers. Cancers that develop in large adenomatous colonic polyps may grow extensively within the epithelium and lamina propria before they gain access to the lymphatic vessels at the level of the muscularis mucosae. Because almost 50% of all adenomatous polyps of the large intestine are located in the rectum and sigmoid colon, they can be detected with rectosigmoidoscopy. As long as the lesion is confined to the mucosa, the endoscopic removal of such polyps is regarded as adequate clinical treatment. However, the final therapeutic decision must be confirmed after careful microscopic examination of the resected specimen.

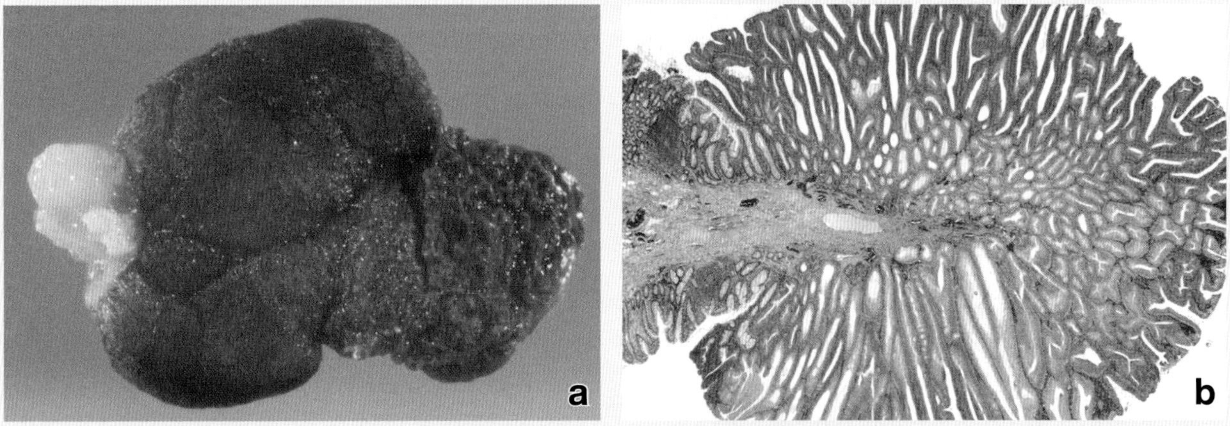

FIGURE F17.6.1. Adenomatous polyp of the large intestine. a. This image shows a macroscopic view of a polyp (about 2 cm in diameter) that was surgically removed from the large intestine during endoscopic colonoscopy. It has a characteristic bosselated surface (with rounded swellings) and a stalk by which it attaches to the wall of the colon. **b.** This photomicrograph was obtained from the center of the polyp. At the tip of the polyp, note the repetitive pattern of tubules covered with neoplastic epithelial cells that have migrated and accumulated on the intestinal surface. The stalk in the center is continuous with the submucosa of the colon. Note also the normal simple columnar epithelium of the large intestine at the base of the stalk. (Reproduced from Mitros FA, Rubin E. The gastrointestinal tract. In Rubin R, Strayer DS, eds. *Rubin's Pathology: Clinicopathologic Foundations of Medicine*. 5th ed. Lippincott Williams & Wilkins; 2008.)

the appendage is filled with fibrous scar tissue. Blockage of the opening between the appendix and the cecum, usually due to scarring, buildup of thick mucus, or stool that enters the lumen of the appendix from the cecum, may cause **appendicitis** (inflammation of the appendix). The appendix is also a common site for **carcinoid**, a type of tumor originating from enteroendocrine cells of lining mucosa (see Folder 17.3).

Rectum and Anal Canal

The **rectum** is the dilated distal portion of the alimentary canal. Its upper part is distinguished from the rest of the large intestine by the presence of folds called **transverse rectal folds**. The mucosa of the rectum is similar to that of the rest of the distal colon, having straight, tubular intestinal glands with many goblet cells.

The most distal portion of the alimentary canal is the **anal canal**. It has an average length of 4 cm and extends from the upper aspect of the pelvic diaphragm to the anus (Fig. 17.32). The upper part of the anal canal has longitudinal folds called **anal columns**. Depressions between the anal columns are called **anal sinuses**. The anal canal is divided into three zones according to the character of the epithelial lining:

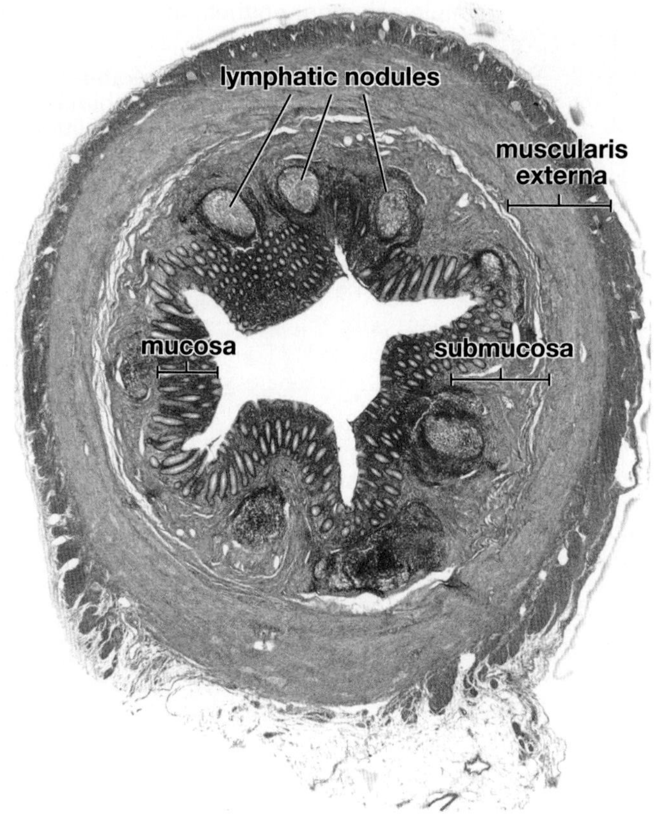

FIGURE 17.31. Photomicrograph of a cross section through the vermiform appendix. The vermiform appendix displays the same four layers as those of the large intestine, except that its diameter is smaller. Typically, lymphatic nodules are seen within the entire mucosa and usually extend into the submucosa. Note the distinct germinal centers within the lymphatic nodules. The muscularis externa is composed of a relatively thick circular layer and a much thinner outer longitudinal layer. The appendix is covered by a serosa that is continuous with the mesentery of the appendix (*lower right*). ×10.

- **Colorectal zone**, which is found in the upper third of the anal canal and contains simple columnar epithelium with characteristics identical to that in the rectum
- **Anal transitional zone (ATZ)**, which occupies the middle third of the anal canal. It represents a transition between the simple columnar epithelium of the rectal mucosa and the stratified squamous epithelium of the perianal skin. The ATZ possesses a stratified columnar epithelium interposed between the simple columnar epithelium and the stratified squamous epithelium, which extends to the cutaneous zone of the anal canal (Fig. 17.33 and Plate 17.11, page 690).
- **Squamous zone**, which is found in the lower third of the anal canal. This zone is lined with stratified squamous epithelium that is continuous with that of the perineal skin.

In the anal canal, **anal glands** extend into the submucosa and even into the muscularis externa. These branched, straight tubular glands secrete mucus onto the anal surface through ducts lined with stratified columnar epithelium. Sometimes, the anal glands are surrounded by diffuse lymphatic tissue. They often lead to the formation of pathologic **fistulas** (an opening between the anal canal and the perianal skin).

Large apocrine glands, the **circumanal glands**, are found in the skin surrounding the anal orifice. In some animals, the secretion of these glands acts as a sex attractant. Hair follicles and sebaceous glands are also found at this site.

The submucosa of the anal columns contains the terminal ramifications of the superior rectal artery and the rectal venous plexus. Enlargements of these submucosal veins constitute **internal hemorrhoids**, which are related to elevated venous pressure in the portal circulation (**portal hypertension**). There are no teniae coli at the level of the rectum; the longitudinal layer of the muscularis externa forms a uniform sheet. The muscularis mucosae disappears at about the level of the ATZ, where the circular layer of the muscularis externa thickens to form the internal anal sphincter. The external anal sphincter is formed by striated muscle of the pelvic floor.

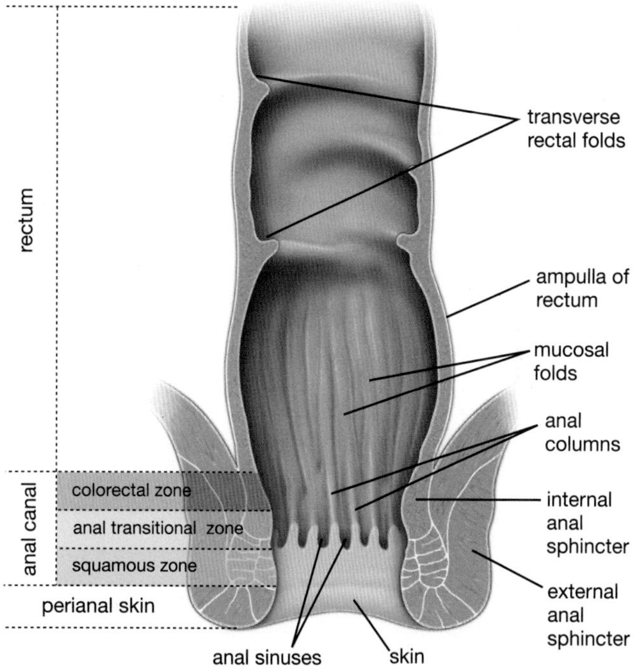

FIGURE 17.32. Drawing of the rectum and anal canal. The rectum and anal canal are the terminal portions of the large intestine. They are lined by the colorectal mucosa that possesses a simple columnar epithelium containing mostly goblet cells and numerous anal glands. In the anal canal, the simple columnar epithelium undergoes transition into a stratified columnar (or cuboidal) epithelium and then to a stratified squamous epithelium. This transition occurs in the area referred to as the *anal transitional zone*, which occupies the middle third of the anal canal between the colorectal zone and the squamous zone of the perianal skin.

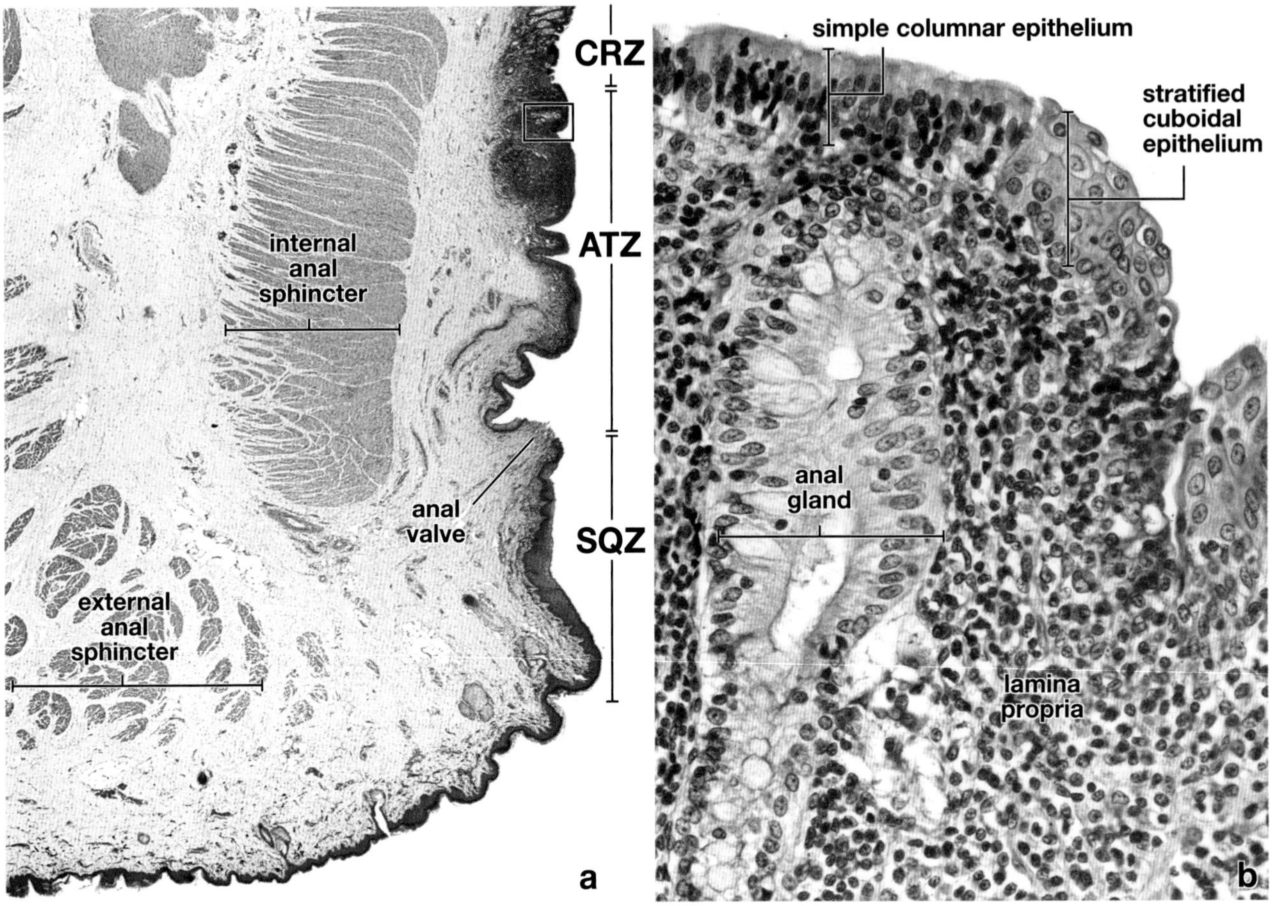

FIGURE 17.33. Photomicrographs of the anal canal. a. This photomicrograph shows a longitudinal section through the wall of the anal canal. Note the three zones in the anal canal: the squamous zone (*SQZ*) containing stratified squamous epithelium; the anal transitional zone (*ATZ*) containing stratified squamous, stratified cuboidal, or columnar epithelium and simple columnar epithelium of the rectal mucosa; and the colorectal zone (*CRZ*) containing only simple columnar epithelium like the rest of the colon. Note the anal valve that demarcates the transition between the *ATZ* and *SQZ*. The internal anal sphincter is derived from the thickening of the circular layer of the muscularis externa. A small portion of the external anal sphincter is seen subcutaneously. ×10. **b.** This high magnification of the area indicated by the *rectangle* in **a** shows the area of the anal transitional zone. Note the abrupt transition between stratified cuboidal and simple columnar epithelium. The simple columnar epithelium of anal glands extends into the submucosa. These straight, mucus-secreting tubular glands are surrounded by diffuse lymphatic tissue. ×200.

FOLDER 17.7

CLINICAL CORRELATION: COLORECTAL CANCER

Colorectal cancer (colon or rectal cancer) is one of the major causes of cancer-related deaths in the United States. Almost 100,000 cases of colon cancer and 40,000 cases of rectal cancers are diagnosed in the United States each year, leading to >50,000 deaths. Colorectal cancer commonly occurs between the ages of 60 and 79 years in individuals with a low-fiber and high-fat diet. Most colorectal cancers (about 98%) are adenocarcinomas and begin as small, benign clumps of cells that arise from the glandular epithelium. They form adenomatous polyps, which typically can be detected by a sigmoidoscopy or colonoscopy. In microscopic examinations, the irregular intestinal glands are lined by one or more layers of dark-stained cancer cells with or without mucus production (Fig. F17.7.1).

Colon cancers vary in distribution throughout the large intestine. Approximately 38% of cancers are found in the cecum and ascending colon, 38% in the transverse colon, 18% in the descending colon, and 8% in the sigmoid colon. It is now thought that chromosomal instability associated with the stepwise accumulation of mutations in proto-oncogenes and suppressor genes plays a vital role in the development of colorectal cancer. Initially, when epithelial cells lose the **APC tumor suppressor gene**, they develop small polyps. Next, mutation in the **K-Ras proto-oncogene** transforms the polyp into a benign adenoma. These cells further undergo mutation and/or deletion of the **p53 tumor suppressor gene** and **DCC gene**, thus leading to the development of the invasive form of adenocarcinoma. The second pathway leading to the development of colorectal cancer is caused by genetic lesions in **DNA-mismatch repair genes** in the epithelial cell of the colon. Colorectal cancer in its early stage usually produces general symptoms, such as changes in bowel movements, persistent constipation or diarrhea, rectal cramping, or rectal bleeding, which may be an indication of a developing malignancy. With early detection, surgery, radiation, and/or chemotherapy can be effective treatments.

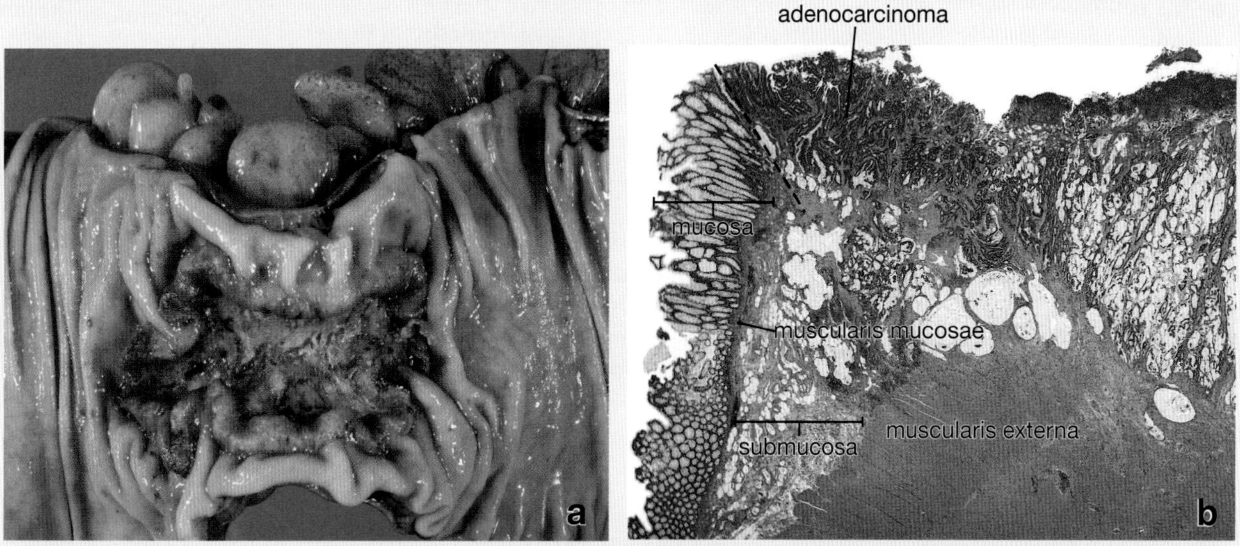

FIGURE F17.7.1. Macroscopic and microscopic features of adenocarcinoma of the colon. a. This photograph shows a surgically resected segment of the colon containing an elevated and centrally ulcerated mass. **b.** This low-magnification photomicrograph shows a section of a tumor that was taken from a free margin of the lesion to show both the typical mucosa of the large intestine (*left*) and the invasive adenocarcinoma (*top left*). The abrupt transition to adenocarcinoma is marked by a *dashed line*. Intestinal glands in the normal part of the epithelium are lined by a single layer of goblet and absorptive cells and occupy the entire thickness of the mucosa. In contrast, tissue invaded by the adenocarcinoma shows an irregular pattern of glands without the presence of mucous production. Cells and their nuclei are intensively stained with hematoxylin (hyperchromatic). Note that muscle fibers derived from the muscularis mucosa travel among colonic glands. ×120. (Both images courtesy of Dr. Thomas C. Smyrk.)

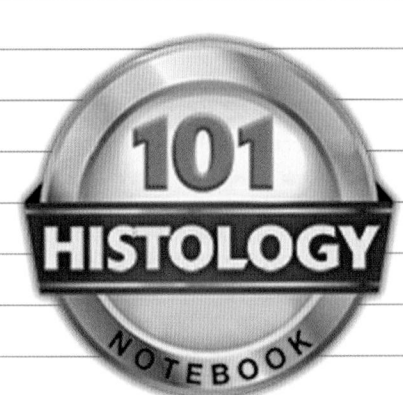

DIGESTIVE SYSTEM II: ESOPHAGUS AND GASTROINTESTINAL TRACT

OVERVIEW OF THE ESOPHAGUS AND GASTROINTESTINAL TRACT

- Extending from the **esophagus** to the **anal canal**, the **alimentary canal** is a hollow tube composed of four distinctive layers (from the lumen going outward): **mucosa, submucosa, muscularis externa**, and **serosa** (when organ is covered by peritoneum) or **adventitia** (when organ is surrounded by connective tissue).
- The **mucosa** is always associated with underlying **lamina propria** (loose connective tissue) and **muscularis mucosae** (smooth muscle layer). The type of mucosal epithelium varies from region to region, as does the thickness of lamina propria and muscularis mucosae.
- The **submucosa** consists of dense irregular connective tissue containing blood and lymphatic vessels, nerve plexus, and occasional glands.
- The **muscularis externa** mixes and propels the content of the canal. It consists of two layers of smooth muscle: The inner layer is circular and the outer layer is longitudinally oriented, with myenteric nerve plexus between them.
- The **serosa** or **adventitia** constitutes the outermost layer of the alimentary canal.

ESOPHAGUS

- The **mucosa** of the esophagus has nonkeratinized stratified squamous epithelium. The **submucosa** contains **esophageal glands proper** that lubricates and protects the mucosal surface. The **muscularis externa** is striated at its upper part and is gradually replaced by a smooth muscle layer in the lower part.
- At the **esophagogastric junction**, nonkeratinized stratified squamous epithelium changes abruptly to simple columnar epithelium of the gastric mucosa. Esophageal cardiac glands are present in the lamina propria at this junction.

STOMACH

- The stomach has three histologic regions: **cardiac** surrounding the esophageal orifice, **pyloric** near the gastroduodenal junction, and **fundic** (anatomically occupied by **fundus** and **body**).
- The **mucosa** of the fundic region forms a number of longitudinal folds (**rugae**). **Surface mucous cells** line the inner surface of the stomach and the **gastric pits**, which are the openings into the branched fundic glands. Surface mucous cells produce an insoluble, viscous, gel-like coat that contains bicarbonate ions to protect against physical and chemical injury of the gastric wall.
- The **fundic glands** produce gastric juice containing four major components: hydrochloric acid (HCl), pepsin (proteolytic enzyme), intrinsic factor (for vitamin B_{12} absorption), and acid-protective mucus.
- The epithelium of the fundic gland has five major cell types: **mucous neck cells**, which produce soluble and low-alkaline mucus secretions; **parietal cells**, which are responsible for the production of HCl within the lumen of their intracellular canalicular system; **chief cells**, which secrete pepsinogen; **enteroendocrine cells**, which produce small regulatory gastrointestinal and paracrine hormones; and **stem cells**, which are precursors to all fundic gland cells.
- **Mucous neck cells** produce soluble and low-alkaline mucus secretions.
- **Parietal cells** are large cells in the middle of the gland and are responsible for the production of HCl within the lumen of their intracellular canalicular system. They also secrete intrinsic factor.
- **Chief cells** reside at the bottom of the fundic gland and secrete the protein pepsinogen. On contact with the low pH of gastric juice, pepsinogen is converted to pepsin, an active proteolytic enzyme.
- **Enteroendocrine cells** are found at every level of the fundic gland. They produce small regulatory gastrointestinal and paracrine hormones.
- **Stem cells** are precursors to all cells in the fundic gland and are located in the neck region and base of the gland.
- **Cardiac glands** are entirely composed of mucus-secreting cells with occasional interspersed enteroendocrine cells.
- **Pyloric glands** are branched and lined with cells resembling surface mucous cells and occasional enteroendocrine cells.

SMALL INTESTINE

- The **small intestine** is the longest component of the digestive tract and is divided into three anatomic regions: **duodenum** (with mucus-secreting Brunner glands in the submucosa), **jejunum**, and **ileum** (with Peyer patches in the submucosa).
- The mucosa of the small intestine is lined by simple columnar epithelium, and its absorptive surface is increased by the **plicae circulares** and **villi**. Simple tubular intestinal glands (or crypts) extend from the muscularis mucosae and open into the lumen at the base of the villi.
- The intestinal mucosal epithelium has at least five types of cells: **enterocytes**, which are absorptive cells specialized for the transport of substances from the lumen to the blood or lymphatic vessels; **goblet cells**, which are unicellular mucin-secreting glands interspersed among other cells of the intestinal epithelium; **Paneth cells**, which secrete antimicrobial substances (e.g., lysozyme, α-defensins); **enteroendocrine cells**, which produce various paracrine and endocrine gastrointestinal hormones; and **M cells**, which are specialized as antigen-transporting cells and cover lymphatic nodules in the lamina propria.
- Cells of the intestinal mucosal epithelium are found both in the intestinal glands and on the surface of the villi, and their ratio changes depending on the region.
- **Enterocytes** are absorptive cells specialized for the transport of substances from the lumen to the blood or lymphatic vessels.
- **Goblet cells** are unicellular mucin-secreting glands interspersed among other cells of the intestinal epithelium.
- **Paneth cells** are found at the bases of the intestinal glands, and their primary function is to secrete antimicrobial substances (e.g., lysozyme, α-defensins).
- **Enteroendocrine cells** produce various paracrine and endocrine gastrointestinal hormones.
- **M cells** (microfold cells) are specialized as antigen-transporting cells. They cover lymphatic nodules in the lamina propria.
- **Stem cells** are precursors to all cells in the intestinal gland and are located near the base of the gland.
- The **muscularis externa** coordinates contractions of the inner circular and the outer longitudinal layers, producing peristalsis that moves the intestinal contents distally. The autonomic **myenteric plexus** (Auerbach plexus) innervates the muscularis externa.

LARGE INTESTINE

- The **large intestine** is composed of the **cecum** (with its projecting **vermiform appendix**), **colon**, **rectum**, and **anal canal**. The appendix has a large number of lymphatic nodules that extend into the submucosa.
- The mucosa of the large intestine contains numerous straight tubular **intestinal glands** (crypts of Lieberkühn) that extend through the full thickness of this layer. The glands are lined by enterocytes (for resorption of water) and goblet cells (for lubrication).
- The **muscularis externa** of the colon has its outer layer condensed into three prominent longitudinal bands, the **teniae coli**, which lead to the formation of sacculations in the wall of the large intestine (haustra coli).
- In the **anal canal**, the simple columnar epithelium becomes stratified in the **anal transitional zone** (middle third of the anal canal). The lower part of the anal canal is covered by stratified squamous epithelium that is continuous with the perineal skin.

PLATE 17.1 ■ ESOPHAGUS

The **esophagus**, the first part of the alimentary canal, represents a muscular tube that conveys food and other substances from the oropharynx to the stomach. The **mucosa** that lines the length of the esophagus has a nonkeratinized stratified squamous epithelium. The underlying **lamina propria** is similar to the lamina propria throughout the alimentary tract; diffuse lymphatic tissue is scattered throughout, and lymphatic nodules are present. The deep layer of the mucosa, the **muscularis mucosae**, is composed of longitudinally organized bundles of smooth muscle fibers. The **submucosa** consists of dense irregular connective tissue that contains the larger blood and lymphatic vessels, nerve fibers, and ganglion cells. The nerve fibers and ganglion cells make up the submucosal plexus (Meissner plexus). The **muscularis externa** consists of two muscle layers, an inner circular layer and an outer longitudinal layer. The upper one-third of muscularis externa consists of striated muscle, a continuation of the muscle of the pharynx. Striated muscle and smooth muscle bundles are mixed and interwoven in the muscularis externa of the middle third of the esophagus. The muscularis externa of the distal one-third consists only of smooth muscle, as in the rest of the digestive tract.

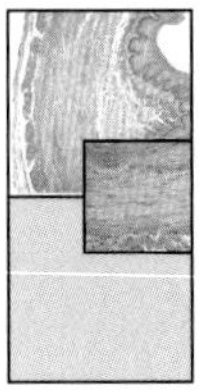

Esophagus, monkey, hematoxylin and eosin (H&E) ×60; inset ×400.

A cross section of the wall of the esophagus is shown here. The **mucosa** (*Muc*) consists of stratified squamous epithelium (*Ep*), **lamina propria** (*LP*), and **muscularis mucosae** (*MM*). The boundary between the epithelium and lamina propria is distinct, although uneven, as a result of the presence of numerous deep connective tissue papillae. The basal layer of the epithelium stains intensely, appearing as a dark band that is relatively conspicuous at low magnification. The intense staining is due, in part, to the cytoplasmic basophilia of the basal cells. The small size of the basal cells results in a high nuclear–cytoplasmic ratio, which further intensifies the hematoxylin staining of this layer.

The **submucosa** consists of dense irregular connective tissue that contains the larger blood vessels and nerves. No glands are seen in the submucosa in this figure, but they are regularly present throughout this layer and are likely to be included in a section of the wall. Whereas the boundary between the epithelium and lamina propria is striking, the boundary between mucosa (*Muc*) and submucosa (*SubM*) is less well marked, although it is readily discernable.

The **muscularis externa** (*ME*) shown here is composed of two muscle layers, an inner circular layer and a much thinner outer longitudinal layer (*L*). In this specimen, the muscularis externa (*ME*) is composed largely of smooth muscle, but it also contains areas of striated muscle. Although the striations are not evident at this low magnification, the more densely stained eosinophilic areas (*asterisks*) prove to be striated muscle when observed at higher magnification. Reference to the *inset*, which is from an area in the *lower half* of the figure, substantiates this identification.

The *inset* shows circularly oriented striated and smooth muscle. The striated muscle stains more intensely with eosin but of greater significance are the distribution and number of nuclei. In the center of the *inset*, numerous elongated and uniformly oriented nuclei are present; this is smooth muscle (*SM*). Above and below, few elongated nuclei are present; moreover, they are largely at the periphery of the bundles. This is striated muscle (*StM*); the cross-striations are just perceptible in some areas. The specimen shown here is from the middle of the esophagus, where both smooth and striated muscles are present. The muscularis externa of the distal third of the esophagus would contain only smooth muscle, whereas that of the proximal third would consist of striated muscle. External to the muscularis externa is the **adventitia** (*Adv*) consisting of dense connective tissue.

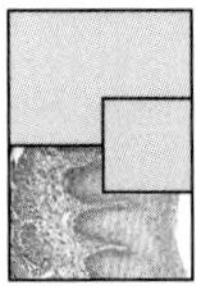

Mucosa, esophagus, monkey, H&E ×300.

As in other stratified squamous epithelia, new cells are produced in the basal layer, from which they move to the surface. During this migration, the shape and orientation of the cells change. This change in cell shape and orientation is also reflected in the appearance of the nuclei. In the deeper layers, the nuclei are spherical; in the more superficial layers, the nuclei are elongated and oriented parallel to the surface. Those nuclei can be seen throughout the epithelial layer, particularly the surface cells, indicating that the epithelium is not keratinized. In some instances, the epithelium of the upper regions of the esophagus may be parakeratinized or, more rarely, keratinized.

As shown in this figure, the **lamina propria** (*LP*) is a very cellular, loose connective tissue containing many lymphocytes (*Lym*), small blood vessels, and lymphatic vessels (*LV*). The deepest part of the mucosa is the muscularis mucosae (*MM*). A layer of smooth muscle defines the boundary between mucosa and submucosa. The nuclei of the smooth muscle cells of the muscularis mucosae appear spherical because the cells have been cut in cross section.

Adv, adventitia
Ep, stratified squamous epithelium
L, longitudinal layer of muscularis externa
LP, lamina propria
LV, lymphatic vessels
Lym, lymphocytes
ME, muscularis externa
MM, muscularis mucosae
Muc, mucosa
SM, smooth muscle
StM, striated muscle
SubM, submucosa
arrows, lower figure, lymphocytes in epithelium
asterisks, upper figure, areas containing striated muscle in the musculatis externa

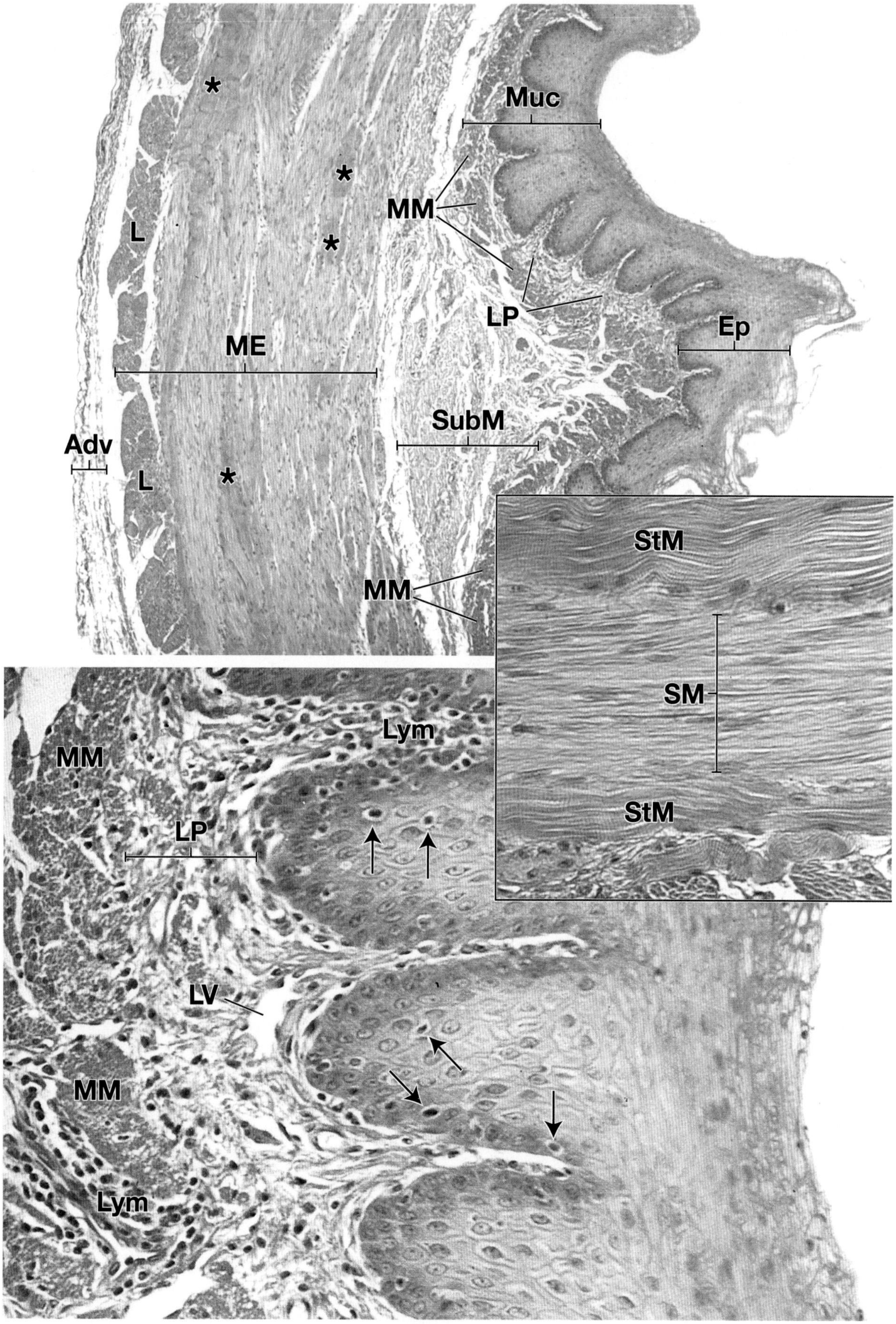
Muc
MM
LP
Ep
ME
L
L
Adv
SubM
MM
StM
SM
StM
MM
Lym
LP
LV
MM
Lym

PLATE 17.2 ■ ESOPHAGUS AND STOMACH, CARDIAC REGION

The **esophagogastric junction** marks a change in function from that of a conduit (esophagus) to that of a digestive organ (stomach). The epithelium of the mucosa changes from stratified squamous (protective) to a simple columnar secretory epithelium that forms mucosal glands that secrete mucinogen, digestive enzymes, and hydrochloric acid. The very cellular lamina propria is rich in diffuse lymphatic tissue, emphasizing the role of this layer in the immune system.

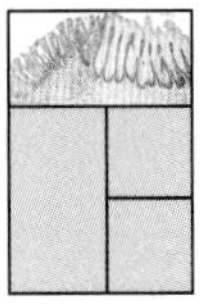

Esophagogastric junction, esophagus-stomach, human, hematoxylin and eosin (H&E) ×100.

The junction between the esophagus and stomach is shown here. The esophagus is on the *right*, and the cardiac region of the stomach is on the *left*. The *large rectangle* marks a representative area of the cardiac mucosa seen at higher magnification in the next figure; the *smaller rectangle* shows part of the junction examined at higher magnification in the figure on the *right*.

As noted in Plate 17.1 (page 670), the esophagus is lined by **stratified squamous epithelium** (*Ep*) that is indented on its undersurface by deep connective tissue papillae. When these are sectioned obliquely (as five of them have been), they appear as islands of connective tissue within the thick epithelium. Under the epithelium are the lamina propria, often infiltrated by lymphocytes (*L*), and the muscularis mucosae (*MM*). At the junction between the esophagus and the stomach (see also *middle right figure*), the stratified squamous epithelium of the esophagus ends abruptly, and the **simple columnar epithelium** of the stomach surface begins.

The surface of the stomach contains numerous and relatively deep depressions called gastric pits (*P*), or foveolae, that are formed by epithelium similar to, and continuous with, that of the surface. **Glands** (*GL*) open into the bottom of the pits; they are cardiac glands. The entire gastric mucosa contains glands. There are three types of gastric glands: cardiac, fundic, and pyloric. Cardiac glands are in the immediate vicinity of the opening of the esophagus, pyloric glands are in the funnel-shaped portion of the stomach that leads to the duodenum, and fundic glands are throughout the remainder of the stomach.

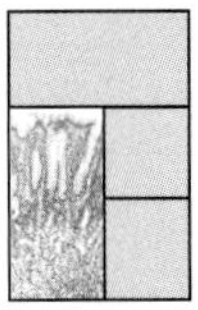

Cardiac region, stomach, human, H&E ×260.

The **cardiac glands** and gastric pits (*P*) seen in the *top figure* are surrounded by a very cellular lamina propria. At this higher magnification, it can be seen that many cells of the lamina propria are lymphocytes and other cells of the immune system. Large numbers of lymphocytes (*L*) may be localized between the smooth muscle cells of the muscularis mucosae (*MM*), and thus, the muscularis mucosae in these locations appears to be disrupted. Also, a few intraepithelial lymphocytes are indicated by the *arrows*.

The cardiac glands (*GL*) are limited to a narrow region around the cardiac orifice. They empty their secretions via ducts (*D*) into the bottom of the gastric pits. They are not sharply delineated from the fundic region of the stomach that contains parietal and chief cells. Thus, at the boundary, occasional parietal cells are seen in the cardiac glands.

In certain animals (e.g., ruminants and pigs), the anatomy and histology of the stomach are different. In these, at least one part of the stomach is lined with stratified squamous epithelium.

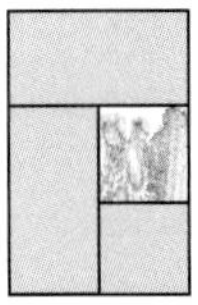

Esophagogastric junction, esophagus-stomach, human, H&E ×440.

The columnar cells of the stomach surface and **gastric pits** (*P*) produce mucus. Each surface and pit cell contains a mucous cup in its apical cytoplasm, thereby forming a glandular sheet of cells named **surface mucous cells** (*SMC*). The content of the mucous cup is usually lost during the preparation of the tissue, and thus, the apical cup portion of the cells appears empty in routine H&E paraffin sections such as the ones shown in this plate. Note the appearance of a loose connective tissue of the lamina propria (*LP*) that separates gastric pits (*P*).

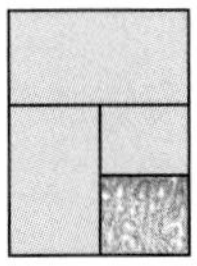

Cardiac region, stomach, human, H&E ×440.

The epithelium of the cardiac glands (*GL*) also consists of **mucous gland cells** (*MGC*). As seen in the photomicrograph, the nucleus of the gland cell is typically flattened; one side is adjacent to the base of the cell, whereas the other side is adjacent to the pale-staining cytoplasm. Again, mucus is lost during processing of the tissue, and this accounts for the pale-staining appearance of the cytoplasm. Although the **cardiac glands** are mostly unbranched, some branching is occasionally seen. The glands empty their secretions via ducts (*D*) into the bottom of the gastric pits. The cells forming the ducts are columnar, and the cytoplasm stains well with eosin. This makes it easy to distinguish the duct cells from mucous gland cells. Among the cells forming the duct portion of the gland are those that undergo mitotic division to replace both surface mucous and gland cells. Cardiac glands also contain enteroendocrine cells, but they are difficult to identify in routine H&E paraffin sections. Interrupted bundles of the muscularis mucosae (*MM*) smooth muscles are visible in close proximity to the gland.

D, ducts of cardiac glands
Ep, epithelium
GL, cardiac glands
L, lymphocytes
LP, lamina propria
MGC, mucous gland cells
MM, muscularis mucosae
P, gastric pits
SMC, surface mucous cells
arrows, intraepithelial lymphocytes

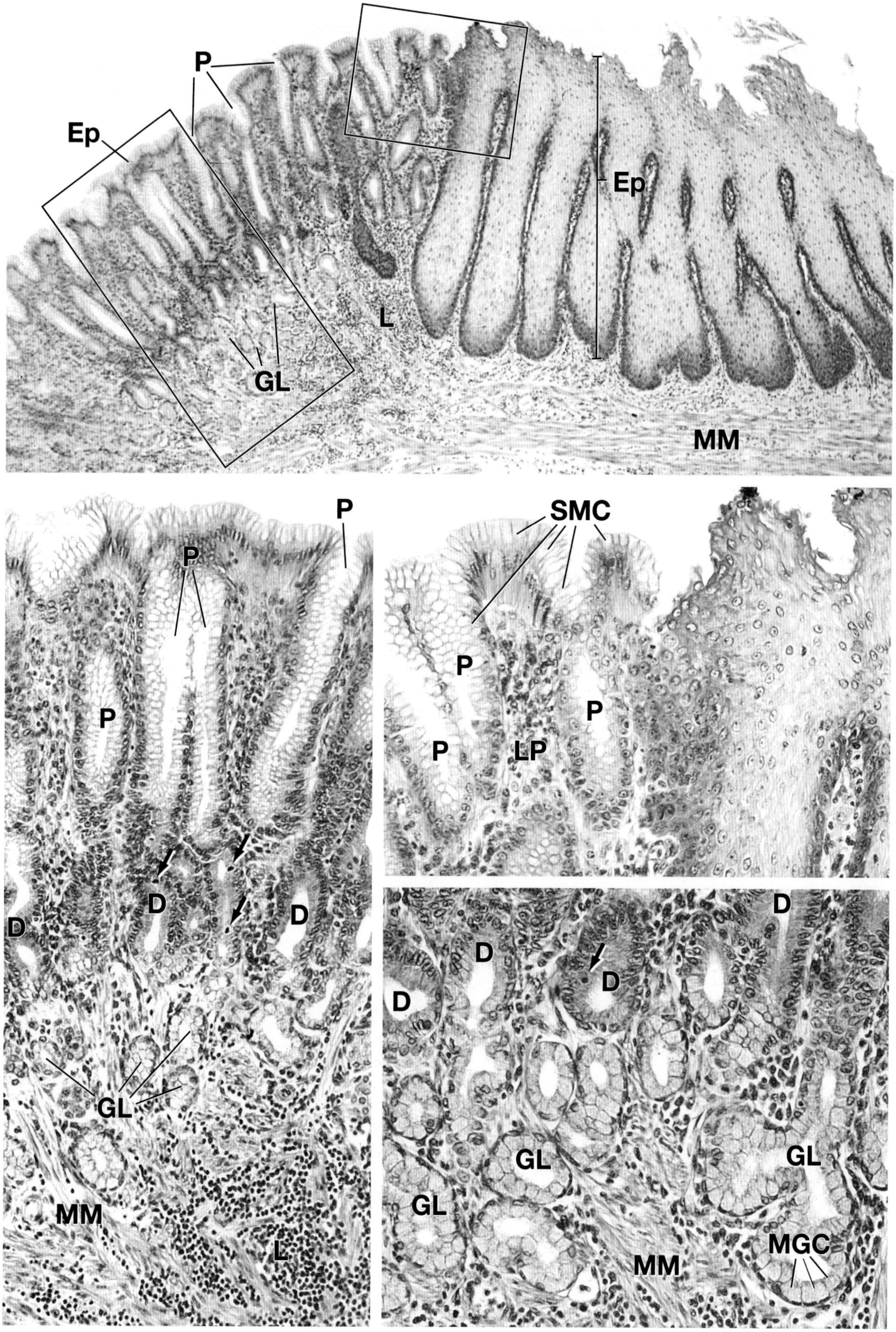
P
Ep
Ep
L
GL
MM
P
P
P
D
D
D
GL
MM
L
SMC
P
P
LP
P
D
D
D
D
GL
GL
GL
MM
MGC

PLATE 17.3 ■ STOMACH I

Histologically, the **stomach** is divided into three regions: The **cardia**, nearest the esophagus, contains cardiac glands that secrete primarily mucinogen; the **pylorus**, proximal to the gastrointestinal (pyloric) sphincter, contains pyloric glands that secrete a mucinogen that resembles that of the *surface mucous cells*; and the **fundus**, the body or largest part of the stomach, contains the fundic (gastric) glands. Fundic glands contain **parietal (oxyntic) cells**, acidophilic cells that secrete 0.16 N HCl, and **chief cells**, basophilic cells that contain acidophilic secretory granules in the apical cytoplasm. The granules contain mostly pepsinogen. The glands in all parts of the stomach contain **enteroendocrine cells**.

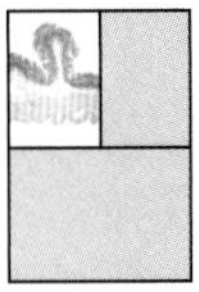

Stomach, human, hematoxylin and eosin (H&E) ×40.

As with other parts of the gastrointestinal tract, the wall of the stomach consists of four layers: mucosa (*Muc*), submucosa (*SubM*), muscularis externa (*ME*), and serosa. The **mucosa** is the innermost layer and reveals three distinctive regions (*arrows*). The most superficial region contains the gastric pits; the middle region contains the necks of the glands, which tend to stain with eosin; and the deepest part of the mucosa stains most heavily with hematoxylin. The cell types of the deep (hematoxylin-staining) portion of the fundic mucosa are considered in the *bottom figure*. The cells of all three regions and their staining characteristics are considered in Plate 17.4 (page 676).

The inner surface of the empty stomach is thrown into long folds referred to as **rugae**. One such cross-sectioned fold is shown here. It consists of mucosa and submucosa (*asterisks*). The rugae are not permanent folds; they disappear when the stomach wall is stretched, as in the distended stomach. Also evident are mamillated areas (*M*), which are slight elevations of the mucosa that resemble cobblestones. The mamillated areas consist only of mucosa without submucosa.

The **submucosa** and **muscularis externa** stain predominantly with eosin; the muscularis externa appears darker. The smooth muscle of the muscularis externa gives an appearance of being homogeneous and uniformly solid. In contrast, the submucosa, being connective tissue, may contain areas with adipocytes and contains numerous profiles of blood vessels (*BV*). The **serosa** is so thin that it is not evident as a discrete layer at this low magnification.

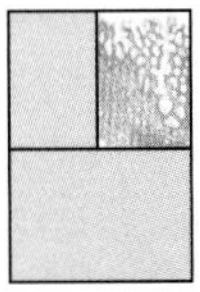

Fundocardiac junction, stomach, human, H&E ×240.

This figure and the next figure show the **fundocardiac junction** between the cardiac and fundic regions of the stomach. This junction can be identified histologically on the basis of the structure of the mucosa. The gastric pits (*P*), some of which are seen opening at the surface (*arrows*), are similar in both regions, but the glands are different. They are composed mostly of mucus-secreting cells and occasional enteroendocrine cells. The boundary between cardiac glands (*CG*) and fundic glands (*FG*) is marked by the *dashed line* in each figure.

The full thickness of the gastric mucosa is shown here, as indicated by the presence of the muscularis mucosae (*MM*) deep into the fundic glands. The muscularis mucosae below the cardiac glands is obscured by a large infiltration of lymphocytes forming a lymphatic nodule (*LN*).

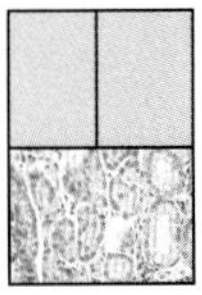

Fundocardiac junction, stomach, human, H&E ×640.

This figure provides a comparison between the cardiac and fundic glands at higher magnification. The **cardiac glands** (*CG*) consist of mucous gland cells arranged as a simple columnar epithelium; the nucleus is in the most basal part of the cell and is somewhat flattened. The cytoplasm appears as a faint network of lightly stained material. The lumina (*L*) of the cardiac glands are relatively wide. On the other hand, the **fundic glands** (*FG*) (*left of the dashed line*) are small, and a lumen is seen readily only in certain fortuitously sectioned glands. As a consequence, most of the glands appear to be cords of cells. Because this is a deep region of the fundic mucosa, most of the cells are chief cells. The basal portion of the chief cell contains the nucleus and extensive rough endoplasmic reticulum (rER), which accounts for its basophilia. The apical cytoplasm, normally occupied by secretory granules that were lost during the preparation of the tissue, stains poorly. Interspersed among the chief cells are parietal cells (*PC*). These cells typically have a round nucleus that is surrounded by eosinophilic cytoplasm. Among the cells of the lamina propria are some with pale elongated nuclei. These are smooth muscle cells (*SM*) that extend into the lamina propria from the muscularis mucosae.

BV, blood vessels
CG, cardiac glands
FG, fundic glands
L, lumen
LN, lymphatic nodule
M, mamillated areas
ME, muscularis externa
MM, muscularis mucosae
Muc, mucosa
P, gastric pits
PC, parietal cells
SM, smooth muscle cells
SubM, submucosa
arrows, top left figure, three differently stained regions of fundic mucosa; top right figure, opening of gastric pits
asterisks, submucosa in rugae
dashed line, boundary between cardiac and fundic glands

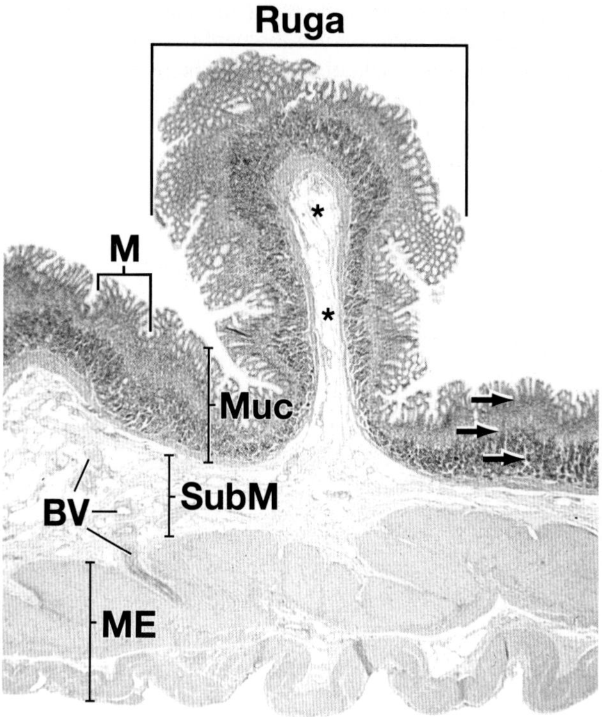
Ruga
M
Muc
SubM
BV
ME

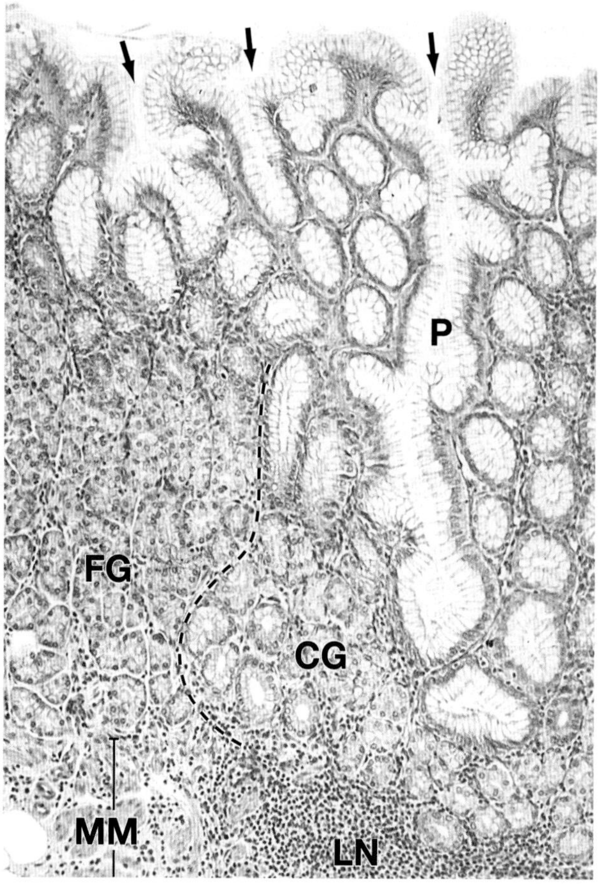
P
FG
CG
MM
LN

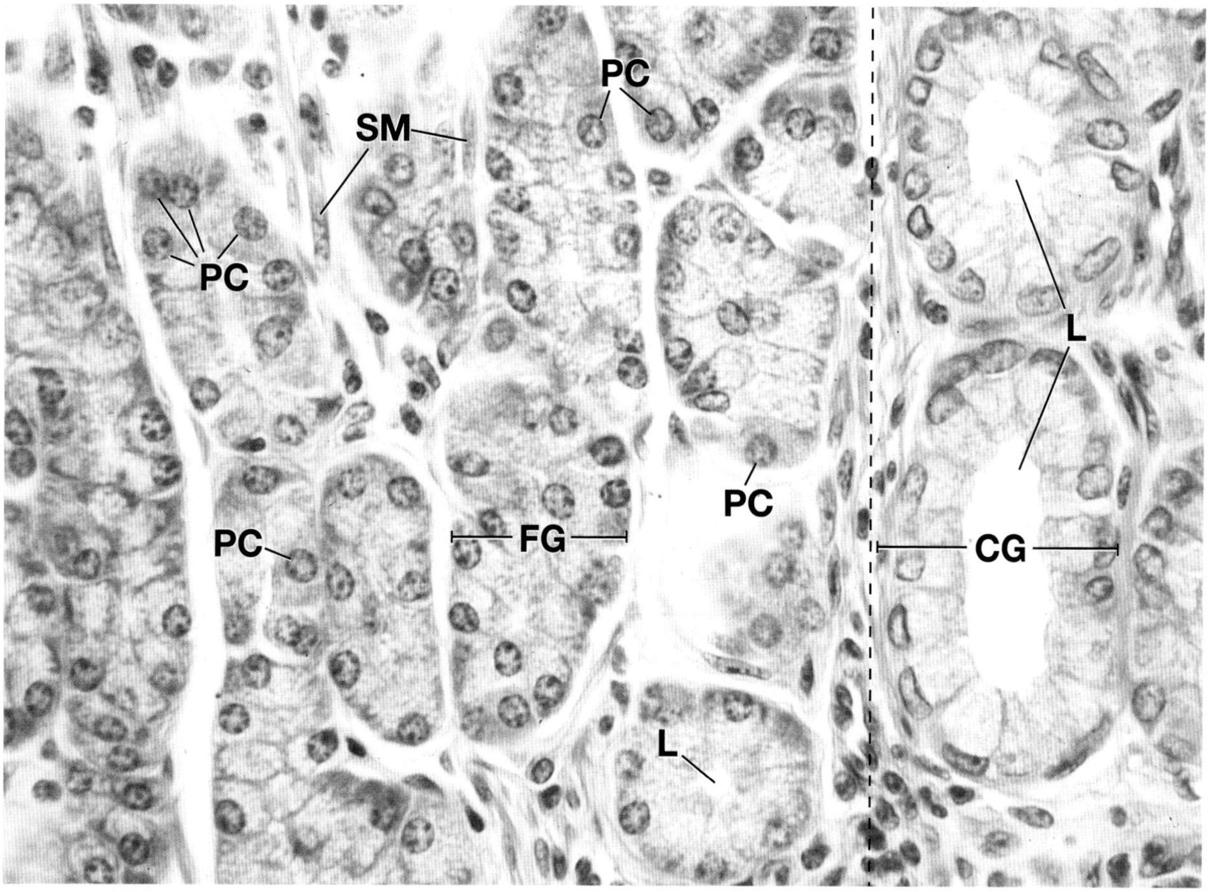
PC
SM
PC
PC
FG
PC
CG
L
L

PLATE 17.4 ■ STOMACH II

The epithelial lining of the alimentary canal is a regularly renewing epithelium; each portion has a characteristic turnover time and stem cell location. In the stomach, stem cells are located in the isthmus (above) the mucous neck cells. Cells that migrate upward to form the mucous cells of the gastric pit and surface have a turnover time of 3–5 days; cells that migrate downward to form the parietal cells, chief cells, and enteroendocrine cells of the glands have a turnover time of about 1 year. Another niche of stem cells is located in the base of the gland.

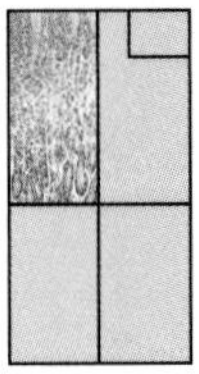

Fundic glands, stomach, monkey, hematoxylin and eosin (H&E) ×320.

This figure shows an area of the **fundic mucosa** that includes the bottom of the gastric pits and the neck and deeper part of the fundic glands. It includes the areas marked by the *arrows* in the *top left* of Plate 17.3 (page 674). The **surface mucous cells** (*SMC*) of the gastric pits are readily identified because the mucous cup in the apical pole of each cell has an empty, washed-out appearance. Just below the gastric pits are the necks (*N*) of the fundic glands, in which **mucous neck cells** (*MNC*) and **parietal cells** (*PC*) can be identified. The mucous neck cells produce a mucous secretion that differs from that produced by the surface mucous cells. As seen here, the mucous neck cells display a cytoplasm that is lightly stained; there are no cytoplasmic areas that stain intensely.

Parietal cells are distinctive primarily because of the pronounced eosinophilic staining of their cytoplasm. Their nucleus is round, like that of the chief cell, but tends to be located closer to the basal lamina of the epithelium than to the lumen of the gland because of the pear-like shape of the parietal cell.

This figure also reveals the significant characteristics of **chief cells** (*CC*), namely, the round nucleus in a basal location; the ergastoplasm, deeply stained with hematoxylin (particularly evident in some of the chief cells where the nucleus has not been included in the plane of section); and the apical, slightly eosinophilic cytoplasm (normally occupied by the secretory granules).

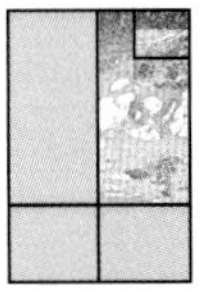

Submucosa, stomach, monkey, H&E ×320.

This figure shows the bottom of the stomach mucosa, the **submucosa** (*SubM*), and part of the muscularis externa (*ME*). The muscularis mucosae (*MM*) is the deepest part of the mucosa. It consists of smooth muscle cells arranged in at least two layers. As seen in the photomicrograph, the smooth muscle cells immediately adjacent to the submucosa have been sectioned longitudinally and display elongated nuclear profiles. Just above this layer, the smooth muscle cells have been cut in cross section and display rounded nuclear profiles.

The submucosa consists of connective tissue of moderate density. Present in the submucosa are adipocytes (*A*), blood vessels (*BV*), and a group of ganglion cells (*GC*). These particular cells belong to the **submucosal plexus** (*Meissner plexus* [*MP*]). The *inset* shows some of the ganglion cells (*GC*) at higher magnification. These are the large cell bodies of the enteric neurons. Each cell body is surrounded by satellite cells intimately apposed to the neuron cell body. The *arrowheads* point to the nuclei of the satellite cells.

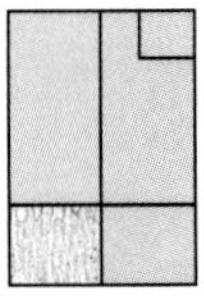

Gastric glands, stomach, silver stain ×160.

Enteroendocrine cells constitute a class of cells that can be displayed with special histochemical or silver-staining methods but that are not readily evident in H&E sections. The distribution of cells demonstrable with special silver-staining procedures is shown here (*arrows*). Because of the staining procedure, these cells are properly designated as **argentaffin cells**. The surface mucous cells (*SMC*) in the section mark the bottom of the gastric pits and establish the fact that the necks of the fundic glands are represented in the section. The argentaffin cells appear *black* in this specimen. The relatively low magnification permits the viewer to assess the frequency of distribution of these cells.

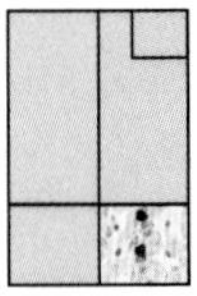

Gastric glands, stomach, silver stain ×640.

At higher magnification, the **argentaffin cells** (*arrows*) are almost totally blackened by the silver staining, although a faint nucleus can be seen in some cells. The silver stains the secretory product lost during the preparation of routine sections, and accordingly, in H&E-stained paraffin sections, the argentaffin cell appears as a clear cell. The special silver staining in this figure and in the figure on the *left* shows that many of the argentaffin cells tend to be near the basal lamina and away from the lumen of the gland.

A, adipocytes
BV, blood vessels
CC, chief cells
GC, ganglion cells
ME, muscularis externa
MM, muscularis mucosae
MNC, mucous neck cells
MP, Meissner plexus
N, neck of fundic glands
PC, parietal cells
SMC, surface mucous cells
SubM, submucosa
arrows, argentaffin cells
arrowheads, nuclei of satellite cells

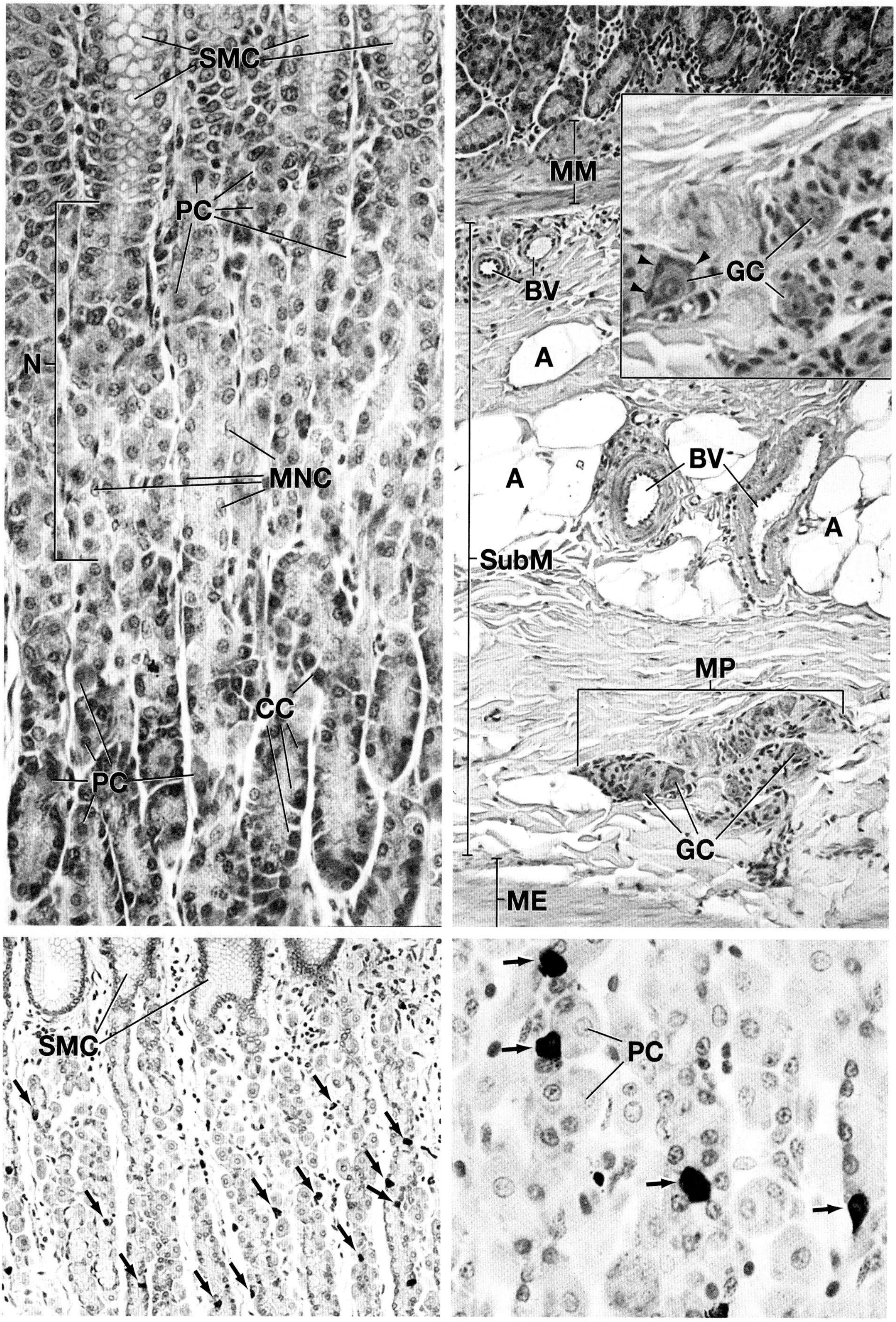
SMC
PC
N
MNC
CC
PC
MM
GC
BV
A
A
BV
A
SubM
MP
GC
ME
SMC
PC

PLATE 17.5 ■ GASTRODUODENAL JUNCTION

The **gastroduodenal junction** marks the entry into the absorptive portion of the alimentary canal. Thickening of the circular layer of muscularis externa at this site forms the pyloric sphincter that regulates the passage of chyme from the stomach to the intestine. The mucous secretion of the pyloric glands helps to neutralize the chyme as it enters the intestine.

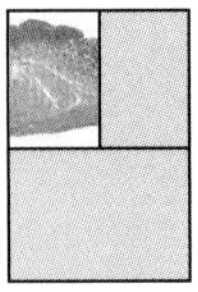

Gastroduodenal junction, stomach-duodenum, monkey, hematoxylin and eosin (H&E) ×40.

The **gastroduodenal junction** between the stomach and the duodenum is shown here. Most of the mucosa in the micrograph belongs to the stomach; it is the **pyloric mucosa** (*PMuc*). The pyloric sphincter appears as a thickened region of smooth muscle below the pyloric mucosa. On the *far right* is the **duodenal mucosa**, the first part of the intestinal mucosa (*IMuc*). The area marked by the *rectangle* is shown at higher magnification in the next figure. It provides a comparison of the two mucosal regions and also shows the submucosal glands (Brunner glands).

The submucosa of the duodenum contains **submucosal (Brunner) glands**. These are below the muscularis mucosae; therefore, this structure serves as a useful landmark in identifying the glands. In the stomach, the **muscularis mucosae** is readily identified as narrow bands of muscular tissue (*MM*). It can be followed toward the right into the duodenum but is then interrupted in the region between the two *asterisks*.

This figure also shows the thickened region of the gastric muscularis externa, where the stomach ends. This is the pyloric sphincter (*PS*). Its thickness, mostly due to the amplification of the circular layer of smooth muscle of the muscularis externa, can be appreciated by comparison with the muscularis externa in the duodenum (*ME*).

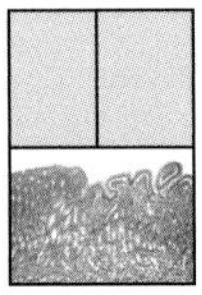

Gastroduodenal junction, stomach-duodenum, monkey, H&E ×120.

Examination of this region at higher magnification reveals that in addition to intestinal glands (*IGl*) within the mucosa, there are glands within the duodenal submucosa. These are **submucosal (Brunner) glands** (*BGl*). Some of the glandular elements (*arrows*) can be seen to pass from the submucosa to the mucosa, thereby interrupting the **muscularis mucosae** (*MM*). The submucosal glands empty their secretions into the duodenal lumen by means of ducts (*D*). In contrast, the pyloric glands (*PGl*) are relatively straight for most of their length but are coiled in the deepest part of the mucosa and are sometimes branched. They are restricted to the mucosa and empty into deep gastric pits. The boundary between the pits and glands is, however, hard to ascertain in H&E sections.

With respect to the mucosal aspects of gastroduodenal histology, as mentioned earlier, the glands of the stomach empty into gastric pits. These are depressions; accordingly, when the pits are sectioned in a plane that is oblique or at right angles to the long axis of the pit, as in this figure, the pits can be recognized as being depressions because they are surrounded by lamina propria. In contrast, the inner surface of the small intestine has villi (*V*). These are projections into the lumen of slightly varying height. When the villus is cross-sectioned or obliquely sectioned, it is surrounded by space of the lumen, as is one of the villi shown here. In addition, the villi have lamina propria (*LP*) in their core.

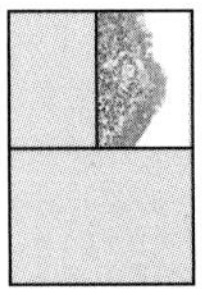

Gastroduodenal junction, stomach-duodenum, monkey, H&E ×640.

The *rectangular area* in the next figure is considered at higher magnification here. It shows how the epithelium of the stomach differs from that of the intestine. In both cases, the epithelium is simple columnar, and the underlying lamina propria (*LP*) is highly cellular because of the presence of large numbers of lymphocytes. The boundary between gastric and duodenal epithelium is marked by the *arrow*. On the stomach side of the *arrow*, the epithelium consists of **surface mucous cells** (*SMC*). The surface cells contain an apical cup of mucous material that typically appears empty in an H&E-stained paraffin section. In contrast, the **absorptive cells** (*AC*) of the intestine do not possess mucus in their cytoplasm. Although goblet cells are found in the intestinal epithelium and are scattered among the absorptive cells, they do not form a complete mucous sheet. The intestinal absorptive cells also possess a striated border, which is shown in Plate 17.7 (page 682).

AC, absorptive cells
BGl, Brunner glands
D, ducts
IGl, intestinal glands
IMuc, intestinal mucosa
LP, lamina propria
ME, muscularis externa
MM, muscularis mucosae
PGl, pyloric glands
PMuc, pyloric mucosa
PS, pyloric sphincter
SMC, surface mucous cells
V, villi
arrows, bottom figure, Brunner gland element that passes from the submucosa to the mucosa; upper right figure, boundary between gastric and duodenal epithelium
asterisks, upper left figure; interruption in muscularis mucosae

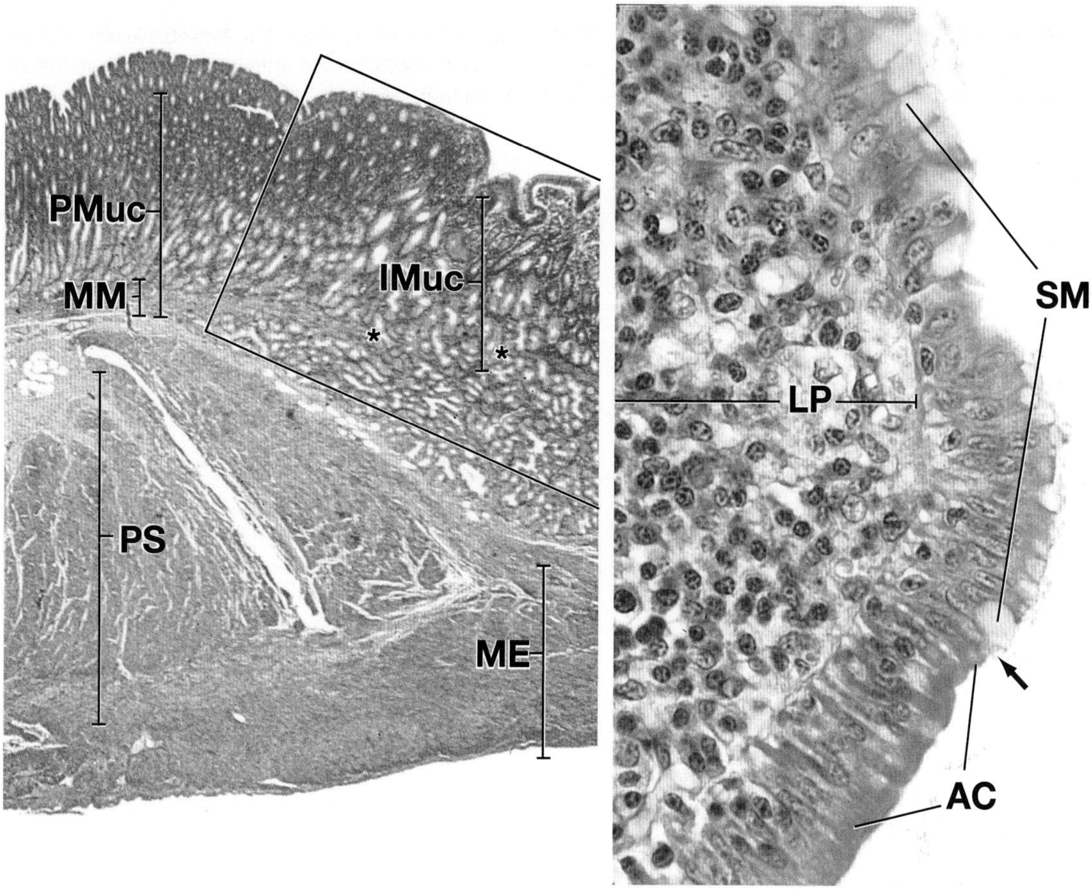
PMuc
MM
IMuc
*
*
PS
ME
SMC
LP
AC

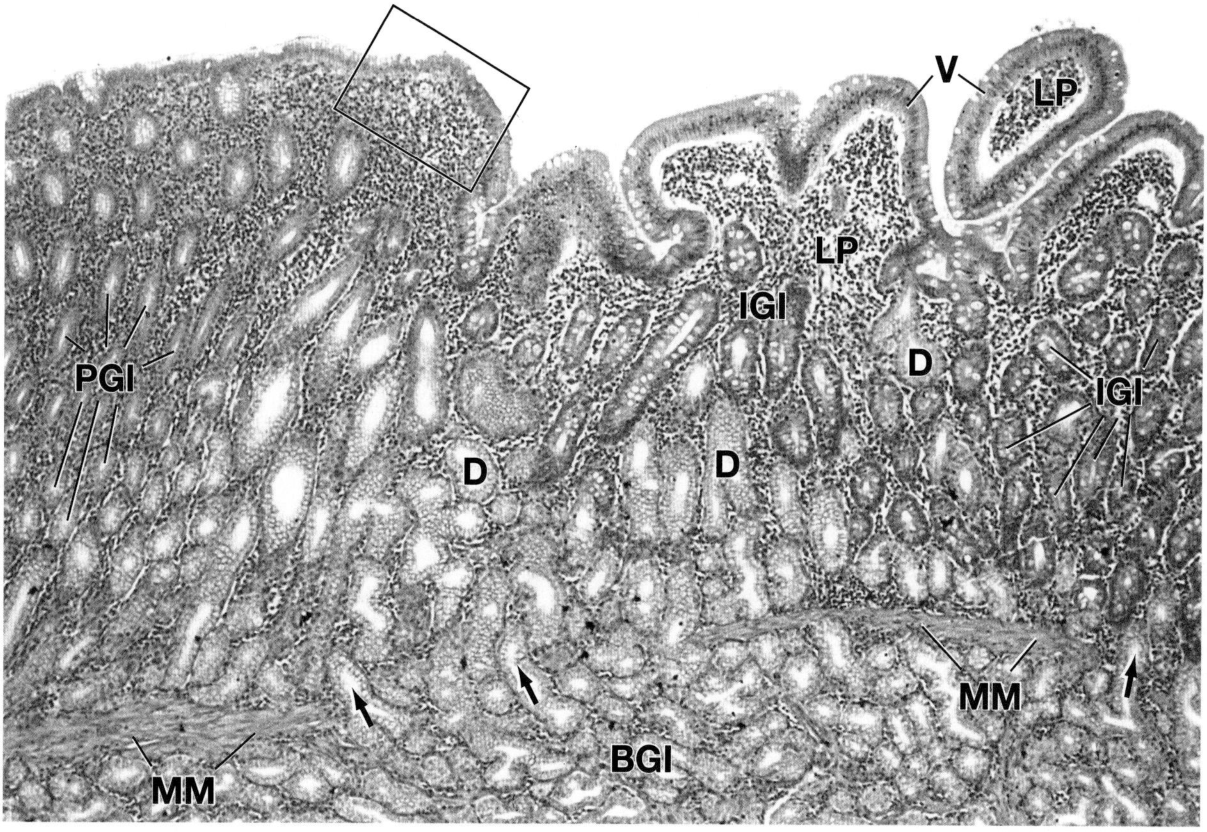
V
LP
LP
IGI
PGI
D
D
D
IGI
MM
BGI
MM

PLATE 17.6 ■ DUODENUM

The **small intestine** is the principal site for the digestion of food and absorption of the products of digestion. It is the longest component of the alimentary canal, measuring over 6 m, and is divided into three segments: **duodenum** (~25 cm), **jejunum** (~2.5 m), and **ileum** (~3.5 m). The first portion, the duodenum, receives a partially digested bolus of food (chyme) from the stomach as well as secretions from the stomach, pancreas, liver, and gallbladder that contain digestive enzymes, enzyme precursors, and other products that aid digestion and absorption.

The small intestine is characterized by **plicae circulares**, permanent transverse folds that contain a core of submucosa, and **villi**, finger- and leaf-like projections of the mucosa that extend into the lumen. Microvilli, multiple finger-like extensions of the apical surface of each intestinal epithelial cell (enterocyte), further increase the surface for absorption of metabolites.

Mucosal glands extend into the lamina propria. They contain the stem cells and developing cells that will ultimately migrate to the surface of the villi. In the duodenum, **submucosal glands (Brunner glands)** secrete an alkaline mucus that helps neutralize the acidic chyme. Enterocytes not only absorb metabolites digested in the intestinal lumen but also synthesize enzymes inserted into the membrane of the microvilli for terminal digestion of disaccharides and dipeptides.

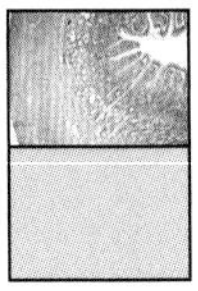

Duodenum, monkey, hematoxylin and eosin (H&E) ×120.

This figure shows a segment of the duodenal wall. As in the stomach, the layers of the wall, in order from the lumen, are the **mucosa** (*Muc*), the **submucosa** (*SubM*), the **muscularis externa** (*ME*), and the **serosa** (*S*). Both longitudinal (*L*) and circular (*C*) layers of the muscularis externa can be distinguished. Although plicae circulares are found in the wall of the small intestine, including the duodenum, none is included in this photomicrograph.

A distinctive feature of the intestinal mucosa is the presence of finger- and leaf-like projections into the intestinal lumen, called **villi**. Most of the villi (*V*) shown here display profiles that correspond to their description as finger like. One villus, however, displays the form of a leaf-like villus (*asterisk*). The *dashed line* marks the boundary between the villi and the **intestinal glands** (also called *crypts of Lieberkühn*). The latter extend as far as the muscularis mucosae (*MM*).

Under the mucosa is the submucosa, containing the **Brunner glands** (*BGl*). These are branched tubular or branched tubuloalveolar glands whose secretory components, shown at higher magnification in the next figure, consist of columnar epithelium. A duct (*D*) through which the glands open into the lumen of the duodenum is shown here and, at higher magnification, in the next figure, where it is marked by an *arrow*.

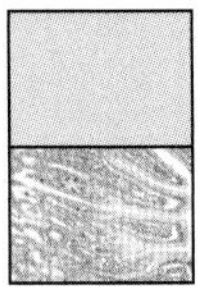

Mucosa, duodenum, monkey, H&E ×240.

The histologic features of the duodenal mucosa are shown at higher magnification here. Two kinds of cells can be recognized in the epithelial layer that forms the surface of the villus: **enterocytes (absorptive cells)** and **goblet cells** (*GC*). Most of the cells are absorptive cells. They have a striated border that will be seen at higher magnification in Plate 17.7 (page 682); their elongated nuclei are located in the basal half of the cell. Goblet cells are readily identified by the presence of the apical mucous cup, which appears empty. Most of the dark round nuclei also seen in the epithelial layer covering the villi belong to lymphocytes.

The **lamina propria** (*LP*) makes up the core of the villus. It contains large numbers of round cells whose individual identity cannot be ascertained at this magnification. Note, however, that these are mostly lymphocytes (and other cells of the immune system), which accounts for the designation of the lamina propria as diffuse lymphatic tissue. The lamina propria surrounding the intestinal glands (*IGl*) similarly consists largely of lymphocytes and related cells. The lamina propria also contains components of loose connective tissue and isolated smooth muscle cells.

The **intestinal glands** (*IGl*) are relatively straight and tend to be dilated at their base. The bases of the intestinal crypts contain the stem cells from which all of the other cells of the intestinal epithelium arise. They also contain Paneth cells. These cells possess eosinophilic granules in their apical cytoplasm. The granules contain lysozyme, a bacteriolytic enzyme thought to play a role in regulating intestinal microbial flora. The main cell type in the intestinal crypt is a relatively undifferentiated columnar cell. These cells are shorter than the enterocytes of the villus surface; they usually undergo two mitoses before they differentiate into absorptive cells or goblet cells. Also present in the intestinal crypts are some mature goblet cells and enteroendocrine cells.

BGl, Brunner glands
C, circular (inner) layer of muscularis externa
D, duct of Brunner gland
GC, goblet cells
IGl, intestinal glands (crypts)
L, longitudinal (outer) layer of muscularis externa
LP, lamina propria
ME, muscularis externa
MM, muscularis mucosae
Muc, mucosa
S, serosa
SubM, submucosa
V, villi
arrow, duct of Brunner gland
asterisk, leaf-like villus
dashed line, top figure, boundary between the base of villi and intestinal glands

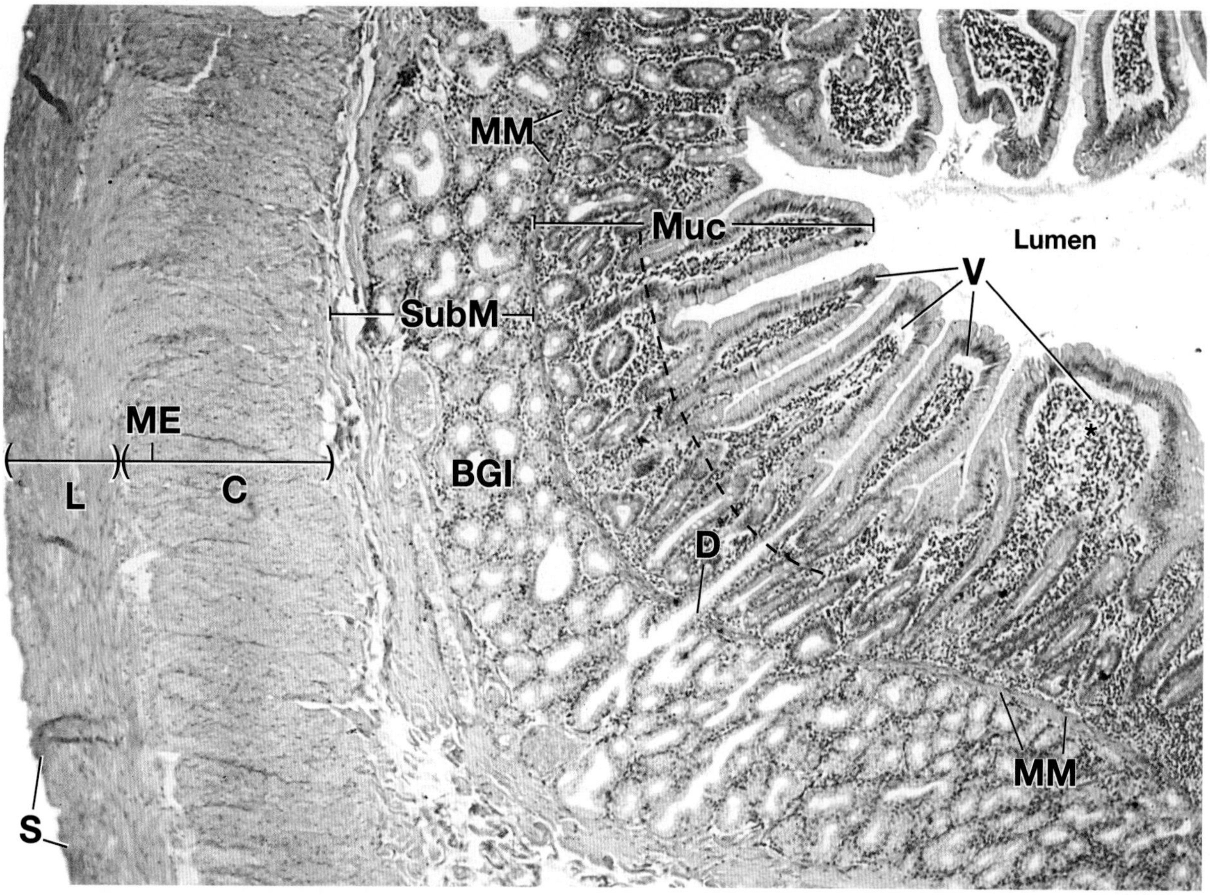
MM
Muc
Lumen
V
SubM
ME
L
C
BGI
D
MM
S

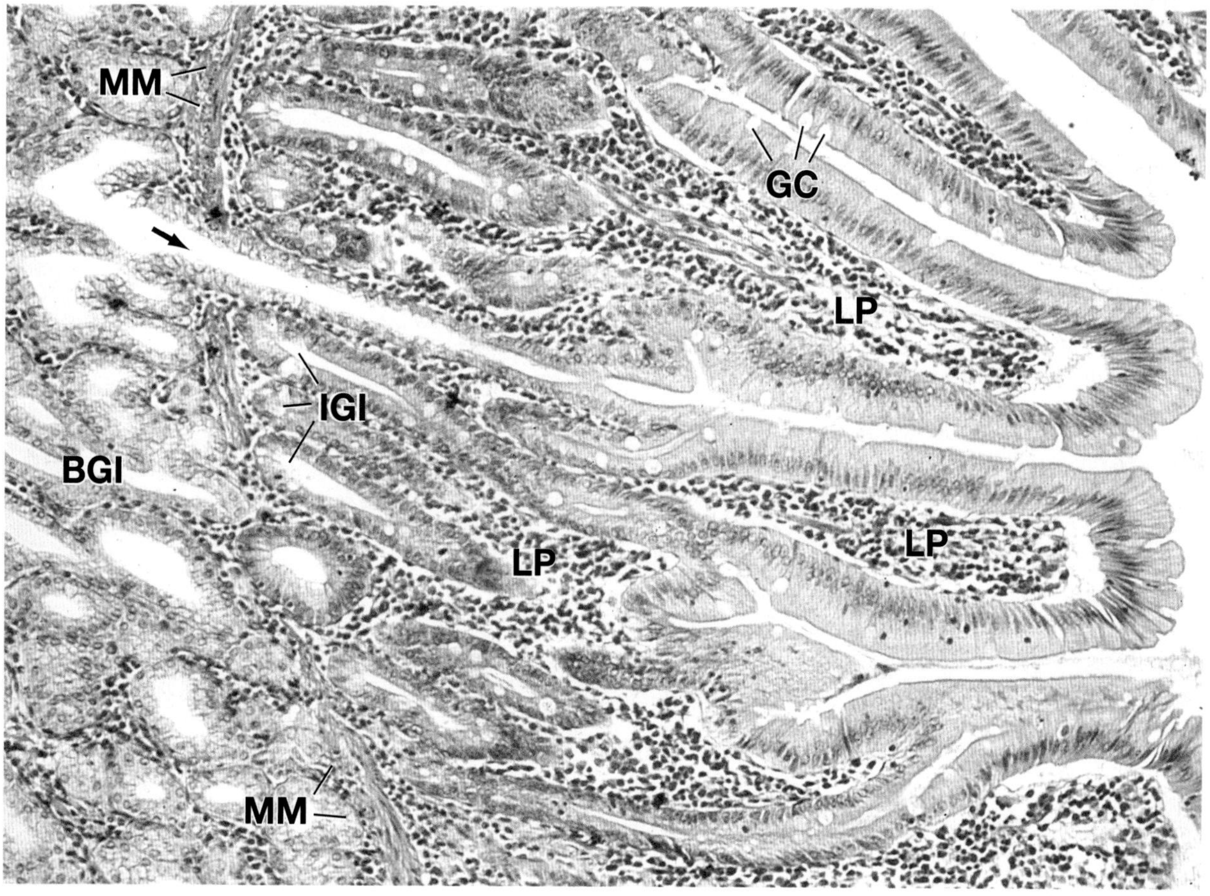
MM
GC
LP
IGI
BGI
LP
LP
MM

PLATE 17.7 ■ JEJUNUM

The **jejunum** is the principal site of absorption of nutrients in the small intestine. The villi are more finger like than leaf like and are covered largely with absorptive columnar epithelial cells (enterocytes), although **goblet cells** and **enteroendocrine cells** are also present. The stem cells for all of these cells and the **Paneth cells** that secrete the antibacterial enzyme lysozyme are found deep into the intestinal gland. Replicating cells line the lower half of the gland.

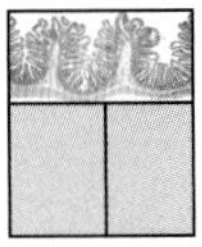

Jejunum, monkey, hematoxylin and eosin (H&E) ×22.

This is a longitudinal section of the jejunum showing the permanent circular folds of the small intestine, the **plicae circulares** (*PC*). These folds or ridges are mostly arranged with their long axis at roughly right angles to the longitudinal axis of the intestine; therefore, the plicae circulares shown here are cut in cross section. The plicae circulares consist of **mucosa** (*Muc*) as well as **submucosa** (*SubM*). The broad band of tissue external to the submucosa is the **muscularis externa** (*ME*) and is not included in the plicae. (The serosa cannot be distinguished at this magnification.) Most of the **villi** (*V*) in this specimen have been cut longitudinally, thereby revealing their full length as well as the fact that some are slightly shorter than others. The shortening is considered to be due to the contraction of smooth muscle cells in the villi. Also seen here are the lacteals (*L*), which, in most of the villi, are dilated. Lacteals are lymphatic capillaries that begin in the villi and carry certain absorbed dietary lipids and proteins from the villi to the larger lymphatic vessels of the submucosa.

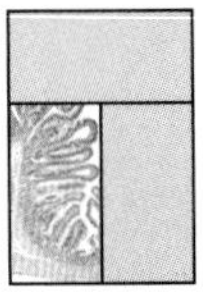

Plica circularis, jejunum, monkey, H&E ×60.

Part of the plica circularis marked by the *bracket* in the previous figure is shown at higher magnification. Note the muscularis mucosae (*MM*), the **intestinal glands** (*GI*), and the **villi** (*V*). The boundary between the glands and the villi is marked by the *dashed line*. Some of the glands are cut longitudinally; some are cut in cross section; most of the villi have been cut longitudinally. In conceptualizing the mucosal structure of the small intestine, it is important to recognize that the glands are epithelial depressions that project into the wall of the intestine, whereas the villi are projections that extend into the lumen. The glands are surrounded by cells of the lamina propria; the villi are surrounded by the space of the intestinal lumen. The lamina propria with its lacteal (*L*) occupies a central position in the villus; the lumen occupies the central position of the gland. Also note that the lumen of the gland tends to be dilated at its base. Studies of enzymatically isolated preparations of mucosa show that the bases of the glands are often divided into two or three finger-like extensions resting on the muscularis mucosae. At this low magnification, the serosa (*S*) and two muscle layers of the muscularis externa (*ME*) are difficult to discern.

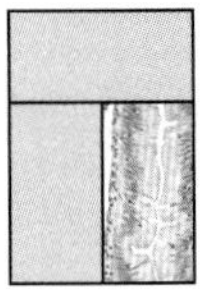

Intestinal villi, jejunum, monkey, H&E ×500.

This figure shows portions of two adjacent villi at higher magnification. The epithelium consists chiefly of **enterocytes**. These are columnar absorptive cells that typically exhibit a **striated border** (*SB*), the light microscopic representation of the microvilli on the apical surface of each enterocyte. The dark band at the base of the striated border is due to the terminal web of the cell, a layer of actin filaments that extends across the apex of the cell to which the actin filaments of the cores of the microvilli attach. The nuclei of the enterocytes have essentially the same shape, orientation, and staining characteristics. Even if the cytoplasmic boundaries were not evident, the nuclei would be an indication of the columnar shape and orientation of the cells. The enterocytes rest on a basal lamina not evident in H&E-stained paraffin sections. The eosinophilic band (*arrow*) at the base of the cell layer, where one would expect a basement membrane, actually consists of flat lateral cytoplasmic processes from the enterocytes. These processes partially delimit the basal–lateral intercellular spaces (*asterisks*) that are dilated, as can be seen here, during active transport of absorbed substrates.

The epithelial cells with an expanded apical cytoplasm in the form of a cup are **goblet cells** (*GC*). In this specimen, the nucleus of almost every goblet cell is just at the base of the cup, and a thin cytoplasmic strand (not always evident) extends to the level of the basement membrane. The scattered round nuclei within the epithelium belong to lymphocytes (*Ly*).

The **lamina propria** (*LP*) and the lacteal (*L*) are located beneath the intestinal epithelium. The cells forming the lacteal are simple squamous epithelium (endothelium). Two nuclei of these cells (*EC*) appear to be exposed to the lumen of the lacteal; another elongated nucleus slightly removed from the lumen belongs to a smooth muscle cell (*M*) accompanying the lacteals.

EC, endothelial cell
GC, goblet cell
GI, intestinal glands (crypts)
L, lacteal
LP, lamina propria
Ly, lymphocytes
M, smooth muscle cell
ME, muscularis externa
MM, muscularis mucosae
Muc, mucosa
PC, plicae circulares
S, serosa
SB, striated border
SubM, submucosa
V, villi
arrow, basal processes of enterocytes
asterisks, basal–lateral intercellular spaces
dashed line, boundary between villi and intestinal glands

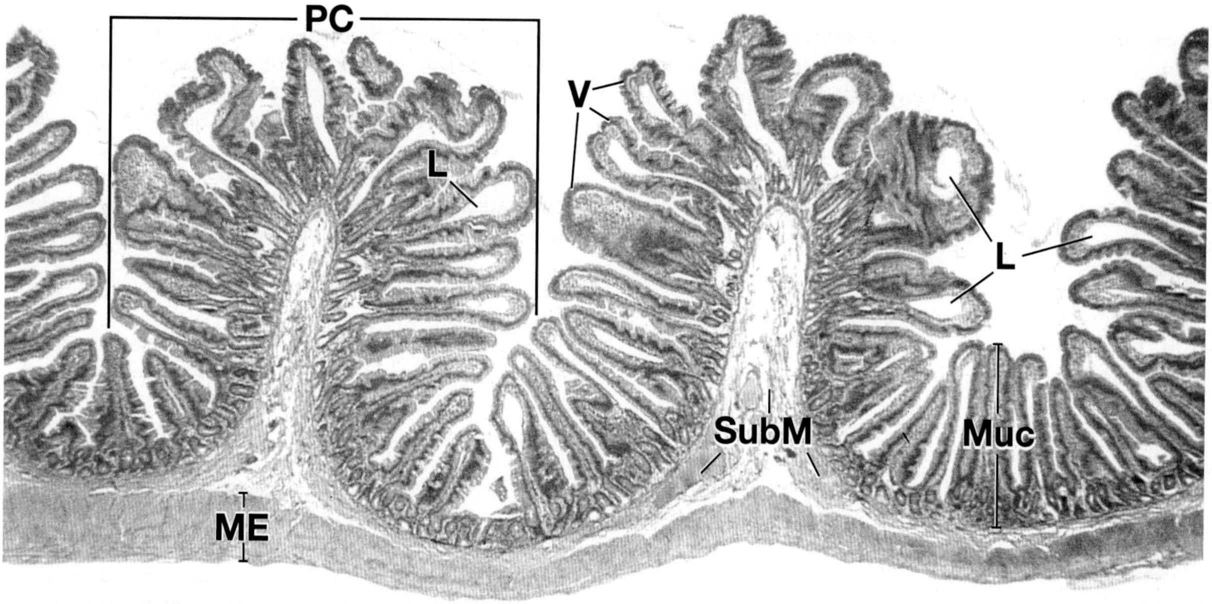
PC
V
L
L
SubM
Muc
ME

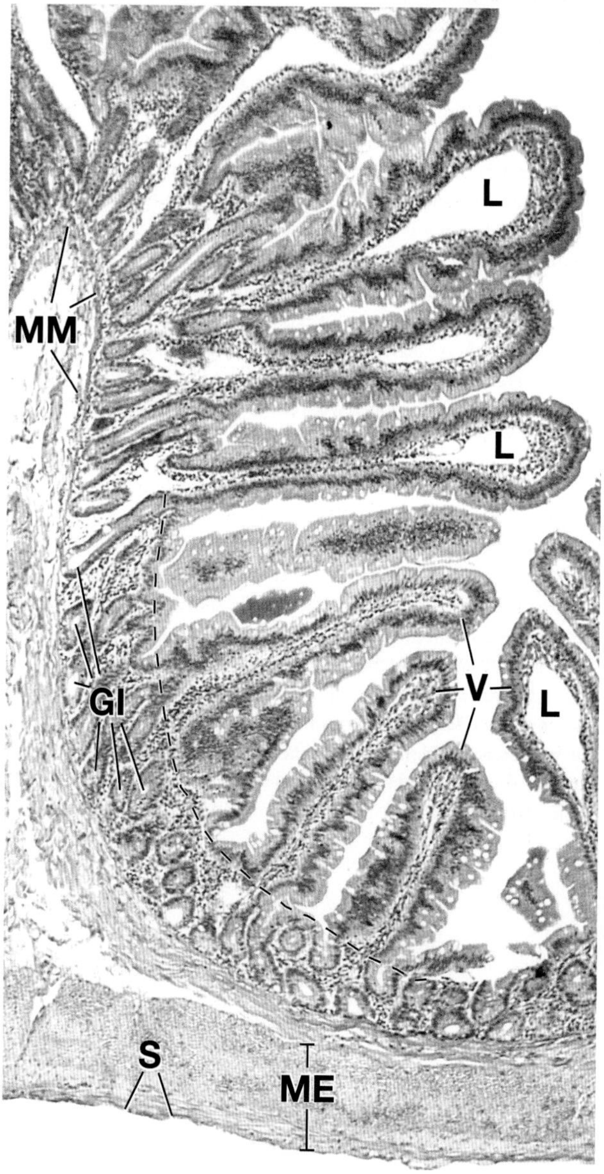
L
MM
L
Gl
V
L
S
ME

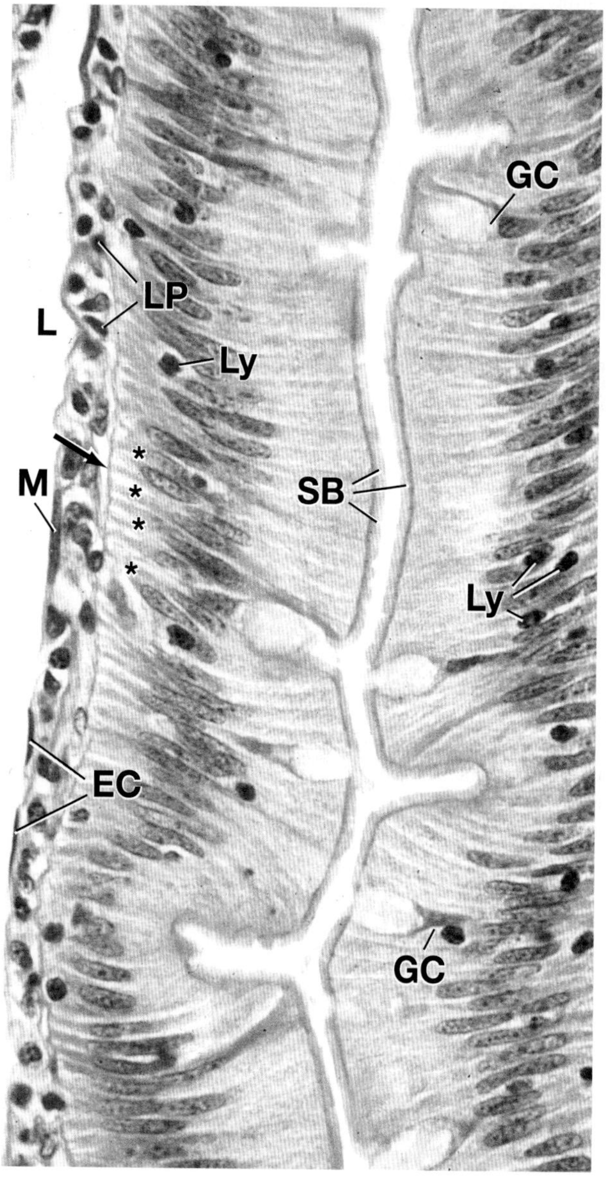
GC
LP
L
Ly
M
SB
Ly
EC
GC

PLATE 17.8 ■ ILEUM

The **ileum** is the principal site of water and electrolyte reabsorption in the small intestine. It has essentially the same histologic features as the jejunum, with some characteristic differences. **Villi** in the ileum are more frequently leaf like, and lymphatic tissue in the lamina propria is organized into numerous small and large nodules found on the antimesenteric side of the ileum. The nodules fuse to form large accumulations of lymphatic tissue called **Peyer patches**.

The surface epithelium of the small intestine renews itself every 5 or 6 days. The stem cells are restricted to the bottom portion of the mucosal gland, and the zone of cell replication is restricted to the lower half of the gland. The cells migrate onto the villus and are lost from its tip. All of the epithelial cells, absorptive cells, and goblet cells, as well as enteroendocrine cells and Paneth cells, derive from the same stem cell population, but enteroendocrine cells migrate slowly, and Paneth cells do not migrate.

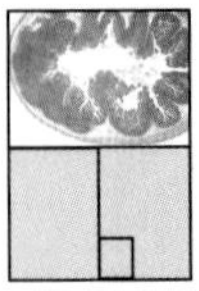

Ileum, monkey, hematoxylin and eosin (H&E) ×20.

For the purposes of orientation, the **submucosa** (*SM*) and **muscularis externa** (*ME*) have been marked in the cross section through the ileum shown here. Just internal to the submucosa is the mucosa; external to the muscularis externa is the serosa. The mucosa reveals several longitudinally sectioned villi (*V*), which have been labeled, and other unlabeled villi, which can be identified easily on the basis of their appearance as islands of tissue completely surrounded by the space of the lumen. They are, of course, not islands because this appearance is due to the plane of section that slices completely through some of the villi obliquely or in cross section, thereby isolating them from their base. Below the villi are the intestinal glands, many of which are obliquely or transversely sectioned and can be readily identified, as was done in the preceding plates, because they are totally surrounded by lamina propria.

There are about 8–10 projections of tissue into the intestinal lumen that are substantially larger than the villi. These are the plicae circulares. As noted earlier, plicae generally have circular orientation, but they may travel in a longitudinal direction for short distances and may branch. In addition, even if all the plicae are arranged in a circular manner, if the section is somewhat oblique, the plicae will be cut at an angle, as appears to be the case with several plicae in this figure. One of the distinctive features of the small intestine is the presence of **single and aggregated lymph nodules** in the intestinal wall. Isolated nodules of lymphatic tissue are common in the proximal end of the intestinal canal. As one proceeds distally through the intestines, however, the lymph nodules occur in increasingly larger numbers. In the ileum, large aggregates of lymph nodules are regularly seen; they are referred to as **Peyer patches**. Several lymphatic nodules (*LN*) forming a Peyer patch are shown in this figure. The nodules are located partly within the mucosa of the ileum and extend into the submucosa. Although not evident in the figure, the nodules are characteristically located opposite to where the mesentery connects to the intestinal tube.

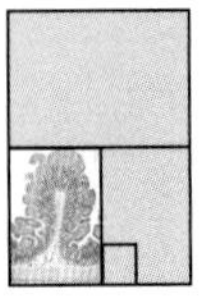

Plica circularis, ileum, monkey, H&E ×40.

Sometimes, in a cross section through the intestine, a plica displays a clear cross-sectional profile such as that shown here. Note, again, that the **submucosa** (*SM*) constitutes from the core of the plica circularis into the muscularis externa (*ME*). Although many of the **villi** in this figure present profiles (*V*) that would be expected if the villus were a finger-like projection, others clearly do not. In particular, one villus (marked with three *asterisks*) shows the broad profile of a longitudinally sectioned leaf-like villus. If this same villus were cut at a right angle to the plane shown here, it would appear as a finger-like villus.

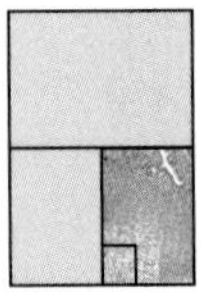

Aggregated lymph nodule, ileum, monkey, H&E ×100; inset ×200.

Part of an aggregated **lymph nodule** and part of the overlying epithelium are shown here at higher magnification. The lymphocytes and related cells are so numerous that they virtually obscure the cells of the muscularis mucosae. Their location, however, can be estimated as being near the presumptive label (*MM??*), inasmuch as the muscularis mucosae is ordinarily adjacent to the base of the intestinal glands (*Gl*). Moreover, on examination of this area at higher magnification (*inset*), groups of smooth muscle cells (*MM*) can be seen separated by numerous lymphocytes close to the intestinal glands (*Gl*). Clearly, the lymphocytes of the nodule are on both sides of the muscularis mucosae and thus within both the mucosa and the submucosa.

In places, the lymph nodule is covered by the intestinal epithelium. Whereas the nature of the epithelium cannot be appreciated fully in the light microscope, electron micrographs (both scanning and transmission) have shown that among the epithelial cells are special cells, designated M cells, that sample the intestinal content (for antigen) and transfer this antigen to the dendritic cells and lymphocytes in the epithelial layer.

Gl, intestinal glands
LN, lymphatic nodules
ME, muscularis externa
MM, muscularis mucosae
MM??, presumptive location of muscularis mucosae
SM, submucosa
V, villi
asterisks, leaf-like villus

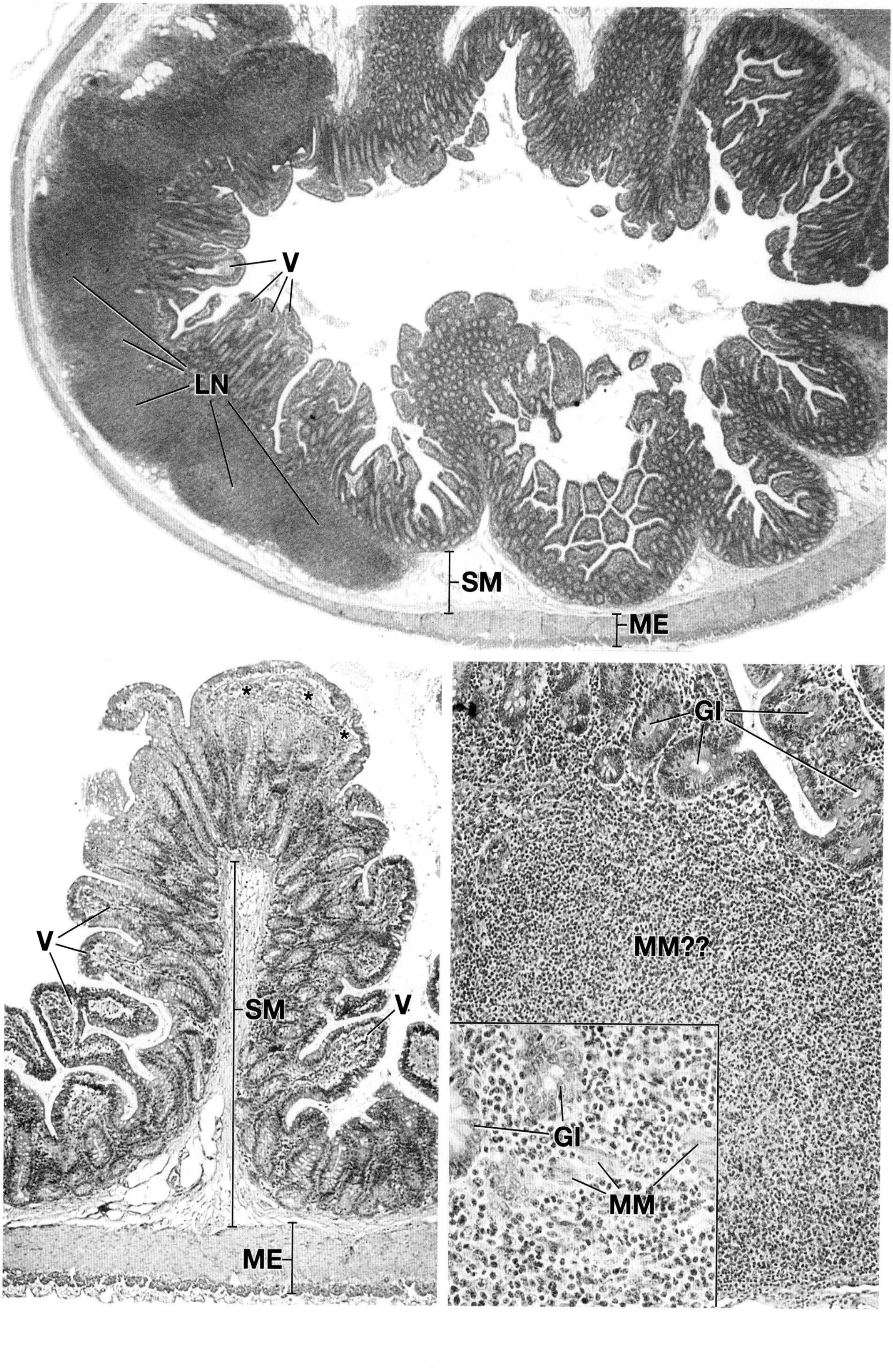
V
LN
SM
ME
*
*
*
V
SM
V
ME
GI
MM??
GI
MM

PLATE 17.9 ■ COLON

The principal functions of the **colon** are reabsorption of electrolytes and water and elimination of undigested food and other waste. The mucosa has a smooth surface; neither plicae circulares nor villi are present. Numerous **simple glands** (crypts of Lieberkühn) extend through the full thickness of the mucosa. The glands, as well as the surface, are lined with a simple columnar epithelium that contains goblet cells, absorptive cells, and enteroendocrine cells but does not normally contain Paneth cells. Here, too, stem cells are restricted to the bottom portions of the glands (crypts), and the normal zone of replication extends about one-third of the height of the crypt.

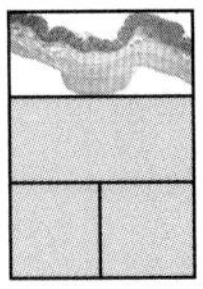

Colon, monkey, hematoxylin and eosin (H&E) ×30.

A cross section through the large intestine is shown at low magnification. It shows the four layers that make up the wall of the colon: the **mucosa** (*Muc*), **submucosa** (*SubM*), **muscularis externa** (*ME*), and **serosa** (*S*). Although these layers are the same as those in the small intestine, several differences should be noted. The large intestine has no villi, nor does it have plicae circulares. On the other hand, the muscularis externa is arranged in a distinctive manner, and this is evident in the photomicrograph. The longitudinal layer (*ME[l]*) is substantially thinner than the circular layer (*ME[c]*), except in three locations where the longitudinal layer of smooth muscle is present as a thick band. One of these thick bands, called a **tenia coli** (*TC*), is shown in this figure. Because the colon is cross-sectioned, the tenia coli is also cross-sectioned. The three teniae coli extend along the length of the large intestine as far as, but not into, the rectum.

The submucosa consists of a rather dense irregular connective tissue. It contains the larger blood vessels (*BV*) and areas of adipose tissue (see *A* in the next figure).

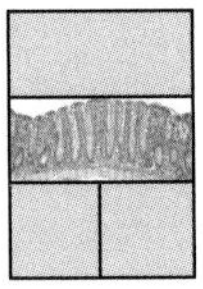

Mucosa, colon, monkey, H&E ×140.

The mucosa (*Muc*), shown at higher magnification, contains straight, unbranched, **tubular glands (crypts of Lieberkühn)** that extend to the muscularis mucosae (*MM*). The *arrows* identify the openings of some of the glands at the intestinal surface. Generally, the lumen of the glands is narrow, except in the deepest part of the gland, where it is often slightly dilated (*asterisks, lower left figure*). Between the glands (*Gl*) is a **lamina propria** (*LP*) that contains considerable numbers of lymphocytes and other cells of the immune system. Note the submucosa (*SubM*) containing dense irregular connective tissue with areas occupied by adipose tissue (*A*). Two *rectangles* mark areas of the mucosa that are examined at higher magnification in the next figures.

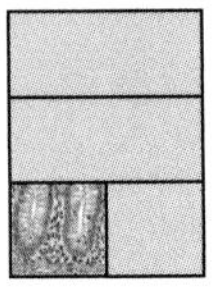

Lamina propria, colon, monkey, H&E ×525.

This figure reveals the **muscularis mucosae** (*MM*) and the cells in the **lamina propria** (*LP*), many of which can be recognized as lymphocytes and plasma cells. The smooth muscle cells of the muscularis mucosae are arranged in two layers. Note that the smooth muscle cells marked by the *arrowheads* show rounded nuclei; however, other smooth muscle cells appear as more or less rounded eosinophilic areas. These smooth muscle cells have been cut in cross section. Just above these cross-sectioned smooth muscle cells are others that have been cut longitudinally; they display elongated nuclei and elongated strands of eosinophilic cytoplasm. Also note the epithelial lining of the lower half of the intestinal glands, the lumens of which are marked by *asterisks*. The majority of the cells are goblet cells (*GC*); however, there are several visible mitotic figures (*M*). These represent dividing intermediate cells (stem cells) that are capable of cell division and differentiation into either absorptive or goblet cells.

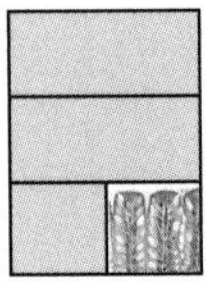

Intestinal glands, colon, monkey, H&E ×525.

The cells that line the surface of the colon and the glands are principally **absorptive cells** (*AC*) and **goblet cells** (*GC*). The absorptive cells have a thin striated border that is evident where the *arrows* show the opening of the glands. Interspersed among the absorptive cells are the goblet cells (*GC*). The number of absorptive cells decreases deeper into the gland, whereas the goblet cells increase in number. Other cells in the gland are enteroendocrine cells, not easily identified in routine H&E-stained paraffin sections, and, in the deep part of the gland, undifferentiated cells of the replicative zone, derived from the stem cells in the base of the crypt. The undifferentiated cells are readily identified if they are undergoing division, by virtue of the mitotic figures (*M*) they display (see figure on the *left*).

A, adipose tissue
AC, absorptive cells
BV, blood vessels
GC, goblet cells
Gl, intestinal glands
LP, lamina propria
M, mitotic figures
ME, muscularis externa
ME(c), circular layer of muscularis externa
ME(l), longitudinal layer of muscularis externa
MM, muscularis mucosae
Muc, mucosa
S, serosa
SubM, submucosa
TC, tenia coli
arrowheads, smooth muscle cells showing rounded nuclei
arrows, opening of intestinal glands
asterisks, lumen of intestinal glands

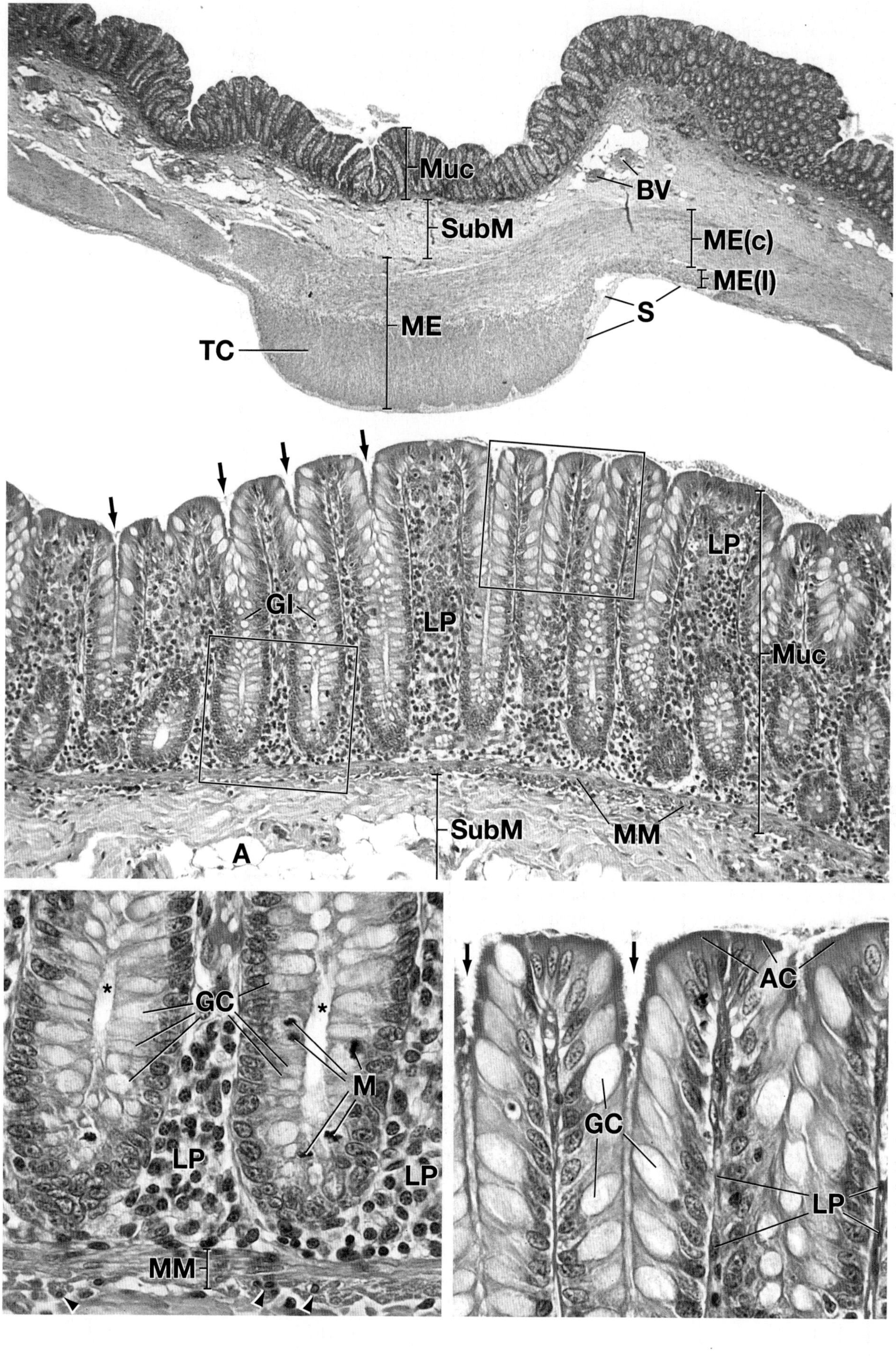
Muc
BV
SubM
ME(c)
ME(l)
S
ME
TC
GI
LP
LP
Muc
SubM
MM
A
GC
M
LP
LP
MM
AC
GC
LP

PLATE 17.10 ■ APPENDIX

The **appendix (vermiform appendix)** is typically described as a worm- or finger-like structure *[L. vermis, worm; forma, form]*. It arises from the cecum (the first segment of the large intestine; the others, in order, are the ascending, transverse, and descending colons; the sigmoid colon; the rectum; and the anal canal) that forms a blind-ending tube ranging from 2.5 cm to as much as 13 cm in length (average length of ~8 cm). Because it is a blind-ended pouch, intestinal contents may be trapped or sequestered in the appendix, often leading to inflammation and infection. In infants and children, it is both relatively and absolutely longer than in adults and contains numerous **lymphatic nodules**, suggesting that it has an immunologic role. Recent evidence indicates that it (and the cecum and terminal ileum) may be the "bursa equivalent" in mammals, that is, the portion of the immature immune system in which potential B lymphocytes achieve immunocompetence (equivalent to the *bursa of Fabricius* in birds).

The wall of the appendix is much like that of the small intestine, having a complete longitudinal layer of muscularis externa, but it lacks both plicae circulares and villi. Thus, the mucosa is similar to that of the colon, having simple glands. Even this resemblance is often obliterated, however, by the large number and size of the lymphatic nodules that usually fuse and extend into the submucosa. In later life, the amount of lymphatic tissue in the appendix regresses, and there is a consequent reduction in size. In many adults, the normal structure is lost, and the appendage is filled with fibrous scar tissue.

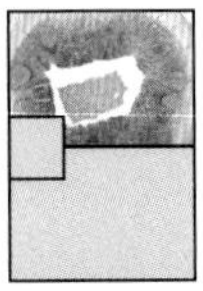

Appendix, human, hematoxylin and eosin (H&E) ×25.

Cross section of an appendix from a preadolescent showing the various structures composing its wall. The lumen (*L*), mucosa (*Muc*), submucosa (*Subm*), muscularis externa (*ME*), and serosa (*S*) are identified.

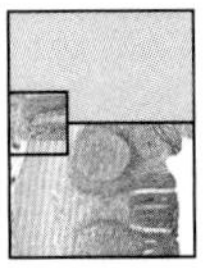

Appendix, human, H&E ×80; inset ×200.

This micrograph is a higher magnification of the *boxed area* in the previous figure. It reveals the straight tubular **glands** (*Gl*) that extend to the muscularis mucosae. Below is the **submucosa** (*Subm*) in which the **lymphatic nodules** (*LN*) and considerable diffuse lymphatic tissue are present. Note the distinct germinal centers (*GC*) of the lymph nodules and the cap region (*Cap*) that faces the lumen. The more superficial part of the submucosa blends and merges with the mucosal lamina propria because of the numerous lymphocytes in these two sites. The deeper part of the submucosa is relatively devoid of lymphocyte infiltration and contains large blood vessels (*BV*) and nerves. The muscularis externa (*ME*) is composed of a relatively thick circular layer and a much thinner outer longitudinal layer. The serosa (*S*) is only partially included in this micrograph.

The *inset* is a higher magnification of the *rectangular area* in the *lower figure*. Note that the epithelium of the glands in the appendix is similar to that of the large intestine. Most of the epithelial cells contain mucin, hence the light appearance of the apical cytoplasm. The lamina propria, as noted, is heavily infiltrated with lymphocytes, and the muscularis mucosae at the base of the glands is difficult to recognize (*arrows*).

BV, blood vessel
Cap, cap of lymphatic nodule
GC, germinal center
Gl, gland
L, lumen
LN, lymphatic nodule
ME, muscularis externa
Muc, mucosa
S, serosa
Subm, submucosa
arrows, muscularis mucosae at the base of glands

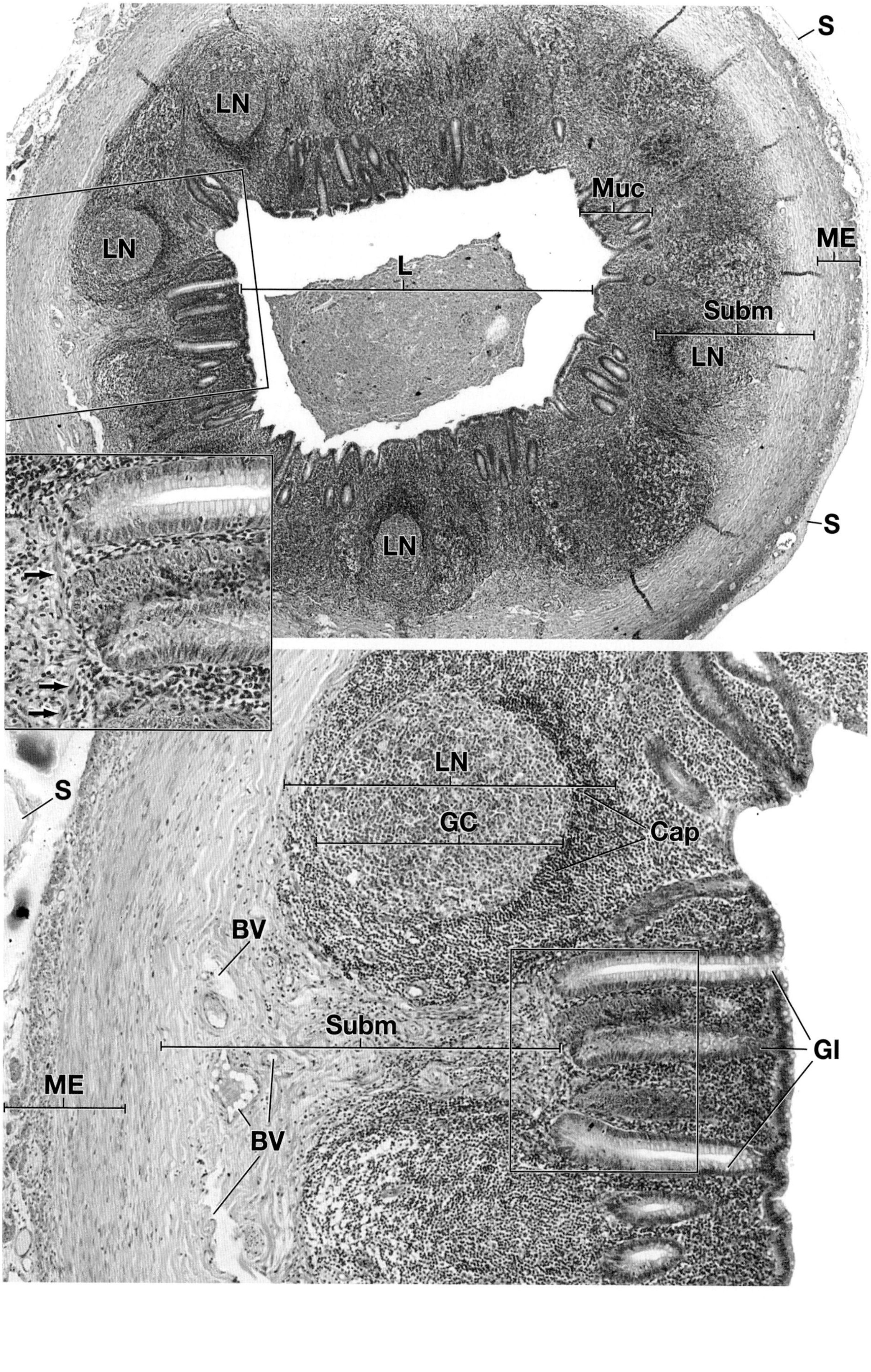
S
LN
Muc
LN
ME
L
Subm
LN
S
LN
S
LN
GC
Cap
BV
Subm
Gl
ME
BV

PLATE 17.11 ■ ANAL CANAL

At the **anal canal**, there is a transition from the simple columnar epithelium of the intestinal mucosa to the keratinized stratified squamous epithelium of the skin. Located between these two distinctly different epithelia is a narrow region (anal transitional zone) where the epithelium is first stratified columnar (or stratified cuboidal) and then nonkeratinized stratified squamous.

At the level of the anal canal, the muscularis mucosae disappears. At the same level, the circular layer of the muscularis externa thickens to become the internal anal sphincter. The external anal sphincter is formed by the striated muscles of the pelvic floor.

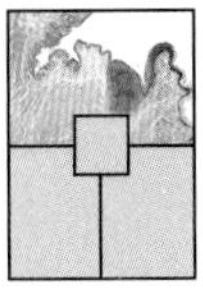

Anal canal, human, hematoxylin and eosin (H&E) ×40.

A view of the anal canal is shown at low magnification. Mucosa characteristic of the large intestine (**colorectal zone**) is seen on the *upper left* of the micrograph. This region is the upper part of the anal canal, and the intestinal glands are the same as those present in the colon. The muscularis mucosae (*MM*) is readily identified as the narrow band of tissue under the glands. Both the intestinal glands and the muscularis mucosae terminate within the *left rectangular area* of the field, and here, at the *diamond*, there is the first major change in the epithelium. This area called the **anal transitional zone** is examined at higher magnification in the *bottom left figure*. The *right rectangular area* includes the stratified squamous epithelium (*StS*) and its transition into stratified squamous keratinized epithelium [*StS(k)*] of the skin in the **squamous zone** of the anal canal and is examined at higher magnification in the *bottom right figure*.

Between the two *diamonds* in the *rectangular areas* shown is epithelium of the lower part of the anal canal. Below this epithelium, there is a lymphatic nodule that has a well-formed germinal center. Isolated lymphatic nodules (*LN*) beneath mucous membranes should not be construed to have fixed locations. Rather, they may or may not be present, according to local demands.

Also, at this low magnification, note the internal anal sphincter muscle (*IAS*), that is, the thickened, most distal portion of the circular layer of smooth muscle of the muscularis externa. Beneath the skin on the right is the subcutaneous part of the external anal sphincter muscle (*EAS*). It is composed of striated muscle fibers, which are seen in cross section.

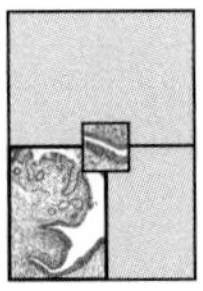

Anal transitional zone, anal canal, human, H&E ×160; inset ×300.

The junction between the simple columnar (*SC*) and the stratified (*ST*) epithelium called the **anal transitional zone** is marked with a *diamond*. The simple columnar epithelium of the upper part of the anal canal contains numerous goblet cells, and as in the mucosa of the colon, this epithelium is continuous with the epithelium of the intestinal glands (*IG*). These glands continue to about the same point as the muscularis mucosae (*MM*). Characteristically, the lamina propria contains large numbers of lymphocytes (*Lym*), particularly so in the region marked. A higher magnification of the stratified columnar epithelium (*StCol*) and stratified cuboidal epithelium (*StC*) found in the transition zone is shown in the *inset*.

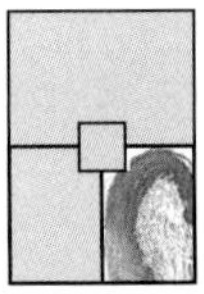

Squamous zone, anal canal, human, H&E ×160.

The final change in epithelial type occurs at the **squamous zone of the anal canal**, which is shown here. On the *right* is the stratified squamous epithelium of skin (*StS[k]*). The keratinized nature of the surface is apparent. Conversely, the stratified squamous epithelium (*StS*) below the level of the *diamond* is not keratinized, and nucleated cells can be seen all the way to the surface. Again, numerous lymphocytes (*Lym*) are located in the underlying connective tissue, and many have migrated into the epithelium in the nonkeratinized area.

EAS, external anal sphincter
IAS, internal anal sphincter
IG, intestinal glands
LN, lymphatic nodules
Lym, lymphocytes
MM, muscularis mucosae
SC, simple columnar epithelium
ST, stratified epithelium
StC, stratified cuboidal epithelium
StCol, stratified columnar epithelium
StS, stratified squamous epithelium
StS(k), stratified squamous epithelium (keratinized)
arrow, termination of muscularis mucosae
diamonds, junctions between epithelial types

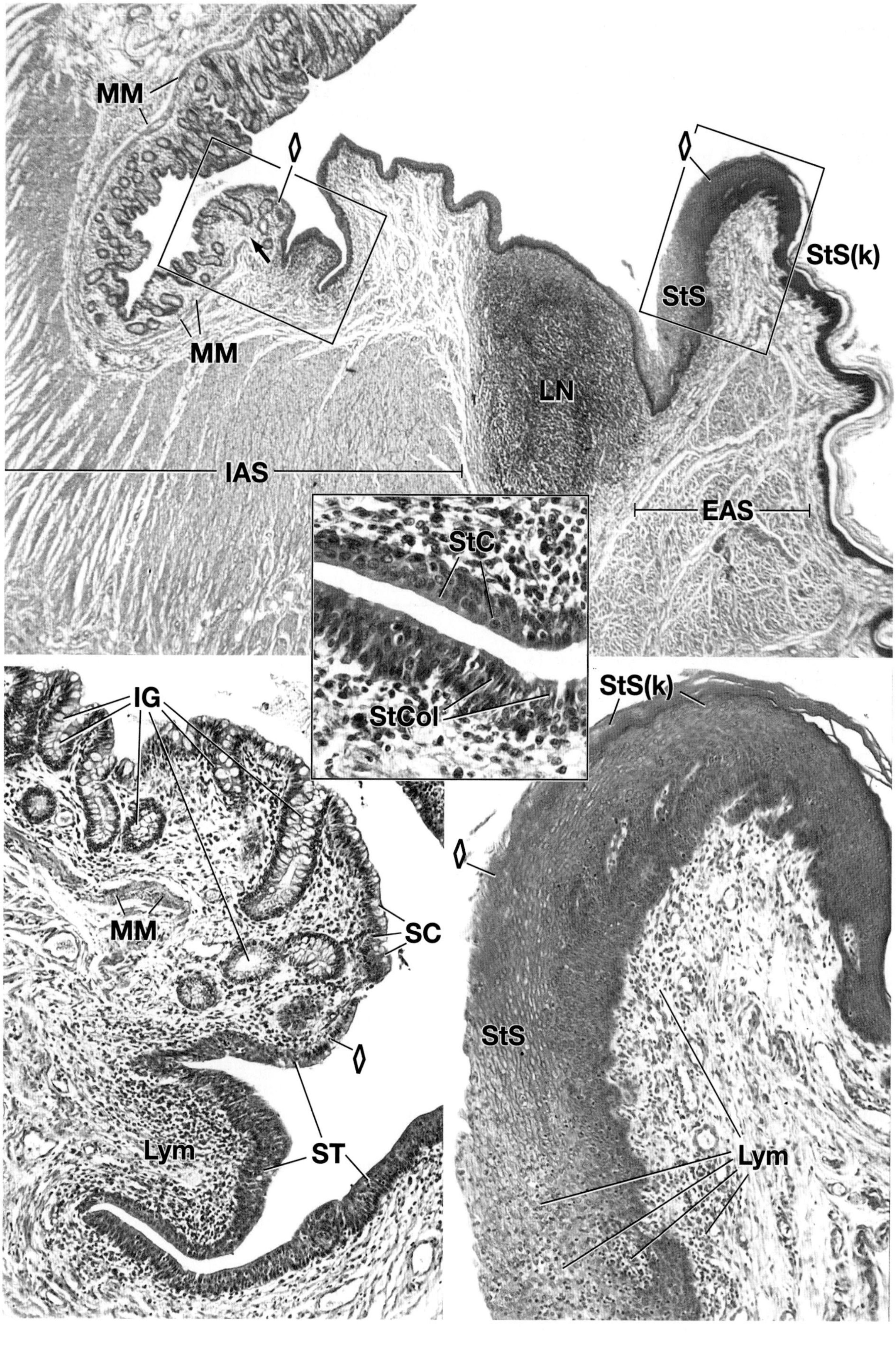
MM
MM
LN
StS
StS(k)
IAS
EAS
StC
StCol
IG
MM
SC
ST
Lym
StS(k)
StS
Lym

18 DIGESTIVE SYSTEM III: LIVER, GALLBLADDER, AND PANCREAS

■ LIVER

Overview

The **liver** is the largest mass of glandular tissue in the body and the largest internal organ, weighing approximately 1,500 g and accounting for nearly 2.5% of adult body weight. It is located in the upper right and partially in the upper left quadrants of the abdominal cavity, protected by the rib cage. The liver is enclosed in a capsule of fibrous connective tissue (Glisson capsule); a serous covering (visceral peritoneum) surrounds the capsule, except where the liver adheres directly to the diaphragm or the other organs.

The liver is anatomically divided by deep grooves into two large lobes (the right and left lobes) and two smaller lobes (the quadrate and caudate lobes; Fig. 18.1). This anatomic division has only topographic significance because it relates the lobes of the liver to other abdominal organs. Division of the liver into functional or surgical segments that correspond to the blood supply and bile drainage is more clinically important.

In the embryo, the liver develops as an **endodermal evagination** from the wall of the foregut (specifically the site that will become the duodenum) to form the **hepatic diverticulum**. The diverticulum proliferates, giving rise to the **hepatocytes**, which become arranged in cellular (liver) cords, thus forming the parenchyma of the liver. The original stalk of the hepatic diverticulum becomes the **common bile duct**. An outgrowth from the common bile duct forms the **cystic diverticulum** that gives rise to the **gallbladder** and **cystic duct**.

Liver Physiology

Many circulating **plasma proteins** are produced and secreted by the liver. The liver plays an important role in the uptake, storage, and distribution of both nutrients and vitamins from the bloodstream. It also maintains the blood glucose level and regulates circulating levels of **very low-density lipoproteins (VLDLs)**. In addition, the liver degrades or conjugates numerous toxic substances and drugs, but overexposure to these toxins can lead to damage. The liver is also an **exocrine organ**; it produces a **bile secretion** that contains bile salts, phospholipids, and cholesterol. Finally, the liver performs important **endocrine-like functions**.

The liver produces most of the body's circulating plasma proteins.

The **circulating plasma proteins** produced by the liver include the following:

- **Albumins**, which are involved in regulating plasma volume and tissue fluid balance by maintaining the plasma colloid osmotic pressure

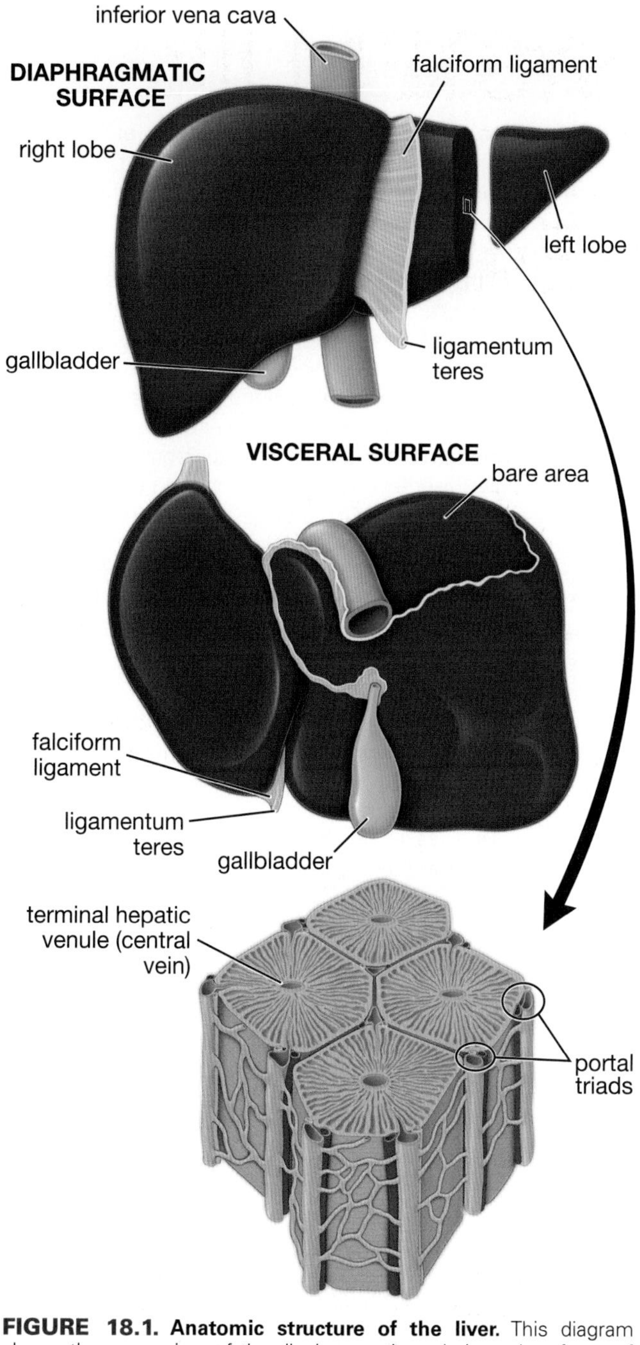

FIGURE 18.1. Anatomic structure of the liver. This diagram shows the gross view of the diaphragmatic and visceral surfaces of the liver, with labeled anatomic landmarks found on both surfaces. The enlarged cross-sectional area of the liver (*bottom*) shows the general microscopic organization of the liver into lobules. Note the presence of hepatic portal triads at the periphery of each lobule, with the terminal hepatic venule (central vein) in the center of the lobule.

- **Lipoproteins**, in particular, VLDLs. The liver synthesizes most VLDLs, which participate in the transport of triglycerides from the liver to other organs. The liver also produces small amounts of other plasma lipoproteins, such as **low-density lipoproteins (LDLs)** and **high-density lipoproteins (HDLs)**. LDLs transport cholesterol esters from the liver to other tissues. HDLs remove cholesterol from the peripheral tissues and transport it to the liver (see Folder 18.1).
- **Glycoproteins**, which include proteins involved in iron transport, such as haptoglobin, transferrin, and hemopexin
- **Prothrombin** and **fibrinogen**, important components of the blood-clotting cascade
- **Nonimmune α-globulins** and **β-globulins**, which also help maintain plasma colloid osmotic pressure and serve as carrier proteins for various substances (see Chapter 10, Blood, page 299)

The liver stores and converts lipid-soluble vitamins.

Several lipid-soluble **vitamins** are taken up from the bloodstream and then stored or biochemically modified by the liver, including:

- **Vitamin A (retinol)**, an important vitamin in vision. Vitamin A is the precursor of retinal, which is required for the synthesis of rhodopsin in the eye. The liver plays a major role in the uptake, storage, and maintenance of circulating levels of vitamin A. When the vitamin A levels in the blood decrease, the liver mobilizes its storage sites in the hepatic stellate cells (see page 702). Vitamin A is then released into the circulation in the form of **retinol** bound to **retinol-binding protein (RBP)**. The liver also synthesizes RBP; RBP synthesis is regulated by the plasma levels of **vitamin A**. **Night blindness** and multiple skin disorders are related to vitamin A deficiency.
- **Vitamin D (cholecalciferol)**, an important vitamin in calcium and phosphate metabolism. Vitamin D is acquired from dietary vitamin D_3 and is also produced in the skin during exposure to ultraviolet light by conversion of 7-dehydrocholesterol. Unlike vitamin A, vitamin D is not stored in the liver but is distributed to skeletal muscles and adipose tissue. The liver plays an important role in vitamin D metabolism by converting vitamin D_3 to **25-hydroxycholecalciferol**, the predominant form of circulating vitamin D. Further conversion takes place in the kidney to 1,25-hydroxycholecalciferol, which is 10 times more active than vitamin D_3. Vitamin D is essential for the development and growth of the skeletal system and teeth. Deficiency of vitamin D is associated with **rickets** and disorders of bone mineralization.
- **Vitamin E**, which represents a group of lipid-soluble tocopherols and tocotrienols. Most vitamin E in the body is in the form of **α-tocopherol**, a powerful, chain-breaking antioxidant that prevents the propagation of free radicals. Vitamin E is transported to the liver in chylomicrons and is bound to α-tocopherol transfer protein (α-TTP). Secretion of α-tocopherol from hepatocytes is linked to VLDL assembly. Individuals with **fatty liver disease** and nonalcoholic steatohepatitis (NASH) have decreased levels of circulating vitamin E.
- **Vitamin K**, which is important in hepatic synthesis of prothrombin and several other clotting factors. Like vitamin D, it is derived from two sources: dietary vitamin K and synthesis in the small intestine by intestinal bacterial flora. Vitamin K is transported to the liver with chylomicrons, where it is rapidly absorbed, partially used, and then partially secreted with the VLDL fraction. Vitamin K deficiency is associated with **hypoprothrombinemia** and bleeding disorders.

The liver is a key organ in the supply, storage, metabolism, and excretion of iron and copper.

The liver functions in the storage, metabolism, and homeostasis of iron and copper. It synthesizes almost all proteins involved in **iron recovery** from damaged or senescent

FOLDER 18.1

CLINICAL CORRELATION: LIPOPROTEINS

Lipoproteins are multicomponent complexes of proteins and lipids that are involved in the transport of cholesterol and triglycerides in the blood. Cholesterol and triglycerides do not circulate freely in the plasma because lipids, on their own, would be unable to remain in suspension. The association of the protein with the lipid-containing core makes the complex sufficiently hydrophilic to remain suspended in the plasma.

Lipoproteins serve a variety of functions in cellular membranes and the transport and metabolism of lipids. Lipoprotein precursors are produced in hepatocytes. The lipid component is produced in the smooth endoplasmic reticulum (sER); the protein component is produced in the rough endoplasmic reticulum (rER). The lipoprotein complexes pass to the Golgi, where secretory vesicles containing electron-dense lipoprotein particles bud off and are then released at the cell surface bordering the perisinusoidal space to reach the bloodstream. Several hormones, such as estrogen and thyroid hormones, regulate the secretion of lipoproteins.

In general, four classes of lipoproteins have been defined by their characteristic density, molecular weight, size, and chemical composition: **chylomicrons**, **VLDLs**, **LDLs**, and **HDLs**. These lipoproteins differ in chemical composition and can be isolated from plasma according to their flotation properties, from largest and least dense to smallest and most dense.

Chylomicrons, the lightest of all lipoproteins, are made only in the small intestine. Their main function is to transport the large amount of absorbed fat to the bloodstream.

VLDLs are denser and smaller than chylomicrons; they are synthesized predominately in the liver and to a lesser extent in the small intestine. The very low-density lipoproteins (VLDLs) are rich in triglycerides. Their function is to transport most of the triglycerides from the liver to other organs. Liver VLDLs are associated with circulating **apolipoprotein B-100**, also synthesized in the liver, which aids in secretion of VLDLs. In congenital liver disease, such as **abetalipoproteinemia**, and, to a lesser degree, in acute and chronic disorders, the liver is unable to produce apolipoprotein B-100, leading to blockage in the secretion of VLDLs. In liver biopsy specimens from these individuals, large lipid droplets occupy most of the hepatocyte cytoplasm.

LDLs and **HDLs** are produced in the plasma; however, small amounts of these fractions are produced by the liver. Low-density lipoproteins (LDLs) are denser than VLDLs, and high-density lipoproteins (HDLs) are denser than LDLs. The function of LDLs is to transport cholesterol esters from the liver to the peripheral organs. The HDLs are involved in the transport of cholesterol from the peripheral tissues to the liver. High levels of LDL are associated with an increased risk of cardiovascular disease; high levels of HDL or low levels of LDL are associated with decreased risk.

red blood cells, including transferrin, haptoglobin, and hemopexin. **Transferrin** is a plasma iron transport protein. **Haptoglobin** binds with high affinity to free hemoglobin in the plasma; this complex is removed by macrophages in the liver (and spleen) to preserve iron. **Hemopexin** is involved in the transport of free heme in the blood. Hepatocytes are the major sites of long-term storage of iron. For details related to iron recovery and its storage in the liver, see pages 701-702.

The liver plays an important role in the disposition of **copper**. Copper is absorbed from the gastrointestinal tract into the portal circulation, where it binds to albumins and amino acids such as histidine. It then passes through the liver, where hepatocytes are the primary site of copper uptake and accumulation in the liver. Copper excretion into bile is regulated by an enzyme called **copper ATPase (Wilson ATPase)**, which promotes incorporation of copper into apoceruloplasmin (an unstable enzyme without the copper) to form **ceruloplasmin**, the major copper-carrying protein in the blood. Ceruloplasmin is a 151-kDa glycoprotein enzyme, contains six copper atoms in its structure, and comprises more than 95% of the copper found in the plasma. Mutations of the **ATP7B gene** encoding Wilson ATPase are responsible for **Wilson disease**, an autosomal recessive disorder characterized by impaired synthesis of ceruloplasmin and biliary excretion of copper. Copper accumulates in the liver and leads to progressive liver damage. In addition, copper accumulates in the brain and other tissues. Affected individuals may show symptoms of **liver failure** and **neuropsychiatric manifestations**. Treatment is lifelong with either an oral chelating agent with copper-binding capacity or zinc salts. Liver transplantation is necessary for patients who do not respond to medical treatment.

The liver degrades drugs and toxins.

Hepatocytes are involved in **degradation of drugs**, **toxins**, and other proteins foreign to the body (**xenobiotics**). Many drugs and toxins are not hydrophilic; therefore, they cannot be eliminated effectively from the circulation by the kidneys. The liver converts these substances into more soluble forms. This process is performed by the hepatocytes in two phases:

- **Phase I (oxidation)** includes hydroxylation (adding an −OH group) and carboxylation (adding a −COOH group) to a foreign compound. This phase is performed in the hepatocyte smooth endoplasmic reticulum (sER) and mitochondria. It involves a series of biochemical reactions with proteins collectively named cytochrome P450.
- **Phase II (conjugation)** includes conjugation with glucuronic acid, glycine, or taurine. This process makes the product of phase I even more water soluble so that it can be easily removed by the kidney.

The liver is involved in many other important pathways related to carbohydrate, lipid, and protein metabolism.

The liver is important in **carbohydrate metabolism** as it maintains an adequate supply of nutrients for cell processes. In **glucose** metabolism, the liver phosphorylates absorb glucose from the gastrointestinal tract to **glucose-6-phosphate**. Depending on energy requirements, glucose-6-phosphate is either stored in the liver in the form of **glycogen** or used in the glycolytic pathways. During fasting, glycogen is broken down by the process of **glycogenolysis**, and glucose is released into the bloodstream.

In addition, the liver functions in **lipid metabolism**. Fatty acids derived from plasma are consumed by hepatocytes using **β-oxidation** to provide energy. The liver also produces **ketone bodies** that are used as fuel by other organs. (The liver cannot use them as an energy source.) The involvement in **cholesterol** metabolism (synthesis and uptake from the blood) is also an important function of the liver. Cholesterol is used in the formation of bile salts, synthesis of VLDLs, and biosynthesis of organelles.

The liver is also involved in **protein metabolism**. It is the site of both protein synthesis and amino acid uptake and metabolism. The liver has also the capacity to deaminate amino acids; thus, it synthesizes most of the **urea** in the body from ammonium ions derived from protein and nucleic acid degradation. Finally, the liver is involved in the synthesis and conversion of **nonessential amino acids**.

Bile production is an exocrine function of the liver.

The liver carries out numerous **metabolic conversions** involving substrates delivered by blood from the digestive tract, pancreas, and spleen. Some of these products are involved in the production of **bile**, an exocrine secretion of the liver. Bile contains conjugated and degraded waste products that are returned to the intestine for disposal as well as substances that bind to metabolites in the intestine to aid in absorption (Table 18.1). Bile is carried from the parenchyma of the liver by bile ducts that fuse to form the **hepatic duct**. The cystic duct then carries the bile into the **gallbladder**, where it is concentrated. Bile is returned, via the cystic duct, to the common bile duct, which delivers bile from the liver and gallbladder to the duodenum (see Fig. 18.17).

The endocrine-like functions of the liver are represented by its ability to modify the structure and function of many hormones.

The **liver modifies the action of hormones** released by other organs. The liver's endocrine-like functions involve modification of the following hormones:

- **Thyroxine**, a hormone secreted by the thyroid gland as tetraiodothyronine (T_4), which is converted in the liver to the biologically active form, **triiodothyronine (T_3)**, by deiodination.
- **Growth hormone (GH)**, a hormone secreted by the pituitary gland. The action of GH is amplified by liver-produced **insulin-like growth factor 1 (IGF-1)** and inhibited by **somatostatin**, which is secreted by enteroendocrine cells of the gastrointestinal tract. Genetic **IGF-1 deficiencies** are found in certain ethnic groups whose members are less than average in height, such as Bayaka pygmies in Central Africa. Hormonal studies indicate that these individuals have normal GH levels; however, the level of IGF-1 in the adolescent population is reduced to one-third of that in control adolescents. Because IGF-1 is the principal factor responsible for normal pubertal growth, members of this ethnic population do not undergo accelerated growth spurt typical of puberty, which results in a short statue of less than 150 cm (5 feet).
- **Insulin** and **glucagon**, both pancreatic hormones. These hormones are degraded in many organs, but the liver and kidney are the most important sites of their degradation.
- In addition, **vitamin D_3** is converted by the liver to **25-hydroxycholecalciferol**, a biologically active metabolite of vitamin D_3 and the predominant form of circulating vitamin D (page 693).

Blood Supply to the Liver

The liver has a **unique dual blood supply** consisting of a venous (portal) supply via the **hepatic portal vein** and an arterial supply via the **hepatic artery**. Both vessels enter the liver at a hilum or **porta hepatis**, the same site at which the common bile duct carries the bile secreted by the liver and the lymphatic vessels leave the liver. Therefore, bile flows in a direction opposite to that of the blood.

The liver receives blood that is initially supplied to the intestines, pancreas, and spleen.

The liver is unique among organs because it receives its major blood supply (about 75%) from the hepatic portal vein, which carries venous blood that is largely depleted of oxygen. The blood delivered to the liver by the **hepatic portal vein** comes from the digestive tract and the major abdominal organs, such as the pancreas and spleen.

The portal blood carried to the liver contains the following substances:

- Nutrients and toxic materials absorbed in the intestine
- Blood cells and breakdown products of blood cells from the spleen
- Endocrine secretions of the pancreas and enteroendocrine cells of the gastrointestinal tract

TABLE 18.1 Composition of Bile

Component	Function
Water	Serves as solvent in which other components are carried
Phospholipids (i.e., lecithin) and cholesterol	Function as metabolic substrates for other cells in the body; act as precursors of membrane components and steroids; largely reabsorbed in the gut and recycled
Bile salts (also called *bile acids*) Primary (secreted by liver): cholic acid, chenodeoxycholic acid Secondary (converted by bacterial flora in the intestine): deoxycholic acid, lithocholic acid	Act as emulsifying agents that aid in the digestion and absorption of lipids from the gut and help to keep the cholesterol and phospholipids of the bile in solution; largely recycled between the liver and gut
Bile pigments, principally the glucuronide of bilirubin produced in the spleen, bone marrow, and liver by the breakdown of hemoglobin	Detoxify bilirubin, the end product of hemoglobin degradation, and carry it to the gut for disposal
Electrolytes: Na^+, K^+, Ca^{2+}, Mg^{2+}, Cl^-, and HCO_3^-	Establish and maintain bile as an isotonic fluid; also largely reabsorbed in the gut

Thus, the liver is placed directly in the pathway of blood vessels that convey substances absorbed from the digestive tract. Although the liver is the first organ to receive metabolic substrates and nutrients, it is also the first exposed to toxic substances that have been absorbed.

The **hepatic artery**, a branch of the celiac trunk, carries oxygenated blood to the liver, providing the remaining 25% of its blood supply. Because blood from the two sources mixes just before it perfuses the hepatocytes of the liver parenchyma, the liver cells are never exposed to fully oxygenated blood.

Within the liver, the distributing branches of the portal vein and hepatic artery, which supply the sinusoidal capillaries (sinusoids) that bathe the hepatocytes, and the draining branches of the bile duct system, which lead to the common hepatic duct, course together in a relationship termed the **portal triad**. Although a convenient term, it is a misnomer because one or more vessels of the lymphatic drainage system of the liver always travel with the vein, artery, and bile duct (Fig. 18.2).

The **sinusoids** are in intimate contact with the hepatocytes and provide for the exchange of substances between the blood and liver cells. The sinusoids lead to a **terminal hepatic venule (central vein)** that, in turn, empties into the **sublobular veins**. Blood leaves the liver through the **hepatic veins**, which empty into the inferior vena cava.

Structural Organization of the Liver

As introduced previously, the liver is made up of the following structures:

- **Parenchyma**, consisting of organized plates of hepatocytes, which, in the adult, are normally one cell thick and are separated by sinusoidal capillaries. In young individuals up to 6 years of age, the liver cells are arranged in plates with two cells thick.
- **Connective tissue stroma** that is continuous with the fibrous capsule of Glisson. Blood vessels, nerves, lymphatic vessels, and bile ducts travel within the connective tissue stroma.
- **Sinusoidal capillaries (sinusoids)**, the vascular channels between the plates of hepatocytes
- **Perisinusoidal spaces (spaces of Disse)**, which lie between the sinusoidal endothelium and the hepatocytes

Liver lobules

There are three ways to describe the structure of the liver in terms of a functional unit: the classic lobule, the portal lobule, and the liver acinus. The classic lobule is the traditional way to describe the organization of the liver parenchyma, and it is relatively easy to visualize. It is based on the distribution of the branches of the portal vein and hepatic artery within the organ and the pathway that blood from them follows as it ultimately perfuses the liver cells.

The classic hepatic lobule is a roughly hexagonal mass of tissue.

The **classic lobule** (Fig. 18.3 and Plate 18.1, page 722) consists of stacks of anastomosing plates of hepatocytes, one cell thick, separated by the anastomosing system of sinusoids that perfuse the cells with the mixed portal and arterial blood. Each lobule measures about 2.0 mm × 0.7 mm. At the center of the lobule is a relatively large venule, the **terminal hepatic venule (central vein)**, into which the sinusoids drain. The plates of cells radiate from the central vein to the periphery of the lobule, as do the sinusoids. At the angles of the hexagon are the **portal canals**, loose stromal connective tissue characterized by the presence of the **portal triads** (hepatic artery, portal vein, and bile duct). This connective tissue is ultimately continuous with the fibrous capsule of the liver. The

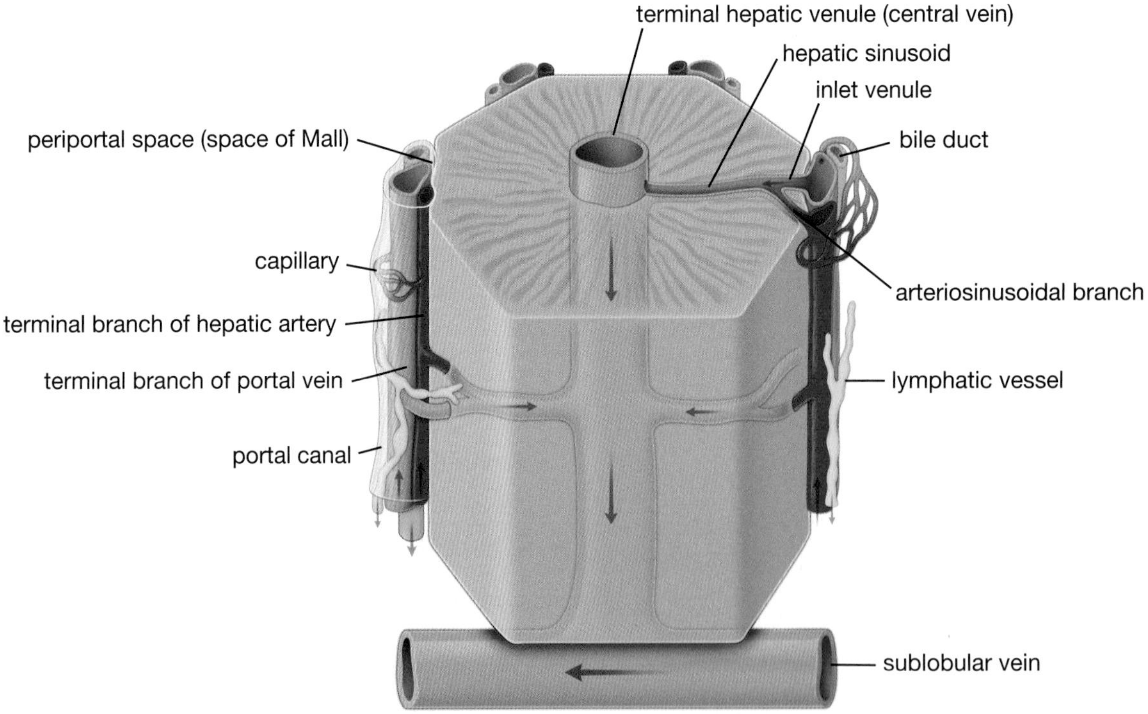

FIGURE 18.2. Blood supply to the liver: the portal triad. The portal triad is composed of the branches of the hepatic artery, portal vein, and bile duct. Blood from the terminal branches of the hepatic artery and portal vein enters the hepatic sinusoids. The mixture of venous and arterial blood is transported by the sinusoids toward the terminal hepatic venule (central vein). Blood then drains into the sublobular veins, the tributaries of the hepatic vein. Note the small vessels and capillary network in the perivascular connective tissue surrounding each hepatic triad within the portal canal. Also note the periportal space (of Mall), located between the portal canal and the outermost hepatocytes. This space is also filled with a small amount of connective tissue in which blind-ended lymphatic capillaries are located; these form larger lymphatic vessels that accompany branches of the hepatic artery.

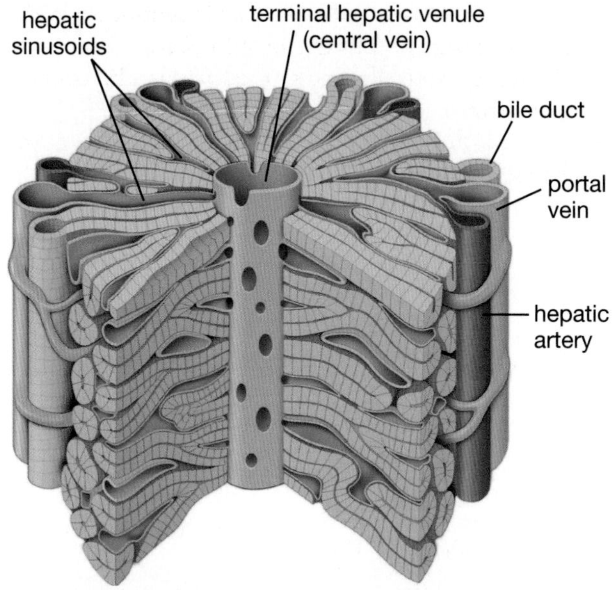

FIGURE 18.3. Diagram of a classic liver lobule. A classic liver lobule can be schematically diagramed as a six-sided polyhedral prism with portal triads (hepatic artery, portal vein, and bile duct) at each corner. The blood vessels of the portal triads send distributing branches along the sides of the lobule, and these branches open into the hepatic sinusoids. The long axis of the lobule is traversed by the terminal hepatic venule (central vein), which receives blood from the hepatic sinusoids. Note that a wedge of the tissue has been removed from the lobule for better visualization of the terminal hepatic venule. Interconnecting sheets or plates of hepatocytes are disposed in a radial pattern from the terminal hepatic venule to the periphery of the lobule.

portal canal is bordered by the outermost hepatocytes of the lobule. At the edges of the portal canal, between the connective tissue stroma and the hepatocytes, is a small space called the **periportal space (space of Mall)**, which in some species (e.g., the rabbit; Fig. 18.4) is easily identified. This space is one of the sites where lymph originates in the liver.

In some species (e.g., the pig; Fig. 18.5a), the classic lobule is easily recognized because the portal areas are connected by relatively thick layers of connective tissue. In humans, however, there is normally very little interlobular connective tissue. For this reason, when examining histologic sections of the liver, it is necessary to draw imaginary lines between portal areas surrounding a central vein to get some sense of the size of the classic lobule (Fig. 18.5b).

The portal lobule emphasizes the exocrine functions of the liver.

The major exocrine function of the liver is bile secretion. Thus, the morphologic axis of the **portal lobule** is the interlobular bile duct of the portal triad of the classic lobule. Its outer margins are imaginary lines drawn between the three central veins that are closest to that portal triad (Fig. 18.6a). These lines define a roughly triangular block of tissue that includes those portions of three classic lobules that secrete the bile that drains into its axial bile duct. This concept allows a description of hepatic parenchymal structure comparable to that of other exocrine glands.

The liver acinus is the structural unit that provides the best correlation between blood perfusion, metabolic activity, and liver pathology.

The **liver acinus** is lozenge shaped and represents the smallest functional unit of the hepatic parenchyma. The **short axis of the acinus** is defined by the terminal branches of the portal triad that lie along the border between two classic lobules. The **long axis of the acinus** is a line drawn between the two central veins closest to the short axis. Therefore, in a two-dimensional view (Fig. 18.6b), the liver acinus occupies parts of adjacent classic lobules. This concept allows a description of the exocrine secretory function of the liver comparable to that of the portal lobule.

The hepatocytes in each liver acinus are described as being arranged in three concentric elliptical zones surrounding the short axis (see Fig. 18.6b):

- **Zone 1** is closest to the short axis and the blood supply from penetrating branches of the portal vein and hepatic artery. This zone corresponds to the periphery of the classic lobules.
- **Zone 3** is farthest from the short axis and closest to the terminal hepatic vein (central vein). This zone corresponds to the most central part of the classic lobule that surrounds the terminal hepatic vein.
- **Zone 2** lies between zones 1 and 3 but has no sharp boundaries.

The zonation is important in the description and interpretation of patterns of degeneration, regeneration, and specific toxic effects in the liver parenchyma relative to the degree or quality of vascular perfusion of the hepatic cells. As a result of the **sinusoidal blood flow**, the oxygen gradient, metabolic activity of the hepatocytes, and distribution of hepatic enzymes vary across the three zones. The distribution of liver damage resulting from ischemia and exposure to toxic substances can be explained using this zonal interpretation.

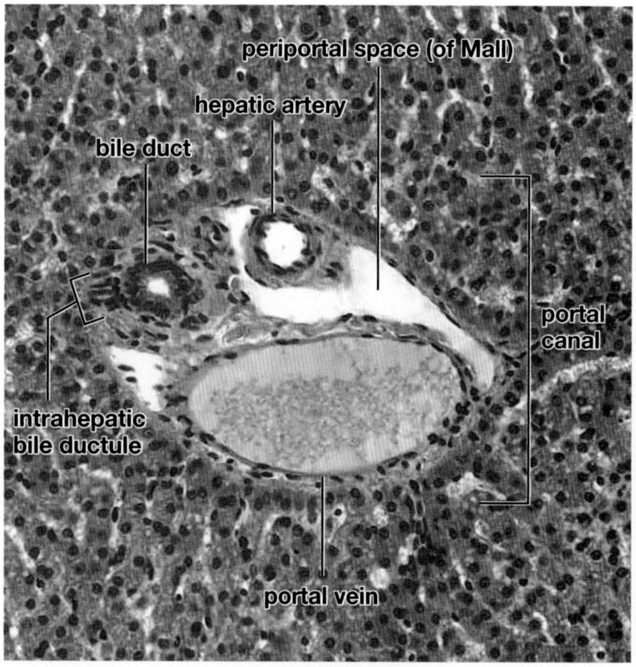

FIGURE 18.4. Photomicrograph of the portal canal in rabbit liver. This high-magnification photomicrograph of rabbit liver from a routine hematoxylin and eosin (H&E) preparation shows the portal canal located at the angles of hepatic lobules. The portal canal is bordered by linearly arranged outermost hepatocytes of the lobule. Each portal is occupied by a portal triad consisting of the portal vein, hepatic artery, and bile duct, all surrounded by loose stromal connective tissue. Note longitudinally sectioned nuclei of cholangiocytes of the intrahepatic bile ductule, which drains into the bile duct. At the periphery of the portal canal, between the connective tissue stroma and the hepatocytes, is a space called the *periportal* space (of Mall), which, in this image, contains two irregular profiles of lymphatic vessels lined by endothelial cells. ×320. (Courtesy of Dr. Nathan Swailes, University of Iowa.)

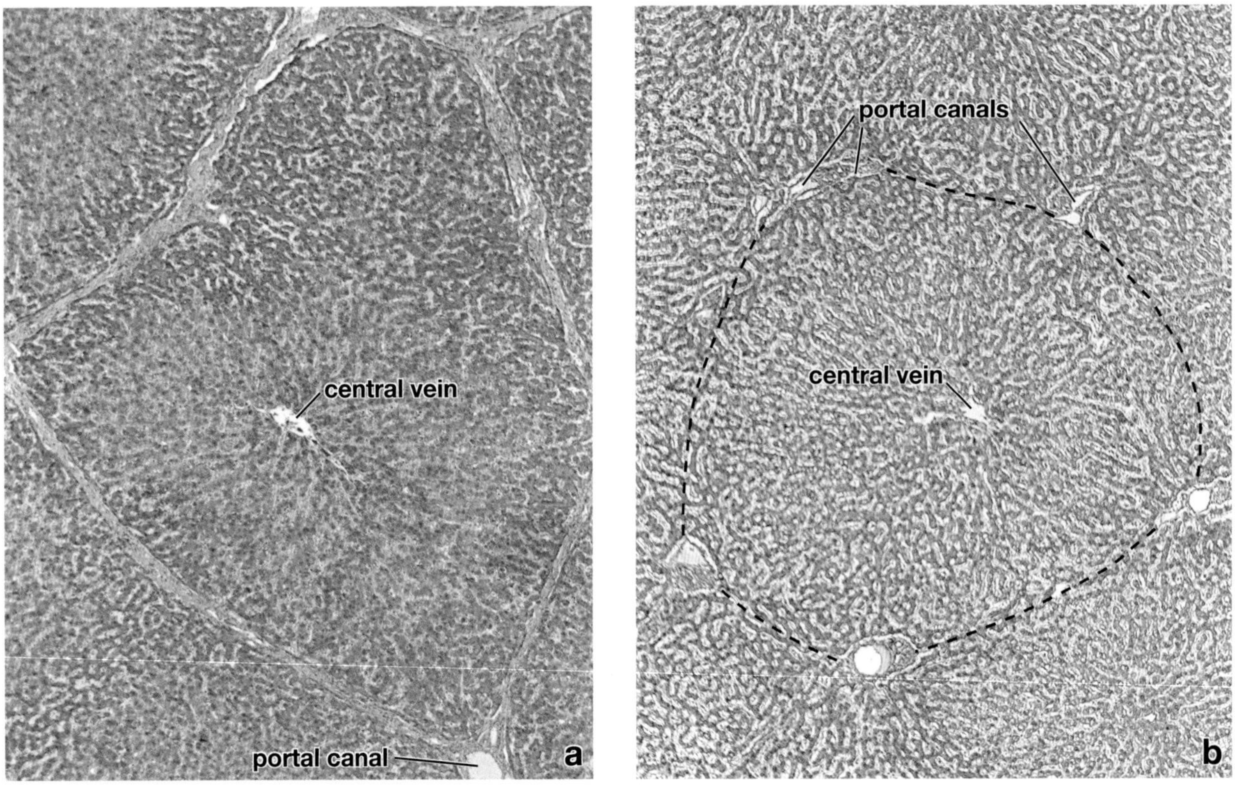

FIGURE 18.5. Photomicrographs of pig and human livers. a. This photomicrograph shows a cross section of a pig liver lobule stained by the Mallory-Azan method to visualize connective tissue components. Note the relatively thick interlobular connective tissue (*stained blue*) surrounding the lobules. The terminal hepatic venule (central vein) is visible in the center of the lobule. ×65. **b.** Photomicrograph of human liver from a routine hematoxylin and eosin (H&E) preparation. Note that in contrast to the pig liver, the lobules of the human liver lack connective tissue septa. The plates of hepatocytes of one lobule merge with those of adjacent lobules. The boundaries of a lobule can be approximated, however, by drawing a line (*dashed line*) from one portal canal to the next, thus circumscribing the lobule. ×65.

Cells in **zone 1** are the first to receive oxygen, nutrients, and toxins from the sinusoidal blood and the first to show morphologic changes after **bile duct occlusion** (bile stasis). These cells are also the last to die if circulation is impaired and the first to regenerate. Conversely, cells in **zone 3** are the first to show ischemic necrosis (**centrilobular necrosis**) in situations of **reduced perfusion** and the first to show fat accumulation. They are the last to respond to toxic substances and bile stasis. Normal variations in enzyme activity, the number and size of cytoplasmic organelles, and the size of cytoplasmic

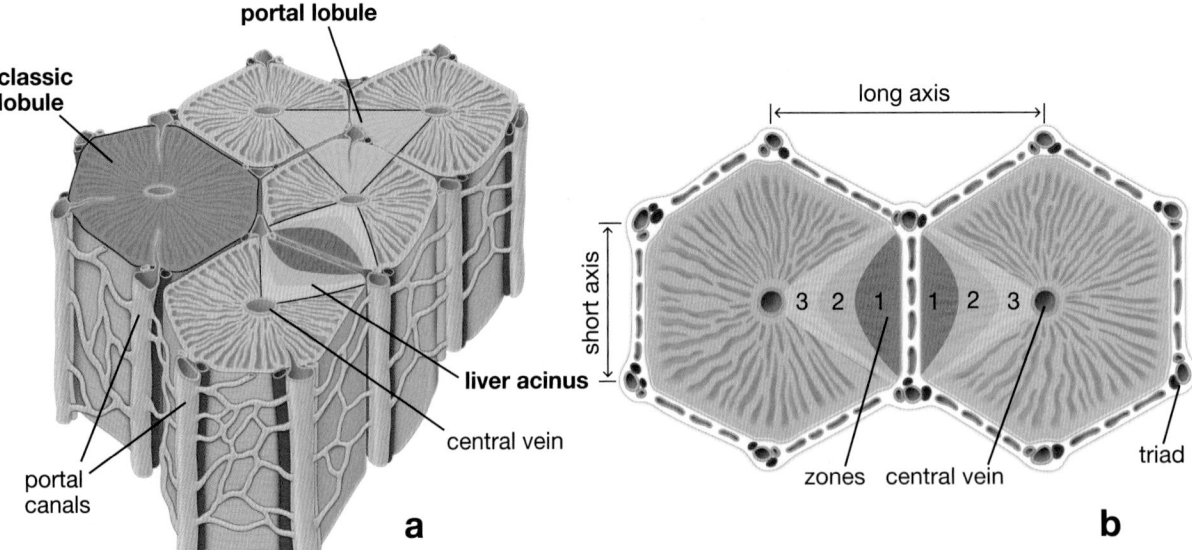

FIGURE 18.6. Comparison of three models of liver organization and function. a. The outlines of a classic hepatic lobule, portal lobule, and liver acinus are visible on this section of the liver tissue. Note that the hexagonal-shaped classic lobule (*red*) has the terminal hepatic venule (central vein) at the center of the lobule and the portal canals containing portal triads at the peripheral angles of the lobule. The triangular portal lobule (*green*) has a portal canal at the center of the lobule and terminal hepatic venules (central veins) at the peripheral angles of the lobule. A diamond-shaped liver acinus (*multicolor*) has distributing vessels at the equator and terminal hepatic venules (central veins) at each pole. **b.** The liver acinus is a functional interpretation of liver organization. It consists of adjacent sectors of neighboring hexagonal fields of classic lobules partially separated by distributing blood vessels. The zones marked 1, 2, and 3 designate areas that receive the most nutrient-dense and oxygenated blood supply (zone 1) to the least (zone 3). The terminal hepatic venules (central veins) in this interpretation are located at the pointed edges of the acinus instead of in the center, as in the classic lobule. The portal triads (terminal branches of the portal vein and hepatic artery) and the smallest bile ducts are shown at the corners of the hexagon that outlines the cross-sectioned profile of the classic lobule.

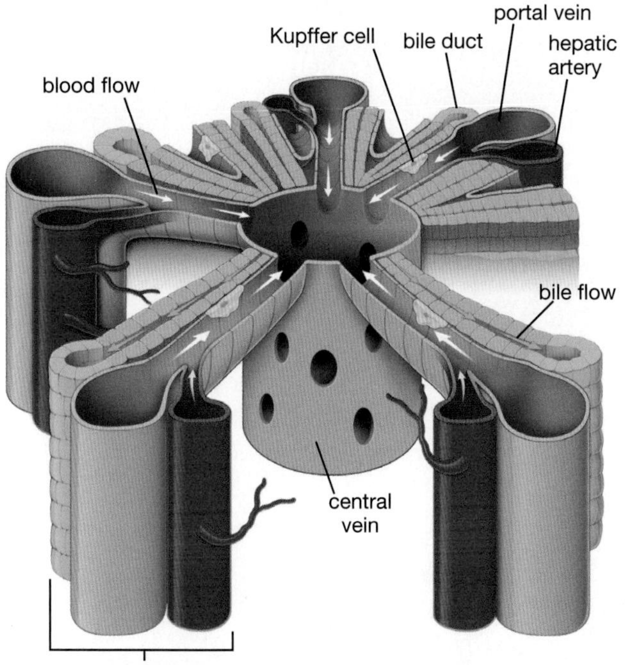

FIGURE 18.7. Diagram of the flow of blood and bile in the liver. This schematic diagram of a part of a classic lobule shows the components of the portal triads, hepatic sinusoids, terminal hepatic venule (central vein), and associated plates of hepatocytes. *White arrows* indicate the direction of the blood flow in the sinusoids. Note that the direction of bile flow (*green arrows*) is opposite that of the blood flow.

glycogen deposits are also seen between zones 1 and 3. Cells in zone 2 have functional and morphologic characteristics and responses intermediate to those of zones 1 and 3.

Blood vessels of the parenchyma

The blood vessels that occupy the **portal canals** are called **interlobular vessels.** Only the interlobular vessels that form the smallest portal triads send blood into the sinusoids. The larger interlobular vessels branch into distributing vessels that are located at the periphery of the lobule. These distributing vessels send inlet vessels to the sinusoids (Fig. 18.7). In the **sinusoids**, the blood flows centripetally toward the central vein. The central vein courses through the central axis of the classic liver lobule, becoming larger as it progresses through the lobule and empties into a sublobular vein. Several sublobular veins converge to form larger hepatic veins that empty into the inferior vena cava.

The structure of the **portal vein** and its branches within the liver is typical of veins in general. The lumen is much larger than that of the artery associated with it. The structure of the **hepatic artery** is like that of other arteries (i.e., it has a thick muscular wall). In addition to providing arterial blood directly to the sinusoids, the hepatic artery provides arterial blood to the connective tissue and other structures in the larger portal canals. Capillaries in these larger portal canals return the blood to the interlobular veins before they empty into the sinusoid.

The **central vein** is a thin-walled vessel receiving blood from the hepatic sinusoids. The endothelial lining of the central vein is surrounded by small amounts of spirally arranged connective tissue fibers. The central vein, so named because of its central position in the classic lobule, is actually the terminal venule of the system of hepatic veins and thus is more properly called the **terminal hepatic venule.** The **sublobular vein**, the vessel that receives blood from the terminal hepatic venules, has a distinct layer of connective tissue fibers, both collagenous and elastic, just external to the endothelium. The sublobular veins and the **hepatic veins**, into which they drain, travel alone. Because they are solitary vessels, they can be readily distinguished in a histologic section from the portal veins that are members of a triad. There are no valves in hepatic veins.

Hepatic sinusoids are lined with a thin discontinuous endothelium.

The **discontinuous sinusoidal endothelium** has a discontinuous basal lamina that is absent over large areas. The discontinuity of the endothelium is evident in two ways:

- **Large fenestrae**, without diaphragms, are present within the endothelial cells.
- Large gaps are present between neighboring endothelial cells.

Hepatic sinusoids differ from other sinusoids in that a second cell type, the **stellate sinusoidal macrophage**, or **Kupffer cell** (Fig. 18.8 and Plate 18.2, page 724), is a regular part of the vessel lining.

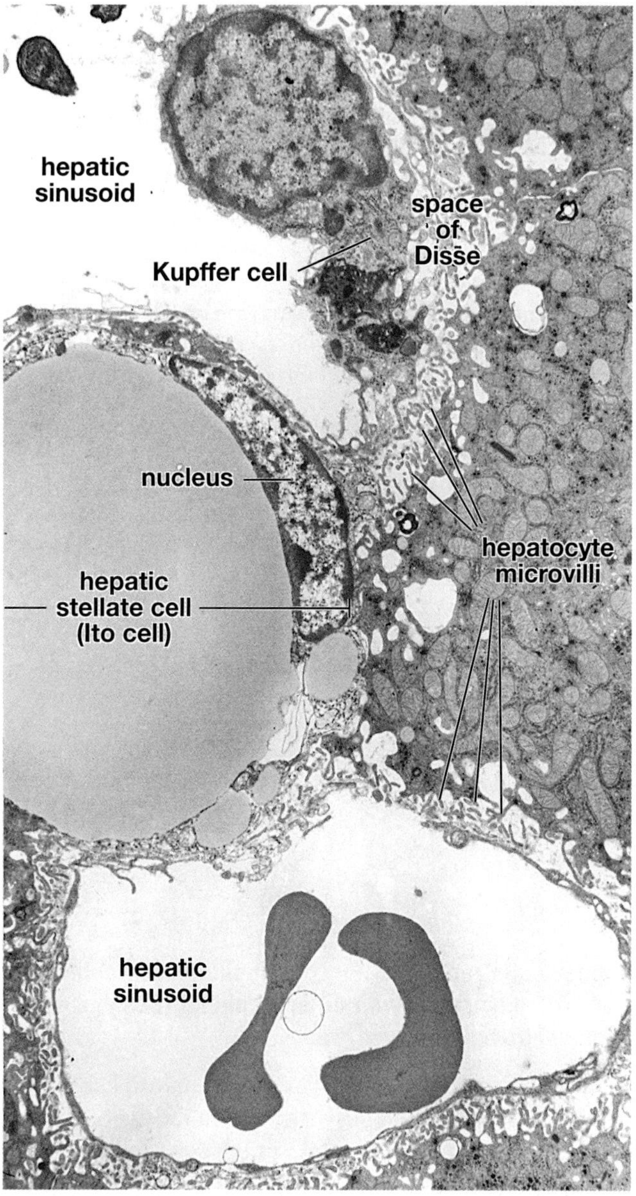

FIGURE 18.8. Electron micrograph of two hepatic sinusoids of the liver. One hepatic sinusoid (*top*) displays a stellate sinusoidal macrophage (Kupffer cell). The remainder of the sinusoid as well as the other sinusoid is lined by thin endothelial cell cytoplasm. Surrounding each sinusoid is the perisinusoidal space (space of Disse), which contains numerous *hepatocyte microvilli.* Also present in the perisinusoidal space is a hepatic stellate cell (Ito cell) with a large lipid droplet and several smaller droplets. Its nucleus conforms to the curve of the lipid droplet. ×6,600.

FOLDER 18.2

CLINICAL CORRELATION: CONGESTIVE HEART FAILURE, ACETAMINOPHEN OVERDOSE, AND LIVER NECROSIS

Liver injury may be triggered by hemodynamic changes in the circulatory system. In congestive heart failure, the heart is unable to provide sufficient oxygenated blood to meet the metabolic requirements of tissues and organs, including the liver, which is readily affected by hypoperfusion and hypoxia (low blood oxygen content). Zone 3 of the liver acinus is the first to be affected by this condition. The hepatocytes in this zone are the last to receive blood as it passes along the sinusoids; as a result, these cells receive a blood supply already depleted in oxygen. Examination of a liver biopsy specimen from an individual with congestive heart failure shows a distinct pattern of liver necrosis. Hepatocytes in zone 3, which is located around the central vein, undergo ischemic necrosis. Typically, no noticeable changes are seen in zones 1 and 2, representing the periphery of a classic lobule. Necrosis of this type is referred to as **centrilobular necrosis**. Figure F18.2.1 shows the centrilobular portion of a classic lobule. The multiple round vacuoles indicate lipid accumulation, and the atrophic changes are the result of dying hepatocytes undergoing autophagocytosis. Centrilobular necrosis as a result of hypoxia is referred to as **cardiac cirrhosis**; however, unlike true cirrhosis, nodular regeneration of hepatocytes is minimal.

Centrilobular necrosis can also occur in individuals who ingest a large amount of **acetaminophen (paracetamol, Tylenol)**, one of the most widely used over-the-counter painkillers. Acetaminophen overdoses, either accidental or intentional, are the leading cause of acute liver failure in the United States, accounting for nearly 500 deaths annually. Ingested acetaminophen is transported to the liver via the portal circulation, where it is converted in hepatocytes with the assistance of cytochromes P450 into a highly reactive toxic intermediate known as *N*-acetyl-p-benzoquinone imine (NAPQI). At therapeutic doses, NAPQI is efficiently detoxified by glutathione, forming an inert acetaminophen–glutathione conjugate that is excreted in the urine. However, at high dosage levels of acetaminophen, excess NAPQI depletes hepatic glutathione. Unconjugated NAPQI covalently binds to proteins and organelles in hepatocytes (mainly in zone 3), causing rapid cell death and centrilobular liver necrosis that can lead to acute liver failure and death.

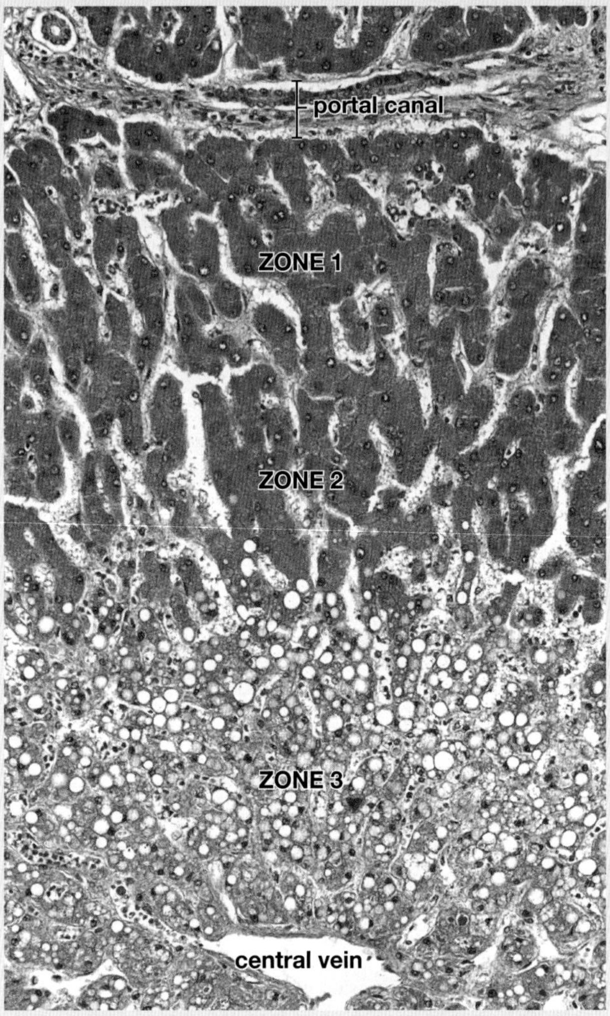

FIGURE F18.2.1. Photomicrograph of centrilobular necrosis in human liver. This photomicrograph shows a routine hematoxylin and eosin (H&E) liver biopsy specimen from an individual with congestive heart failure. Pathologic changes (referred to as *ischemic necrosis*) are most severe in hepatocytes in zone 3. This zone surrounds the terminal hepatic venule (central vein). This type of necrosis is referred to as *centrilobular necrosis*. Note the presence of multiple round vacuoles, which indicates extensive lipid accumulation. No noticeable changes are seen in the periphery of the lobule, which is zone 1 and much of zone 2. ×320.

Stellate sinusoidal macrophages (Kupffer cells)

Kupffer cells represent a mixed population of cells from two different origins with different phenotypes and divergent functionality.

Most tissues have mixed populations of macrophages with different embryologic origins. Microglia in the brain, Kupffer cells in the liver, Langerhans cells in the skin, and mesangial cells in the kidney are examples of **yolk sac–derived macrophages** that originated from erythro-myeloid progenitor cells early in development. In contrast, most intestinal macrophages are **bone marrow–derived macrophages**. These macrophages originate from hematopoietic stem cells, differentiate into **monocytes**, and enter the blood circulation via bone marrow. They travel through the bloodstream to designated tissues and differentiate into macrophages. Recent studies indicate that yolk sac–derived macrophages highly express profibrotic factors, whereas bone marrow–derived macrophages are involved in immune response reactions.

Kupffer cells in the adult liver also represent a mixed population of cells from these two different origins. Both populations of Kupffer cells are phagocytic and demonstrate different phenotypes and divergent functionality. Under experimental conditions, the phagocytic capacity of Kupffer cells can be assessed by measuring the uptake of different molecules, such as colloid carbon injected into the circulation (Fig. 18.9).

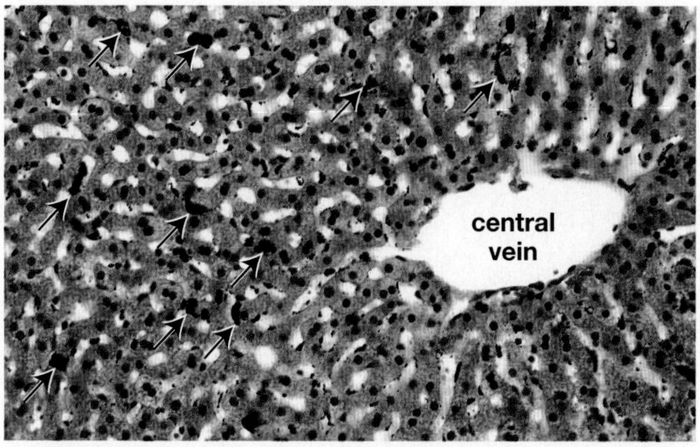

FIGURE 18.9. Photomicrograph of rabbit liver with carbon-labeled Kupffer cells. This high-magnification photomicrograph of the centrilobular area of rabbit liver is stained routinely in hematoxylin and eosin (H&E). To visualize Kupffer cells and test their phagocytic capacity under experimental conditions, colloid carbon was injected into the portal vein 30 minutes before the liver samples were collected for histologic study. Note the terminal hepatic venule (central vein) with plates of hepatocytes radiating from the central vein to the periphery of the hepatic lobule. Cells marked with *arrows* represent Kupffer cells, which have accumulated carbon particles. Note the distribution of Kupffer cells within hepatic sinusoids. ×300. (Courtesy of Dr. Nathan Swailes, University of Iowa.)

The two populations of Kupffer cells are described as follows:

- **Yolk sac–derived cells**. These cells migrate from the yolk sac during early development and colonize the developing liver. Kupffer cells developed from this lineage are self-sustaining and represent a resident **self-renewing phagocytic population** in the liver. They are largely independent of bone marrow hematopoietic stem cell development and, under normal conditions, are not replaced by monocyte-derived macrophages.
- **Bone marrow–derived cells**. These cells represent monocytes that originate from bone marrow. When yolk sack–derived Kupffer cells are damaged (e.g., in liver cirrhosis, hemochromatosis, hepatitis), arriving monocytes undergo environmentally induced changes and replace Kupffer cells. Monocyte-derived Kupffer cells do not divide, and they are replenished by an **influx of circulating monocytes** that enter the liver from the circulation.

The **activation process of Kupffer cells** mirrors that of other antigen-presenting cells, as described in Chapter 14, Immune System and Lymphatic Tissues and Organs (pages 498-500). They follow one of two activation pathways, giving rise to M1 (classically activated) or M2 (alternatively activated) macrophage phenotypes. M1-activated Kupffer cells participate in the inflammatory response, whereas M2-activated Kupffer cells express immune-modulatory properties. Maintaining a balance between both phenotypes of Kupffer cells is important in the course of pathologic changes in the liver. For instance, depletion of M1-activated Kupffer cells and expansion of M2-activated cells may promote healing and tissue repair during active **hepatitis** (an inflammatory process of the liver).

Kupffer cells are antigen-presenting cells that are involved in the immune system response.

Kupffer cells represent liver-resident macrophages that comprise 15% of the cells in the liver and account for 80%–90% of the total macrophages of the body. These antigen-presenting cells serve as the first line of defense against microorganisms and endotoxins that enter the liver via the hepatic portal circulation from the intestines. They initiate an immune response, recruit additional immune cells, and are essential in the clearance of viruses such as hepatitis viruses type B (HBV) and type C (HCV). Kupffer cells capture pathogens by recognizing pathogen-associated molecular patterns (PAMPs) via pattern recognition receptors (PRRs) such as toll-like receptors (TLRs) or nod-like receptors (NLRs) expressed on their surface (see page 309).

The scanning electron microscope (SEM) and transmission electron microscope (TEM) clearly show that the Kupffer cells form part of the lining of the sinusoid. Previously, they had been described as lying on the luminal surface of the endothelial cells. This older histologic description was probably based on the fact that processes of the Kupffer cells occasionally overlap endothelial cells on the luminal side. Cellular processes of Kupffer cells often seem to span the sinusoidal lumen and may even partially occlude it. Kupffer cells do not form junctions with neighboring endothelial cells.

Kupffer cells are involved in removing senescent red blood cells and recovering iron.

The presence of red blood cell fragments and iron (in the form of ferritin) in the cytoplasm of Kupffer cells suggests that they are involved in removing damaged or senescent red blood cells and recovering iron. Together with red pulp macrophages in the spleen and macrophages in bone marrow, Kupffer cells recycle between 90% and 95% of the body's iron necessary to maintain efficient erythropoiesis. The iron recovered from phagocytosed red blood cells is either stored within Kupffer cells, incorporated into iron-containing proteins, or exported from the cell back into the blood. Because free iron is toxic to the cell (water and oxygen in the cell convert Fe^{3+} ions into insoluble rust-like oxides), the stored iron needs to be sheltered from the cytoplasm. **Ferritin**, a 474-kDa multimeric protein in a shape of a hollow sphere (like a tennis ball), performs this function and can protect and store up to 4,500 iron ions. After Fe^{3+} ions enter the ferritin shell, they form small crystallites along with phosphate and hydroxide ions. In this state, Fe^{3+} ions are safely stored in isolation from the cytoplasm within the shell of the ferritin molecule. Ferritin also regulates intracellular iron levels by releasing iron from the core of the protein into the cytoplasm. Fe^{3+} ions are then picked up by **ferroportin (Fpn)-1**, a 62.5-kDa transmembrane protein that mediates iron export from the Kupffer cell directly into the blood of liver sinusoids. Here, Fe^{3+} ions are loaded onto **transferrin**, a 79.5-kDa protein that mediates iron transport through the blood. Each transferrin molecule flows through the blood carrying two Fe^{3+} ions and delivers them to a transferrin receptor on the surface of a target cell.

Some ferritin molecules loaded with iron may be converted into **iron deposition complexes** known as **hemosiderin granules**. These structures are surrounded by lysosomes and represent aggregated forms of partially digested ferritin molecules (Fig. 18.10). The amount of iron stored in Kupffer cells increases following **splenectomy** when the liver becomes essential for red blood cell disposal. Also, multiple blood transfusions may lead to **iron overload**. Excess hemosiderin granules deposited in macrophages and other cells in the body are detectable by magnetic resonance imaging (MRI) techniques owing to their solid crystalline

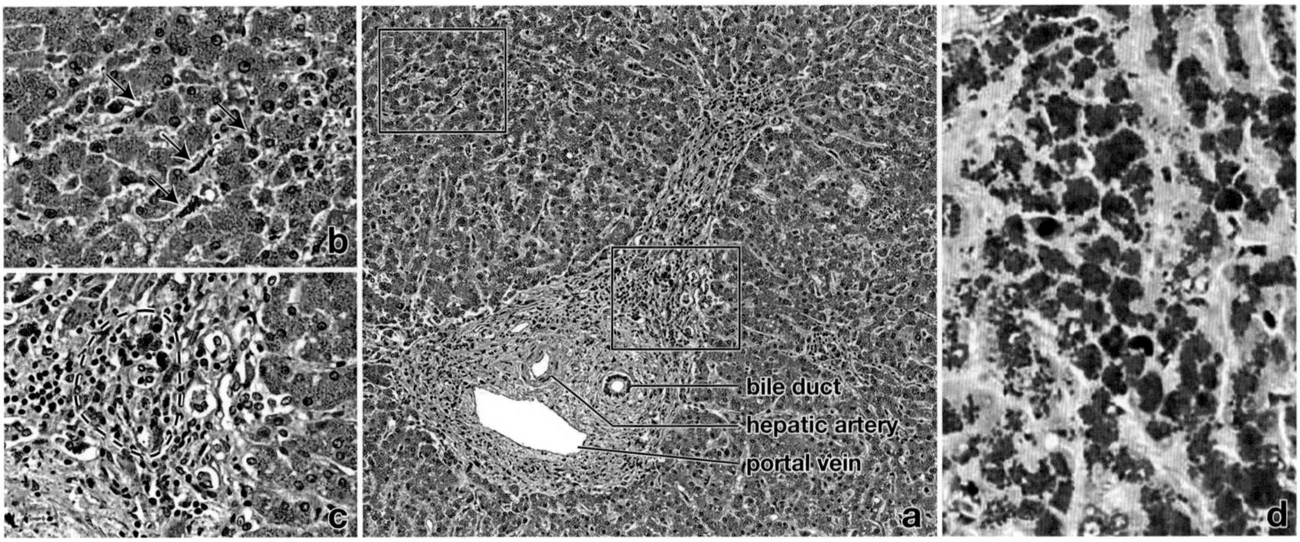

FIGURE 18.10. Hemochromatosis of the liver. a. This photomicrograph of a liver biopsy specimen, from an individual with an iron overload condition called *hemochromatosis*, is routinely stained with hematoxylin and eosin (H&E). It shows the portal canal containing a portal triad (portal vein, hepatic artery, and bile duct) surrounded by an extensive amount of fibrous tissue. Note that at this lower magnification, the hepatocytes have visible coarse golden brown granules of hemosiderin within the cytoplasm. ×85. (Courtesy of Dr. Nathan Swailes, University of Iowa.) **b.** The higher magnification of the area indicated by the *upper rectangle* shows in much better resolution the cytoplasm of hepatocytes filled with the hemosiderin granules. In addition, multiple elongated profiles of Kupffer cells that accumulated hemosiderin are also clearly visible along the liver sinusoids. ×220. **c.** This higher magnification of the area indicated by the *lower rectangle* shows an enlargement of the connective tissue in the portal canal. Note that this area is infiltrated by monocyte-derived macrophages containing hemosiderin granules (encircled by a *dashed line*). In addition, there is an infiltration of lymphocytes that indicates a chronic phase of this disease. ×220. **d.** This high-magnification photomicrograph of a liver biopsy specimen from an individual with hereditary hemochromatosis stained with Prussian blue iron stain. *Blue color* indicates areas with extensive accumulation of hemosiderin within hepatocytes ×320. (Courtesy of Dr. Joseph Grande, Mayo Clinic.)

superparamagnetic iron core that contributes to a decrease in T2 signal intensity. This signal is distinguishable from other soluble paramagnetic iron sources, such as plasma transferrin, ferritin, and hemoglobin. In individuals with an iron overload disorder, such as **hemosiderosis** (excess iron deposition in macrophages of the spleen, bone marrow, and Kupffer cells) or **hemochromatosis** (accumulation of hemosiderin in parenchymal cells of the liver, pancreas, heart, and other organs), noninvasive quantification of iron with MRI techniques has been implemented to replace tissue and organ biopsy. MRI is now considered the standard of care in diagnosing and monitoring iron overload diseases.

Perisinusoidal space (space of Disse)

The perisinusoidal space is the site of exchange of materials between blood and liver cells.

The **perisinusoidal space (space of Disse)** lies between the basal surfaces of hepatocytes and the basal surfaces of endothelial cells and Kupffer cells that line the sinusoids. Small, irregular microvilli project into this space from the basal surface of the hepatocytes (Fig. 18.11).

The microvilli increase the surface area available for exchange of materials between hepatocytes and plasma by as much as 6 times. Because of the large gaps in the endothelial layer and the absence of a continuous basal lamina, no significant barrier exists between the blood plasma in the sinusoid and the hepatocyte plasma membrane. Proteins and lipoproteins synthesized by the hepatocyte are transferred into the blood in the perisinusoidal space; this pathway is for liver secretions other than bile.

In the fetal liver, the space between blood vessels and hepatocytes contains **islands of blood-forming cells**. In cases of chronic anemia in the adult, blood-forming cells may again appear in the perisinusoidal space.

Hepatic stellate cells (Ito cells)

The hepatic stellate cells (Ito cells) store vitamin A; however, in pathologic conditions, they differentiate into myofibroblasts and synthesize collagen.

The other cell type found in the perisinusoidal space is the **hepatic stellate cell** (commonly called an **Ito cell**). These cells of mesenchymal origin are the primary storage site for hepatic **vitamin A** in the form of **retinyl esters** within cytoplasmic lipid droplets (see Fig. 18.8). Vitamin A is released from the hepatic stellate cell as **retinol** (alcohol form) bound to **retinol-binding protein (RBP)**. It is then transported from the liver to the retina, where its stereoisomer 11-*cis*-retinal binds to the protein opsin to form **rhodopsin**, the visual pigment of rods and cones of the retina. Oils derived from the fish livers (e.g., cod liver oil) have been important nutritional sources of vitamin A; today, they are taken in the form of dietary supplements.

In certain pathologic conditions, such as **chronic inflammation** or **liver cirrhosis**, hepatic stellate cells lose their lipid and vitamin A storage capability and differentiate into cells with characteristics of myofibroblasts. These cells appear to play a significant role in **hepatic fibrogenesis**; they synthesize and deposit type I and type III collagen within the perisinusoidal space, resulting in liver fibrosis. This collagen is continuous with the connective tissue of the portal space and the connective tissue surrounding the central vein. An increased amount of perisinusoidal fibrous stroma is an early sign of liver response to toxic substances. The cytoplasm of hepatic stellate cells contains contractile elements, such as desmin and smooth muscle α-actin filaments. During cell contraction, they increase the vascular resistance within the sinusoids by constricting the vascular channels, leading to **portal hypertension**. In addition, hepatic stellate cells

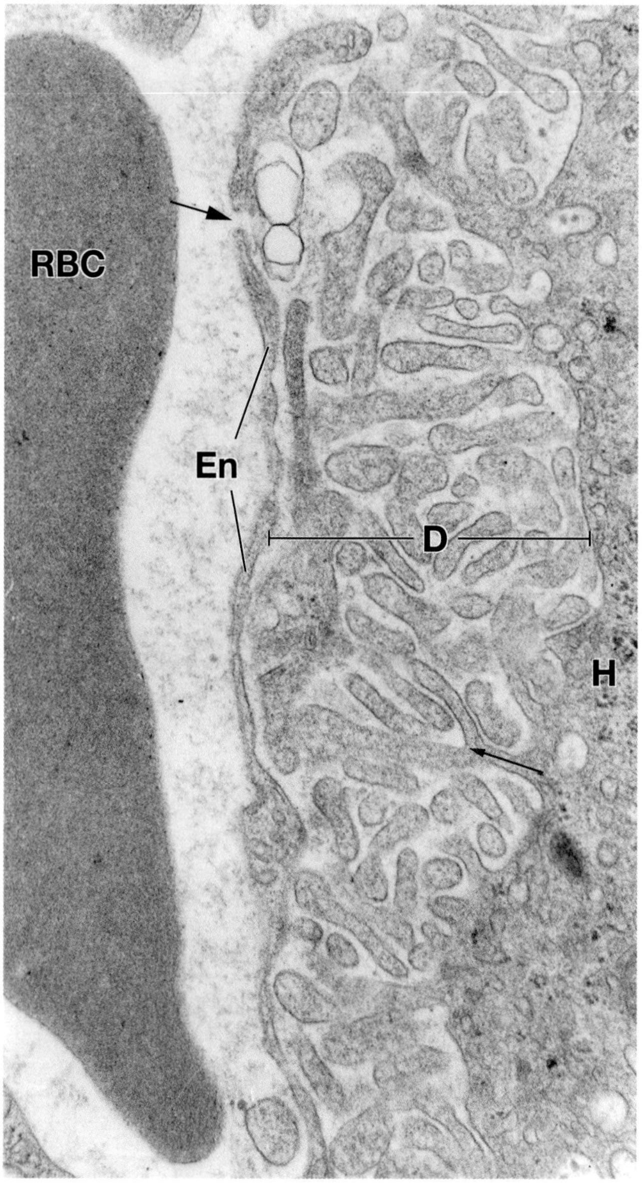

FIGURE 18.11. Electron micrograph showing the perisinusoidal space (of Disse). The perisinusoidal space (*D*) is located between the hepatocytes (*H*) and the sinusoid. A gap (*large arrow*) separates the endothelial cells (*En*) that line the sinusoid. Such gaps allow easy passage of small substances between the sinusoid and the perisinusoidal space. Numerous microvilli extend from the hepatocytes into the perisinusoidal space. These processes are long and frequently branch (*small arrow*). A red blood cell (*RBC*) is within the sinusoid. ×18,000.

play a role in remodeling the extracellular matrix during recovery from liver injury.

Lymphatic Pathway

Hepatic lymph originates in the perisinusoidal space.

Plasma that remains in the perisinusoidal space drains into the periportal connective tissue, where a small space, the **periportal space (space of Mall)** (Fig. 18.12), is described between the stroma of the portal canal and the outermost hepatocytes. From this collecting site, the fluid then enters lymphatic capillaries that travel with the other components of the portal triad.

The lymph moves in progressively larger vessels, in the same direction as the bile (i.e., from the level of the hepatocytes, toward the portal canals and eventually to the hilum of the liver). Approximately 80% of the hepatic lymph follows this pathway and drains into the thoracic duct, forming the major portion of the thoracic duct lymph.

Hepatocytes

Hepatocytes make up the anastomosing cell plates of the liver lobule.

Hepatocytes are large, polygonal cells measuring between 20 and 30 μm in each dimension. They constitute approximately 80% of the cell population of the liver.

Hepatocyte nuclei are large and spherical and occupy the center of the cell. Many cells in the adult liver are binucleate; most cells in the adult liver are tetraploid (i.e., they contain the 4*d* amount of DNA). Heterochromatin is present as scattered clumps in the nucleoplasm and as a distinct band beneath the nuclear envelope. Two or more well-developed nucleoli are present in each nucleus.

Hepatocytes are relatively long-lived for cells associated with the digestive system; their average life span is about 5 months. In addition, liver cells are capable of considerable regeneration when liver tissue is lost to hepatotoxic processes, disease, or surgery.

The **hepatocyte cytoplasm** is generally acidophilic. The following specific cytoplasmic components may be identified by routine and special staining procedures:

- Basophilic regions that represent rough endoplasmic reticulum (rER) and free ribosomes
- Numerous mitochondria; as many as 800–1,000 mitochondria per cell can be demonstrated by vital staining or enzyme histochemistry.
- Multiple small Golgi complexes visible in each cell after specific staining
- Large numbers of peroxisomes demonstrated by immunocytochemistry
- Deposits of glycogen stained by means of the periodic acid–Schiff (PAS) procedure. However, in a well-preserved hematoxylin and eosin (H&E) preparation, glycogen is also visible as irregular spaces, usually giving a fine foamy appearance to the cytoplasm.
- Lipid droplets of various sizes seen after appropriate fixation and Sudan or toluidine blue staining (Plate 18.2, page 724). In routinely prepared histologic sections, round spaces are sometimes seen that represent dissolved lipid droplets. The number of lipid droplets increases after injection or ingestion of certain hepatotoxins, including ethanol.
- Lipofuscin pigment within lysosomes seen with routine H&E staining in various amounts. Well-delineated brown granules can also be visualized by the PAS method.

As noted previously, the hepatocyte is polyhedral; for convenience, it is described as having six surfaces, although there may be more. A schematic section of a cuboidal hepatocyte is shown in Figure 18.13. Two of its surfaces face the perisinusoidal space. The plasma membrane of two surfaces faces a neighboring hepatocyte and a bile canaliculus. Assuming that the cell is cuboidal, the remaining two surfaces, which cannot be seen in the diagram, would also face neighboring cells and bile canaliculi. The surfaces that face the perisinusoidal space correspond to the basal surface of other epithelial cells; the surfaces that face neighboring cells and bile canaliculi correspond to the lateral and apical surfaces, respectively, of other epithelial cells.

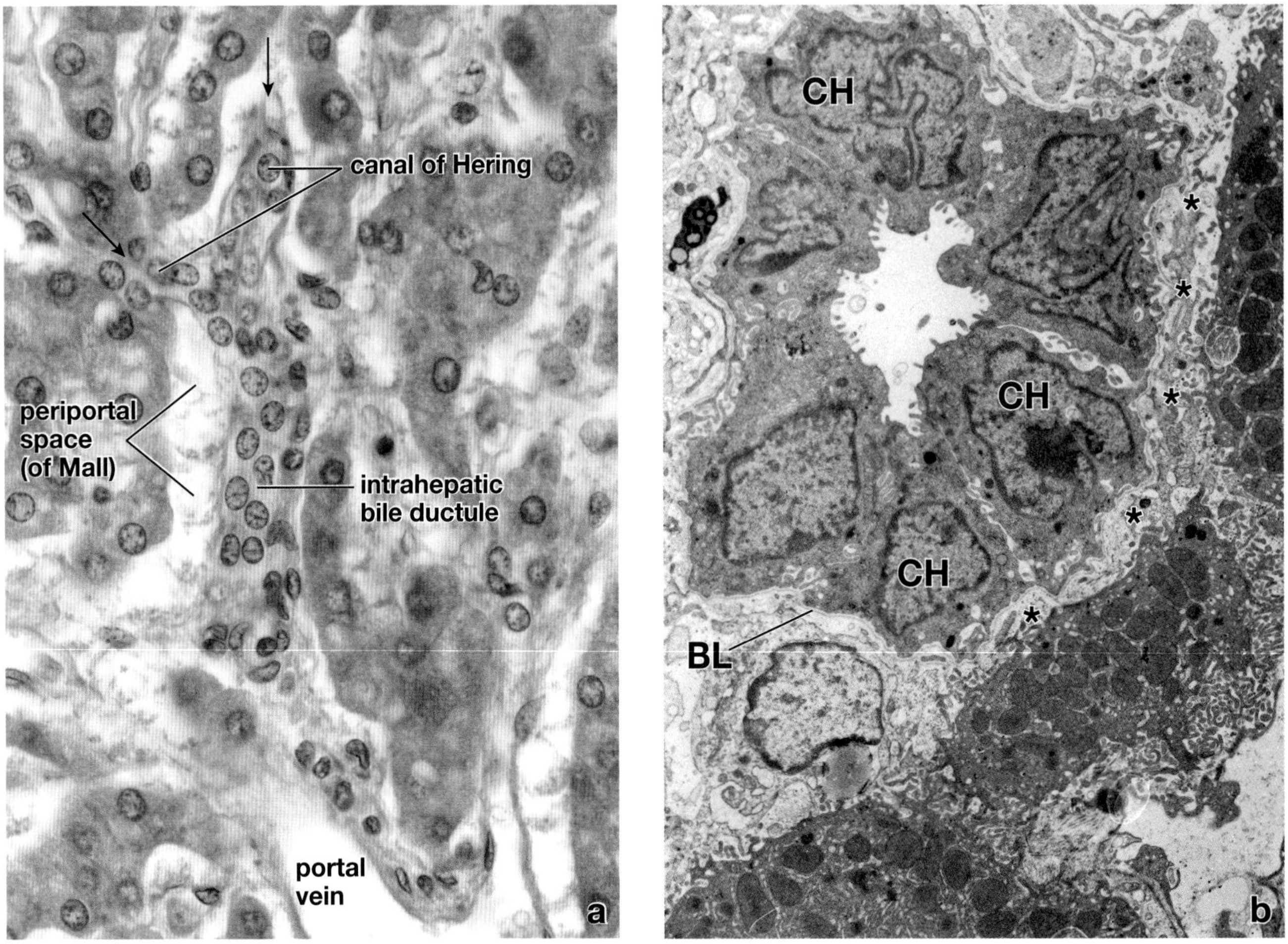

FIGURE 18.12. Canals of Hering and the intrahepatic ductile. a. Photomicrograph showing an area near a portal canal. *Arrows* indicate regions where bile canaliculi are draining into the *canals of Hering.* Note that the canal of Hering is partially lined by hepatocytes and partially by cholangiocytes. It drains into the *intrahepatic bile ductule* surrounded by hepatocytes, in contrast to the interlobular bile duct, which is embedded in the connective tissue of the portal canal. The terminal branch of a *portal vein* (*lower right*) accompanied by a small bile ductule is evident. ×800. **b.** Electron micrograph showing an intrahepatic bile ductule. The ductule collects bile from the canals of Hering. It is close to the hepatocytes, but the actual connection between bile canaliculi and the intrahepatic ductule is not evident in this plane of section. The ductule is composed of cholangiocytes (*CH*) surrounded by a complete basal lamina (*BL*). The narrow space (*asterisks*) into which microvilli of hepatocytes project is the periportal space (of Mall), not the perisinusoidal space (of Disse). ×6,000.

Peroxisomes are numerous in hepatocytes.

Hepatocytes have as many as 200–300 **peroxisomes** per cell. They are relatively large and vary in diameter from 0.2 to 1.0 µm (Fig. 18.14a). Peroxisomes' primary function is lipid metabolism contributing to the breakdown and detoxification of fatty acids. Peroxisomes are also a major site of metabolism of reactive oxygen intermediates (ROIs). They contain many oxidative enzymes that generate toxic **hydrogen peroxide (H_2O_2)**. The enzyme catalase, also residing within peroxisomes, degrades hydrogen peroxide to oxygen and water. These reactions are involved in many detoxification processes occurring in the liver (e.g., detoxification of alcohol). In fact, about one-half of the ethanol that is ingested is converted to acetaldehyde by enzymes contained in liver peroxisomes. In humans, **catalase** and **D-amino acid oxidase**, as well as **alcohol dehydrogenase**, are found in peroxisomes. In addition, peroxisomes almost exclusively metabolize very long-chain fatty acids (**β-oxidation of very long-chain fatty acids**) and branched-chains fatty acids (**α-oxidation of branched-chain fatty acids**) and are also involved in gluconeogenesis and synthesis of bile acids, which are derived from cholesterol. For detailed description of peroxisomes see Chapter 2: Cell Cytoplasm (pages 64-65).

Smooth endoplasmic reticulum (sER) can be extensive in hepatocytes.

The sER in hepatocytes may be extensive but varies with metabolic activity (Fig. 18.14b). The sER contains enzymes involved in the degradation and conjugation of toxins and drugs and synthesis of cholesterol and the lipid portion of lipoproteins. When challenged by drugs, toxins, or metabolic stimulants, a hepatocyte's sER may become the predominant organelle in the cell. In addition to stimulating sER activity, certain drugs and hormones induce the synthesis of new sER membranes and their associated enzymes. The sER undergoes hypertrophy after administration of alcohol, drugs (i.e., phenobarbital, anabolic steroids, and progesterone), and certain chemotherapeutic agents used to treat cancer. Stimulation of the sER by ethanol enhances its ability to detoxify other drugs, certain carcinogens, and some pesticides but increases the hepatocyte-damaging effects of some toxic compounds, such as carbon tetrachloride (CCl4) and 3,4-benzpyrene.

The large Golgi apparatus in hepatocytes consists of as many as 50 Golgi units.

Examination of hepatocytes with the TEM shows the **Golgi apparatus** to be much more elaborate than those seen

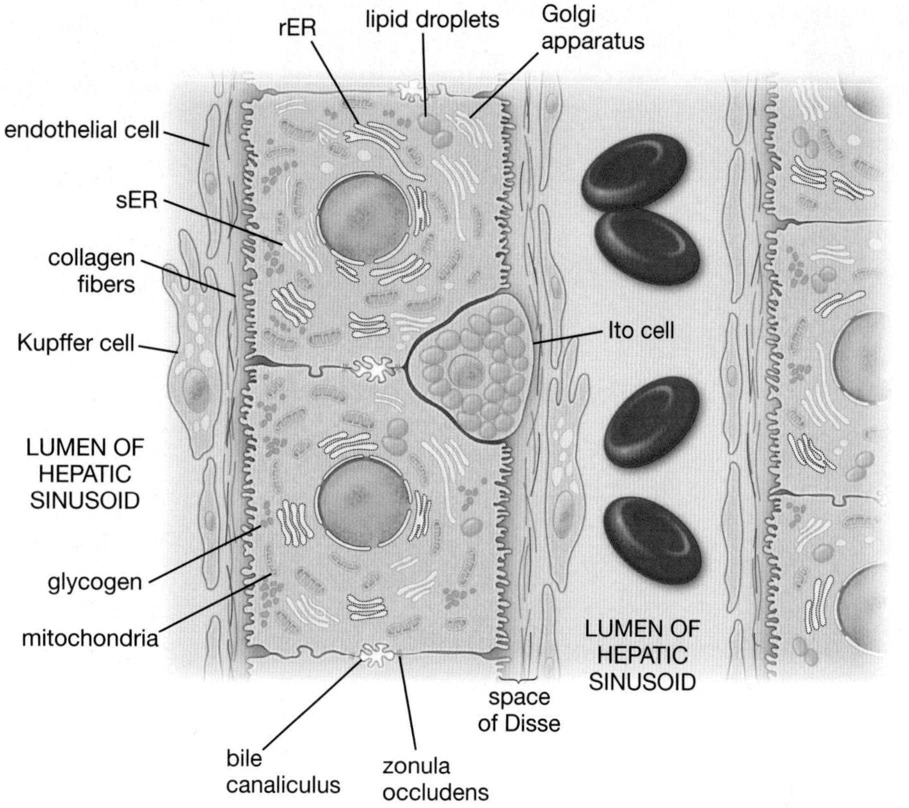

FIGURE 18.13. Schematic diagram of a plate of hepatocytes interposed between hepatic sinusoids. This diagram shows a one-cell-thick plate of hepatocytes interposed between two sinusoids. If it is assumed that the cell is cuboidal, two sides of each cell (shown) would face hepatic sinusoids, two sides of each cell (shown) would face bile canaliculi, and the additional two sides (not shown) would face bile canaliculi. Note the location and features of a hepatic stellate cell (Ito cell) filled with cytoplasmic vacuoles containing vitamin A. The sparse collagen fibers found in the perisinusoidal space (of Disse) are produced by the hepatic stellate cells (Ito cells). In certain pathologic conditions, these cells lose their storage vacuoles and differentiate into myofibroblasts that produce collagen fibers, leading to liver fibrosis. Observe that the stellate sinusoidal macrophage (Kupffer cell) forms an integral part of the sinusoidal lining. *rER*, rough endoplasmic reticulum; *sER*, smooth endoplasmic reticulum.

in routine histologic specimens. Heavy metal preparations (Golgi stains) of thick sections of the liver give an indication of the extent of the Golgi network. As many as 50 Golgi units, each consisting of three to five closely stacked cisternae, plus many large and small vesicles, are found in hepatocytes. These "units" are actually the branches of the tortuous Golgi apparatus seen in heavy metal preparations. Elements of the Golgi apparatus concentrated near the bile canaliculus are believed to be associated with the exocrine secretion of bile. Golgi cisternae and vesicles near the sinusoidal surfaces of the cell, however, contain electron-dense granules 25–80 nm in diameter that are believed to be VLDL and other lipoprotein precursors. These substances are subsequently released into the circulation as part of the endocrine secretory function of the hepatocytes. Similar dense globules are seen in dilated portions of the sER and, occasionally, in the dilated ends of rER cisternae, where they are synthesized.

Lysosomes concentrated near the bile canaliculus correspond to the peribiliary dense bodies seen in histologic sections.

Hepatocyte **lysosomes** are so heterogeneous that they can only be positively identified, even at the TEM level, by histochemical means. In addition to normal lysosomal enzymes, the TEM reveals the following components:

- Pigment granules (lipofuscin)
- Partially digested cytoplasmic organelles
- Myelin figures

Hepatocyte lysosomes may also be a normal storage site for iron (as a ferritin complex) and a site of iron accumulation in certain storage diseases.

The number of lysosomes increases in a variety of pathologic conditions, ranging from simple obstructive bile stasis to viral hepatitis and anemia. However, although the range of normal liver function—particularly the rate of bile secretion—is quite wide, no statistically significant morphologic changes take place in the Golgi apparatus or lysosomes of the peribiliary cytoplasm to correlate with the rate of bile secretion.

Biliary Tree

The **biliary tree** is the three-dimensional system of channels of increasing diameter that bile flows through from the hepatocytes to the gallbladder and then to the intestine. In the adult human liver, there are more than 2 km of interconnecting bile ductules and ducts of different sizes and shapes. These structures are not only passive conduits; they are also capable of modifying bile flow and changing its composition in response to hormonal and neural stimulation.

The biliary tree is lined by cholangiocytes, which monitor bile flow and regulate its content.

Cholangiocytes are epithelial cells that line the biliary tree. Small bile ductules are lined by small cholangiocytes, mainly cuboidal in shape, but as the diameter of the bile duct increases, they become progressively larger and more columnar in shape. When examined in the TEM, cholangiocytes are identified by their organelle-scant cytoplasm, the presence of tight junctions between adjacent cells, and the presence of complete basal lamina. The apical domain of cholangiocytes appears similar to that of hepatocytes with microvilli projecting into the lumen. In addition, each cholangiocyte contains a primary cilium that senses changes

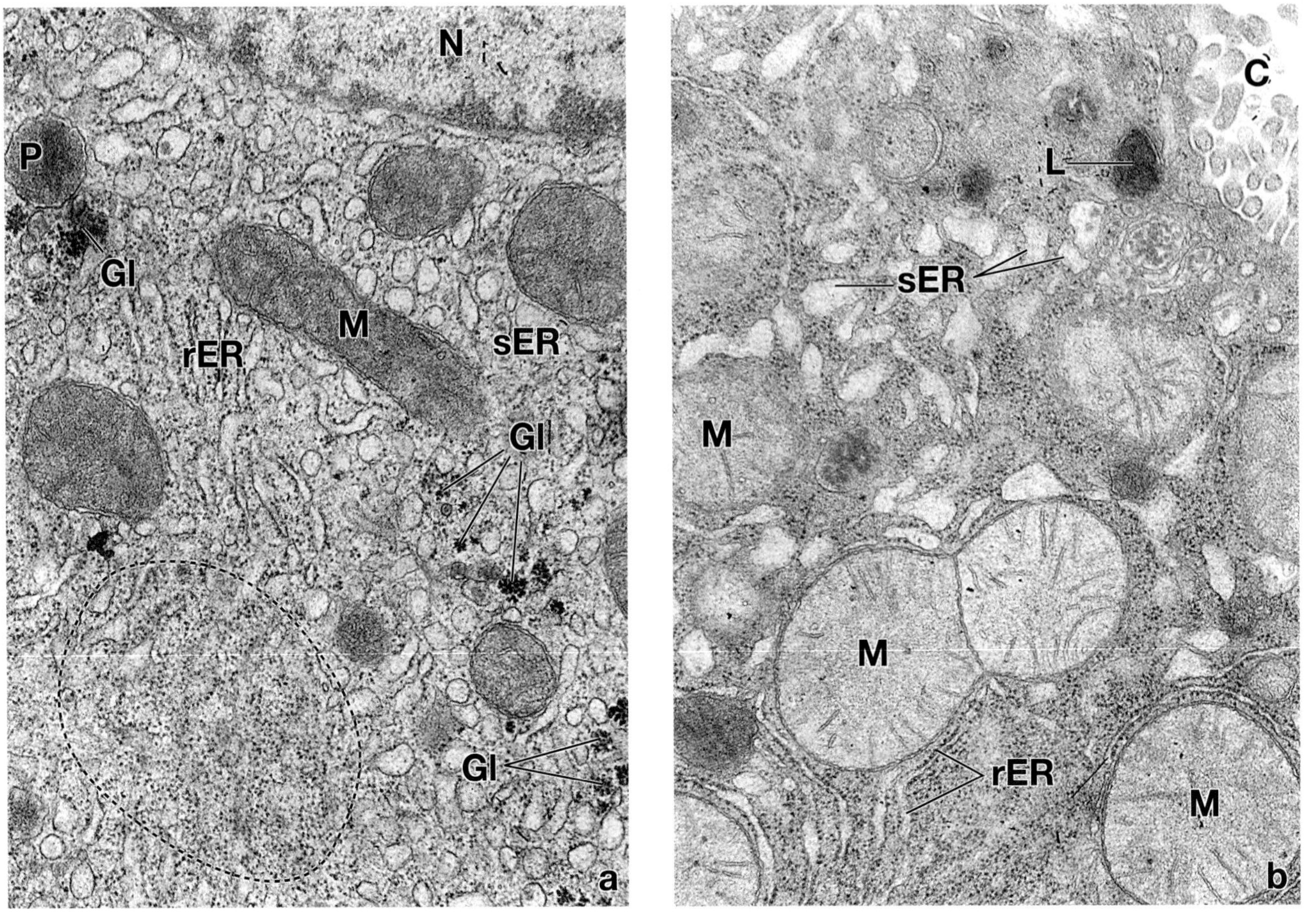

FIGURE 18.14. Electron micrographs of a hepatocyte. a. This electron micrograph shows organelles and other cytoplasmic structures near the nucleus (*N*), including peroxisome (*P*), mitochondrion (*M*), glycogen inclusions (*Gl*), smooth endoplasmic reticulum (*sER*), and rough endoplasmic reticulum (*rER*). In the *lower left*, the membranes of the *rER* have been cut in a tangential plane showing the ribosomes (encircled by a *dashed line*) on the cytoplasmic face of the membrane. ×12,000. **b.** This micrograph shows a region of cytoplasm near a bile canaliculus (*C*). It includes a lysosome (*L*), mitochondria (*M*), and both *sER* and *rER*. Note the microvilli in the bile canaliculus. ×18,000.

in bile flow, resulting in alterations of cholangiocyte secretion (Fig. 18.15).

The bile canaliculus is a small canal formed by apposed grooves on the surface of adjacent hepatocytes.

The smallest branches of the biliary tree are the **bile canaliculi** into which the hepatocytes secrete bile. They form a complete loop around four sides of the idealized six-sided hepatocyte (Fig. 18.16 and Plate 18.2, page 724). They are approximately 0.5 μm in luminal diameter and are isolated from the rest of the intercellular compartment by tight junctions, which form part of a junctional complex that also includes zonulae adherentes and desmosomes. Microvilli of the two adjacent hepatocytes extend into the canalicular lumen. Adenosine triphosphatase (ATPase) and other alkaline phosphatases may be localized on the plasma membranes of the canaliculi, suggesting that bile secretion into this space is an active process. Bile flow is centrifugal, that is, from the region of the terminal hepatic venule (central vein) toward the portal canal (a direction opposite to the blood flow). Near the portal canal but still within the lobule, bile canaliculi transform into the short **canals of Hering**.

A characteristic feature of the canal of Hering is its lining composed of two types of cells, hepatocytes and cholangiocytes.

The **canal of Hering** is a channel partially lined by hepatocytes and partially by cuboidal-shaped cholangiocytes. Similar to cholangiocytes, hepatocytes possess microvilli at their apical surface and tight junctions, and their basal domain rests on a basal lamina, which is characteristic of the entire distal biliary epithelium. Functionally, as demonstrated by video microscopy, the canal of Hering exhibits contractile activity that assists with unidirectional bile flow toward the portal canal. Because the canal

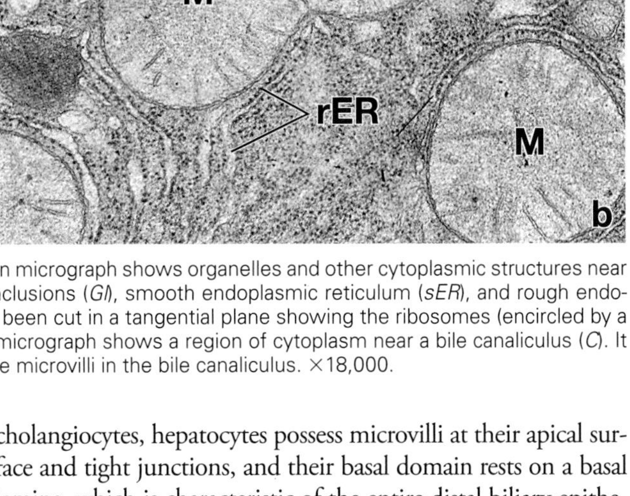

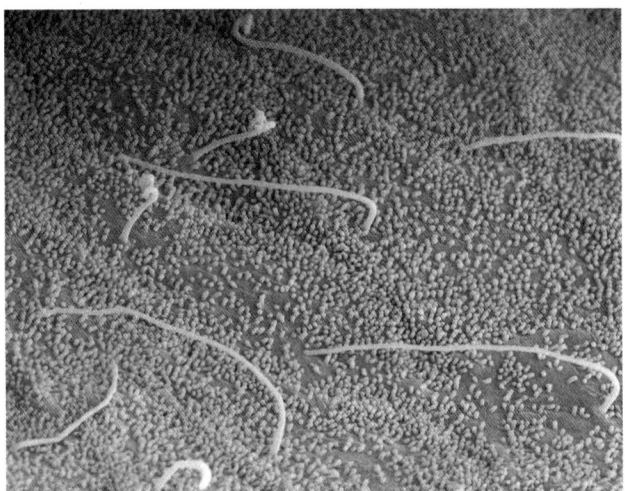

FIGURE 18.15. Scanning electron micrograph of the luminal surface of the bile duct. The bile duct is lined by epithelial lining cells called *cholangiocytes*. Their apical surfaces exhibit numerous short microvilli projecting into the lumen of the bile duct. Each cholangiocyte possesses a long primary cilium, which sense changes in the luminal flow of bile. Note that all cilia are bent in the same direction of bile flow. ×3,600. (Courtesy of Dr. Tetyana V. Masyuk.)

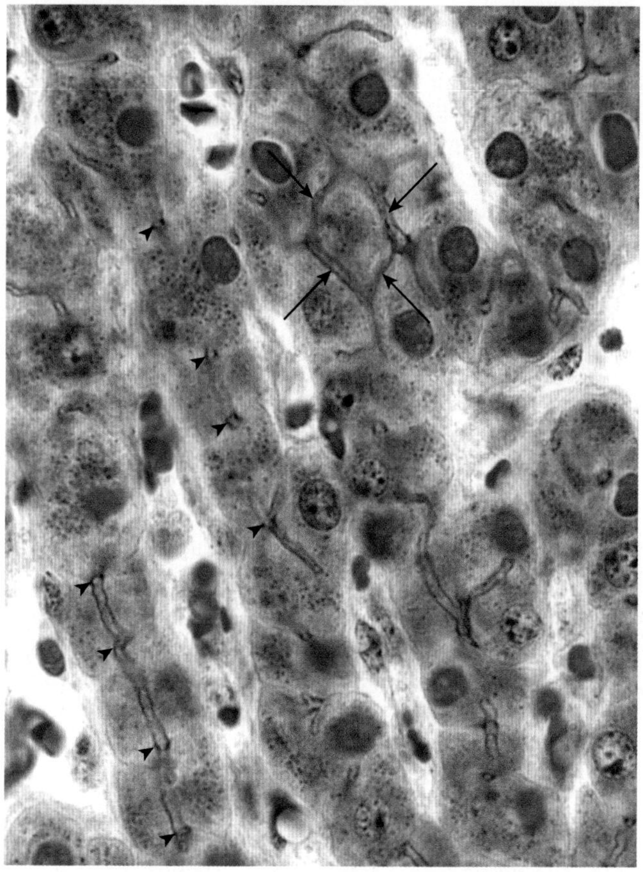

FIGURE 18.16. Photomicrograph of bile canaliculi. This high-magnification photomicrograph shows several one-cell-thick plates of hepatocytes separated by hepatic sinusoids. The plane of section in certain areas is parallel to the bile canaliculi. In this plane, the canaliculi reveal their arrangement on four sides of the hepatocytes (*arrows*). *Arrowheads* indicate those bile canaliculi that appear only in cross-sectional profile. ×1,240.

of Hering represents the smallest and most proximal tributary of the biliary tree containing cholangiocytes, it is often involved in the same diseases that affect small bile ducts. Functional disturbances in contractile activity as well as injury or destruction of the canals of Hering may contribute to **intrahepatic cholestasis** (obstruction of the bile flow).

The canal of Hering serves as a reservoir for liver progenitor cells.

Owing to their location at the crucial interface between hepatocytes and cholangiocytes, it has been proposed that **hepatic stem cells** are present either in the canals of Hering or in their vicinity. This hypothesis is supported by the appearance of liver cell precursors near the canals of Hering in most pathologic conditions characterized by extensive damage to hepatocytes. These cells would then migrate and differentiate into either hepatocytes or bile duct cells. The three-dimensional reconstruction of ductular reactions in liver necrosis suggests that small cholangiocytes lining the canals of Hering proliferate extensively and migrate into the parenchyma of the liver. In immunocytochemical staining, these cells express dual markers of both biliary and hepatocyte antigens and appear to be involved in the repair of liver tissue damaged by chronic pathologic processes. The presence of **hepatic stem cells** in this location has several clinical implications. For example, laboratory studies suggest that in future, hepatic stem cells may ultimately be used therapeutically in the treatment of liver diseases.

The bile ductule is the part of the biliary tree that is lined entirely by cholangiocytes.

Bile from the canal of Hering continues to flow into the **intrahepatic bile ductule** (see Fig. 18.12), which is lined entirely by cholangiocytes. Three-dimensional analysis of immunocytochemical-stained serial sections of the liver reveals that the **canal of Hering** often crosses the boundary of the lobule and continues as a bile ductule in the **periportal space (of Mall)** (see Figs. 18.4 and 18.12). The main distinction between the canal of Hering and the bile ductule is not its location within the lobule but whether the structure is partially or completely lined by cholangiocytes.

Intrahepatic bile ductules carry bile to hepatic ducts.

Intrahepatic **bile ductules** have a diameter of about 1.0–1.5 μm and carry bile to the interlobular **bile ducts** that form part of the portal triad. Interlobular bile ducts range from 15 to 40 μm in diameter and are lined by cholangiocytes that are cuboidal near the lobules and gradually become columnar as the ducts near the porta hepatis. The columnar cells have well-developed microvilli, as do those of the extrahepatic bile ducts and gallbladder. As the bile ducts get larger, they gradually acquire a dense connective tissue investment containing numerous elastic fibers. Smooth muscle cells appear in this connective tissue as the ducts approach the hilum. Interlobular ducts join to form the **right** and **left hepatic ducts**, which, in turn, join at the hilum to form the **common hepatic duct** (Fig. 18.17).

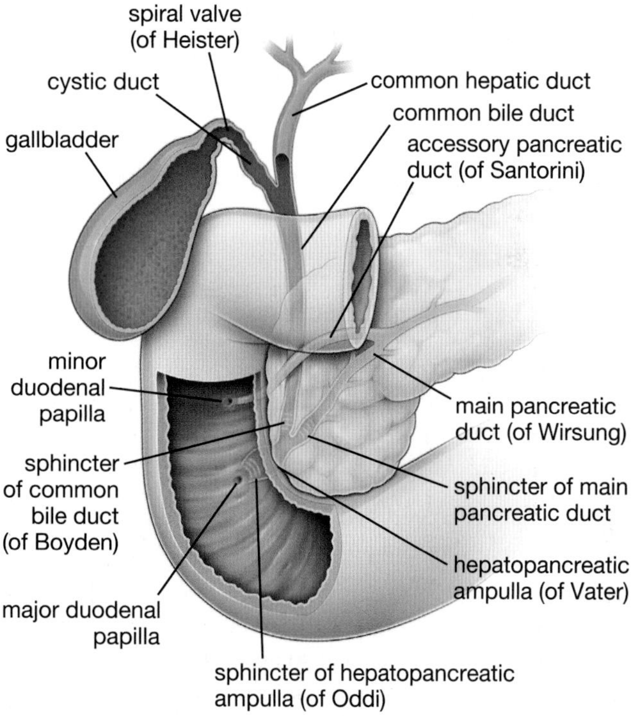

FIGURE 18.17. Diagram showing the relationship of hepatic, pancreatic, and gallbladder ducts. The gallbladder is a blind pouch joined to a single cystic duct in which numerous mucosal folds form the spiral valve (of Heister). The cystic duct joins with the common hepatic duct, and together they form the common bile duct that leads into the duodenum. At the entry to the duodenum, the common bile duct is joined by the main pancreatic duct (of Wirsung) to form the hepatopancreatic ampulla (of Vater), and together they enter the second part of the duodenum. Sphincters can be found at the distal part of these ducts. The sphincters of the common bile duct (of Boyden), the main pancreatic duct, and the hepatopancreatic ampulla (of Oddi) control the flow of bile and pancreatic secretion into the duodenum. When the common bile duct sphincter contracts, bile cannot enter the duodenum; it backs up and flows into the gallbladder, where it is concentrated and stored.

In some individuals, the **ducts of Luschka** are located in the connective tissue between the liver and the gallbladder, near the neck of the gallbladder. These ducts connect with the cystic duct, not with the lumen of the gallbladder. They are histologically similar to the intrahepatic bile ducts and may be remnants of aberrant embryonic bile ducts.

Extrahepatic bile ducts carry bile to the gallbladder and duodenum.

The **common hepatic duct** is about 3 cm long and is lined with tall columnar epithelial cells that closely resemble those of the gallbladder. All of the layers of the alimentary canal (see pages 632-633) are represented in the duct, except the muscularis mucosae. The **cystic duct** connects the common hepatic duct to the gallbladder. It has numerous spirally arranged mucosal folds that form the **spiral valve (of Heister)**. The cystic duct carries bile into and out of the **gallbladder**. The duct and spiral valve contain smooth muscle fibers responsive to pharmacologic, hormonal, and neural stimuli. However, there is no histologic evidence of a sphincter muscle in the cystic duct, which mainly functions as a passive conduit for bile. Distal to the junction with the cystic duct, the fused duct is called the **common bile duct** and extends for about 7 cm to the wall of the duodenum at the **hepatopancreatic ampulla (of Vater)**. Immediately proximal to the hepatopancreatic ampulla, a thickening in the circular layer of smooth muscle fibers, forms the **sphincter of the common bile duct (of Boyden)**, which controls the flow of bile into the ampulla. In addition, a thickening of the muscularis externa of the duodenum at the ampulla constitutes the **sphincter of the hepatopancreatic ampulla (of Oddi)**, which projects into the lumen of the duodenum as the **major duodenal papilla**. Because the hepatopancreatic ampulla (of Vater) contains openings for the common bile duct and the **pancreatic duct**, it acts as a valve to regulate the flow of bile and pancreatic juice into the duodenum.

The adult human liver secretes, on average, about 1 L of bile a day.

The bile fulfills two major functions. It is involved in the **absorption of fat** and is used by the liver as a vehicle for **excretion of cholesterol, bilirubin, iron**, and **copper**. The composition of bile and the specific functions of most of its components are listed in Table 18.1. As noted in the table, the following components of the bile are recycled via the portal circulation:

- About 90% of the **bile salts**, a component of bile, are reabsorbed by the gut and transported back to the liver in the portal blood. The bile salts are then reabsorbed and secreted by hepatocytes. Hepatocytes also synthesize new bile salts to replace those that are lost.
- **Cholesterol** and the phospholipid **lecithin**, as well as most of the **electrolytes** and water delivered to the gut with the bile, are also reabsorbed and recycled.

Bilirubin glucuronide, the detoxified end product of hemoglobin breakdown, is not recycled. It is excreted with the feces and gives them their color. Failure to absorb bilirubin or failure to conjugate it or secrete glucuronide can produce **jaundice**.

Bile flow from the liver is regulated by hormonal and neural control. The rate of blood flow to the liver and the concentration of bile salts in the blood exert regulatory effects on bile flow. Bile flow is increased when hormones such as cholecystokinin (CCK), gastrin, and motilin are released by enteroendocrine cells during digestion. Steroid hormones (i.e., estrogen during pregnancy) decrease bile secretion from the liver. In addition, parasympathetic stimulation increases bile flow by prompting contraction of the gallbladder and relaxation of the sphincter of the hepatopancreatic ampulla (of Oddi). Bile that leaves the liver via the common hepatic duct flows through the cystic duct to the gallbladder. Following stimulation, the gallbladder contracts steadily and delivers the bile to the duodenum via the common bile duct.

The liver has both sympathetic and parasympathetic innervations.

The liver (and gallbladder) receives nerves from both sympathetic and parasympathetic divisions of the autonomic nervous system. The nerves enter the liver at the porta hepatis and ramify through the liver in the portal canals along with the members of the portal triad. **Sympathetic fibers** innervate blood vessels, and increased stimulation in this system causes an increase in vascular resistance, decreased hepatic blood volume, and a rapid increase in serum levels of glucose. **Parasympathetic fibers** are assumed to innervate the large ducts (those that contain smooth muscle in their walls) and possibly blood vessels; their stimulation promotes glucose uptake and utilization. The cell bodies of parasympathetic neurons are often present near the porta hepatis.

■ GALLBLADDER

The **gallbladder** is a pear-shaped, distensible sac with a volume of about 50 mL in humans (see Fig. 18.17). It is attached to the visceral surface of the liver. The gallbladder is a secondary derivative of the embryonic foregut, arising as an evagination of the primitive bile duct that connects the embryonic liver to the developing intestine.

The gallbladder concentrates and stores bile.

The gallbladder is a blind pouch that leads, via a neck, to the cystic duct. Through this duct, it receives dilute bile from the hepatic duct. The gallbladder can store and remove about 90% of the water from the incoming bile, which results in an increase in bile salts, cholesterol, and bilirubin concentrations up to 10-fold. Hormones secreted by the enteroendocrine cells of the small intestine, in response to the presence of fat in the proximal duodenum, stimulate contractions of the smooth muscle of the gallbladder. These contractions help discharge concentrated bile into the common bile duct, which carries it to the duodenum.

The mucosa of the gallbladder has several characteristic features.

The empty or partially filled gallbladder has numerous deep **mucosal folds** (Fig. 18.18). The mucosal surface consists of **simple columnar epithelium** (Fig. 18.19). The tall epithelial cells (cholangiocytes) exhibit the following features:

- Numerous but short and not well-developed apical **microvilli**

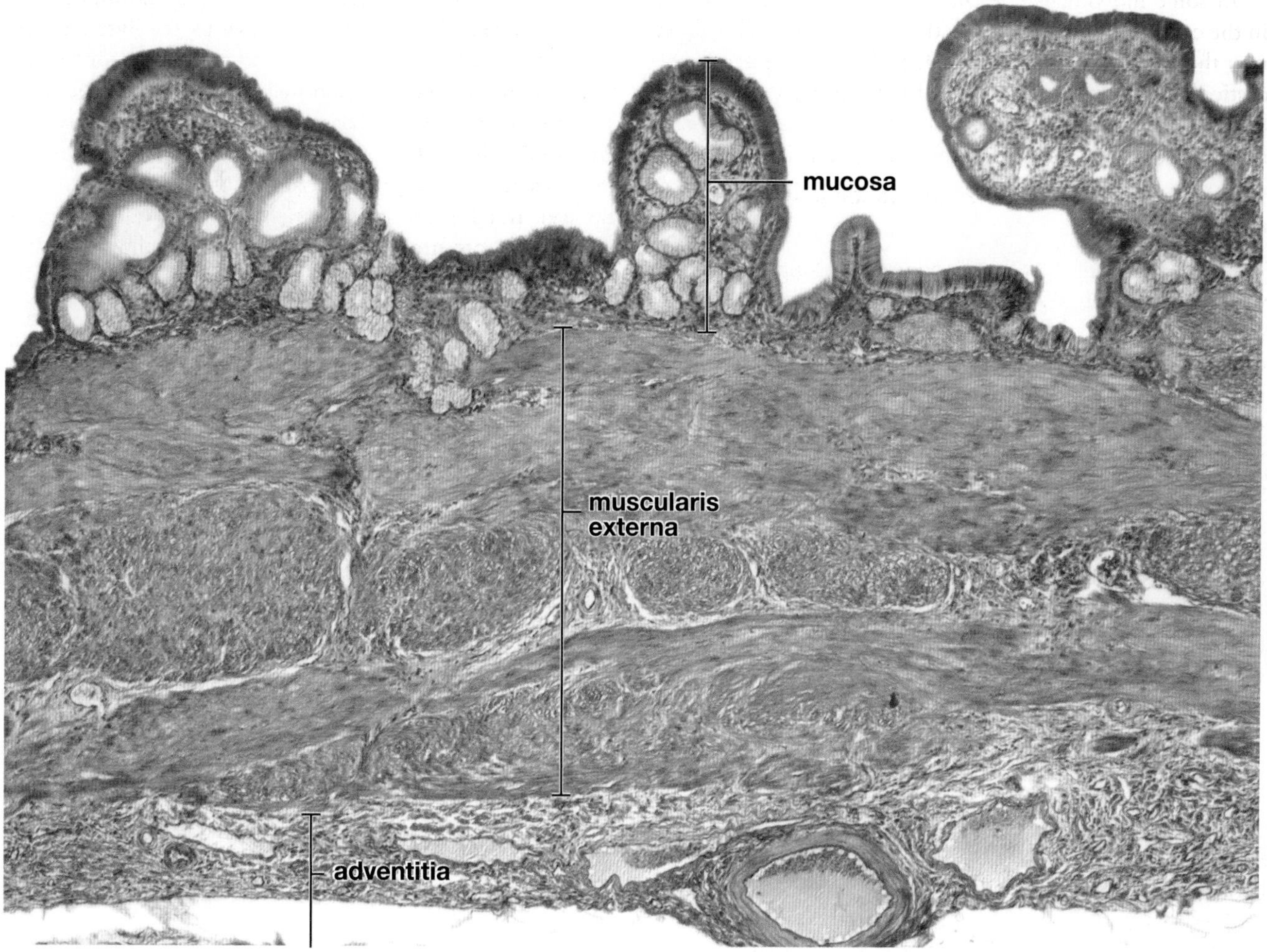

FIGURE 18.18. Photomicrograph of the wall of the gallbladder. The mucosa of the gallbladder consists of a lining of simple columnar epithelial cells and a lamina propria of loose connective tissue, which typically exhibits numerous deep folds in the mucosa. Beneath this layer is a relatively thick layer, the muscularis externa. There is no muscularis mucosa or submucosa. The smooth muscle bundles of the muscularis externa are randomly oriented. External to the muscle is an adventitia containing adipose tissue and blood vessels. The portion of the gallbladder not attached to the liver displays a typical serosa instead of an adventitia. ×175.

- Apical **junctional complexes** that join adjacent cells and form a barrier between the lumen and the intercellular compartment
- Localized concentrations of **mitochondria** in the apical and basal cytoplasm
- Complex **lateral plications**

These cells closely resemble the absorptive cells of the intestine. In addition to sharing the abovementioned characteristics, the lateral plasma membranes of both cells contain Na^+/K^+-activated ATPase and their apical cytoplasms feature secretory vesicles filled with glycoproteins.

The **lamina propria** of the mucosa is particularly rich in fenestrated capillaries and small venules, but there are no lymphatic vessels in this layer. The lamina propria is also very cellular, containing large numbers of lymphocytes and plasma cells. The characteristics of the lamina propria resemble those of the colon, another organ specialized for the absorption of electrolytes and water.

Mucin-secreting glands are sometimes present in the lamina propria in the normal human gallbladder, especially near the neck of the organ, but they are more commonly found in inflamed gallbladders. Cells that appear identical to enteroendocrine cells of the intestine are also found in these glands.

The wall of the gallbladder lacks a muscularis mucosa and submucosa.

External to the lamina propria is a **muscularis externa** that has numerous collagen and elastic fibers among the bundles of smooth muscle cells. Despite its origin as a foregut-derived tube, the gallbladder does not have a muscularis mucosa or submucosa. The smooth muscle bundles are somewhat randomly oriented, unlike the layered organization of the intestine. Contraction of the smooth muscle reduces the volume of the bladder, forcing its contents out through the cystic duct.

External to the muscularis externa is a thick layer of dense connective tissue (see Fig. 18.18). This layer contains large blood vessels, an extensive lymphatic network, and the autonomic nerves that innervate the muscularis externa and the blood vessels (cell bodies of parasympathetic neurons are found in the wall of the cystic duct). The connective tissue is also rich in elastic fibers and adipose tissue. The layer of tissue where the gallbladder attaches to the liver surface is referred to as the **adventitia**. The unattached surface is covered by a **serosa** or visceral peritoneum consisting of a layer of mesothelium and a thin layer of loose connective tissue.

In addition, deep diverticula of the mucosa, called **Rokitansky–Aschoff sinuses**, sometimes extend through

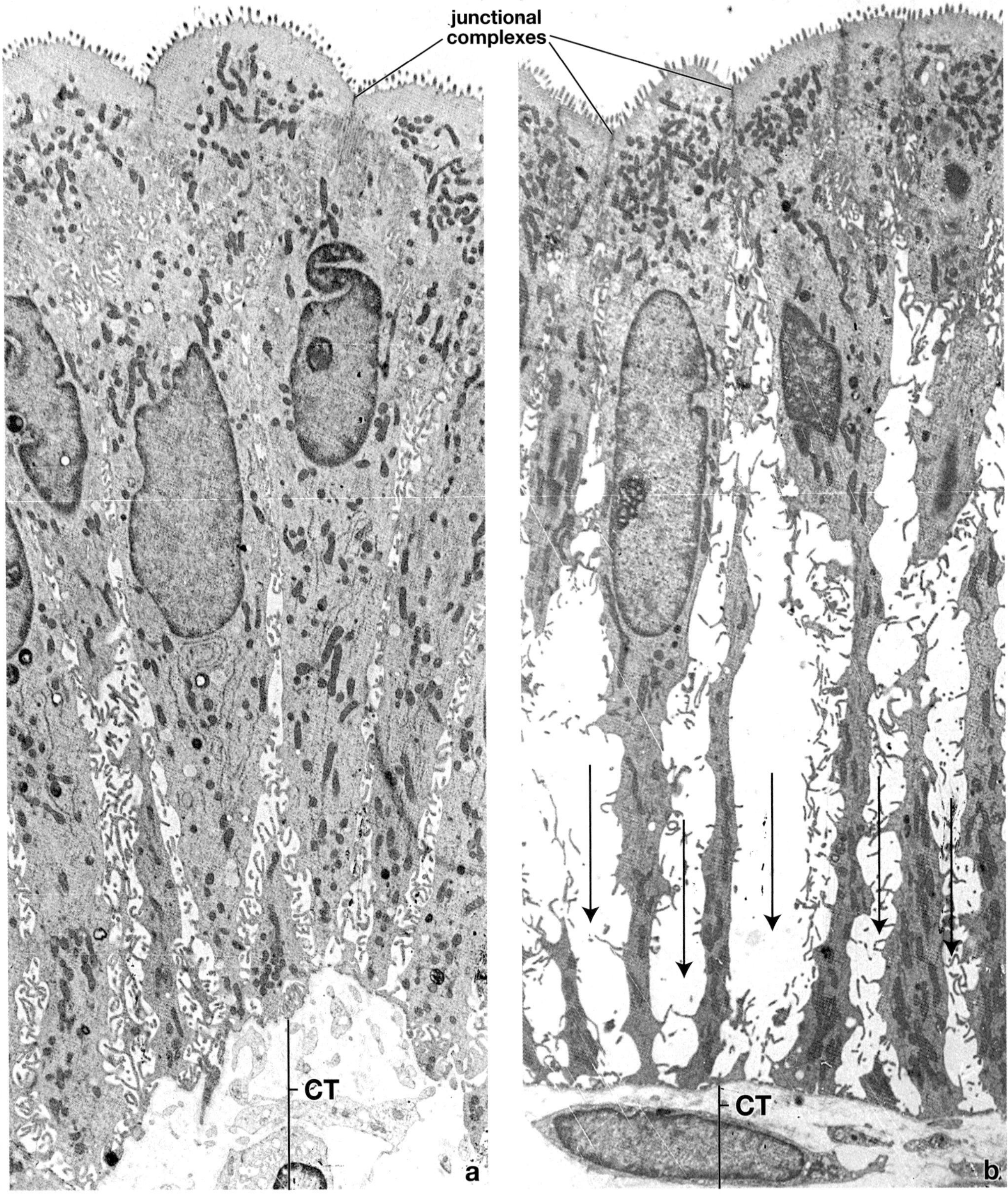

FIGURE 18.19. Electron micrographs of gallbladder epithelium. a. The tall columnar cells display features typical of absorptive cells, with microvilli on their apical surface, an apical junctional complex separating the lumen of the gallbladder from the lateral intercellular space, and numerous mitochondria in the apical portion of the cell. ×3,000. **b.** During active fluid transport, salt is pumped from the cytoplasm into the intercellular space, and water follows the salt. Both salt and water then diffuse into the cell from the lumen. As this process continues, the intercellular space becomes greatly distended (*arrows*). Fluid moves from the engorged intercellular space (*arrows*) across the basal lamina into the underlying connective tissue (*CT*) and then into blood vessels. The increase in the size of the lateral intercellular space during active fluid transport is evident with the light microscope. ×3,000.

the muscularis externa (Fig. 18.20 and Plate 18.3, page 726). They are thought to presage pathologic changes and develop as the result of hyperplasia (excessive growth of cells) and herniation of epithelial cells through the muscularis externa. Also, bacteria may accumulate in these sinuses, causing chronic inflammation that is a risk factor for the formation of **gallstones**.

Concentration of the bile requires the coupled transport of salt and water.

The epithelial cells of the gallbladder **actively transport Na^+, Cl^-, and HCO_3^-** from the cytoplasm into the intercellular compartment of the epithelium. ATPase is located in the lateral plasma membranes of the epithelial cells. This active transport mechanism is essentially identical to that described in

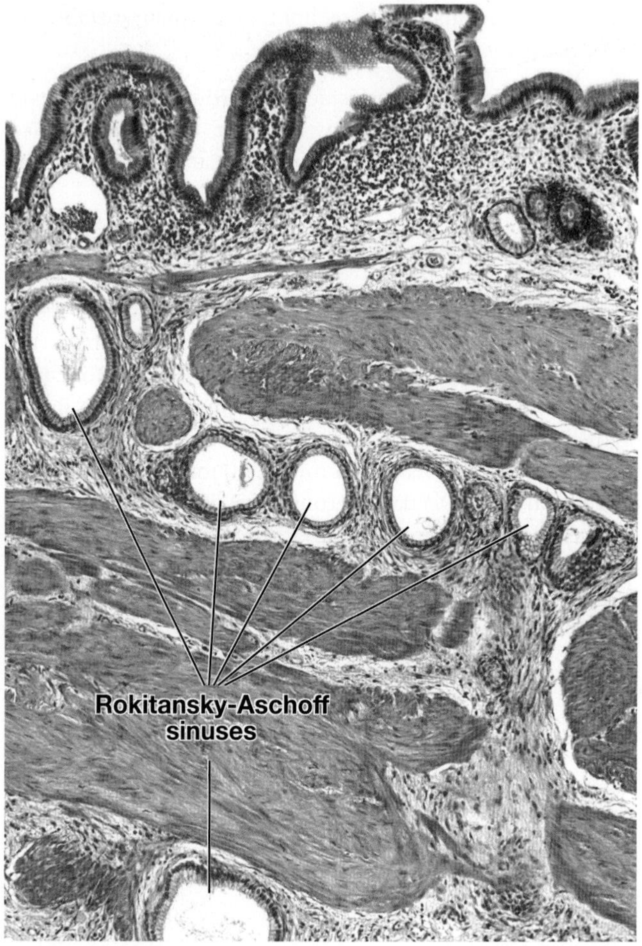

FIGURE 18.20. Photomicrograph of the Rokitansky–Aschoff sinuses in the wall of the gallbladder. This photomicrograph shows deep invaginations of the mucosa extending into the muscularis externa. These invaginations are referred to as *Rokitansky–Aschoff sinuses.* ×120.

Chapter 17, Digestive System II: Esophagus and Gastrointestinal Tract (Folder 17.4, page 648), for the enterocytes of the small intestine and the absorptive cells of the colon. The epithelial cells of the gallbladder also express two types of **aquaporin water channels** (AQP1 and AQP8), integral membrane channel proteins that facilitate rapid passive movement of water (see Chapter 20, Urinary System, Folder 20.5, page 791). The presence of water channels on apical and basolateral plasma membranes of the gallbladder epithelial cells suggests that they may be involved in both water absorption and secretion.

Electrolytes are actively transported across the plasma membrane of epithelial cells of the gallbladder.

Active transport of Na^+, Cl^-, and HCO_3^- across the lateral plasma membrane into the intercellular (paracellular) compartment causes the concentration of electrolytes in the intercellular space to increase. The increased electrolyte concentration creates an osmotic gradient between the intercellular space and the cytoplasm and between the intercellular space and the lumen. Water moves from the cytoplasm and from the lumen into the intercellular space because of the osmotic gradient (i.e., it moves down its concentration gradient; see Fig. 18.19b). Although the intercellular space can distend to a degree often visible with the light microscope, this ability is limited. The movement of electrolytes and water into the space creates hydrostatic pressure that forces a nearly isotonic fluid out of the intercellular compartment into the subepithelial connective tissue (the lamina propria). The fluid that enters the lamina propria quickly passes into the numerous fenestrated capillaries and venules that closely underlie the epithelium.

Studies of fluid transport in the gallbladder first demonstrated the essential role of the intercellular compartment in transepithelial transport of an isotonic fluid from the lumen to the vasculature. The final modification of bile is mainly the result of the active transport of Na^+, Cl^-, and HCO_3^- and the passive, aquaporin-mediated transport of water across the plasma membrane of epithelial cells of the gallbladder.

■ PANCREAS

Overview

The **pancreas** is an elongated gland described as having a head, body, and tail. The **head** is an expanded portion that lies in the C-shaped curve of the duodenum (Fig. 18.21). It is joined to the duodenum by connective tissue. The centrally located **body** of the pancreas crosses the midline of the human body, and the **tail** extends toward the hilum of the spleen. The **pancreatic duct (of Wirsung)** extends through the length of the gland and empties into the duodenum at the **hepatopancreatic ampulla (of Vater)**, through which the common bile duct from the liver and gallbladder also enters the duodenum. The **hepatopancreatic sphincter (of Oddi)** surrounds the ampulla, and it not only regulates the flow of bile and pancreatic juice into the duodenum but also prevents reflux of intestinal contents into the pancreatic duct. In some individuals, an **accessory pancreatic duct (of Santorini)** is present, a vestige of the pancreas' origin from two embryonic endodermal primordia that evaginate from the foregut.

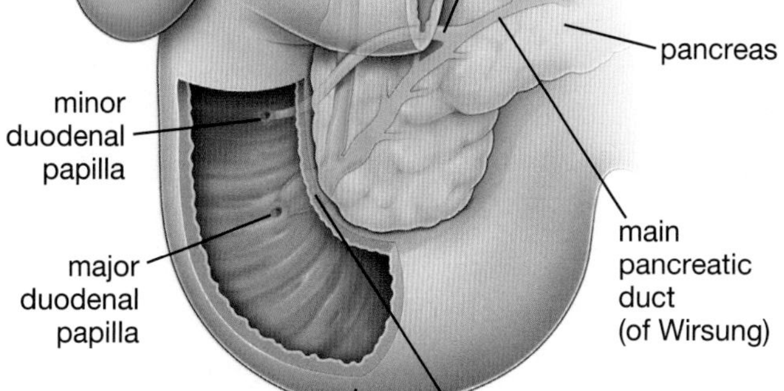

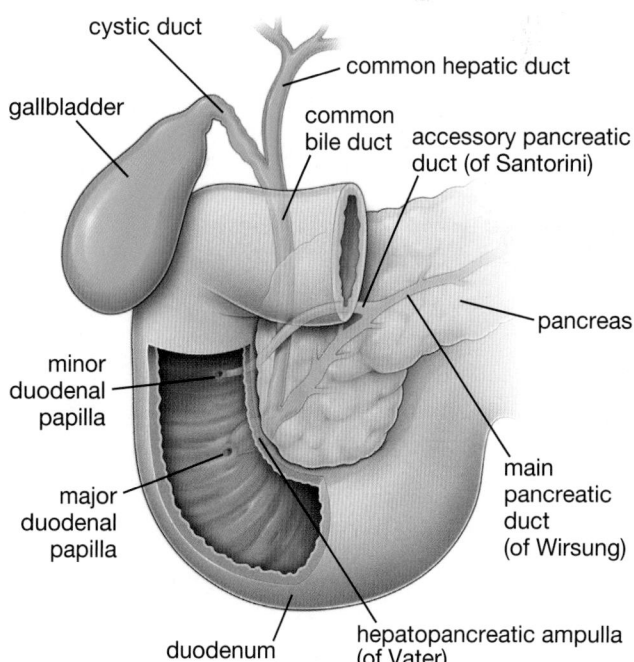

FIGURE 18.21. Diagram of pancreas, duodenum, and associated excretory ducts. The main pancreatic duct (of Wirsung) traverses the length of the pancreas and enters the duodenum after joining with the common bile duct. An accessory pancreatic duct (of Santorini) is commonly present, as shown, and empties into the duodenum at a separate minor duodenal papilla. The site of entry of the common bile duct and main pancreatic duct into the duodenum is typically marked by a major duodenal papilla visible on the inner surface of the duodenum.

A thin layer of loose connective tissue forms a capsule around the gland. From this capsule, septa extend into the gland, dividing it into ill-defined lobules. Within the lobules, a stroma of loose connective tissue surrounds the parenchymal units. Between the lobules, larger amounts of connective tissue surround the larger ducts, blood vessels, and nerves. In the connective tissue surrounding the pancreatic duct, small mucous glands are present that empty into the duct.

The pancreas is an exocrine and endocrine gland.

Unlike the liver, in which the exocrine and secretory (endocrine) functions reside in the same cell, the dual functions of the pancreas are relegated to two structurally distinct components:

- The **exocrine component** synthesizes and secretes enzymes into the duodenum that are essential for digestion in the intestine.
- The **endocrine component** synthesizes and secretes the hormones **insulin** and **glucagon** into the blood. These hormones regulate glucose, lipid, and protein metabolism in the body.

The exocrine pancreas is found throughout the organ; within the exocrine pancreas, distinct cell masses called **islets of Langerhans** are dispersed and constitute the endocrine pancreas.

Exocrine Pancreas

The exocrine pancreas is a serous gland.

Histologically, the **exocrine pancreas** closely resembles the parotid gland, with which it can be confused. The secretory units are acinar or tubuloacinar in shape and are formed by a simple epithelium of pyramidal serous cells (Fig. 18.22a and Plate 18.4, page 728). The cells have a narrow free (luminal) surface and a broad basal surface. Periacinar connective tissue is minimal.

The serous secretory cells of the acinus produce the digestive enzyme precursors secreted by the pancreas. **Pancreatic acini** are unique among glandular acini; the

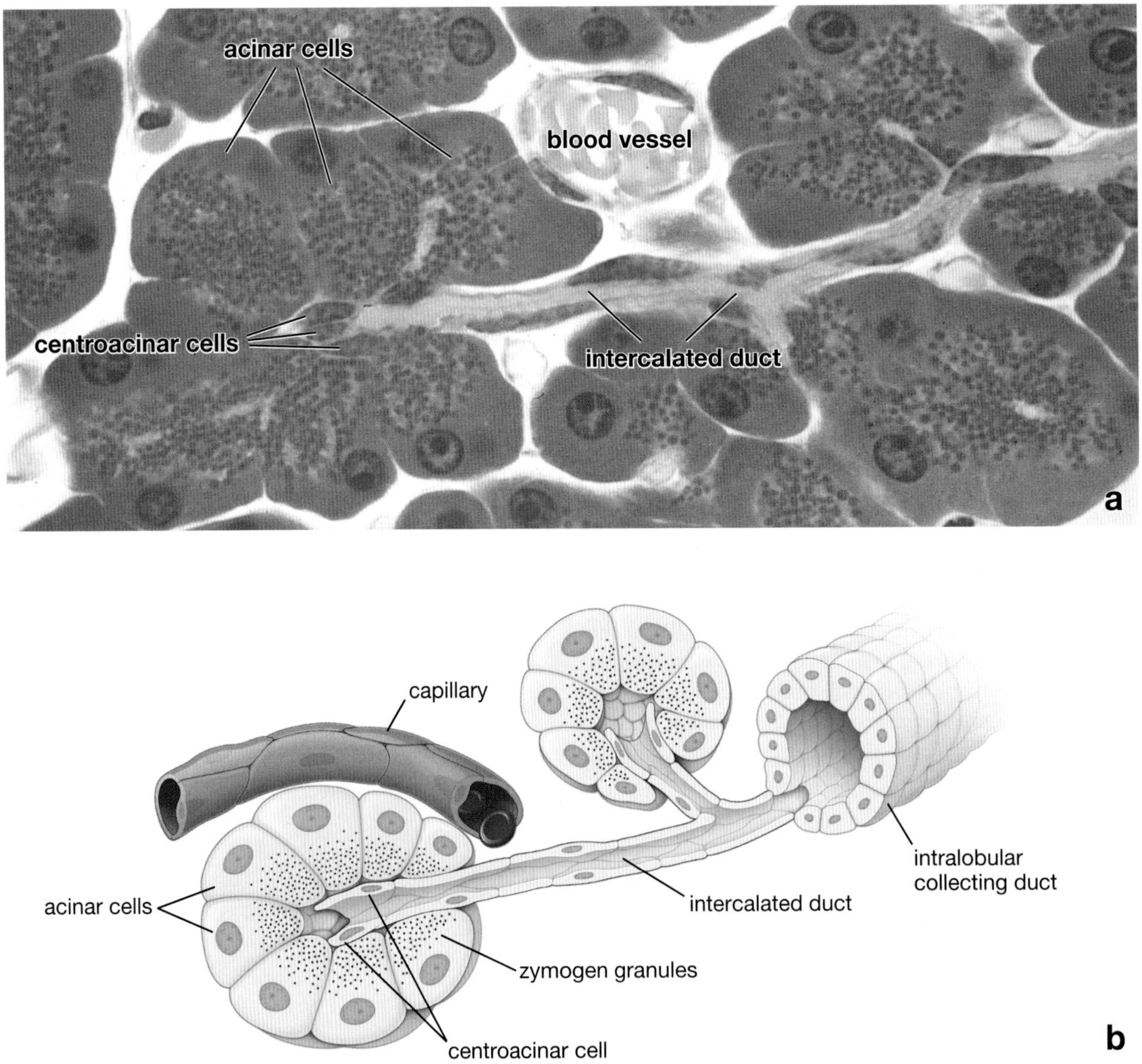

FIGURE 18.22. Pancreatic acinus and its duct system. a. In this photomicrograph of a thin, hematoxylin and eosin (H&E)-stained plastic section, an intercalated duct can be seen originating within a pancreatic acinus. The cells forming the duct within the acinus are the centroacinar cells. The eosinophilic zymogen granules are clearly seen in the apical cytoplasm of the parenchymal cells. ×860. **b.** In this schematic diagram, observe the origin of the intercalated duct. Note the location and shapes of the centroacinar cells within the acinus. They represent the initial lining of the intercalated duct, which drains into an intralobular collecting duct.

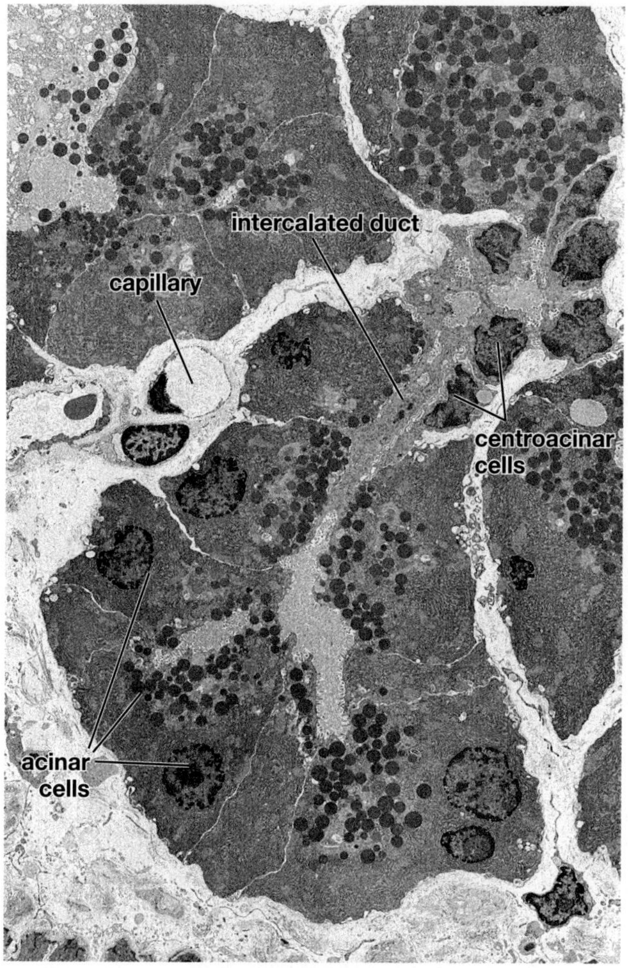

FIGURE 18.23. Electron micrograph of the pancreatic acinus and intercalated duct. Note that the pancreatic acinus is formed from pyramidal acinar cells. Their basal area contains nucleus surrounded by extensive rough endoplasmic reticulum (*rER*) and Golgi apparatus. The apical portion exhibits well-preserved zymogen granules. The origin of the intercalated duct lined by the centroacinar cells is visible on this electron micrograph. ×5,800. (Courtesy of Dr. Holger Jastrow.)

initial duct that leads from the acinus, the **intercalated duct**, actually begins within the acinus (Figs. 18.22b and 18.23). The duct cells located inside the acinus are referred to as **centroacinar cells**.

Acinar cells are characterized by distinct basophilia in the basal cytoplasm and acidophilic **zymogen granules** in the apical cytoplasm (see Figs. 18.22a and 18.23). Zymogen granules are most numerous in the pancreas of fasting individuals. The squamous centroacinar cells lack both ergastoplasm and secretory granules (see Fig. 18.23); thus, they stain very lightly with eosin. This weak staining helps identify them in routine histologic sections.

Zymogen granules contain a variety of digestive enzymes in an inactive form.

Pancreatic enzymes can digest most food substances. The inactive enzymes, or proenzymes, contained in pancreatic zymogen granules are listed here along with the specific substances they digest when activated:

- **Proteolytic endopeptidases** (trypsinogen, chymotrypsinogen) and **proteolytic exopeptidases** (procarboxypeptidase, proaminopeptidase) digest proteins by cleaving their internal peptide bonds (endopeptidases) or by cleaving amino acids from the carboxyl or amino end of the peptide.
- **Amylolytic enzymes** (α-amylase) digest carbohydrates by cleaving the glycosidic linkages of glucose polymers.
- **Lipases** digest lipids by cleaving ester bonds of triglycerides, producing free fatty acids.
- **Nucleolytic enzymes** (deoxyribonuclease and ribonuclease) digest nucleic acids, producing mononucleotides.

The **pancreatic digestive** enzymes are activated only after they reach the lumen of the small intestine. Initially, proteolytic activity of **enterokinases** in the glycocalyx of the microvilli of the intestinal absorptive cells converts trypsinogen to **trypsin**, another potent proteolytic enzyme. Trypsin then catalyzes the conversion of the other inactive enzymes as well as the digestion of proteins in the chyme.

The cytoplasmic basophilia of the pancreatic acinar cells when observed with the TEM appears as an extensive array of rER and free ribosomes. The presence of these numerous organelles correlates with the high level of protein synthetic activity of the acinar cells (Fig. 18.24). A well-developed Golgi apparatus is present in the apical cytoplasm and is involved in concentration and packaging of the secretory products. Mitochondria are small and, although found throughout the cell, are concentrated among the rER cisternae. Acinar cells are joined to one another by **junctional complexes** at their apical poles, thus forming an isolated lumen into which small microvilli extend from the apical surfaces of the acinar cells and into which the zymogen granules are released by exocytosis.

Duct System of the Exocrine Pancreas

The centroacinar cells (see Figs. 18.22a and 18.23) are the sites where the duct system of the exocrine pancreas arises. They have a centrally placed, flattened nucleus and attenuated cytoplasm, which is typical of a squamous cell.

Centroacinar cells are intercalated duct cells located in the acinus.

Centroacinar cells are continuous with the cells of the short intercalated duct that lies outside the acinus. The structural unit of the acinus and centroacinar cells resembles a small balloon (the acinus) into which a drinking straw (the intercalated duct) has been pushed. The **intercalated ducts** are short and drain into intralobular collecting ducts. There are no striated (secretory) ducts in the pancreas.

The complex, branching network of intralobular ducts drains into the larger **interlobular ducts**, which are lined with a low columnar epithelium in which enteroendocrine cells and occasional goblet cells may be found. The interlobular ducts, in turn, drain directly into the **main pancreatic duct (of Wirsung)**, which runs the length of the gland parallel to its long axis, giving this portion of the duct system a herringbone-like appearance (see Fig. 18.21). A second large duct, the **accessory pancreatic duct (of Santorini)**, arises in the head of the pancreas.

The intercalated ducts add bicarbonate and water to the exocrine secretion.

The pancreas secretes about 1 L of fluid per day, about equal to the initial volume of the hepatic bile secretion. Whereas

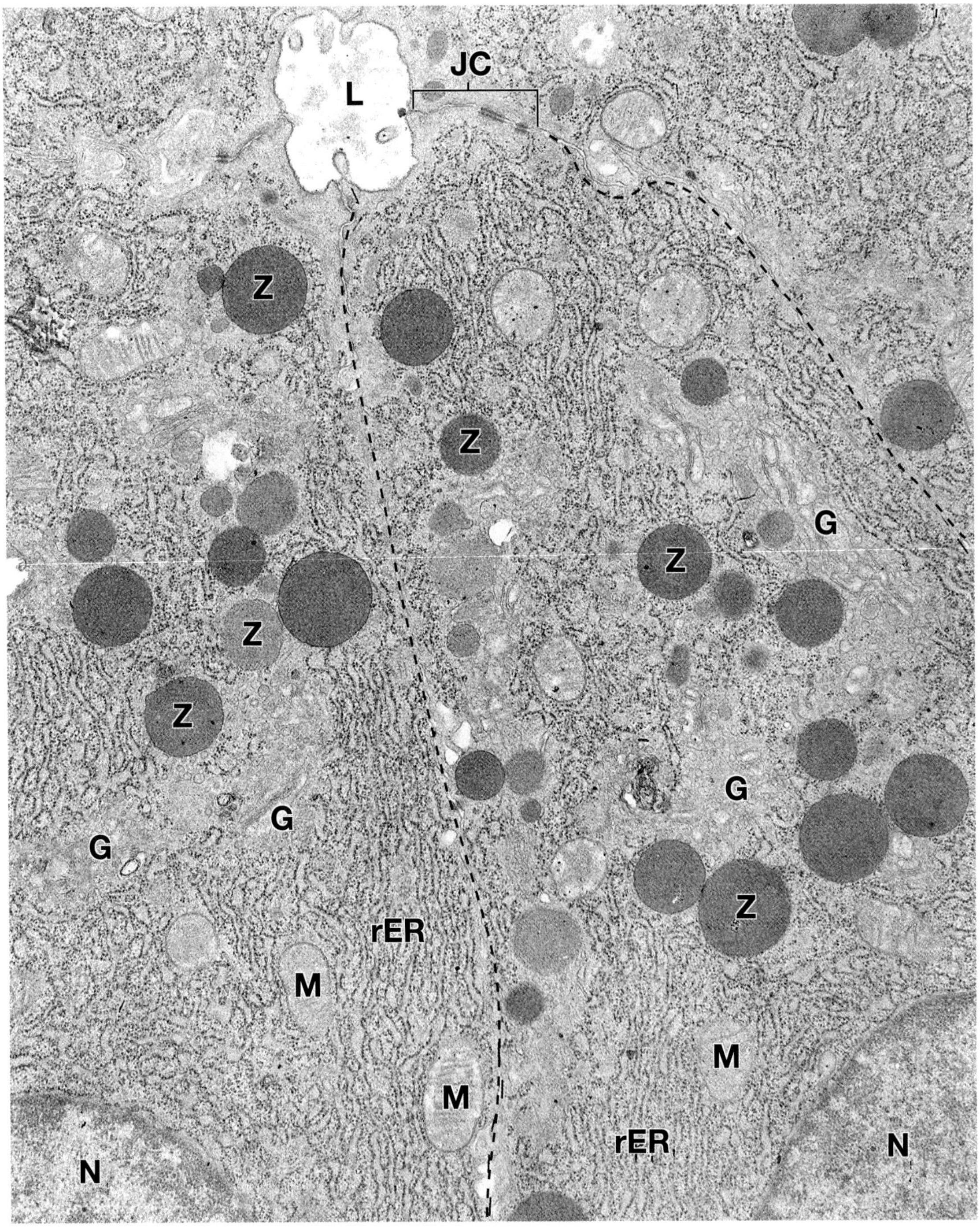

FIGURE 18.24. Electron micrograph of the apical cytoplasm of several pancreatic acinar cells. One pancreatic acinar cell is outlined by the *dashed line*. Nuclei (*N*) of adjoining cells are evident at the *bottom left* and *right* of the electron micrograph. The apical cytoplasm contains extensive rough endoplasmic reticulum (*rER*), mitochondria (*M*), zymogen-containing secretory granules (*Z*), and Golgi profiles (*G*). At the apices of these cells, a lumen (*L*) is present, into which the zymogen granules are discharged. A junctional complex (*JC*) is indicated near the lumen. ×20,000.

bile is concentrated in the gallbladder, the entire volume of the pancreatic secretion is delivered to the duodenum. Although the acini secrete a small volume of protein-rich fluid, the **intercalated duct cells** secrete a large volume of fluid rich in sodium and bicarbonate. The bicarbonate serves to neutralize the acidity of the chyme that enters the duodenum from the stomach and to establish the optimal pH for the activity of the major pancreatic enzymes.

Pancreatic exocrine secretion is under hormonal and neural control.

Two hormones secreted by the enteroendocrine cells of the duodenum, **secretin** and **cholecystokinin (CCK)**, are the principal regulators of the exocrine pancreas (see Table 17.1, page 646). Entry of the acidic chyme into the duodenum stimulates the release of the following hormones into the blood:

- **Secretin**, a polypeptide hormone (27 amino acid residues) that stimulates the duct cells to secrete a large volume of fluid with a high HCO_3^- concentration but little or no enzyme content
- **Cholecystokinin (CCK)**, a polypeptide hormone (33 amino acid residues) that causes the acinar cells to secrete their proenzymes

The coordinated action of the two hormones results in the secretion of a large volume of enzyme-rich, alkaline fluid into

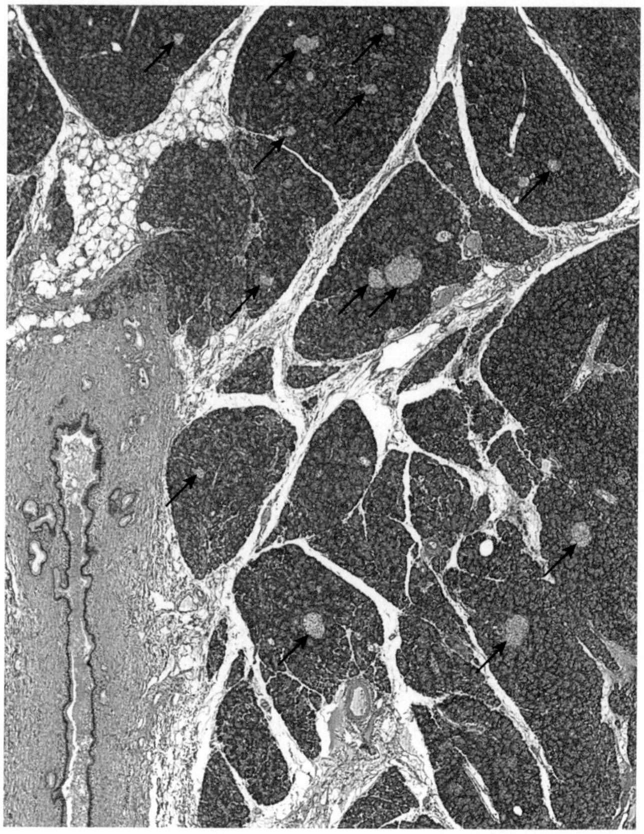

FIGURE 18.25. Photomicrograph of the pancreas. This hematoxylin and eosin (H&E)-stained specimen shows many pancreatic lobules separated by connective tissue septa that are continuous with the thin surrounding capsule of the gland. The pancreatic lobules consist largely of the exocrine acini and their intralobular duct system. Most of the lobules exhibit small, round, lighter staining profiles, which are the islets of Langerhans (*arrows*). Adjacent to the lobules, at the *lower left*, is a large interlobular duct that serves the exocrine pancreas. ×25.

the duodenum. In addition to hormonal influences, the pancreas also receives autonomic innervation. Sympathetic nerve fibers are involved in the regulation of pancreatic blood flow. Parasympathetic fibers stimulate activity of acinar as well as centroacinar cells. Cell bodies of neurons occasionally seen in the pancreas belong to parasympathetic postganglionic neurons.

Endocrine Pancreas

The endocrine pancreas is a diffuse organ that secretes hormones that regulate blood glucose levels.

The **islets of Langerhans**, the **endocrine component** of the pancreas, are scattered throughout the organ in cell groupings of varying size (Fig. 18.25). It is estimated that 1–3 million islets constitute about 1%–2% of the volume of the human pancreas but are most numerous in the tail. Individual islets may contain only a few cells or many hundreds of cells (Plate 18.4, page 728). Their polygonal cells are arranged in short, irregular cords that are profusely invested with a network of fenestrated capillaries. The definitive endocrine cells of the islets develop between 9 and 12 weeks of gestation.

In H&E-stained sections, the islets of Langerhans appear as clusters of pale-staining cells surrounded by more intensely staining pancreatic acini. It is not practical to attempt to identify the several cell types found in the islets in routinely prepared specimens (Fig. 18.26). After Zenker-formol fixation and staining by the Mallory-Azan method, however, it is possible to identify three principal cell types designated **A (α, alpha)**, **B (β, beta)**, and **D (δ, delta) cells** (Table 18.2). With this method, the

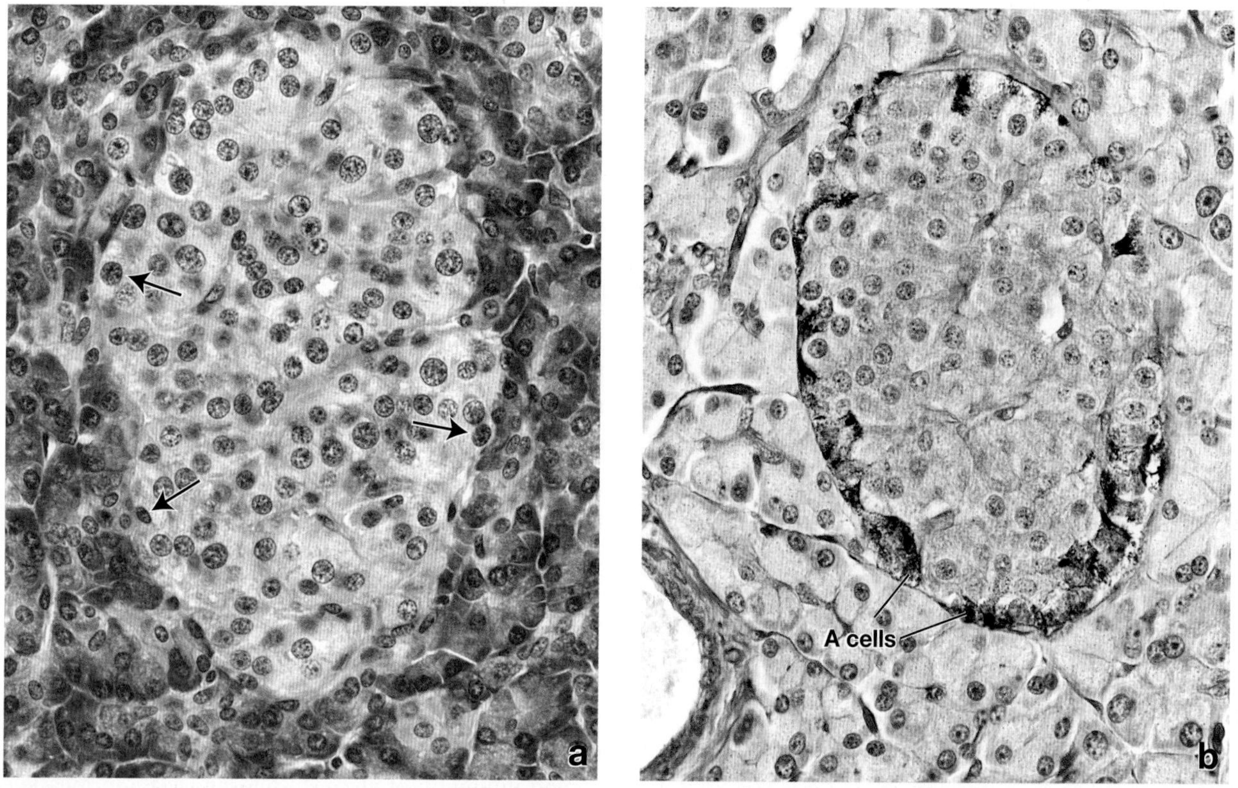

FIGURE 18.26. Photomicrographs of islets of Langerhans. a. In this routine hematoxylin and eosin (H&E) preparation, it is difficult to identify specific islet cell types without special stains. At best, one can identify small cells (*arrows*) at the periphery of the islet that are probably A cells. ×360. **b.** This photomicrograph shows an islet of Langerhans obtained from a rat pancreas stained with a special Grimelius silver stain that reacts with glucagon-secreting cells. The silver-impregnated A cells in the rat pancreas are arranged around the periphery of the islet, which is not the case in the human pancreas. ×360.

TABLE 18.2 Principal Cell Types in Pancreatic Islets

Cell Type	%	Cytoplasmic Staining with Mallory-Azan	Product	Granules (TEM)
A	15–20	Red	Glucagon	About 250 nm; dense, eccentric core surrounded by a light substance
B	60–70	Brownish orange	Insulin	About 300 nm; many with a dense, crystalline (angular) core surrounded by a light substance
D	5–10	Blue	Somatostatin	About 325 nm; homogeneous matrix

TEM, transmission electron microscope.

A cells stain red, the B cells stain brownish orange, and the D cells stain blue. About 5% of the cells appear to be unstained after this procedure. TEM allows identification of the principal cell types by the size and density of their secretory granules. Different makeup of cells in the islets of Langerhans can also be demonstrated by using the immunofluorescence method (Fig. 18.27).

In addition to the three principal islet cells, three minor islet cell types have also been identified by using a combination of the TEM and immunocytochemistry (Table 18.3).

Except for B cells, islet cells are counterparts of the enteroendocrine cells of the gastrointestinal mucosa.

Each islet cell type can be correlated with a specific hormone, and each has a specific location in the islet.

B cells constitute approximately 60%–70% of the total islet cells in humans and are generally located in its central portion. They secrete **insulin** (see Table 18.2). B cells contain numerous secretory granules about 300 nm in diameter with a dense polyhedral core and a pale matrix. The polyhedral core is believed to be crystallized insulin.

A cells constitute approximately 15%–20% of the human islet population and are generally located peripherally in the islets. They secrete **glucagon** (see Table 18.2). A cells contain secretory granules about 250 nm in diameter that are more uniform in size and more densely packed in the cytoplasm than the granules of B cells. The granules are sites of stored glucagon (Fig. 18.28).

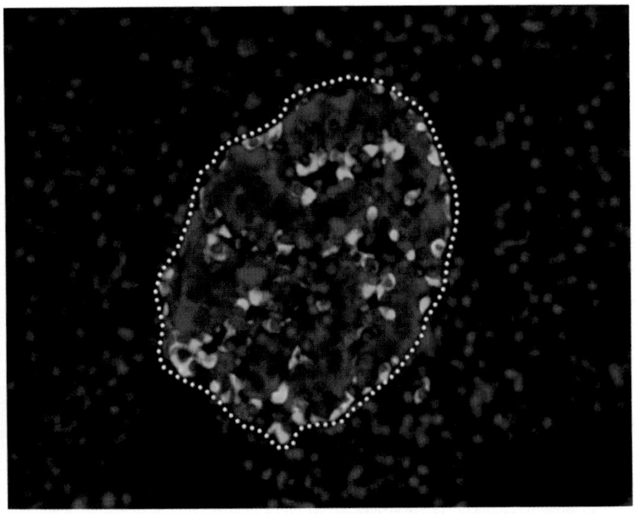

FIGURE 18.27. Islet of Langerhans in human adult pancreas. This immunofluorescence image shows the islet of Langerhans and distribution of glucagon-secreted A cells (*green*) and insulin-secreted B cells (*red*) in the adult pancreas. Cells were counterstained with a 4′,6-diamidino-2-phenylindole (DAPI) stain that reacts with nuclear DNA and exhibits blue fluorescence over the nuclei. Note that B cells comprise most of the islet cells and A cells are scattered throughout the islets. ×280. (From Scharfmann R, Xiao X, Heimberg H, et al. Beta cells within single human islets originate from multiple progenitors. *PLoS ONE*. 2008;2:e3559.)

D cells constitute about 5%–10% of the total pancreatic endocrine tissue and are also located peripherally in the islets. D cells secrete **somatostatin**, which is contained in secretory granules that are larger than those of the A and B cells (300–350 nm) and contain material of low to medium electron density (see Fig. 18.28).

The **minor islet cells** constitute about 5% of the islet tissue and may be represented by the pale cells seen after Mallory-Azan staining. Their characteristics and functions are summarized in Table 18.3.

Evidence suggests that some cells may secrete more than one hormone. Immunocytochemical staining has localized several hormones in addition to glucagon in the A-cell cytoplasm. These include gastric inhibitory peptide (GIP), cholecystokinin (CCK), and adrenocorticotropic hormone (ACTH) endorphin. Although there is no clear morphologic evidence for the presence of G cells (gastrin cells) in the islets, **gastrin** may also be secreted by one or more of the islet cells. Certain pancreatic islet cell tumors secrete large amounts of gastrin, thereby producing excessive acid secretion in the stomach (**Zollinger–Ellison syndrome**).

Functions of pancreatic hormones

Hormones secreted by the endocrine pancreas regulate metabolic functions either systemically, regionally (in the gastrointestinal tract), or locally (in the islet itself).

Insulin, the major hormone secreted by the islet tissue, decreases blood glucose levels.

Insulin is the most abundant endocrine secretion. Its principal effects are on the liver, skeletal muscle, and adipose tissue. Insulin has multiple individual actions in each of these tissues. In general, insulin stimulates the following processes:

- **Uptake of glucose** from the circulation. Specific cell membrane glucose transporters (GLUT4) are upregulated and inserted into the cell membrane of skeletal muscle cells and adipocytes.
- **Storage of glucose** by activation of glycogen synthase and inhibition of glycogen phosphorylase in muscle cells and liver. These actions lead to subsequent **glycogen** synthesis (**glycogenesis**).

TABLE 18.3 Minor Cell Types in Pancreatic Islets

Cell Type	Secretion	Location (in Addition to Islet)	Actions
PP cell (F cell)	Pancreatic polypeptide		Stimulates gastric chief cells Inhibits bile secretion and intestinal motility Inhibits pancreatic enzymes and HCO_3^- secretion
D_1 cell	Vasoactive intestinal peptide (VIP)	Also in exocrine acini and duct epithelium[a]	Similar to those of glucagon (hyperglycemic and glycogenolytic) Affects secretory activity and motility in gut Stimulates pancreatic exocrine secretion
EC cell	Secretin, motilin, substance P	Also in exocrine acini and duct epithelium[a]	Secretin: acts locally to stimulate HCO_3^- secretion in pancreatic juice and pancreatic enzyme secretion Motilin: increases gastric and intestinal motility Substance P: has neurotransmitter properties
Epsilon cell	Ghrelin	Epithelium lining the fundus of the stomach[b]	Stimulates appetite

PP, protein polypeptide; *EC*, enterochromaffin cell.

[a]This localization further emphasizes the ontogeny of the pancreas from the embryonic gut.

[b]Ghrelin is produced in the stomach by P/D_1 (G_r) cells.

- **Utilization of glucose** by promotion of **glycolysis** within cells. This is achieved by activation of pyruvate dehydrogenase and phosphofructokinase in skeletal muscle cells and liver.
- **Breakdown of chylomicrons** and other LDLs into free fatty acids by activation of lipoprotein lipase (LPL). The increased level of free fatty acids increases triglycerides, leading to the formation of lipid droplets (**lipogenesis**).
- **Synthesis of proteins** in skeletal muscle cells and hepatocytes by increasing cellular uptake of amino acids and activation of the mammalian target of rapamycin (mTOR) pathway, which stimulates ribosomal production and decreases cellular proteolysis

Absence or inadequate amounts of **insulin** lead to elevated blood glucose levels and the presence of glucose in the urine, a condition known as **diabetes mellitus**.

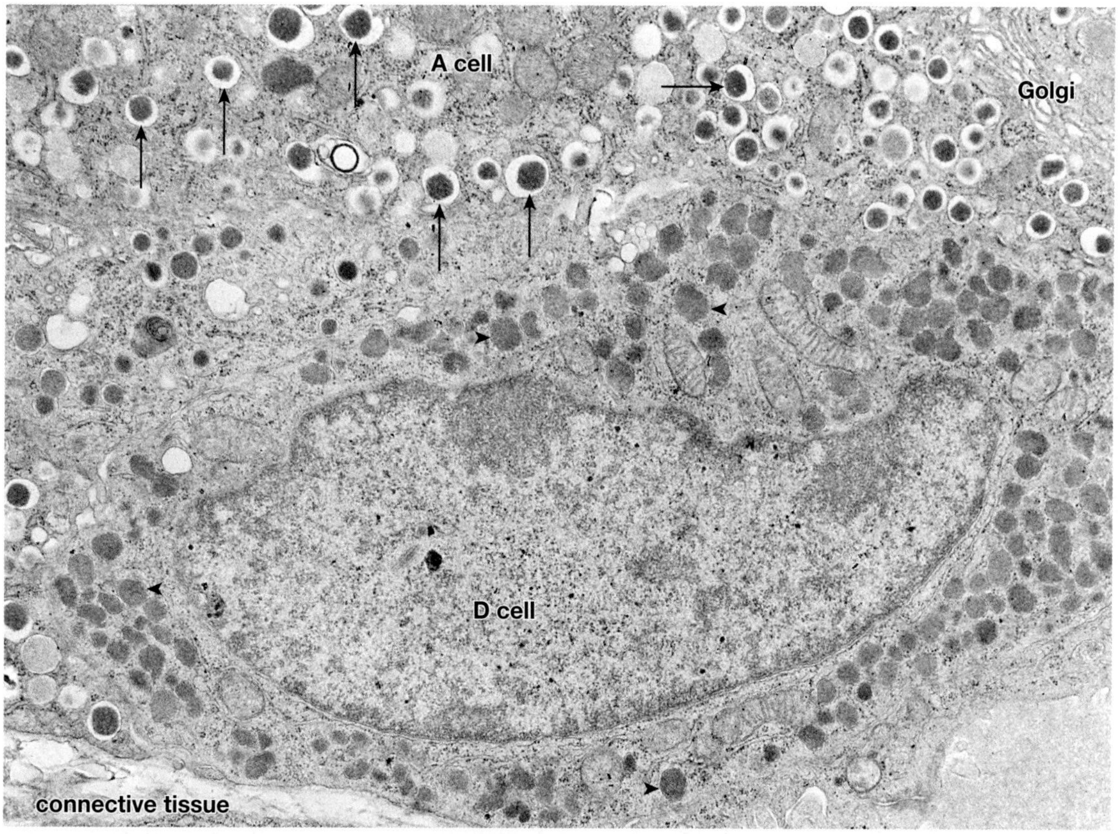

FIGURE 18.28. Electron micrograph of pancreatic islet cells. The portion of the cell in the *upper part* of the illustration is an A cell. It contains characteristic granules (*arrows*) showing a dense spherical core surrounded by a clear area and then a membrane. This cell also displays a characteristically well-developed Golgi apparatus. The cell at the *bottom* of the illustration is a D cell. It contains numerous membrane-bound granules of moderately low density (*arrowheads*). ×15,000.

FOLDER 18.3

CLINICAL CORRELATION: INSULIN PRODUCTION AND ALZHEIMER DISEASE

Insulin and **insulin growth factors (IGF-I and IGF-II)** are expressed by nerve cells in several regions of the brain. Insulin resistance, a characteristic of diabetes mellitus, is linked to neural degeneration, cognitive dysfunction, and dementia. The reduced rate of insulin and IGF production in the brain contributes to the degeneration of brain cells, an early symptom of **Alzheimer disease (AD)**. Postmortem examination of the brain tissue from individuals diagnosed with AD confirms that levels of insulin and IGFs are significantly reduced in the hippocampus (the part of the brain responsible for memory), frontal lobes, and hypothalamus, but not in the cerebellum (which is generally not affected by AD). Further research into these abnormalities in insulin production may lead to the development of novel AD therapies that target insulin and IGF.

Diabetes mellitus is a worldwide public health crisis and affects about 8.3% of the U.S. population. Complications of diabetes mellitus can be cardiovascular (endothelial cells dysfunction with damage to their basement membrane; e.g., hypertension, heart disease, and stroke), renal, retinopathic, or neuropathic. Reduced expression of insulin and insulin growth factors in the central nervous system (CNS) has been linked to Alzheimer disease (Folder 18.3).

Glucagon, secreted in amounts second only to insulin, increases blood glucose levels.

The actions of **glucagon** are essentially reciprocal to those of insulin. Glucagon stimulates the release of glucose into the bloodstream and stimulates **gluconeogenesis** (synthesis of glucose from metabolites of amino acids) and **glycogenolysis** (breakdown of glycogen) in the liver. Glucagon also stimulates proteolysis to promote gluconeogenesis, mobilizes fats from adipose cells (**lipolysis**), and stimulates hepatic lipase.

Somatostatin inhibits insulin and glucagon secretion.

Somatostatin is secreted by the D cells of the islets. It is identical to the hormone secreted by the hypothalamus that regulates somatotropin (GH) release from the anterior pituitary gland. Although the precise role of somatostatin in the islets is unclear, it has been shown to inhibit both insulin and glucagon secretion. It also suppresses the exocrine secretion of the pancreas.

The molecular characteristics of the major and some minor islet hormones are summarized in Table 18.4.

Regulation of islet activity

A **blood glucose level** above the normal 70 mg/100 mL (70 mg/dL) stimulates the release of insulin from β cells, leading to uptake and storage of glucose by the liver and muscle. The resultant decrease in the blood glucose level stops insulin secretion. Some amino acids also stimulate insulin secretion, either alone or in concert with elevated blood glucose levels. Increased blood fatty acid levels also stimulate insulin release, as do circulating gastrin, CCK, and secretin. CCK and glucagon, released in the islet by the A cells, act as paracrine secretions to stimulate B-cell secretion of insulin.

Blood glucose levels below 70 mg/100 mL stimulate the release of glucagon; blood glucose levels significantly above 70 mg/100 mL inhibit glucagon secretion. Glucagon is also released in response to low levels of fatty acids in the blood. Insulin inhibits the release of glucagon by A cells, but because of the cascading circulation in the islet (explained later), this inhibition is affected by a hormonal action of insulin carried in the general circulation.

The islets have both **sympathetic** and **parasympathetic innervations**. About 10% of the islet cells have nerve endings directly on their plasma membrane. Well-developed gap junctions are located between islet cells. Ionic events triggered by synaptic transmitters at the nerve endings are carried from cell to cell across these junctions. Autonomic nerves may have direct effects on hormone secretion by A and B cells.

Parasympathetic (cholinergic) stimulation increases secretion of both insulin and glucagon; sympathetic (adrenergic) stimulation increases glucagon release but inhibits insulin release. This neural control of insulin and glucagon may contribute to the availability of circulating glucose in stress reactions.

TABLE 18.4 Characteristics of Pancreatic Hormones

Hormone	Molecular Weight (Daltons)	Structure
Insulin	5,700–6,000	Two protein chains linked by disulfide bridges: α-chain, 21 amino acids; β-chain, 30 amino acids
Glucagon	3,500	Linear polypeptide: 29 amino acids
Somatostatin	1,638	Cyclic polypeptide: 14 amino acids
VIP	3,300	Linear polypeptide: 28 amino acids
Pancreatic polypeptide	4,200	Linear polypeptide: 36 amino acids

VIP, vasoactive intestinal peptide.

FOLDER 18.4

FUNCTIONAL CONSIDERATIONS: INSULIN SYNTHESIS, AN EXAMPLE OF POST-TRANSLATIONAL PROCESSING

Insulin is produced in B cells of the pancreas. It is a small protein consisting of two polypeptide chains joined by disulfide bridges. Its biosynthesis presents a clear example of the importance of post-translational processing in the achievement of the final, active structure of a protein.

Insulin is originally synthesized as a single 110-amino-acid polypeptide chain with a molecular weight of about 12 kDa. This polypeptide is called **preproinsulin**. Preproinsulin contains an amino-terminus signal sequence (24 amino acids in length) that is required for the precursor hormone to enter the rough endoplasmic reticulum (rER). As the molecule is inserted into the cisternae of the rER, the preproinsulin signal sequence is proteolytically cleaved to form **proinsulin**. Post-translational processing reduces the preproinsulin to a polypeptide with a molecular weight of about 9,000 Da. Proinsulin is a single polypeptide chain of 81–86 amino acids that has the approximate shape of the letter G (Fig. F18.4.1). Two disulfide bonds connect the bar of the G to the top loop.

During packaging and storage of proinsulin in the Golgi apparatus, a cathepsin-like enzyme cleaves most of the side of the loop, leaving the bar of the G as an **A chain** of 21 amino acids cross-linked by the disulfide bridges to the top of the loop, which becomes the **B chain** of 30 amino acids. The 35-amino-acid peptide removed from the loop is called a **C peptide** (connecting peptide). It is stored in the secretory vesicles and released with the insulin in equimolar amounts. No physiologic function has been identified for the C peptide.

Because C peptide has a longer half-life than insulin, higher concentrations of C peptides are detected in the peripheral blood. For these reasons, measurement of circulating levels of C peptides provides important clinical information about the secretory activity of B cells. Because C peptide is cleared from the body by the kidney, measurement of its urinary excretion provides useful information about B-cell insulin secretion. C peptide measurements are frequently used to assess the residual B-cell function in patients treated with insulin, to distinguish between types 1 and 2 diabetes, and in the diagnosis and treatment of **insulinoma (tumor of B cells)**. C peptide levels may also be used to monitor the progress of pancreas or islet cell transplantation.

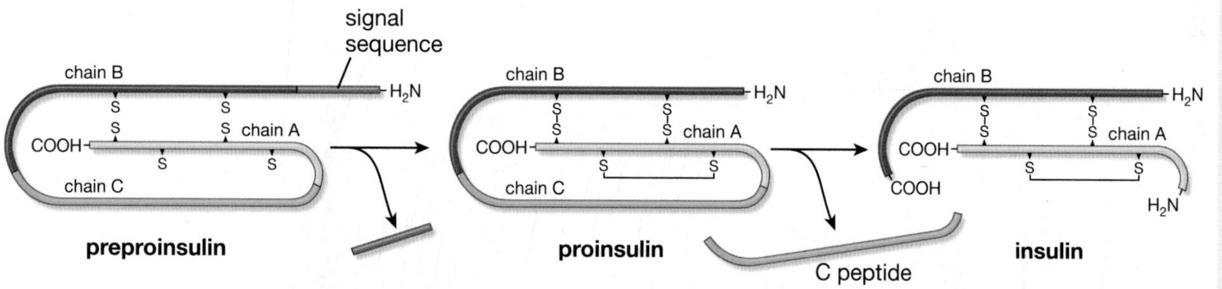

FIGURE F18.4.1. Post-translational processing of insulin. Insulin is synthesized as preproinsulin, a single polypeptide chain that undergoes post-translational modifications. Initially, the signal sequence is removed within the cisternae of the rough endoplasmic reticulum (*rER*). The shortened polypeptide chain, now known as *proinsulin*, is transported to the Golgi apparatus. Here, it is further modified by the formation of internal disulfide bonds and removal of a C chain that produces biologically active insulin.

The blood supply to the pancreas provides a cascading perfusion of the islets and acini.

As mentioned earlier, islets of Langerhans comprise only 1%–2% of the total mass of the pancreas; however, they receive about 10%–15% of the pancreatic blood flow. There are two predominant blood flow patterns in the islets of Langerhans. The most common pattern occurs when blood enters the islets at the center, initially perfusing the core of the islet and then spreading to the periphery. In the second pattern, several arterioles enter the periphery of the islets and branch into fenestrated capillaries to perfuse the core of the islet. In humans, it is likely that the capillaries first perfuse the A and D cells, peripherally, before the blood reaches the B cells, centrally. Larger vessels that travel in septa that penetrate the central portion of the islet are also accompanied by A and D cells so that blood reaching the B cells has always first perfused the A and D cells. Recent in vivo fluorescence imaging studies show distinct blood flow dynamics in the islets of Langerhans. These studies suggest that blood flow is regulated by blood glucose levels in addition to the complex interaction among vasodilators and vasoconstrictors, gastrointestinal peptides, and the autonomic nervous system.

Large **efferent capillaries** leave the islet and branch into the capillary networks that surround the acini of the exocrine pancreas. This cascading flow resembles the portal systems of other endocrine glands (pituitary, adrenal).

Secretions of the islet cells have regulatory effects on the acinar cells.

- Insulin, the vasoactive intestinal peptide (VIP), and cholecystokinin (CCK) stimulate exocrine secretion.
- Glucagon, pancreatic polypeptide (PP), and somatostatin inhibit exocrine secretion.

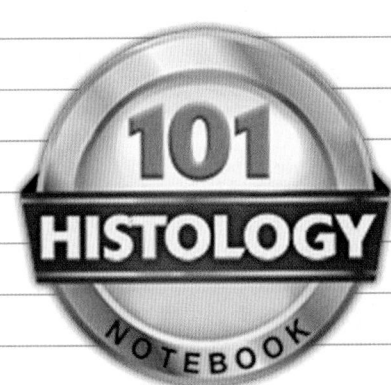

DIGESTIVE SYSTEM III: LIVER, GALLBLADDER, AND PANCREAS

OVERVIEW OF THE LIVER

- The **liver** is the largest internal organ and largest mass of glandular tissue in the body.
- The liver plays an important role in the uptake, storage, and distribution of nutrients. It produces the majority of circulating **plasma proteins** (e.g., albumins), stores iron, converts vitamins, and degrades drugs and toxins.
- The liver also acts as an exocrine organ (produces **bile**) and performs endocrine-like functions.
- The liver has a **dual blood supply**: a venous supply via the **hepatic portal vein** and an arterial supply via the **hepatic artery**.

STRUCTURE OF THE LIVER

- Structural components of the **liver** include **parenchyma** (plates of hepatocytes), **connective tissue stroma**, **sinusoidal capillaries** (hepatic sinusoids), and **perisinusoidal spaces** (of Disse).
- There are three ways to describe the structure of the liver in terms of a functional unit: the **classic lobule** (polygonal in shape), the **portal lobule** (triangular in shape), and the **liver acinus** (a diamond-shaped area that has three zones and best correlates to blood perfusion, metabolic activity, and liver pathology).
- **Hepatocytes** (as seen in the classic lobule) are organized into irregular anastomosing plates that radiate toward a central vein. Corners of the polygonal classic lobule are occupied by the **portal triad**, which contains branches of portal vein, hepatic artery, bile ducts, and small lymphatic vessels.
- **Hepatic sinusoids** form irregular vascular channels that run parallel and between the plates of hepatocytes. They receive mixed blood (~75%) from the venous portal circulation and arterial blood (~25%) from the systemic circulation.
- Hepatic sinusoids are lined with a thin discontinuous endothelium. The **perisinusoidal space (space of Disse)** lies between hepatocytes and the endothelium; it is the site of exchange of materials between the blood and liver cells.
- The sinusoidal endothelium includes specialized **stellate sinusoidal macrophages (Kupffer cells)**, which are part of immune defense system and remove worn-out red blood cells and recycle iron molecules.
- **Hepatic stellate cells (Ito cells)** reside in perisinusoidal spaces and are loaded with lipid droplets for storage of vitamin A. In pathologic conditions, Ito cells may differentiate into myofibroblasts.

HEPATOCYTES

- **Hepatocytes** (constitute 80% of liver cells) are large, polygonal cells with spherical nuclei (often binucleated) and acidophilic cytoplasm containing sER, rER, numerous mitochondria and peroxisomes, and multiple small Golgi complexes.
- The **basal surface** of hepatocytes is in contact with the perisinusoidal space (of Disse), whereas the **apical surface** is connected to the adjacent hepatocyte to form a bile canaliculus.
- **Bile canaliculi** drain into the short **canals of Hering**, which are partially lined by hepatocytes and cuboidal cholangiocytes (cells lining the biliary tree).
- Canals of Hering harbor specific **hepatic stem cells**.

BILIARY TREE

- The **biliary tree** is lined by simple cuboidal or columnar epithelial cells called **cholangiocytes**, which monitor bile flow and regulate its content.
- **Bile** (produced by hepatocytes) is collected by the **bile canaliculi** and drains to the **canals of Hering**. From there, it continues to flow into the **intrahepatic bile ductules** and further into the **interlobular bile ducts** (part of the portal triad). Interlobular ducts eventually merge to form the left and right **hepatic ducts** that exit the liver in the porta hepatis.
- **Extrahepatic bile ducts** carry the bile to the gallbladder and eventually into the duodenum.

OVERVIEW OF THE GALLBLADDER

- The **gallbladder** is a pear-shaped, distensible sac that concentrates (removes 90% of water) and stores bile.
- **Mucosa** of the gallbladder has numerous deep folds (to increase surface area), a **lamina propria** rich in blood vessels, and a well-developed **muscularis externa** (no muscularis mucosae or submucosa).
- The tall columnar **cholangiocytes** are specialized for water uptake from bile. They express aquaporins (water channel proteins) that facilitate a rapid passive movement of water.
- Deep diverticula of the mucosa, called **Rokitansky–Aschoff sinuses**, often extend through the muscularis externa.
- Contraction of the **muscularis externa** reduces the volume of the gallbladder, forcing bile out through the cystic duct and common bile duct to the duodenum.

OVERVIEW OF THE PANCREAS

- The **pancreas** is an **exocrine** and **endocrine** gland located in the retroperitoneal space of the abdomen.
- The **exocrine component** synthesizes and secretes hydrolytic digestive enzymes into the duodenum that are essential for digestion in the intestine. It contains serous acini, which comprise most of the mass of the pancreas.
- **Pancreatic acini** are unique because their intercalated ducts arise within the acinus; therefore, nuclei of duct cells located inside the acinus are referred to as **centroacinar cells** (a characteristic feature of the pancreas).
- The pancreatic acinar cell is pyramidal in shape with **secretory (zymogen) granules** located in the apical cytoplasm. Golgi complexes, rER, and a large nucleus are located at the basal domain of the cell.
- **Intercalated ducts** secrete large amounts of sodium and bicarbonates to neutralize the acidity of the chyme that enters the duodenum from the stomach.
- Intercalated ducts drain pancreatic acini into **intralobular ducts**, larger **interlobular ducts**, and finally into the **pancreatic duct**, which empties into the duodenum.
- The **endocrine component** (islets of Langerhans) synthesizes and secretes hormones into the blood that regulate glucose, lipid, and protein metabolism.
- **Islets of Langerhans** are dispersed in the pancreas and contain three primary types of cells: **A cells** (which produce glucagon), **B cells** (which produce insulin), and **D cells** (which produce somatostatin).

PLATE 18.1 ■ LIVER I

The **liver** is the largest mass of glandular tissue in the body and the largest internal organ. It is unique because it receives its major blood supply from the **hepatic portal vein**, which carries venous blood from the small intestine, pancreas, and spleen. Thus, the liver is directly in the pathway that conveys materials absorbed in the intestine. The liver is the first organ exposed to metabolic substrates and nutrients as well as to noxious and toxic substances absorbed from the intestine. One of the major roles of the liver is to degrade or conjugate toxic substances to render them harmless. It can, however, be seriously damaged by excess exposure to such substances.

Each liver cell has both exocrine and endocrine functions. The exocrine secretion of the liver, called **bile**, contains conjugated and degraded waste products that are delivered back to the intestine for disposal. It also contains substances that bind to metabolites in the intestine to aid absorption. A series of ducts of increasing diameter and complexity, beginning with **bile canaliculi** between individual hepatocytes and ending with the **common bile duct**, delivers bile from the liver and gallbladder to the duodenum.

The endocrine secretions of the liver are released directly into the blood that supplies the liver cells; these secretions include albumin, nonimmune α- and β-globulins, prothrombin, and glycoproteins, including fibronectin. Glucose, released from stored glycogen, and triiodothyronine (T_3), the more active deiodination product of thyroxine, are also released directly into the blood.

Functional units of the liver, described as *lobules* or *acini*, are made up of irregular interconnecting sheets of hepatocytes separated from one another by the blood sinusoids.

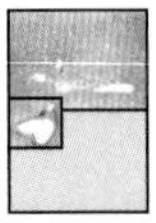

Liver, human, hematoxylin and eosin (H&E) ×65; inset ×65.

At the low magnification shown here, large numbers of hepatic cells appear to be uniformly disposed throughout the specimen. They are organized in discrete lobules (boundaries of a single lobule can be approximated by the *dashed line*) with the central vein (*CV*) in the middle. The **hepatocytes** are arranged in one-cell-thick plates, but when sectioned, they appear as interconnecting cords one or more cells thick, depending on the plane of section. The **sinusoids** appear as light areas between the cords of cells; they are more clearly shown in the next figure (*asterisks*).

Also present in this figure is a **portal canal**. It is a connective tissue septum that carries the branches of the hepatic artery (*HA*) and portal vein (*PV*), bile ducts (*BD*), and lymphatic vessels and nerves. The artery and vein, along with the bile duct, are collectively referred to as a **portal triad**.

The hepatic artery and the portal vein are easy to identify because they are found in relation to one another within the surrounding connective tissue of the portal canal. The vein is typically thin walled; the artery is smaller in diameter and has a thicker wall. The **bile ducts** are composed of a simple cuboidal or columnar epithelium, depending on the size of the duct. Multiple profiles of the blood vessels and bile ducts may be evident in the canal because of either branching or their passage out of the plane of section and then back in again.

The vessel through which blood leaves the liver is the hepatic vein. It is readily identified because it travels alone (*inset*) and is surrounded by an appreciable amount of connective tissue (*CT*) often containing small lymphatic nodules (*L*). If more than one profile of a vein is present within this connective tissue, but no arteries or bile ducts are present, the second vessel will also be a hepatic vein. Such is the case in the *inset*, where a profile of a small hepatic vein is seen just above the larger hepatic vein (*HV*).

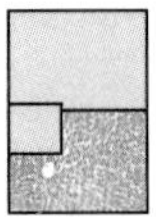

Liver lobule, liver, human, H&E ×160.

The **terminal hepatic venules** or **central veins** (***CV***) are the most distal branches of the hepatic vein, and like the hepatic vein, they also travel alone. Their distinguishing features are the sinusoids (indicated by *asterisks*) that penetrate the wall of the vein and the paucity of surrounding connective tissue. These characteristics are shown to advantage in Plate 18.2 (page 724).

It is best to examine low-magnification views of the liver to define the boundaries of a lobule. A lobule is best identified when it is cut in cross section. The central vein then appears as a circular profile, and the hepatic cells appear as cords radiating from the central vein. Such a lobule is outlined by the *dashed line* in the previous figure.

The limits of the lobule are defined, in part, by the portal canal. In other directions, the plates of the lobule do not appear to have a limit; that is, they have become contiguous with plates of an adjacent lobule. One can estimate the dimensions of the lobule, however, by approximating a circle with the central vein as its center and incorporating those plates that exhibit a radial arrangement up to the point where a portal canal is present. If the lobule has been cross-sectioned, the radial limit is set by the location of one or more of the portal canals as indicated by the bile ducts (*BD*) in this figure.

BD, bile duct
CT, connective tissue
CV, central vein (terminal hepatic venule)
HA, hepatic artery
HV, hepatic vein
L, lymphatic nodule
PV, portal vein
asterisks, bottom figure, blood sinusoids
dashed line, top figure, approximates the limits of a lobule

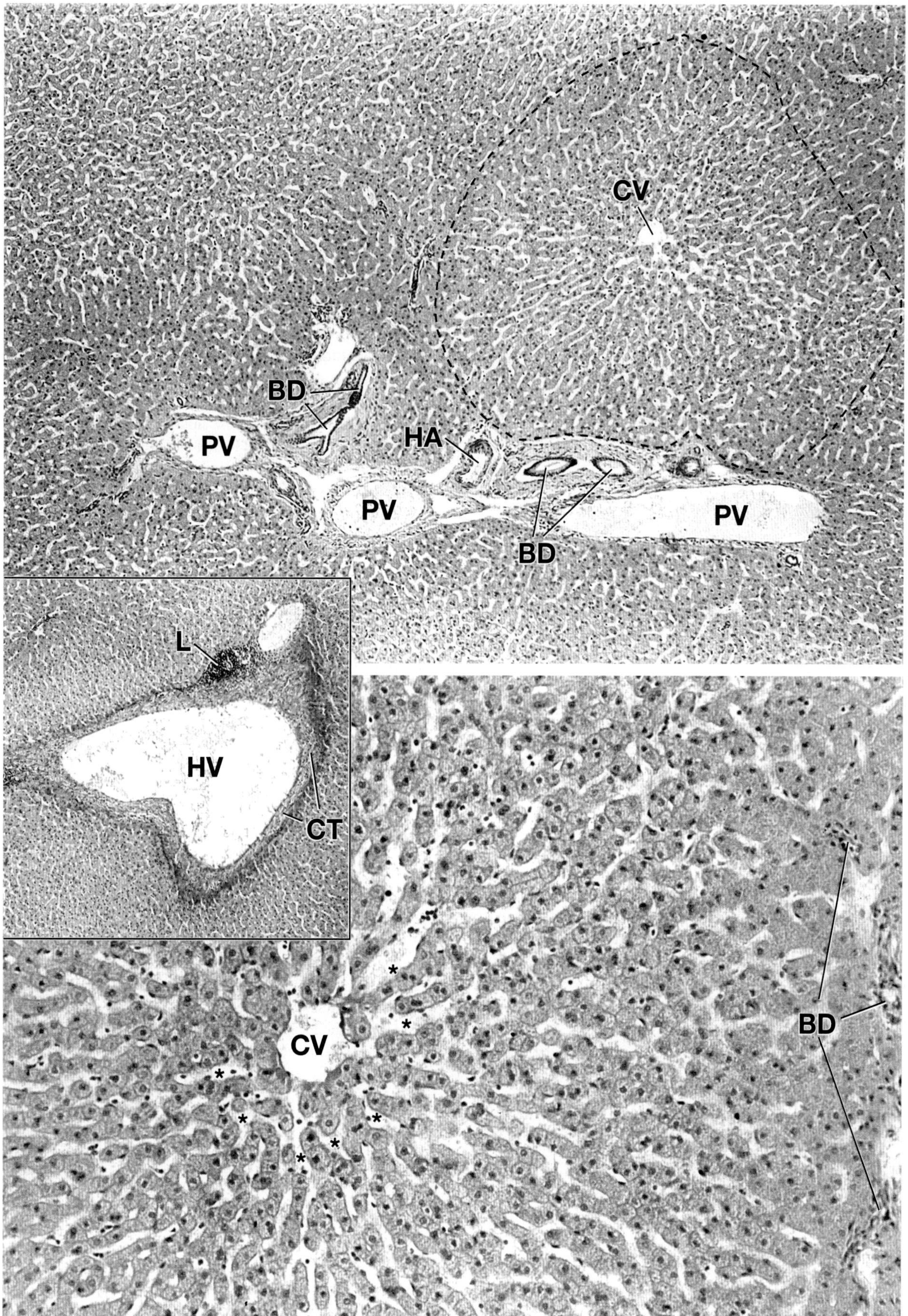
CV
BD
PV
HA
PV
PV
BD
L
HV
CT
*
*
CV
*
*
*
*
*
BD

PLATE 18.2 ■ LIVER II

There are three ways of describing the liver parenchyma in terms of a functional unit, *"classic" lobules, portal lobules*, or *acini*. The **classic lobule** is a roughly hexagonal block of tissue that has at its center the terminal hepatic venule (central vein) and at its six corners the **portal canals.** Each portal canal contains a **portal triad,** each comprising a branch of the portal vein, hepatic artery, and bile duct. The **portal lobule** is a triangular construct that emphasizes the exocrine secretory function. It has as its axis the bile duct of the portal triad of the classic lobule, and its outer margins are imaginary lines drawn between the central veins closest to that portal triad. The **liver acinus** is most closely correlated with blood perfusion, metabolic activity, and liver pathology. The acinus is a small diamond- or lozenge-shaped mass of tissue that has as its short axis the fine branches of the portal triad that lie along the border of two classic lobules and as its long axis a line drawn between the two central veins closest to the short axis. The hepatocytes in each acinus are described as arranged in three concentric elliptical zones around the short axis; zone 1 is closest to, and zone 3 is farthest from, the axis.

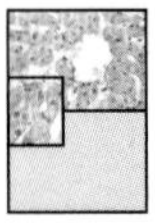

Central vein, liver, human, hematoxylin and eosin (H&E) ×500; inset ×800.

The **central vein** and surrounding hepatocytes from the *lower* figure of Plate 18.1 (page 722) are shown here at higher magnification. The cytoplasm of the **hepatocytes** in this specimen has a foamy appearance because of the extraction of glycogen and lipid during tissue preparation. The boundaries between individual hepatocytes are discernible in some locations, but not between those cells where the knife has cut across the boundary in an oblique plane. Frequently, when cell boundaries are observed at still higher magnification (*inset*), a very small circular or oval profile is observed midway along the boundary. These profiles represent the bile canaliculi (*BC*).

The cells that line the **sinusoids** (*S*) show little, if any, cytoplasmic detail in routine preparations. **Perisinusoidal macrophages** (**Kupffer cells** [*KC*]) are generally recognized by their ovoid nuclei and the projection of the cell into the lumen. The endothelial cell, in contrast, is a squamous cell that has a smaller, attenuated, or elongated nucleus. Some nuclei of this description are evident in the micrograph.

The termination of two of the sinusoids and their union with the central vein (*CV*) is indicated by the *curved arrows*. Note that the wall of the vein is strengthened by connective tissue, mostly collagen, which appears as homogeneous eosin-stained material (*asterisks*). Fibroblasts (*F*) within this connective tissue can be identified and distinguished from the endothelial cell (*EN*) lining of the vein.

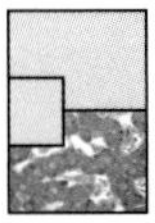

Hepatic sinusoids, liver, rat, glutaraldehyde–osmium fixation, toluidine blue ×900.

This figure shows a plastic-embedded liver specimen fixed by the method normally used for electron microscopy. In contrast to the H&E-stained preparation, it demonstrates to advantage the cytologic detail of the hepatocytes and the sinusoids (*S*). The **hepatocytes** are deeply colored with toluidine blue. Note that the cytoplasm exhibits irregular magenta masses (*arrows*). This is glycogen that has been retained by the glutaraldehyde fixation and stained metachromatically by toluidine blue. Also evident are lipid droplets (*L*) of varying size that have been preserved and stained black by the osmium used as the secondary fixative. The quantities of lipid and glycogen are variable and, under normal conditions, reflect dietary intake. Examination of the hepatocyte cytoplasm also reveals small, punctate, *dark blue* bodies contrasted against the *lighter blue* background of the cell. These are the mitochondria. Another feature of this specimen is the clear representation of the **bile canaliculi** (*BC*) between liver cells. They appear as empty circular profiles when cross-sectioned and as elongated channels (*lower right*) when longitudinally sectioned.

The sinusoidal lining cells are of two distinct types. The **Kupffer cells** (*KC*) are the more prominent cells. They exhibit a large nucleus and a substantial amount of cytoplasm. They protrude into the lumen and may give the appearance of occluding it. However, they do not block the channel. The surface of the Kupffer cell exhibits a very irregular or jagged contour because of the numerous processes that provide the cell with an extensive surface area. The **endothelial cell** (*EN*) has a smaller nucleus, attenuated cytoplasm, and a smooth surface contour.

A third cell type, the less frequently observed perisinusoidal lipocyte (Ito cell), is not seen in this micrograph. This cell would appear as a light cell containing numerous lipid droplets. The lipid droplets contain stored vitamin A.

BC, bile canaliculus
CV, central vein
EN, endothelial cell
F, fibroblast
KC, Kupffer cell
L, lipid droplet
S, sinusoid
arrows, glycogen
asterisks, connective tissue of central vein curved
arrows, opening of sinusoid into central vein

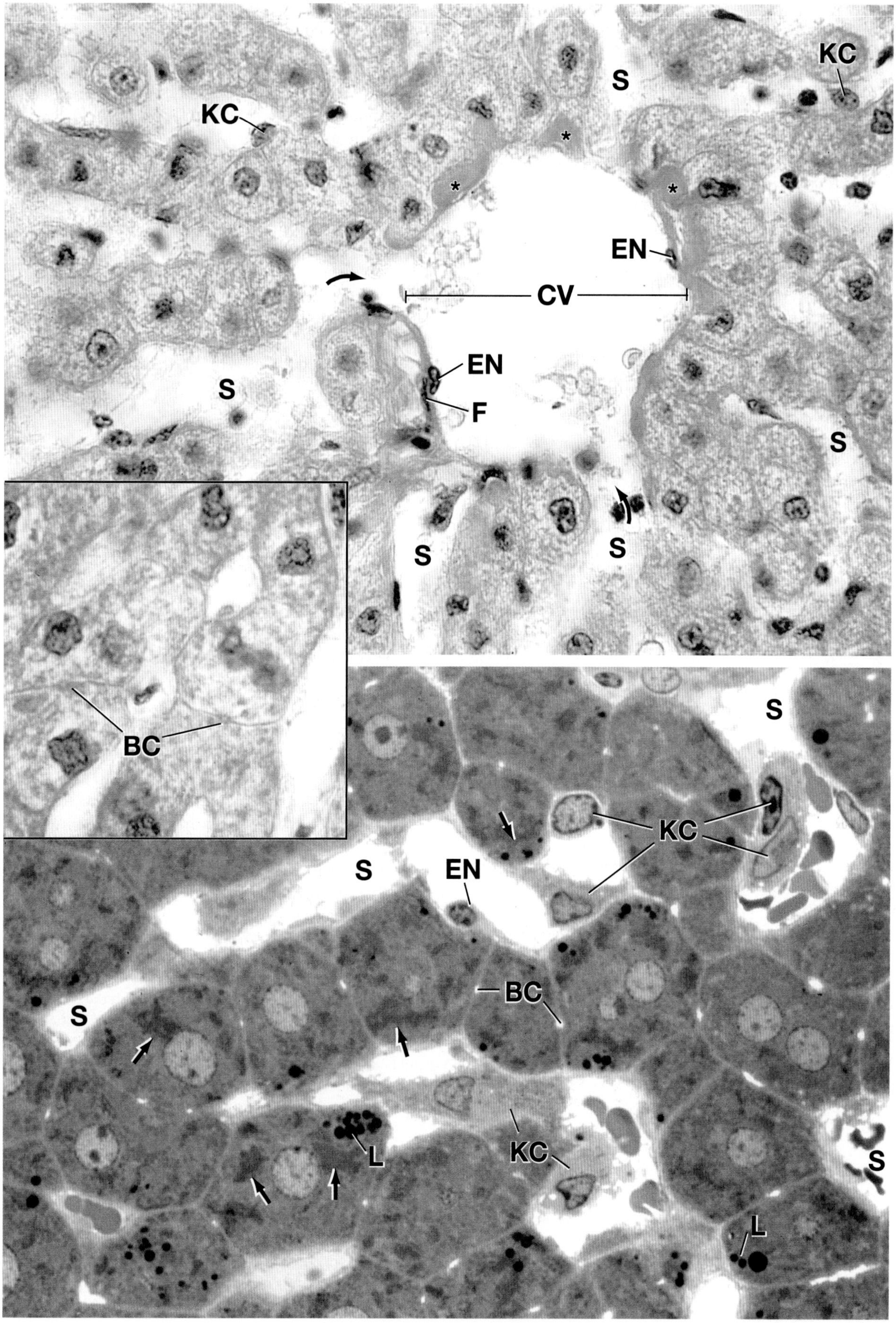
KC
S
KC
*
*
*
*
EN
CV
EN
F
S
S
S
S
S
BC
S
KC
S
EN
BC
S
L
KC
S
L

PLATE 18.3 ■ GALLBLADDER

The **gallbladder** concentrates and stores bile for delivery to the duodenum. Bile is concentrated by the active transport of salt from the bile and the passive movement of water in response to the salt transport. The mucosa is characterized by a tall columnar absorptive epithelium that closely resembles that of the intestine and the colon in both its morphology and function. The epithelial cells are characterized by numerous short apical microvilli, apical junctional complexes, concentrations of mitochondria in the apical and basal cytoplasm, and complex lateral plications. In addition, Na^+/K^+-activated ATPase is localized on the lateral plasma membrane of the epithelial cell.

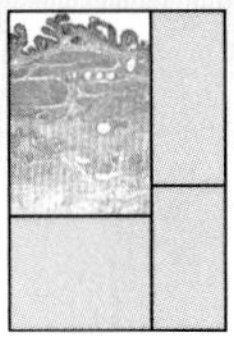

Gallbladder, human, hematoxylin and eosin (H&E) ×45.

The gallbladder is a hollow, pear-shaped organ that concentrates and stores the bile. The full thickness of its wall is shown here. It is composed of a mucosa (*Muc*), muscularis (*Mus*), adventitia (*Adv*), and, on its free surface (not shown), a serosa. The **mucosa** is considered at higher magnification in the next figure. The **muscularis** consists of interlacing bundles of smooth muscle (*SM*). The **adventitia** (*Adv*) consists of irregular dense connective tissue through which the larger blood vessels (*BV*) travel and, more peripherally, of varying amounts of adipose tissue (*AT*).

The mucosa is thrown into numerous folds that are particularly pronounced when the muscularis is highly contracted. Note the presence of several outpouchings of the mucosa, called *Rokitansky–Aschoff sinuses* (RAS). This is the usual histologic appearance of the gallbladder unless, of course, steps are taken to fix and preserve it in a distended state. Occasionally, the section cuts through a recess in a fold, and the recess may then resemble a gland (*arrows*). The mucosa, however, does not possess glands, except in the neck region, where some mucous glands are present (see *lower right figure*).

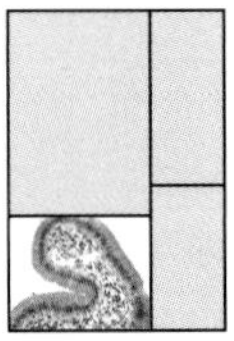

Mucosa, gallbladder, human, H&E ×325.

The **mucosa** consists of a tall simple columnar absorptive epithelium (*Ep*) resting on a lamina propria of loose connective tissue (*CT*) containing blood vessels (*BV*). The epithelium has characteristics that distinguish it from the absorptive epithelium of other organs, such as the intestines. Only one cell type, the tall columnar cell, is present in the epithelial layer (see *upper right figure*). The nuclei are in the basal portion of the cell. The cells possess a thin apical striated border. However, this is not always evident in routine H&E-stained sections. The cytoplasm stains rather uniformly with eosin. This staining pattern reflects the cell's absorptive function and is in contrast to the staining of cells that produce protein. The cells' absorptive function is further demonstrated by their distended intercellular spaces at the basal aspect (see *upper right figure arrows*). This feature is associated with the transport of fluid across the epithelium and, as noted earlier, commonly seen in intestinal absorptive cells.

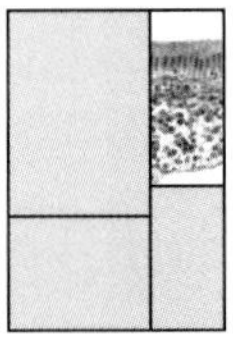

Mucosa, gallbladder, human, H&E ×550.

The **lamina propria** underlying the epithelium is usually very cellular. In this specimen, in addition to lymphocytes (*L*), a relatively common finding, a large number of plasma cells (*PC*) is also present within the lamina propria. (The high concentration of plasma cells suggests chronic inflammation.) Another feature of note in the lamina propria is the presence of several outpouchings of the mucosa, called *Rokitansky–Aschoff sinuses* (*RAS*), other than those seen in the mucosa and noted earlier. These are readily apparent in the *top left* figure, and part of the wall of the Rokitansky–Aschoff sinus is shown at higher magnification in the next figure.

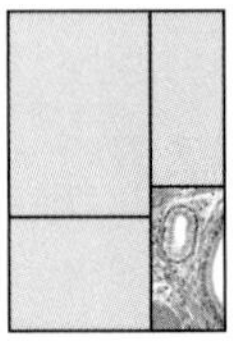

Mucosa, gallbladder neck, human, H&E ×550.

The smaller of the two gland-like structures visible in the connective tissue (*CT*) of lamina propria is composed of **mucous cells** (*MC*) and represents a section through a **mucous gland** (*MG*). This specimen was taken from a site near the neck of the gallbladder where mucous glands are often present. Note the characteristic flattened nuclei at the base of the cell and the lightly stained appearance of the cytoplasm, features characteristic of mucin-secreting cells. In contrast, the epithelium of the large gland-like profile that is only partially included in the micrograph has rounded or ovoid nuclei. This epithelial-lined structure is not a true gland but represents an invagination of the mucous membrane that extends into and often through the thickness of the muscularis. These invaginations are known as **Rokitansky–Aschoff sinuses** (*RAS*).

Adv, adventitia
AT, adipose tissue
BV, blood vessel
CT, connective tissue, lamina propria
Ep, epithelium
L, lymphocytes
MC, mucous cells
MG, mucous gland
Muc, mucosa
Mus, muscularis
PC, plasma cells
RAS, Rokitansky–Aschoff sinus
SM, smooth muscle
arrows, top left figure, recess in luminal surface; top right figure, intercellular spaces

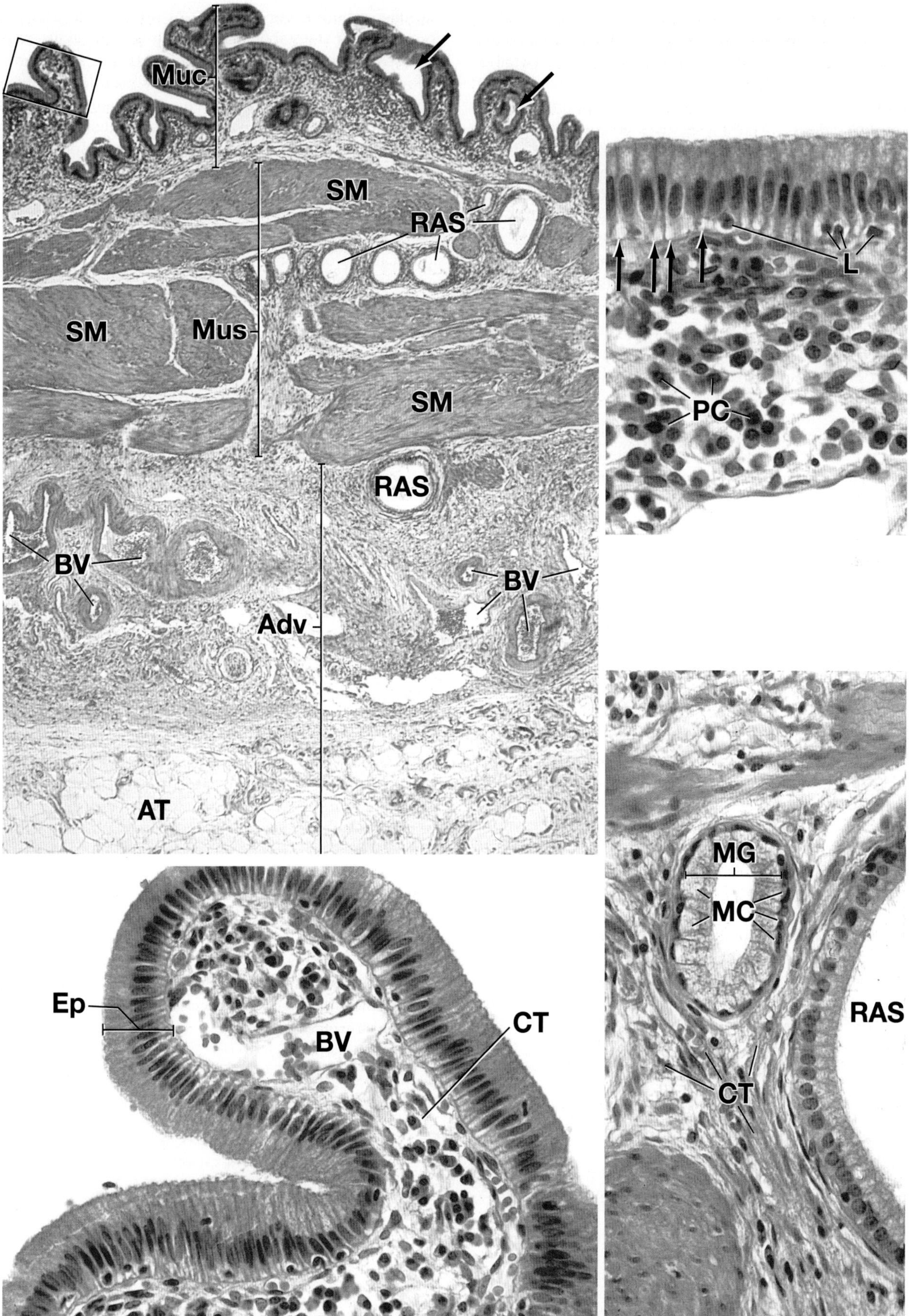
Muc
SM
RAS
SM
Mus
SM
RAS
BV
BV
Adv
AT
L
PC
Ep
BV
CT
MG
MC
CT
RAS

PLATE 18.4 ■ PANCREAS

The **pancreas** is an elongated extramural digestive gland with a head nestled in the C-shaped bend of the duodenum, a body that crosses the midline of the abdomen, and a tail extending across the back of the abdomen. It is a mixed gland containing both an exocrine component and an endocrine component that have distinctive characteristics. The **exocrine component** is a compound tubuloacinar gland with a branching network of ducts that convey the exocrine secretions to the duodenum. These secretions consist primarily of inactive forms of potent proteolytic enzymes as well as amylase, lipase, nucleases, and electrolytes, particularly HCO_3^-.

The **endocrine component** is isolated as highly vascularized islets of epithelioid tissue (islets of Langerhans). The islet cells secrete a variety of polypeptide and protein hormones, most notably insulin and glucagon, which regulate glucose metabolism throughout the other tissues of the body. Other hormones secreted by islet cells include somatostatin, pancreatic polypeptide, vasoactive intestinal peptide, secretin, motilin, and substance P. All of these substances, with the exception of insulin, are also secreted by the population of enteroendocrine cells in the intestine, the organ from which the pancreas is derived during embryonic development. Whereas insulin and glucagon act primarily in the endocrine regulation of distant cells, the other hormones (and glucagon) have significant roles in the paracrine regulation of the insulin-secreting B cells of the pancreatic islet.

Pancreas, human, hematoxylin and eosin (H&E) ×160; inset ×360.

The pancreas is surrounded by a delicate capsule of moderately dense connective tissue. Septa from the capsule divide the pancreas into lobules, one of which is shown here, bounded by connective tissue (*CT*). Larger blood vessels (*BV*) travel in the connective tissue septa; nerves also travel in the septa, but they are seen infrequently. Within the lobule are numerous acini of the exocrine component, an **intralobular duct** (*InD*), intercalated ducts (not readily evident at this low magnification), and **islets of Langerhans** (*IL*; *dashed line*). Also within the lobule are small blood vessels and connective tissue serving as a stroma for the parenchymal elements of the gland.

The islet of Langerhans (*IL*) in this photomicrograph is shown among the far more numerous acini. (Islets are most numerous in the tail of the pancreas and least numerous in the head.) Cells within the islets are arranged as irregular cords. In routine preparations, it is not possible to identify the various cell types within the islets. Note, however, that B cells are the most numerous; these produce insulin. The next most numerous are A cells; these produce glucagon. The *inset* also shows numerous capillaries (*arrows*). The labels *A* and *B* are not intended to identify specific cells but rather to show those parts of the islets where A and B cells are found in greatest number.

Pancreas, human, H&E ×600.

Acini of the pancreas consist of serous cells. In sections, the acini present circular and irregular profiles. The lumen of the acinus is small, and only in fortuitous sections through an acinus is the lumen included (*asterisks*). The nucleus is characteristically in the base of the acinar cell. There is a region of intense basophilia adjacent to the nucleus. This is the ergastoplasm (*Er*), and it reflects the presence of rough endoplasmic reticulum (*rER*) that is active in the synthesis of pancreatic enzymes. Some acini reveal a centrally positioned cell with cytoplasm that shows no special staining characteristics in H&E-stained paraffin sections. These are **centroacinar cells** (*CC*) that represent the origin of the intercalated ducts.

This figure demonstrates particularly well the morphology and relationships of the intercalated ducts. Note, first, the cross-sectioned **intralobular duct** (*InD*) consisting of cuboidal epithelium. (There are no striated ducts in the pancreas.) Leading to the intralobular duct is an **intercalated duct** (*ID*), which is seen in cross section at the furthest distance from the intralobular duct and then, in longitudinal section, in the *center* of the illustration as it travels toward the intralobular duct. The lumen is evident where the intercalated duct is seen in cross section, but is not evident where it is seen in longitudinal section due to the plane of section cutting chiefly through the cells rather than the lumen. As a consequence, this figure provides a good view of the nuclei of the duct cells. They are elongated, with their long axis oriented in the direction of the duct. In addition, they display a staining pattern similar to that of centroacinar cells and different from that of nuclei of the parenchymal cells.

Once the cells of the intercalated duct have been identified in one part of the section, their staining characteristics and location can be used to identify the intercalated ducts in other parts of the lobule, several of which are marked (*ID*).

A, region with most A cells
B, region with most B cells
BV, blood vessels
CC, centroacinar cells
CT, connective tissue
Er, ergastoplasm
ID, intercalated ducts
IL, islets of Langerhans
InD, intralobular duct
rER, rough endoplasmic reticulum
arrows, capillaries
asterisks, lumen of acini

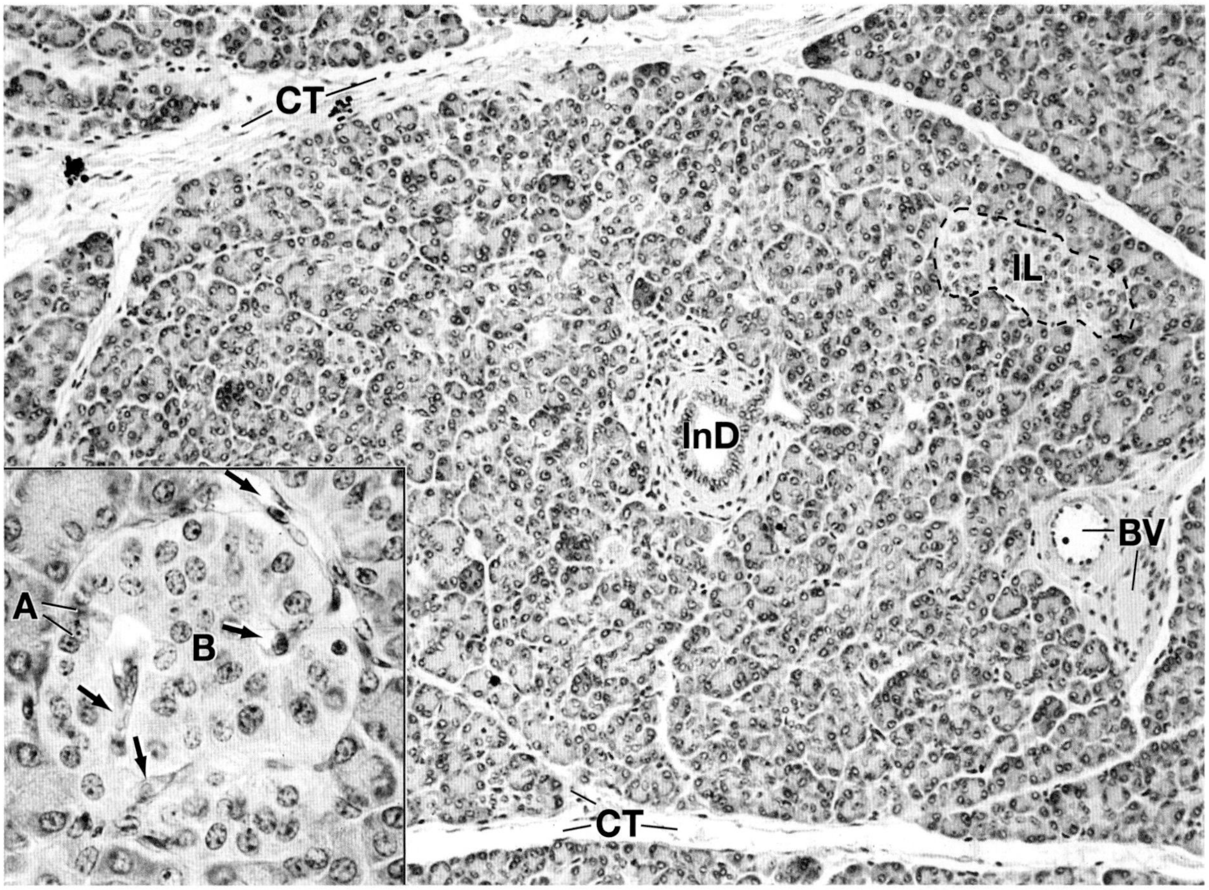
CT
IL
InD
BV
A
B
CT

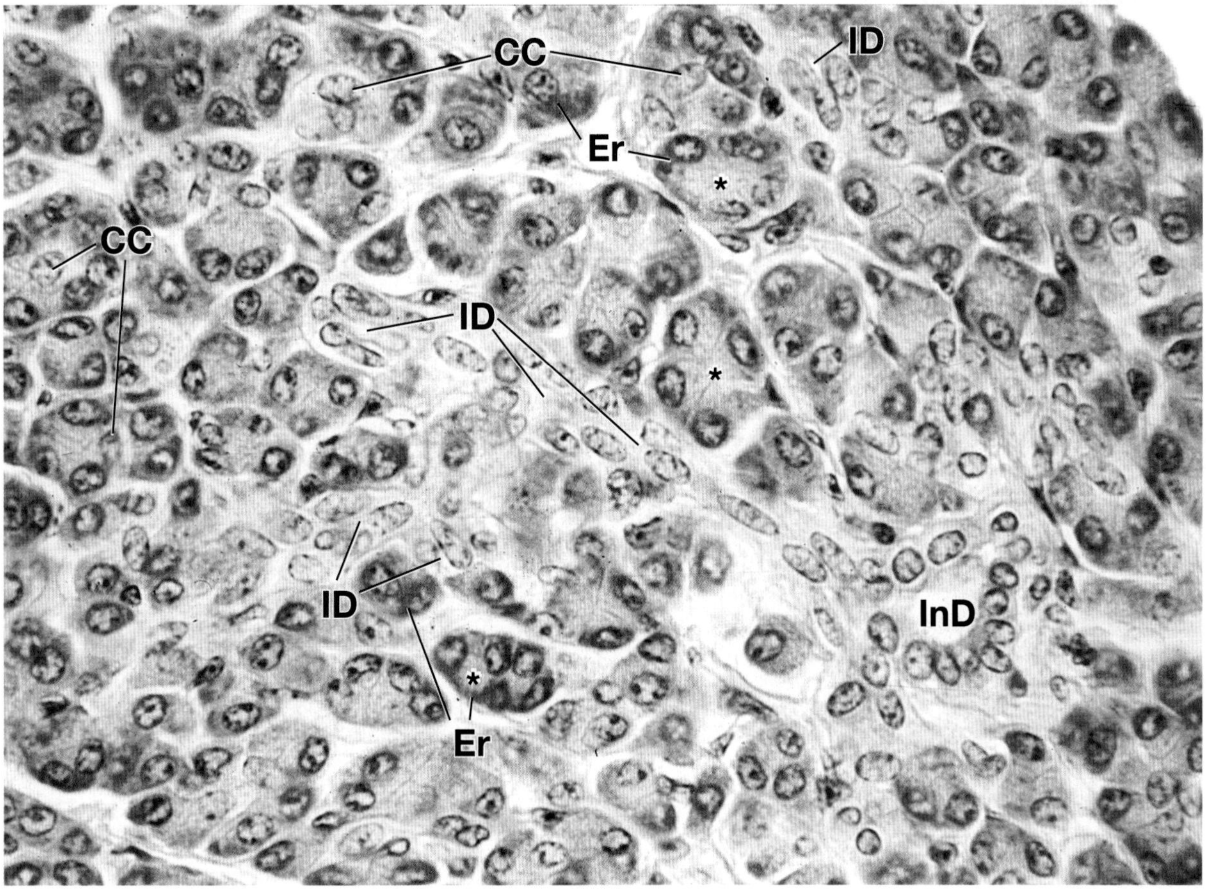
CC
ID
Er
CC
ID
ID
InD
Er

19 RESPIRATORY SYSTEM

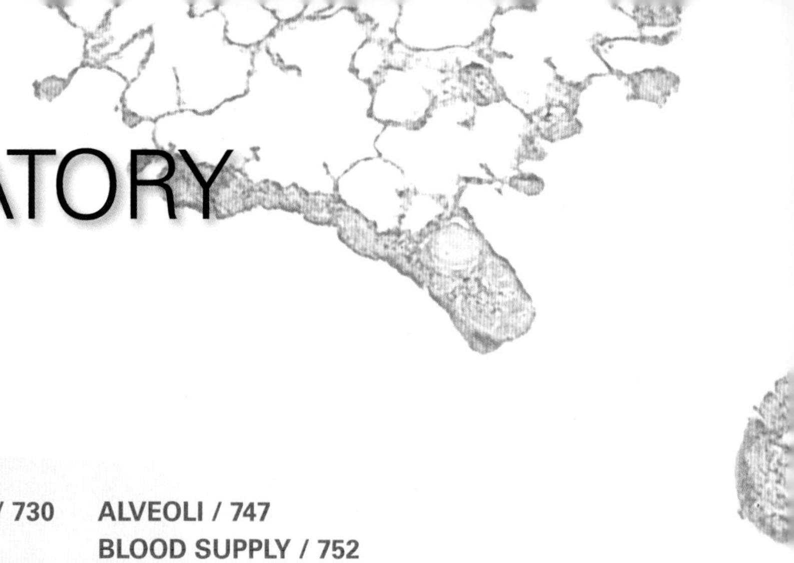

■ OVERVIEW OF THE RESPIRATORY SYSTEM

The **respiratory system** consists of the paired lungs and a series of air passages that lead to and from the lungs. Within the lung, the air passages branch into increasingly smaller tubes until the very smallest air spaces, called **alveoli**, are reached (Fig. 19.1).

Three principal functions are performed by this system: (1) **air conduction**, (2) **air filtration**, and (3) **gas exchange (respiration)**. Gas exchange occurs in the alveoli. In addition, air passing through the **larynx** is used to produce speech, and air passing over the **olfactory mucosa** in the **nasal cavities** carries stimuli for the sense of smell. The respiratory system also participates, to a lesser degree, in endocrine functions (hormone production and secretion) as well as regulation of **immune responses** to inhaled antigens.

Lungs develop from the laryngotracheal diverticulum of the foregut endoderm and its surrounding thoracic splanchnic mesenchyme.

Embryologic development of the **upper part of the respiratory system** containing the nasal cavities, paranasal sinuses, nasopharynx, and oropharynx develops with the oral cavity. The **lower part of the respiratory system** containing the larynx, trachea, bronchi with their divisions, and lungs begins as a ventral evagination of the foregut called the **laryngotracheal (respiratory) diverticulum**. Thus, the epithelium of the respiratory system is of endodermal origin. This initial diverticulum grows into the thoracic splanchnic mesenchyme surrounding the foregut. As its distal end enlarges, the diverticulum forms a bulb-shaped **lung bud**. This lung bud divides into the left and right **bronchial buds**, which enlarge to form the primordium of the left and right **primary bronchi**. Bronchial buds together with the surrounding thoracic mesenchyme differentiate into **lobar bronchi** with subsequent progressive divisions into segmental bronchi. Each **segmental bronchus** with its surrounding mesenchyme further differentiates and divides to form the **bronchopulmonary segments** of the lung. The bronchial cartilages, smooth muscle, and other connective tissue elements are derived from the thoracic mesenchyme.

The air passages of the respiratory system consist of a conducting portion and a respiratory portion.

The **conducting portion of the respiratory system** consists of air passages that lead to the sites of respiration within the lung where gas exchange takes place. The conducting passages include those located outside as well as within the lungs.

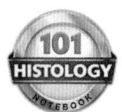

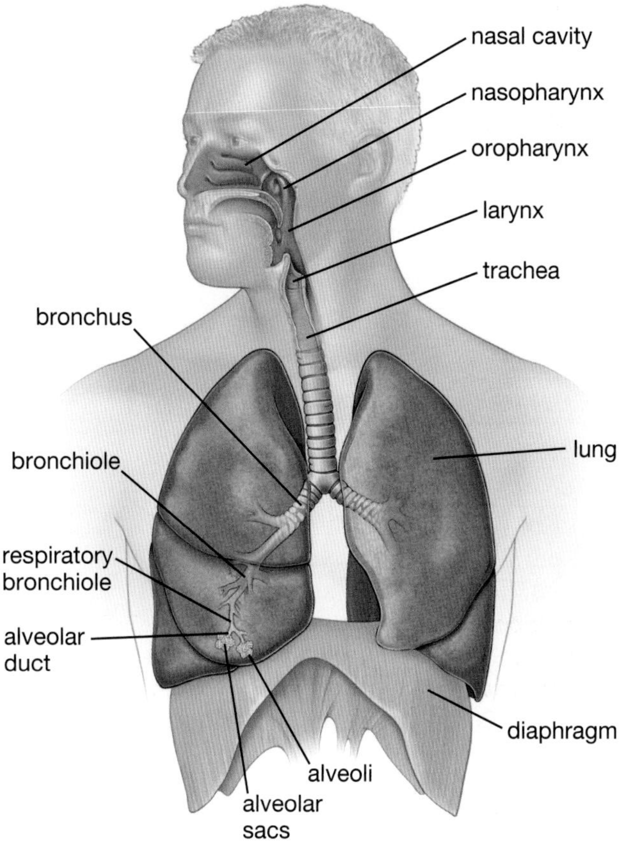

FIGURE 19.1. Diagram of respiratory passages. The nasal cavities, nasopharynx, oropharynx, larynx, trachea, bronchi, and bronchioles constitute the conducting portion of the respiratory system. The respiratory portion of the system, where gas exchange occurs, is composed of respiratory bronchioles, alveolar ducts, alveolar sacs, and alveoli.

The passages external to the lungs consist of the following:

- **Nasal cavities** that represent two large air-filled spaces in the uppermost part of the respiratory system (and, during forced breathing, the **oral cavity** residing inferior to the nasal cavities)
- **Nasopharynx** that lies behind the nasal cavities and above the level of the soft palate and communicates inferiorly with the **oropharynx** that is posterior to the oral cavity
- **Larynx** that is a hollow tubular organ containing the cartilaginous framework responsible for producing sounds
- **Trachea** that is a flexible air tube extending from the larynx to the thorax. It serves as a conduit for air, and in the mediastinum, it bifurcates into paired main bronchi.
- **Paired main (primary) bronchi** that enter the root of the right or left lung

Within the lungs, the **main bronchi** undergo extensive branching (~23 branch generations) to ultimately give rise to the **bronchioles.** The bronchioles represent the terminal part of the conducting passages. Collectively, the internal bronchi and the bronchioles constitute the **bronchial tree.**

The **respiratory portion of the respiratory system** is where gas exchange occurs. Sequentially, it includes the following structures:

- **Respiratory bronchioles** that are involved in both air conduction and gas exchange
- **Alveolar ducts** that are elongated airways that connect the respiratory bronchioles to the alveolar sacs
- **Alveolar sacs** that represent spaces surrounded by clusters of alveoli
- **Alveoli** that are the terminal respiratory units where gas exchange primarily occurs

Blood vessels enter the lung with the bronchi. The arteries branch into smaller vessels as they follow the bronchial tree into the substance of the lung. Capillaries come into intimate contact with the alveoli. This intimate relationship between the alveolar air spaces and the pulmonary capillaries is the structural basis for gas exchange within the lung parenchyma. The essential features of the lung blood supply are described on page 752.

Air passing through the respiratory passages must be conditioned before reaching the terminal respiratory units.

Conditioning or **climatization** of the air occurs in the **conducting portion of the respiratory system,** mainly in the nasal cavities. It includes warming and moistening of the inhaled air in addition to removal of particles. The temperature of inhaled air that passes into the nasopharynx reaches approximately 31°C–34°C (88°F–93°F) with a relative humidity of 90%–95%. Lower parts of the respiratory system only minimally participate in climatization. During expiration, the nasal airways partially extract heat and humidity from the exhaled air, thus reducing the loss of heat and moisture during respiration.

Mucous and **serous secretions** play a major role in climatization. These secretions moisten the air and also trap particles that have managed to slip past the special short thick hairs, called **vibrissae,** in the nasal cavities. Almost 95% of particles with a diameter of more than 15 μm are eliminated from inspired air. Mucus, augmented by these serous secretions, also prevents the dehydration of the underlying epithelium by the moving air. Mucus covers almost the entire luminal surface of the conducting passages and is continuously produced by goblet cells and mucus-secreting glands in the walls of the passages. The mucus and other secretions are moved toward the **pharynx** by means of coordinated sweeping movements of cilia and are then normally swallowed.

■ NASAL CAVITIES

The **nasal cavities** are paired chambers separated by a bony and cartilaginous **nasal septum.** They are elongated spaces with a wide base that rest on the hard and soft palate and a narrow apex that points toward the anterior cranial fossa. The skeletal framework of the nasal cavities is formed by bones and cartilages; most are located centrally in the skull, except for the small anterior region that is enclosed within the **external nose.** Each cavity or chamber communicates anteriorly with the external environment through the **anterior nares** (nostrils); posteriorly with the nasopharynx through the **choanae;** and laterally with the **paranasal sinuses** and **nasolacrimal duct,** which drains tears from the eye into the nasal cavity (Fig. 19.2). The chambers are divided into three regions:

- **Nasal vestibule,** a dilated space of the nasal cavity just inside the nostrils and is lined by skin
- **Respiratory region,** the largest part (inferior two-thirds) of the nasal cavities and is lined by respiratory mucosa
- **Olfactory region,** located at the apex (upper one-third) of each nasal cavity and is lined by specialized olfactory mucosa

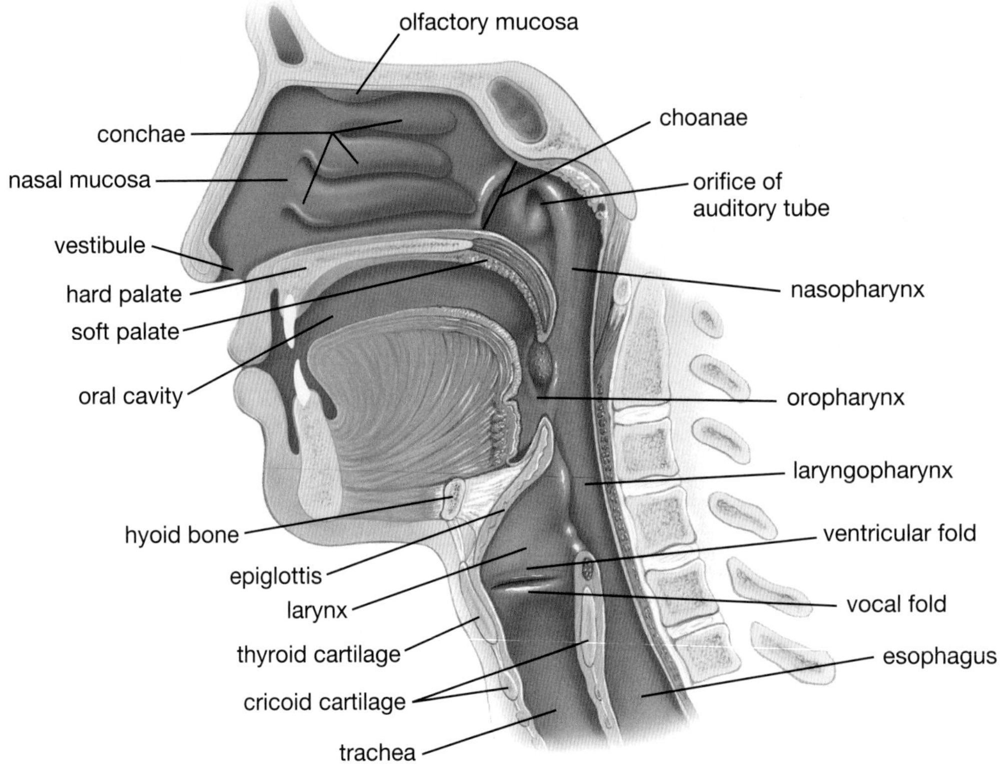

FIGURE 19.2. Diagram of the relationship of the pharynx to the respiratory and digestive systems. The pharynx is divided into three parts: nasopharynx, oropharynx, and laryngopharynx. It is located posterior to the nasal and oral cavities and extends inferiorly past the larynx. The pharynx serves both the respiratory and digestive systems. This midsagittal section also transects the cartilages, forming the skeleton of the larynx (i.e., epiglottis, thyroid cartilage, and cricoid cartilage). Note the ventricular and vocal folds in the middle of the larynx, approximately at the level of the thyroid cartilage. This part of the larynx represents the narrowest portion of the respiratory system and is responsible for producing sound by audible vibration of the vocal folds.

Vestibule of the Nasal Cavity

The **nasal vestibule** forms a part of the external nose and communicates anteriorly with the external environment. It is lined with **stratified squamous epithelium**, a continuation of the skin of the face, and contains a variable number of **vibrissae** that entrap large particulate matter before it is carried in the air stream to the rest of the cavity. Sebaceous glands are also present, and their secretions assist in the entrapment of particulate matter. Posteriorly, where the vestibule ends, the stratified squamous epithelium becomes thinner and undergoes a transition to the pseudostratified epithelium that characterizes the respiratory region. At this site, sebaceous glands are absent.

Respiratory Region of the Nasal Cavity

The **respiratory region** constitutes most of the volume of the nasal cavities. It is lined by the **respiratory mucosa** that contains a ciliated, pseudostratified columnar epithelium on its surface. The surface area of the respiratory mucosa is about 100–200 cm^2. The underlying **lamina propria** is firmly attached to the periosteum and perichondrium of the adjacent bone or cartilage.

The medial wall of the respiratory region, the **nasal septum**, is smooth, but the lateral walls are thrown into folds by the presence of three (rarely four) shelf-like, bony projections called **conchae** or turbinates. The conchae divide each nasal cavity into separate air chambers and play a dual role. They increase surface area and cause turbulence in airflow to allow more efficient conditioning of inspired air.

The **pseudostratified columnar ciliated epithelium** of the respiratory mucosa is composed of five cell types:

- **Ciliated cells**, tall columnar cells with cilia that project into the mucus covering the surface of the epithelium. They are the most abundant cells (up to 70%) in the epithelium.
- **Goblet cells** that synthesize and secrete mucus; they represent 5%–15% of all cells in the epithelium.
- **Brush cells**, a general name for those cells in the respiratory tract that bear short, blunt microvilli; they represent **chemosensory receptor cells** and are intimately connected to sensory nerve fibers.
- **Small granule cells (Kulchitsky cells)** that resemble basal cells but contain secretory granules; they are **endocrine cells** of the diffuse neuroendocrine system (DNES) (see Folder 17.4).
- **Basal cells** that lie on the basement membrane and have no contact with the epithelial surface; they are **stem cells** from which the other cell types arise.

The epithelium of the respiratory region of the nasal cavity is essentially the same as the epithelium lining most of the parts that follow in the conducting system. Because the respiratory epithelium of the trachea is studied and examined in reference to that of the nasal cavity, the abovementioned cell types are discussed in the section on the trachea (page 739).

The mucosa of the respiratory region climatizes and filters inspired air; it also contains cells that provide a local immune response to inhaled foreign antigens.

The **lamina propria** of the respiratory mucosa has a rich, vascular network that includes a complex set of capillary loops. The arrangement of the vessels allows the inhaled air to be warmed by blood flowing through the part of the loop closest to the surface. The capillaries that reside near the surface are arranged in rows; the blood flows perpendicular to the airflow, much as one would find in a mechanical heat exchange system. These same vessels may become engorged and leaky during allergic reactions or viral infections such as the **common cold**. The lamina propria then becomes distended with fluid, resulting in marked swelling of the mucous membrane with consequent restriction of the air passage, making breathing difficult.

The lamina propria also contains mucous glands, many exhibiting serous demilunes. These glands possess ducts opening into small crypts on the epithelial surface. The ducts are lined by a two-layered stratified cuboidal epithelium. Their secretions supplement that of the goblet cells in the respiratory epithelium.

By increasing surface area, the **conchae (turbinates)** increase the efficiency with which the inspired air is warmed. The turbinates also increase the efficiency of filtration of inspired air through the process of **turbulent precipitation**. The air stream is broken into eddies by the turbinates. Particles suspended in the air stream are thrown out of the stream and adhere to the mucus-covered wall of the nasal cavity. Particles trapped in this layer of mucus are transported to the **pharynx** by means of coordinated sweeping movements of cilia and are then swallowed. They may also be forcefully removed from the nasal cavity by sneezing. The **sneeze reflex** is usually provoked by foreign particles trapped in the mucus of nasal cavity. They stimulate sensory receptors that convey impulses to the sneezing center in the medulla. Initially, a rapid inspiration fills the lungs with air; the vocal cords, vestibular folds, and epiglottis of the larynx then close tightly to trap the inspired air in the lung. This is followed by a sudden forceful contraction of the diaphragm and other accessory respiratory muscles, which further increases the pressure in the lungs. Once a sufficiently high pressure is reached, the vocal cords, the vestibular folds, and the epiglottis open suddenly, and the air is pushed out rapidly from the lungs through the nose. Liquid droplets and foreign particles exit the nose at a velocity approaching 50 m/s (180 km/h).

Respiratory mucosa of the nasal cavity also contains cells involved in **mucosal immunity**. These cells are represented by a variety of lymphocyte populations residing in both the respiratory epithelium and the lamina propria. The majority of cells found in these regions are **gamma/delta (γδ) T lymphocytes** expressing the T-cell receptor (TCR) that play an important role in local immunity to inhaled foreign antigens (page 488). Accumulations of other cell types such as helper T lymphocytes, regulatory (suppressor) T lymphocytes, B lymphocytes, neutrophils, macrophages, and mast cells are also found in the lamina propria.

Olfactory Region of the Nasal Cavity

The **olfactory region** is located on part of the dome of each nasal cavity and, to a variable extent, the contiguous lateral and medial nasal walls. It is lined with a specialized **olfactory mucosa**. In living tissue, this mucosa is distinguished by its slight yellowish brown color caused by pigment in the **olfactory epithelium** and the associated **olfactory glands**. In humans, the total surface area of the olfactory mucosa is only about 10 cm^2; in animals with an acute sense of smell, the total surface area of the olfactory mucosa is considerably more extensive. For instance, the surface area of the olfactory mucosa in certain dog species is greater than 150 cm^2.

The lamina propria of the olfactory mucosa is directly contiguous with the periosteum of the underlying bone (Plate 19.1, page 758). This connective tissue contains numerous blood and lymphatic vessels, unmyelinated olfactory nerves, myelinated nerves, and olfactory glands.

The olfactory epithelium, like the epithelium of the respiratory region, is also pseudostratified, but it contains very different cell types. In addition, it lacks goblet cells (Fig. 19.3 and Plate 19.1, page 758).

The **olfactory epithelium** is composed of the following cell types:

- **Olfactory receptor cells** are bipolar olfactory neurons that span the thickness of the epithelium and enter the central nervous system.
- **Supporting (sustentacular) cells** are columnar cells that are similar to neuroglia cells and provide mechanical and metabolic support to the olfactory receptor cells. They synthesize and secrete odorant-binding proteins.
- **Basal cells** are stem cells from which new olfactory receptor cells and supporting cells differentiate.
- **Brush cells** are the same cell type that occurs in the respiratory epithelium.

Olfactory receptor cells are bipolar neurons that possess an apical projection bearing cilia.

The apical domain of each **olfactory receptor cell** has a single **dendritic process** that projects above the epithelial surface as a knob-like structure called the **olfactory vesicle**. A number of long, thin cilia (10–23) with typical basal bodies arise from the olfactory vesicle and extend radially in a plane parallel to the epithelial surface (see Fig. 19.3). The cilia are usually up to 200 μm long and may overlap with cilia of the adjacent olfactory receptor cells. The cilia are regarded as nonmotile, although some research suggests that they may have limited motility. The basal domain of the cell gives rise to an unmyelinated axonal process that leaves the epithelial compartment. Collections of axons from olfactory receptor cells do not come together as a single nerve; instead, they are grouped into bundles that pass through a thin cribriform plate of the ethmoid bone, course through the dura and arachnoid matters, and finally are surrounded by pia matter, entering the olfactory bulb of the brain. The collections of axons from olfactory receptor cells form the **olfactory nerve (cranial nerve I)**. The olfactory axons are very fragile and can be harmed during traumatic head injury. They can be permanently severed, resulting in **anosmia** (loss of the sense of smell).

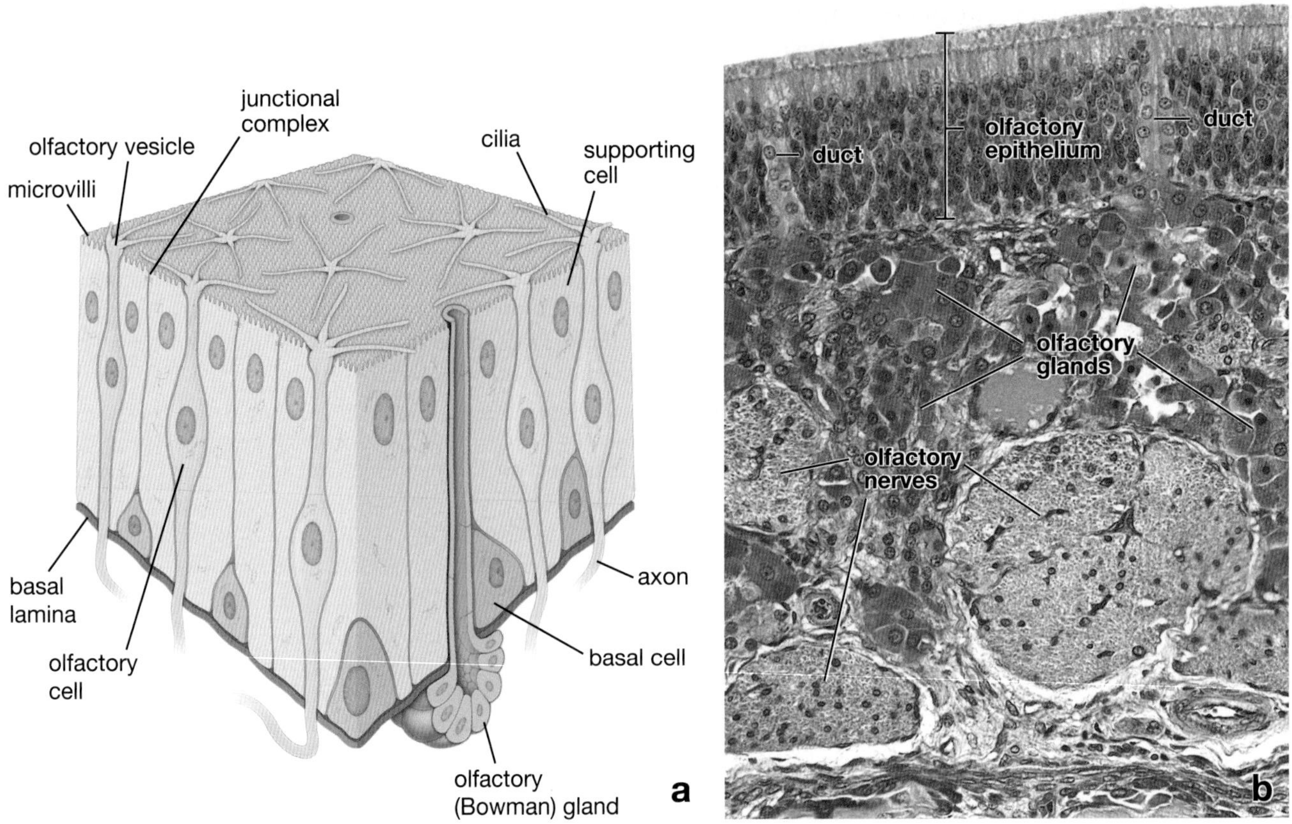

FIGURE 19.3. Olfactory mucosa of the nasal cavity. a. This diagram shows the three major cell types located within the olfactory epithelium: the olfactory cell, supporting (sustentacular) cell, and basal cell. The olfactory cell is the receptor cell; it has an apical expansion, the olfactory vesicle, from which long, nonmotile cilia extend. At its basal surface, it extends an axon into the connective tissue that joins with the axons of other olfactory cells to form an olfactory nerve. The basal cells are small and cuboidal. They are restricted to the basal part of the epithelium. The supporting cells, in contrast, are columnar and extend the full thickness of the epithelium; their nuclei are located in the upper portion of the cell. Note the olfactory (Bowman) gland and its duct that empties on the surface of the mucosa. **b.** Photomicrograph of the olfactory mucosa. The olfactory epithelium exhibits nuclei through much of its thickness, but the individual cell types to which they belong are not discernible. The underlying connective tissue is largely occupied by numerous olfactory (Bowman) glands, olfactory nerves, and blood vessels. Note that the ducts of the olfactory glands extend from the secretory portion of the gland to the epithelial surface. ×240.

Autoradiographic studies show that olfactory receptor cells have a life span of about 1 month. If injured, they are quickly replaced. Olfactory receptor cells (and some neurons of the enteric division of the autonomic nervous system) appear to be the only neurons in the nervous system that are readily replaced during postnatal life.

Entire olfactory transduction pathways occur within the cilia of the olfactory receptor cells.

Molecules involved in **olfactory transduction** are located within long cilia that arise from the olfactory bulb. First, incoming odorant chemicals are solubilized in the olfactory mucus. Next, the odorants selectively bind to **odorant-binding proteins (OBPs)** that are concentrated in the olfactory mucus (Fig. 19.4). The odorant-binding proteins are small (10–30 kDa), water-soluble proteins that are synthesized and secreted by supporting cells. They act as molecular carriers that transport odorants and deliver them to **olfactory receptors** located in the plasma membrane of the cilia.

To date, more than 350 different olfactory receptors have been identified in humans. Olfactory receptors are specific for the olfactory receptor cells and belong to the family of **G-protein–coupled receptors** (known as $\mathbf{G_{olf}}$). When stimulated by odorant molecules, G_{olf} olfactory receptors activate the enzyme adenylyl cyclase and initiate the cyclic adenosine monophosphate (cAMP) cascade of events (see Fig. 19.4). These include binding of cAMP to specific Na^+ and Ca^{2+} channel proteins and influx of Na^+ and Ca^{2+} into the cell, which is responsible for plasma membrane depolarization that generates an action potential.

These 350 different olfactory receptors in humans are able to accurately detect several thousands of known odor molecules by use of a special coding system for different impulses. This is achieved by a **population coding scheme**, in which each olfactory receptor protein binds to different odorants with different sensitivity. Thus, the olfactory system must decode olfactory impulses not from a single cell but from the entire population of cells within the olfactory epithelium.

Supporting cells provide mechanical and metabolic support for the olfactory receptor cells.

Supporting (sustentacular) cells are the most numerous cells in the olfactory epithelium. The nuclei of these tall columnar or sustentacular cells occupy a more apical position in the epithelium than do those of the other cell types, thus aiding in their identification in the light microscope (see Fig. 19.3 and Plate 19.1, page 758). They have numerous microvilli on their apical surface and abundant mitochondria. Numerous profiles of smooth-surfaced endoplasmic reticulum (sER) and, to a more limited extent, rough-surfaced endoplasmic reticulum (rER) are observed in the cytoplasm. They also possess lipofuscin granules. Adhering junctions are present between these cells and the olfactory receptor cells, but gap and tight junctions are absent. The supporting cells function in a manner similar to that of neuroglial

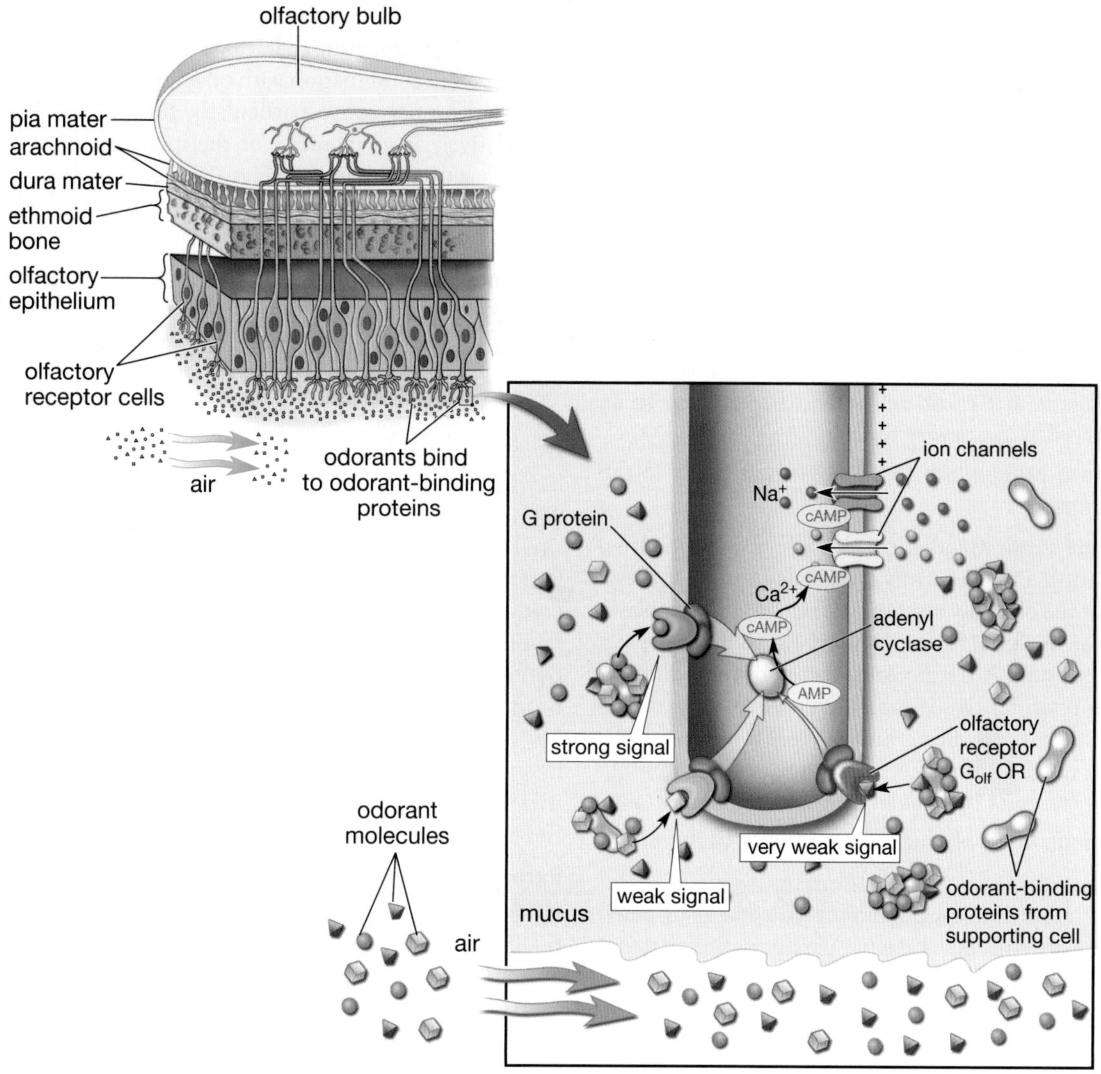

FIGURE 19.4. Diagram of olfactory transduction pathway. This diagram shows interactions of the odorant molecules with proteins associated with olfactory receptor (*OR*) cell. Incoming inhaled air odorant molecules are solubilized in the olfactory mucus and bind to olfactory-binding proteins, which deliver them to the *olfactory receptors*. Note that different odorant molecules bind with different affinity to the olfactory receptors. Strong signal (see *green* G-protein–coupled olfactory receptor) is produced by high-affinity binding where odorant molecule (*green*) matches perfectly the binding site on the receptor. Other olfactory receptors (*yellow* and *pink*) show less affinity binding, thus producing weaker signals. Stimulated by odorant molecules, olfactory receptors activate the enzyme adenylyl cyclase and initiate the cyclic adenosine monophosphate (*cAMP*) cascade of events, leading to the opening of specific Na^+ and Ca^{2+} channels. Influx of Na^+ and Ca^{2+} is responsible for cell depolarization. Generated action potential travels on axons of olfactory receptor cells from the nasal cavity, passing through the ethmoid bone and surrounding brain coverings to the olfactory bulb of the brain.

cells, providing both metabolic support (secretion of odorant-binding protein molecules) and physical support to the olfactory receptor cells. Damage to supporting cells is related to **transient anosmia** (temporary loss of the sense of smell) in individuals infected by the **SARS-CoV-2 virus.** Loss of smell with or without fever (>37.5°C) is one of the most frequently, and perhaps the earliest and often the only, reported symptom in patients who are **COVID-19** positive. SARS-CoV-2 virus gains entry to human cells by binding to **angiotensin-converting enzyme 2 (ACE2)**, and viral uptake is further facilitated by a **transmembrane protease, serine 2 (TmPRSS2)**, which activates the viral spike protein. Cells that highly express these viral cell entry proteins have an increased affinity to binding the virus and are particularly susceptible to infection. A recent study reveals that olfactory receptor cells in the nasal mucosa express neither ACE2 nor TmPRSS2 and thus are not infected by the SARS-CoV-2 virus. However, both enzymes are highly expressed on the **supporting (sustentacular) cells** that provide mechanical and metabolic support to olfactory receptor cells. The virus binds to and subsequently depletes supporting cells in the olfactory epithelium. Although olfactory receptor cells are not directly infected, they do sustain significant damage from the infection of neighboring supporting cells. Depletion of supporting cells is followed by their regeneration about 10 days after infection, and in most cases, the sense of smell is restored.

Brush cells are involved in transduction of general sensation and chemosensation from the mucosa of the nasal cavity.

The olfactory epithelium also contains **brush cells**, which are present in much smaller numbers than ciliated cells. These columnar cells are also present in the epithelium of other parts of the conducting air passages. With the electron microscope (EM), brush cells exhibit large, blunt microvilli at their apical surface, a feature that gives them their name. In addition, the apical plasma membrane contains accumulations of **G-protein–coupled T2R taste receptors** for bitter taste similar to those found in neuroepithelial cells of the taste buds of the tongue. The different T2R chemosensory receptors in brush cells respond to a variety of natural ligands (irritants) that are likely to enter the airways in the form of aerosols and dust particles. The basal surface of a brush cell is in synaptic contact with nerve fibers that penetrate the basal lamina. The nerve fibers are terminal branches of the **trigeminal nerve (cranial nerve V)** that function in general sensation and mediation of reflexes, such as sneezing or coughing in response to inhaled chemical or pathogenic irritants.

In addition, the presence of a microvillus border, vesicles near the apical cell membrane, and a well-defined Golgi apparatus suggests that brush cells might be involved in an absorptive as well as a secretory function.

Basal cells are progenitors to all other cell types in the olfactory mucosa.

Basal cells are small, rounded cells located close to the basal lamina. Their nuclei are frequently invaginated and lie at a level below those of the olfactory receptor cell nuclei. The cytoplasm contains few organelles, a feature consistent with their role as a reserve or **stem cell**. A feature consistent with their differentiation into supporting cells is the observation of processes in some basal cells that partially ensheathe the first portion of the olfactory receptor cell axon. They thus maintain a relationship to the olfactory receptor cell even in their undifferentiated state.

Olfactory glands are a characteristic feature of the olfactory mucosa.

The olfactory epithelium is potentially vulnerable to dehydration by the air entering the nasal passages. The olfactory glands (Bowman glands) and their serous secretion prevent water evaporation and the subsequent increase in ion concentration on the olfactory surface. Maintaining the ion gradients is necessary for proper function (depolarization) of the cilia of the olfactory receptor cells.

The olfactory glands (Bowman glands), a characteristic feature of the olfactory mucosa, are branched tubuloalveolar serous glands that deliver their proteinaceous secretions via ducts onto the olfactory surface (see Fig. 19.3 and Plate 19.1, page 758). Lipofuscin granules are prevalent in the gland cells and, in combination with the lipofuscin granules in the supporting cells of the olfactory epithelium, give the mucosa its natural yellow-brown coloration. Short ducts composed of cuboidal cells lead from the glands and pass through the basal lamina into the olfactory epithelium, where they continue to the epithelial surface to discharge their contents.

Loss of water to evaporation leads to the formation of an osmotic gradient by the remaining ions. Restoring the equilibrium of the mucosa to protect olfactory function requires rapid water transport, which is achieved by the water channels of the **aquaporin pathway**. These channels rapidly transfer water from large superficial venules via the extracellular matrix to the lumen of the Bowman gland. Aquaporin molecules are found in the basolateral (AQP-3 and AQP-4) and apical (AQP-5) cell membrane of the gland's secretory cells. In addition, a similar distribution of aquaporins is present in supporting (sustentacular) and basal cells of the olfactory epithelium.

The serous secretion of the olfactory glands also serves as a trap and solvent for odoriferous substances. The constant flow from the glands rids the mucosa of remnants of detected odoriferous substances so that new odors can be continuously detected as they arise.

The identifying feature of the olfactory region of the nasal mucosa in a histologic preparation is the presence of the olfactory nerves in combination with olfactory glands in the lamina propria. The nerves are particularly conspicuous because of the relatively large diameter of the individual unmyelinated fibers that they contain (see Figs. 19.3 and 19.4).

Paranasal Sinuses

Paranasal sinuses are air-filled spaces in the bones of the walls of the nasal cavity.

The **paranasal sinuses** are extensions of the respiratory region of the nasal cavity and are lined by respiratory epithelium. The sinuses are named for the bone in which they are found (i.e., the ethmoid, frontal, sphenoid, and maxillary bones). The sinuses communicate with the nasal cavities via narrow openings onto the respiratory mucosa. Paranasal sinuses most likely function in voice resonance. The mucosal surface of the sinuses is a thin, ciliated, pseudostratified columnar epithelium with numerous goblet cells. The lamina propria is thin and continuous with the underlying periosteum. It contains only a few small glands. Mucus produced in the sinuses is swept into the nasal cavities by coordinated ciliary movements. The sinuses may become the site of a secondary bacterial infection (**sinusitis**) following viral infection of the upper respiratory tract. Severe infections may require physical drainage.

Paranasal sinuses are the main sites for nitric oxide (NO) production in the airways.

Research conducted in the past decade has shown that the respiratory epithelium of the paranasal sinuses contains large amounts of nitric oxide synthase, an enzyme responsible for **nitric oxide (NO) production**. NO is a potent neurotransmitter and chemical messenger. The concentration levels of NO produced continuously in the paranasal sinuses are several times higher than levels in other parts of the respiratory tract. Because air circulates between the paranasal sinuses and the nasal cavity, high levels of NO enter the nasal cavity and may play an important role in the nasal defense mechanism against invading microorganisms. In addition, NO from the paranasal sinuses reaches the lungs with each inhalation, where it facilitates gas exchange and reduces pulmonary vascular resistance by relaxing vascular smooth muscles.

■ PHARYNX

The **pharynx** connects the nasal and oral cavities to the larynx and esophagus. It serves as a passageway for air and food and acts as a resonating chamber for speech. The pharynx is located posterior to the nasal and oral cavities and is divided regionally into the **nasopharynx** and **oropharynx**, respectively (see Fig. 19.2). The auditory (Eustachian) tubes connect the nasopharynx to each middle ear. Diffuse lymphatic tissue and lymphatic nodules are present in the wall of the nasopharynx. The group of lymphatic nodules concentrated at the junction between the superior and posterior walls of the pharynx is called the **pharyngeal tonsil**.

■ LARYNX

The passageway for air between the oropharynx and the trachea is the **larynx** (see Fig. 19.2). In addition to serving as a conduit for air, the larynx serves as the organ for producing sounds. This complex tubular region of the respiratory system is formed by irregularly shaped plates of **hyaline** and **elastic cartilages** (the epiglottis and the vocal processes of the arytenoid cartilages). Cartilages of the larynx are connected to one another by joints, membranes, and ligaments, and their movements in relation to each other are controlled by **intrinsic laryngeal muscles**. The mucosa of the larynx forms two pairs of shelf-like folds that project into the lumen of the larynx bilaterally. Both folds are oriented in an anteroposterior direction; thus, on the frontal section of the larynx, they are visible in cross section (cut perpendicularly to their length) separated by the invagination of the laryngeal mucosa called **ventricle** (Fig. 19.5). The upper pair of folds, the **vestibular folds**, are immobile, but the lower pair of folds, the **vocal folds**, are mobile and play an important role in producing sounds (phonation).

Vocal folds control the flow of air through the larynx and vibrate to produce sound.

The **vocal folds**, also referred to as *vocal cords* (Fig. 19.6 and Plate 19.2, page 760), define the lateral boundaries of the opening of the larynx, the **rima glottidis**. A supporting ligament and skeletal muscle, the **vocalis muscle**, is contained within each vocal fold. Ligaments and the intrinsic laryngeal muscles join the adjacent cartilaginous plates and are responsible for generating tension in the vocal folds and for opening and closing the rima glottidis. The **extrinsic laryngeal muscles** insert on cartilages of the larynx but originate in extralaryngeal structures. These muscles move the larynx upward and forward during **deglutition** (swallowing).

Expelled air from lungs passing through the narrow space of the **rima glottidis** causes the vocal folds to vibrate against each

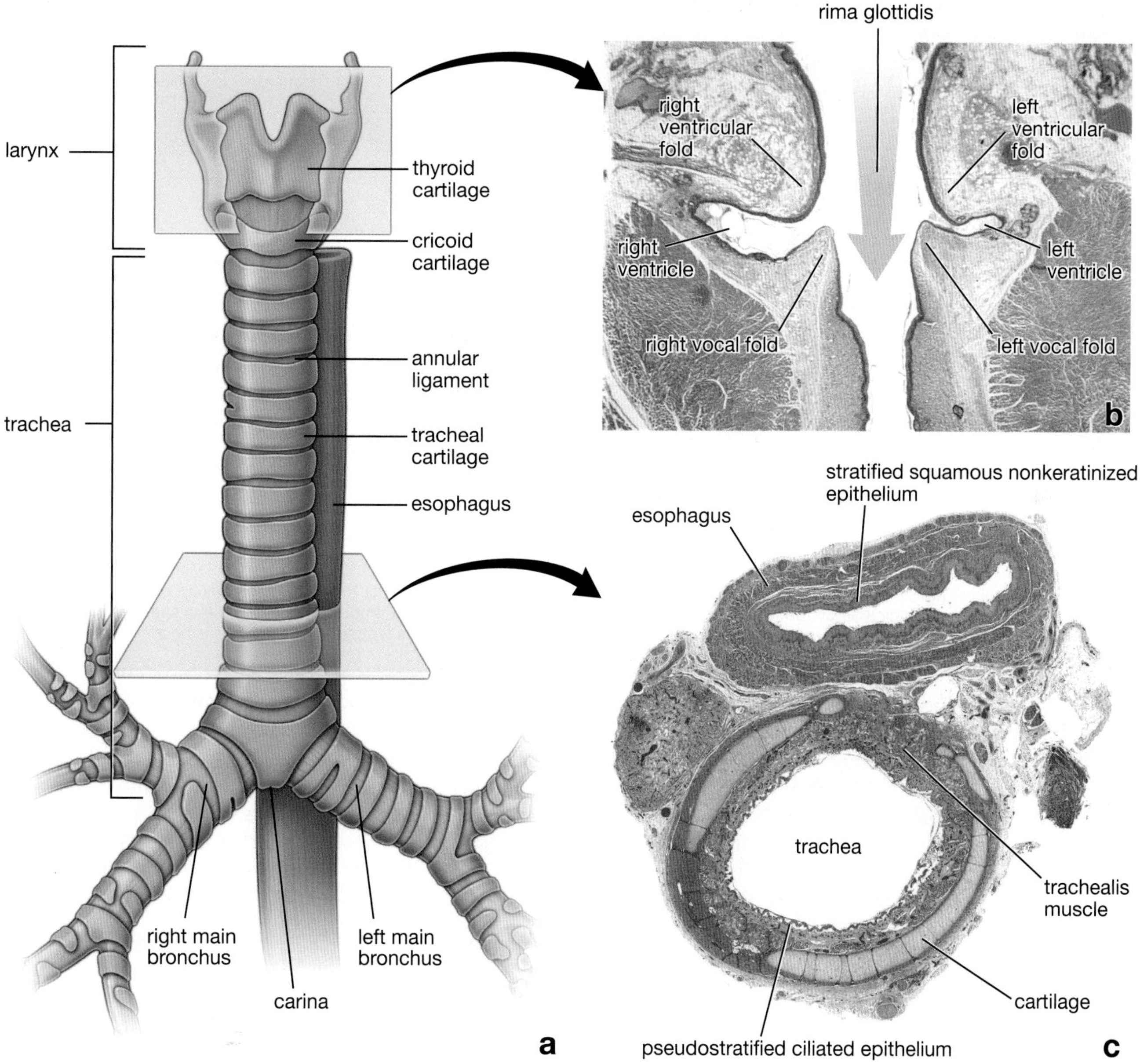

FIGURE 19.5. Topography of the larynx and trachea. a. The larynx is a hollow musculoligamentous structure reinforced by cartilaginous skeleton. It is located in the neck region, and its cavity is continuous inferiorly with the trachea and posteriorly with the oropharynx. The laryngeal cavity contains the vestibular and vocal folds oriented in an anteroposterior direction. The trachea extends from the larynx to the thorax and divides into the two main (primary) bronchi at the level of the T4–T5 thoracic vertebrae. Immediately posterior to the trachea is the esophagus, which continues into the abdomen. **b.** This specimen obtained from a frontal cut through the larynx shows both vocal and ventricular folds in cross section. Note that the vocal and ventricular folds are separated by the ventricle, an invagination of the laryngeal mucosa. ×15. **c.** This photomicrograph shows a horizontal section of the fetal trachea and esophagus and its close relationships in the thorax. The trachealis muscle on the posterior wall of the trachea is adjacent to the anterior wall of the esophagus. The lumen of the trachea is round and remains open due to the arrangement of the cartilaginous rings ×10.

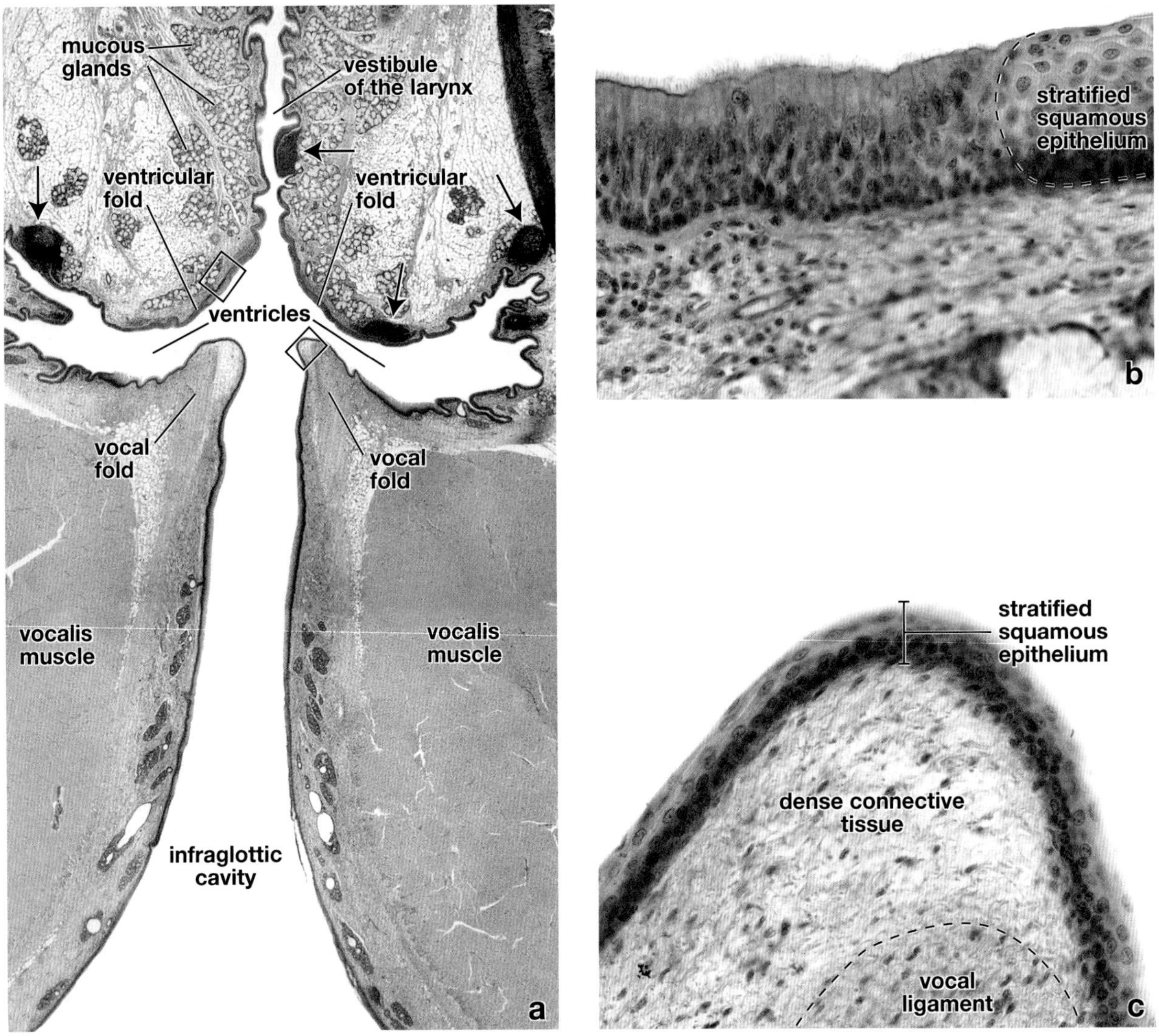

FIGURE 19.6. Photomicrograph of a frontal section of the larynx. a. This photomicrograph shows three parts of the larynx: the vestibule above the ventricular folds, the ventricles between the vestibular folds and superior to the vocal folds, and the infraglottic cavity that extends from the vocal folds to the cricoid cartilage. Note that mucous glands are prominent in the ventricular folds and are covered by the typical pseudostratified ciliated epithelium. The vocal fold is composed of the epithelium, vocal ligament, and underlying vocalis muscle. Numerous lymph nodules are also present within the mucosa of the larynx (*arrows*). ×10. **b.** High magnification of the area of the ventricular fold indicated by the *upper rectangle* in **a** shows on the *left* the pseudostratified ciliated epithelium that lines most of the larynx. Many nonsmoking adults and virtually all smokers exhibit patches of stratified squamous epithelium, as seen on the *right* of the micrograph. ×240. **c.** High magnification of the area of the vocal fold indicated by the *lower rectangle* in **a** reveals normal stratified squamous epithelium at this site. Just beneath the epithelium is the connective tissue known as *Reinke space*. This clinically important site lacks lymphatic vessels and is poorly vascularized. The vocal ligament, inscribed by the *dashed line*, is seen at the *bottom* of the micrograph. ×240.

other. The vibrations are altered by modulating the tension on the vocal folds and by changing the degree of glottal opening. This alteration of vibrations produces sounds of different **pitch**. Relaxed vocal cords produce a deeper pitch, whereas stretched and tense vocal cords produce a higher pitch. Sounds created in the larynx during the process of **phonation** are modified in the upper parts of the respiratory system (nasopharynx, nasal cavities, and paranasal sinuses) and the oral cavity (oropharynx, soft and hard palate, tongue, teeth, lips, etc.) to produce the individual speech sounds (different vowels and consonants).

The ventricular folds located above the vocal folds are the "false vocal cords."

Above the vocal folds is an elongated recess in the larynx called the **ventricle**. Immediately above the ventricle is another pair of mucosal folds, the **ventricular folds** or false vocal cords (see Fig. 19.6 and Plate 19.2, page 760). These folds do not have the intrinsic muscular investment of the true vocal cords and, therefore, do not modulate during phonation. Along with the ventricle, however, they are important in creating **sound resonance.** Inflammation and swelling of the larynx caused by viruses (such as the common cold virus) and other microbial agents is called *acute laryngitis*. Symptoms of **acute laryngitis** may include hoarseness or, in more severe cases, total loss of voice, coughing, and difficulty with swallowing and breathing. **Chronic laryngitis** is usually caused by prolonged exposure to irritating agents, such as tobacco smoke, dust, and/or polluted air.

Stratified squamous and ciliated pseudostratified columnar epithelium line the larynx.

The luminal surface of the **vocal cords** is covered with **stratified squamous epithelium**, as is most of the epiglottis (Plate 19.2, page 760). The epithelium serves to protect the mucosa from abrasion caused by the rapidly moving air stream. The rest of the larynx is lined with the ciliated, pseudostratified columnar epithelium that characterizes the respiratory tract (see Fig. 19.6 and Plate 19.2, page 760). The connective tissue of the larynx contains mixed mucoserous glands that secrete through ducts onto the laryngeal surface.

■ TRACHEA

The **trachea** is a short, flexible air tube approximately 2.5 cm in diameter and 10–12 cm long. It serves as a conduit for air; in addition, its wall assists in the climatization of inspired air. The trachea extends from the larynx to the middle of the thorax and is positioned in the front and adjacent to the esophagus (see Fig. 19.5). In the thorax, it divides into the two **main (primary) bronchi**, which enter the right and left lung. The lumen of the trachea remains open because of the arrangement of the series of cartilaginous rings (see later in this later).

The wall of the trachea consists of four definable layers:

- **Mucosa**, composed of a ciliated, pseudostratified epithelium and an elastic, fiber-rich lamina propria
- **Submucosa**, composed of a slightly denser connective tissue than the lamina propria
- **Cartilaginous layer**, composed of C-shaped hyaline cartilages
- **Adventitia**, composed of connective tissue that binds the trachea to adjacent structures

A unique feature of the trachea is the presence of a series of C-shaped hyaline cartilages that are stacked one on top of each other to form a supporting structure (Fig. 19.7). These cartilages, which might be described as a skeletal framework, prevent the collapse of the tracheal lumen, particularly during expiration. Fibroelastic tissue and smooth muscle, the trachealis muscle, bridge the gap between the free ends of the C-shaped cartilages at the posterior border of the trachea, adjacent to the esophagus.

Tracheal Epithelium

Tracheal epithelium is similar to respiratory epithelium in other parts of the conducting airway.

Ciliated columnar cells, mucous (goblet) cells, and basal cells are the principal cell types in the tracheal **pseudostratified columnar ciliated epithelium** (Figs. 19.8 and 19.9). Brush cells are also present, but in small numbers, as are small granule cells.

- **Ciliated cells**, the most numerous of the tracheal cell types, extend through the full thickness of the epithelium. Cilia appear in histologic sections as short, hair-like profiles projecting from the apical surface (Plate 19.3, page 762). Each cell has approximately 250 cilia. Immediately below the cilia is a dark line formed by the aggregated ciliary basal bodies (Fig. 19.10). The cilia provide a coordinated sweeping motion of the mucous coat from the farthest reaches of the air passages toward the pharynx. In effect, the ciliated cells function as a "**mucociliary escalator**" that serves as an important protective mechanism for removing small inhaled particles from the lungs.
- **Mucous cells** are similar in appearance to intestinal goblet cells and are thus often referred to by the same name. They are interspersed among the ciliated cells and also extend through the full thickness of the epithelium (see Fig. 19.10). They are readily seen in the light microscope after they have accumulated mucinogen granules in their cytoplasm. Although the mucinogen is typically washed out in hematoxylin and eosin (H&E)

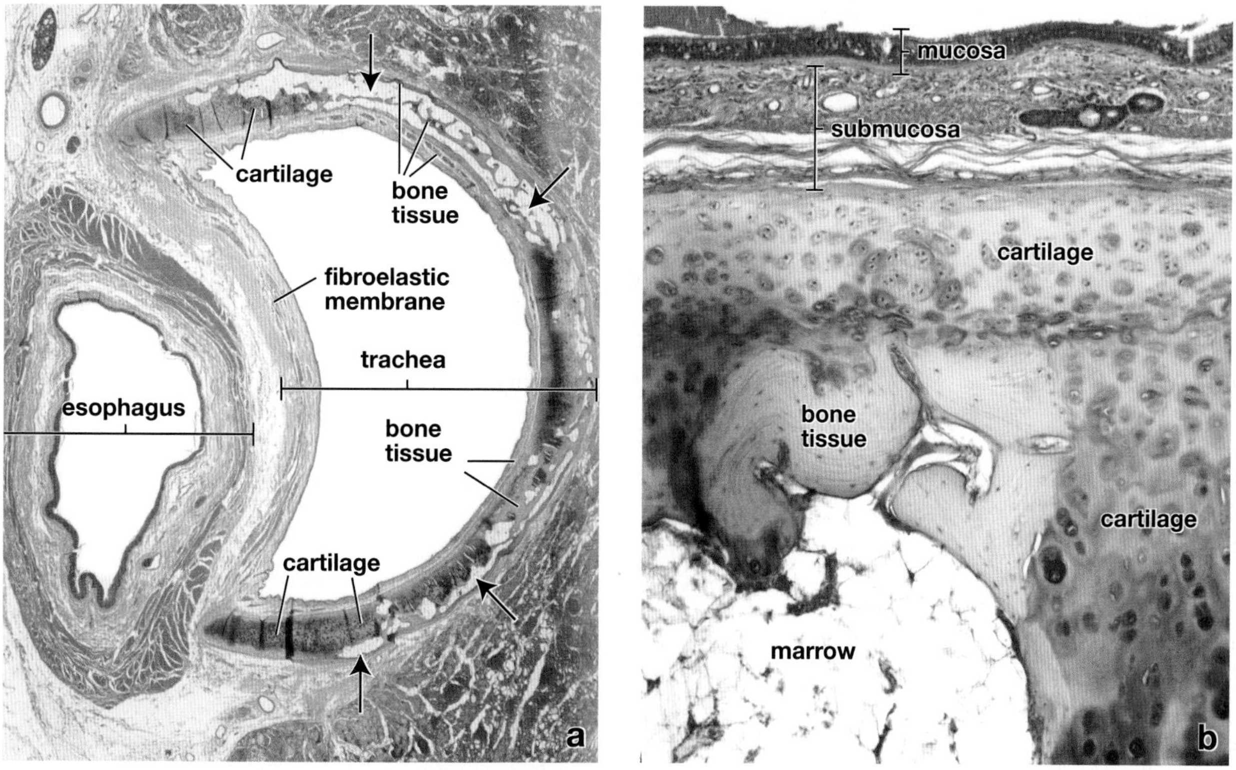

FIGURE 19.7. Photomicrograph of a section of the trachea and esophagus. a. This specimen, obtained from an elderly individual, shows the relationship between the trachea and the esophagus at the base of the neck. The cartilaginous tracheal rings, which keep the trachea patent, have a C-shaped appearance. The cartilage gap, where the trachea is adjacent to the esophageal wall, is spanned by a fibroelastic membrane. It contains the trachealis muscle and numerous seromucous glands. In this specimen, the tracheal ring has been transformed, in part, to bone, a process that occurs in aging. The darker staining material represents cartilage, whereas the lighter staining material has been replaced by bone tissue. The very light areas (*arrows*) are marrow spaces. ×3.25. **b.** This high-magnification photomicrograph shows an area of the tracheal ring that has partially transformed into bone. The *top* of the micrograph shows the tracheal mucosa and submucosa. Below is part of the tracheal ring. In this particular region, however, a substantial portion of the cartilage has been replaced by bone tissue and marrow. The bone tissue exhibits typical lamellae and osteocytes. The cartilage tissue, in contrast, exhibits nests of chondrocytes. ×100.

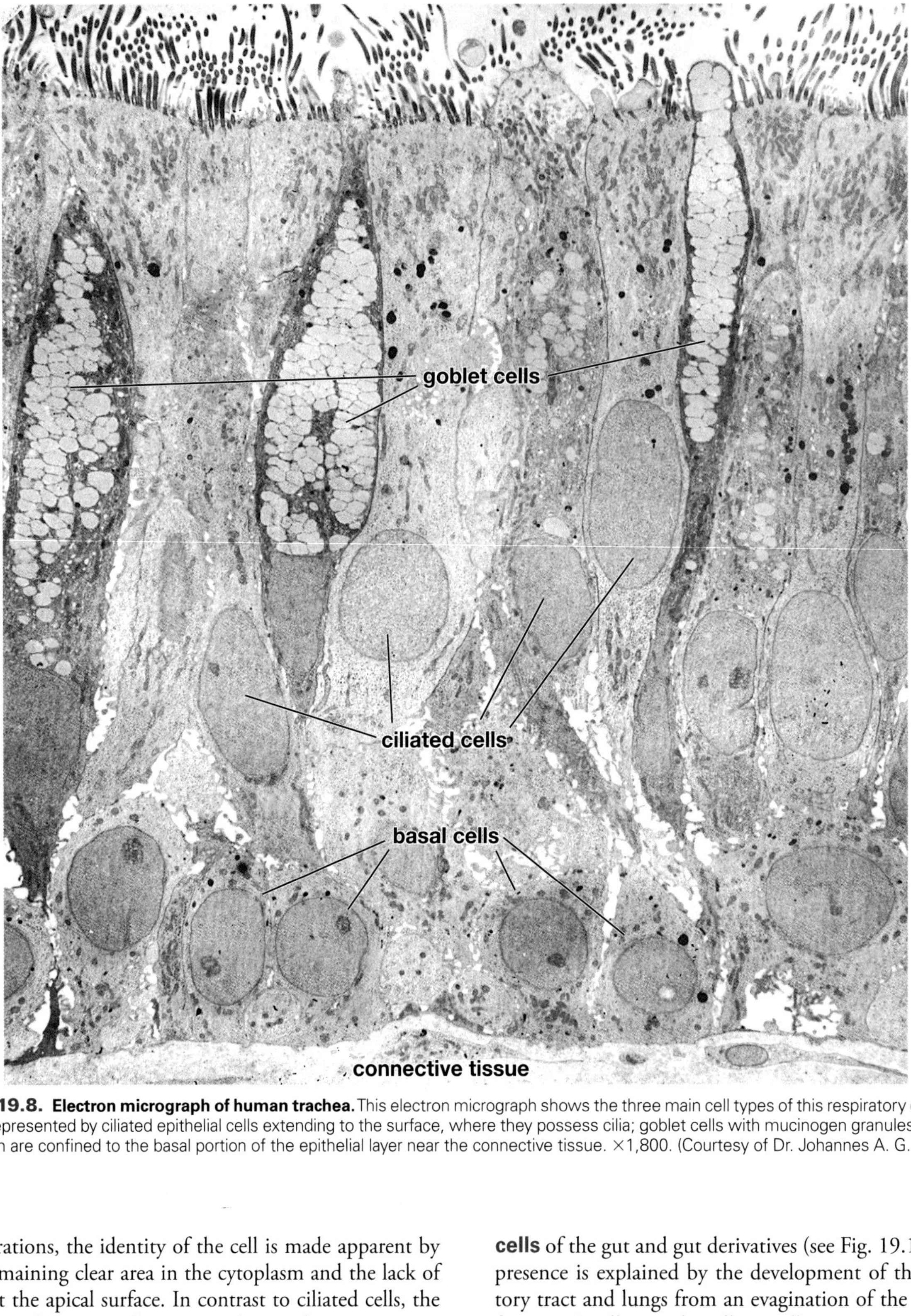

FIGURE 19.8. Electron micrograph of human trachea. This electron micrograph shows the three main cell types of this respiratory epithelium. They are represented by ciliated epithelial cells extending to the surface, where they possess cilia; goblet cells with mucinogen granules; and basal cells, which are confined to the basal portion of the epithelial layer near the connective tissue. ×1,800. (Courtesy of Dr. Johannes A. G. Rhodin.)

preparations, the identity of the cell is made apparent by the remaining clear area in the cytoplasm and the lack of cilia at the apical surface. In contrast to ciliated cells, the number of mucous cells increases during chronic irritation of the air passages.

- **Brush cells** have the same general features as those described for the respiratory epithelium of the nasal cavity (Fig. 19.11). They are columnar cells that bear blunt microvilli. The basal surface of the cells is in synaptic contact with an afferent nerve ending (epitheliodendritic synapse). As discussed earlier, brush cells are regarded as general sensory and chemoreceptor cells.
- **Small granule cells (Kulchitsky cells)** are respiratory representatives of the general class of **enteroendocrine cells** of the gut and gut derivatives (see Fig. 19.11). Their presence is explained by the development of the respiratory tract and lungs from an evagination of the primitive foregut. Small granule cells usually occur singly in the trachea and are sparsely dispersed among the other cell types. They are difficult to distinguish from basal cells in the light microscope without special techniques such as silver staining, which reacts with the granules. The nucleus is located near the basement membrane; the cytoplasm is somewhat more extensive than that of the smaller basal cells. With the transmission electron microscope (TEM), a thin, tapering cytoplasmic process is sometimes observed extending to the lumen. Also, with the TEM, the cytoplasm exhibits numerous, membrane-bound, dense-core

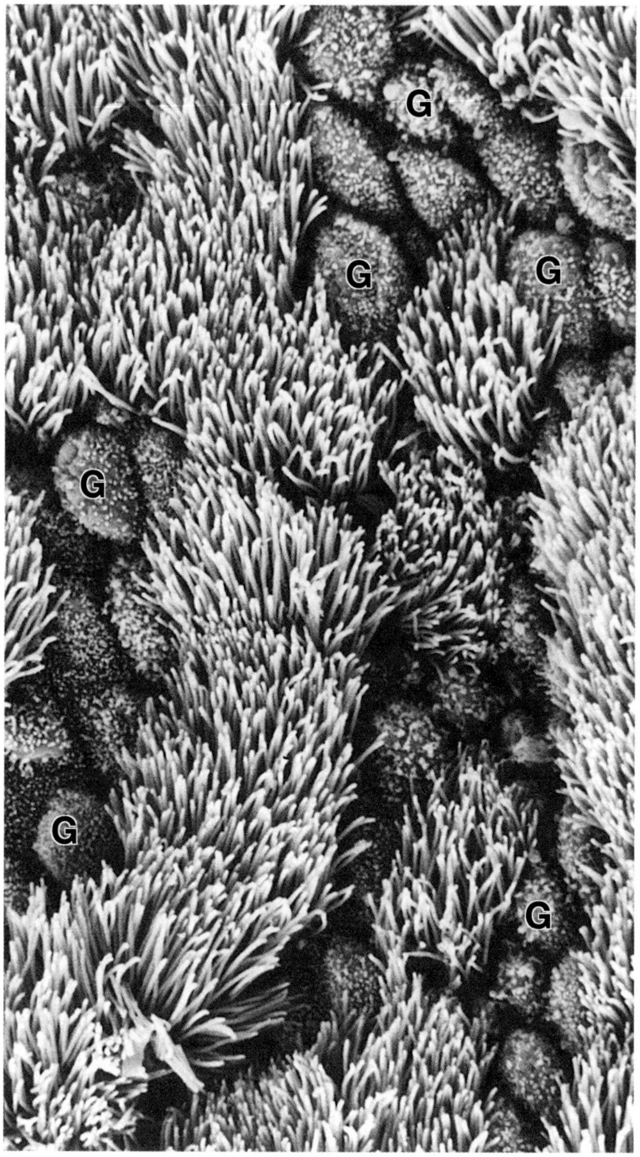

FIGURE 19.9. Scanning electron micrograph of the luminal surface of a bronchus. The nonciliated cells are the goblet cells (*G*). Their surface is characterized by small blunt microvilli that give a stippled appearance to the cell at this low magnification. The cilia of the many ciliated cells occupy the remainder of the micrograph. Note how all are "synchronously" arrayed (i.e., uniformly leaning in the same direction), appearing just as they were when fixed at a specific moment during their wave-like movement. ×1,200.

granules. In one type of small granule cell, the secretion is a **catecholamine**. A second cell type produces polypeptide hormones, such as **serotonin**, **calcitonin**, and **gastrin-releasing peptide (bombesin)**. Some small granule cells appear to be innervated. The function of these cells is not well understood. Some are present in groups in association with nerve fibers, forming neuroepithelial bodies, which are thought to function in reflexes regulating the airway or vascular caliber.

- **Basal cells** represent a stem cell population that maintains individual cell replacement in the epithelium. Basal cells tend to be prominent because their nuclei form a row in close proximity to the basal lamina. Although nuclei of other cells reside at this same general level within the epithelium, they are relatively sparse. Thus, most of the nuclei near the basement membrane belong to basal cells.

Basement Membrane, Lamina Propria, and Submucosa

A thick "basement membrane" is a characteristic feature of the tracheal epithelium.

Located beneath the tracheal epithelium is a distinctive layer typically referred to as a **basement membrane** (see Fig. 19.10). It usually appears as a glassy or homogeneous light-staining layer approximately 25–40 μm thick. EM reveals that it consists of densely packed collagenous fibers that lie immediately under the epithelial basal lamina. Structurally, it can be regarded as an unusually

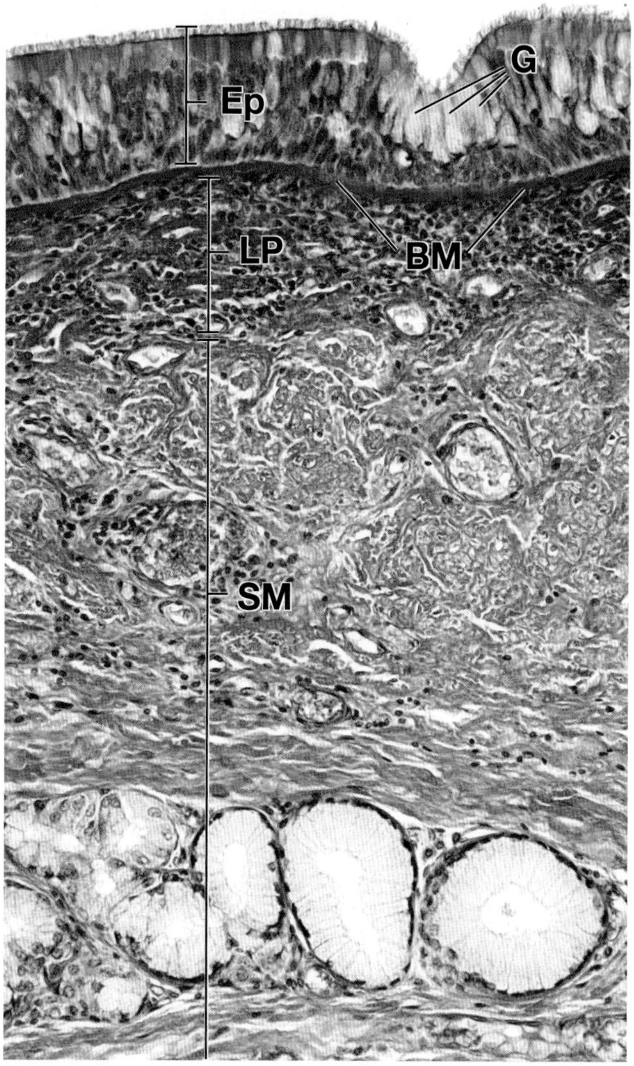

FIGURE 19.10. Photomicrograph of tracheal epithelium. Three major cell types are evident in the tracheal epithelium (*Ep*): ciliated columnar cells; mucus-secreting goblet cells (*G*) interspersed between the ciliated cells; and basal cells, which are close to the basement membrane (*BM*). The ciliated columnar cells extend from the basement membrane to the surface. At their free surface, they contain numerous cilia that, together, give the surface a brush-like appearance. At the base of the cilia is a dense eosinophilic line. This is owing to the linear aggregation of structures referred to as *basal bodies*, located at the proximal end of each cilium. Although basement membranes are not ordinarily seen in hematoxylin and eosin (H&E) preparations, a structure identified as such is seen regularly under the epithelium in the human trachea. The underlying lamina propria (*LP*) consists of loose connective tissue. The more deeply located submucosa (*SM*) contains dense irregular connective tissue with blood and lymphatic vessels, nerves, and numerous mucus-secreting tracheal glands. ×400.

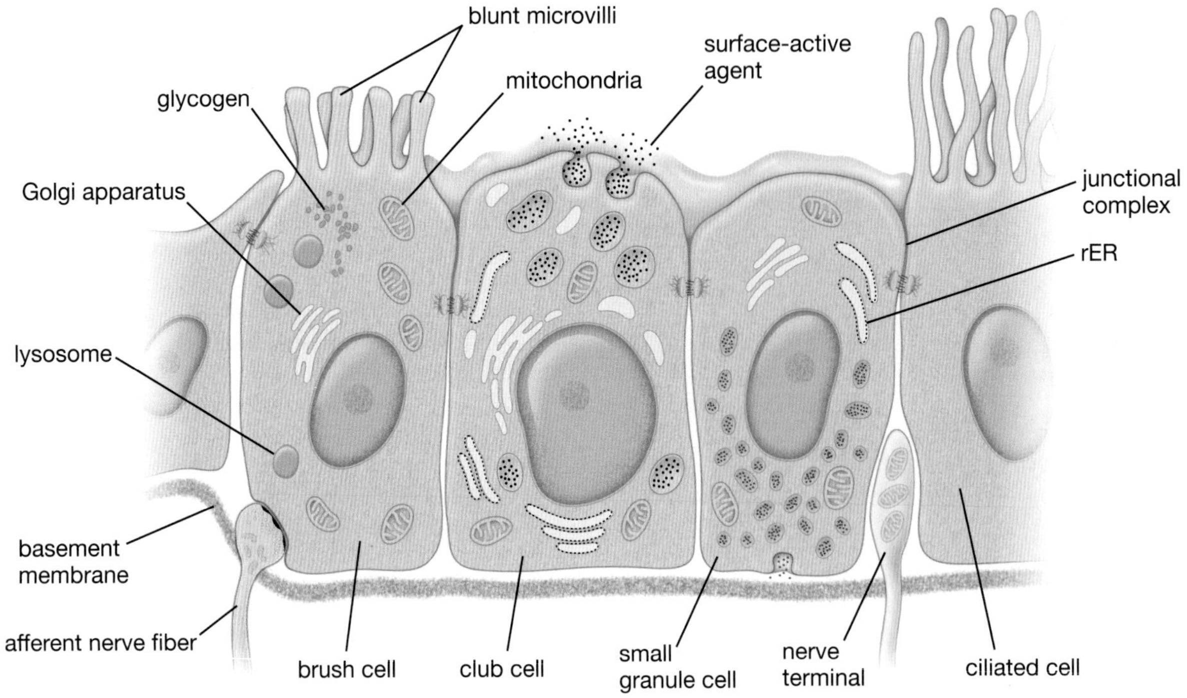

FIGURE 19.11. Diagram of a terminal bronchiolar epithelium. This diagram shows several cells found in the respiratory epithelium. The club cell, as illustrated here, is interposed between the brush cell and the small granule cell. The club cell is a nonciliated cell that has rounded apical surface, well-developed basal rough-surfaced endoplasmic reticulum (*rER*), and Golgi apparatus and contains secretory vesicles filled with a surface-active agent. Adjacent is the brush cell that contains blunt microvilli and makes synaptic contact (epitheliodendritic synapse) with an afferent nerve fiber, which are distinctive features of this cell. Cytoplasm of the brush cell shows a Golgi apparatus, lysosomes, mitochondria, and glycogen inclusions. A small granule cell is shown located between the club cell and the ciliated cell. This cell contains small secretory vesicles, most of which are in the basal portion of the cell. In addition to the vesicles, the most conspicuous organelles of this cell are *rER*, a Golgi apparatus, and mitochondria. A nerve terminal is shown within the epithelium.

thick and dense reticular lamina and, as such, is part of the lamina propria. In smokers, particularly those who experience **chronic coughing**, this layer may be considerably thicker, a response to mucosal irritation. In individuals with **asthma**, the basement membrane is also thicker and more pronounced, especially at the level of the bronchioles.

The boundary between mucosa and submucosa is defined by an elastic membrane.

The **lamina propria**, excluding that part just designated as basement membrane, appears as a typical loose connective tissue. It is very cellular, containing numerous lymphocytes, many of which infiltrate the epithelium. Plasma cells, mast cells, eosinophils, and fibroblasts are the other cell types readily observed in this layer. Lymphatic tissue, in both diffuse and nodular forms, is consistently present in the lamina propria and submucosa of the tracheal wall. It is also present in other parts of the respiratory system involved primarily with air conduction. This lymphatic tissue is the developmental and functional equivalent of the **bronchus-associated lymphatic tissue (BALT)**. Interspersed among the collagenous fibers are numerous elastic fibers. Where the lamina propria ends, the elastic material is more extensive, and in specimens stained for these fibers, a distinct band of elastic material is seen. This band or **elastic membrane** marks the boundary between the lamina propria and submucosa. In H&E preparations, however, the boundary is not obvious.

The **submucosa** is unlike that of most other organs, which is typically a dense connective tissue. In the trachea, the submucosa is a relatively loose connective tissue similar in appearance to the lamina propria, which makes it difficult to determine where it begins. Diffuse lymphatic tissue and lymphatic nodules characteristically extend into this layer from the lamina propria. The submucosa contains the larger distributing vessels and lymphatics of the tracheal wall. Submucosal glands composed of mucus-secreting acini with serous demilunes are also present in the submucosa. Their ducts consist of a simple cuboidal epithelium and extend through the lamina propria to deliver their product, largely glycoproteins, on the epithelial surface. The glands are especially numerous in the cartilage-free gap on the posterior portion of the trachea. Some penetrate the muscle layer at this site and, therefore, also lie in the adventitia. The submucosal layer ends where its connective tissue fibers blend with the perichondrium of the cartilage layer.

The tracheal cartilages and trachealis muscle separate submucosa from adventitia.

The **tracheal cartilages**, which number approximately 16–20 in humans, represent the next layer of the tracheal wall. As noted, the cartilages are C shaped. They sometimes anastomose with adjacent cartilages, but their arrangement provides flexibility to the trachea and also maintains patency of the lumen. With age, the hyaline cartilage may be partially replaced by bone tissue (see Fig. 19.7), causing it to lose much of its flexibility.

FOLDER 19.1

CLINICAL CORRELATION: COMMON CONDITIONS AFFECTING THE NASAL MUCOSA

Inflammation of the nasal mucosa is referred to as **rhinitis**. This inflammatory process may also spread into the paranasal sinuses (**rhinosinusitis**) because of their proximity to and connections with the nasal cavity. Viruses, including rhinoviruses, myxoviruses, coronaviruses, and adenoviruses, are the most common cause of nasal mucosa inflammation, referred to as **viral rhinitis** or the "**common cold**." Viral rhinitis occurs more commonly in children than in adults. Swelling of the nasal mucosa, often called **mucosal inflammation**, may lead to nasal congestion or obstruction, resulting in reduced nasal airflow and increased nasal secretion with simultaneous narrowing of the openings to the paranasal sinuses. Microscopic findings in mucosal inflammation include marked tissue swelling and edema of the respiratory mucosa with significantly increased infiltration of the lamina propria by inflammatory cells, including eosinophils, neutrophils, basophils, mast cells, plasma cells, and lymphocytes (Fig. F19.1.1). Viral infection may lead to secondary bacterial infection (**acute bacterial rhinosinusitis** or **chronic bacterial rhinosinusitis**). The microscopic findings would reveal heavily infiltrated lamina propria and respiratory epithelium with inflammatory cells, including neutrophils and T cells. Acute bacterial rhinosinusitis is usually treated with antibiotic therapy.

Allergic rhinitis, frequently referred to as "**hay fever**," is caused by allergic reactions to airborne particles, such as grass pollens, dust, molds, or animal allergens that are deposited on the nasal mucosa. These particles trigger acute or chronic immune reactions. Allergens in combination with **IgE antibodies** (secreted by the plasma cells in the lamina propria) bind to high-affinity F_c receptors expressed on the surface of mast cells. This triggers activation of **mast cells** with the release of vasoactive agents and inflammatory mediators (e.g., histamine and leukotrienes) from the cell granules (see pages 200-204). Degranulation of mast cells causes rhinorrhea or "runny nose" and nasal congestion. The characteristic microscopic features of allergic rhinitis include infiltration of the nasal mucosa by numerous eosinophils, plasma cells, and mast cells. In chronic allergic rhinitis, an increased number of mast cells and thickening of the basement membrane are often observed. Treatment for allergic rhinitis includes antihistamine agents to suppress immune reactions and anti-inflammatory corticosteroids to control symptoms.

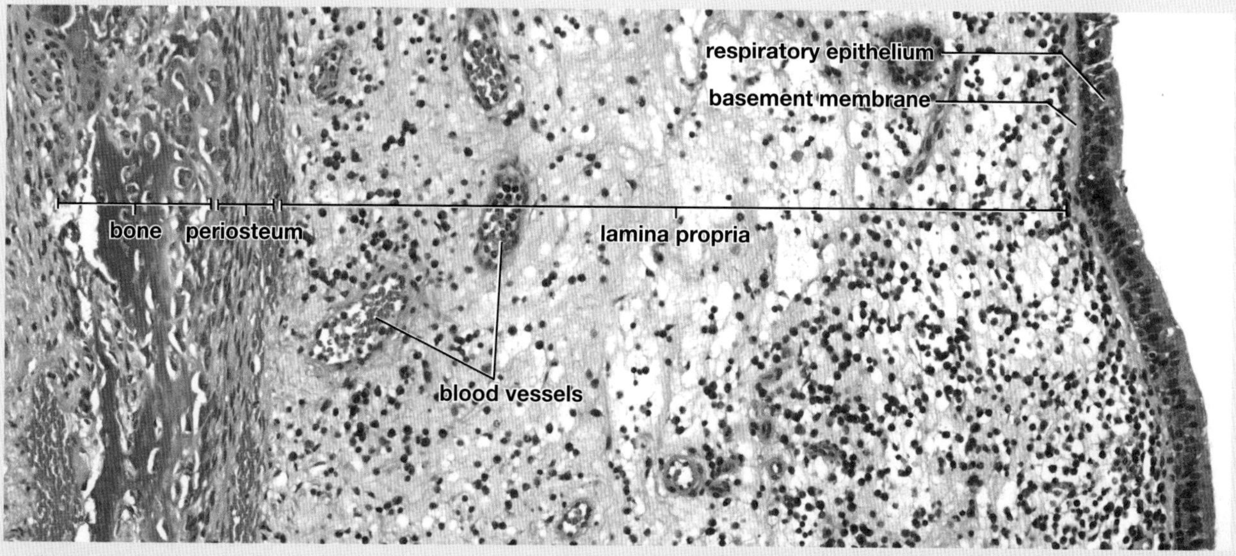

FIGURE F19.1.1. Photomicrograph of a biopsy specimen of the maxillary sinus mucosa from a patient with rhinosinusitis. Microscopic findings in rhinosinusitis include inflammation of the respiratory mucosa of the nasal passages and paranasal sinuses. Note that the respiratory epithelium is separated from the bone of the maxillary sinus by the inflamed lamina propria. In this photomicrograph, the lamina propria is noticeably thickened (edematous) with enlarged blood vessels and is heavily infiltrated by immune cells, mainly lymphocytes, eosinophils, and plasma cells. ×480. (Courtesy of Dr. Joaquin J. Garcia.)

The **adventitia**, the outer layer, lies peripheral to the cartilage rings and trachealis muscle. It binds the trachea to adjacent structures in the neck and mediastinum and contains the largest blood vessels and nerves that supply the tracheal wall as well as the larger lymphatics that drain the wall.

■ BRONCHI

The trachea divides into two branches forming the **main (primary) bronchi**. Anatomically, these divisions are more frequently described as simply the **right and left main bronchi**, terms that are more useful because of the physical difference between the two. The right bronchus is wider and significantly shorter than the left. On entering the hilum of the lung, each main bronchus divides into the **lobar bronchi (secondary bronchi)**. The left lung is divided into two lobes; the right lung is divided into three lobes. Thus, the right bronchus divides into three lobar bronchial branches and the left into two lobar bronchial branches, with each branch supplying one lobe. The left lung is further divided into 8 **bronchopulmonary segments** and the right lung into 10 such segments. Thus, in the right lung, the lobar bronchi give rise to 10 **segmental bronchi (tertiary bronchi)**; the lobar bronchi of the left lung give rise to 8 segmental bronchi.

A **segmental bronchus** and the lung parenchyma that it supplies constitute a bronchopulmonary segment. The significance of the bronchopulmonary segment in the human lung becomes apparent when considering the need for surgical resection, which may be required in certain disease states. The segments, each with their own blood supply and connective tissue septa, are convenient subunits that facilitate surgical resection.

Initially, the bronchi have the same general histologic structure as the trachea. At the point where the bronchi enter the lungs to become intrapulmonary bronchi, the structure of the bronchial wall changes. The cartilage rings are replaced by cartilage plates of irregular shape. The plates are distributed in a linear array around the entire circumference of the wall, giving the bronchi a circular or cylindrical shape in contrast to the ovoid shape with a flattened posterior wall of the trachea. As the bronchi decrease in size because of branching, the cartilage plates become smaller and less numerous. The plates ultimately disappear at the point where the airway reaches a diameter of approximately 1 mm, whereupon the branch is designated a **bronchiole**.

Bronchi can be identified by their cartilage plates and a circular layer of smooth muscle.

The second change observed in the wall of the intrapulmonary bronchus is the addition of **smooth muscle** to form a complete circumferential layer. The smooth muscle becomes an increasingly conspicuous layer as the amount of cartilage diminishes. Initially, the smooth muscle is arranged in interlacing bundles, forming a continuous layer. In the smaller bronchi, the smooth muscle may appear discontinuous.

Because the smooth muscle forms a separate layer, namely, a muscularis, the wall of the bronchus can be regarded as having five layers:

- **Mucosa**, composed of a pseudostratified epithelium with the same cellular composition as the trachea. The height of the cells decreases as the bronchi decrease in diameter. In H&E specimens, the "basement membrane" is conspicuous in the primary bronchi but quickly diminishes in thickness and disappears as a discrete structure in the secondary bronchi. The lamina propria is similar to that of the trachea but is reduced in amount in proportion to the diameter of the bronchi.
- **Muscularis**, a continuous layer of smooth muscle in the larger bronchi. It is more attenuated and loosely organized in smaller bronchi, where it may appear discontinuous because of its spiral course. Contraction of the muscle regulates the appropriate diameter of the airway.
- **Submucosa** remains as a relatively loose connective tissue. Glands are present as well as adipose tissue in the larger bronchi.
- **Cartilage layer** consists of discontinuous cartilage plates that become smaller as the bronchial diameter diminishes.
- **Adventitia** is moderately dense connective tissue that is continuous with that of adjacent structures, such as pulmonary artery and lung parenchyma.

■ BRONCHIOLES

The **bronchopulmonary segments** are further subdivided into **pulmonary lobules**; each lobule is supplied by a bronchiole. Delicate connective tissue septa that partially separate adjacent lobules may be represented on the surface of the lung as faintly outlined polygonal areas. **Pulmonary acini** are smaller units of structure that make up the lobules. Each acinus consists of a **terminal bronchiole** and the **respiratory bronchioles** and **alveoli** that it aerates (Fig. 19.12 and Plate 19.4, page 764). The smallest functional unit of pulmonary structure is thus the **respiratory bronchiolar unit**. It consists of a single respiratory bronchiole and the alveoli that it supplies.

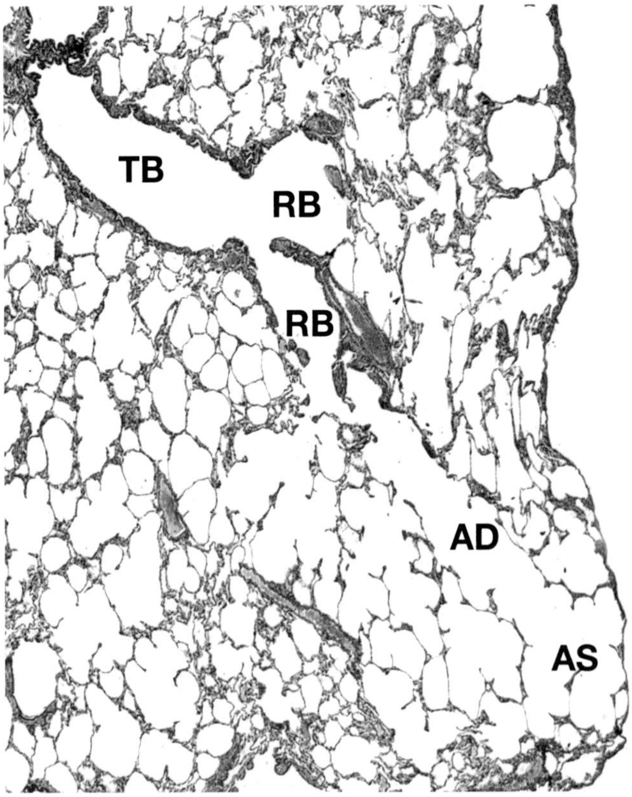

FIGURE 19.12. Photomicrograph showing the respiratory portion of the bronchial tree. In this photomicrograph, a terminal bronchiole (*TB*) is shown longitudinally sectioned as it branches into two respiratory bronchioles (*RB*). The terminal bronchiole is the most distal part of the conducting portion of the respiratory system and is not engaged in gas exchange. The respiratory bronchiole engages in gas exchange and is the beginning of the respiratory portion of the bronchial tree. Respiratory bronchioles give rise to alveolar ducts (*AD*), which are elongated airways that have almost no walls, only alveoli surrounding the duct space. Alveolar sacs (*AS*) are spaces at the termination of the alveolar ducts that, likewise, are surrounded by alveoli. ×120.

Bronchiolar Structure

Bronchioles are air-conducting ducts that measure 1 mm or less in diameter. The larger bronchioles represent branches of the segmental bronchi. These ducts branch repeatedly, giving rise to the smaller **terminal bronchioles** that also branch. The terminal bronchioles finally give rise to the **respiratory bronchioles**.

Cartilage plates and glands are not present in bronchioles.

The larger diameter bronchioles initially have a ciliated, pseudostratified columnar epithelium that gradually transforms into a simple ciliated columnar epithelium as the duct narrows. Goblet cells are still present in the largest bronchioles, but not in the terminal bronchioles that follow. An exception is in smokers and others exposed to irritants in the air. There are no subepithelial glands in bronchioles. Cartilage plates, characteristic of bronchi, are absent in bronchioles. Instead, small elements of cartilage may be present, particularly at branching points. A relatively thick layer of smooth muscle is present in the wall of all bronchioles.

Small bronchioles have a simple cuboidal epithelium. The smallest conducting bronchioles, the **terminal bronchioles**, are lined with a simple cuboidal epithelium in which **club cells** are interspersed among the ciliated cells (Fig. 19.13 and Plate 19.5, page 766). Club cells increase in number as the ciliated cells decrease along the length of the bronchiole. Occasional brush cells and small granule cells are also present. A small amount of connective tissue underlies the epithelium, and a circumferential layer of smooth muscle underlies the connective tissue in the conducting portions.

Club cells are nonciliated cells that have a characteristic rounded or dome-shaped apical surface projection. They display TEM characteristics of protein-secreting cells

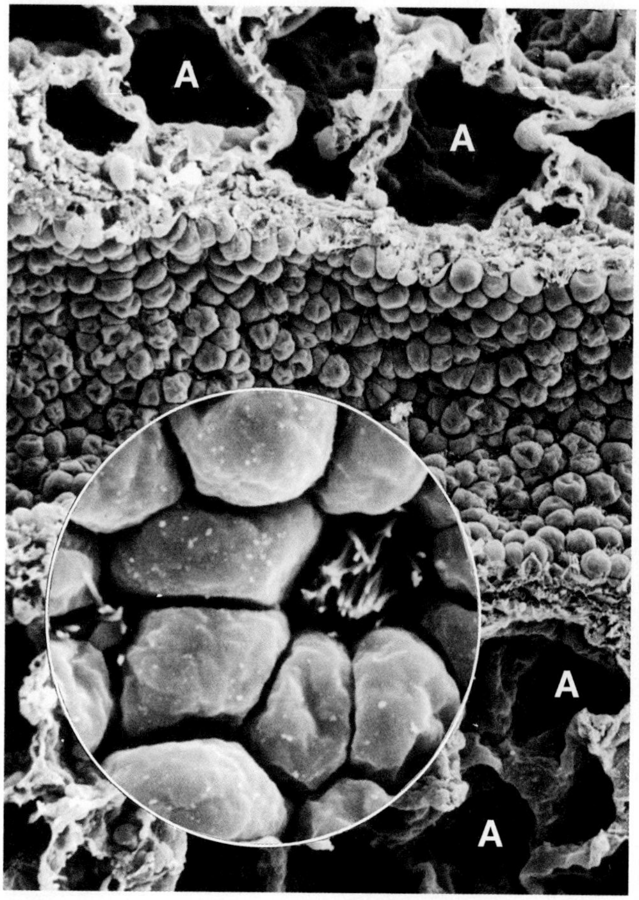

FIGURE 19.13. Scanning electron micrograph of a terminal bronchiole. This scanning photomicrograph shows a longitudinal section throughout the terminal bronchiole and surrounding alveoli (*A*). Note that the apical surfaces of the club cells possess no cilia and have a characteristic dome-shaped appearance. ×150. The *inset* shows some of the club cells at a higher magnification and the cilia of a neighboring ciliated cell, which are present in very small numbers at this level. Note the relatively few cilia present on these small cells. ×1,200.

FOLDER 19.2

CLINICAL CORRELATION: SQUAMOUS METAPLASIA IN THE RESPIRATORY TRACT

In human **respiratory mucosa**, ciliated pseudostratified columnar epithelium may change to stratified squamous epithelium. This change from columnar to squamous epithelium is referred to as **columnar-to-squamous metaplasia** or simply **squamous metaplasia**. Epithelial alterations of this kind are reversible and are characterized by a change from one type of fully differentiated adult cell to a different type of adult cell. A given mature cell does not change to another type of mature cell; rather, basal cell proliferation gives rise to the new differentiated cell type. These cellular changes are considered to be controlled and adaptive.

Squamous metaplasia is a normal occurrence on the rounded, more exposed portions of the turbinates, on the vocal folds, and in certain other regions.

Changes in the character of the respiratory epithelium may, however, occur in other ciliated epithelial sites when the pattern of airflow is altered or when forceful airflow occurs, as in chronic coughing. Typically, in **chronic bronchitis** and **bronchiectasis**, the respiratory epithelium changes in certain regions to a stratified squamous form. The altered epithelium is more resistant to physical stress and insult, but it is less effective functionally. In smokers, a similar epithelial change occurs. Initially, the cilia on ciliated cells lose their synchronous beating pattern as a result of noxious elements in smoke. As a result, removal of mucus is impaired. To compensate, the individual begins to cough, thereby facilitating the expulsion of accumulated mucus in the airway, particularly in the trachea. With time, the number of ciliated cells decreases because of chronic coughing. This reduction in ciliated cells further impairs the normal epithelium and results in its replacement with stratified squamous epithelium at affected sites in the airway. If the factors (i.e., tobacco smoking) that predispose to squamous metaplasia are not eliminated, the metaplastic epithelium may undergo malignant transformation. In this way, one of the two most common forms of cancer of the respiratory tract, **squamous cell carcinoma**, originates from squamous metaplastic cells.

FOLDER 19.3

CLINICAL CORRELATION: ASTHMA

Asthma is a chronic inflammatory disease involving the airways of the lungs and is caused by a combination of genetic and environmental factors. The disease affects people of all ages, races, and ethnic groups worldwide. It is characterized by recurrent **obstruction of airflow** that results from **inflammation** of the bronchioles and **constriction** of their smooth muscles (**bronchospasm**). Obstruction of airways makes it difficult for air to move in and out of the lung alveoli, causing symptoms such as wheezing, coughing, shortness of breath, and chest tightness. Inflammation of the respiratory mucosa, underlying connective tissue, and smooth muscles of bronchioles is found in patients with asthma. It is characterized by infiltration of the bronchiolar wall by eosinophils (in some cases, neutrophils), lymphocytes (mostly activated helper T cells), and mast cells. In individuals with asthma, the bronchiolar epithelium is thick, contains an increased number of goblet cells (thus producing more mucus), and has a thick basement membrane owing to an increased deposition of collagen fibers in the reticular lamina (Fig. F19.3.1). The smooth muscle layer is also more pronounced and contains several layers of hyperplastic smooth muscle cells.

Medications used to treat patients with asthma include **bronchodilators** that cause relaxation of smooth muscle; **anti-inflammatory** medications that suppress inflammatory reactions; and leukotriene modifiers that inhibit the production of leukotrienes, which are lipid mediators linked to increased activity of smooth muscle and mucus secretion. Asthma medications are classified into two general categories according to their time of action in the overall management of this disease: (1) **quick-relief medications**, such as β-adrenergic agonist bronchodilators to reverse smooth muscle constriction, or (2) **long-term control medications**, such as inhaled corticosteroids, long-acting β-agonist bronchodilators, and leukotriene modifiers.

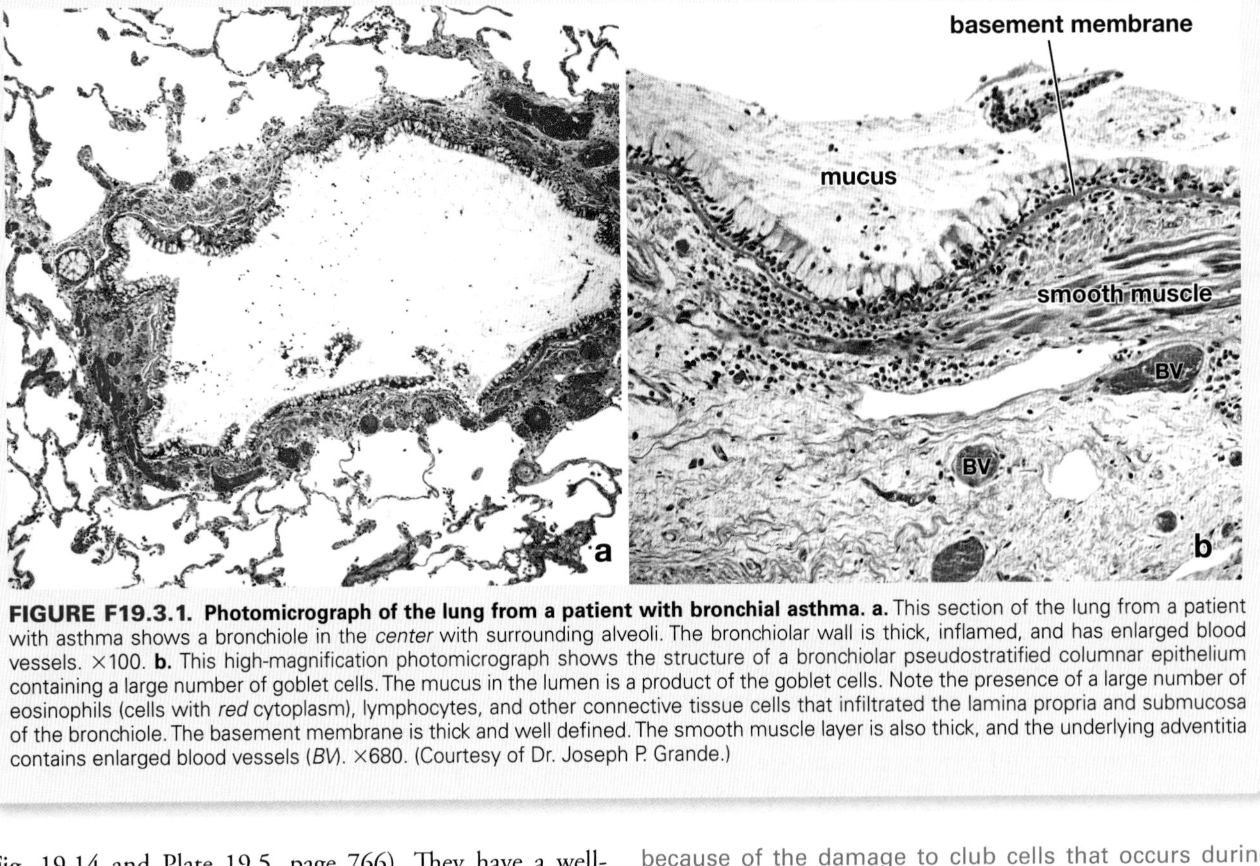

FIGURE F19.3.1. Photomicrograph of the lung from a patient with bronchial asthma. a. This section of the lung from a patient with asthma shows a bronchiole in the *center* with surrounding alveoli. The bronchiolar wall is thick, inflamed, and has enlarged blood vessels. ×100. **b.** This high-magnification photomicrograph shows the structure of a bronchiolar pseudostratified columnar epithelium containing a large number of goblet cells. The mucus in the lumen is a product of the goblet cells. Note the presence of a large number of eosinophils (cells with *red* cytoplasm), lymphocytes, and other connective tissue cells that infiltrated the lamina propria and submucosa of the bronchiole. The basement membrane is thick and well defined. The smooth muscle layer is also thick, and the underlying adventitia contains enlarged blood vessels (*BV*). ×680. (Courtesy of Dr. Joseph P. Grande.)

(Fig. 19.14 and Plate 19.5, page 766). They have a well-developed basal rER, a lateral or supranuclear Golgi apparatus, secretory granules that stain for protein, and numerous cisternae of sER in the apical cytoplasm. Club cells secrete a **surface-active agent**, a lipoprotein that prevents luminal adhesion should the wall of the airway collapse on itself, particularly during expiration. In addition, club cells produce a 16-kDa protein known as **club cell secretory protein (CC16)**, which is an abundant component of airway secretion. Chronic lung diseases, such as **chronic obstructive pulmonary disease (COPD)** and **asthma**, are associated with changes in the levels of CC16 in airway fluid and serum. Secretion of CC16 into the bronchial tree decreases because of the damage to club cells that occurs during lung injury, whereas serum levels of CC16 may increase because of leakage across the air–blood barrier. CC16 can thus be used as a measurable pulmonary marker in bronchoalveolar lavage fluid and serum.

Bronchiolar Function

Respiratory bronchioles are the first part of the bronchial tree that allows gas exchange.

Respiratory bronchioles constitute a transitional zone in the respiratory system; they are involved in both air conduction and gas exchange. They have a narrow diameter and are

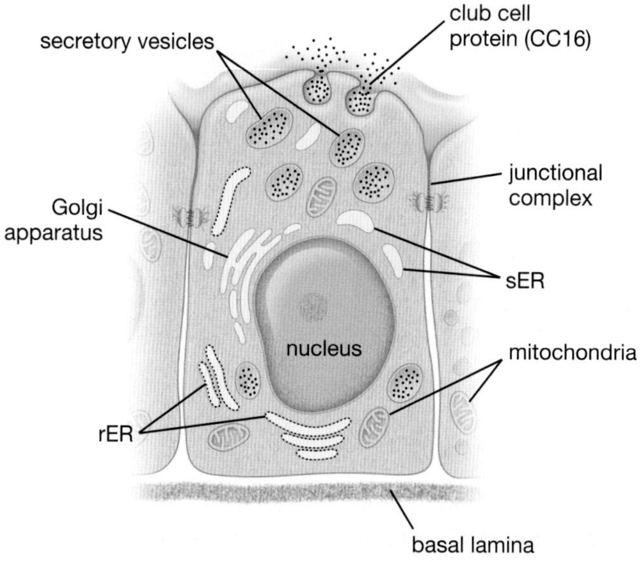

FIGURE 19.14. Diagram of a club cell between bronchiolar ciliated epithelial cells. The nucleus is in a basal location. Rough-surfaced endoplasmic reticulum (*rER*), a Golgi apparatus, and mitochondria are chiefly in basal and paranuclear locations of the cell. Smooth-surfaced endoplasmic reticulum (*sER*) and secretory vesicles are chiefly in the apical cytoplasm. Two of the secretory vesicles are shown discharging its contents onto the surface of the cell.

lined by cuboidal epithelium. The epithelium of the initial segments of the respiratory bronchioles contains both **ciliated cells** and **club cells** (see Fig. 19.13). Distally, club cells predominate. Occasional brush cells and dense-core granule cells are also present along the length of the respiratory bronchiole. Scattered, thin-walled outpocketings, **alveoli**, extend from the lumen of the respiratory bronchioles (see Fig. 19.12). Alveoli are the sites at which air leaves and enters the bronchiole to allow gas exchange.

■ ALVEOLI

Alveoli are the site of gas exchange.

The surface area available for gas exchange is increased by the lung alveoli. **Alveoli** are the terminal air spaces of the respiratory system and are the actual sites of gas exchange between the air and the blood. Each alveolus is surrounded by a network of capillaries that brings blood in close proximity to inhaled air inside the alveolus. About 150–250 million alveoli are found in each adult lung; their combined internal surface area is approximately 75 m^2, roughly the size of a tennis court. Each alveolus is a thin-walled polyhedral chamber approximately 0.2 mm in diameter that is confluent with an alveolar sac (Fig. 19.15 and Plate 19.5, page 766).

- **Alveolar ducts** are elongated airways that have almost no walls, only alveoli, as their peripheral boundary. Rings of smooth muscle are present in the knob-like interalveolar septa (see the next paragraph).
- **Alveolar sacs** are spaces surrounded by clusters of alveoli. The surrounding alveoli open into these spaces.

Alveolar sacs usually occur at the termination of an alveolar duct but may occur anywhere along its length. Alveoli are surrounded and separated from one another by an exceedingly thin connective tissue layer that contains blood capillaries. The tissue between adjacent alveolar air spaces is called the **interalveolar septum** or **septal wall** (Fig. 19.16).

Alveolar epithelium is composed of type I and II alveolar cells and occasional brush cells.

The **alveolar surface** forms a vulnerable biological interface that is subject to many destabilizing surface forces and to continuous exposure to inhaled particles, pathogens, and toxins. The alveolar epithelium is composed of several specialized cells and their products, some of which play defensive and protective roles:

- **Type I alveolar cells**, also known as *type I pneumocytes*, comprise only 40% of the alveolar-lining cells. They are extremely thin squamous cells; they line most (95%) of the surface of the alveoli (see Fig. 19.16). These cells are joined to one another and to the other cells of the alveolar epithelium by occluding junctions (Fig. 19.17). The junctions form an effective barrier between the air space and the components of the septal wall. Type I alveolar cells are not capable of cell division.
- **Type II alveolar cells**, also called *type II pneumocytes* or **septal cells**, are secretory cells. These cuboidal cells are interspersed among the type I cells but tend to congregate at septal junctions. Type II cells account for 60% of the alveolar-lining cells, but because of their different shape, they cover only about 5% of the alveolar air surface. Like club cells, type II cells tend to bulge into the air space (see Fig. 19.17). Their apical cytoplasm is filled with granules that are resolved with the TEM (Fig. 19.18) as stacks of parallel membrane lamellae, the **lamellar bodies**. They are rich in a mixture of phospholipids, neutral lipids, and proteins that are secreted by exocytosis to form an alveolar-lining, surface-active agent called **surfactant**.

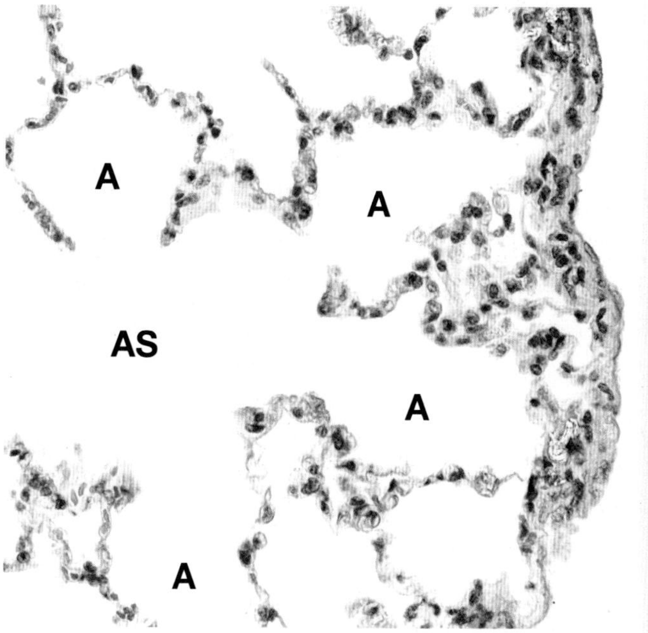

FIGURE 19.15. Photomicrograph showing an alveolar sac with adjacent alveoli. This photomicrograph shows the terminal components of the respiratory system, namely, the alveolar sac (*AS*) and the surrounding alveoli (*A*). The *A* are surrounded and separated from one another by a thin connective tissue layer, the interalveolar septa, containing blood capillaries. On the *right* is the lung surface, which is covered by visceral pleura containing simple squamous epithelium and an underlying layer of connective tissue. ×360.

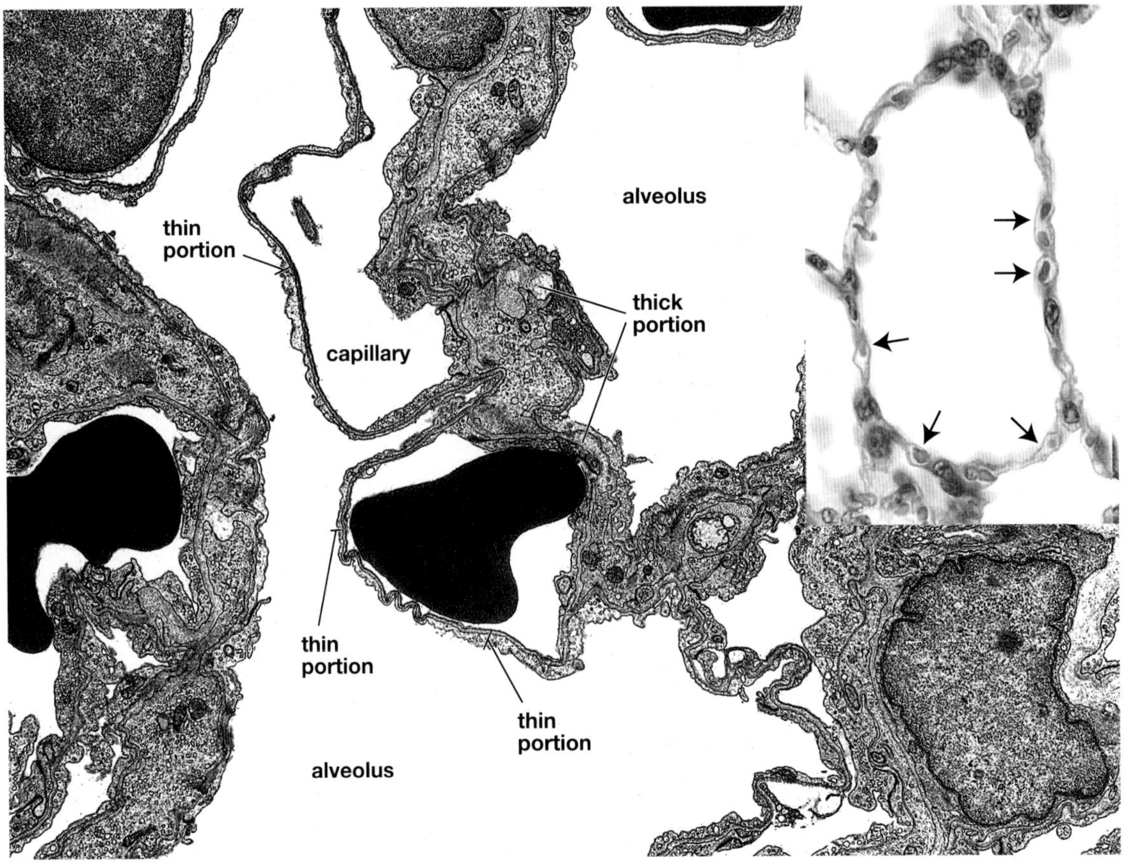

FIGURE 19.16. Electron micrograph of lung alveoli. This electron micrograph shows two alveolar spaces separated by an interalveolar septum containing capillaries, some of which contain red blood cells. Note the areas of thin and thick portions of the interalveolar septum. These are shown at a higher magnification in Figure 19.21. ×5,800. **Inset.** Photomicrograph of an alveolus for comparison with the alveolar wall as seen in an electron micrograph. *Arrows* indicate alveolar capillaries containing red blood cells. ×480.

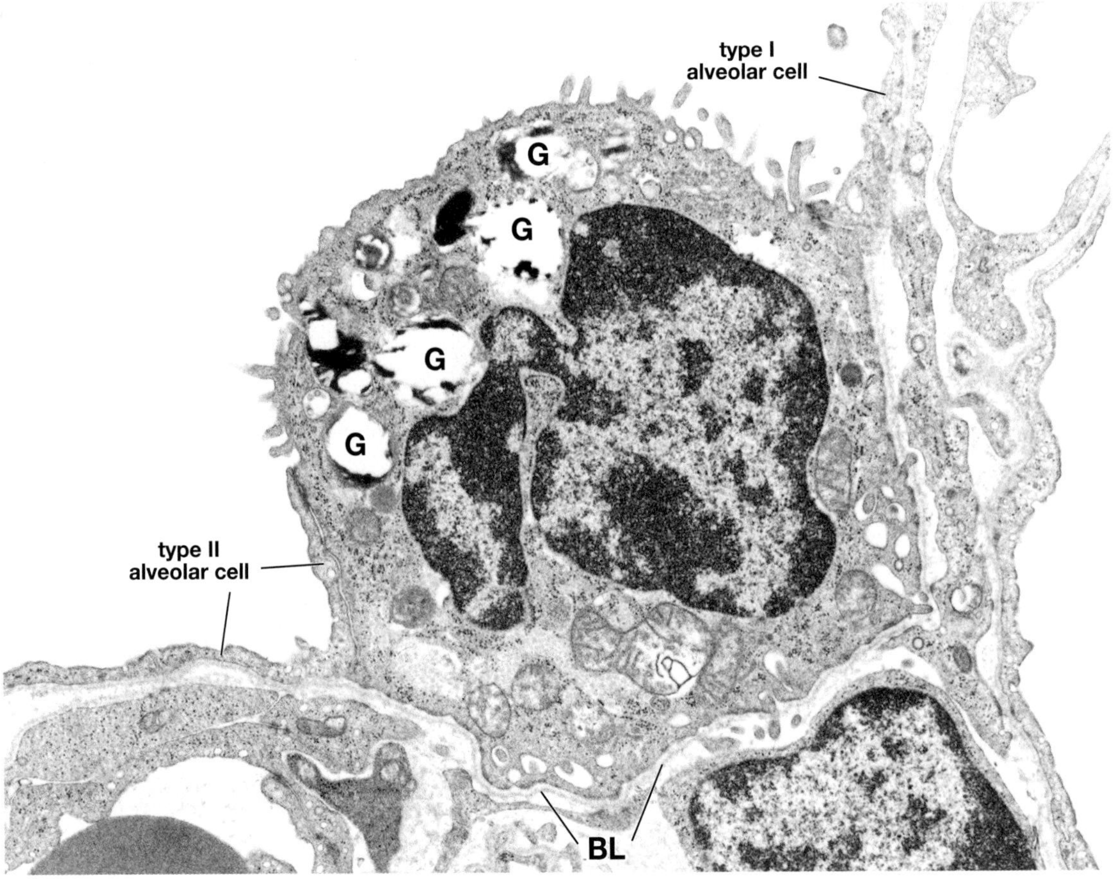

FIGURE 19.17. Electron micrograph of a type II alveolar cell. The type II alveolar cell has a dome-shaped apical surface with a number of short microvilli at its periphery and a relatively smooth-contoured apical center. The lateral cell margins are overlain to a variable degree by the type I alveolar cells that are joined to the type II cell by occluding junctions. Both cell types rest on the basal lamina (*BL*). The secretory vesicles (*G*) in this specimen are largely dissolved, but their lamellar character is shown to advantage in Figure 19.18b. ×24,000.

In addition to secretion of surfactant, type II alveolar cells are progenitor cells for type I alveolar cells. Striking differences in the distribution of both types of alveolar cells can be easily visualized using immunofluorescence techniques (Fig 19.19). Following lung injury, they proliferate and restore both types of alveolar cells within the alveolus. Hyperplasia of type II alveolar cells is an indicator of alveolar injury and repair.

- **Brush cells** are also present in the alveolar wall, but they are few in number. They serve as chemoreceptors that monitor air quality in the lung.

Surfactant decreases the alveolar surface tension and actively participates in the clearance of foreign materials.

The **surfactant** layer produced by type II alveolar cells reduces the surface tension at the air–epithelium interface. The most critical agent for air space stability is a specific phospholipid called **dipalmitoylphosphatidylcholine (DPPC)**, which accounts for almost all surface tension–reducing properties of surfactant. Surfactant synthesis in the fetus occurs after the 35th week of gestation and is modulated by a variety of hormones, including cortisol, insulin, prolactin, and thyroxine. Without adequate secretion of surfactant, the alveoli would collapse on each successive exhalation. Such collapse occurs in preterm infants whose lungs have not developed sufficiently to produce surfactant, which can lead to **neonatal respiratory distress syndrome (RDS)**. Administration of exogenous surfactant at birth to preterm infants reduces the incidence of RDS. In addition, antenatal administration of corticosteroids to women with threatened preterm delivery decreases neonatal mortality.

Surfactant proteins help organize the surfactant layer and modulate alveolar immune responses.

In addition to phospholipids, hydrophobic proteins are necessary for the structure and function of surfactant. These proteins are listed as follows:

- **Surfactant protein A (SP-A)**, the most abundant surfactant protein. SP-A is responsible for surfactant homeostasis (regulating synthesis and secretion of surfactant by type II alveolar cells). It also modulates immune responses to viruses, bacteria, and fungi.
- **Surfactant protein B (SP-B)**, an important protein for the transformation of the lamellar body into the thin surface film of surfactant. SP-B is a critical surfactant-organizing protein responsible for adsorption and spreading of surfactant onto the surface of the alveolar epithelium.
- **Surfactant protein C (SP-C)**, which represents only 1% of the total mass of surfactant protein. Along with SP-B, SP-C aids in orientation of DPPC within the surfactant and maintenance of the thin film layer within the alveoli.
- **Surfactant protein D (SP-D)**, a primary protein involved in host defense. It binds to various microorganisms (e.g., Gram-negative bacteria) and lymphocytes. SP-D participates in a local inflammatory response to acute lung injury and, with SP-A, modulates an immune response to various inhaled antigens.

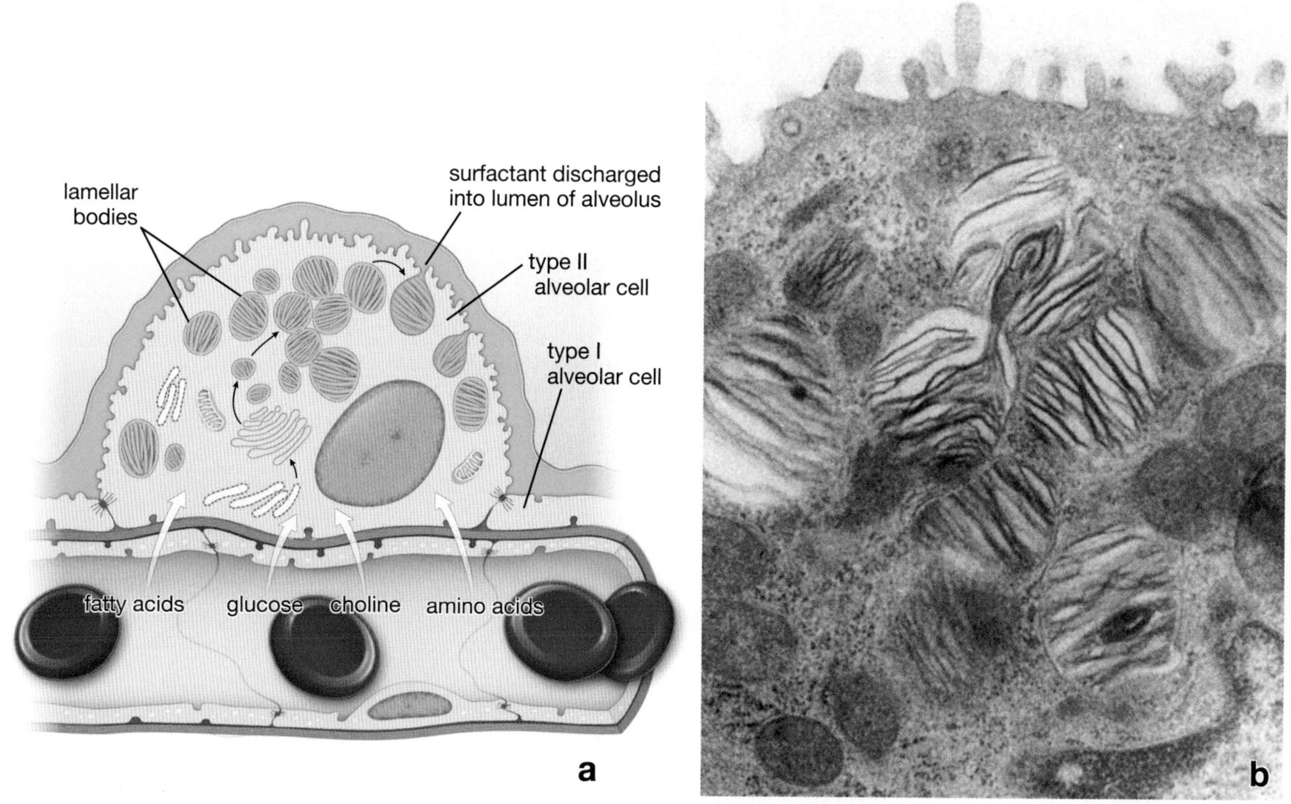

FIGURE 19.18. Diagram of a type II alveolar cell and electron micrograph of lamellar bodies. a. Surfactant is an oily mixture of proteins, phospholipids, and neutral lipids that are synthesized in the rough-surfaced endoplasmic reticulum (*rER*) from precursors in the blood. These precursors are glucose, fatty acids, choline, and amino acids. The protein constituents of surfactant are produced in the *rER* and stored in the cytoplasm within lamellar bodies, which are discharged into the lumen of the alveolus. With the aid of surfactant protein, surfactant is distributed on the surface of epithelial cells lining the alveolus as a thin film that reduces the surface tension. **b.** Higher magnification electron micrograph showing the typical lamellar pattern of the secretory vesicles of type II alveolar cells. These vesicles contain the pulmonary surfactant precursor proteins. ×38,000.

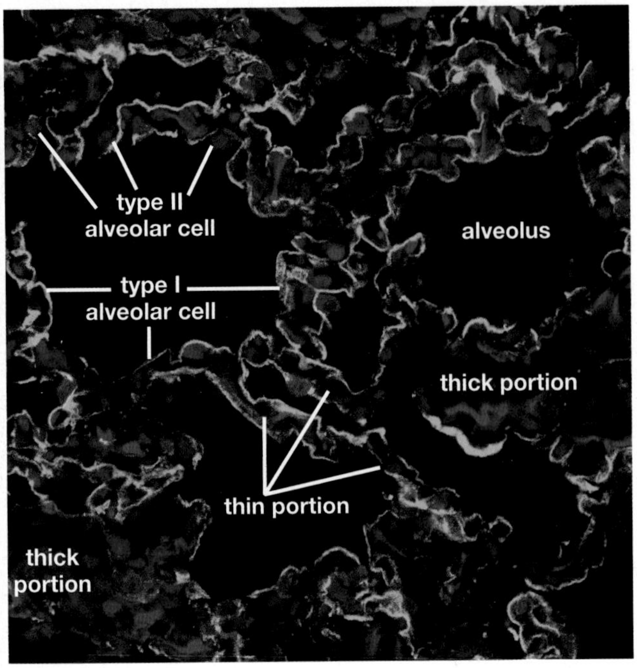

FIGURE 19.19. Immunofluorescent-stained image of the formalin-fixed frozen section of the adult pig lung. This high-magnification image shows the distribution of type I and type II alveolar cells within the alveolar wall. Type I alveolar cells (*green*) are visualized using an indirect immunofluorescence technique that utilizes primary polyclonal goat (IgG) antibodies against the cell membrane receptor for advanced glycation end products (RAGE), followed by secondary anti-goat antibodies conjugated with Alexa Fluor 488 fluorescent stain. The RAGE receptor is a transmembrane protein used as a molecular marker for type I alveolar cells and is localized in their apical cell membrane. Type II alveolar cells (*red*) are visualized using primary polyclonal rabbit (IgG) antibodies against prosurfactant protein C, followed by secondary anti-rabbit antibodies conjugated with Alexa Fluor 555 fluorescent stain. Prosurfactant protein C is synthesized by type II alveolar cells and further processed into mature secreted protein C (SP-C). Note that 95% of the alveolar surface is covered by type I alveolar cells. Nuclei were stained blue by the DAPI stain that reacts with nuclear DNA and exhibits *blue* fluorescence over the nucleus. The nuclei within thin portions of the interalveolar septa belong to both type I and type II alveolar cells and endothelial cells of blood capillaries. Accumulation of septal macrophages and other connective tissue cells is reflected by the accumulation of nuclear stains in thick portions of the interalveolar septa. × 840. (Courtesy Dr. Atta Behfar and Skylar A. Rizzo, Van Cleve Center for Regenerative Medicine, Mayo Clinic.)

The interalveolar septum is the site of the air–blood barrier.

The **air–blood barrier** refers to the cells and cell products across which gases must diffuse between the alveolar and capillary compartments. The thinnest air–blood barrier consists of a thin layer of surfactant, a type I epithelial cell and its basal lamina, and a capillary endothelial cell and its basal lamina. Often, these two basal laminae are fused (Fig. 19.20). Connective tissue cells and fibers that may be present between the two basal laminae widen the air–blood barrier. These two arrangements produce a **thin portion** and a **thick portion** of the barrier (Fig. 19.21). It is thought that most gas exchange occurs across the thin portion of the barrier. The thick portion is thought to be a site in which tissue fluid can accumulate and even cross into the alveolus. Lymphatic vessels in the connective tissue of the terminal bronchioles drain fluid that accumulates in the thick portion of the septum. In acute **interstitial pneumonia,** disruption of the blood–air barrier caused by the injury of type I pneumonocytes or the endothelial epithelium leads to the exudation of plasma proteins into the alveolar space. In **diffuse alveolar damage**, exuded plasma proteins mix with lipids and components of pulmonary surfactant to form hyaline membranes, an elongated, homogeneous, amorphous, and eosinophilic structure that lines the alveolar wall and prevents normal gas exchange.

Alveolar macrophages remove inhaled particulate matter from the air spaces and red blood cells from the septum.

Alveolar macrophages are unusual in that they function in the air space of the alveolus (Fig. 19.22). In air spaces, they scavenge the surface to remove inhaled particulate matter (e.g., dust and pollen), thus giving them one of their alternative names, **dust cells.** Alveolar macrophages are derived from blood monocytes and belong to the mononuclear phagocyte system (see page 203). They phagocytize red blood cells that may enter the alveoli in heart failure (see Fig. 19.22). Some engorged macrophages pass up the bronchial tree in the mucus and are disposed of by swallowing or expectoration when they reach the pharynx. **Septal macrophages** reside in the connective tissue of the interalveolar septa. They represent a population of alveolar macrophages that returned from air spaces of the alveoli or remained stationary in the connective tissue of interalveolar septa. They are filled with accumulated phagocytized material, and they may remain in the septa for much of an individual's life (Fig. 19.23). At autopsy, the lungs of urban dwellers and smokers usually show many **alveolar macrophages** and **septal macrophages** filled with carbon particles, anthracotic pigment, and birefringent needle-like particles of silica. Alveolar macrophages also phagocytose infectious organisms such as *Mycobacterium tuberculosis*, which can be recognized in cells in appropriately stained specimens. These bacilli are not digested by macrophages; however, other infections or conditions that damage alveolar macrophages can cause the release of the bacteria and recurrent tuberculosis. In addition, recent

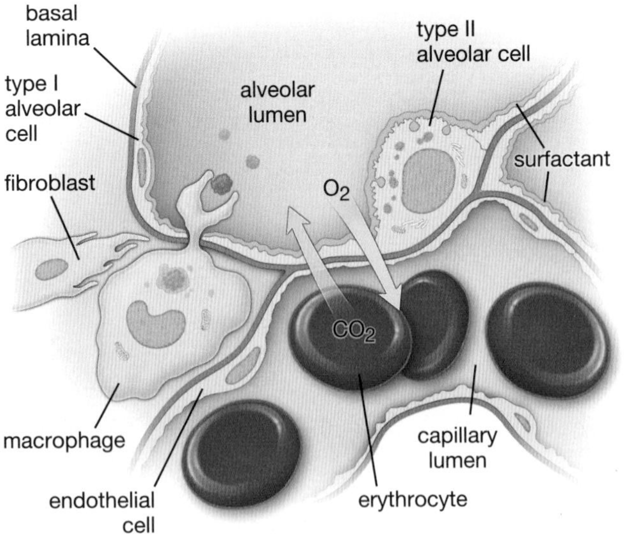

FIGURE 19.20. Diagram of the interalveolar septum. This diagram shows the thick and thin portions of the interalveolar septum. The thin portion forms the air–blood barrier and is responsible for most of the gas exchange that occurs in the lung. *Arrows* indicate the direction of CO_2 and O_2 exchange between the alveolar air space and the blood. The thick portion of the interalveolar septum plays an important role in fluid distribution and its dynamics. It contains connective tissue cells. Note the macrophage in the thick portion that extends its processes into the lumen of the alveolus.

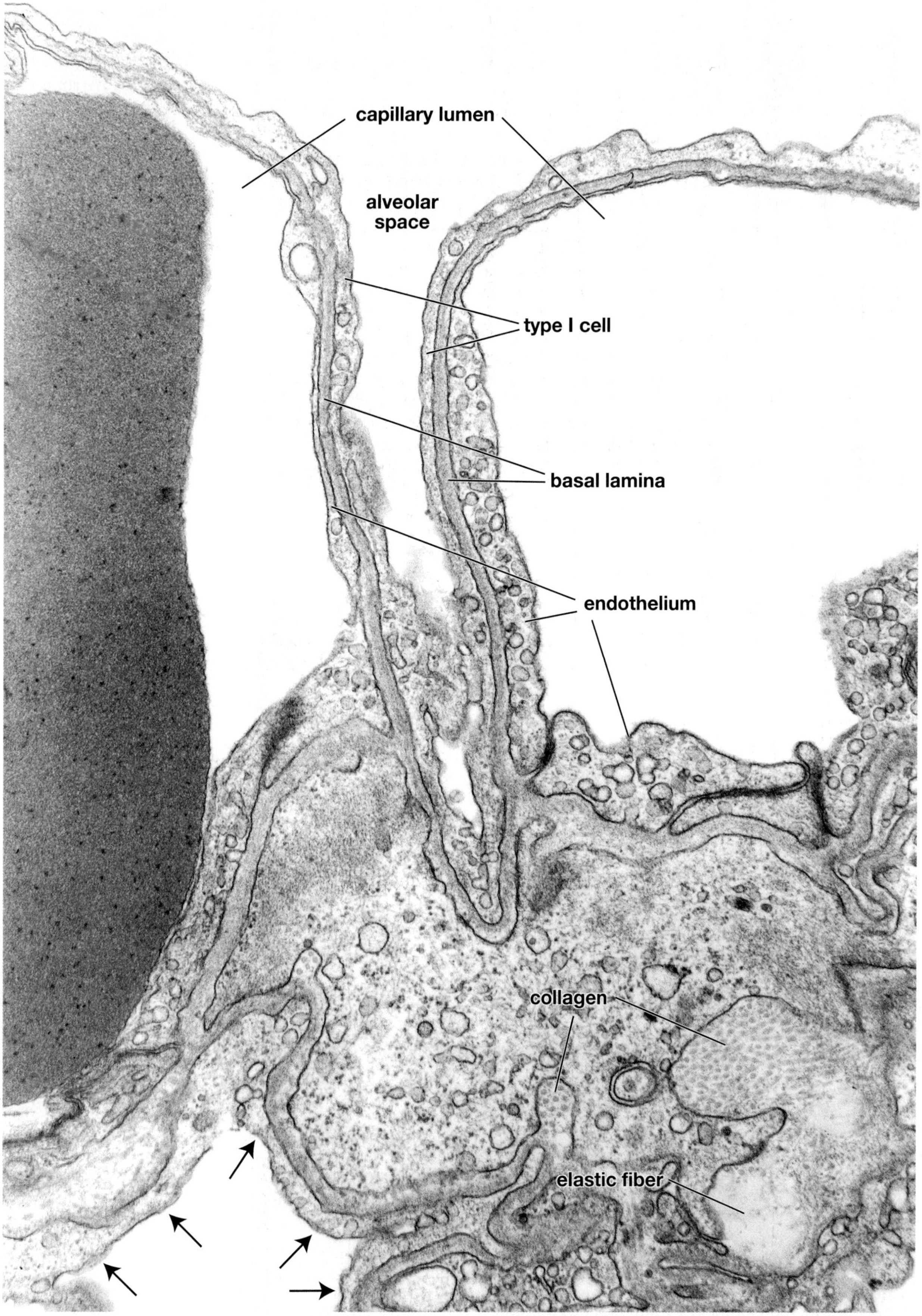

FIGURE 19.21. Electron micrograph of the interalveolar septum. This high-magnification micrograph shows the thin portion of the air–blood barrier where it consists of type I alveolar cells, capillary endothelium, and the fused basal lamina shared by both cells. In the thick portion, the type I alveolar cell (*arrows*) rests on a basal lamina, and on the opposite side is connective tissue in which collagen fibrils and elastic fibers are evident. ×33,000.

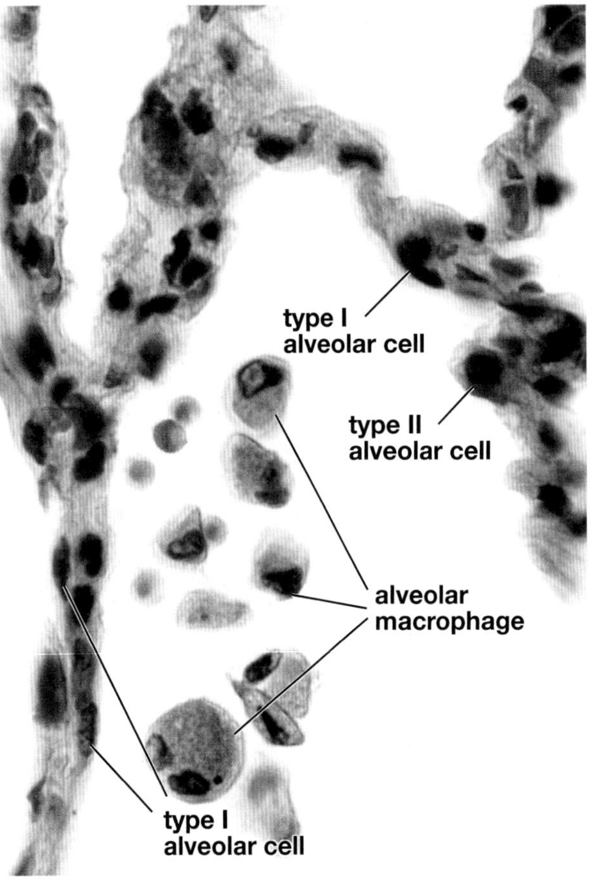

FIGURE 19.22. Photomicrograph of alveoli and alveolar macrophages. This high-magnification photomicrograph shows the structure of the interalveolar septum and the lumen of an alveolus containing alveolar macrophages and red blood cells. The cytoplasm of the alveolar macrophages, when they are present in significant numbers, often contains the brown pigment hemosiderin from phagocytosed red blood cells. These hemosiderin-laden macrophages (often called "heart failure cells") are typically found in heart disease, mostly left ventricular failures that cause pulmonary congestion and edema. This results in enlargement of the alveolar capillaries and small hemorrhages into the alveoli. ×560.

evidence suggests that apoptosis of septal macrophages contributes to the development of emphysema.

Collateral air circulation through alveolar pores allows air to pass between alveoli.

Scanning electron microscopic studies of alveolar structure show openings in the **interalveolar septa** that allow circulation of air from one alveolus to another. These **alveolar pores (of Kohn)** can be of great significance in some pathologic conditions in which obstructive lung disease blocks the normal pathway of air to the alveoli. The alveoli distal to the blockage may continue to be aerated, via the pores, from an adjacent lobule or acinus.

A basic summary of information related to the respiratory system is included in Figure 19.24.

■ BLOOD SUPPLY

The lung has both pulmonary and bronchial circulations.

The **pulmonary circulation** supplies the capillaries of the interalveolar septum and is derived from the pulmonary artery that leaves the right ventricle of the heart. The branches of the pulmonary artery travel with those of the bronchi and bronchioles and carry blood down to the capillary level at the alveoli. This blood is oxygenated and collected by pulmonary venous capillaries that join to form venules. They ultimately form the four pulmonary veins that return blood to the left atrium of the heart. The pulmonary venous system is located at a distance from the respiratory passages at the periphery of the bronchopulmonary segments.

The **bronchial circulation**, via bronchial arteries that branch from the aorta, supplies all of the lung tissue other than the alveoli (i.e., the walls of the bronchi and bronchioles and the connective tissue of the lung other than that of the interalveolar septum). The finest branches of the bronchial arterial tree also open into the pulmonary capillaries. Therefore, the bronchial and pulmonary circulations anastomose at about the level of the junction between the conducting and respiratory passages. Bronchial veins drain only the connective tissue of the hilar region of the lungs. Most of the blood reaching the lungs via the bronchial arteries leaves the lungs via the pulmonary veins.

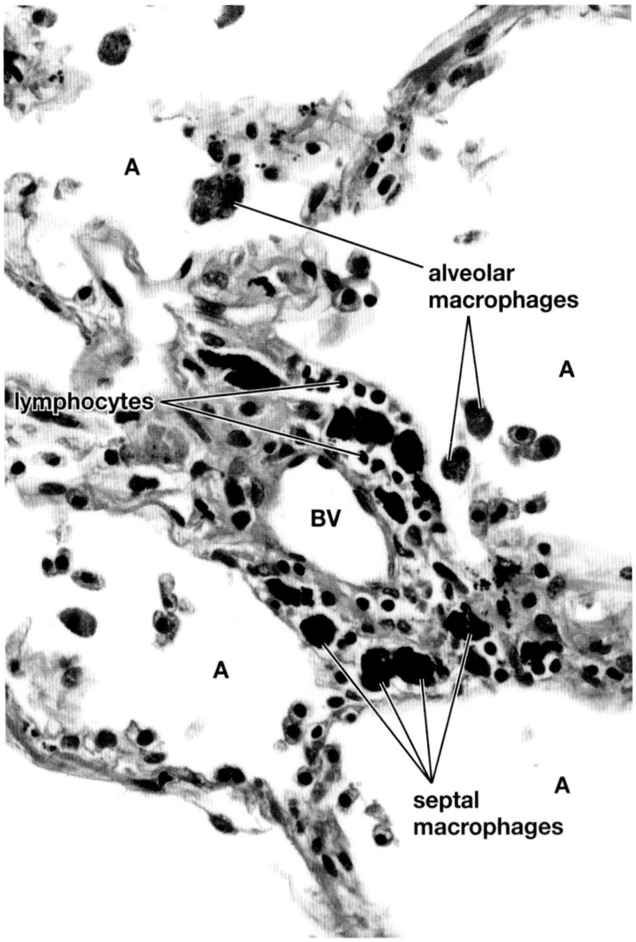

FIGURE 19.23. Photomicrograph of alveolar and septal macrophages. This high-magnification photomicrograph shows interalveolar septa surrounding alveolar air spaces (*A*). The septum in the *middle* contains a larger blood vessel (*BV*). Macrophages that have phagocytosed cellular debris and inhaled environmental pollutants (e.g., dust particles, silica, cigarette tar, and microorganisms) in the alveolar lumen migrate back to the interalveolar septa, where they remain throughout life. These septal macrophages are seen here as large, irregularly shaped cells loaded with black cytoplasmic inclusions that obscure the view of the nucleus. Note that the septal macrophages are surrounded by lymphocytes, a sign of inflammatory response. Alveolar macrophages containing the brown pigment hemosiderin from phagocytosed red blood cells are also present in the lumen of the alveoli. ×560.

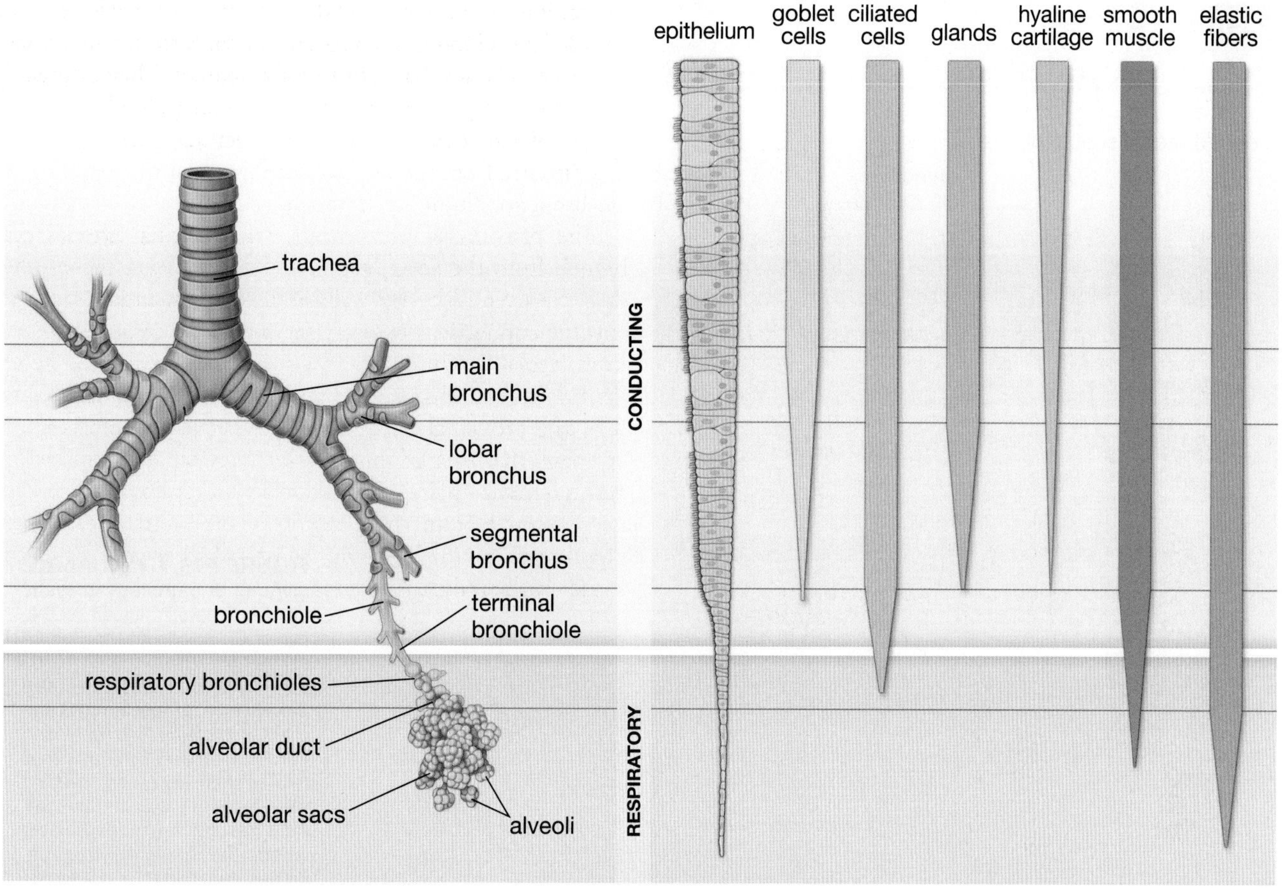

FIGURE 19.24. Divisions of the bronchial tree and summary of its histologic features.

■ LYMPHATIC VESSELS

A dual **lymphatic drainage** of the lungs parallels the dual blood supply. One set of lymphatic vessels drains the parenchyma of the lung and follows the air passages to the hilum. Lymph nodes are found along the route of the larger lymphatic vessels. A second set of lymphatic vessels drains the surface of the lung and travels in the connective tissue of the **visceral pleura**, a serous membrane consisting of a surface mesothelium and the underlying connective tissue. Both of these systems converge in the hilum. Lymph passes through several groups of lymph nodes, including bronchopulmonary, tracheobronchial, and paratracheal, before draining into the venous system via either the thoracic duct on the left side or right lymphatic trunk on the right side of the body.

■ NERVES

Most of the nerves that serve the lung are not visible at the level of the light microscope. They are components of the sympathetic and parasympathetic divisions of the autonomic nervous system and mediate reflexes that modify the dimensions of the air passages (and blood vessels) by contraction of the smooth muscle in their walls. In addition, the autonomic nervous system controls glandular secretion of the respiratory mucosa.

FOLDER 19.4
CLINICAL CORRELATION: CYSTIC FIBROSIS

Cystic fibrosis (CF, mucoviscidosis) is a chronic obstructive pulmonary disease of children and young adults. It is an autosomal recessive disorder caused by a mutation in a gene called the **cystic fibrosis transmembrane conductance regulator (CFTR)** located on chromosome 7. The product of this gene, the **Cl^- channel protein**, is involved in the final alteration of mucus and digestive secretions, sweat, and tears. All mutations of CFTR gene result in abnormal epithelial transport of Cl^- that affects the viscosity of the secretion of the exocrine glands. Almost all exocrine glands secrete abnormally viscid mucus that obstructs the glands and their excretory ducts.

The course of the disease is largely determined by the degree of pulmonary involvement. At birth, the lungs are normal. However, the defective Cl^- channel protein in the bronchial epithelium causes decreased Cl^- secretion and increased Na^+ and water reabsorption from the lumen (Fig. F19.4.1). As a result, the "mucociliary escalator" malfunctions, with consequent accumulation of an unusually thick, viscous mucous secretion. The pulmonary lesion is probably initiated by obstruction of the bronchioles. Bronchiolar obstruction blocks the airways and leads to thickening of the bronchiole walls and other degenerative changes in the alveoli. Because fluids remain trapped in the lungs, individuals with CF have frequent respiratory tract infections.

(continued)

FOLDER 19.4
CLINICAL CORRELATION: CYSTIC FIBROSIS (*continued*)

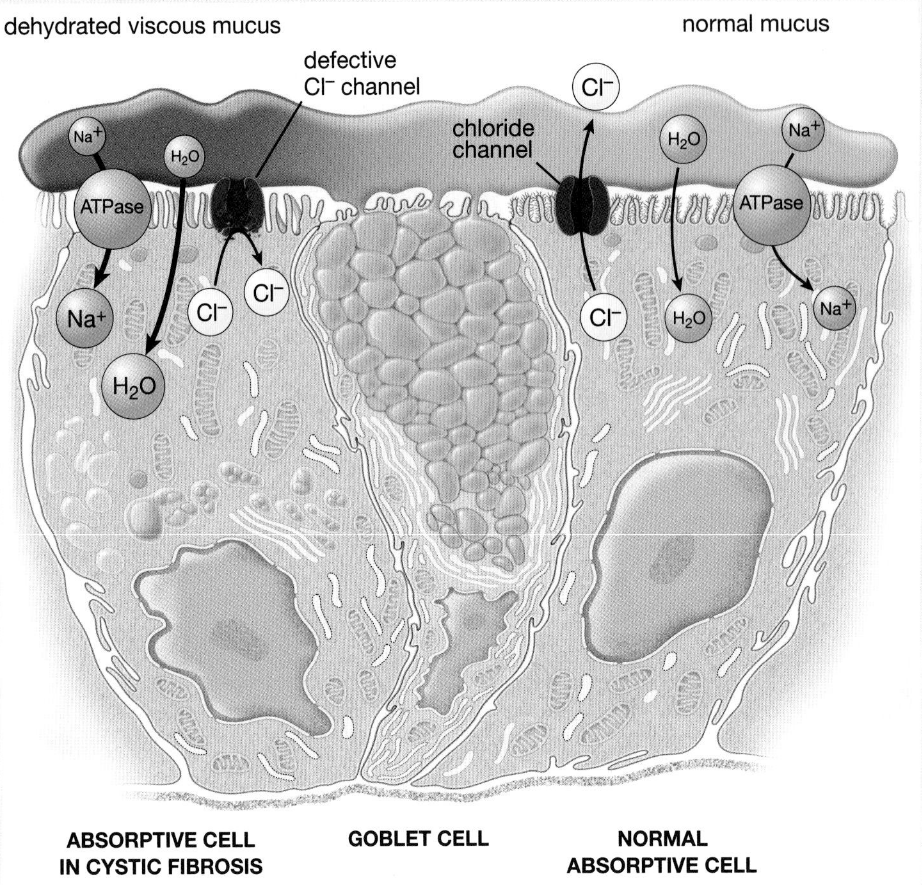

FIGURE F19.4.1. Schematic diagram of pathology in cystic fibrosis. In cystic fibrosis, secretion of Cl^- anions into the lumen of the bronchial tree is markedly decreased because of a defective or nonexistent chloride channel protein. Na^+ resorption from the lumen of the bronchial tree is then increased, causing movement of water into the cell. As a result, the mucous layer within the bronchial tree becomes dehydrated and viscous. This thick mucus is difficult to move by the mucociliary escalator mechanism, and it clogs the lumen of the bronchial tree, obstructing airflow.

FOLDER 19.5
CLINICAL CORRELATION: CHRONIC OBSTRUCTIVE PULMONARY DISEASE AND PNEUMONIA

Chronic obstructive pulmonary disease (COPD) is a pulmonary condition characterized by chronic obstruction of airflow. Several subtypes of COPD have been recognized, including **chronic bronchitis**, **chronic obstructive asthma**, and **emphysema**. The severity of COPD is clinically more important, however, than recognition of the specific subtype.

Emphysema is a condition of the lung characterized by permanent enlargement of the air spaces distal to the terminal bronchiole. This enlargement is accompanied by destruction of the alveolar wall (Fig. F19.5.1a). Thus, significant surface area for gas exchange is lost in this disease. Emphysema is relatively common; it is seen in about half of all autopsies and is easily recognized. Emphysema is often caused by chronic inhalations of foreign particulate material, such as coal dust, textile fibers, and construction dust. The most common cause, however, is cigarette smoking.

The destruction of the alveolar wall may be associated with excess lysis of elastin and other structural proteins in the interalveolar septa. Elastase and other proteases are derived from lung neutrophils, macrophages, and monocytes. A specific genetic disease, **α_1-antitrypsin deficiency**, causes a particularly severe form of emphysema in both heterozygous and homozygous individuals. It is usually fatal in homozygotes if untreated, but its severity can be reduced by supplying the enzyme inhibitor exogenously.

Pneumonia is a generic term that describes inflammation of the lung parenchyma. It is often caused by infection with viruses or bacteria and less often by other microorganisms. Certain drugs (immunosuppressive agents) and autoimmune diseases increase the risk of certain types of pneumonia. Despite the impact of antibiotics, pneumonia caused by *Streptococcus pneumoniae* is quite common (~50% of cases), especially in young and middle-aged adults. Other common bacteria causing pneumonia include *Haemophilus influenzae*, *Chlamydophila pneumoniae*, *Mycoplasma pneumoniae*, *Staphylococcus aureus*, and various Gram-negative microorganisms.

Pneumonia is most commonly acquired by individuals with no primary disorders of the immune system in a community setting (**community-acquired pneumonia**). However, it may be acquired by the infection spread by an organism in the hospital environment (**nosocomial pneumonia**) or as an **opportunistic pneumonia** in individuals with compromised immune systems.

FOLDER 19.5

CLINICAL CORRELATION: CHRONIC OBSTRUCTIVE PULMONARY DISEASE AND PNEUMONIA (*continued*)

In the earliest stage of **bacterial pneumonia**, protein-rich fluid containing numerous microorganisms fills the lung alveoli. Marked enlargement of the capillaries surrounding the alveoli is followed by a massive migration of neutrophils and erythrocytes into the alveolar air space (Fig. F19.5.1b). At this stage, the lung is firm and red and resembles the liver; for this reason, it is often referred to as the **red hepatization stage** of pneumonia. In the next stage, macrophages phagocytose the fragmented neutrophils and other cellular and tissue debris. This stage is called the **gray hepatization stage**; congestion is diminished, but the lung remains firm. The alveolar exudate is then removed, the alveolar spaces gradually become refilled with air, and the lungs return to their normal function.

Respiratory infections caused by **coronavirus 2 (SARS-CoV-2)** range in severity from mild (resembling the common cold) to severe (severe acute respiratory syndrome). The SARS-CoV-2 virus targets cells in the nasal mucosa, bronchial epithelium, and alveolar pneumocytes. Lung examinations from autopsies of individuals who died from SARS-CoV-2 (COVID-19) infection reveal the presence of **diffuse alveolar damage** (characterized by interstitial and alveolar edema, the presence of hyaline membranes composed of condensed plasma proteins that line alveolar walls, proliferation of type II pneumocytes, and progressive interstitial fibrosis), accompanied by extensive **vascular damage** with thrombosis.

The molecular mechanism of SARS-CoV-2 infection is initiated by the virus spike protein (S), which binds to the angiotensin-converting enzyme 2 (ACE2) receptor expressed mainly on type II pneumocytes. This binding activates the virus spike S protein, mediating the entry of the virus into the pneumonocyte. In the later stages of lung infection, the virus spreads into the endothelial cells of pulmonary capillaries and pericytes. In response, an inflammatory reaction involving infiltration by monocytes and neutrophils occurs that eventually leads to diffuse alveolar damage. Accompanied fulminant activation of the coagulation cascade leads to thrombosis, pulmonary emboli, and lung infarcts.

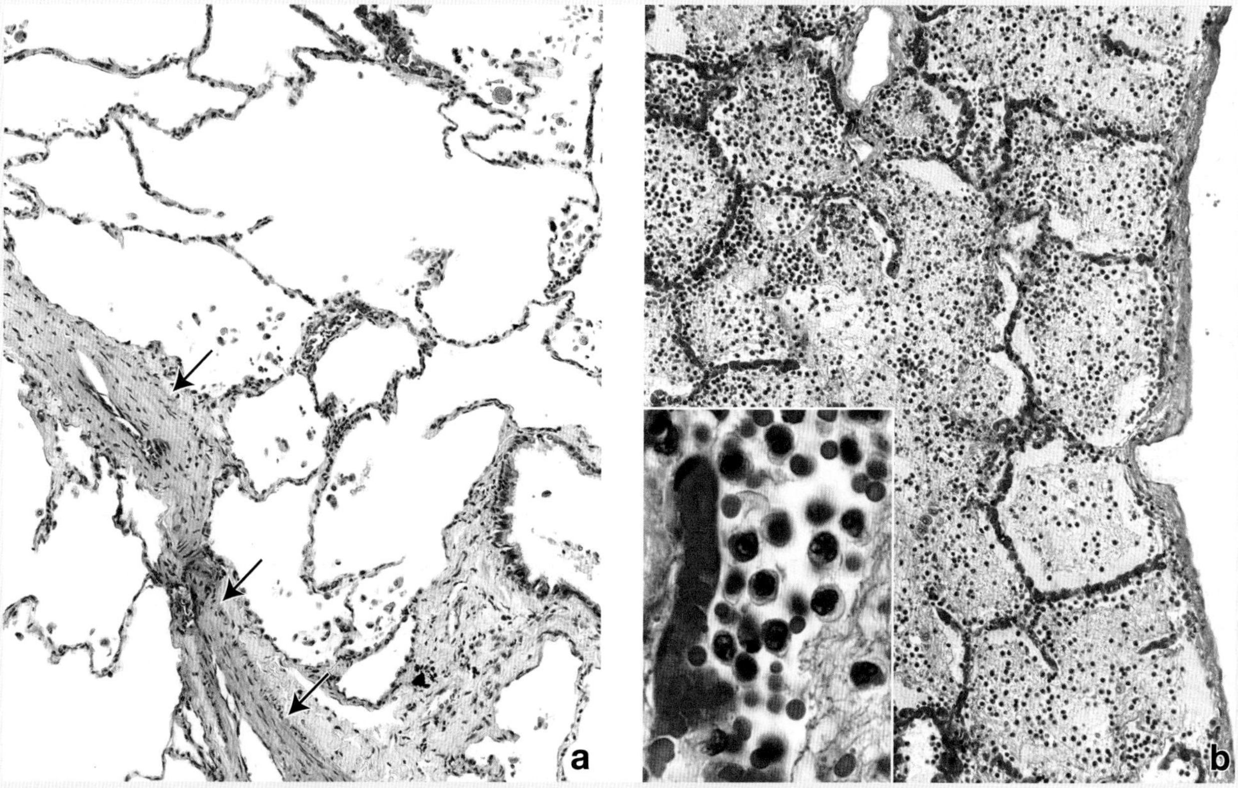

FIGURE F19.5.1. Photomicrographs of emphysema and pneumonia. a. This photomicrograph from the lung of an individual with emphysema shows the partial destruction of interalveolar septa, resulting in permanent enlargement of the air spaces. Note that the changes in the lung parenchyma are accompanied by thickening of the wall of the pulmonary vessels (*arrows*) and the presence of numerous cells within the air spaces. These cells are alveolar macrophages and are shown at higher magnification in Figure 19.22. ×240. **b.** This photomicrograph is from the lung of an individual in the early stages of acute pneumonia (inflammation of the lung). Note that the air spaces are filled with exudate containing white blood cells (mainly neutrophils), red blood cells, and fibrin. The capillaries in the interalveolar septum are enlarged and congested with red blood cells. Pathologists recognize this stage as the red hepatization stage of pneumonia. At this stage, the affected portion of the lung on gross examination appears red (because of enlarged capillaries), firm (because of the lack of air spaces), and heavy (because of the presence of exudate within the alveoli); the term *hepatization* stems from the tissue's resemblance to the liver. ×240. **Inset.** Part of an alveolus at a higher magnification. Note the enlarged, congested capillary within the interalveolar septum. The air space is filled with neutrophils and red blood cells. The *lower right* corner shows early organization of the intra-alveolar exudate; observe that the developing fibrin network contains entrapped neutrophils and several red blood cells. ×420.

RESPIRATORY SYSTEM

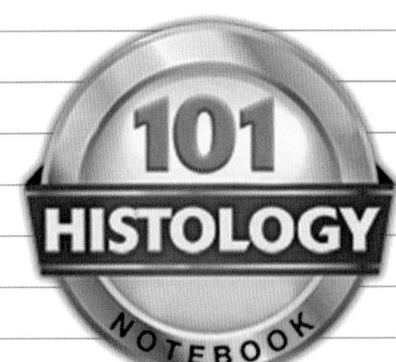

OVERVIEW OF THE RESPIRATORY SYSTEM

- The **respiratory system** consists of the paired lungs and a series of air passages that lead to and from the lungs.
- Three principal functions of the respiratory system are **air conduction, air filtration**, and **gas exchange (respiration).**
- The **upper part of the respiratory system** (nasal cavities, paranasal sinuses, nasopharynx, and oropharynx) develops from the primitive oral cavity.
- The **lower part of the respiratory system** (larynx, trachea, bronchi with their divisions, and lungs) develops from the ventral evagination of the foregut endoderm.
- The **conducting portion** of the respiratory system includes the upper part of the respiratory system, larynx, trachea, bronchi, and most of the bronchioles (up to the terminal bronchioles).
- The **respiratory portion** contains the respiratory bronchioles, alveolar ducts, alveolar sacs, and alveoli.

NASAL CAVITIES

- The paired chambers of the **nasal cavities** are divided into **vestibules** (entrance to nasal cavities), **respiratory regions**, and **olfactory regions.**
- The **respiratory region** is lined by the **respiratory mucosa** that contains **ciliated, pseudostratified columnar epithelium.**
- Respiratory epithelium is composed of tall **columnar cells** with cilia (for movement of secretion and other particles on the mucosal surface), **goblet cells** (to secrete mucus), **brush cells** (for sensory innervation), **small granule cells** (enteroendocrine cells for secreting hormones and cytokines), and **basal cells** (stem cells).
- The **respiratory mucosa** warms, moistens, and filters inspired air. It possesses a rich vascular network in the lamina propria, as well as numerous mucus- and serous-secreting glands.
- The **olfactory region** located at the roof of the nasal cavity is lined by a pseudostratified olfactory epithelium without goblet cells.
- **Olfactory epithelium** is composed of **olfactory receptor cells** (bipolar neurons), **supporting cells, brush cells**, and **basal cells.**
- **Olfactory receptor cells** possess apical immotile cilia, which contain G-protein–coupled receptors involved in the olfactory transduction pathway.
- **Olfactory (Bowman) glands** are a characteristic feature of the olfactory mucosa.

PHARYNX AND LARYNX

- The **pharynx** is a posterior continuation of the oral and nasal cavities. It passes food into the esophagus and air into the larynx.
- The **larynx** is a connection between the pharynx and the trachea. It contains **vocal folds** that control the flow of air through the larynx and vibrate to produce sound.
- The larynx is lined by the **respiratory mucosa**, except for the luminal surface of the vocal cords, which is covered by a **stratified squamous epithelium.**

TRACHEA

- The **trachea** extends from the larynx into the mediastinum, where it divides into the two main (primary) bronchi.
- The wall of the trachea consists of four layers: **mucosa** (composed of a ciliated, pseudostratified epithelium resting on a thick basement membrane), **submucosa** (dense irregular connective tissue), **cartilaginous layer** (composed of C-shaped hyaline cartilages), and **adventitia** (binds the trachea to adjacent structures).

BRONCHI AND BRONCHIOLES

- The trachea divides into **right and left main (primary) bronchi** that enter the lungs and undergo repeated divisions ending with the bronchioles.
- Bronchi are lined by **respiratory mucosa** with the same cellular composition as the trachea. They possess **cartilage plates** and a circular layer of **smooth muscle**.
- **Bronchioles** are branches of segmental bronchi that are 1 mm or less in diameter and do not possess cartilage plates or glands.
- The smallest conducting **terminal bronchioles** are lined with a simple cuboidal epithelium containing **club cells**. These cells produce a surface-acting agent that prevents airway collapse.
- **Respiratory bronchioles** are the first part of the bronchial tree that allows gas exchange.

ALVEOLI

- The **respiratory bronchiole** divides into the alveolar ducts that lead into alveolar sacs surrounded by clusters of alveoli.
- **Alveoli** are the terminal air spaces of the respiratory system. Their septa are the locations for gas exchange between the air and the blood.
- **Alveolar epithelium** is composed of type I and II alveolar cells (pneumocytes) with occasional brush cells.
- **Type I alveolar cells** are extremely thin squamous cells that line 95% of the alveolar surface and form the barrier between the air space and the septal wall.
- **Type II alveolar cells** are secretory cells that produce and secrete surfactant, which lowers surface tension in the alveoli. They have characteristic lamellar bodies visible with EM.
- The **interalveolar septum** is the site of the **air–blood barrier**. It consists of a thin layer of surfactant, a type I epithelial cell with its basal lamina, and a capillary endothelial cell with its basal lamina. Often, these two basal laminae are fused together.
- **Alveolar** and **septal macrophages** are present in alveolar air spaces and septal connective tissue, respectively.

BLOOD SUPPLY, INNERVATION, AND LYMPHATIC DRAINAGE

- The lung has both pulmonary and bronchial circulations.
- **Pulmonary circulation** delivers blood via branches of the pulmonary artery to the capillary network surrounding the alveoli for oxygenation. Blood is collected by pulmonary venous capillaries that eventually form the pulmonary veins.
- **Bronchial circulation**, via bronchial arteries, supplies the walls of the bronchi, bronchioles, and the remaining connective tissue of the lung.
- **Autonomic nerves** follow the branches of pulmonary arteries and innervate the smooth muscle of blood vessels, the bronchial tree, and the respiratory mucosa.
- A dual **lymphatic drainage** of the lungs parallels the dual blood supply. Accumulation of the bronchus-associated lymphatic tissue (**BALT**) and lymph nodes is frequently found near large bronchi.

PLATE 19.1 ■ OLFACTORY MUCOSA

Olfactory mucosa is located in the roof and part of the walls of the nasal cavity. Its pseudostratified epithelium is thicker than that of nonsensory epithelium, and it serves as the receptor for smell. Olfactory epithelium consists of **olfactory cells, supporting (sustentacular) cells, basal cells,** and **brush cells.**

Olfactory cells are bipolar neurons. The apex of the cell is expanded into the olfactory vesicle from which nonmotile cilia, the actual receptors, extend into surface secretions. The base of the cell tapers into an axonal process that enters the lamina propria and joins axons from other receptor cells to form the olfactory nerve. Large, cuboidal Schwann cells are a prominent feature of these axons, giving the nerve an unusual appearance.

Supporting cells are columnar cells with apical microvilli. They attach to the receptor cells through adhering junctions and provide mechanical and metabolic support to the olfactory cells. Basal cells are stem cells from which olfactory and supporting cells differentiate. Brush cells are the same cell type that occurs in nonsensory respiratory epithelium.

The lamina propria is directly contiguous with periosteum. It contains numerous blood and lymphatic vessels, unmyelinated and myelinated nerves, and **olfactory (Bowman) glands.** These are tubuloalveolar serous glands whose watery secretion serves as a trap and solvent for odorant substances and continuously washes the olfactory surface.

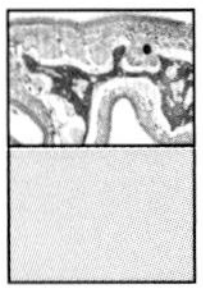

Olfactory mucosa, nasal cavity, human, Azan ×75.

This low-magnification orientation micrograph shows part of the wall of the nasal cavity. The **olfactory mucosa** (*OM*), adjacent ethmoid bone (*EB*), and ethmoid sinus (*ES*) are indicated. The olfactory mucosa is directly attached to the bone tissue; no submucosa is present. In this specimen, however, the mucosa is separated from the bone tissue because of shrinkage, a frequently encountered artifact. The **olfactory epithelium** (*OEp*) is pseudostratified, like respiratory epithelium; however, it is typically thicker. Note the **respiratory epithelium** (*REp*) included in the *lower right* of the micrograph. The feature that is most useful in identifying olfactory mucosa is the presence of numerous large, unmyelinated nerves (*N*) and extensive **olfactory (Bowman) glands** (*BG*) in the connective tissue of the mucosa. Occasional blood vessels (i.e., arteries [*A*] and veins) are also visible. Note that the adjacent respiratory mucosa lacks nerves and exhibits a relative paucity of glands.

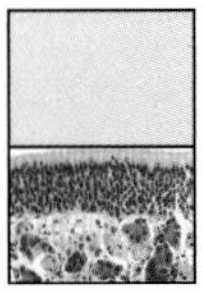

Olfactory mucosa, nasal cavity, human, Azan ×375.

At this higher magnification, it is possible to distinguish in a general way the three principal cell types of the olfactory epithelium on the basis of nuclear location and appearance as well as by certain cytoplasmic characteristics. For example, the nuclei of the **supporting cells** (*SC*) are relatively dense and are located closest to the epithelial surface. They are arranged in an almost discrete single layer. The supporting cell has a cylindrical shape and extends from the basement membrane through the full thickness of the epithelium. Immediately beneath this layer are the cell bodies of the **olfactory receptor cells** (*OC*). They lie at different levels within the thickness of the epithelium. Careful examination of the nuclei of these bipolar neuronal cells reveals that they contain more euchromatin than the nuclei of the supporting cells and often exhibit several nucleoli. In this preparation, the nucleoli appear as small round red bodies. In some cases, particularly when there is shrinkage, the thin tapering dendritic process that extends to the olfactory surface may be observed. Similarly, an axonal process may sometimes be observed extending basally. The **basal cells** (*BC*), the least numerous of the principal cell types, are characterized by their small round nuclei and scant cytoplasm. They are irregularly spaced and lie in proximity to the basement membrane. Note that the olfactory mucosa in contrast to respiratory mucosa lacks goblet cells.

The **lamina propria** contains numerous blood vessels (capillaries [*C*], veins [*V*]), lymphatics, olfactory nerves (*N*), and olfactory (Bowman) glands (*BG*). The **Bowman glands** are branched tubuloalveolar structures. They exhibit a very small lumen (*arrows*). The duct elements extend from the secretory portion of the gland beginning in close proximity to the overlying epithelium (*arrowhead*) and pass directly through the epithelium to deliver their secretions at the surface. The ducts are very short, making it difficult to identify them. The very thin axonal processes (*AP*) of the olfactory cells are sometimes evident within the lamina propria before being ensheathed by Schwann cells to form the prominent olfactory nerves. The nuclei present within the olfactory nerves represent Schwann cell nuclei (*ScC*).

A, artery
AP, axonal process
BC, basal cells
BG, Bowman glands
C, capillary
EB, ethmoid bone
ES, ethmoid sinus
N, olfactory nerves
OC, olfactory cells
OEp, olfactory epithelium
OM, olfactory mucosa
REp, respiratory epithelium
SC, supporting cell nuclei
ScC, Schwann cell nuclei
V, vein
arrows, lumina of Bowman glands
arrowhead, duct of a Bowman gland entering epithelium

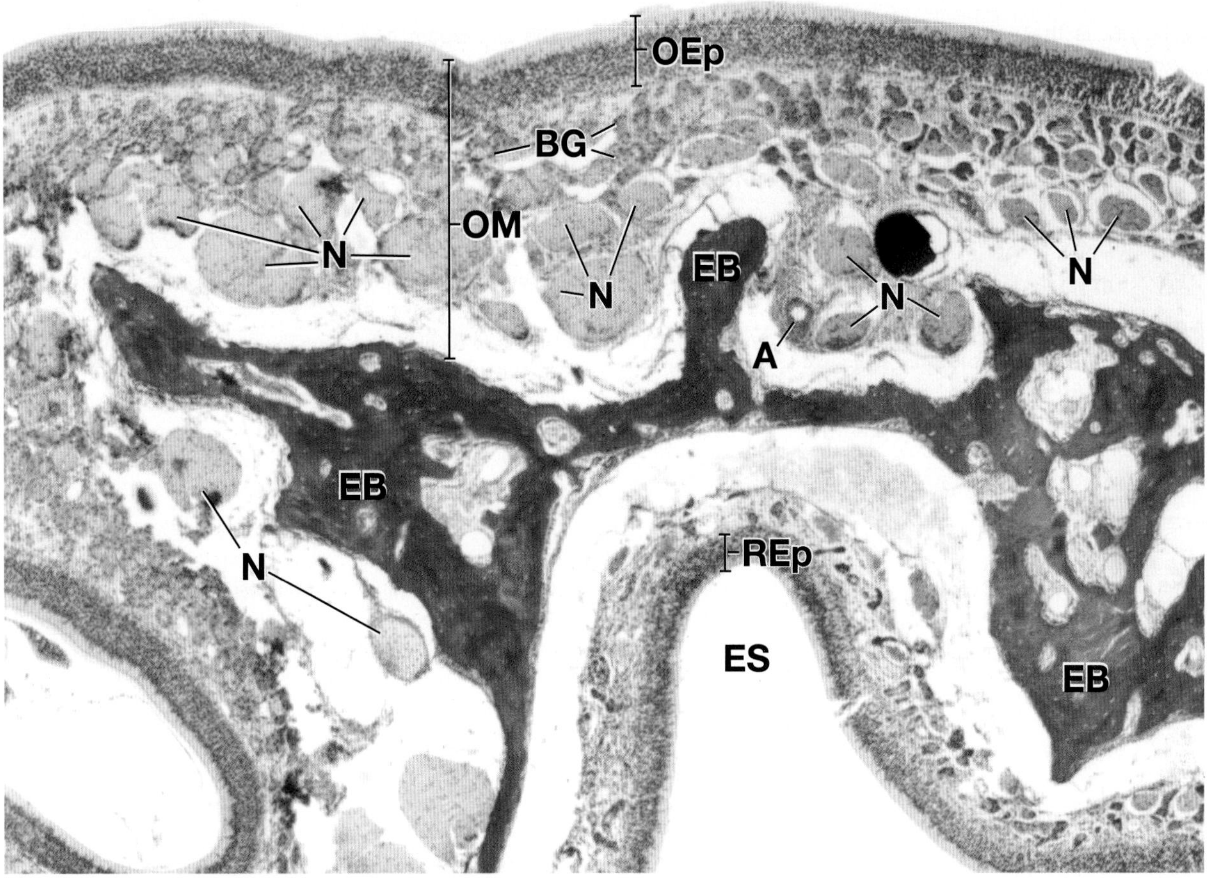
OEp
BG
OM
N
N
EB
N
N
A
EB
N
REp
ES
EB

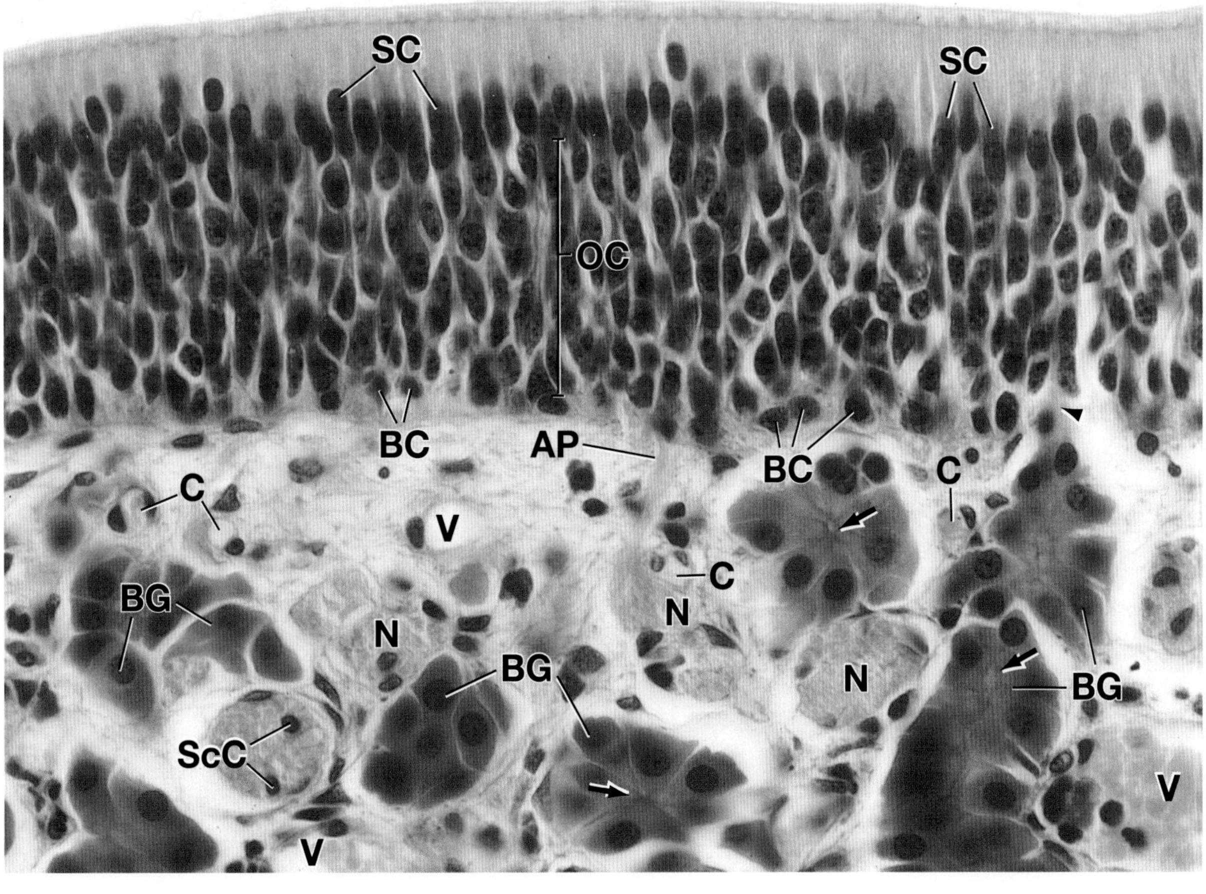
SC
SC
OC
BC
AP
BC
C
C
V
C
BG
N
N
BG
N
BG
ScC
V
V

PLATE 19.2 ■ LARYNX

The **larynx** is the passageway for air between the oropharynx and the trachea that functions in the production of sound. It consists of a cartilaginous framework to which both extrinsic and intrinsic muscles are attached and a mucosal surface that varies in character from pseudostratified to stratified squamous in regions subject to abrasion by the air stream. The muscles move certain cartilages with respect to others, thus increasing or decreasing the opening of the rima glottis and increasing or decreasing the tension on the vocal folds (cords). In this way, vibrations of different wavelengths are generated in the passing air, and sound is produced.

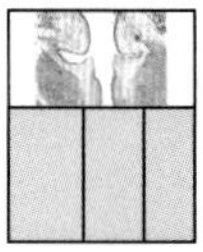

Larynx, monkey, hematoxylin and eosin (H&E) ×15.

The **vocal folds** are ridge-like structures that are oriented in an anteroposterior (ventral-dorsal) direction. In frontal sections, the vocal folds (*VF*) are cross-sectioned, giving the appearance seen here. The two vocal folds and the space between them constitute the glottis. Just above each vocal fold is an elongated recess called the **ventricle** (*V*), and above the ventricle is another ridge called the **ventricular fold** (*VnF*) or, sometimes, the false vocal fold. Below and lateral to the vocal folds are the vocalis muscles (*VM*). Within the vocal fold is a considerable amount of elastic material, although it is usually not evident in routine H&E preparations. This elastic material is part of the vocal ligament. It lies in an anteroposterior direction within the substance of the vocal fold and plays an important role in phonation.

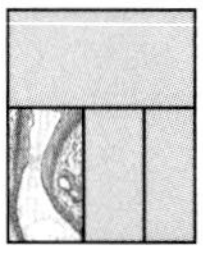

Ventricular and vocal folds, larynx, monkey, H&E ×160.

The surfaces of a **vocal fold** and the facing ventricular fold within *rectangle 1* in the *top figure* are turned 90 degree clockwise and shown at higher magnification in this figure. Medially, both are lined by **stratified squamous epithelium** (*SSE*). Here, the contact between surfaces is considerable. Laterally, the surfaces consist of **stratified columnar epithelium** (*SCE*). The contact between these surfaces is less wearing. Small glands (*Gl*) are in the lamina propria of the laryngeal mucosa.

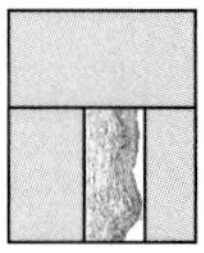

Infraglottic cavity, larynx, monkey, H&E ×160.

Rectangle 2 in the *top figure* is shown at higher magnification in this figure. This area of the larynx below the ventricles and rima glottidis communicates with the trachea and is called the *infraglottic cavity*. It shows the junction between the **stratified squamous epithelium** (*SSE*), with its flat surface cells, and the **stratified columnar epithelium** (*SCE*), with its columnar surface cells. The lamina propria consists of loose connective tissue in which glands (*Gl*) are present.

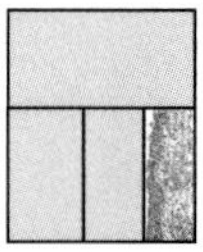

Infraglottic cavity, larynx, monkey, H&E ×160.

Epithelium of the infraglottic cavity of the larynx just below the portion shown in the *top figure* changes again, giving way, below, to the **ciliated pseudostratified columnar epithelium** (*PSE*) shown here. Note the cylinders of cytoplasm that clearly indicate the columnar nature of the surface cells. In the *upper part* of the figure, the epithelium is stratified columnar; in the *lower part* of the figure, it is pseudostratified columnar. This distinction is difficult to make from the examination of a single sample such as that shown here, and other information is needed to make the assessment. The additional information is the presence of cilia on the pseudostratified columnar epithelium; this epithelium is typically ciliated. Although not evident in the photomicrographs, note that stratified columnar epithelium has a very limited distribution, usually occurring between stratified squamous epithelium and some other epithelial types (e.g., pseudostratified columnar here or simple columnar at the anorectal junction; Plate 17.11, page 690). The lamina propria is a loose cellular connective tissue, and it also shows some glands (*Gl*).

Gl, glands
PSE, pseudostratified columnar epithelium
SCE, stratified columnar epithelium
SSE, stratified squamous epithelium
V, ventricles
VF, vocal folds
VM, vocalis muscles
VnF, ventricular folds

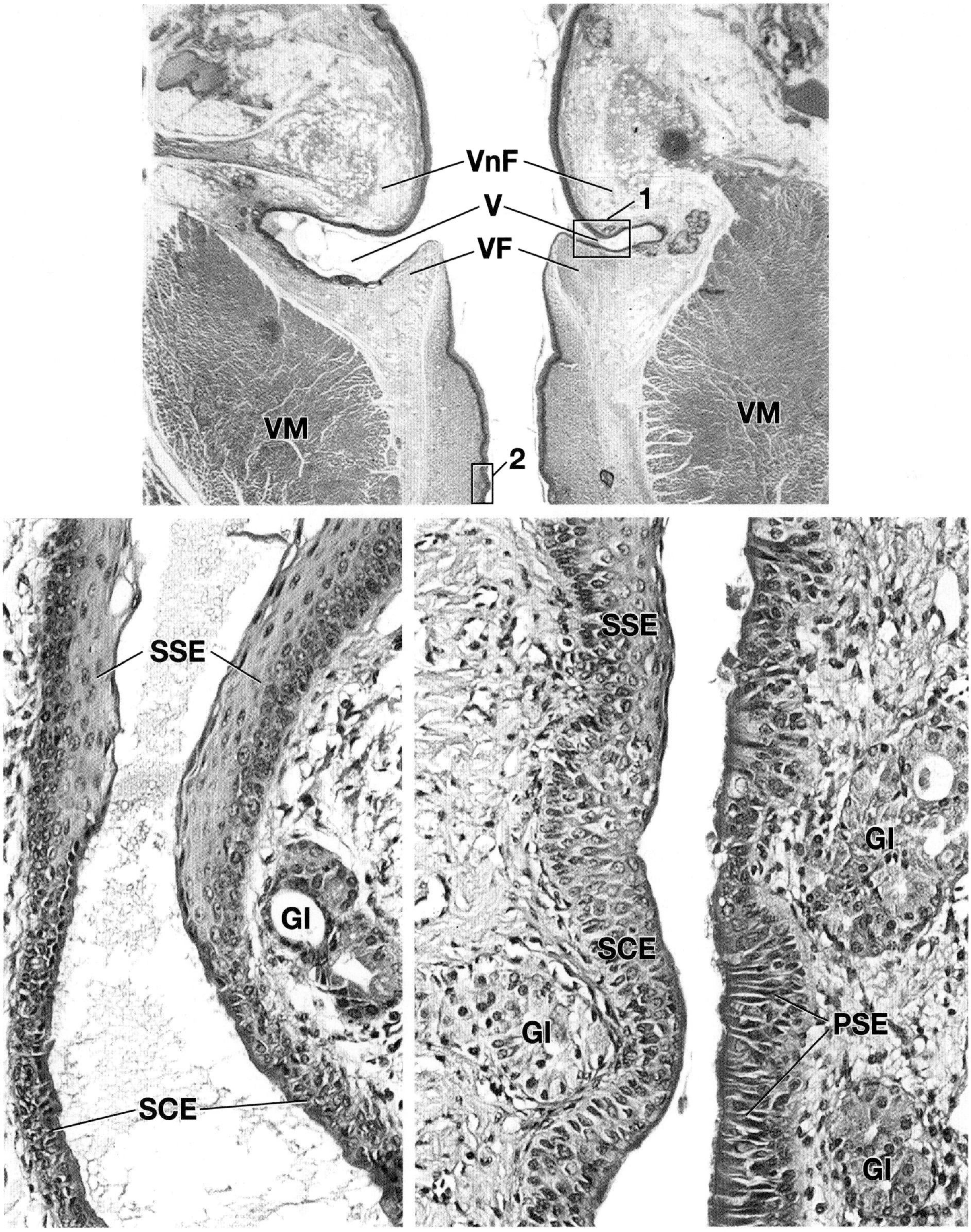
VnF
V
VF
1
VM
VM
2
SSE
GI
SCE
SSE
SCE
GI
GI
PSE
GI

PLATE 19.3 ■ TRACHEA

The **trachea** is a short tube about 2.5 cm in diameter and about 10 cm long. It extends from the larynx to about the middle of the thorax, where it divides into the two main bronchi (**primary bronchi**). Its major function is to serve as a conduit for air. The lumen of the trachea is held open by a series of C-shaped hyaline cartilages that are stacked on one another to form a supporting structure. Fibroelastic tissue and smooth muscle (the **trachealis muscle**) bridge the gap between the free ends of the cartilages at the posterior border of the trachea, adjacent to the esophagus. Typical respiratory (ciliated pseudostratified columnar) epithelium lines the trachea and primary bronchi.

On entering the lungs, the primary bronchi branch immediately to give rise to the **lobar bronchi (secondary bronchi)** that supply the two lobes of the left lung and the three lobes of the right lung. Within the lung, the C-shaped cartilages are replaced by an investment of (sometimes overlapping) cartilaginous plates that completely surround the bronchi.

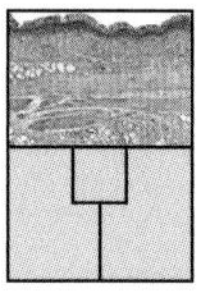

Trachea, human, hematoxylin and eosin (H&E) ×90.

This low-magnification micrograph of the posterior wall of the human trachea shows the **pseudostratified ciliated columnar epithelium** (*EP*) subtended by a well-developed **basement membrane** (*Bm*). The basement membrane, which consists of tightly packed, fine collagen fibers, is actually an unusually thick and dense reticular layer and is thus part of the lamina propria. It is particularly distinct in the human trachea and may thicken with chronic irritation, as in smokers. Numerous goblet cells (*GC*) are evident as clear ovoid spaces in the respiratory epithelium. A thin **lamina propria** (*LP*) and a dense thick submucosa (*SM*) underlie the respiratory epithelium. Seromucous glands (*Gl*) are seen on both sides of the **trachealis muscle** (*TM*), a band of smooth muscle that fills the gap between the posterior ends of the C-shaped tracheal cartilages (not shown) and serves to separate the trachea from the esophagus. Adipose tissue (*Ad*) is also present in the submucosa between the esophagus and the trachea.

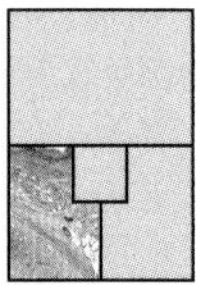

Trachea, human, H&E ×65.

This micrograph shows the wall of the trachea at the level of one end of the C-shaped tracheal cartilage (*TC*). The portion of the **pseudostratified ciliated columnar epithelium** (*EP*) does not exhibit as many goblet cells as are seen in the previous figure. However, the **basement membrane** (*Bm*) is clear, as are the cellular **lamina propria** (*LP*) and the **submucosa** (*SM*) of the trachea. Again, seromucous glands (*Gl*) are evident beneath the submucosa. The ends of the bundles of the trachealis muscle (*TM*) are located toward the posterior midline from the glands. A small lymphatic nodule (*LN*) is located adjacent to the end of one of the bundles. A significant amount of adipose tissue (*Ad*) is found in the connective tissue between the trachealis muscle and the wall of the esophagus (not shown in this figure).

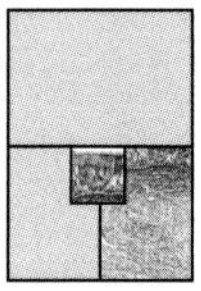

Trachea, human, H&E ×250; inset ×500.

In this higher magnification micrograph of the tracheal wall and in the *inset*, the cilia of the **pseudostratified ciliated columnar epithelium** (*EP*) are particularly well demonstrated, as is the dense line (*BB*) formed by the basal bodies of the cilia (*C*) in the apical cytoplasm of the epithelial cells. **Goblet cells** (*GC*) are easily recognized, and the displacement of the flattened nucleus (*N*) toward the base of the cell is well demonstrated. The thickness and density of the **basement membrane** (*Bm*) are more easily seen here than in the lower magnification views in the other figures. A venule (*V*) containing red cell ghosts is seen in the middle of the submucosa, and some inflammatory cells (*IC*), probably lymphocytes, are seen adjacent to the vein as well as distributed lightly through the submucosa and more densely in the lamina propria. Portions of the seromucous glands (*Gl*) are just visible at the *bottom edge* of the figure.

Ad, adipose tissue
BB, basal bodies
Bm, basement membrane
C, cilia
EP, epithelium
GC, goblet cells
Gl, glands
IC, inflammatory cells
LN, lymphatic nodule
LP, lamina propria
N, nuclei of goblet cells
SM, submucosa
TC, tracheal cartilage
TM, trachealis muscle
V, vein

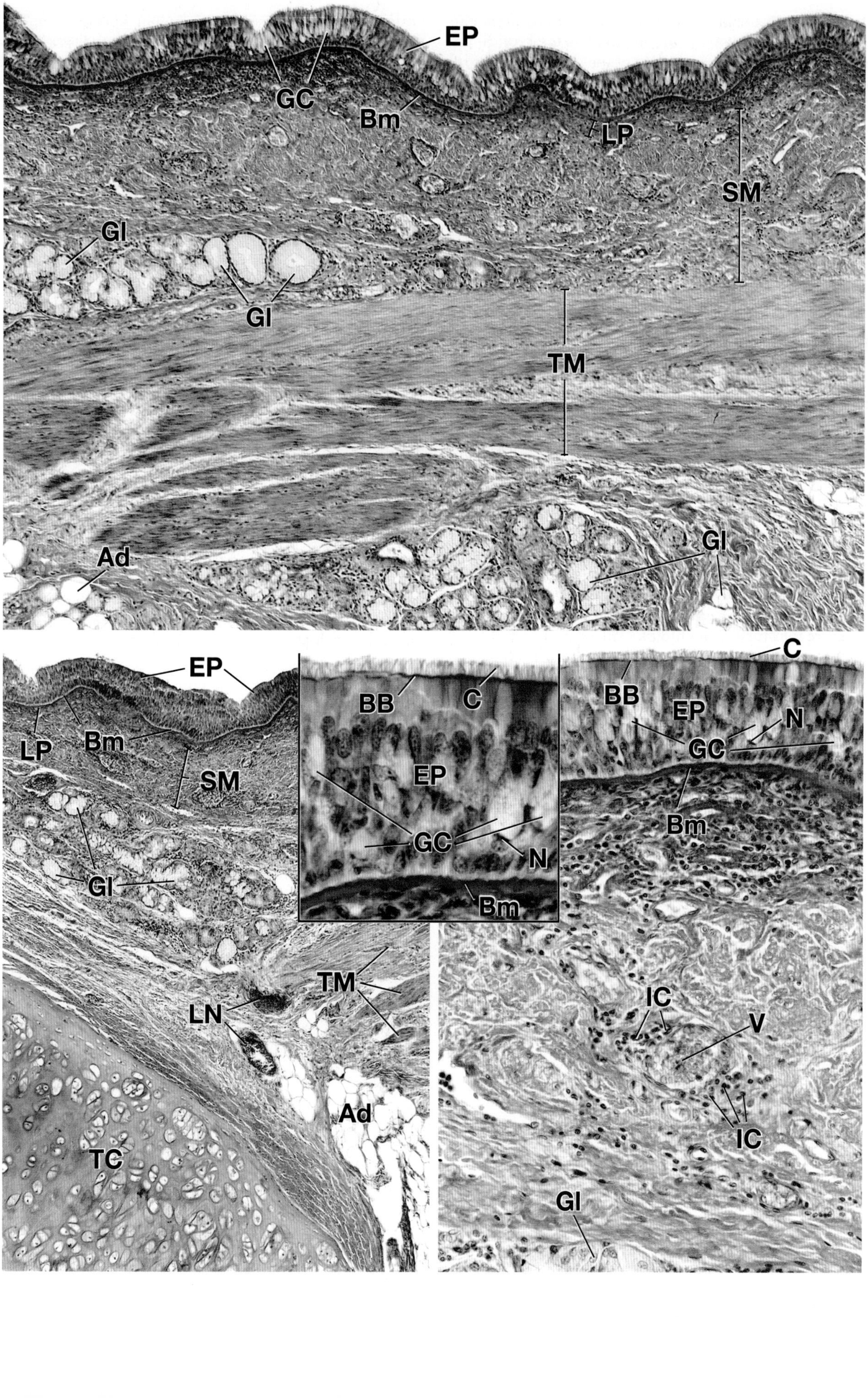
EP
GC
Bm
LP
SM
Gl
Gl
TM
Ad
Gl
EP
LP
Bm
SM
Gl
TM
LN
Ad
TC
BB
C
EP
GC
N
Bm
C
BB
EP
N
GC
Bm
IC
V
IC
Gl

The **primary bronchus** that enters each lung divides into smaller secondary and tertiary bronchi. As the bronchi become smaller, some components of the wall are lost or reduced in amount. Ultimately, the respiratory passage has distinctly different features than those of a bronchus, and it is called a **bronchiole.** The features that characterize the bronchiole are the absence of cartilage, loss of submucosal glands, and gradual disappearance of goblet cells. The epithelium changes from pseudostratified columnar to simple ciliated columnar, and some columnar cells even lack cilia. Smooth muscle occupies a relatively larger portion of the bronchiolar wall than the bronchial wall.

The smallest diameter conducting bronchioles, the **terminal bronchioles**, are lined with simple ciliated cuboidal epithelium in which club cells, cells that secrete a surface-active agent that prevents luminal adhesion of bronchiolar walls during expiration, are found among the ciliated cells. **Respiratory bronchioles** are the first part of the bronchial tree that allows gas exchange to occur. Respiratory bronchioles constitute a transition zone in which both air conduction and gas exchange occur. Scattered, thin-walled evaginations of the lumen of the respiratory bronchiole are called **alveoli**; these are the structures in which gas exchange between the air passages and the blood capillaries occurs.

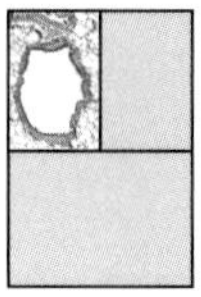

Bronchiole, lungs, human, hematoxylin and eosin (H&E) ×75.

A typical **bronchiole** (*B*) is shown here. Characteristically, blood vessels (*BV*) are adjacent to the bronchiole. The main features of the bronchiolar wall that are evident in the figure are bundles of smooth muscle (*SM*) and the lining epithelium (shown at higher magnification in Plate 19.5, page 766). Higher magnification would reveal that the epithelium is ciliated. The connective tissue is minimal and, at this low magnification, not conspicuous. Nevertheless, it is present and separates the muscle into bundles (i.e., the muscle layer is not a single continuous layer). The connective tissue contains collagenous and some elastic fibers. Glands are not present in the wall of the bronchiole. Surrounding the bronchiole, comprising most of the lung substance, are the air spaces or alveoli of the lung.

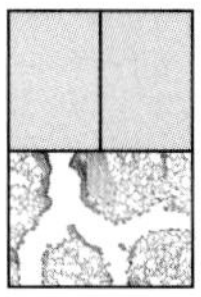

Bronchiole and respiratory bronchioles, lungs, human, H&E ×75.

In this figure, a short length of a bronchiole (*B*) is shown longitudinally sectioned as it branches into two **respiratory bronchioles** (*RB*). The last portion of a bronchiole that leads into respiratory bronchioles is called a **terminal bronchiole**. It is not engaged in exchange of air with the blood; the respiratory bronchiole does engage in air exchange. *Arrows* mark the place where the terminal bronchiole ends. Not uncommonly, as shown here, cartilage (*C*) is found in the bronchiolar wall where branching occurs. Blood vessels (*BV*) and a nodule of lymphocytes (*L*) are adjacent to the bronchiole.

The respiratory bronchiole has a wall composed of two components: One consists of recesses that have a wall similar to that of the alveoli and are thus capable of gas exchange; the other has a wall formed by small cuboidal cells that appear to rest on a small bundle of eosinophilic material. This is smooth muscle surrounded by a thin investment of connective tissue. Both of these components are shown at higher magnification in Plate 19.5 (page 766).

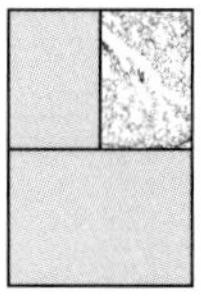

Alveoli, lungs, human, H&E ×75.

The most distal component of the respiratory passage is the alveolus. Groups of alveoli clustered together and sharing a common opening are referred to as an **alveolar sac** (*AS*). Alveoli that form a tube are referred to as **alveolar ducts** (*AD*). The outer surface of lung tissue is the serosa (*S*); it consists of a lining of mesothelial cells resting on a small amount of connective tissue. This is the layer that gross anatomists refer to as the **visceral pleura**.

AD, alveolar ducts
AS, alveolar sacs
B, bronchiole
BV, blood vessels
C, cartilage
L, nodule of lymphocytes
RB, respiratory bronchiole
S, serosa
SM, smooth muscle
arrows, end of terminal bronchiole

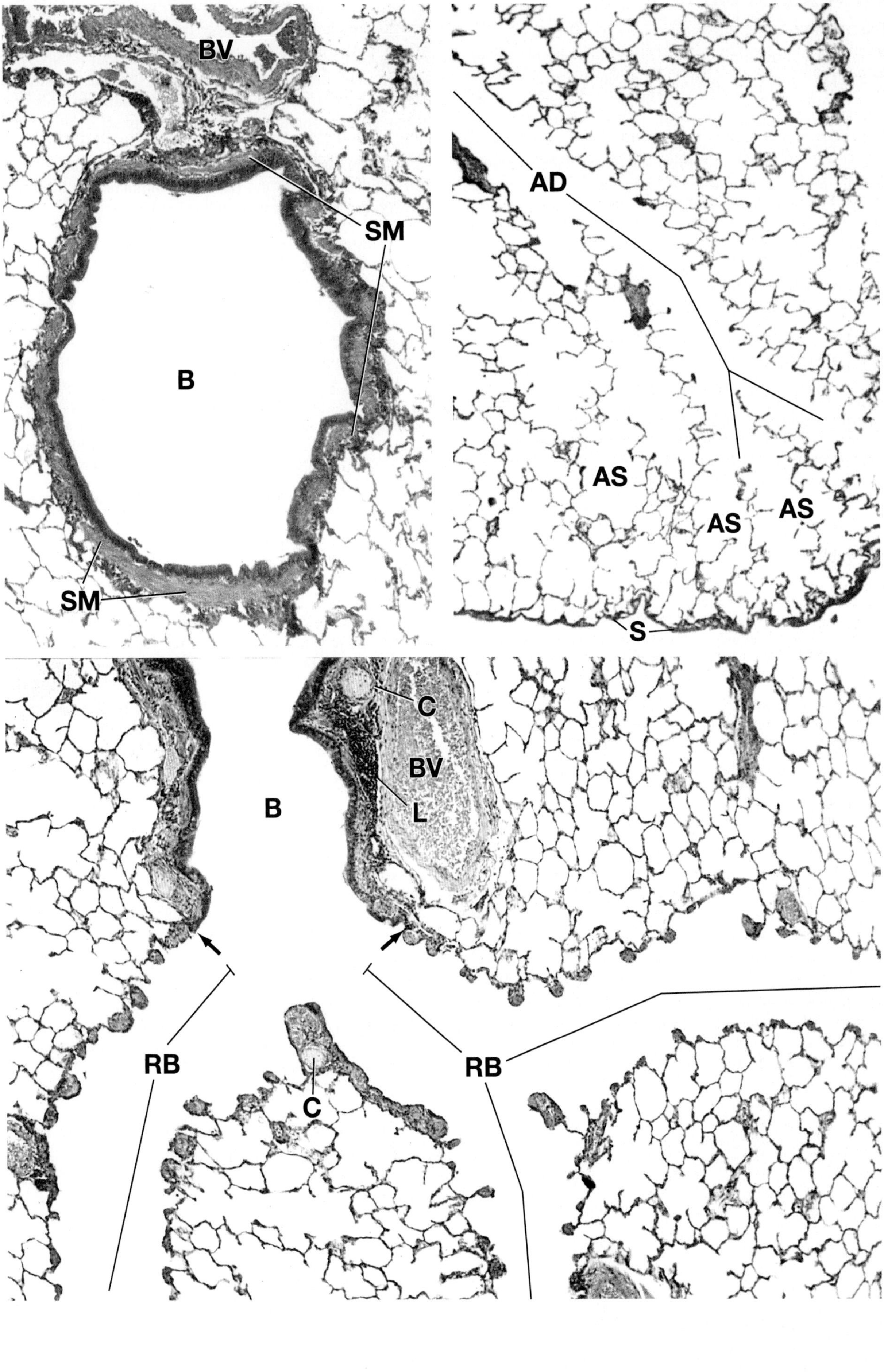
BV
SM
SM
B
SM
AD
AS
AS
AS
S
C
BV
L
B
RB
RB
C

PLATE 19.5 ■ TERMINAL BRONCHIOLE, RESPIRATORY BRONCHIOLE, AND ALVEOLUS

Respiratory bronchioles continue to divide to form **alveolar ducts**, passages lined solely with rows of alveoli that have rings of smooth muscle in knob-like interalveolar septa. The alveolar ducts terminate in **alveolar sacs**, enlarged spaces surrounded by clusters of alveoli that open into the spaces. The alveoli are lined with **type I alveolar cells**, extremely thin squamous cells that cover about 95% of the alveolar surface, and with **type II alveolar cells**, cuboidal cells that secrete **surfactant**, a surface-active agent that reduces surface tension at the air–epithelium surface. The tissue between adjacent alveoli is called the **interalveolar septum**. This consists of the alveolar epithelial cells and their basal lamina, the basal lamina of the underlying capillary endothelium and the endothelial cells, themselves, and any other connective tissue elements that may lie between the two basal laminae. The **interalveolar septum** is the site of the **air–blood barrier**.

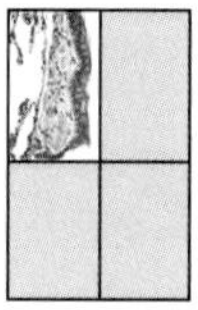

Terminal bronchiole, lungs, human, hematoxylin and eosin (H&E) ×550.

The histologic features of the terminal bronchiolar wall are shown here. Ciliated epithelium extends from the *top* of the figure to the *diamond*. This is **ciliated pseudostratified columnar epithelium** (*PsEp*). Some basal cells are still present, thus the designation pseudostratified columnar. Elsewhere, the epithelium might be ciliated simple columnar, and just before it becomes a respiratory bronchiole, the epithelium may include cuboidal or low columnar nonciliated cells. These nonciliated cells are **club cells** (*CC*, beyond the *diamond*). Club cells produce a surface-active agent that is instrumental in the expansion of the lungs. The smooth muscle (*SM*) in the bronchiolar wall is organized in bundles; other cells under the epithelium and around the smooth muscle belong to the connective tissue.

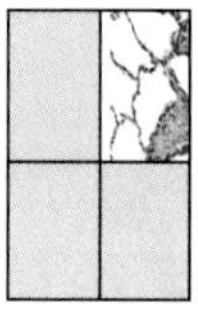

Respiratory bronchiole, lungs, human, H&E ×550.

The wall of a **respiratory bronchiole** is shown here and in the *lower left* figure. The alveoli (*A*) are terminal air spaces on the *left* in each of the two figures. The lumen of the respiratory bronchiole is on the *right*. Characteristically, the wall of the respiratory bronchiole consists of alternating thick and thin regions. The thick regions are similar to the wall of the bronchiole, except that cuboidal club cells, instead of columnar epithelium, form the surface. Thus, as seen here, **club cells** (*CC*) are the surface-lining cells of the thick regions, and **smooth muscle bundles** (*SM*) are under the club cells, with a small amount of intervening connective tissue. The thin regions have a wall similar to the alveolar wall; this is considered in the next figure.

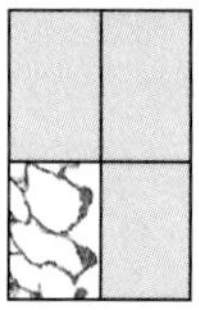

Respiratory bronchiole, lungs, human, H&E ×550.

The **respiratory bronchiole** shown in this figure is slightly more distal than the area seen in the *top right* figure. Structurally, the wall of respiratory bronchiole is surrounded by alveoli (*A*), and it shows essentially the same features as those seen in the *upper right* figure, except that there are fewer club cells and the smooth muscle bundles (*SM*) are somewhat thinner.

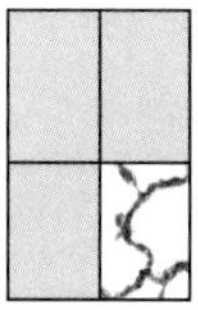

Alveolus, lungs, human, H&E × 800.

The central component of the alveolar wall is the **capillary** (*C*) and, in certain locations, associated connective tissue. On each side, where it faces the alveolus (*A*), a flat squamous cell is interposed between the capillary and the air spaces. This is a **pneumocyte type I cell**. In some places, the type I cell is separated from the capillary endothelial cell by a single basal lamina shared by the two cells. This is the thin portion of the alveolar–capillary complex, readily seen in the *upper part* of the figure (*arrows*). Gas exchange occurs through the thin portion of the alveolar–capillary complex. Elsewhere, connective tissue is interposed between the pneumocyte type I cell and the endothelial cell of the capillary; each of these epithelial cells retains its own basal lamina.

A second cell type, the **pneumocyte type II cell** or septal cell (*SC*), also lines the alveolar air space. This cell typically displays a rounded (rather than flattened) shape, and the nucleus is surrounded by a noticeable amount of cytoplasm, some of which may appear clear. The septal cell produces a surface-active agent different from that of the club cell, which also acts in permitting the lung to expand.

A, alveolus
C, capillary
CC, club cells
PsEp, pseudostratified columnar epithelium
SC, septal cell (pneumocyte type II cell)
SM, smooth muscle
arrows, thin portion of alveolar–capillary complex
diamond, junction between pseudostratified columnar epithelium and club cells

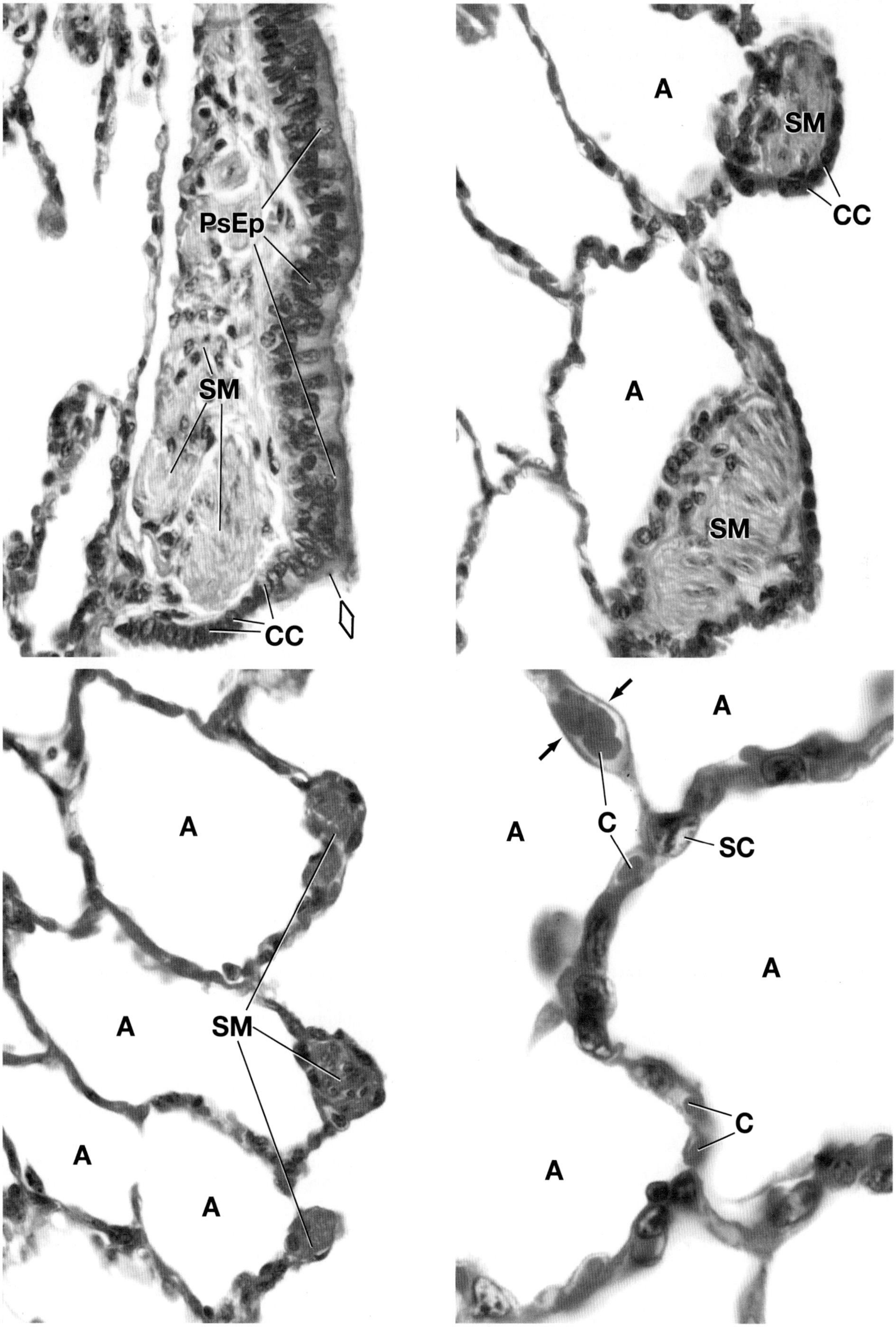
PsEp
SM
CC
A
SM
CC
A
SM
A
A
SM
A
A
A
C
SC
A
C
A

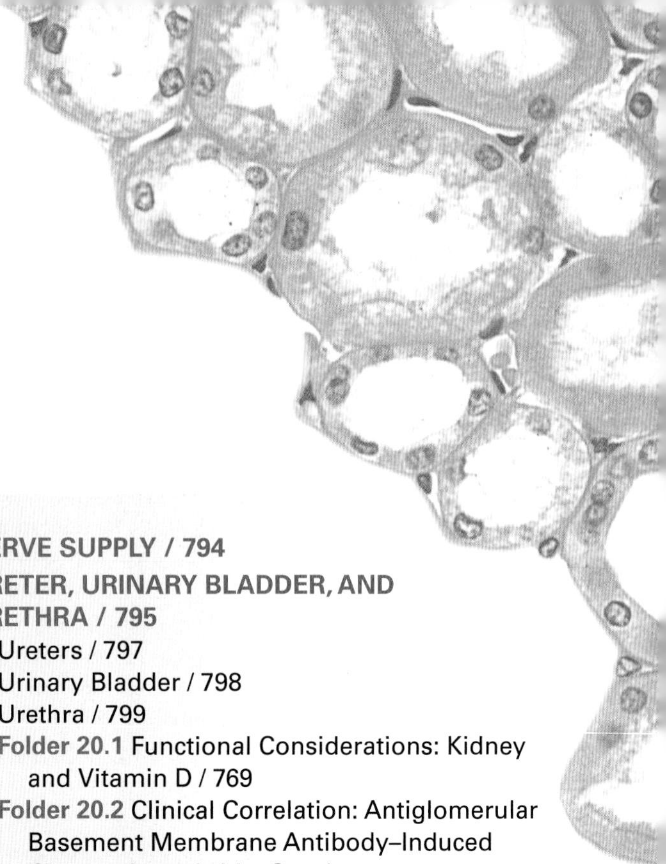

20 URINARY SYSTEM

■ OVERVIEW OF THE URINARY SYSTEM

The urinary system consists of the paired **kidneys**; paired **ureters**, which lead from the kidneys to the **urinary bladder**; and the **urethra**, which leads from the bladder to the exterior of the body.

The kidneys play an important role in body homeostasis by conserving fluids and electrolytes and disposing metabolic waste.

Like the lungs and liver, the **kidneys** retrieve essential materials and dispose of wastes. To maintain **homeostasis**, kidneys conserve water, electrolytes, and certain metabolites. The kidneys are essential in maintaining constant plasma pH by regulating acid–base balance, which is achieved by excreting hydrogen ions when body fluids become too acidic or excreting bicarbonates when body fluids become too basic. The kidneys play an important role in regulating and maintaining the composition and volume of extracellular fluid. Metabolic waste products are discharged from cells into the circulation; within the kidneys, these wastes are removed from the blood by filtration and **excretion** into the urine.

The kidneys are highly vascular organs; they receive approximately 25% of the cardiac output. Both excretory and homeostatic functions of the kidney begin when blood arrives at the **filtration apparatus** in the **glomerulus**. Initially, plasma is separated from the cells and large proteins to produce a **glomerular ultrafiltrate** of the blood or primary urine, which is then modified by selective resorption and specific secretion by the cells of the kidney. The final **urine** is conveyed by the ureters to the urinary bladder, where it is stored until discharged via the urethra.

The final urine contains water and electrolytes as well as waste products, such as urea, uric acid, and creatinine, and breakdown products of various substances.

The kidney also functions as an endocrine organ.

Endocrine activities of the kidneys include the following:

- Synthesis and secretion of the glycoprotein hormone **erythropoietin (EPO)**, which acts on the bone marrow and regulates red blood cell formation in response to decreased blood oxygen concentration. EPO is synthesized by endothelial cells of the peritubular capillaries in the renal cortex and acts on specific receptors expressed on the surface of erythrocyte progenitor (ErP) cells in the bone marrow. **Recombinant human erythropoietin (rhEPO)** is used for the treatment of **anemia** in patients with **end-stage renal disease**. It is also used to treat anemia resulting from **bone marrow suppression** that develops in individuals with AIDS undergoing treatment with antiretroviral drugs, such as azidothymidine (AZT).
- Synthesis and secretion of the acid protease **renin**, an enzyme involved in the control of blood pressure and blood volume. Renin is produced by juxtaglomerular cells and cleaves circulating angiotensinogen to release angiotensin I (see pages 781-784).
- Hydroxylation of **25-OH vitamin D_3**, a steroid precursor produced in the liver, to hormonally active 1,25-$(OH)_2$ vitamin D_3. This step is regulated primarily by parathyroid hormone (PTH), which stimulates the activity of the enzyme **1α-hydroxylase** and increases the production of the active hormone (Folder 20.1).

GENERAL STRUCTURE OF THE KIDNEY

The **kidneys** are large, reddish, bean-shaped organs located on either side of the spinal column in the retroperitoneal space of the posterior abdominal cavity. They extend from the 12th thoracic to the 3rd lumbar vertebrae, with the right kidney positioned slightly lower. Each kidney measures approximately 10 cm long × 6.5 cm wide (from concave to convex border) × 3 cm thick. On the **upper pole** of each kidney, embedded within the renal fascia and a thick protective layer of perirenal adipose tissue, lies an **adrenal gland**. The **medial border** of the kidney is concave and contains a deep vertical fissure, called the **hilum**, through which the renal vessels and nerves pass and the expanded, funnel-shaped origin of the ureter, called the **renal pelvis**, exits. A section through the kidney shows the relationship of these structures as they lie just within the hilum of the kidney in a space called the **renal sinus** (Fig. 20.1). Although not shown in the illustration, the space between and around these structures is filled largely with loose connective tissue and adipose tissue.

Capsule

The kidney surface is covered by a connective tissue **capsule**. The capsule consists of two distinct layers: an outer layer of fibroblasts and collagen fibers and an inner layer with a cellular component of myofibroblasts (Fig. 20.2). The contractility of the myofibroblasts may aid in resisting volume and pressure variations that can accompany variations in kidney function. Its specific role, however, is unknown. The capsule passes inward at the hilum, where it forms the connective tissue covering the sinus and becomes continuous with the

FOLDER 20.1

FUNCTIONAL CONSIDERATIONS: KIDNEY AND VITAMIN D

Despite its name, **vitamin D** is actually an inactive precursor that undergoes a series of transformations to become the fully active hormone that regulates plasma calcium levels. In the human body, vitamin D is derived from two sources:

- **Skin**, in which **vitamin D_3 (cholecalciferol)** is rapidly produced by the action of ultraviolet light on the precursor 7-dehydrocholesterol. The skin is the major source of vitamin D_3, especially in regions where food is not supplemented with vitamin D. Typically, 30 minutes to 2 hours of sunlight exposure per day can provide enough vitamin D to fulfill daily body requirements for this vitamin.
- **Diet**, from which vitamin D_3 is absorbed by the small intestine in association with chylomicrons

In the blood, vitamin D_3 is bound to **vitamin D–binding protein** and transported to the liver. The first transformation occurs in the liver and involves hydroxylation of vitamin D_3 to form **25-OH vitamin D_3**. This compound is released into the bloodstream and undergoes a second hydroxylation in the proximal tubules of the kidney to produce the highly active **1,25-$(OH)_2$ vitamin D_3 (calcitriol)**. The process is regulated indirectly by a decrease in plasma Ca^{2+} concentration, which triggers the secretion of parathyroid hormone (PTH), or directly by a decrease in circulating phosphates, which, in turn, stimulates the activity of 1α-hydroxylase responsible for conversion of 25-OH vitamin D_3 into active 1,25-$(OH)_2$ vitamin D_3. Active 1,25-$(OH)_2$ vitamin D_3 is released into the circulation and stimulates intestinal absorption of Ca^{2+} and phosphate and mobilization of Ca^{2+} from bones. It is, therefore, necessary for the normal development and growth of bones and teeth. The related compound **vitamin D_2 (ergocalciferol)** undergoes the same conversion steps as vitamin D_3 and produces the same biological effects.

Patients with end-stage **chronic kidney disease** have inadequate conversion of vitamin D into active metabolites, resulting in vitamin D_3 deficiency. In adults, vitamin D_3 deficiency is manifested by impaired bone mineralization and reduced bone density. Patients with chronic kidney disease, especially those on prolonged renal hemodialysis, often need vitamin D_3 and calcium supplements to prevent the severe disturbance of calcium homeostasis that results from secondary hyperparathyroidism, a common complication in these patients. Vitamin D_3 deficiency in childhood results in **rickets**, a disease that causes abnormal bone ossification.

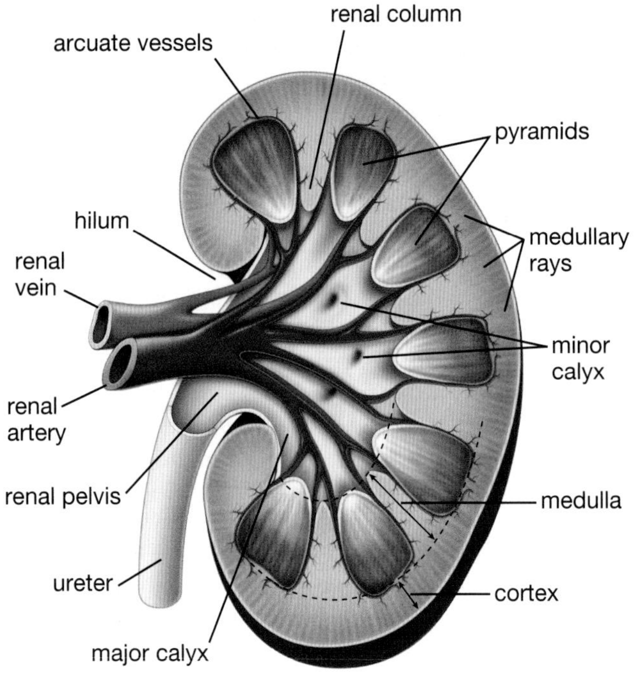

FIGURE 20.1. Diagram of kidney structure. The diagram represents a hemisection of a kidney, revealing its structural organization.

connective tissue, forming the walls of the calyces and renal pelvis (see Fig. 20.1).

Cortex and Medulla

Examination with the naked eye of the cut face of a fresh, hemisected kidney reveals that its substance can be divided into two distinct regions:

- **Cortex**, the outer reddish brown part
- **Medulla**, the much lighter colored inner part

The color seen on the cut surface of the unfixed kidney reflects the distribution of blood in the organ. Approximately 90%–95% of the blood passing through the kidney is in the cortex; 5%–10% is in the medulla.

The cortex is characterized by renal corpuscles and their associated tubules.

The **cortex** consists of **renal corpuscles** along with the **convoluted tubules** and **straight tubules** of the **nephron**, **connecting tubules**, **collecting ducts**, and an extensive vascular supply. The **nephron** is the basic functional unit of the kidney and is described later in this chapter. The renal corpuscles are spherical structures, barely visible with the naked eye. They constitute the beginning segment of the nephron and contain a unique capillary network called a **glomerulus**.

Examination of a section cut through the cortex at an angle perpendicular to the surface of the kidney reveals a series of vertical striations that appear to emanate from the medulla (see Fig. 20.1). These striations are the **medullary rays** (of Ferrein). Their name reflects their appearance, as the striations seem to radiate from the medulla. Approximately 400–500 medullary rays project into the cortex from the medulla.

Each medullary ray is an aggregation of straight tubules and collecting ducts.

Each medullary ray contains **straight tubules** of nephrons and **collecting ducts**. The regions between medullary rays contain the renal corpuscles, the convoluted tubules of the nephrons, and the connecting tubules. These areas are referred to as **cortical labyrinths**. Each nephron and its **connecting tubule** (which connects to a collecting duct in the medullary ray) form the **uriniferous tubule**.

The medulla is characterized by straight tubules, collecting ducts, and a special capillary network, the vasa recta.

The **straight tubules** of the nephrons and the **collecting ducts** continue from the cortex into the medulla. They are accompanied by a capillary network, the **vasa recta**, that runs in parallel with the various tubules. These vessels represent the vascular part of the **countercurrent exchange system** that regulates the concentration of urine.

The **tubules in the medulla**, because of their arrangement and differences in length, collectively form a number of conical structures called **pyramids** (Fig. 20.3). Usually 8–12 but as many as 18 pyramids may be present in the human kidney. The bases of the pyramids face the cortex, and the apices face the renal sinus. The apical portion of each pyramid, which is known as the **papilla**, projects into a minor calyx, a cup-shaped structure that represents an extension of the renal pelvis. The tip of the papilla, also known as the **area cribrosa**, is perforated by the openings of the collecting ducts (Fig. 20.4). The minor calyces are branches of the two or three **major calyces** that, in turn, are major divisions of the renal pelvis (see Fig. 20.1).

Each pyramid is divided into an **outer medulla** (adjacent to the cortex) and an **inner medulla**. The outer medulla is further subdivided into an **inner stripe** and an **outer stripe**. The zonation and stripes are readily recognized

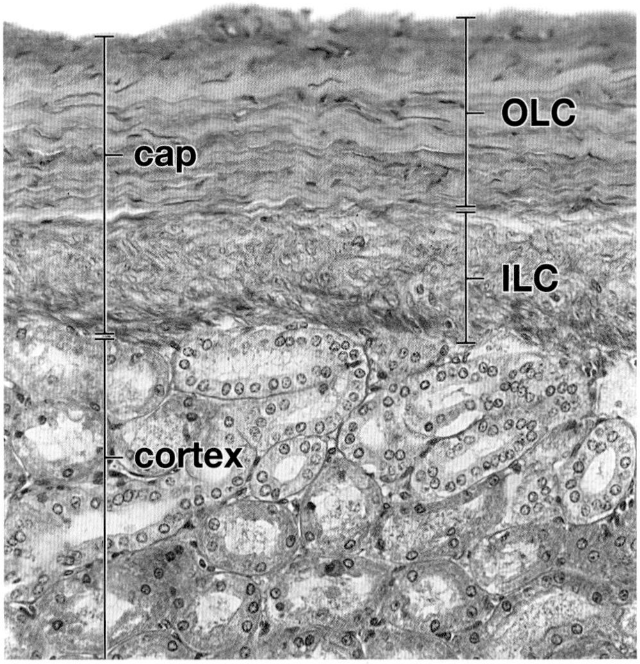

FIGURE 20.2. Photomicrograph of human kidney capsule. This photomicrograph of a Mallory-Azan–stained section shows the capsule (*cap*) and part of the underlying cortex. The outer layer of the capsule (*OLC*) is composed of dense connective tissue. The fibroblasts in this part of the capsule are relatively few in number; their nuclei appear as narrow, elongated, red-staining profiles against a blue background representing the stained collagen fibers. The inner layer of the capsule (*ILC*) consists of large numbers of myofibroblasts whose nuclei appear as round or elongated, red-staining profiles, depending on their orientation within the section. Note that the collagen fibers in this layer are relatively sparse and that the myofibroblast nuclei are more abundant than those of the fibroblasts in the outer layer of the capsule. ×180.

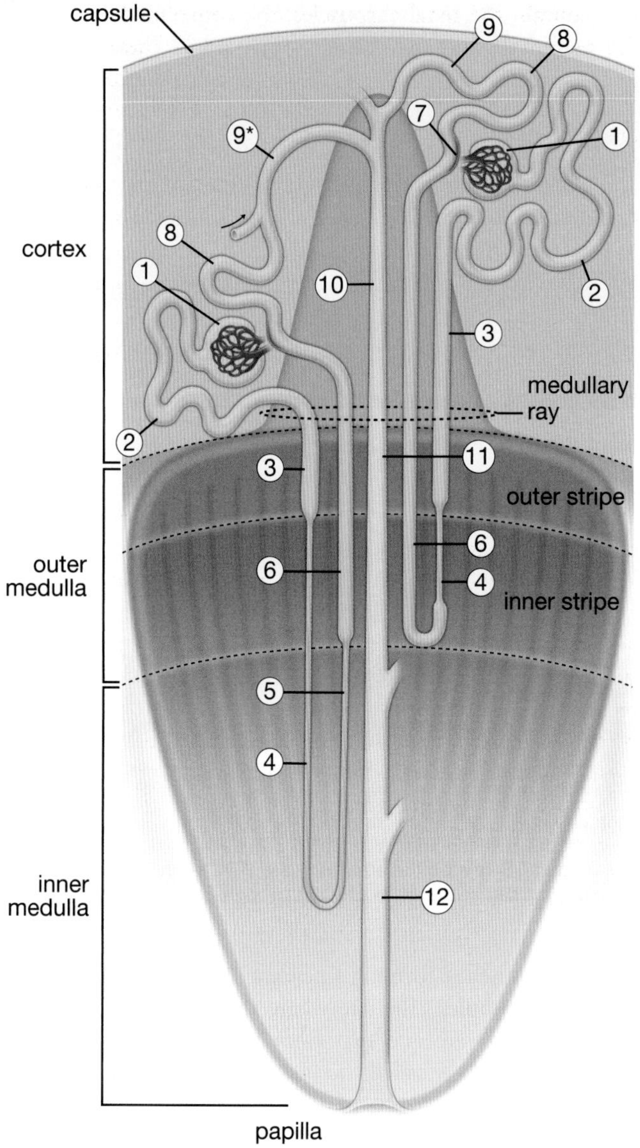

FIGURE 20.3. Diagram showing standard nomenclature for structures in the kidney. The two types of nephrons in the kidney are shown with their associated duct systems. A long-looped nephron is shown on the *left*, and a short-looped nephron is shown on the *right*. The relative position of the cortex, medulla, papilla, and capsule is indicated (not drawn to scale). The inverted cone–shaped area in the cortex represents a medullary ray. The parts of the nephron are indicated by number: *1*, renal corpuscle including the glomerulus and Bowman capsule; *2*, proximal convoluted tubule; *3*, proximal straight tubule (thick descending limb); *4*, descending thin limb; *5*, ascending thin limb; *6*, distal straight tubule (thick ascending limb); *7*, macula densa located in the final portion of the thick ascending limb; *8*, distal convoluted tubule; *9*, connecting tubule; *9**, connecting tubule of the juxtamedullary nephron that forms an arch (arched connecting tubule); *10*, cortical collecting duct; *11*, outer medullary collecting duct; and *12*, inner medullary collecting duct. (Modified from Kriz W, Bankir L. A standard nomenclature for structures of the kidney. The Renal Commission of the International Union of Physiological Sciences. *Kidney Int*. 1988;33:1–7.)

in a sagittal section through the pyramid of a fresh specimen. They reflect the location of distinct parts of the nephron at specific levels within the pyramid (see Fig. 20.3).

The renal columns represent cortical tissue contained within the medulla.

The caps of cortical tissue that lie over the pyramids are sufficiently extensive that they extend peripherally around the lateral portion of the pyramid, forming the **renal columns** (of Bertin). Although renal columns contain the same components as the rest of the cortical tissue, they are regarded as part of the medulla. In effect, the amount of cortical tissue is so extensive that it "spills" over the side of the pyramid much as a large scoop of ice cream extends beyond and overlaps the sides of an ice cream cone.

Kidney Lobes and Lobules

The number of lobes in a kidney equals the number of medullary pyramids.

Each **medullary pyramid** and the associated cortical tissue at its base and sides (one half of each adjacent renal column) constitute a **lobe** of the kidney. The lobar organization of the kidney is conspicuous in the developing fetal kidney (Fig. 20.5). Each lobe is reflected as a convexity on the outer surface of the organ, but they usually disappear after birth. The surface convexities typical of the fetal kidney may persist, however, until the teenage years and, in some cases, into adulthood. Each human kidney contains 8–18 lobes. Kidneys of some animals possess only one pyramid; these kidneys are classified as unilobar, in contrast to the multilobar kidney of the human.

A lobule consists of a collecting duct and all the nephrons that it drains.

The **lobes of the kidney** are further subdivided into **lobules** consisting of a central medullary ray and surrounding cortical material (Fig. 20.6 and Plate 20.2, page 804). Although the center or axis of a lobule is readily identifiable, the boundaries between adjacent lobules are not obviously demarcated from one another by connective tissue septa. The concept of the lobule has an important physiologic basis; the medullary ray containing the collecting duct for a group of nephrons that drain into that duct constitutes the renal secretory unit. It is the equivalent of a glandular secretory unit or lobule.

The Nephron

The nephron is the structural and functional unit of the kidney.

The **nephron** is the fundamental unit of the kidney (see Fig. 20.3). Both human kidneys contain approximately 2 million nephrons. Nephrons are responsible for the production of urine and correspond to the secretory part of glands. The collecting ducts are responsible for the final concentration of the urine and are analogous to the ducts of exocrine glands that modify the concentration of the secretory product. Unlike the typical exocrine gland in which the secretory and duct portions arise from a single epithelial outgrowth, nephrons and their collecting ducts arise from separate primordia and only later become connected.

General organization of the nephron

The nephron consists of the renal corpuscle and a tubule system.

As stated previously, the **renal corpuscle** represents the beginning of the nephron. It consists of the **glomerulus**, a tuft of capillaries composed of 10–20 capillary loops, surrounded by a double-layered epithelial cup, the renal or **Bowman capsule**. The Bowman capsule is the initial portion of the nephron, where blood flowing through the glomerular capillaries undergoes filtration to produce the **glomerular ultrafiltrate**. The glomerular capillaries are supplied by an **afferent arteriole** and are drained by an **efferent arteriole**

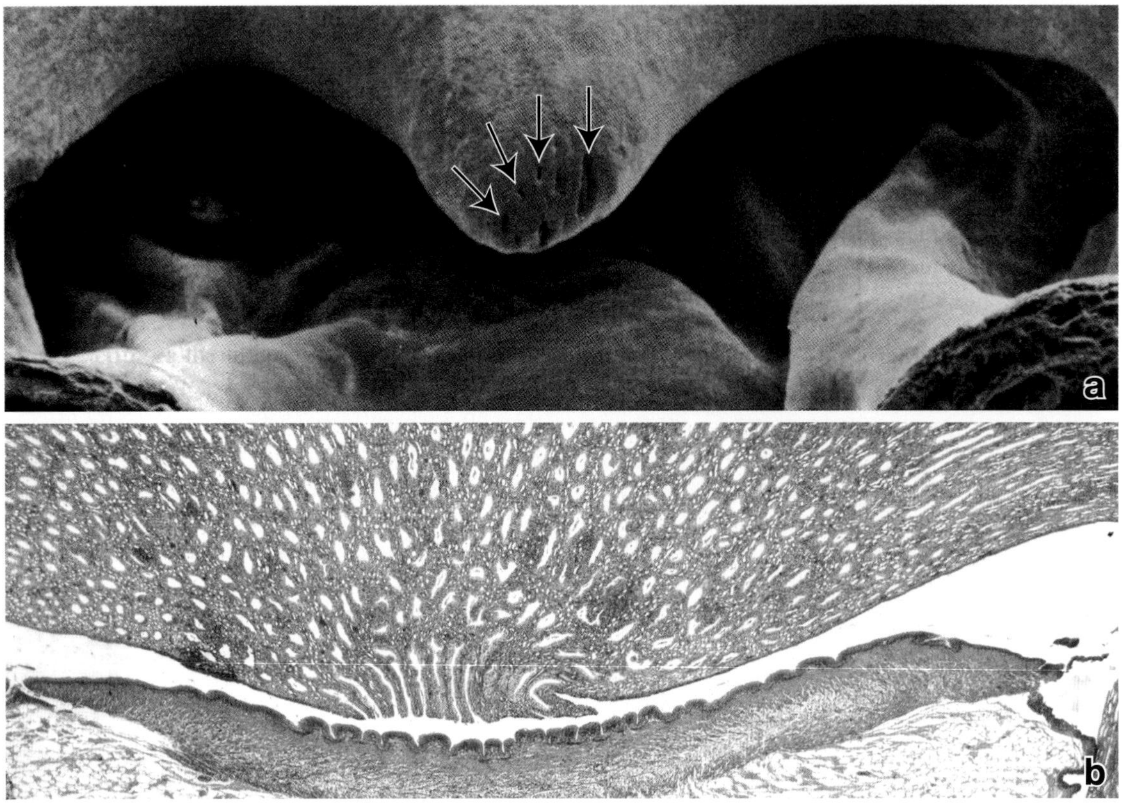

FIGURE 20.4. Renal papilla and calyx. a. This scanning electron micrograph shows the conical structure that represents the renal papilla, projecting into the renal calyx. The apex of the papilla contains openings (*arrows*) of the collecting ducts (of Bellini). These ducts deliver urine from the pyramids to the minor calyx. The surface of the papilla containing the openings is designated the area cribrosa. ×24. **b.** Photomicrograph of a hematoxylin and eosin (H&E)-stained specimen of the papilla showing the distal portion of the collecting ducts opening into the minor calyx. ×120. (Courtesy of Dr. C. Craig Tisher.)

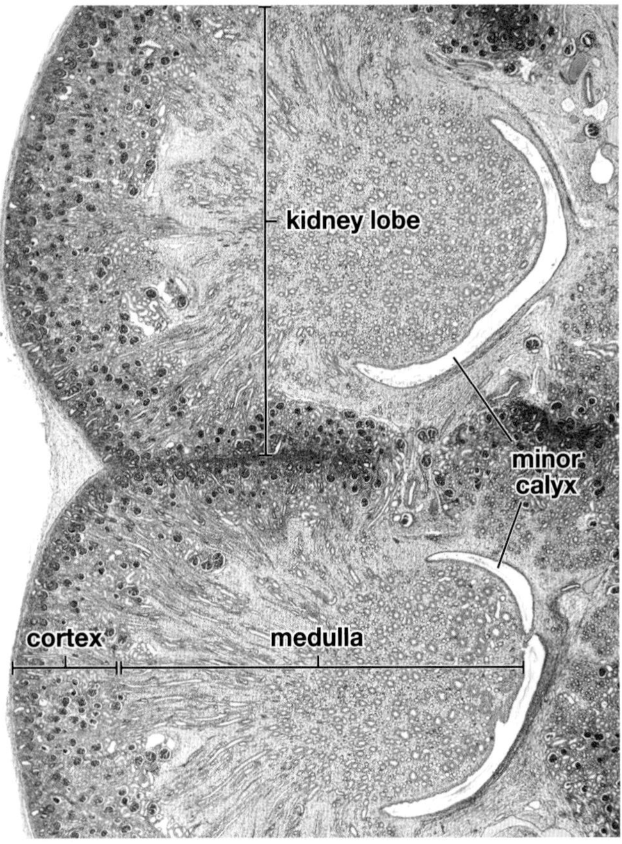

FIGURE 20.5. Photomicrograph of fetal kidney. This photomicrograph of a hematoxylin and eosin (H&E)-stained human fetal kidney shows the cortex, the medulla, and two associated pyramids. Note that each surface convexity corresponds to a kidney lobe. During postnatal life, the lobar convexities disappear, and the kidney then exhibits a smooth surface. ×30.

that then branches, forming a new capillary network to supply the kidney tubules. The site where the afferent and efferent arterioles penetrate and exit from the parietal layer of the Bowman capsule is called the **vascular pole**. Opposite this site is the **urinary pole** of the renal corpuscle, where the proximal convoluted tubule begins (Fig. 20.7).

Continuing from the Bowman capsule, the remaining parts of the nephron (the tubular parts) are as follows:

- **Proximal thick segment**, consisting of the proximal convoluted tubule (pars convoluta) and the proximal straight tubule (pars recta)
- **Thin segment**, which constitutes the thin part of the loop of Henle
- **Distal thick segment**, consisting of the distal straight tubule (pars recta) and the distal convoluted tubule (pars convoluta)

The **distal convoluted tubule** connects to the **cortical collecting duct**, often through a connecting tubule, thus forming the uriniferous tubule (i.e., the nephron plus collecting duct; see Fig. 20.3). The cortical collecting duct continues into the medulla as the **medullary collecting duct** and empties in the papilla of the renal pyramid. In clinical nomenclature, the cortical collecting duct, medullary collecting duct, and, sometimes, the connecting tubule are collectively referred to as the **collecting tubule**, emphasizing the fact that this segment emerges from the confluence of many nephrons. For clarity, the term "collecting tubule" is not used in this chapter because it is easily confused with "connecting tubule" and does not precisely define the cortical versus medullary location of the described segment.

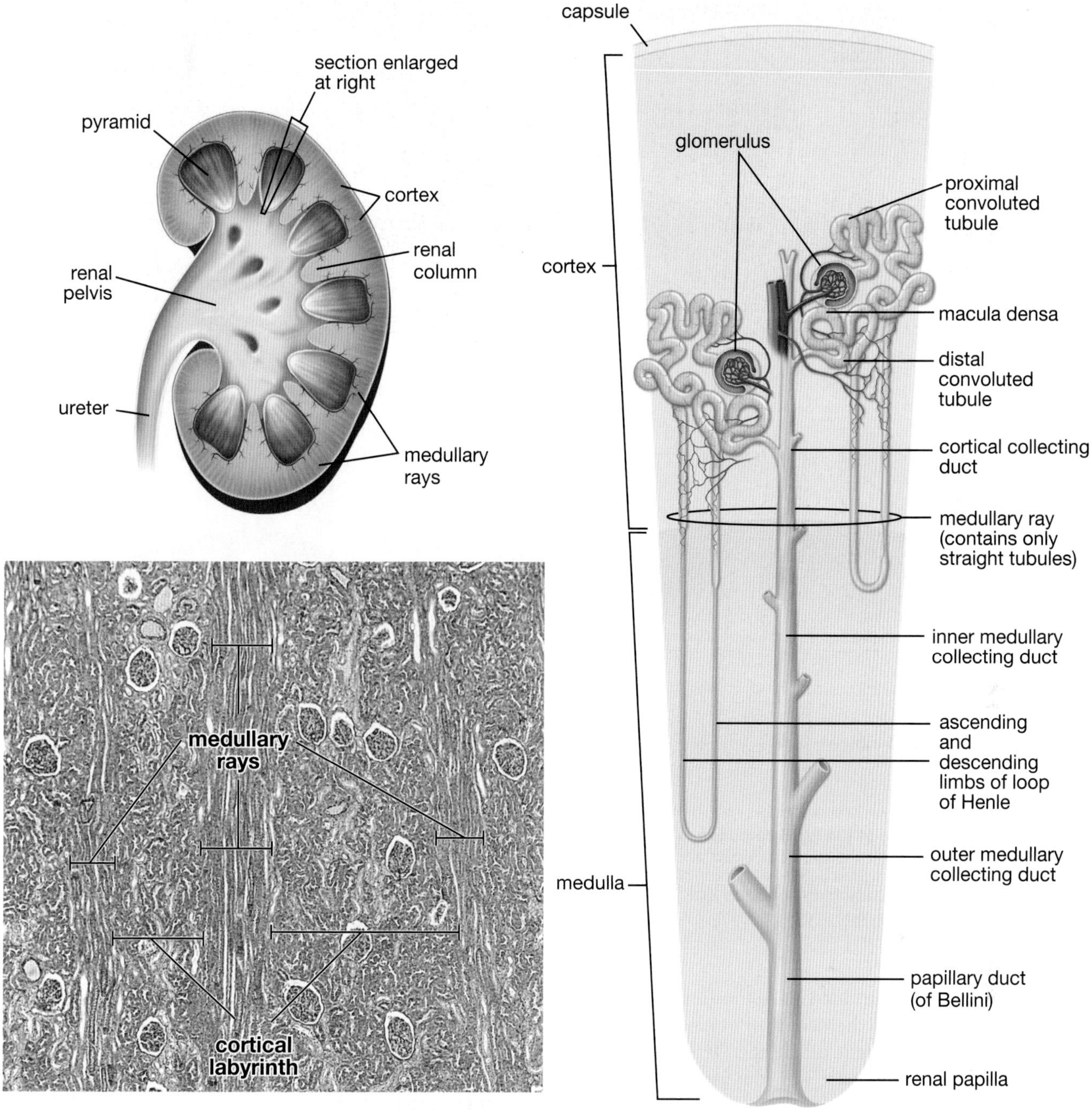

FIGURE 20.6. Diagrams and photomicrograph of an adult human kidney. The *diagram* in the *upper left* is a hemisection of the adult human kidney included for orientation. The *diagram* on the *right* of an enlarged portion of the kidney emphasizes the relationship between two nephrons and their tubules and ducts to the cortex and medulla. The upper nephron, a midcortical nephron, extends only a short distance into the medulla and possesses a short thin segment in the loop of Henle. The lower nephron, a juxtamedullary nephron, has a long loop of Henle that extends deep into the medulla. Both nephrons drain into the cortical collecting ducts in the medullary ray. The photomicrograph shows a section of the cortex. It is organized into a series of medullary rays containing straight tubules and cortical collecting ducts; between the rays are cortical labyrinths containing the renal corpuscles and their associated proximal and distal convoluted tubules. A kidney lobule consists of a medullary ray at its center and half of the adjacent cortical labyrinth on either side. ×60.

Tubules of the nephron

The tubular segments of the nephron are named according to the course that they take (convoluted or straight), location (proximal or distal), and wall thickness (thick or thin).

Beginning from the Bowman capsule, the sequential parts of the **nephron** consist of the following tubules:

- **Proximal convoluted tubule** originates from the urinary pole of the Bowman capsule. It follows a very tortuous or convoluted course and then enters the medullary ray to continue as the proximal straight tubule.
- **Proximal straight tubule**, commonly referred to as the *thick descending limb of the loop of Henle*, descends into the medulla.
- **Thin descending limb** is the continuation of the proximal straight tubule within the medulla. It makes a hairpin turn and returns toward the cortex.
- **Thin ascending limb** is the continuation of the thin descending limb after its hairpin turn.
- **Distal straight tubule**, which is also referred to as the *thick ascending limb of the loop of Henle*, is the continuation of the thin ascending limb. The distal straight tubule

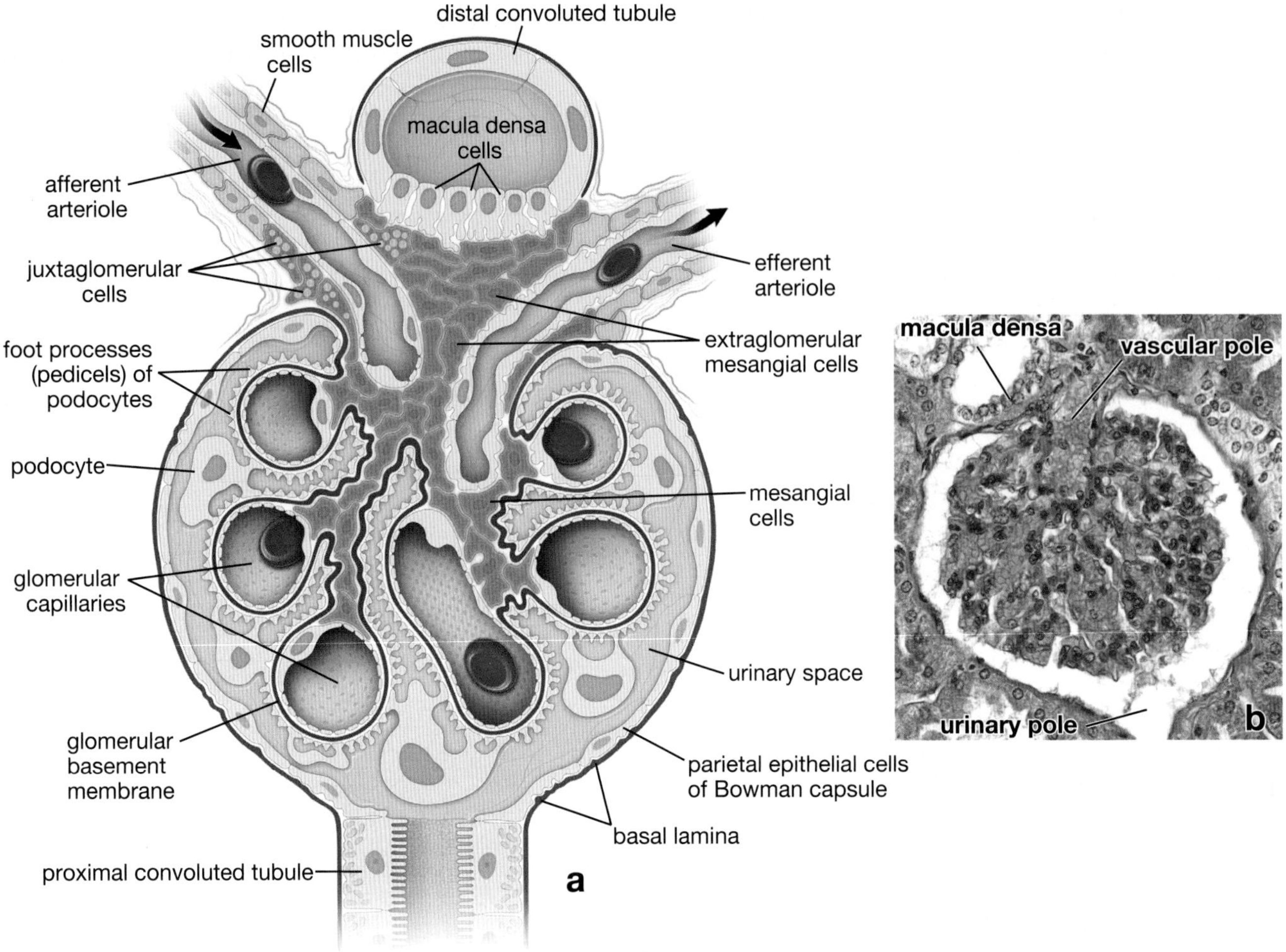

FIGURE 20.7. Structure of the renal corpuscle. a. This schematic diagram shows the organization of the renal corpuscle and associated structures at the vascular and urinary poles. Mesangial cells are associated with the capillary endothelium of the glomerulus and the glomerular basement membrane. The macula densa cells of the distal tubule are shown intimately associated with the juxtaglomerular cells of the afferent arteriole and the extraglomerular mesangial cells. **b.** Photomicrograph of a hematoxylin and eosin (H&E)-stained specimen showing a renal corpuscle. The macula densa is seen in close proximity to the vascular pole. ×160. (Modified from Kriz W, Sakai T. Morphological aspects of glomerular function. In: *Nephrology: Proceedings of the Tenth International Congress of Nephrology.* Bailliere-Tindall; 1987.)

ascends through the medulla and enters the cortex in the medullary ray to reach the vicinity of its renal corpuscle of origin. The distal straight tubule then leaves the medullary ray and makes contact with the vascular pole of its parent renal corpuscle. At this point, the epithelial cells of the tubule adjacent to the afferent arteriole of the glomerulus are modified to form the **macula densa**. The distal tubule then leaves the region of the corpuscle and becomes the distal convoluted tubule.

- **Distal convoluted tubule** is less tortuous than the proximal convoluted tubule; thus, in a section showing the cortical labyrinth, there are fewer distal tubule profiles than proximal tubule profiles. At its termination, the distal convoluted tubule empties into a cortical collecting duct that lies in the medullary ray via either an **arched connecting tubule** or a shorter tubule simply called the **connecting tubule**.

The loop of Henle forms the entire U-shaped portion of a nephron.

The proximal straight tubule, the thin descending limb with its hairpin turn, the thin ascending limb, and the distal straight tubule are collectively called the **loop of Henle**. In some nephrons, the thin descending and ascending segments are extremely short; therefore, the hairpin turn may be made by the distal straight tubule.

Types of nephrons

Several types of nephrons are identified based on the location of their renal corpuscles in the cortex (see Fig. 20.3):

- **Subcapsular nephrons** or **cortical nephrons** have their renal corpuscles located in the outer part of the cortex. They have short loops of Henle, extending only into the outer medulla. They are typical of the nephrons described previously, wherein the hairpin turn occurs in the distal straight tubule.
- **Juxtamedullary nephrons** make up about one-eighth of the total nephron count. Their renal corpuscles occur in proximity to the base of a medullary pyramid. They have long loops of Henle and long ascending thin segments that extend well into the inner region of the pyramid. These structural features are essential to the urine-concentrating mechanism, which is described in a further section.
- **Intermediate nephrons** or **midcortical nephrons** have their renal corpuscles in the midregion of the cortex. Their loops of Henle are of intermediate length.

Collecting Ducts

The **cortical collecting ducts** begin in the cortex from the merger of either **connecting tubules** or **arched connecting tubules** of many nephrons and proceed within the medullary rays toward the medulla. When the cortical collecting ducts reach the medulla, they are referred to as outer or inner **medullary collecting ducts**. These ducts travel to the apex of the pyramid, where they merge into larger collecting ducts (up to 200 μm), the **papillary ducts** (ducts of Bellini), that open into the minor calyx (see Fig. 20.4). The area on the papilla that contains the openings of these collecting ducts is called the **area cribrosa**.

In summary, the gross appearance of the functional tissue of the kidney reflects the structure of the nephron. The renal corpuscle and the proximal and distal convoluted tubules are located in and comprise the substance of the cortical labyrinths. The portions of the straight proximal and straight distal tubules with accompanying cortical collecting ducts in the cortex are located in and comprise the major portion of the medullary rays. The thin descending and thin ascending limbs of the loop of Henle are always located in the medulla and are accompanied by medullary collecting ducts. Thus, the arrangement of the nephrons (and collecting ducts) accounts for the characteristic appearance of the cut surface of the kidney, as seen in Figure 20.6.

Filtration Apparatus of the Kidney

The renal corpuscle contains the filtration apparatus of the kidney, which consists of the glomerular endothelium, underlying glomerular basement membrane, and the visceral layer of the Bowman capsule.

The **renal corpuscle** is spherical and has an average diameter of 200 μm. It consists of the glomerular capillary tuft and the surrounding visceral and parietal epithelial layers of the Bowman capsule (Fig. 20.8). The filtration apparatus, also called **glomerular filtration barrier**, enclosed by the parietal layer of the Bowman capsule, consists of three different components:

- **Endothelium of the glomerular capillaries**, which possesses numerous fenestrations (Fig. 20.9). These fenestrations are larger (70–90 nm in diameter), more numerous, and more irregular in outline than fenestrations in other capillaries. Moreover, the diaphragm that spans the fenestrations in other capillaries is absent in the glomerular capillaries. Endothelial cells of glomerular capillaries possess a large number of aquaporin-1 (AQP-1) water channels that allow the fast movement of water through the epithelium. Secretory products of endothelial cells, such as **nitric oxide (NO)** or **prostaglandins (PGE_2)**, play an important role in the pathogenesis of several **thrombotic glomerular diseases**.
- **Glomerular basement membrane (GBM)**, a thick (300–370 nm) basal lamina that is the joint product of the endothelium and the podocytes, the cells of the visceral layer of the Bowman capsule. Because of its thickness, it is prominent in histologic sections stained with the periodic acid–Schiff (PAS) procedure (see Fig. 1.2, page 6). The GBM is composed of a network consisting of **type IV collagen** (mainly α3-, α4-, and α5-chains), **laminin**, **nidogen**, and **entactin**, together with **heparan sulfate proteoglycans**, such as agrin and perlecan, as well as **multiadhesive glycoproteins** (see pages 195-197). GBM can also be visualized with immunofluorescence techniques using antibodies directed to a specific α-chain of type IV collagen (Fig. 20.10). Mutation in genes encoding the **α3-, α4-, and α5-chains of type IV collagen** gives rise to **Alport syndrome (hereditary glomerulonephritis)**, manifested by hematuria (presence of the red blood cells in the urine), proteinuria (presence of significant amount of protein in the urine), and progressive renal failure. In Alport syndrome, the GBM becomes irregularly thickened with laminated lamina densa and fails to serve as an effective filtration barrier. Collagen type IV is also the target in autoimmune diseases, such as **Goodpasture syndrome** and **Alport post-transplantation disease**. Both diseases are characterized by autoantibodies attacking

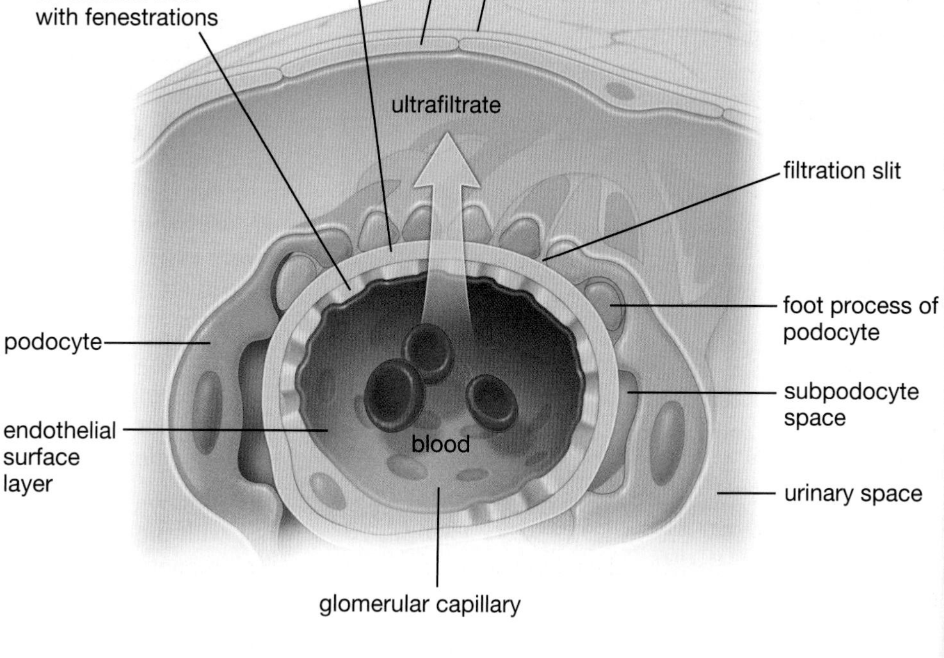

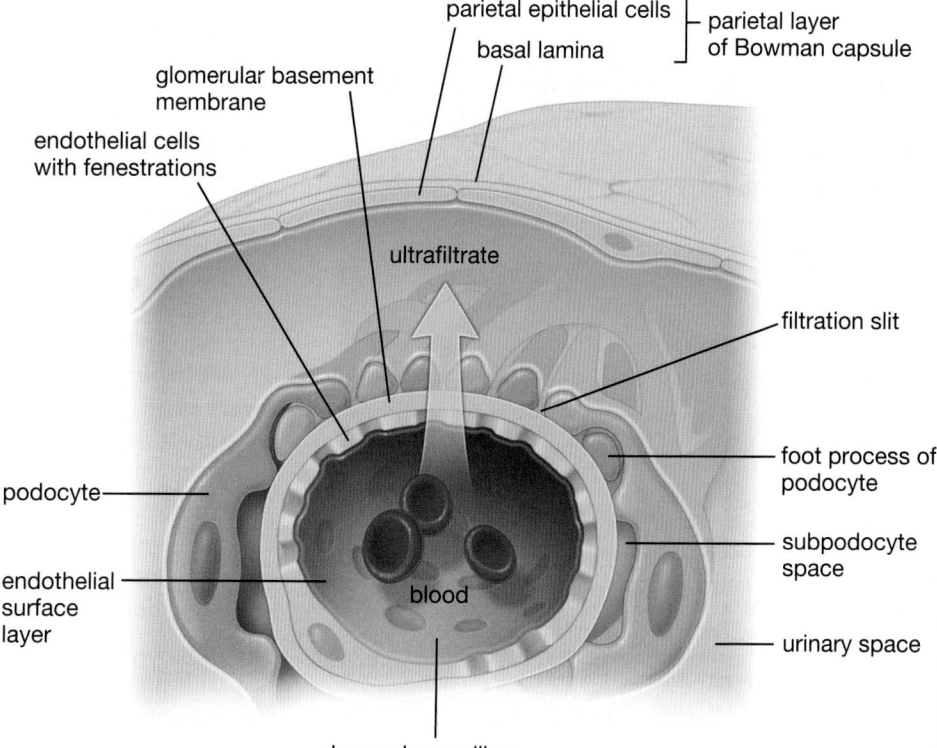

FIGURE 20.8. Schematic diagram of filtration barrier. The *arrow* indicates movement of plasma fluid across the glomerular filtration barrier, forming the glomerular ultrafiltrate (primary urine) that accumulates in the urinary space of the Bowman capsule. Note the layers of the filtration barrier that include fenestrated glomerular endothelial cells, glomerular basement membrane, and podocytes with filtration slit diaphragms spanned between their foot processes. In addition, the endothelial surface layer of glycoproteins and subpodocyte spaces are shown in this diagram.

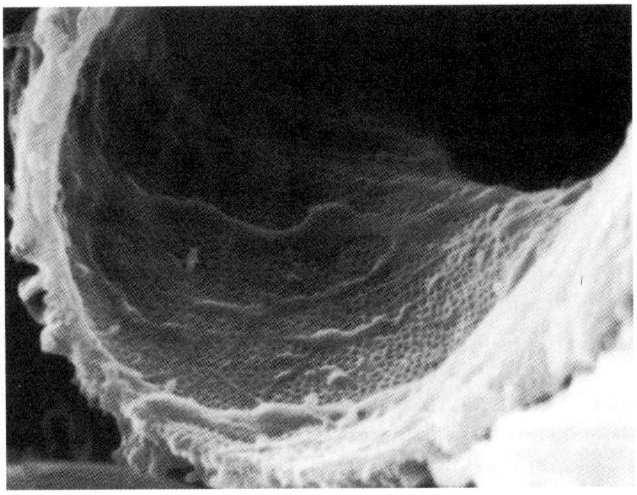

FIGURE 20.9. Scanning electron micrograph of the interior surface of a glomerular capillary. The wall of the capillary shows horizontal ridges formed by the cytoplasm of the endothelial cell. Elsewhere, fenestrations are seen as numerous dark oval and circular profiles. ×5,600. (Courtesy of Dr. C. Craig Tisher.)

the GBM and causing **rapidly progressive glomerulonephritis** (see Folder 20.2).

- **Visceral layer of the Bowman capsule**, which contains specialized cells called **podocytes** or **visceral epithelial cells**. These cells extend processes around the glomerular capillaries (Fig. 20.11 and Plate 20.3, page 806). The podocytes arise during embryonic development from one of the blind ends of the developing nephron through invagination of the end of the tubule to form a double-layered epithelial cup. The inner cell layer (i.e., the visceral cell layer) lies in apposition to a capillary network, the glomerulus, which forms at this site. The outer layer of these cells, the parietal layer, forms the squamous cells of the Bowman capsule. The cup eventually closes to form the spherical structure containing the glomerulus. As they differentiate, the podocytes extend processes around the capillaries and develop numerous primary and secondary processes, giving rise to **pedicels** called **foot processes**. The foot processes interdigitate with foot processes of neighboring podocytes, a feature that can be clearly seen with the scanning electron microscope (SEM; Fig. 20.12). The elongated spaces between the interdigitating foot processes, called **filtration slits**, are about 40 nm wide and covered by an ultrathin **filtration slit diaphragm** that spans the filtration slit slightly above the GBM (Fig. 20.13, *inset*).

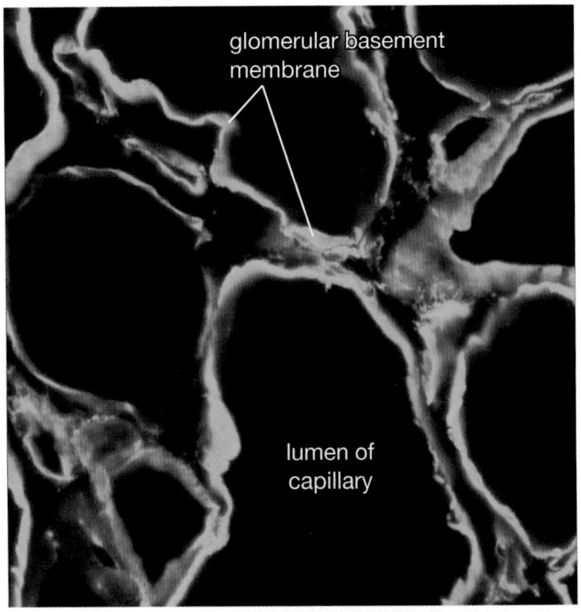

FIGURE 20.10. Immunofluorescent-stained glomerular basement membrane in a human kidney. The glomerular basement membrane (GBM) is composed of five (α1–α5) of the six chains of type IV collagen. This high-magnification micrograph of the GBM within the kidney glomerulus was obtained using primary monoclonal antibodies against the α1-chain of type IV collagen molecules that were visualized by a secondary antibody conjugated with fluorescein dye. ×1,200. (Courtesy of Dr. L. Barisoni.)

Nephrin is an important structural protein of the filtration slit diaphragm.

Studies of the **filtration slit diaphragm** reveal its complex protein structure as a zipper-like sheet configuration with a central density. **Nephrin**, a 185 kDa transmembrane protein, is a key structural and functional component of the slit diaphragm. Nephrin molecules emerging from opposite foot processes interact in the center of the slit (homophilic interactions), forming a central density with pores on both sides (Fig. 20.14). This intercellular protein sheet also contains other adhesion molecules, such as **Neph-1**, **Neph-2**, **P-cadherin**, **FAT1**, and **FAT2**. The filtration slit diaphragm is firmly anchored to numerous actin filaments within the foot processes of podocytes. Regulation and maintenance of the actin cytoskeleton of podocytes has emerged as a critical process for regulating the size, patency, and selectivity of the filtration slits. Mutations in the **nephrin gene (NPHS1)** are associated with congenital **nephrotic syndrome**, a disease characterized by massive proteinuria and edema.

The negative charge of podocalyxin repels the plasma membranes of the neighboring foot processes and maintains open access to the filtration slit diaphragm.

Podocalyxin is a negatively charged transmembrane sialoglycoprotein (55 kDa) that plays a key role in maintaining the structural integrity of the kidney's filtration apparatus. It is synthesized by podocytes and expressed within the glycocalyx covering the apical cell membrane of their foot processes that face the urinary space. Owing to its highly negative charges and location near the filtration slits, podocalyxin acts as an antiadhesive molecule keeping adjacent foot processes separated from each other, thereby maintaining open filtration slits. Podocalyxin acts on actin filaments via actin-associated proteins (i.e., ezrin that links integral membrane proteins with actin filaments), which changes the cytoskeletal architecture of the foot processes. In addition, the negative charges appear to be important in maintaining the urinary space between podocytes and the parietal layer of Bowman capsule. Experimental podocalyxin-deficient mice die within the first 24 hours of life. Their kidneys exhibit severe podocyte malformations characterized by impaired glomerular development and fail to develop podocyte foot processes and slit diaphragms. These changes block the passage of urine, resulting in **renal failure**.

The endothelial surface layer of glomerular capillaries and the subpodocyte space also make important contributions to overall glomerular function.

The filtration apparatus is a complex semipermeable barrier, with properties that allow for a high rate of water filtration, nonrestricted passage of small- and middle-sized molecules, and almost total exclusion of serum albumins

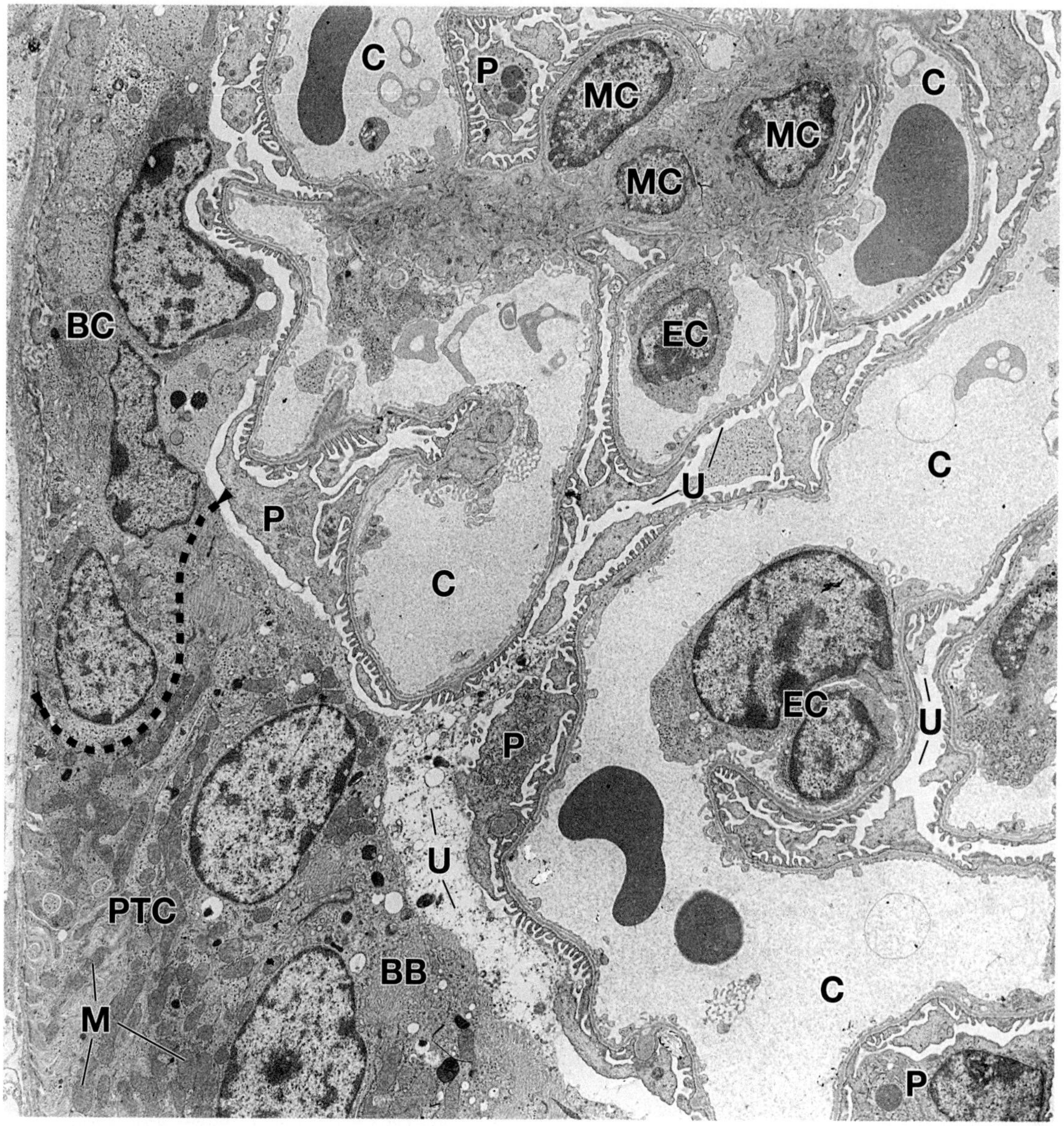

FIGURE 20.11. Transmission electron micrograph of a glomerulus in the region of the urinary pole. The nuclear and perinuclear regions of the endothelial cells (*EC*) that line the glomerular capillaries (*C*) bulge into the vascular lumen. On the outer surface of the capillaries are the processes of the podocytes (*P*). External to the podocytes is the urinary space (*U*). The Bowman capsule (*BC*) is shown on the *left*; it is continuous at the *dashed line* (marked by *arrowheads*) with the tubule cells of the proximal tubule (*PTC*). Note the numerous mitochondria (*M*) in the base of these cells and the brush border (*BB*) at the apex that projects into the urinary space. The nuclei of three adjacent mesangial cells (*MC*) can be seen in the *upper right* of the micrograph. ×4,700.

and other larger proteins. The filtration apparatus may thus be described as a barrier having two discontinuous cellular layers, the **endothelium of glomerular capillaries** and **visceral layer of the Bowman capsule** applied to either side of a continuous extracellular layer of the **glomerular basement membrane.** These three layers have traditionally been considered the glomerular filtration barrier. However, two additional physiologically important layers, the endothelial surface layer of glomerular capillaries and subpodocyte space, are included as part of the filtration apparatus:

- **The endothelial surface layer** of the glomerular capillaries consists of a thick carbohydrate–rich meshwork (200–400 nm) attached to the luminal surface of glomerular endothelial cells. It contains a **glycocalyx**, which refers to plasma membrane–bound negatively charged proteoglycans (such as perlecan, syndecan, and versican) associated with glycosaminoglycan side chains (such as heparan sulfate and chondroitin sulfate) and peripheral membrane proteins. **Plasma proteins** (e.g., albumins) adsorbed from the blood coat the luminal surface of glycocalyx.
- **Subpodocyte space** represents a narrow space between the foot processes with their filtration slit diaphragms on one side and a cell body of the podocyte on the other side (see Fig. 20.13). Recent three-dimensional reconstruction of these spaces revealed their interconnected but structurally restrictive character. They cover approximately 60% of the entire surface area of the glomerular filtration barrier and may function in regulating glomerular fluid flux across the filtration apparatus.

The glomerular basement membrane (GBM) acts as a physical barrier and an ion-selective filter.

As discussed earlier, the **GBM** contains type IV and XVIII collagens, sialoglycoproteins, and other noncollagenous glycoproteins (e.g., laminin, fibronectin, entactin) as well as

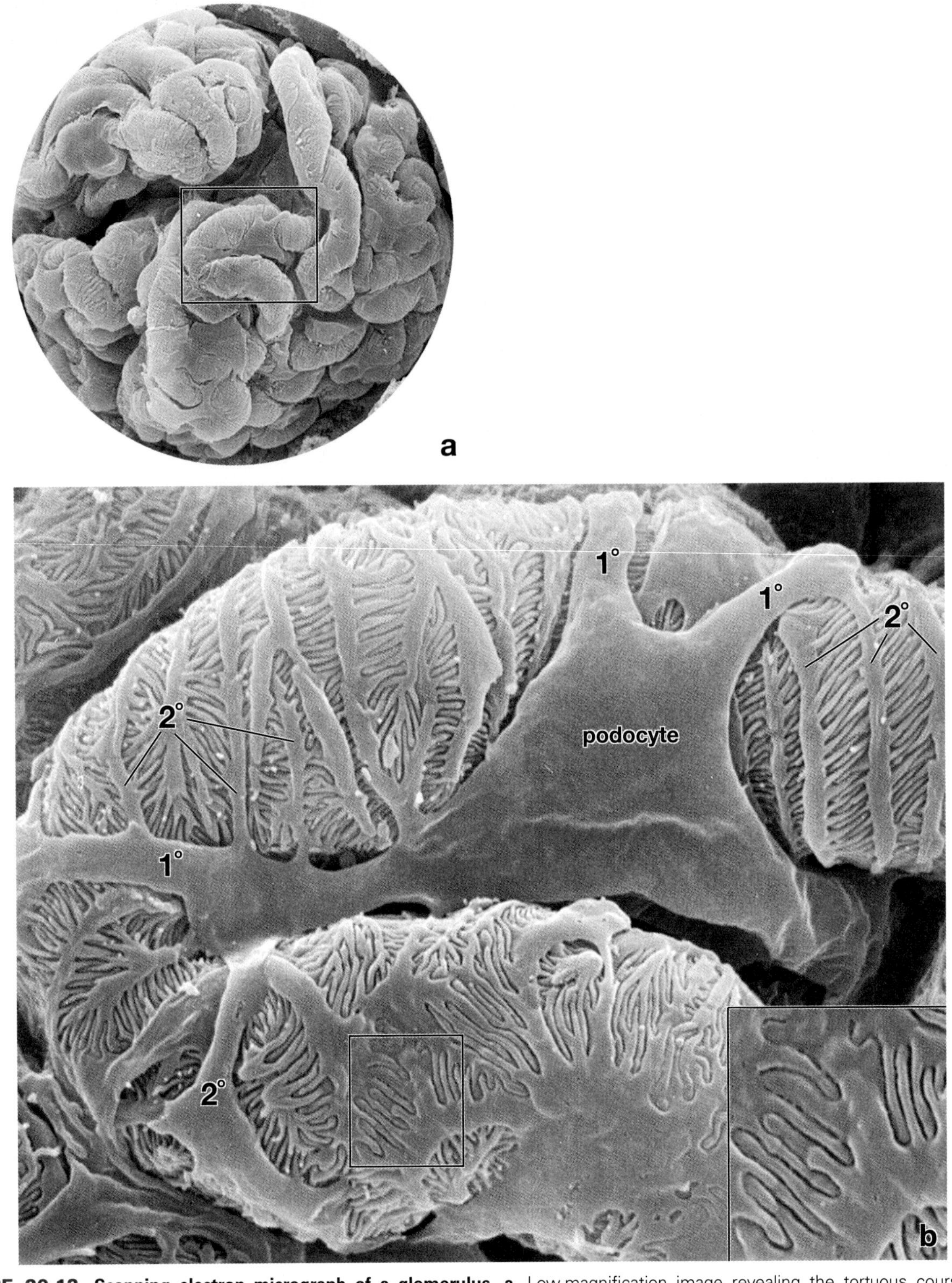

FIGURE 20.12. Scanning electron micrograph of a glomerulus. a. Low-magnification image revealing the tortuous course of the podocyte-covered glomerular capillaries. ×700. **b.** A higher magnification of the area in the *rectangle* in **a**. Note the podocyte and its processes embracing the capillary wall. The primary processes (*1°*) of the podocyte give rise to secondary processes (*2°*), which, in turn, give rise to the pedicels (foot processes). The space between the interdigitating pedicels creates the filtration slits. ×6,000. **Inset.** This higher magnification of the area in the *rectangle* reveals the filtration slits and clearly shows that alternating pedicels belong to the secondary process of one cell; the intervening pedicels belong to the adjacent cell. ×14,000.

proteoglycans (e.g., perlecan, agrin) and glycosaminoglycans, particularly heparan sulfate (Fig. 20.15). These components are localized in particular portions of the GBM:

- The **lamina rara externa**, adjacent to the podocyte processes. It is particularly rich in polyanions, such as heparan sulfate, that specifically impede the passage of negatively charged molecules.
- The **lamina rara interna**, adjacent to the capillary endothelium. Its molecular features are similar to those of the lamina rara externa.
- The **lamina densa**, the overlapping portion of the two basal laminae, sandwiched between the laminae rarae. It contains type IV collagen, which is organized into a network that acts as a physical filter. Type XVIII collagen, perlecan, and

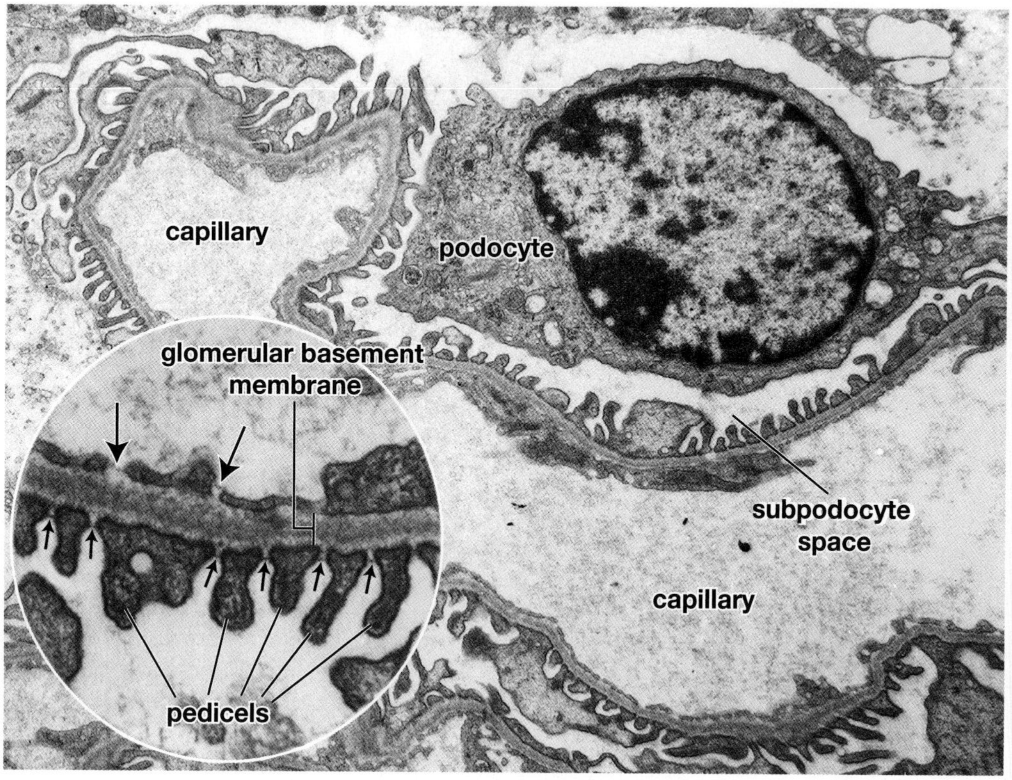

FIGURE 20.13. Transmission electron micrograph of a glomerular capillary and adjacent podocyte. The pedicels of the podocytes rest on the basal lamina adjacent to the capillary endothelium, and together, the three components—capillary endothelium, basal lamina, and podocyte—form a filtration apparatus. ×5,600. **Inset.** The *large arrows* point to the fenestrations in the endothelium. On the other side of the basal lamina are the pedicels of the podocytes. Note the slit diaphragm (*small arrows*) spanning the gap between adjacent pedicels. ×12,000.

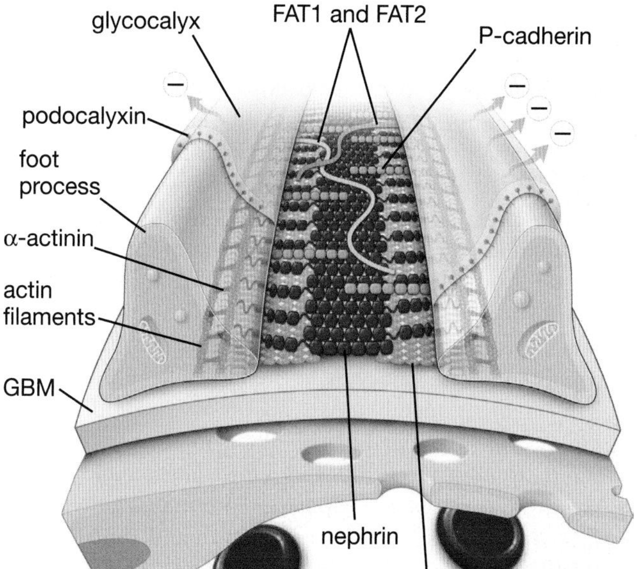

FIGURE 20.14. Diagram of the filtration slit diaphragm. The filtration slit diaphragm is a complex, zipper-like sheet structure formed by the transmembrane protein nephrin. The extracellular domains of the nephrin molecules emerge from the opposite foot processes of neighboring podocytes and interdigitate in the center of the slit, forming a central density with pores on both sides. The intracellular domains of nephrins interact with the actin cytoskeleton within the cytoplasm of foot processes. The sheet of nephrin molecules is reinforced near its attachment to the foot processes by Neph1 and Neph2 proteins that interact with each other and with nephrin. Other adhesion molecules, including P-cadherin, FAT1, and FAT2, are also found in this region. The apical cell membrane of podocytes' foot processes that face the urinary space is covered by the glycocalyx. It contains podocalyxin, a negatively charged membrane–bound sialoglycoprotein that acts as an antiadhesive molecule. The negatively charged podocalyxin keeps adjacent foot processes apart and maintains open filtration slits. Note that the foot processes of the podocytes are separated by the glomerular basement membrane (*GBM*) from the fenestrated endothelial cells lining the glomerular capillaries. (Redrawn from Tryggvason K, Patrakka J, Wartiovaara J. Hereditary proteinuria syndromes and mechanisms of proteinuria. *N Engl J Med.* 2006;354:1387–1401.)

agrin are responsible for the bulk of anionic charges found in GBM. The laminin and other proteins present in the laminae rarae interna and externa are involved in the attachment of the endothelial cells and podocytes to the GBM.

The GBM restricts the movement of particles, usually proteins, larger than approximately **70 kDa** or with a 3.6-nm radius (e.g., albumin or hemoglobin). Although albumin is not a usual constituent, it may sometimes be found in urine, indicating that the size of albumin is close to the effective pore size of the filtration barrier. The polyanionic glycosaminoglycans of the laminae rarae have strong negative charges and restrict the movement of anionic particles and molecules across the GBM, even those smaller than 70 kDa. Despite the ability of the filtration barrier to restrict protein, several grams of protein do pass through the barrier each day. This protein is reabsorbed by endocytosis in the proximal convoluted tubule. **Albuminuria** (presence of significant amounts of albumin in the urine) or **hematuria** (presence of significant amounts of red blood cells in the urine) indicates physical or functional damage to the GBM. In such cases (e.g., **diabetic nephropathy**), the number of anionic sites, especially in the lamina rara externa, is significantly reduced.

The filtration slit diaphragm acts as a size-selective filter.

The narrow **filtration slits** formed by the foot processes of podocytes and the filtration slit diaphragms act as physical barriers to restrict the movement of solutes and solvents across the filtration barrier. The discovery of specific proteins that form the **slit diaphragm** has led to new insights into the function of the filtration apparatus in the kidney. Most of the proteins found in the diaphragm are crucial for the normal development and function of the kidney. The slit diaphragm architecture accounts for true size-selective filter properties, which determine the molecular sieving characteristics of the glomerulus. Several mechanisms prevent clogging of the filtration slit diaphragms.

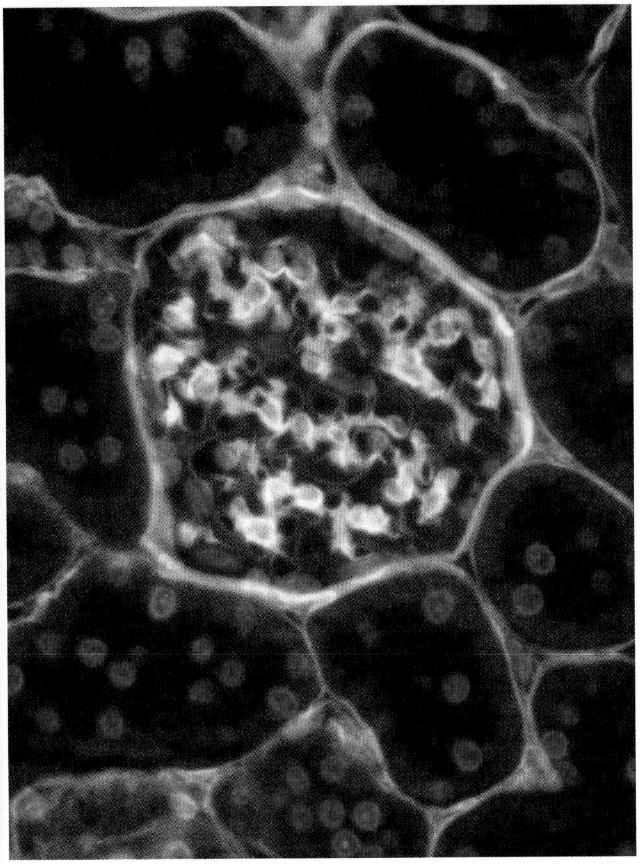

FIGURE 20.15. Immunofluorescent-stained glomerulus. This triple-exposure micrograph of a normal adult rat glomerulus is immunostained with two different antibodies. One antibody recognizes specific extracellular components, namely, basement membrane heparan sulfate proteoglycan (BM-HSPG, rhodamine label). The other antibody recognizes basement membrane chondroitin sulfate proteoglycan (BM-CSPG, fluorescein label). Because it is a triple-exposure micrograph, a yellow color occurs where the two fluorescent labels exactly co-distribute. The blue fluorescence is nuclear counterstaining with Hoechst nuclear stain. The micrograph shows that compartmentalization occurs with respect to glomerular proteoglycan populations. The glomerular capillary basement membrane is composed exclusively of BM-HSPG, whereas the mesangial matrix (*yellow*) contains both BM-HSPG and BM-CSPG. The Bowman capsule appears to be strongly stained by only BM-CSPG antibodies. ×360. (Courtesy of Dr. Kevin J. McCarthy.)

These include the negative charge of glycosaminoglycans in the GBM, negative charge of the podocyte cell membrane (due to sialoglycoproteins such as podocalyxin), and the phagocytic function of mesangial cells in the renal corpuscle.

Changes in individual components of the filtration apparatus influence the functions of other components.

The molecular structure and composition of each component of the glomerular filtration barrier has important consequences for adjacent components of the barrier. For instance, molecular changes in the GBM modify not only the contribution of this layer but also the rate at which solutes and solvents pass through the endothelium of glomerular capillaries on one side and the visceral layer of the Bowman capsule on the other. In addition, it is important to understand that the glomerular filtration barrier is not a passive but an active structure that can remodel itself and modify its own permeability.

Simple squamous epithelium constitutes the parietal layer of the Bowman capsule.

The **parietal layer of the Bowman capsule** contains **parietal epithelial cells** and forms a simple squamous epithelium. At the urinary pole of the renal corpuscle, the parietal layer is continuous with the cuboidal epithelium of the proximal convoluted tubule (see Figs. 20.7 and 20.11). Proliferation of parietal epithelial cells is a typical diagnostic feature in certain types of **glomerulonephritis** (inflammation of the glomerulus). For an example of such a disease, see Folder 20.2.

The space between the visceral and parietal layers of the Bowman capsule is called the **urinary space** or **Bowman space** (see Fig. 20.11). It is the receptacle for the glomerular ultrafiltrate (primary urine) produced by the filtration apparatus of the renal corpuscle. At the urinary pole of the renal corpuscle, the urinary space is continuous with the lumen of the proximal convoluted tubule.

Mesangium

In the renal corpuscle, the GBM is shared among several capillaries to create a space containing an additional group of cells called **mesangial cells**. Mesangial cells are thus enclosed by the GBM (Fig. 20.16). These cells and their extracellular matrix constitute the **mesangium**. The mesangium is most obvious at the vascular stalk of the glomerulus and at the interstices of adjoining glomerular capillaries. The mesangial cells are not confined entirely to the renal corpuscle; some are located outside the corpuscle along the vascular pole, where they are also designated as **lacis cells** and form part of what is called the **juxtaglomerular apparatus** (see Fig. 20.7).

Important functions of the mesangial cells are as follows:

- **Phagocytosis** and **endocytosis**. Mesangial cells remove trapped residues and aggregated proteins from the GBM and filtration slit diaphragm, thus keeping the glomerular filter free of debris. They also endocytose and process a variety of plasma proteins, including immune complexes. Maintaining the structure and function of the glomerular barrier is the primary function of the mesangial cells.
- **Structural support**. Mesangial cells produce components of the extracellular mesangial matrix that provide support for the podocytes in the areas where the epithelial basement membrane is absent or incomplete (see Fig. 20.16). Mesangial matrix differs in composition substantially from the GBM and allows larger molecules to pass from the lumen of capillaries into the mesangium.
- **Secretion**. Mesangial cells synthesize and secrete a variety of molecules such as interleukin-1 (IL-1), PGE_2, and platelet-derived growth factor (PDGF), which play a central role in response to glomerular injury.
- **Modulation of glomerular distension**. Mesangial cells have contractile properties. In the past, it was suggested that contraction of mesangial cells could increase the intraglomerular blood volume and filtration pressure. More recent studies have revealed that mesangial contribution to glomerular filtration rate is minimal and that the mesangial cells may function in regulating glomerular distension in response to increased blood pressure.

Clinically, it has been observed that **mesangial cells** proliferate in certain kidney diseases in which abnormal amounts of protein and protein complexes are trapped in the GBM. Proliferation of mesangial cells is a prominent feature in the **immunoglobulin A (IgA) nephropathy (Berger disease)**, **membranoproliferative glomerulonephritis**, **lupus nephritis**, and **diabetic nephropathy**.

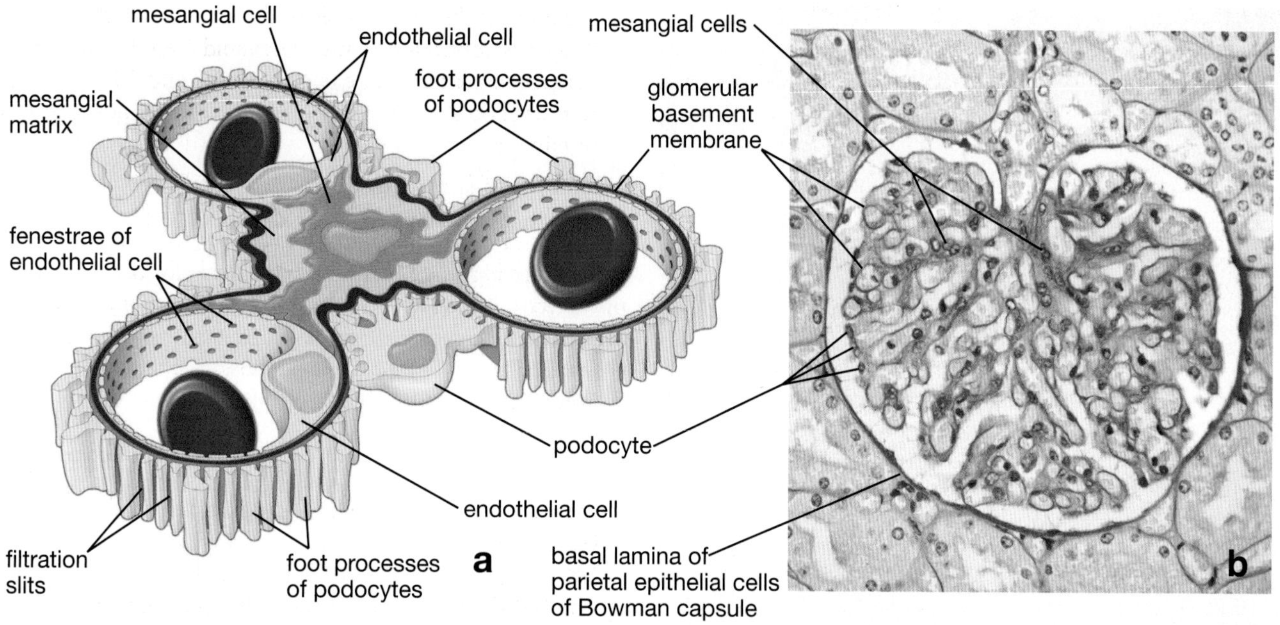

FIGURE 20.16. Diagram and photomicrograph showing the relationship between intraglomerular mesangial cells and glomerular capillaries. a. The mesangial cell and its surrounding matrix are enclosed by the glomerular basement membrane (GBM) of the glomerular capillaries. The mesangial cells are located in the same compartment as the endothelial cells and can be intimately associated with the GBM as well as with the endothelial cells without the intervening GBM. Note that a mesangial cell produces extracellular mesangial matrix, which provides support for the glomerular capillaries. **b.** Photomicrograph of a glomerulus stained by the periodic acid–Schiff (PAS) method. Note that the GBM is well visualized within the glomerulus and surrounds the glomerular capillaries. The GBM reflects at the vascular pole to become the basal lamina of the epithelial cells that form the parietal layer of the Bowman capsule. The nuclei of the PAS-positive mesangial cells are positioned between the loops of capillaries more toward the center of the glomerulus. Specimen was counterstained with hematoxylin. ×360.

Embryologically, mesangial and juxtaglomerular cells (discussed in the following paragraph) are derived from smooth muscle cell precursors from the metanephric mesenchyme. During development, these cells are characterized by expressing **platelet-derived growth factor receptors (PDGFRs).** Their migration into the developing glomeruli is guided by chemotactic effects of the **platelet-derived growth factor-β (PDGFβ)** expressed on the developing podocytes. Although mesangial cells are clearly phagocytotic, they are unusual in the sense that they are not derived from blood-borne monocytes, the usual precursor cells of the mononuclear phagocytotic system.

Juxtaglomerular Apparatus

The juxtaglomerular apparatus includes the macula densa, the juxtaglomerular cells, and the extraglomerular mesangial cells.

Lying directly adjacent to the afferent and efferent arterioles and adjacent to some extraglomerular mesangial cells at the vascular pole of the renal corpuscle is the terminal portion of the **distal straight tubule** of the nephron. At this site, the wall of the tubule contains cells that are referred to collectively as the **macula densa.** When viewed in the light microscope, the cells of the macula densa are distinctive in that they are narrower and usually taller than other distal tubule cells (see Fig. 20.7). The nuclei of these cells appear crowded, even to the extent that they appear partially superimposed over one another, thus the name macula densa.

In this same region, the smooth muscle cells of the adjacent afferent arteriole (and, sometimes, the efferent arteriole) are modified. They contain secretory granules, and their nuclei are spherical, as opposed to the typical elongated smooth muscle cell nucleus. These **juxtaglomerular cells** (see Fig. 20.7) require special stains to reveal the secretory vesicles in the light microscope.

The juxtaglomerular apparatus regulates blood pressure by activating the renin–angiotensin–aldosterone system.

In certain physiologic (low sodium intake) or pathologic conditions (decrease in volume of circulating blood because of hemorrhage or reduction in renal perfusion owing to compression of the renal arteries), juxtaglomerular cells are responsible for activating the **renin–angiotensin–aldosterone system (RAAS).** This system plays an important role in maintaining sodium homeostasis and renal hemodynamics (see Folder 20.3). The granules of the juxtaglomerular cells contain an aspartyl protease called **renin,** which is synthesized, stored, and released into the bloodstream from the modified smooth muscle cells. In the blood, renin catalyzes the hydrolysis of a circulating α_2-globulin, angiotensinogen, to produce the decapeptide angiotensin I. Production of angiotensin I prompt the following sequence of events:

- **Angiotensin I** is converted to the active octapeptide **angiotensin II** by **angiotensin-converting enzyme (ACE)** present in the endothelial cells of lung capillaries.
- Angiotensin II stimulates the synthesis and release of the hormone **aldosterone** from the **zona glomerulosa of the adrenal gland** (see pages 843-844).
- **Aldosterone,** in turn, acts on principal cells of connecting tubules and collecting ducts to increase reabsorption of Na^+ and water, as well as K^+ secretion, thereby raising blood volume and pressure.
- **Angiotensin II** is also a potent vasoconstrictor that has a regulatory role in the control of renal and systemic vascular resistance.

The **juxtaglomerular apparatus** functions not only as an endocrine organ that secretes **renin** but also as a sensor of blood volume and tubular fluid composition. The cells of the macula densa **monitor the Na^+ concentration** in the

FOLDER 20.2

CLINICAL CORRELATION: ANTIGLOMERULAR BASEMENT MEMBRANE ANTIBODY–INDUCED GLOMERULONEPHRITIS; GOODPASTURE SYNDROME

As discussed earlier in the section on the basal lamina assembly (see Chapter 5, Epithelial Tissue), the major building block of any basement membrane, including the **glomerular basement membrane (GBM)**, is the **type IV collagen** molecule. Its core structure is composed of three α-chain monomers, each representing one or more of six types of α-chains (see Table 6.2, page 182). Each molecule has three domains: an amino-terminus 7S domain, a middle collagenous helical domain, and a carboxy-terminus noncollagenous NC1 domain. The molecular architecture of type IV collagen is a key to understanding the pathophysiology of glomerular kidney diseases. For instance, an autoimmune response to the noncollagenous NC1 domain of the α3-chain of type IV collagen (α3[IV]) in the glomerular basement membrane (GBM) is responsible for the development of **anti-GBM antibody–induced glomerulonephritis**. This condition is characterized by a linear deposition of immunoglobulin G (IgG) antibodies in the GBM.

In some individuals, anti-GBM antibodies may cross-react with the alveolar basement membrane in the lungs, producing **Goodpasture syndrome**. A characteristic clinical feature of Goodpasture syndrome is rapidly progressive glomerulonephritis (inflammation in the glomeruli) and pulmonary hemorrhage due to disruption of the air–blood barrier. In response to deposition of IgG in the glomerulus, the complement system is activated and circulating leukocytes elaborate a variety of proteases, leading to disruption of the GBM and deposition of fibrin. Fibrin, in turn, stimulates the proliferation of parietal cells lining the Bowman capsule and causes influx of monocytes from the circulation. The product of these reactions is often seen within the glomerulus as a **crescent**, a characteristic microscopic feature of glomerulonephritis (Fig. F20.2.1). Most patients affected by Goodpasture syndrome have a severe crescentic glomerulonephritis with transiently elevated levels of circulating anti-GBM antibodies. Formation of anti-GBM antibodies is most likely triggered by viruses, cancer, pharmacologic agents, and chemical compounds found in a variety of paints, solvents, and dyes.

Individuals with Goodpasture syndrome present with both respiratory and urinary symptoms, including shortness of breath, cough, and bloody sputum as well as hematuria (blood in urine), proteinuria (proteins in the urine), and other symptoms of progressive kidney failure.

The main therapeutic goal in treating Goodpasture syndrome is to remove the circulating pathogenic antibodies from the blood. This is achieved by plasmapheresis, in which blood plasma is removed from the circulation and replaced by fluid, protein, or donated plasma. In addition, treatment with immunosuppressive drugs and corticosteroids is beneficial to keep the immune system from producing pathogenic autoantibodies.

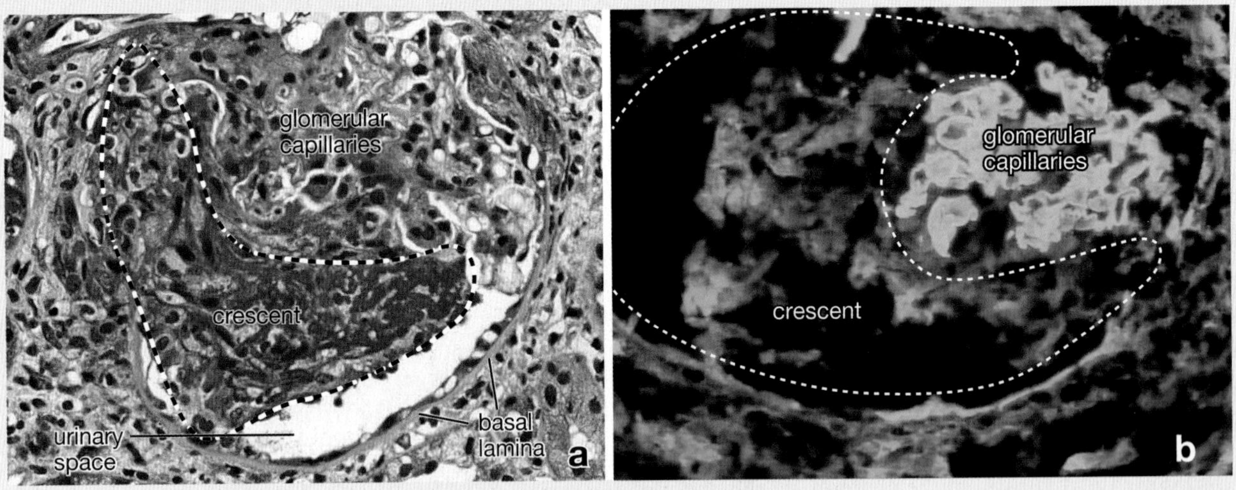

FIGURE F20.2.1. Photomicrograph of a glomerulus in Goodpasture syndrome. a. In this Mallory trichrome–stained specimen obtained from a kidney biopsy, the collagen molecules in the mesangial matrix and glomerular capillaries are stained *dark blue*. The *bright red* stain within the renal corpuscle represents fibrin, which leaked out of the glomerular capillary loops into the urinary space. A cellular crescent (outlined in *dashed line*) is formed by deposition of fibrin infiltrated by macrophages and proliferated parietal cells of the Bowman capsule. The *light blue* color surrounding the glomerulus is reflective of edematous reaction containing cells mediating inflammatory reactions. Note the basal lamina of a parietal layer of the Bowman capsule. ×320. **b.** This immunofluorescence image of the renal corpuscle shows the glomerular basement membrane (GBM) labeled with antibodies directed against human IgG and visualized with secondary antibodies conjugated with fluorescent dye. In Goodpasture syndrome, IgGs bind to the NC1 domain of type IV collagen (α3-chain) found in the GBM. Note the irregular thickness pattern of the GBM surrounding capillary loops. The remaining space is occupied by the cellular crescent. ×360. *IgG*, immunoglobulin G. (Courtesy of Dr. Joseph P. Grande.)

FOLDER 20.3

CLINICAL CORRELATION: RENIN–ANGIOTENSIN–ALDOSTERONE SYSTEM AND HYPERTENSION

The **renin–angiotensin–aldosterone system (RAAS)** plays a key role in Na^+ and blood volume homeostasis as well as in long-term regulation of arterial blood pressure. Renin secreted by the juxtaglomerular apparatus of the kidney converts angiotensinogen to angiotensin I, which is then converted in the lungs by the angiotensin-converting enzyme (ACE) to **angiotensin II**, one of the most potent vasoconstrictors in the human body. Angiotensin II has an important function in stimulating **aldosterone** secretion from the adrenal cortex. Aldosterone reabsorbs Na^+ and excretes K^+; thus, it has an effect on retention of extracellular water volume (Fig. F20.3.1).

For years, cardiologists and nephrologists believed that **chronic essential hypertension**, the most common form of hypertension, was somehow related to an abnormality in the RAAS. However, 24-hour urine renin levels in such patients were usually normal. Not until a factor in the venom of a South American snake (Brazilian pit viper, *Bothrops jararaca*) was shown to be a potent inhibitor of ACE in the lung did investigators have both a clue to the cause of chronic essential hypertension and a new series of drugs with which to treat this common disease.

The "lesion" in chronic essential hypertension is now believed to be excessive production of **angiotensin II** in the lung. Development of the so-called **ACE inhibitors**—captopril, enalapril, and related derivatives of the original snake venom factor—has revolutionized the treatment of chronic essential hypertension. These antihypertensive drugs do not cause the often-dangerous side effects of the diuretics and β-blockers that were previously the most commonly used drugs for the control of this condition.

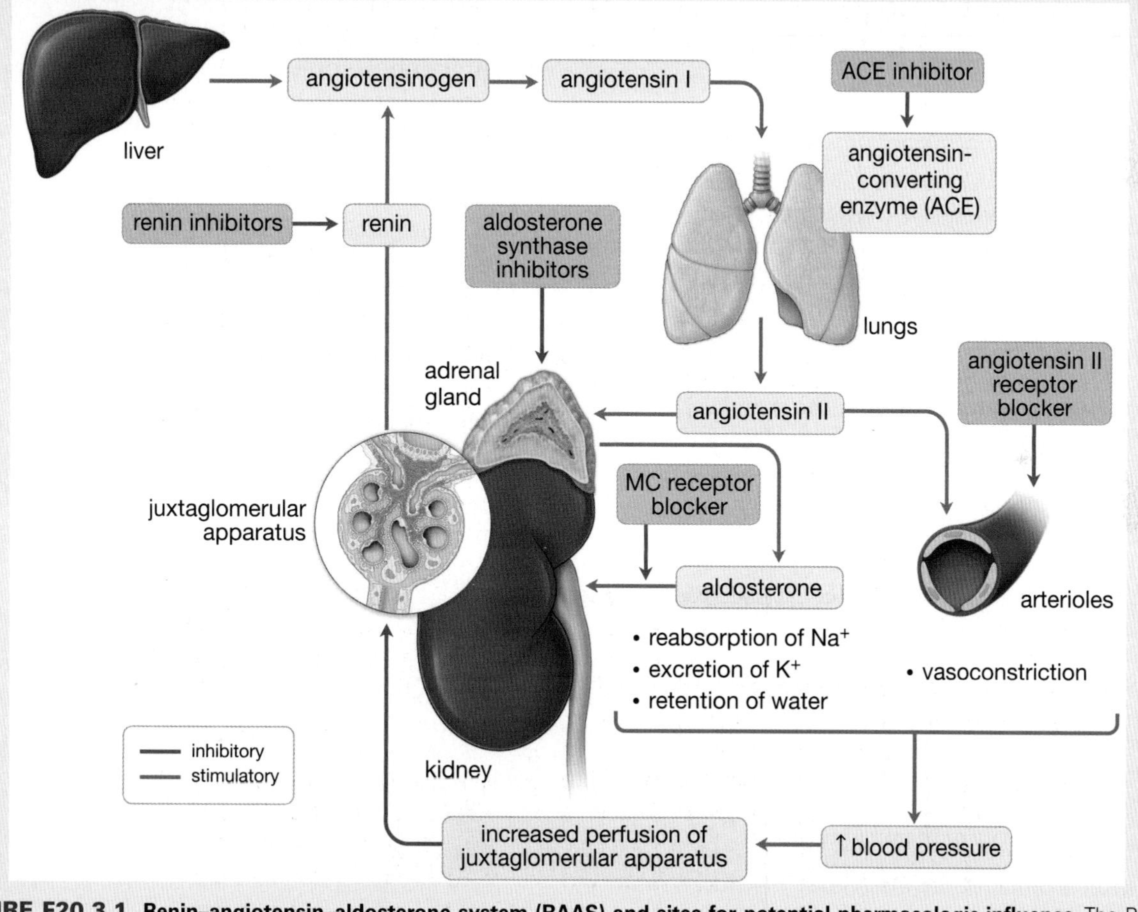

FIGURE F20.3.1. Renin–angiotensin–aldosterone system (RAAS) and sites for potential pharmacologic influence. The RAAS is a multisystem endocrine cascade that regulates electrolyte homeostasis, fluid balance, and blood pressure through action on the kidney and cardiovascular system. Decreased perfusion pressure in the kidney triggers the juxtaglomerular cells to release renin into the bloodstream and begin the cascade. *Blue arrows* indicate stimulatory action on the system; *red arrows* indicate inhibitory feedback and action of pharmaceutical agents. Examples of frequently used pharmaceutical agents that influence RAAS include mineralocorticoid (MC) receptor blockers (e.g., spironolactone, eplerenone), ACE inhibitors (e.g., captopril, enalapril), renin inhibitors (e.g., aliskiren), and angiotensin II receptor blockers (e.g., valsartan, losartan). Aldosterone synthase inhibitors are still in the experimental phase.

FOLDER 20.4

CLINICAL CORRELATION: EXAMINATION OF THE URINE—URINALYSIS

Urinalysis is an important part of the examination of patients with suspected renal disease. It typically includes several measurements of physical, biochemical, and microscopic urine characteristics, such as pH, specific gravity (indirect measurement of ion concentration), bilirubin, concentration of intermediate compounds derived from the fatty acid metabolism known as *ketone bodies*, hemoglobin, and concentration of the proteins. The excretion of excessive amounts of protein in the urine (**proteinuria** or albuminuria) is an important diagnostic sign of renal disease and is a key part of urinalysis. Normally, less than 150 mg of protein is excreted in the urine each day. Although excessive excretion of protein almost always indicates renal disease, extreme exercise, such as jogging, or severe dehydration may produce increased proteinuria in individuals without renal disease. Microscopic examination of the urine may reveal the presence of red and white blood cells, mineral crystals, and pathogenic agents, such as bacteria or fungi. Often, these elements are enclosed within cylindrical structures called **urinary casts**. The matrix of a urinary cast is formed by an 85-kDa protein, **uromodulin (Tamm–Horsfall protein)**, that precipitates in the lumen of distal convoluted tubules and collecting ducts during a disease process.

tubular fluid and regulate both the glomerular filtration rate and the release of renin from the juxtaglomerular cells. The decreased Na^+ concentration in the distal convoluted tubule is believed to be a stimulus for unique ion-transporting molecules expressed on the apical membrane of macula densa cells. These molecules include $Na^+/K^+/2Cl^-$ cotransporters, Na^+/H^+ exchangers, and pH- and calcium-regulated K^+ channels. Activation of membrane transport pathways changes the intracellular ion concentration within the macula densa cells and initiates signaling mechanisms by releasing various mediators, such as adenosine triphosphate (ATP), adenosine, nitric oxide (NO), and prostaglandins (PGE_2). These molecules act in a paracrine manner and signal both the underlying juxtaglomerular cells of the afferent arteriole to secrete renin and the vascular smooth muscle cells to contract. An increase in blood volume sufficient to cause stretching of the juxtaglomerular cells in the afferent arteriole may be the stimulus that closes the feedback loop and stops the secretion of renin.

■ KIDNEY TUBULE FUNCTION

As the **glomerular ultrafiltrate** passes through the uriniferous tubule and collecting ducts of the kidney, it undergoes changes that involve both active and passive absorption and secretion:

- Certain substances within the ultrafiltrate are reabsorbed, some partially (e.g., water, sodium, and bicarbonate) and some completely (e.g., glucose).
- Other substances (e.g., creatinine and organic acids and bases) are added to the ultrafiltrate (i.e., the primary urine) by secretory activity of the tubule cells.

Thus, the volume of the ultrafiltrate is reduced substantially, and the urine is made hyperosmotic. The long loop of Henle and the connecting tubules and collecting ducts that pass parallel to similarly arranged blood vessels, the vasa recta, serve as the basis for the countercurrent multiplier mechanism that is instrumental in concentrating the urine, thereby making it hyperosmotic.

Proximal Convoluted Tubule

The proximal convoluted tubule is the initial and major site of reabsorption.

The **proximal convoluted tubule** receives the ultrafiltrate from the urinary space of the Bowman capsule. The cuboidal cells of the proximal convoluted tubule have elaborate surface specializations associated with cells engaged in absorption and fluid transport. They exhibit the following features:

- A **brush border**, composed of relatively long, closely packed, and straight microvilli (Fig. 20.17)
- A **junctional complex**, consisting of a narrow, tight junction that seals off the intercellular space from the lumen of the tubule and a zonula adherens that maintains the adhesion between neighboring cells
- **Plicae** or **folds** located on the lateral surfaces of the cells, which are large flattened processes, alternating with similar processes of adjacent cells (see Fig. 20.16)
- Extensive **interdigitation of basal processes** of adjacent cells (Figs. 20.18 and 20.19)
- **Basal striations**, consisting of elongated mitochondria concentrated in the basal processes and oriented vertically to the basal surface (see Fig. 20.18)

In well-fixed histologic preparations, the basal striations and the apical brush border help distinguish the cells of the proximal convoluted tubule from those of the other tubules.

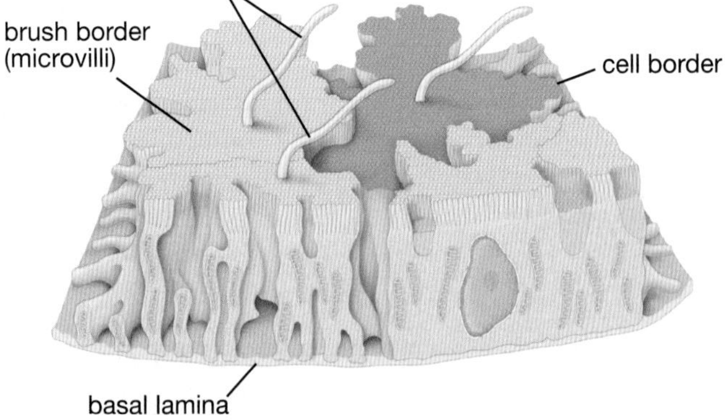

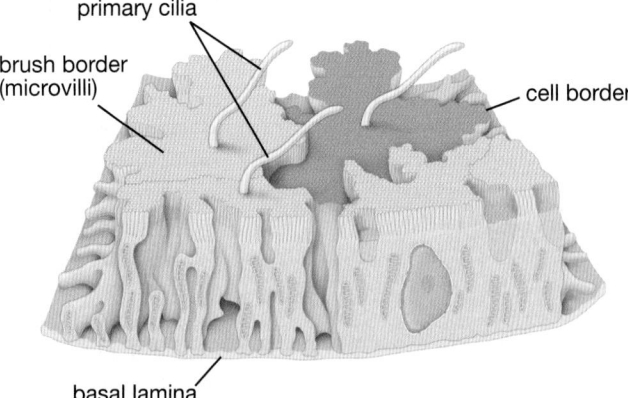

FIGURE 20.17. Diagram of proximal convoluted tubule cells. This diagram is drawn at the electron microscopic level and shows the sectioned face on the *right* and a three-dimensional view of the basolateral surface of a proximal convulsed tubule cell with a partial cut face on the *left*. Here, the interdigitating parts of the adjoining cell have been removed to show the basolateral interdigitations. Some of the interdigitating processes extend the full height of the cell. The processes are long in the basal region and create an elaborate extracellular compartment adjacent to the basal lamina. Apically, the microvilli constitute the brush border. In some locations, the microvilli have been omitted, thereby revealing the convoluted character of the apical cell boundary. (Based on Bulger RE. The shape of rat kidney tubular cells. *Am J Anat.* 1965;116:253.)

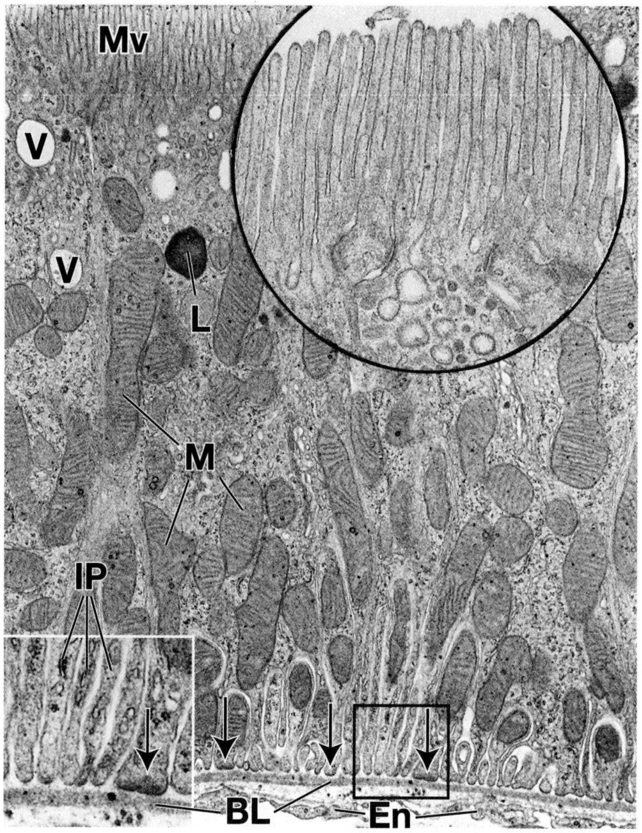

FIGURE 20.18. Electron micrograph of a proximal tubule cell. The apical surface of the cell shows the closely packed microvilli (*Mv*) that collectively are recognized as the brush border in the light microscope. Many vesicles (*V*) are evident in the apical cytoplasm. Also present in the apical region of the cell are lysosomes (*L*). The nucleus has not been included in the plane of section. Extensive numbers of longitudinally oriented mitochondria (*M*) are present in the cell within the interdigitating processes. The mitochondria are responsible for the appearance of the basal striations seen in the light microscope, particularly if the extracellular space is enlarged. The electron micrograph also reveals a basal lamina (*BL*) and a small amount of connective tissue and the fenestrated endothelium (*En*) of an adjacent peritubular capillary. ×15,000. **Upper inset.** This higher magnification of the microvilli shows the small endocytotic vesicles that have pinched off from the plasma membrane at the base of the microvilli. ×32,000. **Lower inset.** A higher magnification of the basal portion of the interdigitating processes (*IP*) below the reach of the mitochondria. The extreme basal aspect of these processes reveals a dense material (*arrows*) that represents bundles of actin filaments (see Fig. 20.16). ×30,000.

At the base of the proximal convoluted tubule cell, in the interdigitating processes, bundles of 6-nm microfilaments are present (see *arrows*, Figs. 20.18 and 20.19). These actin filaments may play a role in regulating the movement of fluid from the basolateral extracellular space across the tubule basal lamina toward the adjacent peritubular capillary.

The proximal convoluted tubule recovers most of the fluid from the ultrafiltrate. Of the 180 L/d of ultrafiltrate entering the nephrons, approximately 120 L/d, or 65% of the ultrafiltrate, is reabsorbed by the proximal convoluted tubule. Two major proteins are responsible for fluid reabsorption in the proximal convoluted tubules:

- **Na^+/K^+-ATPase pumps**, transmembrane proteins that are localized in the lateral folds of the plasma membrane. They are responsible for the *reabsorption of Na+*, which is the major driving force for reabsorption of water in the proximal convoluted tubule. As in the intestinal and gallbladder epithelia, this process is driven by active transport of Na^+ into the lateral intercellular space. Active transport of Na^+ is followed by passive diffusion of Cl^- to maintain electrochemical neutrality. The accumulation of NaCl in the lateral intercellular spaces creates an osmotic gradient that draws water from the lumen into the intercellular compartment. This compartment distends as the amount of fluid in it increases; the lateral folds separate to allow this distension.
- **Aquaporin-1 (AQP-1)**, a small (~30 kDa) transmembrane protein that functions as a molecular water channel in the cell membrane of proximal convoluted tubules. Movement of water through these membrane channels does not require the high energy generated by Na^+/K^+-ATPase pumps. Immunocytochemical methods can be used to demonstrate the presence of these proteins.

The hydrostatic pressure that builds up in the distended intercellular compartment, presumably aided by contractile activity of the actin filaments in the base of the tubule cells,

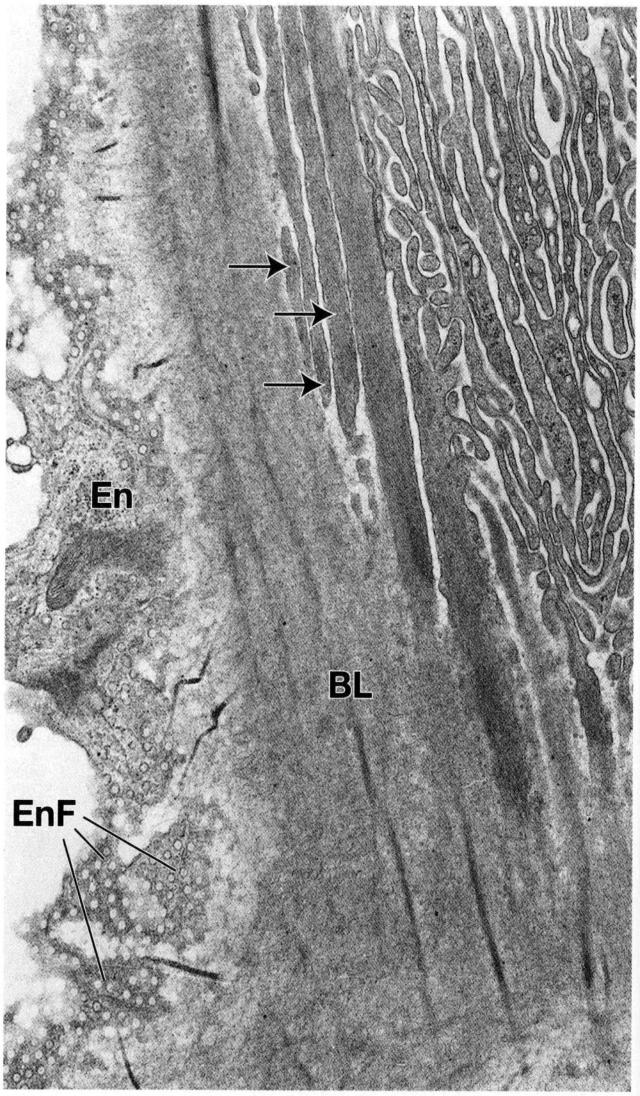

FIGURE 20.19. Electron micrograph of a proximal convoluted tubule cell. This section is almost tangential and slightly oblique to the base of a proximal convoluted tubule cell and the subjacent basal lamina and capillary. In the *left part* of the micrograph is the capillary endothelium (*En*). Characteristically, the endothelium possesses numerous fenestrations (*EnF*), and in this plane of section, the fenestrations are seen en face, displaying circular profiles. The plane of section also makes the basal lamina (*BL*) appears as a broad band of homogeneous material. To the *right* of the basal lamina are the interdigitating basal processes of the proximal tubule cells. The long, straight processes contain longitudinally oriented actin filaments (*arrows*). In this plane of section, the basal extracellular space appears as a maze between the cellular processes. ×32,000.

drives an essentially isosmotic fluid across the tubule basement membrane into the renal connective tissue. Here, the fluid is reabsorbed into the vessels of the peritubular capillary network.

The proximal convoluted tubule also reabsorbs nearly all glucose, amino acids, and small polypeptides.

As in the intestine, the microvilli of the proximal convoluted tubule cells are covered with a well-developed glycocalyx that contains several ATPases, peptidases, and high concentrations of disaccharidases. The proximal convoluted tubule recovers almost 100% of **glucose** using Na^+ glucose cotransporters (SGLT2) that simultaneously absorb Na^+ and glucose from the lumen of the tubule. Glucose uptake by epithelial cells generates a high intracellular concentration of glucose, which activates the family of glucose transporters (GLUT2). GLUT2 transports glucose through the basolateral membrane into the connective tissue, where it enters the lumen of blood vessels. The proximal convoluted tubule also recovers approximately 98% of the filtered **amino acids**. These amino acids are absorbed by several amino acid transporters that either exchange Na^+, H^+, and K^+ ions (acidic amino acid transporters) or Na^+ and H^+ ions (basic and neutral amino acid transporters). The brush border in the proximal convoluted tubule resembles that of a striated border in the small intestine in that it possesses many peptidases that degrade large proteins into smaller proteins and polypeptides. Similar to glucose, **small polypeptides** are recovered in a process that employs apical surface H^+ peptide cotransporters (PepT1 and PepT2). Once inside the cell, polypeptides are rapidly degraded and transported across the basolateral membrane as free amino acids.

Proteins and large peptides are endocytosed in the proximal convoluted tubule.

Deep tubular invaginations are present between the microvilli of the proximal convoluted tubule cells. Proteins in the ultrafiltrate, on reaching the tubule lumen, bind to endocytotic receptors expressed on the plasma membrane. When proteins bind to receptors, the process of endocytosis is initiated and endocytotic vesicles containing the bound protein form large protein-containing early endosomes (see Fig. 20.18). These early endosomes are destined to become lysosomes, and the endocytosed proteins are degraded by acid hydrolases. The amino acids produced in the lysosomal degradation are recycled into the circulation via the intercellular compartment and the interstitial connective tissue.

In addition, the pH of the ultrafiltrate is modified in the proximal convoluted tubule by the reabsorption of bicarbonate and the specific secretion into the lumen of exogenous organic acids and organic bases derived from the peritubular capillary circulation.

Proximal Straight Tubule

The cells of the **proximal straight tubule** (i.e., the thick descending limb of the loop of Henle) are not as specialized for absorption as are those of the proximal convoluted tubule. They are shorter, with a less well-developed brush border and fewer and less complex lateral and basolateral processes. The mitochondria are smaller than those of the cells of the convoluted segment and are randomly distributed in the cytoplasm. There are fewer apical invaginations and endocytotic vesicles as well as fewer lysosomes. Cells in the proximal straight tubule are designed to recover the remaining glucose that escaped recovery in the proximal convoluted tubules before it enters the thin segment of the loop of Henle. They are equipped with high-affinity Na^+ glucose cotransporters (SGLT1) that simultaneously absorb Na^+ and glucose from the lumen of the tubule. These cells also possess complementary GLUT1 glucose transporters in their basolateral membrane to transport glucose out of the cell and into the extracellular matrix.

Thin Segment of Loop of Henle

As noted earlier, the length of the **thin segment** varies with the location of the nephron in the cortex. Juxtamedullary nephrons have the longest limbs; cortical nephrons have the shortest. Furthermore, various cell types are present in the thin segment. In the light microscope, it is possible to detect at least two kinds of thin segment tubules, one with a more squamous epithelium than the other. Electron microscopic examination of the thin segments of various nephrons reveals further differences, namely, the existence of four types of epithelial cells (Fig. 20.20):

- **Type I epithelium** is found in the thin descending and ascending limbs of the loop of Henle of short-looped nephrons. It consists of a thin, simple epithelium. The cells have almost no interdigitations with neighboring cells and few organelles.
- **Type II epithelium**, found in the thin descending limb of long-looped nephrons in the cortical labyrinth, consists of taller epithelium. These cells possess abundant organelles

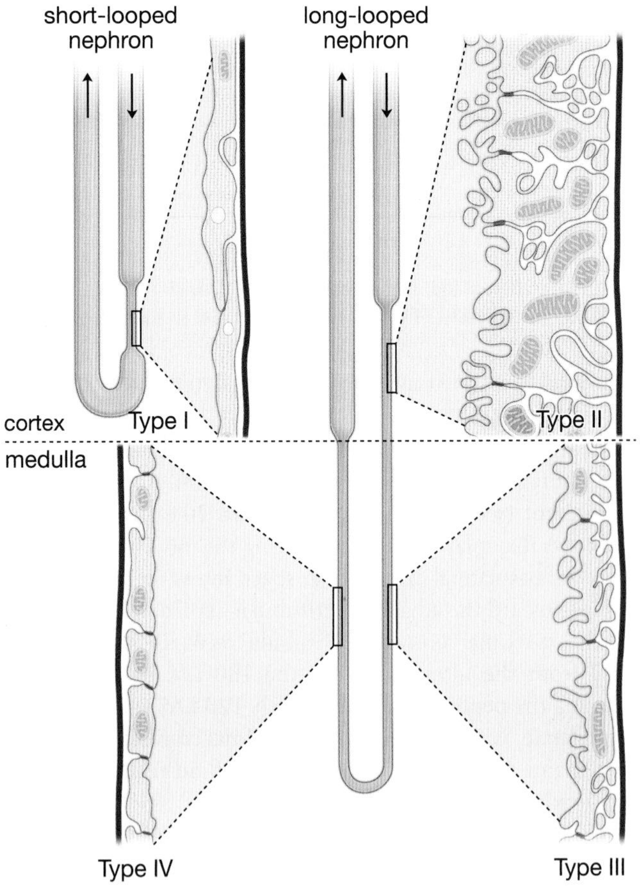

FIGURE 20.20. Schematic diagram of loop of Henle thin limb epithelial cells. This diagram shows the various types of epithelia and the region where they are found in the thin limb of the short and long loops of Henle. The diagrams of the epithelium do not include nuclear regions of the epithelial cells. (Modified from Madsen KM, Tisher CC. Physiologic anatomy of the kidney. In: Fisher JW, ed. *Kidney Hormones*. Academic Press; 1986;3:45–100.)

and have many small, blunt microvilli. The extent of lateral interdigitation with neighboring cells varies by species.

- **Type III epithelium**, found in the thin descending limb in the inner medulla, consists of a thinner epithelium. The cells have a simpler structure and fewer microvilli than type II epithelial cells. Lateral interdigitations are absent.
- **Type IV epithelium**, found at the bend of long-looped nephrons and through the entire thin ascending limb, consists of a low, flattened epithelium without microvilli. The cells possess few organelles.

The specific functional roles of the four cell types are related to their role in the countercurrent exchange system that functions in concentrating tubular fluid. Morphologic differences, such as microvilli, mitochondria, and the degree of cellular interdigitation, probably reflect specific active or passive roles in this process.

The thin descending and ascending limbs of the loop of Henle differ in structural and functional properties.

Studies of the ultrafiltrate that enters the thin descending limb and leaves the thin ascending limb of the loop of Henle reveal dramatic changes in ultrafiltrate osmolality. The ultrafiltrate that enters the **thin descending limb** is **isosmotic**, whereas the ultrafiltrate leaving the **thin ascending limb** is **hyposmotic** to plasma. This change is achieved by reabsorbing more salts than water. The two limbs of the loop of Henle have different permeabilities and thus different functions:

- The **thin descending limb** of the loop of Henle is **highly permeable to water** because of the presence of AQPs that allow for free passage of water. This limb is much less permeable to Na^+ and urea; however, it does permit small amounts to enter the nephron at this site. Urea enters this segment of the nephron via urea transporter A2 (UT-A2). Because the interstitial fluid in the medulla is hyperosmotic, water exits this nephron segment by osmosis, causing the luminal content of Na^+ and Cl^- to become progressively more concentrated. The cells of this limb do not actively transport ions; thus, the *increased tubular fluid osmolality* that occurs in this nephron segment is caused in large part by the passive movement of water into the peritubular connective tissue.
- The **thin ascending limb** of the loop of Henle is **highly permeable to Na^+ and Cl^-** because of the presence of $Na^+/K^+/2Cl^-$ cotransporters in the apical plasma cell membranes. Na^+ is then pumped out of the cells by Na^+/K^+-ATPase, whereas K^+ and Cl^- passively diffuse through their respective channels into the medulla following their concentration gradients. Although the energy from ATP is required to open these channels, the movement of Cl^- is not an example of active transport and does not require Cl^--stimulated ATPase activity. Counter ions, in this case, Na^+ (the majority) and K^+, follow passively to maintain electrochemical neutrality. The hyperosmolarity of the interstitium is directly related to the transport activity of the cells in this nephron segment. Furthermore, the thin ascending limb is largely **impermeable to water**; therefore, Na^+ and Cl^- concentration increases in the interstitium, causing it to become hyperosmotic and the fluid in the lumen of the nephron to become hyposmotic. For this reason, the thin ascending limb is sometimes referred to as the **diluting segment of the nephron**.

In addition, epithelial cells lining the thick ascending limb produce an 85-kDa protein called **uromodulin (Tamm–Horsfall protein)** that influences NaCl reabsorption and urinary concentration ability. **Uromodulin** also modulates cell adhesion and signal transduction by interacting with various cytokines. It also inhibits the aggregation of calcium oxalate crystals (preventing kidney stone formation) and provides a defense against urinary tract infection. In individuals with **inflammatory kidney diseases**, a precipitated uromodulin is detected in urine in the form of **urinary casts** (see Folder 20.4).

Distal Straight Tubule

The distal straight tubule is part of the ascending limb of the loop of Henle.

The **distal straight tubule (thick ascending limb)**, as previously noted, is part of the ascending limb of the loop of Henle and includes both medullary and cortical portions, with the latter located in the medullary rays. The distal straight tubule, like the ascending thin limb, transports ions from the tubular lumen to the interstitium. The apical cell membrane in this segment has electroneutral transporters (synporters) that allow Cl^-, Na^+, and K^+ to enter the cell from the lumen. Na^+ is actively transported across the extensive basolateral plications by the Na^+/K^+-ATPase pumps; Cl^- and K^+ diffuse out from the intracellular space by the Cl^- and K^+ channels. Some K^+ ions leak back into the tubular fluid through K^+ channels, causing the tubular lumen to be positively charged with respect to the interstitium. This positive gradient provides the driving force for the reabsorption of many other ions, such as Ca^{2+} and Mg^{2+}. Note that this significant movement of ions occurs without the movement of water through the wall of the distal straight tubule, resulting in the separation of water from its solutes.

In routine histologic preparations, the large cuboidal cells of the distal straight tubule stain lightly with eosin, and the lateral margins of the cells are indistinct (Plate 20.4, page 808). The nucleus is located in the apical portion of the cell and sometimes, especially in the straight segment, causes the cell to bulge into the lumen. As noted earlier, these cells have extensive basolateral plications, and there are numerous mitochondria associated with these basal folds (Fig. 20.21). They also have considerably fewer and less well-developed microvilli than proximal straight tubule cells (compare Figs. 20.18 and 20.19).

Distal Convoluted Tubule

The structure and function of the distal convoluted tubule depends on the delivery and uptake of Na^+.

The **distal convoluted tubule**, located in the cortical labyrinth, is only about one-third as long (~5 mm) as the proximal convoluted tubule. It begins at a variable distance beyond the macula densa and extends to the connecting tubule, which connects the nephron with the cortical collecting duct. The cells of the distal convoluted tubule resemble those of the distal straight tubule (thick ascending limb) but are considerably taller and lack a well-developed brush border. Similar to the distal straight tubule, the epithelium in the distal convoluted tubule is also relatively impermeable to water. The early part of the distal convoluted tubule is the primary site for PTH-regulated Ca^{2+} reabsorption. The cells in the distal convoluted tubule have the highest Na^+/K^+-ATPase activity

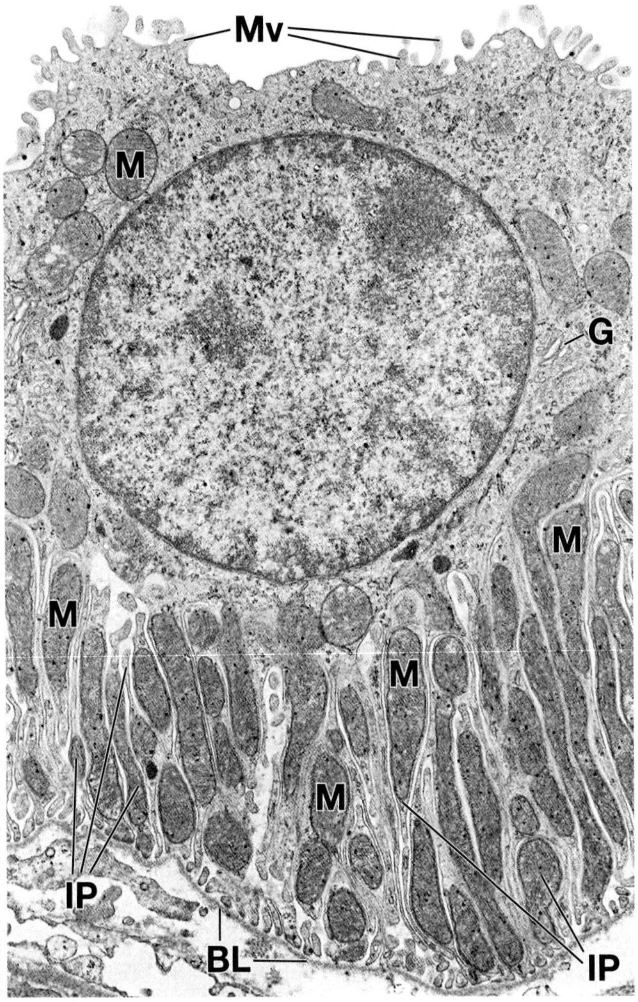

FIGURE 20.21. Electron micrograph of a distal convoluted tubule cell. The apical surface of the cell displays some microvilli (*Mv*), but they are not sufficiently long or numerous to give the appearance of a brush border (compare with Fig. 20.15). The nucleus and Golgi apparatus (*G*) are in the upper portion of the cell. Mitochondria (*M*) are chiefly in the basal region of the cell within the interdigitating processes (*IP*). As in the proximal tubule cell, the mitochondria account for the appearance of basal striations in the light microscope. A basal lamina (*BL*) is seen adjacent to the basal surface of the cell. ×12,000.

in their basolateral membranes than any other segment of the nephron, which provides the driving force for ion transport. This short tubule is responsible for

- **reabsorption of Na^+** and secretion of K^+ into the ultrafiltrate to conserve Na^+;
- **reabsorption of bicarbonate ions**, with concomitant secretion of H^+ ions, leading to further acidification of the urine;
- **reabsorption of chloride (Cl^-)**, which is mediated by thiazide-sensitive Na^+/Cl^- transporters; and
- **secretion of ammonium** in response to the kidneys' need to excrete acid and generate bicarbonate.

Connecting Tubule

The connecting tubule represents a transition region between the distal convoluted tubule and the cortical collecting duct.

Connecting tubules of the subcapsular nephrons join directly to the cortical collecting duct, whereas the connecting tubules from the midcortical and juxtamedullary nephrons merge with other connecting tubules first to form an arched connecting tubule before uniting with the cortical collecting duct. The epithelium of this segment undergoes a gradual transition from the distal convoluted tubule to the collecting duct and consists of intermingling cells from both regions (i.e., principal cells from cortical collecting duct with distal convoluted tubule cells). Both morphologic and physiologic studies demonstrated that the connecting tubules play an important role in K^+ secretion (most likely attributed to the presence of the principal cells), which is, in part, regulated by mineralocorticoids secreted by the adrenal cortex.

Cortical and Medullary Collecting Ducts

The **cortical** and **medullary collecting ducts** determine final urine osmolality by reabsorbing water. The outer medullary collecting duct is also the site of urea reabsorption by facilitated transport utilizing urea transporter A1 (UT-A1). The collecting ducts are composed of simple epithelium. The cortical collecting ducts have flattened cells, somewhat squamous to cuboidal in shape. The medullary collecting ducts have cuboidal cells, with a transition to columnar cells as the ducts increase in size. The collecting ducts are readily distinguished from proximal and distal tubules by virtue of the cell boundaries that can be seen in the light microscope (Fig. 20.22).

Collecting ducts play an essential role in maintaining Na^+/Cl^- balance and acid–base homeostasis.

The epithelium of collecting ducts is composed of light (principal) cells and two different types of dark (intercalated) cells.

- **Light cells**, also called **principal cells** or **collecting duct (CD) cells**, are the predominant cell type of collecting ducts. They are pale-staining cells with true basal infoldings rather than processes that interdigitate with those of adjacent cells. They possess a single primary cilium and relatively few short microvilli (see Fig. 20.22). They contain small, spherical mitochondria. Principal cells express an abundance of cytoplasmic mineralocorticoid receptors (MRs); thus, they are the primary target for **aldosterone** action (see later). Their major function is to reabsorb Na^+ from the lumen of the collecting duct via **epithelial sodium channels (ENaC)** and secrete K^+ via **renal outer medullary potassium (ROMK) channels**. In addition, the apical membrane of these cells possesses an abundance of antidiuretic hormone (ADH)-regulated water channels, **aquaporin-2 (AQP-2)**, which are responsible for the water permeability of the collecting ducts. Aquaporins AQP-3 and AQP-4 are also present within the basolateral membrane of these cells (Fig. 20.23).
- **Dark cells**, also called **intercalated (IC) cells**, occur in considerably smaller numbers than light cells. They make up one-third of the cells in the collecting ducts and mediate acid–base transport. They have many mitochondria, and their cytoplasm appears denser. Microplicae, cytoplasmic folds, are present on their apical surface as well as microvilli. The microplicae are readily observed with the SEM but may be mistaken for microvilli with the TEM (see Fig. 20.22). They do not show basal infoldings but have basally located interdigitations with neighboring cells. Numerous vesicles are present in the apical cytoplasm. Two functionally distinct types of intercalated cells have been identified in the collecting ducts.
- The first type, the **α-intercalated cells**, secretes acid (**H^+ protons**) into the collecting duct lumen via apical H^+-ATPase– and H^+/K^+-ATPase–dependent pumps and releases HCO_3^- via a Cl^-/HCO_3^- exchanger (AE1) located in their basolateral cell membrane. This polarity allows α-intercalated cells to pump H^+ into the lumen of

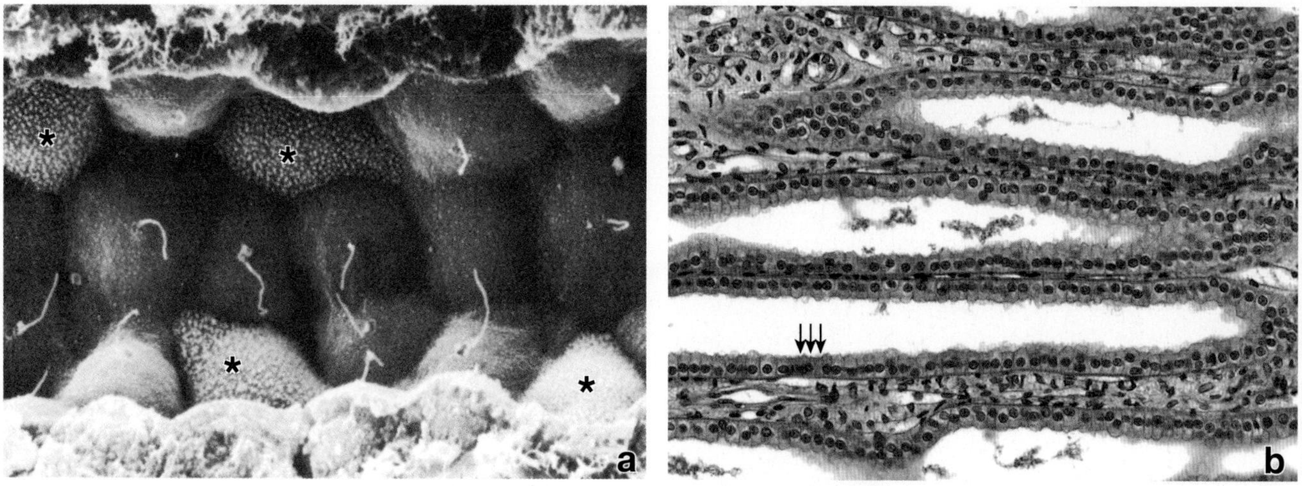

FIGURE 20.22. Scanning electron micrograph and photomicrograph of collecting ducts. a. This scanning electron micrograph shows dark cells (*asterisks*), with numerous short lamellipodia or microridges on their surfaces, and light (principal) cells, each with a primary cilium on its free surface along with small microvilli. The terms *light* and *dark* refer to the staining character of sectioned cells and not to the density differences reflecting charge characteristics of the coated surface of the specimen. (Courtesy of Dr. C. Craig Tisher.) **b.** This photomicrograph of collecting ducts stained with hematoxylin and eosin (H&E) shows several longitudinal profiles of collecting ducts in the medulla of the kidney. Note the simple columnar epithelium lining the lumen of the collecting ducts with characteristically distinct cell boundaries visible between individual cells. Most collecting duct cells stain lightly in H&E and represent light (principal) cells. It is difficult in H&E-stained specimens to differentiate with certainty between light and dark cells. A few more intensely stained cells (*arrows*) most likely represent dark (intercalated) cells. × 240. Source: Kent Christensen, PhD; J. Matthew Velkey, PhD; Lloyd M. Stoolman, MD; Laura Hessler; Diedra Mosley-Brower; and Michael Hortsch, PhD; University of Michigan Medical School. © 2010 The Regents of the University of Michigan. For more information, questions, or permissions requests please contact: Michael Hortsch, PhD, University of Michigan Medical School, hortsch@umich.edu.

the collecting duct, facilitating acid excretion from the body (see Fig. 20.23).

- The second type, the **β-intercalated cells**, has opposite transporter polarities and secretes base (**HCO_3^- bicarbonate anions**) into the collecting duct lumen. The transporters are similar to those in α-intercalated cells but are located on opposite cell membranes. Their apical membranes contain a Cl^-/HCO_3^- exchanger (pendrin) and the Na^+-dependent Cl^-/HCO_3^- exchanger (NDCBE) that facilitate chloride entry into the cells in exchange for bicarbonate excretion into the lumen of the collecting duct (see Fig. 20.23).
- Because of the nature of the diet and thus the need to excrete acid, the epithelium of collecting ducts contains more α- than β-intercalated cells. During metabolic acidosis, the number of β-intercalated cells is reduced and that of α-intercalated cells increases, whereas the total number of intercalated cells in the collecting duct remains unchanged. This finding suggests a **conversion of β- to α-intercalated cells**, giving the kidney a greater ability to secrete H^+ protons and return the pH to the normal range. This conversion event is regulated by an extracellular matrix molecule called **hensin**, (a 230 kDa member of the macrophage scavenger receptor cysteine rich [SRCR] family of proteins), secreted by the β-intercalated cells.

The cells of the collecting ducts gradually become taller as the ducts pass from the outer to the inner medulla and become columnar in the region of the renal papilla. The number of dark cells gradually decreases until there are none in the ducts as they approach the papilla.

Aldosterone does not function at the distal convoluted tubule but rather at the connecting tubules and collecting ducts.

Based on past micropuncture experiments, it was assumed that **aldosterone's** main targets were cells of the distal convoluted tubule. However, more recent molecular research shows that aldosterone acts mainly on the **principal (light) cells** of the **collecting ducts**. As mentioned earlier, the principal cells are not present in the distal convoluted tubule but do have a scattered presence in the connecting tubules. Therefore, aldosterone—similar to ADH—acts on the cortical and medullary collecting ducts, which are lined primarily by the principal cells. The reason for this confusion relates to the fact that the collected tubular fluid during micropuncture experiments often had contact with cells of the connecting tubules and cortical collecting ducts, providing an impression that the experimental treatment with aldosterone had an effect on the distal convoluted tubule. Molecular studies of gene expression provide clear evidence of mineralocorticoid (aldosterone) receptor presence in the principal cells.

Aldosterone bound to mineralocorticoid receptors in the principal cells acts as a transcription factor for proteins involved in exchange of Na^+ for K^+.

Aldosterone is secreted by the adrenal cortex and released under stimulation of angiotensin II or by an increase in blood K^+ concentration (hyperkalemia). It binds to the cytoplasmic mineralocorticoid receptor and then is translocated into the nucleus. The aldosterone–mineralocorticoid receptor complex acts as a transcription factor, upregulating gene expression of several proteins that are involved in the reabsorption of Na^+ and secretion of K^+. These proteins include epithelial sodium channel (ENaC) proteins, renal outer medullary potassium channel (ROMK) proteins, and Na^+/K^+-ATPase. Synthesis of new channel proteins and enzymes takes approximately 6 hours to implement. The net result of aldosterone action is the increase in **reabsorption of Na^+** and **secretion of K^+** by the principal cells. This increases blood serum Na^+ concentration, which, in turn, increases blood volume and blood pressure.

■ INTERSTITIAL CELLS

The connective tissue of the kidney parenchyma, called **interstitial tissue**, surrounds the nephrons, ducts, and blood and lymphatic vessels. This tissue increases considerably in amount from the cortex (where it constitutes ~7% of

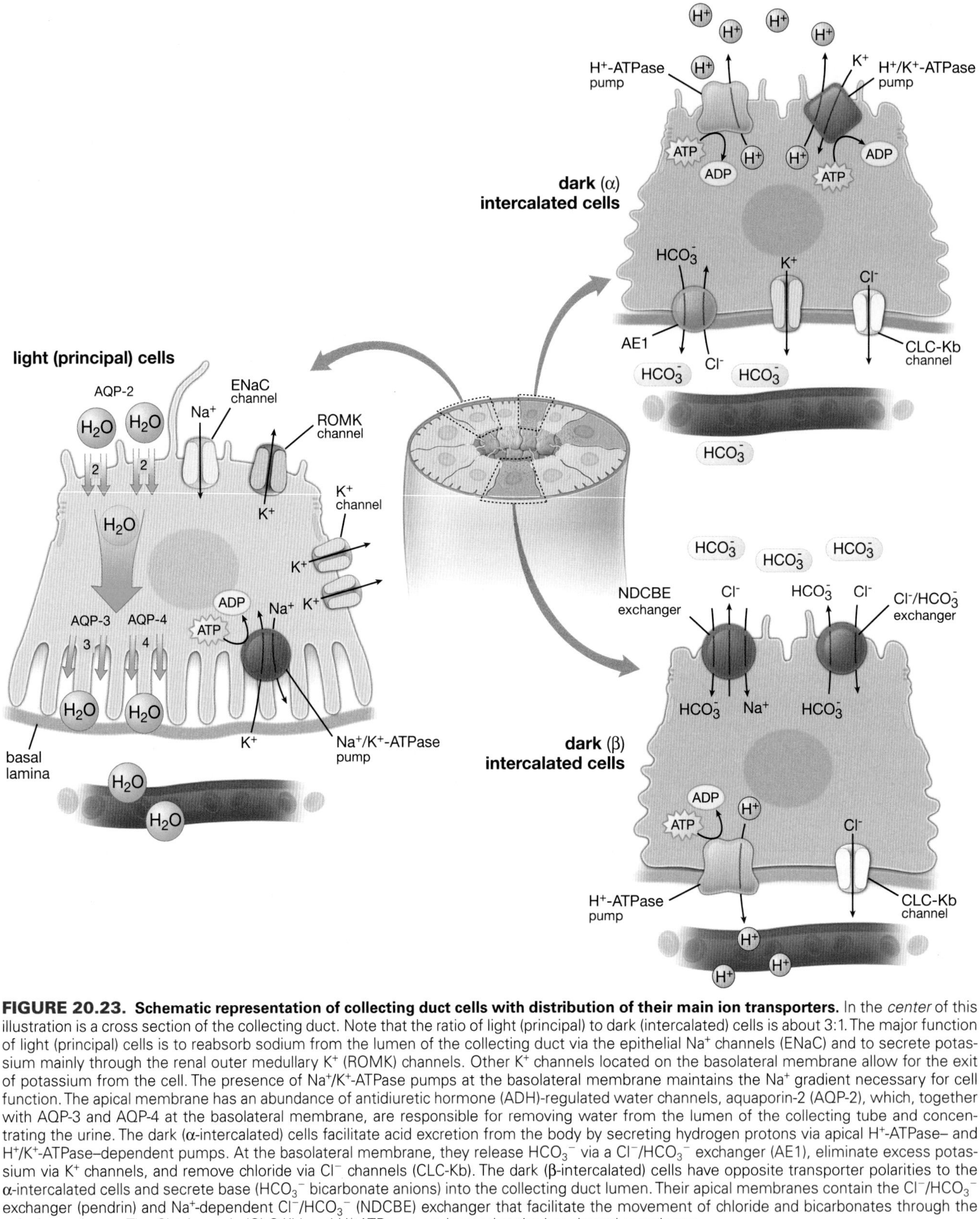

FIGURE 20.23. Schematic representation of collecting duct cells with distribution of their main ion transporters. In the *center* of this illustration is a cross section of the collecting duct. Note that the ratio of light (principal) to dark (intercalated) cells is about 3:1. The major function of light (principal) cells is to reabsorb sodium from the lumen of the collecting duct via the epithelial Na^+ channels (ENaC) and to secrete potassium mainly through the renal outer medullary K^+ (ROMK) channels. Other K^+ channels located on the basolateral membrane allow for the exit of potassium from the cell. The presence of Na^+/K^+-ATPase pumps at the basolateral membrane maintains the Na^+ gradient necessary for cell function. The apical membrane has an abundance of antidiuretic hormone (ADH)-regulated water channels, aquaporin-2 (AQP-2), which, together with AQP-3 and AQP-4 at the basolateral membrane, are responsible for removing water from the lumen of the collecting tube and concentrating the urine. The dark (α-intercalated) cells facilitate acid excretion from the body by secreting hydrogen protons via apical H^+-ATPase– and H^+/K^+-ATPase–dependent pumps. At the basolateral membrane, they release HCO_3^- via a Cl^-/HCO_3^- exchanger (AE1), eliminate excess potassium via K^+ channels, and remove chloride via Cl^- channels (CLC-Kb). The dark (β-intercalated) cells have opposite transporter polarities to the α-intercalated cells and secrete base (HCO_3^- bicarbonate anions) into the collecting duct lumen. Their apical membranes contain the Cl^-/HCO_3^- exchanger (pendrin) and Na^+-dependent Cl^-/HCO_3^- (NDCBE) exchanger that facilitate the movement of chloride and bicarbonates through the apical membrane. The Cl^- channels (CLC-Kb) and H^+-ATPases are located at the basolateral membrane.

the volume) to the inner region of the medulla and papilla (where it may constitute >20% of the volume).

In the cortex, two types of interstitial cells are recognized: **cells that resemble fibroblasts**, found between the basement membrane of the tubules and the adjacent peritubular capillaries, and occasional **macrophages**. In their intimate relationship with the base of the tubular epithelial cells, the fibroblasts resemble the subepithelial fibroblasts of the intestine. These cells synthesize and secrete the collagen and glycosaminoglycans of the extracellular matrix of the interstitium.

In the medulla, the principal interstitial cells resemble **myofibroblasts**. They are oriented to the long axes of the tubular structures and may have a role in compressing these structures. The cells contain prominent bundles of actin filaments, abundant rough endoplasmic reticulum (rER), a well-developed Golgi complex, and lysosomes. Prominent lipid droplets in the cytoplasm appear to increase and decrease in relation to the diuretic state.

FOLDER 20.5

FUNCTIONAL CONSIDERATIONS: STRUCTURE AND FUNCTION OF AQUAPORIN WATER CHANNELS

Aquaporins (AQPs) are small, hydrophobic, transmembrane proteins that mediate water transport in the kidney and other organs (i.e., liver, gallbladder). Thirteen AQPs have been characterized and cloned. The molecular size of AQPs ranges from 26 to 34 kDa. Each protein consists of six transmembrane domains arranged to form a distinct pore. The sites where AQPs are expressed implicate their role in water transport, such as renal tubules (water reabsorption), brain and spinal cord (cerebrospinal fluid reabsorption), pancreatic acinar cells (secretion of pancreatic fluids), lacrimal apparatus (secretion and resorption of tears), and eye (aqueous humor secretion and reabsorption). Most AQPs are selective for the passage of water (AQP-1, AQP-2, AQP-4, AQP-5, AQP-6, and AQP-8), whereas others, such as AQP-3, AQP-7, and AQP-9, called *aquaglyceroporins*, also transport glycerol and other larger molecules in addition to water. Prominent members of the AQP family include:

- **AQP-1**, expressed in kidney (proximal convoluted tubules) and other cell types such as hepatocytes and red blood cells. AQP-1 is also expressed in the lymph nodes, endothelial cells lining lymphatic sinuses, and on the vascular endothelium of high endothelial venules as well as in the endothelial cells of intestinal lacteals.
- **AQP-2**, present in the terminal portion of the distal convoluted tubules, connecting tubules, and the epithelium of collecting ducts. AQP-2 is regulated by antidiuretic hormone (ADH) and is thus known as an *ADH-regulated water channel*. Mutation of the AQP-2 gene has been linked to **congenital nephrogenic diabetes insipidus**.
- **AQP-3** and **AQP-4** have also been detected in the basolateral cell surface of the light (principal) cells of kidney collecting ducts as well in the gastrointestinal epithelium (AQP-3), pancreatic acinar cells (AQP-12), and the brain and spinal cord (AQP-4).

Research into the function and structure of the AQP proteins may lead to the development of water channel blockers that could be used to treat hypertension, congestive heart failure, and brain swelling and to regulate intracranial or intraocular pressure.

Most fibroblasts originate within the interstitial tissue through a mechanism called **epithelial–mesenchymal transition (EMT)**. The EMT is a process in which epithelial cells lose their characteristics and acquire features of mesenchymal cells. During this transition, epithelial cells lose cell-to-cell junctions, apical–basal domain polarity, and epithelial cell markers and acquire cell motility, a spindle cell shape, and mesenchymal cell markers. The reprogramming and conversion of tubular epithelial cells into a mesenchymal phenotype is initiated by an alteration in the balance of local cytokine concentrations (i.e., TGF-β, FGF, EGF) that upregulate specific transcription factors called EMT-TFs. During persistent injury and chronic inflammation of the kidney parenchyma, fibroblasts increase their numbers and, by secreting excess extracellular matrix, destroy the normal interstitial architecture of the kidney. Research studies suggest that in **renal fibrosis**, more than one-third of all disease-related fibroblasts originate from tubular epithelial cells at the site of injury. Proliferation of fibroblasts in response to local mitogens usually leads to irreversible renal failure characterized by **tubulointerstitial nephritis**. Recent therapeutic interventions in renal fibrosis are directed toward inhibiting fibroblast formation by shifting local cytokine balance in favor of **reversal mesenchymal–epithelial transition**.

■ HISTOPHYSIOLOGY OF THE KIDNEY

The countercurrent multiplier system creates hyperosmotic urine.

The term *countercurrent* indicates a flow of fluid in adjacent structures in opposite directions. The ability to excrete hyperosmotic urine depends on the **countercurrent multiplier system** that involves three structures:

- **Loop of Henle**, which acts as a countercurrent multiplier. The ultrafiltrate moves within the descending limb of the thin segment of the loop toward the renal papilla and moves back toward the corticomedullary junction within the ascending limb of the thin segment. The osmotic gradients of the medulla are established along the axis of the loop of Henle.
- **Vasa recta** form loops parallel to the loop of Henle. They act as countercurrent exchangers of water and solutes between the descending part (arteriolae rectae) and ascending part (venulae rectae) of the vasa recta. The vasa recta help maintain the osmotic gradient of the medulla.
- **Collecting duct** in the medulla acts as an **osmotic equilibrating device**. Modified ultrafiltrate in the collecting ducts can be further equilibrated with the hyperosmotic medullary interstitium. The level of equilibration depends on activation of ADH-dependent water channels (AQP-2).

A standing gradient of ion concentration produces hyperosmotic urine by a countercurrent multiplier effect.

The **loop of Henle** creates and maintains a gradient of ion concentration in the medullary interstitium that increases from the corticomedullary junction to the renal papilla. As noted earlier, the thin descending limb of the loop of Henle is freely permeable to water, whereas the ascending limb of the loop of Henle is impermeable to water. Furthermore, the thin ascending limb cells add Na^+ and Cl^- to the interstitium.

Because water cannot leave the thin ascending limb, the interstitium becomes hyperosmotic relative to the luminal contents. Although some of the Cl^- and Na^+ of the interstitium diffuse back into the nephron at the thin descending limb, the ions are transported out again in the thin ascending limb and distal straight tubule (thick ascending limb). This produces the **countercurrent multiplier effect**. Thus, the concentration of NaCl in the interstitium gradually increases down the length of the loop of Henle and, consequently, through the thickness of the medulla from the corticomedullary junction to the papilla.

FOLDER 20.6

FUNCTIONAL CONSIDERATIONS: ANTIDIURETIC HORMONE REGULATION OF COLLECTING DUCT FUNCTION

Water permeability of the epithelium of the collecting ducts is regulated by **antidiuretic hormone (ADH, vasopressin)**, a hormone produced in the **hypothalamus** and released from the posterior lobe of the pituitary gland. ADH increases the permeability of the collecting duct to water, thereby producing more concentrated urine. At the molecular level, ADH acts on the ADH-regulated water channels aquaporin-2 (AQP-2), which is located in the epithelium of the terminal portion of the distal convoluted tubule, connecting tubules, and the epithelium of the collecting ducts. However, the action of ADH is more significant in the collecting ducts. ADH binds to receptors on the cells of these ducts and triggers the following actions:

- **Translocation of the AQP-2–containing intracytoplasmic vesicles** into the apical cell surface—a short-term effect. This results in an increased number of available AQP-2 channels at the cell surface, thus increasing water permeability of the epithelium.
- **Synthesis of AQP-2** and their insertion into the apical cell membrane—a long-term effect

An increase in plasma osmolality or a decrease in blood volume stimulates the release of ADH, as does nicotine.

In the absence of ADH, copious, dilute urine is produced. This condition is called **central diabetes insipidus (CDI)**. Mutation of two genes encoding AQP-2 and ADH receptors is responsible for a form of CDI called **nephrogenic diabetes insipidus**. Because of the loss of normal function of the AQP-2 and ADH receptor proteins synthesized by the collecting duct epithelial cells, the kidney does not respond to ADH. Excess water consumption can also inhibit ADH release, thereby promoting the production of a large volume of hyposmotic urine.

Increased secretion of ADH can produce an extremely hyperosmotic urine, thereby conserving water in the body. Inadequate consumption of water or loss of water because of sweating, vomiting, or diarrhea stimulates the release of ADH. This leads to an increase in the permeability of the epithelium of the distal convoluted tubules and collecting ducts and promotes the production of a small volume of hyperosmotic urine.

Vasa recta containing descending arterioles and ascending venules act as countercurrent exchangers.

To understand the **countercurrent exchange mechanism**, it is necessary to resume the description of the renal circulation at the point at which the efferent arteriole leaves the renal corpuscle.

The **efferent arterioles** of the renal corpuscles of most of the cortex branch to form the capillary network that surrounds the tubular portions of the nephron in the cortex, the **peritubular capillary network**. The efferent arterioles of the juxtamedullary renal corpuscles form several unbranched arterioles that descend into the medullary pyramid. These **arteriolae rectae** make a hairpin turn deep in the medullary pyramid and ascend as the **venulae rectae**. Together, the descending arterioles and the ascending venules are called the **vasa recta**. The arteriolae rectae form capillary plexuses lined by fenestrated endothelium that supply the tubular structures at the various levels of the medullary pyramid.

Interaction between collecting ducts, loops of Henle, and vasa recta is required for concentrating urine by the countercurrent exchange mechanism.

Because the thick ascending limb of the loop of Henle has a high level of transport activity and because it is impermeable to water, the modified ultrafiltrate that ultimately reaches the distal convoluted tubule is *hyposmotic*. When ADH is present, the distal convoluted tubules and the collecting ducts are highly permeable to water. Therefore, within the cortex, in which the interstitium is isosmotic with blood, the modified ultrafiltrate within the distal convoluted tubule equilibrates and becomes isosmotic, partly by loss of water to the interstitium and partly by addition of ions other than Na^+ and Cl^- to the ultrafiltrate. In the medulla, increasing amounts of water leave the ultrafiltrate as the collecting ducts pass through the increasingly hyperosmotic interstitium on their course to the papillae.

As noted previously, the vasa recta also form loops in the medulla that parallel the loop of Henle. This arrangement ensures that the vessels provide circulation to the medulla without disturbing the osmotic gradient established by transport of Cl^- in the epithelium of the ascending limb of the loop of Henle.

The vasa recta form a **countercurrent exchange system** in the following manner: Both the arterial and venous sides of the loop are thin-walled vessels that form plexuses of fenestrated capillaries at all levels in the medulla. As the arterial vessels descend through the medulla, the blood loses water to the interstitium and gains salt from the interstitium so that at the tip of the loop, deep in the medulla, the blood is essentially in equilibrium with the hyperosmotic interstitial fluid.

As the venous vessels ascend toward the corticomedullary junction, the process is reversed (i.e., the hyperosmotic blood loses salt to the interstitium and gains water from the interstitium). This passive countercurrent exchange of water and salt between the blood and the interstitium occurs *without expenditure of energy* by the endothelial cells. The energy that drives this system is the same energy that drives the multiplier system, namely, the movement of Na^+ and Cl^- out of the cells of the water-impermeable ascending limb of the loop of Henle. The countercurrent exchange system and other movements of molecules in different parts of the nephron are shown in Figure 20.24.

■ BLOOD SUPPLY

Some aspects of the **blood supply** of the kidney have been described in relation to specific functions (i.e., glomerular filtration, control of blood pressure, and countercurrent exchange). It remains, however, to provide an overall description of the blood supply of the kidney.

Each kidney receives a large branch from the abdominal aorta, called the **renal artery**. The renal artery branches

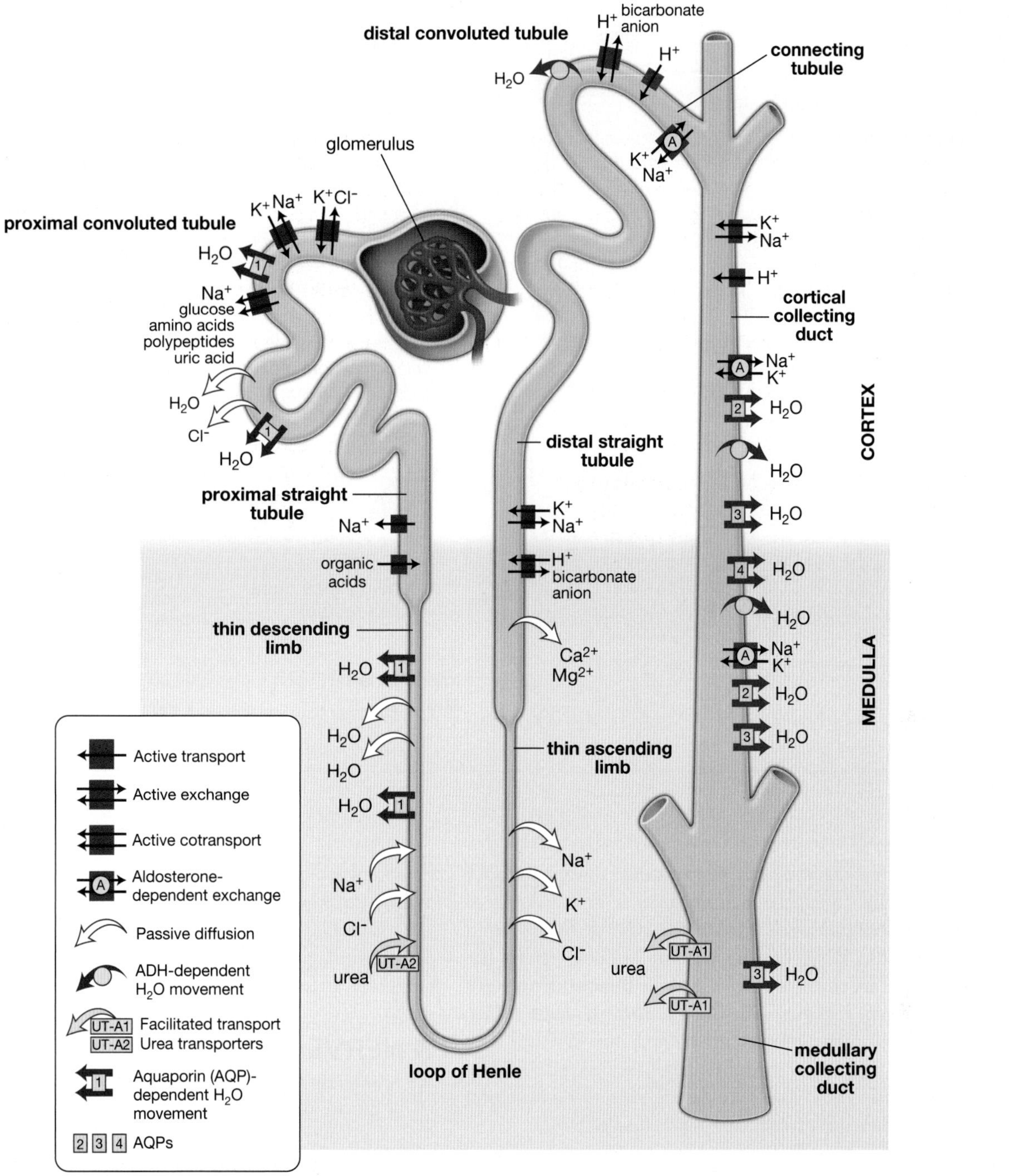

FIGURE 20.24. Diagram showing the movement of substances into and out of the nephron and collecting system. The *symbols* indicate the mode of transport as well as specific molecule-dependent transporters that act on the nephron and collecting ducts (as noted in the key).

within the renal sinus and sends **interlobar arteries** into the substance of the kidney (Fig. 20.25). These arteries travel between the pyramids as far as the cortex and then turn to follow an arched course along the base of the pyramid between the medulla and the cortex. Thus, these interlobar arteries are designated **arcuate arteries**.

Interlobular arteries branch from the arcuate arteries and ascend through the cortex toward the capsule. Although the boundaries between lobules are not distinct, the interlobular arteries, when included in a section cut perpendicular to the vessel, are located midway between adjacent medullary rays, traveling in the cortical labyrinth. As they traverse the cortex toward the capsule, the interlobular arteries give off branches, the **afferent arterioles**, one to each glomerulus (Fig. 20.26). A single afferent arteriole may spring directly from the interlobular artery, or a common stem from the interlobular artery may branch to form several afferent arterioles. Some interlobular arteries terminate near the periphery of the cortex, whereas others enter the kidney capsule to provide its arterial supply.

Afferent arterioles give rise to the capillaries that form the glomerulus. The glomerular capillaries reunite to form an efferent arteriole that, in turn, gives rise to a second network of capillaries, the **peritubular capillaries**. The arrangement of these capillaries differs according to whether they originate from cortical or juxtamedullary glomeruli:

- **Efferent arterioles from cortical glomeruli** lead into a peritubular capillary network that surrounds the local uriniferous tubules (see Fig. 20.25).
- **Efferent arterioles from juxtamedullary glomeruli** descend into the medulla alongside the loop of Henle; they

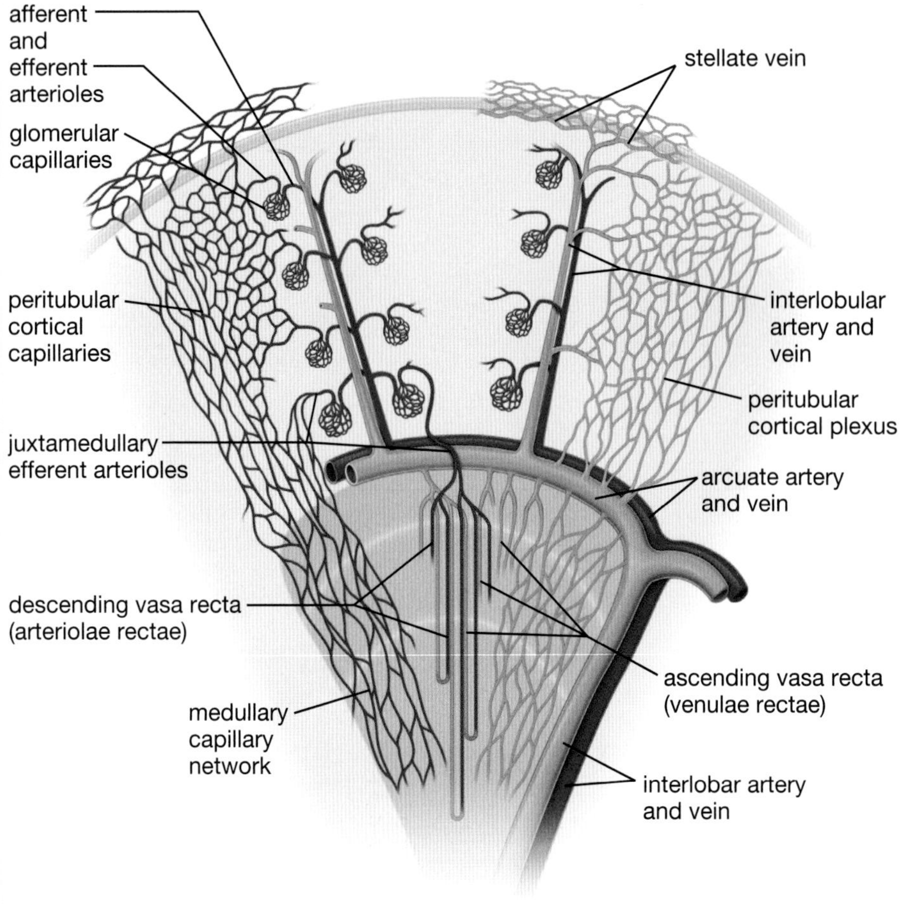

FIGURE 20.25. Schematic diagram of the renal blood supply. The renal artery gives rise to interlobar arteries that branch into arcuate arteries at the border between the medulla and the cortex. Interlobular arteries branch from the arcuate arteries and travel toward the renal capsule, giving off afferent arterioles that contribute to the glomerular capillaries. Glomeruli in the outer part of the cortex send efferent arterioles to the peritubular cortical capillaries that surround the tubules in the cortex. Glomeruli near the medulla, the juxtamedullary glomeruli, send efferent arterioles almost entirely into the medullary network of capillaries that contains the descending vasa recta. Blood returns from the medulla by the ascending vasa recta and the capillary network via veins that enter the arcuate veins. Stellate veins near the capsule drain the capsular network, and the peritubular cortical plexus drains to both the interlobular and arcuate veins.

break up into smaller vessels that continue toward the apex of the pyramid but make hairpin turns at various levels to return as straight vessels toward the base of the pyramid (see Fig. 20.25). Thus, the efferent arterioles from the juxtamedullary glomeruli give rise to the **descending vasa recta**, which, together with the **ascending vasa recta**, are involved in the countercurrent exchange system. They drain via a peritubular medullary capillary network into the arcuate veins. These vessels are described in the explanation of the countercurrent exchange system (page 792).

Generally, venous flow in the kidney follows a reverse course to arterial flow, with the veins running in parallel with the corresponding arteries (see Fig. 20.25). Thus, the venous flow is as follows:

- **Peritubular cortical capillaries** drain into **interlobular veins**, which, in turn, drain into arcuate veins, interlobar veins, and the renal vein.
- The **medullary vascular network** drains into **arcuate veins** and so forth.
- **Peritubular capillaries** near the kidney surface and **capillaries of the capsule** drain into **stellate veins** (so-called for their pattern of distribution when viewed from the kidney surface), which drain into **interlobular veins**, and so forth.

■ LYMPHATIC VESSELS

The kidneys contain two major networks of lymphatic vessels. These networks are not usually visible in routine histologic sections but can be demonstrated by experimental methods. One network is located in the outer regions of the cortex and drains into larger lymphatic vessels in the capsule. The other network is located more deeply in the substance of the kidney and drains into large lymphatic vessels in the renal sinus. There are numerous anastomoses between the two lymphatic networks.

■ NERVE SUPPLY

The fibers that form the **renal plexus** are unmyelinated, derived mostly from the **sympathetic division** of the autonomic nervous system. There is no evidence for parasympathetic innervation of the kidney. The sympathetic postsynaptic nerves that form the renal plexus are adrenergic (secrete **norepinephrine** at their nerve terminals). They travel along the renal artery and vein and are distributed to all segments of the renal vasculature. The highest concentrations of nerves are observed along the afferent arterioles, followed by the efferent arterioles. They cause contraction of vascular smooth muscle and consequent vasoconstriction that regulate urine production as follows:

- Constriction of the afferent arterioles to the glomeruli reduces the filtration rate and decreases the production of urine.
- Constriction of the efferent arterioles from the glomeruli increases the filtration rate and increases the production of urine.
- Loss of sympathetic innervation leads to increased urinary output.

It has been proposed that chronic hyperstimulation of sympathetic nerves in the renal plexus is an important factor in **resistant hypertension**. Therefore, minimally

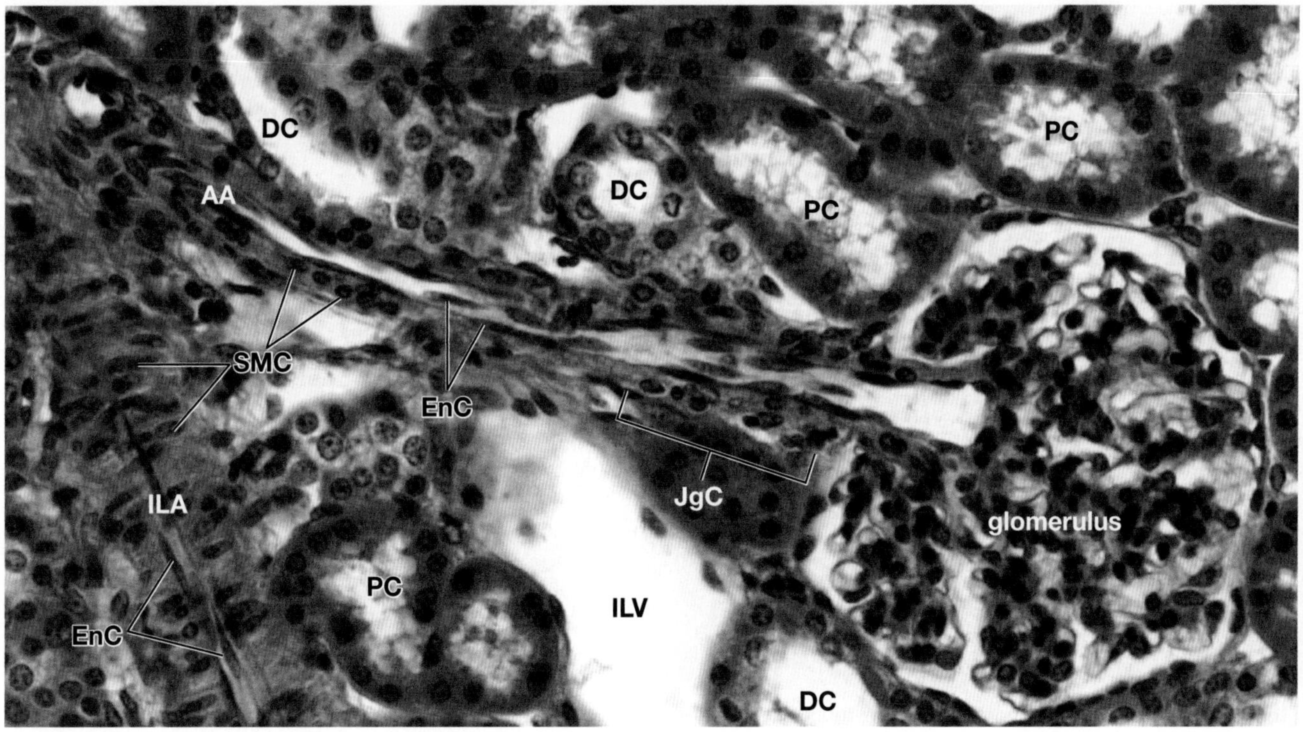

FIGURE 20.26. Photomicrograph of the cortical labyrinth in the kidney from an adult monkey. This high-magnification photomicrograph of a hematoxylin and eosin (H&E)-stained kidney shows the glomerulus with associated tubules and blood vessels. The prominent glomerulus is surrounded by the Bowman capsule and is supplied by an afferent arteriole (*AA*) that originates from the interlobular artery (*ILA*) visible on the *left* side of the image. The afferent arteriole supplying blood to the glomerulus has a distinct circular layer of smooth muscle cells (*SMC*) that was sectioned perpendicularly to the long axis of the arteriole. The modified smooth muscle cells in the terminal portion of the afferent arteriole are termed *juxtaglomerular cells* (*JgC*). In addition to a contractile apparatus, these cells exhibit prominent endoplasmic reticulum, Golgi apparatus, and secretory vesicles containing renin. Macula densa and extraglomerular mesangial cells are not easily discernable. The grazing section of an interlobular artery (*ILA*) reveals a much thicker layer of circular smooth muscle cells with visible nuclei crossing the lumen of the vessel. The elongated endothelial cells (*EnC*) are clearly visible. Note the accompanying intralobular vein (*ILV*) and several profiles of proximal convoluted (*PC*) and distal convoluted (*DC*) tubules of the nephron. ×380. Source: Kent Christensen, PhD; J. Matthew Velkey, PhD; Lloyd M. Stoolman, MD; Laura Hessler; Diedra Mosley-Brower; and Michael Hortsch, PhD; University of Michigan Medical School. © 2010 The Regents of the University of Michigan. For more information, questions, or permissions requests please contact: Michael Hortsch, PhD, University of Michigan Medical School, hortsch@umich.edu.)

invasive techniques targeting the renal plexus are being progressively developed, including intraluminal denervation by radiofrequency ablation, denervation by high-intensity–focused ultrasound, or computed tomography–guided injection of agents (i.e., ethanol or vincristine) that obliterate nerve fibers.

Based on evidence collected from patients who received a **kidney transplant**, it is evident that the extrinsic nerve supply is not necessary for normal renal function. Although the nerve fibers to the kidney are severed during renal transplantation, transplanted kidneys subsequently function normally.

■ URETER, URINARY BLADDER, AND URETHRA

All excretory passages, except the urethra, have the same general organization.

On leaving the collecting ducts at the **area cribrosa**, the urine enters a series of structures that do not modify it but are specialized to store and pass the urine to the exterior of the body. The urine flows sequentially to a **minor calyx**, a **major calyx**, and the **renal pelvis** and leaves each kidney through the **ureter** to the **urinary bladder**, where it is stored. The urine is finally voided through the urethra.

All of these excretory passages, except the urethra, have the same general structures, namely, a mucosa (lined by transitional epithelium), muscularis, and adventitia (or, in some regions, a serosa).

Transitional epithelium lines the calyces, ureters, bladder, and the initial segment of the urethra.

Transitional epithelium (urothelium) lines the excretory passages leading from the kidney and forms the interface between the urinary space and underlying blood vessels, nerves, connective tissue, and smooth muscle cells (Figs. 20.27 and 20.28). This stratified epithelium is essentially impermeable to salts and water. The cells in the transitional epithelium are composed of at least three layers:

- The **superficial layer** contains single or multinucleated large, polyhedral cells (25–250 μm in diameter) that bulge into the lumen. They are frequently described as **dome-shaped** or **umbrella cells** because of their apical surface curvature (see Fig. 20.28). The shape of these epithelial cells depends on the filling state of the excretory passage. For instance, in an empty urinary bladder, dome-shaped cells are roughly cuboidal; however, when the bladder is filled, they are highly stretched and appear flat and squamous. Edges of the cells exhibit ridges, which are formed by the interdigitations of apical surface membranes from adjacent cells. These interdigitations resemble a closed zipper line and contribute to the high-resistance paracellular barrier that reinforces tight junctions.
- The **intermediate cell layer** contains pear-shaped cells that are connected to each other and the overlying dome-shaped cells by desmosomes. The thickness of this layer varies with the state of the urinary tract expansion, which, in humans, may reach up to five layers thick. When the overlying dome-shaped cell is lost, the population of

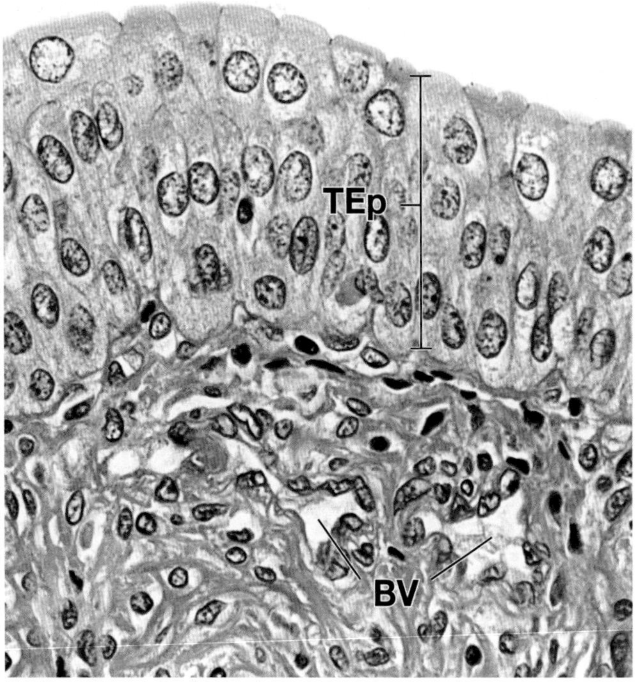

FIGURE 20.27. Photomicrograph of transitional epithelium (urothelium). This hematoxylin and eosin (H&E)-stained specimen shows the four- to five-cell layer thickness of the epithelium in the relaxed ureter. The surface cells exhibit a rounded or dome-shaped profile. The connective tissue (lamina propria) below the epithelium (*TEp*) is relatively cellular and contains a number of lymphocytes. Blood vessels (*BV*) are also abundant in this area. ×450.

intermediate cells rapidly differentiates and replaces the lost surface cell.

- The **basal cell layer** consists of small cells containing a single nucleus that rests on the basement membrane. This layer contains **stem cells** for the urothelium.

The epithelium begins in the minor calyces as two cell layers and increases to four to five layers in the ureter and as many as six or more layers in the empty bladder. However, when the bladder is distended, as few as three layers are seen (see Fig. 20.28). This change reflects the ability of the cells to accommodate distension. The cells in the distended bladder, particularly the large, dome-shaped surface cells, flatten and those in intermediate layers slide past one another to accommodate the increasing surface area. As the individual cells reorganize in the distended bladder, the resulting appearance is the "true" three layers.

The luminal surface of the transitional epithelium is covered by rigid urothelial plaques containing crystalline protein uroplakins, which play an important role in the permeability barrier.

When the wall of a nondistended urinary bladder is examined with the TEM, the **apical plasma membrane** of dome-shaped cells exhibits an unusual scallop-shaped appearance. Most of the apical plasma membrane is covered by the rigid-looking concave **urothelial plaques** separated by intervening narrow **hinge regions** (Fig. 20.29). In cross sections, the outer leaflet of the lipid bilayer is twice as thick as the inner leaflet; thus, the region of the urothelial plaque appears asymmetrical, hence the name **asymmetric unit membrane (AUM)**. The thicker outer leaflet of the urothelial plaque contains a crystalline array of hexagonally arranged 16-nm protein particles composed of a family of five transmembrane proteins called **uroplakins** (UPIa, UPIb, UPII, UPIIIa, and UPIIIb; Fig. 20.30). The crystalline arrangement of the uroplakin particles makes the plaque impermeable to small molecules (water, urea, and protons). In conjunction with tight junctions, urothelial plaques play an important role in the urothelial permeability barrier. The hinge areas of the plasma membrane contain all other nonplaque proteins typically found on the apical cell domain, such as receptors and channels. Approximately 85% of **urinary tract infections** are caused by **uropathogenic *Escherichia coli***, which colonize the transitional epithelium. The initial adhesion to the epithelium allows the bacteria to gain a foothold on the epithelial surface, thus preventing them from being removed during micturition. This binding is mediated by **FimH adhesins** located at the tip of a filamentous attachment apparatus of *E. coli*, which interacts with the **uroplakins** in the asymmetric unit membrane of the urothelial plaques.

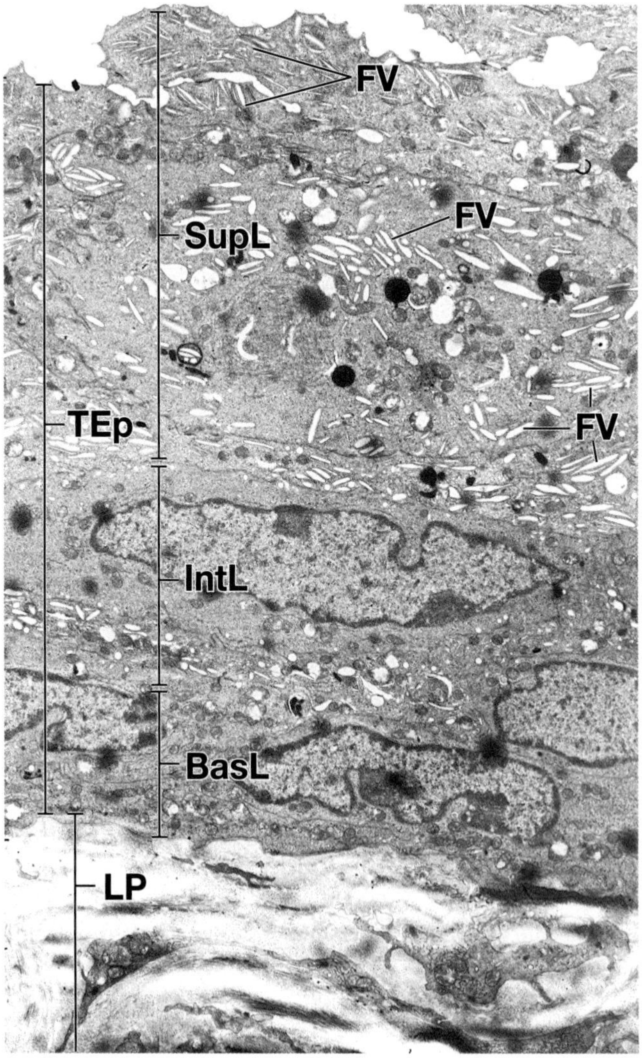

FIGURE 20.28. Transmission electron micrograph of urinary bladder epithelium. The mucous membrane of the urinary bladder consists of transitional epithelium (*TEp*) with an underlying lamina propria (*LP*). The superficial layer (*SupL*) contains dome-shaped cells with unique fusiform vesicles (*FV*), which are evident here at this relatively low magnification. These are seen at higher magnification in Figure 20.29b. The intermediate layer (*IntL*) of variable thickness contains cells that can differentiate and replace lost dome-shaped cells. The basal layer (*BasL*) contains stem cells of the transitional epithelium. ×5,000.

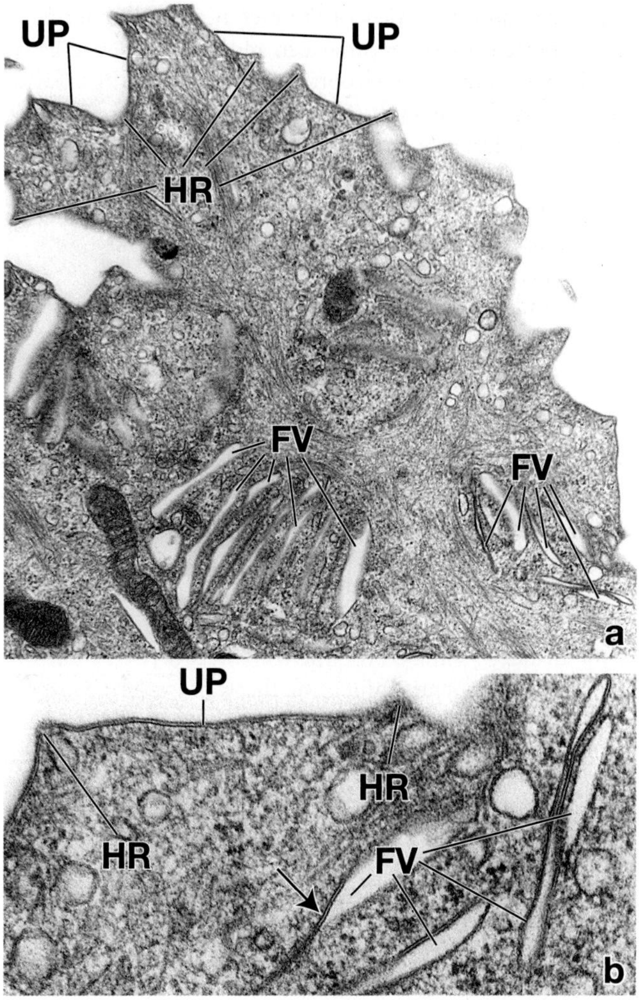

FIGURE 20.29. Transmission electron micrograph of the apical portion of a dome-shaped cell. a. The cytoplasm displays small vesicles, filaments, and mitochondria, but the most distinctive feature of the cell is its fusiform vesicles (*FV*). Note that the apical plasma membrane is covered by the rigid-looking concave urothelial plaques (*UP*) separated by intervening narrow hinge regions (*HR*). ×27,000. **b.** Higher magnification shows that the membrane forming the fusiform vesicles (*arrow*) is similar to the apical plasma membrane of the urothelial plaque (*UP*). Both membranes are thickened and represent an asymmetric unit membrane (*AUM*) in which the outer leaflet of the lipid bilayer is twice as thick as the inner leaflet. Uroplakins, the specific proteins of the urothelial plaque, are produced in the rough endoplasmic reticulum (*rER*) and then transported to the Golgi apparatus, where they undergo oligomerization into 16-nm particles with the final assembly into a crystalline array. The *trans*-Golgi network packages *AUMs* into the fusiform vesicles for delivery to the apical cell membrane. ×60,000.

In addition, the interaction with uroplakins triggers a cascade of events that lead to bacterial invasion into cells of the transitional epithelium.

Transitional epithelium maintains a urothelial permeability barrier despite dynamic changes in the wall of the urinary bladder and other urine-containing organs.

As the bladder or other urine-containing organs distend, the folded surface of the mucosa becomes stretched and expands. Dome-shaped cells also undergo changes in their apical membrane that are associated with the presence of **fusiform vesicles**. When observed with the TEM, the fusiform vesicles are oriented perpendicular and positioned in close proximity to the apical plasma membrane. They are formed by **asymmetric unit membranes** similar to those in the urothelial plaques. In response to the distention of the bladder, the apical membrane expands as a result of exocytosis of the fusiform vesicles that become part of the cell surface (see Fig. 20.28). Most of the fusiform vesicles fuse at the hinge regions to the apical cell surface, whereas the remaining vesicles assume a more parallel position in relation to the apical membrane. During micturition, the process is reversed as the added apical membrane is recovered by endocytosis and the apical membrane of the dome-shaped cells shortens.

Urothelium is an active participant in signaling mechanisms between the external environment facing the urine, nerve fibers, and smooth muscles of the urinary passages.

Experimental studies have shown that urothelium does not act only as a passive permeability barrier but also plays an active role in the signaling mechanisms of the urinary organs. The urothelium responds to chemical and mechanical stimuli and is engaged in autocrine or paracrine communication with nerve fibers and smooth muscles of the urinary passages. Expression of a variety of receptors on its surface (i.e., nicotinic, muscarinic, and adrenergic) and ion channels allows urothelial cells to respond to neurotransmitters released from nerve fibers. In addition, urothelial cells are able to produce and secrete acetylcholine (ACh), nitric oxide (NO), and nerve growth factor (NGF), which regulate the activity of underlying nerve fibers and smooth muscles.

Smooth muscle of the urinary passages is arranged in bundles.

A dense collagenous lamina propria underlies the urothelium throughout the excretory passages. Neither a muscularis mucosae nor a submucosal layer is present in their walls. In the tubular portions (ureters and urethra), usually two layers of **smooth muscle** lie beneath the lamina propria:

- **Longitudinal layer**, the inner layer that is arranged in a loose spiral pattern
- **Circular layer**, the outer layer that is arranged in a tight spiral pattern

Note that this arrangement of the smooth muscle is opposite to that of the muscularis externa of the intestinal tract. The smooth muscle of the urinary passages is mixed with connective tissue so that it forms parallel bundles rather than pure muscular sheets. Peristaltic contractions of the smooth muscle move the urine from the minor calyces through the ureter to the bladder.

Ureters

Each **ureter** conducts urine from the renal pelvis to the urinary bladder and is approximately 24–34 cm long. The distal part of the ureter enters the urinary bladder and follows an oblique path through the wall of the bladder. **Transitional epithelium (urothelium)** lines the luminal surface of the wall of the ureter. The remainder of the wall is composed of smooth muscle and connective tissue. The smooth muscle is arranged in three layers: an inner longitudinal layer, a middle circular layer, and an outer longitudinal layer (Plate 20.5, page 810). However, the outer longitudinal layer is present only at the distal end of the ureter. Usually, the ureter is embedded in the retroperitoneal adipose tissue. The adipose tissue, vessels, and nerves form the adventitia of the ureter.

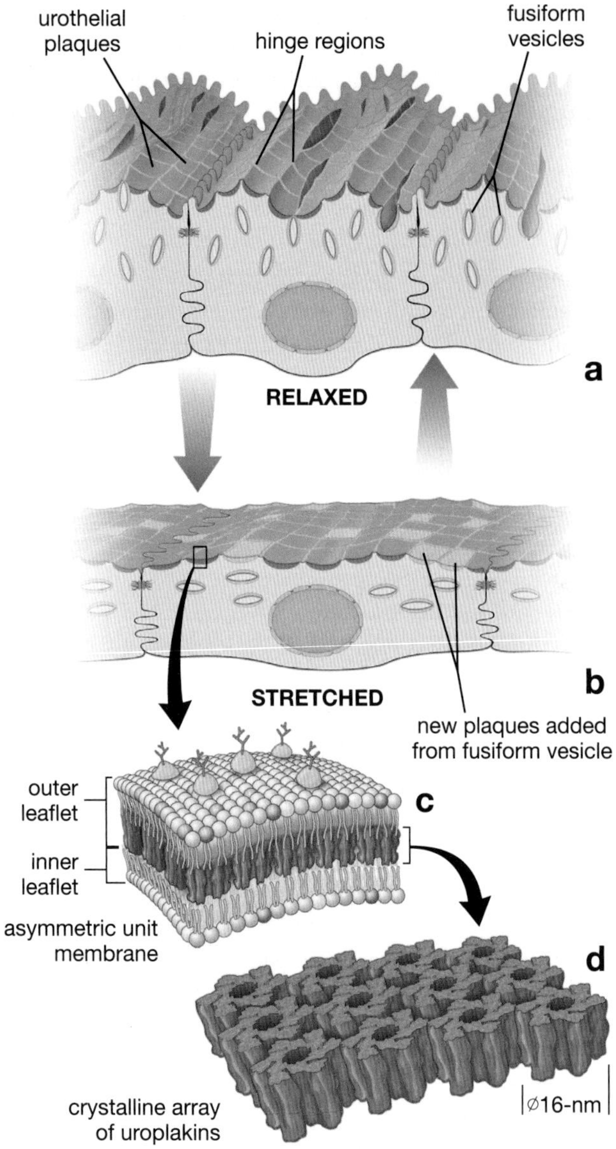

FIGURE 20.30. Diagrams of the luminal surface of dome-shaped cells. a. This drawing depicts a luminal surface of dome-shaped cells in a relaxed bladder. Note the apical plasma membrane of each cell is covered by the ridged concave urothelial plaques that are separated by intervening narrow hinge regions. The fusiform vesicles (*drawn in different color*) containing additional plaque membranes accumulate in the upper part of the cell. Most of them are vertically oriented, and some are attached to hinge regions of the apical cell membrane. **b.** This diagram depicts the same cell shown in **a** as it would appear in a stretched bladder. Note the additional plaques that have been added to the surface from the fusiform vesicles. The remaining vesicles in this stage are visible in a more horizontal position. **c.** The urothelial plaque in cross section exhibits features of the asymmetric unit membrane (*AUM*) in which the outer leaflet of the lipid bilayer is twice as thick as the inner leaflet. The *AUM* is present in both urothelial plaques and fusiform vesicles. **d.** The thicker outer leaflet of the urothelial plaque contains a crystalline array of hexagonally arranged, 16-nm in diameter proteins that is composed of transmembrane proteins called uroplakins.

As the bladder distends with urine, the openings of the ureters are compressed, reducing the possibility of reflux of urine into the ureters. Contraction of the smooth muscle of the bladder wall also compresses the openings of the ureters into the bladder. This action helps prevent the spread of infection from the bladder and urethra, frequent sites of chronic infection (particularly in females), to the kidney.

In the terminal portion of the ureters, a thick outer layer of longitudinal muscle is present in addition to the two listed earlier, particularly in the portion of the ureter that passes through the bladder wall. Most descriptions of the bladder musculature indicate that this longitudinal layer continues into the wall of the bladder to form a principal component of its wall. The smooth muscle of the bladder, however, is not as clearly separated into distinctive layers.

Urinary Bladder

The **urinary bladder** is a distensible reservoir for urine, located in the pelvis, posterior to the pubic symphysis; its size and shape change as it fills. It contains three openings, two for the ureters (**ureteric orifices**) and one for the urethra (**internal urethral orifice**). The triangular region defined by these three openings, the **trigone**, is relatively smooth and constant in thickness, whereas the rest of the bladder wall is thick and folded when the bladder is empty and thin and smooth when the bladder is distended. These differences reflect the embryologic origins of the trigone and the rest of the bladder wall. Because the trigone is derived from the embryonic mesonephric ducts, neither a muscularis mucosae nor a submucosal layer is present. Because the major portion of the bladder wall originates from the cloaca (a part of the hindgut), its wall possesses layers comparable to those found in the gastrointestinal tract.

The smooth muscle of the bladder wall forms the **detrusor muscle**. Toward the opening of the urethra, the muscle fibers form the involuntary **internal urethral sphincter**, a ring-like arrangement of muscle around the opening of the urethra. The smooth muscle bundles of the detrusor muscle are less regularly arranged than that of the tubular portions of the excretory passages; thus, the muscle and collagen bundles are randomly mixed (Plate 20.6, page 812). Contraction of the detrusor muscle of the bladder compresses the entire organ and forces the urine into the urethra.

The **bladder is innervated** by both sympathetic and parasympathetic divisions of the autonomic nervous system:

- **Sympathetic fibers** form a plexus in the adventitia of the bladder wall. These sympathetic postsynaptic fibers originate from the hypogastric plexus and release **noradrenaline (NA)**. NA activates both **β_3-adrenergic receptors** to relax the detrusor muscle and **α_1-adrenergic receptors** to contract smooth muscle fibers of the internal urethral sphincter. In this way, the sympathetic nervous system relaxes the bladder and contracts the internal urethral sphincter simultaneously.
- **Parasympathetic fibers** originate from the S2 to S4 segments of the spinal cord and travel with pelvic splanchnic nerves into the terminal ganglia located in the muscle bundles and adventitia of the bladder. Increased stimulation of parasympathetic postsynaptic nerve fibers releases **acetylcholine (ACh)**, which causes bladder contraction by stimulating **M_3 muscarinic receptors** in the smooth fibers of the detrusor muscle. These nerves also release **nitric oxide (NO)**, which relaxes smooth muscles of the internal urethral sphincter. Therefore, the parasympathetic system provides efferent fibers for the **micturition reflex**.

- **Sensory fibers** from the bladder to the sacral portion of the spinal cord are the afferent fibers of the micturition reflex.

Voluntary control over micturition is provided by the **somatic nerve fibers** from the **pudendal nerve** (S2–S4), which innervate the skeletal (striated) muscle of the external sphincter of the urethra. Somatic axon terminals at the neuromuscular junctions release **acetylcholine (ACh)**, which stimulates contraction of the external sphincter striated muscle by activating **nicotinic cholinergic receptors**. This sphincter surrounds the membranous urethra as it passes through the deep perineal pouch. Innervation from pudendal nerve fibers maintains constant tonic contraction of the skeletal muscle fibers of the external sphincter. During micturition, these fibers are inhibited, causing relaxation of the external sphincter and voiding of urine.

Urethra

The **urethra** is the fibromuscular tube that conveys urine from the urinary bladder to the exterior through the **external urethral orifice**. The size, structure, and functions of the urethra differ in males and females.

In the male, the urethra serves as the terminal duct for both the urinary and genital systems. It is about 20 cm long and has three distinct segments:

- **Prostatic urethra** extends for 3–4 cm from the neck of the bladder through the prostate gland (see pages 885-889). It is lined with transitional epithelium (urothelium). The ejaculatory ducts of the genital system enter the posterior wall of this segment, and many small prostatic ducts also empty into this segment.
- **Membranous urethra** extends for about 1 cm from the apex of the prostate gland to the bulb of the penis. It passes through the **deep perineal pouch** of the pelvic floor as it enters the perineum. Skeletal muscle of the deep perineal pouch surrounding the membranous urethra forms the **external (voluntary) sphincter of the urethra**. Transitional epithelium ends in the membranous urethra. This segment is lined with a stratified or pseudostratified columnar epithelium that resembles the epithelium of the genital duct system more than it resembles the epithelium of the more proximal portions of the urinary duct system.
- **Penile (spongy) urethra** extends for about 15 cm through the length of the penis and opens on the body surface at the **glans penis**. The penile urethra is surrounded by the **corpus spongiosum** as it passes through the length of the penis. It is lined with pseudostratified columnar epithelium, except at its distal end, where it is lined with stratified squamous epithelium continuous with that of the skin of the penis. **Ducts of the bulbourethral glands (Cowper glands)** and mucus-secreting **urethral glands (glands of Littré)** empty into the penile urethra.

In the female, the urethra is short, measuring 3–5 cm in length from the bladder to the vestibule of the vagina, where it normally terminates just posterior to the clitoris (see Chapter 23, Female Reproductive System, page 944). The mucosa is traditionally described as having longitudinal folds. As in the male urethra, the lining is initially transitional epithelium, a continuation of the bladder epithelium, but changes to stratified squamous epithelium before its termination. Some investigators have reported the presence of stratified columnar and pseudostratified columnar epithelium in the midportion of the female urethra.

Numerous small urethral glands, particularly in the proximal part of the urethra, open into the urethral lumen. Other glands, the **paraurethral glands (Skene glands)**, which are homologous to the prostate gland in the male, secrete into the common **paraurethral ducts**. These ducts open on each side of the external urethral orifice. They produce an alkaline secretion. The lamina propria is a highly vascularized layer of connective tissue that resembles the corpus spongiosum in the male. Where the urethra penetrates the urogenital diaphragm (membranous part of the urethra), the striated muscle of this structure forms the external (voluntary) urethral sphincter.

URINARY SYSTEM

HISTOLOGY 101 NOTEBOOK

OVERVIEW OF THE URINARY SYSTEM

- The **urinary system** includes the kidneys, ureters, bladder, and urethra.
- Essential functions of the kidneys include **homeostasis** via control of electrolyte and water balance, plasma pH, tissue osmolality, and blood pressure; **filtration** and **excretion** of metabolic waste products; and **endocrine activities**, such as secretion of hormones to regulate bone marrow erythropoiesis (EPO), blood pressure (renin), and Ca^{2+} metabolism (activation of vitamin D).

GENERAL STRUCTURE OF THE KIDNEY

- Each kidney is surrounded by a connective tissue **capsule** and contains an outer **cortex** and inner **medulla**, which is divided into 8–12 renal **pyramids**. The cortex extends into the medulla to form **renal columns** that separate the renal pyramids from each other.
- The **cortex** is characterized by renal corpuscles and their associated **convoluted** and **straight tubules**. Aggregation of straight tubules and collecting ducts in the cortex forms the **medullary rays.**
- A renal **lobe** includes the renal pyramid and its associated cortical tissue.
- The base of each renal **pyramid** faces the cortex, and the apical portion (**papilla**) projects into the minor calyx, a branch of the **major calyx** that, in turn, is a division of the renal pelvis.
- At the **hilum**, the renal pelvis extends into the ureter, which carries urine into the urinary bladder.
- Each kidney receives blood from the **renal artery**, which branches into the **interlobar arteries** (run between pyramids) that then turn along the base of the pyramid (**arcuate arteries**) and further branch into smaller **interlobular arteries** that supply the cortex.
- In the cortex, the interlobular artery gives off the **afferent arterioles** (one to each glomerulus), which give rise to the capillaries that form the glomerulus. The glomerular capillaries reunite to form a single **efferent arteriole** that, in turn, gives rise to a second network of capillaries, the **peritubular capillaries.**
- Some of the peritubular capillaries form long loops called the **vasa recta**, which accompany the thin segments of the nephrons.
- The peritubular capillaries drain into the **interlobular veins**, which, in turn, drain into the **arcuate veins**, **interlobar veins**, and the **renal vein**.

STRUCTURE AND FUNCTION OF NEPHRONS

- The **nephron** is the structural and functional unit of the kidney.
- The nephron consists of the **renal corpuscle** and a long tubular part that includes a proximal thick segment (**proximal convoluted tubule** and **proximal straight tubule**), thin segment (thin part of the **loop of Henle**), and distal thick segment (**distal straight tubule** and **distal convoluted tubule**). The distal convoluted tubule connects to the **collecting tubule** that opens at the renal papilla.
- The **renal corpuscle** contains the **glomerulus** surrounded by a double layer of the **Bowman capsule.**
- The **filtration apparatus** of the kidney consists of the **glomerular endothelium**, **glomerular basement membrane (GBM)**, and the Bowman capsule **podocytes.**
- The negatively charged **GBM**, which contains type IV and XVIII collagens, sialoglycoproteins, noncollagenous glycoproteins, proteoglycans, and glycosaminoglycans, acts as a physical barrier and an ion-selective filter.
- **Podocytes** extend their processes around the capillaries and develop numerous primary and secondary processes that give rise to **pedicels (foot processes)**, that interdigitate with other foot processes of the neighboring podocytes. The spaces between the interdigitating foot processes form **filtration slits** that are covered by the **filtration slit diaphragm.**
- **Podocalyxin** and **nephrin** play a key role in maintaining the structural and functional integrity of the kidney's filtration apparatus.
- The GBM in the renal corpuscle is shared among several capillaries to create a space for **mesangial cells** and their extracellular matrix.
- **Mesangial cells** are involved in phagocytosis and endocytosis of residues trapped in the filtration slits, secretion of paracrine substances, structural support for podocytes, and modulation of glomerular distention.
- The **juxtaglomerular apparatus** includes the **macula densa** (monitors Na^+ concentration in tubular fluid), **juxtaglomerular cells** (secrete renin), and **extraglomerular mesangial cells.** It regulates blood pressure by activating the **renin–angiotensin–aldosterone system (RAAS).**

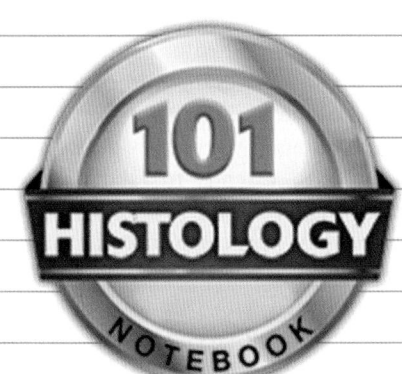

KIDNEY TUBULE FUNCTION

- The **glomerular ultrafiltrate** from the Bowman capsule passes through a series of tubules and collecting ducts lined by epithelial cells that secrete and absorb various substances to produce the final urine.
- The **proximal convoluted tubule** receives the glomerular ultrafiltrate from the Bowman capsule. This tubule is the initial and major site for **reabsorption** of glucose, amino acids, polypeptides, water, and electrolytes.
- Reabsorption of the ultrafiltrate continues as it flows from the proximal convoluted into the **proximal straight tubule** (the thick descending limb of the loop of Henle) that descends into the medulla.
- The **loop of Henle**, with both the descending limb (highly permeable to water) and ascending limb (highly permeable to Na^+ and Cl^-), concentrates the ultrafiltrate.
- The **distal straight tubule** (thick ascending limb) ascends back into the cortex to reach the vicinity of its renal corpuscle, where it makes contact with the afferent arteriole. In this area, the epithelial cells of the tubule form the **macula densa**.
- The **distal convoluted tubule** empties the ultrafiltrate into the **cortical collecting duct** that lies in the medullary ray, which further adjusts the concentration of Na^+ and K^+ in the ultrafiltrate.
- The medullary **collecting duct** is lined by cuboidal cells, with a transition to columnar cells as the duct increases in size. The collecting ducts possess **aquaporins** and **antidiuretic hormone (ADH)-regulated water channels** that regulate water reabsorption.
- The **collecting ducts** open at the renal papilla, and the modified ultrafiltrate, now called **urine**, flows sequentially via the excretory passages.

URETER, URINARY BLADDER, AND URETHRA

- All excretory passages for urine, except the urethra, have the same general organization: They are lined by a mucosa containing **transitional epithelium (urothelium)** and have a smooth muscle layer and a connective tissue adventitia (or serosa).
- **Transitional epithelium** is a specialized stratified epithelium with large **dome-shaped (umbrella) cells** that bulge into the lumen.
- The dome-shaped cells have a modified apical membrane containing **plaques** and **fusiform vesicles** that accommodate the invaginated excess of the plasma membrane, which is needed for the extension of the apical surface when the organ is stretched.
- Transitional epithelium creates a **permeability barrier** and is actively involved in molecular signaling mechanisms.
- The **ureter** conducts urine from the renal pelvis to the urinary bladder. It is lined by transitional epithelium, underlying smooth muscle arranged in three distinct layers, and connective tissue adventitia.
- The **urinary bladder** is also lined by transitional epithelium and possesses many mucosal folds, except in the **trigone** region. Its muscular wall is thick and well developed and forms the **detrusor muscle**.
- The **urethra** conveys urine from the urinary bladder to the **external urethral orifice.**
- The **female urethra** is short and lined by transitional epithelium (upper half), pseudostratified columnar epithelium (lower half), and stratified squamous epithelium (before its termination).
- The **male urethra** is much longer than the female's and is divided into three regions: the **prostatic urethra** (lined by transitional epithelium), a short **membranous urethra** that pierces the external urethral sphincter (lined by stratified or pseudostratified columnar epithelium), and a long **penile urethra** (lined by pseudostratified columnar epithelium).

PLATE 20.1 ■ KIDNEY I

The urinary system consists of the paired **kidneys**; the paired **ureters**, which lead from the kidneys to the **urinary bladder**; and the **urethra**, which leads from the bladder to the exterior of the body. The kidneys conserve body fluid and electrolytes and remove metabolic wastes, such as urea, uric acid, creatinine, and breakdown products of various substances. They produce **urine**, initially an ultrafiltrate of blood that is modified by selective resorption and specific secretion by kidney tubule cells. The kidneys also function as endocrine organs, producing **erythropoietin**, a growth factor that regulates red blood cell formation, and **renin**, a hormone involved in blood pressure and blood volume control. They also hydroxylate vitamin D, a steroid prohormone, to produce its active form.

Each kidney is a flattened, bean-shaped structure ~10 cm long, 6.5 cm wide (from convex to concave border), and 3 cm thick. The concave medial border of each kidney contains a hilum, an indented region through which blood vessels, nerves, and lymphatic vessels enter and leave the kidney. The funnel-shaped origin of the ureter, the **renal pelvis**, also leaves the kidney at the hilum. A cut, hemisected fresh kidney reveals two distinct regions: a **cortex**, the reddish brown outer region, and a **medulla**, a much lighter inner part continuous with the renal pelvis. The cortex is characterized by **renal corpuscles** and their tubules, including the convoluted and straight tubules of the **nephron**, the **cortical collecting ducts**, and an extensive vascular supply.

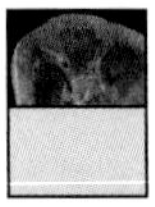

Kidney, human, fresh specimen ×3.

A frontal section through the cortex and medulla of an unembalmed kidney obtained from autopsy is shown here. The visible **hilar region** consists of minor calyces (gray/white) surrounded by *yellow* in appearance adipose tissue. The outer part of the kidney has a *reddish brown* appearance; this is the **cortex**. It is easily distinguished from the inner portion, the medulla, which is further divided into an outer portion (*OM*), identified here by the presence of straight blood vessels, the vasa recta (*VR*), and an inner portion (*IM*), which has a lighter and more homogeneous appearance. The **medulla** consists of renal pyramids, which have their base facing the cortex and their apex in the form of a papilla (*P*) directed toward the hilum. The **pyramids** are separated, sometimes only partially, as in this figure, by cortical material that is designated the **renal columns** (*RCol*). The majority of the outer part of the pyramid on the *left* has not been included in the plane of section. The papillae are free tips of the pyramids that project into the first of a series of large urine–collecting spaces referred to as the **minor calyces** (*MC*); the inner surface of the calyx is white. The minor calyces drain into **major calyces**, and in turn, these open into the **renal pelvis**, which funnels urine into the ureter.

An interesting feature in this specimen is that the blood has been retained in many of the vessels, thereby allowing for visualization of several renal vessels in their geographic location. Among the vessels that can be identified in the cut face of the kidney shown here are the interlobular vessels (*IV*) within the cortex; the arcuate veins (*AV*) and the arcuate arteries (*AA*) at the base of the pyramids; the interlobar arteries (*ILA*) and veins (*ILV*) between renal pyramids; and, in the medulla, the vessels going to and from the capillary network of the pyramid. The latter vessels, both arterioles and venules, are relatively straight and are designated collectively as the vasa recta (*VR*). (Specimen courtesy of Dr. Eric A. Pfeifer.)

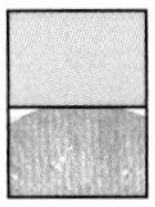

Cortex and medulla, kidney, human, hematoxylin and eosin (H&E) ×20.

A histologic section including the **cortex** and part of the **medulla** is shown here. Located at the boundary between the two (partly marked by the *dashed line*) are numerous profiles of arcuate arteries (*AA*) and arcuate veins (*AV*). The most distinctive feature of the renal cortex, regardless of the plane of section, is the presence of the renal corpuscles (*RC*). These are spherical structures composed of a glomerulus (glomerular vascular tuft) surrounded by the visceral and parietal epithelium of the Bowman capsule. Also seen in the cortex are groups of tubules that are more or less straight and disposed in a radial direction from the base of the medulla (*arrows*); these are the medullary rays. In contrast, the medulla presents profiles of tubular structures that are arranged as gentle curves in the outer part of the medulla, turning slightly to become straight in the inner part of the medulla. The disposition of the tubules (and blood vessels) gives the cut face of the pyramid a slightly striated appearance that is also evident in the gross specimen (see the previous figure).

AA, arcuate arteries
AV, arcuate veins
ILA, interlobar artery
ILV, interlobar vein
IM, inner medulla
IV, interlobular vessels
MC, minor calyx
OM, outer medulla
P, papilla
RCol, renal column
RC, renal corpuscles
VR, vasa recta
arrows, medullary rays
dashed line, boundary between cortex and medulla

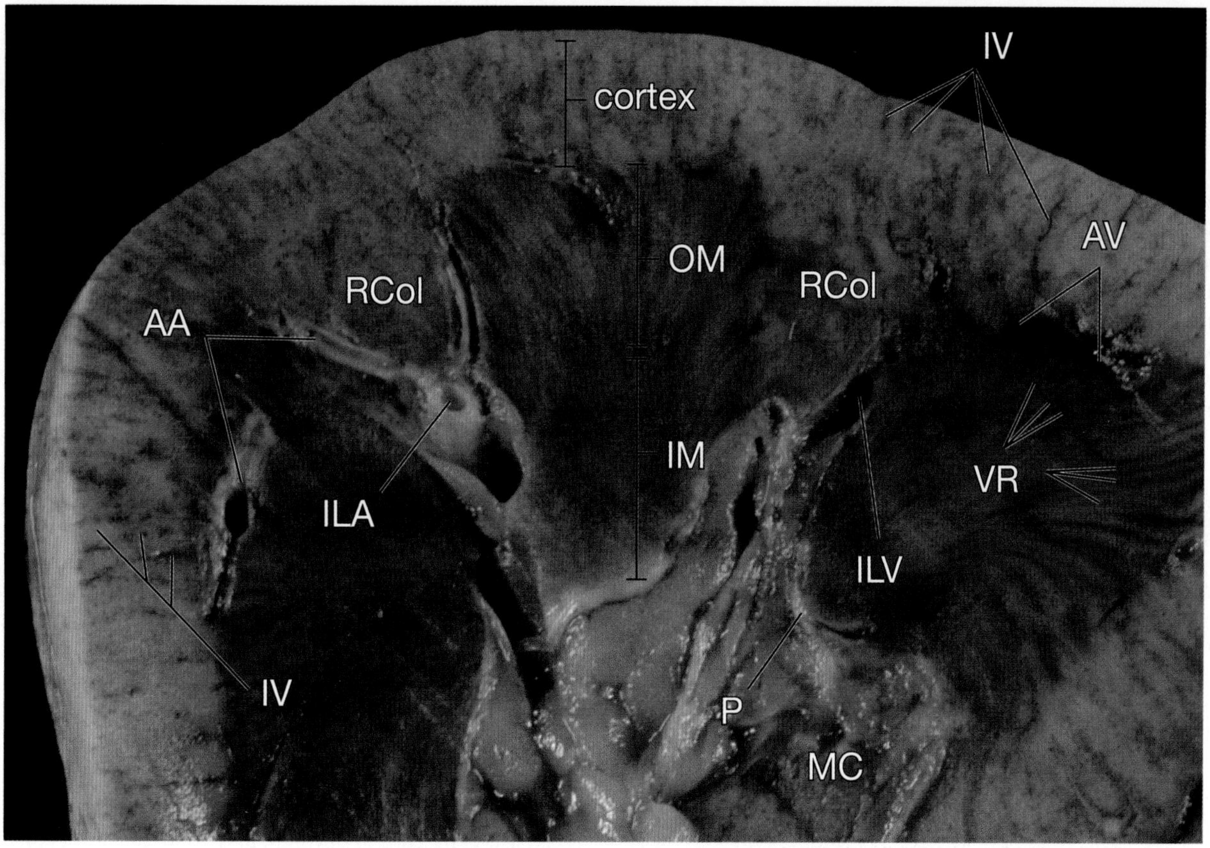
cortex
IV
OM
RCol
RCol
AV
AA
ILA
IM
VR
ILV
IV
P
MC

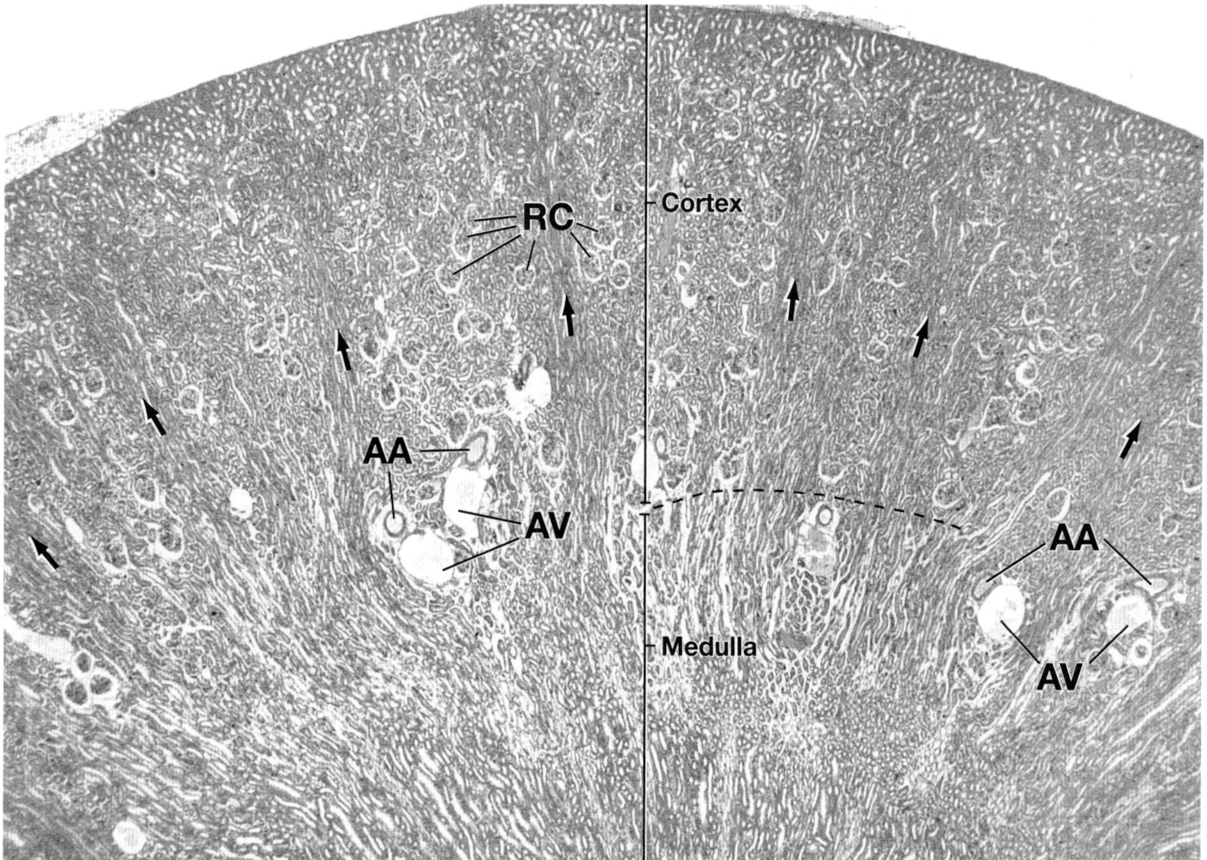
RC
Cortex
AA
AV
AA
AV
Medulla

PLATE 20.2 ■ KIDNEY II

The **nephron** is the functional unit of the kidney. There are about 2 million nephrons in each human kidney. They are responsible for the production of urine and correspond to the secretory part of other glands. The **collecting ducts**, responsible for the final concentration of the urine, are analogous to the ducts of exocrine glands. The nephron is made up of the **renal corpuscle** and the **renal tubule**. The renal corpuscle consists of the **glomerulus**, a tuft of 10–20 capillary loops, surrounded by a double-layered epithelial cup, the **renal or Bowman capsule**. The glomerular capillaries are supplied at the vascular pole of the Bowman capsule by an **afferent arteriole** and drained by an **efferent arteriole** that leaves the Bowman capsule at the vascular pole and then branches to form a new capillary network to supply the kidney tubules. The opposite pole of the Bowman capsule, the urinary pole, is where the filtrate leaves the renal capsule. The tubular parts of the nephron are the **proximal thick segment** (consisting of the **proximal convoluted tubule** and the **proximal straight tubule**); the **thin segment**, which constitutes the *thin* **limb of the loop of Henle**; and the **distal thick segment**, consisting of the **distal straight tubule** and the **distal convoluted tubule**. The loop of Henle is the U-shaped portion of the nephron consisting of the thick straight portions of the proximal and distal tubules and the thin segment between them. The distal convoluted tubule joins the **cortical collecting duct** via either the connecting tubule or arched connecting tubule. The nephron and the connecting tubule constitute the **uriniferous tubule**.

Cortex, kidney, human, hematoxylin and eosin (H&E) ×60.

The **renal cortex** can be divided into regions referred to as the **cortical labyrinth** (*CL*) and the **medullary rays** (*MR*). The cortical labyrinth contains the **renal corpuscles** (*RC*), which appear as relatively large spherical structures. Surrounding each renal corpuscle are the proximal and distal convoluted tubules. They are also part of the cortical labyrinth. The convoluted tubules, particularly the proximal, because of their tortuosity, present a variety of profiles, most of which are oval or circular; others, more elongated, are in the shape of a letter J, a C, or even an S. The medullary rays are composed of groups of straight tubules oriented in the same direction and appear to radiate from the base of the pyramid. When the medullary rays are cut longitudinally, as they are in this figure, the tubules present elongated profiles. The medullary rays contain proximal straight tubules (thick segments; descending limb of loop of Henle), distal straight tubules (thick segments; ascending limbs of loop of Henle), and cortical collecting ducts.

Cortex, kidney, human, H&E ×120.

This figure presents another profile of the **renal cortex**, at a somewhat higher magnification, cut in a plane at a right angle to the section in the previous figure. The peripheral part of the micrograph shows the **cortical labyrinth** in which the tubules display chiefly not only round and oval profiles but also some that are more elongated and curved. The appearance is the same as the cortical labyrinth areas of the previous figure. A **renal corpuscle** (*RC*) is also present in the cortical labyrinth. In contrast, the profiles presented by the tubules of the medullary ray in this figure are quite different from those seen in the previous figure. All of the tubules bounded by the *dashed line* belong to the medullary ray (*MR*), and all are cut in cross section. A general survey of the tubules within the medullary ray reveals that several distinct types can be recognized on the basis of the size of the tubule, shape of the lumen, and size of the tubule cells. These features as well as those of the cortical labyrinth are considered in Plate 20.3 (page 806).

CL, cortical labyrinth
MR, medullary ray
RC, renal corpuscle
dashed line, approximate boundary of the medullary ray

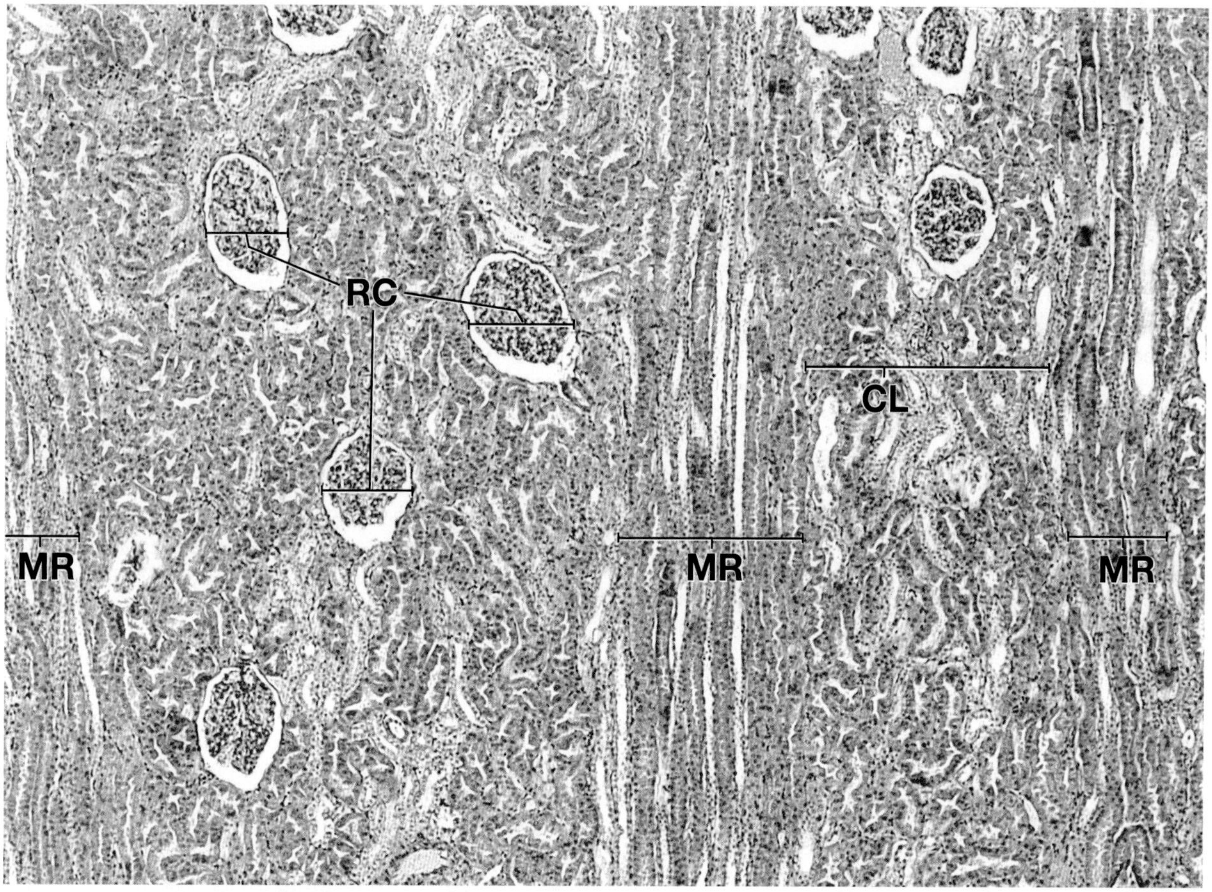
RC
CL
MR
MR
MR

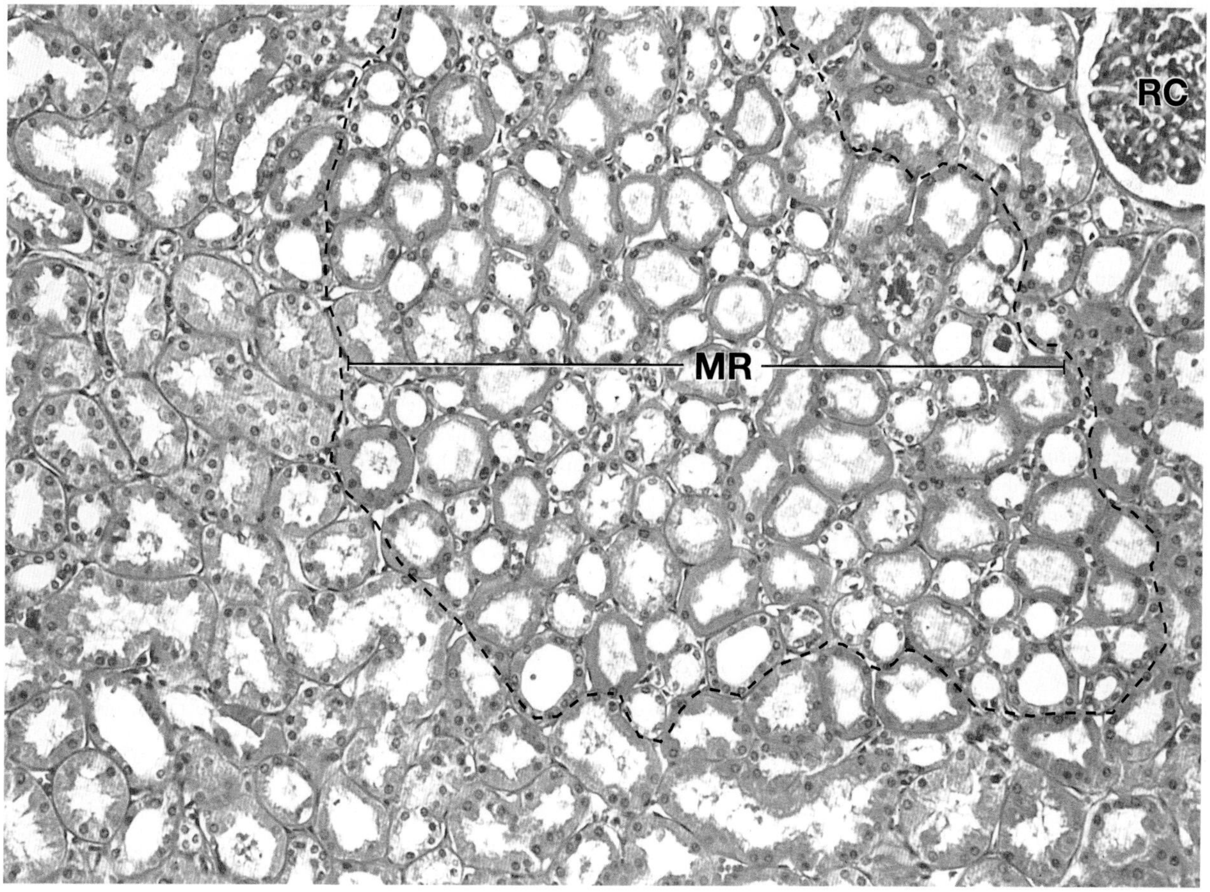
RC
MR

PLATE 20.3 ■ KIDNEY III

Proximal and distal convoluted tubules display features that aid in their identification in hematoxylin and eosin (H&E)-stained paraffin sections. **Proximal convoluted tubules** generally have a larger diameter than distal tubules have; cross sections of the lumen often appear stellate. A brush border (apical microvilli) is often visible on the proximal tubule cells. Also, the proximal convoluted tubule is more than twice as long as the **distal convoluted tubule**; thus, the majority of tubular profiles in the cortical labyrinth will be of proximal tubules.

Mesangial cells and their extracellular matrix constitute the **mesangium** of the renal corpuscle. They underlie the endothelium of the capillaries of the glomerular tuft and extend to the vascular pole, where they become part of the **juxtaglomerular apparatus.** The terminal portion of the distal thick segment of the nephron lies close to the afferent arteriole. Tubule epithelial cells closest to the arteriole are thinner, taller, and more closely packed than other tubule cells and constitute the *macula densa.* Arterial smooth muscle cells opposite the macula densa are modified into **juxtaglomerular cells** that secrete **renin** in response to decreased blood NaCl concentration.

Proximal and distal convoluted tubules, kidney, human, H&E ×240.

In this figure, an area of **cortical labyrinth**, there are six **distal convoluted tubule** (*DC*) profiles. The **proximal convoluted tubules** (unlabeled) have a slightly larger outside diameter than the distal tubules have. The proximal tubules have a brush border, whereas the distal tubules have a cleaner, sharper luminal surface. The lumen of the proximal tubules is often star shaped; this is not the case with distal tubules. Typically, fewer nuclei appear in a cross section of a proximal tubule than in an equivalent segment of a distal tubule.

Most of the abovementioned points can also be utilized in distinguishing the straight portions of the proximal and distal thick segments in the medullary rays, as shown in the figure on the *right*.

Proximal and distal straight tubules, kidney, human, H&E ×240.

In this figure, all of the tubular profiles within the medullary ray are rounded, except for a **proximal convoluted tubule** (*PC*) included in the *lower right corner* of the figure (it belongs to the adjacent cortical labyrinth). Second, the number of proximal straight (*P*) and distal straight (*D*) tubular profiles are about equal in the medullary ray, as is shown by the labeling of each tubule in this figure. Note that, in contrast to the **distal straight tubules**, the **proximal straight tubules** display a brush border and have a larger outside diameter, with many displaying a star-shaped lumen. The medullary ray also contains **cortical collecting ducts** (*CCD*).

Renal corpuscles, kidney, human, H&E ×360.

The **renal corpuscle** appears as a spherical structure whose periphery is composed of a thin capsule that encloses a narrow clear-appearing space, the **urinary space** (*asterisks*), and a capillary tuft or glomerulus that appears as a large cellular mass. The capsule of the renal corpuscle, known as the **renal** or **Bowman capsule**, actually has two parts: a parietal layer, which is marked (*BC*), and a visceral layer. The **parietal layer** consists of simple squamous epithelial cells. The **visceral layer** consists of cells called **podocytes** (*Pod*) that lie on the outer surface of the glomerular capillary. Except where they clearly line the urinary space, as the labeled cells do in the figure on the *left*, podocytes may be difficult to distinguish from the capillary endothelial cells. To complicate matters, the mesangial cells are also a component of the glomerulus. In general, nuclei of podocytes are larger and stain less intensely than do the endothelial and mesangial cell nuclei.

A distal (*DC*) and two proximal (*PC*) convoluted tubules are marked in the figure on the *left*. The cells of the distal tubule are more crowded on one side. These crowded cells constitute the **macula densa** (*MD*) that lies adjacent to the afferent arteriole.

In the figure on the *right*, both the vascular pole and the urinary pole of the renal corpuscle are evident. The **vascular pole** is characterized by the presence of arterioles (*A*), one of which is entering or leaving (*double-headed arrow*) the corpuscle. The afferent arteriole possesses modified smooth muscle cells with granules, the juxtaglomerular cells (not evident in this figure). At the **urinary pole**, the parietal layer of the Bowman capsule is continuous with the beginning of the proximal convoluted tubule (*PC*). Here, the urinary space of the renal corpuscle continues into the lumen of the proximal tubule, and the lining cells change from simple squamous to simple cuboidal or low columnar with a brush border.

A, arteriole
BC, Bowman capsule (parietal layer)
CCD, cortical collecting duct
D, distal straight tubule
DC, distal convoluted tubule
MD, macula densa
P, proximal (straight tubule)
PC, proximal convoluted tubule
Pod, podocyte (visceral layer of Bowman capsule)
asterisks, urinary space **double-headed arrow,** blood vessel at vascular pole of renal corpuscle

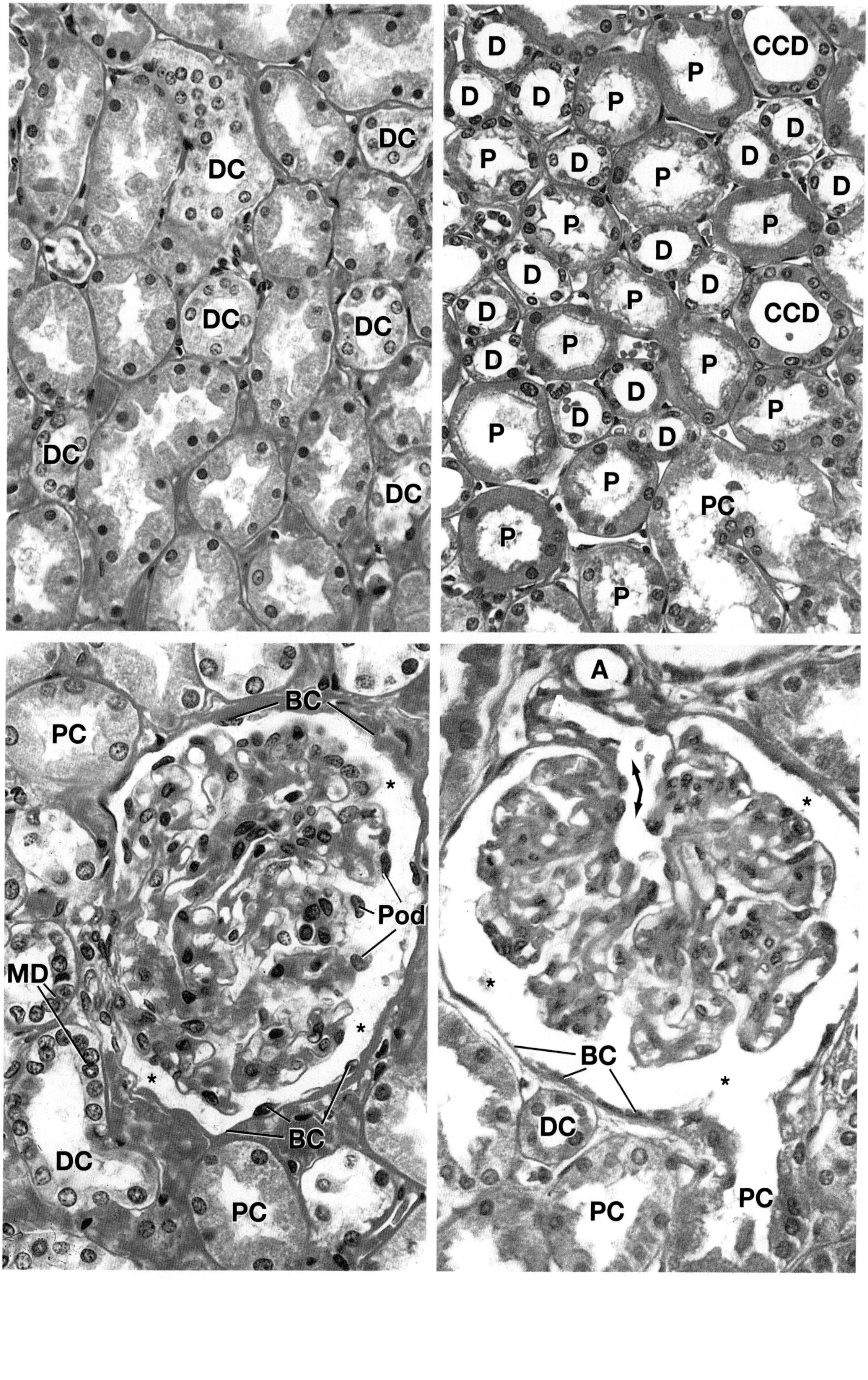
DC
DC
DC
DC
DC
DC
D
CCD
P
P
P
PC
BC
PC
Pod
MD
BC
DC
PC
A
BC
DC
PC
PC

PLATE 20.4 ■ KIDNEY IV

Renal corpuscles are restricted to the cortical labyrinth. The **medulla** contains the thick straight segments of proximal and distal tubules, along with their thin segments, the collecting ducts, and the blood vessels that run in parallel with them. These structures function as the *countercurrent multiplier* and *countercurrent exchange* systems that, ultimately, produce hypertonic urine. The final urine drains from the papillary ducts (of Bellini) into calyces that then empty into the renal pelvis.

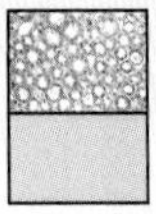

Medulla, kidney, human, hematoxylin and eosin (H&E) ×240.

A section through the **outer portion of the medulla** is shown in this figure. This region contains proximal and distal thick segments, thin segments, and medullary collecting ducts. All of the tubules are parallel, and all are cut in cross section; thus, they present circular profiles. The **proximal straight tubules** (*P*) display typical star-shaped lumina and a brush border (or the fragmented apical cell surface from which the brush border has been partially broken). These tubules have outside diameters that are generally larger than those of the **distal straight tubules** (*D*). As mentioned previously and as shown here, the distal straight tubules display a larger number of nuclei than do comparable segments of proximal straight tubule cells. Note, also, that the lumen of the distal tubule is more rounded and the apical surface of the cells is sharper. The **collecting ducts** (*CD*) have outer diameters that are about the same as those of the proximal tubules and larger than those of distal tubules. The cells forming the collecting ducts are cuboidal and smaller than those of proximal tubules; thus, they also display a relatively larger number of nuclei than do comparable segments of proximal tubule cells. Count them. Finally, boundaries between the cells that constitute the collecting ducts are usually evident (*asterisks*); this serves as one of the most dependable features for the identification of collecting ducts.

The thin segments (*T*) have the thinnest walls of all renal tubules seen in the medulla. They are formed by a low cuboidal or simple squamous epithelium, as seen here, and the lumina are relatively large. Occasionally, a section includes the region of transition from a thick to a thin segment and can be recognized even in a cross section through the tubule. One such junction is evident in this figure (the tubule with *two arrows* in the lumen). On one side, the tubule cell (*left-pointing arrow*) is characteristic of the proximal segment; it possesses a distinctive brush border. The other side of the tubule (*right-pointing arrow*) is composed of low cuboidal cells that resemble the cells forming the thin segments. In addition to the uriniferous tubules and collecting ducts, there are many other small tubular structures in this figure. Thin walled and lined by endothelium, they are small blood vessels.

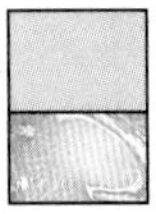

Renal pyramid, kidney, human, H&E ×20.

This figure shows a **renal pyramid** at low magnification. The pyramid is a conical structure composed principally of medullary straight tubules, ducts, and the straight blood vessels (vasa recta). The *dashed line* at the *left* of the micrograph is placed at the junction between cortex and medulla; thus, it marks the base of the pyramid. Note the **arcuate vessels** (*AV*) that lie at the boundary of cortex and medulla. They define the boundary line. The few renal corpuscles (*RC*), *upper left*, belong to the renal column of the medulla. They are referred to as *juxtamedullary corpuscles*.

The pyramid is somewhat distorted in this specimen, as evidenced by regions of longitudinally sectioned tubules, *lower left*, and cross-sectioned and obliquely sectioned tubules in other regions. In effect, part of the pyramid was bent, thus the change in the plane of section of the tubules.

The apical portion of the pyramid (*arrowhead*), known as the **renal papilla**, is lodged in a cup- or funnel-like structure referred to as the *calyx*. It collects the urine that leaves the tip of the papilla from the papillary ducts (of Bellini). (The actual tip of the papilla is not seen within the plane of section, nor are the openings of the ducts at this low magnification.) The surface of the papilla that faces the lumen of the **minor calyx** is simple columnar or cuboidal epithelium (*SCEp*). (In places, this epithelium has separated from the surface of the papilla and appears as a thin strand of tissue.) The calyx is lined by transitional epithelium (*TEp*). Although not evident at the low magnification shown here, the boundary between the columnar epithelium covering the papilla and the transitional epithelium covering the inner surface of the calyx is marked by the *diamonds*.

AV, arcuate vessels
CD, collecting duct
D, distal straight tubule
P, proximal straight tubule
RC, renal corpuscle
SCEp, simple columnar epithelium
T, thin segment
TEp, transitional epithelium
left-pointing arrow (upper panel), proximal tubule cell
right-pointing arrow (upper panel), thin segment cell
arrowhead, location of apex of pyramid
asterisks, boundaries between cells of a collecting duct
diamonds, boundary between a transitional and a columnar epithelium

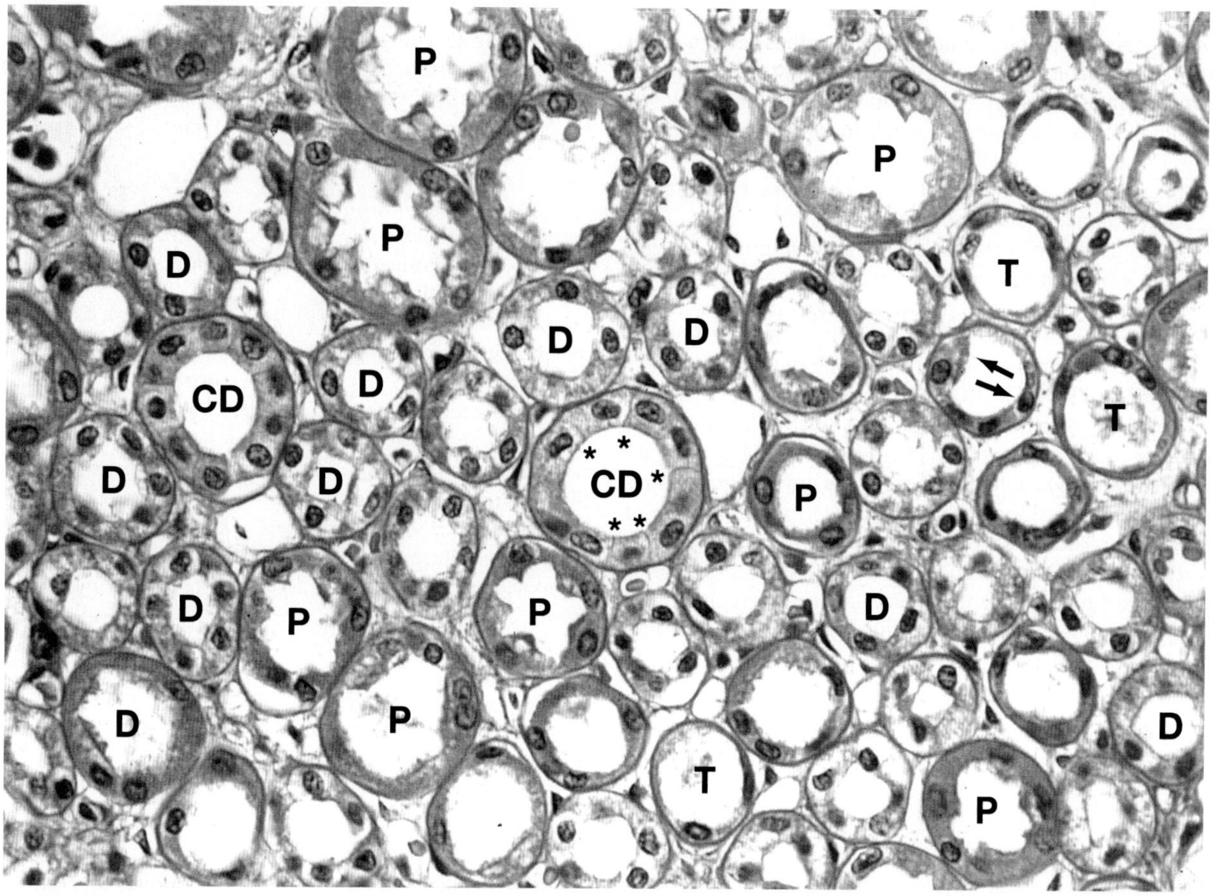
P
P
P
D
D
D
D
D
CD
CD
T
T
D
D
D
P
P
P
D
P
T
P
D
T

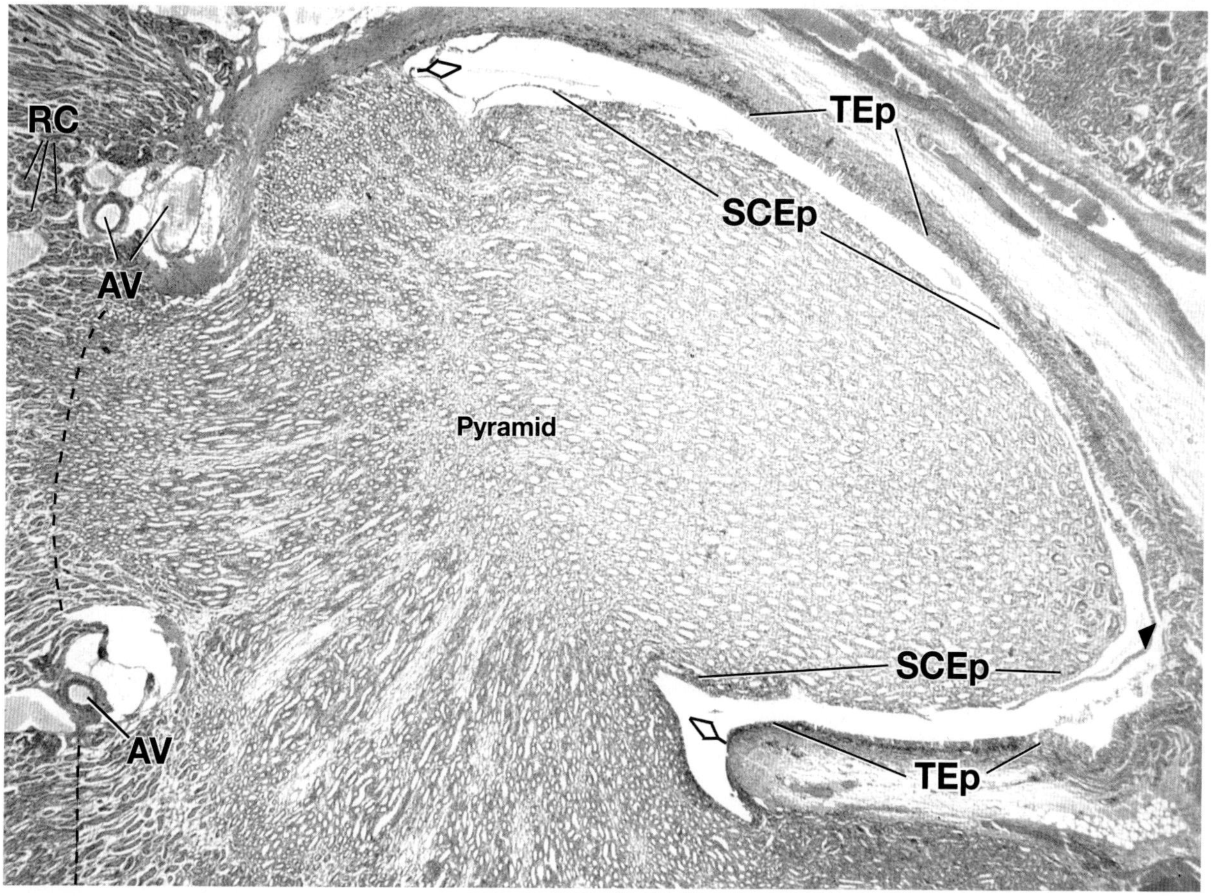
RC
AV
TEp
SCEp
Pyramid
SCEp
AV
TEp

PLATE 20.5 ■ URETER

The **ureters** are paired tubular structures that convey urine from the kidneys to the urinary bladder. They are lined with **transitional epithelium (urothelium)**, an impervious layer that lines the urinary excretory passages from the renal calyces through the urethra. The ability of this epithelium to become thinner and flatter allows all of these passages to accommodate to distension by the urine.

The epithelium rests on a dense collagenous lamina propria, which, in turn, rests on an inner longitudinal and an outer circular layer of smooth muscle. Regular peristaltic contractions of this muscle contribute to the flow of urine from the kidney to the urinary bladder.

ORIENTATION MICROGRAPH: As shown in this low-power orientation micrograph, the wall of the ureter consists of a **mucosa** (*Muc*), a **muscularis** (*Mus*), and an **adventitia** (*Adv*). Note that the ureters are located behind the peritoneum of the abdominal cavity in their course to the bladder. Thus, a **serosa** (*Ser*) may be found covering a portion of the circumference of the tube. Also, because of contraction of the smooth muscle of the muscularis, the luminal surface is characteristically folded, thus creating a star-shaped lumen.

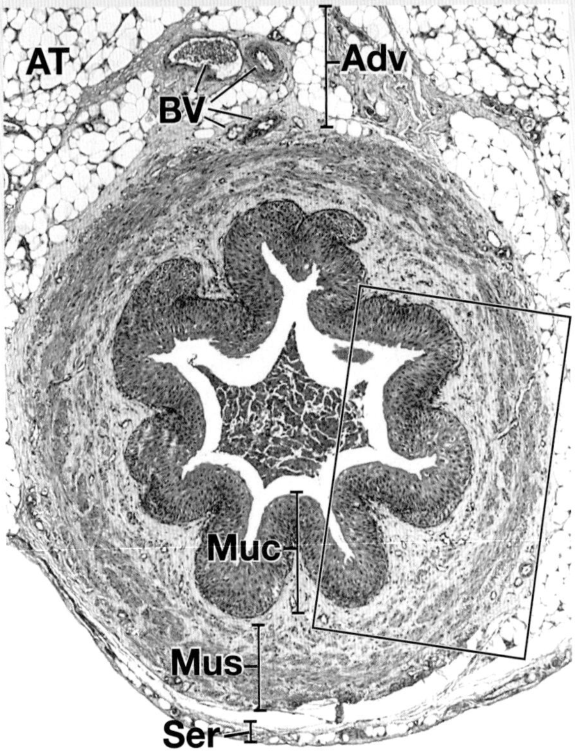

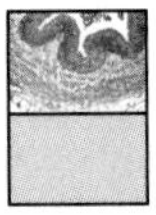

Ureter, monkey, hematoxylin and eosin (H&E) ×160.

The wall of the ureter from the *rectangular area* in the orientation micrograph is examined at higher magnification in this figure. One can immediately recognize the thick epithelial lining, which appears distinct and sharply delineated from the remainder of the wall. This is the **transitional epithelium (urothelium)** (*Ep*). The remainder of the wall is made up of connective tissue (*CT*) and smooth muscle. The latter can be recognized as the darker staining layer. The section also shows some adipose tissue (*AT*), a component of the adventitia.

The transitional epithelium and its supporting connective tissue constitute the **mucosa** (*Muc*). A distinct submucosa is not present, although the term is sometimes applied to the connective tissue that is closest to the muscle.

The **muscularis** (*Mus*) is arranged as an inner longitudinal layer (*SM[l]*), a middle circular layer (*SM[c]*), and an outer longitudinal layer (*SM[l]*). However, the outer longitudinal layer is present only at the lower end of the ureter. In a cross section through the ureter, the inner and outer smooth muscle layers are cut in cross section, whereas the middle circular layer of the muscle cells is cut longitudinally. This is as they appear in this figure.

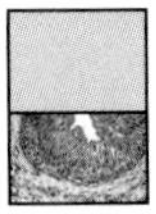

Transitional epithelium, ureter, monkey, H&E ×400.

This figure shows the **inner longitudinal smooth muscle** layer (*SM[l]*) at higher magnification. Note that the nuclei appear as round profiles, indicating that the muscle cells have been cross-sectioned. This figure also shows the **transitional epithelium** (*Ep*) to advantage. The surface cells of the transitional epithelium (urothelium) are characteristically the largest, and some are binucleate (*arrow*). The basal cells are the smallest, and typically, the nuclei appear crowded because of the minimal cytoplasm of each cell. The intermediate cells appear to consist of several layers and are composed of cells larger in size than the basal cells but smaller than the surface cells.

Adv, adventitia
AT, adipose tissue
BV, blood vessels
CT, connective tissue
Ep, transitional epithelium
Muc, mucosa
Mus, muscularis
Ser, serosa
SM(c), circular layer of smooth muscle
SM(l), longitudinal layer of smooth muscle
arrow, binucleate surface cell

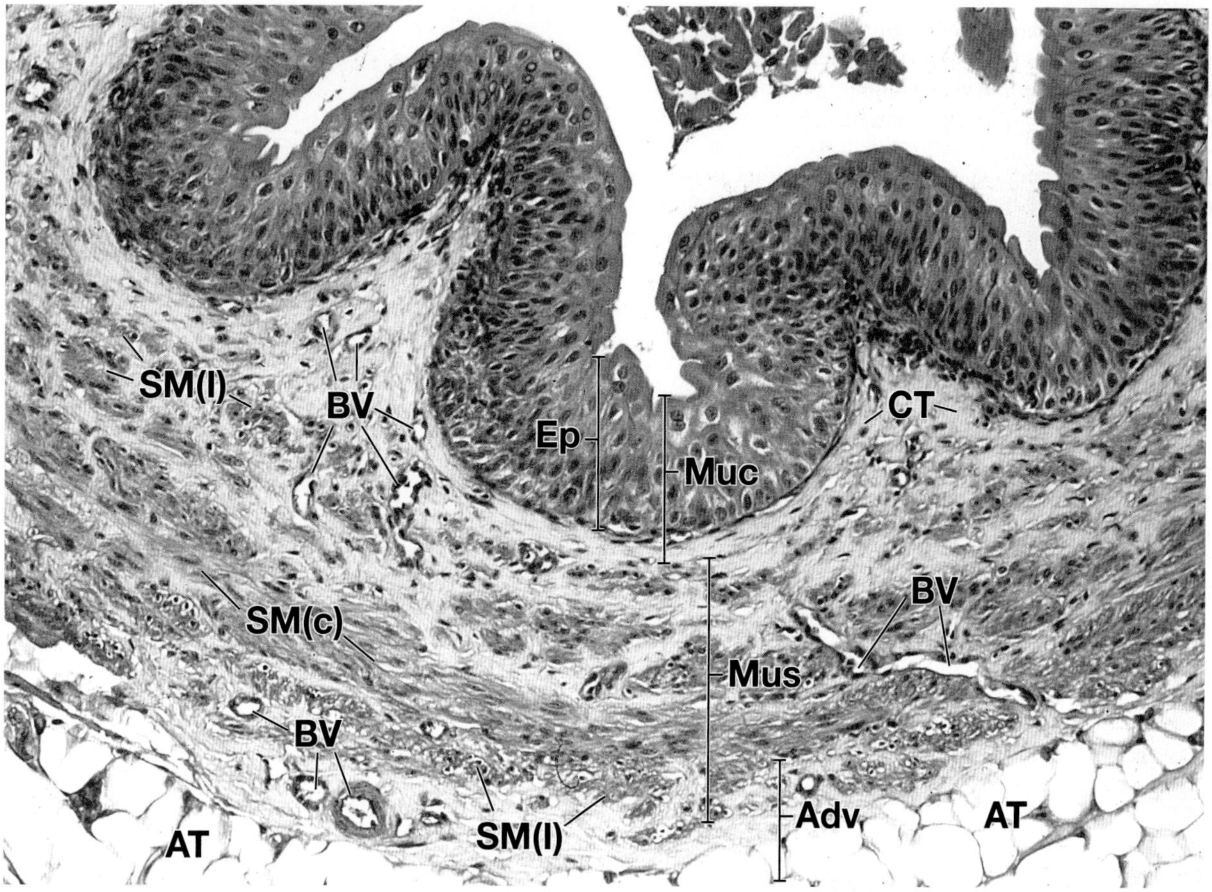
SM(l)
BV
Ep
Muc
CT
BV
SM(c)
Mus
BV
Adv
AT
AT
SM(l)

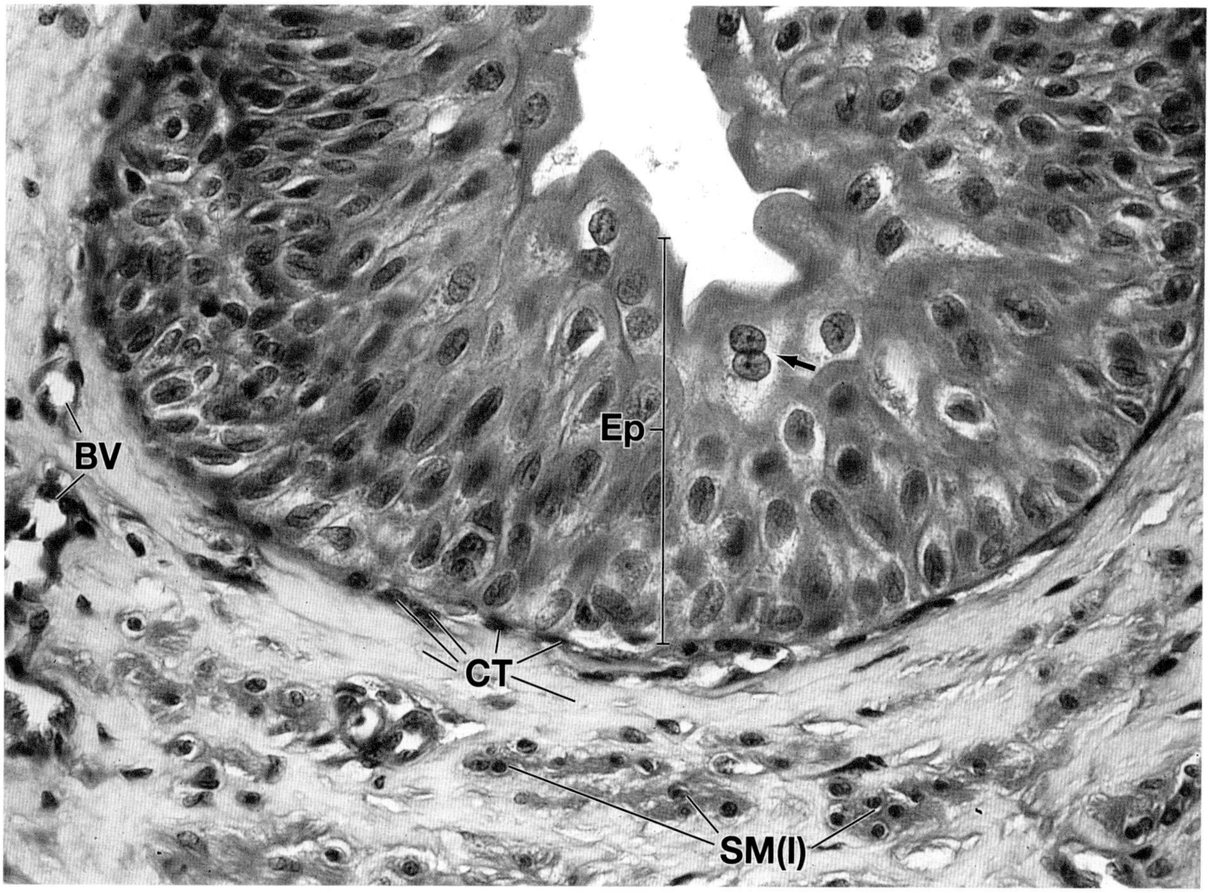
BV
Ep
CT
SM(l)

PLATE 20.6 ■ URINARY BLADDER

The **urinary bladder** receives the urine from the two ureters and stores it until neural stimulation causes it to contract and expel the urine via the urethra. It, too, is lined with **transitional epithelium (urothelium)**. Beneath the epithelium and its underlying connective tissue, the wall of the urinary bladder contains **smooth muscle** that is usually described as being arranged as an inner longitudinal layer, a middle circular layer, and an outer longitudinal layer. As in most distensible hollow viscera that empty their contents through a narrow aperture, the smooth muscle in the wall of the urinary bladder is less regularly arranged than the description indicates, allowing contraction to reduce the volume relatively evenly throughout the bladder.

ORIENTATION MICROGRAPH: This orientation micrograph of the urinary bladder reveals the full thickness of the bladder wall. The luminal surface epithelium is at the *top* of the micrograph. One of the ureters can be seen as it passes through the bladder wall to empty its contents into the bladder lumen. Most of the tissue to the sides and below the ureteral profile is smooth muscle.

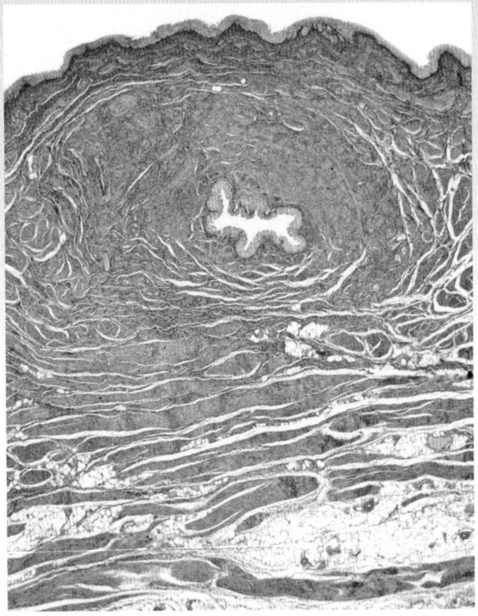

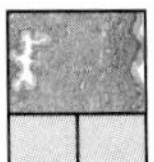

Urinary bladder, human, hematoxylin and eosin (H&E) ×60.

This micrograph shows most of the entire thickness of the urinary bladder. An unusual feature is the presence of one of the ureters (*U*) as it is passing through the bladder wall to empty its contents into the bladder lumen. The **transitional epithelium** (*Ep*) lining the bladder is seen on the *right*. Beneath the epithelium is a relatively thick layer of connective tissue (*CT*) containing blood vessels (*BV*) of various sizes. Note that the connective tissue stains more eosinophilic than the smooth muscle of the underlying **muscularis** (*M*). The epithelium and connective tissue constitute the mucosa of the bladder. The muscularis consists of smooth muscle arranged in three indistinct layers. It should be noted that as the ureter passes through the bladder wall, it carries with it a layer of longitudinally oriented smooth muscle (*SM[L]*). Medium-sized arteries (*A*) and veins (*V*) are occasionally seen in the muscularis.

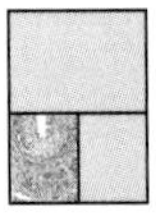

Transitional epithelium, urinary bladder, human, H&E ×250.

This higher magnification of the *left rectangle* of the previous figure shows the **transitional epithelium** (*Ep*) and the underlying connective tissue (*CT*) that represent the mucosa of the ureter. Adjacent to the mucosa are bundles of longitudinally sectioned smooth muscle (*SM[L]*) that belong to the ureter. A small lymphatic vessel (*Lym*) is present in the connective tissue adjacent to the smooth muscle. Note the lymphocytes, identified by their small round densely stained nuclei, within the lumen of the vessel.

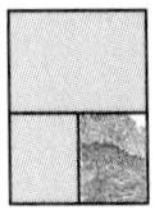

Transitional epithelium, urinary bladder, human, H&E ×250.

This higher magnification of the *right rectangle* of the previous figure shows the bladder **transitional epithelium** (*Ep*) and the underlying connective tissue (*CT*) of the bladder wall. The transitional epithelium is often characterized by the presence of surface cells that are dome shaped. In addition, many of these cells are binucleate (*arrows*). The thickness of transitional epithelium is variable. When the bladder is fully distended, as few as three cell layers are seen. Here, in the contracted bladder, it appears that there are as many as 10 cell layers, a result of the cells folding over one another as the smooth muscle contracts and the lining surface is reduced. The connective tissue consists of bundles of collagen fibers interspersed with varying numbers of lymphocytes identified by their densely stained round nuclei. A vein (*V*) filled with red blood cells is also evident in the mucosal connective tissue.

A, artery
BV, blood vessel
CT, connective tissue
Ep, transitional epithelium
Lym, lymphatic vessel
M, muscularis
SM(L), longitudinally cut smooth muscle
U, ureter
V, vein
arrows, binucleate cells

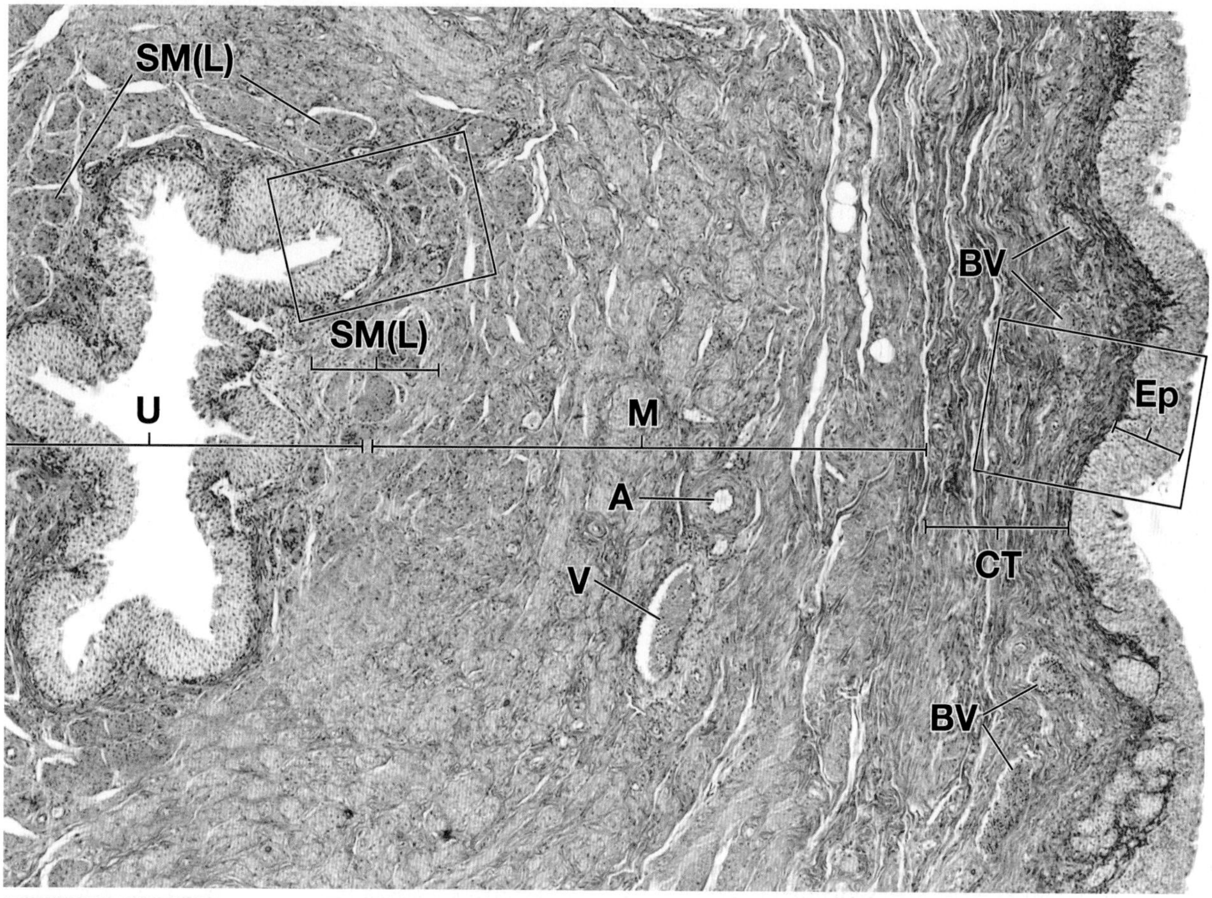
SM(L)
SM(L)
U
M
BV
Ep
A
CT
V
BV

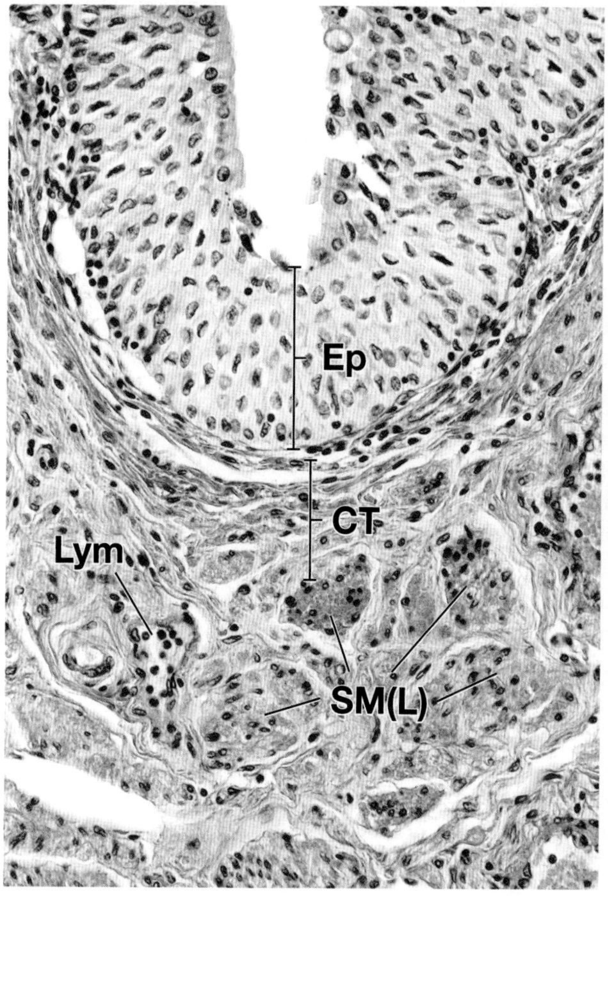
Ep
CT
Lym
SM(L)

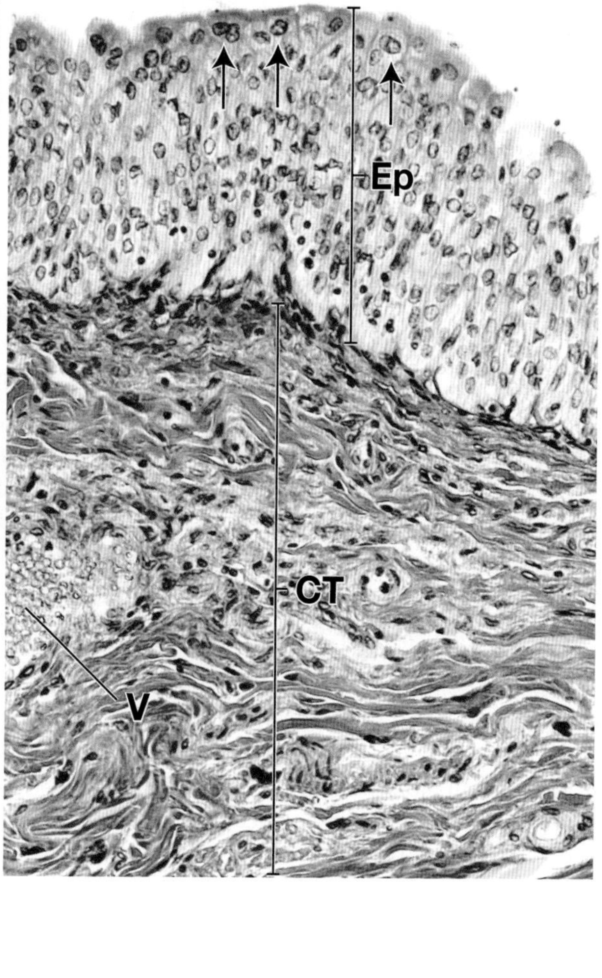
Ep
CT
V

21 ENDOCRINE ORGANS

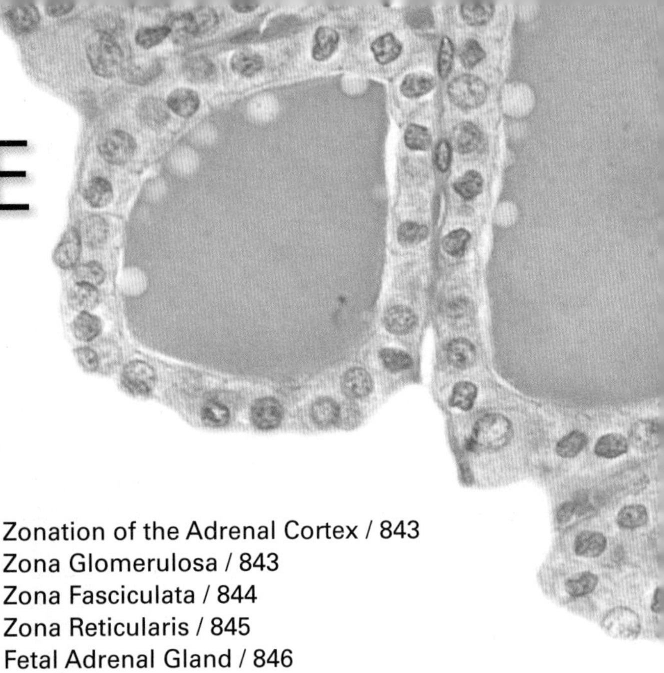

■ OVERVIEW OF THE ENDOCRINE SYSTEM

The **endocrine system** produces various secretions called **hormones** *[Gr. hormaein, to excite, to set in motion]* that serve as effectors to regulate the activities of various cells, tissues, and organs in the body. Its functions are essential in maintaining homeostasis and coordinating body growth and development and are similar to that of the **nervous system**: Both communicate information to peripheral cells and organs. Communication in the nervous system is through transmission of neural impulses along nerve cell processes and the discharge of neurotransmitter. Communication in the endocrine system is through hormones, which are carried to their destination via connective tissue spaces and the vascular system. These two systems are functionally interrelated. The endocrine system produces a slower and more prolonged response than the nervous system. Both systems may act simultaneously on the same target cells and tissues, and some nerve cells secrete hormones.

Endocrine glands possess no excretory ducts, and their secretions are carried to specific destinations via the extracellular matrix of connective tissue and the vascular system.

In general, **endocrine glands** are aggregates of **epithelioid cells** (epithelial cells that lack a free surface) that are embedded within connective tissue. Despite the fact that the endocrine glands vary in size, shape, and location in the body (Fig. 21.1), they still have several common characteristics. Endocrine glands do not possess excretory ducts; therefore, their secretion is discharged into the extracellular matrix of connective tissue, usually near the capillaries. From here, the secretory products (i.e., hormones) are transported into the lumen of the blood (or lymphatic) vessels for body-wide distribution. These secretory products influence target organs or tissues at some distance from the gland. For this reason, endocrine glands are well vascularized and surrounded by rich vascular networks. The exception is the placenta, where

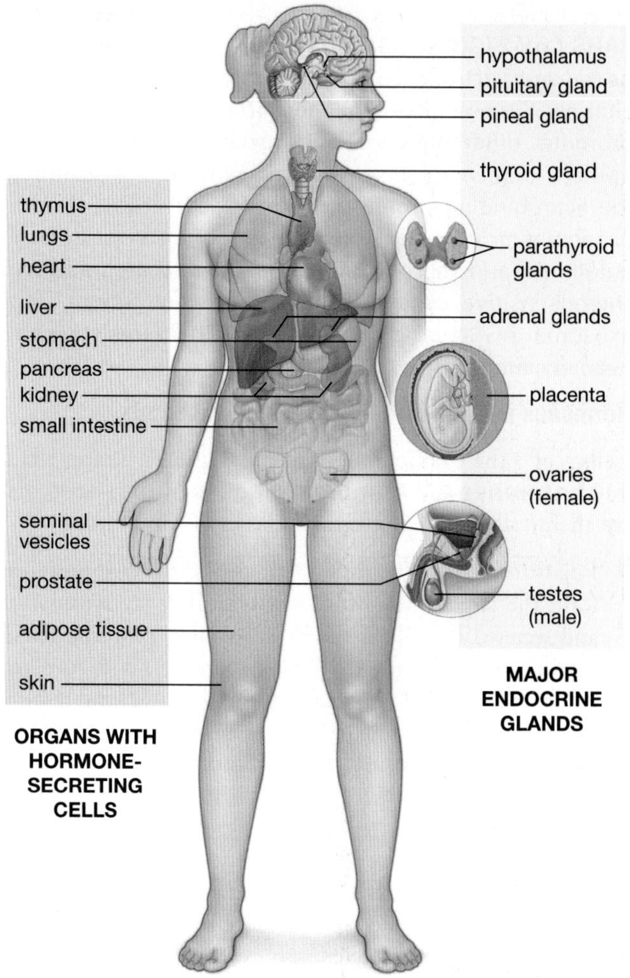

FIGURE 21.1. Location of the major endocrine glands and organs containing hormone-secreting cells. This drawing shows the major endocrine glands in which the hormone-secreting cells constitute the majority of the gland parenchyma. Note that the placenta is a temporary organ developed from maternal and fetal tissues and is also a major endocrine organ that secretes steroid and protein hormones during pregnancy (see Chapter 23, Female Reproductive System, pages 933-938). Hormone-secreting cells, commonly classified as part of the diffuse neuroendocrine system (DNES), are present in many organs to regulate their activity. In addition, adipose tissue is an important hormonally active tissue that secrets a variety of hormones, growth factors, and cytokines, collectively called *adipokines* (see Chapter 9, Adipose Tissue, page 280).

hormones produced by the syncytiotrophoblast pass directly into the maternal blood surrounding the placental villi (see Chapter 23, Female Reproductive System, page 937).

As mentioned earlier, the majority of hormone-producing cells have an **epithelial origin**, either from the **central nervous system (CNS)** (i.e., posterior lobe of pituitary gland, pineal gland), **neural crest** (i.e., medulla of suprarenal gland), or from epithelial lining of the developing **gut tube** (i.e., anterior lobe of pituitary gland, thyroid and parathyroid glands). Only a few endocrine glands/cells have a mesenchymal origin and are derived from the **urogenital ridges** (i.e., cortex of the adrenal gland, Leydig cells in the testis, and steroid-secreting cells of developing follicles in the ovary).

This chapter primarily describes the major **endocrine glands** in which the hormone-secreting cells constitute the majority of the gland parenchyma. Secretory cells in the gland parenchyma form various arrangements, such as follicles (thyroid gland), anastomosing cords (adrenal glands), or nests (parathyroid glands). They are also present in clusters (nuclei in the hypothalamus) or layers surrounding the functional and structural elements of the organ (testis, ovaries, or placenta). These characteristics are useful in the microscopic identification of specific endocrine organs.

Individual hormone-secreting cells are present in many organs to regulate their activity.

The collection of **individual endocrine cells** in various organs constitutes the **diffuse neuroendocrine system (DNES**; see page 644). In addition to their endocrine function, cells of the DNES system exercise autocrine and paracrine control of the activity of their own and adjacent epithelial cells by diffusion of peptide secretions. Other chapters discuss the endocrine function of adipose tissue and individual cells within the liver, pancreas, kidney, and the gastrointestinal, cardiovascular, respiratory, reproductive, lymphatic, and integumentary systems (see Fig. 21.1).

Hormones and Their Receptors

In general, a hormone is described as a biological substance acting on specific target cells.

In the classic definition, a **hormone** is a secretory product of endocrine cells and organs that passes into the circulatory system (bloodstream) for transport to target cells. For many years, this **endocrine control** of target tissues became a central part of endocrinology. However, a variety of hormones and hormonally active substances are not always discharged into the bloodstream but are released into connective tissue spaces. They may act on adjacent cells or diffuse to nearby target cells that express specific receptors for that particular hormone (Fig. 21.2). This type of hormonal action is referred to as **paracrine control**. In addition, some cells express receptors for hormones that they secrete. This type of hormonal action is referred to as **autocrine control**. These hormones regulate the cell's own activity. Figure 21.2 summarizes various hormonal control mechanisms.

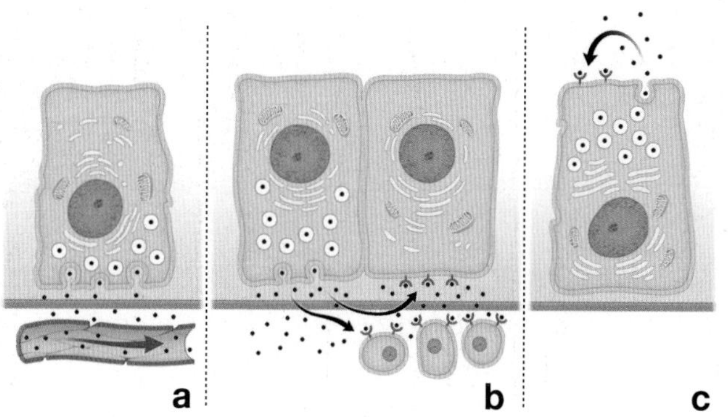

FIGURE 21.2. Hormonal control mechanisms. This schematic diagram shows three basic types of control mechanisms. **a.** In endocrine control, the hormone is discharged from a cell into the bloodstream and is transported to the effector cells. **b.** In paracrine control, the hormone is secreted from one cell and acts on adjacent cells that express specific receptors. **c.** In autocrine control, the hormone responds to the receptors located on the cell that produces it.

New research characterizes exosomes as important components of the endocrine system that provide endocrine, paracrine, and autocrine signals to target cells in the body.

Research over the past decade indicates that in addition to the nervous and endocrine systems, a third system of intercellular or interorgan communication exists that involves **exosomes**. As discussed in Chapter 2, Cell Cytoplasm (pages 47-48), exosomes are small, membrane-bound **cargo vesicles** secreted into the extracellular space by virtually every cell in the body. They are released and detected in all bodily fluids, including blood, lymph, cerebrospinal fluid, vitreous body, interstitial fluids, saliva, breast milk, amniotic fluid, semen, and urine. Most secreted exosomes are disseminated via blood circulation and travel to specific targets in the body. They transfer **messages** and **cargo molecules** from the original (parent) cells to the target destination. The exosomes and their cargo molecules either fuse directly with the plasma membrane of target cells, become endocytosed, or engage in receptor–ligand-mediated interactions (Fig. 21.3). Exosomes can carry a variety of molecules that include **growth factors; lipids; proteins; several forms of DNA molecules**, such as viral DNA (vDNA), mitochondrial DNA (mtDNA), and fragments of double-stranded DNA (dsDNA) or single-stranded DNA (ssDNA); and **several types of RNA molecules**, such as messenger RNA (mRNA), transfer RNA (tRNA), small nuclear RNA (snRNA), small nucleolar RNA (snoRNA), mitochondrial RNA (mtRNA), microRNA (miRNA), viral microRNA (vmiRNA), circular RNA (CircRNA), small noncoding RNA (Y-RNA), toxic small RNA (tsRNA), Piwi-interacting RNA (piRNA), and others. For details on exosomal contents, see Figure 2.21 (page 47).

In disease states, exosomes also carry **viruses** such as **SARS-CoV-2 (COVID-19)** and **HIV-1 (AIDS)**. Their cargo can be transmitted from cell to cell (often in distant locations) to alter cells' metabolism, influence immune cell responses, promote differentiation, and facilitate disease development (e.g., viral diseases and cancer). For example, the actin-binding protein **gelsolin** (pGSN) transported in exosomes promotes ovarian cancer cell survival through autocrine and paracrine mechanisms that transform chemosensitive cancer cells into resistant forms. Thus, exosomal pGSN is a determinant of **chemoresistance** in **ovarian cancer**.

Hormones include three classes of compounds.

Cells of the endocrine system release more than **100 hormones** and **hormonally active substances** that are chemically divided into three classes of compounds:

- **Peptides** (small peptides, polypeptides, and proteins) form the largest group of hormones. They are synthesized and secreted by cells of the hypothalamus, pituitary gland, thyroid gland, parathyroid gland, pancreas, and scattered enteroendocrine cells of the gastrointestinal tract and respiratory system. This group of hormones (**insulin, glucagon, growth hormone [GH], adrenocorticotropic hormone [ACTH], follicle-stimulating hormone [FSH], luteinizing hormone [LH], antidiuretic hormone [ADH], oxytocin, interleukins**, and **various growth factors**), when released into the circulation, dissolve readily in the blood and generally do not require special transport proteins. However, most, if not all, polypeptides and proteins have specific carrier proteins (e.g., **insulin-like growth factor–binding protein [IGFBP]**).

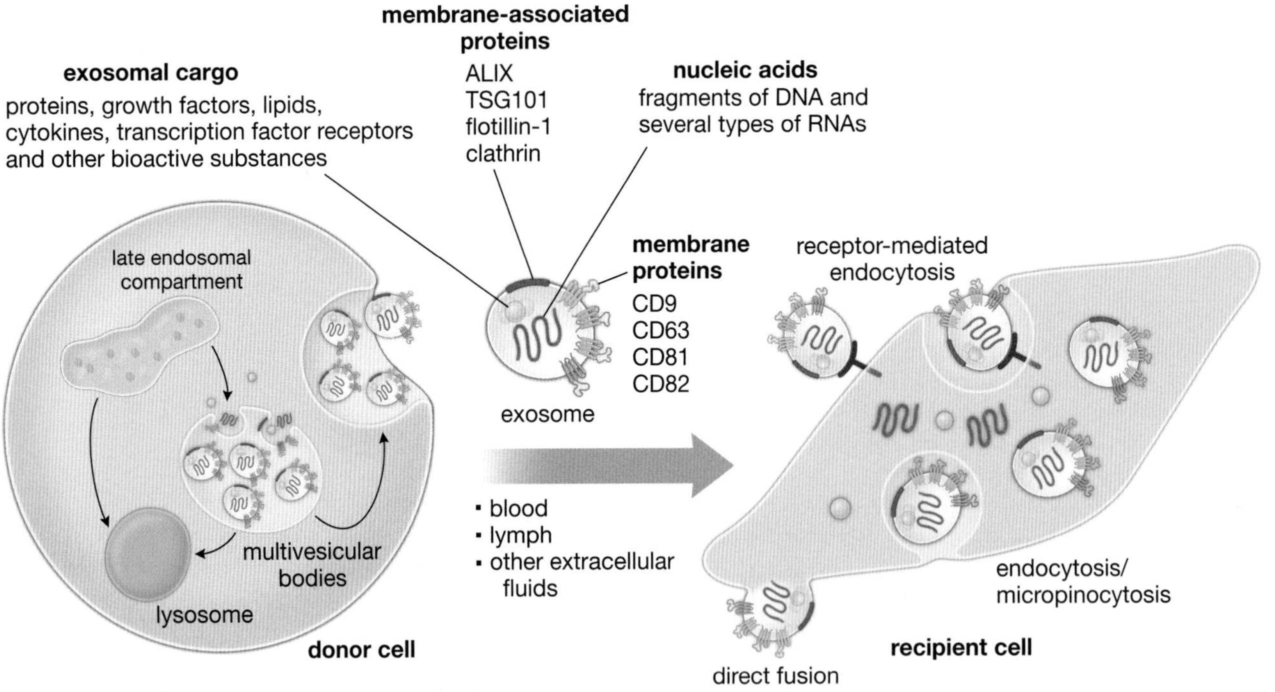

FIGURE 21.3. Exosomal intercellular signaling. This drawing summarizes exosomal signaling, an intercellular communication pathway in which proteins, metabolites, and nucleic acids are delivered to recipient cells using exosomes as transfer vehicles. Exosomes are very small, membrane-bound cargo vesicles derived from multivesicular bodies (MVB) and secreted into the extracellular space. Most exosomes use the blood circulation to reach specific target cells in the body. Exosomes transfer messages in the form of cargo molecules, membrane-associated proteins, and nucleic acids from donor cells to the target destination. Exosomes and their cargo molecules either fuse directly with the plasma membrane of target cells, become endocytosed, or engage in receptor–ligand-mediated interactions. Exosomes then release their contents directly into the cytoplasm of the recipient cell, initiating downstream signaling cascades. Note specific transmembrane proteins (tetraspanins) that serve as exosomal biomarkers.

- **Steroids**, cholesterol-derived compounds, are synthesized and secreted by cells of the ovaries, testes, and adrenal cortex. These hormones (**gonadal** and **adrenocortical steroids**) are released into the bloodstream and transported to target cells with the help of plasma proteins or specialized carrier proteins, such as **androgen-binding protein**. Hormone-binding carrier proteins protect the hormone from degradation during transport to the target tissue. When needed, the hormone is released from the carrier protein to become active.
- **Amino acids** and **arachidonic acid analogs** and their derivatives, including the **catecholamines** (norepinephrine and epinephrine–phenylalanine/tyrosine derivatives) and **prostaglandins**, **prostacyclins**, and **leukotrienes** (arachidonic acid derivatives), are synthesized and secreted by many neurons as well as a variety of cells, including cells of the adrenal medulla. Also included in this group of compounds are **thyroid hormones**, the iodinated derivatives of the amino acid tyrosine that are synthesized and secreted by the thyroid gland. When released into the circulation, catecholamines dissolve readily in the blood, in contrast to thyroid hormones, the majority of which are bound to three carrier proteins: a specialized **thyroxine-binding globulin (TBG)**, prealbumin fraction of serum proteins (**transthyretin**), and a nonspecific fraction of albumins.

Hormones interact with specific hormone receptors to alter biological activity of the target cells.

The first step in hormone action on a target cell is its binding to a **specific hormone receptor**. However, recent studies suggest that some hormones are involved in non–receptor-mediated responses. Hormones interact with their receptors exposed on the surface of the target cell or within its cytoplasm or nucleus. In general, two groups of hormone receptors have been identified:

- **Cell surface receptors** interact with peptide hormones or catecholamines that are unable to penetrate the cell membrane. Activation of these receptors as a result of hormone binding rapidly generates large quantities of small intracellular molecules called **second messengers** (Fig. 21.4a). These molecules amplify the signal initiated by hormone–receptor interaction and are produced by activation of membrane-associated **G-proteins** (named for the ability to hydrolyze guanosine triphosphate [GTP]). Examples of such systems include the **adenylate cyclase/cyclic adenosine monophosphate (cAMP) system** (for most protein hormones and catecholamines), the **guanylyl cyclase/cyclic guanosine monophosphate (cGMP) system** (an antagonistic system for action of cAMP in some protein hormones), the **tyrosine kinase system**

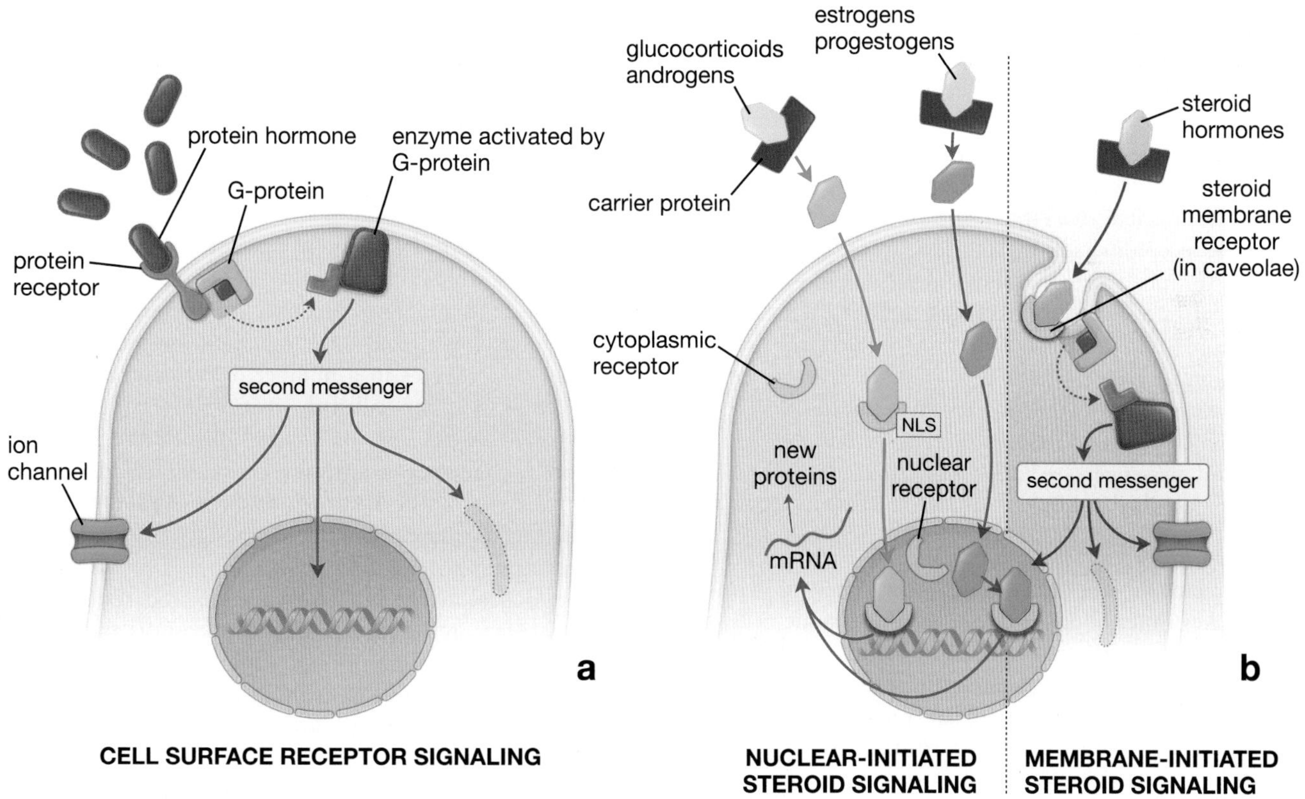

FIGURE 21.4. General mechanisms of protein and steroid hormone actions. a. This schematic diagram shows the basis for protein hormone action involving cell surface receptors. Hormone molecules bind to the cell surface receptors (*orange glow* indicates activated receptor) and initiate a cascade of intracellular signaling reactions that may include G-protein and various protein kinases resulting in the synthesis of second messenger molecules. These molecules, in turn, elicit hormone-specific responses in the stimulated cell that may influence channel proteins, nuclear transcription, and protein synthesis or degradation. **b.** This diagram shows two mechanisms of action for steroid hormones, which include nuclear-initiated steroid signaling (involves intracellular receptors) and membrane-initiated steroid signaling. In the nuclear-initiated steroid signaling (*green arrows*), some steroid hormones (e.g., glucocorticoids, androgens) cross the plasma membrane and bind to specific cytoplasmic receptors. This binding of the hormone causes allosteric transformation of the receptor, and the resulting complex travels to the nucleus guided by the nuclear localization signal (*NLS*), where it binds to DNA and regulates the transcription of specific genes (*orange glow*). Other steroid hormones (e.g., estrogens, progestogens) bind to their specific receptors directly in the nucleus (*blue arrows*). This binding of hormone to the nuclear receptor transforms this complex into the DNA transcription factor (*orange glow*) and leads to mRNA transcription and the subsequent production of new proteins responsible for hormone-specific responses of the stimulated cell. In membrane-initiated steroid signaling (*red arrows*), the steroid receptors are expressed on the cell membrane, usually in the caveolae, and their pathway is similar to that of the cell surface receptor signaling mechanism.

(for insulin and epidermal growth factor [EGF]), the **phosphatidylinositol system** (for certain hormones such as oxytocin, gonadotropin-releasing hormone [GnRH], angiotensin II, and neurotransmitters such as epinephrine), and **activation of ion channels** (as with most neurotransmitters). The majority of second messenger molecules exert a stimulatory function on cell metabolism. Examples of second messenger molecules include **cAMP**, **1,2-diacylglycerol (DAG)**, **inositol 1,4,5-triphosphate (IP_3)**, and **Ca^{2+}**. An inhibitory response is mainly achieved by **cGMP**, which interferes with the production of cAMP. The second messenger molecules produced in the cascade reactions of these systems alter the cell's metabolism and produce hormone-specific responses (see Fig. 21.4a).

- **Intracellular receptors**, which are localized within the cell, are used by **steroid hormones**, **thyroid hormones**, and **vitamins A and D** (Fig. 21.4b). Steroid hormones and vitamins A and D can easily penetrate both plasma and nuclear membranes. In the absence of hormone, steroid receptors for glucocorticoids and gonadocorticoids (adrenal androgens) reside in the cytoplasm, whereas estrogen and progesterone receptors are located in the nucleus. Unoccupied inactive receptors for thyroid hormones and vitamins A and D also reside in the nucleus. Intracellular receptors consist of large multiprotein complexes containing three binding domains: a hormone- or ligand-binding region at the COOH-terminus, a DNA-binding region, and the NH_2-terminus containing the gene regulatory region. Because the receptor–ligand complex must enter the nucleus to regulate transcription, intracellular receptors contain a nuclear localization signal (NLS) for trafficking into the nucleus (see Fig. 21.4b). Binding of the hormone to the receptor causes the allosteric transformation of the receptor into a form that binds to the chromosomal DNA and activates **RNA polymerase activity**. This, in turn, increases transcription of mRNA, resulting in the production of new proteins that regulate cell metabolism. Therefore, hormones acting on the intracellular receptors influence gene expression directly, without the help of a second messenger (see Fig. 21.4b). This type of signaling is often described as **nuclear-initiated steroid signaling**.

Action of steroid hormones on the cell's genome to induce a biological response in the form of new protein synthesis takes time (hours or days). However, some cells react more rapidly (in seconds or minutes) to steroid hormone stimulation by increasing intracellular Ca^+ concentration and activating several intracellular proteins. This finding led to the discovery of **steroid membrane receptors**, which have a similar structure to intracellular receptors but are localized on the plasma membrane most often within the caveolae. Binding to steroid membrane receptors activates the signaling cascade of G-protein, which, in turn, activates protein kinases, causing a rapid change in cell activity (see Fig. 21.4b). This type of signaling is known as **membrane-initiated steroid signaling**. Both nuclear- and membrane-initiated steroid signaling pathways converge to provide a full biological response of the target cell to the steroid hormone stimulation.

Regulation of Hormone Secretion and Feedback Mechanism

Regulation of hormonal function is controlled by feedback mechanisms.

Hormonal production is often controlled through **feedback mechanisms** from the target organ. In general, feedback occurs when the response to a stimulus (action of a hormone) has an effect on the original stimulus (hormone-secreting cell). The nature of this response determines the type of feedback. Two types of feedback are recognized: **Negative feedback** occurs when the response diminishes the original stimulus and is much more common than **positive feedback**, which occurs when the response enhances the original stimulus.

To better understand the function of feedback mechanisms, one can point to an air conditioning system, which also uses a simple negative feedback system. When the compressor produces enough cold air to lower the temperature below the set point of the thermostat, the thermostat is triggered and shuts off the compressor. In this negative feedback system, the lower temperature is then fed back to the compressor and diminishes its response (it shuts off its production of cold air). When the temperature rises back above the set point, the negative feedback is abolished and the compressor comes back on (for more information on negative feedback, see Folder 21.1).

Activities of hormones are constantly monitored on many levels, beginning with molecular biosynthetic processes to the final end points of hormonal action. Several examples of feedback mechanisms are discussed in the sections on the pituitary, hypothalamus, and thyroid glands.

■ PITUITARY GLAND (HYPOPHYSIS)

The **pituitary gland** and the **hypothalamus**, the portion of the brain to which the pituitary gland is attached, are morphologically and functionally linked in the endocrine and neuroendocrine control of other endocrine glands. Because they play central roles in a number of regulatory feedback systems, they are often called the *master organs* of the endocrine system. In the past, the control of pituitary hormone secretion by the hypothalamus was classically regarded as the major function of the **neuroendocrine system**. However, the field of neuroendocrinology today has expanded to encompass multiple reciprocal interactions between the CNS, autonomic nervous system (ANS), endocrine system, and immune system in the regulation of homeostasis and behavioral responses to environmental stimuli. For example, the neuroendocrine axis's role in maintaining energy homeostasis is discussed in Chapter 9, Adipose Tissue (pages 283-285).

Gross Structure and Development

The pituitary gland is composed of glandular epithelial tissue and neural (secretory) tissue.

The **pituitary gland** *[Lat. pituta, phlegm—reflecting its nasopharyngeal origin]* is a pea-sized, compound endocrine gland that weighs 0.5 g in males and 1.5 g in multiparous women (i.e., a woman who has given birth ≥2 times). It is centrally located at the base of the brain, where it lies in a saddle-shaped depression of the sphenoid bone called the **sella turcica**.

FOLDER 21.1

FUNCTIONAL CONSIDERATIONS: REGULATION OF PITUITARY GLAND SECRETION

The **release of hormones from the anterior lobe of the pituitary gland** is carefully regulated by three tiers of control mechanisms that include the following:

- **Tier I: Hypothalamic secretion of hypothalamic-regulating hormones.** The pituitary gland is under significant control by the hypothalamus, which regulates the release of hypothalamic-regulating hormones into the hypophyseal portal veins. The hypothalamic-regulating hormones are produced by the cells of the hypothalamus in response to circulating levels of systemic hormones and impulses from the central nervous system (CNS). These hormones act directly on the highly specific G-protein–linked receptors on the plasma membranes of cells residing in the anterior lobe of the pituitary gland. Activation of receptors elicits positive or negative signals that affect gene transcription and lead to stimulation or inhibition of pituitary hormone secretion. Most of the tropic hormones produced by the anterior lobe of the pituitary gland are regulated by polypeptide-releasing hormones, with the notable exception of dopamine. Prolactin (PRL) production is primarily regulated by the inhibitory effect of dopamine (i.e., PRL secretion is tonically inhibited by the release of dopamine from the hypothalamus).
- **Tier II: Paracrine and autocrine secretions of the pituitary cells.** Release of hormones from the pituitary gland is also regulated by soluble growth factors and cytokines produced by the cells residing in the pituitary gland.
- **Tier III: Feedback effect of circulating hormones.** The level of hormones in the systemic circulation regulates the secretion of cells in the anterior lobe of the pituitary gland. This is primarily achieved by negative feedback regulation of hormones secreted by the pituitary gland by target hormones. For instance, secretion of thyroid-stimulating hormone (TSH) is inhibited by thyroid hormones produced in the thyroid gland under TSH influence.

To better understand the mechanism of negative regulation, consider a simple **negative feedback system** that controls the synthesis and discharge of T_3 and T_4 thyroid hormones (see Fig. 21.18). The secretion of thyroid hormones is controlled by the release of TSH from the anterior lobe of the pituitary gland into the bloodstream. If blood levels of T_3 and T_4 are high, TRH is not produced or released. If blood levels of T_3 and T_4 are low, the hypothalamus discharges TRH into the hypothalamohypophyseal portal system. Release of TRH stimulates specific cells within the anterior lobe of the pituitary gland to produce TSH, which, in turn, stimulates the thyroid to produce and release more thyroid hormones. As the thyroid hormone levels rise, the negative feedback system stops the hypothalamus from discharging thyrotropin-releasing hormone (TRH). Using the same mechanism of negative feedback regulation, thyroid hormones also act on the thyrotropes in the anterior lobe of the pituitary gland to inhibit their secretion of TSH.

A short stalk, the **infundibulum**, and a vascular network connect the pituitary gland to the hypothalamus.

The pituitary gland has two functional components (Fig. 21.5):

- **Anterior lobe (adenohypophysis)**, the glandular epithelial tissue
- **Posterior lobe (neurohypophysis)**, the neural secretory tissue

These two portions are of different embryologic origin. The anterior lobe of the pituitary gland is derived from an evagination of the **ectoderm of the oropharynx** toward the brain **(Rathke pouch)**. The posterior lobe of the pituitary gland is derived from a downgrowth (the future infundibulum) of **neuroectoderm of the floor of the third ventricle** (the diencephalon) of the developing brain (Fig. 21.6).

The **anterior lobe of the pituitary gland** consists of three derivatives of the Rathke pouch:

- **Pars distalis**, which comprises the bulk of the anterior lobe of the pituitary gland and arises from the thickened anterior wall of the pouch
- **Pars intermedia**, a thin remnant of the posterior wall of the pouch that abuts the pars distalis
- **Pars tuberalis**, which develops from the thickened lateral walls of the pouch and forms a collar or sheath around the infundibulum

The embryonic infundibulum gives rise to the posterior lobe of the pituitary gland. The **posterior lobe of the pituitary gland** consists of the following:

- **Pars nervosa**, which contains neurosecretory axons and their endings
- **Infundibulum**, which is continuous with the **median eminence** and contains the neurosecretory axons forming the **hypothalamohypophyseal tracts** (see Fig. 21.5)

Blood Supply

Knowledge of the unusual blood supply of the pituitary gland is important to understanding its functions. The pituitary blood supply is derived from two sets of vessels (Fig. 21.7):

- **Superior hypophyseal arteries** supply the pars tuberalis, median eminence, and infundibulum. These vessels arise from the internal carotid arteries and posterior communicating artery of the circle of Willis.
- **Inferior hypophyseal arteries** primarily supply the pars nervosa. These vessels arise solely from the internal carotid arteries. An important functional observation is that most of the anterior lobe of the pituitary gland has no direct arterial supply.

The hypothalamohypophyseal portal system provides the crucial link between the hypothalamus and the pituitary gland.

The arteries that supply the pars tuberalis, median eminence, and infundibulum give rise to fenestrated capillaries (the primary capillary plexus). These capillaries drain into portal veins, called the **hypophyseal portal veins**, which run along the pars tuberalis and give rise to a second fenestrated sinusoidal capillary network (the secondary capillary plexus).

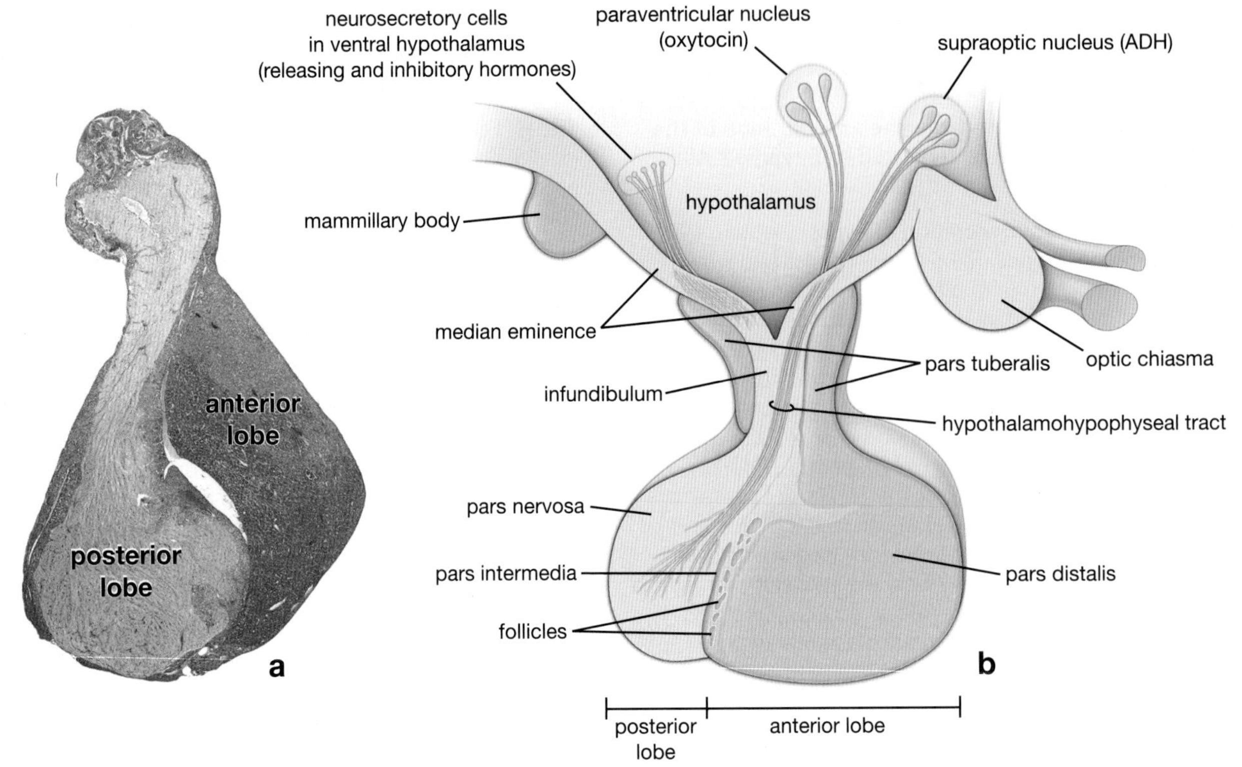

FIGURE 21.5. Pituitary gland. a. Photomicrograph of a pituitary gland. Lobes of the pituitary gland can be identified on the basis of their appearance, location, and relation to each other. ×7. **b.** This drawing shows parts of the pituitary gland and related regions of the hypothalamus. The anterior lobe of the pituitary gland consists of the pars distalis, pars tuberalis, and pars intermedia; the posterior lobe consists of the infundibulum and pars nervosa. Note the distribution of the neurosecretory nuclei in the hypothalamus. The paraventricular nuclei produce oxytocin, and the supraoptic nuclei produce antidiuretic hormone (*ADH*). These hormones are released in the pars nervosa of the posterior lobe. Neurosecretory cells in the ventral nuclei of the hypothalamus secrete releasing and inhibitory hormones that are discharged into capillaries (located in the median eminence and infundibulum) of the hypophyseal portal system to reach pars distalis of the anterior lobe.

This system of vessels carries the neuroendocrine secretions of hypothalamic neurons from their sites of release in the median eminence and infundibulum directly to the cells of the pars distalis.

Most of the blood from the pituitary gland drains into the cavernous sinus at the base of the diencephalon and then into the systemic circulation. Some evidence suggests, however, that blood can flow via short portal veins from the pars distalis to the pars nervosa and that blood from the pars nervosa may flow toward the hypothalamus. These short pathways provide a route by which the hormones of the anterior lobe of the pituitary gland could provide feedback directly to the brain without making the full circuit of the systemic circulation.

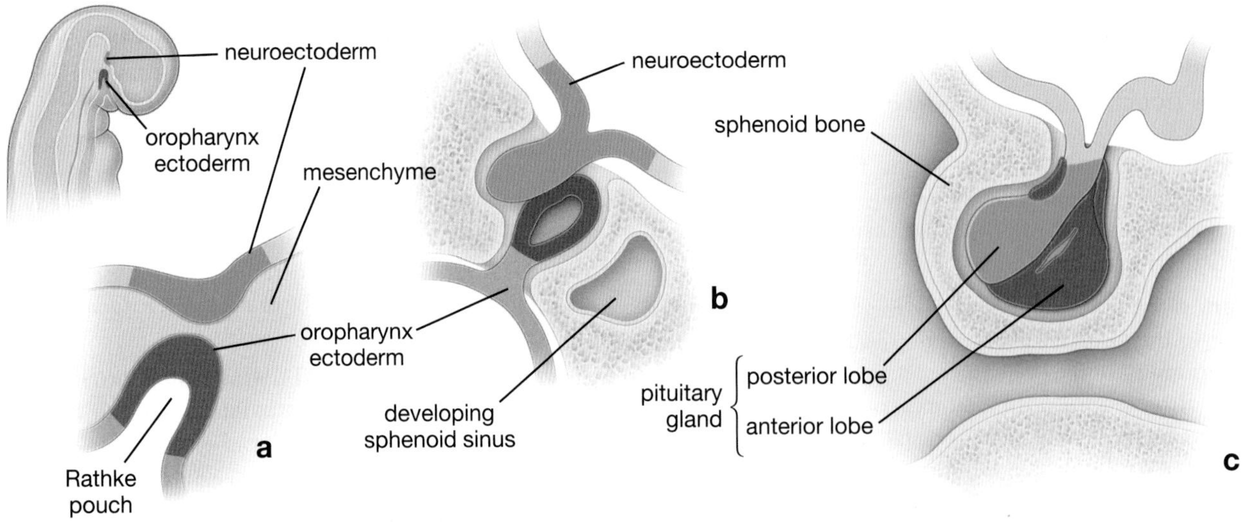

FIGURE 21.6. Development of the pituitary gland. a. The pituitary gland develops from two different structures: an ectodermal diverticulum of the roof of the oropharynx (Rathke pouch) and a downward extension of the neuroectoderm at the floor of diencephalon. This drawing shows the relationship between these two structures in a 6-week-old embryo. **b.** The pituitary gland at 10 weeks of development shows ectodermal tissue from the oropharynx in close proximity to neural tissue. The Rathke pouch is about to lose connection with the oropharynx. **c.** Cells from the Rathke pouch divide and differentiate rapidly into the pars distalis and encircle the infundibulum, which with pars nervosa forms the neuroectodermally derived posterior lobe of the pituitary gland.

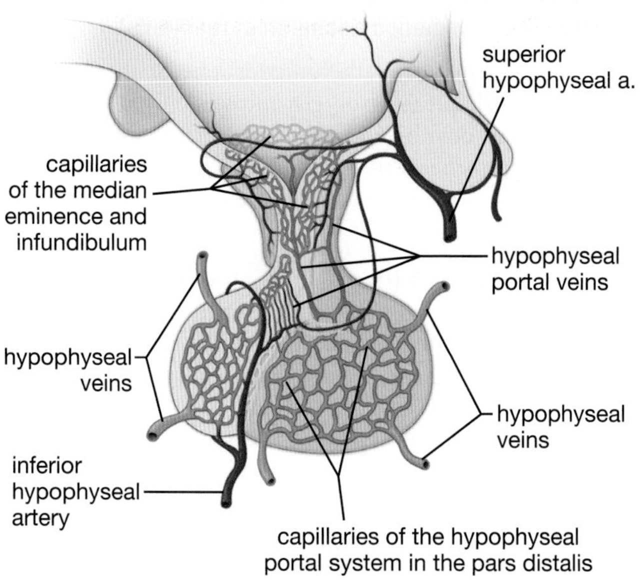

FIGURE 21.7. Diagram of the blood supply and hypothalamohypophyseal portal system of the pituitary gland. The superior and inferior hypophyseal arteries originate from branches of the internal carotid arteries. The superior hypophyseal artery supplies the pars tuberalis, median eminence, and infundibulum of the hypothalamus, where it gives rise to a capillary network that drains into the hypophyseal portal veins. These veins give rise to a second capillary network in the pars distalis, where the neuroendocrine secretions produced in the hypothalamus and collected in the median eminence and infundibulum are released. The inferior hypophyseal artery provides the blood supply to the pars nervosa and has very few (if any) connections with the hypothalamohypophyseal portal system. The blood from the pituitary gland drains into the cavernous sinus and leaves the cranial cavity via the internal jugular veins.

Nerve Supply

The nerves that enter the infundibulum and pars nervosa from the hypothalamic nuclei are components of the posterior lobe of the pituitary gland (see the section that follows on the posterior lobe). The nerves that enter the anterior lobe of the pituitary gland are postsynaptic fibers of the ANS and have vasomotor function.

Anterior Lobe of the Pituitary Gland (Adenohypophysis)

The anterior lobe of the pituitary gland regulates other endocrine glands and some nonendocrine tissues.

Most of the **anterior lobe of the pituitary gland** has the typical organization of endocrine tissue. The cells are organized in clumps and cords separated by fenestrated sinusoidal capillaries of relatively large diameter. These cells respond to signals from the hypothalamus and synthesize and secrete a number of pituitary hormones. Four hormones of the anterior lobe—**adrenocorticotropic hormone (ACTH)**, **thyroid-stimulating (thyrotropic) hormone (TSH; thyrotropin)**, **follicle-stimulating hormone (FSH)**, and **luteinizing hormone (LH)**—are called **tropic hormones** because they regulate the activity of cells in other endocrine glands throughout the body. The two remaining hormones of the anterior lobe, **growth hormone (GH)** and **prolactin (PRL)**, are not considered tropic because they act directly on target organs that are not endocrine. The general character and effects of the pituitary hormones of the anterior lobe are summarized in Table 21.1.

Pars distalis

The cells within the pars distalis vary in size, shape, and staining properties.

The cells within the **pars distalis** are arranged in cords and nests with interweaving capillaries. Early descriptions of the cells within the pars distalis were based solely on the staining properties of secretory vesicles within the cells. Using mixtures of acidic and basic dyes (Fig. 21.8), histologists

TABLE 21.1 Hormones of the Anterior Lobe of the Pituitary Gland

Hormone	Composition	MW (kDa)	Major Functions
Growth hormone (somatotropin, GH)	Straight-chain protein (191 aa)	21,700	Stimulates liver and other organs to synthesize and secrete insulin-like growth factor I (IGF-I), which, in turn, stimulates division of progenitor cells located in growth plates and skeletal muscles, resulting in body growth
Prolactin (PRL)	Straight-chain protein (198 aa)	22,500	Promotes mammary gland development; initiates milk formation; stimulates and maintains secretion of casein, lactalbumin, lipids, and carbohydrates into the milk
Adrenocorticotropic hormone (ACTH)	Small polypeptide (39 aa)	4,000	Maintains structure and stimulates secretion of glucocorticoids and gonadocorticoids (adrenal androgens) by the zona fasciculata and zona reticularis of the adrenal cortex
Follicle-stimulating hormone (FSH)	2-chain glycoprotein[a] (α, 92 aa; β, 111 aa)	28,000	Stimulates follicular development in the ovary and spermatogenesis in the testis
Luteinizing hormone (LH)	2-chain glycoprotein[a] (α, 92 aa; β, 116 aa)	28,300	Regulates final maturation of ovarian follicle, ovulation, and corpus luteum formation; stimulates steroid secretion by follicle and corpus luteum; in males, essential for maintenance of and androgen secretion by the Leydig (interstitial) cells of the testis
Thyroid-stimulating hormone (TSH)	2-chain glycoprotein[a] (α, 92 aa; β, 112 aa)	28,000	Stimulates growth of thyroid epithelial cells; stimulates production and release of thyroglobulin and thyroid hormones

aa, amino acids.

[a]The α-chains of FSH, LH, and TSH are identical and encoded by a single gene; the β-chains are specific for each hormone.

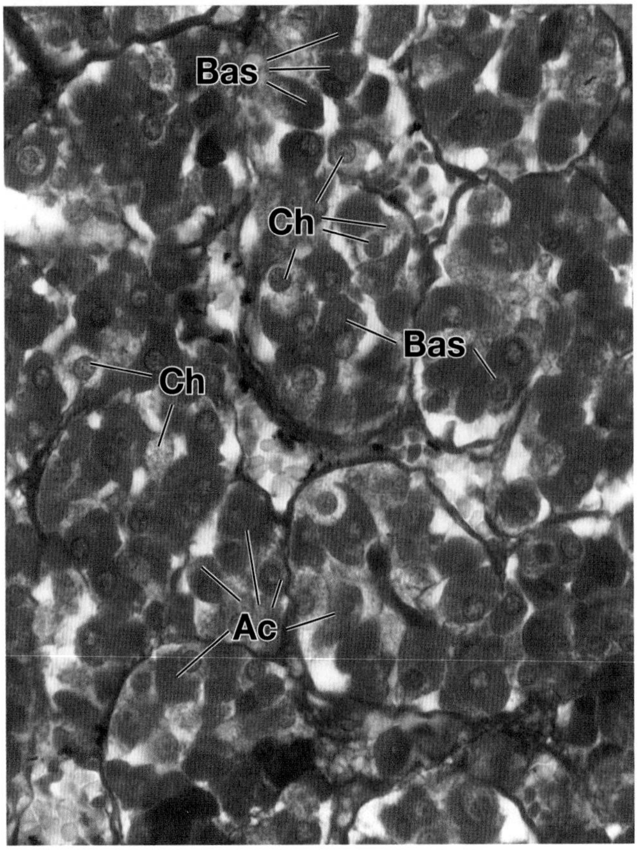

FIGURE 21.8. Pars distalis. This specimen of the pars distalis is stained with brilliant crystal scarlet, aniline blue, and Martius yellow to distinguish the various cell types and connective tissue stroma. The cords of cells are surrounded by a delicate connective tissue stroma stained *blue*. The sinusoidal capillaries are seen in close association with the parenchyma and contain erythrocytes stained *yellow*. In the region shown here, the acidophils (*Ac*) are the most numerous cell type present. Their cytoplasm stains *cherry red*. The basophils (*Bas*) stain *blue*. The chromophobes (*Ch*), although few in number in this particular region, are virtually unstained. ×640.

identified three types of cells according to their staining reaction, namely, **basophils (10%)**, **acidophils (40%)**, and **chromophobes (50%)**. However, this classification provides no information regarding the hormonal secretory activity or functional role of these cells.

Five functional cell types are identified in the pars distalis on the basis of immunocytochemical reactions.

All known hormones of the anterior lobe of the pituitary gland are small proteins or glycoproteins. This important fact has led to definitive identification of specific cell types by immunocytochemistry (Table 21.2). These studies have classified cells of the anterior lobe of the pituitary gland into five cell types:

- **Somatotropes (GH cells)** are most commonly found within the pars distalis and constitute approximately 50% of the parenchymal cells in the anterior lobe of the pituitary gland. These medium-sized, oval cells exhibit round, centrally located nuclei and produce **growth hormone (GH; somatotropin)**. The presence of eosinophilic vesicles in their cytoplasm classifies them as acidophils. Three hormones regulate the release of GH from somatotropes. Two of these hormones are opposing hypothalamic-releasing hormones: **growth hormone–releasing hormone (GHRH)**, which stimulates GH release from the somatotropes, and **somatostatin**, which inhibits GH release from the somatotropes. A third hormone, a 28-amino-acid peptide called **ghrelin**, was isolated from the stomach in 1999. It is a potent stimulator of GH secretion and appears to coordinate food intake with GH secretion. Hormonally active tumors that originate from somatotropes are associated with hypersecretion of GH and cause gigantism in children and acromegaly in adults.
- **Lactotropes (PRL cells, mammotropes)** constitute 15%–20% of the parenchymal cells in the anterior lobe of the pituitary gland. These are large, polygonal cells with oval nuclei. They produce **prolactin (PRL)**. In their storage phase, lactotropes exhibit numerous acidophilic vesicles (the histologic feature of an acidophil). When the contents of these vesicles are released, the cytoplasm of the lactotrope does not stain (the histologic feature of a chromophobe). Secretion of PRL is under inhibitory control by **dopamine**, the catecholamine produced by the hypothalamus. However, **thyrotropin-releasing hormone (TRH)** and **vasoactive inhibitory peptide (VIP)** are known to

TABLE 21.2 Staining Characteristics of Cells Found in the Anterior Lobe of the Pituitary Gland

Cell Type	Percentage of Total Cells	General Staining	Specific Staining	Product
Somatotrope (GH cell)	50	Acidophil	Orange G (PAS−)	Growth hormone (GH)
Lactotrope (PRL cell)	15–20	Acidophil	Orange G (PAS−) Herlant erythrosine Brooke carmoisine	Prolactin (PRL)
Corticotrope (ACTH cell)	15–20	Basophil	Lead hematoxylin (PAS+)	Proopiomelanocortin (POMC), which is cleaved in humans into adrenocorticotropic hormone (ACTH) and β-lipotropic hormone (β-LPH)
Gonadotrope (FSH and LH cells)	10	Basophil	Aldehyde-fuchsin Aldehyde-thionine (PAS+)	Follicle-stimulating hormone (FSH) and luteinizing hormone (LH)
Thyrotrope (TSH cell)	~5	Basophil	Aldehyde-fuchsin Aldehyde-thionine (PAS+)	Thyroid-stimulating hormone (TSH)

PAS, periodic acid–Schiff.

stimulate the synthesis and secretion of PRL. During pregnancy and lactation, these cells undergo hypertrophy and hyperplasia, causing the pituitary gland to increase in size. These processes account for the larger size of the pituitary gland in multiparous women.

- **Corticotropes (ACTH cells)** also constitute 15%–20% of the parenchymal cells in the anterior lobe of the pituitary gland. These polygonal, medium-sized cells with round and eccentric nuclei produce a precursor molecule of **adrenocorticotropic hormone (ACTH)** known as **proopiomelanocortin (POMC)**. Corticotropes stain as basophils and also exhibit a strong positive reaction with periodic acid–Schiff (PAS) reagent because of the carbohydrate moieties associated with POMC. POMC is further cleaved by proteolytic enzymes within the corticotrope into several fragments, namely, ACTH, β-lipotropic hormone (β-LPH), melanocyte-stimulating hormone (MSH), β-endorphin, and enkephalin. ACTH release is regulated by **corticotropin-releasing hormone (CRH)** produced by the hypothalamus.
- **Gonadotropes (FSH and LH cells)** constitute about 10% of the parenchymal cells in the anterior lobe of the pituitary gland. These small, oval cells with round and eccentric nuclei produce both **luteinizing hormone (LH)** and **follicle-stimulating hormone (FSH)**. They are scattered throughout the pars distalis and stain intensely with both basic stains (thus classifying them as the basophil cell type) and PAS reagent. Many gonadotropes are capable of producing both FSH and LH. However, immunocytochemical studies indicate that some gonadotropes may produce only one hormone or the other. The release of FSH and LH is regulated by **gonadotropin-releasing hormone (GnRH)** produced by the hypothalamus. Both FSH and LH play an important role in male and female reproduction, which is discussed in Chapter 22, Male Reproductive System (see pages 869-870 and 879-880), and Chapter 23, Female Reproductive System (see Folder 23.3, pages 926-927).
- **Thyrotropes (TSH cells)** constitute about 5% of the parenchymal cells in the anterior lobe of the pituitary gland. These large, polygonal cells with round and eccentric nuclei produce thyrotropic hormone called **thyroid-stimulating hormone (TSH)**, which acts on the follicular cells of the thyroid gland to stimulate the production of thyroglobulin and thyroid hormones. Thyrotropes exhibit cytoplasmic basophilia (basophils) and stain positively with PAS reagent. Release of TSH is under the hypothalamic control of **thyrotropin-releasing hormone (TRH)**, which also stimulates secretion of PRL. **Somatostatin** has an inhibitory effect on thyrotropes and decreases secretion of the TSH.

Distinctive characteristics of the five cell types of the anterior lobe of the pituitary gland are readily seen with transmission electron microscopy (TEM). These characteristics are summarized in Table 21.3.

In addition to the five types of hormone-producing cells, the anterior lobe of the pituitary gland contains folliculostellate cells.

Folliculostellate cells present in the anterior lobe of the pituitary gland are characterized by a star-like appearance with their cytoplasmic processes encircling hormone-producing cells. They are primarily non–hormone-secreting cells that have the ability to form cell clusters or small follicles and make up about 5%–10% of cells of the anterior lobe of the pituitary gland. Folliculostellate cells are interconnected by gap junctions containing **connexin-43** protein. Based on immunocytochemical and electrophysiologic studies, it is hypothesized that the network of folliculostellate cells interconnected by gap junctions transmits signals from the pars tuberalis to pars distalis. These signals coordinate and modulate hormone release throughout the anterior lobe of the pituitary gland. Discovery of gap junctions interconnecting folliculostellate cells with hormone-producing cells supports this proposed signaling mechanism in the anterior lobe of the pituitary gland. Thus, the **folliculostellate network** appears to have a regulatory function in addition to the hypophyseal portal vein system.

TABLE 21.3 Electron Microscopic Characteristics of Cells Found in the Anterior Lobe of the Pituitary Gland

Cell Type	Size/Shape	Nucleus/Location	Secretory Vesicle Size/ Characteristics	Other Cytoplasmic Characteristics
Somatotrope	Medium/oval	Round/central, with prominent nucleoli	Dense: 350 nm, closely packed	None
Lactotrope	Large/polygonal	Oval/central	Inactive: 200 nm, sparse Active: dense, pleomorphic, 600 nm, sparse	Lysosomes increase after lactation
Corticotrope	Medium/polygonal	Round/eccentric	100–300 nm	Lipid droplets, large lysosomes, perinuclear bundles of intermediate filaments
Gonadotrope	Small/oval	Round/eccentric	Dense: 200–250 nm	Prominent Golgi apparatus, distended rER cisternae
Thyrotrope	Large/polygonal	Round/eccentric	Dense: <150 nm	Prominent Golgi apparatus with numerous vesicles

rER, rough-surfaced endoplasmic reticulum.

Pars intermedia

The pars intermedia surrounds a series of small cystic cavities that represent the residual lumen of the Rathke pouch.

The parenchymal cells of the **pars intermedia** surround colloid-filled follicles. The cells lining these follicles appear to be derived either from folliculostellate cells or various hormone-secreting cells. The TEM reveals that these cells form apical junctional complexes and have vesicles larger than those found in the pars distalis. The nature of this follicular colloid is yet to be determined; however, often, cell debris is found within it. The pars intermedia contains **basophils** and **chromophobes** (Fig. 21.9). Frequently, the basophils and cystic cavities extend into the pars nervosa.

The function of the pars intermedia cells in humans remains unclear. From studies of other species, however, it is known that basophils have scattered vesicles in their cytoplasm that contain either **α- or β-endorphin** (a morphine-related compound). In frogs, the basophils produce **melanocyte-stimulating hormones (MSH)**, which stimulate pigment production in melanocytes and pigment dispersion in melanophores. In humans, MSH is not a distinct, functional hormone but is a by-product of β-LPH post-translational processing. Because MSH is found in the human pars intermedia in small amounts, the basophils of the pars intermedia are assumed to be **corticotropes**.

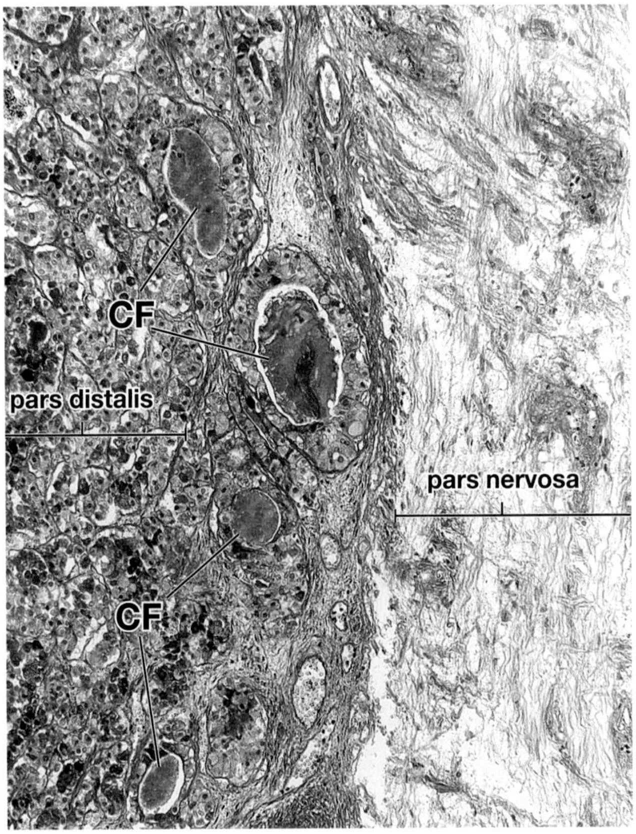

FIGURE 21.9. Photomicrograph of the pars intermedia of an adult human pituitary gland. This photomicrograph of a toluidine blue–stained specimen shows the pars intermedia located between the pars distalis (*on the left*) and the pars nervosa (*on the right*). In humans, this portion of the gland is somewhat rudimentary. However, a characteristic feature of the pars intermedia is the presence of different-sized follicles filled with colloid (*CF*) and small groups of cells consisting of chromophobes and basophils. ×120.

Pars tuberalis

The pars tuberalis is an extension of the anterior lobe along the stalk-like infundibulum.

The **pars tuberalis** is a highly vascular region containing veins of the hypothalamohypophyseal system. The parenchymal cells are arranged in small clusters or cords in association with the blood vessels. Nests of squamous cells and small follicles lined with cuboidal cells are scattered in this region. These cells often show immunoreactivity for ACTH, FSH, and LH.

Posterior Lobe of the Pituitary Gland (Neurohypophysis)

The posterior lobe of the pituitary gland is an extension of the central nervous system (CNS) that stores and releases secretory products from the hypothalamus.

The **posterior lobe of the pituitary gland**, also known as the *neurohypophysis*, consists of the **pars nervosa** and the **infundibulum** that connects it to the hypothalamus. The pars nervosa, the neural lobe of the pituitary, contains the unmyelinated axons and their nerve endings of approximately 100,000 **neurosecretory neurons** whose cell bodies lie in the **supraoptic nuclei** and **paraventricular nuclei** of the hypothalamus. The axons form the **hypothalamohypophyseal tract** and are unique in two respects. First, they do not terminate on other neurons or target cells but end in close proximity to the fenestrated capillary network of the pars nervosa. Second, they contain secretory vesicles in all parts of the cells (i.e., the cell body, axon, and axon terminal). Because of their intense secretory activity, the neurons have well-developed Nissl bodies and, in this respect, resemble ventral horn and ganglion cells.

The posterior lobe of the pituitary gland is *not an endocrine gland*. Rather, it is a **storage site for neurosecretions** of the neurons of the supraoptic and paraventricular nuclei of the hypothalamus. The unmyelinated axons convey neurosecretory products to the pars nervosa. Other neurons from the hypothalamic nuclei (described later in this chapter) also release their secretory products into the fenestrated capillary network of the infundibulum, the first capillary bed of the hypothalamohypophyseal portal system.

Electron microscopy reveals three morphologically distinct neurosecretory vesicles in the nerve endings of the pars nervosa.

Three sizes of membrane-bound vesicles are present in the pars nervosa:

- **Neurosecretory vesicles** with diameters ranging between 10 and 30 nm accumulate in the axon terminals. They also form accumulations that dilate portions of the axon near the terminals (Fig. 21.10). These dilations, called **Herring bodies**, are visible in the light microscope (Plate 21.1, page 850). In the electron microscope, Herring bodies, in addition to abundant neurosecretory vesicles, contain mitochondria, few microtubules, and profiles of smooth-surfaced endoplasmic reticulum (sER) (Fig. 21.11).
- Nerve terminals also contain 30-nm vesicles that contain acetylcholine. These vesicles may play a specific role in the release of neurosecretory vesicles.

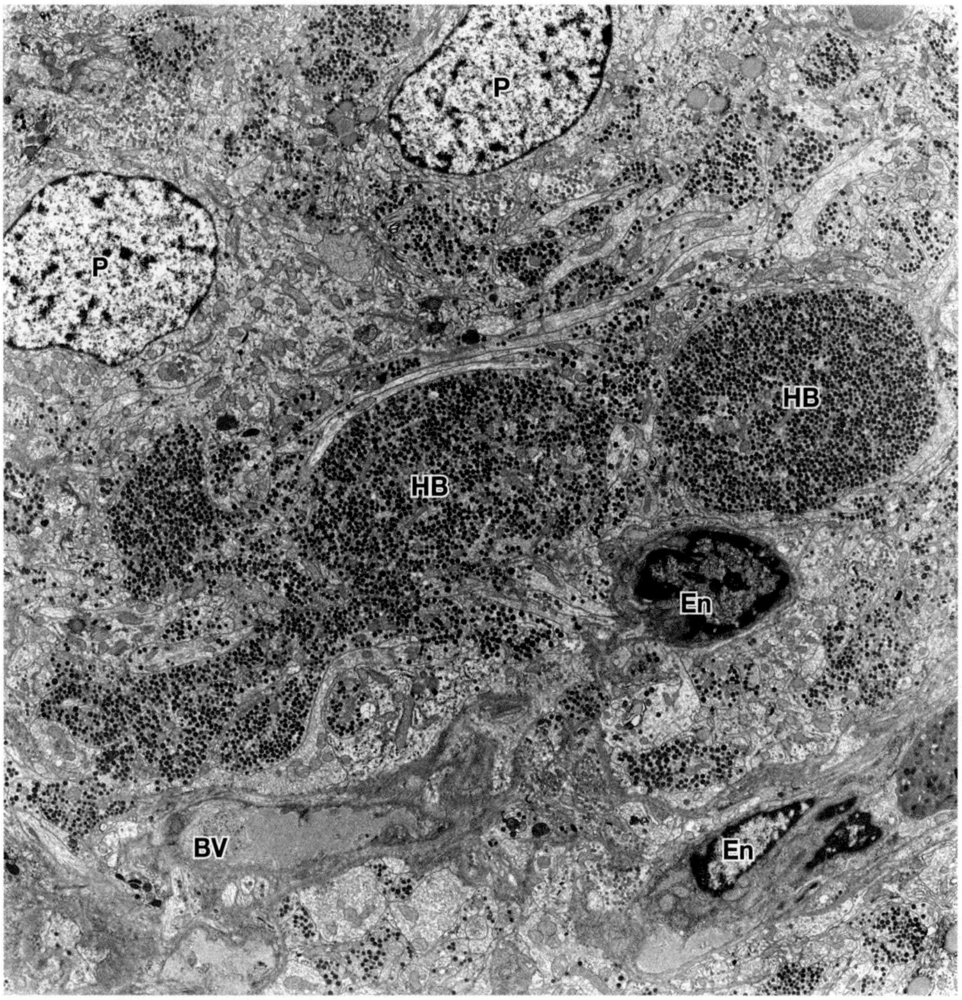

FIGURE 21.10. Electron micrograph of Herring bodies of rat posterior lobe. Dilated portions of axons near their terminals called Herring bodies (*HB*) contain numerous neurosecretory vesicles filled with either oxytocin or antidiuretic hormone (ADH). They are surrounded by the specialized glial cells called pituicytes (*P*). Note that Herring bodies reside in close proximity to blood vessels (*BV*), mainly fenestrated capillaries, lined by endothelial cells (*En*). ×6,000. (Courtesy of Dr. Holger Jastrow.)

- Larger 50- to 80-nm vesicles that resemble the dense-core vesicles of the adrenal medulla and adrenergic nerve endings are present in the same terminal as the other membrane-bound vesicles. The membrane-bound neurosecretory vesicles that aggregate to form Herring bodies contain either **oxytocin** or **antidiuretic hormone** (**ADH**; also called **vasopressin**; Table 21.4). Each hormone is a small peptide of nine amino acid residues. The two hormones differ in only two of these residues. Each vesicle also contains **ATP** and a **neurophysin**, a protein that binds to the hormone by noncovalent bonds. Oxytocin and ADH are synthesized as part of a large molecule that includes the hormone and its specific neurophysin. The large molecule is proteolytically cleaved into the hormone and neurophysin as it travels from the nerve cell body to the axon terminal. Immunocytochemical staining demonstrates that oxytocin and ADH are secreted by different cells in the hypothalamic nuclei.

ADH facilitates reabsorption of water from the distal tubules and collecting ducts of the kidney by altering the permeability of the cells to water.

ADH's original name, vasopressin, was derived from the observation that large nonphysiologic doses increase blood pressure by promoting the contraction of smooth muscle in small arteries and arterioles. However, physiologic levels of ADH have only minimal effects on blood pressure. **ADH** is the main hormone involved in the regulation of **water homeostasis** and **osmolarity of body fluids**. The primary physiologic effect of ADH on the kidney is the insertion of water channels (**aquaporins**) into cells of the distal convoluted tubules and collecting ducts, which increases their permeability for water. Insertion of aquaporin-2 (AQP-2) into the apical domain and AQP-3 into the basolateral domain of these cells is responsible for rapid resorption of water across the tubule epithelium. ADH acts through its specific V2 receptor on the basolateral domain of cells lining the distal convoluted tubules and collecting ducts; mutation of this receptor is responsible for **nephrogenic diabetes insipidus** (Folder 21.3).

Plasma osmolality and blood volume are monitored by specialized receptors of the cardiovascular system (e.g., carotid bodies and juxtaglomerular apparatus). An increase in osmolality or a decrease in blood volume stimulates ADH release. In addition, the cell bodies of the hypothalamic secretory neurons may also serve as osmoreceptors, initiating ADH release. Pain, trauma, emotional stress, and drugs such as nicotine also stimulate the release of ADH.

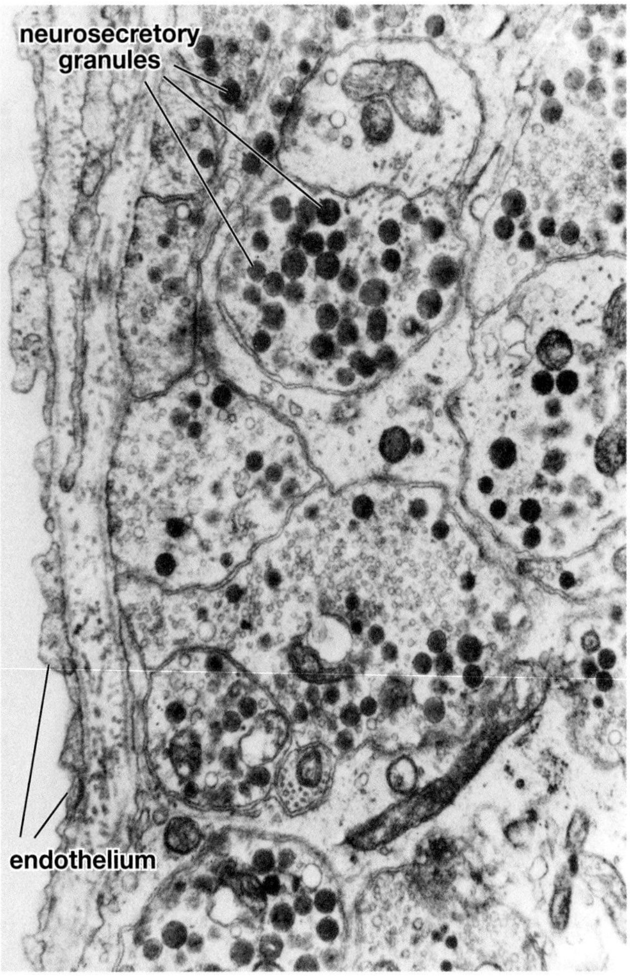

FIGURE 21.11. Electron micrograph of rat posterior lobe. Neurosecretory granules and small vesicles are present in the terminal portions of the axonal processes of the hypothalamohypophyseal tract fibers. Capillaries with fenestrated endothelium are present in close proximity to the nerve endings. ×20,000. (Courtesy of Drs. Sanford L. Palay and P. Orkland.)

Oxytocin promotes contraction of smooth muscle of the uterus and myoepithelial cells of the breast.

Oxytocin is a more potent promoter of smooth muscle contraction than ADH. Its primary effect includes promotion of contraction of the following cells and tissues:

- **Uterine smooth muscle** during orgasm, menstruation, and parturition. As parturition approaches, uterine smooth muscle cells demonstrate about a 200-fold increase in responsiveness to oxytocin. This is accompanied by increased formation of gap junctions between smooth muscle cells and increased density of oxytocin receptors.
- **Myoepithelial cells** of the secretory alveoli and alveolar ducts of the mammary gland. Oxytocin secretion is triggered by neural stimuli that reach the hypothalamus. These stimuli initiate a neurohumoral reflex that resembles a simple sensorimotor reflex. In the uterus, the **neurohumoral reflex** is initiated by distension of the vagina and cervix. In the breast, the reflex is initiated by **breastfeeding (suckling)**. Contraction of the myoepithelial cells that surround the base of the alveolar secretory cells and cells of the larger ducts causes milk to be released and passes through the ducts that open onto the nipple (i.e., milk ejection; see page 947).

Synthetic **analogs of oxytocin** are often used in intravenous infusion pumps to initiate and strengthen uterine contractions during active **labor and delivery**.

The pituicyte is the only cell specific to the posterior lobe of the pituitary gland.

In addition to the numerous axons and terminals of the hypothalamic neurosecretory neurons, the posterior lobe of the pituitary gland contains fibroblasts, mast cells, and specialized glial cells called **pituicytes** associated with the fenestrated capillaries (Plate 21.2, page 852). These cells are irregular in shape, with many branches, and resemble astroglial cells. Their nuclei are round or oval, and pigment vesicles are present in the cytoplasm. Like astroglia, they possess specific intermediate filaments assembled from **glial fibrillary acidic proteins (GFAP)**. Pituicytes often have processes that terminate in the perivascular space. Because of their many processes and relationships to the blood, the pituicyte serves a supporting role similar to that of astrocytes in the rest of the CNS (see pages 410-412).

■ HYPOTHALAMUS

The hypothalamus regulates pituitary gland activity.

The **hypothalamus** is located in the middle of the base of the brain, and it encapsulates the ventral portion of the third ventricle. It coordinates most endocrine functions of the body and serves as one of the major controlling centers of the ANS. Some of the functions that it regulates include

TABLE 21.4 Hormones of the Posterior Lobe of the Pituitary Gland

Hormone	Composition	Source	Major Functions
Oxytocin	Polypeptide containing nine amino acids	Cell bodies of neurons located in the supraoptic and paraventricular nuclei of the hypothalamus[a]	Stimulates activity of the contractile cells around the ducts of the mammary glands to eject milk from the glands; stimulates contraction of smooth muscle cells in the pregnant uterus
Antidiuretic hormone (ADH; vasopressin)	Polypeptide containing nine amino acids; two forms: arginine-ADH (most common in humans) and lysine-ADH	Cell bodies of neurons located in the supraoptic and paraventricular nuclei of the hypothalamus[a]	Decreases urine volume by increasing reabsorption of water by collecting ducts of the kidney; decreases the rate of perspiration in response to dehydration; increases blood pressure by stimulating contractions of smooth muscle cells in the wall of arterioles

[a]Immunocytochemical studies indicate that oxytocin and ADH are produced by separate sets of neurons within the supraoptic and paraventricular nuclei of the hypothalamus. Biochemical studies have demonstrated that the supraoptic nucleus contains equal amounts of both hormones, whereas the paraventricular nucleus contains more oxytocin than ADH but less than the amount found in the supraoptic nucleus.

FOLDER 21.2

CLINICAL CORRELATION: PRINCIPLES OF ENDOCRINE DISEASES

Abnormalities in the signaling mechanisms that coordinate and control the function of multiple organs and biological processes are the bases of many endocrine diseases. Classic biochemistry, physiology, and advances in cell and molecular biology and genetics combined with clinical observations are able to explain the mechanisms of hormonal action and endocrine diseases. Endocrine diseases can be classified into four major categories:

- **Hormone overproduction**. The most common cause of hormone overproduction is an increase in the total number of cells producing a specific hormone. An example of this mechanism is hyperthyroidism (Graves disease; see Folder 21.4). Briefly, the presence of abnormal antibodies that mimic the action of thyroid-stimulating hormone (TSH) stimulates a dramatic increase in the number of thyroid cells. In some instances, increased hormone secretion is related to genetic abnormality that affects the regulation of hormone synthesis and release. In addition, mutation in tumor suppressor genes and proto-oncogenes may lead to proliferation of mutant cells that produce the specific hormone. This commonly occurs in cells of the anterior lobe of the pituitary gland.
- **Hormone underproduction**. Underproduction of hormones may result from destruction of an endocrine organ by a disease process (e.g., tuberculosis of the adrenal glands) or autoimmunity (e.g., Hashimoto disease in which abnormal antibodies target and destroy thyroid hormone–producing cells). Also, genetic abnormalities that lead to abnormal development of endocrine glands (e.g., hypogonadotropic hypogonadism), abnormal hormone synthesis (e.g., deletion of the GH gene), or abnormal regulation of hormone secretion (e.g., hypoparathyroidism associated with mutation of the calcium-sensing receptor expressed on parathyroid cells) can cause decreased serum levels or lack of active hormones. Iatrogenic injury to endocrine glands such as occurs when the parathyroid gland is removed during thyroidectomy (thyroid gland removal) may also be responsible.
- **Altered tissue responses to hormones**. This category of endocrine disease is often caused by a variety of genetic mutation in hormone receptors (e.g., TSH, luteinizing hormone [LH], and parathyroid hormone [PTH]). In diabetic patients, the resistance to insulin in muscles and the liver is mainly caused by signals originating from adipose tissue (see Chapter 9, Adipose Tissue, page 280).
- **Tumors of endocrine glands**. Most of the tumors of endocrine gland are hormonally active and are responsible for hormone overproduction. However, some tumors of endocrine glands do not produce hormones but compress neighboring organs or cause destructions of other organs due to metastasis. An example of such a tumor is thyroid cancer that can metastasize throughout the body without presenting signs of thyroid hormone overproduction (hyperthyroidism).

Hormones are used to treat endocrine diseases. A common use is as **hormone replacement therapies** when a specific endocrine gland is not developed or ceases to produce the required hormone. Hormones and their synthetic analogs can be used to suppress the effects of other hormones. In general, thyroid and steroid hormones can be administered orally, whereas protein hormones (e.g., insulin, growth hormone [GH]) need to be injected. Recent technological innovations, including computerized mini-pumps and depot intramuscular injections, have made therapy more manageable for patients.

blood pressure, body temperature, fluid and electrolyte balance, body weight, and appetite. The hypothalamus produces numerous neurosecretory products. In addition to **oxytocin** and **ADH**, hypothalamic neurons secrete polypeptides that promote and inhibit the secretion and release of hormones from the anterior lobe of the pituitary gland (Table 21.5). These **hypothalamic polypeptides** also accumulate in nerve endings near the median eminence and infundibulum and are released into the capillary bed of the **hypothalamohypophyseal portal system** for transport to the pars distalis of the pituitary gland.

A feedback system regulates endocrine function at two levels: hormone production in the pituitary gland and hypothalamic-releasing hormone production in the hypothalamus.

The circulating level of a specific secretory product of a target organ, a hormone or its metabolite, may act directly on the cells of the anterior lobe of the pituitary gland or the hypothalamus to regulate the secretion of hypothalamic-releasing hormones (see Fig. 21.19 for a diagram of the hypothalamus–pituitary–thyroid feedback loop). The two levels of feedback allow exquisite sensitivity in the control of secretory function. The hormone itself normally regulates the secretory activity of the cells in the hypothalamus and pituitary gland that regulate its secretion.

In addition, information from most physiologic and psychological stimuli that reach the brain also reaches the hypothalamus. The **hypothalamohypophyseal feedback loop** provides a regulatory pathway whereby general information from the CNS contributes to the regulation of the anterior lobe of the pituitary gland and, consequently, to the regulation of the entire endocrine system. The secretion of hypothalamic regulatory peptides is the primary mechanism by which changes in emotional state are translated into changes in the physiologic homeostatic state.

■ PINEAL GLAND

The **pineal gland** (pineal body, epiphysis cerebri) is an endocrine or neuroendocrine gland that regulates daily body rhythm. It develops from neuroectoderm of the posterior portion of the roof of the diencephalon and remains attached to the brain by a short stalk. In humans, it is located at the posterior wall of the third ventricle near the center of the brain. The pineal gland is a flattened, pine cone–shaped structure, hence its name (Fig. 21.12). It measures 5–8 mm high and 3–5 mm in diameter and weighs between 100 and 200 mg.

FOLDER 21.3

CLINICAL CORRELATION: PATHOLOGIES ASSOCIATED WITH ANTIDIURETIC HORMONE SECRETION

The absence or reduced production of antidiuretic hormone (ADH) leads to a condition known as **diabetes insipidus**, which is characterized by polyuria (production of large volumes of diluted urine—up to 20 L/d) with hypotonic and tasteless (insipid) urine. Individuals with this condition have extreme thirst, which allows them to counteract the loss of water by drinking large amounts of fluids. This disease commonly results from head injuries, tumors, or other lesions that can damage the hypothalamus or posterior lobe of the pituitary gland. This form of the disease is classified as **hypothalamic diabetes insipidus** in contrast to **nephrogenic diabetes insipidus**, in which secretion of the ADH is normal or elevated, but there is a lack of renal response to circulating levels of ADH. Nephrogenic diabetes is usually a congenital disorder related to the mutation of the aquaporin-2 (AQP-2) water channel gene or different ADH V2 receptor mutations in kidney tubules. Hypothalamic diabetes insipidus is usually treated by administration of synthetic analogs of ADH (desmopressin), whereas the treatment of the nephrogenic type of this disease is aimed at reducing the volume of urine output.

Abnormally high levels of ADH are found in the **syndrome of inappropriate antidiuretic hormone secretion (SIADH)**, which is characterized by hyponatremia (low serum levels of sodium), decreased serum osmolality associated with excessive urine sodium excretion and elevated urine osmolality. In SIADH, the elevated level of ADH increases the absorption of water, thereby leading to the production of concentrated urine, inability to excrete water, and hyponatremia that results from excess water rather than sodium deficiency. The increase in ADH secretion may be related to central nervous system (CNS) disorders (tumors, injuries, infections, or cerebrovascular accidents), pulmonary diseases (pneumonia, chronic obstructive pulmonary disease, a lung abscess, or tuberculosis), tumors that secrete ADH (small cell carcinoma of the lung, tumors of the pancreas, thymoma, or lymphomas), and certain drugs (anti-inflammatories, nicotine, diuretics, and many others). Treatment of SIADH depends on the underlying etiology and includes fluid restrictions as well as pharmacologic treatment. An ADH V2–receptor antagonist (conivaptan) is now available to improve hyponatremia and to increase the free water diuresis without loss of other ions in the urine of patients with SIADH.

The pineal gland contains two types of parenchymal cells: pinealocytes and interstitial (glial) cells.

Pinealocytes are the chief cells of the pineal gland. They are arranged in clumps or cords within lobules formed by connective tissue septa that extend into the gland from the pia mater that covers its surface. These cells have a large, deeply infolded nucleus with one or more prominent nucleoli and contain lipid droplets within their cytoplasm. When examined with the TEM, pinealocytes show typical cytoplasmic organelles along with numerous, dense-core, membrane-bound vesicles in their elaborate, elongated cytoplasmic processes. The processes also contain numerous parallel bundles of microtubules. The expanded, club-like endings of the processes are associated with the blood capillaries. This feature strongly suggests neuroendocrine activity.

TABLE 21.5 Hypothalamic-Regulating Hormones

Hormone	Composition	Source	Major Functions
Growth hormone–releasing hormone (GHRH)	Two forms in humans: polypeptides containing 40 and 44 amino acids	Cell bodies of neurons located in the arcuate nucleus of hypothalamus	Stimulates secretion and gene expression of GH by somatotropes
Somatostatin	Two forms in humans: polypeptides containing 14 and 28 amino acids	Cell bodies of neurons located in the periventricular, paraventricular, and arcuate nuclei of the hypothalamus	Inhibits secretion of GH by somatotropes and TSH by thyrotropes; inhibits insulin secretion by B cells of pancreatic islets
Dopamine	Catecholamine (amino acid derivative)	Cell bodies of neurons located in the arcuate nucleus of hypothalamus	Inhibits secretion of PRL by lactotropes
Corticotropin-releasing hormone (CRH)	Polypeptide containing 41 amino acids	Cell bodies of neurons located in the arcuate, periventricular, and medial paraventricular nuclei of hypothalamus	Stimulates secretion of ACTH by corticotropes; stimulates gene expression for POMC in corticotropes
Gonadotropin-releasing hormone (GnRH)	Polypeptide containing 10 amino acids	Cell bodies of neurons located in the arcuate, ventromedial, dorsal, and paraventricular nuclei of hypothalamus	Stimulates secretion of LH and FSH by gonadotropes
Thyrotropin-releasing hormone (TRH)	Polypeptide containing 3 amino acids	Cell bodies of neurons located by the ventromedial, dorsal, and paraventricular nuclei of hypothalamus	Stimulates secretion and gene expression of TSH by thyrotropes; stimulates synthesis and secretion of PRL

ACTH, adrenocorticotropic hormone; *FSH*, follicle-stimulating hormone; *GH*, growth hormone; *LH*, luteinizing hormone; *POMC*, proopiomelanocortin; *PRL*, prolactin; *TSH*, thyroid-stimulating hormone.

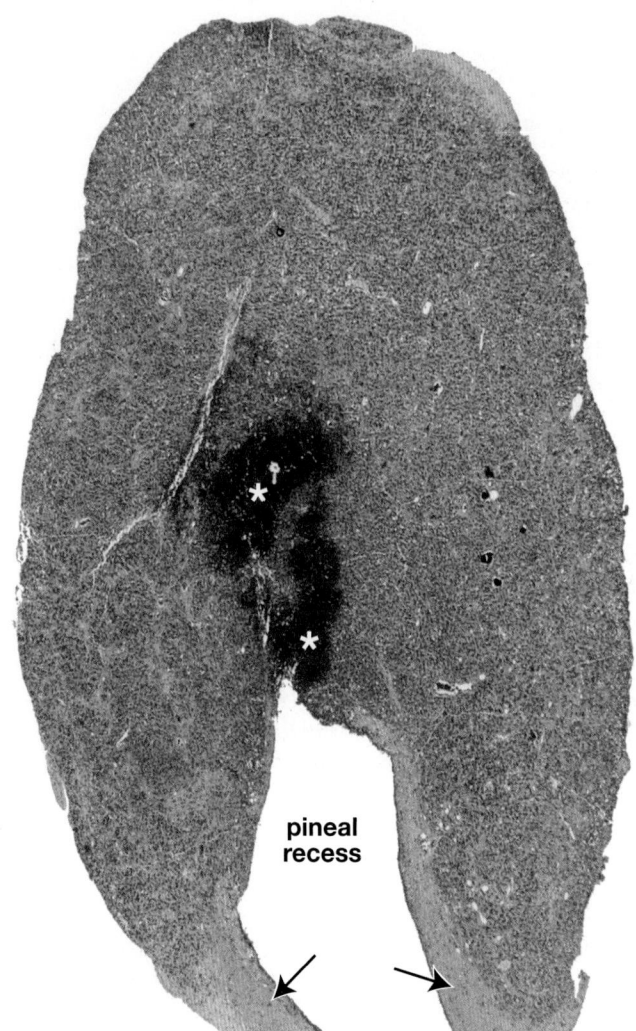

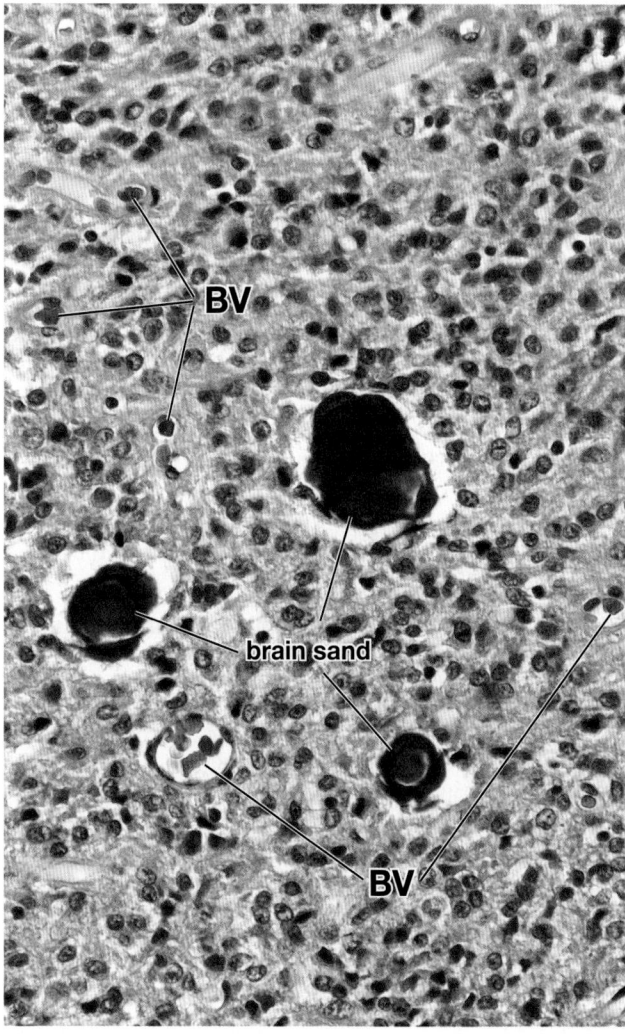

FIGURE 21.12. Photomicrograph of infant pineal gland. This hematoxylin and eosin (H&E)-stained section is obtained from a median cut through the pine cone–shaped gland. The conical anterior end of the gland is at the *top* of the micrograph. The *arrows* indicate the part of the gland that connects with the posterior commissure. The gland is formed by an evagination of the posterior portion of the roof of the third ventricle (diencephalon). The dark areas indicated by *asterisks* are caused by bleeding within the gland. ×25.

The **interstitial (glial) cells** constitute about 5% of the cells in the gland. They have staining and ultrastructural features that closely resemble those of astrocytes and are reminiscent of the pituicytes of the posterior lobe of the pituitary gland.

In addition to the two cell types, the human pineal gland is characterized by the presence of calcified concretions, called **corpora arenacea** or **brain sand** (Fig. 21.13 and Plate 21.3, page 854). These concretions appear to be derived from precipitation of calcium phosphates and carbonates on carrier proteins that are released into the cytoplasm when the pineal secretions are exocytosed. The **concretions** are recognizable in childhood and increase in number with age. Because they are opaque to x-rays and located in the midline of the brain, they serve as convenient **markers** in radiographic and **computed tomography (CT) studies**.

The human pineal gland relates light intensity and duration to endocrine activity.

The pineal gland is a photosensitive organ and an important timekeeper and regulator of the day/night cycle (circadian rhythm). It obtains information about light and dark cycles from the retina via the **retinohypothalamic tract**, which connects the suprachiasmatic nucleus with sympathetic neural tracts traveling into the pineal gland. During the day, light impulses inhibit the production of the major pineal gland hormone, **melatonin**. Therefore, pineal activity, as measured by changes in the plasma level of melatonin, increases during darkness and decreases during light. In humans, these circadian changes of melatonin secretion play an important role in regulating **daily body (circadian) rhythms**.

Melatonin is released in the dark and regulates reproductive function in mammals by inhibiting the steroidogenic activity of the gonads (Table 21.6). Production of **gonadal steroids** is decreased by the inhibitory action of melatonin on neurosecretory neurons located in the hypothalamus (arcuate nucleus) that produce GnRH. Inhibition of GnRH causes a decrease in the release of FSH and LH from the anterior lobe of the pituitary gland. In addition to melatonin, extracts of pineal glands from many animals contain numerous neurotransmitters, such as

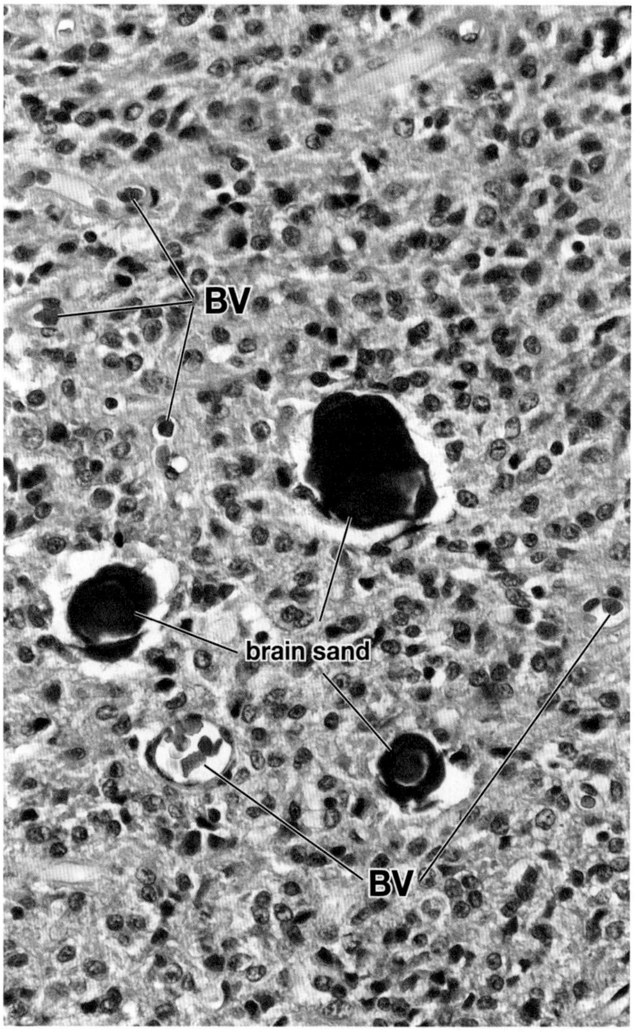

FIGURE 21.13. Photomicrograph of human pineal gland. This higher magnification photomicrograph shows the characteristic concretions called *brain sand* or *corpora arenacea*. Pinealocytes (chief cells of the pineal gland) account for the majority of the cells seen in the specimen. They are arranged in clumps or cords. Those blood vessels (*BV*) that contain red blood cells are readily apparent; numerous other blood vessels are also present but are not recognized at this magnification without evidence of the blood cells. ×250.

TABLE 21.6 Hormones of the Pineal Gland

Hormone	Composition	Source	Major Functions
Melatonin	Indolamine (*N*-acetyl-5-methoxytryptamine)	Pinealocytes	Regulates daily body rhythms and day/night cycle (circadian rhythms); inhibits secretion of GnRH and regulates steroidogenic activity of the gonads particularly as related to the menstrual cycle; in animals, influences seasonal sexual activity

GnRH, gonadotropin-releasing hormone.

serotonin, **norepinephrine**, **dopamine**, and **histamine**, and hypothalamic-regulating hormones, such as **somatostatin** and **TRH**. Clinically, tumors that destroy the pineal gland are associated with **precocious (early-onset) puberty**.

Animal studies demonstrate that information relating to the length of daylight reaches the pineal gland from photoreceptors in the retina. The pineal gland thus influences seasonal sexual activity. The pineal gland has a role in adjusting to sudden changes in day length, such as those experienced by travelers who suffer from **jet lag**. In addition, the pineal gland plays a role in **altering emotional responses** to the reduced length of day during winter in temperate and subarctic zones known as **seasonal affective disorder (SAD)**.

■ THYROID GLAND

The thyroid gland is located in the anterior neck region adjacent to the larynx and trachea.

The **thyroid gland** is a bilobate endocrine gland located in the anterior neck region and consists of two large **lateral lobes** connected by an **isthmus**, a thin band of thyroid tissue. The two lobes, each approximately 5 cm in length, 2.5 cm in width, and 20–30 g in weight, lie on either side of the larynx and upper trachea. The isthmus crosses the anterior surface of the second and third tracheal cartilages. A **pyramidal lobe** often extends upward from the isthmus. A thin connective tissue capsule surrounds the gland (Fig. 21.14). It sends trabeculae into the parenchyma that partially outlines irregular lobes and lobules. **Thyroid follicles** constitute the functional units of the gland.

The thyroid gland develops from the endodermal lining of the floor of the primitive pharynx.

The **thyroid gland** begins to develop during the fourth week of gestation from a primordium originating as an endodermal thickening of the floor of the primitive pharynx. The primordium grows caudally and forms a duct-like invagination known as the **thyroglossal duct**. The thyroglossal duct descends through the tissue of the neck to its final destination in front of the trachea, where it divides into two lobes. During this downward migration, the thyroglossal duct undergoes atrophy, leaving an embryologic remnant, the pyramidal lobe of the thyroid, which is present in about 40% of the population.

At about the ninth week of gestation, endodermal cells differentiate into plates of **follicular cells** that become arranged into follicles. By week 14, well-developed follicles lined by the follicular cells contain colloid in their lumens. During week 7, parallel to the development of thyroid follicles, epithelial cells lining the invagination of the fourth pharyngeal (branchial) pouches, known as the **ultimobranchial bodies**, start their migration toward the developing thyroid gland and become incorporated into the lateral lobes. After fusing with the thyroid, ultimobranchial body cells disperse among the follicles, giving rise to **parafollicular cells** that become incorporated into the follicular epithelium.

The thyroid follicle is the structural and functional unit of the thyroid gland.

A **thyroid follicle** is a roughly spherical cyst-like compartment with a wall formed by a simple cuboidal or low columnar epithelium, the **follicular epithelium**. Hundreds of thousands of follicles that vary in diameter from about 0.2 to 1.0 mm constitute nearly the entire mass of the human thyroid gland. The follicles contain a gel-like mass called **colloid**

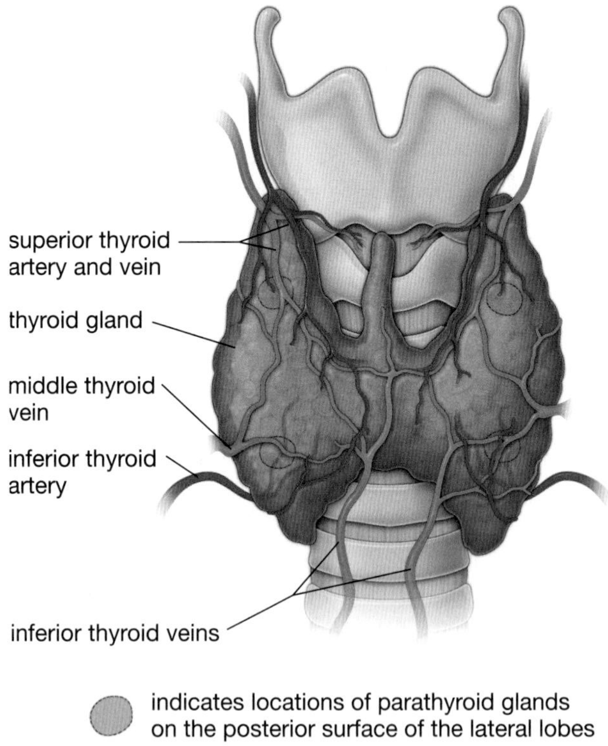

FIGURE 21.14. Topography and blood supply of the thyroid gland. This drawing shows the location of the thyroid gland in the anterior region of the neck in close proximity to the trachea and laryngeal cartilages. The gland consists of two lateral lobes connected by an isthmus. In about 40% of cases, the thyroid gland exhibits a pyramidal lobe, which is a remnant of the thyroglossal duct, a developmental connection with the base of the tongue. The thyroid gland is supplied by blood from the superior and inferior thyroid arteries, and blood from the gland is drained by the superior, middle, and inferior thyroid veins. On the posterior (deep) surface of the lateral lobes, there are two pairs of small ovoid structures that are designated as superior and inferior parathyroid glands. Note the outlined areas of the parathyroid glands' location visible from the anterior view.

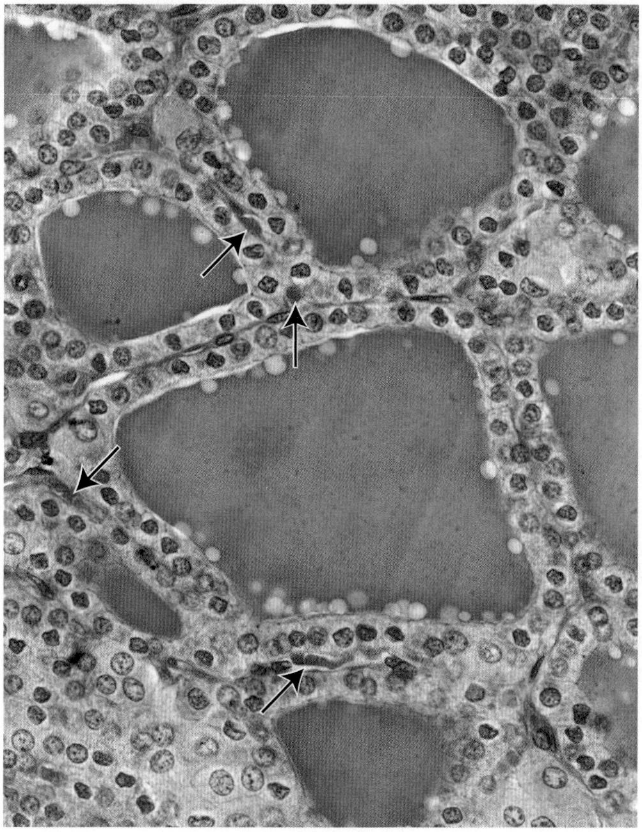

FIGURE 21.15. Thyroid gland. This photomicrograph of a human thyroid is from a section stained with hematoxylin and eosin (H&E). It shows the colloid-containing follicles of the gland. Each follicle consists of a single layer of epithelial cells surrounding a central mass of colloid. The *arrows* indicate some of the blood capillaries between the follicles. ×500.

(Fig. 21.15 and Plate 21.4, page 856). The apical surfaces of the follicular cells are in contact with the colloid, and the basal surfaces rest on a typical basal lamina.

Follicular epithelium contains two types of cells: follicular and parafollicular cells.

The parenchyma of the thyroid gland is composed of epithelium containing two types of cells:

- **Follicular cells (principal cells)** are responsible for the production of the thyroid hormones T_4 and T_3. These cells vary in shape and size according to the functional state of the gland. In routine hematoxylin and eosin (H&E) preparations, follicular cells exhibit a slightly basophilic basal cytoplasm with spherical nuclei containing one or more prominent nucleoli. The Golgi apparatus has a supranuclear position. Lipid droplets and PAS-positive droplets can be identified with appropriate staining. At the ultrastructural level, the follicle cells reveal organelles commonly associated with both secretory and absorptive cells (Fig. 21.16), including typical junctional complexes at the apical end of the cell and short microvilli on the apical cell surface. Numerous profiles of rough-surfaced endoplasmic reticulum (rER) are present in the basal region. Small vesicles present in the apical cytoplasm are morphologically similar to vesicles associated with the Golgi apparatus. Abundant endocytic vesicles, identified as **colloidal resorption droplets**, and lysosomes are also present in the apical cytoplasm.
- **Parafollicular cells (C cells)** are located in the periphery of the follicular epithelium and lie within the follicle basal lamina. These cells have no exposure to the follicle lumen. They secrete **calcitonin**, a hormone that regulates calcium metabolism. In routine H&E preparations, C cells are pale staining and occur as solitary cells or small clusters of cells. Human parafollicular cells are difficult to identify with light microscopy. At the electron microscope level, the parafollicular cells reveal numerous small secretory vesicles, which range in diameter from 60 to 550 nm, and a prominent Golgi apparatus (Fig. 21.17).

An extensive network of fenestrated capillaries derived from the superior and inferior thyroid arteries surrounds the follicles. Blind-ended lymphatic capillaries are present in the interfollicular connective tissue and may also provide a second route for conveying the hormones from the gland.

Thyroid gland function is essential to normal growth and development.

The thyroid gland produces three hormones, each of which is essential to normal metabolism and homeostasis (Table 21.7):

- **Thyroxine (3,3′,5,5′-tetraiodothyronine, T_4)** and **3,3′,5-triiodothyronine (T_3)** are synthesized and secreted by **follicular cells**. Both hormones regulate cell and tissue basal metabolism and heat production and influence body growth and development. Secretion of these hormones is regulated by TSH released from the anterior lobe of the pituitary gland.

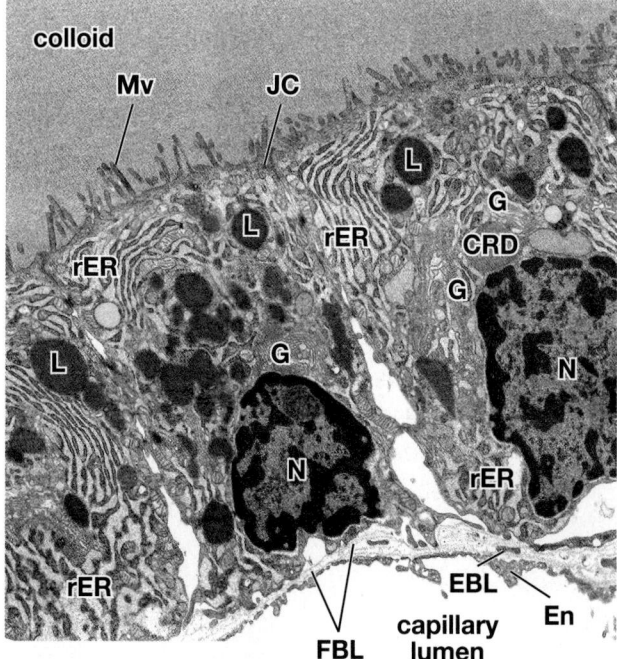

FIGURE 21.16. Electron micrograph of follicular cells in rat thyroid gland. This electron micrograph shows a single layer of epithelium containing low columnar follicular cells. The apical surfaces with visible microvilli (*Mv*) are in contact with the colloid, whereas basal surfaces of follicular cells rest on the basal lamina (*FBL*). A narrow extracellular connective tissue space separates the follicular cells from the lumen of the capillary. Note that the fenestrated endothelial cells (*En*) lining the capillary lumen rest on the basal lamina (*EBL*). Accumulation of lysosomes (*L*) and colloid resorption droplets (*CRD*), extensive Golgi apparatus (*G*), rough-surfaced endoplasmic reticulum (*rER*), and the presence of enlarged intercellular spaces are indicative of intensive activity of follicular cells. *JC*, junctional complex; *N*, nucleus. ×14,000. (Courtesy of Dr. Holger Jastrow.)

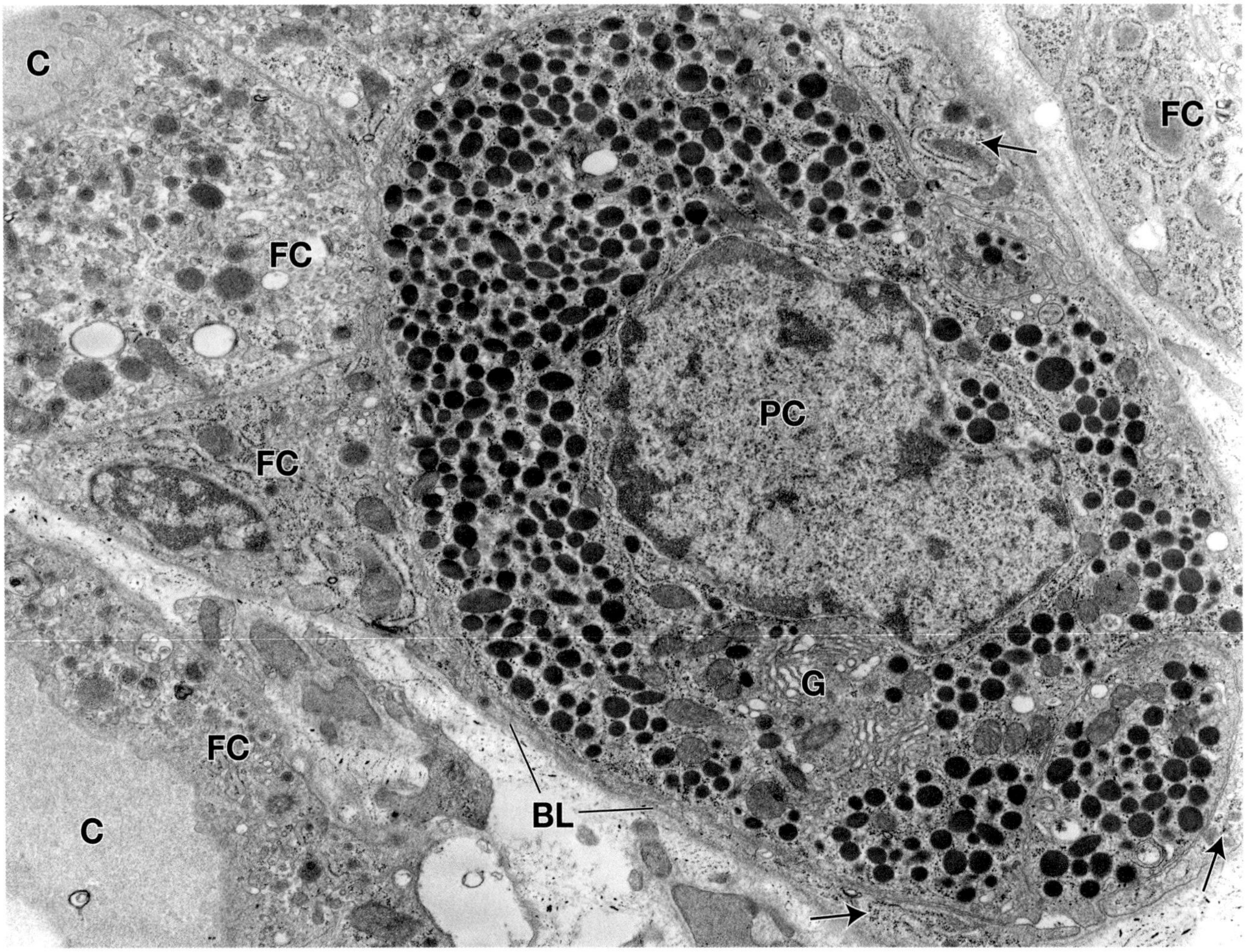

FIGURE 21.17. Electron micrograph of a parafollicular cell. Cytoplasmic processes of follicular cells (*arrows*) partially surround the parafollicular cell (*PC*), which contains numerous electron-dense granules and a prominent Golgi apparatus (*G*). A basal lamina (*BL*) is associated with the follicular cells (*FC*). A portion of the central mass of colloidal material (*C*) in two adjacent follicles can be seen in the *left corners* of the micrograph. ×12,000. (Courtesy of Dr. Emmanuel-Adrien Nunez.)

- **Calcitonin (thyrocalcitonin)** is synthesized by the **parafollicular cells (C cells)** and is a physiologic antagonist to parathyroid hormone (PTH). Calcitonin has an important role in regulating serum calcium levels in lower animals; however, its physiologic role in humans remains elusive. Calcitonin lowers blood calcium levels by suppressing the resorptive action of osteoclasts and promotes calcium deposition in bones by increasing the rate of osteoid calcification. Secretion of calcitonin is regulated directly by blood calcium levels. High levels of calcium stimulate secretion; low levels inhibit it. Secretion of calcitonin is unaffected by the hypothalamus and pituitary gland. Calcitonin is secreted by several endocrine tumors (e.g., **medullary carcinoma of the thyroid**);

TABLE 21.7 Hormones of the Thyroid Gland

Hormone	Composition	Source	Major Functions
Thyroxine (tetraiodothyronine, T_4 and triiodothyronine, T_3)[a]	Iodinated tyrosine derivatives	Follicular cells (principal cells)	Regulates tissue basal metabolism (increases rate of carbohydrate use, protein synthesis and degradation, and fat synthesis and degradation), regulates heat production, influences body and tissue growth and development of the nervous system in the fetus and young child,[b] increases absorption of carbohydrates from the intestine
Calcitonin (thyrocalcitonin)	Polypeptide containing 32 amino acids	Parafollicular cells (C cells)	Decreases blood calcium levels by inhibiting bone resorption and stimulating absorption of calcium by the bones

[a]Thyroid gland secretes substantially more T_4 than T_3; however, about 40% of T_4 is peripherally converted to T_3, which acts more rapidly and is a more potent hormone.

[b]Deficiency of T_3 and T_4 during development results in fewer and smaller neurons, defective myelination, and severe intellectual disability.

therefore, it is used as a tumor marker to monitor the progress of recovery after surgical resection of the tumor. Although calcitonin is used to treat patients with several disorders associated with excess bone resorption (e.g., **osteoporosis** and **Paget disease**), no clinical disease has been associated with its deficiency or even its absence after total thyroidectomy.

The principal component of colloid is thyroglobulin, an inactive storage form of thyroid hormones.

The principal component of colloid is a large (660 kDa), iodinated glycoprotein called **thyroglobulin** containing about 120 tyrosine residues. Colloid also contains several enzymes and other glycoproteins. It stains with both basic and acidic dyes and is strongly PAS positive. Thyroglobulin is not a hormone. It is an inactive storage form of thyroid hormones. Active thyroid hormones are liberated from thyroglobulin and released into the fenestrated blood capillaries that surround the follicles only after further cellular processing. The thyroid is unique among endocrine glands because it stores large amounts of its secretory product extracellularly.

Synthesis of thyroid hormone involves several steps.

The **synthesis** of the two major thyroid hormones, **thyroxine (T_4)** and **triiodothyronine (T_3)**, takes place in the thyroid follicle in a series of discrete steps (Fig. 21.18):

1. **Synthesis of thyroglobulin**. The precursor of thyroglobulin is synthesized in the rER of the follicular epithelial cells. Thyroglobulin is post-translationally glycosylated in the rER and the Golgi apparatus before it is packaged into vesicles and secreted by exocytosis into the lumen of the follicle.
2. **Resorption, diffusion, and oxidation of iodide**. Follicular epithelial cells actively transport **iodide** from the blood into their cytoplasm using ATPase-dependent **sodium/iodide symporters (NIS)**. The NIS is the 87-kDa transmembrane protein that mediates active iodide uptake in the basolateral membrane of the follicular epithelial cells. These cells are capable of establishing an intracellular concentration of iodide that is 30–40 times greater than that of the serum. Iodide ions then diffuse rapidly toward the apical cell membrane. From here, iodide ions are transported to the lumen of the follicle by the 86-kDa **iodide/chloride transporter** called **pendrin** located in the apical cell membrane. Iodide is then immediately oxidized to **iodine**, the active form of iodide. This process occurs in the colloid and is catalyzed by membrane-bound **thyroid peroxidase (TPO)**.
3. **Iodination of thyroglobulin**. One or two iodine atoms are then added to the specific tyrosine residues of thyroglobulin. This process occurs in the colloid at the microvillar surface of the follicular cells and is also

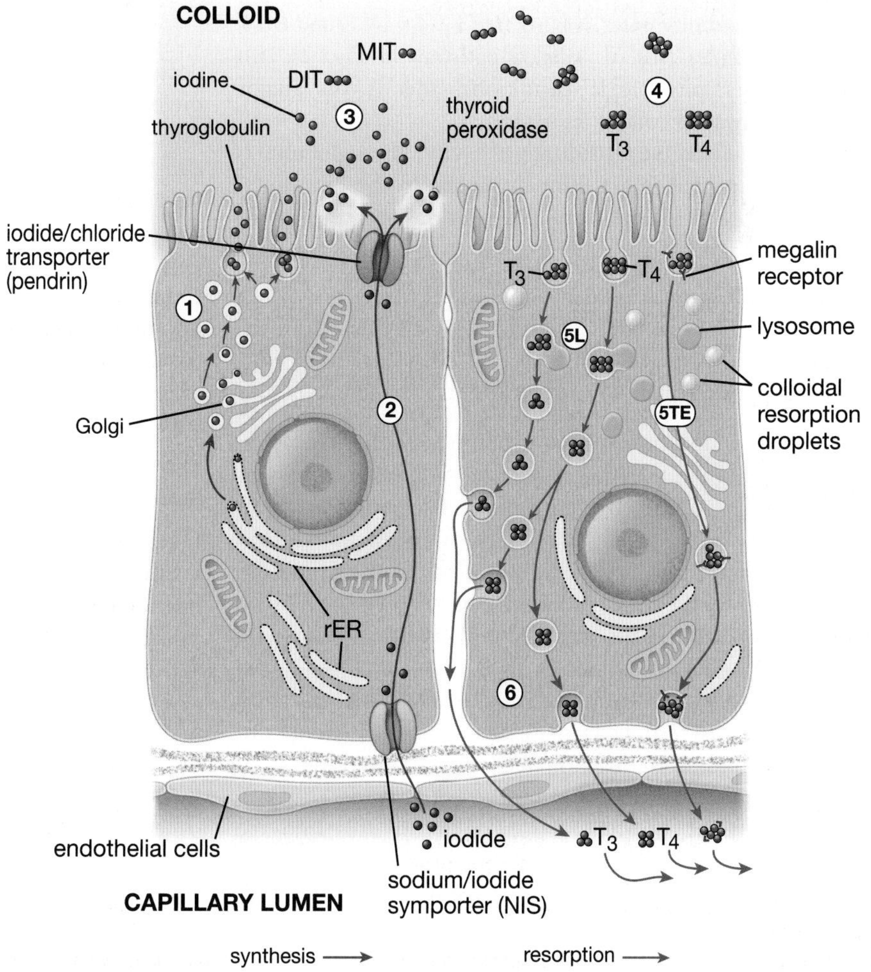

FIGURE 21.18. Diagram of steps in thyroid hormone synthesis. This diagram depicts two follicular cells: one in the process of thyroglobulin synthesis (*on the left with red pathways*) and the other in the process of thyroglobulin resorption (*on the right with blue pathways*). The *numbers*, which are described more fully in the text, indicate the sequential steps that occur: *1*, synthesis and secretion of thyroglobulin; *2*, uptake and concentration of iodide from the blood by sodium/iodide symporters (*NIS*), release of iodide into the colloid via iodide/chloride (pendrin) transporters, and oxidation of iodide to iodine by thyroid peroxidase; *3*, iodination of thyroglobulin in the colloid; *4*, formation of T_3 and T_4 hormones in the colloid by oxidative coupling reactions; *5L*, resorption of colloid via lysosomal pathway (major pathway); *5TE*, resorption of colloid via megalin receptor–mediated transepithelial pathway; and *6*, release of T_4 and T_3 from the cell into the circulation. *DIT*, diiodotyrosine; *MIT*, monoiodotyrosine; *rER*, rough-surfaced endoplasmic reticulum.

catalyzed by **thyroid peroxidase (TPO)**. Addition of one iodine atom to a single tyrosine residue forms **monoiodotyrosine (MIT)**. Addition of a second iodine atom to the MIT residue forms a **diiodotyrosine (DIT)**.

4. **Formation of T_3 and T_4** by oxidative coupling reactions. Thyroid hormones are formed by oxidative coupling reactions of two iodinated tyrosine residues in close proximity. For example, when neighboring DIT and MIT residues undergo a coupling reaction, T_3 is formed; when two DIT residues react with each other, T_4 is formed. After iodination, T_4 and T_3 as well as the DIT and MIT residues that are still linked to a thyroglobulin molecule are stored as the colloid within the lumen of the follicle.
5. **Resorption of colloid**. In response to TSH, follicular cells take up thyroglobulin from the colloid by a process of receptor-mediated endocytosis. If the levels of TSH remain high, the amount of colloid in the follicle is reduced because it is synthesized, secreted, iodinated, and resorbed too rapidly to accumulate. After endocytosis, thyroglobulin follows at least two different intracellular pathways.
   - In the **lysosomal pathway**, thyroglobulin is internalized and transported within endocytic vesicles to early endosomes. They eventually mature into lysosomes or fuse with existing lysosomes. Resorption of thyroglobulin at this stage can be confirmed by the presence of large endocytic vesicles called **colloidal resorption droplets** in the apical region of the follicular cells. Thyroglobulin is then degraded by lysosomal proteases into constituent amino acids and carbohydrates, leaving free T_4, T_3, DIT, and MIT molecules (see 5L labeled pathway in Fig. 21.18). Under physiologic conditions, this is the major pathway of colloid resorption.
   - In the **transepithelial pathway**, thyroglobulin is transported intact from the apical to the basolateral surface of follicular cells. To enter this pathway, thyroglobulin binds to its receptor, **megalin**, a 330-kDa member of the low-density lipoprotein (LDL) endocytic receptor family. Megalin is a transmembrane protein expressed at the apical surface of follicular epithelial cells directly facing colloid. Thyroglobulin internalized by megalin avoids the lysosomal pathway, and endocytic vesicles are delivered to the basolateral membrane of follicular cells (see 5TE labeled pathway in Fig. 21.18). In pathologic conditions of high TSH or TSH-like stimulation, **megalin** expression is increased, and large amounts of thyroglobulin follow the transepithelial pathway. This pathway may reduce the extent of T_4 and T_3 release by diverting thyroglobulin away from the lysosomal pathway. Individuals with **Graves disease** and other thyroid diseases have detectable amounts of circulating thyroglobulin that contains portions of megalin receptor.
6. **Release of T_4 and T_3** from follicular cells into the circulation. Follicular cells predominately produce T_4 in a T_4-to-T_3 ratio of 20:1. Most of the T_4 and T_3 produced is liberated from thyroglobulin in the lysosomal pathway, and only negligible amounts of T_4 and T_3 are released bound to thyroglobulin. Both T_4 and T_3 cross the basal membrane and enter the blood and lymphatic capillaries. Most of the released hormones are immediately bound to a specific plasma protein (54 kDa), **thyroxine-binding globulin (TBG)** (~70%), or a prealbumin fraction of serum protein called **transthyretin** (~20%). T_4 has a stronger bond to TBG, whereas T_3 has a stronger bond to transthyretin. Less than approximately 10% of released hormones are bound to a nonspecific fraction of **albumin**, leaving only small amounts (~1%) of free circulating hormones that are metabolically active. The free circulating hormones also function in the feedback system that regulates the secretory activity of the thyroid (Fig. 21.19). One-third of circulating T_4 is converted to T_3 in peripheral organs, such as the kidney, liver, and heart. T_3 is five times more potent than T_4 and is mainly responsible for biological activity by binding to the thyroid nuclear receptors in the target cells.

Transport across the cell membrane is essential for thyroid hormone action and metabolism.

Based on the biochemical structure of thyroid hormones, it was long thought that thyroid hormones can enter the cell by simple diffusion. However, it is now well established that thyroid hormones are transported across cell membranes by several **thyroid hormone transporter molecules**. Within the CNS, T_3 and T_4 are transported via the blood–brain barrier to the nerve and glial cells by **monocarboxylate transporter-8 (MCT8)** and **MCT10** as well as a family of **organic anion–transporting polypeptides (OATPs)**. For example, the OATP1C1 transporter is exclusively expressed on the endothelial cells forming the blood–brain barrier and is responsible for T_4 uptake into the brain. The MCT8 is also found in the heart, kidney, liver, and skeletal muscle. Mutations in the MCT8 gene cause severe psychomotor and intellectual disability associated with high serum T_3 levels in affected male individuals, a condition known as **Allan–Herndon–Dudley syndrome**. Defective MCT8 transporters are unable to transport T_3 into nerve cells, which disrupts normal brain development. Because T_3 is not utilized by nerve cells, excessive amounts of this hormone continue to circulate in the blood, causing signs and symptoms of **thyroid hormone toxicity**.

The triiodothyronine (T_3) hormone is more biologically active than thyroxine (T_4).

Once T_3 and T_4 molecules enter the cell, they interact with a specific **thyroid nuclear receptor** that is similar to the nuclear-initiated steroid signaling pathway (see Fig. 21.4b). T_3 binds to nuclear receptors much faster and with higher affinity than T_4; thus, T_3 is more rapidly and biologically active than T_4. In addition, T_3 binds to mitochondria, increasing the production of adenosine triphosphate (ATP). Therefore, **biological activity** and metabolic effect of the thyroid hormone are largely determined by the intracellular concentration of T_3.

Several factors impact the intracellular concentration of T_3. These include serum concentration of circulating T_3, which depends on the conversion rate of T_4 to T_3 in the peripheral organs; transport of thyroid hormones across the

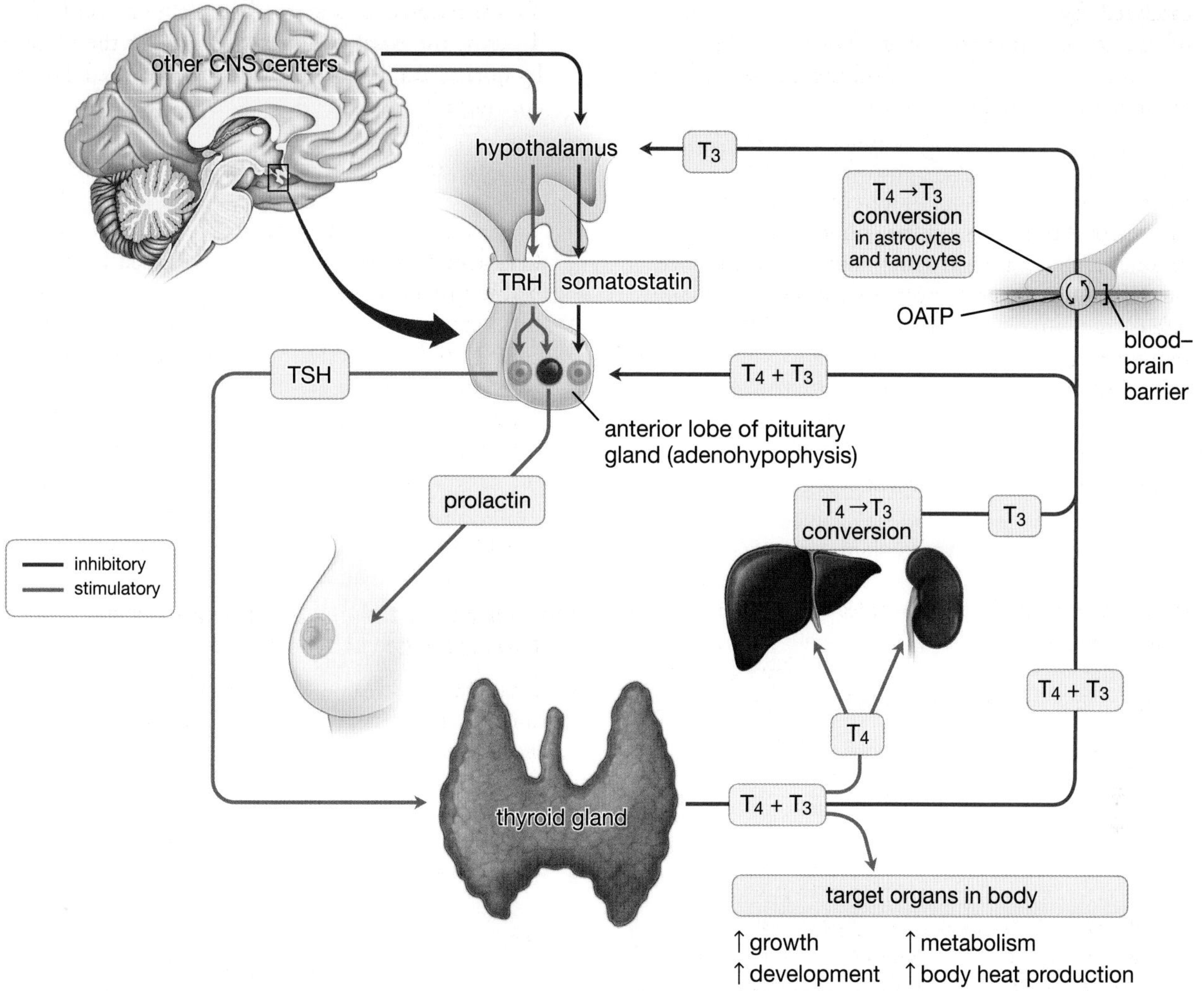

FIGURE 21.19. Production, transport, and regulation of thyroid hormones. Production of T_4 and T_3 is regulated through a negative feedback system. The follicular cells of the thyroid gland predominately produce about 20 times more T_4 than T_3; however, T_4 is converted in the peripheral organs (e.g., liver, kidney) to a more active form of T_3. Approximately 99% of T_4 and T_3 released from the thyroid gland into the circulation bind to specific plasma proteins. The remaining free (unbound) T_4 and T_3 exert negative feedback on the system and inhibit the further release of T_4 and T_3. This inhibition occurs at the level of the anterior lobe of the pituitary gland and the hypothalamus. At the pituitary level, T_4 and T_3 inhibit secretion of TSH by thyrotropes. To elicit an inhibitory effect on the hypothalamus, both T_4 and T_3 need to cross the blood–brain barrier by utilizing the OATP thyroid hormone transporter expressed on the membrane of the endothelial cells. Increased concentration of T_4 and T_3 reduces expression of OATP transporters as part of the negative feedback loop, thus decreasing the amount of available thyroid hormones in the brain. After crossing the blood–brain barrier, T_4 and T_3 are transferred into neighboring astrocytes, where T_4 is converted to T_3. Note that T_3 is the predominant hormone that enters the neurons. T_4 and T_3 are also secreted into the cerebrospinal fluid and are taken up by the tanycytes (specialized ependymal cells) and astrocytes, where T_4 is converted to T_3. In addition to TRH, which also stimulates the production of prolactin in lactotropes, the hypothalamus secretes somatostatin that has an inhibitory effect on TSH production by thyrotropes. The feedback system is activated in response to low thyroid hormone levels in the blood or metabolic needs. In addition to chemical control mechanisms, a variety of nerve endings in the hypothalamus regulate secretion of TRH. For example, cold stress increases secretion of TRH, whereas increased body temperature inhibits TRH secretion. *CNS*, central nervous system; *TRH*, thyrotropin-releasing hormone; *TSH*, thyroid-stimulating hormone (thyrotropin); *OATP*, organic anion–transporting polypeptides.

cell membrane by specialized thyroid hormone transporters; and the presence of **iodothyronine deiodinase** enzymes, which activate or inactivate thyroid hormones. For instance, two deiodinase enzymes called D_1 and D_2 convert T_4 to the more active T_3, whereas the third enzyme called D_3 degrades T_4 to the inactive form of rT_3 (reverse T_3) and DIT. Both T_3 and T_4 are deiodinated and deaminated in the target tissues, conjugated in the liver, and then passed into the bile, where they are excreted into the intestine. Conjugated and free hormones are also excreted by the kidney.

Thyroid hormones play an essential role in normal fetal development.

In humans, **thyroid hormones** are essential to normal growth and development. In normal pregnancy, both T_3 and T_4 cross the placental barrier and are critical in the early stages of brain development. In addition, the fetal thyroid gland begins to function during the 14th week of gestation and also contributes additional thyroid hormones. Thyroid hormone deficiency during **fetal development** results in irreversible damage to the central nervous system (CNS), causing reduced numbers of neurons, defective myelination, and intellectual disability. If maternal thyroid deficiency is present before the development of the fetal thyroid gland, intellectual disability can be severe. Recent studies reveal that thyroid hormones also stimulate gene expression for GH in the somatotropes. Therefore, in addition to neural abnormalities, a generalized stunted body growth is typical. The combination of these two abnormalities is called **congenital hypothyroidism**.

FOLDER 21.4

CLINICAL CORRELATION: ABNORMAL THYROID FUNCTION

The most common symptom of thyroid disease is **goiter**, the enlargement of the thyroid gland. It may indicate either hypothyroidism or hyperthyroidism.

Hypothyroidism can be caused by insufficient dietary iodine (**iodine-deficiency goiter, endemic goiter**) or by one of several inherited autoimmune diseases, such as **autoimmune thyroiditis (Hashimoto thyroiditis)**. Autoimmune thyroiditis is characterized by the presence of abnormal autoimmunoglobulins directed against thyroglobulin (TgAb), thyroid peroxidase (TPOAb), and the thyroid-stimulating hormone (TSH) receptor (TSHAb). The results are thyroid cell apoptosis and follicular destruction. The low levels of circulating thyroid hormone stimulate release of excessive amounts of TSH, which cause hypertrophy of the thyroid through synthesis of more thyroglobulin. Adult **hypothyroidism**, formerly called *myxedema* (due to the puffy appearance of the skin), is characterized by mental and physical sluggishness. The edema that occurs in the severe stages of hypothyroidism is caused by the accumulation of large amounts of hyaluronan in the extracellular matrix of the connective tissue of the dermis.

In **hyperthyroidism (toxic goiter or Graves disease)**, excessive amounts of thyroid hormones are released into the circulation. Individuals with Graves disease have detectable levels of autoantibodies. These abnormal immunoglobulins G (IgG) bind to the TSH receptors on the follicular cells and stimulate adenylate cyclase activity. As a result, increased levels of cyclic adenosine monophosphate (cAMP) in follicular cells lead to continuous stimulation of the cells and increased thyroid hormone secretion. Because of negative feedback, the levels of TSH in the circulation are usually normal. However, under such stimulation, the thyroid gland undergoes hypertrophy, and thyroid hormone is secreted at abnormally high rates, causing increased metabolism. Most of the clinical features are associated with increased metabolic rate and increased sympathetic nerve activities. These include weight loss, excessive sweating, tachycardia, and nervousness. Noticeable signs include protrusion of the eyeballs and retraction of the eyelids, resulting from increased sympathetic activity and increased deposition of extracellular matrix in the adipose tissue located behind the eyeball (Fig. F21.4.1a). The thyroid gland is enlarged. Microscopic features include the presence of columnar follicular cells lining the thyroid follicles. Because of the high utilization of colloid, the colloid tends to be depleted in the areas of contact with the apical surface of follicular cells (Fig. F21.4.1b). Treatment for Graves disease is either surgery to remove the thyroid gland or radiotherapy by ingestion of radioactive iodine (^{131}I), which destroys most active follicular cells.

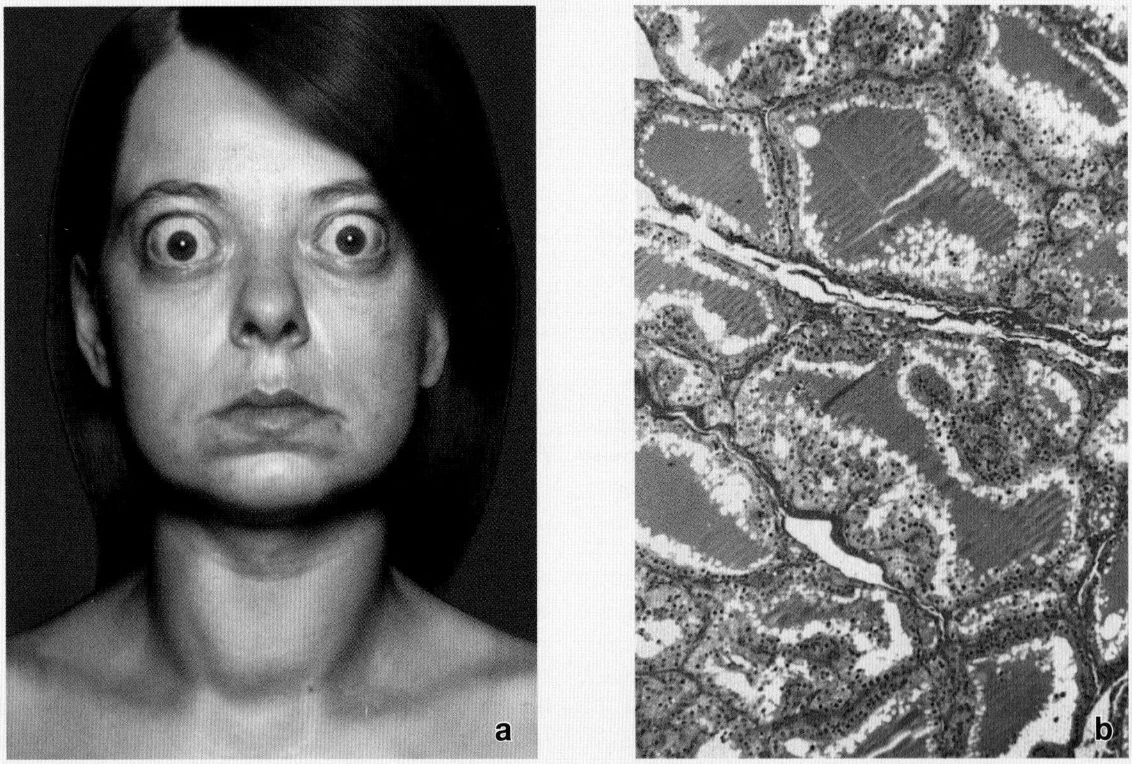

FIGURE F21.4.1. Hyperthyroidism. a. A young woman with signs of hyperthyroidism. Note the enlarged mass on the neck and the typical ocular symptoms known as *exophthalmos*. **b.** Photomicrograph of a thyroid gland specimen from an individual with Graves disease. Owing to the increased utilization of colloid, there is a lack of staining at the periphery of the colloid near the apical surface of the follicular cell. Note that the majority of the cells are columnar in shape. (Reprinted with permission from Rubin E, Gorstein F, Rubin R, et al. *Rubin's Pathology, Clinicopathologic Foundations of Medicine*. 4th ed. Lippincott Williams & Wilkins; 2005.)

■ PARATHYROID GLANDS

The **parathyroid glands** are small endocrine glands closely associated with the thyroid. They are ovoid, a few millimeters in diameter, and arranged in two pairs, constituting the **superior** and **inferior parathyroid glands**. They are usually located in the connective tissue on the posterior surface of the lateral lobes of the thyroid gland (see Fig. 21.14 and Plate 21.4, page 856). However, the number and location may vary. In 2%–10% of individuals, additional glands are associated with the thymus.

Structurally, each parathyroid gland is surrounded by a thin connective tissue capsule that separates it from the thyroid. Septa extend from the capsule into the gland to divide it into poorly defined lobules and to separate the densely packed cords of cells. The connective tissue is more evident in the adult, with the development of fat cells that increase with age and ultimately constitute as much as 60%–70% of the glandular mass.

The glands receive their blood supply from the inferior thyroid arteries or anastomoses between the superior and inferior thyroid arteries. Typical of endocrine glands, rich networks of fenestrated blood capillaries and lymphatic capillaries surround the parenchyma of the parathyroids.

Parathyroid glands develop from the endodermal cells derived from the third and fourth pharyngeal pouches.

Embryologically, the **inferior parathyroid glands** (and the thymus) are derived from the superiorly located third pharyngeal pouch; the **superior parathyroid glands** (and ultimobranchial body) are derived from the fourth pharyngeal pouch. Initially, the inferior parathyroid glands descend with the thymus. Later, the inferior parathyroid glands separate from the thymus and come to lie below the superior parathyroid glands. Failure of these structures to separate results in the atypical association of the parathyroid glands with the thymus in the adult. The principal (chief) cells differentiate during embryonic development and are functionally active in regulating fetal calcium metabolism. The oxyphil cells differentiate later at puberty.

Principal cells and oxyphil cells constitute the epithelial cells of the parathyroid gland.

- **Principal (chief) cells**, the more numerous of the parenchymal cells of the parathyroid (Fig. 21.20), are responsible for regulating the synthesis, storage, and secretion of large amounts of **PTH**. They are small, polygonal cells, with a diameter of 7–10 μm and a centrally located nucleus. The pale-staining, slightly acidophilic cytoplasm contains lipofuscin-containing vesicles, large accumulations of glycogen, and lipid droplets. Small, dense, membrane-limited vesicles seen with the TEM or after using special stains with

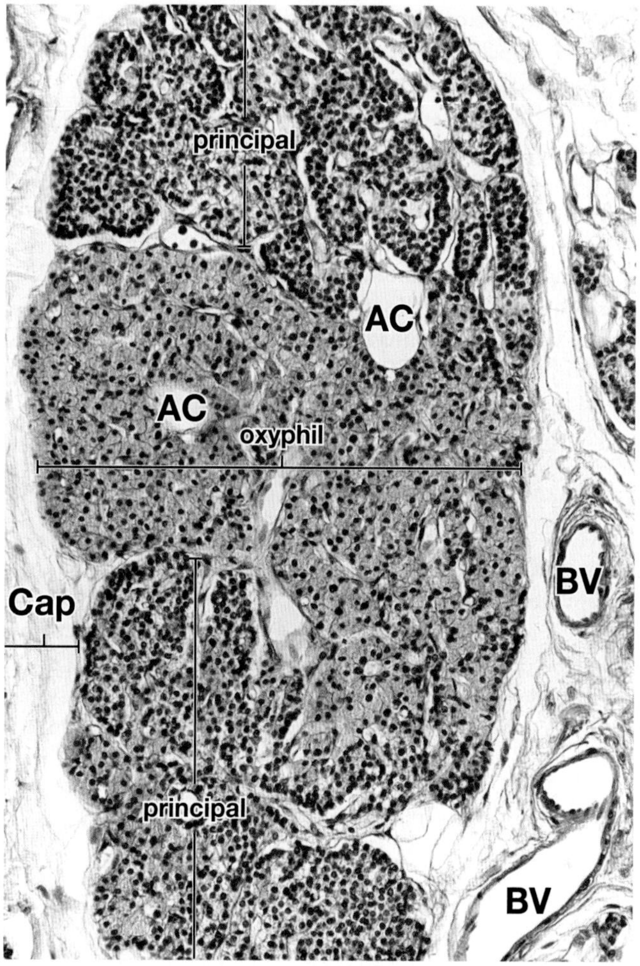

FIGURE 21.20. Photomicrograph of human parathyroid gland. This hematoxylin and eosin (H&E)-stained specimen shows the gland with part of its connective tissue capsule (*Cap*). The blood vessels (*BV*) are located in the connective tissue septum between the lobes of the gland. The principal cells are arranged in two masses (*top* and *bottom*) and are separated by a large cluster of oxyphil cells (*center*). The oxyphil cells are the larger cell type with prominent eosinophilic cytoplasm. They may occur in small groups or larger masses, as seen here. The principal cells are more numerous. They are smaller, have less cytoplasm, and consequently exhibit closer proximity to their nuclei. Adipose cells (*AC*) are present in variable, although limited, numbers. ×175.

TABLE 21.8 Parathyroid Hormone

Hormone	Composition	Source	Major Functions
Parathyroid hormone (PTH)	Polypeptide containing 84 amino acids	Principal (chief) cells[a]	Increases blood calcium level in three ways: (1) promotes calcium release from bone (acting on osteoblasts via RANK-RANKL signaling system, it increases the relative number of osteoclasts); (2) acts on the kidney to stimulate calcium reabsorption by the distal tubule while inhibiting phosphate reabsorption in the proximal tubule; and (3) increases formation of hormonally active 1,25-dihydroxycholecalciferol (1,25-$[OH]_2$ vitamin D_3) in the kidney, which promotes tubular reabsorption of calcium

[a]Some evidence suggests that oxyphil cells, which first appear in the parathyroid gland at about 4–7 years of age and increase in number after puberty, may also produce PTH.

RANK-RANKL, receptor activator of NF-κB–receptor activator NF-κB ligand.

the light microscope are thought to be the storage form of PTH. Principal cells can replicate when they are chronically stimulated by changes in blood calcium levels.

- **Oxyphil cells** constitute a minor portion of the parenchymal cells and are not known to have a secretory role. They are found either singly or in clusters; the cells are more rounded, considerably larger than the principal cells, and have a distinctly acidophilic cytoplasm (see Fig. 21.20). Mitochondria, often with bizarre shapes and sizes, almost fill the cytoplasm and are responsible for the strong acidophilia of these cells. No secretory vesicles and little, if any, rER are present. Cytoplasmic inclusion bodies consist of occasional lysosomes, lipid droplets, and glycogen distributed among the mitochondria.

Parathyroid hormone regulates calcium and phosphate levels in the blood.

The parathyroids function in the regulation of calcium and phosphate levels. **Parathyroid hormone (PTH)** is essential for life. Therefore, care must be taken during **thyroidectomy** to leave some functioning parathyroid tissue. If the glands are totally removed, death will ensue because muscles, including the laryngeal and other respiratory muscles, go into **tetanic contraction** as the blood calcium level falls.

PTH is an 84-amino-acid linear peptide (Table 21.8). It binds to a specific PTH receptor on target cells that interacts with G-protein to activate a second messenger system. PTH release causes the **level of calcium in the blood to increase**. Simultaneously, it reduces the concentration of serum phosphate. Secretion of PTH is regulated by the serum calcium level through a simple feedback system. When parathyroid calcium-sensing receptors on principal cells detect low serum calcium levels, they stimulate secretion of PTH; high levels of serum calcium inhibit its secretion.

PTH functions at several sites:

- **Action on bone tissue**. Until recently, bone resorption had been considered the major effect of PTH action on bone. However, the actions of PTH on bone are more complicated. PTH acts directly and indirectly on several cell types. Receptors for PTH are found on osteoprogenitor cells, osteoblasts, osteocytes, and bone-lining cells. Surprisingly, the bone-resorbing osteoclasts do not have PTH receptors; thus, they are indirectly activated by the RANK-RANKL signaling mechanism of osteoblasts (pages 250-251). The prolonged continuous exposure of PTH increases local RANK production in the osteoblasts and decreases osteoprotegerin (OPG) secretion. These changes then stimulate osteoclast differentiation, which leads to increased bone resorption and release of calcium and phosphates into the extracellular fluid. Briefly, intermittent exposure to PTH

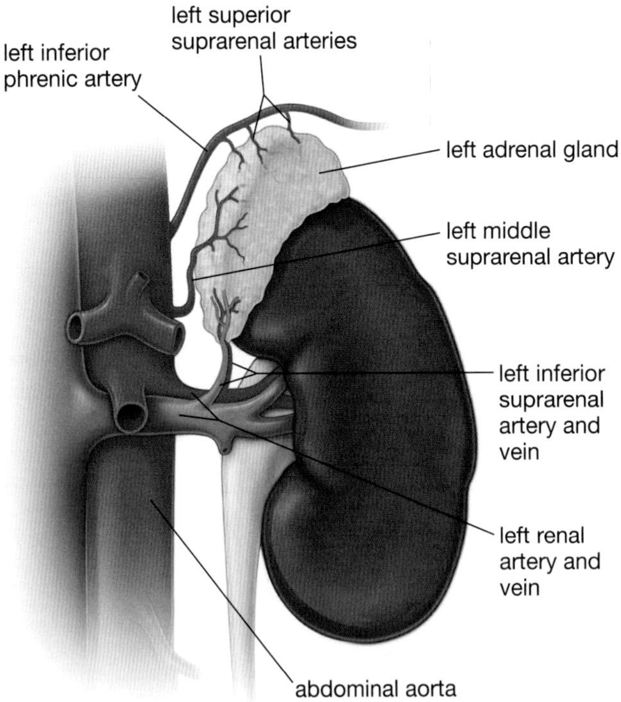

FIGURE 21.21. Topography and blood supply of the adrenal (suprarenal) gland. This drawing shows the location of the left adrenal gland at the superior pole of the left kidney. The perirenal fat has been removed from this image to show blood supply to the organ. Note that the adrenal gland is supplied by three arteries. The middle suprarenal artery originates directly from the aorta, whereas the superior and inferior suprarenal arteries originate from the left inferior phrenic and left renal arteries, respectively. Blood drains into the suprarenal vein, which, on the *left* side, empties into the left renal vein and, on the *right* side, directly into the inferior vena cava.

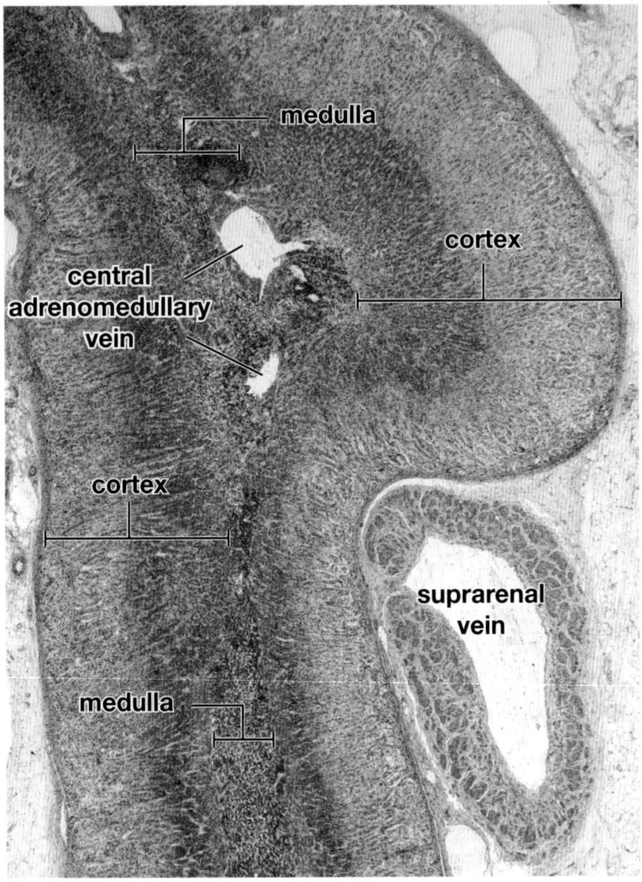

FIGURE 21.22. Photomicrograph of the adrenal gland. This low-power micrograph of a hematoxylin and eosin (H&E)-stained specimen shows the full thickness of the adrenal gland with the cortex seen on both surfaces and a central region containing the medulla. Within the medulla are profiles of the central vein. Note that the deeper portion of the cortex stains darker than the outer portion, a reflection of the washed-out lipid in the zona glomerulosa and outer region of the zona fasciculata. This section also includes a cross section of the adrenal vein, which is characterized by the longitudinally arranged bundles of smooth muscle in its wall. ×20.

increases bone mass through the cAMP/IGF-I pathway in osteocytes and osteoblasts. This anabolic effect of increasing bone mass by intermittent dosing of PTH is utilized in the treatment of osteoporosis (see Folder 8.2 in Chapter 8, Bone, pages 263-264).

- **Kidney excretion of calcium** is decreased by PTH stimulation of tubular reabsorption, thus conserving calcium.
- **Urinary phosphate excretion** is increased by PTH secretion, thus lowering phosphate concentration in the blood and extracellular fluids.
- **Kidney conversion of 25-OH vitamin D_3** to hormonally active **1,25-$(OH)_2$ vitamin D_3** is regulated primarily by PTH, which stimulates the activity of 1α-hydroxylase and increases the production of active hormone.
- **Intestinal absorption of calcium** is increased under the influence of PTH. Vitamin D_3, however, has a greater effect than PTH on the intestinal absorption of calcium.

PTH and calcitonin have reciprocal effects in the regulation of blood calcium levels.

Although **PTH** increases blood calcium levels, the peak increase after its release is not reached for several hours. PTH appears to have a rather slow, long-term homeostatic action. **Calcitonin**, however, rapidly lowers blood calcium levels and has its peak effect in about 1 hour; therefore, it has a rapid, acute homeostatic action.

■ ADRENAL GLANDS

The **adrenal (suprarenal) glands** are paired organs located in the retroperitoneal space of the abdominal cavity. The right gland is flattened and triangular, and the left gland is semilunar in shape. They are both embedded in the perirenal fat at the superior poles of the kidneys (Fig. 21.21). The adrenal glands secrete steroid hormones and catecholamines.

The adrenal glands are covered with a thick connective tissue **capsule** from which trabeculae extend into the parenchyma, carrying blood vessels and nerves. The secretory parenchymal tissue is organized into two distinct regions (Fig. 21.22 and Plate 21.5, page 858):

- The **cortex** is the steroid-secreting portion. It lies beneath the capsule and constitutes nearly 90% of the gland by weight.
- The **medulla** is the catecholamine-secreting portion. It lies deep into the cortex and forms the center of the gland.

Parenchymal cells of the cortex and medulla are of different embryologic origin.

Embryologically, the cortical cells originate from **mesodermal mesenchyme**, whereas the medulla originates from **neural crest** cells that migrate into the developing gland (Fig. 21.23). Although embryologically distinct, the two portions of the adrenal gland are functionally related (see later). The parenchymal cells of the adrenal cortex are controlled in part by the anterior lobe of the pituitary gland and function in regulating metabolism and maintaining normal electrolyte balance (Table 21.9).

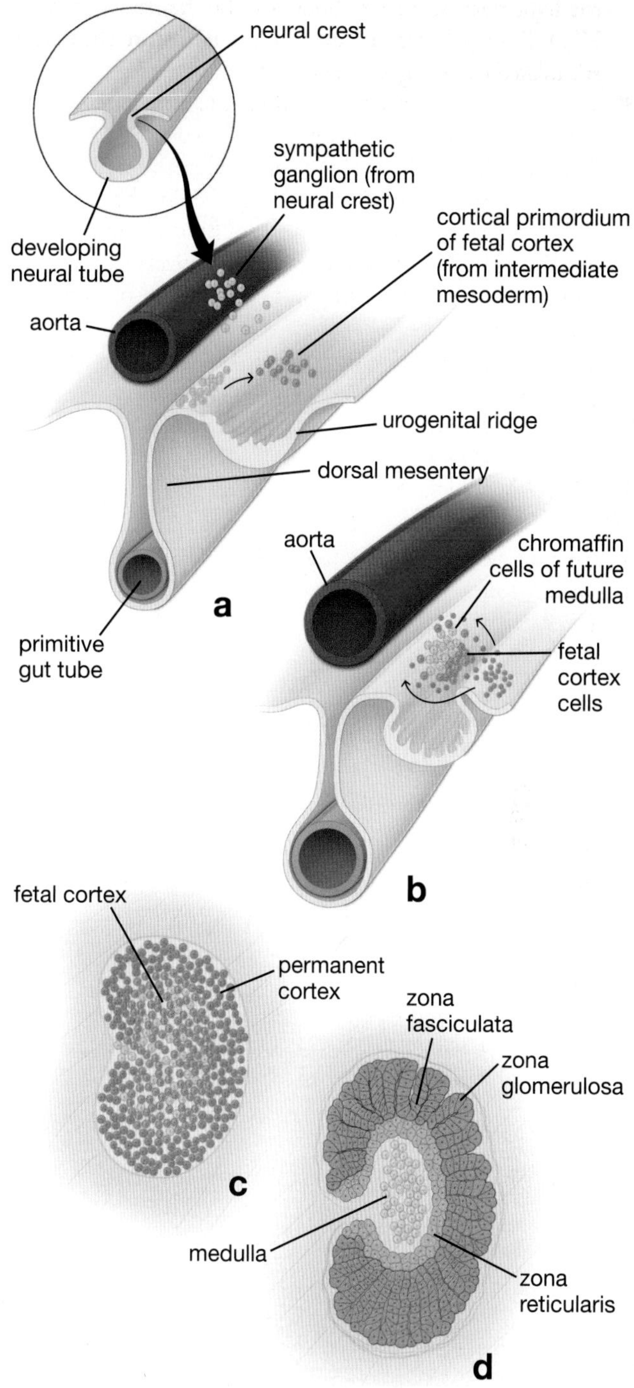

FIGURE 21.23. Development of the adrenal gland. a. In this early stage, the cortex is shown developing from cells of the intermediate mesoderm, and the medulla is shown differentiating from cells in the neural crest and migrating from the neighboring sympathetic ganglion. The cells that form the fetal cortex originate from mesothelial cells located between the root of the dorsal mesentery and the developing urogenital ridges (future gonads). They divide and differentiate into fetal cortex cells. **b.** Mesodermal cells from the fetal cortex surround the cells of the developing medulla. Later, more mesenchymal cells arrive from the mesothelium of the posterior abdominal wall. They surround the original mass of cells containing the fetal cortex cells and chromaffin cells. These cells later give rise to the permanent cortex. **c.** At this stage (about 7 months of development), the fetal cortex occupies about 70% of the cortex. The permanent cortex develops outside the fetal cortex. **d.** The fully developed adrenal cortex is visible at the age of 4 months. The permanent cortex replaces the fetal cortex, which at this age has completely disappeared. Note the fully developed zonation of the permanent cortex.

TABLE 21.9 Hormones of the Adrenal Glands

Hormone	Composition	Source	Major Functions
Adrenal Cortex			
Mineralocorticoids: aldosterone (95% of mineralocorticoid activity in aldosterone)	Steroid hormones (cholesterol derivatives)	Parenchymal cells of the zona glomerulosa	Aid in controlling electrolyte homeostasis (act on distal tubule of kidney to increase sodium reabsorption and decrease potassium reabsorption); function in maintaining the osmotic balance in the urine and in preventing serum acidosis
Glucocorticoids: corticosterone and cortisol (95% of glucocorticoid activity is in cortisol)	Steroid hormones (cholesterol derivatives)	Parenchymal cells of the zona fasciculata (and, to a lesser extent, of the zona reticularis)	Promote normal metabolism, particularly carbohydrate metabolism (increase rate of amino acid transport to live, promote removal of protein from skeletal muscle and its transport to liver, reduce rate of glucose metabolism by cells and stimulate glycogen synthesis by liver, stimulate mobilization of fats from storage deposits for energy use); provide resistance to stress; suppress inflammatory response and some allergic reactions
Gonadocorticoids (adrenal androgens): dehydroepiandrosterone (DHEA), dehydroepiandrosterone sulfate (DHEAS), and androstenedione (produced in both men and women)	Steroid hormones (cholesterol derivatives)	Parenchymal cells of the zona reticularis (and, to a lesser, extent of the zona fasciculata)	As weak androgens, they induce development of axillary and pubic hair at puberty in women; cause masculinizing effect; at normal serum levels, usually their function is insignificant
Adrenal Medulla			
Norepinephrine and epinephrine (in humans, 80% epinephrine)	Catecholamines (amino acid derivatives)	Chromaffin cells	Sympathomimetic (produce effects similar to those induced by the sympathetic division of the autonomic nervous system)[a]; increase heart rate, increase blood pressure, reduce blood flow to viscera and skin; stimulate conversion of glycogen to glucose; increase sweating; induce dilation of bronchioles; increase rate of respiration; decrease digestion; decrease enzyme production by digestive system glands; decrease urine production

[a]The catecholamines influence the activity of glandular epithelium, cardiac muscle, and smooth muscle located in the walls of blood vessels and viscera.

Blood Supply

Each **adrenal gland** is supplied with blood by the **superior**, **middle**, and **inferior suprarenal arteries** and drained by the **suprarenal veins** (see Fig. 21.21). On the left side, the suprarenal vein drains into the left renal vein, whereas on the right side, the suprarenal vein drains directly into the inferior vena cava. These vessels branch before entering the capsule to produce many small arteries that penetrate the capsule. In the capsule, the arteries branch to give rise to three principal patterns of blood distribution (Fig. 21.24). The vessels form a system that consists of the following:

- **Capsular capillaries** that supply the capsule
- **Fenestrated cortical sinusoidal capillaries** that supply the cortex and then drain into the fenestrated medullary capillary sinusoids
- **Medullary arterioles** that traverse the cortex, traveling within the trabeculae, and bring arterial blood to the **medullary capillary sinusoids**

The medulla thus has a dual blood supply: arterial blood from the medullary arterioles and venous blood from the cortical sinusoidal capillaries that have already supplied the cortex. The venules that arise from the cortical and medullary sinusoids drain into the small adrenomedullary collecting veins that join to form the large **central adrenomedullary vein**, which then drains directly as the suprarenal vein into the inferior vena cava on the right side and into the left renal vein on the left side (see Fig. 21.21). In humans, the central adrenomedullary vein and its tributaries are unusual in that they have a tunica media containing conspicuous, longitudinally oriented bundles of smooth muscle cells (Fig. 21.25).

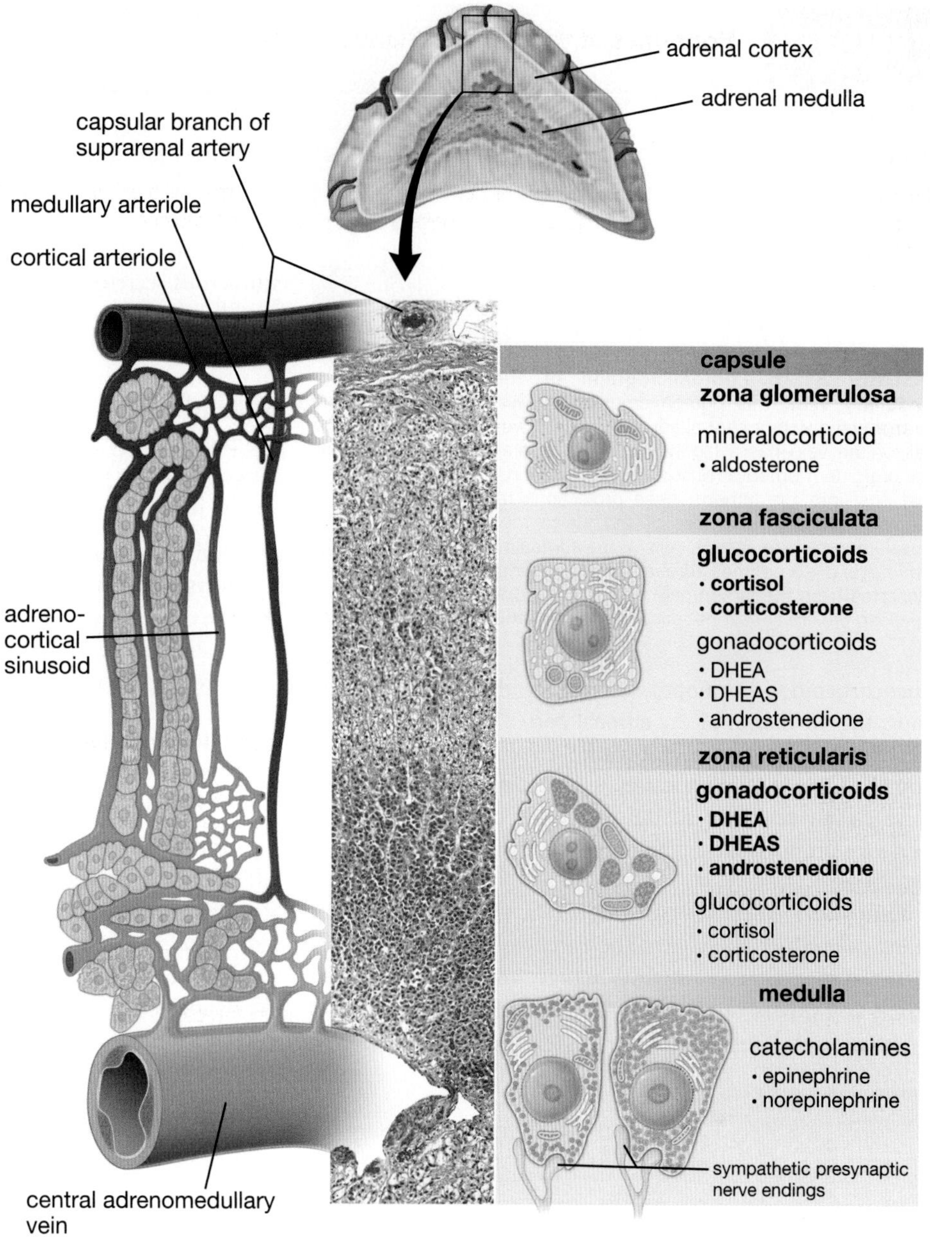

FIGURE 21.24. Organization and blood supply of the human adrenal gland. This diagram shows the blood supply to the adrenal cortex and medulla. The cortical arterioles form a cortical network of capillaries, which drain into a second capillary network in the medulla. The medullary capillary network is formed primarily by the medullary arterioles and drains into the central medullary vein. Adrenal medulla, zones of the cortex, and features of basic cell types and their secretory products are noted. *DHEA*, dehydroepiandrosterone; *DHEAS*, dehydroepiandrosterone sulfate.

Synchronous contraction of longitudinal smooth muscle bundles along the central adrenomedullary vein and its tributaries causes the volume of the adrenal gland to decrease. This decreased volume enhances the efflux of hormones from the adrenal medulla into the circulation, an action comparable to squeezing a wet sponge.

Lymphatic vessels are present in the capsule and the connective tissue around the larger blood vessels in the gland. They also have been found in the parenchyma of the adrenal medulla. The lymphatic vessels have an important role in distributing **chromogranin A**, a secretory product of chromaffin cells. Chromogranin A is a 48-kDa intracellular storage protein complex for epinephrine and norepinephrine and is also a precursor molecule for several regulatory peptides, including vasostatin 1 and 2 (VST I, VST II), pancreastatin (PST), catestatin (CST), and parastatin (PARA). These peptides negatively modulate the neuroendocrine function of the chromaffin cells (autocrine effect) and other hormone-producing cells in distant organs.

Cells of the Adrenal Medulla

Chromaffin cells located in the adrenal medulla are innervated by presynaptic sympathetic neurons.

The central portion of the adrenal gland, the **medulla**, is composed of a parenchyma of large, pale-staining epithelioid cells called **chromaffin cells (medullary cells)**, connective tissue, numerous sinusoidal blood capillaries, and nerves. The chromaffin cells are, in effect, modified neurons (Folder 21.5). Numerous myelinated, presynaptic sympathetic nerve fibers pass directly to the chromaffin cells of the medulla (see Chapter 12, Nerve Tissue, page 421). When nerve impulses carried by the sympathetic fibers reach the catecholamine-secreting chromaffin cells, they release their secretory products. Therefore, chromaffin cells are considered the equivalent of postsynaptic neurons. However, they lack axonal processes. Experimental studies reveal that when chromaffin cells are grown in culture, they extend axon-like processes. However, axonal growth can be inhibited by

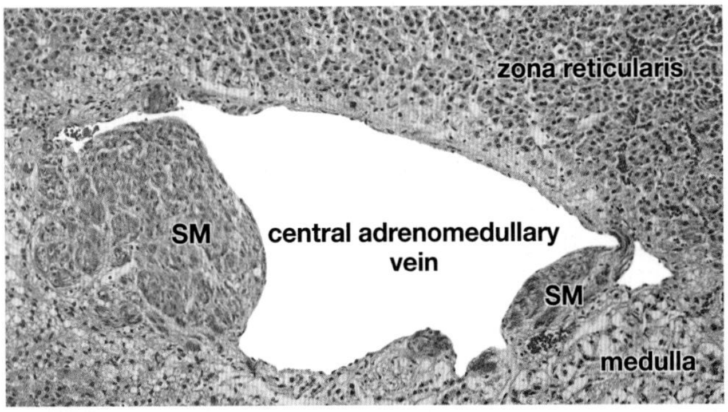

FIGURE 21.25. Photomicrograph of the central adrenomedullary vein. This photomicrograph shows the center of the adrenal gland with a central adrenomedullary vein in the *middle*. The wall of the vein has a highly irregular appearance, containing several prominent smooth muscle (*SM*) projections (also called *muscle cushions*) into the lumen. These projections represent longitudinal bundles of smooth muscles of the tunica media. In areas where muscle bundles are absent, cells of the adrenal medulla (*lower part of the image*) or sometimes adrenal cortex (*upper part of the image*) are separated from the lumen only by a thin layer of tunica intima. Note the close proximity of zona reticularis to the lumen of the vein. ×180.

glucocorticoids—hormones secreted by the adrenal cortex. Thus, the hormones of the adrenal cortex exert control over the morphology of the chromaffin cells and prevent them from forming neural processes. Chromaffin cells, therefore, more closely resemble typical endocrine cells, in that their secretory product enters the bloodstream via the fenestrated capillaries.

Ganglion cells are also present in the medulla. Their axons extend peripherally to the parenchyma of the adrenal cortex to modulate its secretory activity and innervate blood vessels and extend outside the gland to the splanchnic nerves innervating abdominal organs.

Chromaffin cells of the adrenal medulla have a secretory function.

Chromaffin cells are organized in ovoid clusters and short interconnecting cords (Plate 21.6, page 860). The blood capillaries are arranged in intimate relation to the parenchyma. They originate either from the cortical capillaries or, as branches, from the cortical arterioles.

Ultrastructurally, the chromaffin cells are characterized by numerous secretory vesicles with diameters of 100–300 nm, profiles of rER, and a well-developed Golgi apparatus. The secretory material in the vesicles can be stained specifically to demonstrate histochemically that the catecholamines epinephrine and norepinephrine secreted by the chromaffin cells are produced by different cell types (Fig. 21.26). The TEM also reveals two populations of chromaffin cells distinguished by the nature of their membrane-bound vesicles:

- One population of cells contains only large **dense-core vesicles.** These cells secrete norepinephrine.
- The other population of cells **contains vesicles** that are smaller, more homogeneous, and less dense. These cells secrete epinephrine.

Exocytosis of the secretory vesicles is triggered by the release of acetylcholine from presynaptic sympathetic axons that synapse with each chromaffin cell.

Epinephrine and **norepinephrine** account for less than 20% of the contents of the medullary secretory vesicles. The vesicles also contain large amounts of soluble 48-kDa proteins, called **chromogranins**, that appear to impart the density of the vesicles' contents. These proteins, along with ATP and Ca^{2+}, may help bind the low-molecular-weight catecholamines and are released with the hormones during

FOLDER 21.5

CLINICAL CORRELATION: CHROMAFFIN CELLS AND PHEOCHROMOCYTOMA

Chromaffin cells (so named because they react with chromate salts) of the adrenal medulla are part of the amine precursor uptake and decarboxylation (APUD) system of cells. The chromaffin reaction is thought to involve oxidation and polymerization of the catecholamines contained within the secretory vesicles of these cells. Classically, chromaffin cells have been defined as being derived from neuroectoderm, innervated by presynaptic sympathetic nerve fibers, and capable of synthesizing and secreting catecholamines.

A rare tumor derived from chromaffin cells, called **pheochromocytoma**, produces excessive amounts of catecholamines. Because chromaffin cells are also found outside the adrenal medulla in paravertebral and prevertebral sympathetic ganglia and other locations, tumors may arise from outside the adrenal gland. These extra-adrenal pheochromocytomas are called **paragangliomas** because scattered groups of chromaffin cells located among or near the components of the autonomic nervous system (ANS) are called *paraganglia.* Pheochromocytomas may cause episodic symptoms related to the pharmacologic effects of excessive catecholamine secretion and are often described according to the "**rule of 10s**":

- 10% are extra-adrenal (paragangliomas), and of those, 10% reside outside the abdomen.
- 10% occur in children.
- 10% are multiple or bilateral.
- 10% are not associated with hypertension.
- 10% are malignant.
- 10% are familial.
- 10% recur after surgical removal.
- 10% are found incidentally during unrelated imaging studies.

Pheochromocytomas may precipitate life-threatening hypertension, cardiac arrhythmias, anxiety, and fear of impending death. Most pheochromocytomas contain predominantly chromaffin cells that secrete norepinephrine compared with the normal adrenal medulla that comprises about 85% epinephrine-secreting cells. Stimulation of α-adrenergic receptors results in elevated blood pressure, increased cardiac contractility, glycogenolysis, gluconeogenesis, and intestinal relaxation. Stimulation of β-adrenergic receptors results in an increased heart rate and contractility. Surgical resection of the tumor is the treatment of choice. Careful monitoring with α- and β-blockers is required during surgery to prevent hypertensive crises.

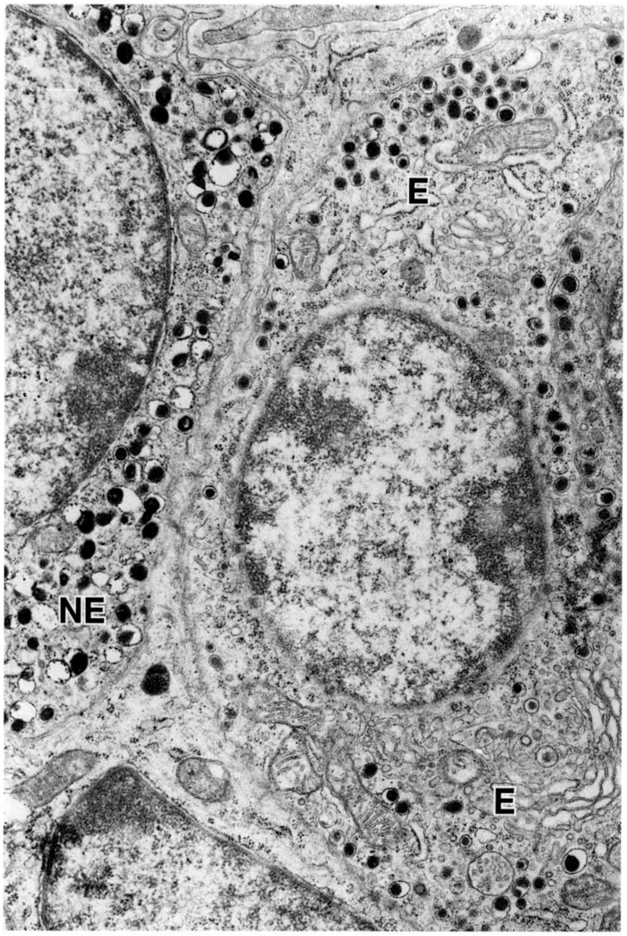

FIGURE 21.26. Electron micrograph of medullary cells. Two types of medullary cells are present. The norepinephrine-secreting cells (*NE*) are identified by their vesicles, which contain a very dense core. The epinephrine-secreting cells (*E*) possess vesicles with less intensely staining granules. ×15,000.

exocytosis. The catecholamines, synthesized in the cytosol, are transported into the vesicles through the action of a magnesium-activated ATPase in the membrane of the vesicle. Drugs such as **reserpine**, which cause depletion of catecholamines from the vesicles, may act by inhibiting this transport mechanism.

Glucocorticoids secreted in the cortex induce the conversion of norepinephrine to epinephrine in chromaffin cells.

Glucocorticoids produced in the adrenal cortex reach the medulla directly through the continuity of the cortical and medullary sinusoidal capillaries. They induce the enzyme that catalyzes the methylation of norepinephrine to produce epinephrine. The nature of the blood flow correlates with regional differences in the distribution of norepinephrine- and epinephrine-containing chromaffin cells. The epinephrine-containing cells are more numerous in areas of the medulla supplied with blood that has passed through the cortical sinusoids and thus contains secreted glucocorticoids. In some species, the norepinephrine-containing cells are more numerous in those regions of the medulla supplied by capillaries derived from the cortical arterioles.

The catecholamines, in concert with the glucocorticoids, prepare the body for the "fight-or-flight" response.

The **sudden release of catecholamines** establishes conditions for maximum use of energy and thus maximum physical effort. Both epinephrine and norepinephrine stimulate glycogenolysis (release glucose into the bloodstream) and mobilization of free fatty acids from adipose tissue. The release of catecholamines also causes an increase in blood pressure, dilation of the coronary blood vessels, vasodilation of vessels supplying skeletal muscle, vasoconstriction of vessels conveying blood to the skin and gut, an increase in heart rate and output, and an increase in the rate and depth of breathing.

Zonation of the Adrenal Cortex

The **adrenal cortex** is divided into three zones on the basis of the arrangement of its cells (Fig. 21.27):

- **Zona glomerulosa**, the narrow outer zone that constitutes up to 15% of the cortical volume
- **Zona fasciculata**, the thick middle zone that constitutes nearly 80% of the cortical volume
- **Zona reticularis**, the inner zone that constitutes only 5%–7% of the cortical volume but is thicker than the glomerulosa because of its more central location

Zona Glomerulosa

The cells of the **zona glomerulosa** *[Lat. glomus, ball]* are arranged in closely packed ovoid clusters and curved columns that are continuous with the cellular cords in the zona fasciculata (see Fig. 21.27a). Cells of the zona glomerulosa are relatively small and columnar or pyramidal (see Fig. 21.24). Their spherical nuclei appear closely packed and stain densely. In humans, some areas of the cortex may lack a recognizable zona glomerulosa. A rich network of fenestrated sinusoidal capillaries surrounds each cell cluster. The cells have abundant sER, multiple Golgi complexes, large mitochondria with shelf-like cristae, free ribosomes, and some rER. Lipid droplets are sparse.

The zona glomerulosa secretes aldosterone, which functions in the control of blood pressure.

The cells of the zona glomerulosa secrete the primary **mineralocorticoid** called **aldosterone**, a compound that functions in the regulation of sodium and potassium homeostasis and water balance. Aldosterone acts on the principal cells in the distal tubules of the nephron in the kidney, the gastric mucosa, and the salivary and sweat glands to stimulate resorption of sodium at these sites as well as to stimulate excretion of potassium by the kidney. Aldosterone is produced from **cholesterol** by a series of enzymatic reactions controlled by angiotensin II (see later). The final step of aldosterone biosynthesis is facilitated by **aldosterone synthase**, which is exclusively expressed in cells of the zona glomerulosa. Cells of the zona glomerulosa lack the enzyme 17α-hydrolase and, therefore, are unable to produce other adrenal steroid hormones, such as cortisol or adrenal androgens.

The renin–angiotensin–aldosterone system provides feedback control for the zona glomerulosa.

The zona glomerulosa is under feedback control of the **renin–angiotensin–aldosterone system (RAAS)**. The **juxtaglomerular cells** in the kidney release **renin** in response to a decrease in blood pressure or a low blood sodium level. Circulating renin catalyzes the conversion of

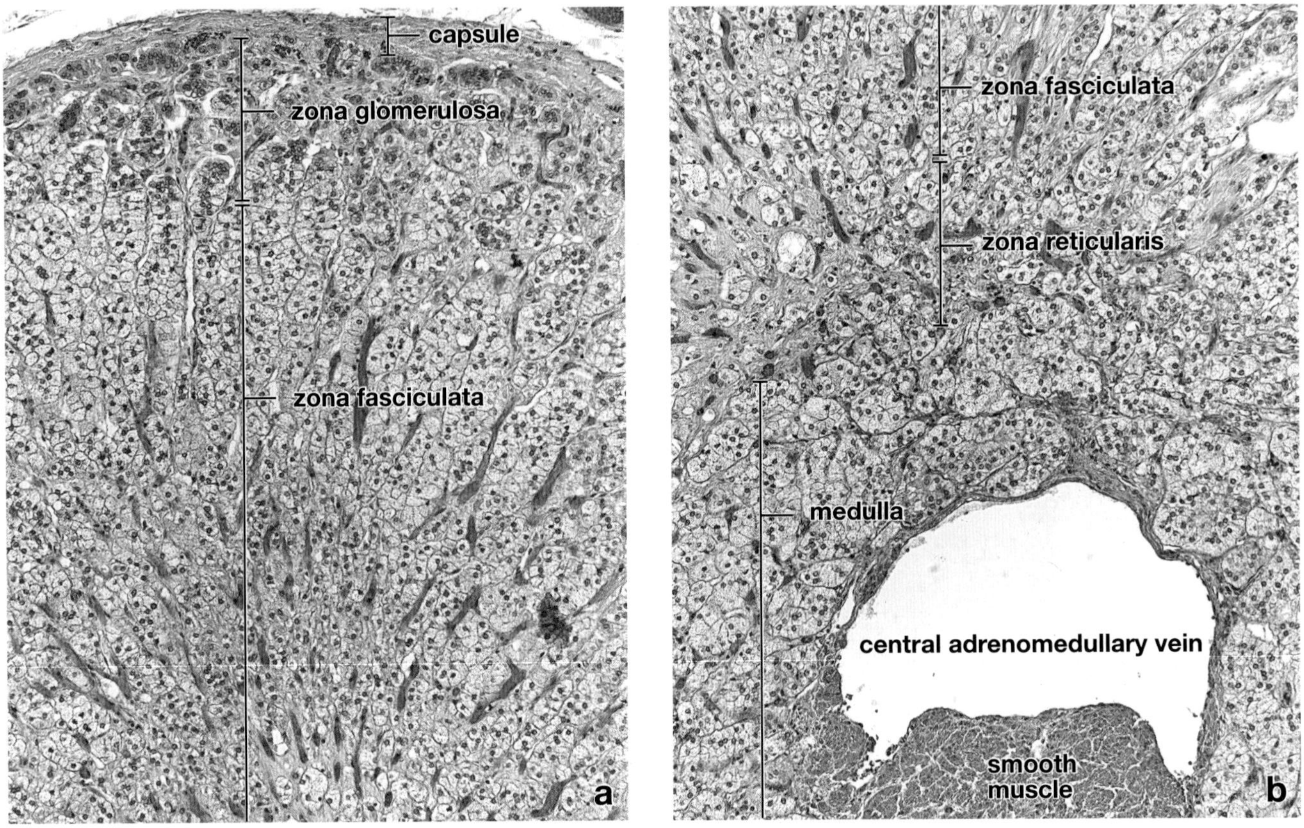

FIGURE 21.27. Photomicrographs of the cortex and medulla of the human adrenal gland. a. This photomicrograph shows a hematoxylin and eosin (H&E)-stained specimen of the outer cortex. It includes the connective tissue capsule, the zona glomerulosa, and the zona fasciculata. Continuous with the zona glomerulosa are the straight cords of cells that characterize the zona fasciculata. Between the cords are the capillaries and the less numerous arterioles. The *red* linear stripes represent capillaries that are engorged with red blood cells. ×120. **b.** The deep parts of the zona fasciculata, zona reticularis, and medulla are shown here. Note that the linear arrays of the cords in the zona fasciculata give way to irregular groups of cells of the zona reticularis. The medulla, in contrast, consists of ovoid groups of cells and short interconnecting cords of cells. A central adrenomedullary vein is also seen here. Note a cross section of the thick longitudinally arranged smooth muscle bundle in part of its wall. ×120.

circulating **angiotensinogen** to **angiotensin I**, which, in turn, is converted by angiotensin-converting enzyme (ACE) in the lung to **angiotensin II**. Angiotensin II then stimulates the cells of the zona glomerulosa to produce and secrete **aldosterone.** As the blood pressure, sodium concentration, and blood volume increase in response to aldosterone, the release of renin from the juxtaglomerular cells is inhibited. Drugs that inhibit ACE in the lung are effective in the treatment of **chronic essential hypertension**.

Zona Fasciculata

The cells of the **zona fasciculata** *[Lat. fascis, bundle]* are large and polyhedral. They are arranged in long straight cords, one or two cells thick, that are separated by sinusoidal capillaries (see Fig. 21.27a). The cells of the zona fasciculata have a lightly staining spherical nucleus. Binucleate cells are common in this zone. TEM studies reveal characteristics typical of steroid-secreting cells, that is, a highly developed sER (more so than cells of the zona glomerulosa) and mitochondria with tubular cristae. They also have a well-developed Golgi apparatus and numerous profiles of rER that may give a slight basophilia to some parts of the cytoplasm (Fig. 21.28). In general, however, the cytoplasm is acidophilic and contains numerous lipid droplets, although it usually appears vacuolated in routine histologic sections because of the extraction of lipid during dehydration. The lipid droplets contain neutral fats, fatty acids, cholesterol, and phospholipids that are precursors for the steroid hormones secreted by these cells.

The principal secretion of the zona fasciculata is glucocorticoids that regulate glucose and fatty acid metabolism.

Cells in the zona fasciculata cannot produce aldosterone because they lack the enzyme aldosterone synthase. However, they do possess two other important enzymes, 17α-hydrolase and 17,20-lyase, to produce **glucocorticoids** and small amounts of **gonadocorticoids (adrenal androgens)**. Glucocorticoids are named for their role in regulating **gluconeogenesis** (glucose synthesis) and **glycogenesis** (glycogen polymerization). One of the major glucocorticoids secreted by the zona fasciculata, **cortisol**, acts on many different cells and tissues to increase the metabolic availability of glucose and fatty acids, both of which are immediate sources of energy. The other glucocorticoid, **corticosterone**, is secreted and circulates in the blood at 10- to 20-fold lower levels than cortisol. Within this broad function, glucocorticoids may have different, even opposite, effects in different tissues:

- In the **liver**, glucocorticoids stimulate conversion of amino acids to glucose, stimulate the polymerization of glucose to glycogen, and promote the uptake of amino acids and fatty acids.

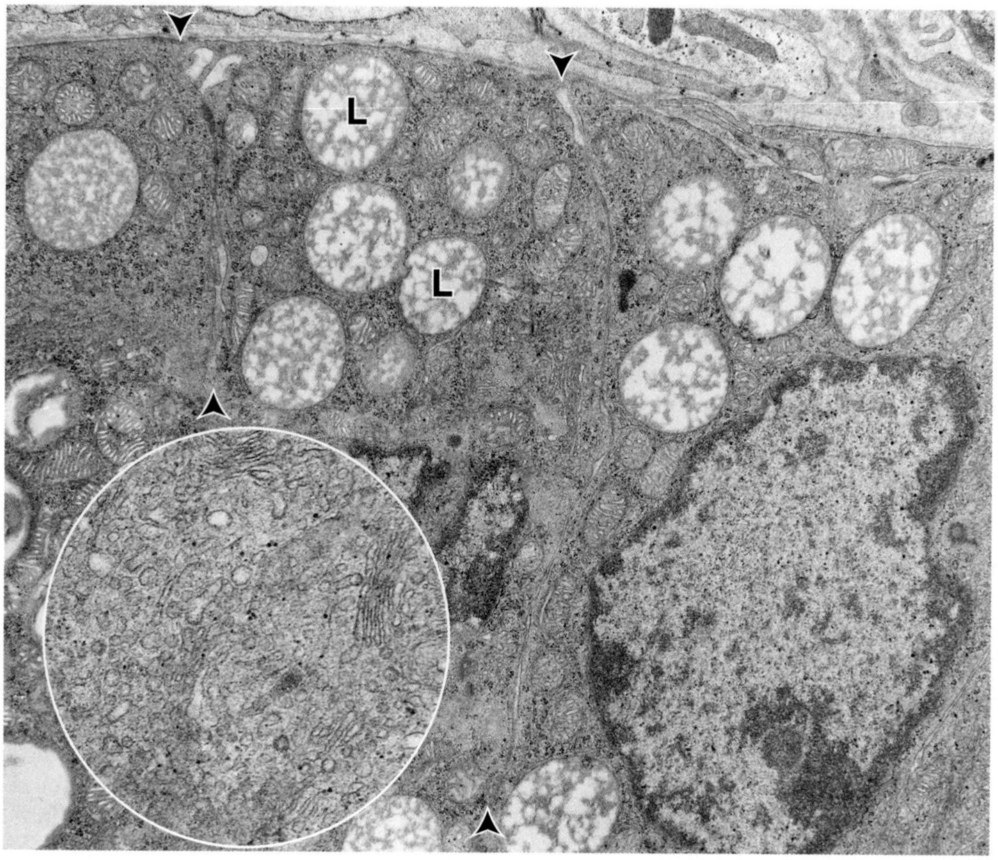

FIGURE 21.28. Electron micrograph of cells in the zona fasciculata. The boundary between adjacent cells of the cord is indicated by the *arrowheads*. Lipid droplets (*L*) are numerous (the lipid has been partially extracted). ×15,000. **Inset.** A higher magnification of an area in the cell at the *top* of the micrograph reveals the extensive sER that is characteristic of steroid-secreting cells. Portions of the Golgi apparatus are also evident. ×40,000. *sER*, smooth-surfaced endoplasmic reticulum.

- In **adipose tissue**, glucocorticoids stimulate the breakdown of lipids to glycerol and free fatty acids.
- In **other tissues**, they reduce the rate of glucose use and promote the oxidation of fatty acids.
- In **cells** such as fibroblasts, they inhibit protein synthesis and even promote protein catabolism to provide amino acids for conversion to glucose in the liver.

Glucocorticoids also depress the immune and inflammatory responses and, as a result of the latter, inhibit wound healing. **Hydrocortisone**, a synthetic form of cortisol, is used in the treatment of **allergies** and **inflammation**. It depresses the inflammatory response by suppressing interleukin-1 (IL-1) and IL-2 production by lymphocytes and macrophages. Glucocorticoids also stimulate destruction of lymphocytes in lymph nodes and inhibit mitosis in transformed lymphoblasts.

ACTH regulates secretion of the zona fasciculata.

The secretion and production of glucocorticoids and sex steroids by the zona fasciculata is under feedback control of the **CRH–ACTH system**. ACTH is necessary for cell growth and maintenance and also stimulates steroid synthesis and increases blood flow through the adrenal gland. In animals, administration of ACTH causes hypertrophy of the zona fasciculata.

Circulating glucocorticoids may act directly on the pituitary gland, but they most commonly exert their feedback control on neurons in the arcuate nucleus of the hypothalamus, causing the release of corticotropin-releasing hormone (CRH) into the hypothalamohypophyseal portal circulation. Evidence also suggests that circulating glucocorticoids and the physiologic effects that they produce stimulate higher brain centers that, in turn, cause the hypothalamic neurons to release CRH.

Zona Reticularis

The cells of the **zona reticularis** *[Lat. rete, net]* are noticeably smaller than those of the zona fasciculata, and their nuclei are more deeply stained (see Fig. 21.24). They are arranged in anastomosing cords separated by fenestrated capillaries. The cells have relatively few lipid droplets. Both light and dark cells are seen. Dark cells have abundant large lipofuscin pigment granules, and deeply staining nuclei are evident. The cells in this zone are small because they have less cytoplasm than the cells in the zona fasciculata; thus, the nuclei appear more closely packed. They exhibit features of steroid-secreting cells, namely, a well-developed sER and numerous elongated mitochondria with tubular cristae, but they have little rER.

The principal secretion of the zona reticularis is gonadocorticoids (adrenal androgens).

The principal secretion of the cells in the zona reticularis consists of **gonadocorticoids (adrenal androgens)**, mostly **dehydroepiandrosterone (DHEA)**, **dehydroepiandrosterone sulfate (DHEAS)**, and **androstenedione**. The cells also secrete some glucocorticoids but in much smaller amounts than those of the zona fasciculata. Here, too, the principal glucocorticoid secreted is **cortisol**.

DHEA and DHEAS are less potent than androgens produced by the gonads, but they do have an effect on the development of **secondary sex characteristics**. In men, adrenal androgens have negligible importance because testosterone produced by the testis is a much more powerful androgen. However, in women, adrenal androgens stimulate the growth of axillary and pubic hair during puberty and adolescence. DHEA can be converted into androstenedione and then more potent androgens, such as testosterone and estrogens in peripheral tissues. The key enzyme that facilitates the conversion of androstenedione to testosterone is **17-ketosteroid reductase (17KSR)**, and this reaction represents a major pathway in testosterone production in women.

The zona reticularis is also regulated by the feedback control of the CRH–ACTH system and atrophies after **hypophysectomy**. Exogenous ACTH maintains the structure and function of the zona reticularis after hypophysectomy.

Fetal Adrenal Gland

The fetal adrenal gland consists of an outer narrow permanent cortex and an inner thick fetal cortex or fetal zone.

Once fully established, the **fetal adrenal gland** is unusual in terms of its organization and its large size relative to other developing organs. The gland arises from mesothelial cells of mesodermal origin located between the root of the mesentery and the developing urogenital ridges (see Fig. 21.23a). The mesodermal cells penetrate the underlying mesenchyme and give rise to a large eosinophilic cell mass that will become the functional fetal cortex (see Fig. 21.23b). Later, a second wave of cells derived from the mesothelium of the posterior abdominal wall surrounds the primary cell mass (see Fig. 21.23b). By the fourth fetal month, the adrenal gland reaches its maximum mass in terms of body weight and is only slightly smaller than the adjacent kidney (see Fig. 21.23c). At term, the adrenal glands are equivalent in size and weight to those of the adult and produce 100–200 mg of steroid compounds per day, about twice that of the adult glands.

The histologic appearance of the fetal adrenal gland is superficially similar to that of the adult adrenal gland. During late fetal life, most of the gland consists of cords of large eosinophilic cells that constitute approximately 80% of its mass. This portion of the gland, referred to as the **fetal cortex** (also called **fetal zone**), arises from the initial mesodermal cell migration. The remainder of the gland is composed of the peripheral layer of small cells with scanty cytoplasm. This portion, referred to as the **permanent cortex**, arises from the secondary mesodermal cell migration. The narrow permanent cortex, when fully established in the embryo, appears similar to the adult zona glomerulosa. The cells are arranged in arched groups that extend into short cords. They, in turn, become continuous with the cords of the underlying fetal zone (Fig. 21.29). In H&E preparations, the cytoplasm of

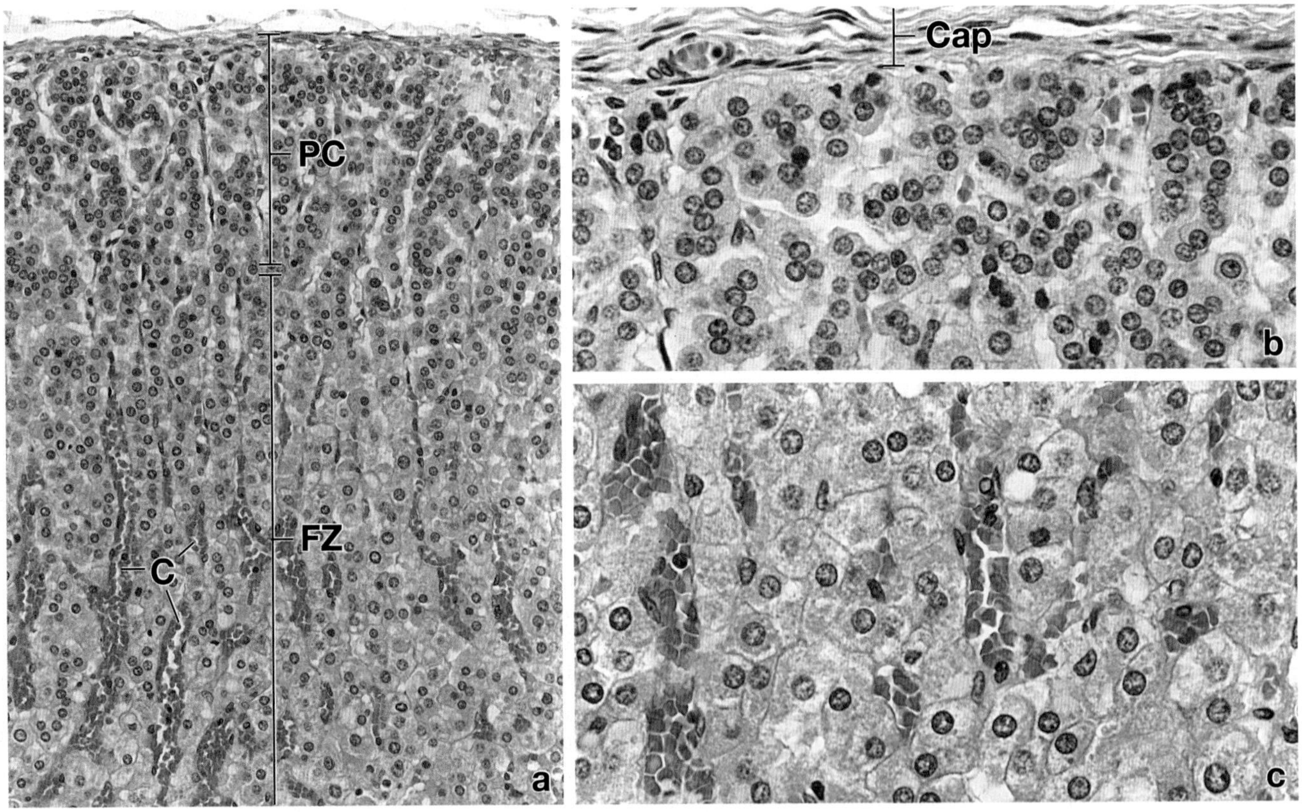

FIGURE 21.29. Photomicrographs of a human fetal adrenal gland. a. Low-power micrograph of a hematoxylin and eosin (H&E)-strained section of a fetal adrenal gland. The permanent cortex (*PC*) is indicated in the *upper portion* of the micrograph. Below is the fetal zone (*FZ*) in which the cells are arranged in anastomosing linear cords. Some of the capillaries (*C*) are engorged with red blood cells, thereby making them more apparent. ×100. **b.** Higher power micrograph of the same specimen showing the capsule (*Cap*) and the underlying permanent cortex. The cells are arranged in arched groups that extend into short cords. Note the close proximity of the nuclei and the small amount of cytoplasm in these cells. ×200. **c.** This micrograph shows the cells of the fetal zone at the same magnification as in **b**. Note the slightly larger size of the nuclei and the considerable amount of cytoplasm in each of the fetal zone cells. Also note the eosinophilia of the cytoplasm, compared with the more basophilic cytoplasm of the cells of the permanent cortex. ×200. (Original specimen courtesy of Dr. William H. Donnelly.)

FOLDER 21.6

FUNCTIONAL CONSIDERATIONS: BIOSYNTHESIS OF ADRENAL HORMONES

Cholesterol is the basic precursor of several steroid hormones, namely, corticosteroids, sex hormones, bile acids, and vitamin D. About one-half of the cholesterol in the body comes from the diet, and the other one-half derives from de novo biosynthesis. Cholesterol synthesis occurs in the cytoplasm and organelles from acetyl-CoA. Biosynthesis in the liver accounts for ~10%, and in the intestines, ~15% of the amount is produced each day. In addition, a small portion of cholesterol is synthesized by the adrenal cortical cells. Both dietary cholesterol and that synthesized de novo are transported within **low-density lipoproteins (LDLs)**. Cholesterol is stored in lipid droplets within the cytoplasm of adrenal cortical cells in the form of cholesterol esters.

Steroid hormones in adrenal glands are synthesized from cholesterol esters by removal of part of the side chain and modifications at specific sites on the remainder of the molecule. The enzymes catalyzing these modifications are located in different zones of the cortex as well as in different cytoplasmic sites within the cells. For instance, cleavage of the cholesterol side chain is catalyzed by **P450-linked side chain cleavage enzyme (P450scc)** or desmolase, which is found only in the mitochondria of steroid-producing cells. This enzyme is induced by angiotensin II in the zona glomerulosa and by ACTH in the zona fasciculata and zona reticularis. The other enzymes necessary for steroid production are located within smooth-surfaced endoplasmic reticulum (sER), cytosol, and mitochondria. Thus, a precursor molecule may move from the sER to a mitochondrion and back again several times before the definitive molecular structure of a given corticosteroid is obtained.

Cholesterol esters removed from cytoplasmic lipid droplets and used in steroid hormone synthesis are quickly replenished from the cholesterol esters contained within LDL carried in the bloodstream. These esters are the primary source of the cholesterol used in corticosteroid synthesis. Under conditions of short-term or prolonged ACTH stimulation, the lipid stores in adrenal cortical cells are recruited for corticosteroid synthesis.

the cells in the permanent cortex exhibits some basophilia; in combination with the closely packed nuclei, this gives this part of the gland a blue appearance, in contrast to the eosinophilic staining of the fetal zone.

With the TEM, the cells of the permanent cortex exhibit small mitochondria with shelf-like cristae, abundant ribosomes, and small Golgi profiles. The cells of the fetal zone, in contrast, are considerably larger and are arranged in irregular cords of varying width. With the TEM, these cells exhibit spherical mitochondria with tubular cristae, small lipid droplets, an extensive sER that accounts for the eosinophilia of the cytoplasm, and multiple Golgi profiles. Collectively, these features are characteristic of steroid-secreting cells.

The development of the fetal adrenal gland is part of a complex process of maturation and preparation of the fetus for extrauterine life.

The fetal adrenal gland **lacks a definitive medulla**. Chromaffin cells are present but are scattered among the cells of the fetal zone and are difficult to recognize in H&E preparations. The chromaffin cells originate from the neural crest (see Fig. 21.23a) and invade the fetal zone at the time of its formation (see Fig. 21.23b). They remain in this location in small, scattered cell clusters during fetal life (see Fig. 21.23c).

The blood supply to both the permanent cortex and the fetal zone is through sinusoidal capillaries that course between the cords and join to form larger venous channels in the center of the gland. Unlike the postnatal adrenal, arterioles are absent in the parenchyma of the fetal adrenal gland.

Functionally, the fetal adrenal gland is under the control of the CRH–ACTH feedback system through the fetal pituitary. It interacts with the placenta to function as a steroid-secreting organ because it lacks certain enzymes necessary for steroid synthesis that are present in the placenta. Similarly, the placenta lacks certain enzymes necessary for steroid synthesis that are present in the fetal adrenal gland. Thus, the fetal adrenal gland is part of a **fetal–placental unit**. Precursor molecules are transported back and forth between the two organs to enable the synthesis of glucocorticoids, aldosterone, androgens, and estrogens.

At birth, the fetal cortex undergoes a rapid involution that reduces the gland within the first postnatal month to about a quarter of its previous size. The permanent cortex grows and matures to form the characteristic zonation of the adult cortex. With the involution and disappearance of the fetal zone cells, the chromaffin cells aggregate to form the medulla. If the adrenal glands fail to develop properly, **congenital adrenal hyperplasia (CAH)** may result. CAH represents a group of autosomal recessive disorders characterized by a deficiency of an enzyme involved in the synthesis of cortisol and/or aldosterone. Deficiency of **enzyme 21-hydroxylase** involved in the aldosterone synthesis pathway is the most common form of CAH, accounting for more than 90% of cases.

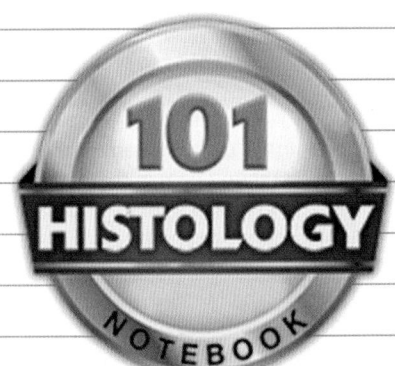

ENDOCRINE ORGANS

OVERVIEW OF THE ENDOCRINE SYSTEM

- The **endocrine system** produces various secretions called **hormones** and hormonally active substances that enter the circulatory system for transport to target cells.
- Hormones and hormonally active substances are divided into three classes of compounds: **peptides** (e.g., insulin, GH, ACTH), **steroids** (gonadal and adrenocortical steroids), and **amino acids** and **arachidonic acid analogs** (e.g., catecholamines, prostaglandins).
- Hormones interact with specific **cell surface receptors** (peptide hormones or catecholamines) or **intracellular receptors** (steroids and thyroid hormones).
- Regulation of hormonal function is controlled by **feedback mechanisms** from the target organs.

PITUITARY GLAND (HYPOPHYSIS)

- The **pituitary gland** is composed of two parts: the **anterior lobe (adenohypophysis)**, which is composed of glandular epithelial tissues, and the **posterior lobe (neurohypophysis)**, which is composed of neural secretory tissue that developed from the neuroectoderm of the CNS.
- The **anterior lobe** of the pituitary gland consists of three parts: **pars distalis**, **pars intermedia**, and **pars tuberalis**, which surrounds the infundibulum.
- The **hypothalamohypophyseal portal system** provides the blood supply to the pituitary gland and serves as the link between the hypothalamus and the pituitary gland.
- **Portal circulation** involves a network of fenestrated capillaries in the infundibulum and median eminence of the hypothalamus as well as hypophyseal portal veins and a secondary network of capillaries in the pars distalis. Circulation carries **releasing hormones** from the hypothalamic neurons to the cells in the pars distalis, where cell secretion is controlled.
- Based on staining reactions of endocrine cell secretory granules, cells in the pars distalis are identified as **basophils** (10%), **acidophils** (40%), and **chromophobes** (50%).
- Based on immunocytochemical reactions, five functional cell types are identified in the pars distalis: **somatotropes (GH cells)** produce **growth hormone (GH; somatotropin)**; **lactotropes (PRL cells, mammotropes)** produce **prolactin (PRL)**; **corticotropes (ACTH cells)** produce **proopiomelanocortin (POMC)**, a precursor molecule of **adrenocorticotropic hormone (ACTH)**; **gonadotropes (FSH and LH cells)** produce both **luteinizing hormone (LH)** and **follicle-stimulating hormone (FSH)**; and **thyrotropes (TSH cells)** produce **thyroid-stimulating hormone (TSH)**.
- The **posterior lobe** of the pituitary gland (pars nervosa and the infundibulum) is an extension of the CNS. It releases hormones produced in the **supraoptic nuclei** (**antidiuretic hormone [ADH]** or **vasopressin**) and **paraventricular nuclei** (**oxytocin**) of the hypothalamus.
- The **hypothalamohypophyseal tract** delivers ADH and oxytocin to the posterior lobe, where they are stored in axon terminals (**Herring bodies**) and released into circulation.

PINEAL GLAND

- The **pineal gland** is a neuroendocrine gland that develops from the neuroectoderm and remains attached to the brain. Because the pineal gland has connections with the eye via the retinohypothalamic tract, it is an important regulator of **circadian rhythm**.
- The pineal gland contains two types of parenchymal cells: **pinealocytes** that secrete **melatonin** and supporting **interstitial (glial) cells**. It also possesses characteristic calcified concretions called **corpora arenacea** or **brain sand**.

THYROID GLAND

- The **thyroid gland** is located in the neck and develops from the endodermal lining of the floor of the primitive pharynx.
- The thyroid gland consists mainly of **thyroid follicles**, which generally are formed from simple cuboidal **follicular epithelium**. The lumen of the follicles is filled with a gel-like mass called **colloid**, which contains thyroglobulin, an inactive storage form of thyroid hormones.
- Follicular epithelium contains two types of cells: **follicular cells** that produce thyroid hormones T_4 and T_3 and **parafollicular cells** that produce calcitonin.
- **Synthesis** of T_4 and T_3 takes place in follicular cells and the lumen of the follicle. It involves a series of steps, from the synthesis of thyroglobulin, to the uptake and oxidation of iodide, to iodination of the thyroglobulin to form T_4 and T_3.
- In response to **TSH stimulation**, follicular cells resorb colloid and transport T_4 and T_3 into circulation.

PARATHYROID GLANDS

- The **parathyroid glands** (two pairs) are located on the posterior surface of the thyroid gland. They develop from the third and fourth pharyngeal pouches.
- Parathyroid glands consist of two major epithelial cells: **principal cells**, which are the most numerous and secrete **parathyroid hormone (PTH)**, and **oxyphil cells**.
- **PTH** regulates calcium and phosphate levels in the blood. It binds to the PTH receptors on target cells and increases the Ca^{2+} level in the blood.

ADRENAL (SUPRARENAL) GLANDS

- The **adrenal glands** are paired triangular organs embedded in the perirenal fat at the upper poles of the kidneys.
- Adrenal glands are organized into two distinct regions: the **cortex**, a steroid-secreting portion that developed from the mesoderm, and the **medulla**, a catecholamine-secreting portion that developed from neural crest cells.
- During development, the **fetal adrenal gland** is composed of the fetal cortex without a definitive medulla.
- The **adrenal medulla** contains chromaffin cells that synthesize epinephrine and norepinephrine to prepare the body for a "fight-or-flight" response.
- The **adrenal cortex** is divided into three zones: **zona glomerulosa** (outer); **zona fasciculata** (thick middle); and **zona reticularis** (inner), which communicates with the medulla.
- **Zona glomerulosa** cells form ovoid clusters and produce **mineralocorticoids** (e.g., aldosterone). The **renin–angiotensin–aldosterone system** provides the feedback mechanism to control secretion of the zona glomerulosa cells.
- **Zona fasciculata** cells are arranged in long straight cords and produce **glucocorticoids** (e.g., cortisol) that regulate gluconeogenesis (glucose synthesis) and glycogenesis (glycogen polymerization). ACTH regulates secretion of the zona fasciculata cells.
- **Zona reticularis** cells are arranged in anastomosing cords separated by fenestrated capillaries and produce weak **androgens** (mostly DHEA). ACTH regulates secretion of the zona reticularis cells.

PLATE 21.1 ■ PITUITARY I

The **pituitary gland** is located at the base of the brain and rests in a depression of the sphenoid bone called the *sella turcica* on the floor of the middle cranial fossa. It is connected by a short stalk to the hypothalamus. Although joined to the brain, only the **posterior lobe** of the gland, the **neurohypophysis**, develops from neuroectoderm. The larger **anterior lobe** of the gland, the **adenohypophysis**, develops from oropharyngeal ectoderm as a diverticulum of the buccal epithelium, called the **Rathke pouch**.

The anterior lobe regulates other endocrine glands. It is composed of clumps and cords of epithelioid cells, separated by large-diameter fenestrated capillaries. The posterior lobe is a nerve tract whose terminals store and release secretory products synthesized by their cell bodies located in the **supraoptic** and **paraventricular nuclei**. The secretions contain either **oxytocin** or **antidiuretic hormone (ADH)**. Other neurons from the hypothalamus release secretions into the fenestrated capillaries of the infundibulum, the first capillary bed of the **hypophyseal portal system** that carries blood to the fenestrated capillaries of the anterior lobe. These hypothalamic secretions regulate the activity of the anterior lobe of the pituitary gland.

Pituitary, human, hematoxylin and eosin (H&E) ×50.

This specimen is a sagittal section of the pituitary gland. The **posterior lobe** of the gland is delineated by the *dashed line* (indicated by *arrows*) that separates it from the anterior lobe. The **pars nervosa** (*PN*) is the expanded portion of the posterior lobe that is continuous with the infundibulum. The **pars tuberalis** (*PT*) of the **anterior lobe** is located around the infundibular stem but may cover the pars nervosa to a variable extent. The **pars intermedia** (*PI*) is a narrow band of tissue that lies between the **pars distalis** (*PD*) and the pars nervosa. It borders a small cleft (*Cl*) that constitutes the remains of the lumen of the Rathke pouch. The pars distalis, the anterior lobe of the gland, is its largest part. It contains a variety of cell types that are not uniformly distributed. This accounts for differences in staining (light- and dark-staining areas) that are seen throughout the pars distalis. The pituitary gland contains a connective tissue capsule (*Caps*) that separates the gland from the surrounding meninges.

Each of the components of the anterior lobe (i.e., the pars distalis, pars tuberalis, and pars intermedia), when examined at higher magnification, exhibit features at the cellular level that aid in their identification. These features are described in the following figures as well as those in Plate 21.2 (page 852).

Pars distalis, pituitary, human, H&E ×375.

This photomicrograph shows a region of the **pars distalis** of the anterior lobe that is rich in **acidophils** (*A*). **Basophils** (*B*) are present in this area in lesser numbers. The acidophils are readily identified by the acidophilic staining of their cytoplasm, in contrast to the basophils whose cytoplasm is clearly basophilic. **Chromophobes** (*C*) are also very numerous in this field. The cytoplasm stains poorly in contrast to that of the acidophils and basophils. The cells are arranged in cords and clumps, between which are capillaries (*Cap*), some of which can be recognized, but most are in a collapsed state and difficult to visualize at this magnification.

Pars distalis, pituitary, human, H&E ×375.

This photomicrograph shows a region of the **pars distalis** of the anterior lobe that is rich in basophils (*B*). At this particular site, there are no recognizable acidophils (at other sites, it is possible to find a more equal distribution of acidophils and basophils, although, typically, one cell type outnumbers the other in a given region). **Chromophobes** (*C*) are also relatively numerous at this site. In this particular region, the chromophobe nuclei are readily apparent, but the cytoplasm of the cells is difficult to discern.

Pars intermedia, pituitary, human, periodic acid–Schiff (PAS)/aniline blue black ×380.

This photomicrograph shows a small portion of the **pars distalis** (*PD*); the remainder reveals the **pars intermedia** (*PI*) of the anterior lobe. The pars distalis shown here contains numerous capillaries filled with red blood cells, thus producing a bright red appearance. The pars intermedia contains a number of small cysts (*Cy*). The cells that make up the pars intermedia, which is relatively small in humans, consist of small basophils and chromophobes. The basophils have taken up the blue stain, thus making them prominent. To the extreme *right* is a less cellular area, the **pars nervosa** (*PN*).

A, acidophils
B, basophils
C, chromophobes
Cap, capillaries
Caps, capsule
Cl, cleft
Cy, cysts
PD, pars distalis
PI, pars intermedia
PN, pars nervosa
PT, pars tuberalis

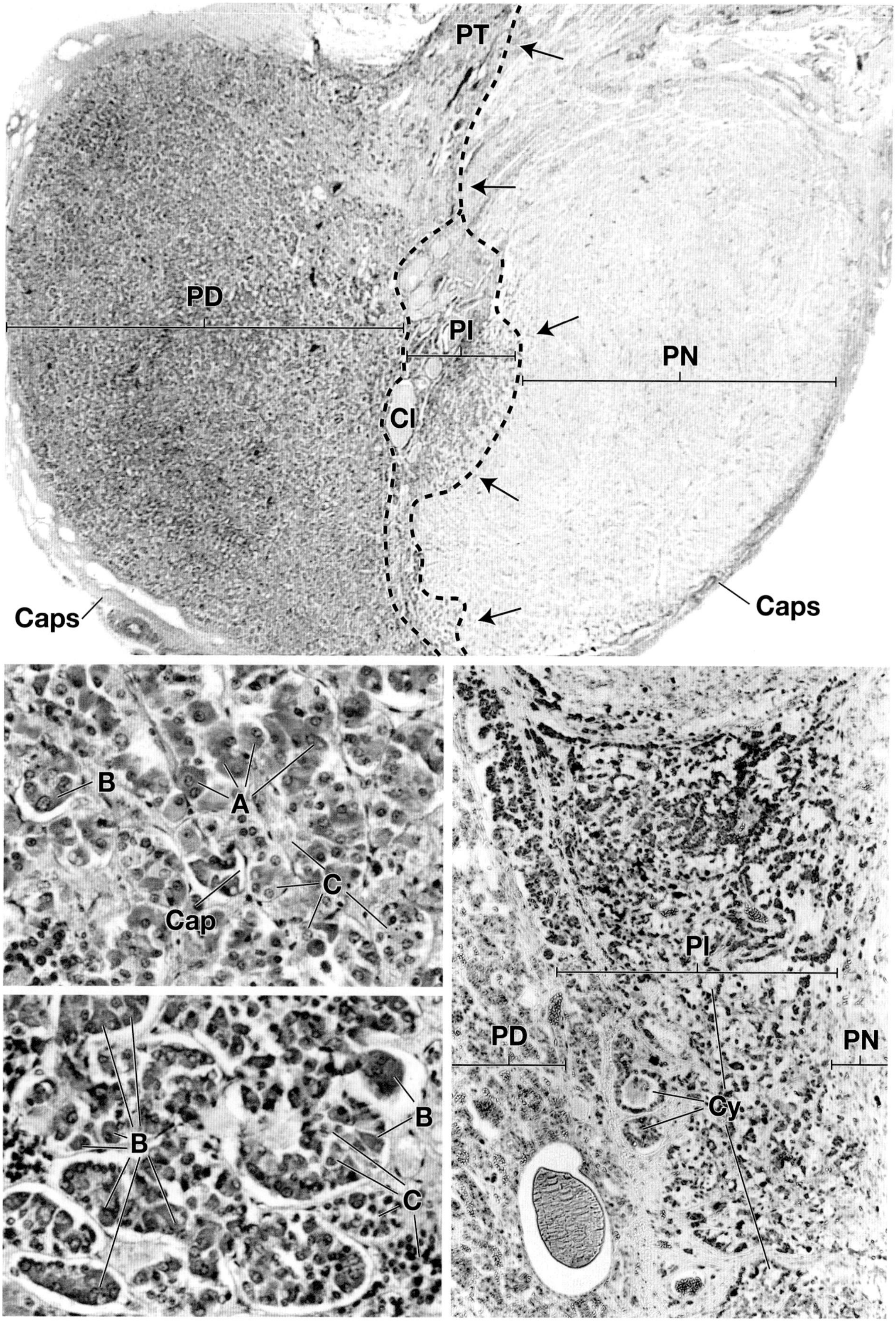
PT
PD
PI
PN
Cl
Caps
Caps
B
A
C
Cap
B
B
C
PI
PD
PN
Cy

PLATE 21.2 ■ PITUITARY II

The parenchyma of the **pars distalis** consists of two general cell types: **chromophobes** and **chromophils**. Chromophobes stain poorly; chromophils stain well. Chromophils are further subdivided into **acidophils** and **basophils**. Basophils stain with basic dyes or hematoxylin, whereas the cytoplasm of the acidophil stains with acid dyes such as eosin. The cytoplasm of basophils also stains with the periodic acid–Schiff (PAS) reaction because of the glycoprotein in its secretory granules.

Acidophils can be further subdivided into two groups on the basis of special cytochemical and ultrastructural features. One group, called **somatotropes**, produces the growth hormone, *somatotropic hormone* (STH); the other group of acidophils, called **lactotropes**, produces *prolactin* (PRL).

The groups of basophils can also be distinguished with the electron microscope and with special cytochemical procedures. One group of **thyrotropes** produces *thyroid-stimulating hormone* (TSH); another group of **gonadotropes** produces the gonadotropic hormones *follicle-stimulating hormone* (FSH), and *luteinizing hormone* (LH); and a third group of **corticotropes** produces *adrenocorticotropic hormone* (ACTH) and *lipotropic hormone* (LPH).

Chromophobes are also a heterogeneous group of cells. Many are considered to be depleted acidophils or basophils.

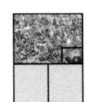

Pars distalis, pituitary, human, Mallory trichrome ×360; inset ×1,200.

This photomicrograph of the pars distalis is from an area where there is an almost equal distribution of **acidophils** (*A*) and **basophils** (*B*). The clumps and cords of cells are delineated by strands of connective tissue (*stained blue*) that surround them. A number of engorged capillaries (*Cap*) containing red blood cells (*stained yellow*) are also seen. The acidophil's cytoplasm in this preparation stains a reddish or rust color. The basophils stain a *reddish blue to deep blue*, and the **chromophobes** (*C*) exhibit a *pale blue* color. The *inset* shows the three general cell types at higher magnification. The secretory granules of the acidophils (*A*) and basophils (*B*) are just discernible. It is the granules that stain and provide the overall coloration to the two cell types. In contrast, the chromophobe (*C*) lacks granules and simply reveals a *pale blue* background color.

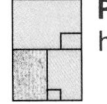

Pars nervosa, pituitary, human, hematoxylin and eosin (H&E) ×325.

The **pars nervosa** of the posterior lobe seen here contains cells called *pituicytes,* and unmyelinated nerve fibers form the supraoptic and paraventricular nuclei of the hypothalamus. The **pituicytes** (*P*) are comparable with neuroglial cells of the central nervous system. The nuclei are round to oval; the cytoplasm extends from the nuclear region of the cell as long processes. In H&E preparations such as this, the cytoplasm of the pituicyte cannot be distinguished from the unmyelinated nerve fibers. The hormones of the posterior lobe, oxytocin, and antidiuretic hormone (ADH; also called *vasopressin*) are formed in the hypothalamic nuclei and pass via the fibers of the hypothalamohypophyseal tract to the posterior lobe, where they are stored in the expanded nerve terminal portion of the nerve fibers. The stored neurosecretory material appears as **Herring bodies** (*HB*). In H&E preparations, the Herring bodies simply appear as small islands of eosin-stained substance. Interspersed among the nerve fibers are capillaries (*Cap*).

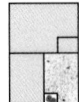

Pars nervosa, pituitary, human, periodic acid–Schiff (PAS)/aniline blue black ×250; inset ×700.

In this specimen from the pars nervosa, the *aniline blue* has stained the nuclei of the **pituicytes** (*P*); the nerve fibers have taken up some of the stains to give a *light blue* background. With this staining technique, the **Herring bodies** (*HB*) appear as *dark black islands*. The *inset* shows a Herring body near the *bottom* of the micrograph at high magnification. The granular texture of the Herring body as seen here is a reflection of the accumulated secretory granules in the nerve terminals. Also of note in this specimen are the capillaries (*Cap*), which are prominent as a result of the contrasting red staining of the red blood cells within them.

A, acidophils
B, basophils
C, chromophobes
Cap, capillaries
HB, Herring bodies
P, pituicytes

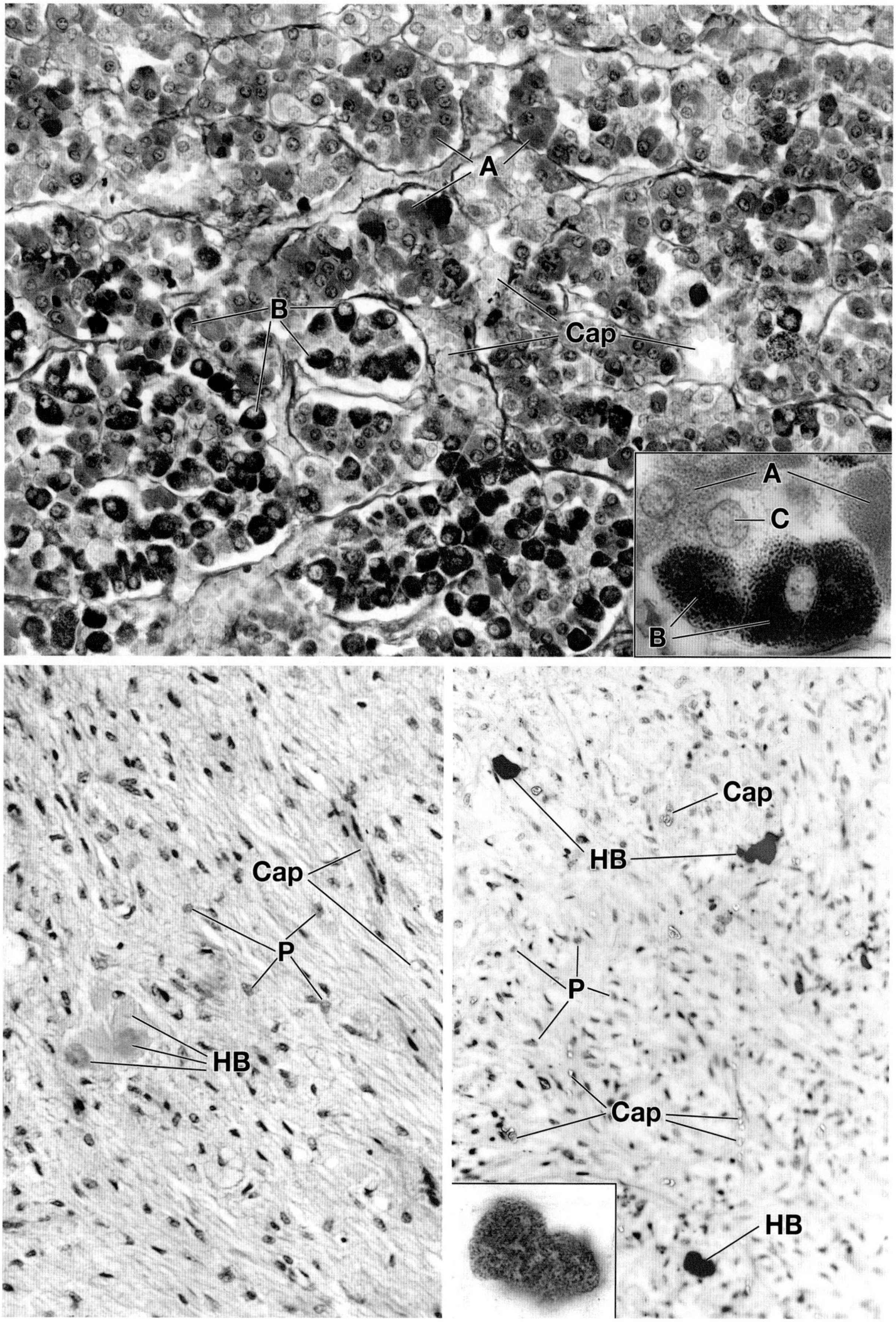
A
B
Cap
A
C
B
Cap
P
HB
Cap
HB
P
Cap
HB

PLATE 21.3 ■ PINEAL GLAND

The **pineal gland** (*pineal body, epiphysis cerebri*) is located in the brain above the superior colliculi. It develops from neuroectoderm but, in the adult, bears little resemblance to nerve tissue.

Two cell types have been described within the pineal gland: **pinealocytes (parenchymal) cells** and **glial cells**. The full extent of these cells cannot be appreciated without the application of special staining methods. These would show that the glial cells and the pinealocytes have processes that are expanded at their periphery. The pinealocytes are more numerous. In a hematoxylin and eosin (H&E) preparation, the nuclei of the pinealocytes are pale staining. The nuclei of the glial cells, on the other hand, are smaller and stain more intensely.

The secretion of the pineal gland has an antigonadal effect: It decreases the production of gonadal steroids. For example, hypogenitalism has been reported with pineal tumors that consist chiefly of pinealocytes, whereas sexual precocity (puberty that occurs at an unusually early age) is associated with glial cell tumors (presumably, the pinealocytes have been destroyed). In addition, experiments with animals indicate that the pineal gland has a neuroendocrine function, whereby the pineal gland serves as an intermediary that relates endocrine function (particularly gonadal function) to cycles of light and dark. The external photic stimuli reach the pineal gland via optical pathways that connect with the superior cervical ganglion. In turn, the superior cervical ganglion sends postganglionic nerve fibers to the pineal gland. The pineal gland has a role in adjusting to sudden changes in day length, such as those experienced by travelers who suffer from jet lag, and a role in regulating emotional responses to reduced day length during winter in temperate and subarctic zones (seasonal affective disorder [SAD]).

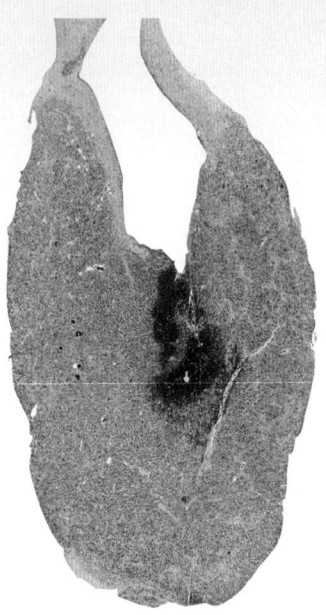

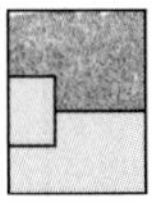

Pineal gland, human, H&E ×180.

The pineal gland is surrounded by a very thin **capsule** (*Cap*) that is formed by the pia mater. Connective tissue trabeculae (*CT*) extend from the capsule into the substance of the gland dividing it into lobules. The **lobules** (*L*) appear often as indistinct groups of cells of varying size surrounded by the connective tissue. Blood vessels, generally small arteries (*A*) and veins (*V*), course through the connective tissue. The arteries give rise to capillaries that surround and penetrate the lobules to supply the parenchyma of the gland. In this specimen and even at this low magnification, the capillaries (*C*) are prominent as a consequence of the red blood cells present in their lumina.

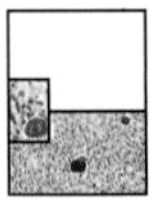

Pineal gland, human, H&E ×360; inset ×700.

This micrograph shows at higher magnification the parenchyma of the pineal gland as well as a component called **brain sand** (*BS*) or **corpora arenacea**. When viewed at even higher magnification, the corpora arenacea are seen to have an indistinct lamellated structure. Typically, they stain heavily with hematoxylin. The presence of these structures is an identifying feature of the pineal gland. A careful examination of the cells within the gland at the light microscopic level reveals two specific cell types. One cell type represents the pinealocytes (or chief cells of the pineal gland), which are by far the most numerous. Pinealocytes are modified neurons. Their nuclei are spherical and are relatively lightly stained because of the amount of euchromatin that they contain. The second cell type is the interstitial cell or glial cell that constitutes a relatively small percentage of the cells in the gland. Their nuclei are smaller and more elongated than those of the pinealocytes. The *inset* reveals several **glial cells** (*G*) that can be identified by their more densely staining nuclei. The majority of the nuclei of the other cells seen here belong to pinealocytes. Also seen in the **inset** are several fibroblasts (*F*) that are present within a trabecula.

A, artery	**Cap,** capsule	**G,** glial cell
BS, brain sand	**CT,** connective tissue	**L,** lobule
C, capillary	**F,** fibroblast	**V,** vein

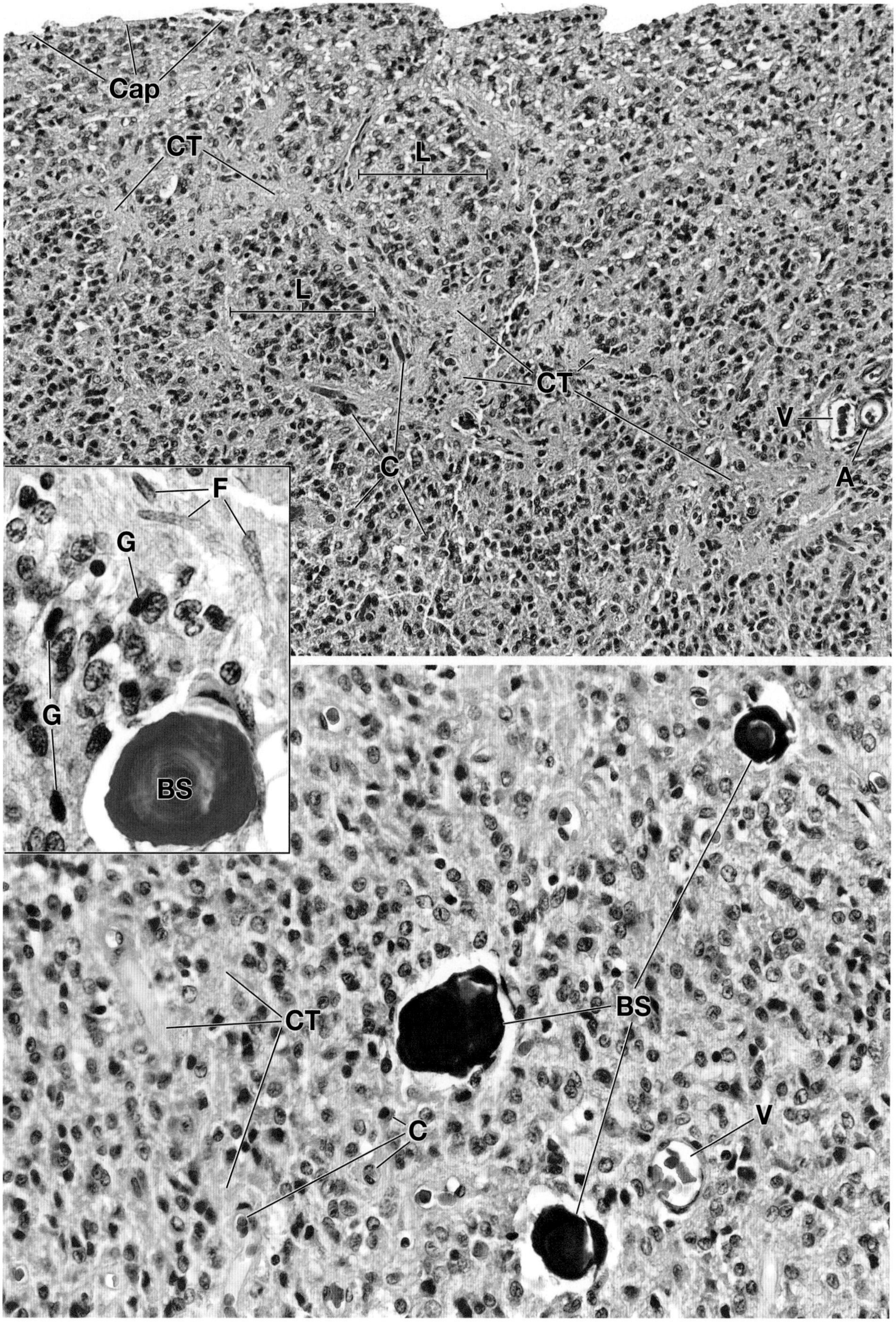
Cap
CT
L
L
CT
V
C
A
F
G
G
BS
BS
CT
C
V

PLATE 21.4 ■ PARATHYROID AND THYROID GLANDS

The **parathyroid glands** are usually four in number. Each is surrounded by a capsule and lies on or is partially embedded in the thyroid gland. Connective tissue trabeculae extend from the capsule into the substance of the gland.

The **parathyroid glands** elaborate a hormone that influences calcium and bone metabolism. Injection of parathyroid hormone into laboratory animals results in the release of calcium from bone by the action of osteocytes (osteocytic osteolysis) and osteoclasts. Removal of the parathyroid glands results in a rapid drop in blood calcium levels.

The **thyroid gland** is located in the neck in close relation to the upper part of the trachea and the lower part of the larynx. It consists of two lateral lobes that are joined by a narrow isthmus. The follicle, which consists of a single layer of cuboidal or low columnar epithelium surrounding a colloid-filled space, is the functional unit of the thyroid gland. A rich capillary network is present in the connective tissue that separates the follicles. The connective tissue also contains lymphatic capillaries.

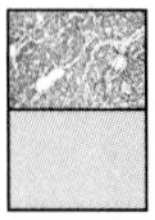

Parathyroid gland, human, hematoxylin and eosin (H&E) ×320.

As seen here, the larger blood vessels are associated with the trabeculae (*BV*) and, occasionally, adipose cells (*A*). The parenchyma of the parathyroid glands appears as cords or sheets of cells separated by capillaries and delicate connective tissue septa.

Two parenchymal cell types can be distinguished in routine H&E sections: chief cells (principal cells) and oxyphil cells. The **chief cells** (*CC*) are more numerous. They contain a spherical nucleus surrounded by a small amount of cytoplasm. **Oxyphil cells** (*OC*) are less numerous. They are conspicuously larger than chief cells but have a slightly smaller and more intensely staining nucleus. Their cytoplasm stains with eosin, and the boundaries between the cells are usually well marked. Moreover, the oxyphils are arranged in groups of variable size that appear scattered about in a much larger field of chief cells. Even with low magnification, it is often possible to identify clusters of oxyphil cells because a unit area contains fewer nuclei than a comparable unit area of chief cells, as is clearly evident in this figure. Oxyphil cells appear during the end of the first decade of life and become more numerous around puberty. A subsequent increase may be seen in older individuals.

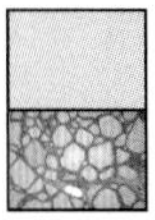

Thyroid gland, human, H&E ×240.

A histologic section of the thyroid gland is shown here. The **thyroid follicles** (*F*) vary somewhat in size and shape and appear closely packed. The homogeneous mass in the center of each follicle is the colloid. The follicular cells of the gland appear to form a simple cuboidal epithelium enclosing the colloid. Careful examination of the apical surface of follicular cells reveals small vacuoles, an indication of colloid resorption. Although the individual cells are difficult to distinguish at this magnification, the nuclei of the cells serve as an indication of their location and arrangement. The thyroid is well vascularized: Larger **blood vessels** (*BV*) are found in the connective tissue (*CT*), and the capillary network surrounds follicles.

This specimen has few areas of large groups of cells with nuclei that are of the same size, shape, and staining characteristics as follicular cells. These areas represent **tangentially sectioned follicles** (*tsF*).

A, adipose cells
BV, blood vessels
CC, chief cells
CT, connective tissue
F, follicles
OC, oxyphil cells
tsF, tangentially sectioned follicle

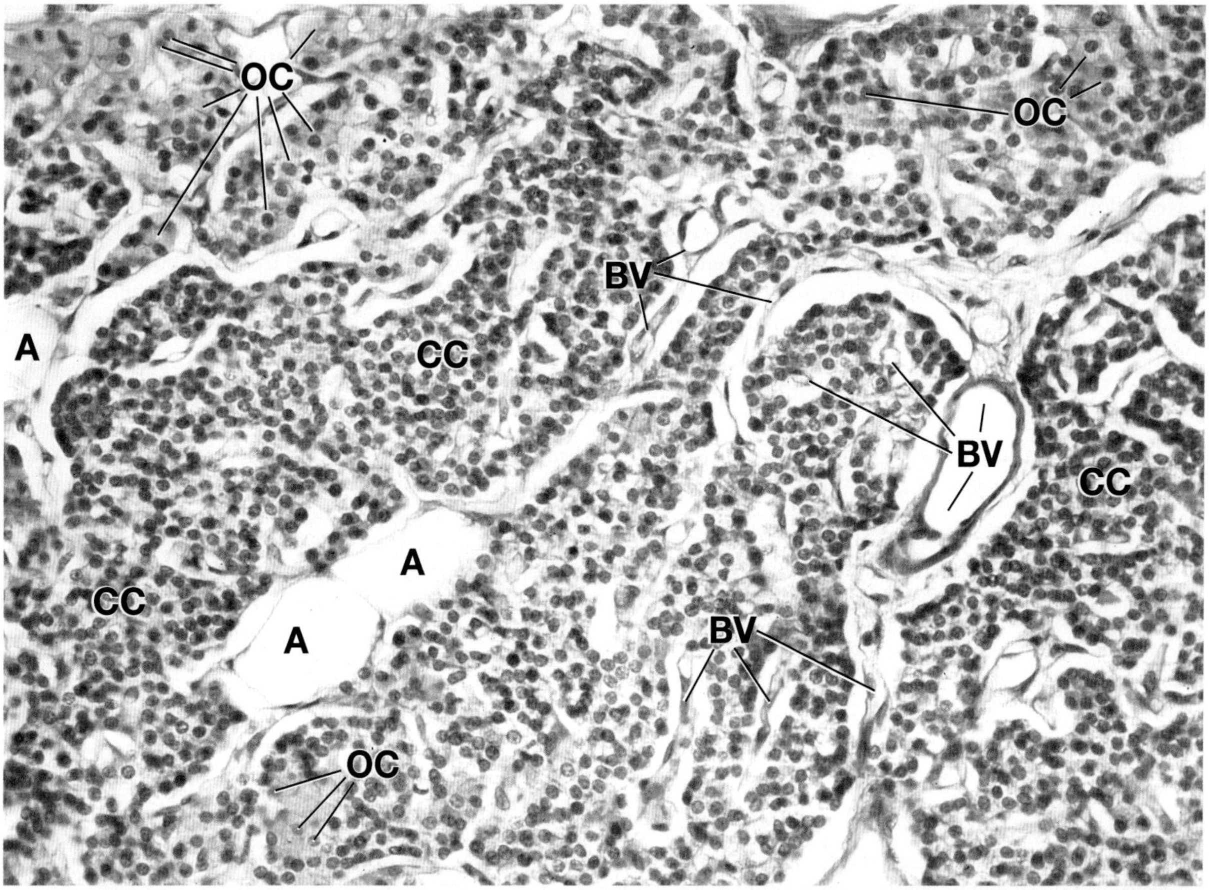
OC
OC
BV
A
CC
BV
CC
A
CC
A
BV
OC

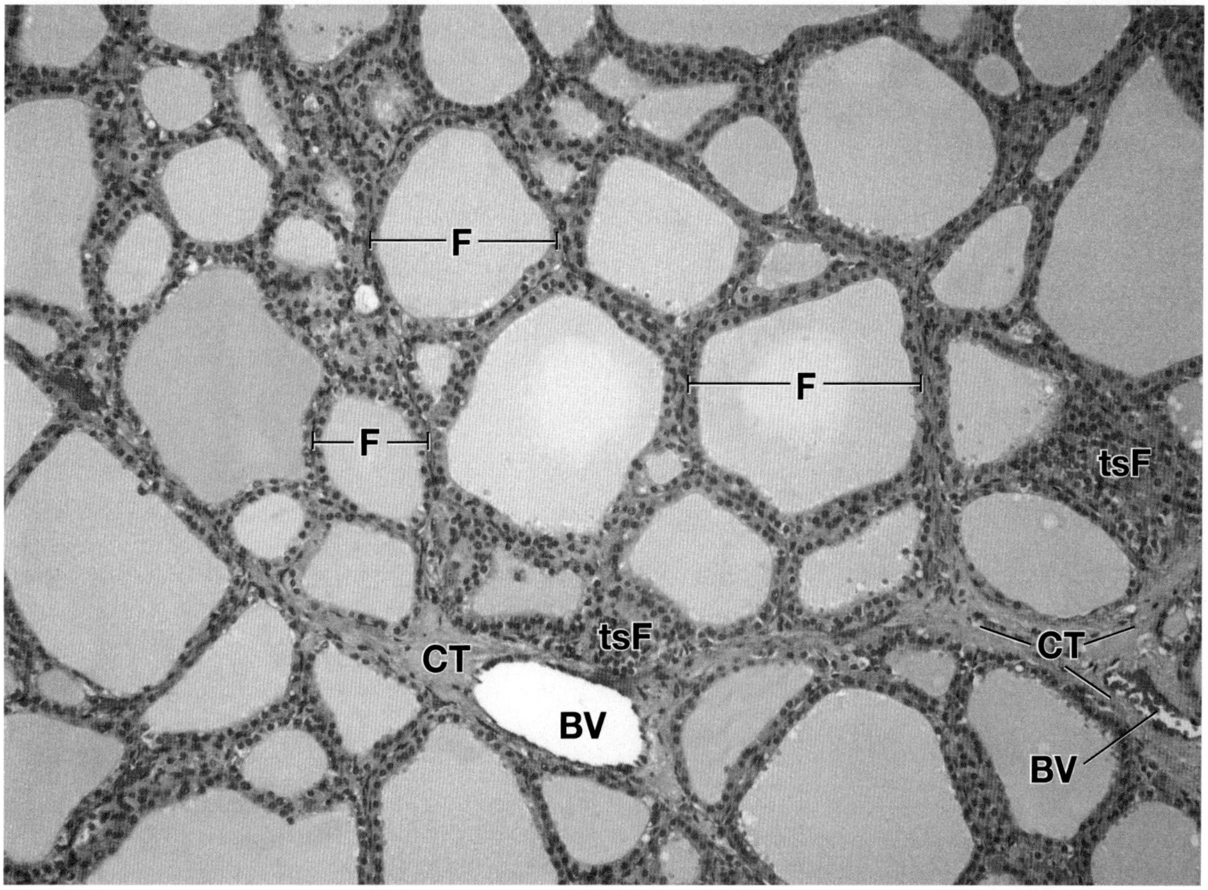
F
F
F
tsF
CT
tsF
CT
BV
BV

PLATE 21.5 ■ ADRENAL GLAND I

There are two **adrenal glands**, one at the upper pole of each kidney. The gland is a composite of two distinct structural and functional components: a **cortex** and a **medulla**. The cortex develops from mesoderm and secretes *steroid hormones*; the medulla develops from neuroectoderm of the neural crest and secretes *catecholamines*.

The adrenal cortex is divided into three zones according to the type and arrangement of its parenchymal cells. These are designated as **zona glomerulosa, zona fasciculata**, and **zona reticularis**. The zona glomerulosa constitutes 15% of the cortical volume. It secretes *mineralocorticoid* (*aldosterone*). The zona fasciculata constitutes nearly 80% of the cortical volume. It secretes *glucocorticoids* (*cortisol* and *corticosterone*) and a small amount of adrenal androgens. The zona reticularis (5%–7% of cortical volume) produces most of the adrenal androgens.

The zona fasciculata and the zona reticularis are regulated by *adrenocorticotropic hormone* (ACTH) secreted by the anterior lobe of the pituitary gland in response to *corticotropin-releasing factor* (CRF) produced by the hypothalamus. The zona glomerulosa is not regulated by ACTH but by angiotensin II, which is part of feedback control of the *renin–angiotensin–aldosterone system* that also regulates blood pressure.

Adrenal gland, human, hematoxylin and eosin (H&E) ×45.

This low-magnification micrograph of a section through the partial thickness of an adrenal gland shows the outer capsule (*Cap*), the **cortex** (*Cort*) from one surface of the gland, the underlying **medulla** (*Med*), and a very small portion of the cortex from the other surface of the gland (*Cort, bottom center*). The cortex has a distinctly different appearance in both structural organization and staining characteristics. From the inner portion, the medulla, note the lighter appearance of the medullary tissue. A small amount of adipose tissue (*AT*) in which the gland is partially embedded is seen at the *upper center* of the micrograph. The corticomedullary boundary (*dashed lines*) has a wave-like contour, a reflection of the irregular shape of the gland. Within the medulla are a number of relatively large blood vessels (*BV*). These are the adrenomedullary collecting veins that drain both the cortex and the medulla.

Cortex, adrenal gland, human, H&E ×180.

This is a higher magnification of a portion of the capsule and the full thickness of the **cortex** from an area in the previous figure. The capsule consists of dense connective tissue in which the larger arteries (*A*) travel to give rise to smaller vessels that will supply the cortex and medulla. The **zona glomerulosa** (*ZG*) is located at the outer part of the cortex, immediately under the capsule. The parenchyma of this zone consists of small cells that appear as arching cords or as oval groups of cells.

The **zona fasciculata** (*ZF*) consists of radially oriented cords and sheets of cells, usually two cells in width, that extend toward the medulla. The cells of the outer part of the zona fasciculata are generally larger than those of the inner portion of this zone and typically stain poorly because of the large number of lipid droplets that they contain. The cells of the **zona reticularis** (*ZR*) are relatively small and contain little or no lipid droplets and, consequently, stain prominently with eosin. Because of their small size, the nuclei are in close proximity to one another, much like the cells of the zona glomerulosa.

Cortex, adrenal gland, human, H&E ×245.

This is a higher magnification of the area inscribed by the *left rectangle* in the previous figure. It shows the **zona glomerulosa** (*ZG*) and the outer portion of the **zona fasciculata** (*ZF*). Note the smaller size of the cells in the zona glomerulosa than those in the zona fasciculata. In addition, cells of the zona glomerulosa contain fewer lipid droplets than those of the zona fasciculata. Typically, the cells in this part of the zona fasciculata are filled with lipid droplets, thus the very poor staining characteristic of their cytoplasm. Delicate connective tissue trabeculae (*arrows*) extend from the capsule to surround the glomerular groups of cells and extend between the cords of cells in the zona fasciculata. Capillaries and arterioles are located within the connective tissue trabeculae. Usually, the capillaries are collapsed and, without the presence of red blood cells in their lumina, are thus difficult to identify.

Cortex, adrenal gland, human, H&E ×245.

This is a higher magnification of the area inscribed by the *right rectangle* in the previous figure. This deep portion of the **zona fasciculata** (*ZF*) reveals smaller cells, although they are still arranged in cords and contain lipid droplets, although in lesser amounts. The cells of the **zona reticularis** (*ZR*) are arranged in irregular anastomosing cords and contain only a small amount of lipid and, consequently, their cytoplasm stains with eosin.

A, arteries
AT, adipose tissue
BV, blood vessels
Cap, capsule
Cort, cortex
Med, medulla
ZF, zona fasciculate
ZG, zona glomerulosa
ZR, zona reticularis
arrows, connective tissue trabeculae
dashed line, corticomedullary boundary

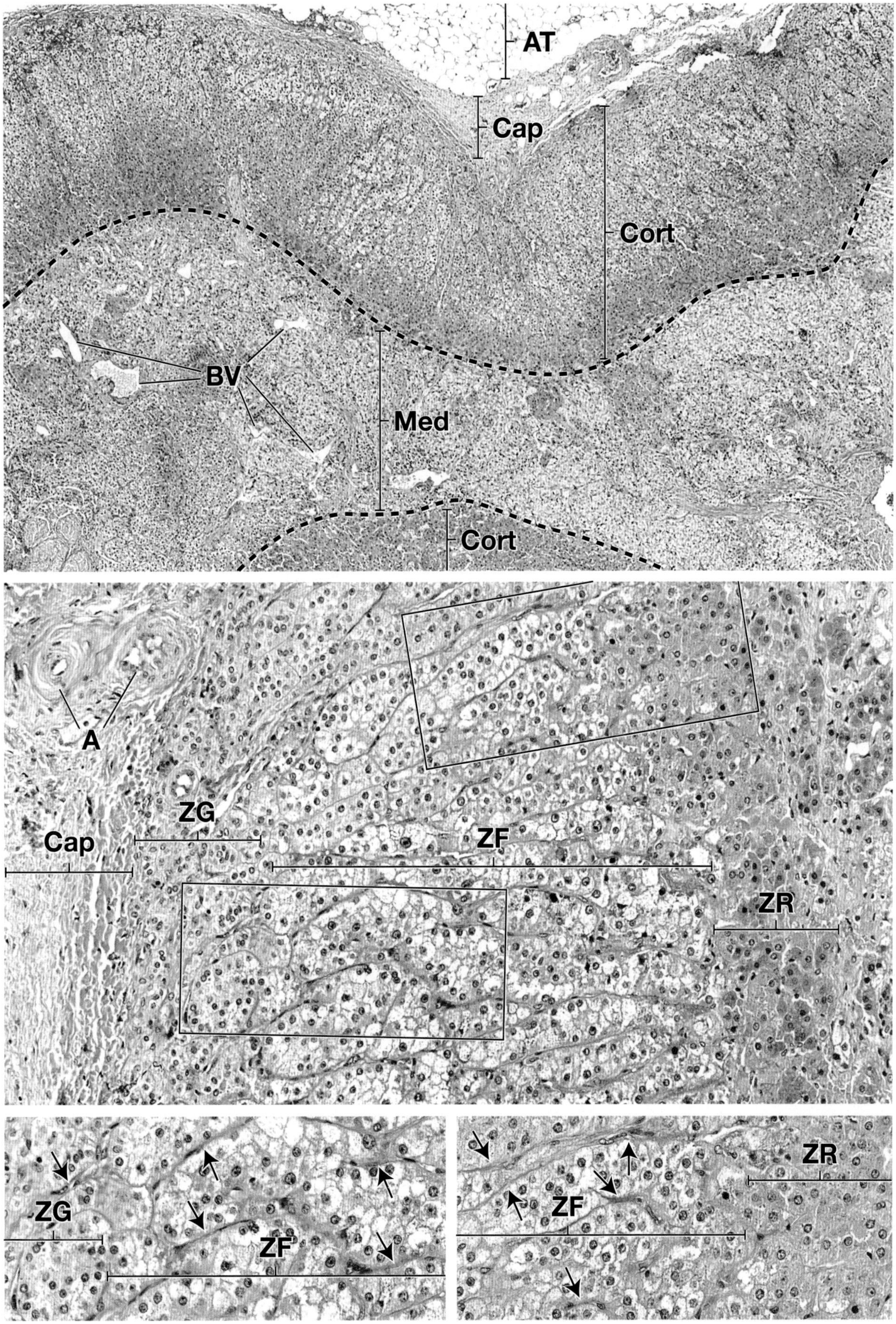
AT
Cap
Cort
BV
Med
Cort
A
ZG
Cap
ZF
ZR
ZG
ZF
ZF
ZR

PLATE 21.6 ■ ADRENAL GLAND II

The cells of the **adrenal medulla** develop from the same source as the postganglionic cells of the sympathetic nervous system. They are directly innervated by preganglionic cells of the sympathetic system and may be regarded as modified postganglionic cells that are specialized to secrete. These cells produce the catecholamines *epinephrine* and *norepinephrine*.

The adrenal medulla receives its blood supply via two routes: by arterioles that pass through the cortex and by capillaries that continue from the cortex, a type of portal circulation. Thus, some of the blood supplying the medulla contains cortical secretions that regulate medullary function. Blood leaves the medulla via the central adrenomedullary vein. Its structure is unusual in that the tunica media of the vessel contains prominent bundles of longitudinally oriented smooth muscle, the contraction of which facilitates rapid outflow of blood when medullary catecholamines are released.

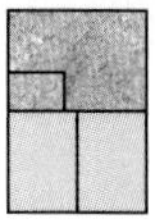

Medulla, adrenal gland, human, hematoxylin and eosin (H&E) ×175; inset ×250.

This moderately low-power photomicrograph shows the cells of the **adrenal medulla**. The medullary cells are organized in ovoid groups and short interconnecting cords. The cytoplasm of the medullary cells may stain with different intensity. The cytoplasm of some cells is very poorly stained, appearing almost clear, whereas others show greater intensity of eosin staining. In this photomicrograph, a portion of the wall, namely, the tunica media (*TM*) of the central adrenomedullary vein, can be seen. The nature of the central adrenomedullary vein is described in the *lower left* figure. The *inset* shows the ovoid groups of medullary cells at a higher magnification. Between these groups of cells are capillaries (*Cap*) that, as in the cortex, can be identified when they contain red blood cells as shown here.

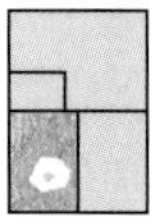

Medulla, adrenal gland, human, H&E ×125.

This micrograph shows a **central adrenomedullary vein** (*AMV*) that drains the adrenal medulla. The tunica media (*TM*) is unusually thick. The smooth muscle that constitutes this part of the vessel wall is in the form of bundles that are arranged longitudinally, that is, in the same direction as the vessel. Thus, the muscle seen here is cut in cross section, as is the vein. Whereas the central adrenomedullary vein occupies most of the micrograph, **medullary cells** (*MC*) can be seen in several locations surrounding the vein. The portion of the figure outlined by the *rectangle* is seen at higher magnification in the *bottom right* figure.

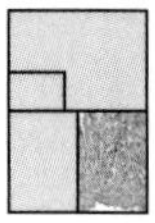

Central adrenomedullary vein, adrenal gland, human, H&E ×350.

This higher magnification view of the *rectangle* in the *bottom left* figure shows part of the lumen (*L*) of the **central adrenomedullary vein** (*AMV*) at the bottom of the field. The tunica intima (*TI*) of the vessel is relatively thin but may contain a variable amount of connective tissue. The smooth muscle (*SM*) of the tunica media (*TM*) is readily seen here as being arranged in bundles and appears in cross section. There is no discrete tunica adventitia in this vein. Instead, its connective tissue blends in with surrounding structures. **Ganglion cells** (*GC*) are frequently found in proximity to the wall of the central adrenomedullary vein. They are large cells with a moderately basophilic cytoplasm. Because of the large size of the cell, the nucleus is often missed in the section, and only the cell cytoplasm is seen.

AMV, central adrenomedullary vein
Cap, capillary
GC, ganglion cells
L, lumen of central adrenomedullary vein
MC, medullary cells
SM, smooth muscle
TI, tunica intima
TM, tunica media

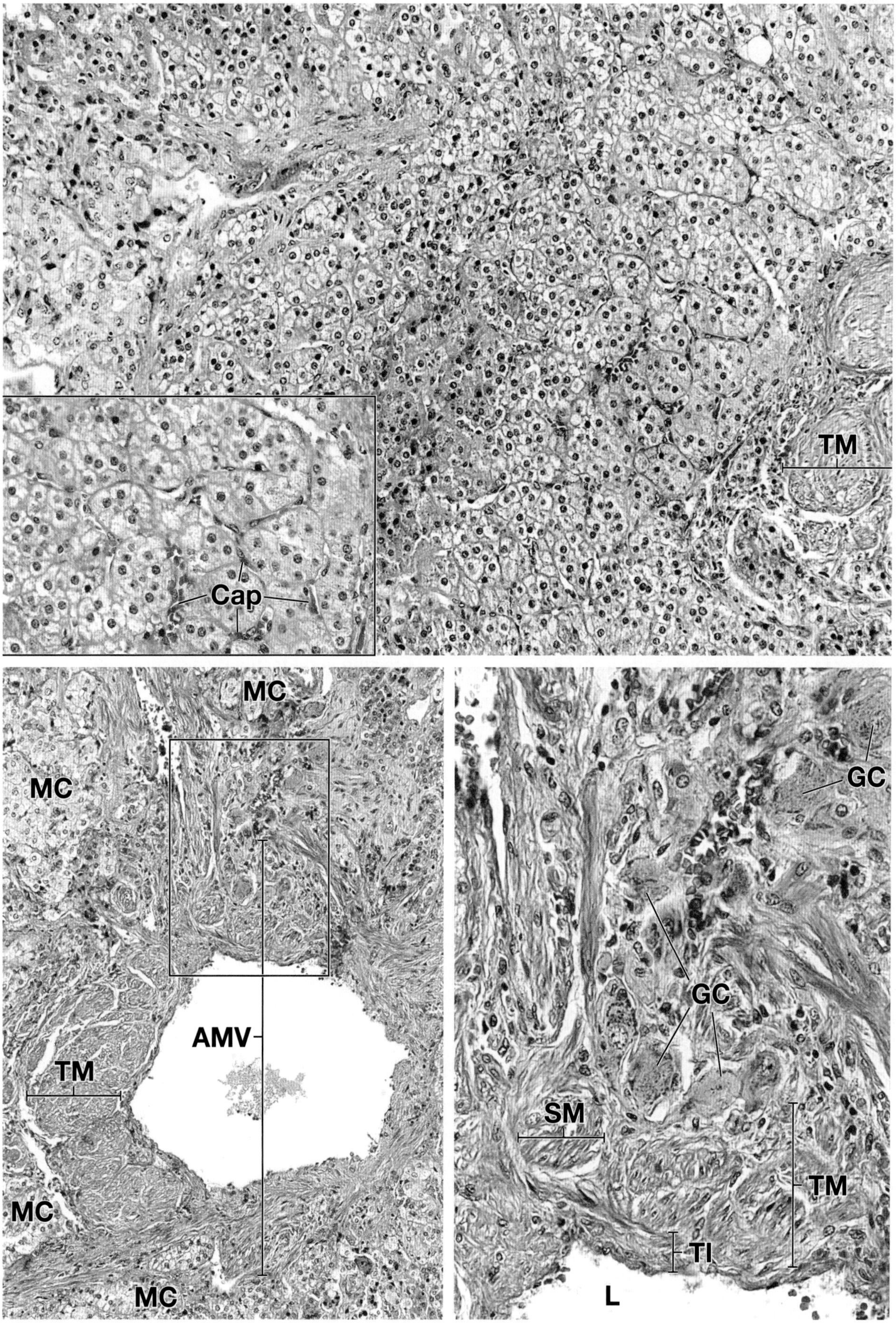
TM
Cap
MC
MC
AMV
TM
MC
MC
GC
GC
SM
TM
TI
L

22 MALE REPRODUCTIVE SYSTEM

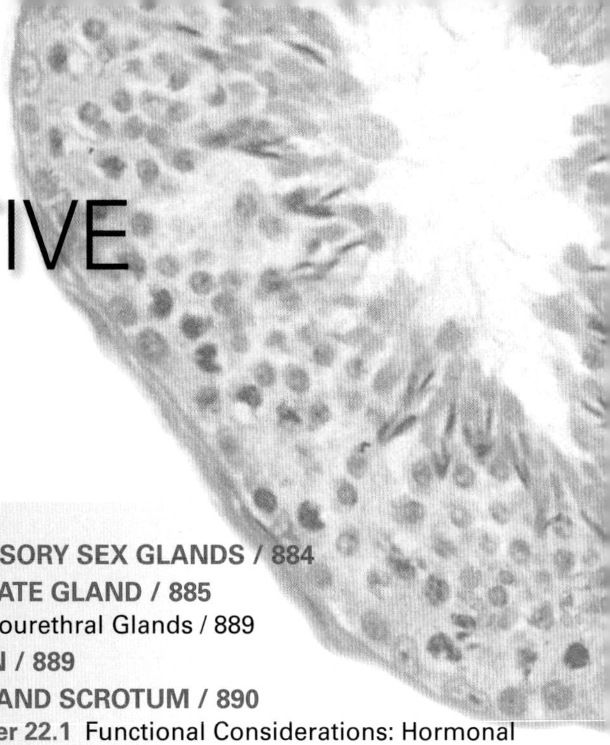

OVERVIEW OF THE MALE REPRODUCTIVE SYSTEM

The **male reproductive system** consists of the testes, genital excurrent ducts, accessory sex glands, and external genitalia containing the penis and scrotum (Fig. 22.1). The accessory sex glands include the seminal vesicles, the prostate, and bulbourethral glands. The two primary functions of the testis are **spermatogenesis** (the production of sperm, called *male gametes*) and **steroidogenesis** (synthesis of androgens, also called *sex hormones*). Androgens, mainly testosterone, are essential for spermatogenesis. They also play an important role in embryonic development of the male embryo into the phenotypic male fetus and are responsible for sexual dimorphism (male physical and behavioral characteristics). The events of cell division that occur during the production of male gametes, as well as those of the female (the ova), involve both normal division (mitosis) and reduction division (meiosis).

A brief description of mitosis and meiosis is included in Chapter 3, The Cell Nucleus (pages 99-103). A basic understanding of these processes is essential to understanding the production of gametes in both sexes.

TESTIS

The adult **testes** are paired ovoid organs that lie within the **scrotum**, located outside the body. Each testis is suspended within the end of an elongated musculofascial pouch, which is continuous with the layers of the anterior abdominal wall that projects into the scrotum. Testes are connected by the spermatic cords to the abdominal wall and tethered to the scrotum by scrotal ligaments, the remnants of the gubernaculum (see discussion later in this chapter).

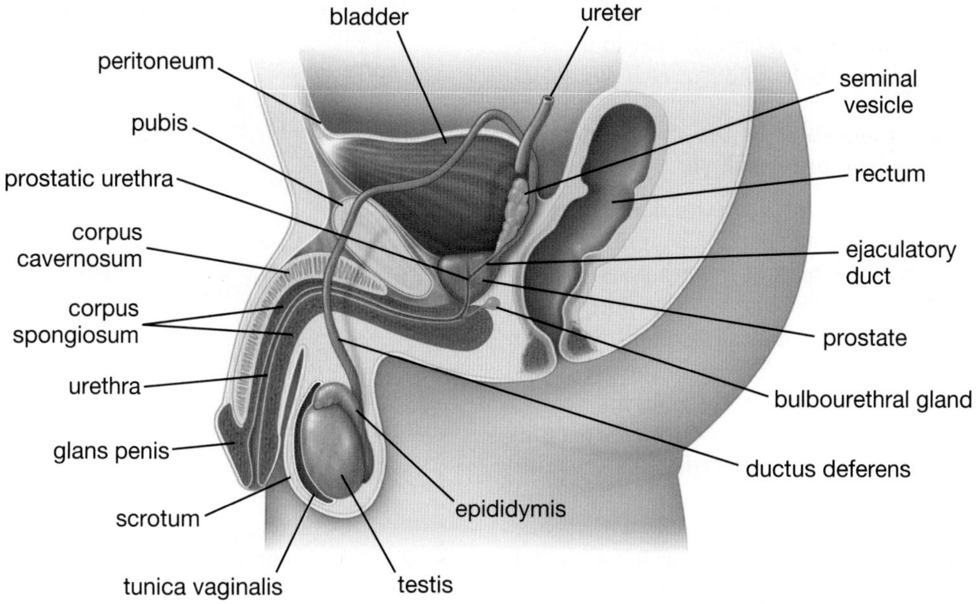

FIGURE 22.1. Schematic diagram demonstrating the components of the male reproductive system. Midline structures are depicted in sagittal section; bilateral structures, including the testis, epididymis, ductus deferens, and seminal vesicle, are shown intact.

Sex Determination and Development of the Testis

Sex differentiation is accomplished through a cascade of gene activations.

Genetic sex is determined at fertilization by the presence or absence of the Y chromosome. The testes, however, do not form until the seventh week of development. **Gonadal sex** is determined by the presence of the **SRY gene** located in the **sex-determining region Y** of the short arm of the Y chromosome. SRY gene expression in early embryonic development triggers the differentiation of the gonads into the testis. Mutations in this gene give rise to **XY female embryo with gonadal dysgenesis**, a condition known as **Swyer syndrome**. Females with Swyer syndrome have an X and Y chromosome and functional female genitalia, including the vagina, uterus, and uterine tubes. However, they lack female sex gonads (ovaries). Females with this syndrome do not produce sex hormones. Treatment with hormone therapy is necessary to induce puberty.

The genetic information encoded in the Y chromosome itself is not sufficient to guide the complex development of the male gonads. Instead, the SRY gene operates as a **master switch** that controls the cascade of several gene activations on autosomes 9, 11, 17, and 19 and the X chromosome. A transcription factor called the **testis-determining factor (TDF)**, encoded by the SRY gene, contains a molecular domain that binds to a specific region of DNA and alters its structure. The affected DNA forms a loop that permits binding of other transcription factors. These factors, in turn, cause the expression of other genes that initiate male sex determination (formation of the testes and other male sex organs). These genes include the following:

- **WT-1 gene** (Wilms tumor 1 gene), which is required for the development of the urogenital system and regulation of the SRY transcription. Mutations of the WT-1 gene are present in children with **familial Wilms tumor** and in children with accompanied **genitourinary malformations.**
- **SOX-9 gene** (SRY [sex-determining region Y]-box 9 gene) activates the **AMH gene** (anti-Müllerian hormone gene) that is responsible for Müllerian-inhibiting factor (MIF) synthesis. Mutation of the SOX9 gene is linked the formation of ambiguous or female sex organs in a genetically male individual (46,XY).
- **SF-1 gene** (steroidogenic factor-1 gene) that regulates the expression of a number of steroidogenic genes
- **DAX-1 gene** (dosage-sensitive sex reversal, adrenal hypoplasia critical region, on chromosome X, gene 1) that encodes nuclear receptor DAX-1. Activation of this receptor suppresses the SRY gene during gonadal sex differentiation, and its mutation is responsible for **congenital adrenal hypoplasia**.

The testes develop on the posterior wall of the abdomen and later descend into the scrotum.

The **testes** develop in close association with the urinary system retroperitoneally on the posterior wall of the abdominal cavity. Testes (like ovaries) are derived from three sources:

- **Intermediate mesoderm** forms the urogenital ridges on the posterior abdominal wall, giving rise to Leydig cells (interstitial cells) and myoid cells (peritubular contractile cells).
- **Mesodermal epithelium (coelomic mesothelium)** lines the urogenital ridges and gives rise to finger-like epithelial cords called *primary sex cords*. These cords grow into the underlying intermediate mesoderm and become colonized by primordial germ cells. The primary sex cords also give rise to Sertoli cells.
- **Primordial germ cells** migrate from the yolk sac into developing gonads, where they are incorporated into the **primary sex cords**. They differentiate into **gonocytes**, which are the precursors of the definitive germ cells called **spermatogonia**. At this stage, the cords are composed of primordial germ cells, pre-Sertoli cells, and a surrounding

layer of myoid cells. Later, primary sex cords differentiate into the **seminiferous cords**, which give rise to the seminiferous tubules, straight tubules, and rete testis (Fig. 22.2).

SRY expression is responsible for the development of male sex organs in the indifferent embryo.

In the first stage of development, the testes develop on the posterior abdominal wall from indifferent primordia of **urogenital ridges** that are identical in both sexes. During this **indifferent stage**, an embryo has the potential to develop into either a male or female. However, expression of the SRY gene, which occurs exclusively in the pre-Sertoli cells, orchestrates male development of the embryo.

Early in male development, mesenchyme separating the seminiferous cords gives rise to **Leydig (interstitial) cells** that produce **testosterone** to stimulate the development of the indifferent primordium into a testis. Testosterone is also responsible for the growth and differentiation of the mesonephric (Wolffian) ducts that develop into the male genital excurrent ducts. Also during this early stage, the **Sertoli (sustentacular) cells** that develop within the seminiferous cords produce another important hormonal substance, called **Müllerian-inhibiting factor (MIF)**. The molecular structure of MIF is similar to that of transforming growth factor-β (TGF-β). It is a large glycoprotein that inhibits cell division of the paramesonephric (Müllerian) ducts, which, in turn, inhibits the development of female reproductive organs (Fig. 22.3).

Development and differentiation of the external genitalia (also from the sexually indifferent stage) occur at the same time and result from the action of **dihydrotestosterone (DHT)**, a product of the conversion of testosterone by 5α-reductase. Without DHT, regardless of the genetic or gonadal sex, the external genitalia will develop along the female template. The appearance of testosterone, MIF, and DHT is the trigger that determines the development of male sex organs in the embryo (Folder 22.1).

The testes descend from the abdomen into the scrotum along the inguinal canal at approximately 26 weeks of gestation.

At approximately 26 weeks of gestation, the testes descend from the abdomen into the scrotum. This migration of the testes is caused by differential growth of the abdominal cavity combined with the action of testosterone that causes shortening of the **gubernaculum**, the testosterone-sensitive ligament connecting the inferior pole of each testis to the developing scrotum. The testes descend into the scrotum by passing through the inguinal canal, the narrow passage between the abdominal cavity and the scrotum. During descent, the testes carry their blood vessels, lymphatic vessels, and nerves as well as their principal excurrent duct system, the ductus deferens, with them. Descent of the testis is sometimes obstructed, resulting in **cryptorchidism**, or **undescended testes**. This condition is common (30%) in premature newborns and approximately 1% of full-term newborns. Cryptorchidism can lead to irreversible histologic changes in the testis and increases the risk of testicular cancer. An undescended testis requires surgical correction. **Orchiopexy** (placement in the scrotal sac) should preferably be performed before histologic changes become irreversible at approximately 2 years of age.

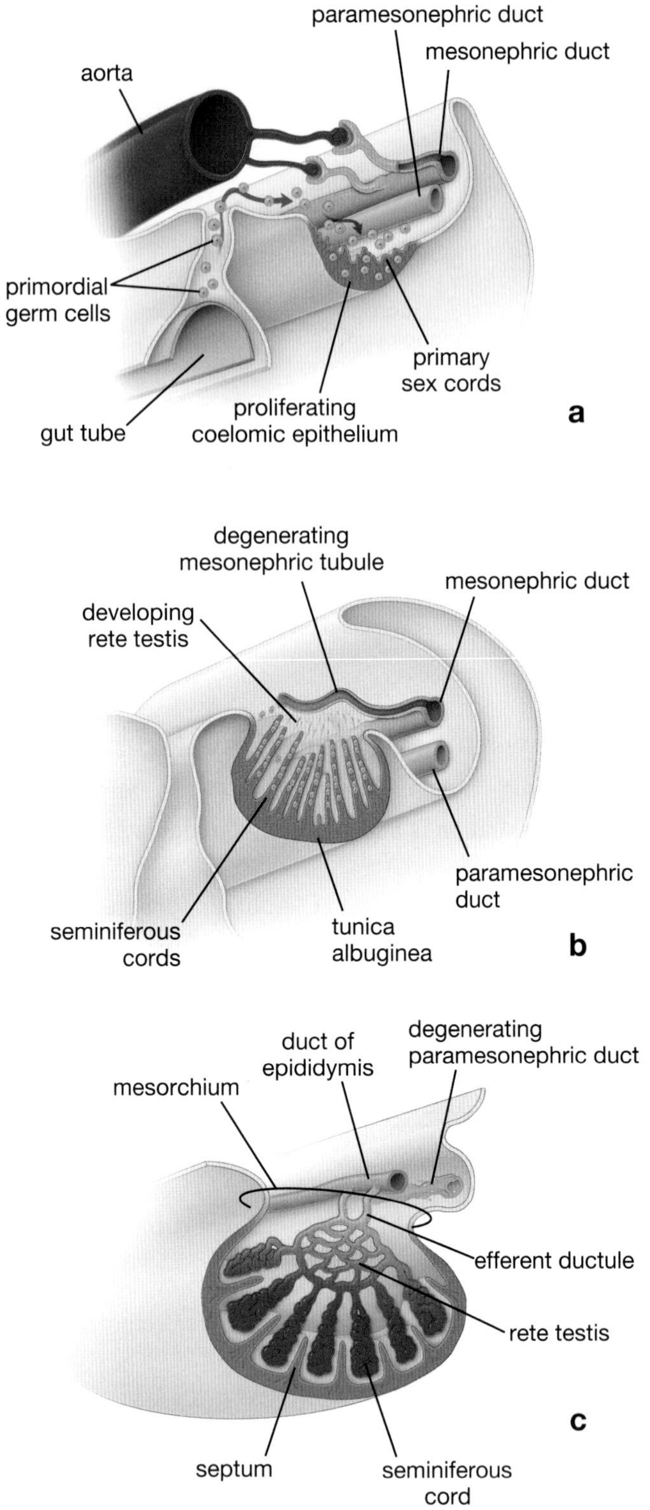

FIGURE 22.2. Schematic diagram of the stages of testicular development. a. This diagram shows the 5-week embryo in the stage of indifferent gonads. The gonadal ridges visible on the posterior abdominal wall are being infiltrated by primordial germ cells (*green*) that migrate from the yolk sac. Most of the developing gonad is formed by mesenchyme derived from the coelomic epithelium. The primordial germ cells become incorporated into the primary sex cords. **b.** At a later stage, under hormonal influence of testis-determining factor (TDF), the developing gonad initiates the production of testosterone. This is followed by differentiation of the primary sex cords into seminiferous cords. At the same time, the developing gonad produces Müllerian-inhibiting factor (MIF), which causes regression of the paramesonephric duct and those structures derived from it. Note that the mesonephric tubules come in close contact with the developing rete testis. **c.** Final stages of testicular development. The tunica albuginea surrounding the testis contributes to the development of the testicular septa. The rete testis connects with the seminiferous cords and with the excurrent duct system that develops from the mesonephric duct and tubules.

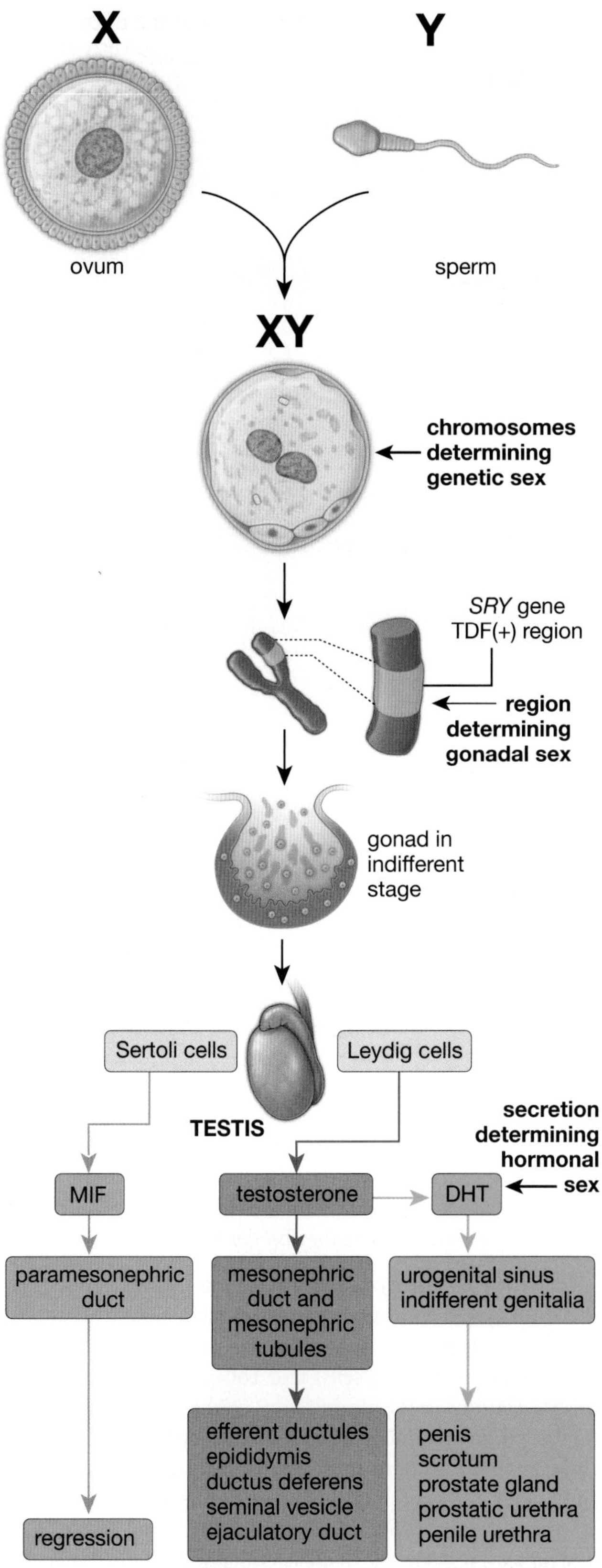

FIGURE 22.3. Schematic diagram of male sex development and hormonal influence on developing reproductive organs. This diagram illustrates three levels at which the sex of the developing embryo is determined. Genetic sex is determined at the time of fertilization; gonadal sex is determined by activation of the sex-determining region Y (*SRY*) gene located on the short arm of chromosome Y; and hormonal sex is determined by a hormone secreted by the developing gonad. The diagram shows the influence of Müllerian-inhibiting factor (*MIF*), testosterone, and dihydrotestosterone (*DHT*) on the developing structures. *TDF*, testis-determining factor.

Spermatogenesis requires that the testes be maintained below normal body temperature.

As the **testes descend** from the abdominal cavity into the scrotum, they carry blood vessels, lymphatic vessels, autonomic nerves, and an extension of the abdominal peritoneum called the **tunica vaginalis**, which covers their anterolateral surface. Within the scrotum, the temperature of the testes is 2°C–3°C below body temperature. This lower temperature is essential for spermatogenesis but is not required for hormone production (steroidogenesis), which can occur at normal body temperature. An increase in the testicular temperature of more than 37°C can induce testicular **heat stress** that alters spermatogenesis, especially the differentiation and maturation of spermatocytes and spermatids. Heat stress decreases DNA synthesis, causes DNA damage, and increases the degradation of messenger RNAs (mRNAs) and denaturation of cytoplasmic proteins in spermatocytes and spermatids, triggering their apoptosis and autophagy. Several factors that increase the temperature of the testis, such as fever, prolonged exposure to high temperatures (e.g., saunas), obesity, varicocele (enlargement of veins within the scrotum), and cryptorchidism (failure of the testis to descend into the scrotum) may lead to infertility.

Each testis receives blood through a **testicular artery**, a direct branch of the abdominal aorta. It is highly convoluted near the testis, where it is surrounded by the **pampiniform venous plexus**, which carries blood from the testis to the abdominal veins. This arrangement allows heat exchange between the blood vessels and helps maintain the testes at a lower temperature. The cooler venous blood returning from the testis cools the arterial blood before it enters the testis through a **countercurrent heat exchange mechanism**. In addition, the **cremaster muscle**, whose fibers originate in the internal abdominal oblique muscle of the anterior abdominal wall, responds to changes in ambient temperature. Its contraction moves the testes closer to the abdominal wall, and its relaxation lowers the testes within the scrotum. Cold temperatures also cause contraction of a thin sheet of smooth muscle (**dartos muscle**) in the superficial fascia of the scrotum. Contraction of the dartos muscles causes the scrotum to wrinkle when cold to help regulate heat loss (Folder 22.2).

Structure of the Testis

The testes have an unusually thick connective tissue capsule, the tunica albuginea.

An unusually thick, dense connective tissue capsule, the **tunica albuginea**, covers each testis (Fig. 22.4). The inner part of this capsule, the **tunica vasculosa**, is a loose connective tissue layer that contains blood and lymphatic vessels. Each testis is divided into approximately 250 lobules by incomplete **connective tissue septa** that project from the capsule. Along the posterior surface of the testis, the tunica albuginea thickens and projects inward as the mediastinum testis. Blood vessels, lymphatic vessels, and the genital excurrent ducts pass through the mediastinum as they enter or leave the testis.

Each lobule consists of several highly convoluted seminiferous tubules.

Each lobule of the testis consists of one to four **seminiferous tubules**, in which sperm are produced, and a connective

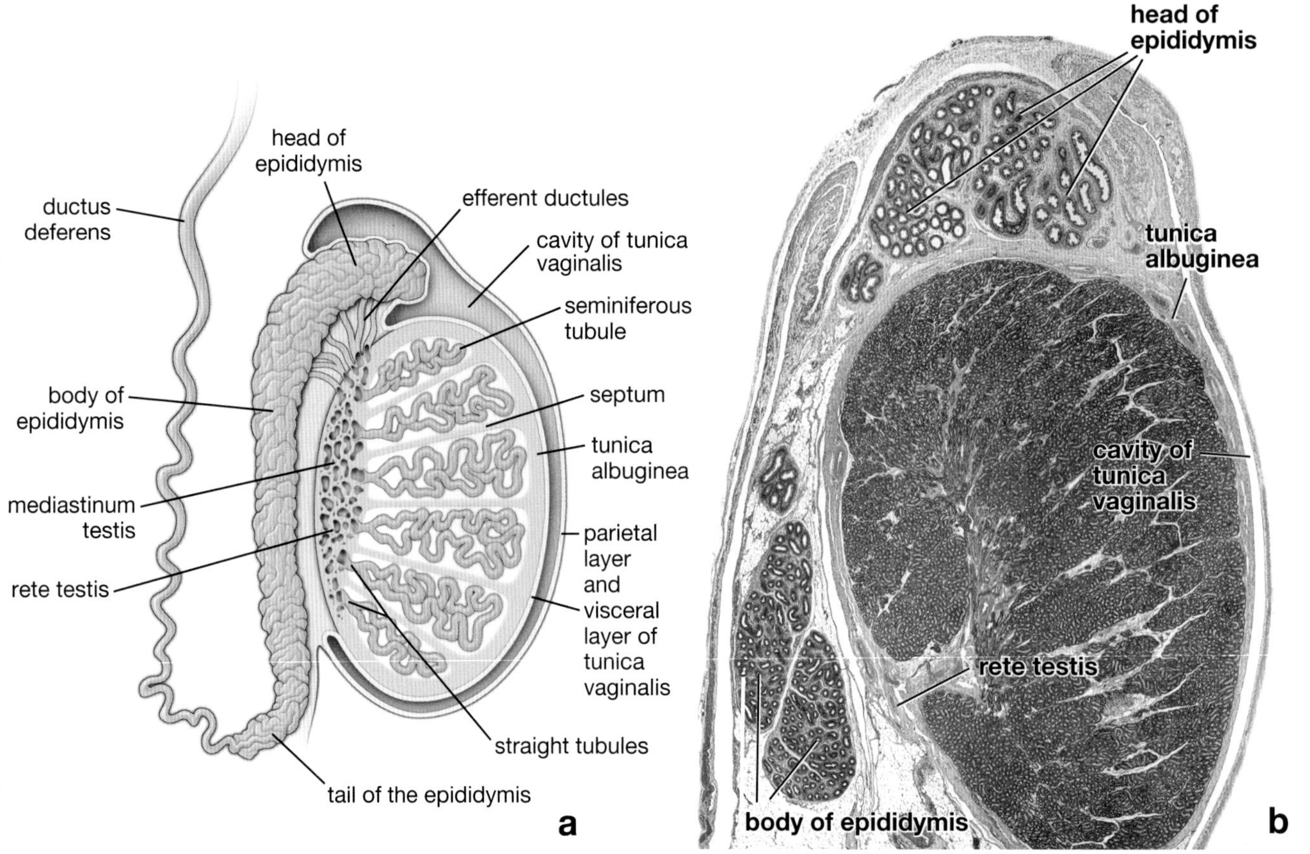

FIGURE 22.4. Sagittal section of the human testis. a. This schematic diagram shows a midsagittal section of the human testis. The genital duct system, which includes the tubuli recti, rete testis, efferent ducts, duct of the epididymis, and ductus deferens, is also shown. Note the thick connective tissue covering, the tunica albuginea, and the surrounding tunica vaginalis. (Modified from Dym M. In: Weiss L, ed. *Cell and Tissue Biology: A Textbook of Histology*. 6th ed. Urban & Schwarzenberg; 1988.) **b.** Sagittal section of a hematoxylin and eosin (H&E)-stained section of the testis and the head and body of the epididymis. Again, note the surrounding tunica albuginea and tunica vaginalis. Only a small portion of the rete testis is visible in this section. Its connection with the excurrent duct system is not evident in the plane of this section. ×3.

tissue stroma, in which testosterone-producing **Leydig (interstitial) cells** are contained (Fig. 22.5 and Plate 22.1, page 896). Each tubule within the lobule forms a loop and, because of its considerable length, is highly convoluted, actually folding on itself within the lobule. The ends of the loop are located near the **mediastinum** of the testis, where they assume a short straight course. This part of the seminiferous tubule is called the **straight tubule (tubulus rectus)**. It becomes continuous with the **rete testis**, an anastomosing channel system within the mediastinum.

The seminiferous tubules consist of a seminiferous epithelium surrounded by a tunica propria.

Each **seminiferous tubule** is approximately 50 cm long (range, 30–80 cm) and 150–250 μm in diameter. The seminiferous epithelium is an unusual and complex stratified epithelium composed of two basic cell populations:

- **Sertoli cells**, also known as *supporting*, or *sustentacular*, *cells*. These cells do not replicate after puberty. Sertoli cells are columnar cells with extensive apical and lateral processes that surround the adjacent spermatogenic cells and occupy the spaces between them. However, this elaborate configuration of the Sertoli cells cannot be seen distinctly in routine hematoxylin and eosin (H&E) preparations. Sertoli cells give structural organization to the tubules as they extend through the full thickness of the seminiferous epithelium.
- **Spermatogenic cells**, which regularly replicate and differentiate into mature sperm. These cells are derived from primordial germ cells originating in the yolk sac that colonize the gonadal ridges during the early development of the testis. Spermatogenic cells are organized in poorly defined layers of progressive development between adjacent Sertoli cells (Fig. 22.6). The most immature spermatogenic cells, called **spermatogonia**, rest on the basal lamina. The most mature cells, called **spermatids**, are attached to the apical portion of the Sertoli cell, where they border the lumen of the tubule.

The **tunica (lamina) propria**, also called *peritubular tissue*, is a multilayered connective tissue that lacks typical fibroblasts. In humans, it consists of three to five layers of **myoid cells** (peritubular contractile cells) and collagen fibrils, external to the basal lamina of the seminiferous epithelium (see Fig. 22.6). At the ultrastructural level, myoid cells demonstrate features associated with smooth muscle cells, including a basal lamina and large numbers of actin filaments. They also exhibit a significant amount of rough endoplasmic reticulum (rER), a feature indicating their role in collagen synthesis in the absence of typical fibroblasts. Rhythmic contractions of the myoid cells create peristaltic waves that help move spermatozoa and testicular fluid through the seminiferous tubules to the excurrent duct system. Blood vessels and extensive lymphatic vasculature as well as Leydig cells are present external to the myoid layer.

As a normal consequence of aging, the tunica propria increases in thickness. This thickening is accompanied by a decreased rate of sperm production and an overall reduction in the size of the seminiferous tubules. Excessive thickening of the tunica propria earlier in life is associated with infertility.

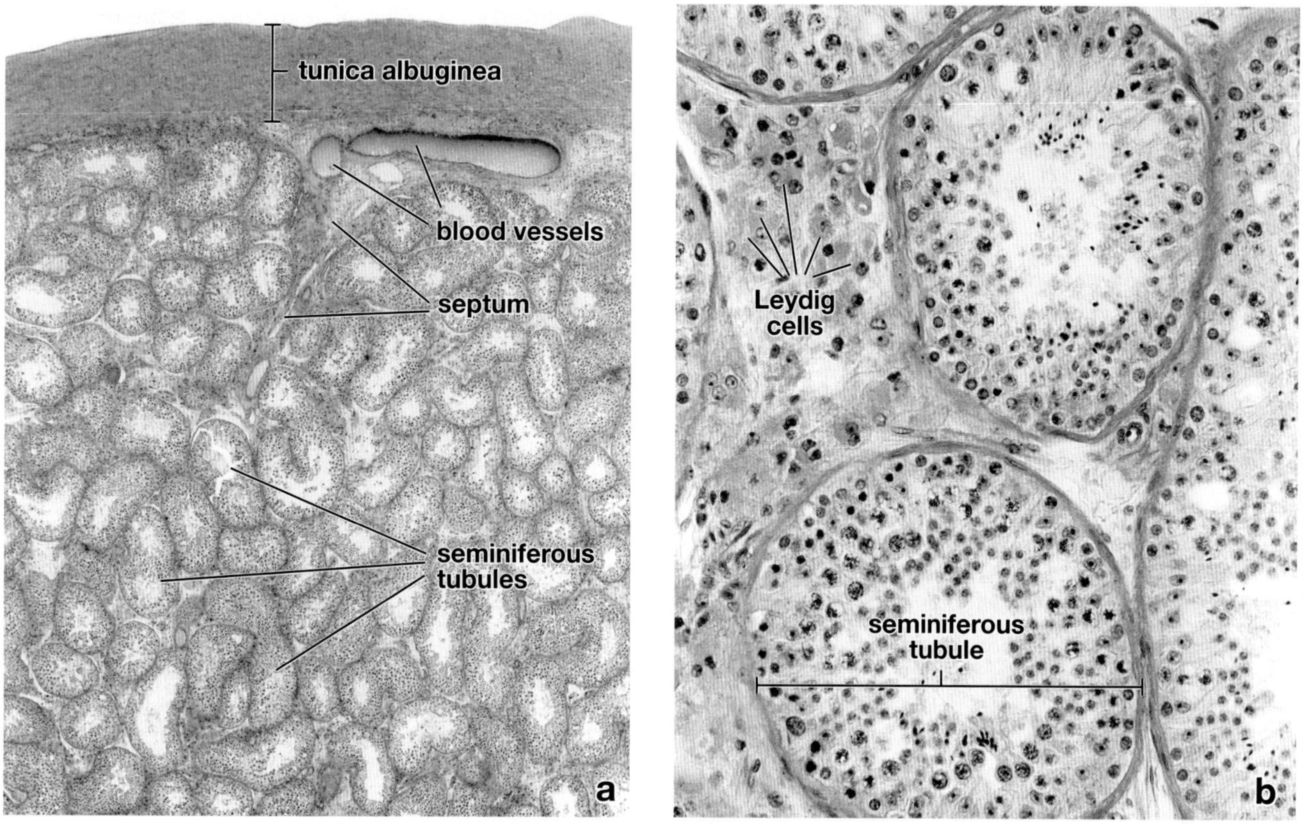

FIGURE 22.5. Photomicrographs of human testis. a. This low-magnification photomicrograph of a hematoxylin and eosin (H&E)-stained section of human testis shows seminiferous tubules and the tunica albuginea. The larger blood vessels are present in the inner aspect of the tunica albuginea. The seminiferous tubules are highly convoluted; thus, the profiles that they present in the section are variable in appearance. ×30. **b.** A higher magnification of the previous specimen shows several seminiferous tubules. Note the population of Leydig (interstitial) cells that occur in small clusters in the space between adjoining tubules. ×250.

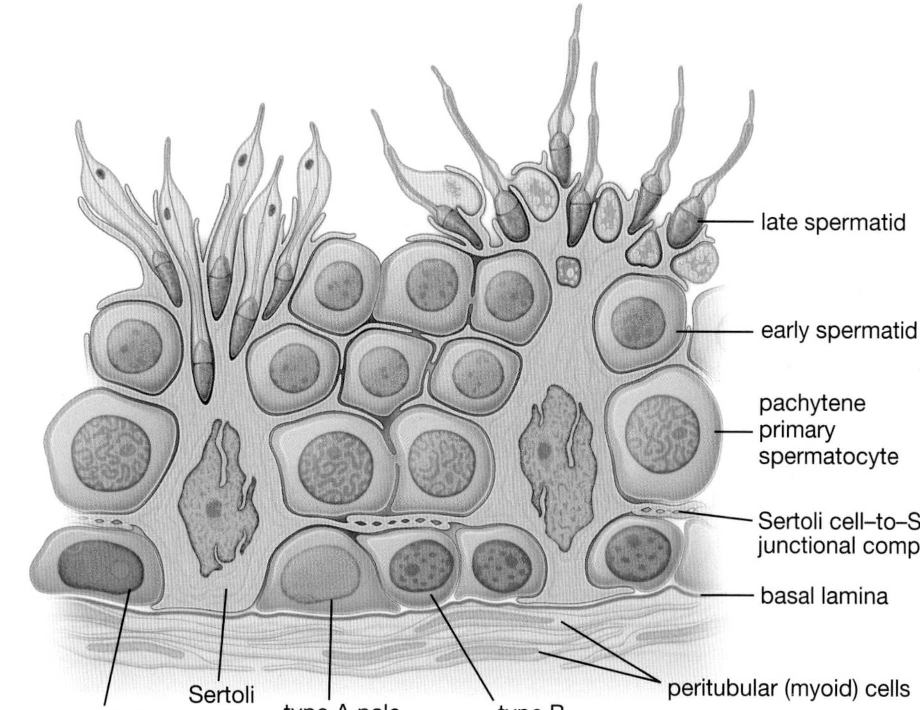

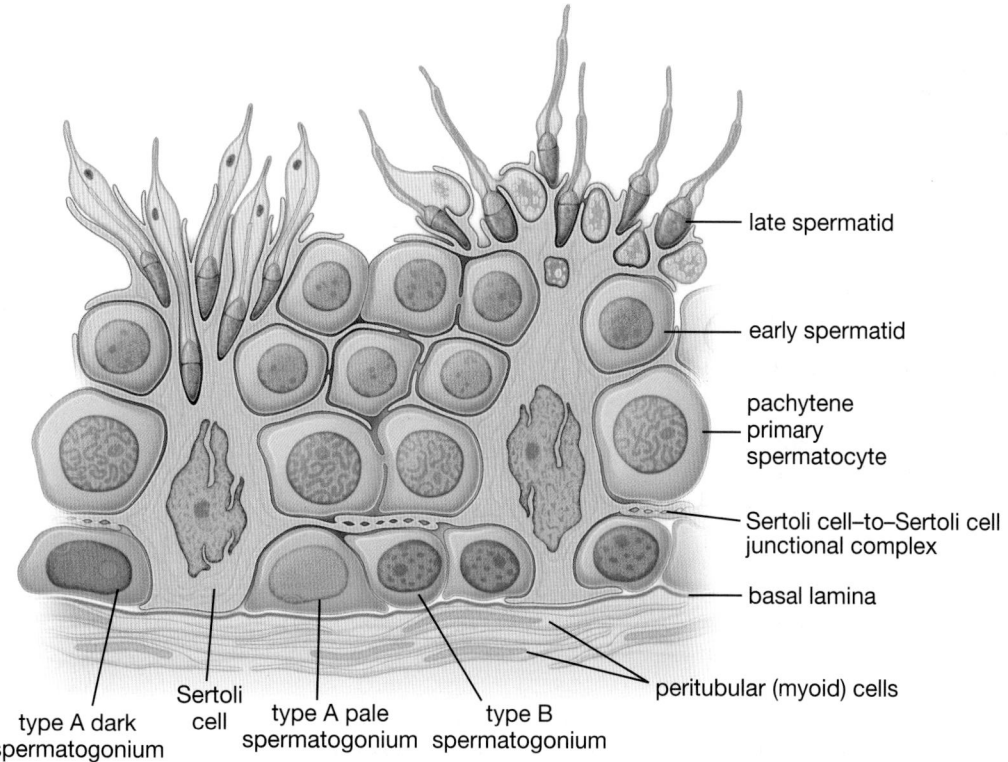

FIGURE 22.6. Schematic drawing of human seminiferous epithelium. This drawing shows the relationship of the Sertoli cells to the spermatogenic cells. The seminiferous epithelium rests on a basal lamina, and a layer of peritubular cells surrounds the seminiferous tubule. The spermatogonia—type A pale, type A dark, and type B—and preleptotene spermatocytes are located in the basal compartment of the seminiferous epithelium below the junctional complex, between adjacent Sertoli cells. Pachytene primary spermatocytes, early spermatids, and late spermatids, with partitioning residual cytoplasm that becomes the residual body, are seen above the junctional complex in the abluminal compartment. (Redrawn from Clermont Y. The cycle of the seminiferous epithelium in man. *Am J Anat.* 1963;112:35.)

Leydig Cells

Leydig cells (interstitial cells) are large, polygonal, eosinophilic cells that typically contain lipid droplets (Fig. 22.7). Lipofuscin pigment is also frequently present in these cells as well as distinctive, rod-shaped cytoplasmic crystals, the **crystals of Reinke** (Fig. 22.8). In routine histologic preparations, these crystals are refractile and measure approximately 3 × 20 μm. Although their exact nature and function remain unknown, they probably represent a protein product of the cell.

Like other steroid-secreting cells, Leydig cells have an elaborate smooth endoplasmic reticulum (sER), a feature that accounts for their eosinophilia (see Fig. 22.7). The enzymes necessary for the synthesis of testosterone from cholesterol are associated with the sER. Mitochondria with tubulovesicular cristae, another characteristic of steroid-secreting cells, are also present in Leydig cells.

Leydig cells differentiate and secrete **testosterone** during early fetal life. Secretion of testosterone is required during embryonic development, sexual maturation, and reproductive function:

- In the **embryo**, secretion of testosterone and other androgens is essential for the normal development of the gonads in the male fetus. In addition to testosterone, Leydig cells secrete **insulin-like protein 3 (INSL3)** that stimulates the descent of the testis during development.
- At **puberty**, secretion of testosterone is responsible for the initiation of sperm production, accessory sex gland secretion, and development of secondary sex characteristics. Secretion of INSL3 also promotes meiotic divisions in the seminiferous tubules.
- In the **adult**, secretion of testosterone is essential for the maintenance of spermatogenesis and secondary sex characteristics, genital excurrent ducts, and accessory sex glands. **Leydig cells** in the adult testes are the chief source of circulating **insulin-like factor-3 (INSL3) protein**. Measurement of INSL3 is utilized in clinical tests to establish the Leydig cell **steroidogenetic capacity index**. In addition to the secretion of INSL3, Leydig cells produce and secrete **oxytocin**. Testicular oxytocin stimulates contraction of myoid cells that surround the seminiferous tubules, moving the spermatozoa toward the efferent ductules.

The Leydig cells are active in the early differentiation of the male fetus and then undergo a period of inactivity beginning at about 5 months of fetal life. Inactive Leydig cells are difficult to distinguish from fibroblasts. When Leydig cells are exposed to gonadotropic stimulation at puberty, they again become androgen-secreting cells and remain active throughout life.

Leydig cell tumors are usually benign tumors and occur during two distinct periods (in childhood and adults between

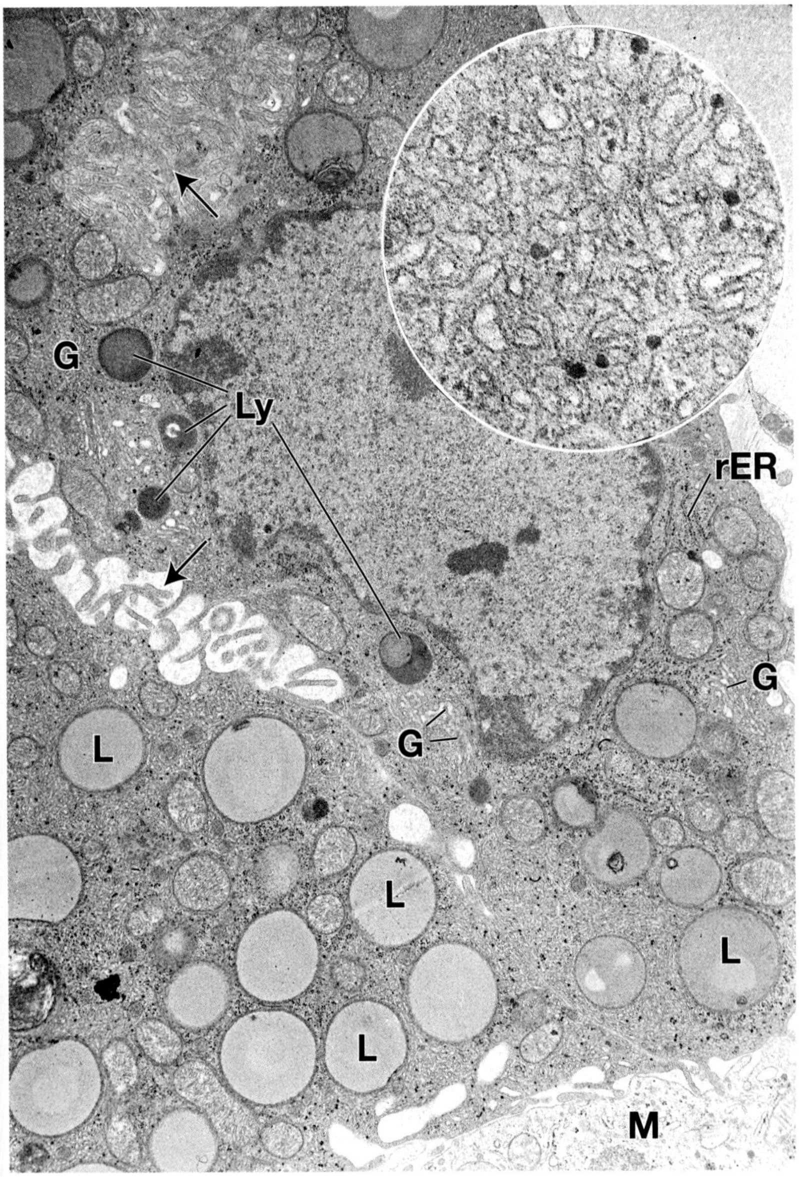

FIGURE 22.7. Electron micrograph of Leydig cells. This electron micrograph shows portions of several Leydig cells. The cytoplasm contains an abundance of smooth endoplasmic reticulum (sER), a characteristic of Leydig cells. Other features characteristic of the Leydig cell seen in the lower power micrograph are the numerous lipid droplets (*L*), the segmented profiles of the Golgi apparatus (*G*), and the presence of variable numbers of lysosomes (*Ly*). Occasional profiles of rough endoplasmic reticulum (*rER*) are also seen. Note also the microvilli along portions of the cell surface (*arrows*). *M*, cytoplasm of adjacent macrophage. ×10,000. **Inset.** sER at higher magnification. The very dense particles are glycogen. ×60,000.

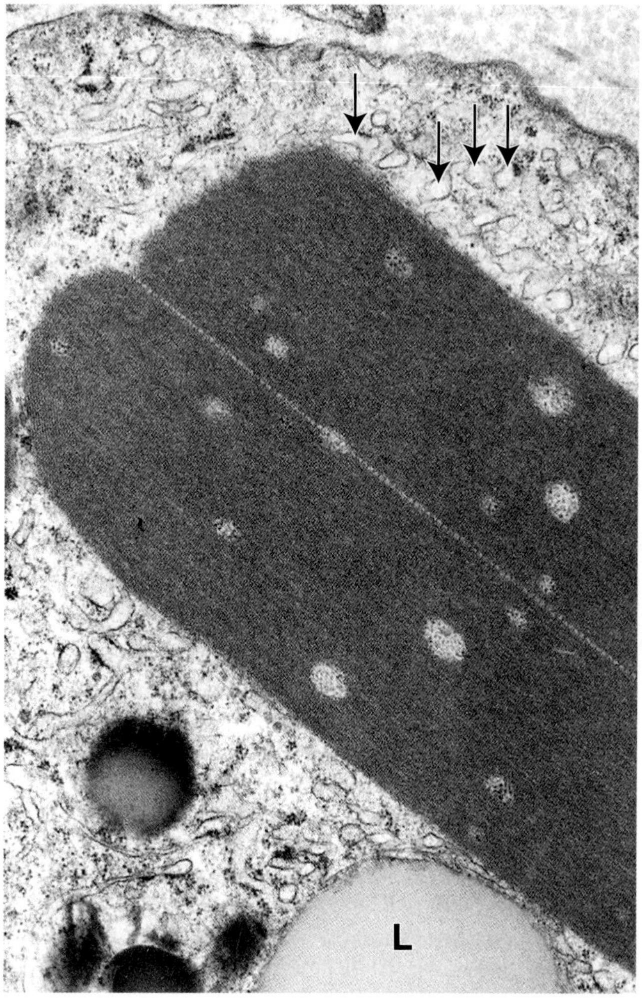

FIGURE 22.8. Electron micrograph of a Reinke crystal. This electron micrograph shows the internal structure of a Reinke crystal in the cytoplasm of a human Leydig cell. Also note the smooth endoplasmic reticulum (sER) (*arrows*) and a lipid droplet (*L*) in the cytoplasm. ×16,000. (Courtesy of Dr. Don F. Cameron.)

20 and 60 years old). They are hormonally active and secrete androgens or a combination of androgens and estrogens. Commonly, they are composed of uniform cells that have all of the characteristics of steroid hormone–secreting cells, including Reinke crystals. Initial symptoms of these benign tumors, besides testicular enlargement, are usually related to an abnormal level of hormone production. In prepubertal individuals, this leads to **sexual precocity** (unexpected pubertal changes in early age), whereas in adults, it may be observed as **feminization** (development of female sexual characteristics) and **gynecomastia** (development of breast in males).

■ SPERMATOGENESIS

Spermatogenesis is the process by which spermatogonia develop into sperm.

Spermatogenesis, the process by which sperm are produced, involves a complex and unique series of events. It begins shortly before puberty, under the influence of rising levels of pituitary gonadotropins, and continues throughout life. For descriptive purposes, spermatogenesis is divided into three distinct phases:

- **Spermatogonial phase**, in which spermatogonia divide by mitosis to replace themselves as well as provide a population of committed spermatogonia that will eventually give rise to primary spermatocytes
- **Spermatocyte phase (meiosis)**, in which primary spermatocytes undergo two meiotic divisions to reduce both the chromosome number and amount of DNA to produce haploid cells called *spermatids*
- **Spermatid phase (spermiogenesis)**, in which spermatids differentiate into mature sperm cells

At the conclusion of spermatogenesis, spermatids undergo their final maturation and are released during a process called **spermiation** from the supporting Sertoli cells into the lumen of the seminiferous tubule.

FOLDER 22.1

FUNCTIONAL CONSIDERATIONS: HORMONAL REGULATION OF SPERMATOGENESIS

Normal function of the testis is dependent on hormones acting through endocrine and paracrine pathways. The endocrine function of the testis resides primarily in the Leydig cell population that synthesizes and secretes the principal circulating androgen, **testosterone**. Nearly all of the testosterone is produced by the testis; less than 5% is produced by the adrenal glands. It is estimated in humans that the total Leydig cell population produces about 7 mg of testosterone per day. As testosterone leaves the Leydig cells, it enters the bloodstream and lymphatic capillaries and crosses into the peritubular tissue to reach the seminiferous epithelium.

High local levels of testosterone within the testis (estimated to be as much as 200 times the circulating levels) are necessary for the proliferation and differentiation of spermatogenic cells. This high testicular level of testosterone can be significantly decreased by negative feedback from exogenous testosterone. Intensive research in this area has focused on the development of the male testosterone-based contraceptive drugs. In early clinical studies, these drugs have been shown to cause a significant decrease in the testicular testosterone concentration and inhibition of spermatogenesis. Recovery of spermatogenesis occurs after discontinuation of contraceptive use. However, in some individuals, this type of contraceptive does not cause spermatogenic suppression. It also can cause significant side effects, including acne and depression.

Peripheral testosterone has the following effects:

- Differentiation of the **central nervous system** (CNS) and the genital apparatus and genital excurrent duct system
- Growth and maintenance of **secondary sexual characteristics** (such as the beard, male distribution of pubic hair, and low-pitched voice)
- Growth and maintenance of the **accessory sex glands** (seminal vesicles and prostate and bulbourethral glands), genital excurrent duct system, and the external genitalia (mainly byproducts of testosterone conversion to dihydrotestosterone [DHT])

(*continued*)

FOLDER 22.1

FUNCTIONAL CONSIDERATIONS: HORMONAL REGULATION OF SPERMATOGENESIS (*continued*)

- **Anabolic and general metabolic processes**, including skeletal growth, skeletal muscle growth, distribution of subcutaneous fat, and kidney function
- **Behavioral effects**, including libido

The steroidogenic and spermatogenic activities of the testis are regulated by hormonal interaction between the hypothalamus, anterior lobe of the pituitary gland, and gonadal cells (i.e., Sertoli, spermatogenic, and Leydig cells). The anterior lobe of the pituitary gland produces three hormones involved in this process: luteinizing hormone (LH), which, in the male, is sometimes referred to as interstitial cell–stimulating hormone (ICSH); follicle-stimulating hormone (FSH); and prolactin (PRL). In response to LH release by the pituitary, Leydig cells produce increasing amounts of testosterone. PRL acts in combination with LH to increase the steroidogenic activity of Leydig cells. Because FSH and testosterone receptors are found in Sertoli cells, these cells are the primary regulators of spermatogenesis.

Spermatogonial Phase

In the spermatogonial phase, stem cells divide to replace themselves and provide a population of committed spermatogonia.

Spermatogonial stem cells undergo multiple divisions and produce **spermatogonia** that can be differentiated into three types based on the appearance of their nuclei in routine H&E preparations:

- **Type A dark (Ad) spermatogonia** have ovoid nuclei with intensely basophilic, finely granular chromatin. These spermatogonia are thought to be the stem cells of the seminiferous epithelium. They divide at irregular intervals to give rise to either a pair of type Ad spermatogonia that remain as **reserve stem cells** or to a pair of type Ap spermatogonia.
- **Type A pale (Ap) spermatogonia** have ovoid nuclei with lightly staining, finely granular chromatin. Ap spermatogonia are committed to the differentiation process that produces the sperm. They undergo several successive mitotic divisions, thereby increasing their number. Type Ap spermatogonia are also called **renewing stem cells**.

FOLDER 22.2

CLINICAL CORRELATION: FACTORS AFFECTING SPERMATOGENESIS

Spermatogenic cells are sensitive to noxious agents. Degenerative changes, such as apoptosis, premature sloughing of cells, or formation of multinucleated giant cells, are readily apparent after exposure to such agents. Factors that negatively affect spermatogenesis include the following:

- **Dietary deficiencies.** Reduced dietary intake is known to impair spermatogenesis. Vitamins, coenzymes, and microelements such as vitamin A, vitamin B_{12}, vitamin C, vitamin E, β-carotenes, zinc, and selenium have been shown to affect sperm formation.
- **Environmental/lifestyle factors.** A recent study conducted in Denmark compared the sperm count in two groups of young men from rural and urban populations. A higher median sperm count (24%) was found in the men from the rural group compared with those from the urban group.
- **Developmental disorders.** Cryptorchidism, hypospadias, and factors such as low birth weight have been found to be important risk factors for testicular cancer associated with reduced semen quality and reduced fertility.
- **Systemic diseases or local infections.** Infections involving the testis (orchitis) may have an effect on spermatogenesis. Systemic diseases that can impair spermatogenesis include fever, kidney diseases, HIV and other viral infections, and metabolic disorders.
- **Elevated testicular temperature.** A sedentary lifestyle may impair the ability to maintain the lower temperature in the scrotum necessary for sperm production. A higher-than-average scrotal temperature has been linked to the failure of spermatogenesis.
- **Steroid hormones and related medications.** Exposure to synthetic estrogen (diethylstilbestrol) and other sex steroids can exert negative feedback on follicle-stimulating hormone (FSH) secretion, resulting in decreased spermatogenesis. Prenatal exposure to estrogens can potentially inhibit fetal gonadotropin secretion and inhibit Sertoli cell proliferation.
- **Toxic agents.** Mutagenic agents, antimetabolites, and some pesticides, such as dibromochloropropane (DBCP), can drastically affect spermatogenesis and production of normal sperm. DBCP is a nematocide pesticide that is still used in some developing countries. It has been shown to cause a major decrease in sperm count and infertility after human exposure. Other agents that may affect fertility include chemicals in plastics (e.g., phthalates), pesticides (e.g., DDT), products of combustion (e.g., dioxins), polychlorinated biphenyls (PCBs), and others. Most of these chemicals possess weak estrogen properties and are known as **endocrine-disrupting chemicals (EDCs)**. Direct toxicity to the spermatogonia is linked to changes in sperm quality.
- **Ionizing radiation and alkylating agents.** Nitrogen mustard gas and procarbazine have been found to have toxic effects on spermatogonia. **Electromagnetic** and **microwave radiation** also affect sperm count and motility.

Proliferating cells are particularly sensitive to mutagenic agents and the absence of essential metabolites. Therefore, nondividing Sertoli cells, Leydig cells, and reserve stem cells, which demonstrate low mitotic activity, are much less vulnerable than actively dividing, differentiating spermatogenic cells.

- **Type B spermatogonia** have generally spherical nuclei with chromatin that is condensed into large clumps along the nuclear envelope and around a central nucleolus (see Fig. 22.6).

An unusual feature of the division of an Ad spermatogonium into two types Ap spermatogonia is that the daughter cells remain connected by a thin cytoplasmic bridge. This same phenomenon occurs with each subsequent mitotic and meiotic division of the progeny of the original pair of Ap spermatogonia (Fig. 22.9). Thus, all of the progeny of an initial pair of Ap spermatogonia are connected, much like a strand of pearls. These cytoplasmic connections remain intact until the last stages of spermatid maturation and are essential for the synchronous development of each clone from an original pair of Ap cells.

After several divisions, type A spermatogonia differentiate into type B spermatogonia. The appearance of type B spermatogonia represents the last event in the spermatogonial phase.

Spermatocyte Phase (Meiosis)

In the spermatocyte phase, primary spermatocytes undergo meiosis to reduce both the chromosome number and the amount of DNA.

The mitotic division of type B spermatogonia produces **primary spermatocytes**. They replicate their DNA shortly after they form and before meiosis begins so that each primary spermatocyte contains the normal chromosomal number (2n). Because each chromosome consists of two sister chromatids, primary spermatocytes contain double the amount of DNA (4d).

Meiosis I results in reduction of both the number of chromosomes (from 2n to 1n) and the amount of DNA to the haploid number (from 4d to 2d); thus, secondary spermatocytes have a haploid number of chromosomes (1n) and 2d amount of DNA. Because no DNA replication precedes **meiosis II**, the spermatids, which are formed after this division, will also have the haploid (1n) number of chromosomes, each containing a single chromatid (1d). Meiosis is described in detail in Chapter 3, The Cell Nucleus (pages 102-103); a brief description of spermatocyte meiosis follows.

Each spermatocyte undergoes meiosis to form four haploid spermatids.

Prophase of the first meiotic division, during which the chromatin condenses into visible chromosomes, lasts up to 22 days in human primary spermatocytes. At the end of prophase, 44 autosomes and an X and a Y chromosome, each having two chromatin strands (chromatids), can be identified. Homologous chromosomes are paired as they line up on the metaphase plate.

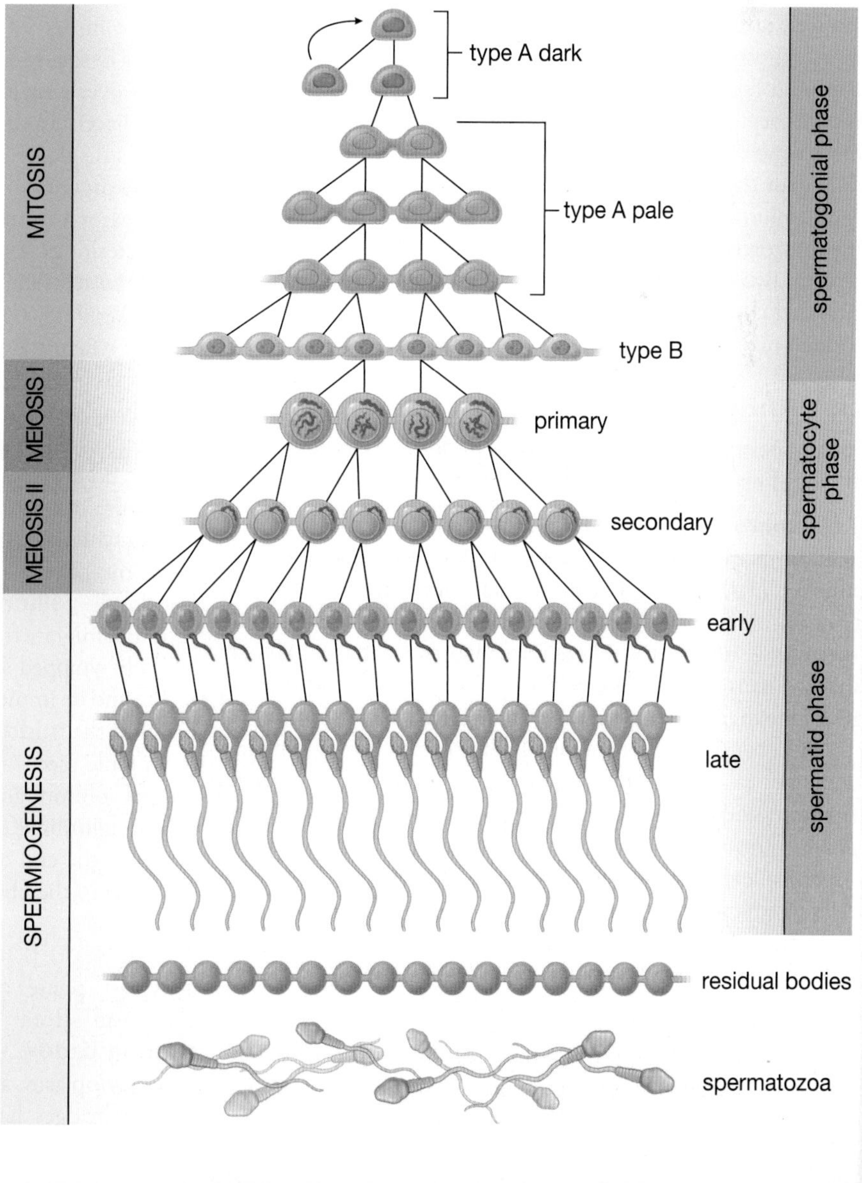

FIGURE 22.9. Schematic diagram illustrating the generations of spermatogenic cells. This diagram shows the clonal nature of the successive generations of spermatogenic cells. Type A dark spermatogonia are recognized as the reserve stem cells in the testis, whereas type A pale spermatogonia are the renewing stem cells. Type A pale spermatogonia undergo a series of synchronized cell divisions to either produce new type A pale cells or form more differentiated type B spermatogonia that undergo further divisions into primary spermatocytes. Note that cytoplasmic division is complete only in the type A dark spermatogonia. All other spermatogenic cells remain connected by intercellular bridges as they undergo mitotic and meiotic division and differentiation of the spermatids. Note also that primary spermatocytes undergo meiosis I and secondary spermatocytes undergo meiosis II. The cells separate into individual spermatozoa as they are released from the seminiferous epithelium. The residual bodies remain connected and are phagocytosed by the Sertoli cells. (Based on Dym M, Fawcett DW. Further observations on the numbers of spermatogonia, spermatocytes, and spermatids connected by intercellular bridges in the mammalian testis. *Biol Reprod.* 1971;4:195–215.)

The **paired homologous chromosomes**, called **tetrads** because they consist of four chromatids, exchange genetic material in a process called **crossing-over**. During this exchange, the four chromatids rearrange into a tripartite structure called a **synaptonemal complex**. This process ensures genetic diversity. Through genetic exchange, the four spermatids produced from each spermatocyte differ from each other and from every other spermatid.

After crossing-over is complete, the homologous chromosomes separate and move to the opposite poles of the meiotic spindle. Thus, the tetrads, which have been modified by crossing-over, separate and become dyads again. The two chromatids of each original chromosome (although modified by crossing-over) remain together.

The movement of a particular chromosome of a homologous pair to either pole of the spindle is random (i.e., maternally derived chromosomes and paternally derived chromosomes do not sort themselves out at the metaphase plate). This random sorting is another source of genetic diversity in the resulting sperm.

The cells derived from the first meiotic division are called **secondary spermatocytes**. These cells immediately enter the prophase of the second meiotic division *without synthesizing new DNA* (i.e., without passing through an S phase; see pages 102-103). The second meiotic division is short and lasts only several hours. Each secondary spermatocyte has a reduced number of chromosomes (1n), which is represented by 22 autosomes, and an X or a Y chromosome. Each of these chromosomes consists of two sister chromatids. The secondary spermatocyte has the (2d) diploid amount of DNA. During the metaphase of the second meiotic division, the chromosomes line up at the metaphase plate, and the sister chromatids separate and move to opposite poles of the spindle. As the second meiotic division is completed and the nuclear membranes reform, two haploid **spermatids**, each containing 23 single-stranded chromosomes (1n) and the 1d amount of DNA, are formed from each secondary spermatocyte (Fig. 22.10).

Spermatid Phase (Spermiogenesis)

In the spermatid phase, spermatids undergo extensive cell remodeling as they differentiate into mature sperm.

Each **spermatid** that results from the second meiotic division is haploid in DNA content **(1d)** and chromosome number **(1n)** represented by 22 autosomes and an X or Y chromosome. No further division occurs. The haploid spermatids undergo a differentiation process that produces mature sperm, which are also haploid. The 2d condition is restored when a sperm fertilizes an oocyte.

The extensive cell remodeling that occurs during differentiation of the spermatid population into mature sperm (spermiogenesis) consists of four phases: the Golgi phase, cap phase, acrosome phase, and maturation phase. These phases occur while the spermatids are physically attached to the Sertoli cell's plasma membrane by specialized junctions. The morphologic changes in all four phases that occur during spermiogenesis are described here and summarized in Figure 22.11.

Golgi phase

This phase is characterized by the presence of periodic acid–Schiff (PAS)-positive granules that accumulate in the numerous Golgi complexes of the spermatid. These **proacrosomal granules**, rich in glycoproteins, coalesce into a membrane-bound vesicle, the **acrosomal vesicle**, adjacent to the nuclear envelope. The vesicle enlarges and its contents increase during this phase. The position of the acrosomal vesicle determines the anterior pole of the developing sperm. Also during this phase, the centrioles migrate from the juxtanuclear region to the posterior pole of the spermatid, where the mature centriole aligns at right angles to the plasma membrane. The centriole initiates the assembly of the nine peripheral microtubule doublets and two central microtubules that constitute the **axoneme** of the sperm tail.

Cap phase

In this phase, the acrosomal vesicle spreads over the anterior half of the nucleus. This reshaped structure is called the **acrosomal cap**. The portion of the nuclear envelope beneath the acrosomal cap loses its pores and becomes thicker. The nuclear content also condenses. DNA in the spermatid is about 6 times smaller than the DNA in mitotic chromosomes. This high condensation of nuclear DNA is achieved by the presence of small, highly basic proteins called **protamines** that become incorporated into the chromatin during spermiogenesis, replacing the core histones.

Acrosome phase

In this phase, the spermatid reorients itself so that the head becomes deeply embedded in the Sertoli cell and points toward the basal lamina. The developing flagellum extends into the lumen of the seminiferous tubule. The condensed nucleus of the spermatid flattens and elongates, the nucleus and its overlying acrosome also move to a position immediately adjacent to the anterior plasma membrane, and the cytoplasm is displaced posteriorly. The cytoplasmic microtubules become organized into a cylindrical sheath, the **manchette**, which extends from the posterior rim of the acrosome toward the posterior pole of the spermatid.

The **centrioles**, which had earlier initiated the development of the flagellum, now move back to the posterior surface of the nucleus where the immature centriole becomes attached to a shallow groove in the nucleus. They are then modified to form the connecting piece, or neck region, of the developing sperm. Nine coarse fibers develop from the centrioles attached to the nucleus and extend into the tail, becoming the outer dense fibers peripheral to the microtubules of the axoneme. These fibers unite the nucleus with the flagellum; hence, the name **connecting piece**.

As the plasma membrane moves posteriorly to cover the growing **flagellum**, the manchette disappears, and the mitochondria migrate from the rest of the cytoplasm to form a tight, helically wrapped sheath around the coarse fibers in the neck region and its immediate posterior extension (Fig. 22.12). This region is the **middle piece** of the tail of the sperm. Distal to the middle piece, a **fibrous sheath** consisting of two longitudinal columns and numerous connecting ribs surrounds the nine longitudinal fibers of the **principal piece** and extends nearly to the end of the flagellum. This short segment of the tail distal to the fibrous sheath is called the **end piece**.

Maturation phase

This last phase of spermatid remodeling reduces excess cytoplasm from around the flagella to form mature **spermatozoon**. The Sertoli cells then phagocytose this excess cytoplasm, also termed the **residual body**. The intercellular bridges have characterized the developing gametes

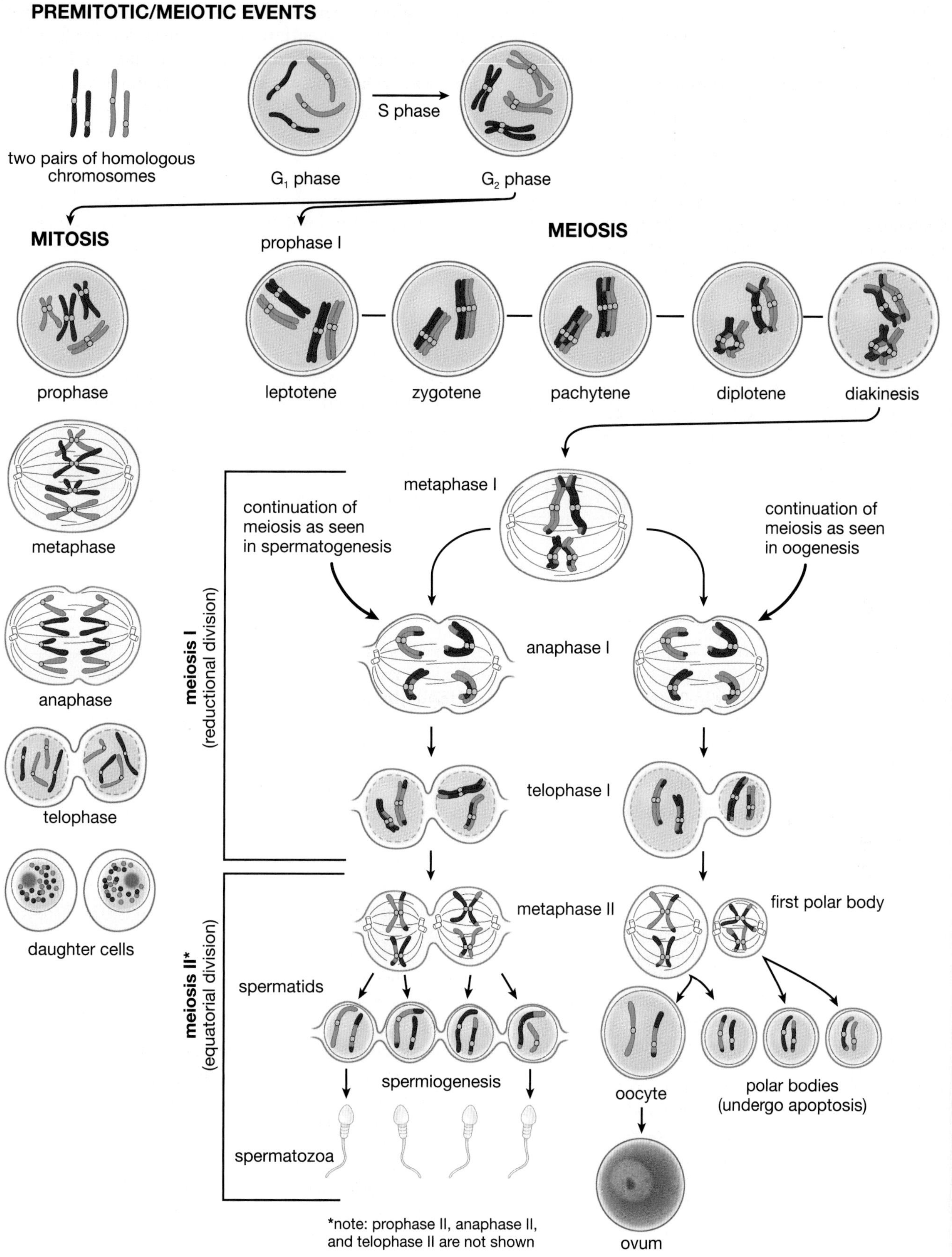

FIGURE 22.10. Comparison of mitosis and meiosis in spermatogenesis and oogenesis. The two pairs of chromosomes (2n) of maternal and paternal origin are depicted in *red* and *blue*, respectively. Mitotic division produces daughter cells that are genetically identical to the parental (2n) cell. Meiotic division, which has two components, a reductional division and an equatorial division, produces a cell that has only half the number of chromosomes (n). In addition, during the chromosome pairing in prophase I of meiosis, chromosome segments are exchanged, a process called *crossing-over*, creating genetic diversity. In humans, the first polar body does not divide, but it does so in other species.

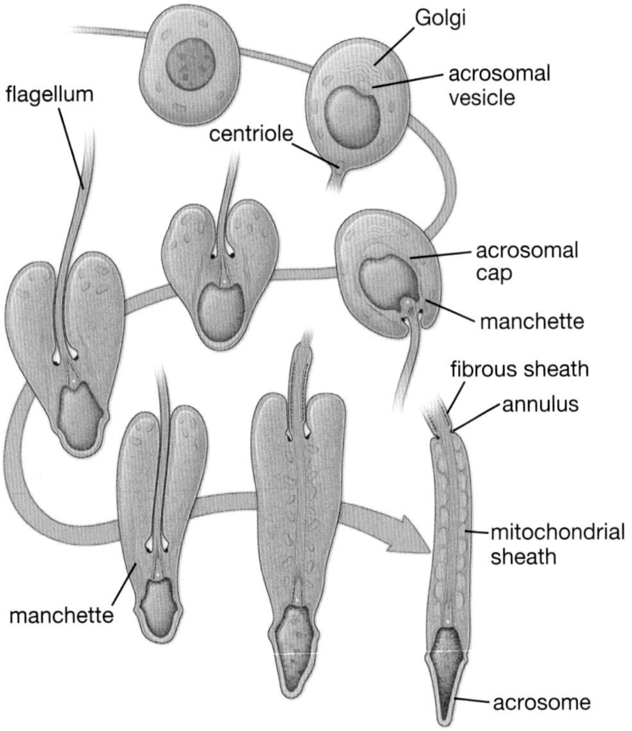

FIGURE 22.11. Schematic diagram of spermiogenesis in the human. The basic changes in the structure of the key organelles of the spermatid are illustrated (see text for detailed explanation). (Modified from Dym M. In: Weiss L, ed. *Cell and Tissue Biology: A Textbook of Histology*. 6th ed. Urban & Schwarzenberg; 1988.)

because the prespermatocyte stages remain with the residual bodies. Spermatids are no longer attached to each other and are released from the Sertoli cells.

Spermatids are released into the lumen of the seminiferous tubules during the process called spermiation.

Toward the end of the maturation phase of spermatogenesis, elongated spermatids are released from Sertoli cells into the lumen of seminiferous tubule. This complex process called **spermiation** involves the progressive removal of specialized Sertoli-to-spermatid junctional complexes and disengagement of spermatids from the Sertoli cell. The presence of β1-integrins in the Sertoli-to-spermatid junctions, as well as increased activity of integrin-linked kinase at the time of spermiation, suggests enzymatic control of spermatid release. The rate of spermiation in the testis determines the number of sperm cells in the ejaculate of semen. Various pharmacologic treatments, toxic agents, and gonadotropin suppression result in **spermiation failure**, in which spermatids are not released but instead are retained and phagocytosed by the Sertoli cell.

Structure of the Mature Sperm

The events of spermiogenesis result in a structurally unique cell.

The **mature human sperm** is about 60 μm long. The **sperm head** is flattened and pointed and measures 4.5 μm long by 3 μm wide by 1 μm thick (see Fig. 22.12). The **acrosomal cap** that covers the anterior two-thirds of the nucleus contains **hyaluronidase, neuraminidase, acid phosphatase**, and a **trypsin-like protease** called **acrosin**. These acrosomal enzymes are essential for penetration of the zona pellucida of the ovum. The release of acrosomal enzymes as the sperm makes contact with the egg is the first step in the **acrosome reaction**. This complex process facilitates sperm penetration and subsequent fertilization and prevents the entry of additional sperm into the ovum.

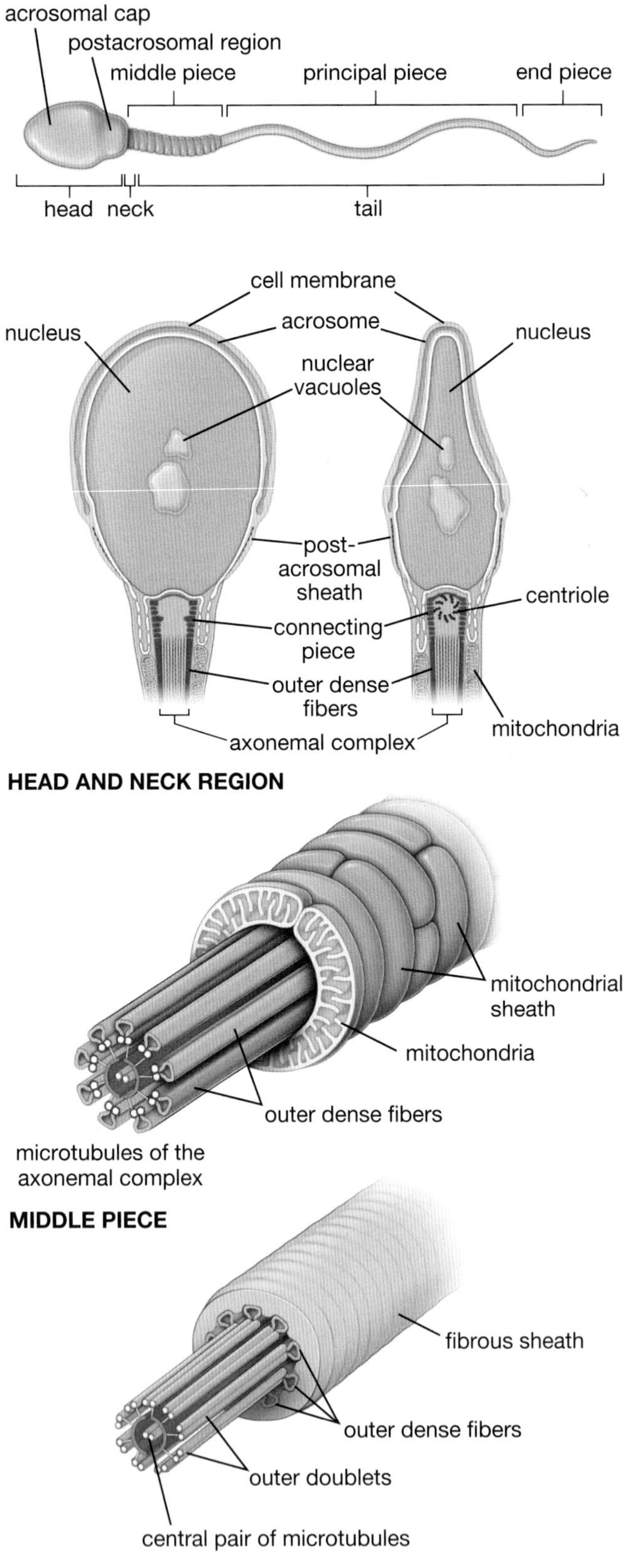

FIGURE 22.12. Diagram of a human spermatozoon. Regions of the spermatozoon are indicated on the *top*. Key structural features of the head (viewed in frontal and sagittal planes), the middle piece, and the principal piece of the spermatozoon are illustrated on the *bottom*. (Modified from Pederson PL, Fawcett DW. In: Hafez ESE, ed. *Human Semen and Fertility Regulation in the Male*. CV Mosby; 1976.)

The **sperm tail** is subdivided into the neck, middle piece, principal piece, and end piece. The short neck contains the centrioles and the origin of the coarse fibers. The middle piece is approximately 7 μm long and contains mitochondria, helically wrapped around the coarse fibers and the axonemal complex. These mitochondria provide the energy for movement of the tail and thus are responsible for the motility of the sperm. The principal piece is approximately 40 μm long and contains the fibrous sheath external to the coarse fibers and the axonemal complex. The end piece, approximately the last 5 μm of the flagellum in the mature sperm, contains only the axonemal complex.

Newly released sperm cells are processed in the epididymis where they acquire motility and undergo further maturation.

Newly released sperm cells are **nonmotile** and are transported from the seminiferous tubules in a fluid secreted by the Sertoli cells. The fluid and sperm flow through the **seminiferous tubules**, facilitated by peristaltic contractions of the peritubular contractile cells of the lamina propria. They then enter the **straight tubules**, a short segment of the seminiferous tubule where the epithelium consists only of Sertoli cells. At the mediastinum testis, the fluid and sperm enter the **rete testis**, an anastomosing system of ducts lined by simple cuboidal epithelium (Plate 22.2, page 898). From the rete testis, they move into the extratesticular portion of the **efferent ductules** (ductuli efferentes), the first part of the excurrent duct system, and then into the proximal portion of the **duct of the epididymis** (ductus epididymis). As the sperm cells move through 4–5 m of the highly coiled duct of the epididymis, they acquire motility and undergo several maturational changes. These changes include the following:

- Further condensation of nuclear DNA due to a series of chromatin remodeling events, leading to replacement of histones by protamines. The head of the sperm decreases in size.
- Additional reduction of cytoplasm. The sperm cells become more slender.
- Changes in plasma membrane lipids, proteins, and glycosylation
- Alterations in the outer acrosomal membrane (decapacitation). The surface-associated decapacitation factor is added to inhibit the fertilizing ability of the sperm cells (page 883).

Initiation of sperm cell motility during cell transit through the epididymis is most likely related to changes in the intracellular levels of cyclic adenosine monophosphate (cAMP), calcium ions (Ca^{2+}), and intracellular pH. These factors regulate flagellar activity through changes in **protein phosphorylation**, resulting from activities of **protein kinases** and **protein phosphatases**. For instance, pharmacologic stimulation of **protein kinase A** activity increases motility of sperm cells, whereas inhibition of **protein phosphatase** activity may initiate or stimulate such motility. This suggests that phosphatases have an important role in the regulation of **sperm kinetic activity**.

Contractions of the smooth muscle that surrounds the progressively distal and larger ducts continue to move the sperm by peristaltic action until they reach the distal portion of the duct of the epididymis, where they are stored before ejaculation.

Sperm can *live* for several weeks in the male excurrent duct system, but they will *survive* only 2–3 days in the female reproductive tract. They acquire the ability to fertilize the ovum only after some time in the female tract. This process, which involves removal and replacement of glycocalyx components (glycoconjugates) on the sperm membrane, is called **capacitation**. Capacitation of spermatozoa is described in detail in Chapter 23, The Female Reproductive System (pages 919-920).

■ SEMINIFEROUS TUBULES

Cycle of the Seminiferous Epithelium

Differentiating spermatogenic cells are not arranged at random in the seminiferous epithelium; specific cell types are grouped together. These groupings or associations occur because intercellular bridges are present between the progeny of each pair of **type Ap spermatogonia** and because the synchronized cells spend specific amounts of time in each stage of maturation. All phases of differentiation occur sequentially at any given site in a seminiferous tubule as the progeny of stem cells remain connected by cytoplasmic bridges and undergo synchronous mitotic and meiotic divisions and maturation (see Fig. 22.10).

Each recognizable grouping, or **cell association**, is considered a **stage** in a cyclic process. The series of stages that appears between two successive occurrences of the same cell association pattern at any given site in the seminiferous tubule constitutes a **cycle of the seminiferous epithelium**. The cycle of the seminiferous epithelium has been most thoroughly studied in rats, in which 14 successive stages occur in a linear sequence along the tubule. In humans, six stages or cell associations are defined in the cycle of the seminiferous epithelium (Fig. 22.13). These stages are not as clearly delineated as those in rodents because in humans, the cellular associations occur in irregular patches that form a mosaic pattern.

Duration of spermatogenesis in humans is approximately 74 days.

After injecting a pulse of tritiated thymidine, a specific generation of cells can be followed by sequential biopsies of the seminiferous tubules. In this way, the time required for the labeled cells to go through the various stages can be determined. Several generations of developing cells may be present in the thickness of the seminiferous epithelium at any given site and at any given time, which produces the characteristic cell associations. Autoradiographic studies have revealed that the duration of the **cycle of the seminiferous epithelium** is constant, lasting about 16 days in humans. In humans, it would require about 4.6 cycles (each 16 days long), or **approximately 74 days**, for a spermatogonium produced by a stem cell to complete the process of spermatogenesis. It would then require approximately **12 days** for the spermatozoon to **pass through the epididymis**. Approximately 300 million sperm cells are produced daily in the human testis. The length of the cycle and the time required for spermatogenesis are constant and specific in each species. Therefore, in any pharmacologic intervention (e.g., therapy for male infertility), if a drug is given that affects the initial phases of spermatogenesis, approximately **86 days** are required to see the effect of that compound on sperm production.

Waves of the Seminiferous Epithelium

As indicated earlier, the cycle of the seminiferous epithelium describes changes that occur with time at any given site in the tubule. In addition, the **wave of the seminiferous**

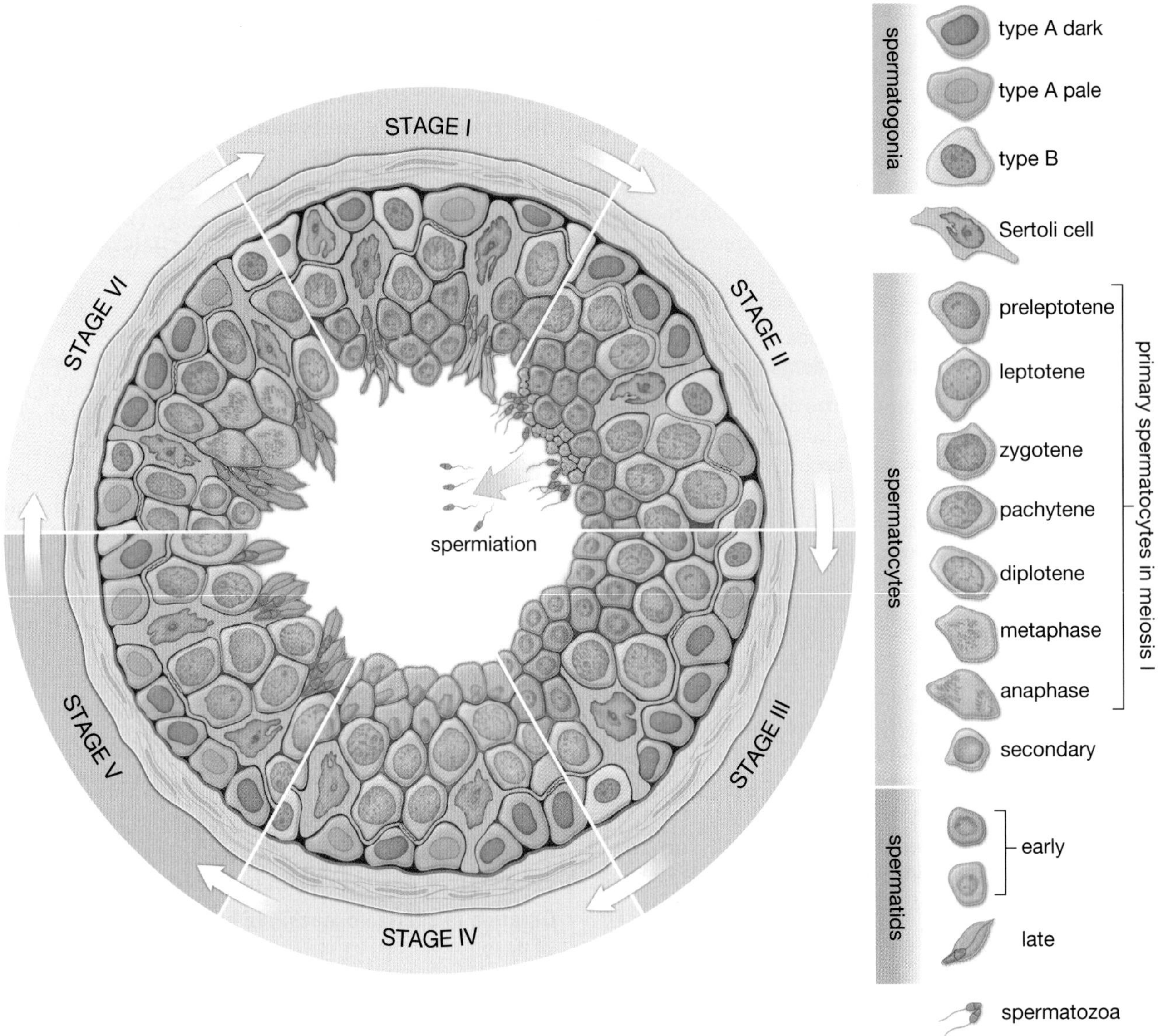

FIGURE 22.13. Schematic drawing of the stages of the human seminiferous epithelium. This diagram shows each of the six recognizable cell associations (stages) that occur in the cycle of the human seminiferous epithelium. These stages of spermatogenesis are artificially defined according to changes observed in the spermatids during their various steps of differentiation. In 1952, six stages of human seminiferous epithelium were first described by Leblond and Clermont and, since then, have been adopted by most researchers. Stages are labeled with Roman numerals I to VI. (Cell associations depicted in this drawing are based on Clermont Y. The cycle of the seminiferous epithelium in man. *Am J Anat.* 1963;112:35–51.)

epithelium describes the distribution of patterns of cellular association (**spermatogenic stages**) along the length of the tubule. In rodents and other mammals that have been studied, including subhuman primates, each stage occupies a significant length of the seminiferous tubule, and the stages appear to occur sequentially along the length of the tubule. In the rat, there are approximately 12 waves in each tubule. A transverse section through the tubule usually reveals only one pattern of cell associations. There are no waves in the human seminiferous epithelium, and the arrangement of spermatogenic stages along the seminiferous tubule is random. Each pattern of cellular associations (spermatogenic stage) has a **patch-like distribution in the human** seminiferous tubule (Fig. 22.14). Patches do not extend around the circumference of the tubule, nor are they in sequence. Therefore, a transverse section through a human seminiferous tubule may reveal as many as six different stages of the cycle arranged in a pie-wedge manner around the circumference of the tubule.

Sertoli Cells

Sertoli cells constitute the true epithelium of the seminiferous epithelium.

Sertoli cells (sustentacular cells) are tall, columnar, nonreplicating epithelial cells that rest on the thick, multilayered basal lamina of the seminiferous epithelium (Fig. 22.15). They are the supporting cells for the developing spermatozoa that attach to their surface after meiosis. Sertoli cells contain an extensive sER, a well-developed rER, and stacks of annulate lamellae. They have numerous spherical and elongated mitochondria, a well-developed Golgi apparatus, and varying numbers of lysosomes, lipid droplets, vesicles, and glycogen granules.

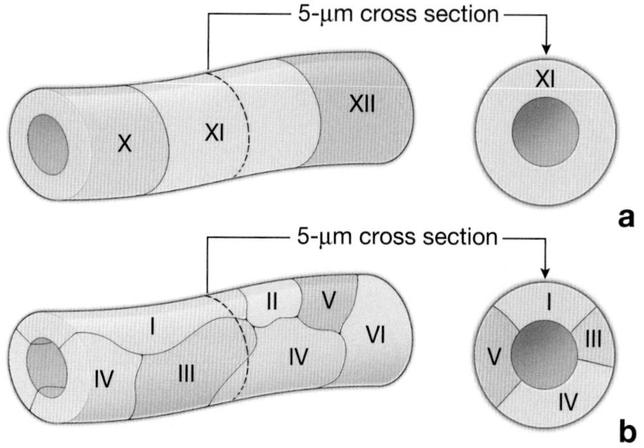

FIGURE 22.14. Diagram of organization of seminiferous epithelium in humans and other species. a. In mice and other rodent species, a specific cellular association occupies varying lengths along the tubule. Therefore, in a typical cross section, only a single cellular association is observed. **b.** In humans, cellular associations occur in irregularly shaped areas along the tubule, and therefore, a cross section typically shows two or more cellular associations.

The cytoskeleton of the Sertoli cell is one of the most elaborate in the human body and contains the following components:

- **Microtubules** that are abundant and predominately oriented parallel to the long axis of the cell. Unlike in many other cells, microtubules are nucleated at the periphery of the Sertoli cell and not from the microtubule-organizing center (MTOC). They are all oriented with their minus (−) ends toward the apex and plus (+) ends toward the base of the cell. In addition to their role in vesicular transport, recent evidence suggests that microtubules and microtubule-associated motor proteins are responsible for repositioning of the embedded elongated spermatids in the Sertoli cell's cytoplasm.
- **Intermediate filaments** that are a major component of the Sertoli cell's cytoskeleton and consist mainly of **vimentin** (class III of intermediate filament proteins). They form a perinuclear sheath that surrounds and separates the nucleus from other cytoplasmic organelles. Intermediate filaments extend from the perinuclear sheath to the desmosome-like junctions between the adjacent Sertoli cells and the hemidesmosomes.
- **Actin filaments** that are concentrated beneath the plasma membrane near the intercellular junctions. Actin filaments reinforce and stabilize the Sertoli intercellular junction specializations of plasma membrane.

The euchromatic Sertoli cell nucleus, a reflection of this very active cell, is generally ovoid or triangular and may have one or more deep infoldings. Its shape and location vary. It may be flattened, lying in the basal portion of the cell near and parallel to the base of the cell, or it may be triangular or ovoid, lying near or some distance from the base of the cell. In some species, the Sertoli cell's nucleus contains a unique tripartite structure that consists of an RNA-containing nucleolus flanked by a pair of DNA-containing bodies called **karyosomes** (Fig. 22.16).

In humans, characteristic **inclusion bodies of Charcot–Böttcher** are found in the basal cytoplasm. These slender fusiform crystalloids measure 10–25 μm long by 1 μm wide and are visible in routine histologic preparations. With transmission electron microscopy, they are resolved as bundles of poorly ordered, parallel or converging, straight, dense 15-nm-diameter filaments (see Fig. 22.15). Their chemical composition and function are unknown; however, recent studies detect an accumulation of lipoprotein receptor (CLA-1) proteins. This suggests that inclusion bodies may be involved in lipid transport and their utilization by the Sertoli cells.

The Sertoli cell-to-Sertoli cell junctional complex consists of a structurally unique combination of membrane and cytoplasmic specializations.

Sertoli cells are bound to one another by an unusual **Sertoli cell-to-Sertoli cell junctional complex** (Fig. 22.17). This complex is characterized, in part, by an exceedingly tight junction (zonula occludens) that includes more than 50 parallel fusion lines in the adjacent membranes. In addition, two cytoplasmic components characterize this unique junctional complex:

- A **flattened cisterna of sER** lies parallel to the plasma membrane in the region of the junction in each cell.
- **Actin filament bundles**, hexagonally packed, are interposed between the sER cisternae and the plasma membranes.

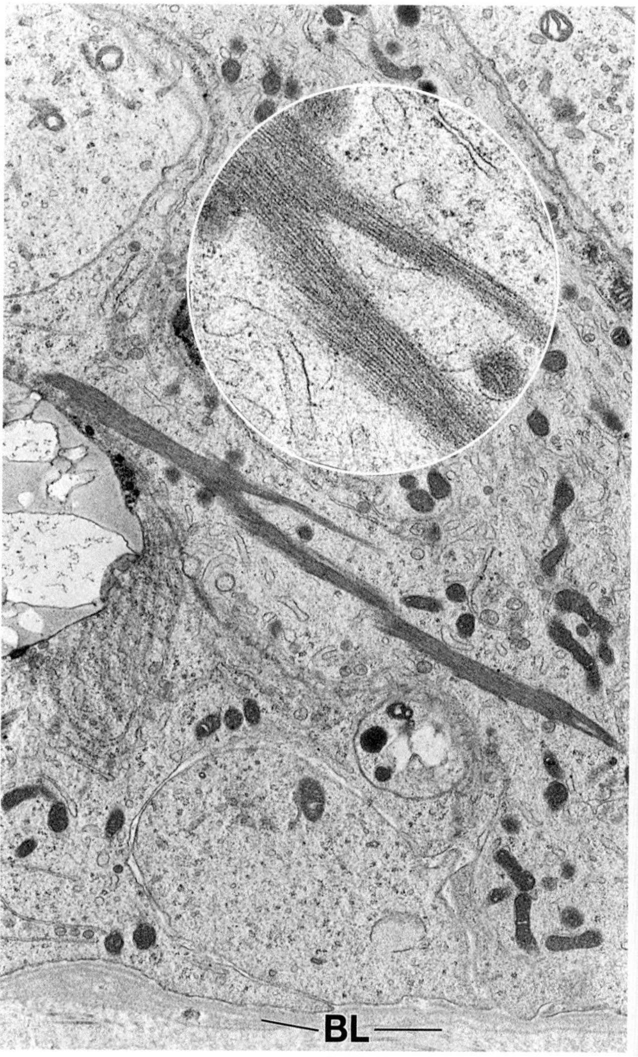

FIGURE 22.15. Electron micrograph of a human Sertoli cell. This electron micrograph shows characteristic crystalloid inclusion bodies of Charcot–Böttcher in the basal cytoplasm of the Sertoli cell. The basal lamina (*BL*) is indicated for orientation. ×9,000. **Inset.** This higher magnification shows filaments of the crystalloid. ×27,000. (Courtesy of Dr. Don F. Cameron.)

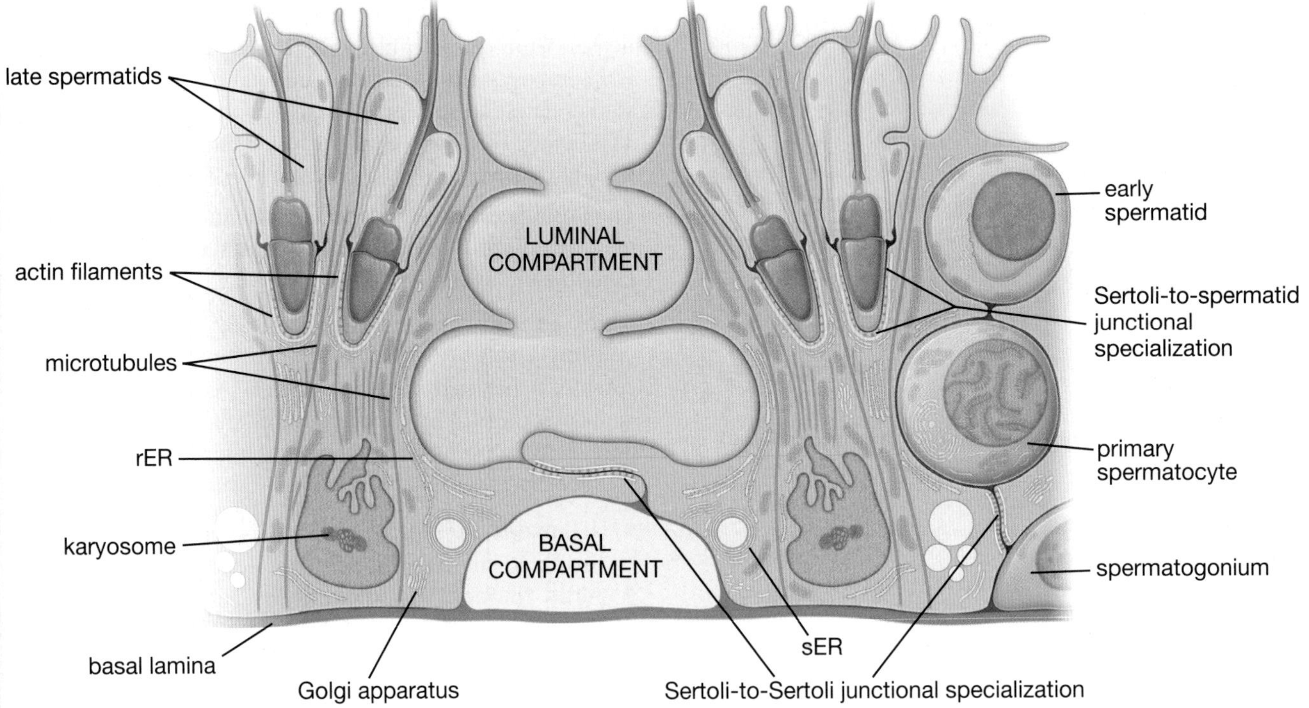

FIGURE 22.16. Schematic drawing of the Sertoli cell and its relationship to adjacent spermatogenic cells. This drawing shows the Sertoli-to-Sertoli junctional specialization between adjacent Sertoli cells and the Sertoli-to-spermatid junctional specialization between the Sertoli cell and late spermatids. The Sertoli-to-Sertoli junctional complex is an adhesion device that includes a tight junction that contributes to the blood–testis barrier. The junctional specialization between the Sertoli cell and late spermatids residing in deep recesses within the apical cytoplasm is an adhesion device only. Lateral processes of the Sertoli cells extend over the surface of the spermatocytes and spermatids. Note the ultrastructural features of the Sertoli cell, including the microtubule arrays and characteristic shape of the nucleus and its karyosome. *rER*, rough endoplasmic reticulum; *sER*, smooth endoplasmic reticulum. (Reprinted with permission from Bloom W, Fawcett DW. *A Textbook of Histology*. WB Saunders; 1975.)

A similar-appearing junctional complex in the Sertoli cell is also present at the site where the spermatids are attached. However, no tight junction is present, and the spermatid lacks flattened cisternae of sER and actin filament bundles (see Figs. 22.16 and 22.17). Other junctional specializations of the Sertoli cells include gap junctions between Sertoli cells, desmosome-like junctions between Sertoli cells and early-stage spermatogenic cells, and hemidesmosomes at the Sertoli cell–basal lamina interface.

The Sertoli cell-to-Sertoli cell junctional complex divides the seminiferous epithelium into basal and luminal compartments, segregating postmeiotic germ cell development and differentiation from the systemic circulation.

The Sertoli cell-to-Sertoli cell junctions establish two epithelial compartments, a **basal epithelial compartment** and a **luminal compartment** (see Fig. 22.16). Spermatogonia and early primary spermatocytes are restricted to the basal compartment (i.e., between the Sertoli cell-to-Sertoli cell junctions and the basal lamina). More mature spermatocytes and spermatids are restricted to the luminal side of the Sertoli cell-to-Sertoli cell junctions. **Early spermatocytes** produced by mitotic division of type B spermatogonia **must pass through the junctional complex** to move from the basal compartment to the luminal compartment. This movement occurs via the formation of a new junctional complex between Sertoli cell processes that extends beneath the newly formed spermatocytes, followed by the breakdown of the junction above them. Thus, in the differentiation of the spermatogenic cells, meiosis and spermiogenesis take place in the luminal compartment.

In both compartments, spermatogenic cells are surrounded by complex processes of the Sertoli cells. Because of the unusually close relationships between Sertoli cells and differentiating spermatogenic cells, it has been suggested that Sertoli cells serve as "nurse," or supporting, cells (i.e., they function in the exchange of metabolic substrates and wastes between the developing spermatogenic cells and the circulatory system).

In addition, Sertoli cells phagocytose and break down the residual bodies formed in the last stage of spermiogenesis. They also phagocytose any spermatogenic cells that fail to differentiate completely.

The Sertoli cell-to-Sertoli cell junctional complex is the site of the blood–testis barrier.

In addition to the physical compartmentalization described earlier, the Sertoli cell-to-Sertoli cell junctional complex also creates a permeability barrier called the **blood–testis barrier**. This barrier is essential in creating a physiologic compartmentalization within the seminiferous epithelium with respect to ionic, amino acid, carbohydrate, and protein composition. Therefore, the composition of the fluid in the seminiferous tubules and excurrent ducts differs considerably from the composition of the blood plasma and testicular lymph.

Plasma proteins and circulating antibodies are excluded from the lumen of the seminiferous tubules. The exocrine secretory products of the Sertoli cells (particularly **androgen-binding protein [ABP]**, which has a high

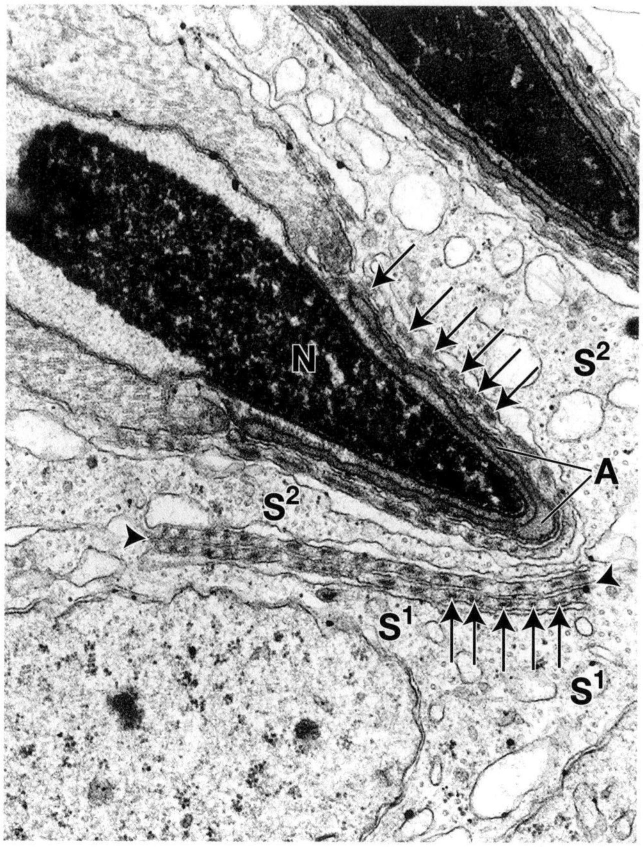

FIGURE 22.17. Electron micrograph of Sertoli cell junctions. This electron micrograph demonstrates a Sertoli-to-Sertoli junctional complex and, in close proximity, a Sertoli-to-spermatid junctional specialization. Condensation and shaping of the spermatid nucleus (*N*) are well advanced. The acrosome (*A*) of the spermatid appears as a V-shaped profile, and in close association with it is the Sertoli cell junctional specialization characterized by bundles of microfilaments that are cut in cross section (*arrows*). The associated profile of endoplasmic reticulum resides immediately adjacent to the microfilament bundles. The Sertoli-to-Sertoli junction lies below, joining one Sertoli cell (S^1) to the adjacent Sertoli cell (S^2). The *arrowheads* indicate the limits of the junction. Note that the junction here reveals the same elements, the microfilament bundles (*arrows*) and a profile of endoplasmic reticulum, as are seen in the Sertoli-to-spermatid junctional specialization. Not evident at this magnification is the tight junction associated with the Sertoli-to-Sertoli junctional complex. ×30,000.

binding affinity for testosterone and DHT) are highly concentrated in the lumen of the seminiferous tubules and maintain a high concentration of testosterone, which provides a favorable microenvironment for the differentiating spermatogenic cells.

Most importantly, the blood–testis barrier isolates the genetically different and, therefore, antigenic haploid germ cells (secondary spermatocytes, spermatids, and sperm) from the immune system of the adult male. Antigens produced by, or specific to, the sperm are prevented from reaching the systemic circulation. Conversely, γ-globulins and specific sperm antibodies found in some individuals are prevented from reaching the developing spermatogenic cells in the seminiferous tubule (Folder 22.3). Therefore, the **blood–testis barrier** serves an essential role in isolating the spermatogenic cells from the immune system.

Sertoli cells have both exocrine and endocrine secretory functions.

In addition to secreting fluid that facilitates passage of the maturing sperm along the seminiferous tubules to the intratesticular ducts, **Sertoli cells** produce critical factors necessary for the successful progression of spermatogonia into spermatozoa. They secrete a 90-kDa **androgen-binding protein (ABP)**. ABP concentrates testosterone in the luminal compartment of the seminiferous tubule, where high concentrations of testosterone are essential for the normal maturation of the developing sperm.

Follicle-stimulating hormone (FSH) receptors and testosterone receptors are present in Sertoli cells; therefore, their secretory function is regulated by both FSH and testosterone (Fig. 22.18). Sertoli cells secrete several endocrine substances, such as **inhibin**, a 32-kDa glycoprotein hormone involved in the feedback loop that inhibits FSH release from the anterior pituitary gland. In addition, Sertoli cells synthesize **plasminogen activator**, which converts plasminogen to the active proteolytic hormone plasmin, **transferrin** (an iron-transporting protein), and **ceruloplasmin** (a copper-transporting protein). Furthermore, the Sertoli cells secrete other glycoproteins that function as growth factors or paracrine factors, such as MIF, stem cell factor (SCF), and glial cell line–derived neurotrophic factor (GDNF).

FOLDER 22.3

CLINICAL CORRELATION: SPERM-SPECIFIC ANTIGENS AND THE IMMUNE RESPONSE

Two basic facts are well established about the immunologic importance of the **blood–testis barrier**:

- Spermatozoa and spermatogenic cells possess molecules that are unique to these cells and are recognized as "foreign" (not self) by the immune system.
- Spermatozoa are first produced at puberty, long after the individual has become immunocompetent (i.e., capable of recognizing foreign molecules and producing antibodies against them).

Failure of the spermatogenic cells and spermatozoa to remain isolated results in the production of sperm-specific antibodies. Such an immune response is sometimes seen after **vasectomy** and in some cases of **infertility**. After vasectomy, sperm-specific antibodies are produced as the cells of the immune system are exposed to the spermatozoa that may leak from the severed ductus deferens. Thus, sperm no longer remain isolated from the immune system within the reproductive tract. In some cases of infertility, sperm-specific antibodies have been found in the semen. These antibodies cause the sperm to agglutinate, preventing movement and interaction with the ovum.

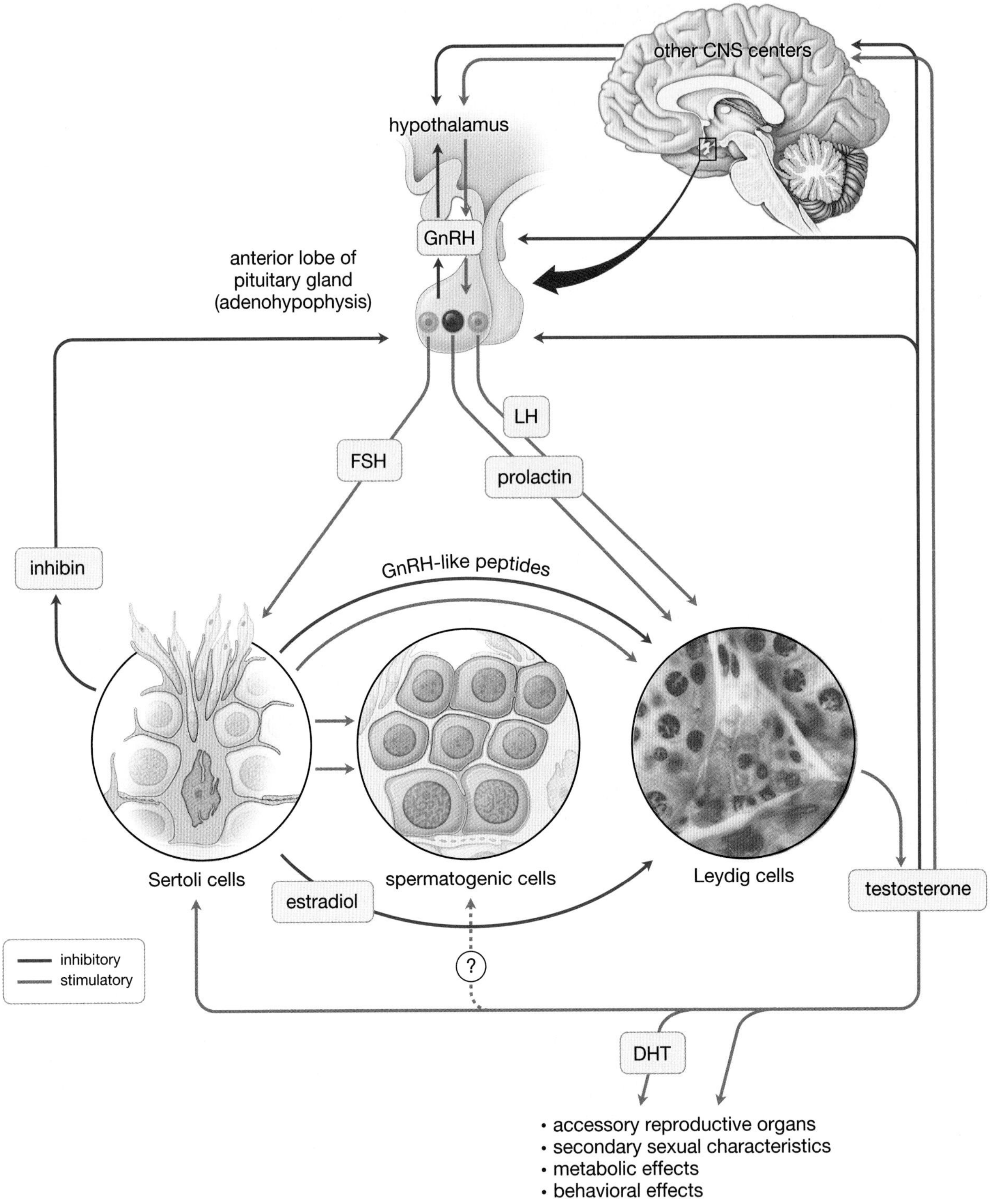

FIGURE 22.18. Diagram depicting the hormonal regulation of male reproductive function. *Blue arrows* indicate stimulatory action on the system; *red arrows* indicate inhibitory feedback. See text for explanation. *CNS*, central nervous system; *DHT*, dihydrotestosterone; *FSH*, follicle-stimulating hormone; *GnRH*, gonadotropin-releasing hormone; *LH*, luteinizing hormone.

■ INTRATESTICULAR DUCTS

At the end of each seminiferous tubule, there is an abrupt transition to the **straight tubules**, or **tubuli recti**. This short terminal section of the seminiferous tubule is lined only by Sertoli cells (Plate 22.2, page 898). Near their termination, the straight tubules narrow, and their lining changes to a simple cuboidal epithelium.

The straight tubules empty into the **rete testis**, a complex series of interconnecting channels within the highly vascular connective tissue of the mediastinum (Fig. 22.19). A simple cuboidal or low columnar epithelium lines the channels of the rete testis. These cells have a single apical cilium and relatively few short apical microvilli.

■ EXCURRENT DUCT SYSTEM

The excurrent duct system develops from the mesonephric (Wolffian) duct and mesonephric tubules.

The initial development of Leydig cells and initiation of testosterone secretion stimulate the mesonephric (Wolffian) duct to differentiate into the excretory duct system for the developing testis (Fig. 22.20). The portion of the mesonephric duct adjacent

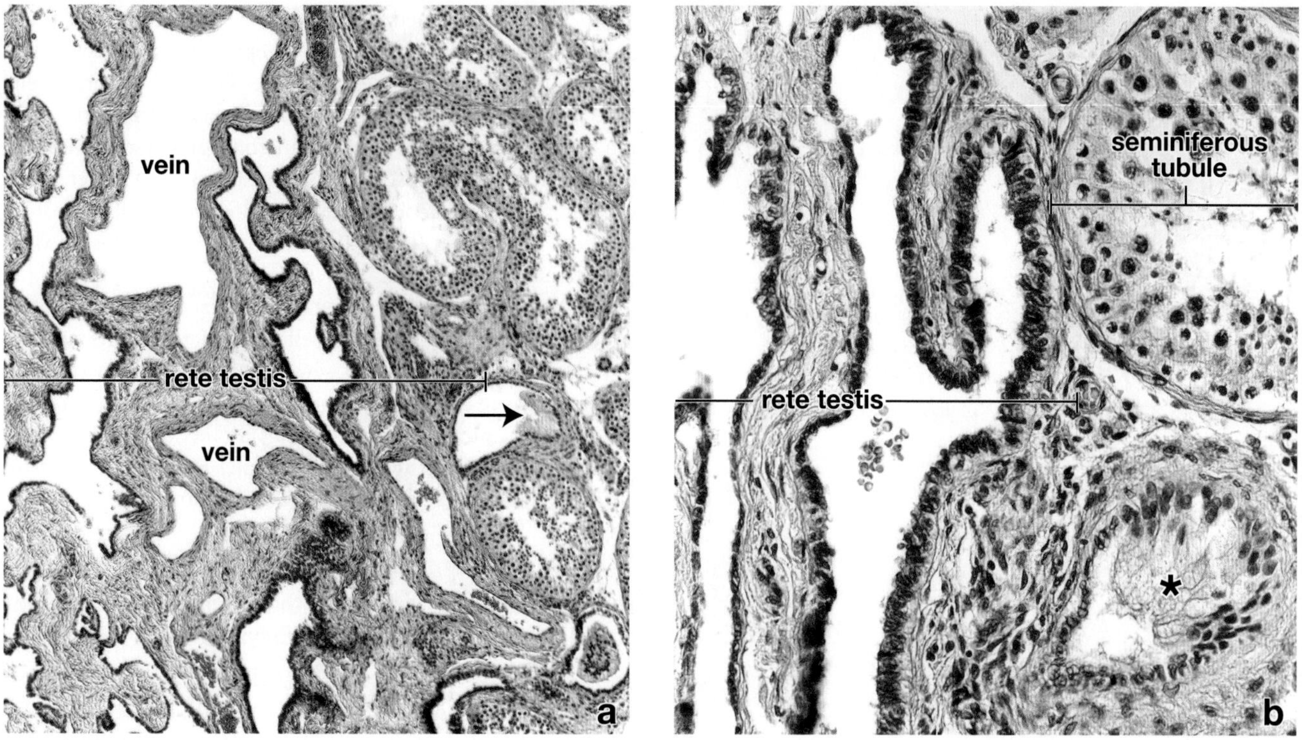

FIGURE 22.19. Photomicrograph of human testis. a. This hematoxylin and eosin (H&E)-stained specimen shows the site that includes the mediastinum of the testis. On the *right* are seminiferous tubules, and on the *left* are the anastomosing channels of the rete testis. The *arrow* indicates termination of a straight tubule that is lined only by Sertoli cells. It is at this site that the tubule contents enter the rete testis and the channels are then lined by a simple cuboidal epithelium. ×70. **b.** This higher magnification from a slightly deeper section of the same specimen shows the rete testis (*left*), a cross section of a seminiferous tubule (*upper right*), and a terminating straight tubule (*asterisk*) where it is entering the rete testis. Note the abrupt change in the epithelial lining at this site. As noted, the lining epithelium of the rete testis is simple cuboidal. ×275.

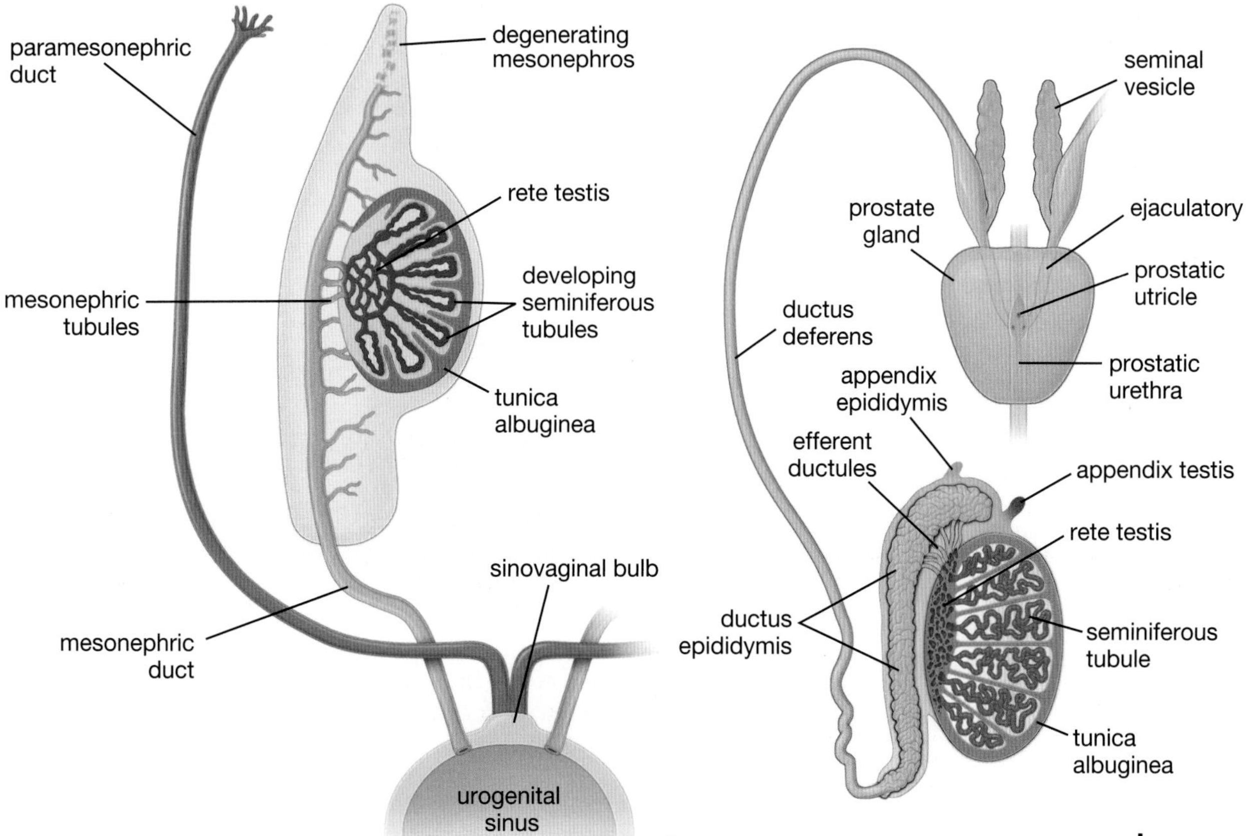

FIGURE 22.20. Schematic diagram of development of intratesticular and excurrent duct systems. a. This diagram shows the testis in the seventh week of development before it descends into the scrotal sac. Note that the mesonephric duct and its tubules give rise to the excurrent duct system for the developing testis. **b.** Sagittal section of a fully developed testis positioned within the scrotum. Note that the seminal vesicles, ejaculatory ducts, ductus deferens, and epididymis are all developed from the mesonephric duct. Efferent ductules originated from mesonephric tubules. The seminiferous tubules, straight tubules, and rete testis develop from the indifferent gonads. The prostate gland develops from the multiple outgrowths that originate from the pelvic urethra (a urogenital sinus derivative).

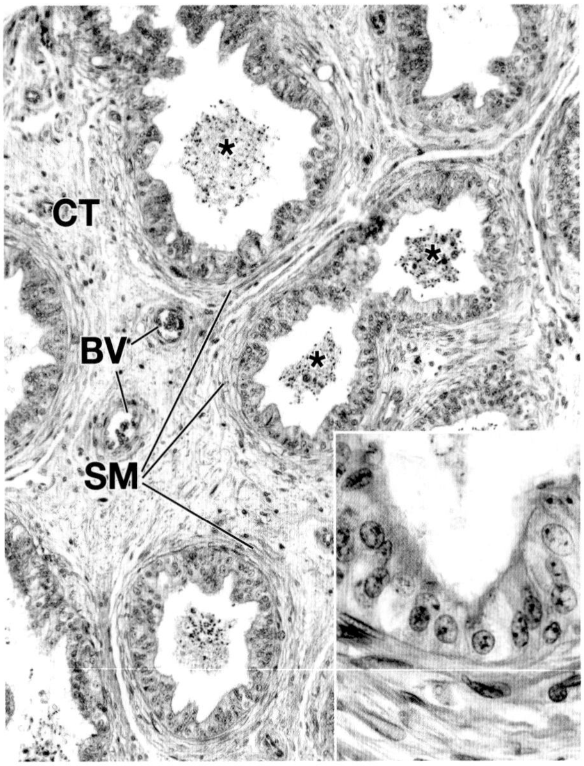

FIGURE 22.21. Photomicrograph of efferent ductules. The specimen in this photomicrograph was stained with picric acid and hematoxylin to better visualize the epithelial components of the efferent ductules. The efferent ductules are lined by pseudostratified columnar epithelium. The luminal surface has an uneven or wavy appearance because of the presence of alternating groups of tall columnar cells and cuboidal cells. The ductules are surrounded by several layers of circularly arranged smooth muscle (*SM*). Within the ductule lumina are clumped spermatozoa (*asterisks*). Connective tissue (*CT*) makes up the stroma of the organ and contains blood vessels (*BV*) of various sizes. ×120. **Inset.** This higher magnification of the pseudostratified epithelium shows columnar and cuboidal cells that contain sparse cilia. ×500.

to the developing testis becomes convoluted and differentiates into the **duct of the epididymis**. In addition, a number (about 20) of the remaining mesonephric tubules in this region make contact with the developing seminiferous cords and finally develop into the **efferent ductules** (Fig. 22.21 and Plate 22.3, page 900). They connect the developing rete testis with the duct of the epididymis. The distal part of the mesonephric duct acquires a thick, smooth muscle coat and becomes the **ductus deferens**. The end of the distal mesonephric duct gives rise to the **ejaculatory duct** and **seminal vesicles**.

The efferent ductules are lined with pseudostratified columnar epithelium.

In humans, approximately 20 **efferent ductules** connect the channels of the **rete testis** at the superior end of the mediastinum to the proximal portion of the **duct of the epididymis**. As the efferent ductules exit the testis, they become highly coiled and form 6–10 conical masses, the **coni vasculosi**, whose bases form part of the head of the epididymis. The coni vasculosi, each about 10 mm in length, contain highly convoluted ducts that measure 15–20 cm in length. At the base of the cones, the efferent ductules open into a single channel, the duct of the epididymis (see Fig. 22.4).

The efferent ductules are lined with a pseudostratified columnar epithelium that contains clumps of tall and short cells, giving the luminal surface a saw-tooth appearance (see Fig. 22.21). Interspersed among the columnar cells are occasional basal cells that serve as epithelial stem cells. The tall columnar cells are ciliated. The short nonciliated cells have numerous microvilli and canalicular invaginations of the apical surface as well as numerous pinocytotic vesicles, membrane-bound dense bodies, lysosomes, and other cytoplasmic structures associated with endocytic activity. Most of the fluid secreted in the seminiferous tubules is reabsorbed in the efferent ductules.

A **smooth muscle layer** in the excurrent ducts first appears at the beginning of the efferent ductules. The smooth muscle cells form a layer of several cells thick in which the cells are arrayed as a circular sheath in the wall of the ductule. Interspersed among the muscle cells are elastic fibers. Transport of the sperm in the efferent ductules is affected largely by both ciliary action and contraction of this fibromuscular layer.

Epididymis

The epididymis is an organ that contains the efferent ductules and the duct of the epididymis.

The **epididymis** is a crescent-shaped structure that lies along the superior and posterior surfaces of the testis. It measures about 7.5 cm in length and consists of the **efferent ductules** and the **duct of the epididymis** and associated vessels, smooth muscles, and connective tissue coverings (Fig. 22.22 and Plate 22.3, page 900). The duct of the epididymis is a highly coiled tube measuring 4–6 m in length. The epididymis is

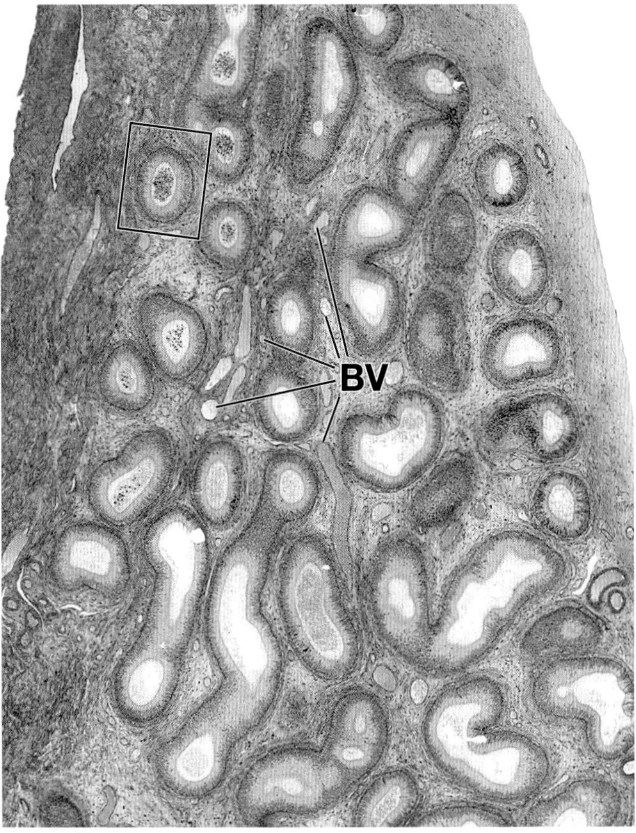

FIGURE 22.22. Photomicrograph of human epididymis. This photomicrograph of a hematoxylin and eosin (H&E)-stained section shows the highly coiled ductus epididymis. Its coiled nature is reflected in the variously shaped profiles of the duct. Within the connective tissue are numerous profiles of blood vessels (*BV*). The vessels tend to follow the duct; thus, they too reflect multiple profiles of several vessels. The section of the duct within the *rectangle* is shown at higher magnification in Figure 22.23. ×30.

divided into a **head**, a **body**, and a **tail** (see Fig. 22.4). The efferent ductules occupy the head, and the duct of the epididymis occupies the body and tail. Newly produced sperm, which enter the epididymis from the testis, mature during their passage through the duct of the epididymis, acquiring motility and the ability to fertilize an oocyte. During this androgen-dependent maturation process, the head of the sperm is modified by the addition of **surface-associated decapacitation factor** containing epididymal fluid glycoconjugates. This process, called **decapacitation**, inhibits the fertilizing ability of the sperm in a reversible manner. The surface-associated decapacitation factor is later released during **capacitation** that occurs in the female reproductive tract just before fertilization. After maturation in the epididymis, sperm can transport their haploid content of DNA to the ovum, and after capacitation, they can bind to sperm receptors on the zona pellucida of the ovum. This binding triggers the acrosome reaction in which the sperm uses its acrosomal enzymes to penetrate the outer covering of the oocyte.

The principal cells in the pseudostratified epithelium of the epididymis are characterized by stereocilia.

Like most of the excurrent duct system, the duct of the epididymis is also lined with a pseudostratified columnar epithelium (Fig. 22.23). In general, it contains two types of cells:

- **Principal cells** that vary from approximately 80 μm in height in the head of the epididymis to approximately 40 μm in height in the tail. Numerous long, modified microvilli called **stereocilia** extend from the luminal surface of the principal cells (Plate 22.3, page 900). The stereocilia vary in height from 25 μm in the head to approximately 10 μm in the tail.
- **Basal cells** that represent small, round cells resting on the basal lamina. They are the stem cells of the duct epithelium.

In addition, **migrating lymphocytes** called **halo cells** are often found within the epithelium. Under normal conditions, the epithelium of the epididymis represents the most proximal level of the excurrent duct system in which lymphocytes are present.

Epididymal cells function in both absorption and secretion.

Most of the fluid that is not reabsorbed by the efferent ductules is reabsorbed in the proximal portion of the epididymis. The epithelial cells also phagocytose any residual bodies not removed by the Sertoli cells as well as sperm that degenerate in the duct. The apical cytoplasm of the principal cells contains numerous invaginations at the bases of the stereocilia, along with coated vesicles, multivesicular bodies, and lysosomes (Fig. 22.24).

The principal cells secrete glycerophosphocholine, sialic acid, and glycoproteins, which, in addition to the glycocalyx and steroids, aid in the **maturation of the sperm**. They have numerous cisternae of rER surrounding the basally located nucleus and a remarkably large supranuclear Golgi apparatus. Profiles of sER and rER are also present in the apical cytoplasm.

The smooth muscle coat of the duct of the epididymis gradually increases in thickness to become three layered in the tail.

In the head of the epididymis and most of the body, the smooth muscle coat consists of a thin layer of circular smooth muscle, resembling that of the efferent ductules. In the tail, inner and outer longitudinal layers are added. These three layers are then continuous with the three smooth muscle layers of the ductus deferens, the next component of the excurrent duct system (Plate 22.4, page 902).

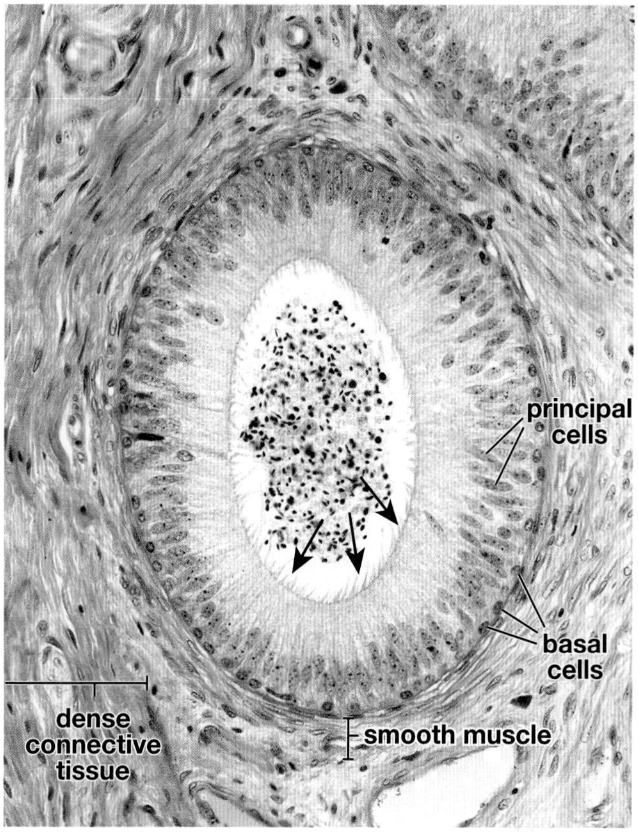

FIGURE 22.23. Photomicrograph of human ductus epididymis. This higher magnification of the *rectangular area* in Figure 22.22 reveals the two cell types of the epididymal epithelium, the principal cells and the basal cells. Stereocilia (*arrows*) extend from the apical surface of the principal cells. The nuclei of the basal cells are spherical and are located in close proximity to the basement membrane, whereas the nuclei of the principal cells are cylindrical and conform to the columnar shape of the cell. Surrounding the duct epithelium is a layer of circularly arranged smooth muscle cells. The duct lumen contains numerous sperm. ×250.

Differences in smooth muscle function parallel these morphologic differences. In the head and body of the epididymis, spontaneous, rhythmic peristaltic contractions serve to move the sperm along the duct. Few peristaltic contractions occur in the tail of the epididymis, which serves as the principal reservoir for mature sperm. These sperm are forced into the ductus deferens by intense contractions of the three smooth muscle layers after appropriate neural stimulation associated with ejaculation.

Ductus Deferens

The ductus deferens is the longest part of the excurrent duct system.

The **ductus deferens (vas deferens)** is a direct continuation of the tail of the epididymis (see Fig. 22.1). In the scrotum, the ductus deferens ascends along the posterior border of the testis, close to the testicular vessels and nerves. It then enters the abdomen as a component of the spermatic cord by passing through the inguinal canal. The **spermatic cord** contains all of the structures that pass to and from the testis. In addition to the ductus deferens, the spermatic cord contains the testicular artery, small arteries to the ductus deferens and cremaster muscle, the pampiniform plexus, lymphatic vessels, sympathetic nerve fibers, and the genital branch of the genitofemoral nerve. All of these structures are surrounded by fascial coverings

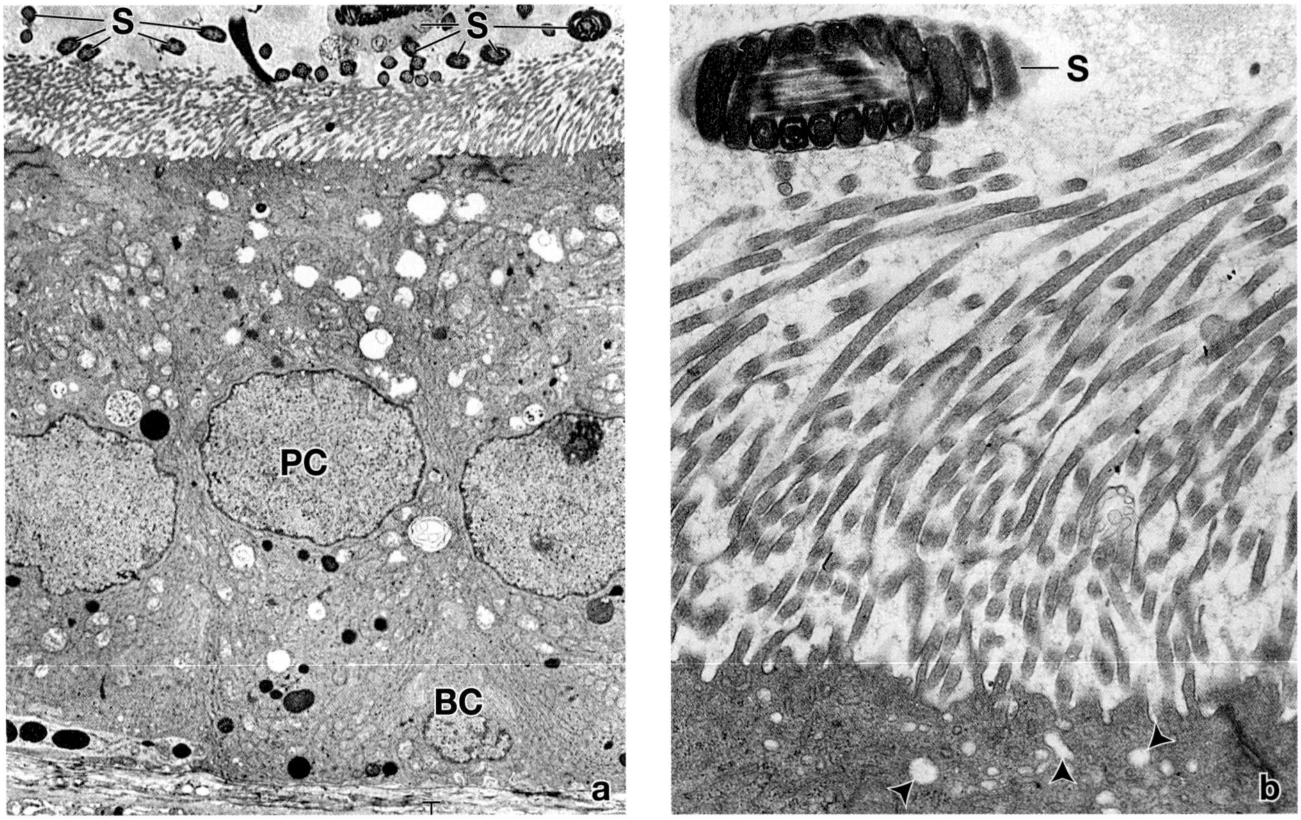

FIGURE 22.24. Electron micrograph of epididymis. a. Electron micrograph of the epididymal epithelium showing principal cells (*PC*) extending to the lumen and a basal cell (*BC*) limited to the basal portion of the epithelium. Profiles of sperm (*S*) are seen in the lumen. The apical cytoplasm of the principal cells exhibits numerous long microvilli (stereocilia). ×3,000. **b.** Apical surface of the epithelial cell with its numerous long microvilli (stereocilia). The middle piece of a sperm (*S*) is evident in the lumen. The small, light circular profiles (*arrowheads*) are endocytotic vesicles. ×13,000.

derived from the anterior abdominal wall. After leaving the spermatic cord, the ductus deferens descends into the pelvis to the level of the bladder, where its distal end enlarges to form the **ampulla of ductus deferens**. The ampulla is joined there by the **duct of the seminal vesicle** and continues through the prostate gland to the prostatic urethra as the **ejaculatory duct**.

The ductus deferens is lined with a pseudostratified columnar epithelium that closely resembles that of the epididymis (Plate 22.4, page 902). The tall columnar cells also have stereocilia that extend into the lumen. The rounded basal cells rest on the basal lamina. Unlike the epididymis, however, the lumen of the duct does not appear smooth. In histologic preparations (Fig. 22.25), it appears to be thrown into deep longitudinal folds throughout most of its length, probably because of the contraction of the thick (1–1.5 mm) muscular coat of the duct during fixation.

As the **vas deferens** passes through the spermatic cord, it can be easily palpable during physical examination of the scrotum. The easy access to this structure is advantageous during **vasectomy**, a male option for sterilization. Vasectomy is a safe and relatively simple method of sterilization and has lower rates of morbidity and mortality than female sterilization (uterine tube occlusion). During a vasectomy, small incisions in the skin of the scrotum are made and the vas deferens from each testis is exposed, clamped, and severed, preventing passage of the sperm cells into the ejaculatory duct and prostatic urethra. Following vasectomy, both testes continue to produce sperm cells. In 10%–30% of vasectomy cases, increased intraluminal pressure causes distension of the epididymis and pressure-mediated damage to the seminiferous epithelium, followed by **sperm granuloma** formation at the vasectomy site, epididymis, or rete testis. A sperm granuloma is a site of spermatozoa phagocytosis by large, activated macrophages. Degradation products of macrophages are absorbed by the epididymal epithelium. Sperm granulomas are rarely symptomatic. In addition, owing to the constant leak of spermatozoal antigens into the tissues, mechanisms of humoral immunity may be activated, resulting in the production of **IgA antisperm antibodies**. Although these antibodies develop in a significant proportion of patients postvasectomy, they do not increase the risk of immune complex or atherosclerotic heart disease. About 500,000 vasectomies are performed each year in the United States, with up to 6% of patients requesting **vasectomy reversal** in the form of vasovasostomy or vasoepididymostomy for various reasons. Research indicates that after vasectomy reversal microsurgery, the patency of vas deference can be achieved at about 89% and successful pregnancy rates follow at approximately 73%.

The **ampulla of ductus deferens** has taller, branched mucosal folds that often show glandular diverticula. The muscle coat surrounding the ampulla is thinner than that of the rest of the ductus deferens, and the longitudinal layers disappear near the origin of the ejaculatory duct. The epithelium of the ampulla and ejaculatory duct appears to have a secretory function. The cells contain large numbers of yellow pigment granules. The wall of the ejaculatory duct does not have a muscularis layer; the fibromuscular tissue of the prostate substitutes for it.

■ ACCESSORY SEX GLANDS

The paired seminal vesicles secrete a fluid rich in fructose.

The **seminal vesicles** are paired, elongated, and highly folded tubular glands located on the posterior wall of the

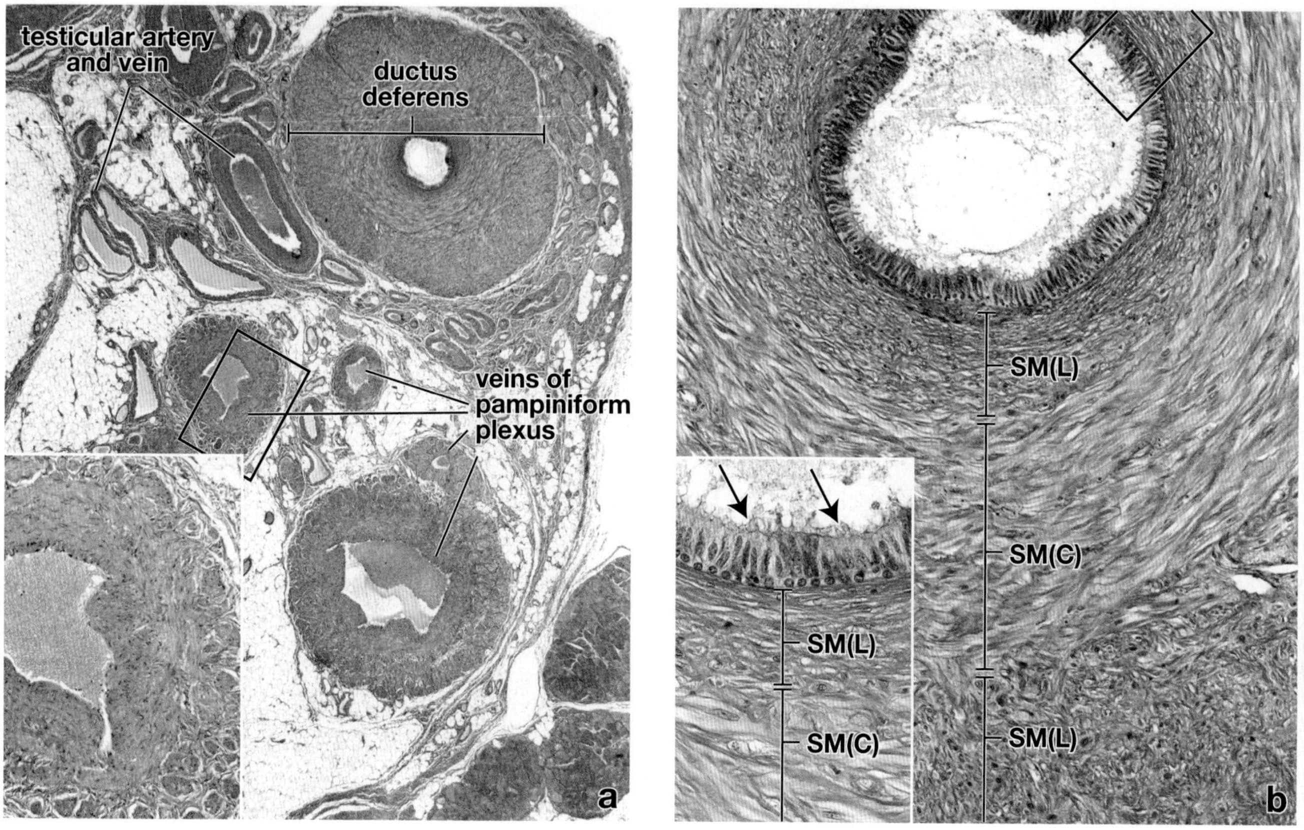

FIGURE 22.25. Photomicrograph of human spermatic cord. a. This low-magnification photomicrograph shows a cross section of the spermatic cord containing several structures. These include the ductus deferens, the accompanying testicular artery and vein, and veins of the pampiniform plexus. ×15. **Inset.** A higher magnification of a pampiniform vein. Note the bundles of longitudinal smooth muscles (cut in cross section) in the tunica adventitia and tunica intima. ×55. **b.** This cross section of the ductus deferens shows the thick muscular wall organized in three distinct smooth muscle layers: an inner longitudinal (*SM[L]*), middle circular (*SM[C]*), and outer longitudinal (*SM[L]*). ×100. **Inset.** A higher magnification shows the pseudostratified epithelium lining the ductus deferens. The tall principal cells possess long microvilli (stereocilia; *arrows*). The basal cells are in close proximity to the basement membrane and possess spherical nuclei. ×215.

urinary bladder, parallel to the ampulla of the ductus deferens. A short excretory duct from each seminal vesicle combines with the ampulla of the ductus deferens to form the **ejaculatory duct**. Seminal vesicles develop as evaginations of the mesonephric (Wolffian) ducts in the region of future ampullae. The wall of the seminal vesicles contains a mucosa, a thin layer of smooth muscle, and a fibrous coat (Fig. 22.26). The mucosa is thrown into numerous primary, secondary, and tertiary folds that increase the secretory surface area (Plate 22.6, page 906). All of the irregular spaces thus formed, however, communicate with the lumen.

The pseudostratified columnar epithelium contains tall, nonciliated columnar cells and short, round cells that rest on the basal lamina. The short cells appear identical to those of the rest of the excurrent duct system. They are the stem cells from which the columnar cells are derived. The columnar cells have the morphology of protein-secreting cells, with a well-developed rER and large secretory vacuoles in the apical cytoplasm.

The **secretion of the seminal vesicles** is a whitish yellow, viscous material. It contains fructose, which is the principal metabolic substrate for sperm, along with other simple sugars, amino acids, ascorbic acid, and prostaglandins. Although prostaglandins were first isolated from the prostate gland (hence the name), they are actually synthesized in large amounts in the seminal vesicles. Contraction of the smooth muscle coat of the seminal vesicles during ejaculation discharges their secretion into the ejaculatory ducts and helps to flush sperm out of the urethra. The secretory function and morphology of the seminal vesicles are under the control of testosterone.

■ PROSTATE GLAND

The prostate, the largest accessory sex gland, is divided into several morphologic and functional zones.

The **prostate** is the largest **accessory sex gland** of the male reproductive system. Its size and shape are commonly compared to those of a walnut. The main function of the prostate gland is to secrete a clear, slightly alkaline (pH 7.29) fluid that contributes to the formation of seminal fluid. The gland is located in the pelvis, inferior to the bladder, where it surrounds the prostatic part of the urethra. It consists of 30–50 tubuloalveolar glands arranged in three concentric layers: an inner **mucosal layer**, an intermediate submucosal layer, and a peripheral layer containing the main prostatic glands (Fig. 22.27). The glands of the mucosal layer secrete directly into the urethra; the other two layers have ducts that open into the prostatic sinuses located on either side of the urethral crest on the posterior wall of the urethra.

The **adult prostatic parenchyma** is divided into four anatomically and clinically distinct zones:

- The **central zone** surrounds the ejaculatory ducts as they pierce the prostate gland. This zone comprises approximately 25% of the glandular tissue of the prostate gland and is resistant to both carcinoma and inflammation. In comparison to the other zones, cells in the central zone have distinctive morphologic features (a more prominent and slightly basophilic cytoplasm and larger nuclei displaced at different levels in adjacent cells). Recent findings suggest

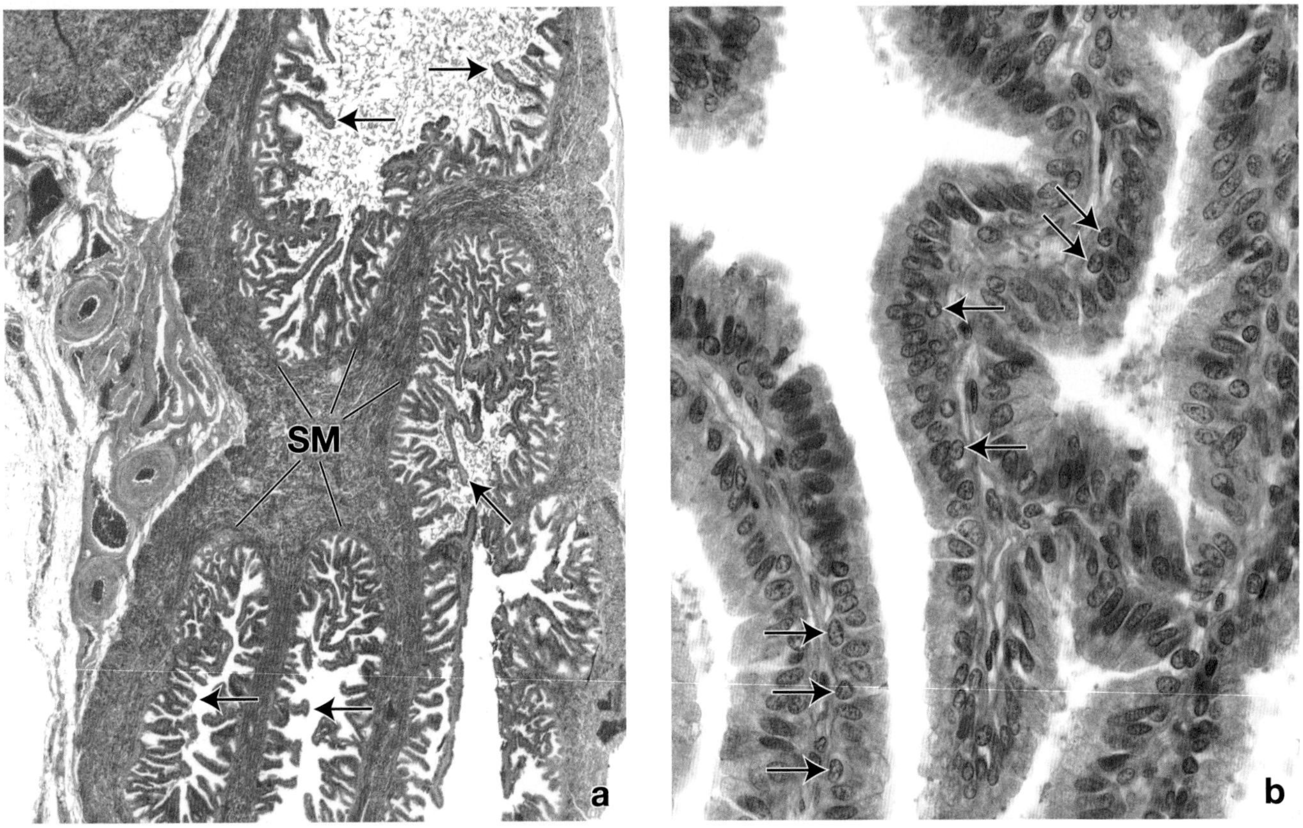

FIGURE 22.26. Photomicrograph of human seminal vesicle. a. This low-magnification photomicrograph shows part of a hematoxylin and eosin (H&E)-stained section of a human seminal vesicle. This gland is a tortuous tubular structure and in a section exhibits what appear to be a number of isolated lumina. In actuality, there is only one lumen. The mucosa is characterized by extensive folding (*arrows*). It rests on a thick smooth muscle (*SM*) investment that is organized in two layers: an inner circular layer and an outer longitudinal layer. ×20. **b.** This higher magnification shows the mucosal folds surfaced by a pseudostratified epithelium. *Arrows* indicate the basal cells. ×500.

that this zone originates embryologically from the inclusion of mesonephric duct cells into the developing prostate.

- The **peripheral zone** comprises 70% of the glandular tissue of the prostate. It surrounds the central zone and occupies the posterior and lateral parts of the gland. Most **prostatic carcinomas** arise from the **peripheral zone** of the prostate gland. The peripheral zone is palpable during digital examination of the rectum. This zone is also the most susceptible to inflammation.
- The **transitional zone** surrounds the prostatic urethra; it comprises about 5% of the prostatic glandular tissue and contains the mucosal glands. In older individuals, the parenchymal cells of this zone frequently undergo extensive division (hyperplasia) and form nodular masses of epithelial cells. Because the **transitional zone** is proximate to the prostatic urethra, these nodules can compress the prostatic urethra, causing difficult urination. This condition is known as **benign prostatic hyperplasia (BPH)** and is discussed in Folder 22.4 (pages 887–888).
- The **periurethral zone** contains mucosal and submucosal glands. In the later stages of BPH, this zone may undergo pathologic growth but mainly from the stromal components. Together with the glandular nodules of the transitional zone, this growth causes increased **urethral compression** and further retention of urine in the bladder.

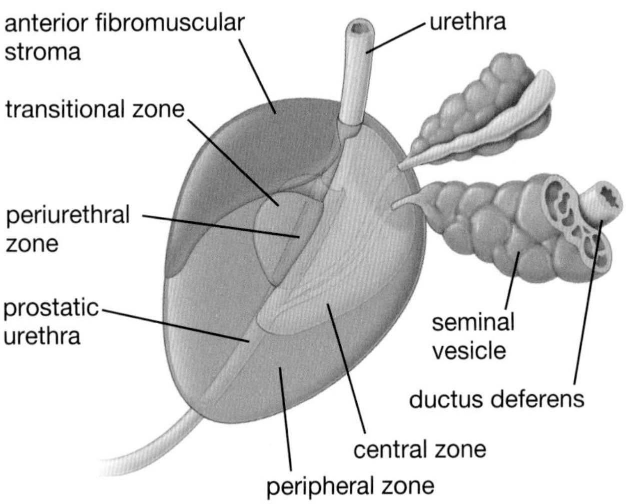

FIGURE 22.27. Schematic drawing of the zones of the human prostate gland. This drawing illustrates the relative location, by color, of the four zones of the prostate gland and anterior fibromuscular stroma of the gland.

In addition, **fibromuscular stroma** occupies the anterior surface of the prostate gland anterior to the urethra and is composed of dense irregular connective tissue with a large amount of smooth muscle fibers.

The growth of the prostatic glandular epithelium is regulated by the hormone dihydrotestosterone.

Within each prostate zone, the **glandular epithelium** is generally simple columnar, but there may be patches that are simple cuboidal, squamous, or occasionally pseudostratified (Fig. 22.28). The alveoli of the prostatic glands, especially those in older individuals, often contain **prostatic concretions (corpora amylacea)** of varied shape and size, often up to 2 mm in diameter (see Fig. 22.28 and Plate 22.5, page 904). They appear in sections as concentric lamellated bodies and are believed to be formed by precipitation of secretory material around cell fragments. They may become partially calcified.

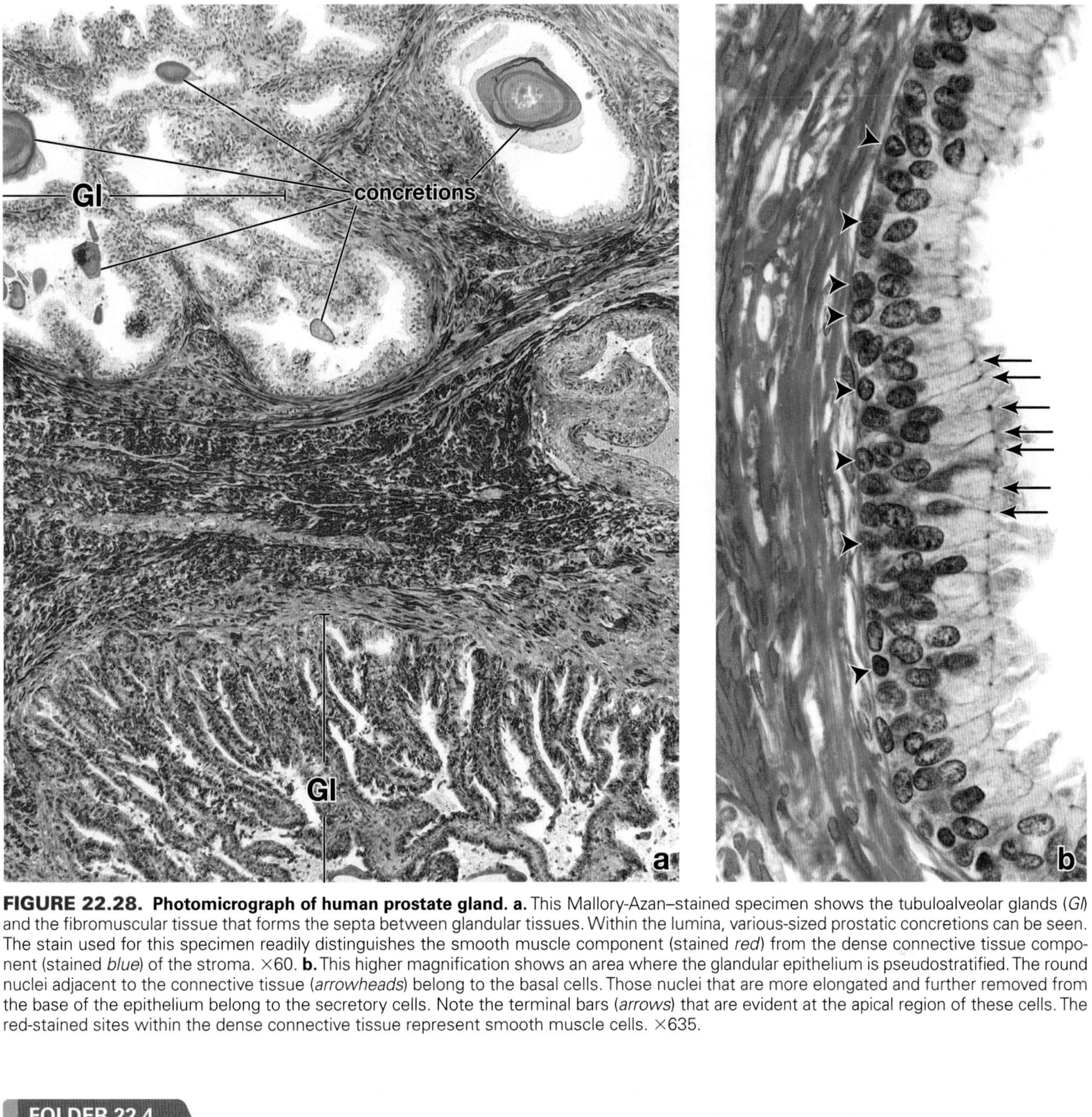

FIGURE 22.28. Photomicrograph of human prostate gland. a. This Mallory-Azan–stained specimen shows the tubuloalveolar glands (*Gl*) and the fibromuscular tissue that forms the septa between glandular tissues. Within the lumina, various-sized prostatic concretions can be seen. The stain used for this specimen readily distinguishes the smooth muscle component (stained *red*) from the dense connective tissue component (stained *blue*) of the stroma. ×60. **b.** This higher magnification shows an area where the glandular epithelium is pseudostratified. The round nuclei adjacent to the connective tissue (*arrowheads*) belong to the basal cells. Those nuclei that are more elongated and further removed from the base of the epithelium belong to the secretory cells. Note the terminal bars (*arrows*) that are evident at the apical region of these cells. The red-stained sites within the dense connective tissue represent smooth muscle cells. ×635.

FOLDER 22.4

CLINICAL CORRELATION: BENIGN PROSTATIC HYPERTROPHY AND CANCER OF THE PROSTATE

Benign prostatic hypertrophy (nodular hyperplasia, BPH) occurs almost exclusively in the transitional and periurethral zones, leading to partial or total obstruction of the urethra (Fig. F22.4.1a). A widely accepted theory of the pathogenesis of BPH is related to the action of dihydrotestosterone (DHT). DHT is synthesized in the stromal cells by conversion from circulating testosterone in the presence of 5α-reductase. Once synthesized, DHT acts as an autocrine agent on the stromal cells and as a paracrine hormone on the glandular epithelial cells, causing them to proliferate (Fig. F22.4.1b). BHP is believed to occur to some extent in all male individuals by age 80.

Several options are available to treat BHP. **Noninvasive treatment** includes medications (α-receptor blockers) to relax the prostate smooth muscles and relieve pressure on the compressed urethra. Clinical trials have shown that inhibitors of 5α-reductase reduce the DHT concentration and thus decrease the size of the prostate and reduce urethral obstruction.

Minimally invasive treatment options use laser, microwave, or radiofrequency energy to destroy the prostate tissue causing urethral obstruction. These include interstitial laser coagulation (ILC), microwave hyperthermia, and transurethral needle ablation (TUNA). Finally, a variety of **surgical procedures** are used to remove hypertrophied regions of the prostate gland. They include transurethral incision of the prostate (TUIP), a more extensive transurethral resection of the prostate (TURP), and

(*continued*)

FOLDER 22.4

CLINICAL CORRELATION: BENIGN PROSTATIC HYPERTROPHY AND CANCER OF THE PROSTATE (*continued*)

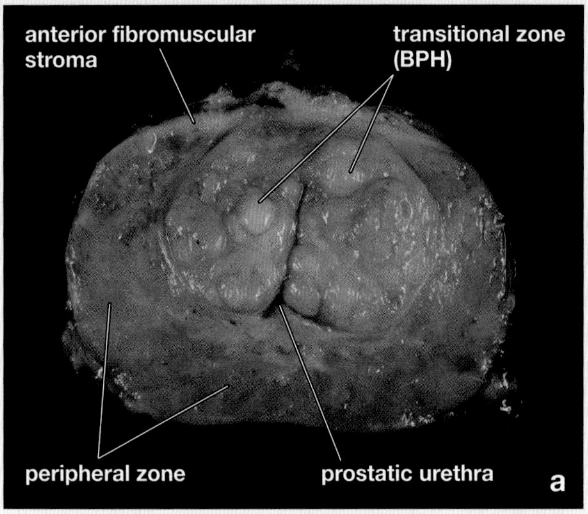

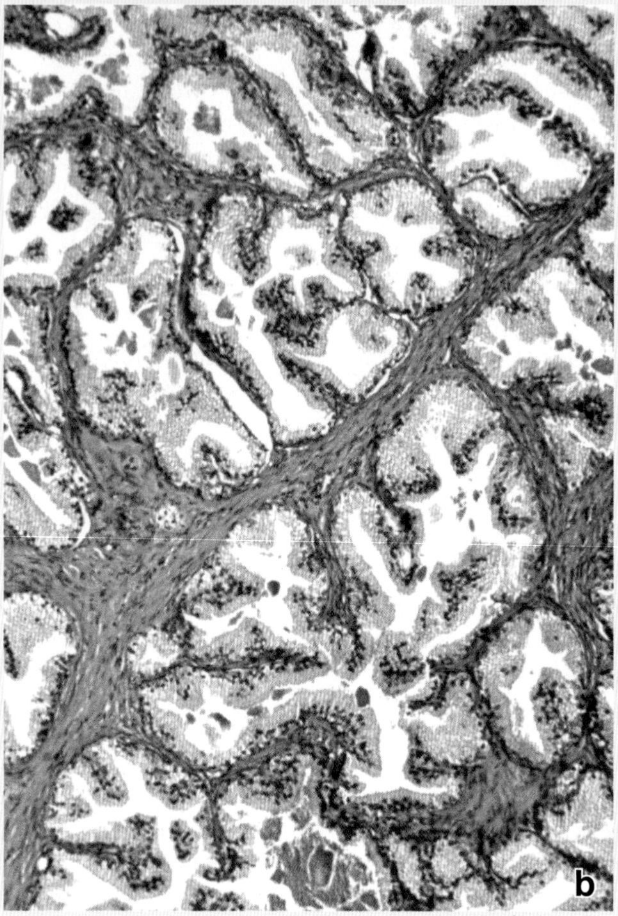

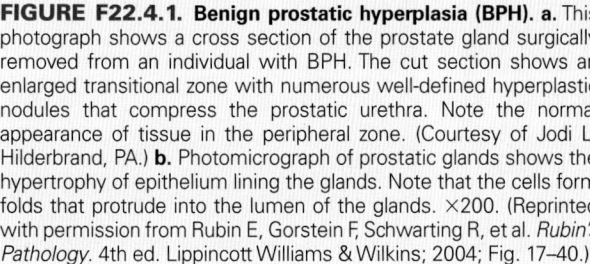

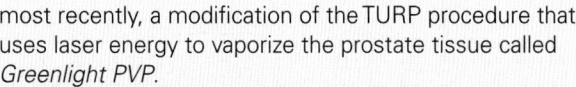

FIGURE F22.4.1. Benign prostatic hyperplasia (BPH). a. This photograph shows a cross section of the prostate gland surgically removed from an individual with BPH. The cut section shows an enlarged transitional zone with numerous well-defined hyperplastic nodules that compress the prostatic urethra. Note the normal appearance of tissue in the peripheral zone. (Courtesy of Jodi L. Hilderbrand, PA.) **b.** Photomicrograph of prostatic glands shows the hypertrophy of epithelium lining the glands. Note that the cells form folds that protrude into the lumen of the glands. ×200. (Reprinted with permission from Rubin E, Gorstein F, Schwarting R, et al. *Rubin's Pathology*. 4th ed. Lippincott Williams & Wilkins; 2004; Fig. 17–40.)

most recently, a modification of the TURP procedure that uses laser energy to vaporize the prostate tissue called *Greenlight PVP*.

Cancer of the prostate is one of the most common cancers in the male: The lifetime risk of developing prostate cancer is 16.7% (one in six men). The incidence of prostatic cancer increases with age, and it is estimated that 70% of men between the ages of 70 and 80 years will develop this disease. Tumors usually develop in the peripheral zone of the gland. In the past, early detection was uncommon because the abnormal growth of the tumor did not impinge on the urethra to produce symptoms that demanded prompt attention. Therefore, prostatic cancer was often inoperable by the time it was discovered. In the late 1980s, universal screening for prostate-specific antigen (PSA) for prostate cancer was introduced. Its use with annual digital rectal examination in prostate cancer screening programs has significantly increased the early detection of the disease.

Screening with PSA to detect prostate cancer is debatable. Recently, large epidemiologic studies revealed that the proportion of men who are diagnosed with prostate cancer but never develop associated clinical problems may range from 23% to 66%. The current view is that the value of screening for prostate cancer in most cases is low because in most cases, the chances of harm from screening (repeated testing, aggressive therapy, and patient anxiety) outweigh the chances of benefit. Therefore, screening for prostate cancer using the PSA test is **currently regarded as controversial** among health professionals and organizations who publish screening guidelines and recommendations for health care professionals.

The most common prostate cancer grading system known as the **Gleason score** is used to predict tumor behavior and patient survival rate. Tissue obtained from two biopsies from the largest areas of prostate cancer is evaluated and grades ranging from 1 to 5 are assigned. A ranking of 1 indicates well-differentiated cells, which form the slowest growing and the least aggressive form of cancer. The ranking 5 is given to poorly differentiated cells characteristic of the fastest growing cancers. These grades, when added together, represent a Gleason score or sum between 2 and 10. The higher the score, the more likely the cancer will grow and spread rapidly.

Treatment of the cancer is by surgery, radiotherapy, or both for patients with localized disease. Hormonal therapy is the treatment of choice for advanced cancer with metastases. Because prostatic cancer cells depend on androgens, the goal of therapy is to deprive the cells of testosterone by performing orchiectomy (removal of the testis) or by administration of estrogens or gonadotropin-releasing hormone (GnRH) agonists to suppress testosterone production. Despite treatment, patients with metastasis have a poor prognosis.

The **glandular epithelium** is influenced by sex hormones, such as testosterone and adrenal androgens. These hormones enter the secretory cells of the glandular epithelium and are converted to **dihydrotestosterone (DHT)** by the enzyme **5α-reductase**. DHT is approximately 30 times more potent than testosterone. Binding of DHT to the **androgen receptor (AR)** results in a conformational change of the receptor and its relocation from the cytosol to the cell nucleus. Here, the phosphorylated dimers of the AR complex bind to a specific sequence of DNA known as a **hormone-response element** residing in the promoter regions of target genes. The primary function of AR is direct upregulation or downregulation of specific genes. DHT stimulation is a factor in both proliferation and growth of BPH and androgen-dependent prostate cancer.

The prostate gland secretes prostatic acid phosphatase (PAP), fibrinolysin, citric acid, and prostate-specific antigen (PSA).

The epithelial cells in the prostate gland produce several enzymes, particularly prostate-specific antigen (PSA), prostatic acid phosphatase (PAP), fibrinolysin, and citric acid.

- **Prostate-specific antigen (PSA)**, a 33-kDa serine protease, is one of the most clinically important tumor markers. In normal conditions, PSA is secreted into prostatic gland alveoli and ultimately incorporated into seminal fluid. The alveolar secretion from the prostate gland is pumped into the prostatic urethra during ejaculation by contraction of the fibromuscular tissue of the prostate. Because PSA is predominately released into the prostatic secretion, only a very small amount of PSA (usually <4 ng/mL) normally circulates in the blood of a healthy individual. However, in **prostate cancer**, serum concentration of PSA increases; large amounts of PSA are produced and misdirected into the circulation by the transformed prostatic epithelium. An increased **PSA serum level** is used as a **clinical marker** for progression of the disease. Recently, it has become widely accepted that small amounts of PSA are also present in many nonprostatic tissues, including breast, ovary, salivary gland, and liver tissue, and in various tumors. In addition, high circulating levels of PSA are also associated with benign (noncancerous) conditions such as prostatitis (infection of the prostate gland), interrupted blood flow to the prostate, or BPH (for more details on PSA screening, see Folder 22.4).
- **Prostatic acid phosphatase (PAP)** (100 kDa) regulates cell growth and metabolism of the prostate glandular epithelium. Because elevated **serum levels of PAP** are found in patients with metastatic prostate cancer, this enzyme is routinely used as an **alternate marker** to PSA for **prostatic tumors**. Measurements of PAP and PSA are useful in assessing the prognosis of prostate cancer.
- **Fibrinolysin**, secreted from the prostate gland, liquefies semen.

Bulbourethral Glands

The bulbourethral glands secrete preseminal fluid.

The paired **bulbourethral glands (Cowper glands)** are pea-sized structures located in the urogenital diaphragm (see

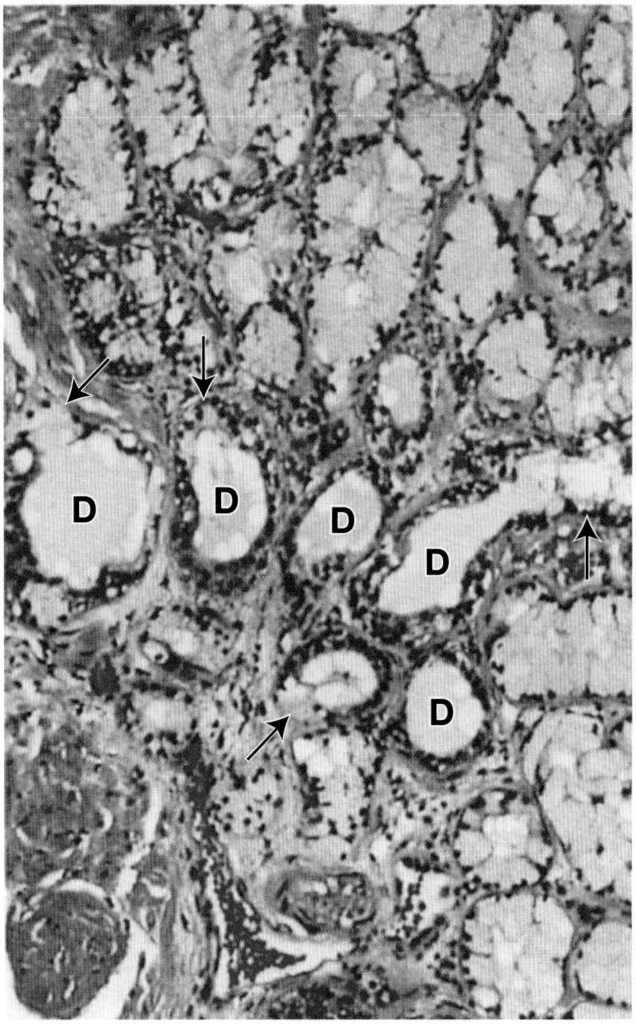

FIGURE 22.29. Photomicrograph of human bulbourethral gland. This photomicrograph shows a hematoxylin and eosin (H&E)-stained section of the compound tubuloalveolar bulbourethral gland. The epithelium consists of columnar mucus-secreting cells. The nuclei are displaced to the base of the cells by the accumulated secretory material that they contain. The cytoplasm has an appearance similar to typical mucus-secreting cells. Note several ducts (*D*) lined by a simple columnar epithelium. The ducts will merge to form a single excretory duct. In some sites, the ducts contain mucus-secreting cells (*arrows*). ×40.

Fig. 22.1). The duct of each gland passes through the inferior fascia of the urogenital diaphragm and joins the initial portion of the penile urethra. The glands are compound tubuloalveolar glands that structurally resemble mucus-secretory glands (Fig. 22.29). The simple columnar epithelium, which varies considerably in height depending on the functional state of the gland, is under the control of testosterone.

The clear, mucus-like glandular secretion contains considerable amounts of galactose, galactosamine, galacturonic acid, sialic acid, and methylpentose. Sexual stimulation causes the release of this secretion, which constitutes the major portion of the preseminal fluid and serves to lubricate the penile urethra, neutralizing any traces of acidic urine.

■ SEMEN

Semen contains fluids and sperm cells from the testis and secretory products from the epididymis, ductus deferens, prostate, seminal vesicles, and bulbourethral glands. The seminal fluid provides nutrients (e.g., amino acids, citrates, and fructose) and protection for the sperm cells during their passage through the excurrent duct system. Semen is alkaline (pH 7.7) and helps to neutralize the acid environment of the urethra and vagina. The major components of semen can be traced to the secretion from the seminal vesicles (65%–75%) and prostate gland (25%–30%). Additional components include testicular fluid (2%–5%) that was not completely absorbed in the straight tubules as well as secretions from the bulbourethral (Cowper) glands that account for less than 1%. Semen also contains prostaglandins (produced by seminal vesicles) that may influence sperm transit in both the male and female reproductive tracts and may have a role in implantation of a fertilized ovum.

The average **ejaculate** of semen has a volume of about 3 mL and normally contains up to 100 million sperm cells per milliliter. It is estimated that 20% of the sperm in any ejaculate are morphologically abnormal and nearly 25% are immotile.

■ PENIS AND SCROTUM

Erection of the penis involves filling of the vascular spaces of the corpora cavernosa and corpus spongiosum.

The **penis** consists principally of two dorsal masses of erectile tissue, the **corpora cavernosa**, and a ventral mass of erectile tissue, the **corpus spongiosum**, in which the spongy part of the urethra is embedded. A dense, fibroelastic layer, the **tunica albuginea**, binds the three together and forms a capsule around each (Fig. 22.30). The corpora cavernosa contain numerous wide, irregularly shaped vascular spaces lined with vascular endothelium. These spaces are surrounded by a thin layer of smooth muscle that forms trabeculae within the tunica albuginea interconnecting and crisscrossing the corpus cavernosum. Irregular smooth muscle bundles are observed frequently as "subendothelial cushions" surrounding irregular vascular spaces (Fig. 22.31).

The interstitial connective tissue contains many nerve endings and lymphatic vessels. The vascular spaces increase in size and rigidity by filling with blood, principally derived from the **deep artery of the penis** that divides into branches called the **helicine arteries.** These arteries dilate during erection (Folder 22.5) to increase blood flow to the penis. An arteriovenous (AV) anastomosis exists between the deep artery of the penis and the peripheral venous system (see Folder 22.5).

Skin of the penis shows a thin epidermis with minimal keratinization.

The **skin of the penis** is thin and loosely attached to the underlying connective tissue, except at the **glans penis**, where it is very thin and tightly attached. The skin of the glans is so thin that blood within its large, muscular anastomosing veins that drain the corpus spongiosum may give it a bluish color. The epithelium of the glans penis in uncircumcised individuals is stratified squamous nonkeratinized; however, after circumcision, the epithelium becomes keratinized. There is no adipose tissue in the subcutaneous tissue. There is, however, a thin layer of smooth muscle that is continuous with the dartos layer of the scrotum. The **dartos layer** in the skin of the penis is composed of smooth muscle fibers arranged in superficial (longitudinal) and deep (transverse) layers. These two layers are separated by the dense irregular connective tissue and are comparable to the hypodermis of

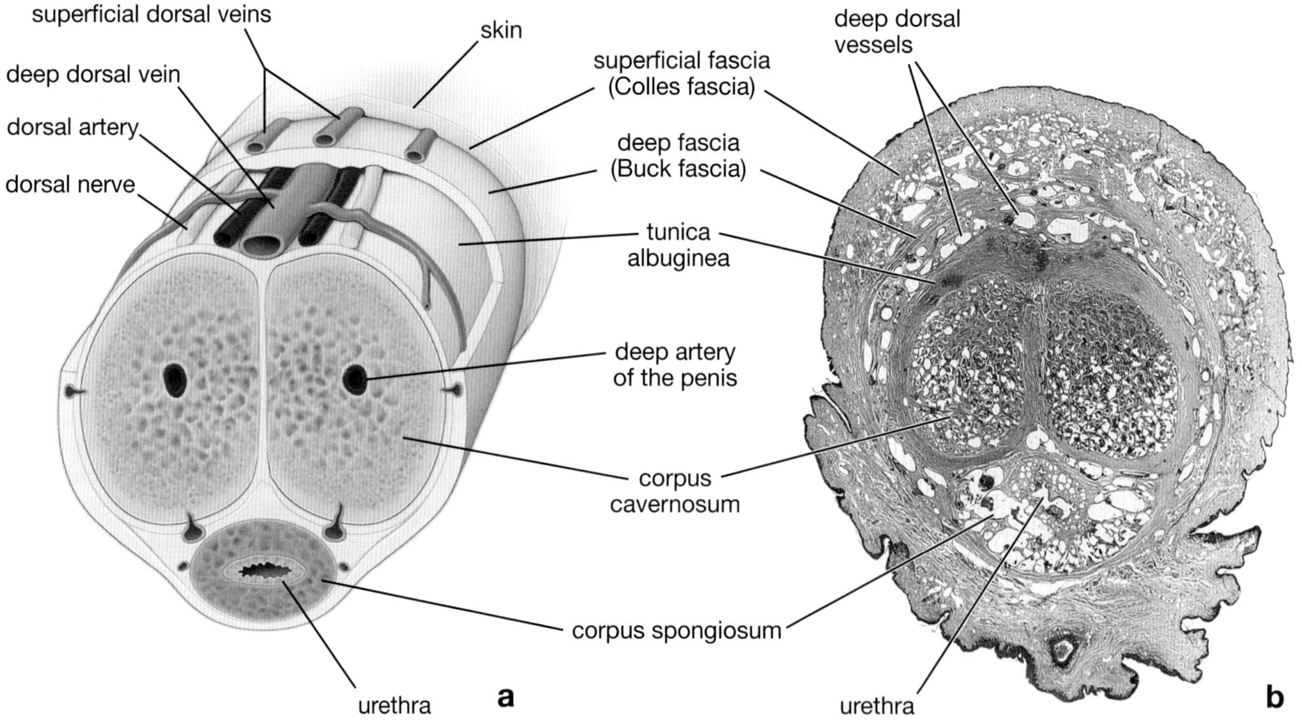

FIGURE 22.30. Transverse section of the penis. a. This diagram shows a cross section of the penis with the location of major vessels and nerves and their relationships to the fascial layers and erectile tissues. **b.** This photomicrograph shows a hematoxylin and eosin (H&E)-stained specimen of a cross section of the penis near the base of the organ. Note the arrangement of the corpora cavernosa and corpus spongiosum; the latter contains the urethra. ×3.

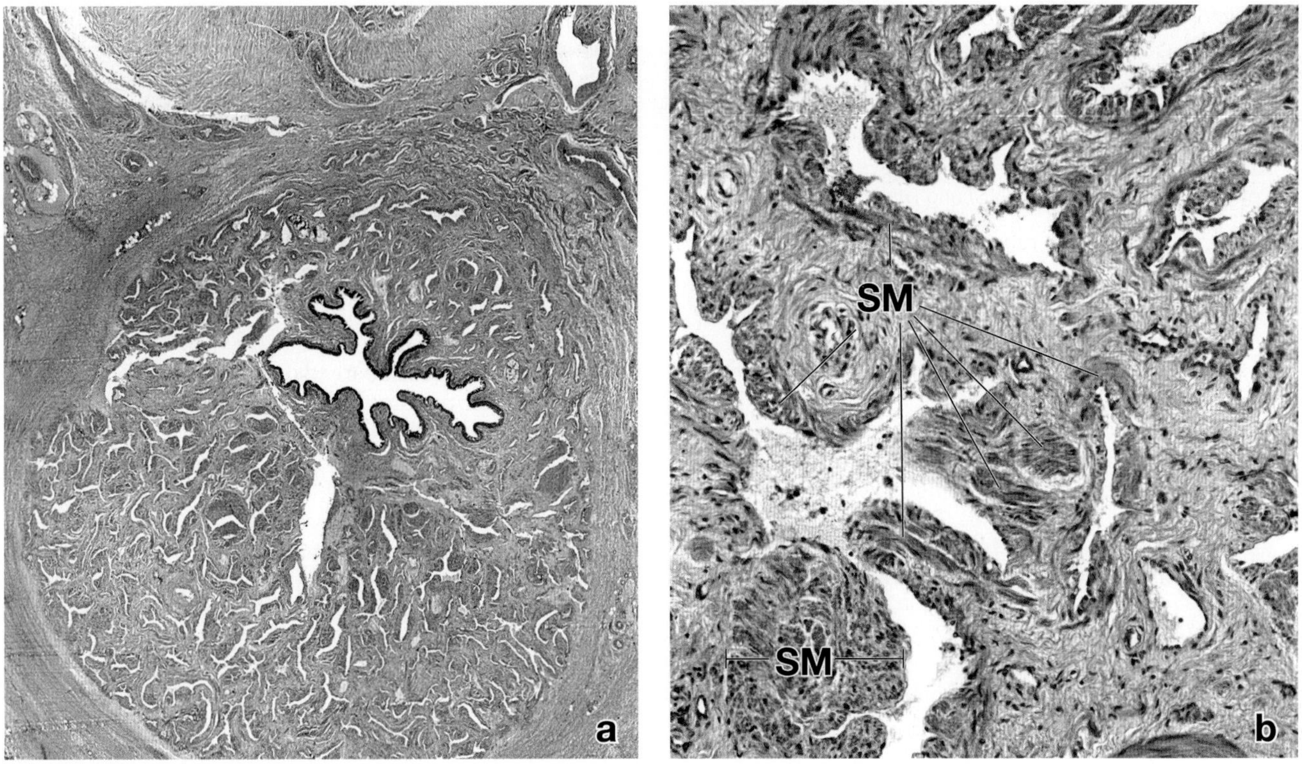

FIGURE 22.31. Photomicrograph of corpus spongiosum. a. This photomicrograph of a hematoxylin and eosin (H&E)-stained section shows the corpus spongiosum and urethra. ×20. **b.** This higher magnification of the corpus spongiosum shows the numerous irregularly shaped vascular spaces. Note the surrounding layer of smooth muscle (*SM*) forming the "subendothelial cushions." ×135.

the skin but without adipose tissue. In uncircumcised males, the glans is covered with a fold of skin, the **prepuce**, which resembles a mucous membrane on its inner aspect and the skin of the penis on the outer aspect. Numerous sebaceous glands not related to hair follicles are present in the skin of the penis just proximal to the glans. The **deep fascia of the penis (Buck fascia)** is visible underneath the dartos layer. It is composed of a continuous fibroelastic membrane that encircles both the corpora cavernosa and the corpus spongiosum.

The penis is innervated by somatic and visceral motor (sympathetic and parasympathetic) fibers. Many sensory nerve endings are distributed throughout the tissue of the penis. The visceral motor fibers innervate the smooth muscle of the trabeculae of the tunica albuginea and the blood vessels. Both sensory and visceral motor fibers play essential roles in erectile and ejaculatory responses. **Parasympathetic stimulation** initiates **erection**, whereas **sympathetic stimulation** terminates erection and causes **ejaculation**, a rhythmic contraction of smooth muscle that ejects semen from the spongy urethra (see Folder 22.5).

The wall of the scrotum reflects the layers of the abdominal wall that were pulled into the developing scrotum during the descent of the testis.

The **scrotum** represents a musculocutaneous pigmented pouch located inferior to the shaft of the penis and pubic symphysis. The scrotum is embryologically derived from the fusion of the labioscrotal folds and is homologous to the labia majora in the female. The **medium raphe** (and the septum inside the scrotum) divides the left and right parts of the scrotum and extends from the ventral surface of the penis anteriorly to the anus posteriorly. Each part of the scrotum contains a testis, epididymis, and proximal part of the spermatic cord.

The wall of the scrotum is complex and contains several layers that are extensions of the anterior abdominal wall layers. This arrangement can be traced to the descent of the testis in fetal life. The descending testes travel into the developing scrotum taking with them the blood and lymphatic vessels, nerves, attached peritoneum, and the muscular and aponeurotic layers of the abdominal wall. As discussed earlier, the temperature within the scrotum is about 2°C–3°C lower than body temperature, creating an optimal environment for the thermosensitive testes to maintain spermatogenesis.

The **wall of the scrotum** consists of the following layers, starting from the most superficial:

- **Skin of the scrotum**. The skin is thin, corrugated (wrinkled), and darker than the skin of neighboring regions. It consists of an epidermis made of the keratinized stratified squamous epithelium. The basal layer of the epidermis contains a high concentration of melanocytes (about one melanocyte to four basal cells). Most of the pigment resides in the stratum basale but is also present in cells progressing toward the surface. The dermis comprises a papillary layer (loose connective tissue) and a reticular layer (dense irregular connective tissue). It contains small, smooth muscle fibers and myofibroblasts embedded in the extracellular matrix that is rich in elastic fibers. The dermis also contains hair follicles, apocrine and eccrine sweat glands, and sebaceous glands. The subcutaneous adipose tissue is absent in the hypodermis and is replaced by the dartos layer of smooth muscles (Fig 22.32).

FOLDER 22.5

CLINICAL CORRELATION: MECHANISM OF ERECTION AND ERECTILE DYSFUNCTION

Erection of the penis is a vascular event initiated by the central nervous system (CNS) and maintained by complex interactions between vascular and neurologic events. The CNS responds to external or internal stimuli (sensory impulses, perception, desire, etc.) that involve the sympathetic and parasympathetic innervation of the penis.

Parasympathetic stimulation initiates erection by relaxation of the trabecular smooth muscle cells and dilation of the helicine arteries. This leads to expansion of the corpora cavernosa and, to a lesser degree, the corpus spongiosum. Arterial blood accumulates in these erectile tissues by compression of the venules against the nondistensible tunica albuginea. This process is referred to as the **corporal veno-occlusive mechanism**. The tunica albuginea also compresses the larger veins that drain blood from the corpora cavernosa so that venous outflow is also blocked, resulting in tumescence and rigidity of the penis.

Two neuromediators, acetylcholine and nitric oxide, are involved in the relaxation of smooth muscle during the initiation and maintenance of penile erection.

- **Acetylcholine** is released by the parasympathetic nerve endings and acts primarily on the endothelial cells that line the vascular spaces of the corpora cavernosa. This causes the release of vasoactive intestinal peptide (VIP) and, more importantly, nitric oxide.
- **Nitric oxide (NO)** activates guanylate cyclase in the trabecular smooth muscle cells to produce cyclic guanosine monophosphate (cGMP). cGMP causes the smooth muscle cells to relax.

Sympathetic stimulation terminates penile erection by causing contraction of the trabecular smooth muscle cells of the helicine arteries. These events decrease the flow of blood to the corpora cavernosa, reducing blood pressure in the erectile tissue to normal venous pressure. The lower pressure within the corpus cavernosum allows the veins leading from the corpora cavernosa to open and drain the excess blood.

Erectile dysfunction (ED) is an inability to achieve and maintain sufficient penile erection to complete satisfactory intercourse. Adequate arterial blood supply is critical for erection; therefore, any disorder that decreases blood flow into the corpora cavernosa may cause erectile failure.

Many cases of ED that do not involve parasympathetic nerve damage can now be treated effectively with drugs known as *phosphodiesterase* inhibitors (i.e., sildenafil citrate [Viagra], tadalafil [Cialis], vardenafil [Levitra], and others). These compounds enhance the relaxing effect of NO on smooth muscle cells of the corpora cavernosa by inhibiting phosphodiesterase, which is responsible for degradation of cGMP. As noted earlier, cGMP causes smooth muscle relaxation, which, in turn, allows inflow of blood into the corpus cavernosum to initiate erection.

However, when parasympathetic nerve damage has occurred (e.g., as a complication of prostatic surgery), phosphodiesterase inhibitors have no effect because the event involving parasympathetic stimulation and release of acetylcholine cannot occur. Without acetylcholine, NO cannot produce cGMP, and without cGMP, smooth muscle cells cannot relax to allow inflow of blood to fill the erectile tissue. In these cases of ED, **prostaglandin E1 (PGE1)** (alprostadil) can be used in a direct intracavernous injection (or as intraurethral suppository). PGE1 is produced endogenously to relax vascular smooth muscle and cause vasodilation. In adult males, after injections into erectile tissue, the PGE1 causes relaxation of smooth muscles of the helicine arteries and the trabecular smooth muscles, resulting in rapid inflow of blood and expansion of the vascular spaces within the corpora cavernosa. As the pressure within the corpora cavernosa is increasing, the venous outflow through the subtunical vessels is compressed (the corporal veno-occlusive mechanism) and penile rigidity develops. The alternative option in the treatment of ED is the use of special pumps that draw blood into the erectile tissues using negative pressure.

- **Dartos layer**. This smooth muscle layer replaces the hypodermis and is firmly attached to the dermis. There are two distinct perpendicularly arranged layers of the dartos muscle, the superficial (longitudinal) and deep (transverse), as shown in Figure 22.32. As the layers contract, this crisscrossing organization of the dartos layer is responsible for the reduction of the scrotal skin surface, giving the scrotum a wrinkled appearance. Apocrine and eccrine sweat glands, as well as roots of hair follicles, are often visible between these two layers. The **dartos muscle** contracts in response to cold, exercise, and sexual stimulation. In a cold environment, the contraction of the dartos layer causes elevation (retraction) of the testes, bringing them toward the abdominal wall. In a hot environment, the dartos layer relaxes, providing a larger skin surface for heat dissipation and preventing testicular hyperthermia.
- **External spermatic fascia**. This extension of the external abdominal oblique aponeurosis is thin and more organized than the typical irregular connective tissue layer. Thick bundles of collagen fibers, nerve fibers, and blood vessels are clearly visible; a few smooth muscle fibers on the outer surface are also detectable.
- **Cremaster muscle and cremasteric fasciae**. The cremaster muscle (*Gr. Κρεμαστήρ, suspender*) is an elongation of the internal oblique muscle into the scrotal wall. It consists of loosely arranged striated muscle fascicles surrounded by cremasteric fascia. They are predominately type I fibers (slow oxidative fibers) that contract slowly but are fatigue resistant. They differ from skeletal muscle by having multiple motor end plates and several nerve endings that terminate on a single muscle fiber. A few smooth muscle fibers, nerve cells, and nerve plexuses can be found between skeletal fibers in this layer. Because

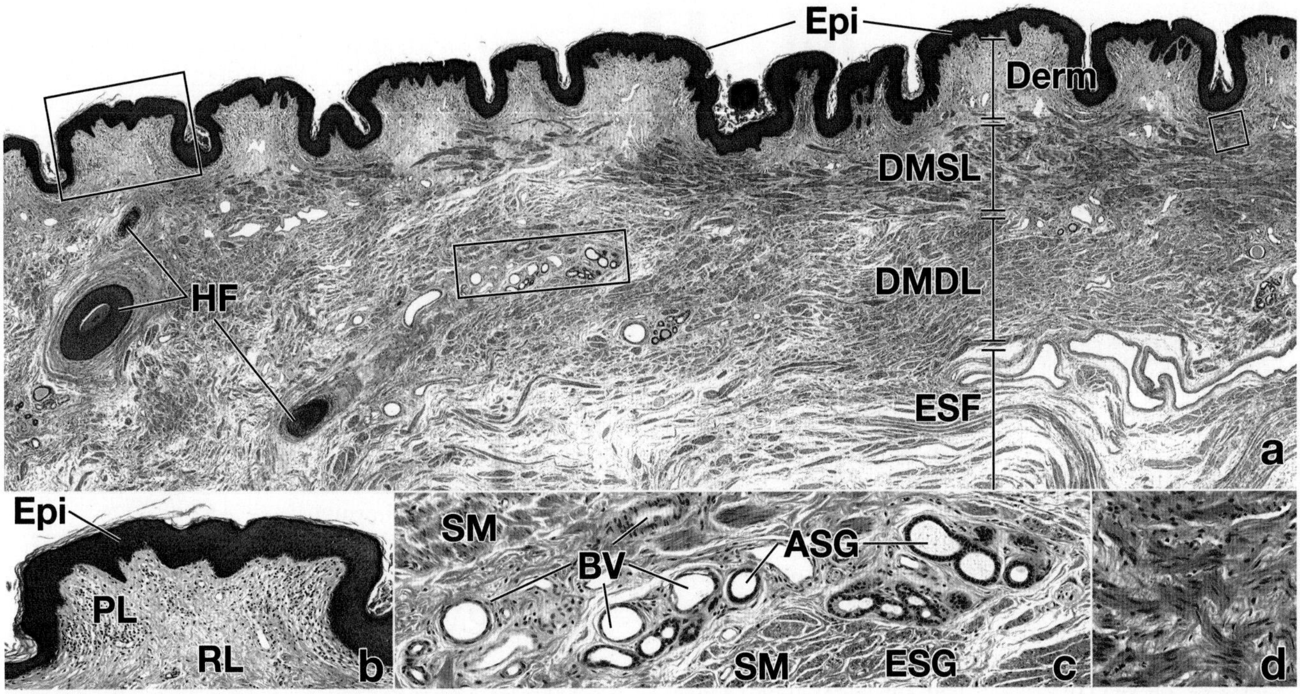

FIGURE 22.32. Photomicrograph of the wall of the scrotum. a. This photomicrograph of a hematoxylin and eosin (H&E)-stained specimen shows the superficial layers of the scrotum. Note the wrinkled appearance of the skin that shows the stratified squamous keratinized epithelium (*Epi*) on the surface. The underlying dermis (*Derm*) contains a few small smooth muscle fibers and myofibroblasts embedded in the elastic-rich extracellular matrix. These structures are not visible at this magnification. The subcutaneous adipose tissue is absent in the hypodermis and is replaced by the two layers of dartos smooth muscle: the superficial layer (*DMSL*) and deep layer (*DMDL*). The apocrine and eccrine sweat glands as well as roots of hair follicles (*HF*) are often visible between these two layers. Deep to the dartos muscle is a layer of the external spermatic fascia (*ESF*), which is an extension of the external abdominal oblique aponeurosis. ×55. **b.** A higher magnification of the epidermis (*Epi*) taken from the *left rectangular area* shows loose connective tissue in the papillary layer (*PL*) and reticular layer (*RL*) of dense irregular connective tissue with rich elastic fiber content. Note the dark brown appearance of the basal layer of the epithelium, which gives the skin of the scrotum its dark appearance. ×150. **c.** A higher magnification view of glandular tissue from the *center rectangular box*. Note both the apocrine (*ASG*) and eccrine (*ESG*) sweat glands surrounded by layers of dartos smooth muscle (*SM*). Large blood vessels (*BV*) also pass between these layers. ×220. **d.** A higher magnification photomicrograph of smooth muscle bundles from the *right rectangular area* that form an interlocking network of the dartos layer. ×320. (Courtesy of Dr. Robert A. Bloodgood, University of Virginia School of Medicine.)

the muscle has a weak somatic innervation (by the genital branch of the genitofemoral nerve), these plexuses provide autonomic innervations, leading to involuntary contraction of the cremaster muscle. The **cremaster muscle reflex** can be elicited to assess spinal cord injury at levels L1 and L2 and provide evidence of successful spinal anesthesia. It is also used to assess scrotal pain in testicular torsion, which is unilateral and absent on the side of the torsion.

- **Internal spermatic fascia**. This layer is positioned between the parietal layer of the tunica vaginalis and the cremaster muscle. It originates from and represents the elongation of the transversalis fascia, which resides deep into the transversus abdominis muscle. This layer is mostly composed of dense irregular connective tissue containing nerves and blood and lymphatic vessels.
- **Parietal layer of tunica vaginalis**. This layer of the serous membrane forms the inner surface of the scrotal wall. It represents the mesothelial layer that originated from the parietal peritoneum of the abdominal cavity. A thin, submesothelial layer of connective tissue supports the simple squamous epithelium lining its surface. The parietal layer, together with the visceral layer (which is attached to the testis), defines the **cavity of the tunica vaginalis**. A small amount of a lubricating fluid essential for the smooth movement of the testis is found in the cavity of the tunica vaginalis. An abnormal collection of peritoneal fluid in the cavity of the tunica vaginalis is referred as a **hydrocele**. Hydrocele can either be congenital (processus vaginalis is patent and communicates with the peritoneal cavity) or acquired (i.e., infections, injury, and malignancy). Hydrocele is caused by an imbalance between secretion and reabsorption of peritoneal fluid by the tunica vaginalis.

The scrotum receives its main blood supply from the anterior scrotal arteries (branches of external pudendal arteries) and posterior scrotal arteries (branches of internal pudendal arteries). The additional blood supply of the scrotum comes from small branches of the cremasteric and testicular arteries that traverse the spermatic cords. Venous drainage accompanies the arteries. Lymphatic drainage of the scrotum is to the superficial inguinal nodes. The ilioinguinal and genitofemoral nerves provide the innervation of the skin of the anterior part of the scrotum. Posterior scrotal nerves (branches of the pudendal nerve) supply innervation to the posterior part of the scrotum.

101 HISTOLOGY NOTEBOOK

MALE REPRODUCTIVE SYSTEM

OVERVIEW OF THE MALE REPRODUCTIVE SYSTEM

- The **male reproductive system** consists of the testes, genital excurrent ducts, accessory sex glands, and external genitalia containing the penis and scrotum.
- Testes lie within the scrotum and are responsible for **spermatogenesis** (production of sperm) and **steroidogenesis** (synthesis of steroid hormones called *androgens*).

TESTIS

- Development of the male reproductive system is guided by a cascade of gene activations triggered in response to the presence of the **Y chromosome** (chromosome-determining genetic sex).
- Activation of the **SRY gene** in the sex-determining region of the Y chromosome results in the production of **testis-determining factor (TDF)**, which activates several other genes required for the development of the male reproductive organs (**region-determining gonadal sex**).
- Hormonal secretion from the developing testis allows for the growth and differentiation of the male reproductive organs (**secretion-determining hormonal sex**).
- The testes develop on the posterior abdominal wall from three sources: **intermediate mesoderm** (which forms urogenital ridges), **mesodermal epithelium** (which gives rise to primary sex cords), and **primordial germ cells** (which migrate from the yolk sac).
- Under the influence of **testosterone** and **Müllerian-inhibiting factor (MIF)**, the testes develop from indifferent gonads to fully developed organs that descend into the scrotum during fetal development.
- **Dihydrotestosterone (DHT)** is responsible for the development of the external genitalia and accessory sex glands.
- Scrotal position of the testes allows for spermatogenesis to occur. This process requires lower-than-normal body temperature.
- Each testis has approximately 250 lobules containing one to four highly convoluted **seminiferous tubules**, which are surrounded by a lamina propria containing blood, lymphatic vessels, and Leydig (interstitial) cells.
- **Leydig (interstitial) cells** produce testosterone and other hormones (e.g., androgens, insulin-like protein 3) that guide the development and descent of the testis.
- The seminiferous tubules consist of a **seminiferous epithelium** that contains **Sertoli cells** and **spermatogenic cells.** The walls of the tubules consist of connective tissue that contains **myoid cells** (peritubular contractile cells).

SPERMATOGENESIS

- **Spermatogenesis** is the process by which spermatogonia develop into sperm. It begins before puberty and continues throughout life.
- Spermatogenesis occurs in the seminiferous tubules in two compartments established by Sertoli cells: a **basal compartment** containing diploid (2d) cells (i.e., spermatogonia) and a **luminal compartment** containing haploid (1d) cells (i.e., spermatocytes and spermatids).
- These compartments are separated by **Sertoli cell-to-Sertoli cell junctional complexes** that represent the site of the blood–testis barrier.
- Spermatogenesis in humans lasts approximately 74 days and is divided into three distinct phases.
- During the **spermatogonial phase**, spermatogonia (stem cells) undergo mitosis to replace themselves and provide a population of committed cells that eventually give rise to primary spermatocytes.
- During the **spermatocyte phase**, primary spermatocytes undergo a first meiotic division (lasts up to 22 days) to produce secondary spermatocytes. Then they undergo a second meiotic division (only a few hours long) to produce haploid cells called **spermatids** that have a reduced number of chromosomes (1n) and amount of DNA (1d).
- During the **spermatid phase** (spermiogenesis), spermatids undergo extensive cell remodeling in association with Sertoli cells, including condensation of DNA content in the nucleus, formation of an acrosomal cap, and development of a long flagellum.
- Spermatids then differentiate into **spermatozoa**, which are released during spermiation into the lumen of the seminiferous tubule.
- The mature sperm cell contains a flattened **head** covered by the **acrosomal cap** (contains hydrolytic enzymes for penetration of the ovum) and an axonemal complex in the sperm **tail** that is helically wrapped by mitochondria.
- Newly released sperm cells are nonmotile. Their travel from the **seminiferous tubules** is facilitated by myoid cell contractions. Sperm cells first enter the short straight tubules and then the **rete testis**, which is connected via **efferent ductules** to the head of the **epididymis**.

EXCURRENT DUCT SYSTEM

- The **excurrent duct system** develops from the mesonephric (Wolffian) duct (epididymis, ductus deferens, ejaculatory duct) and mesonephric tubules (efferent ductules).
- **Efferent ductules** connect the rete testis with the **duct of the epididymis**, which forms the head, body, and tail of the epididymis. Sperm cells acquire motility, undergo further maturation, and are stored in the epididymis before ejaculation.
- The **duct of the epididymis** is lined with a pseudostratified columnar epithelium containing stereocilia and is surrounded by a smooth muscle coat that gradually increases in thickness.
- The **ductus (vas) deferens** is a direct continuation of the tail of the epididymis. It is lined with a pseudostratified columnar epithelium with stereocilia that is surrounded by a thick (1–1.5 mm) muscular coat.
- During **ejaculation**, sperm cells are forcefully squeezed from the epididymis to the ductus deferens and are propelled into the **ejaculatory duct**.

ACCESSORY SEX GLANDS

- The **seminal vesicles** are lined by a mucosa that forms numerous thin folds. They produce a fluid rich in fructose that becomes a constituent of semen.
- The excretory duct of each seminal vesicle unites with the ampulla of the ductus deferens to form the **ejaculatory duct**, which pierces the prostate to enter the prostatic urethra.
- The **prostate** is a tubuloalveolar gland that lies beneath the bladder and surrounds the prostatic urethra. Parenchyma of the prostate is divided into several distinct anatomic and clinical zones.
- **Glandular epithelium** of prostatic alveoli is simple columnar with characteristic **prostatic concretions** that are often located within the lumen of the glands.
- The prostate gland secretes several enzymes, including **prostatic acid phosphatase (PAP)** and **prostate-specific antigen (PSA)**.
- **Bulbourethral (Cowper) glands** are located within the urogenital diaphragm and discharge their secretion directly to the penile urethra. They lubricate and protect the urethra.
- **Semen** contains fluids and sperm cells from the testis and secretory products from the epididymis, ductus deferens, prostate, seminal vesicles, and bulbourethral glands.

PENIS AND SCROTUM

- The **penis** consists of three erectile tissues: two **corpora cavernosa** at the dorsum of the penis and the **corpus spongiosum** that contains the spongy part of the urethra.
- **Erectile tissues** contain vascular spaces that increase in size and rigidity by filling with blood during erection.
- The wall of the **scrotum** reflects the layers of the abdominal wall that were pulled into the developing scrotum during the descent of the testis.
- The **temperature** within the scrotum is about **2°C–3°C lower** than body temperature, creating an optimal environment for **spermatogenesis**.
- Layers of the scrotum include **skin** of the scrotum, **dartos layer**, **external spermatic fascia**, **cremaster muscle**, and **cremasteric fasciae**, **internal spermatic fascia**, and **parietal layer of tunica vaginalis.**

PLATE 22.1 ■ TESTIS I

The **male reproductive system** consists of the paired **testes, epididymides,** and **genital ducts** as well as accessory reproductive glands and the penis. The functions of the testis are the production of **sperm** and the synthesis and secretion of **androgens**, especially **testosterone.** The events of cell division that lead to the production of mature sperm involve both normal cell division, **mitosis**, and reduction division, **meiosis**, to yield a haploid chromosome number and haploid DNA content. Androgen secretion by the testis begins early in fetal development and is essential for the continued normal development of the male fetus. At puberty, androgen production resumes and is responsible for initiation and maintenance of sperm production (**spermatogenesis**), secretion by accessory sex glands (e.g., **prostate** and **seminal vesicles**), and development of secondary sex characteristics.

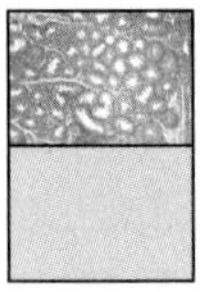

Testis, monkey, hematoxylin and eosin (H&E) ×65.

This section of the testis shows the **seminiferous tubules** and the **tunica albuginea** (*TA*), the capsule of the organ. Extending from the very thick capsule are connective tissue septa (*S*) that divide the organ into compartments. Each compartment contains several seminiferous tubules and represents a lobule (*L*). Blood vessels (*BV*) are present within the inner portion of the capsule, the part referred to as the *tunica vasculosa*, and in the connective tissue septa.

The seminiferous tubules are convoluted; thus, the profiles they present in a section are variable in appearance. Not infrequently, the wall of a tubule is sectioned tangentially, thus obscuring the lumen and revealing what appears to be a solid mass of cells (*X*).

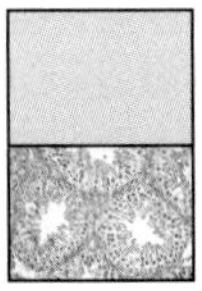

Seminiferous tubules, testis, monkey, H&E ×400.

Examination at higher magnification, as in this figure, reveals a population of interstitial cells that occur in small clusters and lie in the space between adjoining tubules. They consist mostly of **Leydig cells** (*LC*), the chief source of testosterone in male. They are readily identified by virtue of their location and by their small round nucleus and eosinophilic cytoplasm. Macrophages are also found, in close association with the Leydig cells, but in lesser numbers. They are, however, difficult to identify in H&E sections.

A layer of closely apposed squamous cells forms a sheath-like investment around the **tubule epithelium** of each seminiferous tubule. In humans, several layers of cells invest the tubule epithelium. The cells of this peritubular investment exhibit myoid features and account for the slow peristaltic activity of the tubules. Peripheral to the myoid layer is a broad lymphatic channel that occupies an extensive space between the tubules. In routine histologic sections, however, the lymphatic channels are usually collapsed and thus unrecognizable. The cellular elements that surround the tubule epithelium are generally referred to as a **lamina propria** (*LP*) or a *boundary tissue*. As a lamina propria, it is atypical. It is not a loose connective tissue. Indeed, under normal circumstances, lymphocytes and other cell types related to the immune system are conspicuously absent.

Examination of the tubule epithelium reveals two kinds of cells: a proliferating population of spermatogenic cells and a nonproliferating population, the sustentacular, or Sertoli, cells. The Sertoli cells are considerably fewer and can be recognized by their elongated, pale-staining nuclei (*Sn*) and conspicuous nucleolus. The Sertoli cell cytoplasm extends from the periphery of the tubule to the lumen.

The **spermatogenic cells** consist of successive generations arranged in concentric layers. Thus, the **spermatogonia** (*Sg*) are found at the periphery. The **spermatocytes** (*Sc*), most of which have large round nuclei with visible chromatin arranged in a distinctive pattern, lie above the spermatogonia. The spermatid population (*Sp*) consists of one or two generations and occupies the site closest to the lumen. The tubules in this figure have been identified according to their stage of development. The tubule at the *upper right* can be identified as stage *VI*. At this stage, the mature population of **spermatids** (identified by their dark blue heads and eosinophilic thread-like flagella protruding into the lumen) are in the process of being released (spermiogenesis). The younger generation of spermatids is composed of round cells and exhibits round nuclei. Moving clockwise, the tubule indicated as stage *VII* is slightly more advanced. The mature spermatids are now gone. Progressing to stage *VIII*, the tubule at the *bottom* of the micrograph reveals that the spermatid population is undergoing a change in nuclear shape. Note the tapered nuclei (*arrows*). Further maturation of the spermatids is reflected in the tubule at the *top* of the micrograph, stage *XI*. Finally, the tubule marked stage *II*, on the *left*, reveals slightly greater maturation of the luminal spermatids, and with the start of the new cycle (stage *I*), a newly formed spermatid population is now present. By examining the spermatid population and assessing the number of generations present (i.e., one or two) and the degree of maturation, it is possible to approximate the stage of a tubule (see Fig. 22.14).

BV, blood vessels
L, lobule
LC, Leydig cells
LP, lamina propria
S, connective tissue septa
Sc, spermatocytes
Sg, spermatogonia
Sn, Sertoli nuclei
Sp, spermatids
TA, tunica albuginea
X, tangential section of tubule with lumen obscured
arrows, spermatid nuclei displaying early shape change
roman numerals, stages of seminiferous tubule epithelium

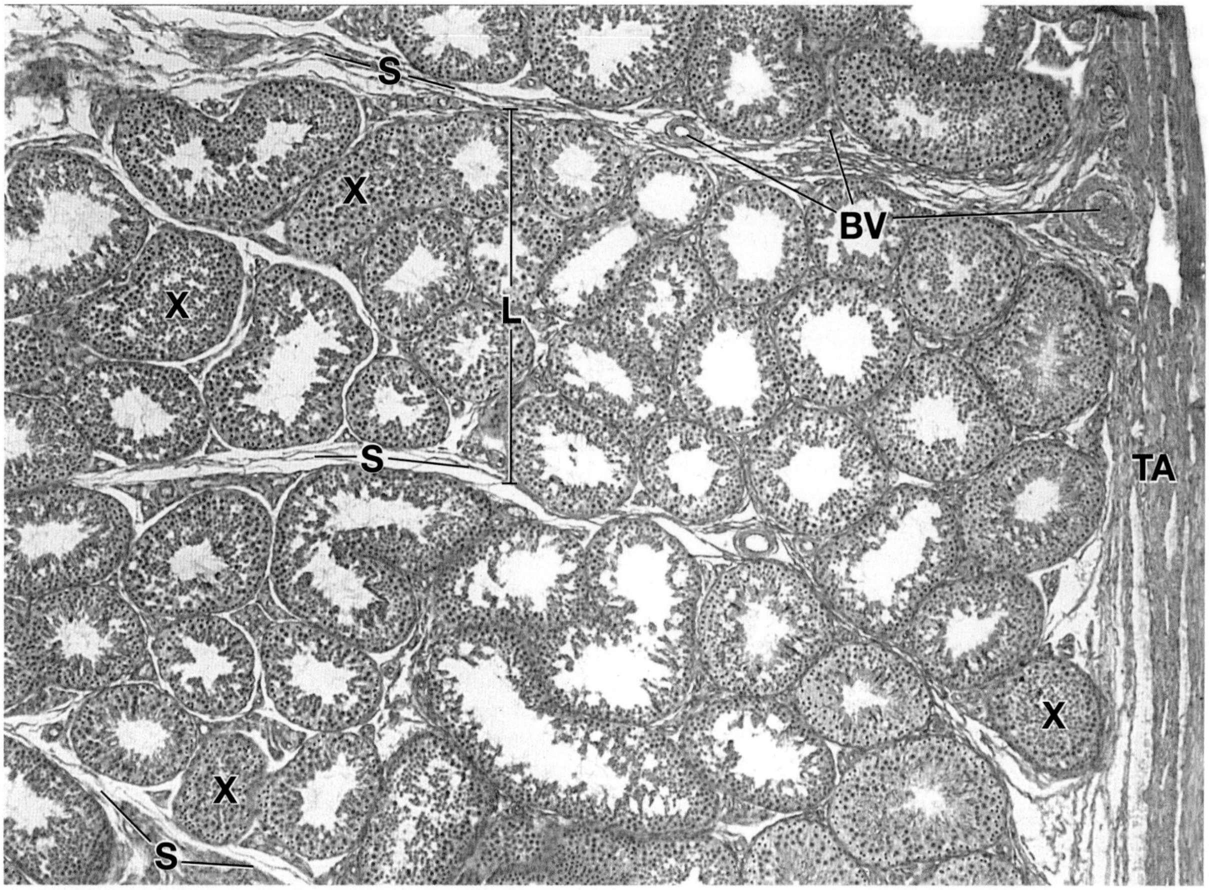
S
L
X
X
BV
S
TA
X
X
S

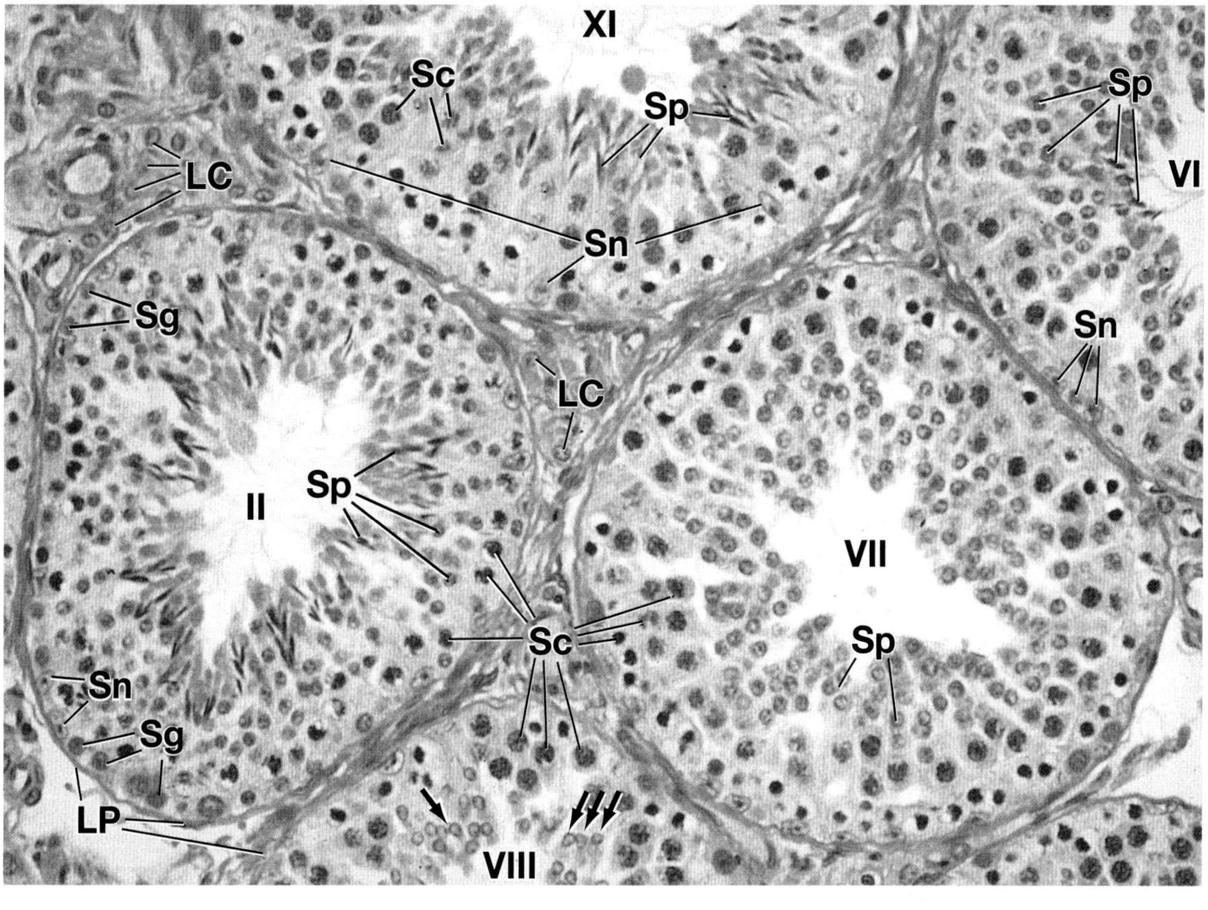
XI
Sc
Sp
Sp
LC
VI
Sn
Sg
Sn
LC
Sp
II
VII
Sc
Sp
Sn
Sg
LP
VIII

PLATE 22.2 ■ TESTIS II

Although the mature testis is characterized by seminiferous tubules, the **immature testis** is characterized by cords of cells consisting of an epithelium of **sustentacular (Sertoli) cells** surrounding occasional **gonocytes**, precursors of spermatogonia that are derived from the primordial germ cells that invaded the developing gonad in the embryo. At puberty, these cords become canalized, and the gonocytes begin the multiple divisions that give rise to the **spermatogonia** that, in turn, will divide and differentiate into mature sperm. The **seminiferous tubules** terminate as **straight tubules (tubuli recti)** that are lined only by Sertoli cells. The tubuli recti lead to the **rete testis**, a complex series of anastomosing channels in the mediastinum testis that signifies the termination of the intratesticular tubule system.

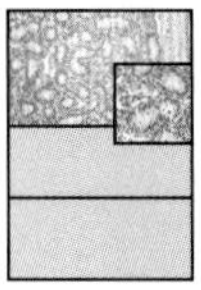

Prepubertal testis, newborn human, hematoxylin and eosin (H&E) ×180; inset ×360.

The various germ cell types representative of spermatogenesis in the mature seminiferous tubules is not present in the testis before puberty or in the postpubertal undescended testis. Instead, the "tubules" are represented by cords of cells in which a lumen is lacking. The **seminiferous cords** display the same tortuosity as in the adult; the tunica albuginea (*TA*) of the testis, although thinner, is of the same relative thickness.

The seminiferous cords are of considerably smaller diameter than the tubules of the adult and are composed of two cell types: the gonocyte, or first-generation spermatogonium, derived from the primordial germ cell that migrates from the yolk sac to the developing gonad in the embryo, and a cell that resembles the Sertoli cell of the adult. The latter cell type predominates and constitutes the bulk of the cord. The cells are columnar, and their nuclei are close to the basement membrane. The **gonocytes** (*G, inset*) are the precursors of the definitive germ cells, or spermatogonia. They are round cells that have a centrally placed, spherical nucleus. The cytoplasm takes little stain and usually appears as a light ring around the nucleus. This gives the gonocyte a distinctive appearance in histologic sections. Generally, the gonocytes are found at the periphery of the cord, but many are also found more centrally. The gonocytes give rise to spermatogonia that begin to proliferate in males between the ages of 10 and 13 years. The seminiferous epithelium then becomes populated with cells at various stages of spermatogenesis, as seen in the adult.

The seminiferous cords are surrounded by one or two layers of cells with long processes and flat nuclei. They resemble fibroblasts at the ultrastructural level and give rise to the myoid peritubular cells of the adult.

The interstitial cells (of Leydig) are conspicuous in the newborn, a reflection of the residual effects of maternal hormones. Leydig cells, however, regress and do not become conspicuous again until puberty. In this preparation, the **Leydig cells** (*LC, inset*) can be seen between the cords. They are ovoid or polygonal and are closely grouped so that adjacent cells are in contact with each other. Overall, they have the same appearance as the Leydig cells of the adult.

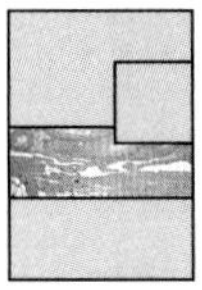

Mediastinum testis, testis, monkey, H&E ×65.

In the posterior portion of the testis, the connective tissue of the tunica albuginea extends more deeply into the organ. This inward extension of connective tissue is called the **mediastinum testis**. It contains a network of anastomosing channels called the **rete testis**. Only a small portion of the mediastinum testis (*MT*) is evident in the figure. The area includes, however, a few seminiferous tubules (*ST*) in the *upper portion* of the micrograph and, fortuitously, the site where one of the seminiferous tubules terminates and joins the rete testis (*RT*). This can be recognized in the area delineated by the *rectangle*, which is shown at higher magnification in the next figure. As noted earlier, the seminiferous tubules are arranged in the form of a loop, with each end joining the rete testis. The seminiferous tubules open into the rete testis by way of a straight tubule. Straight tubules are very short and are lined by Sertoli-like cells; no germ cell component is present. The connective tissue of the mediastinum is very dense but exhibits no other special features, nor is smooth muscle present. Adipose cells (*AC*) and blood vessels (*BV*), particularly veins of varying size, are present within the connective tissue.

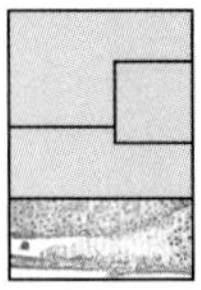

Straight tubule, testis, monkey, H&E ×400.

This photomicrograph is a higher magnification of the *boxed* area on the image immediately above. The **seminiferous tubule** (*ST*) is seen in continuity with a **straight tubule** or tubulus rectus (*TR*). Straight tubule is relatively short and terminates at the point where it enters a channel of the **rete testis** (*RT*). The rete testis is identified by its simple cuboidal epithelium. Note that because of the angle at which the straight tubule was sectioned, it appears that the cuboidal epithelium characterizing the rete testis begins on the upper side of the tubule before it is seen on the lower side of the tubule. The rete testis (*RT*) constitutes an anastomosing system of channels that lead to the efferent ductules. The epithelial cells lining the rete testis are sometimes more squamous than cuboidal or, occasionally, may be low columnar in appearance. Typically, they possess a single (primary) cilium; however, this is difficult to see in routine H&E preparations.

AC, adipose cells
BV, blood vessels
G, gonocytes
LC, Leydig cells
MT, mediastinum testis
RT, rete testis
ST, seminiferous tubules
TA, tunica albuginea
TR, tubulus rectus

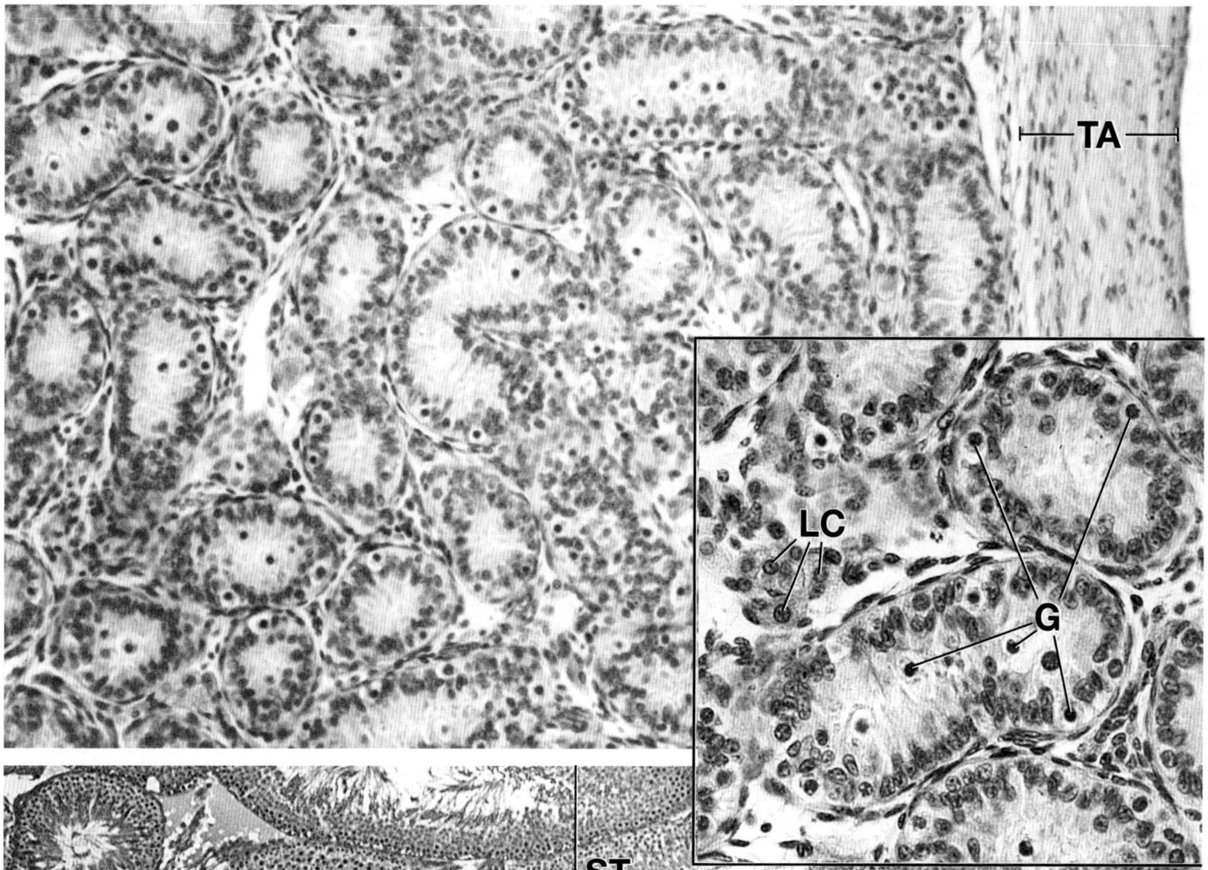
TA
LC
G

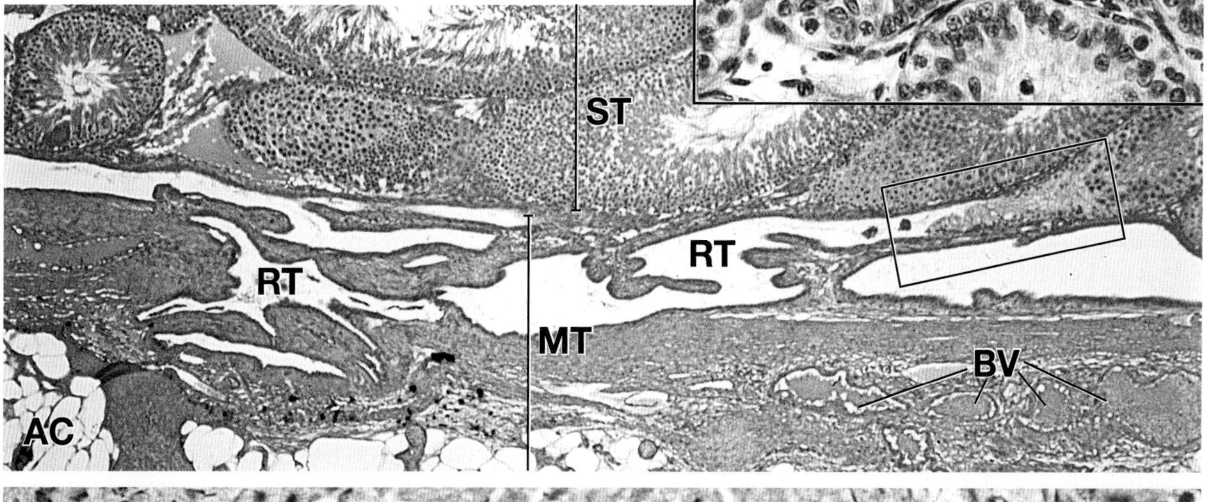
ST
RT
RT
MT
BV
AC

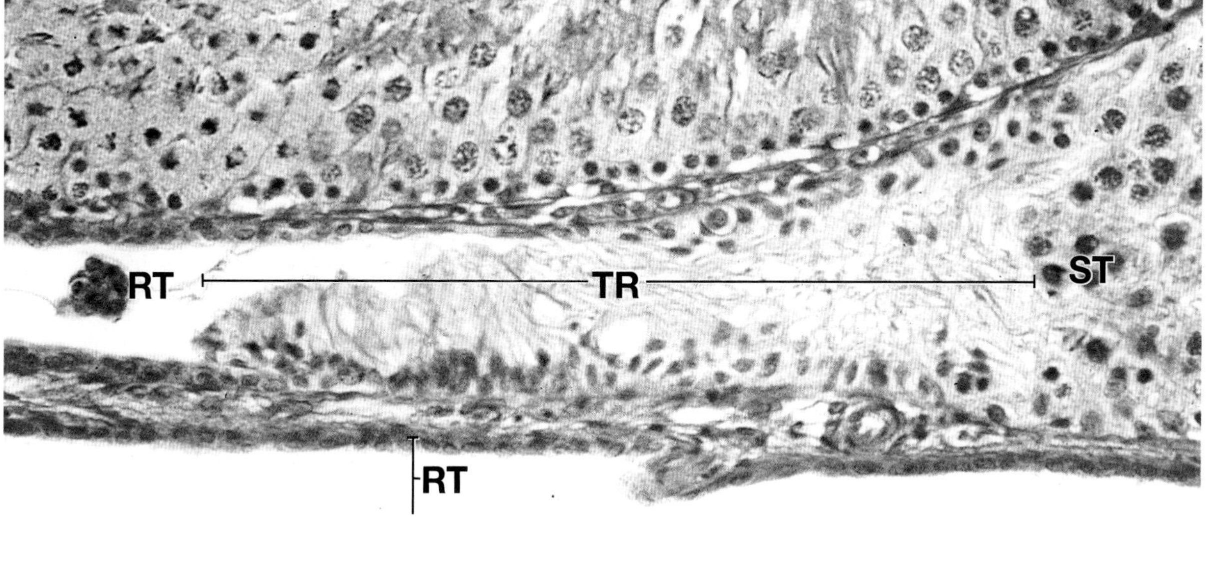
RT
TR
ST
RT

PLATE 22.3 ■ EFFERENT DUCTULES AND EPIDIDYMIS

The **rete testis** is connected via ~20 **efferent ductules** (*ductuli efferentes*; remnants of nephrons of the fetal mesonephric kidney) to the **ductus epididymis.** These are the first elements of the excurrent duct system of the male genital system. Most of the fluid secreted in the seminiferous tubules is reabsorbed in the efferent ductules. The muscular coat characteristic of the excurrent duct system first appears at the beginning of the efferent ductules. The ductus epididymis is a highly coiled tube, 4–6 m long; sperm mature during their passage along its length, acquiring motility as well as the ability to fertilize an egg. This maturation is also androgen dependent and involves changes in the sperm plasma membrane and addition to the glycocalyx of glycoproteins secreted by the epididymal epithelial cells.

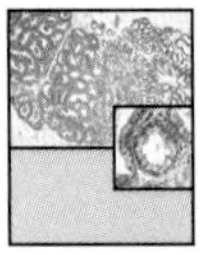

Efferent ductules, testis-epididymis, monkey, hematoxylin and eosin (H&E) ×60; inset ×360.

About 12–20 **efferent ductules** leave the testis and serve as channels from the rete testis to the ductus epididymis. Each of the efferent ductules undergoes numerous spiral windings and convolutions to form a group of conical structures; together, they constitute the initial part of the head of the epididymis. When examined in a tissue section, the ductules exhibit a variety of irregular profiles owing to their twisting and turning. This is evident on the *right side* of this micrograph.

The epithelium that lines the efferent ductules is distinctive in that groups of tall columnar cells alternate with groups of cuboidal cells, giving the luminal surface an unevenly contoured appearance. Thus, small cup–like depressions are created where the epithelium contains groups of cuboidal or low columnar cells. Typically, these shorter cells exhibit a brush border–like apical surface because of the microvilli that they possess (*arrowhead, inset*). The basal surface of the ductule, in contrast, has a smooth contour (see next figure and *inset*). Some of the cells, generally the tall columnar cells, possess cilia (*C*) (*inset*). Whereas the ciliated cells aid in moving the contents of the tubule toward the epididymis, the cells with the microvilli are largely responsible for absorbing fluid from the lumen. In addition to the columnar and cuboidal cells, basal cells are also present; thus, the epithelium is designated pseudostratified columnar. The basal cells possess little cytoplasm and presumably serve as stem cells.

The efferent ductules possess a thin layer of circularly arranged smooth muscle cells (*SM, inset*). The muscle is close to the basal surface of the epithelial cells, being separated from it by only a small amount of connective tissue (*CT, inset*). Because of this close association, the smooth muscle may be overlooked or misidentified as connective tissue. Smooth muscle facilitates the movement of luminal contents of the ductule to the ductus epididymis.

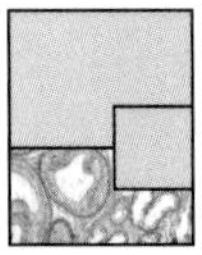

Epididymis, monkey, H&E ×180.

The **epididymis**, by virtue of its shape, is divided into a head, body, and tail. The initial part of the head contains the **ductus epididymis**, a single convoluted duct into which the efferent ductules open. The duct is, at first, highly convoluted but becomes less tortuous in the body and tail. A section through the **head of the epididymis**, as shown in the previous figure, cuts the ductus epididymis in numerous places, and as in the efferent ductules, different-shaped profiles are observed.

The epithelium contains two distinguishable cell types: tall columnar cells and basal cells similar to those of the efferent ductules. The epithelium is, therefore, also pseudostratified columnar. The columnar cells are tallest in the head of the epididymis and diminish in height as the tail is reached. The free surface of the cell possesses **stereocilia** (*SC*). These are extremely long, branching microvilli. They evidently adhere to each other during the preparation of the tissue to form the fine tapering structures that are characteristically seen with the light microscope. The nuclei of the **columnar cells** are elongated and are located a moderate distance from the base of the cell. They are readily distinguished from the spherical nuclei of the **basal cells** that lie close to the basement membrane. Other conspicuous features of the columnar cells include a very large supranuclear Golgi apparatus (not seen at the magnification offered here), pigment accumulations (*P*), and numerous lysosomes, demonstrable with appropriate techniques.

Because of the unusual height of the columnar cells and the tortuosity of the duct, an uneven lumen appears in some sites; indeed, even "islands" of epithelium can be encountered in the lumen (see *arrows*, previous figure). Such profiles are accounted for by sharp turns in the duct where the epithelial wall on one side of the duct is partially cut. For example, a cut in the plane of the *double-headed arrow* indicated in this figure would create such an isolated epithelial island.

A thin layer of smooth muscle circumscribes the duct and appears similar to that associated with the efferent ductules. In the terminal portion of the epididymis, however, the smooth muscle acquires a greater thickness, and longitudinal fibers are also present. Beyond the smooth muscle coat, there is a small amount of connective tissue (*CT*) that binds the loops of the duct together and carries the blood vessels (*BV*) and nerves.

AT, adipose tissue
BV, blood vessel
C, cilia
CT, connective tissue
P, pigment
SC, stereocilia
SM, smooth muscle
arrowhead (inset), brush border
arrows, "islands" of epithelium in the lumen

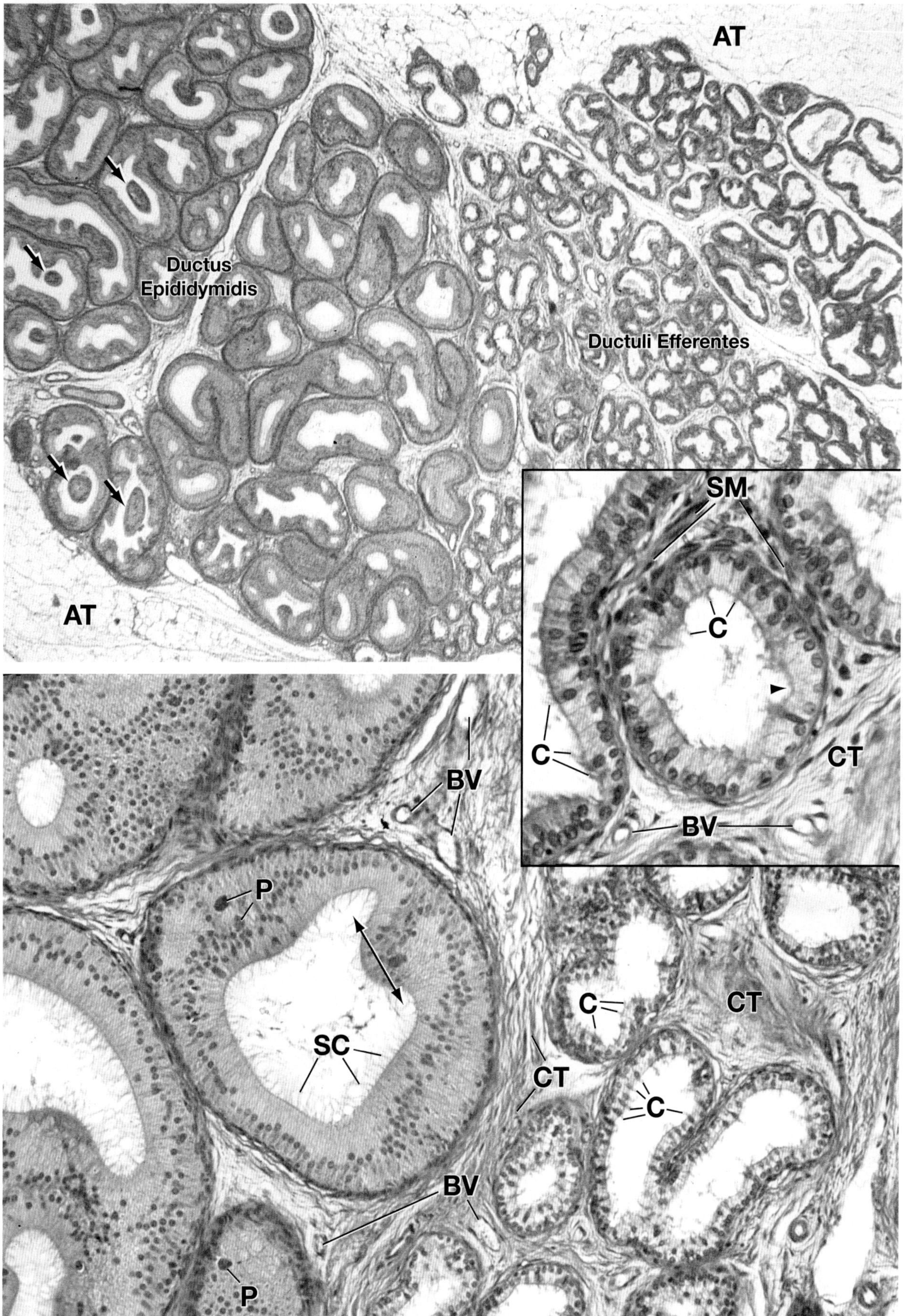
AT
Ductus Epididymidis
Ductuli Efferentes
AT
SM
C
C
CT
BV
BV
P
SC
C
CT
CT
C
BV
P

The **ductus (vas) deferens** continues from the duct of the epididymis as a thick-walled muscular tube that leaves the scrotum and passes through the inguinal canal as a component of the spermatic cord. At the deep inguinal ring, it continues into the pelvis and, behind the urinary bladder, joins with the excretory duct from the seminal vesicle to form the **ejaculatory duct**. The ejaculatory duct then pierces the prostate gland and opens into the **urethra**.

Mature sperm are stored in the terminal portion (tail) of the ductus epididymis. These sperm are forced into the ductus deferens by intense contractions of the three smooth muscle layers of the ductus deferens following appropriate neural stimulation. Contraction of the smooth muscle of the ductus deferens continues the movement of the sperm through the ejaculatory duct into the urethra during the ejaculatory reflex. The seminal vesicles (see Plate 22.6, page 906) are not storage sites for sperm but, rather, secrete a fructose-rich fluid that becomes part of the ejaculated semen. Fructose is the principal metabolic substrate for sperm.

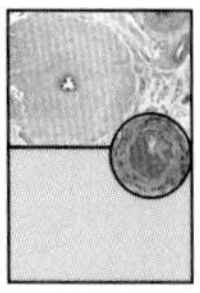

Spermatic cord, human, hematoxylin and eosin (H&E) ×80.

A cross section through the **ductus deferens** and some of the vessels and nerves that accompany the duct in the spermatic cord is shown in this figure. The wall of the ductus deferens is extremely thick, mostly because of the presence of a large amount of smooth muscle. The muscle contracts when the tissue is removed, causing the mucosa to form longitudinal folds. For this reason, in histologic sections, the lumen (*L*) usually appears irregular in cross section.

The smooth muscle of the ductus deferens is arranged as a thick outer longitudinal layer (*SM[L]*), a thick middle circular layer (*SM[C]*), and a thinner inner longitudinal layer (*SM[L]*). Between the epithelium and the inner longitudinal smooth muscle layer, there is a moderately thick cellular layer of loose connective tissue, the lamina propria (*LP*). The connective tissue immediately surrounding the ductus deferens contains nerves and some of the smaller blood vessels that supply the duct. In fact, some of these vessels can be seen penetrating the outer longitudinal smooth muscle layer (*asterisks*).

A unique feature of the spermatic cord is the presence of a plexus of atypical veins **(pampiniform plexus)** that arise from the spermatic veins. These vessels receive the blood from the testis. (The pampiniform plexus also receives tributaries from the epididymis.) The plexus is an anastomosing vascular network that constitutes the bulk of the spermatic cord. Portions of several of these veins (*BV*) are evident in the *upper right* of the previous figure along with a number of nerves (*N*). The unusual feature of the veins is their thick muscular wall that, at a glance, gives the appearance of an artery rather than a vein. Careful examination of these vessels (*inset*) shows that the bulk of the vessel wall is composed of two layers of smooth muscle—an outer circular layer *SM(C)* and an inner longitudinal layer *SM(L)*.

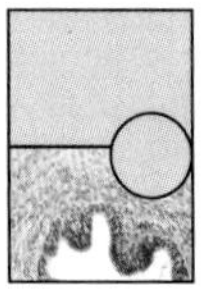

Ductus deferens, human, H&E ×320; inset ×250.

The epithelial lining of the **ductus deferens** consists of pseudostratified columnar epithelium with stereocilia (*arrowheads*). It resembles the epithelium of the epididymis, but the cells are not as tall. The elongated nuclei of the columnar cells are readily distinguished from the spherical nuclei of the **basal cells** (*arrows*). The epithelium rests on a loose connective tissue known as the lamina propria (*LP*) that extends to the smooth muscle; no submucosa is described.

BV, blood vessels	**N,** nerve	**arrowheads,** stereocilia
L, lumen of ductus deferens	**SM(C),** circular layer of smooth muscle	**arrows,** basal cell nucleus
LP, lamina propria	**SM(L),** longitudinal layer of smooth muscle	**asterisks,** small arteries supplying ductus deferens
Lu, lumen of blood vessel		

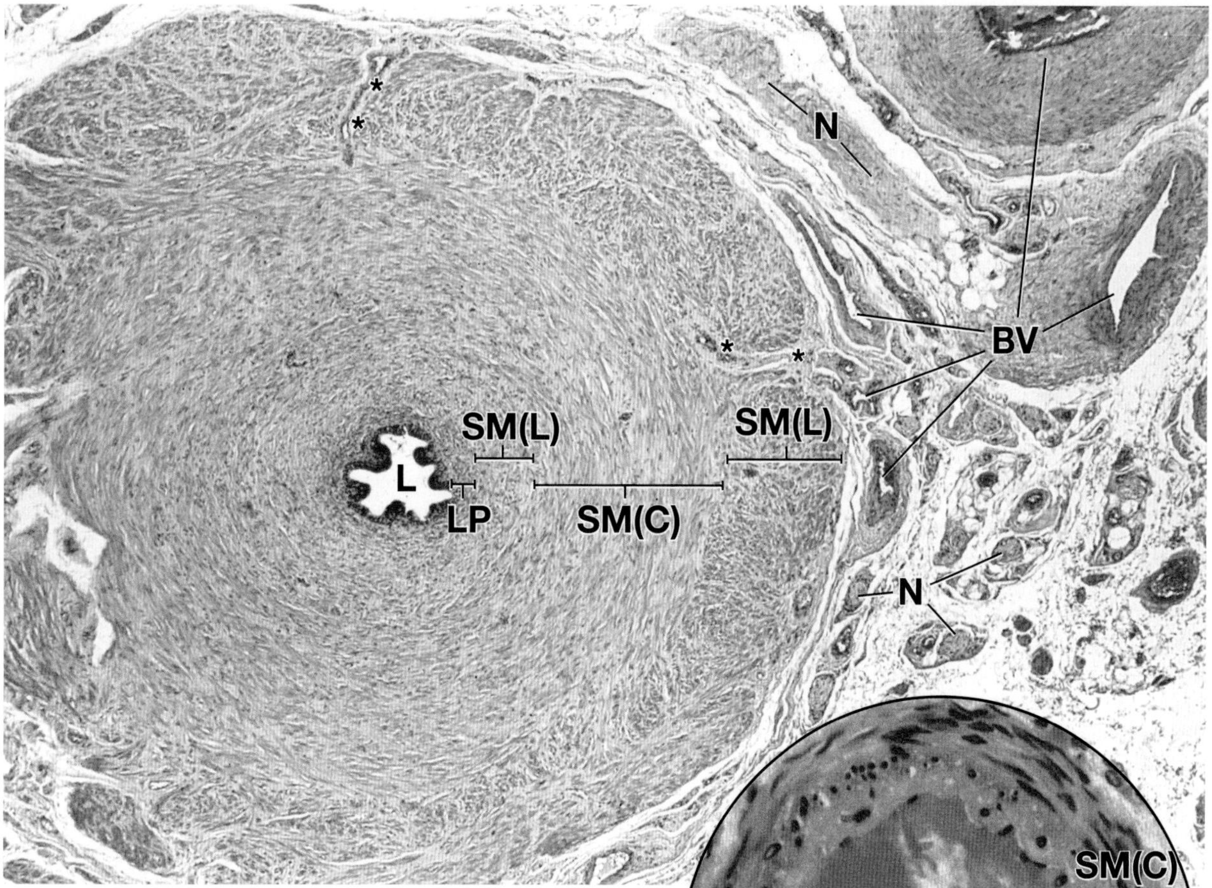
*
*
N
BV
*
*
SM(L)
SM(L)
L
LP
SM(C)
N

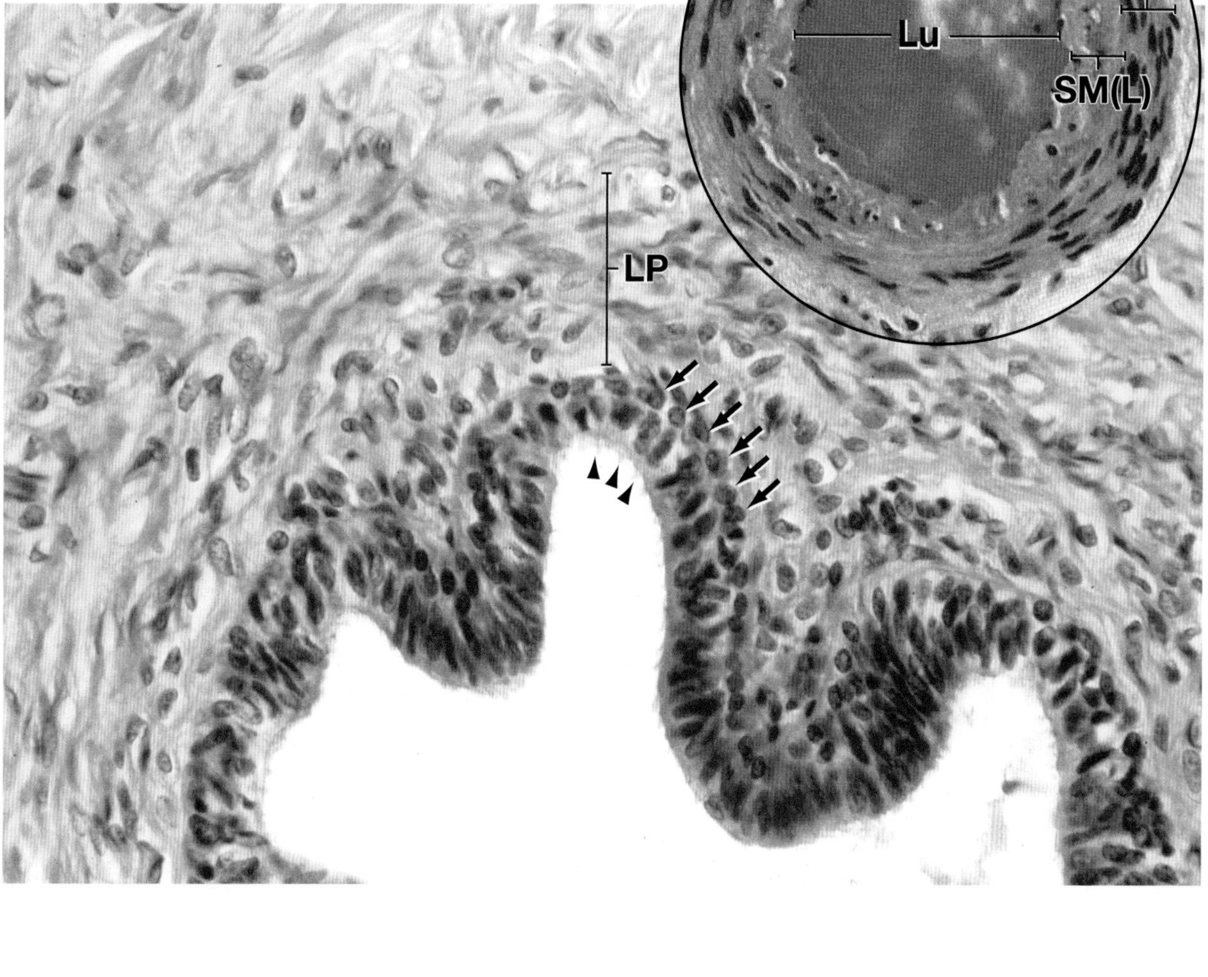
SM(C)
Lu
SM(L)
LP

PLATE 22.5 ■ PROSTATE GLAND

The **prostate gland** is the largest accessory sex gland. It consists of 30–50 **tubuloalveolar glands** that surround the proximal urethra. Because of this relationship, a common condition in later life, benign prostatic hyperplasia, can result in partial or total obstruction of the urethra.

The prostatic glands are arranged in three concentric layers: a mucosal layer, a submucosal layer, and a peripheral layer containing the main prostatic glands. The mucosal glands secrete directly into the urethra; the other two sets of glands deliver their secretions through ducts that open into the prostatic sinuses on the posterior wall of the urethra. All of the glands are made up of a pseudostratified columnar epithelium that secretes several components of the semen, including acid phosphatase, citric acid (a nutrient for sperm), and fibrinolysin (which keeps the semen liquified). Aggregations of dead epithelial cells and precipitated secretory products form **prostatic concretions** in the alveoli of the glands; these are a characteristic feature that aids in recognition of the prostate.

The stroma is characterized by numerous small bundles of smooth muscle so that it can also be described as a **fibromuscular stroma**. Contraction of this muscle occurs at ejaculation, forcing the secretion into the urethra. Surrounding the gland is a fibroelastic capsule that also contains small bundles of smooth muscle.

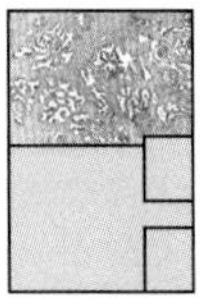

Prostate gland, human, hematoxylin and eosin (H&E) ×47.

A portion of the **prostate gland** is shown in this low-magnification micrograph. A small section of the capsule (*Cap*) of the gland is seen in the *upper left* corner. The rest of the field is filled with the glandular and stromal components of the prostate. The secretory tubuloalveoli of the prostate gland vary greatly in form, as is evident in the figure. They may appear as tubes, as isolated alveoli, as alveoli with branches, or as tubes with branches. Tangential sections through alveoli may even produce the appearance of "epithelial islands" (*arrowheads*) in the lumen of the alveoli. This is due to the extremely uneven contour of the epithelial surface. It should also be noted that many of the alveoli may appear rudimentary in structure (*arrows*). These are simply in an inactive state and are increasingly observed in older individuals. As noted earlier, aggregations of dead epithelial cells and precipitated secretions form **prostatic concretions** (*C*) in the lumina of the alveoli; these gradually increase in number and size with age. The concretions stain with eosin and may have a concentric lamellar appearance, as is clearly shown in the concretion in the *lower right*. With time, they may become impregnated with calcium salts and can thus be easily recognized in x-rays of the lower abdomen.

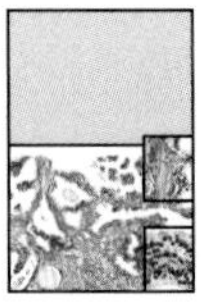

Glands and fibromuscular stroma, prostate, human, H&E ×178; upper inset ×350; lower inset ×650.

In this higher magnification view of a portion of the prostate gland, the **fibromuscular stroma** is clearly seen both immediately subtending the secretory epithelium of the tubuloalveoli as well as in deeper, nonsecretory areas. In the *upper inset*, corresponding to the *larger rectangle*, the intensity of the staining of the **smooth muscle** (*SM*) clearly distinguishes it from the fibrous stromal connective tissue with which it is intimately intermingled. There are no clearly outlined bundles or layers of smooth muscle in the prostate; rather, it is randomly arrayed throughout the stroma. **Prostatic concretions** (*C*) are again evident in the lumina of alveoli, in one instance compressing the epithelium to a degree that makes it nearly unrecognizable. The *lower inset*, corresponding to the *smaller rectangle*, clearly demonstrates the pseudostratified columnar nature of the prostatic epithelium (*Ep*). Well-delineated basal cells (*arrowheads*) are seen along with the taller columnar secretory cells. A small blood vessel (*BV*) immediately subtending the epithelium is recognizable by the red blood cells in its lumen. A lymphocytic infiltration (*L*) appears to fill the stroma along the *lower border* of this image, suggesting an inflammatory process occurring in the prostate gland.

BV, blood vessel
C, prostatic concretion
Cap, capsule
Ep, epithelium
L, lymphocytes
SM, smooth muscle
arrows, inactive alveoli
arrowheads, top figure, "epithelial islands;" lower inset figure, basal cells

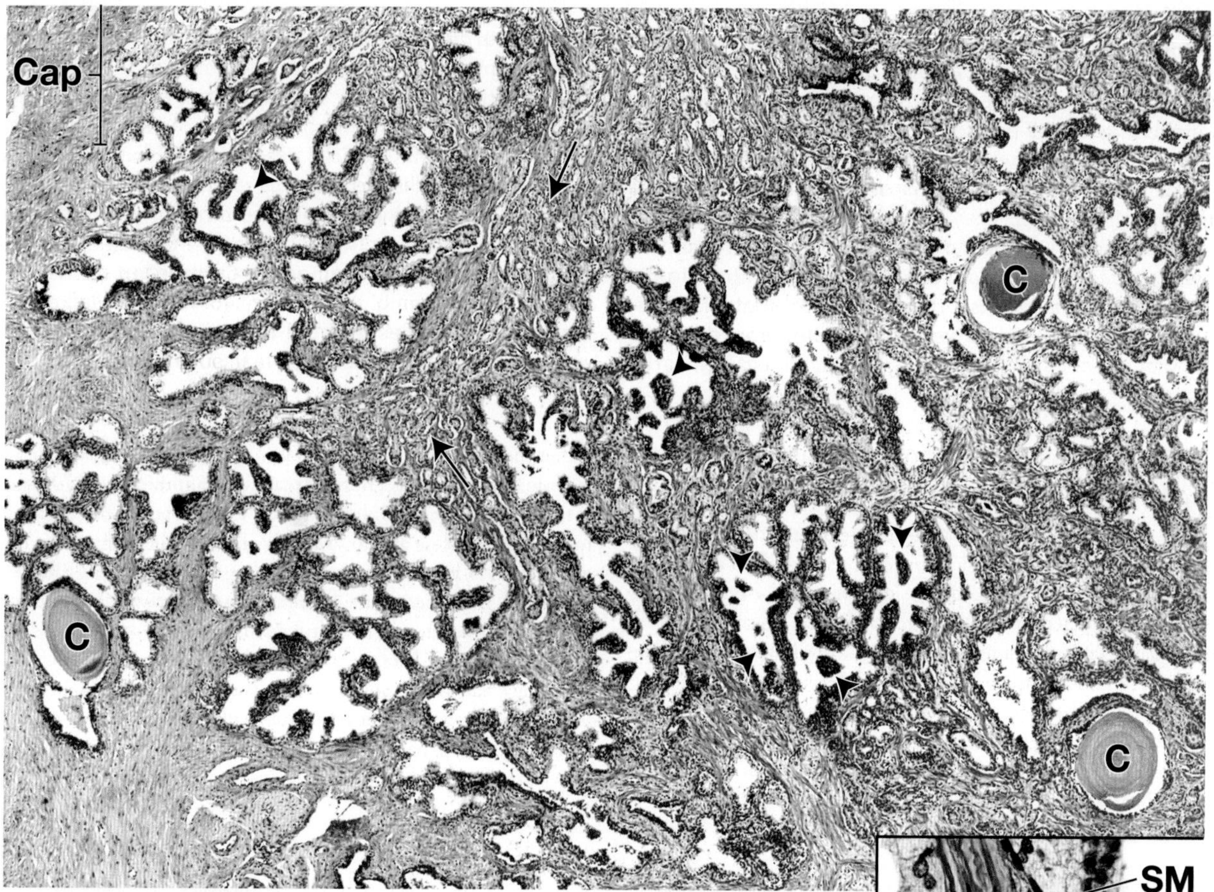
Cap
C
C
C

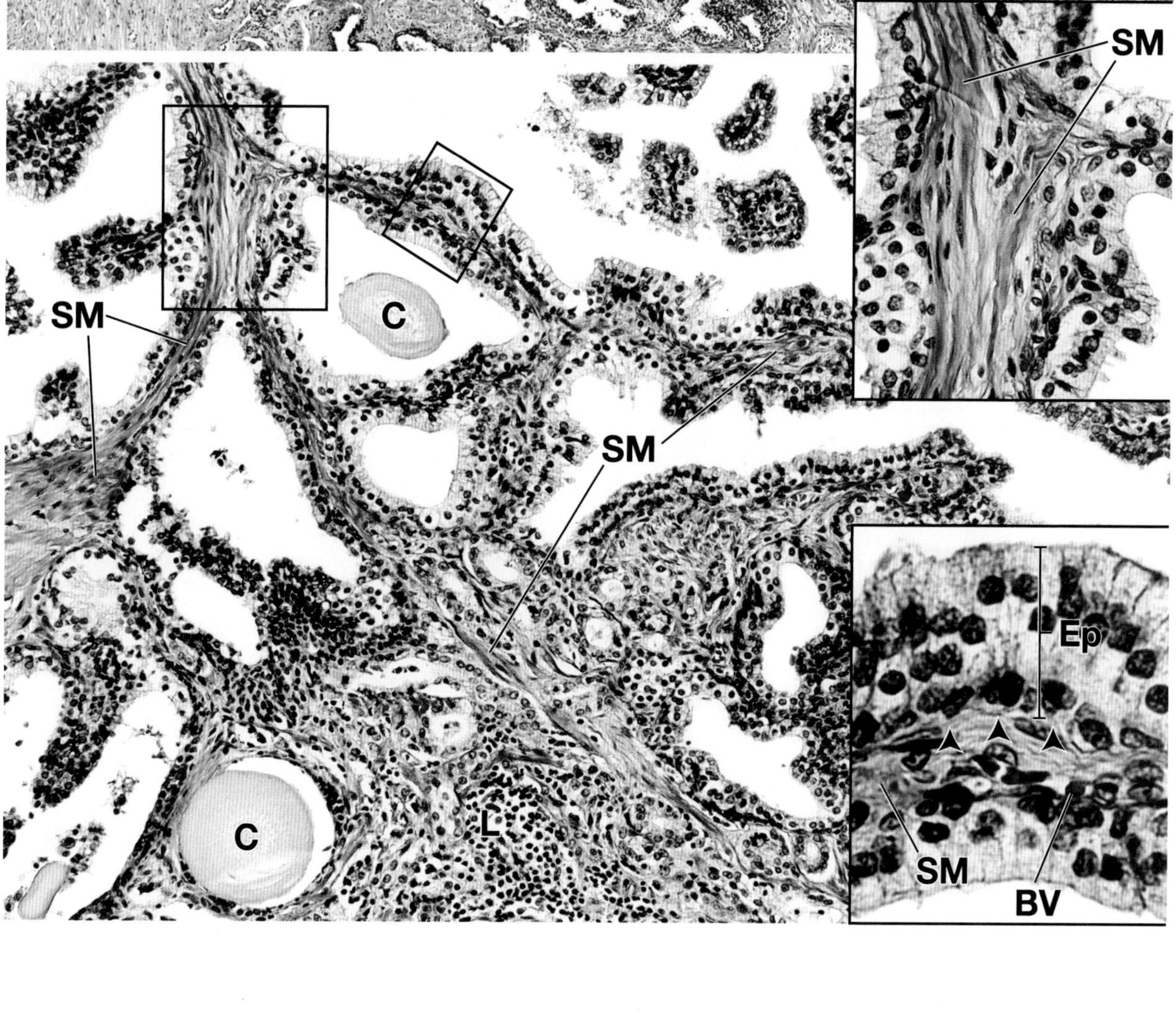
SM
SM
C
SM
C
L
SM
Ep
SM
BV

PLATE 22.6 ■ SEMINAL VESICLE

The **seminal vesicles** are evaginations from the end of each ductus deferens that form tightly coiled tubes. Although sections through this structure may show many lumina, they are all profiles of a single continuous tubular lumen. The seminal vesicles are lined with a pseudostratified columnar epithelium that closely resembles that of the prostate gland.

The secretion of the seminal vesicles is a whitish yellow viscous material that contains fructose, other simple sugars, amino acids, ascorbic acid, and prostaglandins. Although prostaglandins were first isolated from the prostate gland (hence the name), they are synthesized in large amounts in the seminal vesicles. Fructose is the primary nutrient source for the sperm in the semen.

The **mucosa** rests on a thick layer of smooth muscle that is directly continuous with that of the ductus deferens, from which the seminal vesicle evaginates. The smooth muscle consists of an indistinct inner circular layer and an outer longitudinal layer (compare with the three layers of the ductus epididymis and the ductus deferens; Plate 22.3, page 900), which are difficult to distinguish. Contraction of the smooth muscle coat during ejaculation forces the secretions of the seminal vesicles into the ejaculatory ducts. Beyond the smooth muscle is the connective tissue of the adventitia.

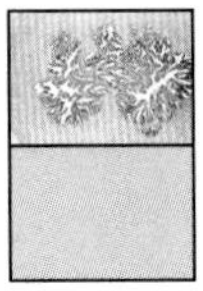

Seminal vesicle, human, hematoxylin and eosin (H&E) ×30.

This figure shows a cross section of a **seminal vesicle**. Because of the coiled nature of the vesicle, two almost distinct lumina, lying side by side, appear to be present. They are, however, connected so that, in effect, all of the internal spaces are continuous and what is seen here is actually a two-dimensional configuration reflecting the coiling of the tube.

The **mucosa** of the seminal vesicles is characterized by extensive folds or ridges. The ridges vary in size and typically branch and interconnect with one another. The larger ridges may form recesses that contain smaller ridges, and when cut obliquely, these appear as mucosal arches that enclose the smaller folds (*arrows*). When the plane of section is normal to the surface, the mucosal ridges appear as "villi." In some areas, particularly the peripheral region of the lumen, the interconnecting folds of the mucosa appear as alveoli. Each of these chambers is, however, simply a pocket-like structure that is open and continuous with the lumen. The mucosa is subtended by a very cellular loose connective tissue (*CT*) that, in turn, is surrounded by smooth muscle (*SM*).

The seminal vesicles are paired, elongated sacs. Each vesicle consists of a single tube folded and coiled on itself with occasional diverticula in its wall. The upper extremity ends as a cul-de-sac; the lower extremity is constricted into a narrow straight excretory duct that joins and empties into its corresponding ductus deferens.

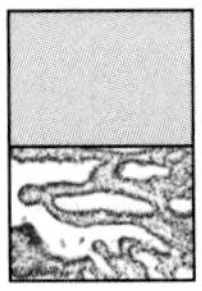

Mucosal folds, seminal vesicle, human, H&E ×220.

This higher magnification of the mucosal folds reveals the **epithelium** (*Ep*) and the underlying loose connective tissue or **lamina propria** (*LP*). The epithelium is described as pseudostratified. It is composed of low columnar or cuboidal cells and small, round basal cells. The latter are randomly interspersed between the larger principal cells, but they are relatively sparse. For this reason, the epithelium may not be readily recognized as pseudostratified. In some areas, the epithelium appears thick (*arrowhead*) and, based on the disposition of the nuclei, would seem to be multilayered. This is due to a tangential section of the epithelium and is not a true stratification. The lamina propria of the mucosa is composed of a very cellular connective tissue containing some smooth muscle cells and is rich in elastic fibers.

CT, connective tissue
Ep, epithelium
LP, lamina propria
SM, smooth muscle
arrowhead, oblique section of epithelium
arrows, mucosal arches

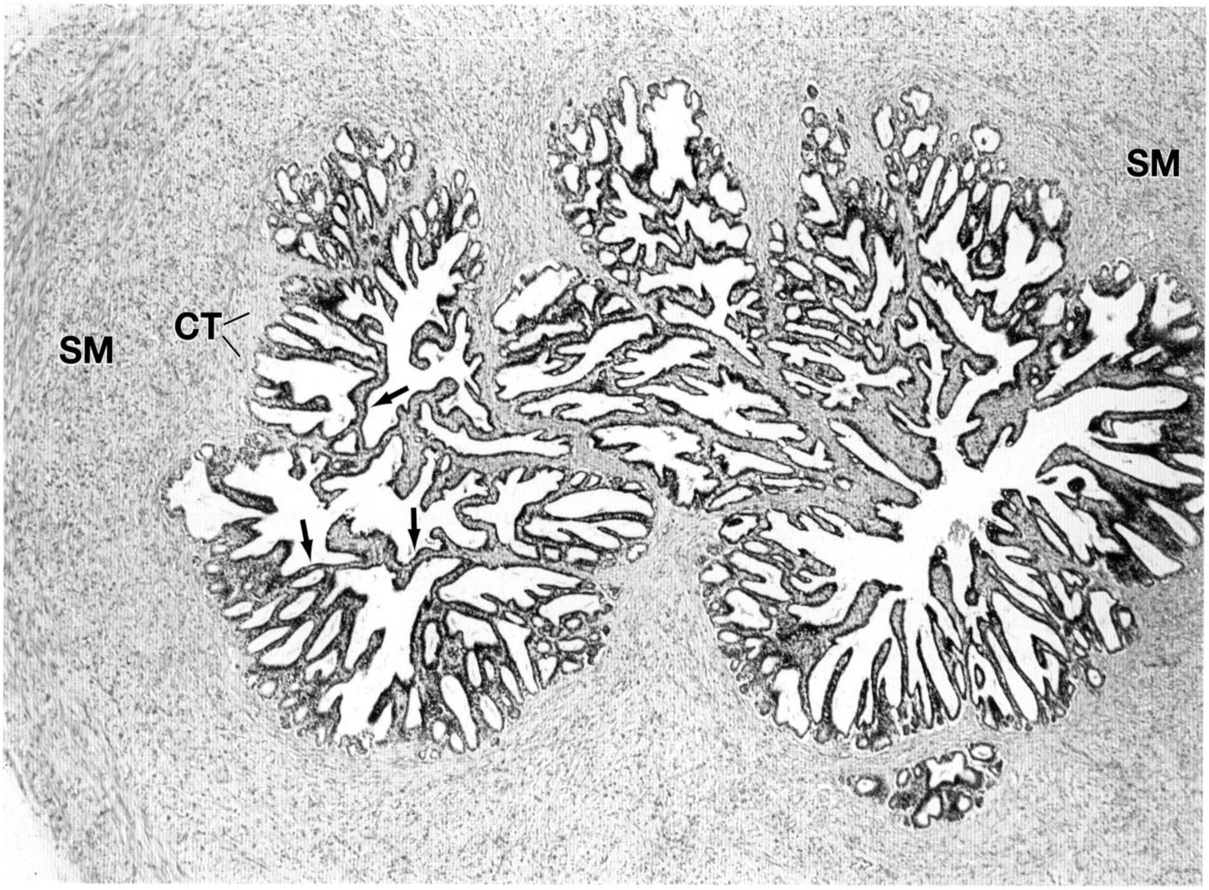
SM
CT
SM

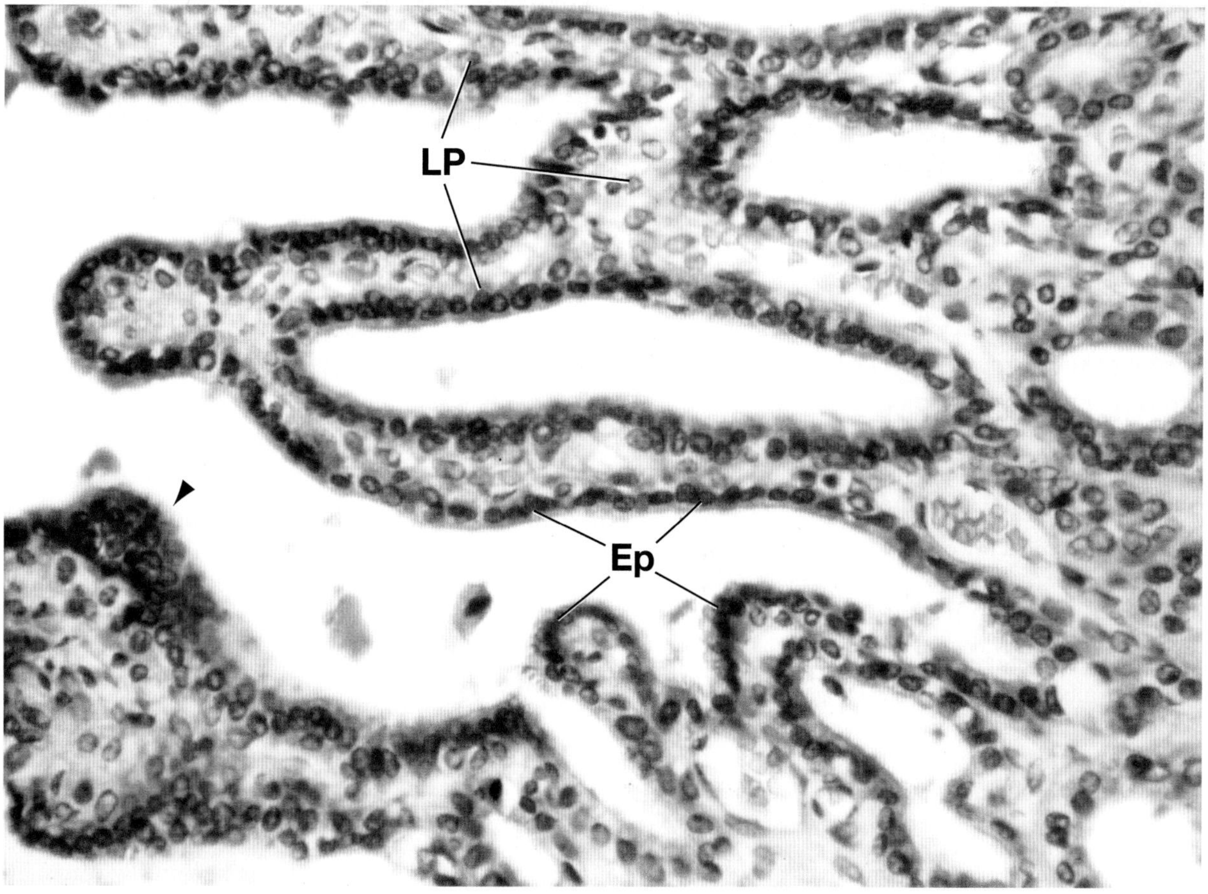
LP
Ep

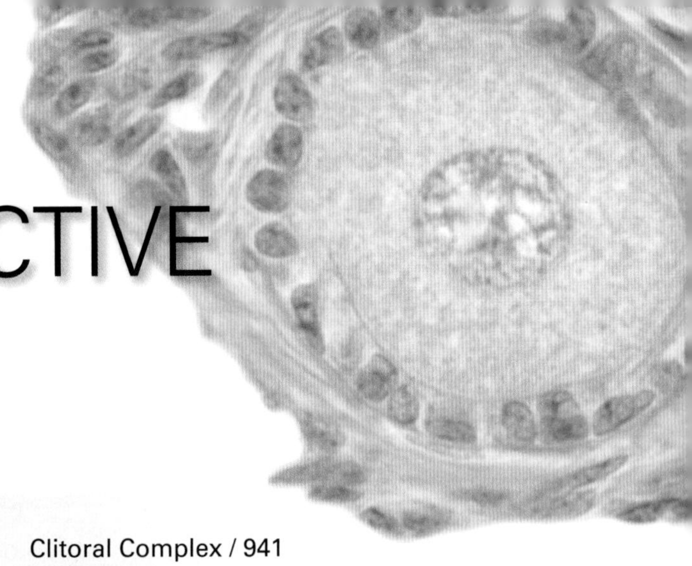

23 FEMALE REPRODUCTIVE SYSTEM

■ OVERVIEW OF THE FEMALE REPRODUCTIVE SYSTEM

The female reproductive system consists of internal sex organs and external genital structures.

The internal female reproductive organs are located in the pelvis, and the external genital structures (external genitalia) are situated in the anterior part of the perineum known as the **vulva**.

- The **internal female reproductive organs** are the ovaries, uterine tubes, uterus, and vagina (Fig. 23.1). They are contained mainly within the pelvic cavity and in the perineum.
- The **external genitalia** include the mons pubis, labia majora and minora, clitoris, vestibule and opening of the vagina, hymen, and external urethral orifice.

The mammary glands are included in this chapter because their development and functional state are directly related to the hormonal activity of the female reproductive system. Similarly, the placenta is included because of its functional and physical relationship to the uterus in pregnancy.

Female reproductive organs undergo regular cyclical changes from puberty to menopause.

The **ovaries**, **uterine tubes**, and **uterus** of the sexually mature female undergo marked structural and functional changes related to neural activity and changes in hormone levels during each **menstrual cycle** and during **pregnancy**. These mechanisms also regulate the early development of the female reproductive system. The initiation of menstruation, referred to as **menarche**, occurs in females between 9 and 14 years of age (the mean age of menarche is 12.4 years) and marks the beginning of the reproductive life span. During this phase of life, the menstrual cycle averages 21–34 days in length. Between 45 and 55 years of age (the mean age is 51.4 years), the menstrual cycle becomes irregular and eventually ceases. This change in reproductive function is referred to as **menopause** or *climacteric*. The ovaries cease their reproductive function of

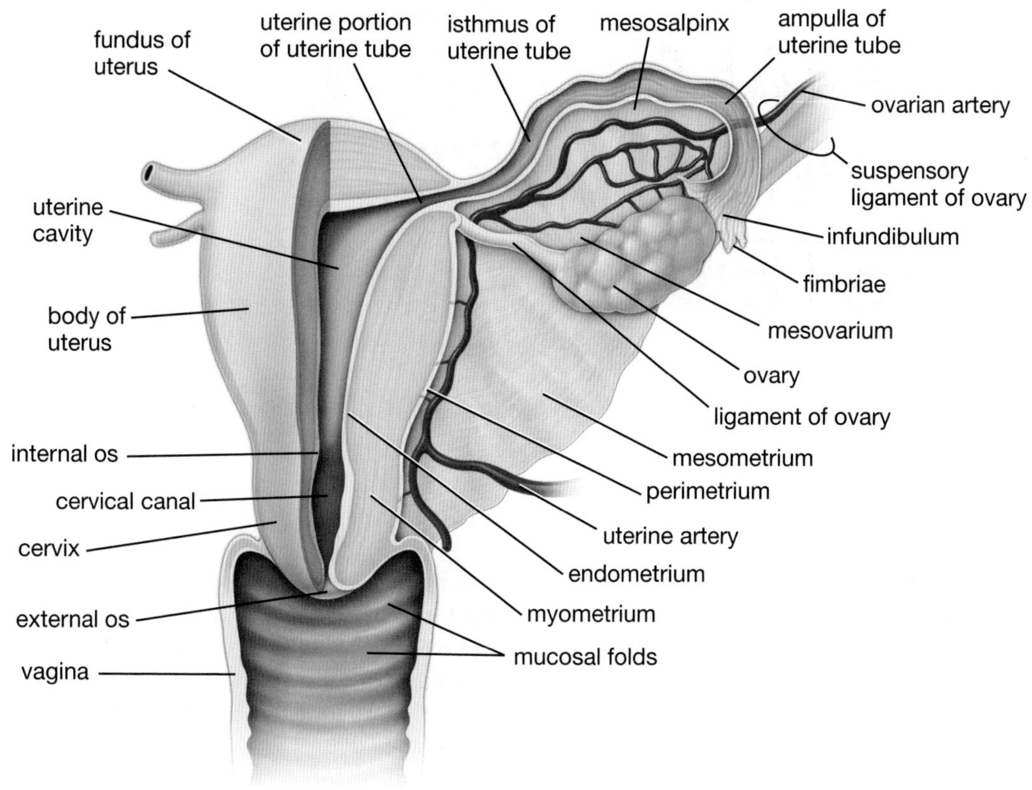

FIGURE 23.1. Schematic drawing of female internal sex organs. This drawing shows the posterior view of the female internal sex organs. Part of the wall of the uterus, uterine tube, and vagina has been removed to reveal their internal structure. Note the three distinct layers of the uterine wall: the inner layer, the endometrium lining the uterine cavity; the middle and thickest layer, the myometrium; and the outer layer, the perimetrium, which is the peritoneal covering of the uterus.

producing oocytes and their endocrine function of producing hormones that regulate reproductive activity. Other organs (e.g., the vagina and mammary glands) show varying degrees of reduced function, particularly secretory activity.

■ OVARY

Production of gametes and steroid hormones are the two major functions of the ovary.

The **ovaries** have two interrelated functions: **gametogenesis** (the production of gametes; oocytes for fertilization and successful propagation of the species) and **steroidogenesis** (the production of steroids that allow the development of female secondary sexual characteristics and support of oocyte development and pregnancy). The production of female gametes is called **oogenesis.** Developing gametes are called **oocytes**; mature gametes are called **ova**.

Two major groups of **steroid hormones**—estrogens and progestogens—are secreted by the ovaries.

- **Estrogens** promote the growth and maturation of internal and external sex organs and are responsible for the female sex characteristics that develop at puberty. Estrogens also act on mammary glands to promote breast development by stimulating ductal and stromal growth and accumulation of adipose tissue.
- **Progestogens** prepare the internal sex organs, mainly the uterus, for pregnancy by promoting secretory changes in the endometrium (discussed in the section on cyclical changes in the endometrium). Progestogens also prepare the mammary gland for lactation by promoting lobular proliferation.

Both hormones play an important role in the menstrual cycle by preparing the uterus for implantation of a fertilized ovum. If implantation does not occur, the endometrium of the uterus degenerates and menstruation follows.

Ovarian Structure

In nulliparous female (individuals who have not given birth), the **ovaries** are paired, almond-shaped, pinkish white structures measuring about 3 cm in length, 1.5 cm in width, and 1 cm in thickness. Each ovary is attached to the posterior surface of the **broad ligament** by a peritoneal fold, the **mesovarium** (see Fig. 23.1). The superior (or tubal) pole of the ovary is attached to the pelvic wall by the **suspensory ligament of the ovary**, which carries the ovarian vessels and nerves. The inferior (or uterine) pole is attached to the uterus by the **ovarian ligament.** This ligament is a remnant of the **gubernaculum**, the embryonic fibrous cord that attaches the developing gonad to the floor of the pelvis. Before puberty, the surface of the ovary is smooth, but during reproductive life, it becomes progressively scarred and irregular because of repeated ovulation. After menopause, the ovaries are about one-fourth the size observed during the reproductive period.

The ovary is composed of a cortex and a medulla.

A section through the ovary reveals two distinct regions:

- The **medulla** or **medullary region** is located in the central portion of the ovary and contains loose connective tissue, a mass of relatively large contorted blood vessels, lymphatic vessels, and nerves (Fig. 23.2).
- The **cortex** or **cortical region** is found in the peripheral portion of the ovary surrounding the medulla. The cortex contains the **ovarian follicles** embedded in a richly cellular connective tissue (Plate 23.1, page 956). Scattered smooth muscle fibers are present in the stroma around the follicles. The boundary between the medulla and the cortex is indistinct.

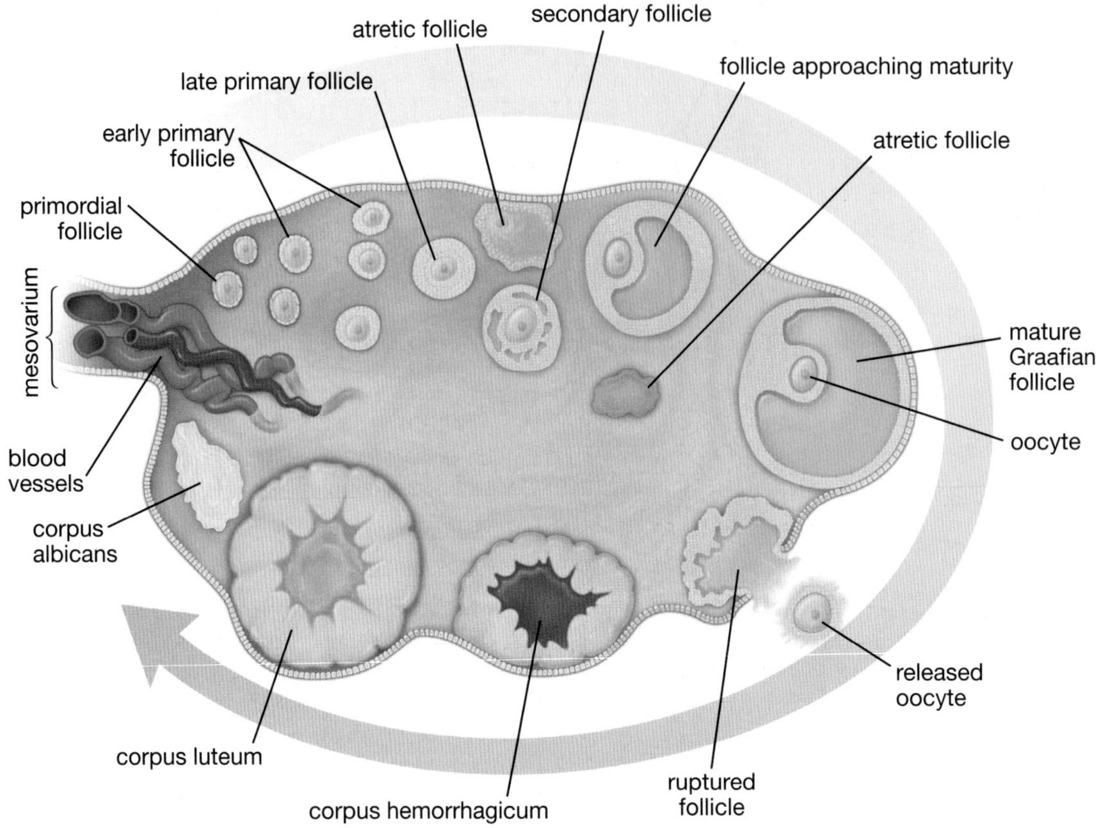

FIGURE 23.2. Schematic drawing of a section through the ovary. This drawing shows stages of follicular development from the early primary follicle to the mature (Graafian) follicle. The maturation of the follicles occurs in the direction of the *arrow*. Changes in the follicle after ovulation lead to the development of the corpus luteum and eventually the corpus albicans. Note the highly coiled blood vessels in the hilum and medulla of the ovary.

"Germinal epithelium" instead of mesothelium covers the ovary.

The **surface of the ovary** is covered by a single layer of cuboidal and, in some parts, almost squamous cells. This cellular layer, known as the **germinal epithelium**, is continuous with the mesothelium that covers the mesovarium. The term *germinal epithelium* is a carryover from the past when it was incorrectly thought to be the site of germ cell formation during embryonic development. It is now known that the **primordial germ cells** (both male and female) are of extragonadal origin and that they migrate from the embryonic yolk sac into the cortex of the embryonic gonad, where they differentiate and induce differentiation of the ovary. A dense connective tissue layer, the **tunica albuginea**, lies between the germinal epithelium and the underlying cortex (Plate 23.1, page 956). Tumors that arise from the epithelial surface of the ovary account for more than 70% of **ovarian cancers**. The origin of surface epithelial tumors may be related to repeated disruption and repair of the germinal epithelium that occurs during ovulation.

Ovarian follicles provide the microenvironment for the developing oocyte.

Ovarian follicles of various sizes, each containing a single oocyte, are distributed in the stroma of the cortex. The size of a follicle indicates the developmental state of the oocyte. Early stages of oogenesis occur during fetal life when mitotic divisions massively increase the number of oogonia (see the section on oogenesis). The oocytes present at birth remain arrested in development in the diplotene stage of prophase of the first meiotic division (see page 917). During puberty, small groups of follicles undergo **cyclic growth and maturation**. Ovulation may occur irregularly throughout adolescence. Usually by the third year after menarche, a regular, cyclic pattern of follicular maturation and ovulation is established.

Normally, only one oocyte reaches full maturity and is released from the ovary during each menstrual cycle. Obviously, the maturation and release of more than one egg at ovulation may lead to multiple zygotes. During the reproductive life span, only about **400 mature ova** are produced. Most of the estimated 600,000–800,000 primary oocytes present at birth do not complete maturation and are gradually lost through atresia, spontaneous death, and subsequent resorption of immature oocytes. This process begins as early as the fifth month of fetal life and is mediated by apoptosis of cells surrounding the oocyte. Atresia reduces the number of primary oocytes in a logarithmic manner throughout life from as many as 5 million in the fetus to less than 20% of that number at birth. The oocytes that remain at menopause degenerate within a few years.

Follicle Development

Histologically, three basic types of **ovarian follicles** can be identified on the basis of developmental state:

- **Primordial follicles**
- **Growing follicles**, which are further subcategorized as primary and secondary (or antral) follicles
- **Mature follicle** or **Graafian follicles**

Some histologists and clinicians identify additional stages in the continuum of follicular development. In the ovary, follicles are found at all stages of development, but primordial follicles predominate. The fate of each follicle is controlled by endocrine as well as paracrine factors.

The primordial follicle is the earliest stage of follicular development.

Primordial follicles first appear in the ovaries during the third month of fetal development. Early growth of the primordial follicles is independent of gonadotropin stimulation. The primordial follicles do not express follicle-stimulating hormone (FSH) receptors. In the mature ovary, primordial follicles are found in the stroma of the cortex just beneath the tunica albuginea. A single layer of **squamous follicle cells** surrounds the oocyte (Fig. 23.3 and Plate 23.1, page 956). The outer surface of the follicle cells is bounded by a basal lamina. At this stage, the oocyte and the surrounding follicle cells are closely apposed to one another. The oocyte in the follicle measures about 30 μm in diameter and has a large, eccentric nucleus that contains finely dispersed chromatin and one or more large nucleoli. The cytoplasm of the oocyte, referred to as *ooplasm*, contains a **Balbiani body** (Fig. 23.3a). At the ultrastructural level, the Balbiani body is revealed as a localized accumulation of Golgi membranes and vesicles, endoplasmic reticulum, centrioles, numerous mitochondria, and lysosomes. In addition, human oocytes contain **annulate lamellae**, and numerous small vesicles are scattered throughout the cytoplasm along with small, spherical mitochondria. Annulate lamellae resemble a stack of nuclear envelope profiles. Each layer of the stack includes pore structures that are morphologically identical to nuclear pores.

The primary follicle is the first stage in the development of the growing follicle.

As a **primordial follicle** develops into a **growing follicle**, changes occur in the oocyte, follicle cells, and adjacent stroma. Initially, the oocyte enlarges, and the surrounding flattened follicle cells proliferate and become cuboidal. At this stage—that is, when the follicle cells become cuboidal—the follicle is identified as a **primary follicle**. As the oocyte grows, it secretes specific proteins that are assembled into an extracellular coat called the **zona pellucida**.

The zona pellucida is composed of glycoproteins that bind to the capacitated spermatozoa and induce the acrosome reaction.

The **zona pellucida (ZP)** appears between the oocyte and the adjacent follicle cells (Fig. 23.4). In humans, it is composed of four classes of sulfated acidic **zona pellucida (ZP) glycoproteins** termed **ZP-1** (638 amino acids), **ZP-2** (745 aa), **ZP-3** (424 aa), and **ZP-4** (540 aa). Human glycoproteins of zona pellucida are heavily glycosylated. ZP-3 and ZP-4 function as the primary spermatozoa-binding receptors. Their binding is detected in the acrosomal cap of the spermatozoon. ZP-1 and ZP-2 act as secondary spermatozoa-binding proteins that interact mainly with the equatorial segment of the spermatozoon head. In addition, ZP-1, ZP-3, and ZP-4 are responsible for the induction of the **acrosome reaction** in capacitated spermatozoa (see page 920). Subsequent to the fusion of the spermatozoon membrane with the plasma membrane of the oocyte (oolemma), zona pellucida glycoproteins are cleaved by metalloendoproteases, which are released from cortical granules, thus making zona pellucida proteins nonrecognizable for binding with other spermatozoa.

In the light microscope, the zona pellucida is clearly visible as a homogeneous and refractile layer that stains deeply with acidophilic stains and with the periodic acid–Schiff (PAS) reagents (Plate 23.1, page 956). It is first apparent when the oocyte, surrounded by a single layer of cuboidal or columnar follicle cells, has grown to a diameter of 50–80 μm.

Follicle cells undergo stratification to form the granulosa layer of the primary follicle.

Through rapid mitotic proliferation, the single layer of follicle cells gives rise to a stratified epithelium, the **membrana granulosa (stratum granulosum)**, surrounding the oocyte. The follicle cells are now identified as **granulosa cells**. The basal lamina retains its position between the

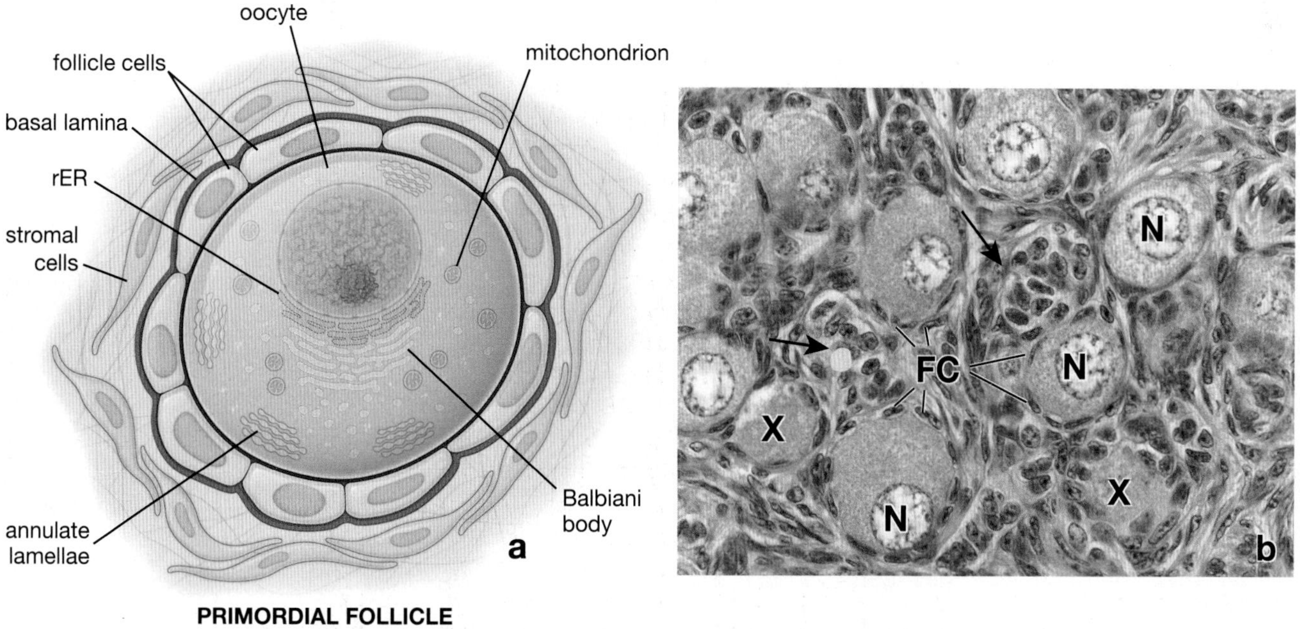

PRIMORDIAL FOLLICLE

FIGURE 23.3. Primordial follicle. a. Schematic drawing of a primordial follicle shows the oocyte arrested in prophase of the first meiotic division. The oocyte is closely surrounded by a single layer of squamous follicle cells. The outer surface of these cells is separated from the connective tissue by a basal lamina. The ooplasm contains characteristic organelles, as seen with the electron microscope, including a Balbiani body, annulate lamellae, and small spherical mitochondria. *rER*, rough-surfaced endoplasmic reticulum. **b.** This photomicrograph of primordial follicles shows the oocytes surrounded by a single layer of flattened follicle cells (*FC*). Usually, the nucleus (*N*) of the oocyte is in an eccentric position. Two oocytes in which the nucleus is not included in the plane of section are indicated (*X*). Similarly, there are two follicles (*arrows*) in which the follicle cells are revealed en face or tangential view and the enclosed oocytes are not included in the section. ×640.

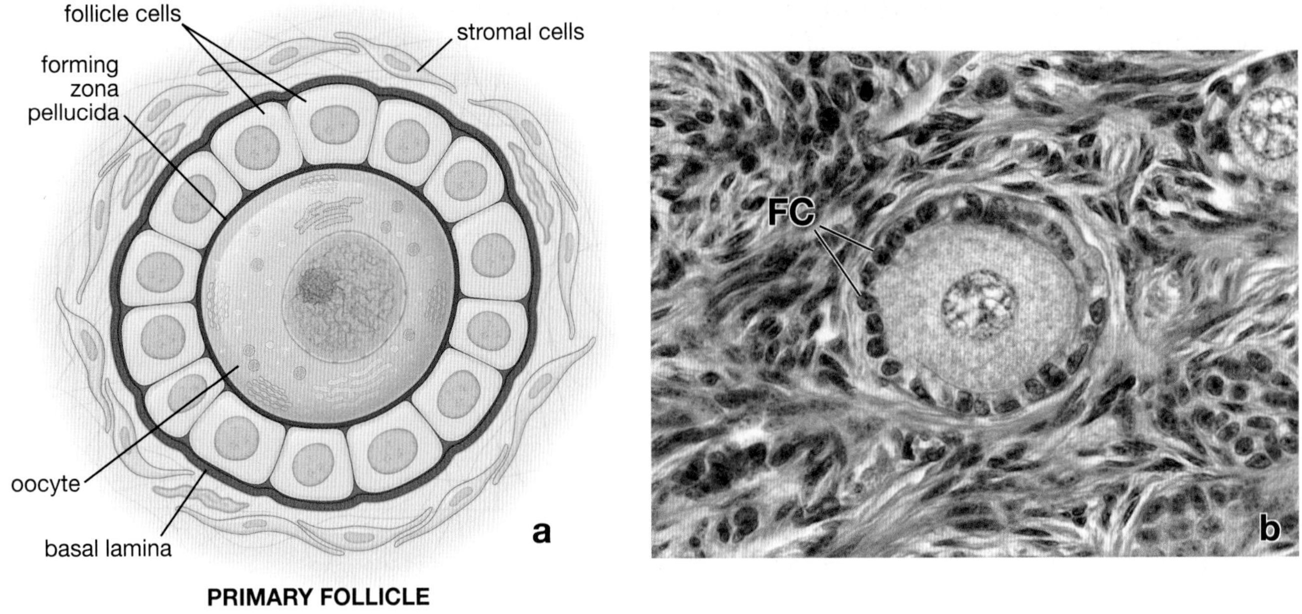

FIGURE 23.4. Early primary follicle. a. Schematic drawing of a primary follicle in an early stage of development. Note the formation of the zona pellucida between the oocyte and the adjacent follicle cells. A single layer of cuboidal follicle cells surrounds the growing oocyte. **b.** Photomicrograph of a primary follicle. Note the distinct layer of follicle cells (*FC*) surrounding the oocyte. ×640.

outermost layer of the follicle cells, which become columnar, and the connective tissue stroma.

During follicular growth, extensive gap junctions develop between granulosa cells. Unlike Sertoli cells in the testis, however, the basal layer of the granulosa cells does not possess elaborate tight junctions (zonulae occludentes), indicating the absence of a blood–follicle barrier. Movement of nutrients and small informational macromolecules from the blood into the follicular fluid is essential for the normal development of the ovum and follicle.

Connective tissue cells form the theca layers of the primary follicle.

As the granulosa cells proliferate, **stromal cells** immediately surrounding the follicle form a sheath of connective tissue cells, known as the **theca folliculi**, just external to the basal lamina (Fig. 23.5). The theca folliculi further differentiates into two layers:

- The **theca interna** is the inner, highly vascularized layer of cuboidal secretory cells (Plate 23.2, page 958). The fully differentiated cells of the theca interna possess ultrastructural

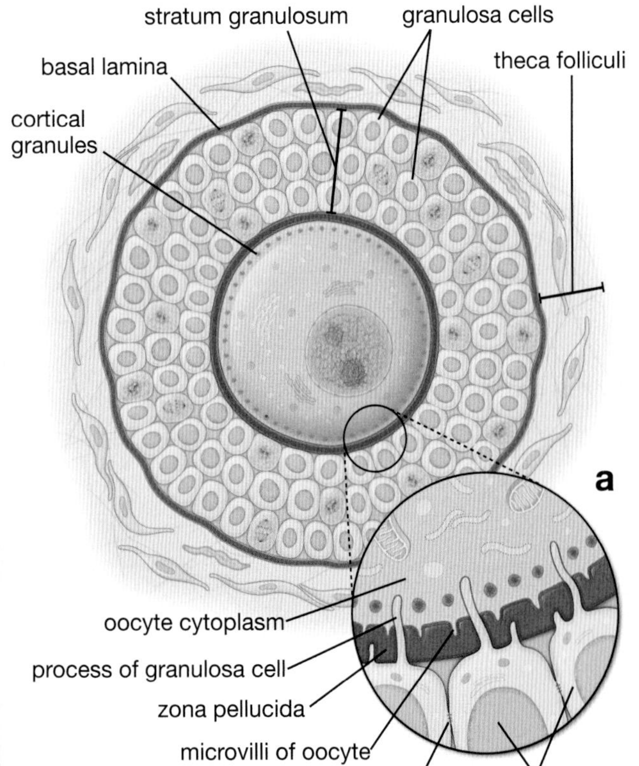

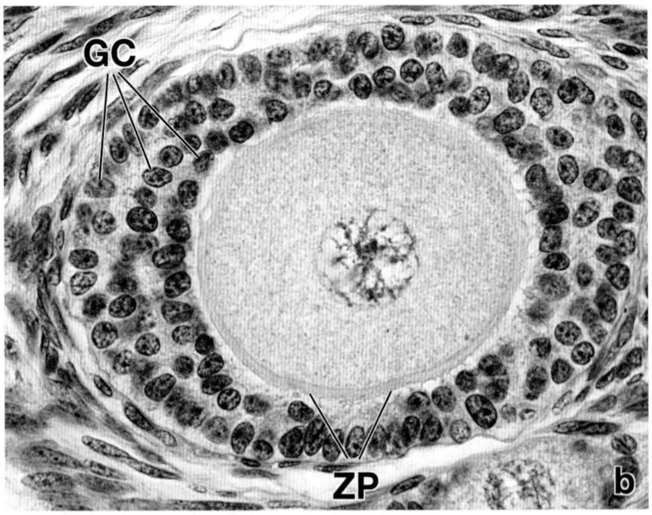

FIGURE 23.5. Late primary follicle. a. Schematic drawing of a late primary follicle shows a multilayered mass of granulosa cells (differentiated from follicle cells) surrounding the oocyte. Note that the innermost layer of granulosa cells is adjacent to the zona pellucida, and the outermost layer of these cells rests on the basal lamina, which is adjacent to the stromal cells now called the *theca folliculi*. The Balbiani body at this stage reorganizes into multiple Golgi units, and cortical granules appear in the cytoplasm. The *circle-shaped enlargement* depicts the ultrastructure of an oocyte and adjacent follicle cells. Numerous microvilli from the oocyte and slender processes from the granulosa cells extend into the zona pellucida that surrounds the oocyte. Processes of the granulosa cells contact the plasma membrane of the oocyte. **b.** Photomicrograph of a late primary follicle (monkey). Multiple layers of granulosa cells (*GC*) can be seen surrounding the primary oocyte. The zona pellucida (*ZP*) is present between the oocyte and follicle cells. ×640.

features characteristic of steroid-producing cells. Cells of the theca interna possess a large number of **luteinizing hormone (LH) receptors**. In response to LH stimulation, they synthesize and secrete the androgens that are the precursors of estrogens. In addition to secretory cells, the theca interna contains fibroblasts, collagen bundles, and a rich network of small vessels typical of endocrine organs.

- The **theca externa** is the outer layer of connective tissue cells. It contains mainly smooth muscle cells and bundles of collagen fibers.

Boundaries between the thecal layers and between the theca externa and surrounding stroma are not distinct. However, the **basal lamina** between the granulosa layer and the theca interna establishes a distinct boundary between these layers. It separates the rich capillary bed of the theca interna from the granulosa layer, which is avascular during the period of follicular growth. The basal lamina boundary between granulosa layer and the theca interna restricts the entry of leukocytes and high-molecular-weight substances (such as low-density lipoproteins) into the follicle.

Maturation of the oocyte occurs in the primary follicle.

The distribution of organelles changes as the oocyte matures. Multiple, dispersed Golgi elements derived from the single Balbiani body of the primordial oocyte become scattered in the cytoplasm. The number of free ribosomes, mitochondria, small vesicles, and multivesicular bodies and the amount of rough-surfaced endoplasmic reticulum (rER) increase. Occasional lipid droplets and masses of lipochrome pigment may also be seen. The oocytes of many species, including mammals, exhibit specialized secretory vesicles known as **cortical granules** (see Fig. 23.5a). They are located just beneath the **oolemma**. The granules contain proteases that are released by exocytosis when the ovum is activated by the sperm (discussed in the section on fertilization).

Numerous irregular microvilli project from the oocyte into the **perivitelline space** between the oocyte and the surrounding granulosa cells as the zona pellucida is deposited (see Fig. 23.5). At the same time, slender processes from the granulosa cells develop and project toward the oocyte, intermingling with oocyte microvilli and, occasionally, invaginating into the oocyte plasma membrane. They form gap junctions with the plasma membrane of the oocyte. **Cyclic guanosine monophosphate (cGMP)** that is produced by granulosa cells enters the oocyte via gap junctions and **maintains maturational arrest** of oocytes in the first meiotic division by inhibiting hydrolysis of **cyclic adenosine monophosphate (cAMP)** by phosphodiesterase (PDE3A). This inhibition maintains a high concentration of cAMP in the oocyte and thus blocks meiotic progression.

The secondary follicle is characterized by a fluid-containing antrum.

The primary follicle initially moves deeper into the cortical stroma as it increases in size, mostly through proliferation of the granulosa cells. Several factors are required for oocyte and follicular growth:

- **Follicle-stimulating hormone (FSH)**
- **Growth factors** (e.g., epidermal growth factor [EGF], insulin-like growth factor I [IGF-I])
- **Calcium ions (Ca^{2+})**

When the stratum granulosum reaches a thickness of 6–12 cell layers, **fluid-filled cavities** appear among the granulosa cells (Fig. 23.6). As the hyaluronan-rich fluid called

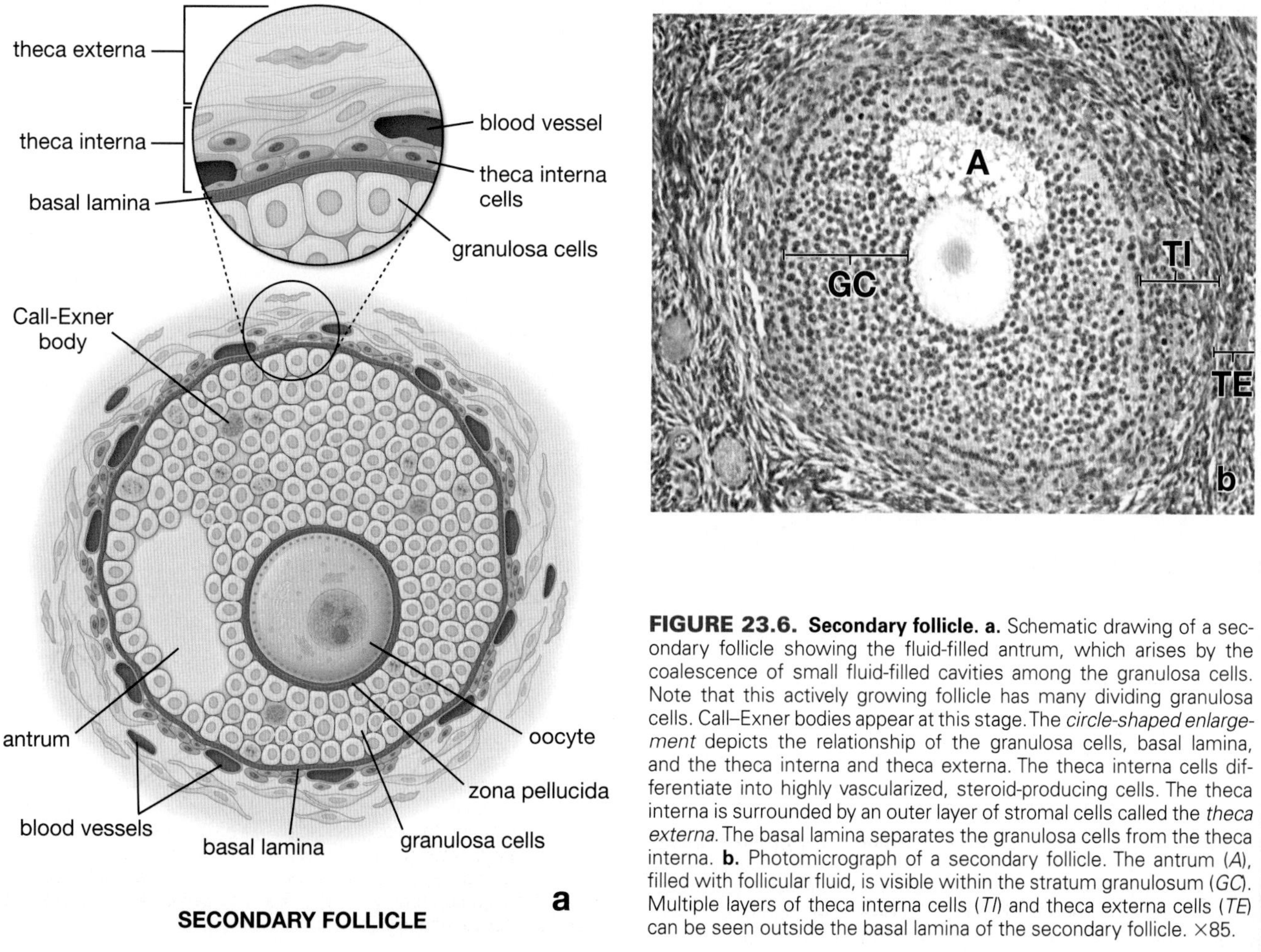

FIGURE 23.6. Secondary follicle. a. Schematic drawing of a secondary follicle showing the fluid-filled antrum, which arises by the coalescence of small fluid-filled cavities among the granulosa cells. Note that this actively growing follicle has many dividing granulosa cells. Call–Exner bodies appear at this stage. The *circle-shaped enlargement* depicts the relationship of the granulosa cells, basal lamina, and the theca interna and theca externa. The theca interna cells differentiate into highly vascularized, steroid-producing cells. The theca interna is surrounded by an outer layer of stromal cells called the *theca externa*. The basal lamina separates the granulosa cells from the theca interna. **b.** Photomicrograph of a secondary follicle. The antrum (*A*), filled with follicular fluid, is visible within the stratum granulosum (*GC*). Multiple layers of theca interna cells (*TI*) and theca externa cells (*TE*) can be seen outside the basal lamina of the secondary follicle. ×85.

liquor folliculi continues to accumulate among the granulosa cells, the cavities begin to coalesce, eventually forming a single, crescent-shaped cavity called the **antrum**. The follicle is now identified as a **secondary follicle** or **antral follicle** (Plate 23.2, page 958). The eccentrically positioned oocyte, which has attained a diameter of about 125 μm, undergoes no further growth. At the secondary follicle stage, most follicles undergo atresia, whereas only a few follicles, under the cyclic gonadotropin stimulation, reach the stage of readiness for ovulation.

Cyclic nucleotides play a key role in maintaining meiotic arrest of the oocyte during follicle growth and maturation.

The cyclic nucleotides **cGMP** and **cAMP**, produced in the granulosa and oocyte, are the principal molecules responsible for **maintaining oocyte meiotic arrest**. In addition, the inhibition of growth and maturation of the oocyte is also controlled by the natriuretic peptide family. Its representative, a small molecular weight peptide called **C-type natriuretic peptide (CNP)**, is secreted by the granulosa cells into the antral fluid and functions as **oocyte maturation inhibitor**. A direct correlation is observed between the size of the secondary follicle and CNP concentration. The concentration is highest in small follicles and lowest in mature follicles. The follicle, which was 0.2 mm in diameter as an early secondary follicle when the fluid first appeared, continues to grow and reaches 10 mm or more in diameter.

Cells of the cumulus oophorus form a corona radiata around the secretory follicle oocyte.

As the **secondary follicle** increases in size, the antrum, lined by several layers of granulosa cells, also enlarges (Fig. 23.7). The stratum granulosum has a relatively uniform thickness, except for the region associated with the oocyte. Here, the granulosa cells form a thickened mound, the **cumulus oophorus**, which projects into the antrum. The cells of the cumulus oophorus that immediately surround the oocyte and remain with it at ovulation are referred to as the **corona radiata**. The corona radiata is composed of cumulus cells that send penetrating microvilli throughout the zona pellucida to communicate via gap junctions with microvilli of the oocyte. During follicular maturation, the number of surface microvilli of granulosa cells increases and is correlated with an increased number of LH receptors on the free antral surface. Extracellular, densely staining, PAS-positive material called **Call–Exner bodies** (see Fig. 23.6a) may be seen between the granulosa cells. These bodies are secreted by granulosa cells and contain hyaluronan and proteoglycans.

The mature or Graafian follicle contains the mature secondary oocyte.

The **mature follicle**, also known as a **Graafian follicle**, has a diameter of 10 mm or more. Because of its large size, it extends through the full thickness of the ovarian cortex and causes a bulge on the surface of the ovary. As the follicle nears its maximum size, the mitotic activity of the granulosa cells decreases. The stratum granulosum appears to become thinner as the antrum increases in size. As the spaces between the granulosa cells continue to enlarge, the oocyte and cumulus cells are gradually loosened from the rest of the granulosa cells in preparation for ovulation. The cumulus cells immediately surrounding the oocyte now form a single layer of cells of the corona radiata. These cells and loosely attached cumulus cells remain with the oocyte at ovulation.

During this period of follicle maturation, the thecal layers become more prominent. Lipid droplets appear in the cytoplasm of the theca interna cells, and the cells demonstrate ultrastructural features associated with steroid-producing cells.

The synthesis of estrogens in the ovary requires a collaborative relationship between theca interna and granulosa cells.

Cooperative interaction of both **theca interna cells** and **granulosa cells** is required for estrogen (i.e., estrone, estradiol) production in the developing follicles. Neither granulosa nor

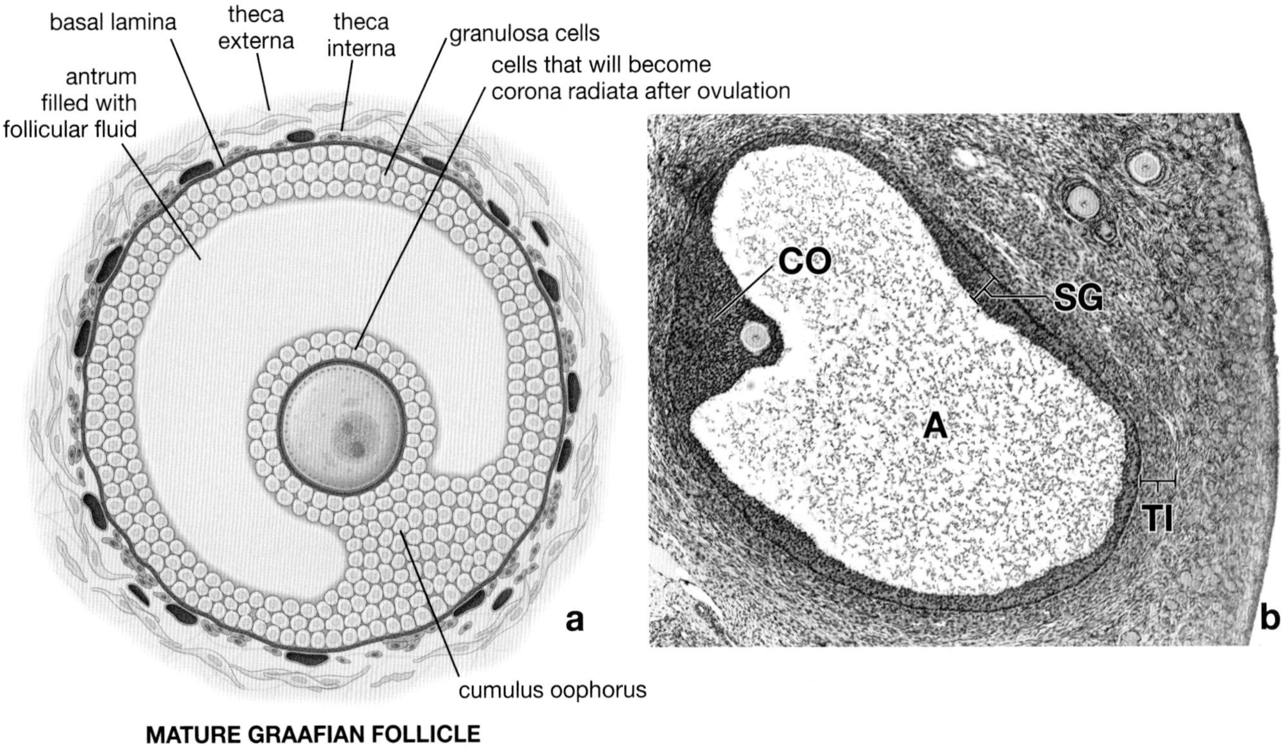

FIGURE 23.7. Secondary follicle in a late stage of development. a. Schematic drawing of a mature (Graafian) follicle with a large antrum containing an oocyte embedded within the cumulus oophorus. The cells of the cumulus oophorus immediately surrounding the oocyte remain with it after ovulation and are referred to as the *corona radiata*. **b.** Photomicrograph of a mature secondary follicle. Note the large fluid-filled antrum (*A*) and the cumulus oophorus (*CO*) containing the oocyte. The remaining cells that surround the lumen of the antrum make up the membrana granulosa (stratum granulosum, *SG*). The surface of the ovary is visible on the *right*. Note the presence of two primary follicles (*upper right*). *TI*, theca interna. ×45.

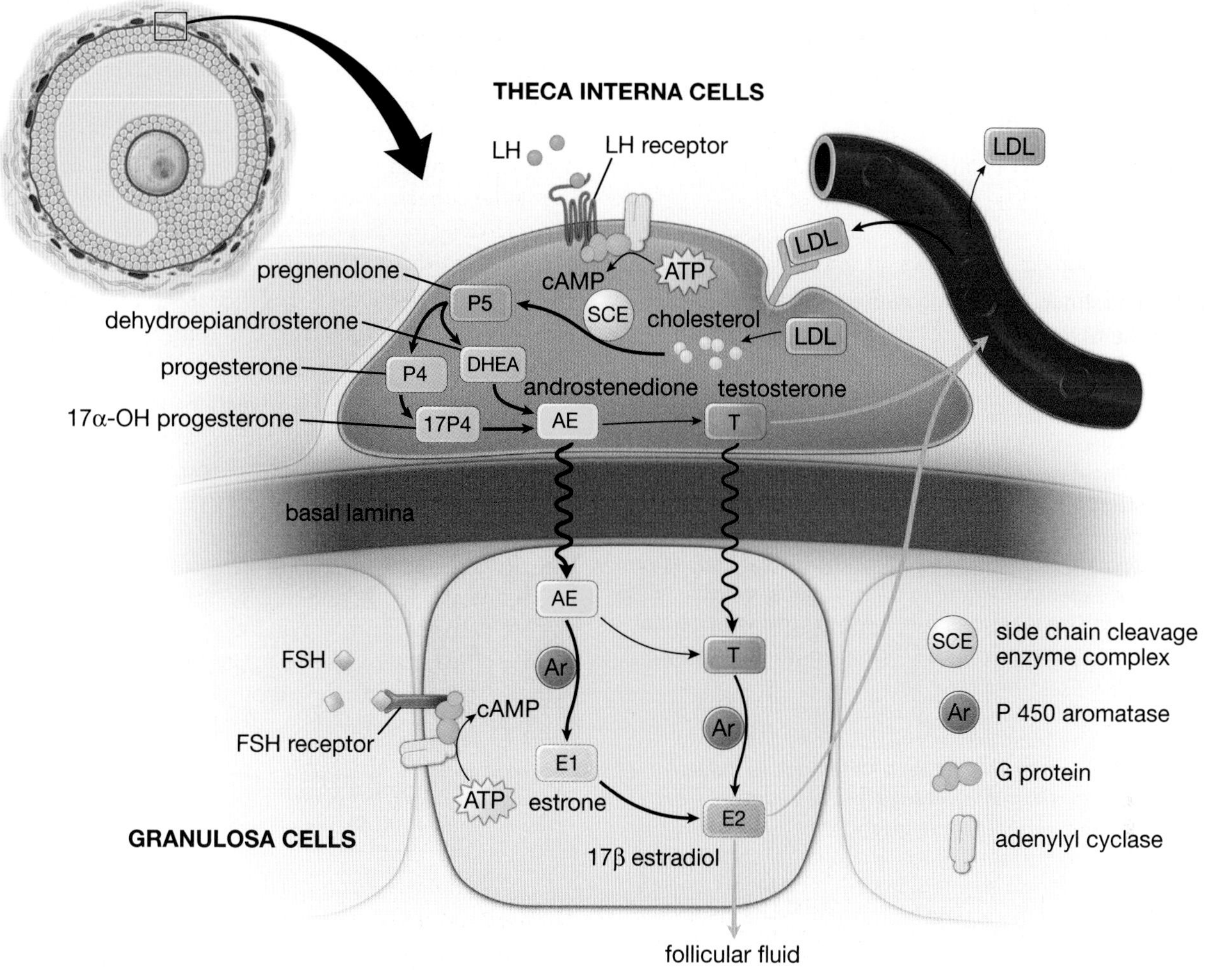

FIGURE 23.8. Synthesis of estrogens in the ovarian follicle. Synthesis of estrogens in the ovary requires collaboration between theca interna and granulosa cells. Theca interna cells express both luteinizing hormone (*LH*) and low-density lipoprotein (*LDL*) receptors on their surface. *LH* stimulation of theca interna cells facilitates conversion of cholesterol (liberated from lactate dehydrogenase [*LDH*]) to pregnenolone (*P5*) and then via further intermediates into androgens (androstenedione and testosterone). These androgens diffuse into neighboring granulosa cells where they are converted to estrogens by the enzyme P450 aromatase. Granulosa cells express follicle-stimulating hormone (*FSH*) receptors and their activation by *FSH* is a primary stimulator of P450 aromatase activity. *FSH* also promotes the conversion of estrone to 17β-estradiol. *ATP*, adenosine triphosphate; *cAMP*, cyclic adenosine monophosphate.

theca cells express the full complement of enzymes needed for synthesis of estradiol, the primary female sex hormone. Theca interna cells reside in a highly vascularized layer of the follicle and express both LH and low-density lipoprotein (LDL) receptors on their surface. LDL receptors in these cells expedite the uptake of LDL molecules from which cholesterol is liberated and becomes the main substrate in steroid hormone synthesis (Fig. 23.8).

When stimulated by LH, theca interna cells facilitate conversion of **cholesterol** to pregnenolone and then via further intermediates to **androgens** (i.e., dehydroepiandrosterone [DHEA], androstenediol, androstenedione, testosterone) (see Fig. 23.8). Owing to the lack of the enzyme **P450 aromatase**, the theca interna cells are not able to produce estrogens. In contrast, neighboring granulosa cells are equipped with P450 aromatase. Thus, androgens secreted by theca interna cells enter granulosa cells where they are converted in the cells' smooth-surfaced endoplasmic reticulum (sER) by P450 aromatase to **estrogens** in response to FSH stimulation (see Fig. 23.8).

FSH is the primary stimulator of P450 aromatase gene expression in granulosa cells. However, not all granulosa cells have the same capacity to produce estrogens. The highest levels of aromatase activity are found in the peripheral cells near the theca interna, whereas the lowest levels are in the cells bordering the antrum. Almost all (99%) of the aromatization capacity (conversion of androgens to estrogens) in the developing follicles occur in granulosa cells and are thus the only source of estradiol in the follicular phase of the ovarian cycle. Estrogens secreted by granulosa cells stimulate their own proliferation and thereby increase the size of the follicle.

Aromatase inhibitors (AIs) are a class of drug used in the treatment of estrogen-sensitive breast cancer. This type of breast cancer grows in response to estrogen. AIs bind to different sites on the aromatase enzyme and prevent the conversion of androgens to estrogens, thus lowering the level of estrogen in the body and decreasing the potential for growth of cancer cells.

Increased estrogen levels from both follicular and systemic sources are correlated with increased sensitization of gonadotropes to gonadotropin-releasing hormone. A surge in the release of LH (and a smaller surge of FSH) is induced in the adenohypophysis approximately 24 hours before ovulation. In response to the LH surge, LH receptors are downregulated (desensitized), and granulosa cells no longer produce estrogens. Triggered by this surge, the first meiotic division of the primary oocyte resumes. This event occurs between 12 and 24 hours after the LH surge, resulting in the formation of the secondary oocyte and the first polar body. Both the granulosa and thecal cells then undergo luteinization and produce progesterone (see pages 918-919, section on the corpus luteum).

FOLDER 23.1

CLINICAL CORRELATION: POLYCYSTIC OVARY DISEASE

Polycystic ovary disease is a syndrome characterized by a variety of clinical signs and symptoms, including bilaterally enlarged ovaries with numerous follicular cysts, irregular menstrual periods, anovulation that may lead to infertility, obesity, and excess hair growth on the face, acne, and oily skin. Morphologically, the ovaries resemble a small, white balloon filled with tightly packed marbles. Affected ovaries, often called *oyster ovaries*, have a smooth, pearl-white surface but do not show surface scarring because no ovulations have occurred. Their appearance is attributable to the large number of fluid-filled follicular cysts and atrophic secondary follicles that lie beneath an unusually thick tunica albuginea.

Although the pathogenesis of polycystic ovary syndrome (PCOS) is not clear, it may be related to a defect in the regulation of androgen biosynthesis that causes production of excessive amounts of androgens, which inhibits ovulation and causes abnormal hair growth and acne that are often associated with PCOS. Insulin resistance also appears to play a role in PCOS.

Treatments of PCOS are individualized based on a patient's desire for childbearing. For those wishing to have children, drugs that sensitize the body to insulin and promote weight loss may reduce insulin resistance and result in the resumption of ovulation. If these measures fail, ovulation-stimulating drugs and laparoscopic surgical procedures are implemented. In vitro fertilization may also be an option. For those who do not wish to have children, combined contraception (containing both estrogen and progesterone) may regulate the menstrual cycle and reduce acne and abnormal hair growth (Fig. F23.1.1).

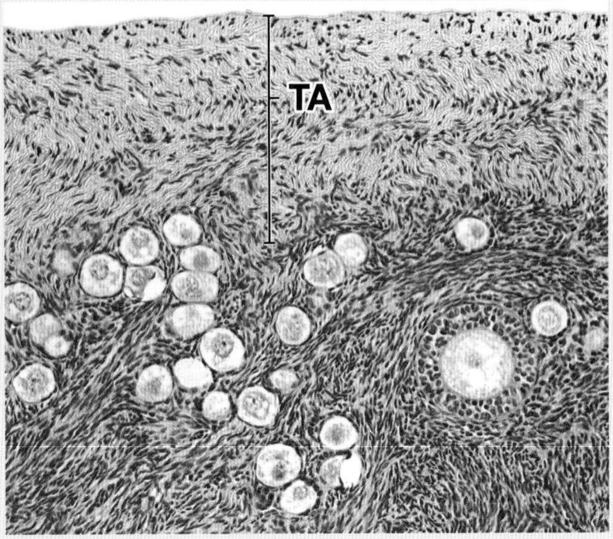

FIGURE F23.1.1. Polycystic ovary disease. This photomicrograph shows a section through the cortex of the ovary from an individual with polycystic ovary disease. Note the unusually thick tunica albuginea (*TA*) that overlies numerous follicles. The thickness of the tunica albuginea prevents ovulation of the mature (Graafian) follicles. Note that one of the follicles has developed to the primary follicle stage. ×45.

Ovulation

Ovulation is a hormone-mediated process resulting in the release of the secondary oocyte.

Ovulation is the process by which a **secondary oocyte** is released from the Graafian follicle. The follicle destined to ovulate in any menstrual cycle is recruited from a cohort of several primary follicles in the first few days of the cycle. During ovulation, the oocyte traverses the entire follicular wall, including the germinal epithelium.

A combination of hormonal changes and enzymatic effects is responsible for the actual release of the **secondary oocyte**, which occurs 14 days before the start of the next menstrual cycle (i.e., on the 14th day of a 28-day cycle). These factors include

- increase in the volume and pressure of the follicular fluid;
- enzymatic proteolysis of the follicular wall by activated plasminogen;
- hormonally directed deposition of glycosaminoglycans between the oocyte–cumulus complex and the stratum granulosum; and
- contraction of the smooth muscle fibers in the theca externa layer, triggered by prostaglandins.

Just before ovulation, blood flow stops in a small area of the ovarian surface overlying the bulging follicle. This area of the germinal epithelium, known as the **macula pellucida** or **follicular stigma**, becomes elevated and then ruptures (Fig. 23.9a). The oocyte, surrounded by the corona radiata and cells of the cumulus oophorus, is released from the ruptured follicle. At the time of ovulation, the fimbriae of the uterine tube become closely apposed to the surface of the ovary, and the **cumulus mass** containing the oocyte is gently swept by the fimbriae into the abdominal ostium of the uterine tube. The cumulus mass firmly adheres to the fimbriae and is actively transported by the ciliated cells lining the uterine tube, preventing its passage into the peritoneal cavity. Nonsurgical ultrasound technology can be used to monitor ovarian follicle development. **Transvaginal ultrasound** examination

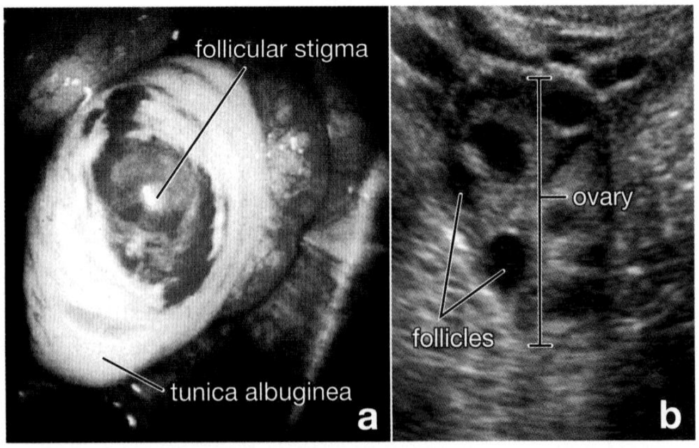

FIGURE 23.9. Endoscopic and ultrasound examination of the ovary. a. This photograph shows a view of the human ovary during endoscopic oocyte harvest surgery. The ovary is in the stage just before ovulation. Note the area of the bulging follicle with the follicular stigma clearly visible. The germinal epithelium covering the tunica albuginea is ruptured in the area of imminent ovulation. **b.** Development of nonsurgical techniques such as ultrasound imaging helps in monitoring of follicular growth and is useful as a method for determining the time for harvesting preovulatory oocytes. (Courtesy of Dr. Charles C. Coddington, III, Mayo Clinic.)

can provide detailed information about the number and size of developing follicles, which is useful during infertility assessment and treatment (Fig. 23.9b). After ovulation, the secondary oocyte remains viable for approximately 24 hours. If fertilization does not occur during this period, the secondary oocyte degenerates as it passes through the uterine tube.

Oocytes that fail to enter the uterine tube usually degenerate in the peritoneal cavity. Occasionally, however, an oocyte may be fertilized and implant in the peritoneal cavity on the surface of the ovary or intestine or inside the rectouterine (Douglas) pouch. A pregnancy that develops at any site other than the endometrium of the uterine cavity is called an **ectopic pregnancy**. An ectopic pregnancy is not viable and must be removed surgically or with the use of certain medications (e.g., methotrexate). Ectopic pregnancy that develops at any site other than the endometrium of the uterine cavity continues to be the most common cause of maternal mortality in the first half of pregnancy.

Normally, only one follicle completes maturation in each cycle and ruptures to release its secondary oocyte. Rarely, oocytes are released from other follicles that have reached full maturity during the same cycle, leading to the possibility of multiple zygotes. Drugs such as clomiphene citrate or gonadotropins that stimulate ovarian activity greatly increase the possibility of multiple births by causing simultaneous maturation of several follicles.

The primary oocyte is arrested for 12–50 years in the diplotene stage of prophase of the first meiotic division.

The **primary oocytes** within the primordial follicles begin the first meiotic division in the embryo, but the process is **arrested at the diplotene stage of meiotic prophase** (see the section on meiosis in Chapter 3, The Cell Nucleus, page 102). The first meiotic prophase is not completed until just before ovulation. Therefore, the primary oocytes remain arrested in the first meiotic prophase for 12–50 years. This long period of **meiotic arrest** exposes the primary oocyte to adverse environmental influences and may contribute to errors in meiotic division, such as nondisjunction. Such errors result in an abnormal number of chromosomes (aneuploidy), such as **trisomy of chromosome 21 (Down syndrome)**.

As the first meiotic division (reduction division) is completed in the mature follicle (Fig. 23.10), each daughter cell of the **primary oocyte** receives an equal share of chromatin, but one daughter cell receives most of the cytoplasm and becomes the **secondary oocyte**. It measures 150 μm in diameter. The other daughter cell receives a minimal amount of cytoplasm and becomes the **first polar body**.

The secondary oocyte is arrested at metaphase in the second meiotic division just before ovulation.

As soon as the first meiotic division is completed, the **secondary oocyte** begins the second meiotic division. As the secondary oocyte surrounded by the cells of the corona radiata leaves the follicle at ovulation, the second meiotic division (equatorial division) is in progress. This division is **arrested at metaphase** and completed only if the secondary oocyte is fertilized by a spermatozoon. If fertilization occurs, the secondary oocyte completes the second meiotic division and forms a mature **ovum** with the **female (maternal) pronucleus** containing a set of 23 chromosomes. The other cell produced at this division is a **second polar body**.

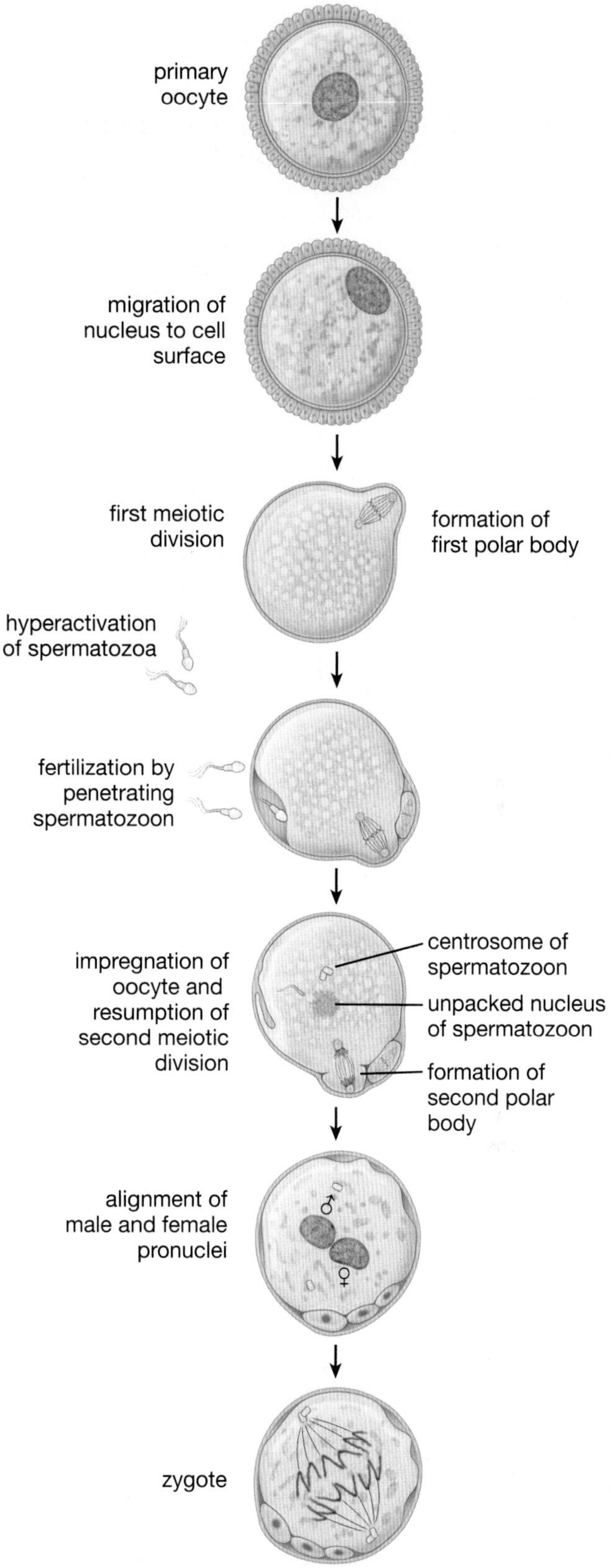

FIGURE 23.10. Diagram illustrating changes that occur during growth, maturation, and fertilization of the oocyte. The primary oocyte remains arrested in prophase I of meiosis. The first meiotic or reductional division is completed only after the oocyte progresses to ovulation. The second meiotic or equatorial division is not completed unless the secondary oocyte is impregnated by a spermatozoon. Note the formation of the first and second polar bodies. In some mammals, the first polar body divides (as shown in this drawing) so that there are four total meiotic products. However, in humans, the first polar body does not divide but persists for about 20 hours; therefore, the fertilized egg can be recognized by the presence of two polar bodies.

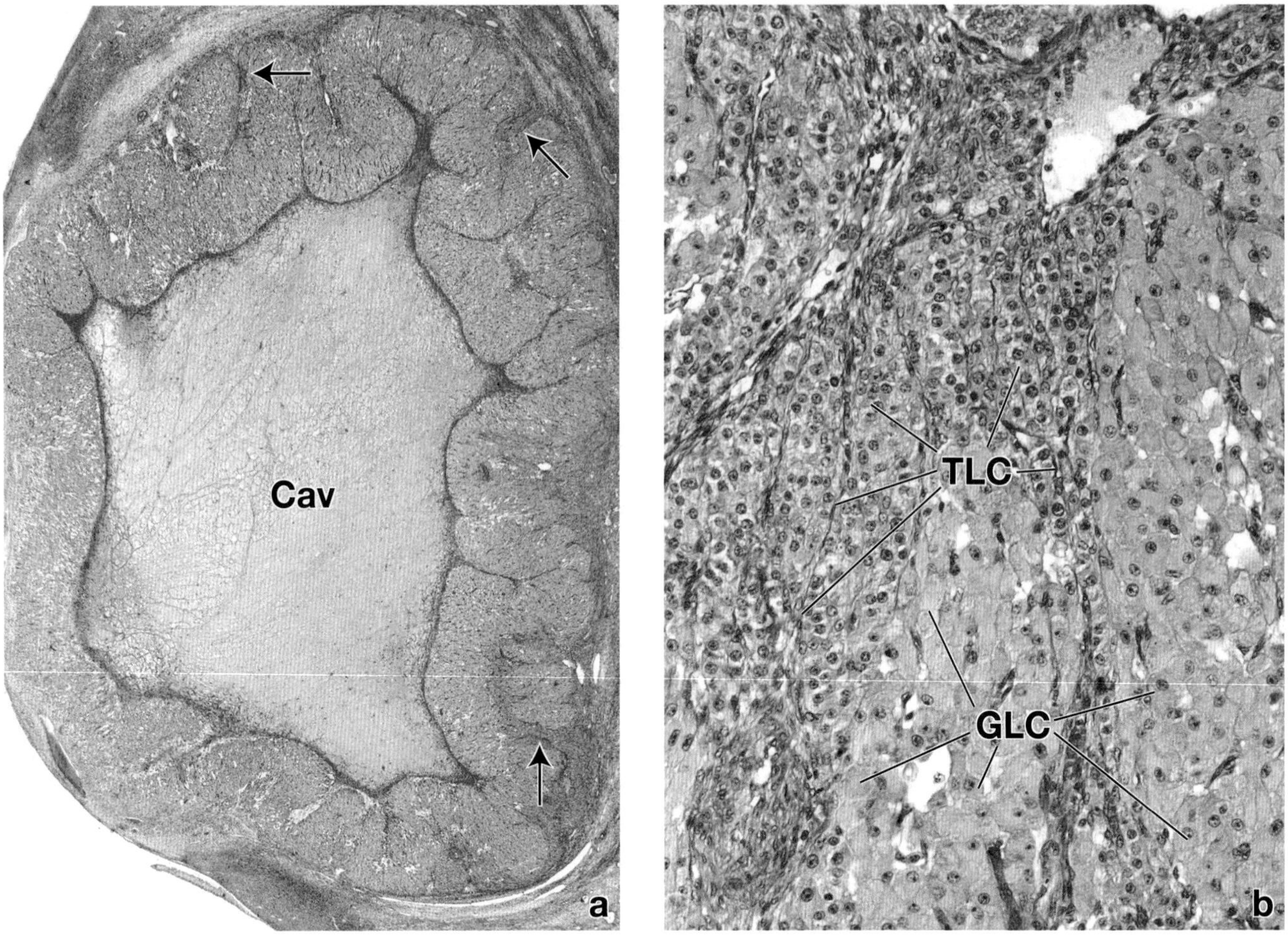

FIGURE 23.11. Photomicrograph of human corpus luteum. a. The corpus luteum is formed from the collapsed follicle wall that contains the granulosa and theca cells. The granulosa lutein cells form a thick, folded layer around the former follicular cavity (*Cav*). Within the folds are cells of the theca interna (*arrows*). ×12. **b.** This photomicrograph shows the wall of the corpus luteum at higher magnification. The main cell mass is composed of granulosa lutein cells (*GLC*). These cells have a large spherical nucleus and a large amount of cytoplasm. The theca lutein cells (*TLC*) also have a spherical nucleus, but the cells are considerably smaller than the granulosa lutein cells. ×240.

In humans, the first polar body persists for more than 20 hours after ovulation and does not divide; therefore, the fertilized egg can be recognized by the presence of two polar bodies (diploid first polar body and haploid second polar body). In some mammals, the first polar body can divide, so the final outcome of meiosis consists of one oocyte and three haploid polar bodies (see Fig. 23.10). The polar bodies, which are not capable of further development, undergo apoptosis.

Corpus Luteum

The collapsed follicle undergoes reorganization into the corpus luteum after ovulation.

At ovulation, the **follicular wall**, composed of the remaining granulosa and thecal cells, is thrown into deep folds as the follicle collapses and is transformed into the **corpus luteum** (yellow body) or **luteal gland** (Fig. 23.11a and Plate 23.3, page 960). At first, bleeding from the capillaries in the theca interna into the follicular lumen leads to the formation of the **corpus hemorrhagicum** with a central clot. Connective tissue from the stroma then invades the former follicular cavity. Cells of the granulosa and theca interna layers then differentiate into granulosa luteal and theca luteal cells in a process called **luteinization**. These luteal cells undergo dramatic morphologic changes, increasing in size and filling with lipid droplets (Fig. 23.11b). A lipid-soluble pigment, lipochrome, in the cytoplasm of the cells gives them a yellow appearance in fresh preparations (Fig. 23.12). At the

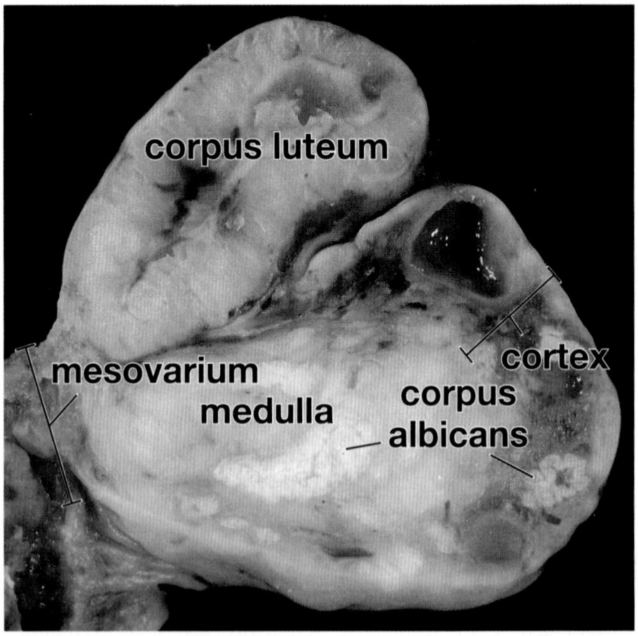

FIGURE 23.12. Human corpus luteum of menstruation. This photograph shows a section of a normal ovary that was surgically removed during an oophorectomy. The corpus luteum is fully developed in the cortex of the ovary, which indicates the midluteal phase of the ovarian cycle. The cortex of the ovary contains atretic follicles, a small ovarian cyst, and a few corpora albicantia that represent remnants of corpora lutea from previous ovarian cycles. Note that the medulla of the ovary contains a larger corpus albicans, which is most likely a remnant of the corpus luteum of pregnancy. ×2. (Courtesy of Dr. Edward Uthman.)

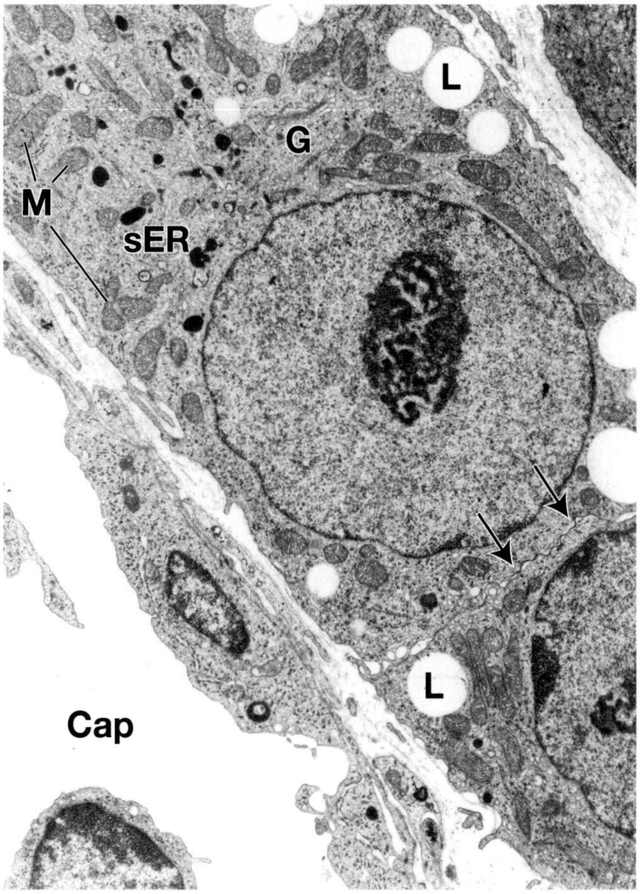

FIGURE 23.13. Electron micrograph of theca lutein cells from the corpus luteum of a monkey. At this early implantation stage (day 11 of gestation), membrane-bound dense bodies are clustered near the Golgi apparatus (*G*); most of the cytoplasm is packed with tubules of smooth-surfaced endoplasmic reticulum (*sER*), lipid droplets (*L*), and mitochondria (*M*). Note the capillary (*Cap*) and the closely apposed cell membranes of the theca lutein cells (*arrows*). ×10,000. (Courtesy of Dr. Carolynn B. Booher.)

ultrastructural level, the cells demonstrate features associated with steroid-secreting cells, namely, abundant sER and mitochondria with tubular cristae (Fig. 23.13).

Two types of luteal cells are identified:

- **Granulosa lutein cells** are large (about 30 μm in diameter), centrally located cells derived from granulosa cells. They constitute about 80% of the corpus luteum and synthesize **estrogens**, **progesterone**, and **inhibin**. The latter regulates the production and secretion of FSH from the anterior lobe of the pituitary gland.
- **Theca lutein cells** are smaller (about 15 μm), more deeply staining, and peripherally located cells derived from the cells of the theca interna layer (Plate 23.3, page 960). They represent the remaining 20% of cells in the corpus luteum and secrete **androgens** and **progesterone**.

As the **corpus luteum** begins to form, blood and lymphatic vessels from the theca interna rapidly grow into the granulosa layer. A rich vascular network is established within the corpus luteum. This highly vascularized structure located in the cortex of the ovary secretes progesterone and estrogens. These hormones stimulate the growth and secretory activity of the lining of the uterus, the endometrium, to prepare it for the implantation of the developing zygote in the event that fertilization occurs.

The corpus luteum of menstruation is formed in the absence of fertilization.

If fertilization and implantation do not occur, the corpus luteum remains active only for the next 10 days. In this case, it is called the **corpus luteum of menstruation**. In the absence of human chorionic gonadotropin (hCG) and other luteotropins, the rate of secretion of progestogens and estrogens declines, and the corpus luteum begins to degenerate about 10 days after ovulation.

The **corpus luteum degenerates** and undergoes a slow involution after pregnancy or menstruation. The cells become loaded with lipid, decrease in size, and undergo autolysis. A white scar, the **corpus albicans**, is formed as intercellular hyaline material accumulates among the degenerating cells of the former corpus luteum (Fig. 23.14). The corpus albicans sinks deeper into the ovarian cortex as it slowly disappears over a period of several months.

Capacitation and Fertilization

During capacitation, the mature spermatozoa acquire the ability to fertilize the oocyte.

Following their maturation in the epididymis, spermatozoa must be activated within the female reproductive tract for fertilization to occur. During this activation process, called **capacitation**, structural and functional changes take place in the spermatozoon that results in its increased affinity to bind to zona pellucida receptors. Processes leading to the acrosome reaction are

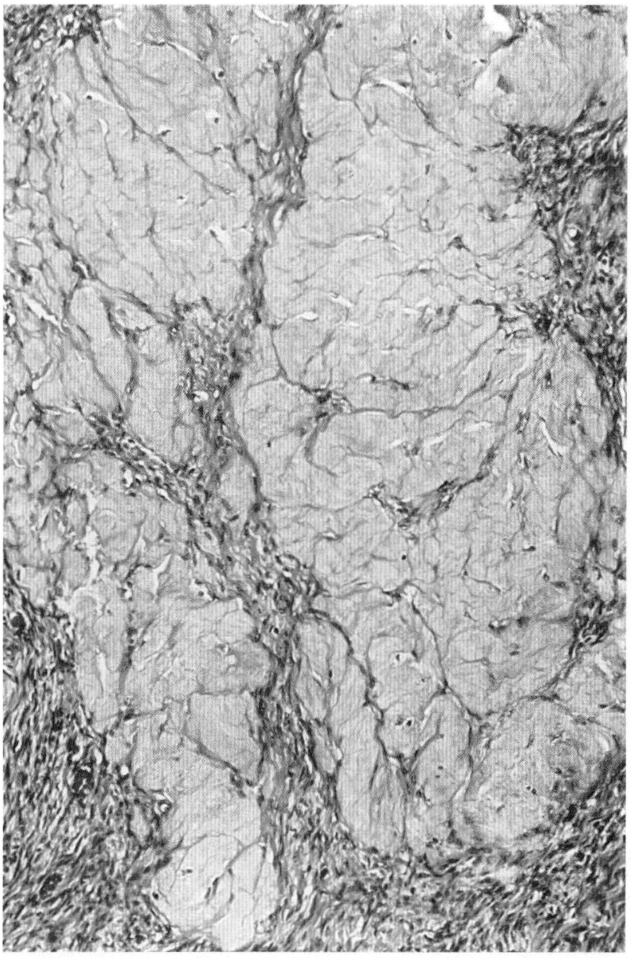

FIGURE 23.14. Photomicrograph of the corpus albicans of a human ovary. Large amounts of hyaline material can be seen among the degenerating cells of the former corpus luteum. The corpus albicans is surrounded by ovarian stroma. ×125.

associated with the sperm head, whereas those related to sperm motility occur in the tail. Successful capacitation is confirmed by **hyperactivation** of the spermatozoa, which manifests as a vigorous, whiplash-like beating pattern of their flagella.

Capacitation involves several biochemical changes and modifications to the spermatozoon and its plasma membrane, including:

- Increased activity of adenylyl cyclase leads to increasing levels of cAMP.
- The rate of tyrosine phosphorylation by the Src kinase family increases (measurement of tyrosine phosphorylation is used clinically as a biochemical marker of capacitation).
- Serine/threonine (Ser/Thr) phosphatase activity is inhibited.
- Increase in pH and plasma membrane hyperpolarization activates Ca^{2+} channels, resulting in increased intracellular Ca^{2+} levels essential for the acquisition of hyperactivated motility.
- Seminal fluid glycoconjugates are released from the surface of the head of the spermatozoon. These surface glycosides (also called *decapacitation factors*) added during sperm maturation in the epididymis inhibit binding to the zona pellucida receptors.
- The plasma membrane of the spermatozoon is extensively modified by removal of cholesterol, the predominant inhibitor of capacitation, and redistribution of phospholipids and carbohydrate moieties.

Fertilization normally occurs in the ampulla of the uterine tube.

Usually, only a few hundred of the millions of spermatozoa in an ejaculate reach the site of fertilization, typically the ampulla of the uterine tube. On arrival, spermatozoa encounter the secondary oocyte surrounded by the corona radiata. **Spermatozoa must penetrate the corona radiata** to gain access to the zona pellucida. Although several spermatozoa may penetrate the zona pellucida only one spermatozoon completes the fertilization process. Capacitation is complete when spermatozoa are able to **bind to the zona pellucida receptors**. Binding to the ZP-1, ZP-3, or ZP-4 receptors on the zona pellucida triggers the **acrosome reaction** in which enzymes (mainly hyaluronidases) released from the acrosome enable a single spermatozoon to penetrate the zona pellucida. Penetration is accomplished by limited **proteolysis of the zona pellucida** in front of the advancing hypermotile spermatozoon. During penetration, the spermatozoon must maintain its adherence to the oocyte coat via transient secondary binding supported by the ZP-1 and ZP-2 receptors.

After penetrating the zona pellucida the spermatozoon enters the **perivitelline space** between the zona pellucida and the oocyte plasma membrane (or oolemma). Here, the spermatozoon plasma membrane **binds to the oolemma** via fertilin (PH-30) and subsequently **fuses** with it. Fusion of both membranes occurs by lipid mixing that transforms the two gamete membrane bilayers into a single layer. After fusion, the nucleus of the sperm head is finally incorporated into the oocyte. It forms the **male (paternal) pronucleus** containing 23 paternal chromosomes. After the alignment and dissolution of nuclear membranes of the two pronuclei, the paternal and maternal chromosomes are united in the first mitotic spindle. The resulting **zygote**, with its diploid (2n) complement of 46 chromosomes, undergoes a mitotic division or first cleavage. This two-cell stage marks the beginning of embryonic development.

Before spermatozoa can fertilize the secondary oocyte, they must acquire more thrust to penetrate the corona radiata and zona pellucida.

When approaching a secondary oocyte, a **spermatozoon** becomes hyperactivated: It swims faster, and its tail movements become more forceful and erratic. Recent studies indicate that this **hyperactivation reaction** is caused by a sudden influx of Ca^{2+} into the tails of spermatozoa. The plasma membrane of the sperm tail contains large numbers of transmembrane Ca^{2+} channel proteins called **CatSpers** (cation channels of sperm). CatSper proteins are expressed exclusively in membranes of the tail. Influx of Ca^{2+} causes the tail to be more active and bend more forcefully, resulting in faster sperm movement through the viscous environment of the uterine tube. Together with limited proteolysis of the zona pellucida, hyperactivation is responsible for the physical penetration of the oocyte. **Sperm hyperactivity** is necessary for breaking physical barriers that protect the secondary oocyte from fertilization. Thus, **activation of CatSpers** is required for male fertility.

Impregnation of the oocyte allows structures lying inside the spermatozoon to enter the cytoplasm of the oocyte.

After penetrating the zona pellucida, the **spermatozoon enters the perivitelline space** between the zona pellucida and the oolemma. Here, after binding to the oolemma, the spermatozoon plasma membrane fuses with it. This process, called the **impregnation of the oocyte**, allows the nucleus of the sperm (containing highly concentrated DNA), the centrosome, the midpiece with the mitochondria, and the kinocilium to be incorporated into the cytoplasm of the oocyte. The tail plasma membrane remains as an appendage to the oolemma.

An impregnating spermatozoon generates a molecular signal for resumption and termination of the **second meiotic division**. Currently, diffusion of sperm-derived phospholipase C zeta 1 (PLCz1) into the oocyte cytoplasm is the most promising candidate for this signaling mechanism. This second meiotic division transforms the secondary oocyte into a mature oocyte and triggers the expulsion of the second polar body into the perivitelline space. The **female pronucleus** resides in the cytoplasm adjacent to the second polar body.

The male genetic material carried within the nucleus of incorporated sperm head is unpacked and used for building the **male pronucleus**, which contains 23 paternal chromosomes. Both female and male pronuclei migrate toward the center to unite maternal and paternal DNA, as well as for the development of mitotic spindle. Nuclear membranes of both female and male pronuclei dissolve (without fusion), and the chromosomes align themselves within the first mitotic spindle. The resulting **zygote** contains a diploid **(2n)** complement of 46 chromosomes and later undergoes the first mitotic division or cleavage. The male centrosome is essential for the alignment of the mitotic spindle that divides chromosomes into the first two cells of the embryo. Only centrosomes from the father are used in building the first and subsequent mitotic spindles. The incorporated kinocilium is finally dissolved, and all **sperm mitochondria are eliminated** from the cytoplasm of the oocyte. Note that all mitochondria in human cells normally derive from the mother's oocyte, but all centrosomes originate from the father's sperm cell.

Several spermatozoa may penetrate the zona pellucida, but only one spermatozoon completes the fertilization process.

Preventing polyspermy, or the fertilization of an oocyte by more than one spermatozoon, is essential for normal embryonic development. Polyspermy causes severe chromosomal defects and embryonic mortality. As the fertilizing spermatozoon penetrates the ooplasm, at least three types of **postfusion reactions** occur to prevent other spermatozoa from entering the secondary oocyte. These events include the following:

- **Fast block to polyspermy**. A large and long-lasting (up to 1 minute) depolarization of the oolemma creates a transient electrical block to polyspermy. It is most likely achieved by the fertilization-evoked activation of Ca^{2+}-activated Cl^- channel proteins.
- **Cortical reaction**. Changes in the polarity of the oolemma then trigger the release of Ca^{2+} from ooplasmic stores. The Ca^{2+} propagates a cortical reaction wave in which cortical granules move to the surface and fuse with the oolemma, leading to a transient increase in the surface area of the ovum and reorganization of the membrane. The contents of the cortical granules are released into the perivitelline space.
- **Zona reaction**. The released enzymes (proteases) of the cortical granules not only degrade the glycoprotein oocyte plasma membrane receptors for sperm binding but also form the **perivitelline barrier** by cross-linking proteins on the surface of the zona pellucida. This event creates the final and permanent block to polyspermy.

The corpus luteum of pregnancy is formed after fertilization and implantation.

If fertilization and implantation occur, the corpus luteum increases in size to form the **corpus luteum of pregnancy**. The existence and function of the corpus luteum depend on a combination of paracrine and endocrine secretions, collectively described as luteotropins.

Paracrine luteotropins are locally produced by the ovary. They include

- **estrogens**,
- **IGF-I** and **IGF-II**.

Endocrine luteotropins are produced at a distance from their target organ, the corpus luteum. They include

- **hCG**, a 37-kDa glycoprotein secreted by the trophoblast of the chorion, which stimulates LH receptors on the corpus luteum and prevents its degeneration (page 919);
- **LH** and **prolactin**, both secreted by the pituitary gland; and
- **insulin**, produced by the pancreas.

High levels of **progesterone**, produced from cholesterol by the corpus luteum, block the cyclic development of ovarian follicles. In early pregnancy, the corpus luteum measures 2–3 cm, thus filling most of the ovary. Its function begins to decline gradually after 8 weeks of pregnancy, although it persists throughout pregnancy. Although the corpus luteum remains active, the placenta produces sufficient amounts of estrogens and progestogens from maternal and fetal precursors to take over the function of the corpus luteum after 6 weeks of pregnancy. **Human chorionic gonadotropin (hCG)** can be detected in the serum as early as 6 days after fertilization and in the urine as early as 10–14 days after fertilization. Detection of hCG in the urine by specific antibodies forms the basis of **pregnancy tests**. In addition, the rapid increase in circulating level of hCG in early pregnancy is responsible for "**morning sickness**," a condition characterized by nausea and vomiting. These symptoms usually occur in the early hours of the morning and are often among the first signs of pregnancy.

Atresia

Most ovarian follicles are lost by atresia mediated by apoptosis of granulosa cells.

As stated, very few of the ovarian follicles that begin their differentiation in the embryonic ovary are destined to complete their maturation. Most of the follicles degenerate and disappear through a process called **ovarian follicular atresia**. Atresia is mediated by apoptosis of granulosa cells. Large numbers of follicles undergo atresia during fetal development, early postnatal life, and puberty. After puberty, groups of follicles begin to mature during each menstrual cycle; normally, only one follicle completes its maturation. Atresia is now thought to be a mechanism whereby a few follicles are stimulated to maintain their development through the programmed death of the other follicles. Thus, at any stage of its maturation, a follicle may undergo atresia. The process becomes more complex as the follicle progresses toward maturation.

In atresia of primordial and small, growing follicles, the immature oocyte becomes smaller and degenerates; similar changes occur in the granulosa cells. **Atretic follicles** shrink and eventually disappear from the stroma of the ovary as a result of repeated apoptosis and phagocytosis by granulosa cells (Plate 23.2, page 958). As the cells are reabsorbed and disappear, the surrounding stromal cells migrate into the space previously occupied by the follicle, leaving no trace of its existence.

In atresia of large, growing follicles, the degeneration of the mature oocyte is delayed and appears to occur secondary to degenerative changes in the follicular wall (Plate 23.2, page 958). This delay indicates that once the oocyte has achieved its maturity and competence, it is no longer sensitive to the same stimuli that initiate atresia in granulosa cells. The follicular changes include the following sequential events:

- Initiation of apoptosis within the granulosa cells, indicated by cessation of mitosis and expression of endonucleases and other hydrolytic enzymes within the granulosa cells
- Invasion of the granulosa layer by neutrophils and macrophages
- Invasion of the granulosa layer by strands of vascularized connective tissue
- Sloughing of the granulosa cells into the antrum of the follicle
- Hypertrophy of the theca interna cells
- Collapse of the follicle as degeneration continues
- Invasion of connective tissue into the cavity of the follicle

Several gene products regulate the process of follicular atresia. One of these products is the gonadotropin-induced **neural apoptosis inhibitory protein (NAIP)**, which inhibits and delays apoptotic changes in the granulosa cell. NAIP gene expression is present in all stages of the growing follicle but absent in follicles undergoing atresia. A high level of gonadotropins inhibits apoptosis in ovarian follicles by increasing the expression of NAIP in the ovaries.

FOLDER 23.2

CLINICAL CORRELATION: IN VITRO FERTILIZATION

There are several indications for **in vitro fertilization (IVF)**, but the primary one is infertility as a result of surgically uncorrectable damage to, or absence of, the uterine tubes. Individuals choosing IVF must first undergo controlled hyperstimulation of the ovaries to induce multiple follicle development and maturation. Hyperstimulation for IVF is usually achieved by different hormonal therapies using human gonadotropins, with or without follicle-stimulating hormone (FSH).

Mature preovulatory oocytes are collected from the Graafian follicles by either laparoscopic or ultrasound-guided percutaneous aspiration or transvaginal aspiration. Before insemination, the oocytes are preincubated in a specialized medium with serum complements for a time determined by their stage of maturity.

The collected semen is placed in a special medium. The oocytes are then added to the medium containing the collected semen for fertilization. Twelve to 16 hours later, the oocytes are examined with the differential interference contrast microscope to determine the presence of female and male pronuclei, which indicates successful fertilization (Fig. F23.2.1a). At this stage, a fertilized oocyte may be frozen for future IVF transfers.

Generally, 80% of mature oocytes cultured in vitro are fertilized. The embryo is transferred to a special growth medium for 24–48 hours, where it is allowed to grow to the stage of four to six cells (Fig. F23.2.1b). Embryos are then transferred under ultrasound guidance into the uterus via the vagina and cervical canal on the third or fourth day after the initial aspiration of the oocyte. Before embryo transfer, the uterus is prepared to receive the embryo by administration of appropriate hormones. Embryos are, therefore, placed into a hormonally prepared uterus under conditions equivalent to those in normal implantation (see pages 930-931). Intensive progesterone treatment is usually begun just after the transfer to mimic the function of the corpus luteum of pregnancy.

In recent years, existing treatment protocols have been optimized to such an extent that success rates of pregnancy and delivery with IVF programs have reached >30% per embryo transfer. Further improvements in pregnancy rates may be achieved by the introduction of new drugs, such as recombinant FSH or gonadotropin-releasing hormone (GnRH) antagonists that provide individualized hormonal treatment. In addition, the occurrence of multiple pregnancies, which is the main complication of IVF, may be limited by reducing the number of transferred embryos.

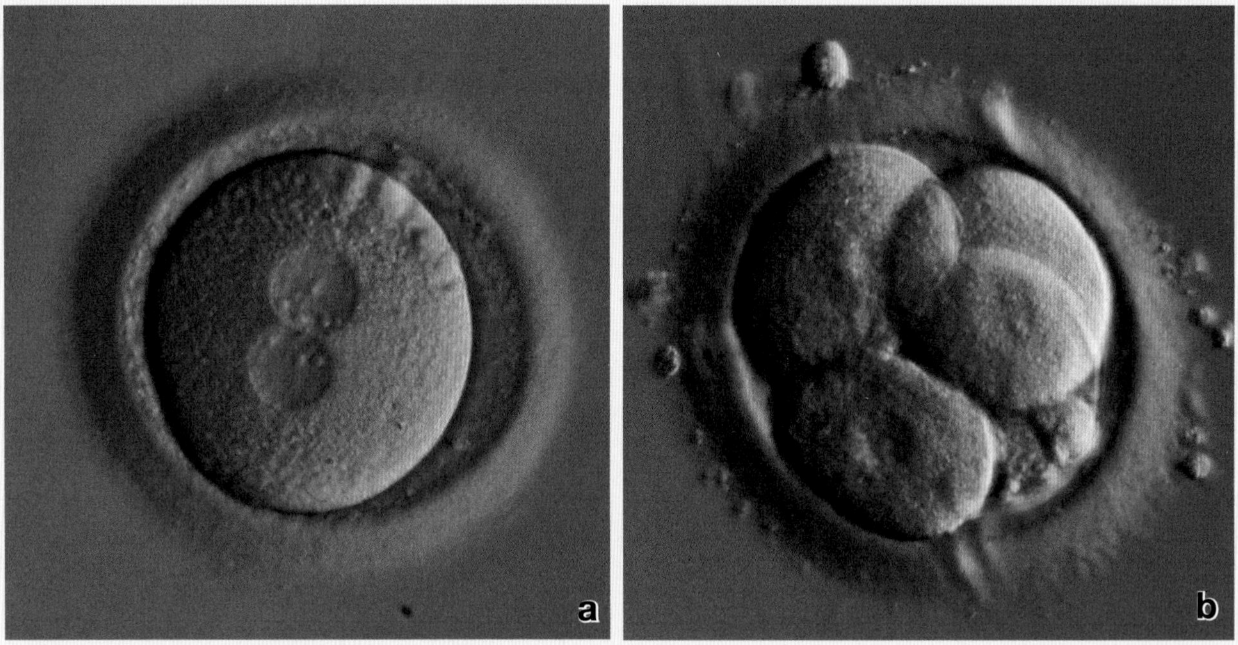

FIGURE F23.2.1. Early developmental stages of the human embryo. a. This image, obtained with an interference contrast microscope equipped with Nomarski optics, shows a human fertilized oocyte with two pronuclei. The zygote develops after alignment and dissolution of nuclear membranes of both female and male pronuclei. The resulting cell will contain a diploid complement of 46 chromosomes. ×400. **b.** This image shows a 48-hour-old human embryo growing in a special growth medium. At this stage, the embryo consists of four cells. In in vitro fertilization (IVF) procedures, it is at this stage that the embryo is usually transferred into the uterine cavity. ×400. (Courtesy of Dr. Peter Fehr.)

The oocyte undergoes typical changes associated with degeneration and autolysis, and the remnants are phagocytosed by invading macrophages. The zona pellucida which is resistant to the autolytic changes occurring in the cells associated with it, becomes folded and collapses as it is slowly broken down within the cavity of the follicle. Macrophages in the connective tissue are involved in the phagocytosis of the zona pellucida and the remnants of the degenerating cells.

The basement membrane between the follicle cells from the theca interna may separate from the follicle cells and increase in thickness, forming a wavy hyaline layer called the **glassy membrane**. This structure is characteristic of follicles in the late stages of atresia.

Enlargement of the cells of the theca interna occurs in some atretic follicles. These cells are similar to theca lutein cells and become organized into radially arranged strands separated by connective tissue. A rich capillary network develops in the connective tissue. These atretic follicles, which resemble an old corpus luteum, are called **corpora lutea atretica**.

The interstitial gland arises from the theca interna of the atretic follicle.

As **atretic follicles** continue to degenerate, a scar with hyaline streaks develops in the center of the cell mass, giving it the appearance of a small corpus albicans. This structure eventually disappears as the ovarian stroma invades the degenerating follicle. In the ovaries of a number of mammals, the strands of luteal cells do not degenerate immediately but become broken up and scattered in the stroma. These cords of cells contribute to the **interstitial gland** of the ovary and produce steroid hormones. The development of the interstitial gland is most extensive in animal species that have large litters.

In the human ovary, there are relatively few interstitial cells. They occur in the largest numbers in the first year of life and during the early phases of puberty, corresponding to times of increased follicular atresia. At menarche, involution of the interstitial cells occurs; therefore, few are present during the reproductive life span and menopause. It has been suggested that in humans, the interstitial cells are an important source of the estrogens that influence the growth and development of the secondary sex organs during the early phases of puberty. In other species, the interstitial cells have been shown to produce progesterone.

In humans, cells called **ovarian hilar cells** are found in the hilum of the ovary in association with vascular spaces and unmyelinated nerve fibers. These cells, which appear to be structurally related to the interstitial cells of the testis, contain **Reinke crystalloids**. The hilar cells appear to respond to hormonal changes during pregnancy and at the onset of menopause. Research suggests that the hilar cells secrete androgens; hyperplasia or tumors associated with these cells usually lead to masculinization.

Blood Supply and Lymphatics

Blood supply to the ovaries comes from two different sources: ovarian and uterine arteries.

The **ovarian arteries** are the branches of the abdominal aorta that pass to the ovaries through the suspensory ligaments and provide the principal arterial supply to the ovaries and uterine tubes. These arteries anastomose with the second blood source to the ovary, the **ovarian branches of the uterine arteries**, which arise from the internal iliac arteries. Relatively large vessels arising from this region of anastomosis pass through the mesovarium and enter the hilum of the ovary. These large arteries are called **spiral arteries** because they branch and become highly coiled as they pass into the ovarian medulla (see Fig. 23.2).

Veins accompany the arteries and form a plexus called the **pampiniform plexus** as they emerge from the hilum. The ovarian vein is formed from the plexus.

In the cortical region of the ovary, networks of lymphatic vessels in the thecal layers surround the large developing and atretic follicles and corpora lutea. The lymphatic vessels follow the course of the ovarian arteries as they ascend to para-aortic lymph nodes in the lumbar region.

Innervation

Ovaries are innervated by the autonomic ovarian plexus.

Autonomic nerve fibers that supply the ovary are conveyed mainly by the ovarian plexus. Although it is clear that the ovary receives both sympathetic and parasympathetic fibers, little is known about their actual distribution. Groups of parasympathetic ganglion cells are scattered in the medulla. Nerve fibers follow the arteries, supplying the smooth muscle in the walls of these vessels, as they pass into the medulla and cortex of the ovary. Nerve fibers associated with the follicles do not penetrate the basal lamina. Sensory nerve endings are scattered in the stroma. The sensory fibers convey impulses via the ovarian plexus and reach the dorsal root ganglia of the first lumbar spinal nerves. Therefore, ovarian pain is referred over the cutaneous distribution of these spinal nerves.

At ovulation, about 45% of females experience **midcycle pain** ("mittelschmerz"). It is usually described as a sharp, lower abdominal pain that lasts from a few minutes to as long as 24 hours and may be accompanied by a small amount of bleeding from the uterus. It is believed that this pain is related to smooth muscle cell contraction in the ovary and its ligaments. These contractions are in response to an increased level of prostaglandin $F_{2\alpha}$ mediated by the surge of LH.

■ UTERINE TUBES

The **uterine tubes** are paired tubes that extend bilaterally from the uterus toward the ovaries (see Fig. 23.1). Also commonly referred to as the **fallopian tubes**, the uterine tubes transport the ovum from the ovary to the uterus and provide the necessary environment for fertilization and initial development of the zygote to the morula stage. One end of the tube is adjacent to the ovary and opens into the peritoneal cavity; the other end communicates with the uterine cavity.

Each **uterine tube** is approximately 10–12 cm long and can be divided into four segments by gross inspection:

- The **infundibulum** is the funnel-shaped segment of the tube adjacent to the ovary. At the distal end, it opens into the peritoneal cavity. The proximal end communicates with the ampulla. Fringed extensions, or **fimbriae**, extend from the mouth of the infundibulum toward the ovary.
- The **ampulla** is the longest segment of the tube, constituting about two-thirds of the total length, and is the site of fertilization.
- The **isthmus** is the narrow, medial segment of the uterine tube adjacent to the uterus.
- The **uterine** or **intramural** part, measuring about 1 cm in length, lies within the uterine wall and opens into the cavity of the uterus.

The wall of the uterine tube is composed of three layers.

The **uterine tube** wall resembles the wall of other hollow viscera, consisting of an external serosal layer, an intermediate muscular layer, and an internal mucosal layer. However, there is no submucosa.

- The **serosa** or peritoneum is the outermost layer of the uterine tube and is composed of mesothelium and a thin layer of connective tissue.

- The **muscularis**, throughout most of its length, is organized into an inner, relatively thick circular layer and an outer, thinner longitudinal layer. The boundary between these layers is often indistinct.
- The **mucosa**, the inner lining of the uterine tube, exhibits relatively thin longitudinal folds that project into the lumen of the uterine tube throughout its length. The folds are most numerous and complex in the ampulla (Fig. 23.15 and Plate 23.4, page 962) and become smaller in the isthmus.

The **mucosal lining** is simple columnar epithelium composed of two kinds of cells—ciliated and nonciliated (Fig. 23.15b). They represent different functional states of a single cell type.

- **Ciliated cells** are most numerous in the infundibulum and ampulla. The wave of the cilia is directed toward the uterus.
- **Nonciliated, peg cells** are secretory cells that produce the fluid that provides nutritive material for the ovum.

The epithelial cells undergo cyclic hypertrophy during the follicular phase and atrophy during the luteal phase in response to changes in hormonal levels, particularly estrogens. Also, the ratio of ciliated to nonciliated cells changes during the hormonal cycle. Estrogen stimulates ciliogenesis, and progesterone increases the number of secretory cells. At about the time of ovulation, the epithelium reaches a height of approximately 30 μm and is then reduced to about one-half that height just before the onset of menstruation.

Bidirectional transport occurs in the uterine tube.

The **uterine tube** demonstrates active movements just before ovulation as the fimbriae become closely apposed to the ovary and localize over the region of the ovarian surface where rupture will occur. As the oocyte is released, the ciliated cells in the infundibulum sweep it toward the opening of the uterine tube and thus prevent it from entering the peritoneal cavity. The oocyte is transported along the uterine tube by peristaltic contractions. The mechanisms by which spermatozoa and the oocyte are transported from opposite ends of the uterine tube are not fully understood. Research suggests that both **ciliary movements** and **peristaltic muscular activity** are involved in the movements of the oocyte. The movement of the spermatozoa is much too rapid, however, to be accounted for by intrinsic motility. **Fertilization usually occurs in the ampulla**, near its junction with the isthmus. The ovum remains in the uterine tube for about 3 days before it enters the uterine cavity. Several conditions that may alter the integrity of the tubal transport system (e.g., inflammation, use of intrauterine devices, surgical manipulation, tubal ligation) may cause a tubal **ectopic pregnancy**. Most ectopic pregnancies (98%) occur in the **uterine tube**

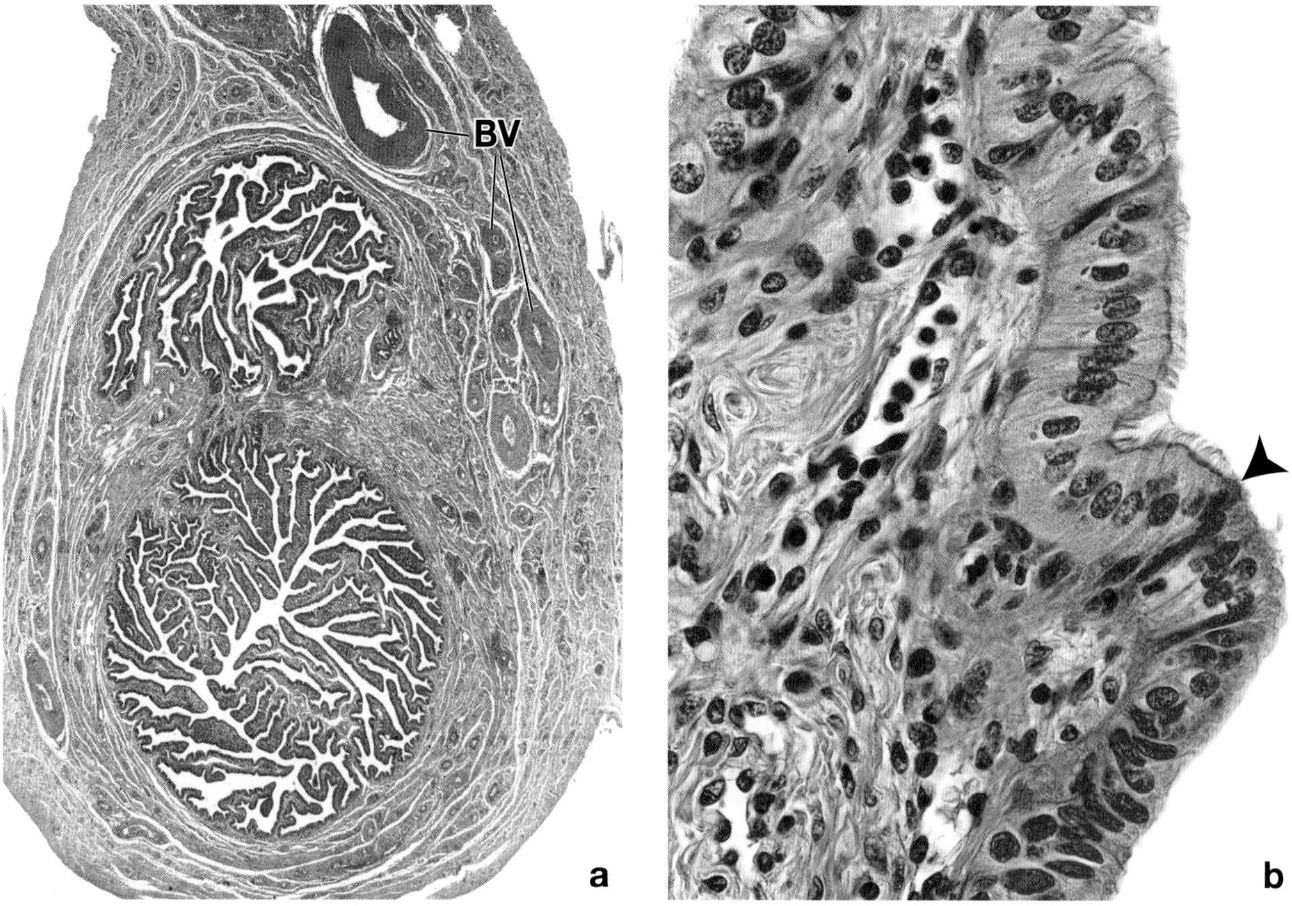

FIGURE 23.15. Photomicrograph of a human uterine tube. a. This cross section is near the ampulla region of the uterine tube. The mucosa is thrown into extensive folds that project into the lumen of the tube. The muscularis is composed of a thick inner layer of circularly arranged fibers and an outer layer of longitudinal fibers. Note several branches of the uterine and ovarian arteries (*BV*) that travel along the uterine tube. ×16. **b.** The lumen of the tube is lined by a simple columnar epithelium composed of ciliated cells (above the point of the *arrowhead*) and nonciliated cells (below the point of the *arrowhead*). ×640.

(tubal pregnancies). An ectopic pregnancy that occurs in the uterine tube can cause life-threatening bleeding if the tube ruptures. Prompt treatment with surgery to remove the tube or medication to stop the growth of the fertilized ovum is needed.

■ UTERUS

The uterus receives the rapidly developing morula from the uterine tube. All subsequent embryonic and fetal development occurs within the uterus, which undergoes dramatic increases in size and development. The human uterus is a hollow, pear-shaped organ located in the pelvis between the bladder and the rectum. In a nulliparous female, it weighs 30–40 g and measures 7.5 cm in length, 5 cm in width at its superior aspect, and 2.5 cm in thickness. Its lumen, which is also flattened, is continuous with the uterine tubes and the vagina.

Anatomically, the **uterus** is divided into two regions:

- The **body** is the large upper portion of the uterus. The anterior surface is almost flat; the posterior surface is convex. The upper, rounded part of the body that expands above the attachment of the uterine tubes is called the **fundus**.
- The **cervix** is the lower, barrel-shaped part of the uterus separated from the body by the **isthmus** (see Fig. 23.1). The lumen of the cervix, the **cervical canal**, has a constricted opening at each end. The **internal os** communicates with the cavity of the uterus; the **external os** with the vagina.

Organization of the Uterine Wall

The uterine wall is composed of three layers (Fig. 23.16). From the lumen outward, they are as follows:

- The **endometrium** is the mucosa of the uterus.
- The **myometrium** is the thick muscular layer. It is continuous with the muscle layer of the uterine tube and vagina. The smooth muscle fibers also extend into the ligaments connected to the uterus.
- The **perimetrium**, the outer serous layer or visceral peritoneal covering of the uterus, is continuous with the pelvic and abdominal peritoneum and consists of a mesothelium and a thin layer of loose connective tissue. Beneath the mesothelium, a layer of elastic tissue is usually prominent. The perimetrium covers the entire posterior surface of the uterus but only part of the anterior surface. The remaining part of the anterior surface consists of connective tissue or adventitia.

Both myometrium and endometrium undergo cyclic changes each month to prepare the uterus for implantation of an embryo. These changes constitute the menstrual cycle. If an embryo implants, the cycle stops, and both layers undergo considerable growth and differentiation during pregnancy (described in the next section).

The myometrium forms a structural and functional syncytium.

The **myometrium** is the thickest layer of the uterine wall. It is composed of three indistinctly defined layers of smooth muscle:

- The middle muscle layer contains numerous large blood vessels (venous plexuses) and lymphatics and is called the **stratum vasculare**. It is the thickest layer and has interlaced smooth muscle bundles oriented in a circular or spiral pattern.

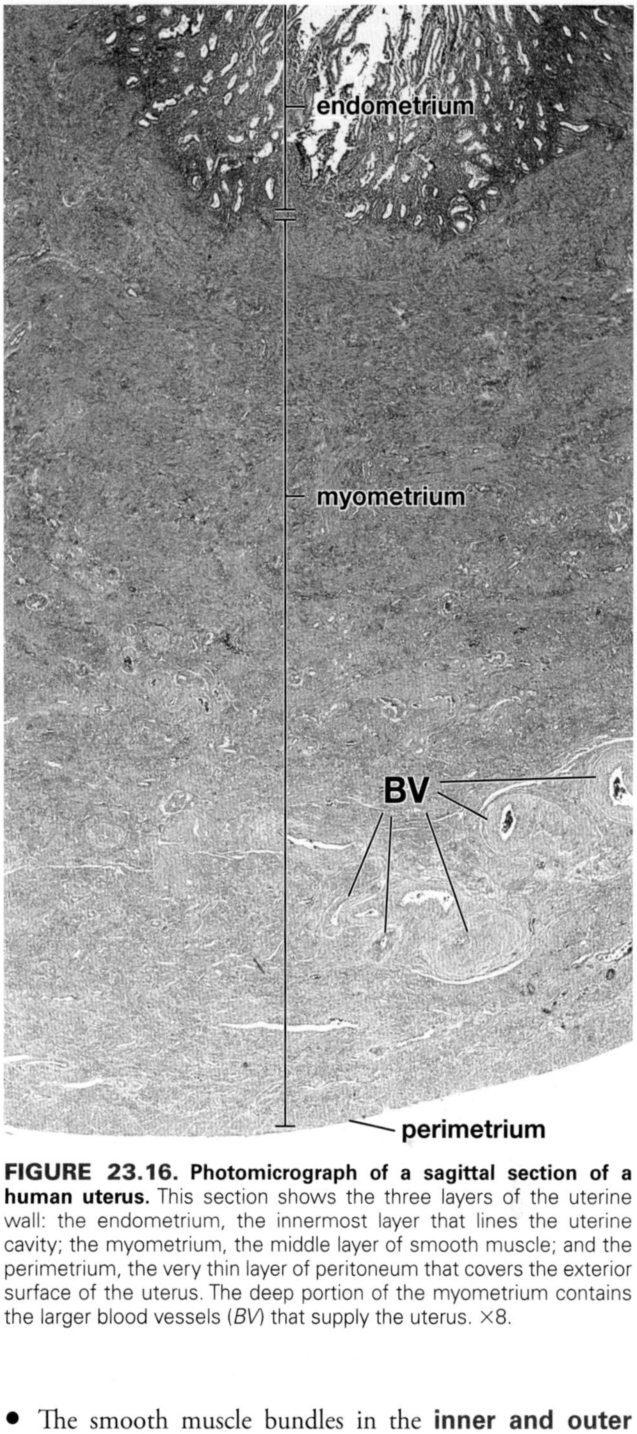

FIGURE 23.16. Photomicrograph of a sagittal section of a human uterus. This section shows the three layers of the uterine wall: the endometrium, the innermost layer that lines the uterine cavity; the myometrium, the middle layer of smooth muscle; and the perimetrium, the very thin layer of peritoneum that covers the exterior surface of the uterus. The deep portion of the myometrium contains the larger blood vessels (*BV*) that supply the uterus. ×8.

- The smooth muscle bundles in the **inner and outer layers** are predominantly oriented parallel to the long axis of the uterus.

As in most bulb-shaped hollow organs, such as the gallbladder and urinary bladder, muscular orientation is not distinctive. The muscle bundles seen in routine histologic sections appear to be randomly arrayed. During uterine contraction, all three layers of the myometrium work together as a functional syncytium expelling the contents of the lumen through a narrow orifice.

In the nonpregnant uterus, the smooth muscle cells are about 50 µm long. During pregnancy, the uterus undergoes enormous enlargement. The growth is primarily owing to the hypertrophy of existing smooth muscle cells, which may reach more than 500 µm in length, and secondarily attributable to the development of new fibers through the division of existing muscle cells and the differentiation of undifferentiated mesenchymal cells. The amount of connective tissue also increases. As **pregnancy** proceeds, the uterine wall becomes progressively thinner as it stretches because of the growth of the fetus. After parturition, although some muscle fibers degenerate, the uterus returns to almost its original size. The collagen produced during pregnancy to strengthen the myometrium is then enzymatically degraded by the cells that secreted it. The uterine cavity remains larger and the muscular wall remains thicker than before pregnancy.

Compared with the body of the uterus, the cervix has more connective tissue and less smooth muscle. Elastic fibers are abundant in the cervix but are found in appreciable quantities only in the outer layer of the myometrium of the body of the uterus.

The endometrium proliferates and then degenerates during a menstrual cycle.

Throughout the reproductive life span, the **endometrium undergoes cyclic changes** each month that prepare it for the implantation of the embryo and the subsequent events of embryonic and fetal development. Changes in the secretory activity of the endometrium during the cycle are correlated with the maturation of the ovarian follicles (see Folder 23.3). The end of each cycle is characterized by the partial destruction and sloughing of the endometrium, accompanied by bleeding from the mucosal vessels. The discharge of tissue and blood from the vagina, which usually continues for 3–5 days, is referred to as **menstruation** or **menstrual flow**. The **menstrual cycle** is defined as beginning on the day when menstrual flow begins.

During reproductive life, the endometrium consists of two layers or zones that differ in structure and function (Fig. 23.17 and Plate 23.5, page 964):

- The **stratum functionale** or **functional layer** is the thick part of the endometrium, which is sloughed off at menstruation.
- The **stratum basale** or **basal layer** is retained during menstruation and serves as the source for the regeneration of the stratum functionale.

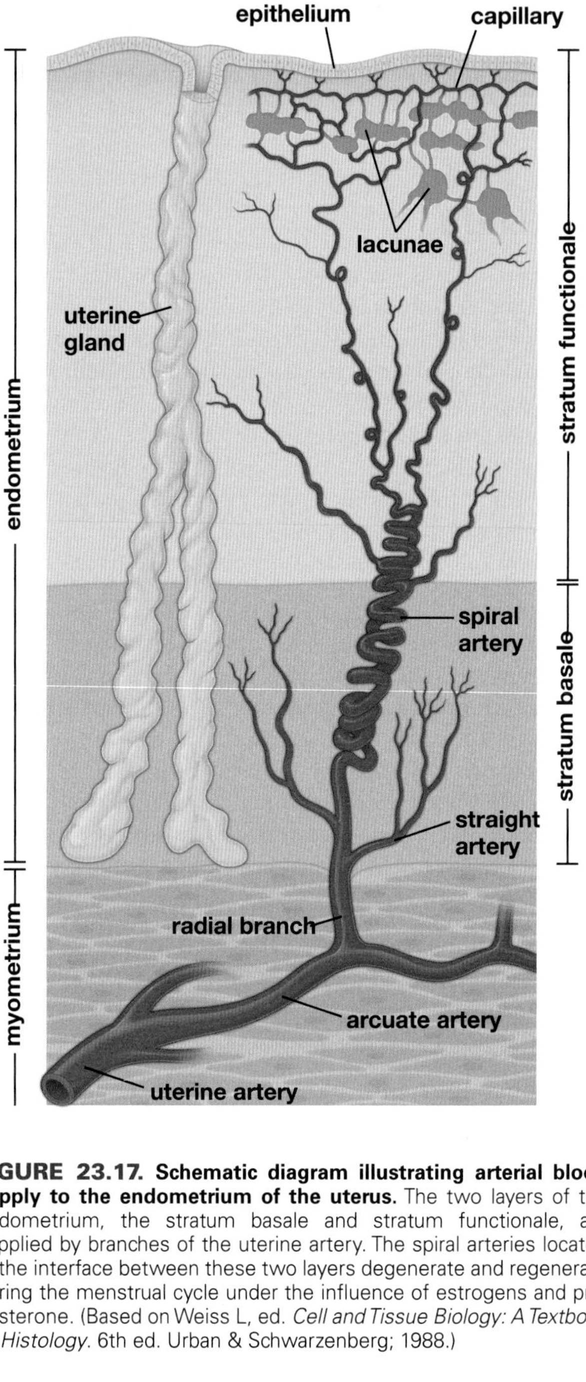

FIGURE 23.17. Schematic diagram illustrating arterial blood supply to the endometrium of the uterus. The two layers of the endometrium, the stratum basale and stratum functionale, are supplied by branches of the uterine artery. The spiral arteries located at the interface between these two layers degenerate and regenerate during the menstrual cycle under the influence of estrogens and progesterone. (Based on Weiss L, ed. *Cell and Tissue Biology: A Textbook of Histology*. 6th ed. Urban & Schwarzenberg; 1988.)

FOLDER 23.3

FUNCTIONAL CONSIDERATIONS: SUMMARY OF HORMONAL REGULATION OF THE OVARIAN CYCLE

During each **menstrual cycle**, the ovary undergoes cyclic changes that involve two phases:

- Follicular phase
- Luteal phase

Ovulation occurs between the two phases (Fig. F23.3.1).

The **follicular phase** begins with the development of a small number of primary follicles (10–20) under the influence of follicle-stimulating hormone (FSH) and luteinizing hormone (LH). Selection of dominant follicles occurs by days 5–7 of the menstrual cycle. During the first 8–10 days of the cycle, FSH is the principal hormone influencing the growth of the follicles. It stimulates the granulosa and thecal cells, which begin to secrete steroid hormones, principally estrogens, into the follicular lumen. As estrogen production from the dominant follicle increases, FSH production is inhibited by a negative feedback loop from the pituitary gland. Estrogens continue to accumulate in the follicular lumen, finally reaching a level that allows the follicle to be independent of FSH for its continued growth and development.

FOLDER 23.3

FUNCTIONAL CONSIDERATIONS: SUMMARY OF HORMONAL REGULATION OF THE OVARIAN CYCLE (*continued*)

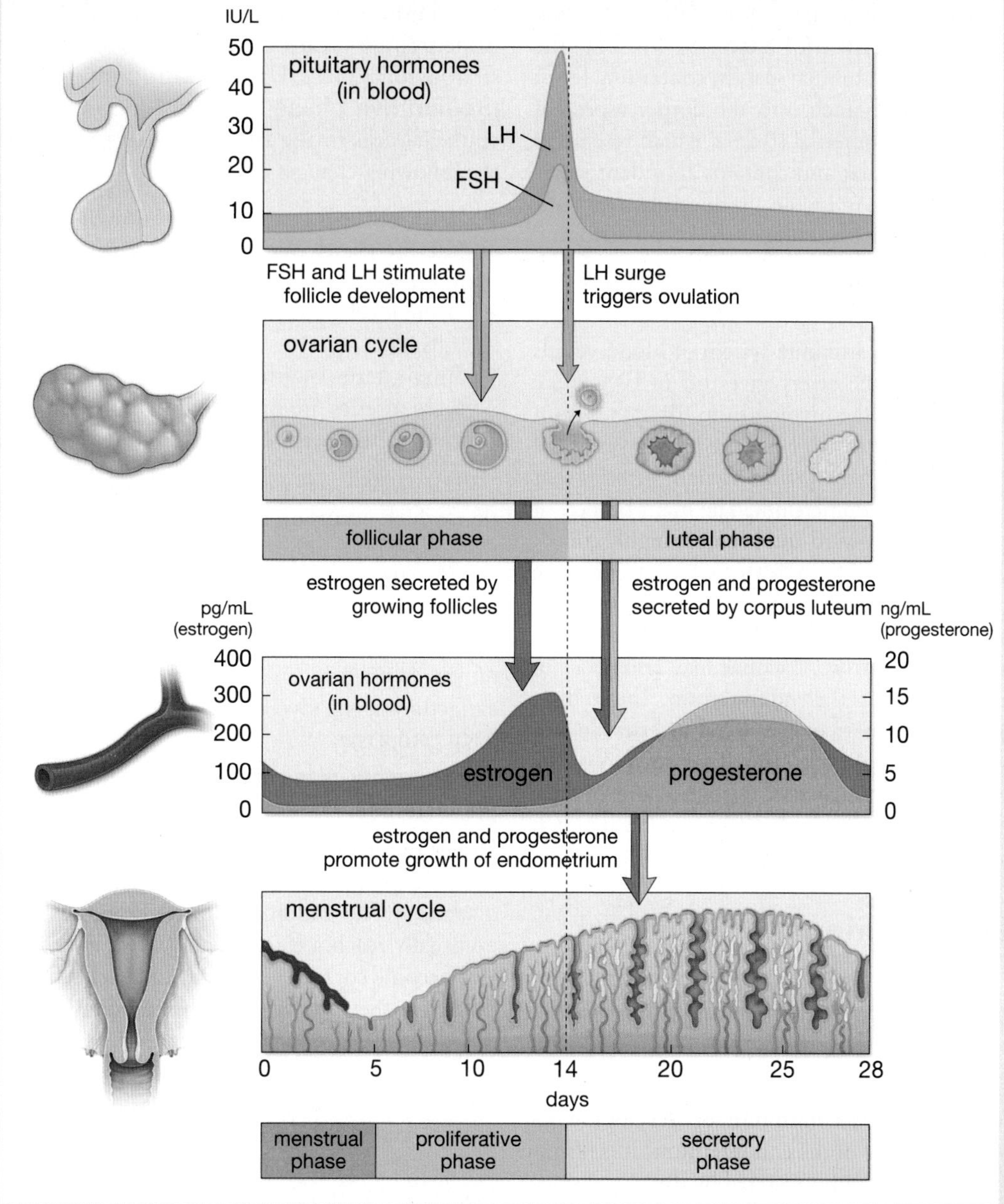

FIGURE F23.3.1. Relationship of morphologic and physiologic events that occur in the menstrual cycle. This diagram illustrates the relationship of the morphologic changes in the endometrium and ovary to the pituitary and ovarian blood hormone levels that occur during the menstrual cycle. The pituitary and ovarian hormones and their plasma concentrations are indicated in arbitrary units. *FSH*, follicle-stimulating hormone; *LH*, luteinizing hormone.

Late in the follicular phase, before ovulation, progesterone levels begin to increase under the influence of LH. The amount of estrogens in the circulating blood inhibits further production of FSH by the adenohypophysis. Ovulation is induced by a surge in the LH level, which occurs concomitantly with a smaller increase in the FSH level. It occurs ~34–36 hours after the start of the LH surge or about 10–12 hours after the peak of the LH surge.

The **luteal phase** begins immediately after ovulation as the granulosa and thecal cells of the ruptured follicle undergo rapid morphologic transformation to form the corpus luteum. Estrogens and large amounts of progesterone are secreted by the corpus luteum. Under the influence of both hormones, but primarily progesterone, the endometrium begins its secretory phase, which is essential for the preparation of the uterus for implantation in the event that the egg is fertilized. LH appears to be responsible for the development and maintenance of the corpus luteum during the menstrual cycle. If fertilization does not occur, the corpus luteum degenerates within a few days as hormone levels drop. If fertilization does occur, the corpus luteum is maintained and continues to secrete progesterone and estrogens. Human chorionic gonadotropin (hCG), which is initially produced by the embryo and later by the placenta, stimulates the corpus luteum and is responsible for its maintenance during pregnancy.

The stratum functionale is the layer that proliferates and degenerates during the menstrual cycle.

During the **phases of the menstrual cycle**, the endometrium varies from 1 to 6 mm in thickness. It is lined by a simple columnar epithelium with a mixture of secretory and ciliated cells. The surface epithelium invaginates into the underlying lamina propria, the **endometrial stroma**, forming the uterine glands. These simple tubular glands, containing fewer ciliated cells, occasionally branch into the deeper aspect of the endometrium. The endometrial stroma, which resembles mesenchyme, is highly cellular and contains abundant intercellular ground substance. As in the uterine tube, no submucosa separates the endometrium from the myometrium.

The vasculature of the endometrium also proliferates and degenerates during each menstrual cycle.

The endometrium contains a unique system of blood vessels (see Fig. 23.17). The uterine artery gives off 6–10 arcuate arteries that anastomose in the myometrium. Branches from these arteries, the **radial arteries**, enter the basal layer of the endometrium where they give off small straight arteries that supply this region of the endometrium. The main branch of the radial artery continues upward and becomes highly coiled; it is, therefore, called the **spiral artery**. Spiral arteries give off numerous arterioles that often anastomose as they supply a rich capillary bed. The capillary bed includes thin-walled dilated segments called **lacunae**. Lacunae may also occur in the venous system that drains the endometrium. The straight arteries and the proximal part of the spiral arteries do not change during the menstrual cycle. The distal portion of the spiral arteries, under the influence of estrogens and progesterone, undergoes degeneration and regeneration with each menstrual cycle.

Cyclic Changes During the Menstrual Cycle

Cyclic changes of the endometrium during the menstrual cycle are represented by the proliferative, secretory, and menstrual phases.

The **menstrual cycle** is a continuum of developmental stages in the functional layer of the endometrium. It is ultimately controlled by gonadotropins secreted by the pars distalis of the pituitary gland that regulate the steroid secretions of the ovary. The cycle normally repeats every 28 days, during which the endometrium passes through a sequence of morphologic and functional changes. It is convenient to describe the cycle as having three successive phases:

- The **proliferative phase** occurs concurrently with follicular maturation and is influenced by ovarian estrogen secretion.
- The **secretory phase** coincides with the functional activity of the corpus luteum and is primarily influenced by progesterone secretion.
- The **menstrual phase** commences as hormone production by the ovary declines with the degeneration of the corpus luteum (see Folder 23.3).

The phases are part of a continuous process; there is no abrupt change from one to the next.

The proliferative phase of the menstrual cycle is regulated by estrogens.

At the end of the menstrual phase, the endometrium consists of a thin band of connective tissue, about 1 mm thick, containing the basal portions of the uterine glands and the lower portions of the spiral arteries (see Fig. 23.17). This layer is the stratum basale; the layer that was sloughed off was the stratum functionale. Under the **influence of estrogens**, the **proliferative phase** is initiated. Stromal, endothelial, and epithelial cells in the stratum basale proliferate rapidly, and the following changes can be seen:

- Epithelial cells in the basal portion of the glands reconstitute the glands and migrate to cover the denuded endometrial surface.
- Stromal cells proliferate and secrete collagen and ground substance.
- Spiral arteries lengthen as the endometrium is reestablished; these arteries are only slightly coiled and do not extend into the upper third of the endometrium.

The proliferative phase continues until 1 day after ovulation, which occurs on day 14 of a 28-day cycle. At the end of this phase, the endometrium has reached a thickness of about 3 mm. The glands have narrow lumina and are relatively straight but have a slightly wavy appearance (Fig. 23.18a). Accumulations of glycogen are present in the basal portions of the epithelial cells. In routine histologic preparations, extraction of the glycogen gives an empty appearance to the basal cytoplasm.

The secretory phase of the menstrual cycle is regulated by progesterone.

Under the **influence of progesterone**, dramatic changes occur in the stratum functionale, beginning a day or 2 after ovulation. The endometrium becomes edematous and may eventually reach a thickness of 5–6 mm. The glands enlarge and become corkscrew shaped, and their lumina become sacculated as they fill with secretory products (Fig. 23.18b). The mucoid fluid produced by the gland epithelium is rich in nutrients, particularly glycogen, required to support development if implantation occurs. Mitoses are now rare. The growth seen at this stage results from hypertrophy of the epithelial cells, an increase in vascularity, and edema of the endometrium. The spiral arteries, however, lengthen and become more coiled. They extend nearly to the surface of the endometrium (Plate 23.6, page 966).

The sequential influence of estrogens and progesterone on the **stromal cells** enables their transformation into **decidual cells**. The stimulus for transformation is the implantation of the blastocyst. Large, pale cells rich in glycogen result from this transformation. Although the precise function of these cells is not known, it is clear that they provide a favorable environment for the nourishment of the embryo and that they create a specialized layer that facilitates the separation of the placenta from the uterine wall following parturition.

The menstrual phase results from a decline in the ovarian secretion of progesterone and estrogen.

The **corpus luteum** actively produces hormones for about 10 days if fertilization does not occur. As hormone levels rapidly decline, changes occur in the blood supply to the

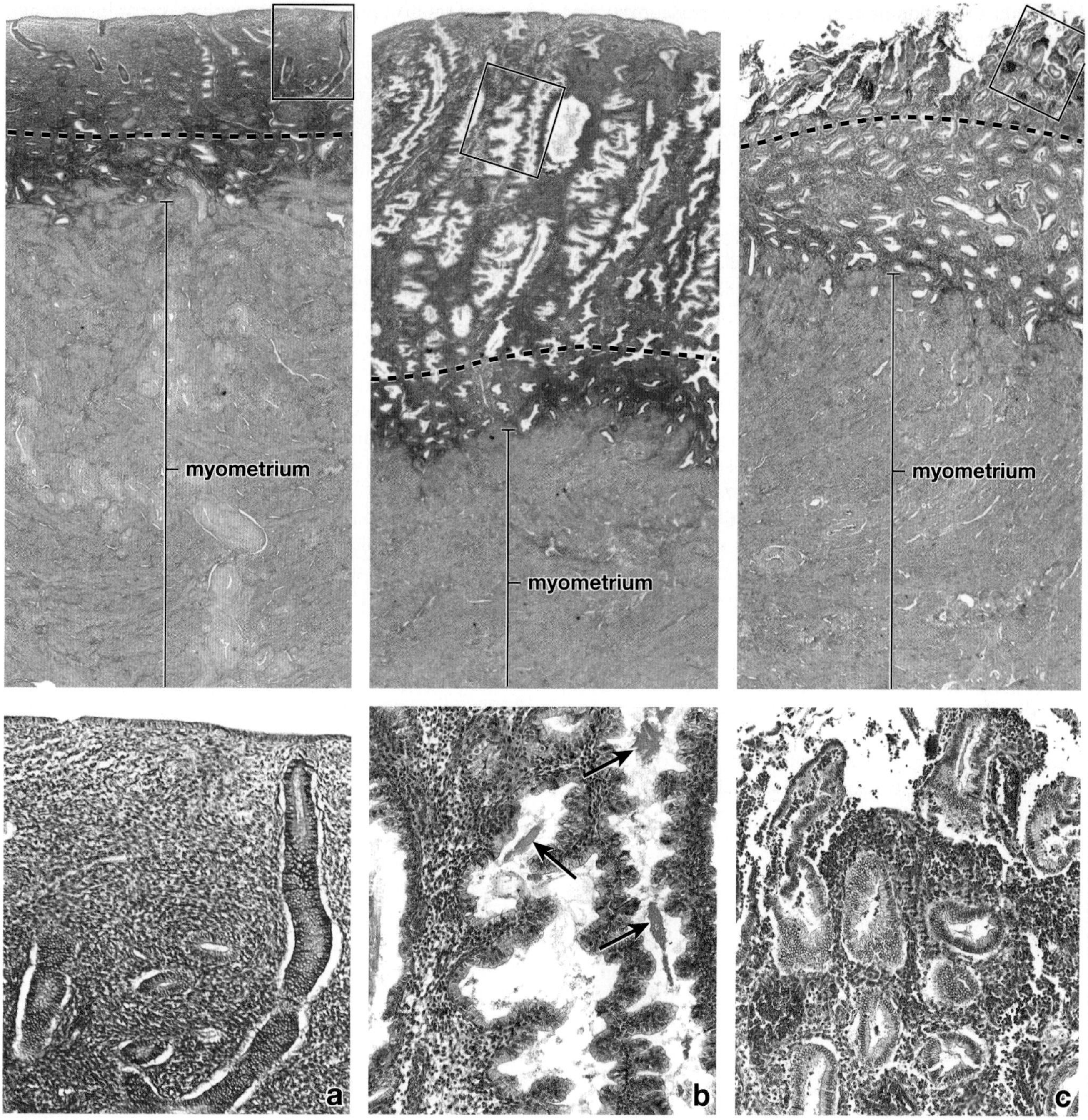

FIGURE 23.18. Photomicrographs of the uterine lining in proliferative, secretory, and menstrual phases of the menstrual cycle. a. The *upper panel* shows the endometrium at the proliferative phase of the cycle. During this phase, the stratum functionale (separated by the *dashed line* from the stratum basale) greatly thickens. ×15. The *lower panel* shows at higher magnification the endometrial glands that extend from the stratum basale to the surface. ×55. **b.** The *upper panel* shows the endometrium at the secretory phase of the cycle. The glands have acquired a corkscrew shape as the endometrium increases further in thickness. The stratum basale (below the *dashed line*) exhibits less dramatic changes in morphology. ×20. The *lower panel* shows uterine glands that have been cut in a plane that is close to their long axes. Note the pronounced corkscrew shape of the glands and mucus secretion (*arrows*). ×60. **c.** The *upper panel* shows the stratum functionale (above the *dashed line*). Much of the stratum functionale has degenerated and sloughed away. ×15. The *lower panel* shows the extravasated blood and necrosis of the stratum functionale. ×55.

stratum functionale. Initially, periodic contractions of the walls of the spiral arteries, lasting for several hours, cause the **stratum functionale** to become **ischemic**. The glands stop secreting, and the endometrium shrinks in height as the stroma becomes less edematous. After about 2 days, extended periods of arterial contraction, with only brief periods of blood flow, cause disruption of the surface epithelium and rupture of the blood vessels. When the spiral arteries close off, blood flows into the stratum basale, but not into the stratum functionale. Blood, uterine fluid, and stromal and epithelial cells from the stratum functionale constitute the menstrual discharge. As patches of tissue separate from the endometrium, the torn ends of veins, arteries, and glands are exposed (Fig. 23.18c). The desquamation continues until only the stratum basale remains. Clotting of blood is inhibited during this period of menstrual flow. Arterial blood flow is restricted, except for the brief periods of relaxation of the walls of the spiral arteries. Blood continually seeps from the open ends of the veins. The period of **menstrual flow** normally lasts about 5 days. The average blood loss in the menstrual phase is

35–50 mL. Blood flow through the straight arteries maintains the stratum basale.

As noted, this process is cyclic. Figure F23.3.1 in Folder 23.3 shows a single cycle of the endometrium. In the absence of fertilization, cessation of bleeding accompanies the growth and maturation of new ovarian follicles. The epithelial cells rapidly proliferate and migrate to restore the surface epithelium as the proliferative phase of the next cycle begins.

In the absence of ovulation (a cycle referred to as an **anovulatory cycle**), a corpus luteum does not form, and progesterone is not produced. In the absence of progesterone, the endometrium does not enter the secretory phase and continues in the proliferative phase until menstruation. In cases of **infertility**, biopsies of the endometrium can be used to diagnose **anovulatory cycles** as well as other disorders of the ovary and endometrium.

Implantation

If fertilization and implantation occur, a gravid phase replaces the menstrual phase of the cycle.

If fertilization and subsequent **implantation** occur, decline of the endometrium is delayed until after parturition. As the blastocyst becomes embedded in the uterine mucosa in the early part of the second week, cells in the chorion of the developing placenta begin to secrete **hCG** and other luteotropins. These hormones maintain the corpus luteum and stimulate it to continue the production of progesterone and estrogens. Thus, the decline of the endometrium is prevented, and the endometrium undergoes further development during the first few weeks of pregnancy.

Implantation is the process by which the blastocyst settles into the endometrium.

The **fertilized human ovum (zygote)** undergoes a series of changes as it passes through the uterine tube into the uterine cavity in preparation for becoming embedded in the uterine mucosa. The developing embryo initiates an embryo–maternal dialogue, which is critical for further implantation and development. Shortly after fertilization, the viable embryo secretes **preimplantation factor (PIF)**, an embryo-specific 15-amino-acid peptide (MVRIKPGSANKPSDD) that promotes adhesion of the embryo to the endometrium. At the time of implantation, PIF stimulates proliferation and invasion of the trophoblast into the decidua basalis (see page 931).

The zygote undergoes cleavage, followed by a series of mitotic divisions without cell growth, resulting in a rapid increase in the number of cells in the embryo. Initially, the embryo is under the control of maternal informational macromolecules that have accumulated in the cytoplasm of the ovum during oogenesis. Later development depends on activation of the embryonic genome, which encodes various growth factors, cell junction components, and other macromolecules required for normal progression to the blastocyst stage. The cell mass resulting from the series of mitotic divisions is known as a **morula** *[L. morum, mulberry]*, and the individual cells are known as **blastomeres.** During the third day after fertilization, the morula, which now contains 12–16 cells is still surrounded by the zona pellucida enters the uterine cavity. The morula remains free in the uterus for about a day while continued cell division and development occur. The early embryo gives rise to a blastocyst, a hollow sphere of cells with a centrally located clump of cells. This **inner cell mass** will give rise to the tissues of the embryo proper; the surrounding layer of cells, the **outer cell mass,** will form the trophoblast and then the placenta (Fig. 23.19).

Fluid passes inward through the zona pellucida during this process, forming a fluid-filled cavity, the **blastocyst cavity**. This event defines the beginning of the **blastocyst**. As the blastocyst remains free in the uterine lumen for 1 or 2 days and undergoes further mitotic divisions, the zona pellucida disappears. The outer cell mass is now called the **trophoblast**, and the inner cell mass is referred to as the **embryoblast**.

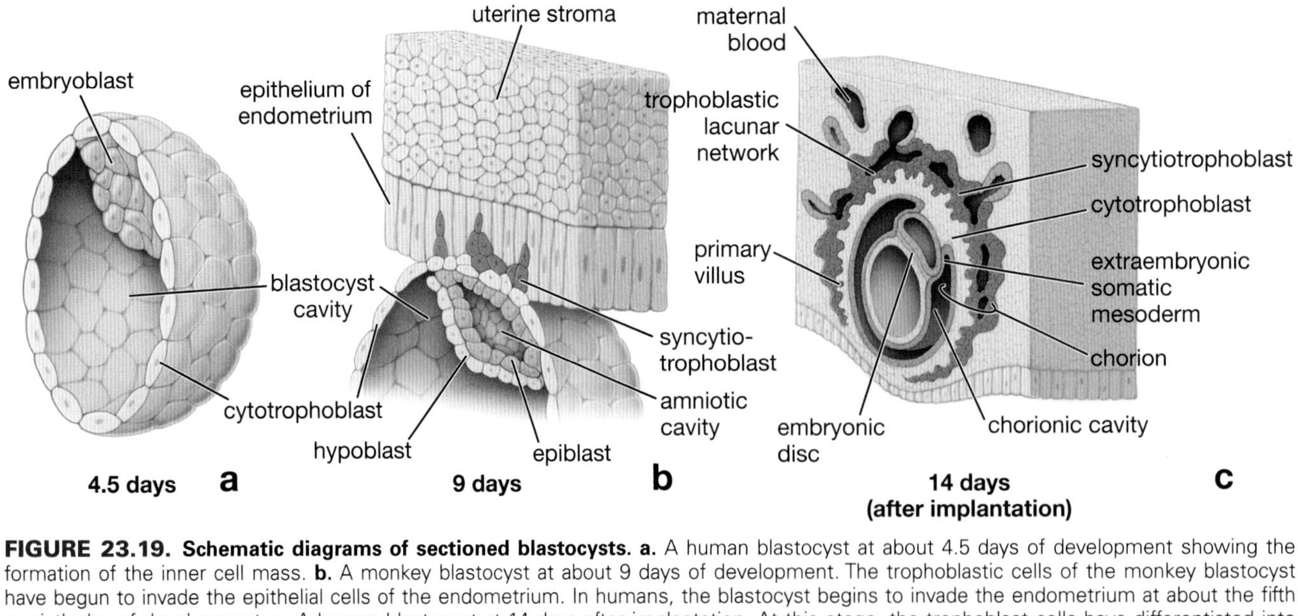

FIGURE 23.19. Schematic diagrams of sectioned blastocysts. a. A human blastocyst at about 4.5 days of development showing the formation of the inner cell mass. **b.** A monkey blastocyst at about 9 days of development. The trophoblastic cells of the monkey blastocyst have begun to invade the epithelial cells of the endometrium. In humans, the blastocyst begins to invade the endometrium at about the fifth or sixth day of development. **c.** A human blastocyst at 14 days after implantation. At this stage, the trophoblast cells have differentiated into syncytiotrophoblasts and cytotrophoblasts.

Implantation occurs during a short period known as the implantation window.

The attachment of the blastocyst to the endometrial epithelium occurs during the **implantation window**, the period when the uterus is receptive for implantation of the blastocyst. This short period results from a series of programmed actions of progesterone and estrogens on the endometrium. **Antiprogesterone drugs** such as mifepristone (RU-486) and its derivatives compete for the receptors in the endometrial epithelium, thus blocking hormone binding. The failure of progesterone to gain access to its receptors prevents implantation, thus effectively closing the window. In human, the implantation window begins on day 6 after the LH surge and is completed by day 10.

As contact is made with the uterine wall by the **trophoblastic cells** over the embryoblast pole, the trophoblast rapidly proliferates and begins to invade the endometrium. The invading **trophoblast** differentiates into the syncytiotrophoblast and the cytotrophoblast.

- The **cytotrophoblast** is a mitotically active inner cell layer producing cells that fuse with the syncytiotrophoblast, the outer erosive layer. The fusion of the cytotrophoblast with the overlying multinucleated syncytiotrophoblast may be triggered by programmed cell death (apoptosis).
- The **syncytiotrophoblast** is not mitotically active and consists of a multinucleate cytoplasmic mass; it actively invades the epithelium and underlying stroma of the endometrium.

Through the activity of the trophoblast, the blastocyst is entirely embedded within the endometrium on about the 11th day of development. (Further development of the syncytiotrophoblast and cytotrophoblast is described in the section on the placenta.)

The syncytiotrophoblast has well-developed Golgi complexes, abundant sER and rER, numerous mitochondria, and relatively large numbers of lipid droplets. These features are consistent with the secretion of progesterone, estrogens, hCG, and lactogens by this layer. Recent evidence indicates that cytotrophoblast cells may also be a source of steroid hormones and hCG.

After implantation, the endometrium undergoes decidualization.

During pregnancy, the portion of the **endometrium** that undergoes morphologic changes is called the **decidua** or **decidua graviditatis**. As its name implies, this layer is shed with the placenta at parturition. The decidua includes all but the deepest layer of the endometrium. During the **decidualization process**, which typically takes at least 8–10 days, the stromal cells differentiate into large, rounded **decidual cells** in response to the elevated progesterone levels (see page 935). The uterine glands enlarge and become more coiled during the early part of pregnancy and then become thin and flattened as the growing fetus fills the uterine lumen.

Three different regions of the decidua are identified by their relationship to the site of implantation (Fig. 23.20):

- The **decidua basalis** is the portion of the endometrium that underlies the implantation site.
- The **decidua capsularis** is a thin portion of endometrium that lies between the implantation site and the uterine lumen.
- The **decidua parietalis** includes the remaining endometrium of the uterus.

By the end of the third month of gestation, the fetus grows to the point that the overlying decidua capsularis fuses with the decidua parietalis of the opposite wall, thereby obliterating the uterine cavity.

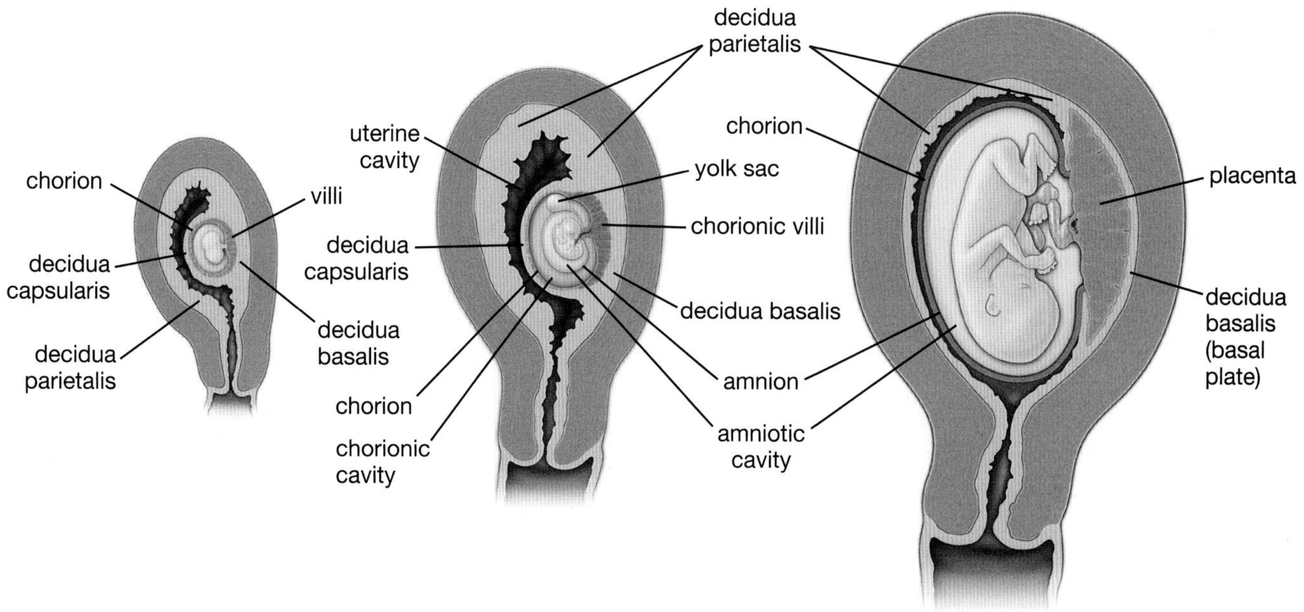

FIGURE 23.20. Development of the placenta. This schematic drawing shows growth of the uterus during human pregnancy and development of the placenta and its membranes. Note that there is a gradual obliteration of the uterine lumen and disappearance of the decidua capsularis as the definitive placenta is established. (Modified from Williams J. Placenta circumvallata. *Am J Obstet Gynecol.* 1927;13:1–16.)

By the 13th day of development, an extraembryonic space, the **chorionic cavity**, has been established (Fig. 23.19c). The cell layers that form the outer boundary of this cavity (i.e., the syncytiotrophoblast, cytotrophoblast, and extraembryonic somatic mesoderm) are collectively referred to as the **chorion**. The innermost membranes enveloping the embryo are called the **amnion** (see Fig. 23.20).

Cervix

The endometrium of the cervix differs from the rest of the uterus.

The **cervical mucosa** measures about 2–3 mm in thickness and differs dramatically from the rest of the uterine endometrium in that it contains large, branched glands (Fig. 23.21

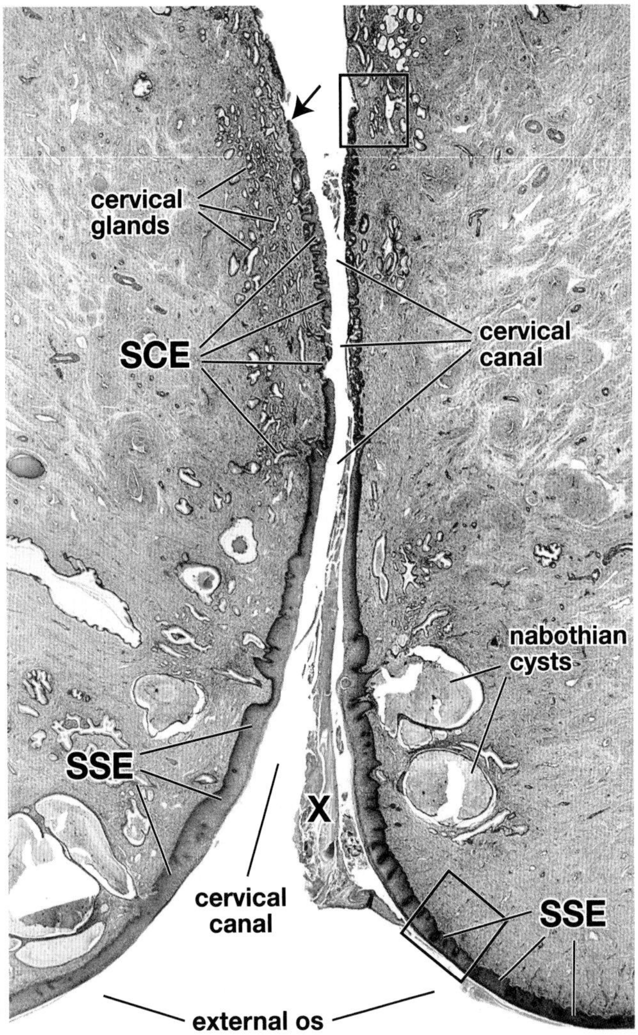

FIGURE 23.21. Photomicrograph of a human cervix. This hematoxylin and eosin (H&E)-stained specimen is from a postmenopausal female. Its lower portion projects into the upper vagina where an opening, the external os, leads to the uterus through the cervical canal. The surface of the cervix is covered by stratified squamous epithelium (*SSE*) that is continuous with the epithelial lining of the vagina. An abrupt transition from stratified squamous epithelium to simple columnar epithelium (*SCE*) occurs at the entry to the cervical canal. In this specimen, the stratified epithelium has extended into the canal, an event that occurs with aging. Mucus-secreting cervical glands are seen along the cervical canal. These are simple branched tubular glands that arise as invaginations of the epithelium lining the canal. Frequently, the glands develop into nabothian cysts as a result of retention of mucus secretion by blockage of the gland opening. The material marked by the *X* is mucus secreted from the cervical glands. ×10.

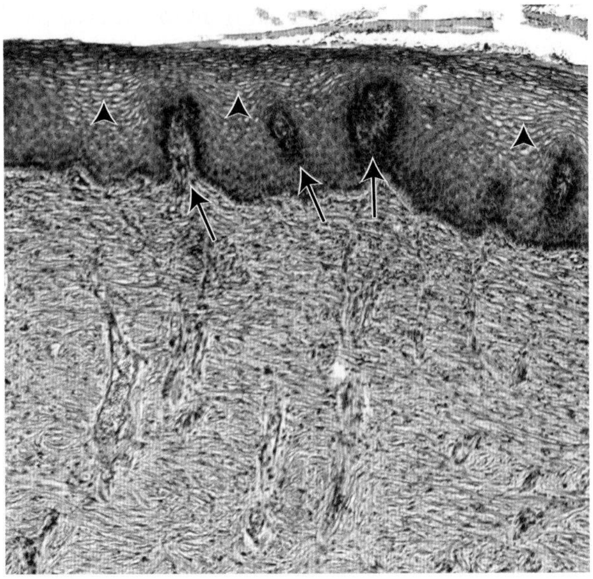

FIGURE 23.22. Stratified squamous epithelium of the ectocervix. The stratified squamous epithelium and underlying fibrous connective tissue within the *lower rectangle* in Figure 23.21 are shown here at higher magnification. The more mature epithelial cells have a clear cytoplasm (*arrowheads*), a reflection of their high glycogen content. Also, note the connective tissue papillae protruding into the epithelium (*arrows*). The bulk of the cervix is made up of dense, fibrous connective tissue with relatively little smooth muscle. ×120.

and Plate 23.7, page 968). It also lacks spiral arteries. The cervical mucosa undergoes little change in thickness during the menstrual cycle and is not sloughed during the period of menstruation. During each menstrual cycle, however, the **cervical glands** undergo important functional changes that are related to the transport of spermatozoa within the cervical canal. The amount and properties of the mucus secreted by the gland cells vary during the menstrual cycle under the influence of ovarian hormones. At midcycle, the amount of mucus produced increases 10-fold. This mucus is less viscous and appears to provide a more favorable environment for sperm migration. The cervical mucus at other times in the cycle restricts the passage of sperm into the uterus. Thus, hormonal mechanisms ensure that ovulation and changes in the cervical mucus are coordinated, thereby increasing the possibility that fertilization will occur if spermatozoa and the ovum arrive simultaneously at the site of fertilization in the uterine tube.

Blockage of the openings of the mucosal glands results in the retention of their secretions, leading to the formation of dilated cysts within the cervix called **nabothian cysts**. Nabothian cysts develop frequently but are clinically important only if numerous cysts produce marked enlargement of the cervix.

The transformation zone is the site of transition between vaginal stratified squamous epithelium and cervical simple columnar epithelium.

The portion of the cervix that projects into the vagina, the **vaginal part** or **ectocervix**, is covered with a stratified squamous epithelium (Fig. 23.22). An abrupt transition between this squamous epithelium and the mucus-secreting columnar epithelium of the **cervical canal**, the **endocervix**, occurs in the **transformation zone** that during reproductive age is located just outside the **external os** (Plate 23.7, page 968). Before puberty and after menopause, the transformation

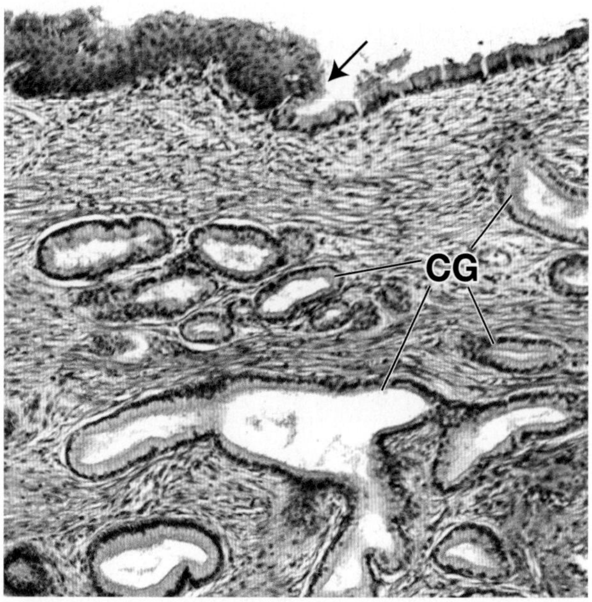

FIGURE 23.23. Transformation zone of the cervix. The site of the squamocolumnar junction from the *upper rectangle* in Figure 23.21 is shown here at higher magnification. Note the abrupt change from stratified squamous epithelium to simple columnar epithelium (*arrow*). Neoplastic changes leading to the development of cervical cancer most frequently begin in this transformation zone. Within the connective tissue are the branched, mucus-secreting cervical glands (*CG*) composed of a simple columnar epithelium that is continuous with the lining epithelium of the cervical canal. ×120.

zone resides in the cervical canal (Fig. 23.23). **Metaplastic changes** in this transformation zone constitute precancerous lesions of the cervix. Metaplasia *[Gr. change in form]* represents an adoptive and reversible response to persistent injury of the epithelium caused by chronic infection. It results from a reprogramming of epithelial stem cells that begin to differentiate into new cell lineage. Within the cervical canal (endocervix), it is manifested as a replacement of the simple columnar epithelium with fully mature stratified squamous epithelium (Fig. 23.24). The cervical epithelial cells are constantly exfoliated into the vagina. Samples of the cervical cells may be stained and examined for morphologic changes (**Papanicolaou [Pap] test**) or tested for the presence of high-risk strains of human papillomavirus (HPV), the leading cause of cervical cancer. These tests are used routinely to screen for precancerous and cancerous lesions of the cervix.

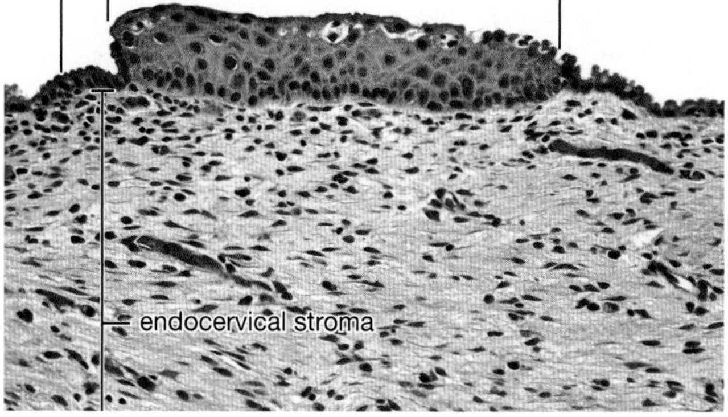

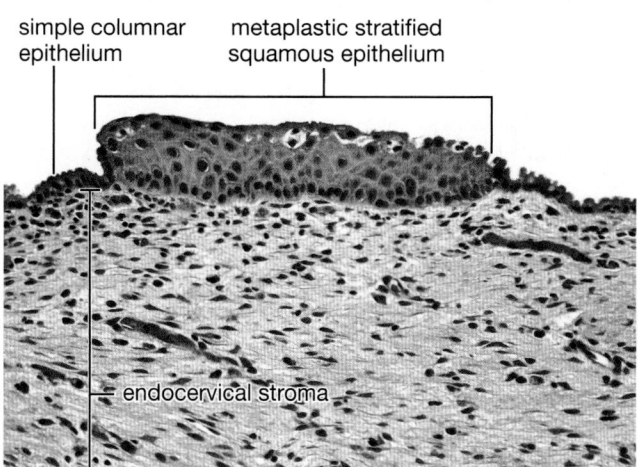

FIGURE 23.24. Metaplastic stratified squamous epithelium of the cervical canal. This photomicrograph shows an island of the fully mature stratified squamous epithelium surrounded by the simple columnar epithelium normally found in the cervical canal. ×450. (Courtesy of Dr. Fabiola Medeiros.)

■ PLACENTA

The developing fetus is maintained by the placenta, which develops from fetal and maternal tissues.

The placenta consists of a fetal portion, formed by the chorion, and a maternal portion, formed by the decidua basalis. The two parts are involved in physiologic exchange of substances between the maternal and fetal circulations.

The **uteroplacental circulatory system** begins to develop around day 9 after fertilization, with the development of vascular spaces called **trophoblastic lacunae** within the syncytiotrophoblast. Maternal sinusoids, which develop from capillaries of the maternal side, anastomose with the trophoblastic lacunae (Fig. 23.25). The differential pressure between the arterial and venous channels that communicate with the lacunae establishes directional flow from the arteries into the veins, thereby establishing a primitive uteroplacental circulation. Numerous pinocytotic vesicles present in the syncytiotrophoblast indicate the transfer of nutrients from the maternal vessels to the embryo.

Proliferation of the **cytotrophoblast**, growth of **chorionic mesoderm**, and blood vessel development successively give rise to the chorionic villi (Fig. 23.26). They undergo the following changes:

- **Primary chorionic villi** are formed by the rapidly proliferating cytotrophoblast. They send cords or masses of cells into the blood-filled trophoblastic lacunae within the syncytiotrophoblast (see Figs. 23.19b and 23.27). The primary villi appear between days 11 and 13 of development.
- **Secondary chorionic villi** are composed of a central core of mesenchyme surrounded by an inner layer of cytotrophoblast and an outer layer of syncytiotrophoblast (see Fig. 23.26). They develop at about day 16 when the primary chorionic villi become invaded by loose connective tissue from chorionic mesenchyme. The secondary villi cover the entire surface of the chorionic sac.
- **Tertiary chorionic villi** are formed by the end of the third week as the secondary villi become vascularized by blood vessels that have developed in their connective tissue cores (see Fig. 23.25b and Plate 23.9, page 972).

As the tertiary villi are forming, cytotrophoblastic cells in the villi continue to grow out through the syncytiotrophoblast. When they meet the maternal endometrium, they grow laterally and meet similar processes growing from neighboring villi. Thus, a thin layer of cytotrophoblastic cells called the **trophoblastic shell** is formed around the syncytiotrophoblast. The trophoblastic shell is interrupted only at sites where maternal vessels communicate with the intervillous spaces.

Chorionic villi continuously form out of the trophoblastic sprouts throughout pregnancy. The chorionic villi can remain either free (**floating villi**) in the intervillous space or grow into the maternal side of the placenta (basal plate) to form **main stem villi** or **anchoring villi**. Future growth

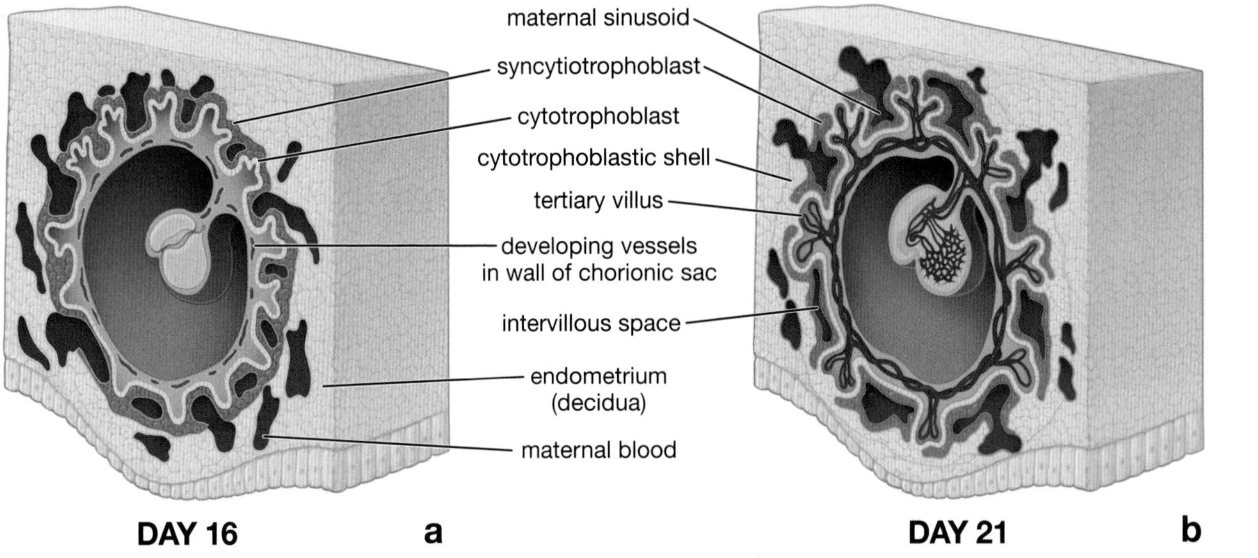

FIGURE 23.25. Schematic diagrams of sections through a developing human embryo. a. This drawing shows the chorionic sac and placenta at 16 days of development. **b.** The same embryo at 21 days of development. The diagrams illustrate the separation of the fetal and maternal blood vessels by the placental membrane, which is composed of the endothelium of the capillaries, mesenchyme, cytotrophoblast, and syncytiotrophoblast.

of the placenta is accomplished by interstitial growth of the trophoblastic shell. During pregnancy, the villi mature and become smaller in diameter. The layer of cytotrophoblast appears to be discontinuous, and in some areas, nuclei of the syncytiotrophoblast are gathered in clusters to form irregularly dispersed **syncytial knots** (see Fig. 23.26 and Plate 23.9, page 972). The number of syncytial knots increases with gestational age of the placenta and can be used to evaluate **villous maturity**. An increased number of syncytial knots is also associated with some pathologic conditions, such as **uteroplacental malperfusion**.

Several types of cells are recognized in the connective tissue stroma of the villi: mesenchymal cells, reticular cells, fibroblasts, myofibroblasts, smooth muscle cells, and **fetal placental antigen–presenting cells (placental macrophages)**, historically also known as **Hofbauer cells** (Plate 23.9, page 972). Fetal placental antigen–presenting cells are the specific villous macrophages of fetal origin that participate in placental innate immune reactions. In response to an antigen, they proliferate and upregulate specific surface receptors that recognize and bind to a variety of pathogens. Like other antigen-presenting cells, if stimulated, they increase the number of major histocompatibility complex II (MHC II) molecules on their surface. They are more common in the early placenta. The vacuoles in these cells contain lipids, glycosaminoglycans, and glycoproteins.

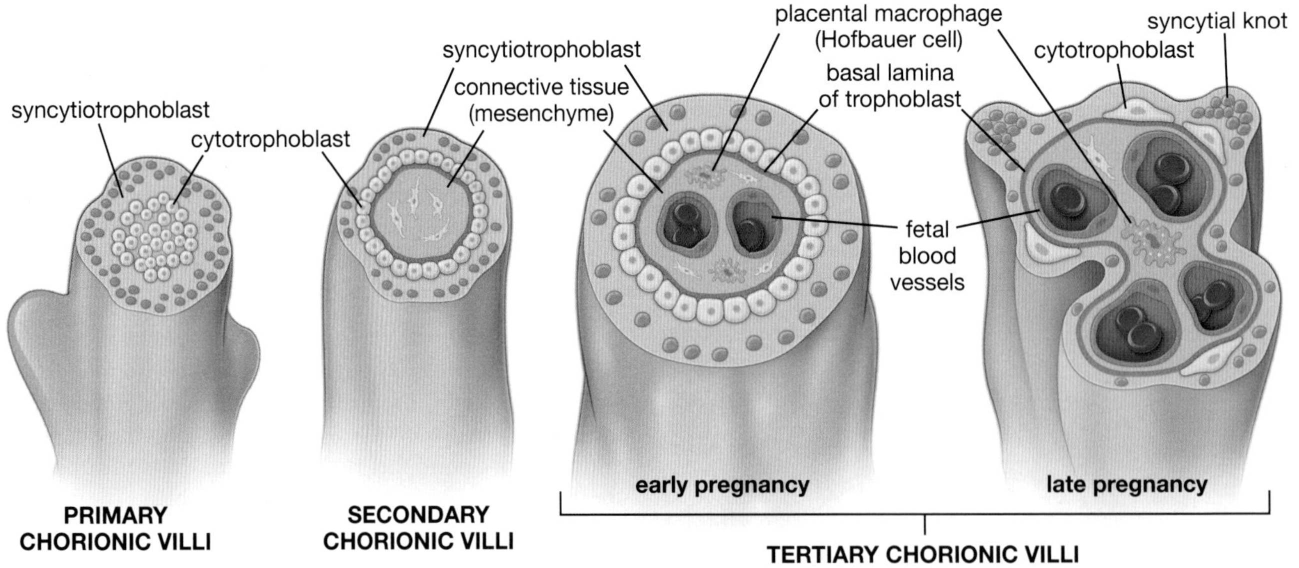

FIGURE 23.26. Schematic diagram of chorionic villi in various stages of development. This drawing shows the developmental stages of chorionic villi. Primary villi represent the first stage of development in which the syncytiotrophoblast and cytotrophoblast form finger-like extensions into the maternal decidua. In secondary chorionic villi, the extraembryonic connective tissue (mesenchyme) grows into the villi and is surrounded by a layer of cytotrophoblast. In tertiary chorionic villi, blood vessels and supportive cells differentiate within the mesenchymal core. In early pregnancy, villi are large and edematous with few blood vessels surrounded by many cells of connective tissue. They are covered by a thick layer of syncytiotrophoblast and a continuous layer of cytotrophoblast cells. In late pregnancy, the layer of cytotrophoblast appears to be discontinuous, and nuclei of the syncytiotrophoblast aggregate to form irregularly dispersed projections called *syncytial knots.* More fetal blood vessels are found in the connective tissue core, which becomes less cellular and contains fewer placental macrophages.

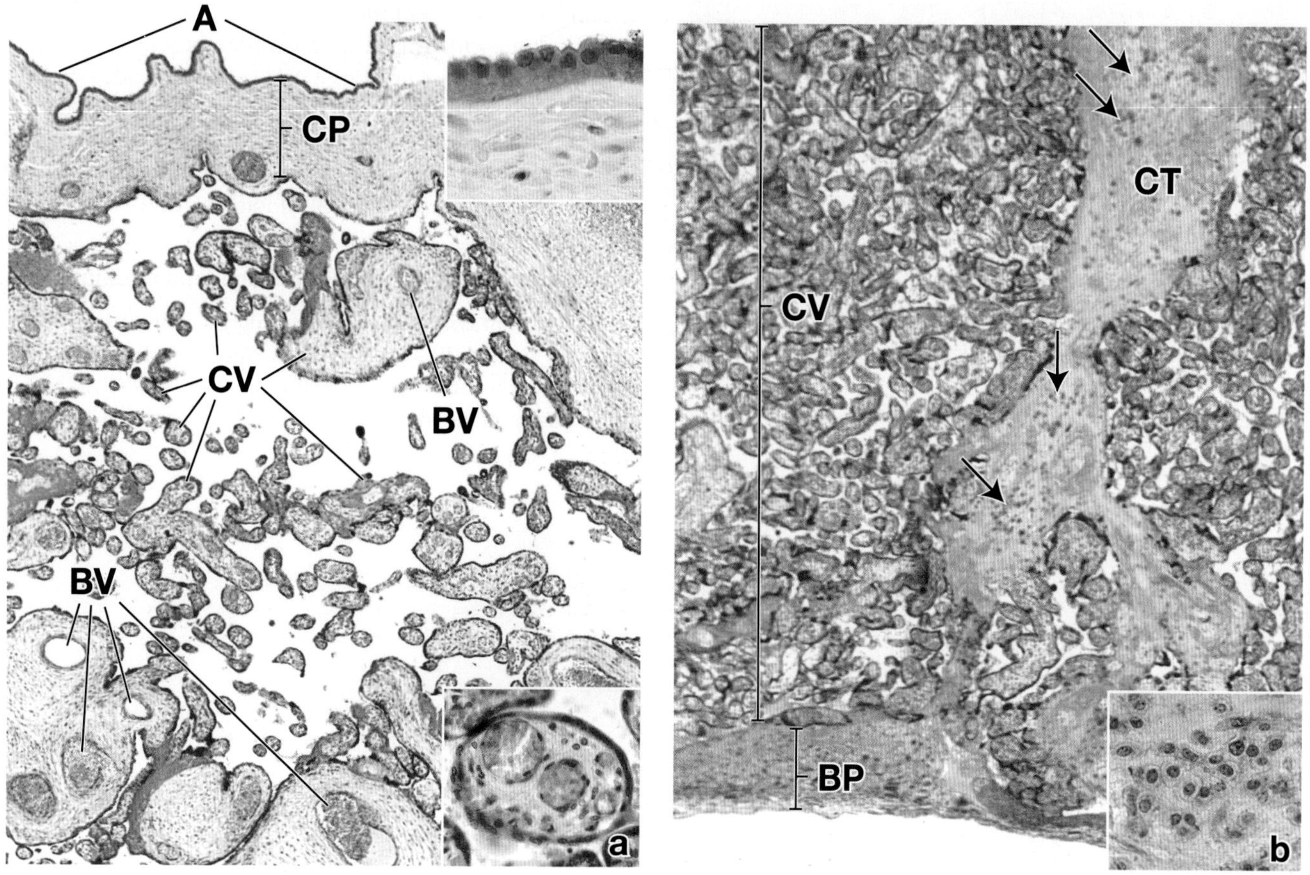

FIGURE 23.27. Photomicrographs of a human placenta. a. This hematoxylin and eosin (H&E)-stained specimen shows the amniotic surface (*A*), the chorionic plate (*CP*), and, below, the various-sized profiles of the chorionic villi (*CV*). These villi emerge from the chorionic plate as large stem villi and branch into increasingly smaller villi. Blood vessels (*BV*) are evident in the larger villi. The smallest villi contain capillaries where exchange takes place. ×60. **Upper inset.** This higher magnification shows the simple cuboidal epithelium of the amnion and the underlying connective tissue. ×200. **Lower inset.** This higher magnification shows a cross-sectioned villus containing several larger blood vessels and its thin surface syncytiotrophoblast layer. ×200. **b.** This H&E-stained specimen shows the maternal side of the placenta. The basal plate (*BP*), the part of the uterus to which some of the chorionic villi (*CV*) anchor, is seen at the *bottom* of the micrograph. Also evident is a stromal connective tissue (*CT*) component, part of the basal plate, to which many of the chorionic villi are also attached. Within the basal plate and the connective tissue stroma are clusters of cells, the decidual cells (*arrows*), which arose from connective tissue cells. ×60. **Inset.** Decidual cells seen at higher magnification. ×200.

Studies of **HIV-infected placentas** indicate that HIV is primarily localized within the fetal placental antigen-presenting cells and in the syncytiotrophoblast.

Early in development, the blood vessels of the villi become connected with vessels from the embryo.

Blood begins to circulate through the embryonic cardiovascular system and the villi at about 21 days. The intervillous spaces provide the site for exchange of nutrients, metabolic products and intermediates, and wastes between the maternal and fetal circulatory systems.

During the first 8 weeks, villi cover the entire chorionic surface, but as growth continues, villi on the decidua capsularis begin to degenerate, producing a smooth, relatively avascular surface called the **chorion laeve**. The villi adjacent to the decidua basalis rapidly increase in size and number and become highly branched. This region of the chorion, which is the fetal component of the placenta, is called the **chorion frondosum** or **villous chorion**. The layer of the placenta from which the villi project is called the **chorionic plate** (Plate 23.8, page 970).

During the period of rapid growth of the chorion frondosum, at about the fourth to fifth month of gestation, the fetal part of the placenta is divided by the **placental (decidual) septa** into 15–25 areas called **cotyledons**. Wedge-like placental septa form the boundaries of the cotyledons, and because they do not fuse with the chorionic plate, maternal blood can circulate easily between them. Cotyledons are visible as the bulging areas on the maternal side of the basal plate.

The **decidua basalis** forms a compact layer that is the maternal component of the placenta (see Fig. 23.27). The **basal plate**, the outer part of the placenta that is in contact with the uterine wall, consists of embryonic tissues (trophoblastic shell containing a thin layer of syncytiotrophoblast and cytotrophoblast) and maternal tissues (decidua basalis). Vessels within this part of the endometrium supply blood to the intervillous spaces. With rare exceptions, fetal blood and maternal blood do not mix.

Fetal and maternal blood are separated by the placental barrier.

Separation of the fetal and maternal blood, referred to as the **placental barrier**, is maintained primarily by the layers of fetal tissue (Fig. 23.28). Starting at the fourth month, these layers become very thin to facilitate the exchange of products across the placental barrier. The thinning of the wall of the villus is caused in part by surface and volume expansion of the villi as well as by the degeneration of the inner cytotrophoblast layer (see Fig. 23.27). However, although the cytotrophoblast layer indeed becomes much thinner, it does not become discontinuous.

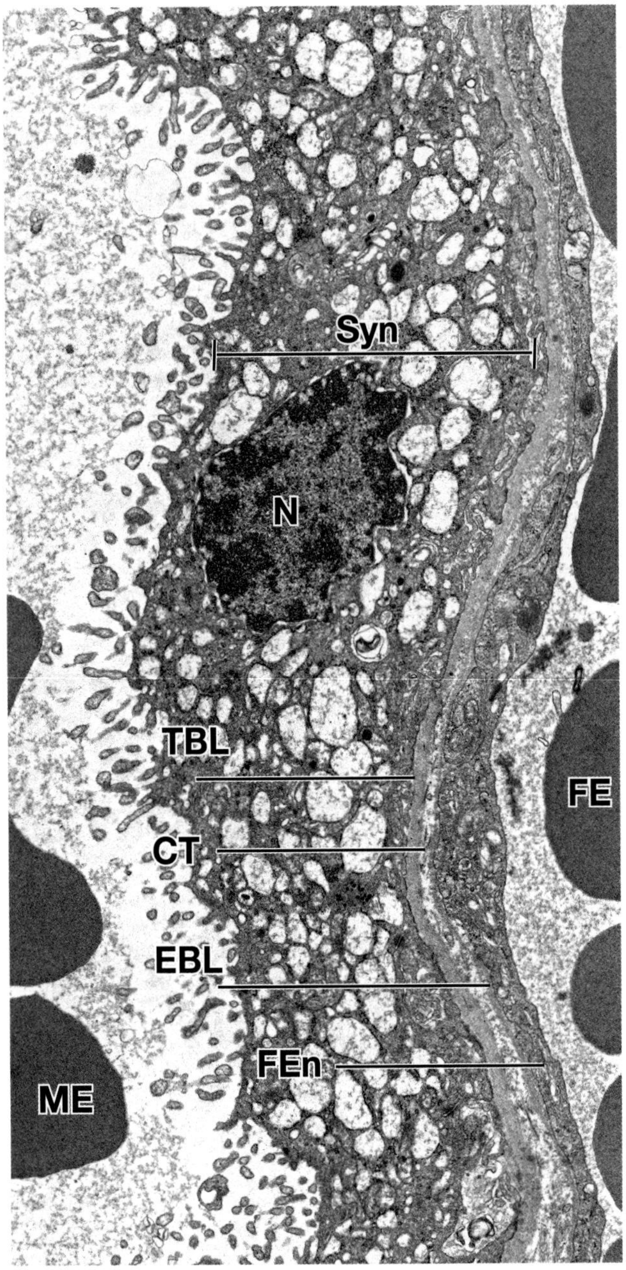

FIGURE 23.28. Human placental barrier in the third trimester of pregnancy. This high-magnification electron micrograph shows the thinnest layer of a fully developed placental barrier (section does not include cytotrophoblast cells that form a thin [or discontinuous] layer in the human placenta). The lumen of intervillous space containing maternal erythrocytes (*ME*) (*to the left*) is separated from the fetal capillary space containing fetal erythrocytes (*FE*) (*to the right*). The intervillous space is lined by the multinucleated syncytiotrophoblast (*Syn*). Its surface contains microvilli projecting into maternal blood space. The cytoplasm of the syncytiotrophoblast contains multiple nuclei (*N*) and has an abundance of transport vesicles, rER, sER, mitochondria, and occasional lipid droplets. The syncytiotrophoblast rests on the basal lamina (*TBL*), which is separated by a thin layer of the connective tissue (*CT*) from the basal lamina (*EBL*) of the fetal endothelial cells (*FEn*). ×11,000. *rER*, rough-surfaced endoplasmic reticulum; *sER*, smooth-surfaced endoplasmic reticulum. (Courtesy of Dr. Holger Jastrow.)

At its thinnest, the **placental barrier consists** of

- syncytiotrophoblast,
- thin (or discontinuous) inner cytotrophoblast layer,
- basal lamina of the trophoblast,
- connective (mesenchymal) tissue of the villus,
- basal lamina of the endothelium, and
- endothelium of the fetal placental capillary in the tertiary villus.

This barrier bears a strong resemblance to the air–blood barrier of the lung, with which it has an important parallel function, namely, the exchange of oxygen and carbon dioxide—in this case, between the maternal blood and the fetal blood. It also resembles the air–blood barrier by having a particular type of macrophage in its connective tissue—in this instance, the fetal placental antigen–presenting cells (Hofbauer cell).

The placenta is the site of exchange of gases and metabolites between the maternal and fetal circulation.

Fetal blood enters the placenta through a pair of **umbilical arteries** (Fig. 23.29). As they pass into the placenta, these arteries branch into several radially disposed vessels that give numerous branches in the chorionic plate. Branches from these

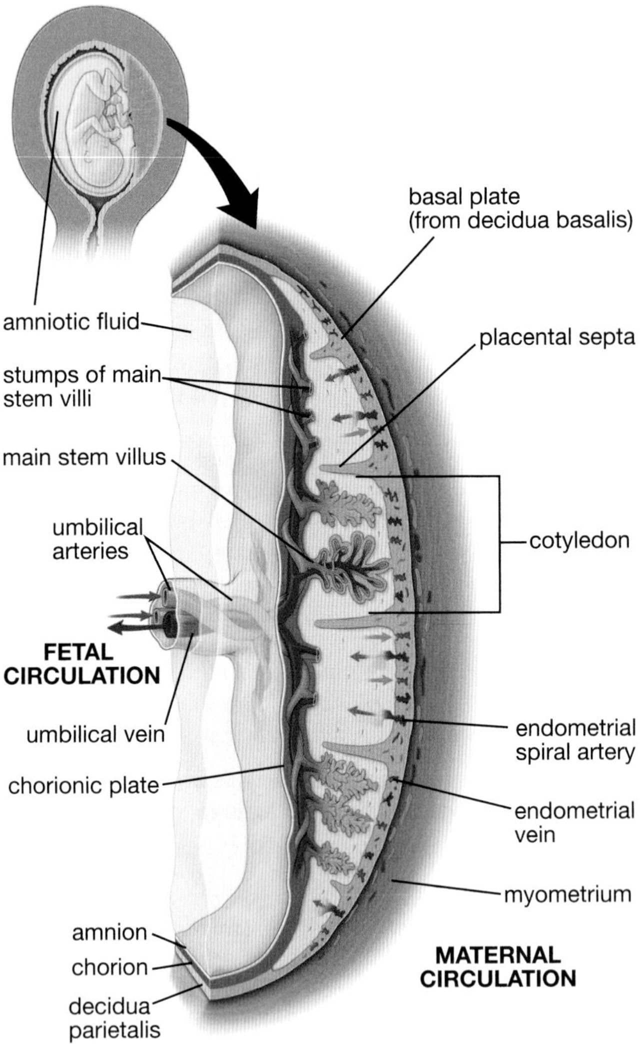

FIGURE 23.29. Schematic diagram of mature human placenta. The sagittal section of the uterus (*above*) with the developing embryo shows the most common location of the placenta. The mature placenta (*below*) is divided into cotyledons by placental septa that are formed by outgrowths of the decidua basalis. Maternal blood enters the placenta through numerous endometrial spiral arteries that penetrate the basal plate. As the blood enters the cotyledon, it is directed deep into the intervillous spaces (*red arrows*). It then passes over the surface of the villi, where exchange of gases and metabolic products occurs. The maternal blood finally leaves the intervillous space (*blue arrows*) through endometrial veins. The fetal blood enters the placenta through the umbilical arteries that divide into a series of radially disposed arteries within the chorionic plate. Branches from the vessels pass into the main stem villi and there form extensive capillary networks. The veins within the villi then carry the blood back through a system of veins that parallels that of the fetal arteries.

vessels pass into the villi, forming extensive capillary networks in close association with the intervillous spaces. Gases and metabolic products are exchanged across the thin fetal layers that separate the two bloodstreams at this level. Antibodies can also cross this layer and enter the fetal circulation to provide passive immunity against a variety of infectious agents—for example, those of diphtheria, smallpox, and measles. Fetal blood returns through a system of veins that parallel the arteries, except that they converge on a single **umbilical vein**.

Maternal blood is supplied to the placenta through 80–100 spiral endometrial arteries that penetrate the basal plate. Blood from these spiral arteries flows into the base of the intervillous spaces, which contain about 150 mL of maternal blood that is exchanged 3–4 times per minute. The blood pressure in the spiral arteries is much higher than that in the intervillous spaces. As blood is injected into these spaces at each pulse, it is directed deep into the spaces. As the pressure decreases, the blood flows back over the surfaces of the villi and eventually enters endometrial veins also located in the base of the spaces.

Exchange of gases and metabolic products occurs as the blood passes over the villi. Normally, water, carbon dioxide, metabolic waste products, and hormones are transferred from the fetal blood to the maternal blood; water, oxygen, metabolites, electrolytes, vitamins, hormones, and some antibodies pass in the opposite direction. The placental barrier does not exclude many potentially dangerous agents, such as alcohol, nicotine, viruses, drugs, exogenous hormones, and heavy metals. Therefore, during pregnancy, exposure to or ingestion of such agents should be avoided to reduce the risk of injury to the embryo or fetus.

Before the establishment of blood flow through the placenta, the growth of the embryo is supported in part by metabolic products that are synthesized by or transported through the trophoblast. The syncytiotrophoblast synthesizes glycogen, cholesterol, and fatty acids as well as other nutrients used by the embryo.

The placenta is a major endocrine organ producing steroid and protein hormones.

The **placenta** also functions as an **endocrine organ**, producing steroid and peptide hormones as well as prostaglandins that play an important role in the onset of labor. Immunocytochemical studies indicate that the **syncytiotrophoblast** is the site of synthesis of these hormones. Hormones produced by syncytiotrophoblast are secreted directly into the maternal blood surrounding the placental villi.

The **steroid hormones** progesterone and estrogen have essential roles in the maintenance of pregnancy. As pregnancy proceeds, the placenta takes over the major role in the secretion of these steroids from the corpus luteum. The placenta produces enough progesterone by the end of the eighth week to maintain pregnancy if the corpus luteum is surgically removed or fails to function. In the production of placental estrogen, the fetal adrenal cortex plays an essential role, providing the precursors needed for estrogen synthesis. Because the placenta lacks the enzymes needed for the production of estrogen precursors, a cooperative **fetoplacental (endocrine) unit** is established. Clinically, monitoring of estrogen production during pregnancy can be used as an **index of fetal development** in certain situations.

The following **peptide hormones** are secreted by the placenta:

- **Human chorionic gonadotropin (hCG)** is required for implantation and maintenance of the pregnancy. Its synthesis begins around day 6 after fertilization, even before the syncytiotrophoblast is formed. hCG exhibits extensive (about 85%) sequence homology to LH, which is required for ovulation and maintenance of the corpus luteum during the menstrual cycle. Similar to the function of LH during the menstrual cycle, hCG maintains the corpus luteum during early pregnancy. hCG also possesses marked homology to thyroid-stimulating hormone (TSH),

FOLDER 23.4

CLINICAL CORRELATION: THE PLACENTA

The placenta is a temporary organ made by the body only during pregnancy. The mature **placenta** measures about 15–20 cm in diameter and 2–3 cm in thickness, covers 25%–30% of the uterine surface, and weighs 500–600 g at term. The surface area of the villi of human placenta is estimated to be about 10 m^2. The microvilli on the syncytiotrophoblast increase the effective area for metabolic exchange to >90 m^2. After childbirth, the uterus continues to contract, reducing the luminal surface and inducing placental separation from the uterine wall. The entire fetal portion of the placenta, fetal membranes, and the intervening projections of decidual tissue are released. During uncomplicated labor, the placenta separates from the uterine wall and is delivered ~30 minutes after birth.

One of the most severe complications of labor results from **abnormal placentation** (abnormal attachment of the placenta on uterine wall). If decidual tissue during implantation is disrupted, the placenta invades deep into the uterine wall. This may cause one of the three clinical conditions: placenta accreta, placenta increta, or placenta percreta. Classification depends on the severity and deepness of the placental attachment. **Placenta accreta**, accounting for ~75% of all cases, occurs when the placenta attaches too deeply into the uterine wall but does not penetrate the myometrium. **Placenta increta** (about 15% of all cases) occurs when the placental villi penetrate deep into the muscular layer of the myometrium. In the remaining 10% of all cases, **placenta percreta** penetrates through the entire uterine wall and attaches to another organ, such as the bladder, rectum, intestines, or large blood vessels. It is the most serious complication of placentation and may cause rupture of the uterus and other complications related to its attachment. A retained abnormal placenta or placental fragments may cause massive postpartum bleeding and need to be manually removed. Placenta increta and percreta may need to be treated by emergency hysterectomy.

After physiologic delivery of the placenta, the endometrial glands and stroma of the decidua basalis regenerate. Endometrial regeneration is completed by the end of the third week postpartum, except at the placental site, where regeneration usually extends for another 3 weeks. During the first week after delivery, remnants of the decidua are shed and constitute the red-brown uterine discharge known as **lochia rubra.**

which may account for **hyperthyroidism in pregnancy** by stimulating the maternal thyroid gland to increase the secretion of tetraiodothyronine (T_4). Measurement of hCG is used to detect early pregnancy and assess pregnancy viability. Two other clinical conditions that increase the blood levels of hCG include **trophoblastic diseases** and **ectopic pregnancies**.

- **Human chorionic somatomammotropin (hCS)**, also known as **human placental lactogen (hPL)**, is closely related to human growth hormone. Synthesized in the syncytiotrophoblast, it promotes general growth, regulates glucose metabolism, and stimulates mammary duct proliferation in the maternal breast. The effects of hCS on maternal metabolism are significant, but the role of this hormone in fetal development remains unknown.
- **IGF-I** and **IGF-II** are produced by and stimulate proliferation and differentiation of the cytotrophoblast.
- **Endothelial growth factor (EGF)** exhibits an age-dependent dual action on the early placenta. In the 4- to 5-week-old placenta, EGF is synthesized by the cytotrophoblast and stimulates proliferation of the trophoblast. In the 6- to 12-week-old placenta, synthesis of EGF is shifted to the syncytiotrophoblast; it then stimulates and maintains the function of the differentiated trophoblast.
- **Relaxin** is synthesized by decidual cells and is involved in the "softening" of the cervix and the pelvic ligaments in preparation for parturition.
- **Leptin** is synthesized by the syncytiotrophoblast, particularly during the last month of gestation. Leptin appears to regulate maternal nutrient storage to the nutrient requirements of the fetus. It is also involved in transporting nutrients across the placental barrier from the mother to the fetus.
- **Other growth factors** stimulate cytotrophoblastic growth (e.g., fibroblast growth factor [FGF], colony-stimulating factor [CSF-1], platelet-derived growth factor, and interleukins [IL-1 and IL-3]) or inhibit trophoblast growth and proliferation (e.g., tumor necrosis factor).

■ VAGINA

The vagina is a fibromuscular tube that joins internal reproductive organs to the external environment.

The **vagina** is a fibromuscular sheath extending from the cervix to the vestibule, which is the area between the labia minora. The opening into the vagina may be surrounded by the **hymen**, folds of mucous membrane extending into the vaginal lumen. The hymen or its remnants are derived from the endodermal membrane that separated the developing vagina from the cavity of the definitive urogenital sinus in the embryo.

The **vaginal wall** (Fig. 23.30) consists of the following:

- An inner **mucosal layer** has numerous transverse folds or rugae (see Fig. 23.1) and is lined with stratified squamous epithelium (Fig. 23.31). Connective tissue papillae from the underlying lamina propria project into the epithelial layer. In humans and other primates, keratohyalin granules may be present in the epithelial cells, but under normal conditions, keratinization does not occur. Therefore, nuclei can be seen in epithelial cells throughout the thickness of the epithelium.

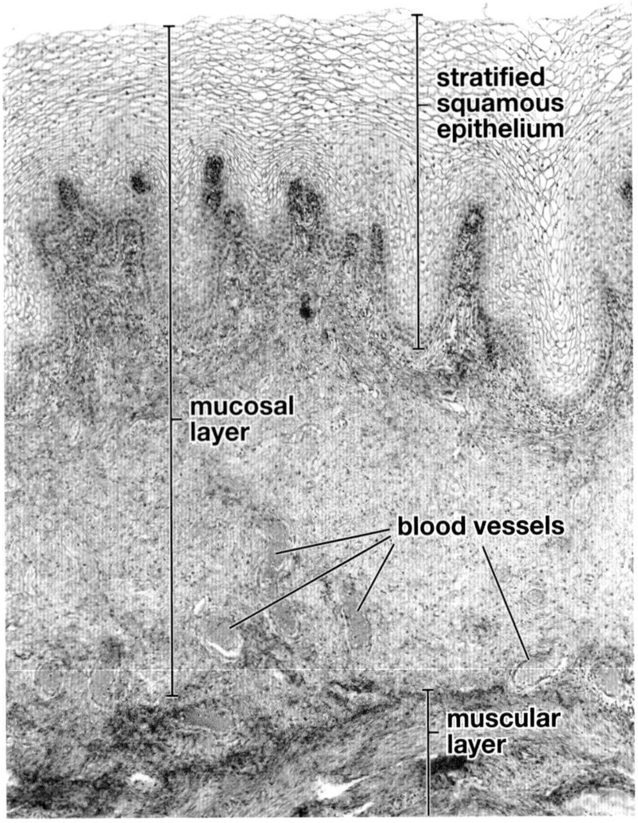

FIGURE 23.30. Photomicrograph of a human vagina. This low-magnification hematoxylin and eosin (H&E)-stained specimen of the vaginal wall shows two of three layers of the vagina: the mucosal layer and the muscular layer (the outer layer, the adventitia, is not included). The mucosal layer consists of a stratified squamous epithelium and the underlying connective tissue. The epithelial–connective tissue boundary is typically very irregular, with prominent papillae projecting into the undersurface of the epithelium. The muscular layer is seen only in part; it consists of irregularly arranged bundles of smooth muscle cells. Also, the deep region of the connective tissue contains a rich supply of blood vessels that supply the various layers of the vaginal wall. ×40.

- An intermediate **muscular layer** is organized into two sometimes indistinct, intermingling smooth muscle layers, an outer longitudinal layer and an inner circular layer. The outer layer is continuous with the corresponding layer in the uterus and is much thicker than the inner layer. Striated muscle fibers of the bulbospongiosus muscle are present at the vaginal opening (Plate 23.10, page 974).
- An outer **adventitial layer** is organized into an inner dense connective tissue layer adjacent to the muscularis and an outer loose connective tissue layer that blends with the adventitia of the surrounding structures. The inner layer contains numerous elastic fibers that contribute to the elasticity and strength of the vaginal wall. The outer layer contains numerous blood and lymphatic vessels and nerves.

The vagina possesses a stratified, squamous nonkeratinized epithelium and lacks glands.

The lumen of the vagina is lined by **stratified squamous, nonkeratinized epithelium**. Its surface is lubricated mainly by mucus produced by the cervical glands. The greater and lesser vestibular glands located in the wall of the vaginal vestibule produce additional mucus that lubricates the vagina. Glands are not present in the wall of the vagina. The epithelium of the vagina undergoes **cyclic changes** during the menstrual cycle. Under the influence of estrogens, during the follicular phase, the epithelial cells synthesize and

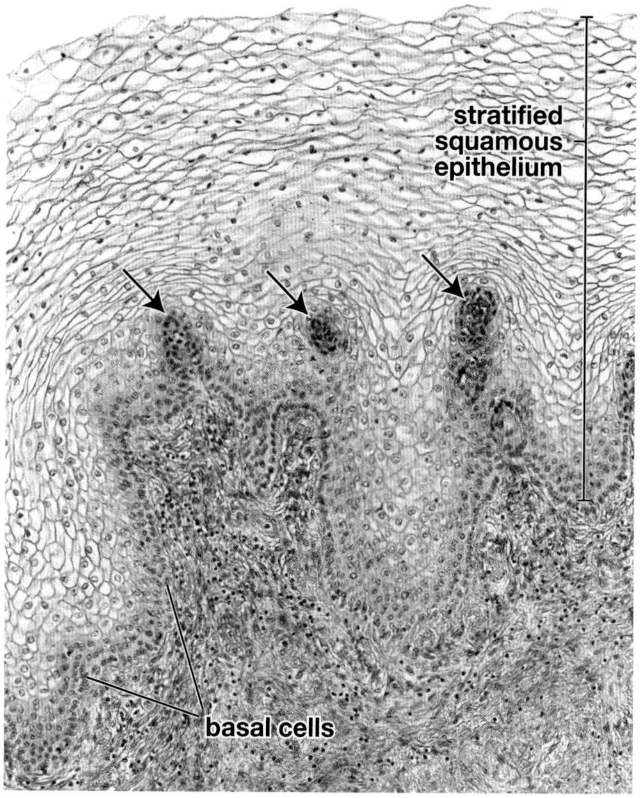

FIGURE 23.31. Photomicrograph of the vaginal mucosa. This micrograph, a higher magnification of Figure 23.30, shows the stratified squamous epithelium and mature cells with small pyknotic nuclei. Note a single layer of basal cells and two or three layers of cells undergoing differentiation (with eosinophilic cytoplasm). Projections of the connective tissue papillae into the epithelium give the connective tissue–epithelial junction an uneven appearance. The tips of these projections often appear as isolated structures surrounded by epithelium (*arrows*). ×180.

accumulate glycogen as they migrate toward the surface. Cells are continuously desquamated, but near or during the menstrual phase, the superficial layer of the vaginal epithelium may be shed.

The **lamina propria** exhibits two distinct regions. The outer region immediately below the epithelium is a highly cellular loose connective tissue. The deeper region, adjacent to the muscular layer, is denser and may be considered a submucosa. The deeper region contains many thin-walled veins that simulate erectile tissue during sexual arousal. Numerous elastic fibers are present immediately below the epithelium, and some of the fibers extend into the muscular layer. Many lymphocytes and leukocytes (particularly neutrophils) are found in the lamina propria and migrate into the epithelium. Solitary lymphatic nodules may also be present. The number of lymphocytes and leukocytes in the mucosa and vaginal lumen dramatically increases around the time of menstrual flow. The vagina has few general sensory nerve endings. The sensory nerve endings that are more plentiful in the lower third of the vagina are probably associated primarily with pain and stretch sensations.

■ EXTERNAL GENITALIA

The **female external genitalia** consist of the structures located within the anterior (urogenital) triangle of the female perineum. These structures are collectively referred to as the **vulva** [*Lat., volva, womb, female sexual organ; Lat., volvere, to turn, twist, roll, revolve, wrap*]. As the etymology of the word "vulva" implies, this region appears to be wrapped by skin folds. Structures included in the vulva consist of the **mons pubis**, **labia majora**, **labia minora**, **clitoral complex**, **vestibule** and **opening of the vagina**, **hymen** (or hymenal caruncles after it is ruptured), and **external urethral orifice** (Fig. 23.32). The vulva and its components extend from the mons pubis anteriorly to the **perineal body** posteriorly, which is a fibromuscular structure located in the midline of the perineum (anterior to the anus).

Mons Pubis

Mons pubis is the rounded prominence over the pubic symphysis.

The **mons pubis** is the rounded prominence over the pubic symphysis formed by an accumulation of subcutaneous **adipose tissue**. The mons pubis becomes more prominent with the onset of puberty. Hair in the pubic area exhibits a characteristic growth pattern during puberty that can be used to evaluate the developmental stages of external genitalia. **Tanner staging**, also known as sexual maturity rating (SMR), is an objective system to track the development of secondary sex characteristics during puberty. **Pubic hair** follicle depth in the mons pubis is the greatest compared with other parts of the vulva. The skin in this area is rich in **sebaceous** and **apocrine glands** that secret pheromone-like chemicals. In addition, the skin of the mons pubis contains an abundance of **nerve endings**, including Meissner and Merkel corpuscles, free nerve endings, and Pacinian corpuscles.

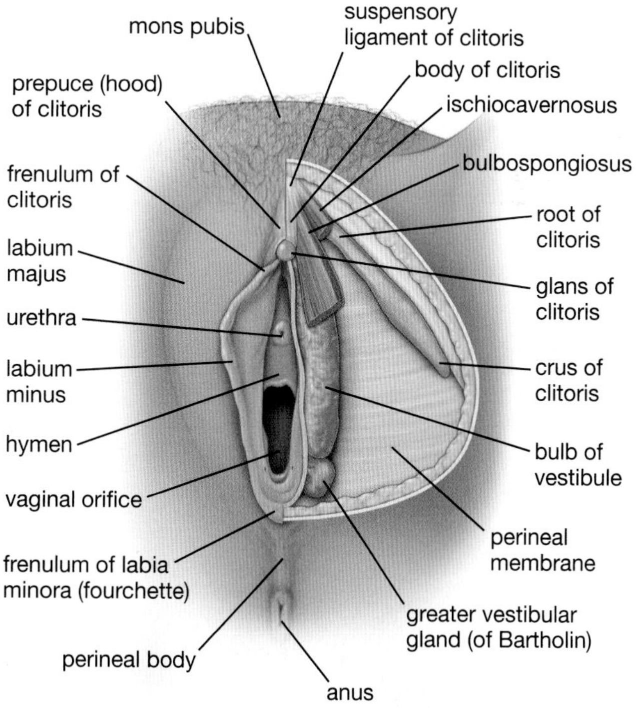

FIGURE 23.32. Schematic diagram illustrating the components of the female external genitalia (vulva). The left side of the vulva shows intact structures that consist of the mons pubis, labium majus, labium minus, glans of the clitoris with associated prepuce and frenulum, vestibule and opening of the vagina, hymen, and external urethral orifice. The right side of the vulva is dissected and shows structures after the removal of skin and superficial fascia. Note the deep structures of the clitoral complex (body, crus of the clitoris, and the bulb of vestibule). The major vestibular (of Bartholin) gland is in close proximity to the distal ends of the bulbs of the vestibule.

Labia Majora and Labia Minora

The labia majora and labia minora represent two folds of skin that form the lateral boundaries of the vestibule of the vagina.

As mentioned earlier, during clinical examination, the vulva appears to be wrapped by two paired skin folds called the **labia majora** and **labia minora**. The labia majora and labia minora develop around cloacal membrane from the proliferating mesenchyme that forms the cloacal folds. These folds unite in the cranial portion to produce the **genital tubercle** (future clitoris). With the division of the cloaca into urogenital sinus and anorectal canal, the cloacal folds are likewise subdivided into **urogenital folds** and anal folds. At the same time, **labioscrotal swellings** develop on both sides of the urogenital folds. Labioscrotal swellings in the female embryo develop into labia majora, and the urogenital folds do not fuse (as they do in the male embryo) and instead develop into the labia minora that border urogenital cleft (the vertical fissure of the vulva that develops into the vestibule of vagina). The development of external genitalia is a complex process driven by the sequential expression of regulatory **Wnt genes** encoding growth factors, especially **fibroblast growth factor (FGF)**.

- The **labia majora** [*sing. labium majus*] are two prominent longitudinal folds of skin that extend from the mons pubis anteriorly and to the perineal body posteriorly. The anterior parts of the labia majora unite beneath the mons pubis to form the **anterior labial commissure**. The posterior parts of the labia majora gradually merge with the surrounding skin of the perineum at their **posterior labial commissure** (see Fig. 23.32). The labia majora form the outer lateral boundaries of the urogenital cleft and are separated by the interlabial sulci from the labia minora. The size and contour of the labia are related to the amount of underlying adipose tissue deposits. During puberty, the labia majora increase in size, and after menopause, the labia atrophy due to decreased estrogen and loss of adipose tissue.

The skin of the labia majora is covered by **stratified squamous keratinized epithelium**. Sebaceous, eccrine, and apocrine sweat glands are present on both surfaces. The **outer surface** of the labium majus is darker than the inner surface and, like that of the mons pubis, has deeply imbedded **hair follicles** (Fig. 23.33a). Sebaceous glands associated with hair follicles are prominent, and they discharge their holocrine secretion into pilosebaceous canals. An abundance of apocrine sweat glands in the skin of labia majora discharge their secretion directly into the hair follicles (Fig 23.33b). In addition to sebaceous and apocrine sweat glands, the labia majora have many eccrine sweat glands. The thin skin of the **inner surface** is smooth and devoid of hair. An abundance of **sebaceous glands** is found on the inner surface of labia majora. Their ducts open directly on the surface of the epithelium (Fig. 23.34). The skin of the labia majora is rich in **sensory receptors**, including Markel and Meissner corpuscles for touch, Ruffini corpuscles for stretch and torque, Pacinian corpuscles for pressure, and free nerve endings for pain. Below the skin surface, the labia majora contain a thin layer of smooth muscle (dartos tunic) resembling the dartos muscle of the scrotum (see Fig. 23.33a) and a large amount of subcutaneous adipose tissue. The **bulbs of the vestibule** lie deep into the adipose tissue beneath the labia majora (page 942). They are homologous to the bulb of the penis in males and represent erectile tissue. They are covered by the bulbospongiosus muscle, a striated muscle that belongs to superficial muscles of the perineum.

The oval **major vestibular (Bartholin) glands** are in close proximity to the distal ends of the bulbs of the vestibule. This paired tubuloalveolar gland corresponds to the male bulbourethral (Cowper glands). The secretory acini are lined by simple columnar cells that produce mucus secretions (Fig. 23.35) that lubricate the vestibulum and distal end of the vagina during sexual intercourse. The basal domain of secretory acini is ensheathed by myoepithelial cells. The secretion of the gland is discharged into the long (~2.5 cm) **Bartholin gland duct** that opens into the 4 o'clock and 8 o'clock positions (posterior lateral aspect) of the vestibule of the vagina. The epithelium of the duct transitions from simple cuboidal (near the acini) to stratified cuboidal and stratified

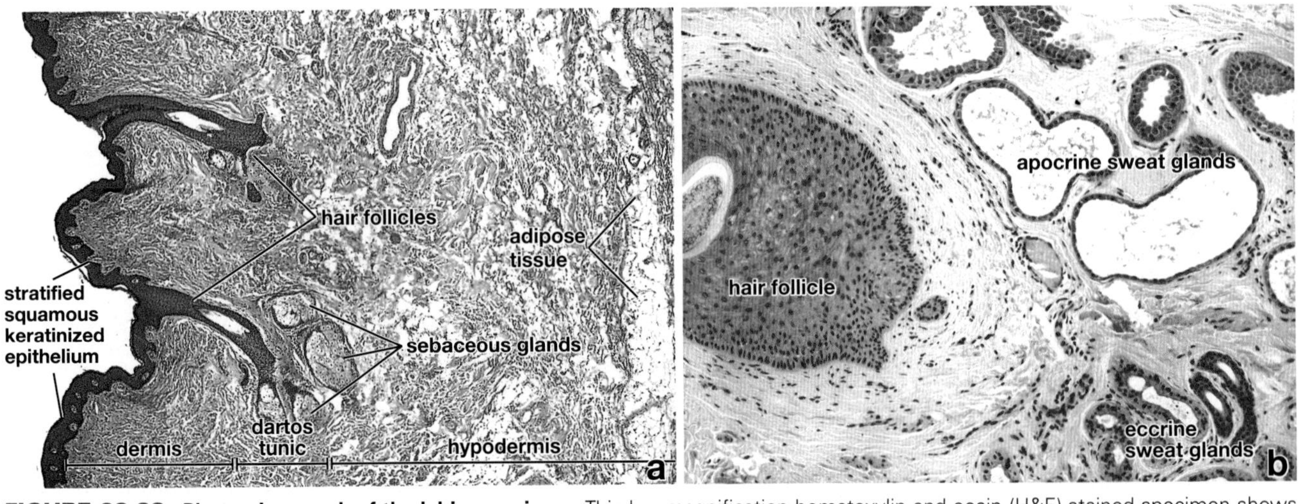

FIGURE 23.33. Photomicrograph of the labium majus. a. This low-magnification hematoxylin and eosin (H&E)-stained specimen shows tissue excised from the midportion of the outer surface of the labium majus. This surface shows the stratified squamous keratinized epithelium with two deeply embedded hair follicles. Sebaceous glands associated with the hair follicles are prominent, and they discharge their holocrine secretion into pilosebaceous canals. Below the skin surface, the labia majora contain a thin layer of smooth muscle resembling the dartos muscle of the scrotum. At this low magnification, dispersed smooth muscles bundle are difficult to identify in this layer. Note accumulations of subcutaneous adipose tissue in the hypodermis. ×25. **b.** In addition to sebaceous glands, the labia majora have many eccrine sweat glands and an abundance of apocrine sweat glands that discharge their secretion directly into the hair follicles. ×260. (Reprinted with permission from Hanley KZ. Vulva. In: Mills SM, ed. *Histology for Pathologists*. Wolters Kluwer; 2020:1031–1046.)

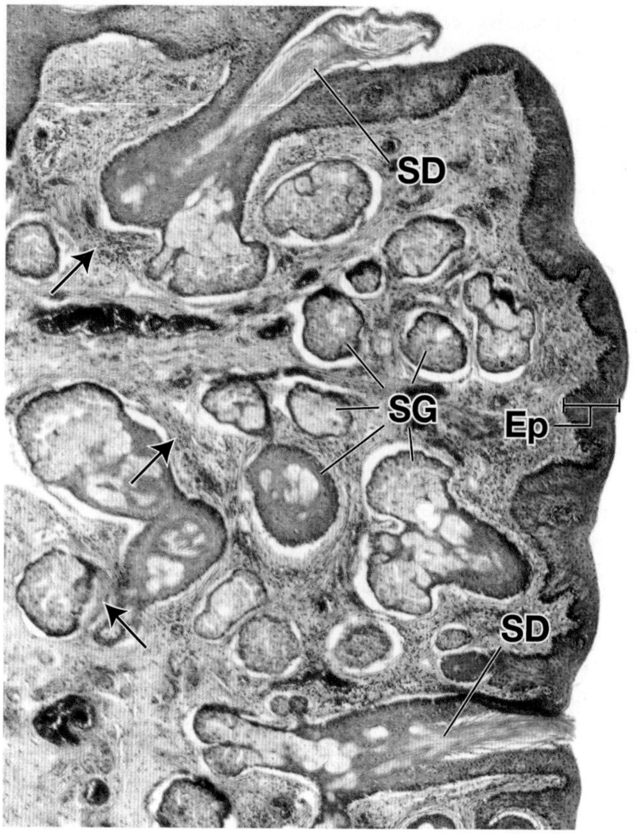

FIGURE 23.34. Photomicrograph of the inner surface of the labia majora. This low-power hematoxylin and eosin (H&E)-stained specimen of the labia majora's inner surface shows its stratified squamous epithelium (*Ep*) with no visible signs of keratinization and abundant sebaceous glands (*SG*). Two sebaceous ducts (*SD*) are also evident. Note the continuity of the duct epithelium with the epithelium of the skin and the sebaceous gland epithelium. At this magnification, several smooth muscle bundles can just barely be discerned (*arrows*).

squamous epithelium at the opening into the vestibule (see Fig. 23.35). **Bartholinitis** is a condition in which the major vestibular glands become infected and inflamed, and it may lead to the development of bacterial cysts or abscesses. If the duct of the Bartholin gland becomes obstructed, it usually dilates and fills with a secretion produced by the gland that may form a **Bartholin cyst.** Symptoms include severe pain, redness, swelling of the involved labium majus, and, sometimes, fever. On physical examination, the affected labium majus appears red and enlarged. A large abscess requires surgical incision with drainage or complete excision.

- The **labia minora** [*sing. labium minus*] are paired, hairless folds of skin that border the vestibule. They lie immediately lateral to the vaginal vestibule and medial to the labia majora. Upon reaching the clitoris, the anterior end of the labia minora splits into two parts. The more anterior part travels above (anterior) to the body of the clitoris, forming the **prepuce (hood) of the clitoris**, whereas the posterior part crossing below the clitoris forms the **frenulum of the clitoris**. The posterior ends of the labia minora terminate as they fuse into a skin fold called the **frenulum of the labia minora**, or fourchette. In most cases, the labia minora are not symmetrical and may protrude beyond the labia majora.
- The skin of the labia minora contains **stratified squamous epithelium** that exhibits a small degree of keratinization (Fig. 23.36). The epithelium lacks skin appendages; however, the lateral surface of the labia minora may contain sweat glands. In some individuals, large sebaceous glands are present in the stroma; their secretion is directly released on the surface of the labia minora. Abundant **melanin pigment** is present in the deep cells of the epithelium. The core of connective tissue within each fold is devoid of adipose tissue but does contain numerous blood vessels and fine **elastic fibers.** The labia minora are highly innervated structures that directly connect to the glans of the clitoris and the erectile tissues of the bulb of the vestibule located deep into the labia majora. The labia minora have the highest concentration of Meissner and Merkel corpuscles for sensitivity to light touch of the entire vulva (see Fig. 23.36). A high density of Pacinian corpuscles for pressure reception and free nerve endings are also found in the labia minora. Enlarged **labia minora** can cause functional problems related to menstrual hygiene and irritation from clothing. In specific conditions, labial alteration procedures (e.g., **labiaplasty**) for medical indications (e.g., treatment of labial hypertrophy or asymmetrical labial growth or chronic irritation) can be performed. These procedures are sometimes performed for cosmetic purposes despite the lack of high-quality data about their safety and long-term outcomes. Potential complications of labiaplasty include pain, infection, and scarring. Patients who are dissatisfied with the appearance of their labia minora can be counseled about normal variations in the color, size, and shape of external genitalia.

Clitoral Complex

The clitoral complex, composed of the glans, body, crura of the clitoris, and bulbs of the vestibule, is a female erectile organ that is sexually responsive.

The **clitoral complex** is composed of the **glans of the clitoris**, **body of the clitoris**, **left and right crus of the clitoris**, and **two bulbs of the vestibule**. In recent

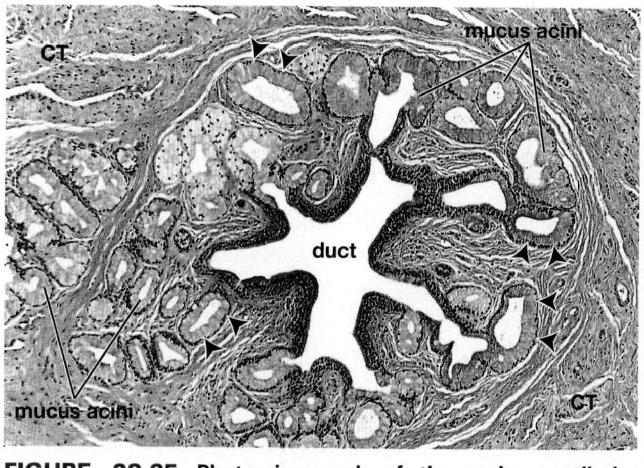

FIGURE 23.35. Photomicrograph of the major vestibular (Bartholin) gland. This low-magnification hematoxylin and eosin (H&E)-stained specimen shows mucus acini lined by simple columnar cells that produce mucus secretions. Note that nuclei of secretory mucus cells are positioned at their basal domain (*arrowheads*). The basal domain of secretory acini is ensheathed by myoepithelial cells (not visible at this magnification). The gland's secretion is discharged into the Bartholin gland duct, visible in the *center* of the image. The epithelium of the duct transitions from simple cuboidal (near the acini) to stratified cuboidal and stratified squamous epithelium at the opening into the vestibule. The gland is embedded in the dense irregular connective tissue (*CT*) of the labia majora. ×60. (Reprinted with permission from Hanley KZ. Vulva. In: Mills SM, ed. *Histology for Pathologists*. Wolters Kluwer; 2020:1031–1046.)

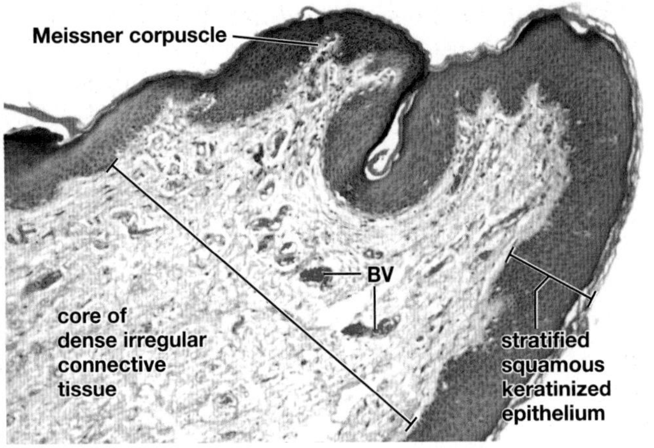

FIGURE 23.36. Photomicrograph of a labium minus. This low-magnification hematoxylin and eosin (H&E)-stained specimen shows a section through the labium minus that includes both the lateral and medial surfaces. Each labium minus represents a fold of thin skin with a stratified squamous epithelium demonstrating a small degree of keratinization on the surface. The epithelium lacks skin appendages. Abundant melanin pigment is present in the cells in the basal layer of the epithelium; however, it is difficult to discern them at this low magnification. The core of dense regular connective tissue within the labia minora is devoid of adipose tissue but does contain numerous blood vessels (*BV*), elastic fibers, and nerves. Note a Meissner corpuscle residing in the dermal papilla. ×60. (Reprinted with permission from Hanley KZ. Vulva. In: Mills SM, ed. *Histology for Pathologists*. Wolters Kluwer; 2020:1031–1046.)

descriptions, the clitoral complex is often compared to the "tip of the iceberg" because the glans of the clitoris, the only visible part of this complex, represents only 10% of the complex's total size; the remainder is embedded deep into the vulva. The clitoral complex is well innervated, containing many nerve endings, especially Pacinian corpuscles. Other touch receptors (Meissner and Merkel corpuscles) are present in reduced numbers compared with the mons pubis or labia majora. Free nerve endings (pain receptors) are present in relatively high concentrations. The clitoral complex comprises two histologically distinct types of **specialized vascular tissue** that consist of:

- **Erectile tissue**, which is found in the body and crura of the clitoris and bulbs of the vestibule. The body of the clitoris (as seen in cross section in Fig. 23.37) contains numerous wide, irregularly shaped vascular spaces lined with vascular endothelium. These spaces are surrounded by connective tissue trabeculae with a thin layer of smooth muscle. Irregular smooth muscle bundles are frequently observed as "subendothelial cushions" surrounding irregular vascular spaces. During sexual arousal, the erectile tissue allows for distension with blood and volume expansion. The vascular spaces increase in size and rigidity by filling with blood, principally derived from the divisions of internal pudendal arteries. These include deep dorsal artery of the clitoris that is positioned at the dorsal aspect of the body of the clitoris, deep artery of the clitoris running within the erectile tissue of the body of the clitoris, and artery to the bulb of the vestibule that enters the deep surface of the bulb.
- **Nonerectile vascular tissue**, which is found in the glans of the clitoris. This tissue is characterized by a high density of blood vessels dispersed within a dense irregular connective tissue stroma containing a minimal amount of smooth muscle. During sexual arousal, increased blood flow is observed; however, the tissue does not undergo physical expansion. This type of nonerectile, sexually responsive vascular tissue also surrounds the urethral orifice and is present within the labia minora and the adventitia of the vaginal wall.

The **body of the clitoris** is composed of paired conjoined **erectile bodies**, which originate from extensions of the crura of the clitoris. These bodies are surrounded by **tunica albuginea**, a thin fibroelastic connective tissue sheath (see Fig. 23.37). A connective tissue septum between the paired erectile bodies is incomplete, and vascular spaces communicate with each other at the dorsal aspect of the clitoris. The adventitia of the **deep arteries of the clitoris** blends on both sides with the connective tissue of the septum. The body of the clitoris with investing tunica albuginea is surrounded by the inner layer of the fascia, called the **fascia of the clitoris**, that is continuous with the deep perineal fascia investing the perineal muscles, vestibule of vagina, and crura of the clitoris. **Deep dorsal arteries, deep dorsal veins**, and **dorsal nerves of the clitoris** course between the tunica albuginea and the fascia of the clitoris (see Fig. 23.37). The outer layer is a part of the superficial (Colles) fascia of the perineum and may contain the superficial dorsal vein of the clitoris. The body of the clitoris is attached to the pubic symphysis by the connective tissue **suspensory ligaments.** They attach to the clitoral complex at the angle of the clitoris, a transition point (>90 degree) between the crura and the body of the clitoris. As mentioned in the section on the labia minora (see page 941), the body of the clitoris does not have circumferential skin coverage; instead, the skin of the prepuce and the frenulum of the clitoris flare laterally to the labia minora (see Fig. 23.37).

The **glans clitoris**, an oval tubercle at the tip of the corpora cavernosa (average length 8 mm and width 4 mm), is formed by nonerectile vascular tissue. The skin over the glans is very thin, forms the prepuce of the clitoris, and as discussed earlier, contains numerous sensory nerve endings (see page 941).

The two **crura of the clitoris** are extensions of erectile tissues of the body of the clitoris that firmly anchor the clitoris to the pubic rami. They are about 36 mm in length and 7 mm in width (as measured in magnetic resonance imaging [MRI] scans) and are composed of erectile tissue surrounded by tunica albuginea, consistent with that of the body of the clitoris. At the place of bony attachment, the tunica albuginea fuses with the fibrous layer of the periosteum of pubic rami. The unattached surface of the crura is invested by a thin layer of ischiocavernosus muscle (a superficial striated muscle of the perineum) that is covered by a deep layer of the perineal fascia.

The **bulbs of the vestibule** are paired structures formed from the erectile tissue similar to that described in the body of the clitoris with some modifications. The erectile tissue of a bulb has more pronounced fibromuscular trabeculae and more prominent bundles of smooth muscles located just under the epithelium of the vascular spaces. In addition, a distinct tunica albuginea is often missing in the bulbs. They have a single origin from the inferior aspect of the body of the clitoris. After splitting into right and left structures, they travel posteriorly on the lateral side of the urethra and vagina and medially to the crura of the clitoris. They are firmly attached to the perineal membrane just deep into the labia majora and are covered by the thin layer of the bulbospongiosus muscle (a superficial striated muscle of the perineum). During sexual excitation, the bulb of the vestibule becomes engorged with blood. This significant enlargement of the bulbs of vestibule during sexual arousal is a result of the tunica albuginea absence.

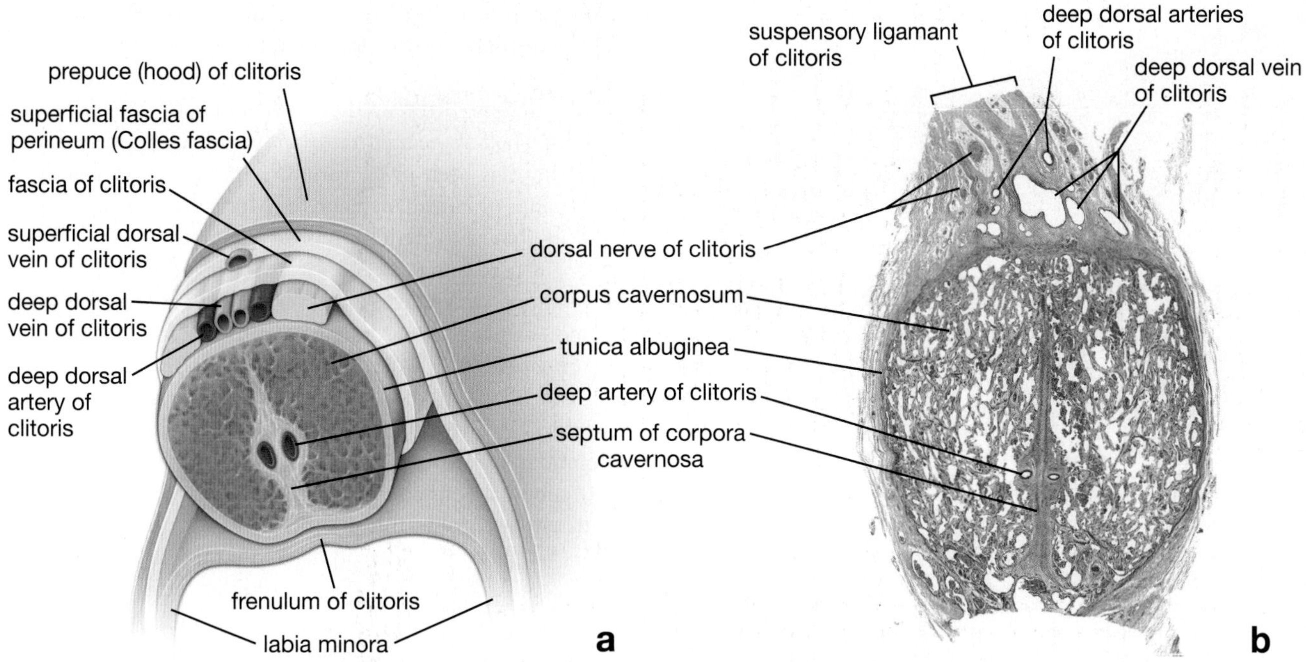

FIGURE 23.37. Schematic diagram and a photomicrograph of the body of the clitoris in cross section. a. The diagram shows a midsection through the body of the clitoris. The body of the clitoris is not completely surrounded by the skin; instead, it has contact with divisions originating from the proximal ends of the labia minora. On the dorsal and lateral surfaces, the body is covered by the prepuce of the clitoris (hood), which emerged from the anterior division of the labia minora. The ventral part of the body is in close proximity to the frenulum that originated from the posterior division of the labia minora. Corpora cavernosa, the erectile tissue of the clitoris, is surrounded by a thick fibrous layer of tunica albuginea. Note that the corpora cavernosa are separated by the incomplete septum, which is closely associated with deep arteries of the clitoris; they are visible on both sides of the septum. The fascia of the clitoris surrounds the corpora cavernosa and the neurovascular bundle located at the dorsal aspect of the clitoris. Note the arrangement of deep dorsal arteries, deep dorsal veins, and dorsal nerves of the clitoris, which lie between the tunica albuginea and the fascia of the clitoris. The superficial dorsal vein of the clitoris resides in the superficial fascia. **b.** This low-power photomicrograph hematoxylin and eosin (H&E)-stained specimen shows the body of the clitoris that corresponds to the drawing. The specimen has been removed through the incision of the prepuce and separated from the skin and fascial layers. Note the well-defined tunica albuginea and erectile vascular spaces incompletely separated by the septum. Vascular spaces contain numerous irregularly shaped channels lined by vascular endothelium. These spaces are defined by the connective tissue trabeculae with a thin layer of smooth muscle. The neurovascular bundle is visible on the dorsal aspect of the body of the clitoris. ×10. (Courtesy of Dr. Karen Pinder from the University of British Columbia, Vancouver, Canada.)

Vestibule of the Vagina

The vestibule of the vagina is the middle part of the vulva that contains the external urethral orifice, opening of the vagina, and multiple openings of a variety of secretory glands.

The vestibule of the vagina is a somewhat concave space positioned in the middle part of the vulva that extends from the frenulum of the clitoris anteriorly to the frenulum of the labia minora posteriorly. Its lateral borders are formed by the labia minora and majora. The vestibule is lined with endodermally derived **stratified squamous nonkeratinized epithelium,** which, on the lateral sides, blends with ectodermally derived stratified squamous keratinized epithelium of the labia minora and majora, prepuce of the clitoris, and frenulum of the labia minora. The epithelium of the vestibule is rich in **glycogen** and is similar to that found in the vagina. The vestibule of the vagina contains the vaginal opening, which may be partially covered by the hymen, and the external urethral meatus. Numerous small mucous glands, the **lesser vestibular glands** (often incorrectly called Skene glands), open directly into the mucosa of the vestibule. They are simple tubular glands lined by mucous-secreting columnar cells that merge with the stratified squamous nonkeratinized epithelium of the vestibule. In addition, as discussed earlier, the ducts of the major vestibular (Bartholin) glands (see page 940 and Fig. 23.35) and glands surrounding the urethra with prominent paraurethral (Skene) glands (see page 944) discharge their secretions into the vestibule. The mucosa of the vestibule has multiple sensory and pain receptors similar to those found in other regions of the vulva. The **lesser vestibular glands** may undergo **squamous metaplasia** similar to that described for the cervix (see page 126). Metaplastic epithelium may completely replace the glandular epithelium, forming **vestibular clefts**. Obstruction of the glands may also produce a **vulvar mucous cyst** due to the accumulation of the mucous secretion.

The hymen is a thin mucous membrane at the entrance to the vagina.

The **hymen** is the thin, fibrous tissue plate that surrounds and partially covers the entrance to the vagina, leaving an opening for vaginal and menstrual discharge. When it is ruptured, small tag–like elevations known as **hymenal caruncles** are present at the opening of the vagina. Embryologically, the hymen is derived from the **endodermal membrane** that separates the developing vagina from the cavity of the **definitive urogenital sinus** in the embryo. Thus, it marks the inferior boundary of the vagina and the superior boundary of the vestibule. Both vaginal and vestibular surfaces of the hymen are covered by a **mucosa** containing stratified squamous nonkeratinized epithelium, which is similar to that of the vaginal epithelium (Fig. 23.38). The lighter staining of epithelium on the vaginal surface reflects larger amounts of glycogen stored in the epithelial cells. The border between epithelium and underlying lamina propria is clearly defined by the closely packed small cells of the stratum basale (see Fig.23.38). Deep connective tissue

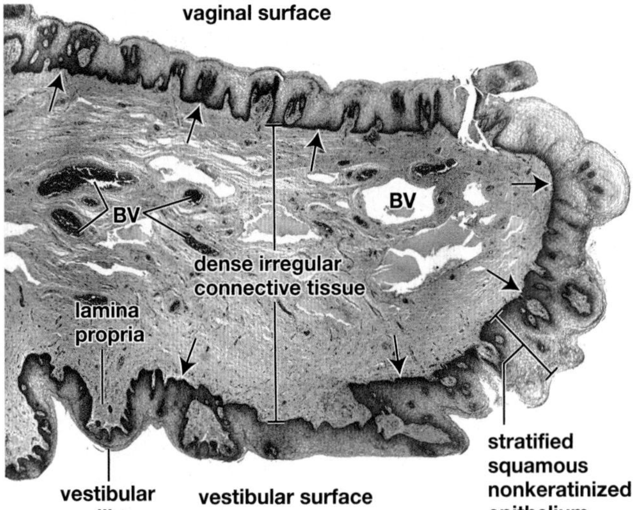

FIGURE 23.38. Photomicrograph of the hymen. This low-magnification hematoxylin and eosin (H&E)-stained specimen shows the section of the hymen that includes the free edge of the hymenal ring. Note a gradual transition of the stratified squamous nonkeratinized epithelium from the vaginal surface (vaginal mucosa) to the vestibular surface (vestibular mucosa). The lighter staining of epithelium on the vaginal surface reflects larger amounts of glycogen stored in the epithelial cells. The vaginal surface also appears smooth. The vestibular surface stains darker (less glycogen content) and may contain vestibular papillae, small surface projections caused by projections of underlying lamina propria into the epithelium. The border between epithelium and underlying lamina propria is clearly defined by closely packed small cells of the stratum basale (*arrows*). Dense irregular connective tissue containing blood vessels is present in the core of the hymen. ×45. (Reprinted with permission from Hanley KZ. Vulva. In: Mills SM, ed. *Histology for Pathologists*. Wolters Kluwer; 2020:1031–1046.)

papillae are present on both vaginal and vestibular surfaces and are formed by invaginations of underlying lamina propria into the epithelium. The vaginal surface appears smooth; however, the vestibular surface may contain small projections, known as *vestibular papillae* (see Fig. 23.38). Dense irregular connective tissue containing a rich network of blood vessels with a few nerve fibers is present in the core of the hymen. The hymen has a limited number of nerve receptors. Only Merkel corpuscles and free nerve endings are present in the hymenal ring. The size, shape, and degree of the hymenal opening vary greatly among individuals. The hymen may be imperforate, round, annular, septate, or cribriform. In cases of **imperforate hymen**, the hymen lacks the opening between the vagina and the vestibulum. If this condition is diagnosed during puberty, it may lead to progressive accumulation of menstrual discharge that results in distension of the vagina (**hematocolpos**).

Glandular tissue surrounding the female urethra shares immunohistochemical characteristics with the prostate gland in males.

The **external urethral orifice** is part of the vestibulum of the vagina and is located between the glans of the clitoris and the opening of the vagina. In most cases, the lumen of the urethra is lined by transitional epithelium (urothelium) that changes at the external urethra orifice into stratified squamous nonkeratinized epithelium of the vaginal vestibule. However, stratified columnar and pseudostratified epithelium have also been reported in the female urethra.

The glandular tissue around the urethra is represented by small **periurethral glands**. These glands are present in the wall of the urethra and open with the short ducts throughout the entire length of the urethral lumen being more numerous at the distal half of the urethra. Glandular tissue associated with the urethra has been given various names, such as glands of Littré, glands of Huffman, glands of Morgani, intermural glans of the urethra, and periurethral or paraurethral glans. These names are used interchangeably, reflecting the lack of consensus among researchers. However, two larger accumulations of glandular tissue often described in the literature, known as the **paraurethral glands (of Skene)**, are located near the distal end of the urethra. They have longer and more prominent ducts (1.5 cm in length) that empty in the distal part of the urethra. These ducts are lined by the stratified (two layers thick) cuboidal epithelium. In multiparas, where the urethral meatus can be considerably distended, the duct of Skene glands appears visible on the side and deep into the urethral orifice.

The entire glandular tissue complex surrounding the urethra exhibits a similar histologic appearance. All glands are of mixed branched tubuloalveolar type lined by the simple columnar epithelium with occasional nests of pseudocolumnar epithelium with basal cells. A prominent fibromuscular stroma separates glandular profiles. Immunohistochemical analysis reveals that all glandular tissue surrounding the lumen of the urethra stain positively for prostate-specific antigen (PSA), prostatic acid phosphatase (PAP), prostate-specific alkaline phosphatase (PSAkP), and androgen receptor (AR), leading some researchers to characterize the periurethral glandular tissue as the **female prostate**. Also, physiologic studies determined that the urethra is the source of secretions that can occur during sexual excitement. Biochemical analysis suggests that this secretion is similar in composition to male ejaculate.

■ MAMMARY GLANDS

The **mammary glands**, or breasts, are a distinguishing feature of mammals. They are structurally dynamic organs, varying with age, menstrual cycle, and reproductive status of the female. During embryologic development, growth and development of breast tissue occur in both sexes. Multiple glands develop along paired epidermal thickenings called **mammary ridges (milk lines)** that extend from the developing axilla to the developing inguinal region. In humans, normally, only one group of cells develops into a breast on each side. An extra breast (**polymastia**) or nipple (**polythelia**) may occur as an inheritable condition in about 1% of the female population. These relatively rare conditions may also occur in men.

In females, mammary glands develop under the influence of sex hormones.

Until puberty, both females' and males' mammary glands develop in similar manner. At the onset of puberty in males, testosterone acts on the mesenchymal cells to inhibit further growth of the mammary gland. At the same time, the mammary glands undergo further development under hormonal influence of estrogen and progesterone. Estrogen stimulates further development of mesenchymal cells. The mammary gland increases in size, mainly due to the growth of interlobular adipose tissue. The ducts extend and branch into the expanding connective tissue stroma. Proliferation of

FOLDER 23.5

CLINICAL CORRELATION: CERVICAL CYTOLOGY: THE PAP TEST

The examination of samples of cervical cells is a valuable diagnostic tool in evaluating the vaginal and cervical mucosae (Fig. F23.5.1). Superficial epithelial cells are removed from the mucosa, added to a liquid medium, and sent to a laboratory for microscopic examination. Before the advent of liquid-based cervical cytology, cervical cell samples were spread on glass slides and stained with the Papanicolaou (Pap) stain (a combination of hematoxylin, orange G, and eosin azure). Cervical cytology provides valuable diagnostic information about the epithelium regarding pathologic changes, response to hormonal changes during the menstrual cycle, and the microbial environment of the vagina.

Cervical cytology results are reported using the Bethesda system. This system stratifies results into three major categories:

- **Negative for intraepithelial lesions or malignancy**: This category includes both normal results and results that indicate infectious organisms or other nonneoplastic changes.
- **Other**: This category is used to report the presence of benign-appearing endometrial cells in a female aged 45 years or older. This finding may indicate an endometrial abnormality.
- **Epithelial cell abnormalities**: This category is used to report both squamous and glandular cell abnormalities.

Nonneoplastic Changes

The synthesis and release of glycogen by the epithelial cells of the uterus and vagina are directly related to changes in the pH of vaginal fluid. The pH of the fluid, which is normally low, around pH 4, becomes more acid near midcycle as *Lactobacillus acidophilus*, a lactic acid–forming bacterium in the vagina, metabolizes the secreted glycogen. An alkaline environment can favor the growth of infectious agents such as *Staphylococci*, *Corynebacterium vaginale*, *Trichomonas vaginalis*, and *Candida albicans*, causing an abnormal increase in vaginal transexudates and inflammation of the vaginal mucosa and vulvar skin known as **vulvovaginitis**. These pathologic conditions are readily diagnosed with cervical cytology. Specific antimicrobial agents (antibiotics, sulfonamides, and antifungals) may be used together with nonspecific therapy (acidified 0.1% hexetidine gel) to restore the normal low pH in the vagina and thus prevent the growth of these agents.

Epithelial Cell Abnormalities

Cervical cytology is widely used to screen for precancer stages of the cervix. Because precancerous cervical lesions may exist for as long as 20 years, the abnormal cells shed from the epithelium are easily detected with cervical cytology. Microscopic examination of these cells permits differentiation between normal and abnormal cells, determines their site of origin, and allows classifying cellular changes related to the spread of the disease.

In the Bethesda system, epithelial lesions are differentiated as either squamous or glandular into the following categories:

- Squamous cells
  - Atypical squamous cells
  - Low-grade squamous intraepithelial lesion
  - High-grade squamous intraepithelial lesion
  - Squamous cell carcinoma
- Glandular cells
  - Atypical (endocervical, endometrial, or glandular cells)
  - Endocervical adenocarcinoma in situ
  - Adenocarcinoma

The Pap test is an extremely effective and inexpensive screening method for preventing cervical cancer. Because most of the cell abnormalities detected by Pap tests are in the precancerous stage, it allows prompt treatment and follow-up that is able to prevent the onset of invasive cervical cancer. Since the 1950s, when cervical cytology was first introduced, deaths from cervical cancer in the United States have declined ~70%. However, in areas where cervical cancer screening is not as widely used, cervical cancer deaths remain high.

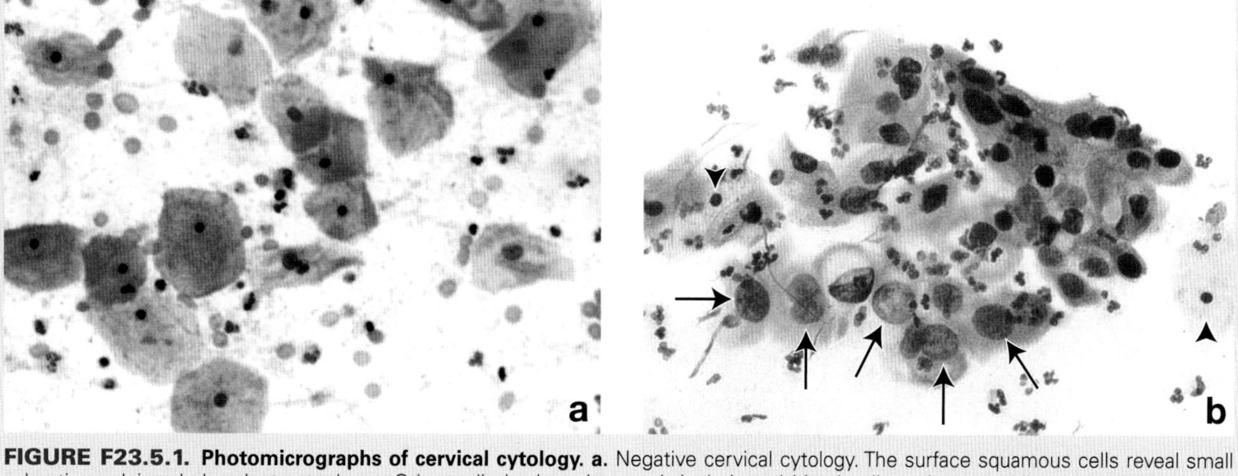

FIGURE F23.5.1. Photomicrographs of cervical cytology. a. Negative cervical cytology. The surface squamous cells reveal small pyknotic nuclei and abundant cytoplasm. Other cells in the micrograph include red blood cells and neutrophils. ×600. **b.** Abnormal cytology. Many of the cells in this specimen contain large nuclei with no evidence of pyknosis (*arrows*). The cytoplasm is relatively scant. Other cells exhibit a more normal appearance with pyknotic nuclei and more surrounding cytoplasm (*arrowheads*). Neutrophils are also present. ×600.

epithelial cells is controlled by interactions between the epithelium and the specialized intralobular hormone–sensitive loose connective tissue stroma. By adulthood, the complete ductal architecture of the gland has been established.

The mammary glands remain in an **inactive state** until pregnancy, during which the mammary glands assume their complete morphologic and functional maturation. This occurs in response to estrogens and progesterone initially secreted from the corpus luteum and later from placenta, prolactin (PRL) from pituitary gland, and gonadocorticoids produced by the adrenal cortex. By the end of pregnancy, secretory vesicles are found in the epithelial cells, but milk production is inhibited by high levels of progesterone. The actual initiation of **milk secretion** occurs immediately after birth and is induced by **prolactin (PRL)** secreted by the adenohypophysis. The ejection of milk from the breast is stimulated by **oxytocin** released from the neurohypophysis. With the change in the hormonal environment at menopause, the glandular component of the breast regresses or involutes and is replaced by fat and connective tissue. In men, some additional development of the mammary glands normally occurs after puberty, and the glands remain rudimentary.

Hormonal exposure and genetic predisposition are the major risk factors for the development of **breast cancer**. It is the most common malignancy in women in the United States. Each year, an estimated nearly 270,000 women (and also 2,500 men) are diagnosed with breast cancer. Most breast cancers are linked to hormonal exposure (which increases with age, early menarche, late menopause, and with older age of a first full-term pregnancy). About 5%–10% of all breast cancers are attributable to mutation in autosomal dominant **breast cancer genes (BRCA1 and BRCA2)**.

Mammary glands are modified tubuloalveolar apocrine sweat glands.

The tubuloalveolar **mammary glands**, derived from modified sweat glands in the epidermis, lie in the subcutaneous tissue. The inactive adult mammary gland is composed of 15–20 irregular lobes separated by fibrous bands of connective tissue. They radiate from the **mammary papilla**, or **nipple**, and are further subdivided into numerous lobules known as **terminal duct lobular units (TDLUs)** (Fig. 23.39). Some of the fibrous bands, called **suspensory** or **Cooper ligaments**, connect with the dermis. Abundant adipose tissue is present in the dense connective tissue of the interlobular spaces.

Each gland ends in a **lactiferous duct** that opens through a constricted orifice into the nipple. Beneath the **areola**, the pigmented area surrounding the **nipple**, each duct has a dilated portion, the **lactiferous sinus**. Near their openings, the lactiferous ducts are lined with stratified squamous keratinized epithelium. The epithelial lining of the duct shows a gradual transition from stratified squamous to two layers of cuboidal cells in the lactiferous sinus and finally to a single layer of columnar or cuboidal cells through the remainder of the duct system.

The epidermis of the adult nipple and areola is highly pigmented and somewhat wrinkled and has long dermal papillae invading its deep surface (Fig. 23.40). It is covered by keratinized stratified squamous epithelium. The pigmentation of the nipple increases at puberty, and the nipple becomes more prominent. During pregnancy, the areola becomes larger, and the degree of pigmentation increases further. Deep to the areola and nipple, bundles of smooth muscle fibers are arranged

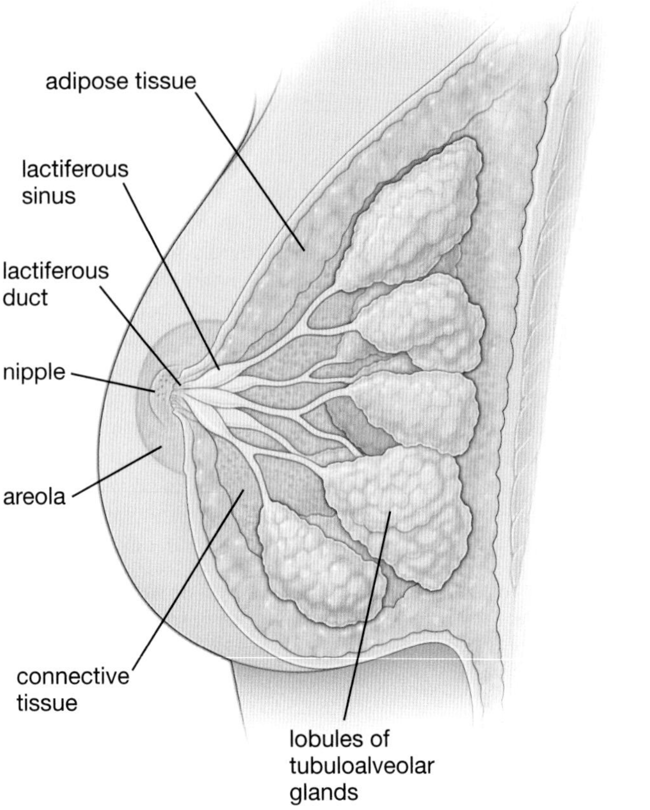

FIGURE 23.39. Schematic drawing of the human breast as seen during lactation. The breast is composed largely of terminal duct lobular units (TDLUs) containing branched tubuloalveolar glands. TDLUs are contained within an extensive connective tissue stroma and variable amounts of adipose tissue.

radially and circumferentially in the dense connective tissue and longitudinally along the lactiferous ducts. These muscle fibers allow the nipple to become erect in response to various stimuli.

The **areola** contains sebaceous glands, sweat glands, and modified mammary glands (**Montgomery glands**). These glands have a structure intermediate between that of sweat glands and true mammary glands, and they produce small elevations on the surface of the areola. It is believed that Montgomery glands produce a lubricating and protective secretion that changes the skin's pH and discourages microbial growth. Numerous sensory nerve endings are present in the nipple; the areola contains fewer sensory nerve endings.

The terminal duct lobular unit (TDLU) of the mammary gland represents a cluster of small secretory alveoli (in a lactating gland) or terminal ductules (in an inactive gland) surrounded by intralobular stroma.

Successive branching of lactiferous ducts leads to the **terminal duct lobular unit (TDLU)**. Each TDLU represents a grape-like cluster of small alveoli that forms a lobule (Fig. 23.41) and consists of the following:

- **Terminal ductules** are present in the inactive gland. During pregnancy and after childbirth, the epithelium of the terminal ductules, which is lined by secretory cells, differentiates into fully functional secretory alveoli that produce milk.
- The **intralobular collecting duct** carries alveolar secretions into the lactiferous duct.
- The **intralobular stroma** is a specialized, hormonally sensitive loose connective tissue that surrounds the terminal ductules and alveoli. The intralobular connective tissue contains few adipose cells.

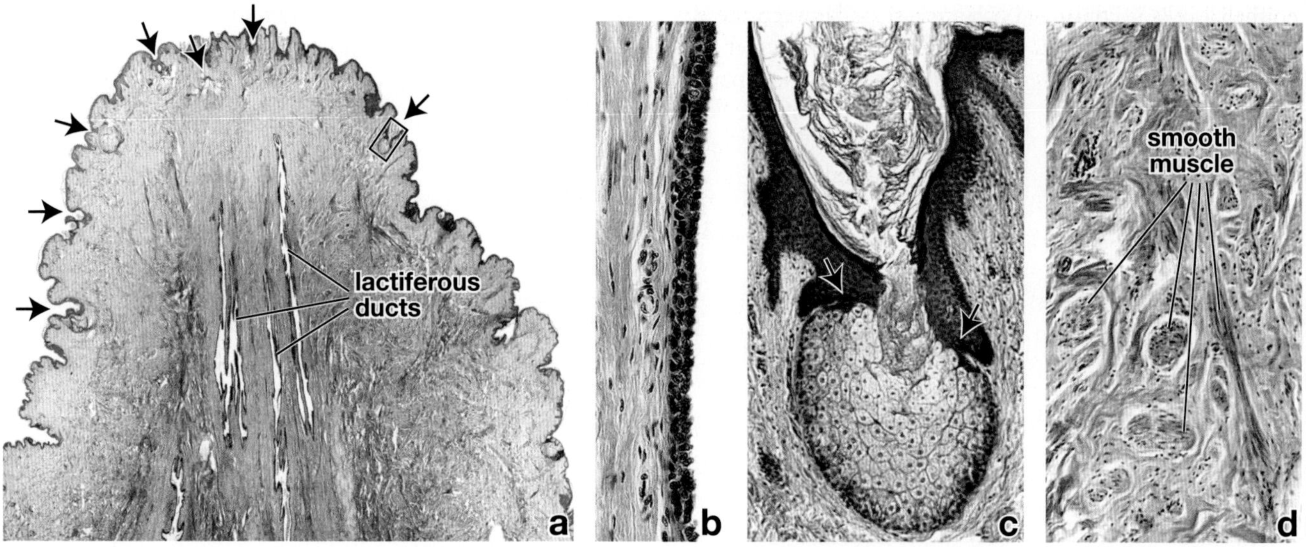

FIGURE 23.40. Photomicrographs of a section through the female nipple. a. This low-magnification micrograph of a hematoxylin and eosin (H&E)-stained sagittal section through the nipple shows the wrinkled surface contour, a thin stratified squamous epithelium, and associated sebaceous glands (*arrows*). The core of the nipple consists of dense connective tissue, smooth muscle bundles, and the lactiferous ducts that open at the nipple surface. ×6. **b.** The wall of one of the lactiferous ducts is shown here at higher magnification. Its epithelium is stratified cuboidal, consisting of two-cell layers. As it approaches the tip of the nipple, it changes to a stratified squamous epithelium and becomes continuous with the epidermis. ×175. **c.** A higher magnification of the sebaceous gland from the *rectangle* in **a**. Note how the glandular epithelium is continuous with the epidermis (*arrows*), and the sebum is being secreted onto the epidermal surface. ×90. **d.** A higher magnification showing bundles of smooth muscle in longitudinal and cross-sectional profiles. ×350.

Glandular epithelial and myoepithelial cells are the most important cells associated with mammary ducts and lobules. **Glandular epithelial cells** line the duct system, whereas **myoepithelial cells** lie deep within the epithelium between the epithelial cells and the basal lamina. These cells, arranged in a basket-like network, are present in the secretory portions of the gland. In a routine hematoxylin and eosin (H&E) preparation, the myoepithelial cells are more apparent in the larger ducts. However, in an immunocytochemical preparation, their discontinuous, basket-like arrangement is better visualized within the alveoli (Fig. 23.42). Contraction of myoepithelial cells assists in **milk ejection** during lactation. Recent immunofluorescence studies have proven that breast progenitor cells found in the ductular epithelium give rise to both glandular cells of the alveoli and myoepithelial cells.

The morphology of the secretory portion of the mammary gland varies with the menstrual cycle.

In the **inactive gland**, the glandular component is sparse and consists chiefly of duct elements (Fig. 23.43 and Plate 23.11, page 976). During the menstrual cycle, the inactive breast undergoes slight cyclic changes. Early in the follicular phase, the intralobular stroma is less dense, and terminal ductules appear as cords formed by the cuboidal-shaped epithelial cells with little or no lumen. During the luteal phase, the epithelial cells increase in height, and lumina appear in the ducts as small amounts of secretions accumulate. Also, fluid accumulates in the connective tissue. This is followed by abrupt involution and apoptosis during the last few days of the menstrual cycle before the onset of menstruation.

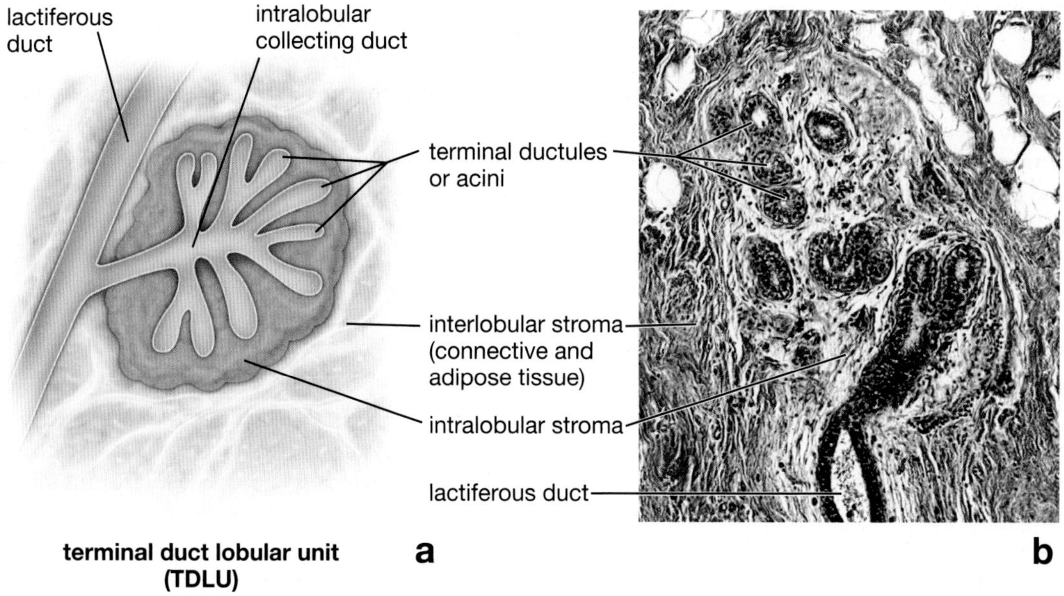

FIGURE 23.41. Terminal duct lobular unit. a. This schematic diagram shows components of the terminal duct lobular unit (*TDLU*). Terminal ductules and the intralobular collecting duct are surrounded by a specialized hormonally sensitive loose connective tissue called *intralobular stroma*. *TDLUs* are separated from each other by interlobular stroma containing a variable amount of dense irregular connective tissue and adipose tissue. In active mammary glands, terminal ductules differentiate into milk-producing alveoli. **b.** This photomicrograph shows the *TDLU* from an inactive mammary gland. The clear area in the *upper part* of the image represents adipose cells. ×120.

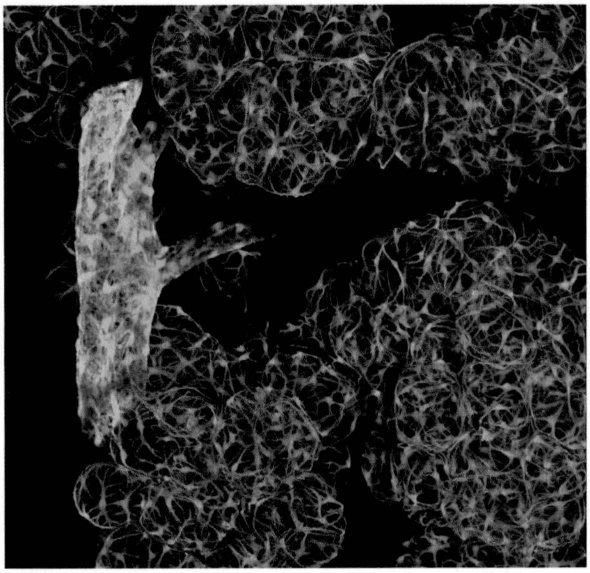

FIGURE 23.42. Myoepithelial cells in the mammary gland. This immunofluorescence image is obtained from the mammary gland of a lactating mouse 2 days postparturition. The mouse carries a transgene composed of the smooth muscle α-actin promoter conjugated to enhance the green fluorescent protein (GFP) reaction. Three-dimensional organization of myoepithelial cells is visualized in *green color* due to the expression of the promoter transgene in myoepithelial cells. The tissue was also stained *red* with antibody against smooth muscle α-actin conjugated directly with CY3 fluorescent dye. The *orange color* staining results from overlapping of the *green* and *red* staining. The cells on the surface of the terminal duct lobular unit are stained *orange*, whereas those deeper in the tissue stained only *green* because the antibody did not penetrate deep into the tissue. Note a small intralobular duct that merges into the larger lactiferous duct. ×600. (Courtesy Dr. James J. Tomasek, University of Oklahoma Health Science Center.)

Mammary glands undergo dramatic proliferation and development during pregnancy.

The **mammary glands** exhibit a number of changes in preparation for lactation. These can be examined during the trimester of pregnancy.

- **First trimester** is characterized by elongation and branching of the terminal ductules. The lining epithelial and myoepithelial cells proliferate and differentiate from breast progenitor cells found in the epithelium of terminal ductules. Myoepithelial cells proliferate between the base of the epithelial cells and the basal lamina in both the alveolar and ductal portions of the gland.
- **Second trimester** is characterized by differentiation of alveoli from the growing ends of the terminal ductules. The development of the glandular tissue is not uniform, and variation in the degree of development is seen even within a single lobule. The cells vary in shape from flattened to low columnar. Plasma cells, lymphocytes, and eosinophils infiltrate the intralobular connective tissue stroma as the breast develops (Plate 23.12, page 978). At this stage, the amount of glandular tissue and mass of the breast increase, mainly due to the growth of the alveoli (Fig. 23.44).
- **Third trimester** commences maturation of the alveoli. The epithelial glandular cells become cuboidal, with nuclei positioned at the basal cell surface. They develop an extensive rER; secretory vesicles and lipid droplets appear in the cytoplasm. The actual proliferation of the interlobular stromal cells declines, and subsequent enlargement of the breast occurs through hypertrophy of the secretory cells and accumulation of secretory product in the alveoli.

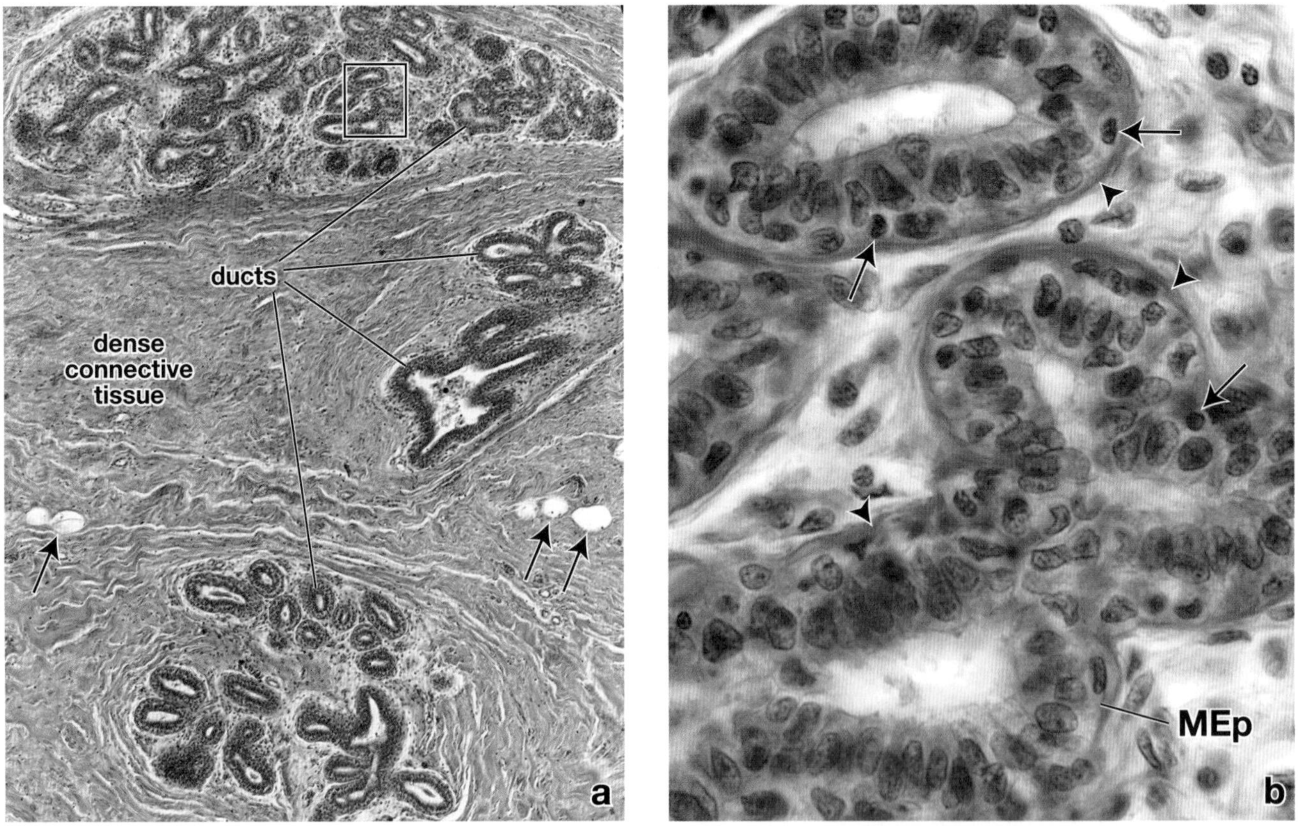

FIGURE 23.43. Photomicrograph of an inactive mammary gland. a. This low-magnification hematoxylin and eosin (H&E)-stained specimen shows several lobules within the dense connective tissue of the breast. The epithelial component consists of a branching duct system that makes up the lobule. The clear areas (*arrows*) are adipose cells. ×60. **b.** A higher magnification of the area in the *rectangle* of **a**. The epithelial cells of the ducts are columnar and exhibit interspersed lymphocytes (*arrows*) that have entered the epithelium. The surrounding stained material (*arrowheads*) represents the myoepithelial cells (*MEp*) and collagen bundles in the adjacent connective tissue. ×700.

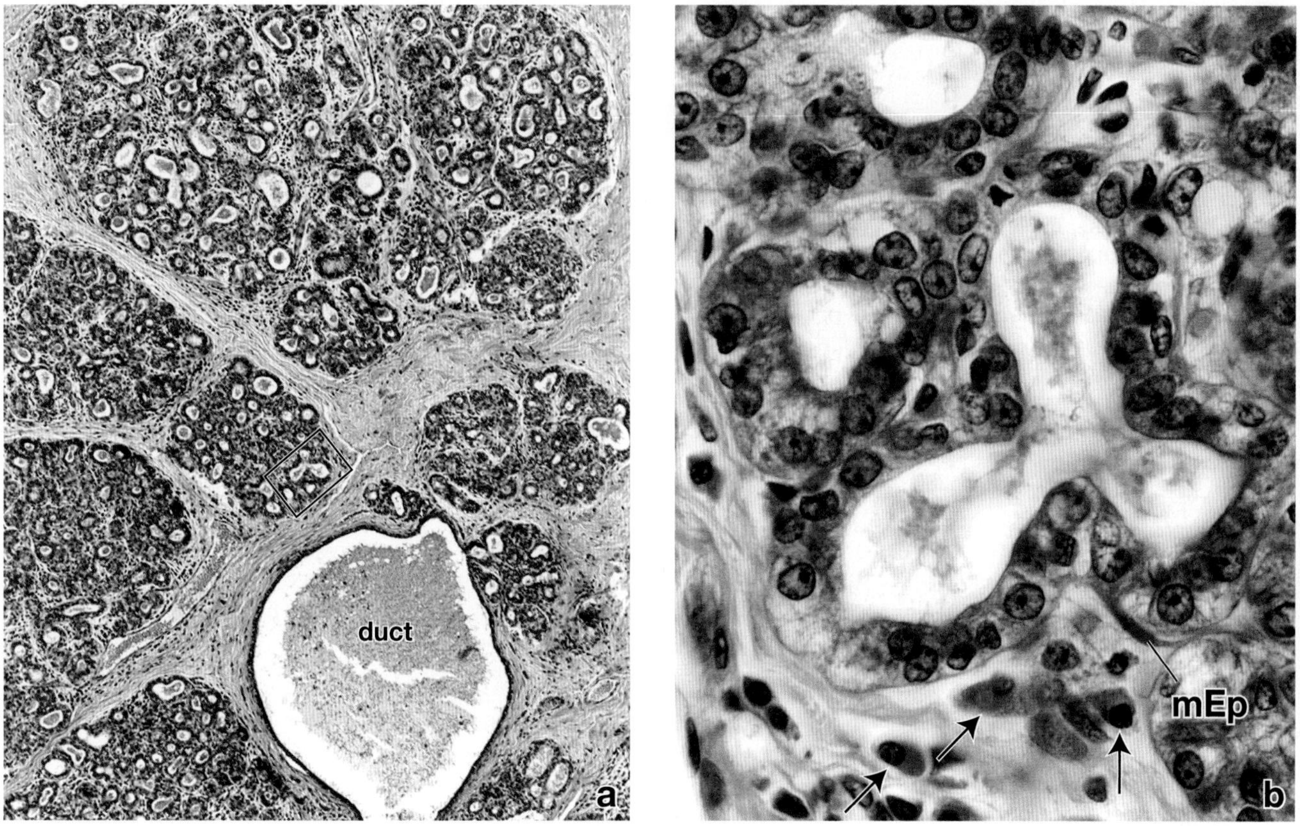

FIGURE 23.44. Photomicrograph of an active mammary gland during late pregnancy. a. This low-magnification hematoxylin and eosin (H&E)-stained specimen shows the marked proliferation of the duct system giving rise to the secretory alveoli that constitute the major portion of the lobules. The intralobular ducts are difficult to identify because their epithelium also secretes. Outside the lobules is a large excretory duct. ×60. **b.** A higher magnification of an area in **a**. The secretory alveolar cells are mostly cuboidal here. A myoepithelial cell (*mEp*) as well as a number of plasma cells (*arrows*) can be identified in the adjacent loose connective tissue. ×700.

The changes in glandular tissue during pregnancy are accompanied by a decrease in the amount of connective tissue and adipose tissue.

Both merocrine and apocrine secretion are involved in the production of milk.

The secreting cells contain abundant granular endoplasmic reticulum, a moderate number of large mitochondria, a supranuclear Golgi apparatus, and a number of dense lysosomes (Fig. 23.45). Depending on the secretory state, large lipid droplets and secretory vesicles may be present in the apical cytoplasm. The secretory cells produce two distinct products that are released by different mechanisms.

- **Merocrine secretion**. The protein component of the milk is synthesized in the rER, packaged into membrane-limited secretory vesicles for transport in the Golgi apparatus, and released from the cell by fusion of the vesicle's limiting membrane with the plasma membrane.
- **Apocrine secretion**. The fatty or lipid component of the milk arises as lipid droplets that are free in the cytoplasm. The lipid coalesces to form large droplets that pass to the apical region of the cell and project into the lumen of the acinus. The droplets are invested with an envelope of plasma membrane as they are released. A thin layer of cytoplasm is trapped between the plasma membrane and lipid droplet and is released with the lipid, but the cytoplasmic loss in this process is minimal.

The secretion released in the first few days after childbirth is known as **colostrum**. This premilk is an alkaline, yellowish secretion with a higher protein, vitamin A, sodium, and chloride content and a lower lipid, carbohydrate, and potassium content than milk. It contains considerable amounts of antibodies (mainly **secretory IgA**) that provide the newborn with some degree of passive immunity. The antibodies in the colostrum are believed to be produced by the lymphocytes and plasma cells that infiltrate the loose connective tissue of the breast during its proliferation and development and are secreted across the glandular cells as in salivary glands and intestine. As these wandering cells decrease in number after parturition, the production of colostrum stops, and lipid-rich milk is produced.

Hormonal Regulation of the Mammary Gland

The initial growth and development of the mammary gland at puberty occur under the influence of estrogens and progesterone produced by the maturing ovary. Under hormonal influence, the TDLUs develop and differentiate into dynamic functional units. Subsequent to this initial development, slight changes in the morphology of the glandular tissue occur during each ovarian cycle. During the follicular phase of the menstrual cycle, **estrogen** in the circulation stimulates **proliferation of the lactiferous duct components**. After ovulation in the luteal phase, **progesterone** stimulates the **growth of alveoli**; intralobular stroma becomes edematous. Clinically, during the luteal phase, tenderness and a progressive increase in breast tissue mass may be felt. During pregnancy, the corpus luteum and placenta continuously produce estrogens and progesterone, causing a massive increase in TDLUs. It is now believed that the growth of the mammary glands also depends on the presence of PRL, which is produced by the anterior lobe of the pituitary gland (adenohypophysis); hCS, which is produced by the placenta; and adrenal glucocorticoids.

FOLDER 23.6
CLINICAL CORRELATION: CERVICAL CANCER AND HUMAN PAPILLOMAVIRUS INFECTION

Human papillomavirus (HPV) is the most common sexually transmitted virus in the United States. Most individuals will become infected with HPV during their lifetime. More than 30 HPV types are known to infect the urogenital and anal regions of both sexes, targeting the stratified squamous epithelium of the perineal skin or mucous membranes. About 12 types of HPV, called *low-risk* HPV types, cause **genital warts**. Most cases of genital warts are caused by HPV types 6 and 11. Approximately 13 types of HPV, called *high-risk* HPV types, can cause cancer of the cervix, anus, vagina, vulva, penis, and head and neck. Most cases of HPV-associated cancer are caused by HPV types 16 and 18.

HPV infection usually resolves on its own. Persistent infection develops in only a small percentage (5%–10%) of cases. Risk factors for persistent infection include older age and smoking. Persistent infection with high-risk HPV types is associated with an increased risk of cervical cancer.

Most HPV-associated lesions can be diagnosed by cervical cytology. In difficult cases, ancillary techniques such as in situ hybridization can help confirm the diagnosis (Fig. F23.6.1). An HPV vaccine, called *Gardasil 9*, is available for the prevention of HPV. Gardasil 9 protects against types 6, 11, 16, and 18 and five other high-risk HPV types. Vaccinations against HPV virus are recommended for both sexes between the ages of 9 and 26 years.

None of the vaccines are therapeutic (i.e., they do not clear prior infection), but both lead to the development of specific immunity against HPV infections. The vaccines are most effective in those who have had no prior HPV exposure and who are immunized before initiation of sexual activity.

Cervical cancer screening now includes HPV testing in addition to cervical cytology for certain age groups. The following are the most current **cervical cancer screening recommendations** for people who have no other risks factors for cervical cancer from the American College of Obstetricians and Gynecologists:

- Age 21 years and younger: no screening
- Ages 21–29 years: cervical cytology (Pap test) every 3 years
- Ages 30–65 years: primary HPV testing alone every 5 years or HPV testing plus cervical cytology every 5 years OR cervical cytology every 3 years

The increased interval between screening tests (as opposed to annual testing) and the avoidance of HPV testing in younger individuals are recommended to decrease the number of false-positive results and unnecessary diagnostic procedures. HPV infection usually resolves spontaneously in younger patients. When infections do persist, they usually do so for many years before precancerous changes can be detected.

Diagnosis of precancer of the cervix includes **colposcopy**, in which a colposcope (a specifically designed microscope to magnify the view of the cervix) is used to examine the cervix for lesions and to perform cervical biopsy. Treatment for precancerous lesions is accomplished by removal of the precancerous cells by **cone biopsy (conization)**, a procedure in which a cone-shaped tissue of the cervix containing part of ectocervix, transformation zone, and cervical canal is excised or destroyed. Conization can be performed with a scalpel (cold-knife conization), laser, electrosurgical loop, or freezing (cryoconization).

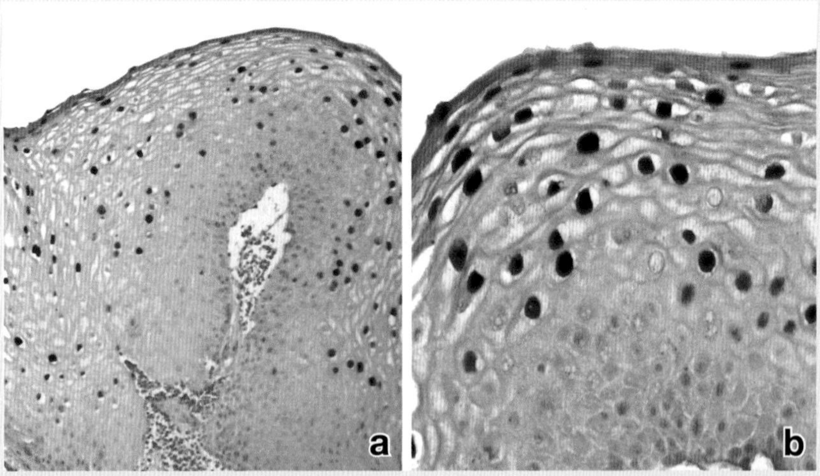

FIGURE F23.6.1. Photomicrograph of in situ hybridization of a human cervical biopsy showing human papillomavirus (HPV) infection. a. This low-magnification photomicrograph shows stratified squamous epithelium of the cervix hybridized with DNA probes to HPV types 6 and 11 and counterstained with nuclear fast red. Note that the majority of infected cells are mature cells located in the upper layers of the stratified squamous epithelium of the ectocervix. ×120. **b.** This higher magnification photomicrograph shows viral particles stained *purple* within the nuclei of infected cells. ×225. (Courtesy of Dr. Fabiola Medeiros.)

Lactation is under the neurohormonal control of the adenohypophysis and hypothalamus.

Although estrogen and progesterone are essential for the physical development of the breast during pregnancy, both of these hormones also suppress the effects of PRL and hCS, the levels of which increase as pregnancy progresses. Immediately after childbirth, however, the sudden loss of estrogen and progesterone secretion from the placenta and corpus luteum allows PRL to assume its lactogenic role. Production of milk also requires adequate secretion of

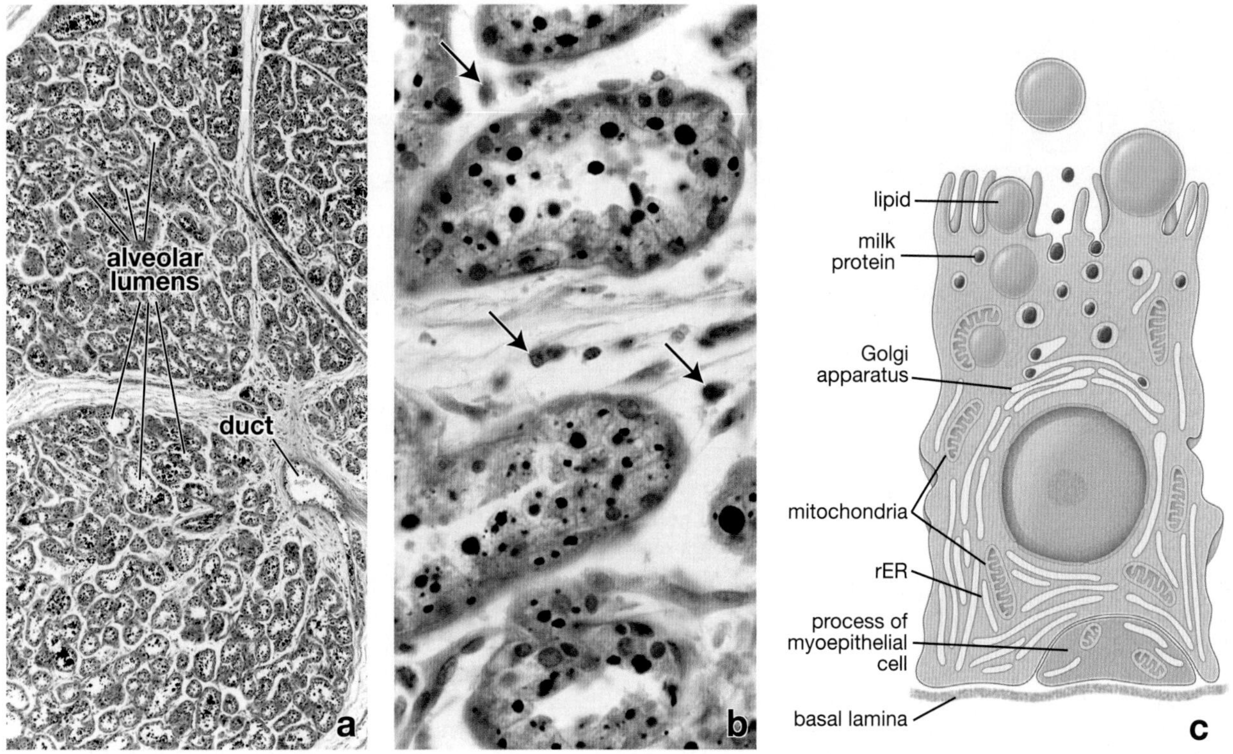

FIGURE 23.45. Photomicrographs and diagram of a lactating mammary gland. a. Low-magnification micrograph of a fast-green osmium–stained section of a lactating mammary gland. Portions of several large lobules and an excretory duct are seen. Many of the alveoli exhibit a prominent lumen, even at this magnification. ×60. **b.** A higher magnification of an area in **a** shows lipid droplets (*black* circular profiles) within the secretory cells of the alveoli as well as in the alveolar lumina. The *arrows* indicate plasma cells within the interstitial spaces. ×480. **c.** Diagram of a lactating mammary gland epithelial cell. *rER*, rough-surfaced endoplasmic reticulum. (Redrawn after Bloom W, Fawcett DW. *A Textbook of Histology*. 10th ed. WB Saunders; 1975.)

growth hormones, adrenal glucocorticoids, and parathyroid hormones.

The act of **suckling** during breastfeeding initiates sensory impulses from receptors in the nipple to the hypothalamus. The impulses inhibit the release of prolactin-inhibiting factor, and **prolactin** is then released from the adenohypophysis. The sensory impulses also cause the release of **oxytocin** in the neurohypophysis. Oxytocin stimulates the myoepithelial cells that surround the base of the alveolar secretory cells and the base of the cells in the larger ducts, causing them to contract and eject the milk from the alveoli and the ducts. In the **absence of suckling**, secretion of milk ceases, and the mammary glands begin to regress and atrophy. The glandular tissue then returns to an inactive condition.

Involution of the Mammary Gland

After menopause, the specialized stroma of the mammary gland **involutes**, causing the gland to atrophy. In the absence of ovarian hormone stimulation, the secretory cells of the TDLUs degenerate and disappear, leaving only ducts to create a histologic pattern that resembles that of the male breast. The connective tissue also demonstrates degenerative changes, marked by a decrease in the number of fibroblasts and collagen fibers and loss of elastic fibers.

Blood Supply and Lymphatics

The arteries that supply the breast are derived from the thoracic branches of the **axillary artery**, the **internal thoracic artery**, and anterior intercostal arteries. Branches of the vessels pass primarily along the path of the alveolar ducts as they reach capillary beds surrounding the alveoli. In general, veins basically follow the path of the arteries as they return to the axillary and internal thoracic veins.

Lymphatic capillaries are located in the connective tissue surrounding the alveoli. The larger lymphatic vessels drain into **axillary**, **supraclavicular**, or **parasternal lymph nodes**.

Innervation

The nerves that supply the breast are anterior and lateral cutaneous branches from the second to sixth **intercostal nerves**. The nerves convey afferent and sympathetic fibers to and from the breast. The secretory function is primarily under hormonal control, but afferent impulses associated with suckling are involved in the reflex secretion of PRL and oxytocin.

FOLDER 23.7

FUNCTIONAL CONSIDERATIONS: LACTATION AND INFERTILITY

Almost 50% of females who fully breastfeed exhibit **lactational amenorrhea** (lack of menstruation during lactation) and infertility. This effect is caused by high levels of serum prolactin, which inhibit secretion of pulsatile gonadotropin-releasing hormone (GnRH), thus suppressing secretion of the luteinizing hormone (LH). Ovulation usually resumes after 6 months or earlier with a decrease in suckling frequency.

101 HISTOLOGY NOTEBOOK

FEMALE REPRODUCTIVE SYSTEM

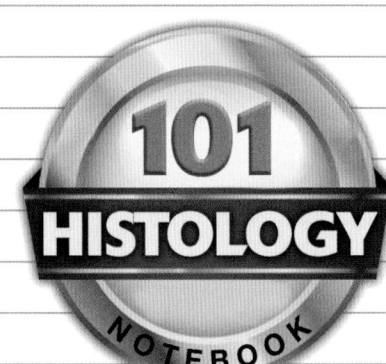

OVERVIEW OF THE FEMALE REPRODUCTIVE SYSTEM

- The female reproductive system consists of **internal female reproductive organs** (ovaries, uterine tubes, uterus, and vagina) and **external genitalia** (vulva).
- Internal female reproductive organs undergo regular cyclic changes during each **menstrual cycle**, from **puberty** to **menopause**, that reflect changes in hormone levels.

OVARY

- The major functions of the ovaries are the production of gametes (**oogenesis**) and the production of steroid hormones (estrogen and progesterone; **steroidogenesis**).
- Ovaries have a **medulla** in their center that contains loose connective tissue, nerves, blood and lymphatic vessels, and a **cortex** on their periphery that contains a large number of **ovarian follicles** that provide a microenvironment for developing oocytes.
- The surface of the ovary is covered by **germinal epithelium**, which is a single cuboidal epithelium that overlies a dense layer of connective tissue called **tunica albuginea**.

OVARIAN FOLLICLE DEVELOPMENT

- There are three basic developmental stages of an **ovarian follicle: primordial**, **growing** (both primary and secondary), and **mature (Graafian) follicle**.
- Before puberty, the cortex of an ovary is occupied only by **primordial follicles**. They contain a single primary oocyte that is arrested in the first meiotic prophase and is surrounded by a single layer of **squamous follicle cells**.
- After puberty following cyclic hormonal changes, a selected cohort of primary follicles develops into **growing follicles**. Follicle cells surrounding the oocyte become cuboidal and undergo further stratification to form the **primary follicle**.
- Cells of the growing follicle develop into **granulosa cells**; connective tissue surrounding the follicle differentiates into the **theca interna** and **theca externa**; and the oocyte grows and produces the **zona pellucida** (ZP) that contains specific ZP glycoproteins involved in the fertilization process.
- As **granulosa cells** proliferate, they become involved in steroid hormone metabolism (conversion of androgens produced by the theca interna into estrogens) and actively secrete follicular fluid that accumulates in cavities between the granulosa cells.
- A growing follicle that contains a single fluid cavity (**antrum**) is called the **secondary (antral) follicle**. It still contains the primary oocyte arrested in the first prophase of meiotic division.
- As the **secondary follicle** enlarges and undergoes further maturation, the thin layer of granulosa cells that is associated with the oocyte forms the **cumulus oophorus** and **corona radiata**.
- The **mature (Graafian) follicle** has a large antrum and a prominent, steroid-producing theca interna layer. Triggered by an LH surge just before ovulation, the oocyte resumes its first meiotic division and becomes the **secondary oocyte**.

OVULATION

- During the ovarian cycle, usually, only one Graafian follicle undergoes **ovulation**. All other follicles in the developing cohort undergo **follicular atresia**, a process of degeneration involving apoptosis.
- During ovulation, a **secondary oocyte** is released from the ruptured Graafian follicle. The released oocyte is arrested in the metaphase of the second meiotic division.
- At ovulation, the **follicular wall**, composed of the remaining granulosa and thecal cells, is transformed into the **corpus luteum**. Under the influence of LH in the process of **luteinization**, the **granulosa lutein cells** (produce estrogen) and the **theca lutein cells** (produce progesterone) are formed.
- The **corpus luteum of menstruation** is formed in the absence of fertilization; it degenerates 10–12 days after ovulation to become the **corpus albicans**.
- The **corpus luteum of pregnancy** is formed after fertilization and implantation; it is a major source of **progesterone** and **luteotropins** (estrogen, insulin-like growth factor) during the first 8 weeks of pregnancy, after which it degenerates and leaves a permanent scar in the ovary.

CAPACITATION AND FERTILIZATION

- During **capacitation**, the mature spermatozoa acquire the ability to fertilize the oocyte within the female reproductive tract.
- **Fertilization** normally occurs in the ampulla of the uterine tube; it involves the capacitation of spermatozoa and their penetration of the corona radiata to reach the oocyte.
- After capacitation, the spermatozoa bind to the **zona pellucida receptors**, which trigger the **acrosome reaction**. Enzymes released from the acrosome allow a single spermatozoon to penetrate the zona pellucida and **impregnate the oocyte**.
- During impregnation, the entire spermatozoon, except for the tail plasma membrane, becomes incorporated into the ooplasm, which triggers resumption of the **second meiotic division** (transforms the secondary oocyte into a mature oocyte).
- At least three types of **postfusion reactions** prevent other spermatozoa from entering the oocyte: fast depolarization of the oolemma, the cortical reaction (changes of polarity of the oolemma), and the zona reaction (which forms a **perivitelline barrier** by cross-linking proteins on the oocyte surface and degrading ZP receptors).
- The sperm head within the oocyte cytoplasm undergoes changes to form the **male pronucleus**. Nuclear membranes of both **male and female pronuclei** break down without fusion to form a diploid **zygote**. The zygote immediately enters its first mitotic division.

UTERINE TUBES

- The **uterine tubes** are paired bilateral structures that connect the uterus with the ovaries.
- Each uterine tube has four segments: **infundibulum** (a funnel-shaped end surrounded by **fimbriae** adjacent to the ovary), **ampulla** (common site of fertilization), **isthmus** (narrow segment adjacent to the uterus), and **intramural** part (traversing the uterine wall).
- The uterine tube wall consists of three layers: external **serosa**, thick **muscularis**, and highly folded **mucosa**.
- The **mucosal lining** is simple columnar epithelium composed of two cell types: **ciliated** and **nonciliated (peg) cells.**
- The oocyte (and zygote after fertilization) is propelled into the uterine cavity by a coordinated movement of cilia on the surface of mucosa and peristaltic muscular contractions of the uterine tube.

UTERUS

- The **uterus** is divided into the **body** (upper portion containing **fundus**) and the **cervix** (lower portion that projects into the vagina).
- The uterine wall is composed of **endometrium** (lining mucosa of the uterus), **myometrium** (smooth muscular layer), and **perimetrium** (a serous layer of visceral peritoneum).
- The **endometrium** is lined by simple columnar epithelium that invaginates into the underlying lamina propria (**endometrial stroma**), forming **uterine glands.**
- The endometrium consists of **stratum basale** and **stratum functionale**, which undergoes cyclic changes due to fluctuating levels of estrogens and progesterone during the menstrual cycle.
- The thickness of the endometrium, its glandular activity, and its vascular pattern are unique for each of the three phases (**proliferative**, **secretory**, and **menstrual**) of the **menstrual cycle**, which lasts an average of 28 days.
- The **proliferative phase** is influenced by estrogens produced by the growing follicles; the **secretory phase** is influenced by progesterone secreted from the corpus luteum; and if no implantation occurs, the **menstrual phase** represents ischemia of the stratum functionale that is being sloughed off during menses.
- If the embryo implants successfully, the **endometrium** undergoes **decidualization** (the process of conversion to **decidua**) and, together with the trophoblastic cells from the embryo, initiates the development of the **placenta.**
- The endometrium of the **cervix** differs from the rest of the uterus in that it is not sloughed off during menstruation. **Cervical glands** modify the viscosity of the secreted mucus during each menstrual cycle.
- The part of the cervix projecting into the vagina has a **transformation zone** where simple columnar epithelium of the cervix changes abruptly into stratified squamous epithelium of the vagina.

PLACENTA

- The **placenta** allows for exchange of gases and metabolites between the maternal and fetal circulations; it consists of a **fetal portion** (**chorion**) and a **maternal portion** (**decidua basalis**).
- After implantation, the invading **trophoblast** differentiates into the **syncytiotrophoblast** (multinucleate cytoplasmic mass that actively invades the decidua) and the **cytotrophoblast** (a mitotically active layer producing cells that fuse with the syncytiotrophoblast).
- Fetal and maternal blood remain separated by the **placental barrier**, which develops in the **tertiary chorionic villi** (projections of chorion containing syncytiotrophoblast, occasional cytotrophoblast cells, mesenchymal connective tissue, and fetal blood vessels).
- Villi are immersed in the maternal blood that fills vascular spaces in the placenta (**cotyledons**).
- The placenta is a major **endocrine organ** that supports the development of the fetus; it produces both **steroid hormones** (mainly progesterone) and **protein hormones** (e.g., hCG, hCS, relaxin, and leptin).

VAGINA AND EXTERNAL GENITALIA

- The **vagina** extends from the cervix to the vestibule; it is lined with **stratified squamous nonkeratinized epithelium** and lacks glands.
- **Female external genitalia (vulva)** consist of the **mons pubis** (formed by underlying adipose tissue), **labia majora** (longitudinal folds of skin containing adipose tissue, a thin layer of smooth muscle, and sebaceous and sweat glands), **labia minora** (core of connective tissue devoid of adipose tissue but contains large sebaceous glands), **clitoral complex**, **vestibule** (lined with stratified squamous epithelium with numerous small mucous glands), **opening of the vagina**, **hymen**, and **external urethral orifice.**
- The **clitoral complex** is composed of the **glans of the clitoris**, **body of the clitoris**, **left and right crus of the clitoris**, and two **bulbs of the vestibule**. They possess erectile and nonerectile vascular tissue homologous to the penis.

MAMMARY GLANDS

- The **mammary glands** develop in both sexes from **mammary ridges** in the embryo, but they undergo further development after puberty due to the hormonal influence of estrogen and progesterone.
- **Mammary glands** are modified tubuloalveolar apocrine sweat glands consisting of **terminal duct lobular units (TDLUs)**. Each TDLU is connected to collecting duct systems, which form the **lactiferous ducts** that open at the **nipple.**
- The TDLU of the mammary gland represents a cluster of small **secretory alveoli** (in active lactating gland) or **terminal ductules** (in inactive gland) surrounded by a hormonally sensitive **intralobular stroma.**
- The morphology of the secretory portion of the **inactive mammary gland** varies with the menstrual cycle.
- Mammary glands undergo dramatic proliferation and development during pregnancy in preparation for **lactation** under the influence of estrogen (proliferation of duct components) and progesterone (growth of alveoli).
- The protein component of milk is released by alveolar cells using **merocrine secretion**, whereas the lipid component of milk is released by **apocrine secretion.**

PLATE 23.1 ■ OVARY I

The **ovaries** are small, paired, ovoid structures that exhibit a **cortex** and **medulla** when sectioned. On one side is a hilum for the transit of neurovascular structures; on this same side is a mesovarium that joins the ovary to the broad ligament. The functions of the ovary are the production of *ova* and the synthesis and secretion of **estrogen** and **progesterone**.

In the cortex are numerous **primordial follicles** that are present at the time of birth and that remain unchanged until sexual maturation. The oogonia in these follicles are arrested in prophase of the first meiotic division. At puberty, under the influence of pituitary gonadotropins, the ovaries begin to undergo the cyclical changes designated the **ovarian cycle**. During each cycle, the ovaries normally produce a single oocyte that is ready for fertilization.

At the beginning of the ovarian cycle, under the influence of pituitary follicle-stimulating hormone (FSH), some of the primordial follicles begin to undergo changes that lead to the development of a **mature (Graafian) follicle**. These changes include proliferation of follicle cells and enlargement of the follicle. Although several primordial follicles begin these developmental changes, usually, only one reaches maturity and yields an oocyte. Occasionally, two follicles will mature and ovulate, leading to the possibility of dizygotic twin development. The discharge of the oocyte and its adherent cells is called **ovulation**. At ovulation, the oocyte completes the first meiotic division. Only if fertilization occurs does the oocyte complete the second meiotic division. Whether or not fertilization occurs, the other follicles that began to proliferate in the same cycle degenerate, a process referred to as **atresia**.

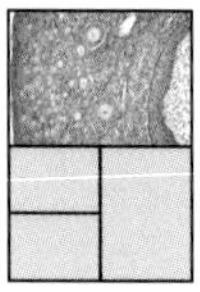

Cortex, ovary, monkey, hematoxylin and eosin (H&E) ×120.

The **cortex** of an ovary from a sexually mature individual is shown here. On the surface, there is a single layer of epithelial cells designated the **germinal epithelium** (*GEp*). This epithelium is continuous with the serosa (peritoneum) of the mesovarium. Contrary to its name, the epithelium does not give rise to the germ cells. The germinal epithelium covers a dense fibrous connective tissue layer, the **tunica albuginea** (*TA*); under the tunica albuginea are the **primordial follicles** (*PF*). It is not unusual to see follicles at various stages of development or atresia in the ovary. In this figure, along with the large number of primordial follicles, there are four **growing follicles** (*GF*), with a clearly visible eosinophilic layer of the zona pellucida (*ZP*), an atretic follicle (*AF*), and part of a large follicle on the *right*. The region of the large follicle shown in the figure includes the theca interna (*TI*), granulosa cells (*GC*), and part of the antrum (*A*).

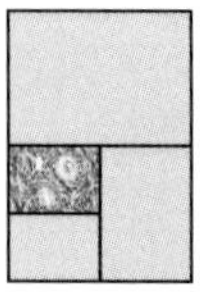

Early primary follicles, ovary, monkey, H&E ×450.

When a **primordial follicle** begins the changes leading to the formation of a mature follicle, the layer of squamous follicle cells becomes cuboidal (*FC*), as in this figure. In addition, the follicle cells proliferate and become multilayered. A follicle undergoing these early changes is called a **primary follicle**. Thus, an early primary follicle may still be unilaminar, but it is surrounded by cuboidal cells, and this distinguishes it from the more numerous unilaminar primordial follicles that are surrounded by squamous cells. Note the large nucleus (*N*) of the oocyte in the primary follicle. Some oocytes may not have visible nuclei (see cell label *X*) due to the plane of section.

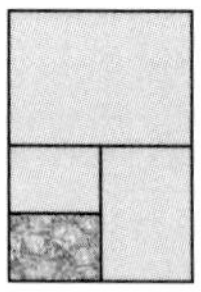

Primordial follicles, ovary, monkey, H&E ×450.

This figure shows several **primordial follicles** at higher magnification. Each follicle consists of an oocyte surrounded by a single layer of squamous follicle cells (*F*). The nucleus (*N*) of the oocyte is typically large, but the oocyte itself is so large that the nucleus is often not included in the plane of section, as in the oocyte marked *X*. The group of epithelioid-appearing cells (*arrowhead*) are follicle cells of a primordial follicle that has been sectioned in a plane that just grazes the follicular surface. In this case, the follicle cells are seen en face.

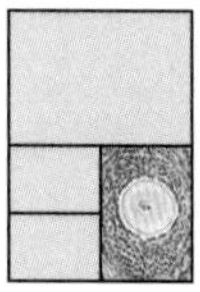

Late primary follicle, ovary, monkey, H&E ×450.

The **primary follicle** in this figure shows a multilayered mass of **follicle cells** (*FC*) surrounding the oocyte with a clearly visible large nucleus (*N*). The innermost layer of follicle cells is adjacent to a thick eosinophilic layer of extracellular homogeneous material called the **zona pellucida** (*ZP*). At this stage of development, the oocyte has also enlarged slightly. The entire structure surrounded by the zona pellucida is actually the oocyte.

Surrounding the follicles are elongate cells of the highly cellular connective tissue, referred to as *stromal cells*. The stromal cells surrounding a secondary follicle become disposed into two layers designated the theca interna and the theca externa. As seen in the previous figure, stromal cells become epithelioid in the cell-rich theca interna (*TI*).

A, antrum
AF, atretic follicle
F, follicle cells, primordial
FC, follicle cells
GC, granulosa cells
GEp, germinal epithelium
GF, growing follicles
N, nucleus of oocyte
PF, primordial follicles
TA, tunica albuginea
TI, theca interna
X, oocyte showing only cytoplasm
ZP, zona pellucida
arrowhead, follicle cells seen en face

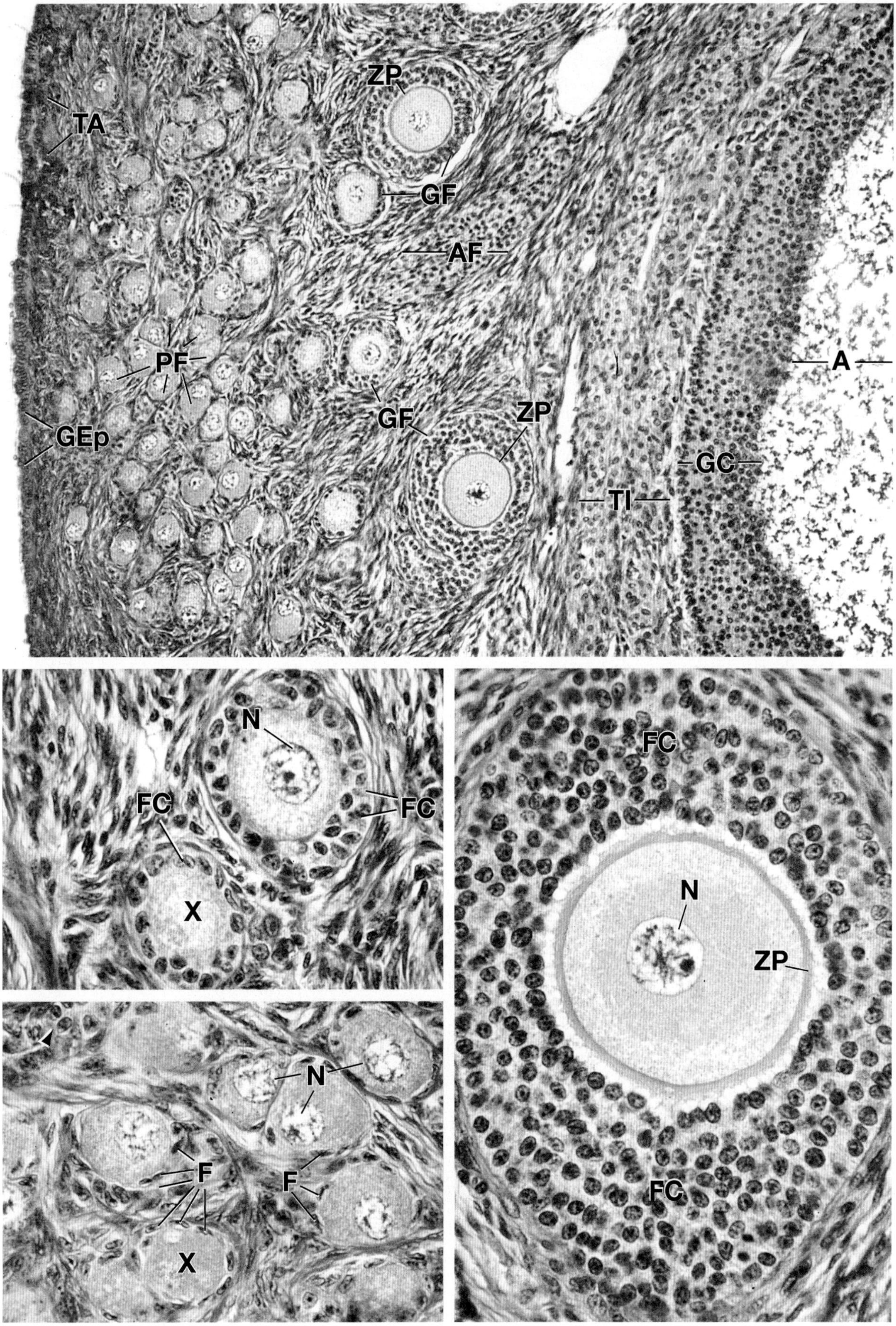
ZP
TA
GF
AF
PF
A
GEp
GF
ZP
GC
TI
N
FC
FC
FC
X
N
ZP
FC
N
F
F
X

PLATE 23.2 ■ OVARY II

Atresia of follicles is a regular event in the ovary, beginning in embryonic life. In any section through the postpubertal ovary, follicles of various stages can be seen undergoing atresia. In atresia, the initial changes involve pyknosis of the nuclei of the follicle cells and dissolution of their cytoplasm. The follicle is then invaded by macrophages and other connective tissue cells. The oocyte degenerates, leaving behind the prominent zona pellucida. This may fold inward or collapse, but it usually retains its thickness and staining characteristics. When included in the plane of section, a distorted zona pellucida serves as a reliable diagnostic feature of an **atretic follicle**.

In atresia of large, nearly mature follicles, cells of the theca interna remain to form clusters of epithelioid cells in the ovarian cortex. These are referred to collectively as *interstitial glands* and continue to secrete steroid hormones.

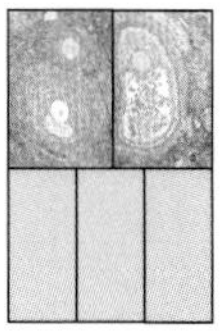

Secondary follicles, ovary, monkey, hematoxylin and eosin (H&E) ×120.

Two follicles growing under the influence of follicle-stimulating hormone (FSH) are shown in the figure on the *left*. The more advanced follicle is a **secondary follicle**. The oocyte in this follicle is surrounded by several layers of **follicle cells** (*FC*) that, at this stage, are identified as granulosa cells. At a slightly earlier time, small lakes of fluid formed between the follicle cells, and these lakes have now fused into a well-defined larger cavity called the **follicular antrum** (*FA*), which is evident in the figure. The antrum is also filled with fluid and stains with the periodic acid–Schiff (PAS) reaction, although only lightly. The substance that stains with the PAS reaction has been retained as an eosinophilic precipitate in the antra of the secondary follicles shown here and in the figure on the *right*. Immediately above the obvious secondary follicle is a slightly smaller follicle. Because no antral spaces are evident between the follicle cells, it is appropriate to classify it as a **primary follicle**. In both follicles, but particularly in the larger follicle with the antrum, the surrounding stromal cells have become altered to form two distinctive layers designated **theca interna** (*TI*) and **theca externa** (*TE*). The theca interna is a more cellular layer, and the cells are epithelioid. When seen with the electron microscope, they display the characteristics of endocrine cells, particularly steroid-secreting cells. In contrast, the theca externa is a connective tissue layer. Its cells are more or less spindle shaped.

In the figure on the *right*, a later stage in the growth of the secondary follicle is shown. The antrum (*FA*) is larger, and the oocyte is off to one side, surrounded by a mound of follicle cells called the *cumulus oophorus*. The remaining follicle cells that surround the antral cavity are referred to as the *membrana granulosa* (*MG*), or simply granulosa cells.

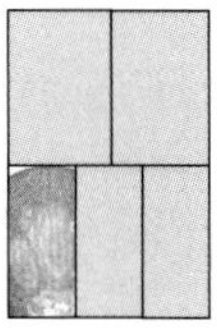

Atretic follicle, ovary, monkey, H&E ×65.

Atretic follicles (*AF*) are shown here and at higher magnification in the adjacent figure on the *right*. The two smaller atretic follicles can be identified by virtue of the retained zona pellucida (*ZP*) labeled on the adjacent figure to the *right*. The two larger, more advanced follicles do not display the remains of a zona pellucida, but they do display other features of follicular atresia.

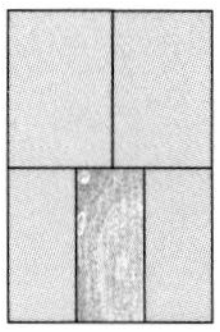

Atretic follicles, ovary, monkey, H&E ×120.

During atresia of a more advanced follicle, the follicle cells tend to degenerate more rapidly than the cells of the theca interna, and the basement membrane separating the two becomes thickened to form a hyalinized membrane, the glassy membrane. Thus, the **glassy membrane** (*arrows*) separates an outer layer of remaining theca interna cells from the degenerating inner follicle cells. The remaining theca interna cells may show cytologic integrity (*RTI*); these intact theca cells remain temporarily functional in steroid secretion.

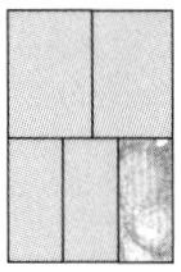

Atretic follicles, ovary, monkey, H&E ×120.

Additional **atretic follicles** (*AF*) are shown here. Again, some show remnants of a zona pellucida (*ZP*), and two show a glassy membrane (*arrows*). Note that although the atresia in these follicles is well advanced, some of the cells external to one of the glassy membranes still retain their epithelioid character (*arrowhead*). These are persisting theca interna cells.

AF, atretic follicle
FA, antrum of follicle
FC, follicle cells
MG, membrana granulosa
RTI, remaining theca interna cells
TE, theca externa
TI, theca interna
ZP, zona pellucida
arrowhead, persisting theca interna cells
arrows, glassy membrane

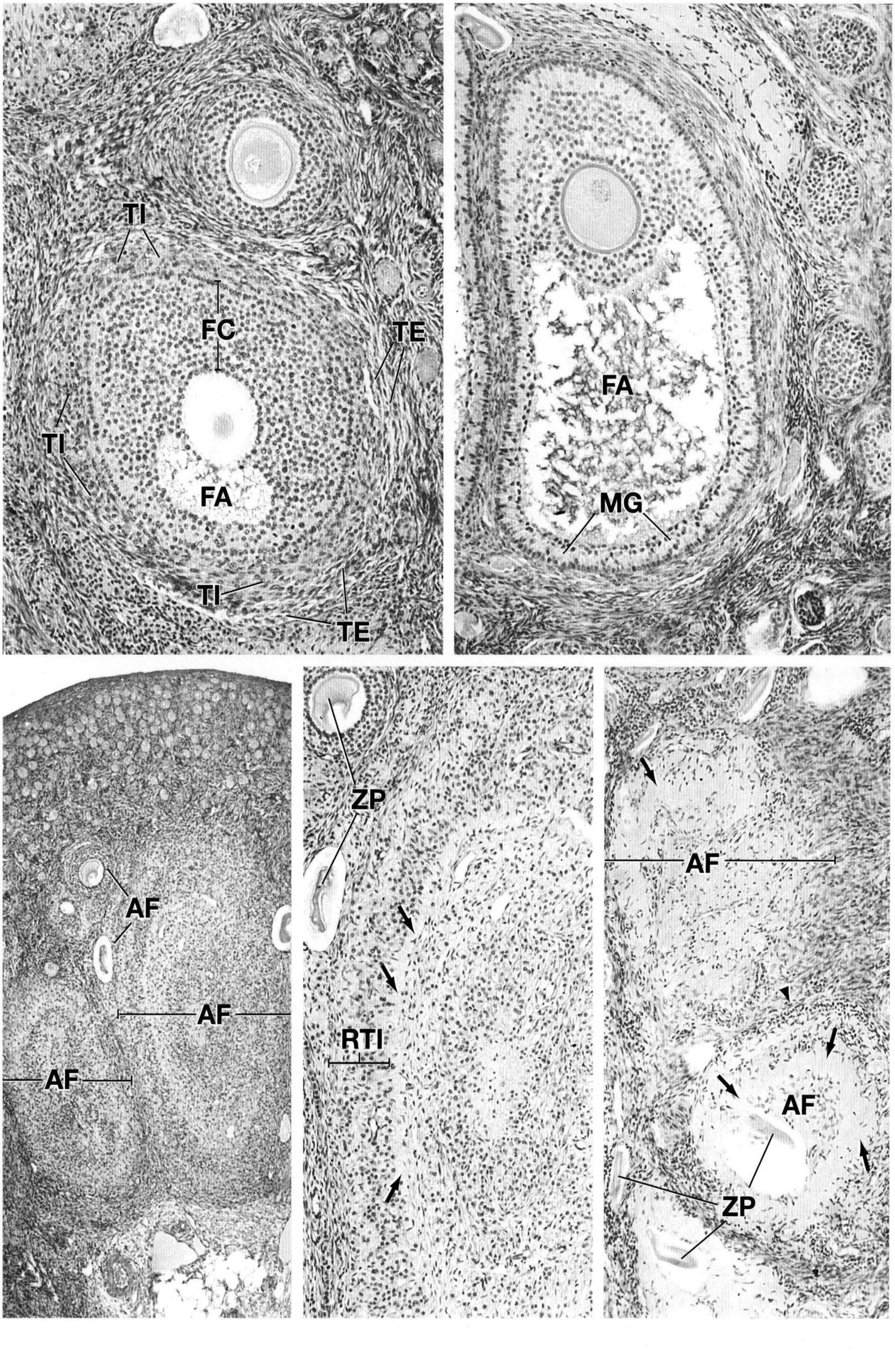
TI
FC
TE
TI
FA
TI
TE
FA
MG
AF
AF
AF
ZP
RTI
AF
AF
ZP

PLATE 23.3 ■ CORPUS LUTEUM

After the oocyte and its immediately surrounding cells (i.e., the cells of the cumulus oophorus) are discharged from the mature ovarian follicle (ovulation), the remaining follicle cells (membrana granulosa) and the adjacent theca interna cells differentiate into a new functional unit, the **corpus luteum**.

The cells of the corpus luteum, luteal cells, rapidly increase in size and become filled with lipid droplets. A lipid-soluble pigment in the cytoplasm of the cells, lipochrome, gives them their yellow appearance in fresh tissue. Electron micrographs of the luteal cells demonstrate that they have features typical of steroid-secreting cells, namely, abundant smooth-surfaced endoplasmic reticulum and mitochondria with tubular cristae. Two types of luteal cells are identified: Large, centrally located **granulosa lutein cells** are derived from the granulosa cells; smaller, peripherally located **theca lutein cells** are derived from the theca interna. A rich vascular network is established in the corpus luteum into which progesterone and estrogen are secreted by the lutein cells. These hormones stimulate the growth and differentiation of the uterine endometrium to prepare it for implantation of a fertilized ovum.

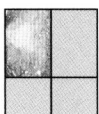

Corpus luteum, ovary, human, hematoxylin and eosin (H&E) ×20.

This figure shows ovarian **cortex** shortly after ovulation. The *arrowhead* points toward the surface of the ovary at the site of ovulation. The cavity (*FC*) of the former follicle has been invaded by connective tissue (*CT*). The membrana granulosa has become plicated, and the granulosa cells, now transforming into cells of the corpus luteum, are called **granulosa lutein cells** (*TC*). The plication of the membrana granulosa begins just before ovulation and continues as the corpus luteum develops. As the corpus luteum becomes more plicated, the former follicular cavity becomes reduced in size. At the same time, blood vessels (*BV*) from the theca of the follicle invade the former cavity and the transforming membrana granulosa cells. Cells of the theca interna follow the blood vessels into the outermost depressions of the plicated structure. These theca interna cells become transformed into cells of the corpus luteum called *theca lutein cells*.

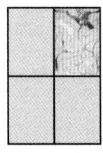

Corpus luteum, ovary, human, H&E ×20.

A portion of a fully formed **corpus luteum** is shown here. Most endocrine cells are the **granulosa lutein cells** (*GLC*). These form a folded cell mass that surrounds the remains of the former follicular cavity (*FC*). External to the corpus luteum is the connective tissue of the ovary (*CT*) with a large quantity of blood vessels (*BV*). Keep in mind that the theca interna is derived from the connective tissue stroma of the ovary. The location of **theca lutein cells** (*TLC*) reflects this origin, and these cells can be found in the deep outer recesses of the glandular mass, adjacent to the surrounding connective tissue.

Corpus luteum, ovary, human, H&E ×65 (on left) and ×240 (on right).

A segment of the plicated **corpus luteum** is shown in the figure on the *left* at slightly higher magnification. As noted earlier, the main cell mass is composed of **granulosa lutein cells** (*GLC*). On one side of this cell mass is the connective tissue (*CT*) within the former follicular cavity; on the other side are the theca lutein cells. The same arrangement of cells is shown in the figure on the *right* at much higher magnification. The granulosa lutein cells contain a large, spherical nucleus (see also *GLC*, in the figure on that *right*) and a large amount of cytoplasm. The cytoplasm contains a yellow pigment (usually not evident in routine H&E sections), hence the name, corpus luteum. **Theca lutein cells** (*TLC*) also contain a spherical nucleus, but the cells are smaller than the granulosa lutein cells. Thus, when identifying the two cell types, aside from location, note that the nuclei of adjacent theca lutein cells generally appear to be closer to each other than nuclei of adjacent granulosa lutein cells. The connective tissue (*CT*) and small blood vessels that invaded the mass of granulosa lutein cells can be identified as the flattened and elongated components between the granulosa lutein cells.

The changes whereby the ruptured ovarian follicle is transformed into a corpus luteum occur under the influence of pituitary luteinizing hormone. In turn, the corpus luteum itself secretes progesterone, which has a profound effect on the estrogen-primed uterus. If pregnancy occurs, the corpus luteum remains functional; if pregnancy does not occur, the corpus luteum regresses after having reached a point of peak development, roughly 2 weeks after ovulation. The regressing cellular components of the corpus luteum are replaced by fibrous connective tissue, and the structure is then called a *corpus albicans*.

BV, blood vessels
CT, connective tissue
FC, former follicular cavity
GLC, granulosa lutein cells
TC, granulosa cells transforming into corpus luteum cells
TLC, theca lutein cells

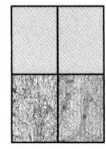

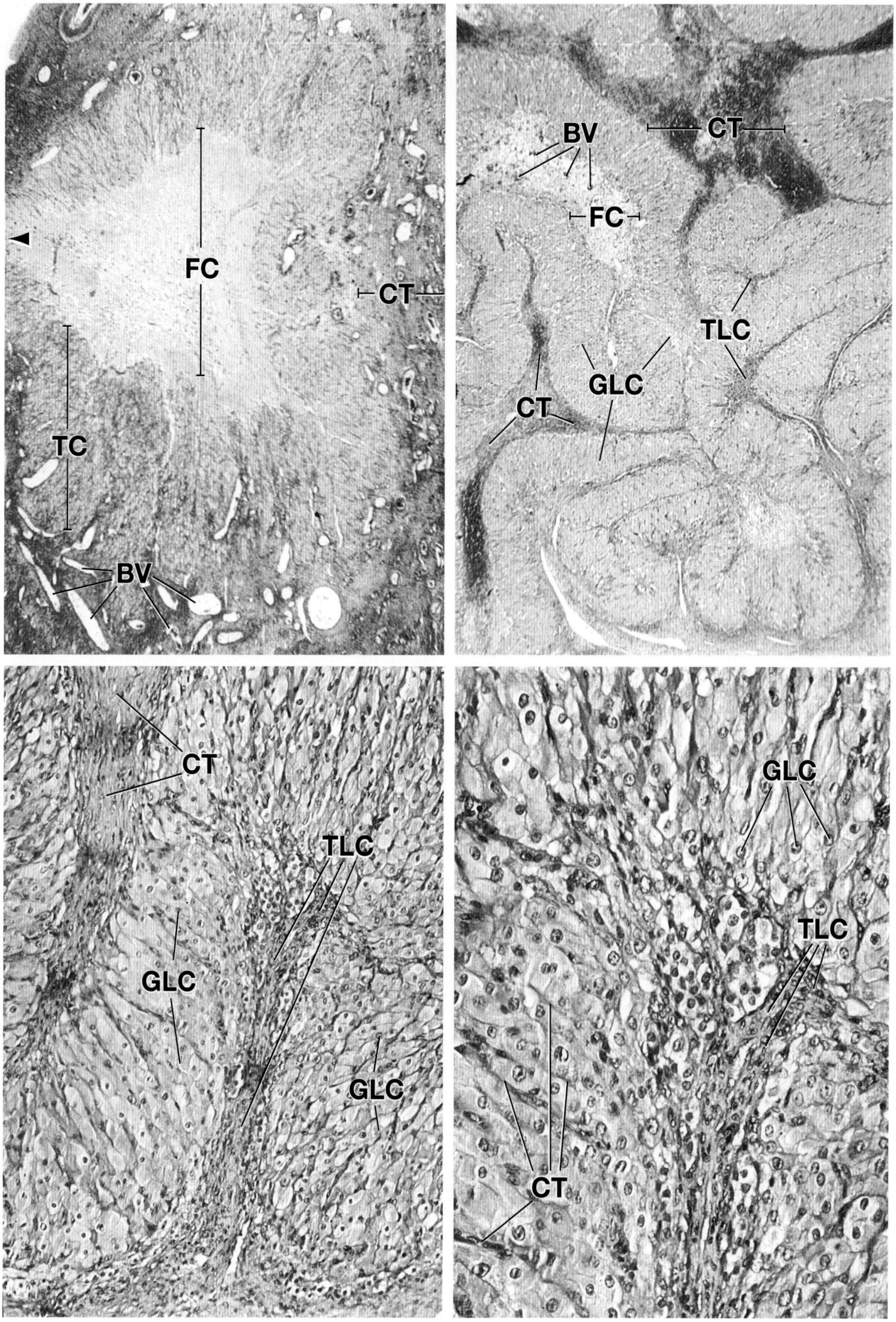
FC
CT
TC
BV
BV
CT
FC
TLC
GLC
CT
CT
TLC
GLC
GLC
GLC
TLC
CT

PLATE 23.4 ■ UTERINE TUBE

The **uterine tubes** (oviducts, fallopian tubes) are joined to the uterus and extend to the ovaries, where they present an open flared end (abdominal ostium) for entry of the ovum at ovulation. The oviduct undergoes cyclical changes along with those of the uterus, but these are not nearly as pronounced. The epithelial cells increase in height during the middle of the cycle, just about the time the ovum will be passing through the tube and become reduced during the premenstrual period. Some of the epithelial cells are ciliated. The epithelial cells depend on the ovaries for their viability. Not only does the number of ciliated cells increase during the follicular phase of the ovarian cycle, but removal of the ovaries leads to atrophy of the epithelium and loss of ciliated cells.

The uterine tube varies in size and degree of mucosal folding along its length. The mucosal folds are evident in its distal portion, the infundibulum, as it nears the open end. Near the opening, the tube flares outward and is called the **infundibulum**. It has fringed folded edges called **fimbria**. The infundibulum leads proximally to the **ampulla**, which constitutes about two-thirds of the length of the oviduct, has the most numerous and complex mucosal folds, and is the site of fertilization. Mucosal folds are least numerous at the proximal end of the oviduct, near the uterus, where the tube is narrow and referred to as the **isthmus**. A **uterine** or **intramural** portion measures about 1 cm in length and passes through the uterine wall to empty into the uterine cavity.

Fertilization of the ovum usually occurs in the distal portion of the ampulla. For the first several days of development, as it navigates the complex pathway created by the mucosal folds, the embryo is transported proximally by the beating of the cilia of the ciliated epithelial cells and by peristaltic contractions of the well-developed muscularis layer that underlies the mucosa.

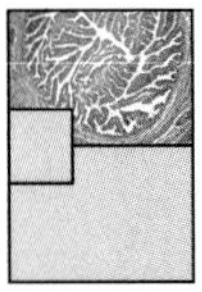

Uterine tube, human, hematoxylin and eosin (H&E) ×40.

A cross section through the **ampulla** of the uterine tube is shown here. Many mucosal folds project into the lumen (*L*), and the complicated nature of the folds is evident by the variety of profiles that are seen. In addition to the **mucosa** (*Muc*), the remainder of the wall consists of a **muscularis** (*Mus*) and connective tissue.

The muscularis consists of smooth muscle that forms a relatively thick layer of circular fibers and a thinner outer layer of longitudinal fibers. The layers are not clearly delineated, and no sharp boundary separates them.

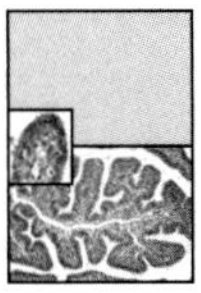

Mucosal fold, uterine tube, human, H&E ×160; inset ×320.

The area enclosed by the *rectangle* in the previous figure is shown here at higher magnification. The specimen shows a longitudinal section through a lymphatic vessel (*Lym*). In other planes of section, the lymphatic vessels are difficult to identify. The fortuitously sectioned lymphatic vessel is seen in the core of the **mucosal fold**, along with a highly cellular connective tissue (*CT*) and the blood vessels (*BV*) within the connective tissue. The epithelium (*Ep*) lining the mucosa is shown in the *inset*. The ciliated cells are readily identified by the presence of well-formed cilia (*C*). Nonciliated cells, also called *peg cells* (*PC*), are readily identified by the absence of cilia; moreover, they have elongate nuclei and sometimes appear to be squeezed between the ciliated cells. The connective tissue (*CT*) contains cells whose nuclei are arranged typically in a random manner. They vary in shape, being elongated, oval, or round. Their cytoplasm cannot be distinguished from the intercellular material (*inset*). The character of the connective tissue is essentially the same from the epithelium to the muscularis, and for this reason, no submucosa is described.

BV, blood vessels
C, cilia
CT, connective tissue
Ep, epithelium
L, lumen
Lym, lymphatic vessel
Muc, mucosa
Mus, muscularis
PC, peg cells

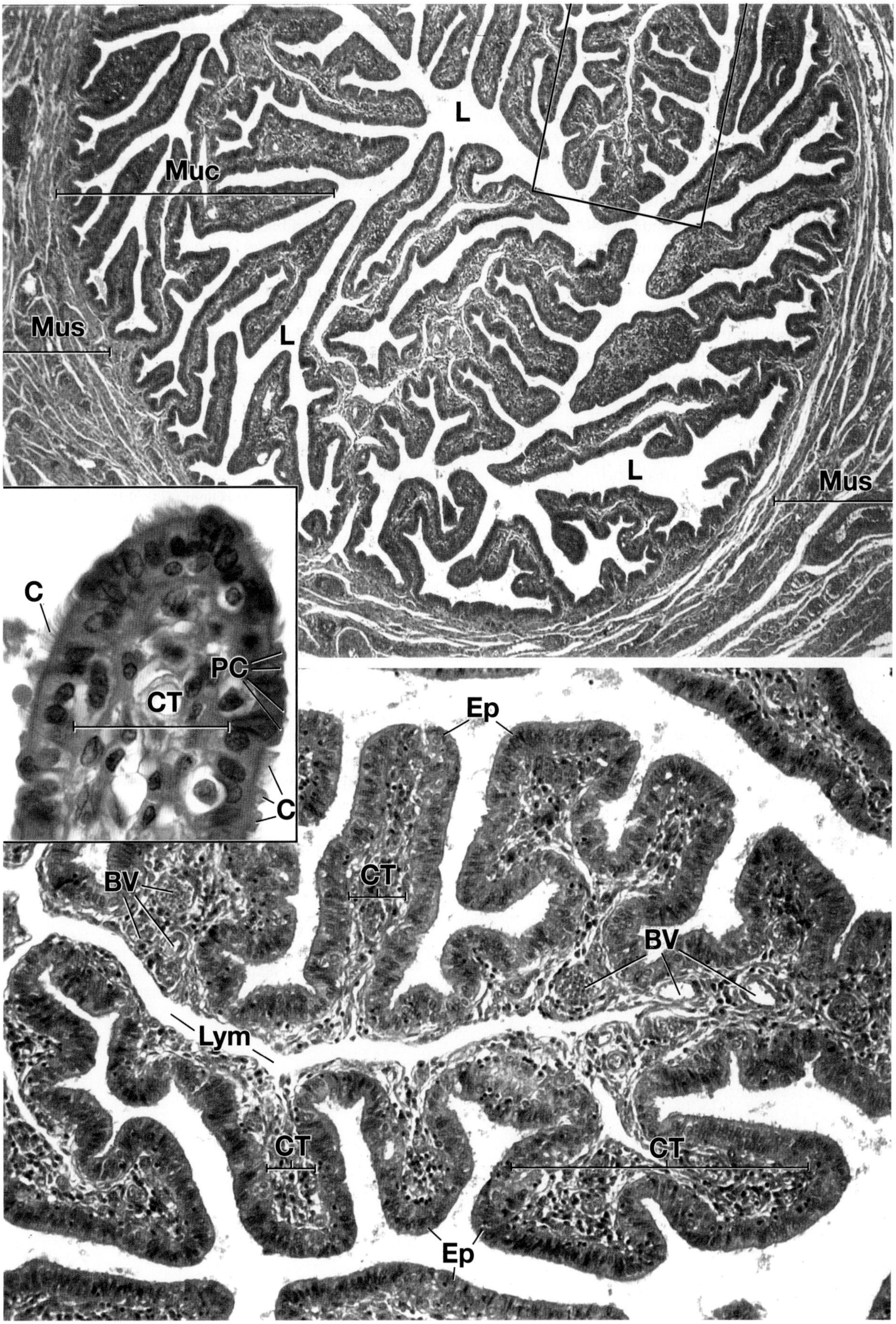
L
Muc
Mus
L
L
Mus
C
PC
CT
C
Ep
CT
BV
BV
Lym
CT
CT
Ep

PLATE 23.5 ■ UTERUS I

The **uterus** is a hollow, pear-shaped organ with a thick wall and, in the nonpregnant state, a narrow cavity. The uterine wall is composed of a mucosa, referred to as the **endometrium**; a muscularis, referred to as the **myometrium**; and, externally, a serosal cover, the **perimetrium**. The myometrium consists of smooth muscle and connective tissue and contains the large blood vessels that give rise to the vessels that supply the endometrium.

The uterus undergoes cyclical changes that are largely manifested by changes that occur in the endometrium. If implantation of a fertilized ovum does not occur after preparation for this event, the state of readiness is not maintained, and much of the endometrium degenerates and is sloughed off, constituting the menstrual flow. The part of the endometrium that is lost is referred to as the **stratum functionale**; the part that is retained is called the **stratum basale**. The stratum basale is the deeper part of the endometrium and adjoins the myometrium.

The myometrium also undergoes changes associated with implantation of a zygote. In the nonpregnant uterus, the smooth muscle cells are about 50 μm in length; during pregnancy, they undergo enormous hypertrophy, often reaching >500 μm in length. In addition, new muscle fibers develop after division of existing muscle cells and division and differentiation of undifferentiated mesenchymal cells. The connective tissue also increases to strengthen the uterine wall. Fibroblasts increase by division and secrete additional collagen and elastic fibers. After parturition, the uterus nearly returns to its normal size. Most muscle fibers return to their normal size, and some degenerate. Collagen secreted during pregnancy is digested by the very cells that secreted it, the fibroblasts. Similar, but less pronounced, proliferation and degeneration of fibroblasts and collagen occur in each menstrual cycle.

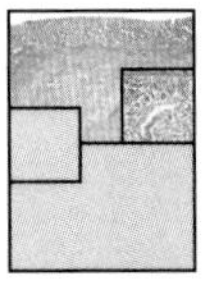

Uterus, human, hematoxylin and eosin (H&E) ×25; inset ×120.

After the **stratum functionale** (*SF*) is sloughed off, resurfacing of endometrium occurs. The epithelial resurfacing comes from the glands that remain in the **stratum basale** (*SB*). The gland epithelium simply proliferates and grows over the surface. This figure shows the endometrium as it appears when resurfacing is complete. The area inscribed in the *upper small rectangle* is shown at higher magnification in the *inset* on the *right*. Note the simple columnar epithelium (*SEp*) that covers the endometrial surface and its similarity to the glandular epithelium (*Gl*). The endometrium is relatively thin at this phase, and over half of it consists of the stratum basale. The area inscribed by the *lower small rectangle*, located in the region of the stratum basale, is shown at higher magnification in the *inset* in the next figure. The glandular epithelium of the deep portion of the glands is similar to that of the endometrial surface. Below the endometrium is the myometrium (*M*), in which a number of large blood vessels (*BV*) are present.

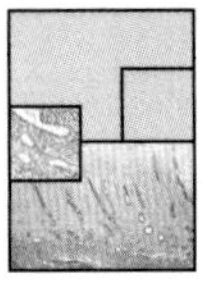

Endometrium, proliferative phase, uterus, human, H&E ×25; inset ×120.

Under the influence of estrogen, the various components of the endometrium proliferate (proliferative phase) so that the total thickness of the endometrium is increased. As shown in this figure, the endometrial glands (*Gl*) become rather long and follow a fairly straight course within the **stratum functionale** (*SF*) to reach the surface. Several profiles of blood vessels (*BV*) that represent spiral arteries are visible in the lower two-thirds of the stratum functionale. The **stratum basale** (*SB*) remains essentially unaffected by the estrogen and appears much the same as in the previous figure. Below the stratum basale is the myometrium (*M*). In this figure, the stratum functionale (*SF*), on the other hand, has increased in thickness and constitutes about four-fifths of the endometrial thickness.

BV, blood vessels	**M,** myometrium	**SEp,** surface epithelium
Gl, endometrial glands	**SB,** stratum basale	**SF,** stratum functionale

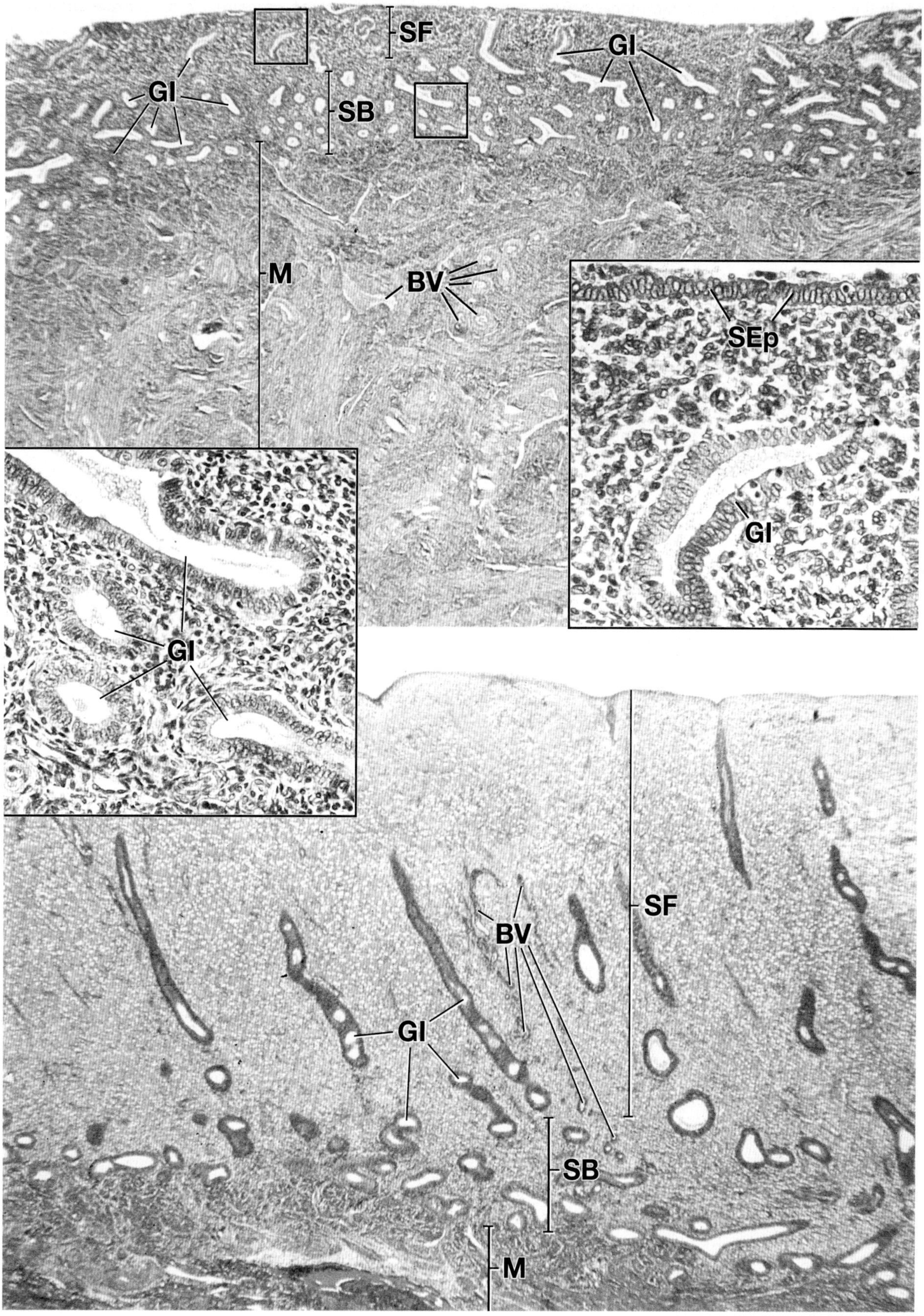
SF
GI
GI
SB
M
BV
SEp
GI
GI
SF
BV
GI
SB
M

After **estrogen** brings about the uterine events designated the proliferative phase, another hormone, progesterone, influences uterine changes that constitute the secretory phase of the uterine cycle. This hormone brings the endometrium to a state of readiness for implantation, and as a consequence of its actions, the thickness of the endometrium increases further. There are conspicuous changes in the glands, primarily in the stratum functionale, where the glands take on a more pronounced corkscrew shape and secrete mucus that accumulates in sacculations along their length.

The **vasculature** of the endometrium also proliferates and degenerates in each menstrual cycle. **Radial arteries** enter the stratum basale of the endometrium from the myometrium and give rise to small, straight arteries that supply the stratum basale and continue into the endometrium to become the highly coiled **spiral arteries**. Arterioles derived from the spiral arteries supply the stratum functionale. The distal portion of the spiral arteries and the arterioles are sloughed with the stratum functionale during menstruation. Alternating contraction and relaxation of the basal portions of the spiral arteries prevent excessive blood loss during menstruation.

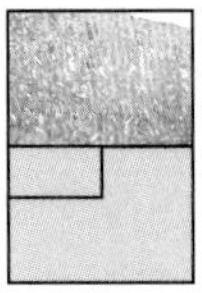

Uterus, human, hematoxylin and eosin (H&E) ×25.

This view of the endometrium in the secretory phase shows the **stratum functionale** (*SF*), the **stratum basale** (*SB*), and, in the *lower left* of the photomicrograph, a small amount of the **myometrium** (*M*). The uterine glands have been cut in a plane that is close to their long axes, and one gland (*arrow*) is seen opening at the uterine surface. Except for a few glands *near the center* of the figure that resemble those of the proliferative phase, most of the glands (*Gl*) in this figure, including those that are labeled, show numerous shallow sacculations that give the profile of the glandular epithelium a serrated appearance. This is one of the distinctive features of the secretory phase. It is seen most advantageously in areas where the plane of section is close to the long axis of the gland. In contrast to the characteristic sinuous course of the glands in the stratum functionale, glands of the stratum basale more closely resemble those in the proliferative phase. They are not oriented in any noticeable relationship to the uterine surface, and many of their long profiles are even parallel to the plane of the surface.

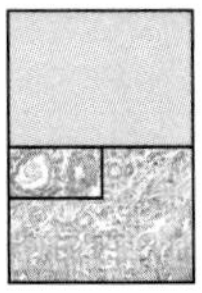

Endometrium, secretory phase, uterus, human, H&E ×30; inset ×120.

This slightly higher magnification view of the **stratum functionale** shows essentially the same characteristics of the **endometrial glands** (*Gl*) described earlier; it also shows other modifications that occur during the secretory phase. One of these is that the endometrium becomes edematous. The increase in endometrial thickness because of edema is reflected by the presence of empty spaces between cells and other formed elements. Thus, many areas of this figure, especially the area within and near the *rectangle*, show histologic signs of edema. In addition, in this phase, the glandular epithelial cells begin to secrete a mucoid fluid that is rich in glycogen. This product is secreted into the lumen of the glands, causing them to dilate. Typically, the glands of the secretory endometrium are more dilated than those of the proliferative endometrium.

The *rectangle* in this figure highlights two glands that are shown at higher magnification in the *inset*. Each of these glands contains some substance within the lumen. The mucoid character of the substance within one of the glands can be surmised from its blue staining. Although not evident in routine H&E paraffin sections, the epithelial cells also contain glycogen during the secretory phase, and as mentioned earlier, this becomes part of the secretion. The *arrowheads* indicate stromal cells; some of these cells undergo enlargement late in the secretory phase. These modified stromal cells, called *decidual cells*, play a role in implantation.

Gl, endometrial glands
M, myometrium
SB, stratum basale
SF, stratum functionale
arrow, glandular opening at uterine surface
arrowheads, stromal cells

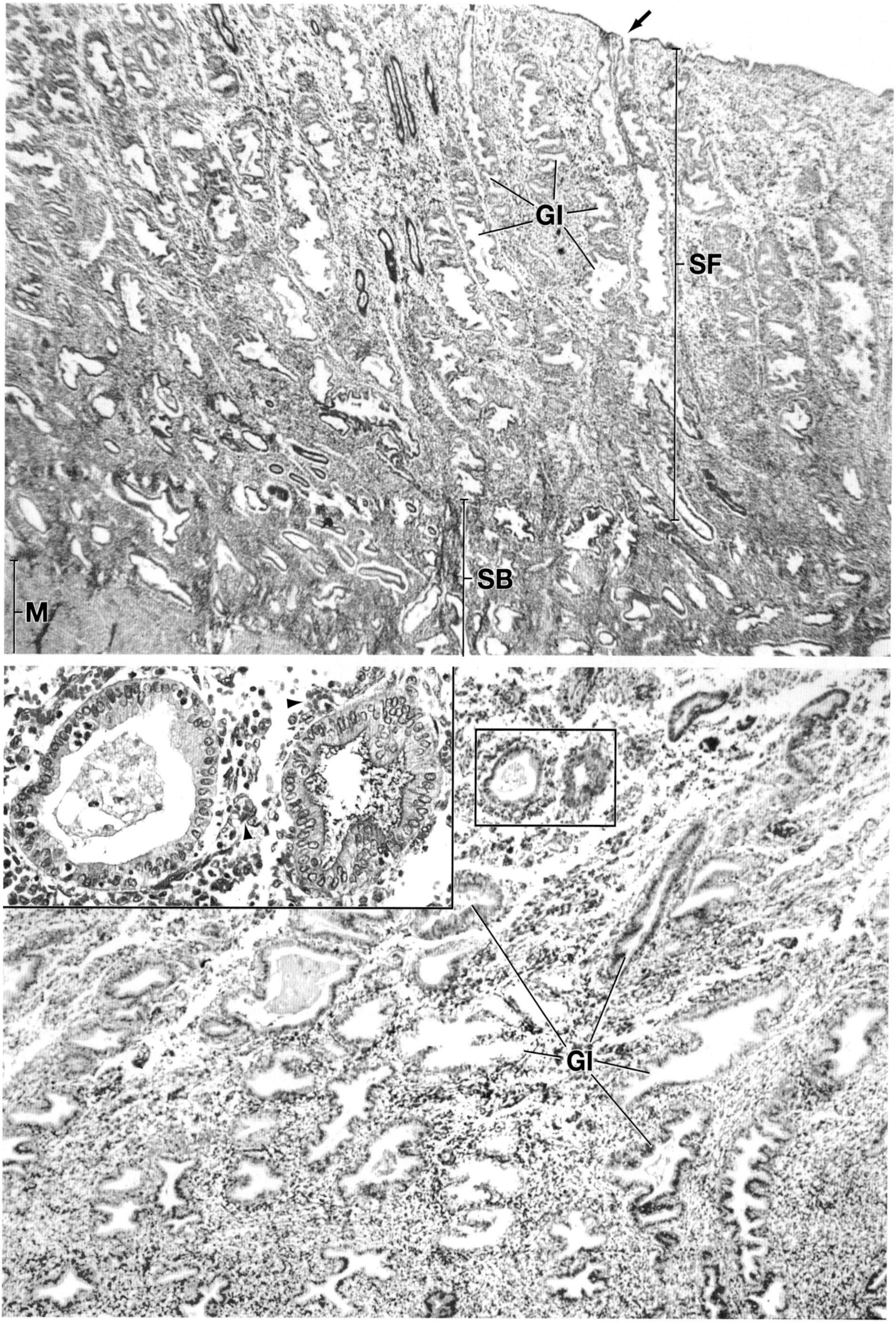
GI
SF
SB
M
GI

PLATE 23.7 ■ CERVIX

The **cervix** is the narrow or constricted inferior portion of the uterus, part of which projects into the vagina. The cervical canal traverses the cervix and provides a channel connecting the vagina and the uterine cavity. The structure of the cervix resembles the rest of the uterus in that it consists of a mucosa (endometrium) and a myometrium. There are, however, some important differences in the mucosa.

The **endometrium** of the cervix does not undergo the cyclical growth and loss of tissue that is characteristic of the body and fundus of the uterus. Rather, the amount and character of the mucus secretion of its simple columnar epithelium vary at different times in the uterine cycle under the influence of ovarian hormones. At midcycle, there is a 10-fold increase in the amount of mucus produced; this mucus is thin and provides a favorable environment for sperm migration. At other times in the cycle, the mucus is thick and restricts the passage of sperm into the uterus.

The **myometrium** forms the major thickness of the cervix. It consists of interweaving bundles of smooth muscle cells in an extensive, continuous network of fibrous connective tissue.

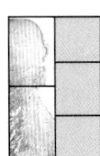

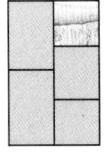

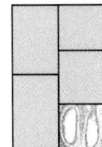

Cervix, uterus, human, hematoxylin and eosin (H&E) ×15.

The portion of the cervix that projects into the vagina, the **vaginal part** or **ectocervix**, is represented by the upper two-thirds of the *top* figure. The lower third of the micrograph reveals the portion of the **cervical canal** (*CC*). The *lower* figure shows the continuation of the cervical canal (*CC*). The plane of section in both figures passes through the long axis of the cervical canal, which is narrowed and cone shaped at its two ends. The upper end, the **internal os**, communicates with the uterine cavity, and the lower end, the **external os** (*Os*), communicates with the vagina. (For purposes of orientation, realize that only one side of the longitudinal section of the cervix is shown in these figures and that the actual specimen, as seen in a section, would present a similar image on the other side of the cervical canal.)

The **mucosa** (*Muc*) of the cervix differs according to the cavity it faces. The *two rectangles* in the *upper* figure delineate representative areas of the mucosa that are shown at higher magnification in the *upper right* and *middle right* figures, respectively.

The *bottom* figure emphasizes the nature of the **cervical glands** (*Gl*). The glands differ from those of the uterus in that they branch extensively. They secrete mucus into the cervical canal that serves to lubricate the vagina.

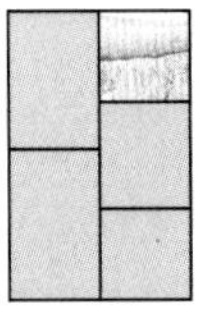

Ectocervix, uterus, human, H&E ×240.

The surface of the **vaginal part of the cervix**, the **ectocervix**, is covered by stratified squamous epithelium (*SSEp*). The epithelium–connective tissue junction presents a relatively even contour in contrast to the irregular profile seen in the vagina. In other respects, the epithelium has the same general features as the vaginal epithelium. Another similarity is that the epithelial surface of the ectocervix undergoes cyclical changes similar to those of the vagina in response to ovarian hormones. The mucosa of the ectocervix, like that of the vagina, is devoid of glands.

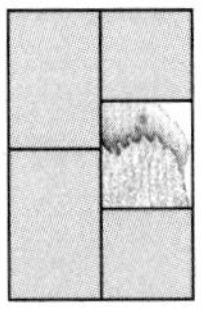

Transformation zone, cervix, uterus, human, H&E ×240.

The mucosa of the cervical canal is covered with columnar epithelium. An abrupt change from **stratified squamous epithelium** (*SSEp*) to **simple columnar epithelium** (*CEp*) occurs within the **transformation zone** (*TZ*) at the vaginal opening of the cervical canal (external os). The *lower rectangle* in the *top left* figure marks this site, known as the *transformation zone*, which is shown at a higher magnification here. Note the abrupt change in the epithelium at the transformation zone as well as the large number of lymphocytes and blood vessels (*BV*) present in this region.

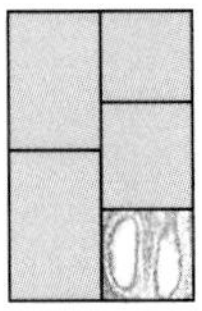

Cervical glands, cervix, uterus, human, H&E ×500.

This figure shows, at high magnification, portions of the **cervical gland** identified in the *rectangle* in the figure on the *left*. Note the tall epithelial cells and the lightly staining supranuclear cytoplasm, a reflection of the mucin that dissolved out of the cell during tissue preparation. The crowding and the change in shape of the nuclei (*asterisk*) seen at the *upper part* of one of the glands in this figure are due to a tangential cut through the wall of the gland as it passed out of the plane of section. (It is not uncommon for cervical glands to develop into cysts as a result of obstruction in the duct. Such cysts are referred to as **nabothian cysts**.)

BV, blood vessels
CC, cervical canal
CEp, columnar epithelium
Gl, cervical glands
Muc, mucosa
Os, ostium of the uterus
SSEp, stratified squamous epithelium
TZ, transformation zone
asterisk, tangential cut of the epithelial surface

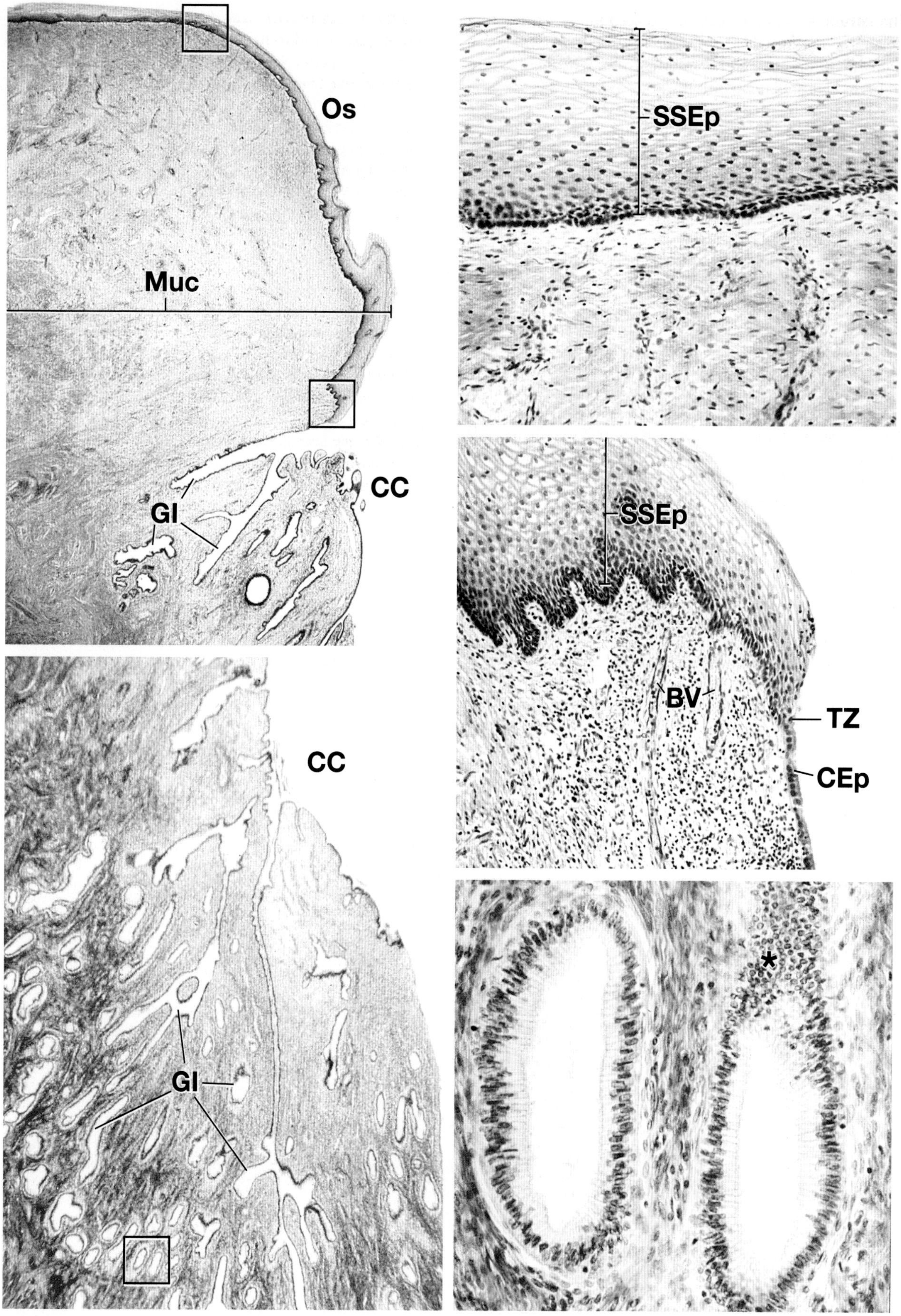
Os
Muc
CC
Gl
SSEp
SSEp
BV
TZ
CEp
CC
Gl
*

PLATE 23.8 ■ PLACENTA I

The **placenta** is a disc-shaped organ that serves for the exchange of materials between the fetal and maternal circulations during pregnancy. It develops primarily from embryonic tissue, the **chorion frondosum**. One side of the placenta is embedded in the uterine wall at the basal plate. The other side faces the amniotic cavity that contains the fetus. After childbirth, the placenta separates from the wall of the uterus and is discharged along with the contiguous membranes of the amniotic cavity.

The **umbilical cord** connects the fetus to the placenta. It contains two arteries that carry blood from the fetus to the placenta and a vein that returns blood from the placenta to the fetus. The umbilical arteries have thick muscular walls. These are arranged as two layers, an inner longitudinal layer and an outer circular layer. Elastic lamellae are poorly developed in these vessels and, indeed, may be absent. The umbilical vein is similar to the arteries, also having a thick muscular wall arranged as an inner longitudinal and an outer circular layer.

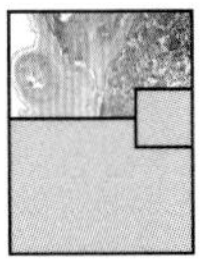

Placenta, human, hematoxylin and eosin (H&E) ×16.

A section extending from the amniotic surface into the substance of the placenta is shown here. This includes the **amnion** (*A*), the **chorionic plate** (*CP*), and the **chorionic villi** (*CV*). The amnion consists of a layer of simple cuboidal epithelium and an underlying layer of connective tissue. The connective tissue of the amnion is continuous with the connective tissue of the chorionic plate as a result of their fusion at an earlier time. The plane of fusion, however, is not evident in H&E sections; the separation (*asterisks*) in parts of this figure in the vicinity of the fusion is an artifact.

The chorionic plate is a thick connective tissue mass that contains the ramifications of the umbilical arteries and vein. These vessels (*BVp*) do not have the distinct organizational features characteristic of arteries and veins; rather, they resemble the vessels of the umbilical cord. Although their identification as blood vessels is relatively simple, it is difficult to distinguish which vessels are branches of an umbilical artery and which are tributaries of the vein.

The main substance of the placenta consists of chorionic villi of different sizes (see Plate 23.9, page 972). These emerge from the chorionic plate as large stem villi that branch into increasingly smaller villi. Branches of the umbilical arteries and vein (*BVv*, in the next figure) enter the stem villi and ramify through the branching villous network. Some villi extend from the chorionic plate to the maternal side of the placenta and make contact with the maternal tissue; these are called **anchoring villi**. Other villi, the **free villi**, simply arborize within the substance of the placenta without anchoring onto the maternal side.

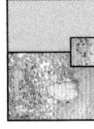

Placenta, human, H&E ×70; inset ×370.

The maternal side of the placenta is shown in this figure. The **basal plate** (*BP*) is on the *right side* of the illustration. This is the part of the uterus to which the chorionic villi anchor. Along with the usual connective tissue elements, the basal plate contains specialized cells called **decidual cells** (*DC*). The same cells are shown at higher magnification in the *inset*. Decidual cells are usually found in clusters and have an epithelial appearance. Because of these features, they are easily identified.

Septa from the basal plate extend into the portion of the placenta that contains the chorionic villi. The septa do not contain the branches of the umbilical vessels and, on this basis, can frequently be distinguished from stem villi or their branches.

A, amnion
BP, basal plate
BVp, blood vessels in chorionic plate
BVv, blood vessels in chorionic villi
CP, chorionic plate
CV, chorionic villi
DC, decidual cells
asterisks, separation that is actually an artifact

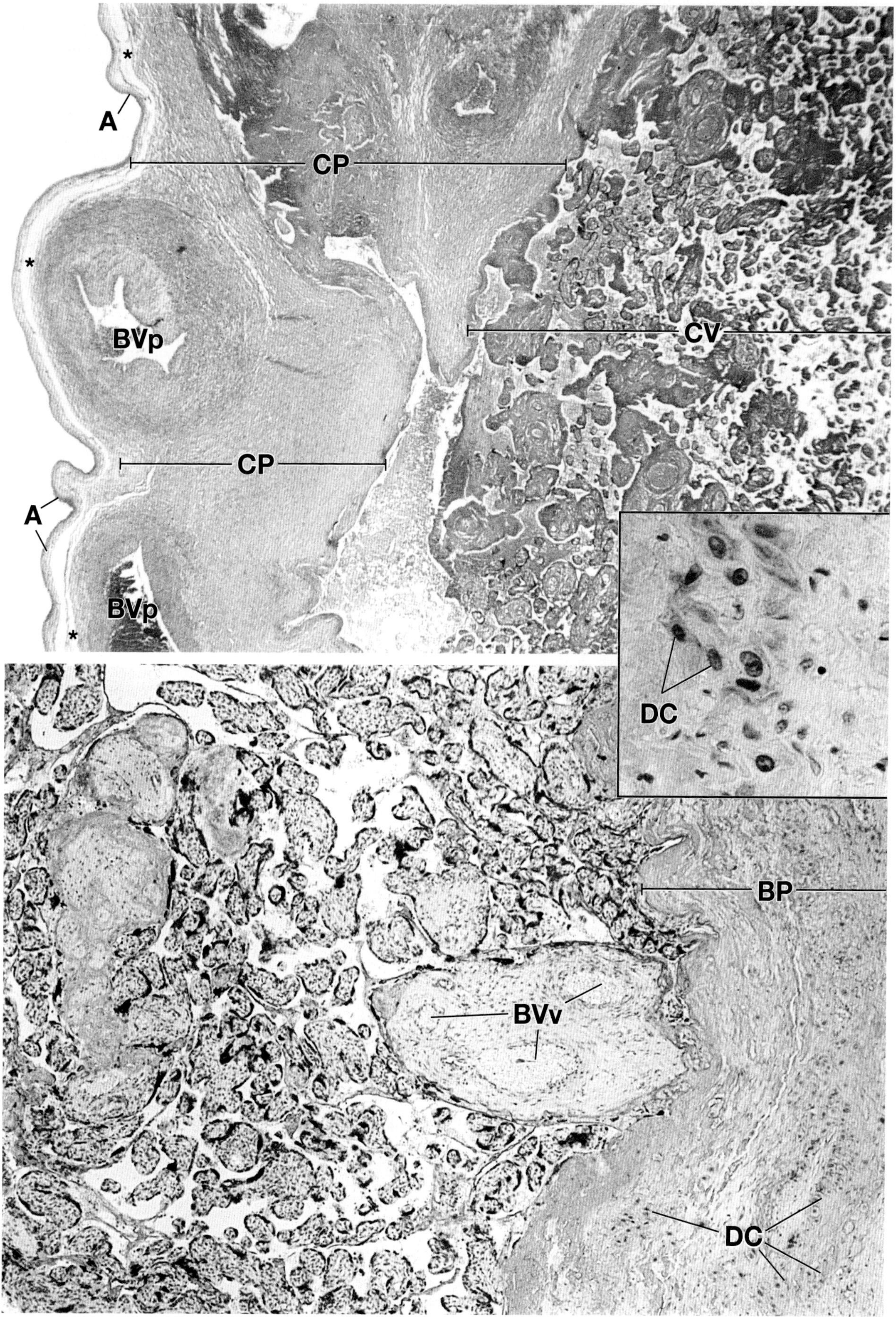

*
A
CP
*
BVp
CV
CP
A
A
BVp
*
DC
BP
BVv
DC

PLATE 23.9 ■ PLACENTA II

As the embryo develops, the invasive activity of the syncytiotrophoblast erodes the maternal capillaries and anastomoses them with the trophoblast lacunae, forming the maternal blood sinusoids. These communicate with each other and form a single blood compartment, lined by syncytiotrophoblasts, called the *intervillous space*. At the end of the second week of development, cytotrophoblast cells form **primary chorionic villi.** They project into the maternal blood space. In the third week of development, invasion of the extraembryonic mesenchyme into the primary chorionic villi creates **secondary chorionic villi.** At the end of the third week, core mesenchyme differentiates into connective tissue and blood vessels that connect with the embryonic circulation. These **tertiary chorionic villi** constitute functional units for exchange of gases, nutrients, and waste products between maternal and fetal circulation without direct contact with each other. This separation of fetal and maternal blood is referred to as the *placental barrier*. Each tertiary villus consists of a connective tissue core surrounded by two distinct layers of trophoblast-derived cells. The outermost layer consists of the syncytiotrophoblast; immediately beneath it is a layer of cytotrophoblast cells. Starting at the fourth month, these layers become very thin to facilitate the exchange of products across the placental barrier. The thinning of the wall of the villus is due to the loss of the inner, cytotrophoblastic layer. At this stage, the syncytiotrophoblast forms numerous trophoblastic buds that resemble the primary chorionic villi; however, the cytotrophoblast and the connective tissue grow very rapidly into these structures, transforming them into tertiary villi. At term, the **placental barrier** consists of the syncytiotrophoblasts; a spare, thin (or discontinuous), inner cytotrophoblast layer; the basal lamina of the trophoblast; the connective tissue of the villus; the basal lamina of the endothelium; and the endothelium of the fetal placental capillary in the tertiary villus.

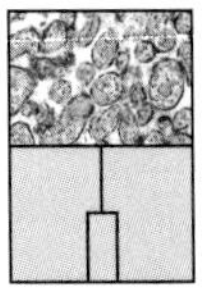

Tertiary chorionic villi, placenta, full-term, human, hematoxylin and eosin (H&E) ×280.

This photomicrograph shows a section through the intervillous space of the placenta at term. It includes **chorionic villi** (*CV*) of different sizes and the surrounding **intervillous space** (*IS*). The connective tissue of the villi contains branches and tributaries of the umbilical vein (*UV*) and arteries. The intervillous space usually contains maternal blood (only a few maternal blood cells are seen here). The outermost layer of each chorionic villus derives from the fusion of cytotrophoblast cells. This layer, known as the **syncytiotrophoblast** (*S*), has no intercellular boundaries, and its nuclei are rather evenly distributed, giving this layer an appearance similar to that of cuboidal epithelium. In some areas, nuclei are gathered in clusters forming **syncytial knots** (*SK*); in other regions, the syncytiotrophoblast layer appears relatively free of nuclei (*arrows*). These stretches of the syncytiotrophoblast may be so attenuated in places that the villous surface appears devoid of a covering. The syncytiotrophoblast contains microvilli that project into the intervillous space. In well-preserved specimens, they may appear as a striated border (see *inset below*). The cytotrophoblast consists of an irregular layer of mononucleated cells that lies beneath the syncytiotrophoblast. In immature placentas, the cytotrophoblasts form an almost complete layer of cells. In this full-term placenta, only occasional **cytotrophoblast cells** (*C*) can be discerned. Most of the cells within the core of the villus are typical connective tissue fibroblasts and endothelial cells. Other cells have a visible amount of cytoplasm that surrounds the nucleus. These are considered to be fetal placental antigen–presenting cells or placental macrophages (*PM*) historically known as *Hofbauer cells*.

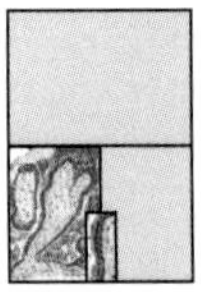

Secondary chorionic villi, placenta, midterm, human, H&E ×320; inset ×640.

This micrograph shows the **secondary chorionic villi** in the third week of embryonic development. These villi are composed of a **mesenchymal core** (*MC*) surrounded by two distinct layers of the trophoblast. Secondary villi have a much larger number of **cytotrophoblast cells** (*C*) than the mature tertiary villi and form an almost complete layer of cells immediately deep into the **syncytiotrophoblast** (*S*) (see *inset*). The syncytiotrophoblast not only covers the surface of the chorionic villi but also extends into the chorionic plate. Maternal red blood cells are present in the intervillous space.

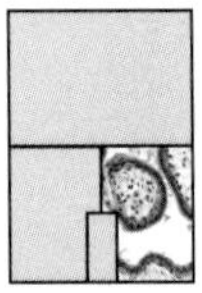

Tertiary chorionic villi, placenta, full-term, human, H&E ×320.

This higher magnification photomicrograph shows a cross section through **immature chorionic tertiary villi** surrounded by the intervillous space (*IS*). At this stage, chorionic villi are growing by proliferation of their core mesenchyme, syncytiotrophoblast (*S*), and fetal endothelial cells. Note a discontinued layer of cytotrophoblast cells (*C*). The syncytiotrophoblast surrounding the chorionic villus (*center of the image*) forms **syncytial knots** (*SK*), which are present in the full-term mature placenta. They represent aggregation of syncytiotrophoblast nuclei on the surface of mature terminal villi. In addition to fibroblasts, several fetal placental **antigen–presenting cells (placental macrophages)** (*PM*) can be identified by the amount of cytoplasm surrounding their nuclei.

C, cytotrophoblast cells
CV, chorionic villi
IS, intervillous space
MC, mesenchymal core
PM, placental macrophages
S, syncytiotrophoblast
SK, syncytial knot
UV, umbilical vein

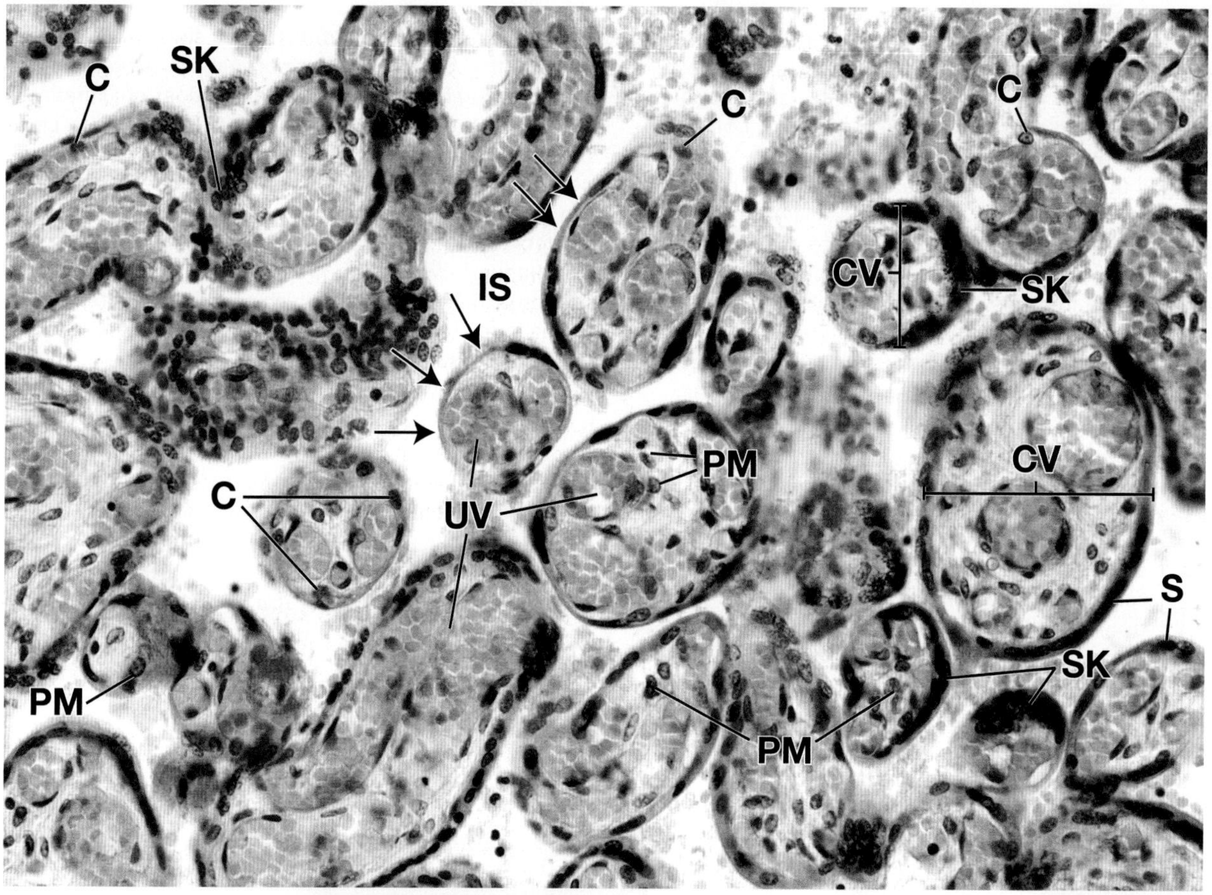
C
SK
C
C
IS
CV
SK
PM
C
UV
CV
S
SK
PM
PM

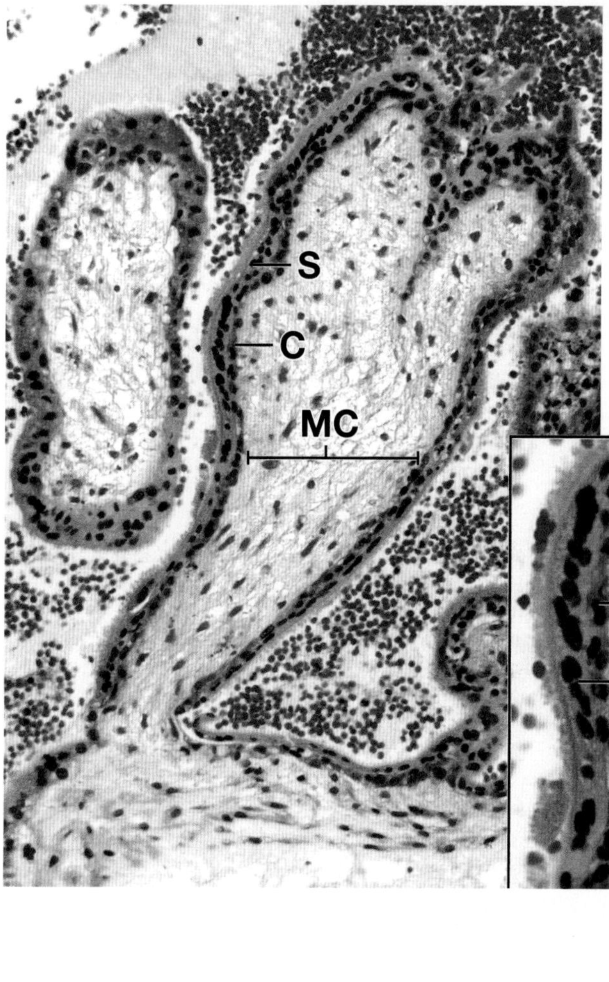
S
C
MC
C
S
MC

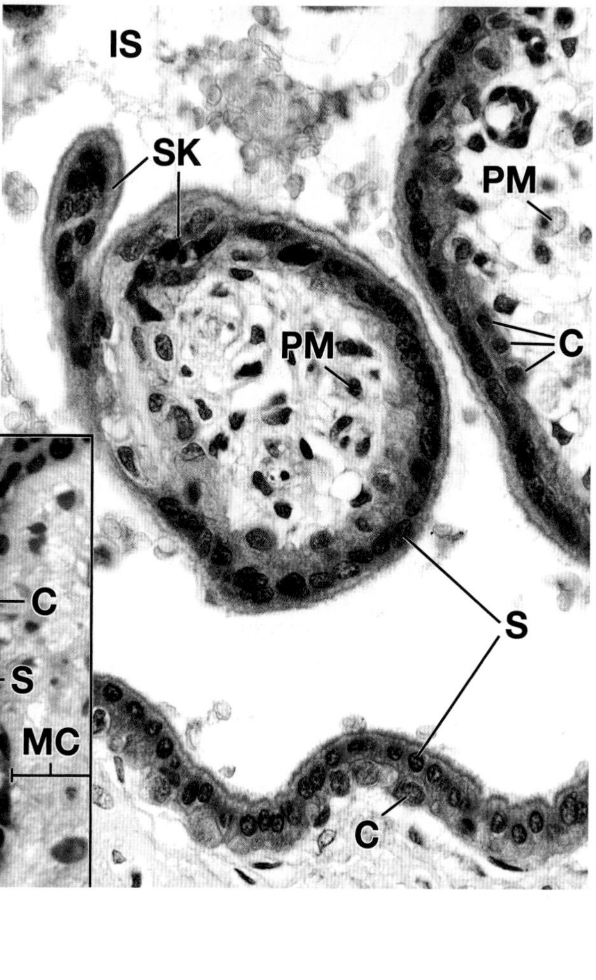
IS
SK
PM
PM
C
S
C

PLATE 23.10 ■ VAGINA

The **vagina** is the fibromuscular tube of the female reproductive tract that leads to the exterior of the body. The wall of the vagina consists of three layers: a **mucosa**, a **muscularis**, and an **adventitia**. The epithelium of the mucosa is nonkeratinized stratified squamous. It undergoes changes that correspond to the ovarian cycle. The amount of glycogen stored in the epithelial cells increases under the influence of **estrogen**, whereas the rate of desquamation increases under the influence of **progesterone**. The glycogen liberated from the desquamated cells is fermented by **lactobacilli vaginalis**, producing lactic acid that acidifies the vaginal surface and inhibits colonization by yeasts and potentially harmful bacteria.

The vagina has certain histologic similarities to the proximal portion of the alimentary canal but is distinguished by the following features: The epithelium does not keratinize, and except for the deepest layers, the cells appear to be empty in routine hematoxylin and eosin (H&E) sections; the mucosa contains neither glands nor a muscularis mucosae; and the muscle is smooth and not well ordered. This can be contrasted with the oral cavity, pharynx, and upper part of the esophagus in which the muscle is striated. The more distal portion of the esophagus, which contains smooth muscle, can be distinguished easily from the vagina because it has a muscularis mucosae.

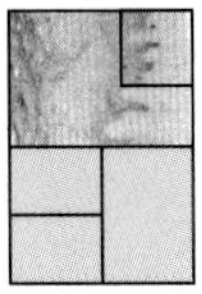

Vagina, human, H&E ×90.

The mucosa of the vagina consists of a **stratified squamous epithelium** (*Ep*) and an underlying fibrous connective tissue (*CT*) that often appears more cellular than other fibrous connective tissue. The boundary between the two is readily identified because of the conspicuous staining of the closely packed small cells of the basal layer (*B*) of the epithelium. Connective tissue papillae project into the underside of the epithelium, giving the epithelial–connective tissue junction an uneven appearance. The papillae may be cut obliquely or in cross section and thus may appear as connective tissue islands (*arrows*) within the lower portion of the epithelium. The epithelium is characteristically thick, and although keratohyalin granules may be found in the superficial cells, keratinization does not occur in the human vaginal epithelium. Thus, nuclei can be observed throughout the entire thickness of the epithelium despite the fact that the cytoplasm of most of the cells above the basal layers appears empty. These cells are normally filled with large deposits of glycogen that are lost in the processes of fixation and embedding of the tissue. The *rectangle* outlines a portion of the epithelium and connective tissue papillae that is examined at higher magnification (next figure). The muscular layer of the vaginal wall consists of smooth muscle arranged in two ill-defined layers. The outer layer is generally said to be longitudinally arranged (*SML*), and the inner layer is generally said to be circularly arranged (*SMC*), but the fibers are more usually organized as interlacing bundles surrounded by connective tissue. Many blood vessels (*BV*) are seen in the connective tissue.

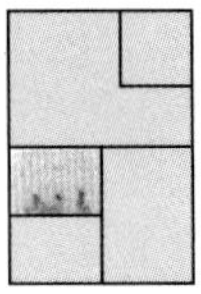

Mucosa, vagina, human, H&E ×110.

This is a higher magnification of the epithelium (*Ep*) that includes the area outlined by the *rectangle* in the *upper* figure (turned 90 degree). The obliquely cut and cross-sectioned portions of connective tissue papillae that appear as connective tissue islands in the epithelium are more clearly seen here (*arrows*), in some instances, outlined by the surrounding closely packed cells of the basal epithelial cell layer. Note, again, that the epithelial cells even at the surface still retain their nuclei and there is no evidence of keratinization.

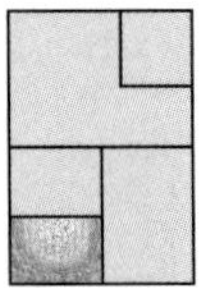

Mucosa, vagina, human, H&E ×225.

This is a higher magnification micrograph of the basal portion of the epithelium (*Ep*) between connective tissue papillae. Note the regularity and dense packing of the basal epithelial cells. They are the stem cells for the stratified squamous epithelium. Daughter cells of these cells migrate toward the surface and begin to accumulate glycogen and become less regularly arranged as they move toward the surface. The highly cellular connective tissue (*CT*) immediately beneath the basal layer (*B*) of the epithelium typically contains many lymphocytes (*L*). The number of lymphocytes varies with the stage of the ovarian cycle. Lymphocytes invade the epithelium around the time of menstruation and appear along with the epithelial cells in vaginal smears.

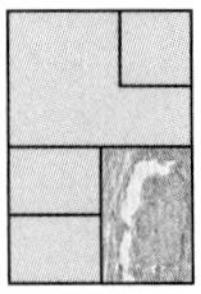

Muscularis, vagina, human, H&E ×125.

This higher magnification micrograph of the smooth muscle of the vaginal wall emphasizes the irregularity of the arrangement of the muscle bundles. At the *right edge* of the figure is a bundle of smooth muscle cut in a longitudinal section (*SML*). Adjacent to this is a bundle of smooth muscle cut in cross section (*SMC*). This bundle abuts on a longitudinally sectioned lymphatic vessel (*LV*). To the left of the lymphatic vessel is another longitudinal bundle of smooth muscle (*SML*). A valve (*Va*) is seen in the lymphatic vessel. A small vein (*V*) is present in the circular smooth muscle close to the lymphatic vessel.

B, basal layer of vaginal epithelium
BV, blood vessels
CT, connective tissue
Ep, epithelium
L, lymphocytes
LV, lymphatic vessel
SMC, smooth muscle, cross section
SML, smooth muscle, longitudinal section
V, vein
Va, valve in lymphatic vessel
arrows, connective tissue islands in epithelium

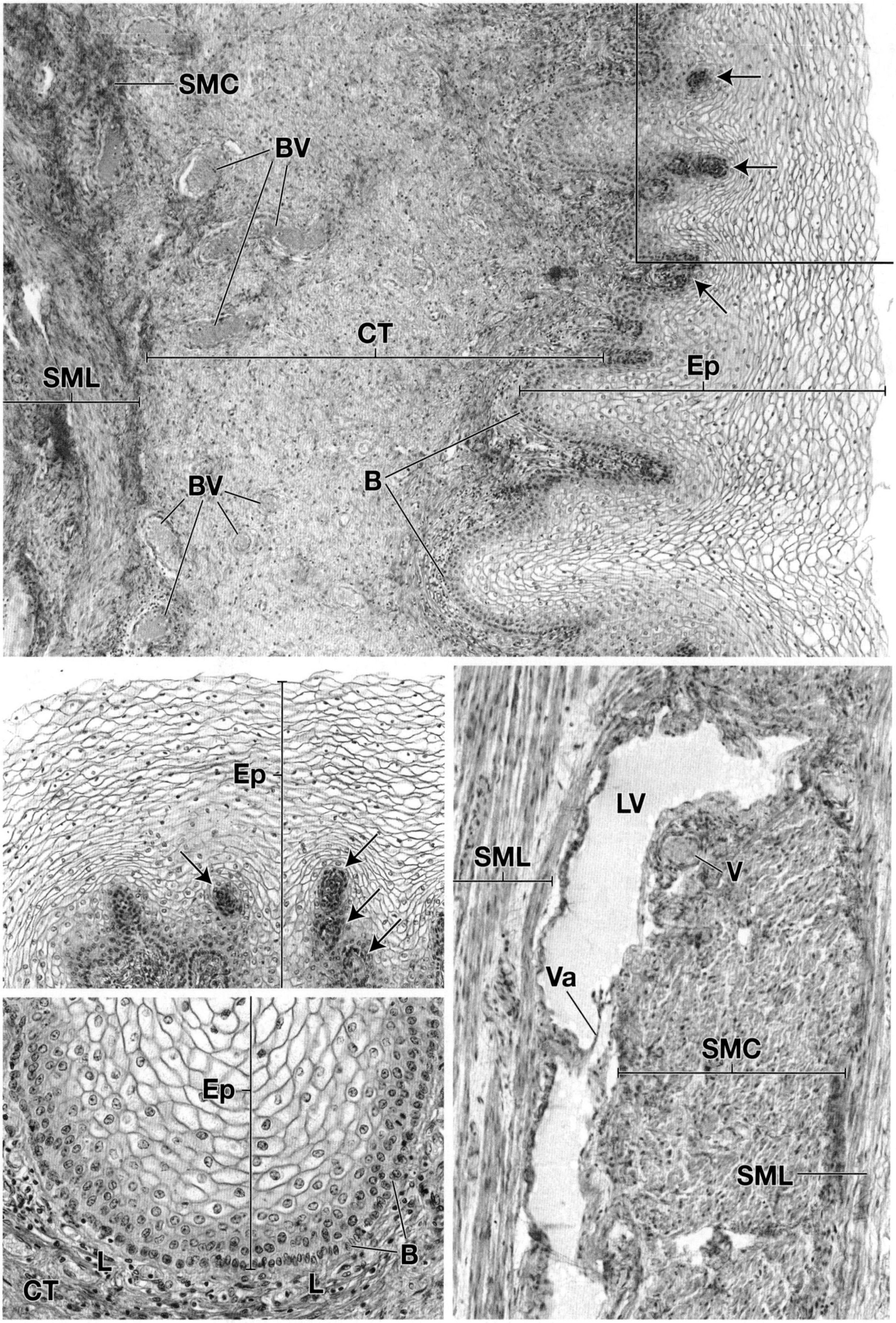
SMC
BV
CT
SML
Ep
B
BV
Ep
Ep
B
L
L
CT
LV
SML
V
Va
SMC
SML

PLATE 23.11 ■ MAMMARY GLAND INACTIVE STAGE

The **mammary glands** are branched tubuloalveolar glands that develop from epidermis and come to lie in the subcutaneous tissue (superficial fascia). They begin to develop at puberty in the female but do not reach a fully functional state until after pregnancy. The glands also develop in the male at puberty; the development is limited, however, and the glands usually remain in a stabilized state.

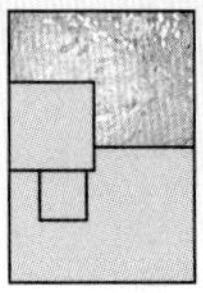

Mammary gland, inactive stage, human, hematoxylin and eosin (H&E) ×80.

This figure is a section through an **inactive gland**. The parenchyma is sparse and consists mainly of duct elements. Several ducts (*D*) are shown in the *center* of the field. A small lumen can be seen in each. The ducts are surrounded by loose connective tissue (see *CT[L]*, in the next figure), and together, the ducts and surrounding connective tissue constitute a lobule. Two terminal duct lobular units (*TDLU*) are bracketed in this figure. Beyond the **lobular unit**, the connective tissue is more dense (*CT[D]*) and contains adipocytes (*A*). The two types of connective tissues can be distinguished at the low magnification of this figure.

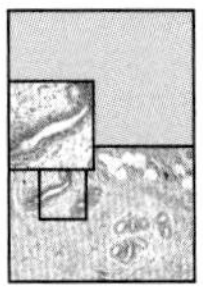

Mammary gland, inactive stage, human, H&E ×200; inset ×400.

Additional details are evident at higher magnification. In distinguishing between the loose and dense connective tissue, recall that both extracellular and cellular features show differences that are evident in both the figure and the *inset*. Note the thicker collagenous fibers in the dense connective tissue in contrast to the much thinner fibers of the loose connective tissue. The loose connective tissue (*CT[L]*) contains far more cells per unit area and a greater variety of cell types. This figure shows a cluster of **lymphocytes** (*L*) and, at still higher magnification (*inset*), **plasma cells** (*P*) and individual lymphocytes (*L*). Both plasma cells and lymphocytes are cells with a rounded shape, but plasma cells are larger and show more cytoplasm. In addition, regions of plasma cell cytoplasm display basophilia. Elongate nuclei in spindle-shaped cells belong to fibroblasts. In contrast, although the cell types in the dense connective tissue may also be diverse, a simple examination of equal areas of loose and dense connective tissue will, by far, show fewer cells in the dense connective tissue. Characteristically, the dense connective tissue contains numerous aggregates of adipocytes (*A*).

The epithelial cells within the resting lobular units are regarded as being chiefly duct elements (*D*). Usually, alveoli are not found; their precursors, however, are represented as cellular thickenings of the duct wall. The epithelium of the resting lobule is cuboidal; in addition, myoepithelial cells are present. Reexamination of the *inset* shows a thickening of the epithelium in one location, presumably the precursor of an alveolus, and **myoepithelial cells** (*M*) at the base of the epithelium. As elsewhere, the myoepithelial cells are on the epithelial side of the basement membrane. During pregnancy, the glands begin to proliferate. This can be thought of as a dual process in which ducts proliferate and alveoli grow from the ducts.

A, adipocytes
CT(D), dense connective tissue
CT(L), loose connective tissue
D, ducts
L, lymphocytes
M, myoepithelial cells
P, plasma cells
TDLU, terminal duct lobular unit

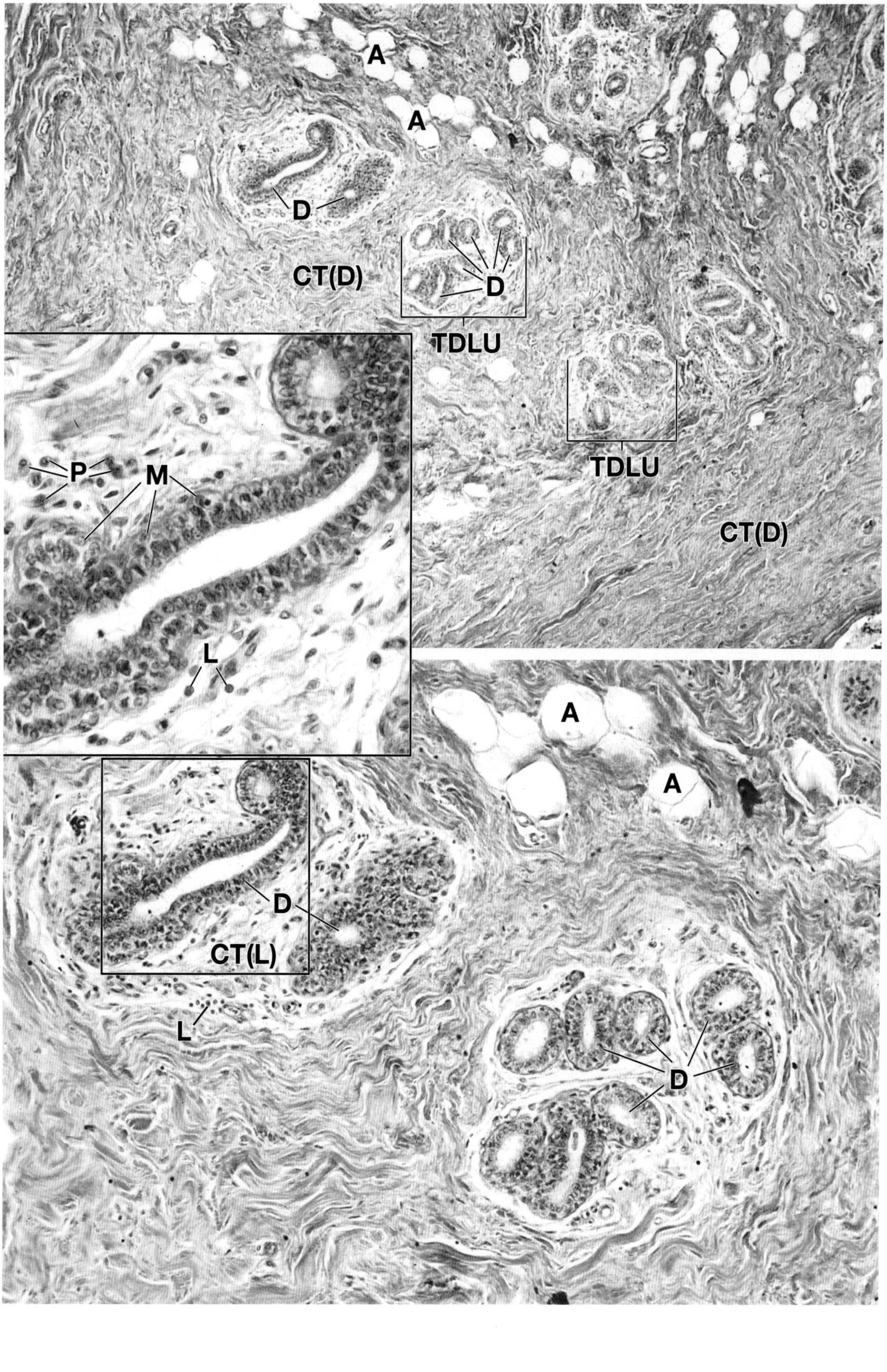
A
A
D
CT(D)
D
TDLU
TDLU
CT(D)
P
M
L
A
A
D
CT(L)
L
D

PLATE 23.12 ■ MAMMARY GLAND, LATE PROLIFERATIVE AND LACTATING STAGES

Mammary glands exhibit a number of changes during pregnancy in preparation for lactation. Lymphocytes and plasma cells infiltrate the loose connective tissue as the glandular tissue develops. As the cells of the glandular portion proliferate by mitotic division, the ducts branch and alveoli begin to develop at their growing ends. Alveolar development becomes most prominent in the later stages of pregnancy, and accumulation of secretory product takes place in the alveoli. At the same time, lymphocytes and plasma cells become prominent in the loose connective tissue of the developing lobules. Myoepithelial cells proliferate between the base of the epithelial cells and the basal lamina in both the alveolar and the ductal portion of the glands. They are most prominent in the larger ducts.

Both **merocrine** and **apocrine secretion** are involved in the production of milk. The protein component is synthesized, concentrated, and secreted by exocytosis in a manner typical for protein secretion. The lipid component begins as droplets in the cytoplasm that coalesce into large droplets in the apical cytoplasm of the alveolar cells and cause the apical plasma membrane to bulge into the alveolar lumen. The droplets are surrounded by a thin layer of cytoplasm and are enveloped in plasma membrane as they are released.

The initial secretion in the first days after birth is called **colostrum**. This premilk is an alkaline secretion with a higher protein, vitamin A, sodium, and chloride content than milk and a lower lipid, carbohydrate, and potassium content. Considerable amounts of antibodies are contained in colostrum, and these provide the newborn with passive immunity to many antigens. The antibodies are produced by the plasma cells in the stroma of the breast and are carried across the glandular cells in a manner similar to that for secretory immunoglobulin A (IgA) in the salivary glands and intestine. A few days after parturition, the secretion of colostrum stops and lipid-rich milk is produced.

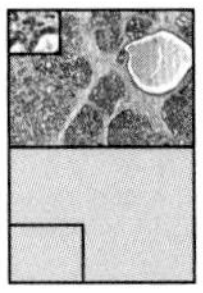

Mammary gland, late proliferative stage, human, hematoxylin and eosin (H&E) ×90; inset ×560.

Whereas the development of the duct elements in the mammary gland occurs during the **early proliferative stage**, the development of the alveolar elements becomes conspicuous in the late proliferative stage. This figure shows the **terminal duct lobular units** (*TDLU*) at the late proliferative stage. Individual lobular units are separated by narrow, dense **connective tissue septa** (*S*). The connective tissue within the lobular unit is a typical loose connective tissue that is now more cellular, containing mostly plasma cells and lymphocytes. The alveoli are well developed, and many exhibit precipitated secretory product. Each of the alveoli is joined to a duct, although that relationship can be difficult to identify. The epithelium of the intralobular ducts is similar in appearance to the alveolar epithelium. The cells of both components are secretory. The alveoli as well as the intralobular ducts consist of a single layer of cuboidal epithelial cells subtended by myoepithelial cells. Often, what appear to be several alveoli are seen merging with one another (*asterisks*). Such profiles represent alveolar units opening into a duct. **Interlobular ducts** (*D*) are easy to identify as they are surrounded by dense connective tissue. In one instance, an intralobular duct can be seen emptying into an interlobular duct (*arrow*). The *inset* shows the secretory epithelium at a much higher magnification. Note that it is a simple columnar epithelium. The nucleus of a **myoepithelial cell** (*M*) is seen at the base of the epithelium. Generally, these cells are difficult to recognize. Also, as noted earlier, numerous plasma cells (*P*) and lymphocytes (*Ly*) are present in the loose connective tissue of the lobule.

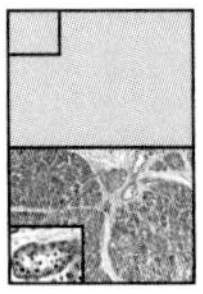

Mammary gland, lactating stage, human, methyl green–osmium ×90; inset ×700.

The specimen shown here is from a **lactating mammary gland**. It is similar in appearance to the gland at the late proliferative stage but differs mainly to the extent that the alveoli are more uniform in appearance and their lumina are larger. As in the late proliferative stage, several alveoli can be seen merging with one another (*asterisks*). The use of osmium in this specimen stains the lipid component of the secretion. The *inset* reveals the lipid droplets within the epithelial cell cytoplasm as well as lipid that has been secreted into the lumen of the alveolus. The lipid first appears as small droplets within the epithelial cells. These droplets become larger and ultimately are secreted into the alveolar lumen along with milk proteins. The milk proteins are present in small vacuoles in the apical part of the cell but cannot be seen by light microscopic methods. They are secreted by exocytosis. The lipid droplets, in contrast, are large and surrounded by the apical cell membrane as they are pinched off to enter the lumen; thus, it is an apocrine secretion. Several **interlobular ducts** (*D*) are evident. One of these ducts reveals a small branch, an ending intralobular duct (*arrows*) joining the interlobular duct.

D, interlobular duct
Ly, lymphocyte
M, myoepithelial cell
P, plasma cell
S, connective tissue septa
TDLU, terminal duct lobular unit
arrows, union of intralobular duct with interlobular duct
asterisks, sites of merging alveoli

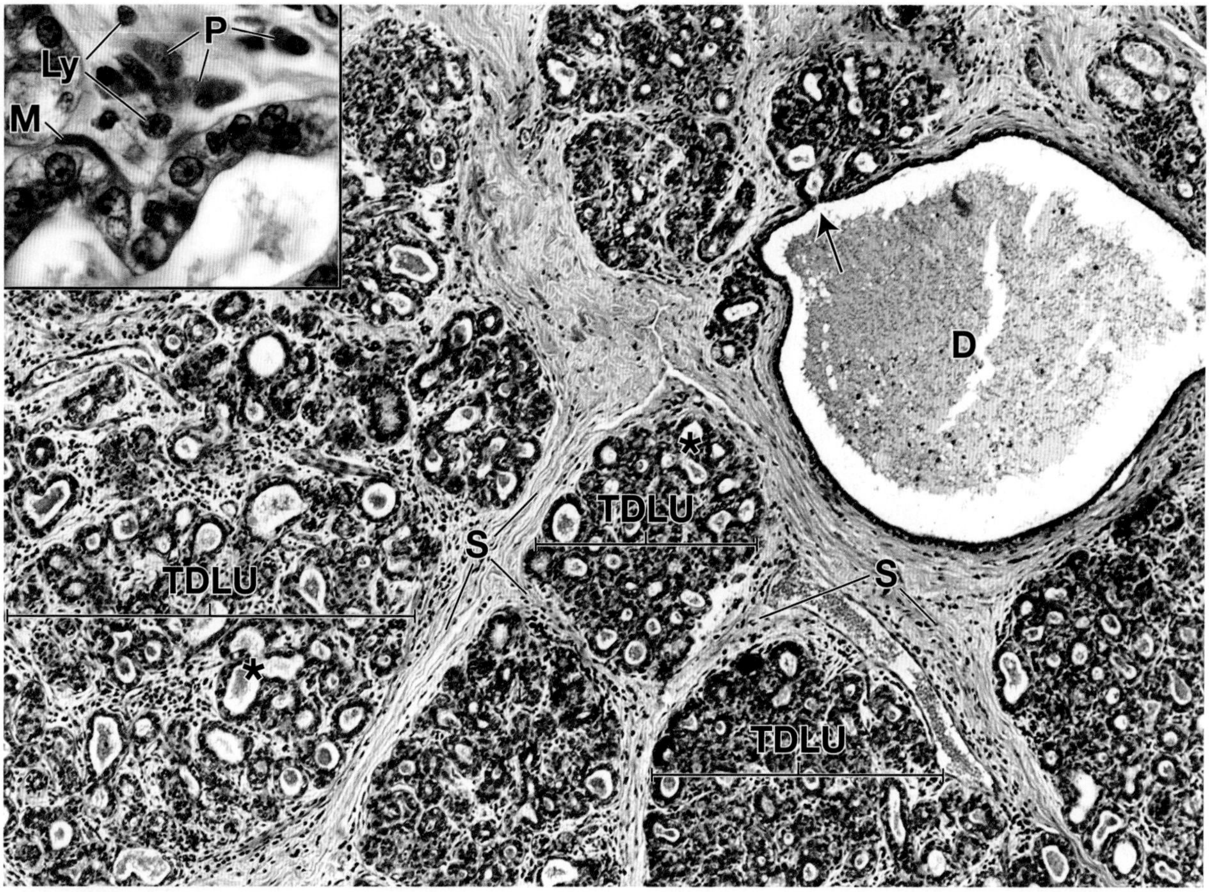
P
Ly
M
D
*
TDLU
S
TDLU
S
*
TDLU

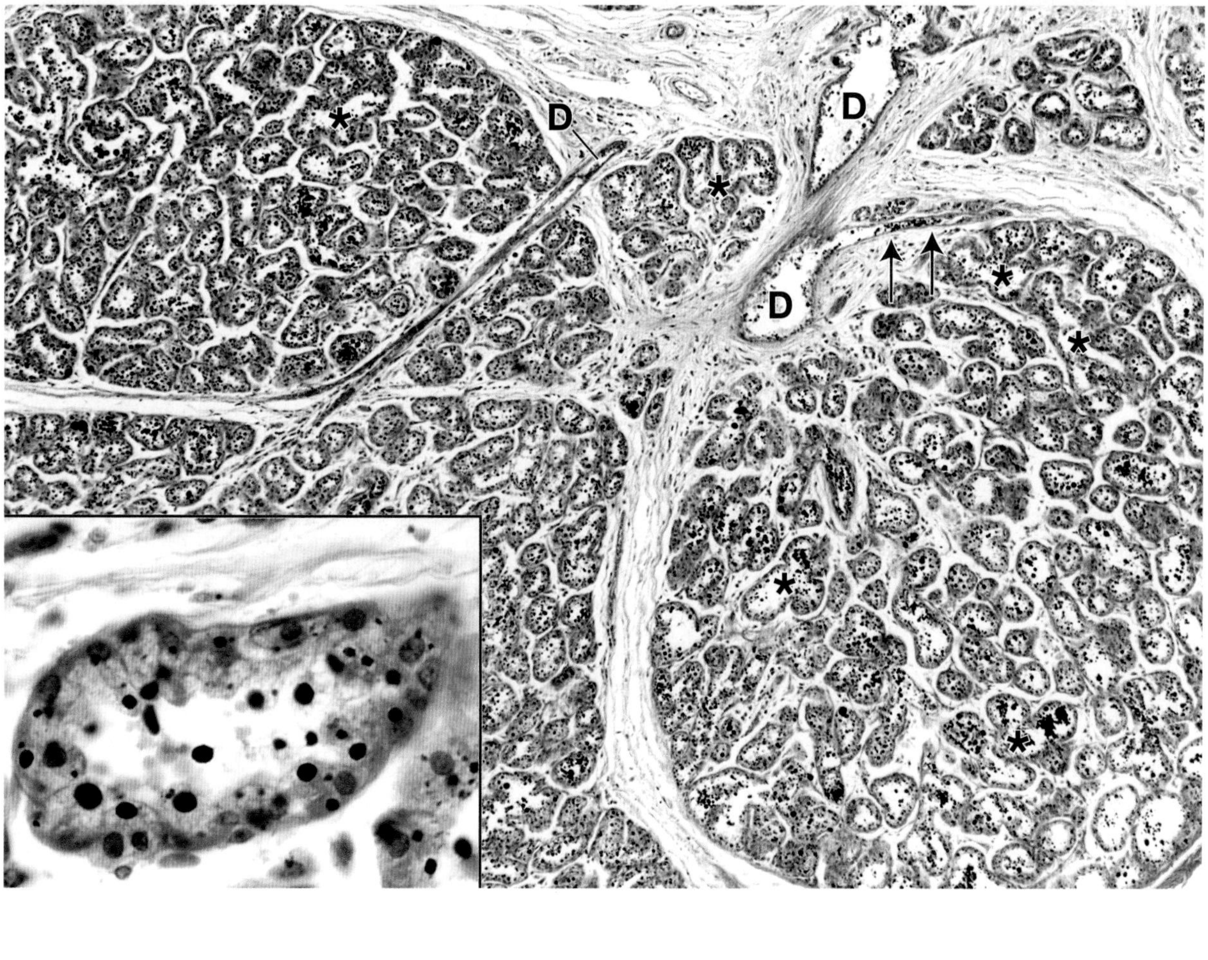
D
D
*
*
D
*
*
*
*

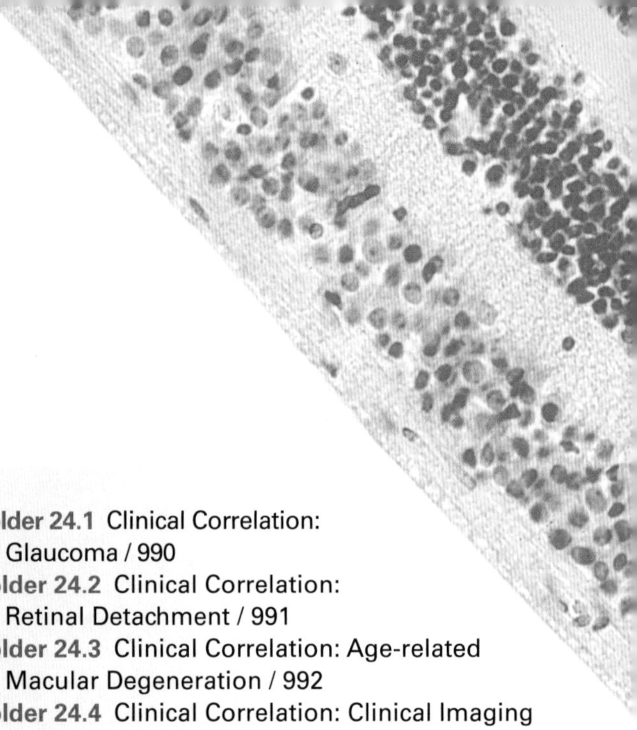

24 EYE

■ OVERVIEW OF THE EYE

The **eye** is a complex sensory organ that provides the sense of sight. In many ways, the eye is similar to a digital camera. Like the optical system of a camera, the **cornea** and **lens** of the eye capture and automatically focus light, whereas the iris automatically adjusts the diameter of the pupil to differences in illumination. The light detector in a digital camera, the charge-coupled device (CCD), consists of closely spaced photodiodes that capture, collect, and convert the light image into a series of electrical impulses. Similarly, the **photoreceptor cells** in the **retina** of the eye detect light intensity and color (wavelengths of visible light that are reflected by different objects) and encode these parameters into electrical impulses for transmission to the brain via the **optic nerve**. The retina has other capabilities beyond those of a CCD: It can extract and modify specific impulses from the visual image before sending them to the central nervous system (CNS).

In other ways, the optical system of the eye is far more elaborate and complex than a camera. For example, the eye is able to track moving objects with coordinated eye movements. The eye can also protect, maintain, self-repair, and clean its transparent optical system.

Because the eyes are paired and spatially separated, two slightly different and overlapping views (visual fields) are sent to the brain. The brain integrates these two slightly different images from each eye into a single **three-dimensional (3D) image** in a process called **stereopsis**. The primary visual cortex located in the occipital lobes processes the differences between the two images to create the perception of depth. The final image is then projected onto the visual cortex. In addition, other complex neural mechanisms coordinate eye movements, enabling refinements in the perception of depth and distance. Therefore, the way in which we see the world around us largely depends on impulses processed within the retina and the analysis and interpretation of these impulses by the CNS.

■ GENERAL STRUCTURE OF THE EYE

The eye measures approximately 25 mm in diameter. It is suspended in the bony orbital socket by six extrinsic muscles that control its movement. A thick layer of adipose tissue partially surrounds and cushions the eye as it moves within the orbit. The extraocular muscles are coordinated so that the eyes move symmetrically around their own central axes.

Layers of the Eye

The wall of the eye consists of three concentric layers or coats.

The eyeball is composed of three concentric structural layers (Fig. 24.1):

- The **corneoscleral coat**, the outer or fibrous layer, includes the **sclera**, the white portion, and the **cornea**, the transparent portion.

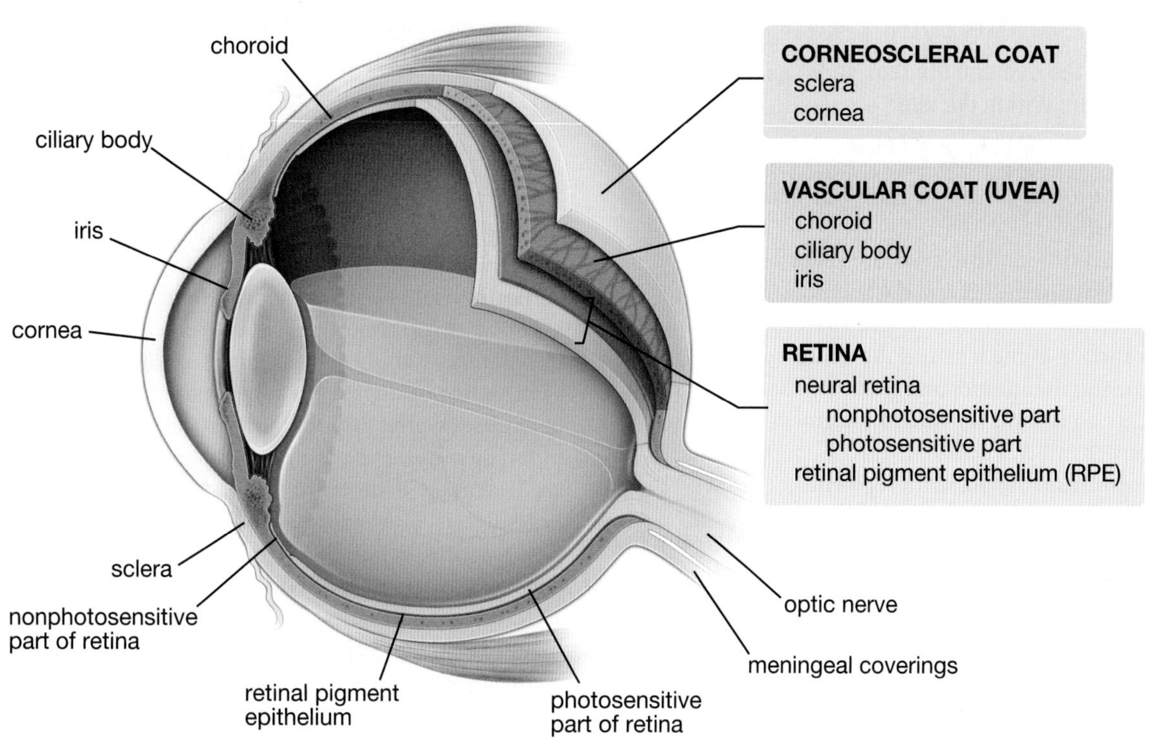

FIGURE 24.1. Schematic diagram of the layers of the eye. The wall of the eyeball is organized in three separate concentric layers: an outer supporting fibrous layer, the corneoscleral coat; a middle vascular coat or uvea; and an inner layer consisting of the retina. Note that the retina has two layers: a neural retina (*yellow*) and a retinal pigment epithelium (*orange*). The photosensitive and nonphotosensitive parts of the neural retina occupy different regions of the eye. The photosensitive part of the retina is found in the posterior part of the eye and terminates anteriorly along the ora serrata. The nonphotosensitive region of the retina is located anterior to the ora serrata and lines the inner aspect of the ciliary body and the posterior surface of the iris. The vitreous body (*partially removed*) occupies considerable space within the eyeball.

- The **vascular coat**, the middle layer, or **uvea**, includes the **choroid** and the stroma of the **ciliary body** and **iris**.
- The **retina**, the inner layer, includes an outer pigment epithelium, the inner neural retina, and the epithelium of the ciliary body and iris. The neural retina is continuous with the CNS through the **optic nerve**.

The corneoscleral coat consists of the transparent cornea and the white opaque sclera.

The **cornea** covers the anterior one-sixth of the eye (see Fig. 24.1). In this window-like region, the surface of the eye has a prominence or convexity. The cornea is continuous with the **sclera** *[Gr. skleros, hard]*. The sclera is composed of dense fibrous connective tissue that provides attachment for the extrinsic muscles of the eye. The corneoscleral coat encloses the inner two layers, except where it is penetrated by the optic nerve. The sclera constitutes the "white" of the eye. In children, it has a slightly blue tint because of its thinness; in elderly people, it is yellowish because of the accumulation of lipofuscin in its stromal cells. A noticeable feature of patients with **jaundice** is a yellow discoloration of the sclera (**scleral icterus**) caused by a high level of circulating bilirubin.

The uvea consists principally of the choroid, the vascular layer that provides nutrients to the retina.

Blood vessels and melanin pigment give the **choroid** an intense dark brown color. The pigment absorbs scattered and reflected light to minimize glare within the eye. The choroid contains numerous venous plexuses and layers of capillaries and is firmly attached to the retina (see Fig. 24.1). The anterior rim of the uveal layer continues forward, where it forms the stroma of the **ciliary body** and **iris**.

The **ciliary body** is a ring-like thickening that extends inward just posterior to the level of the corneoscleral junction. Within the ciliary body is the **ciliary muscle**, a smooth muscle that is responsible for lens **accommodation**. Contraction of the ciliary muscle changes the shape of the lens, which enables it to bring light rays from different distances to focus on the retina.

The **iris** is a contractile diaphragm that extends over the anterior surface of the lens. It also contains smooth muscle and melanin-containing pigment cells scattered in the connective tissue. The **pupil** is the central circular aperture of the iris. It appears black because one looks through the lens toward the heavily pigmented back of the eye. In the process of **adaptation**, the iris contracts or expands, changing the size of the pupil in response to the amount of light that passes through the lens to reach the retina.

The retina consists of two components: the neural retina and pigment epithelium.

The **retina** is a thin, delicate layer (see Fig. 24.1) consisting of two components:

- The **neural retina** is the inner layer that contains light-sensitive receptors and complex neuronal networks.
- The **retinal pigment epithelium (RPE)** is the outer layer composed of simple cuboidal melanin-containing cells.

Externally, the retina rests on the choroid; internally, it is associated with the vitreous body. The neural retina consists largely of **photoreceptor cells**, called retinal **rods** and **cones**, and interneurons. Visual information encoded by the rods and cones is sent to the brain via impulses conveyed along the optic nerve.

Chambers of the Eye

The layers of the eye and the lens serve as boundaries for three chambers within the eye.

The chambers of the eye are as follows:

- The **anterior chamber** is the space between the cornea and the iris.
- The **posterior chamber** is the space between the posterior surface of the iris and the anterior surface of the lens.
- The **vitreous chamber** is the space between the posterior surface of the lens and the neural retina (Fig. 24.2). The cornea, the anterior and posterior chambers, and their contents constitute the anterior segment of the eye. The vitreous chamber, visual retina, RPE, posterior sclera, and uvea constitute the posterior segment.

The refractile media components of the eye alter the light path to focus it on the retina.

As light rays pass through the components of the eye, they are refracted. Refraction focuses the light rays on the photoreceptor cells of the retina. Four transparent components of the eye, called the **refractile (or dioptric) media**, alter the path of the light rays:

- The **cornea** is the anterior window of the eye.
- The **aqueous humor** is the watery fluid located in the anterior and posterior chambers.
- The **lens** is a transparent, crystalline, biconvex structure suspended from the inner surface of the ciliary body by a ring of radially oriented fibers, the **zonule of Zinn**.
- The **vitreous body** is composed of a transparent gel-like substance that fills the vitreous chamber. It acts as a "shock absorber" that protects the fragile retina during rapid eye movement and helps maintain the shape of the eye. The vitreous body is almost 99% water with soluble proteins, hyaluronan, glycoproteins, widely dispersed collagen fibrils, and traces of other insoluble proteins. The fluid component of the vitreous body is called the **vitreous humor**.

The **cornea** is the chief refractive element of the eye. It is the single most powerful focusing element of the eye and has a refractive index of 1.376 (air has a refractive index of 1.0). The cornea provides about 80% of the eye's refractive power and is almost twice as powerful as the lens. The lens is second in importance to the cornea in refracting light rays. It is responsible for fine-tuning and focusing light onto the retina. Because of its elasticity, the shape of the **lens** can undergo slight changes in response to the tension of the ciliary muscle. These changes are important in **accommodation** for proper focusing on near objects. The aqueous humor and vitreous body have only minor roles in refraction. However, the aqueous humor plays an important role in providing nutrients to two avascular structures, the lens and cornea. In addition to transmitting light, the vitreous body helps maintain the position of the lens and helps keep the neural retina in contact with the RPE.

Development of the Eye

To appreciate the unusual structural and functional relationships in the eye, it is helpful to understand how it forms in the embryo.

The tissues of the eye are derived from neuroectoderm, surface ectoderm, and mesoderm.

By the 22nd day of development, the **eyes** are evident as shallow grooves—the **optic sulci** or **optic grooves**—located in the neural folds at the cranial end of the embryo. As the neural tube closes, the paired grooves form

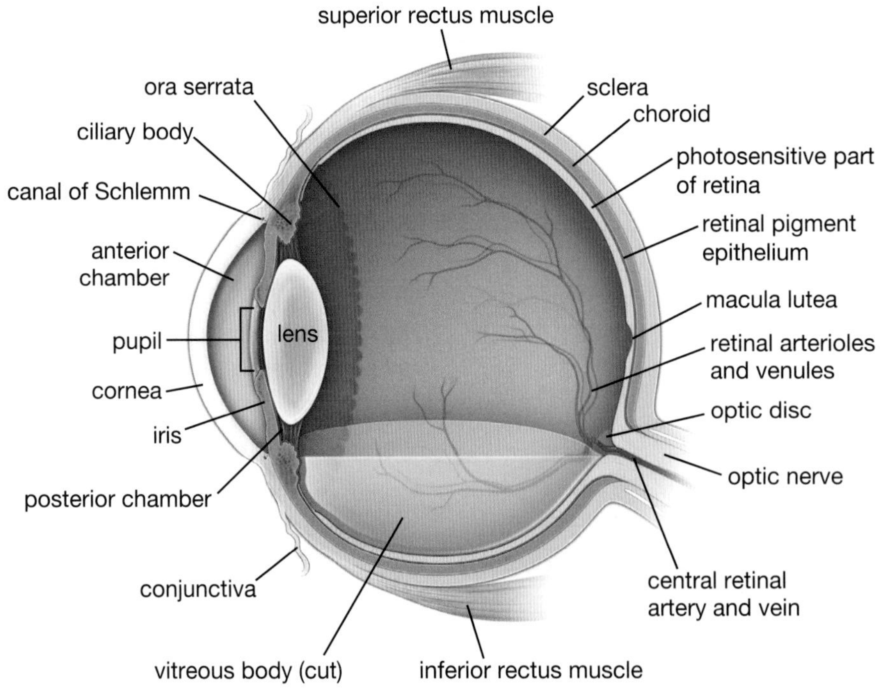

FIGURE 24.2. Schematic diagram illustrating the internal structures of the human eye. This diagram shows the relationship between the layers of the eye and internal structures. The lens is suspended between the edges of the ciliary body. Note the posterior chamber of the eye, which is a narrow space between the anterior surface of the lens and the posterior surface of the iris. It communicates through the pupil with the larger anterior chamber that is bordered by the iris and the cornea. These spaces are filled with the aqueous humor produced by the ciliary body. The large cavity posterior to the lens, the vitreous chamber, is filled with a transparent jelly-like substance called the *vitreous body*. In this figure, most of the vitreous body has been removed to illustrate the distribution of the central retinal vessels on the surface of the retina. The other layers of the eyeball and the attachment of two of the extraocular muscles to the sclera are also shown.

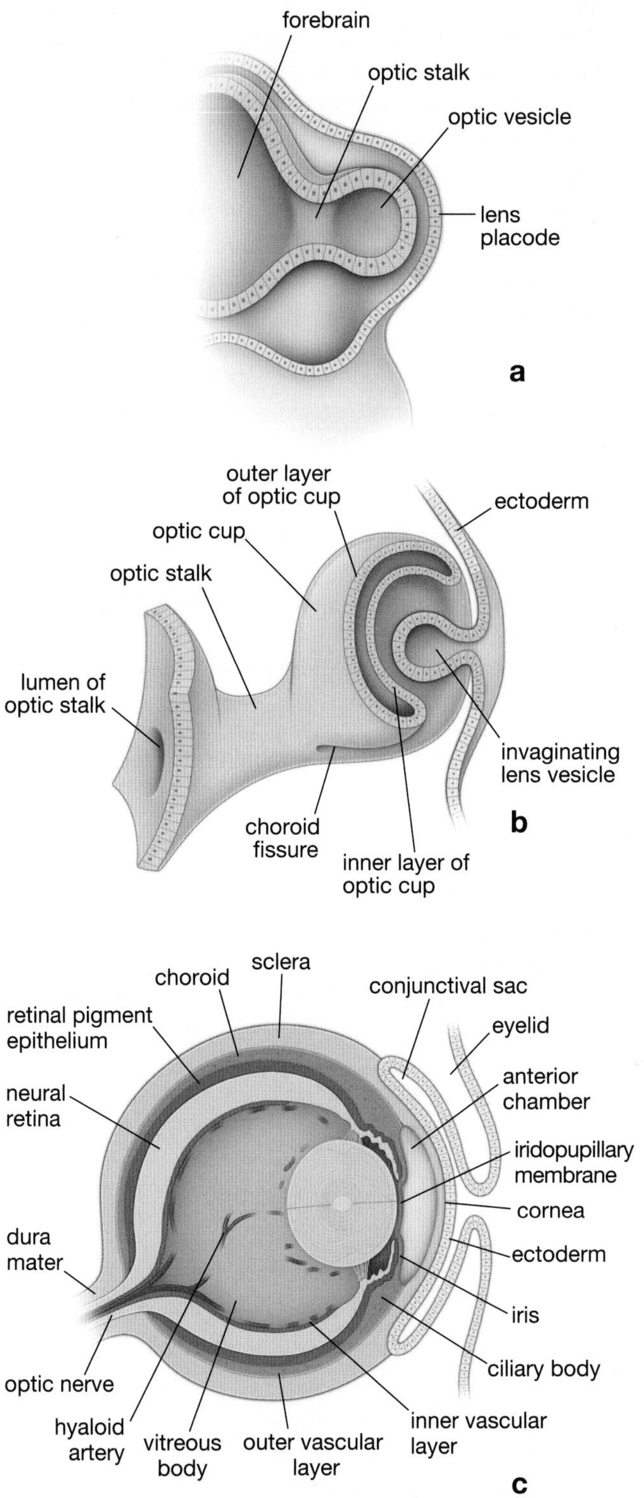

FIGURE 24.3. Schematic drawing illustrating the development of the eye. a. Forebrain and developing optic vesicles as seen in a 4-mm embryo. **b.** Bilayered optic cup and invaginating lens vesicle as seen in a 7.5-mm embryo. The optic stalk connects the developing eye to the brain. **c.** The eye as seen in a 15-week fetus. All the layers of the eye are established, and the hyaloid artery traverses the vitreous body from the optic disc to the posterior surface of the lens.

outpocketings called **optic vesicles** (Fig. 24.3a). As each optic vesicle grows laterally, the connection to the forebrain becomes constricted into an optic stalk, and the overlying surface ectoderm thickens and forms a **lens placode**. These events are followed by concomitant invagination of the optic vesicles and the lens placodes. The invagination of the optic vesicle results in the formation of a double-layered **optic cup** (Fig. 24.3b). The inner layer becomes the **neural retina**. The outer layer becomes the **RPE**. The mesenchyme surrounding the optic cup gives rise to the **sclera**.

Invagination of the central region of each **lens placode** results in the formation of the **lens vesicle**. By the fifth week of development, the lens vesicle loses contact with the surface ectoderm and comes to lie in the mouth of the optic cup. After the lens vesicle detaches from the surface ectoderm, this same site again thickens to form the corneal epithelium. **Mesenchymal cells** from the periphery then give rise to the **corneal endothelium** and the **corneal stroma**.

Grooves containing blood vessels derived from mesenchyme develop along the inferior surface of each optic cup and stalk. Called the **choroid fissures**, the grooves enable the hyaloid artery to reach the inner chamber of the eye. This artery and its branches supply the inner chamber of the optic cup, lens vesicle, and mesenchyme within the optic cup. The hyaloid vein returns blood from these structures. The distal portions of the hyaloid vessels degenerate, but the proximal portions remain as the **central retinal artery** and **central retinal vein**. By the end of the seventh week, the edges of the choroid fissure fuse, and a round opening, the future pupil, forms over the lens vesicle.

The **outer layer of the optic cup** forms a single layer of pigmented cells (Fig. 24.3c). Pigmentation begins at the end of the fifth week. The **inner layer** undergoes a complex differentiation into the nine layers of the **neural retina**. The photoreceptor cells (rods and cones) as well as the bipolar, amacrine, and ganglion cells and nerve fibers are present by the seventh month. The macular depression, a future site of fovea centralis, begins to develop during the eighth month and is not complete until about 6 months after birth.

During the third month, the growth of the optic cup gives rise to the **ciliary body** and the future **iris**, which forms a double row of epithelium in front of the lens. The mesoderm located external to this region becomes the stroma of the ciliary body and iris. Both epithelial layers of the iris become pigmented. In the ciliary body, however, only the outer layer is pigmented. At birth, the iris is light blue in fair-skinned people because the pigment is usually not present. The dilator and sphincter pupillary muscles develop during the sixth month as derivatives of the neuroectoderm of the outer layer of the optic cup.

The embryonic origins of the individual eye structures are summarized in Table 24.1.

■ MICROSCOPIC STRUCTURE OF THE EYE

The three layers of the eye—the **corneoscleral coat**, the **vascular coat**, and the **retina**—are in turn composed of complex molecular layers and structures that reflect their various functions.

Corneoscleral Coat

The cornea is a unique tissue and the most powerful focusing element of the eye. It forms part of the anterior segment of the eye, protecting structures within the eye from the external environment. The most important characteristics of the cornea include its mechanical strength and transparency to incoming light.

TABLE 24.1 Embryonic Origins of the Individual Structures of the Eye

Source	Derivative
Surface ectoderm	Lens Epithelium of the cornea, conjunctiva, and lacrimal gland and its drainage system
Neural ectoderm	Vitreous body (derived partly from neural ectoderm of the optic cup and partly from mesenchyme) Epithelium of the retina, iris, and ciliary body Sphincter pupillae and dilator papillae muscles Optic nerve
Mesoderm	Sclera Stroma of the cornea, ciliary body, iris, and choroids Extraocular muscles Eyelids (except epithelium and conjunctiva) Hyaloid system (most of which degenerates before birth) Coverings of the optic nerve Connective tissue and blood vessels of the eye, bony orbit, and vitreous body

The cornea consists of five layers: three cellular layers and two noncellular layers.

The transparent **cornea** (see Figs. 24.1 and 24.2) is only 0.5 mm thick at its center and about 1 mm thick peripherally. It consists of three cellular layers that are distinct in both appearance and origin. These layers are separated by two important membranes that appear homogeneous when viewed in the light microscope. Thus, the **five layers of the cornea** seen in a transverse section are the following:

- **Corneal epithelium**
- **Bowman membrane** (anterior basement membrane)
- **Corneal stroma**
- **Descemet membrane** (posterior basement membrane)
- **Corneal endothelium**

The corneal epithelium is a nonkeratinized stratified squamous epithelium.

The **corneal epithelium** (Fig. 24.4) represents **nonkeratinized stratified squamous epithelium** that

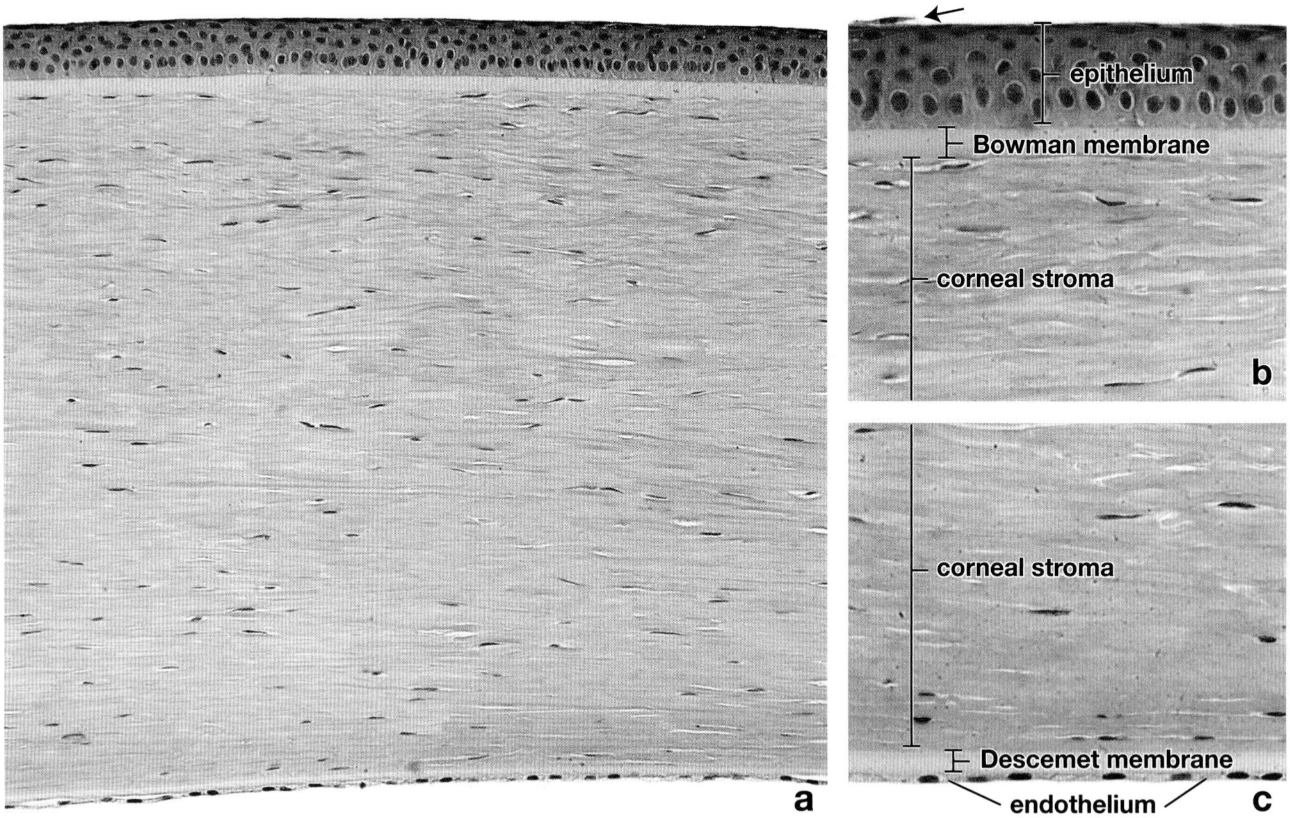

FIGURE 24.4. Photomicrograph of the cornea. a. This photomicrograph of a section through the full thickness of the cornea shows the corneal stroma and the two corneal surfaces covered by different types of epithelia. The corneal stroma does not contain blood or lymphatic vessels. ×140. **b.** A higher magnification of the anterior surface of the cornea showing the *corneal stroma* covered by a stratified squamous (corneal) *epithelium*. The basal cells that rest on *Bowman membrane*, which is a homogeneous condensed layer of corneal stroma, are low columnar in contrast to the squamous surface cells. Note that one of the surface cells is in the process of desquamation (*arrow*). ×280. **c.** A higher magnification photomicrograph of the posterior surface of the cornea covered by a thin layer of simple squamous epithelium (corneal *endothelium*). These cells are in direct contact with the aqueous humor of the anterior chamber of the eye. Note the very thick *Descemet membrane* (basal lamina) of the corneal endothelial cells. ×280.

consists of approximately five layers of cells and measures about 50 μm in average thickness. It is continuous with the conjunctival epithelium that overlies the adjacent sclera. The epithelial cells adhere to neighboring cells via desmosomes that are present in short interdigitating processes. Like other stratified epithelia, such as that of the skin, the cells proliferate from a basal layer and become squamous at the surface. The basal cells are low columnar with round, ovoid nuclei; the surface cells acquire a squamous or discoid shape, and their nuclei are flattened and pyknotic (Fig. 24.4b). As the cells migrate to the surface, the cytoplasmic organelles gradually disappear, indicating a progressive decline in metabolic activity. The corneal epithelium has a remarkable regenerative capacity with a turnover time of approximately 7 days.

The actual stem cells for the corneal epithelium, called **corneolimbal stem cells**, reside at the **corneoscleral limbus**, the junction of the cornea and sclera. The microenvironment of this stem cell niche is important in maintaining the stem cell population. It also acts as a barrier that prevents migration of conjunctival epithelial cells to the corneal surface. The **corneolimbal stem cells** may be partially or totally depleted by disease or extensive injury, resulting in abnormalities of the corneal surface that lead to **conjunctivalization** of the cornea, which is characterized by vascularization, appearance of goblet cells, and an irregular and unstable epithelium. These changes cause ocular discomfort and reduced vision. Minor injuries of the corneal surface heal rapidly by inducing stem cell proliferation and migration of cells from the corneoscleral limbus to fill the defect.

Numerous free nerve endings in the corneal epithelium provide it with extreme sensitivity to touch. Stimulation of these nerves (e.g., by small foreign bodies) elicits blinking of the eyelids, flow of tears, and, sometimes, severe pain. Microvilli present on the surface epithelial cells help retain the tear film over the entire corneal surface. Drying of the corneal surface may cause ulceration.

DNA in the corneal epithelial cells is protected from UV light damage by nuclear ferritin.

Despite constant exposure of the corneal epithelium to ultraviolet (UV) light, cancer of the corneal epithelium is extremely rare. Unlike the epidermis, which is also exposed to UV light, melanin is not present as a defense mechanism in the corneal epithelium. The presence of melanin in the cornea would diminish light transmission. Instead, it has recently been shown that corneal epithelial cell nuclei contain **ferritin**, an iron-storage protein. Experimental studies with avian corneas have shown that **nuclear ferritin** protects the DNA in the corneal epithelial cells from free radical damage caused by UV light exposure.

Bowman membrane is a homogeneous-appearing layer on which the corneal epithelium rests.

Bowman membrane (anterior basement membrane) is a homogeneous, faintly fibrillar lamina that is approximately 8–10 μm thick. It lies between the corneal epithelium and the underlying corneal stroma and ends abruptly at the corneoscleral limbus. The collagen fibrils of Bowman membrane have a diameter of about 18 nm and are randomly oriented. Bowman membrane imparts some strength to the cornea, but more significantly, it acts as a barrier to the spread of infections. It does not regenerate. Therefore, if damaged, an opaque scar forms that may impair vision. In addition, changes in Bowman membrane are associated with **recurrent corneal erosions**.

The corneal stroma constitutes 90% of the corneal thickness.

The **corneal stroma**, also called **substantia propria**, is composed of about 60 thin lamellae. Each lamella consists of parallel bundles of collagen fibrils. Located between the lamellae are nearly complete sheets of slender, flattened fibroblasts. The collagen fibrils are very uniform, measuring approximately 23 nm in diameter and as long as 1 cm in length, and are arranged at approximately right angles to those in adjacent lamellae (Fig. 24.5). The ground substance of cornea contains **small leucine-rich proteoglycans (SLRPs)**, which comprise sulfated glycosaminoglycans—chiefly, keratan sulfate proteoglycan (**lumican**) and chondroitin sulfate proteoglycan (**decorin**). They are responsible for the 3D organization of collagen fibrils. Lumican regulates the normal collagen fibril assembly in the cornea and is critical to the development of a highly organized collagenous matrix.

Corneal transparency is achieved by the regular arrangement of small collagen fibrils and the spaces between them that are smaller than one-half of a wavelength of visible light.

The **transparency of the cornea** is directly related to the spaces between collagen fibrils containing glycosaminoglycans and the size of the collagen fibrils. If these spaces are smaller than one-half of a wavelength of visible light, the cornea is clear and transparent. The uniform spacing of type I collagen fibrils and lamellae, as well as the **orthogonal array** of the lamellae (alternating layers at right angles), helps maintain corneal transparency. Proteoglycans (**lumican**), along with **type V collagen**, regulate the precise diameter and spacing of the type I collagen fibrils, maintaining corneal clarity. The necessity for uniformity of collagen fibrils explains the ratio of

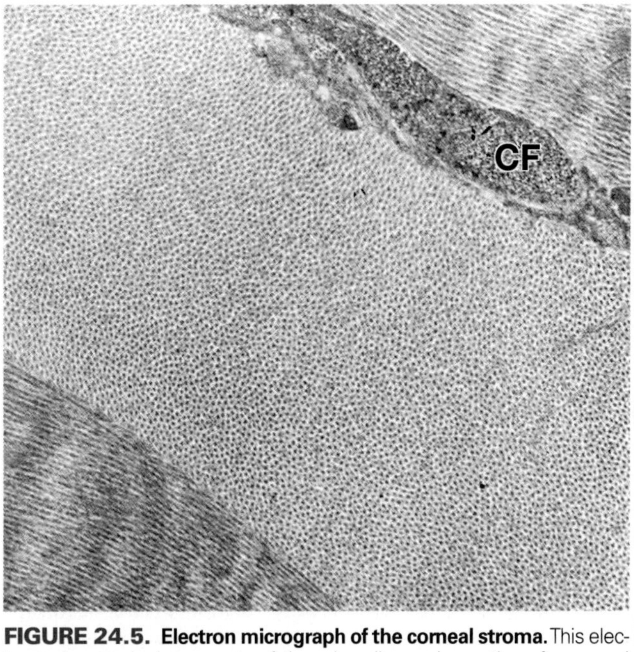

FIGURE 24.5. Electron micrograph of the corneal stroma. This electron micrograph shows parts of three lamellae and a portion of a corneal fibroblast (*CF*) between two of the lamellae. Note that the collagen fibrils in adjacent lamellae are oriented at right angles to one another. ×16,700.

type V to type I collagen, which is much higher in the corneal stroma than in other tissues. **Corneal swelling** after injury to the epithelium or endothelium disrupts this precise array and leads to translucency or opacity of the cornea. The hazy appearance of the cornea is related to the enlargement of the spaces between collagen fibers. Lumican is overexpressed during the wound healing process following corneal injury. Normally, the cornea contains no blood vessels or pigments. During an inflammatory response involving the cornea, large numbers of neutrophils and lymphocytes migrate from the blood vessels of the corneoscleral limbus and penetrate the stromal lamellae.

Descemet membrane is an unusually thick basal lamina.

Descemet membrane (posterior basement membrane) is the basal lamina of corneal endothelial cells. It is intensely positive to periodic acid–Schiff (PAS) and can be as thick as 10 μm. Descemet membrane has a felt-like appearance and consists of an interwoven meshwork of fibers and pores. It separates the corneal endothelium from the adjacent corneal stroma. Unlike Bowman membrane, Descemet membrane readily regenerates after injury. It is produced continuously but slowly thickens with age. Descemet membrane also contributes to the diagnosis of **Wilson disease**, a rare inherited disorder of copper metabolism that causes excessive deposition of copper in organs and other tissues. A common ophthalmologic finding in individuals with Wilson disease is the presence of **Kayser–Fleischer rings**. These are caused by increased depositions of copper within Descemet membrane. A Kayser–Fleischer ring usually appears as a gold brown ring located in the periphery of the cornea.

Descemet membrane extends peripherally beneath the sclera as a trabecular meshwork forming the **pectinate ligament**. Strands from the pectinate ligament penetrate the ciliary muscle and sclera and may help maintain the normal curvature of the cornea by exerting tension on Descemet membrane.

The corneal endothelium provides for metabolic exchange between the cornea and the aqueous humor.

The **corneal endothelium** is a single layer of squamous cells covering the surface of the cornea that faces the anterior chamber (Fig. 24.4c). The cells are joined by well-developed zonulae adherentes, relatively leaky zonulae occludentes, and desmosomes. Virtually, all of the metabolic exchanges of the cornea occur across the endothelium. The endothelial cells contain many mitochondria and vesicles and an extensive rough-surfaced endoplasmic reticulum (rER) and Golgi apparatus. They demonstrate endocytotic activity and are engaged in active transport. Na^+/K^+-activated ATPase is located on the lateral plasma membrane.

Transparency of the cornea requires precise regulation of the water content of the stroma. Physical or metabolic damage to the endothelium leads to rapid **corneal swelling** and, if the damage is severe, corneal opacity. Restoration of endothelial integrity is usually followed by deturgescence (dehydration necessary to maintain the transparency), although corneas can swell beyond their ability for self-repair. Such swelling can result in permanent focal opacities caused by aggregation of collagen fibrils in the swollen cornea. Essential sulfated glycosaminoglycans that normally separate the corneal collagen fibers are extracted from the swollen cornea.

Human **corneal endothelium** has a **limited proliferative capacity**. Severely damaged endothelium can be repaired only by transplantation of a donor cornea. Recent studies indicate that the periphery of the cornea represents a regenerative zone of the corneal endothelial cells. However, soon after **corneal transplantation**, endothelial cells exhibit contact inhibition when exposed to the extracellular matrix of Descemet membrane. The discovery that inhibitory factors released by Descemet membrane prevent proliferation of endothelial cells has focused current corneal research on the reversal or prevention of this inhibition with exogenous growth factors.

The sclera is an opaque layer that consists predominantly of dense connective tissue.

The **sclera** is a thick fibrous layer containing flat collagen bundles that pass in various directions and in planes parallel to its surface. Both the collagen bundles and the fibrils that form them are irregular in diameter and arrangement. Interspersed between the collagen bundles are fine networks of elastic fibers and a moderate amount of ground substance. Fibroblasts are scattered among these fibers (Plate 24.4, page 1016).

The opacity of the sclera, like that of other dense connective tissues, is primarily attributable to the irregularity of its structure. The sclera is pierced by blood vessels, nerves, and the optic nerve (see Fig. 24.2). It is 1 mm thick posteriorly, 0.3–0.4 mm thick at its equator, and 0.7 mm thick at the corneoscleral margin or limbus.

The sclera is divided into three rather ill-defined layers:

- The **episcleral layer (episclera)**, the external layer, is the loose connective tissue adjacent to the periorbital fat.
- The **substantia propria** (**sclera proper**, also called **Tenon capsule**) is the investing fascia of the eye and is composed of a dense network of thick collagen fibers.
- The **suprachoroid lamina (lamina fusca)**, the inner aspect of the sclera, is located adjacent to the choroid and contains thinner collagen fibers and elastic fibers as well as fibroblasts, melanocytes, macrophages, and other connective tissue cells.

In addition, the **episcleral space (Tenon space)** is located between the episcleral layer and substantia propria of the sclera. This space and the surrounding periorbital fat allow the eye to rotate freely within the orbit. The tendons of the extraocular muscles attach to the substantia propria of the sclera.

The corneoscleral limbus is the transitional zone between the cornea and the sclera that contains corneolimbal stem cells.

At the **junction of the cornea and sclera** (Fig. 24.6 and Plate 24.4, page 1016), Bowman membrane ends abruptly. The overlying epithelium at this site thickens from the 5 cell layers of the cornea to the 10–12 cell layers of the conjunctiva. The surface of the limbus is composed of two distinct types of epithelial cells: One type constitutes the conjunctival cells, and the other constitutes the corneal epithelial cells. The basal layer of the limbus contains the **corneolimbal stem cells** that generate and maintain the corneal epithelium. These cells proliferate, differentiate, and migrate to the surface of the limbus and then toward the center of the cornea to replace damaged epithelial cells. As mentioned

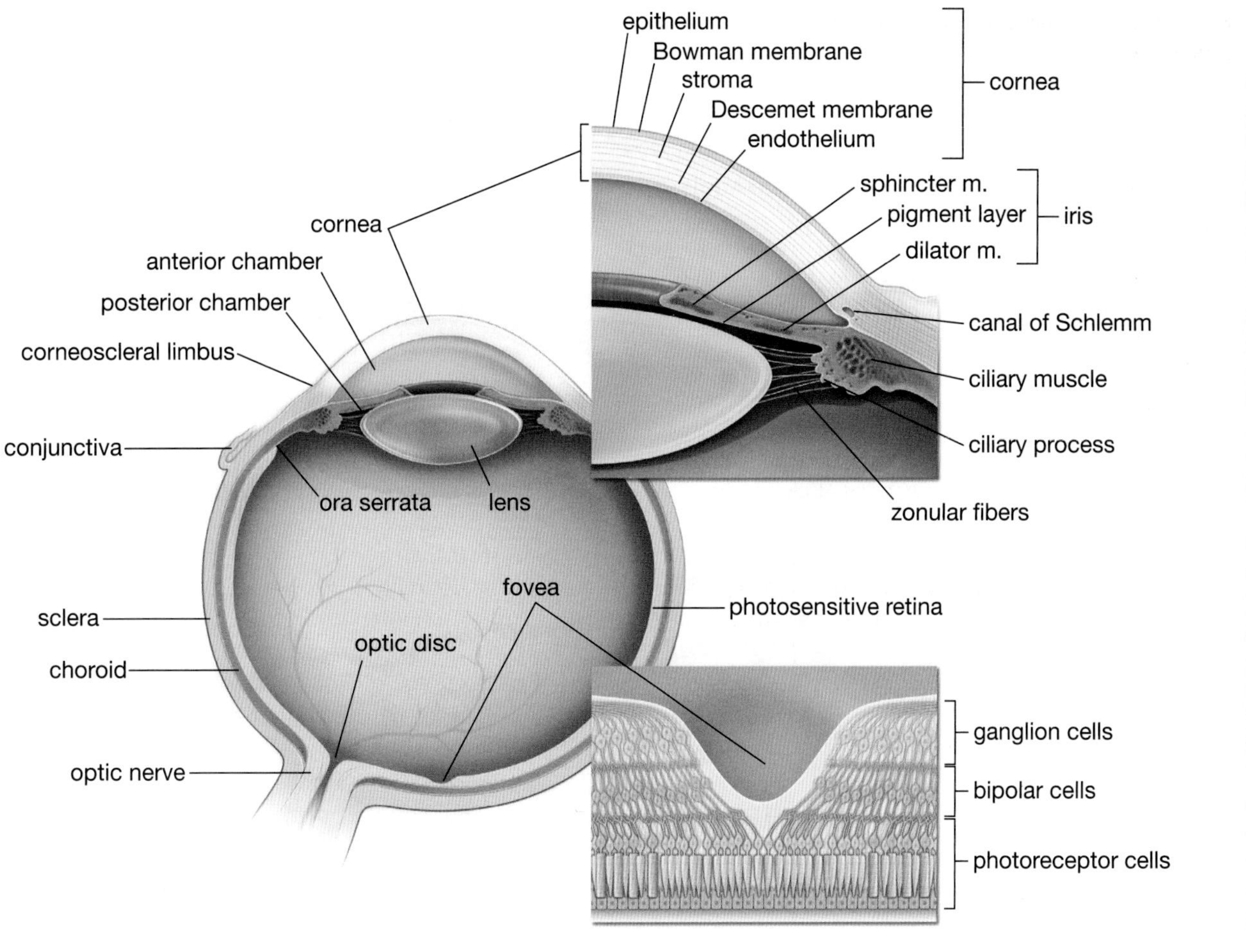

FIGURE 24.6. Schematic diagram of the structure of the eye. This drawing shows a horizontal section of the eyeball with color-coded layers of its wall. **Upper inset.** Enlargement of the anterior and posterior chambers is shown in more detail. Note the location of the iridocorneal angle and canal of Schlemm (scleral venous sinus), which drains the aqueous humor from the anterior chamber of the eye. **Lower inset.** Typical organization of the cells and nerve fibers of the fovea.

previously, this movement of cells at the corneoscleral limbus also creates a barrier that prevents conjunctival epithelium from migrating onto the cornea. At this junction, the corneal lamellae become less regular as they merge with the oblique bundles of collagen fibers of the sclera. An abrupt transition from the avascular cornea to the well-vascularized sclera also occurs here.

The limbus region, specifically, the **iridocorneal angle**, contains the apparatus for the outflow of aqueous humor (Fig. 24.7). In the stromal layer, endothelium-lined channels called the **trabecular meshwork** (or **spaces of Fontana**) merge to form the **scleral venous sinus (canal of Schlemm)**. This sinus encircles the eye (see Figs. 24.6 and 24.7). The aqueous humor is produced by the ciliary processes that border the lens in the posterior chamber of the eye. The fluid passes from the posterior chamber into the anterior chamber through the valve-like potential opening between the iris and lens. The fluid then passes through the openings in the trabecular meshwork in the limbus region as it continues its course to enter the scleral venous sinus. Collecting vessels in the sclera, called **aqueous veins** (of Ascher) because they convey aqueous humor instead of blood, transport the aqueous humor to episcleral and conjunctival (blood) veins located in the sclera. Changes in the **iridocorneal angle** may lead to blockage in the drainage of aqueous humor, causing **glaucoma** (see Folder 24.1, page 990). The iridocorneal angle can be visualized during eye examination using a **gonioscope**, a specialized optical device that uses mirrors or prisms to reflect the light from the iridocorneal angle into the direction of the observer. In conjunction with a slit lamp or operating microscope, the ophthalmologist can examine this region to monitor various eye conditions associated with glaucoma. The iridocorneal angle can be also visualized using the **ultrasound biomicroscopy (UBM)**. This high-resolution imaging technique utilizes a high-frequency ultrasound transducer to visualize the narrowed iridocorneal angle in primary angle-closure glaucoma.

Vascular Coat (Uvea)

The iris, the most anterior part of the vascular coat, forms a contractile diaphragm in front of the lens.

The **iris** arises from the anterior border of the ciliary body (see Fig. 24.7) and is attached to the sclera about 2 mm posterior to the corneoscleral junction. The **pupil** is the central aperture of this thin disc. The iris is pushed slightly forward as it changes in size in response to light intensity. It consists of a highly vascularized connective tissue stroma that is covered on its posterior surface by highly pigmented cells, the **posterior pigment epithelium** (Fig. 24.8). The basal lamina of these cells faces the posterior chamber of the eye. The degree of pigmentation is so great that neither the nucleus nor the character of the cytoplasm can be seen in the light microscope. Located beneath this layer

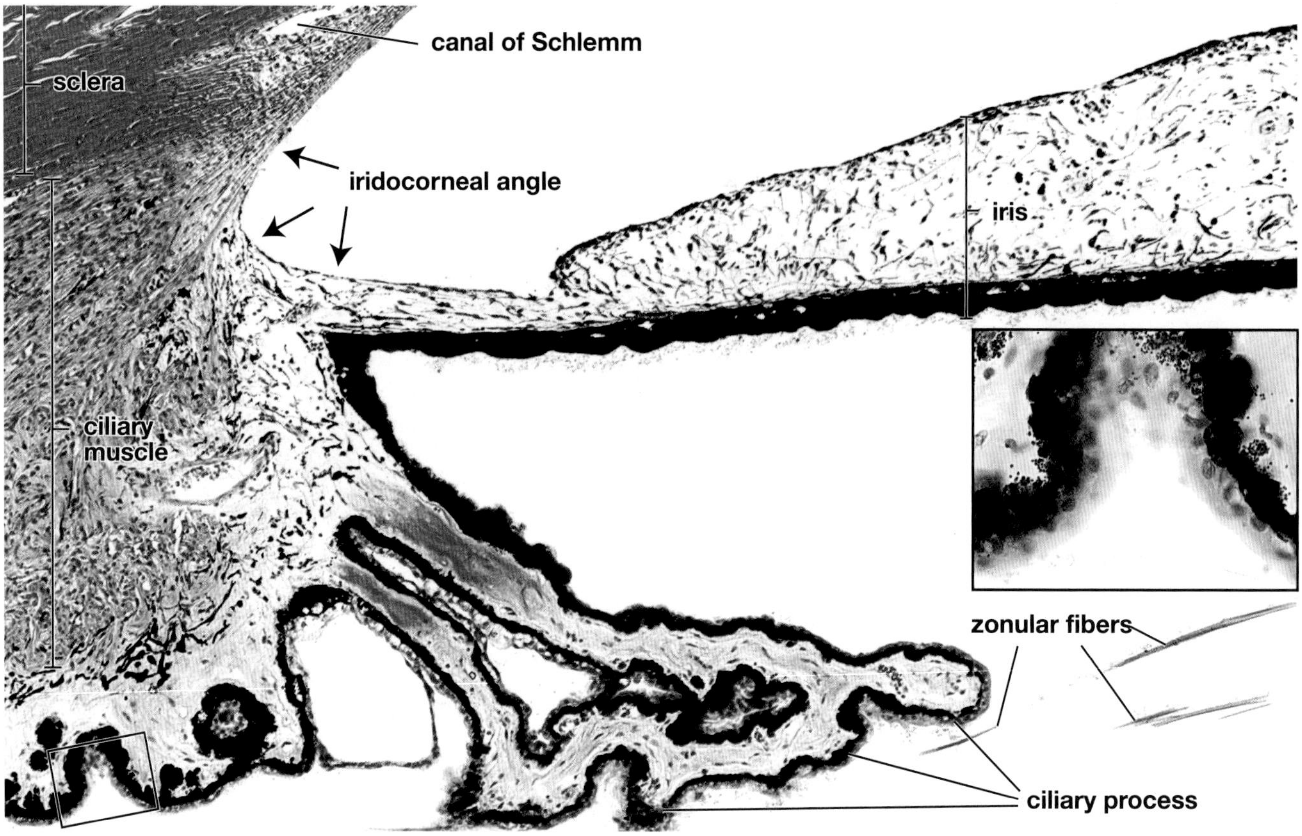

FIGURE 24.7. Photomicrograph of the ciliary body and iridocorneal angle. This photomicrograph of the human eye shows the anterior portion of the ciliary body and parts of the *iris* and *sclera.* The inner surface of the ciliary body forms radially arranged, ridge-shaped elevations, the *ciliary processes*, to which the *zonular fibers* are anchored. The ciliary body contains the *ciliary muscle*, connective tissue with blood vessels of the vascular coat, and the ciliary epithelium, which is responsible for the production of aqueous humor. Anterior to the ciliary body, between the iris and the cornea, is the *iridocorneal angle.* The scleral venous sinus (*canal of Schlemm*) is located in close proximity to this angle and drains the aqueous humor to regulate intraocular pressure. ×120. The *inset* shows that the ciliary epithelium consists of two layers, the outer pigmented layer and the inner nonpigmented layer. ×480.

is a layer of myoepithelial cells, the **anterior pigment myoepithelium**. The apical (posterior) portions of these myoepithelial cells are laden with melanin granules, which effectively obscure their boundaries with the adjacent posterior pigment epithelial cells. The basal (anterior) portions of myoepithelial cells possess processes containing contractile elements that extend radially and collectively make up the **dilator pupillae muscle** of the iris. The contractile processes are enclosed by a basal lamina that separates them from the adjacent stroma.

Constriction of the pupil is produced by smooth muscle cells located in the stroma of the iris near the pupillary margin of the iris. These circumferentially oriented cells collectively compose the **sphincter pupillae muscle**.

The anterior surface of the iris reveals numerous ridges and grooves that can be seen in clinical examination with the ophthalmoscope. When this surface is examined in the light microscope, it appears as a discontinuous layer of fibroblasts and melanocytes. The number of melanocytes in the stroma is responsible for variation in eye color. The function of these **pigment-containing cells** in the iris is to absorb light rays. If there are few melanocytes in the stroma, the color of the iris is derived from light reflected from the pigment present in the cells of the iris's posterior surface, giving it a blue appearance. With increasing amounts of pigment present in the stroma, the iris color changes from blue to shades of greenish blue, gray, and, finally, brown.

The sphincter pupillae is innervated by parasympathetic nerves; the dilator pupillae muscle is under sympathetic nerve control.

The **size of the pupil** is controlled by contraction of the sphincter pupillae and dilator pupillae muscles. The process of **adaptation** (increasing or decreasing the size of the pupil) ensures that only the appropriate amount of light enters the eye. Two muscles are actively involved in adaptation:

- The **sphincter pupillae muscle**, a circular band of smooth muscle cells (Plate 24.3, page 1014), is innervated by parasympathetic nerves carried in the oculomotor nerve (cranial nerve III) and is responsible for reducing pupillary size in response to bright light. Failure of the pupil to respond when light is shined into the eye—"**pupil fixed and dilated**"—is an important clinical sign showing a lack of nerve or brain function.
- The **dilator pupillae muscle** is a thin sheet of radially oriented contractile processes of pigmented myoepithelial cells constituting the anterior pigment epithelium of the iris. This muscle is innervated by sympathetic nerves from the superior cervical ganglion and is responsible for increasing pupillary size in response to dim light.

Just before **ophthalmoscopic examination**, mydriatic agents such as **atropine** are given as eye drops to cause dilation of the pupil. Acetylcholine (ACh) is the neurotransmitter of the parasympathetic nervous system (it innervates the sphincter pupillae muscle); the addition of

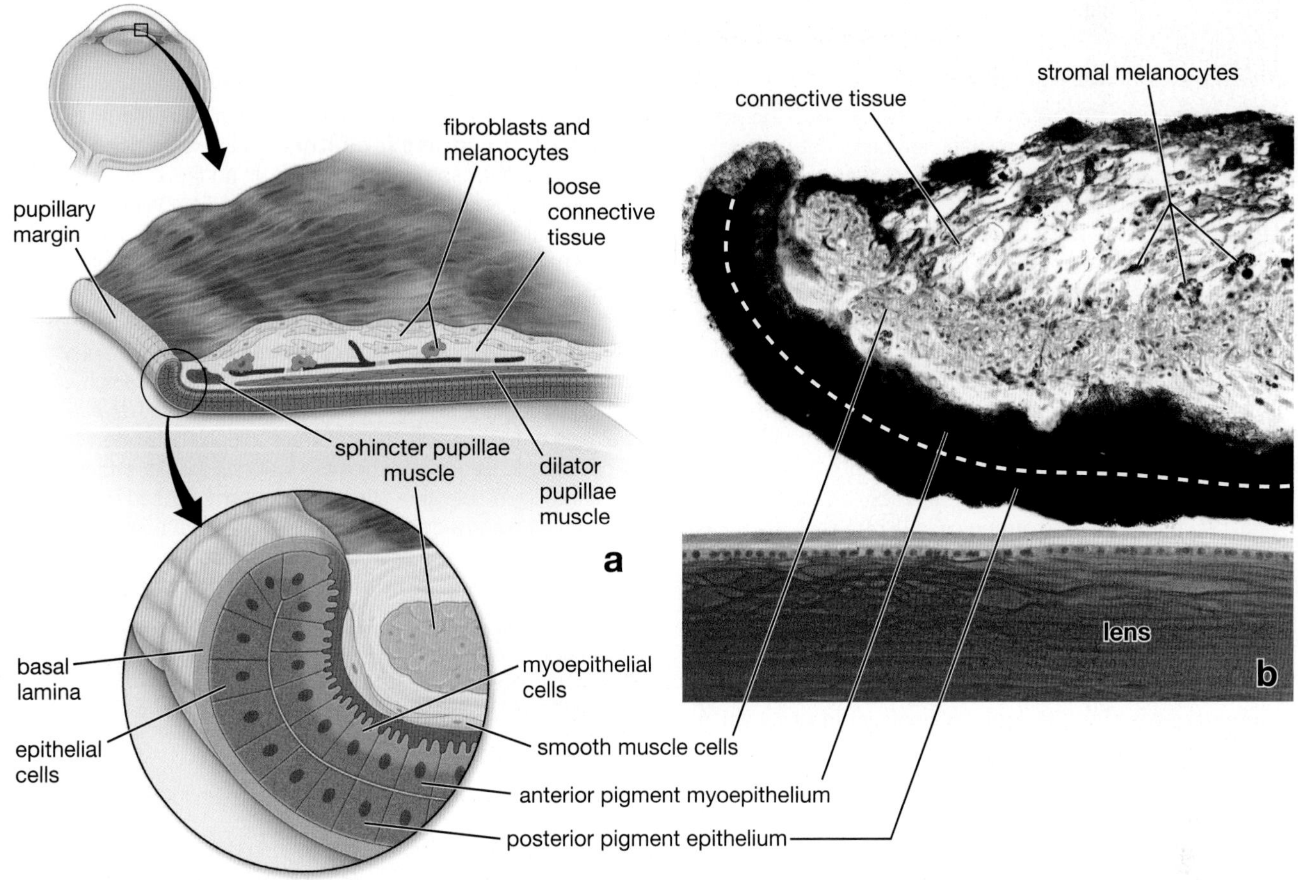

FIGURE 24.8. Structure of the iris. a. This schematic diagram shows the layers of the iris. Note that the pigmented epithelial cells are reflected as occurs at the pupillary margin of the iris. The two layers of pigmented epithelial cells are in contact with the dilator pupillae muscle. The incomplete layer of fibroblasts and stromal melanocytes is indicated on the anterior surface of the iris. **b.** Photomicrograph of the iris showing the histologic features of this structure. The *lens*, which lies posterior to the iris, is included for orientation. The iris is composed of a *connective tissue* stroma covered on its posterior surface by the posterior pigment epithelium. The basal lamina (not visible) faces the posterior chamber of the eye. Because of intense pigmentation, the histologic features of these cells are not discernible. Just anterior to these cells is the anterior pigment myoepithelium layer (the *dashed line* separates the two layers). Note that the posterior portion of the myoepithelial cells contains melanin, whereas the anterior portion contains contractile elements forming the dilator pupillae muscle of the iris. The sphincter pupillae muscle is evident in the stroma. The color of the iris depends on the number of *stromal melanocytes* scattered throughout the connective tissue stroma. At the *bottom*, note the presence of the lens. ×570.

atropine blocks muscarinic acetylcholine receptors, temporally blocking the action of the sphincter muscle, and leaving the **pupil wide open** and unreactive to light originating from ophthalmoscope.

The ciliary body is the thickened anterior portion of the vascular coat and is located between the iris and the choroid.

The **ciliary body** extends about 6 mm from the root of the iris posterolaterally to the **ora serrata** (see Fig. 24.2). As seen from behind, the lateral edge of the ora serrata bears 17–34 grooves or crenulations. These grooves mark the anterior limit of both the retina and the choroid. The anterior third of the ciliary body has approximately 75 radial ridges or **ciliary processes** (see Fig. 24.7). The fibers of the zonule arise from the grooves between the ciliary processes.

The layers of the ciliary body are similar to those of the iris and consist of a stroma and an epithelium. The stroma is divided into two layers:

- An **outer layer** of smooth muscle, the **ciliary muscle**, makes up the bulk of the ciliary body.
- An **inner vascular region** extends into the ciliary processes.

The epithelial layer covering the internal surface of the ciliary body is a direct continuation of the two layers of the retinal epithelium (see Fig. 24.1).

The ciliary muscle is organized into three functional portions or groups of smooth muscle fibers.

The smooth muscle of the ciliary body has its origin in the scleral spur, a ridge-like projection on the inner surface of the sclera at the corneoscleral junction. The muscle fibers spread out in several directions and are classified into three functional groups on the basis of their direction and insertion:

- The **meridional (or longitudinal) portion** consists of the outer muscle fibers that pass posteriorly into the stroma of the choroid. These fibers function chiefly in stretching the choroid. It also may help open the iridocorneal angle and facilitate drainage of the aqueous humor.
- The **radial (or oblique) portion** consists of deeper muscle fiber bundles that radiate in a fan-like manner to insert into the ciliary body. Its contraction causes the lens to flatten and thus focus on distant vision.
- The **circular (or sphincteric) portion** consists of inner muscle fiber bundles oriented in a circular pattern that forms a sphincter. It reduces the tension on the lens, causing the lens to accommodate for near vision.

FOLDER 24.1

CLINICAL CORRELATION: GLAUCOMA

Glaucoma is a clinical condition resulting from increased intraocular pressure over a sustained period of time. It can be caused by excessive secretion of aqueous humor or impedance of the drainage of aqueous humor from the anterior chamber. The internal tissues of the eye, particularly the retina, are nourished by the diffusion of oxygen and nutrients from the intraocular vessels. Blood flows normally through these vessels (including the capillaries and veins) when the hydrostatic pressure within the vessels exceeds the intraocular pressure. If the drainage of the aqueous humor is impeded, the intraocular pressure increases because the layers of the eye do not allow the wall to expand. This increased pressure interferes with normal retinal nourishment and function, causing the retinal nerve fiber layer to atrophy (Fig. F24.1.1).

There are two major types of glaucoma:

- **Open-angle glaucoma** is the most common type of glaucoma and the leading cause of blindness among adults. The removal of aqueous humor is obstructed because of reduced flow through the trabecular meshwork of the iridocorneal angle into the scleral venous sinus (canal of Schlemm).
- **Angle-closure glaucoma (acute glaucoma)** is less common and is characterized by a narrowed iridocorneal angle that obstructs the inflow of the aqueous humor into the scleral venous sinus. Usually, it is associated with a sudden, painful, complete blockage of the scleral venous sinus and can result in permanent blindness if not treated promptly.

Visual deficits associated with glaucoma include blurring of vision and impaired dark adaptation (symptoms that indicate loss of normal retinal function) and halos around lights (a symptom indicating corneal endothelial damage). If the condition is not treated, the retina will be permanently damaged, and blindness will occur. Treatment is directed toward lowering the intraocular pressure by decreasing the rate of production of aqueous humor or eliminating the cause of the obstruction of normal drainage. Topical **prostaglandin analogs** (i.e., latanoprost, bimatoprost, travoprost) are the first line of treatment for open-angle glaucoma. They are very effective in reducing intraocular pressure by increasing the drainage of aqueous humor into the canal of Schlemm. **Carbonic anhydrase inhibitors**, which were used in the past to decrease the production of aqueous humor, have largely been replaced by prostaglandin analogs that have fewer systemic side effects.

There are two main types of laser surgery to treat glaucoma. They facilitate drainage of aqueous humor from the iridocorneal angle. Laser **trabeculoplasty** utilizes a laser beam to induce focal scarring of the trabecular meshwork. This results in mechanical stretching of the surrounding untreated regions of the meshwork, which facilitates drainage of the aqueous humor. Trabeculoplasty is often used in open-angle glaucoma when medications are not effective or cause intolerable side effects. **Iridotomy** is used in patients with angle-closure glaucoma. The laser beam incises a small opening at the base of the iris, which widens the iridocorneal angle to allow better drainage of aqueous humor.

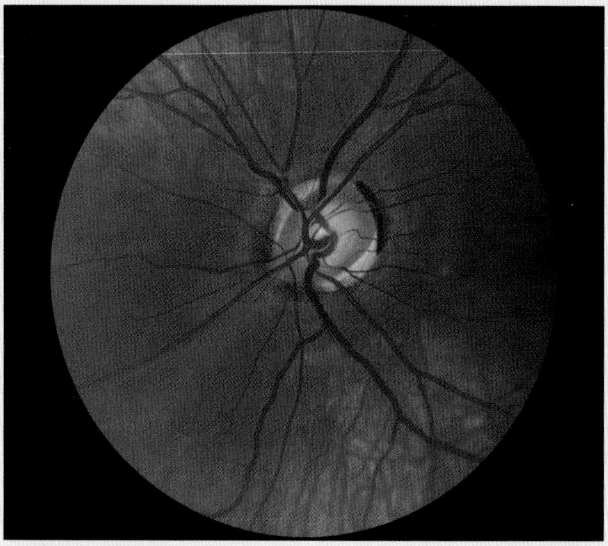

FIGURE F24.1.1. Glaucoma. This image shows a view of the fundus of the left eye in a patient with advanced glaucoma. As a result of the increased intraocular pressure, retinal nerve fibers undergo atrophy and shrink in size. Note a pale optic disc in the *center* of the image with a less pronounced rim due to atrophy of nerve fibers. Enlargement of the optic nerve cup (central area of the optic disc) is also visible and a characteristic finding for glaucoma. Compare this image to a normal retina in Figure 24.15. (Courtesy of Dr. Renzo A. Zaldivar.)

Examination of a histologic preparation does not clearly reveal the arrangement of the muscle fibers. Rather, the organizational grouping is based on microdissection techniques.

Ciliary processes are ridge-like extensions of the ciliary body from which zonular fibers emerge and extend to the lens.

Ciliary processes are thickenings of the inner vascular region of the ciliary body. They are continuous with the vascular layers of the choroid. Scattered macrophages containing melanin pigment granules and elastic fibers are present in these processes (Plate 24.3, page 1014). The processes and the ciliary body are covered by a double layer of columnar epithelial cells, the **ciliary epithelium**, which was originally derived from the two layers of the optic cup. The ciliary epithelium has three principal functions:

- Secretion of **aqueous humor**
- Participation in the **blood–aqueous barrier** (part of the **blood–ocular barrier**)
- Secretion and anchoring of the **zonular fibers** that form the **suspensory ligament of the lens**

The inner cell layer of the ciliary epithelium has a basal lamina facing the posterior and vitreous chambers. The cells in this layer are nonpigmented. The cell layer that has its basal lamina facing the connective tissue stroma of the ciliary body is heavily pigmented and is directly continuous with the pigmented epithelial layer of the retina. The **double-layered ciliary epithelium** continues over the iris, where it becomes the posterior pigmented epithelium and anterior pigmented myoepithelium. The zonular fibers extend from the basal lamina of the nonpigmented epithelial cells of the ciliary processes and insert into the lens capsule (the thickened basal lamina of the lens).

The blood–aqueous barrier separates the interior environment of the eye from the blood entering the ciliary body.

The **cells of the nonpigmented layer** have all the characteristics of a fluid-transporting epithelium, including complex cell-to-cell junctions with a well-developed zonula occludens, extensive lateral and basal plications, and localization of Na^+/K^+-ATPase in the lateral plasma membrane. In addition, they have an elaborate rER and Golgi complex, consistent with their role in the secretion of zonular fibers. Tight junctions (zonulae occludentes) between the nonpigmented ciliary epithelial cells are responsible for maintaining the **blood–aqueous barrier**. This barrier restricts free diffusion across the ciliary epithelium to maintain the unique environment of the aqueous humor, which is quite different from that of blood vessels and stroma of the ciliary body. The blood–aqueous barrier contributes to the nutrition and function of the cornea and the lens. **Disruption of the blood–aqueous barrier** may be observed in ocular inflammation, intraocular surgery, trauma, or vascular diseases. The aqueous humor becomes cloudy because of the leakage of plasma proteins (fibrinogen) and migration of inflammatory cells from the stroma of the ciliary body and iris into the posterior and anterior chambers of the eye.

The **cells of the pigmented layer** have a less developed junctional zone and often exhibit large, irregular lateral intercellular spaces. Both desmosomes and gap junctions hold together the apical surfaces of the two cell layers, creating discontinuous "luminal" spaces called **ciliary channels**.

The aqueous humor is derived from plasma and maintains intraocular pressure.

The **aqueous humor** is secreted by the double-layered ciliary epithelium and originates from blood capillaries. It is similar in ionic composition to plasma but contains less than 0.1% protein (compared to 7% protein in plasma). The main functions of the aqueous humor are to maintain **intraocular pressure** and to provide nutrients and remove metabolites from the avascular tissues of the cornea and lens. The aqueous humor passes from the ciliary body toward the lens and then between the iris and the lens, before it reaches the anterior chamber of the eye (see Fig. 24.6). In the anterior chamber of the eye, the aqueous humor passes laterally to the angle formed between the cornea and the iris. Here, it penetrates the tissues of the limbus as it enters the labyrinthine spaces of the limbus's trabecular meshwork in the iridocorneal angle and finally reaches the **canal of Schlemm**, which communicates with the veins of the sclera (see Folder 24.1). Normal turnover of the aqueous humor in the human eye is approximately once every 1.5–2 hours.

The choroid is the portion of the vascular coat that lies deep into the retina.

The **choroid** is a dark brown vascular sheet only 0.25 mm thick posteriorly and 0.1 mm thick anteriorly. It lies between the sclera and the retina (see Fig. 24.1).

Two layers can be identified in the choroid:

- **Choriocapillary layer**, an inner vascular layer
- **Bruch membrane**, a thin, amorphous hyaline membrane

FOLDER 24.2

CLINICAL CORRELATION: RETINAL DETACHMENT

A potential space exists in the retina as a vestige of the space between the apical surfaces of the two epithelial layers of the optic cup. If this space expands, the neural retina separates from the retinal pigment epithelium (RPE), which remains attached to the choroid layer. This condition is called **retinal detachment**. As a result of retinal detachment, the photoreceptor cells are no longer supplied by nutrients from the underlying vessels in the choriocapillary plexus of the choroid.

Clinical symptoms of retinal detachment include visual sensations commonly described as a "shower of pepper" or floaters. These are caused by red blood cells extravasated from the capillary vessels that have been injured during the retinal tear or detachment. In addition, some individuals describe sudden flashes of light as well as a "web" or "veil" in front of the eye in conjunction with the onset of floaters. A detached retina can be observed and diagnosed during ophthalmoscopic eye examination (Fig. F24.2.1).

Another common retinal condition occurs with aging. As the vitreous body ages (in the sixth and seventh decades of life), it tends to shrink and pull away from the neural retina, which causes single or multiple tears in the neural retina.

If not repositioned quickly, the detached area of the retina will undergo necrosis, resulting in blindness. An argon laser is often used to repair retinal detachment by photocoagulating the edges of the detachment and producing scar tissue. This method prevents the retina from further detachment and facilitates the repositioning of photoreceptor cells.

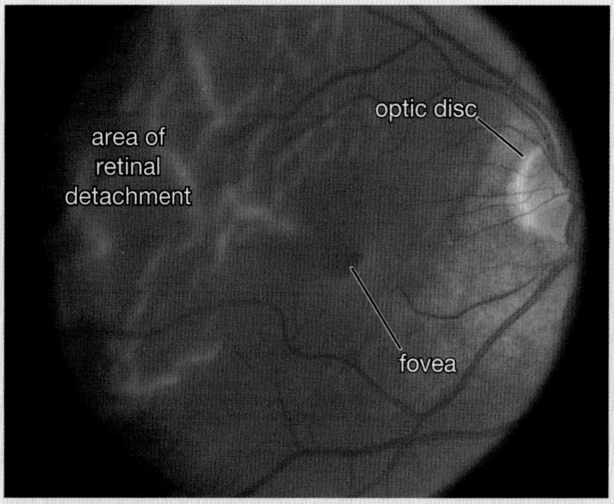

FIGURE F24.2.1. Retinal detachment. This image shows a view of the fundus of the right eye in a patient with retinal detachment. The central retinal vessels emerging from the optic disc are in focus, but in the *area of the retinal detachment,* they appear to be out of focus. Because the area of retinal detachment is elevated (note multiple ridges and shadows), it is located anterior to the plane of focus of the ophthalmoscope. (Courtesy of Dr. Renzo A. Zaldivar.)

FOLDER 24.3

CLINICAL CORRELATION: AGE-RELATED MACULAR DEGENERATION

Age-related macular degeneration (ARMD) is the most common cause of blindness in older individuals. Although the cause of this disease is still unknown, evidence suggests both genetic and environmental (ultraviolet [UV] irradiation, drugs) components. The disease causes loss of central vision, although peripheral vision remains unaffected. Two forms of ARMD are recognized: a dry (atrophic, nonexudative) form and a wet (exudative, neovascular) form. The latter is considered a complication of the first. **Dry ARMD** is the most common form (90% of all cases) and involves degenerative lesions localized in the area of the macula lutea. The degenerative lesions include **drusen**, which are focal thickenings of Bruch membrane, atrophy, depigmentation of the RPE, and obliteration of capillaries in the underlying choroid layer. These changes lead to the deterioration of the overlying photosensitive retina, resulting in the formation of blind spots in the visual field (Fig. F24.3.1). **Wet ARMD** is a complication of dry ARMD caused by neovascularization of blind spots of the retina in the large drusen. These newly formed, thin, fragile vessels frequently leak and produce exudates and hemorrhages in the space just beneath the retina, resulting in fibrosis and scarring. These changes are responsible for the progressive loss of central vision over a short time. The treatment of wet ARMD includes conventional **laser photocoagulation** therapy and pharmacologic therapy with intravitreal injection of ranibizumab, a **vascular endothelial growth factor (VEGF) inhibitor**. Other surgical methods, such as **macular translocation**, have been recently introduced. In this procedure, the retina is detached, translocated, and reattached in a new location, away from the choroid neovascular tissue. Conventional laser treatment is then applied to destroy pathologic vessels without destroying central vision.

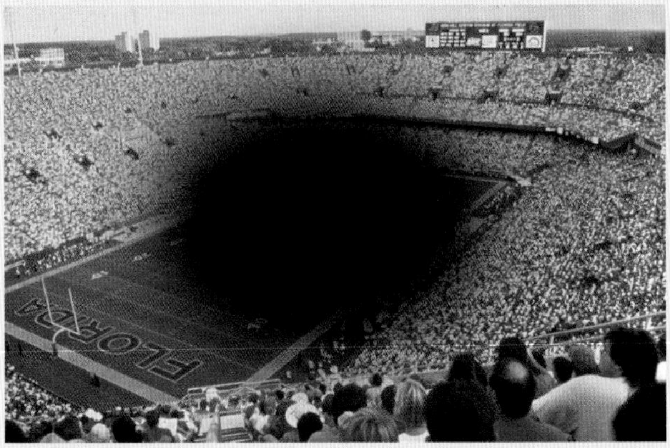

FIGURE F24.3.1. Photograph depicting the visual field in individuals with age-related macular degeneration. Note that central vision is absent because of the changes in the macula region of the retina. To maximize their remaining vision, individuals with this condition are instructed to use eccentric fixation of their eyes.

The choroid is attached firmly to the sclera at the margin of the optic nerve. A potential space, the **perichoroidal space** (between the sclera and the retina), is traversed by thin, ribbon-like branching lamellae or strands that pass from the sclera to the choroid. These lamellae originate from the **suprachoroid lamina** (lamina fusca) and consist of large, flat melanocytes scattered between connective tissue elements, including collagen and elastic fibers, fibroblasts, macrophages, lymphocytes, plasma cells, and mast cells. The lamellae pass inward to surround the vessels in the remainder of the choroid layer. Free smooth muscle cells, not associated with blood vessels, are present in this tissue. Lymphatic channels called **epichoroid lymph spaces**, long and short posterior ciliary vessels, and nerves on their way to the front of the eye are also present in the suprachoroid lamina.

Most of the blood vessels decrease in size as they approach the retina. The largest vessels continue forward beyond the ora serrata into the ciliary body. These vessels can be seen with an ophthalmoscope. The large vessels are mostly veins that course in whorls before passing obliquely through the sclera as vortex veins. The inner layer of vessels, arranged in a single plane, is called the **choriocapillary layer**. The vessels of this layer provide nutrients to the cells of the retina. The fenestrated capillaries have lumina that are large and irregular in shape. In the region of the fovea, the choriocapillary layer is thicker, and the capillary network is denser. This layer ends at the ora serrata.

Bruch membrane, also called the **lamina vitrea**, measures 1–4 μm in thickness and lies between the choriocapillary layer and the pigment epithelium of the retina. It runs from the optic nerve to the ora serrata, where it undergoes modifications before continuing into the ciliary body. Bruch membrane is a thin, amorphous refractile layer. The transmission electron microscope (TEM) reveals that it consists of a multilaminar sheet containing a center layer of elastic and collagen fibers. Five different layers are identified in Bruch membrane:

- The basal lamina of the endothelial cells of the choriocapillary layer
- A layer of collagen fibers approximately 0.5 μm thick
- A layer of elastic fibers approximately 2 μm thick
- A second layer of collagen fibers (thus forming a "sandwich" around the intervening elastic tissue layer)
- The basal lamina of the RPE cells

At the ora serrata, the collagenous and elastic layers disappear into the ciliary stroma, and Bruch membrane becomes continuous with the basal lamina of the RPE of the ciliary body.

Retina

The retina represents the innermost layer of the eye.

The **retina**, derived from the inner and outer layers of the optic cup, is the innermost of the three concentric layers of the eye (see Fig. 24.1). It consists of two basic layers:

- The **neural retina** or **retina proper** is the inner layer that contains the photoreceptor cells.
- The **retinal pigment epithelium (RPE)** is the outer layer that rests on and is firmly attached through the Bruch membrane to the choriocapillary layer of the choroid.

A potential space exists between the two layers of the retina. The two layers may be separated mechanically in the preparation of histologic specimens. Separation of the layers, "**retinal detachment**" (see Folder 24.2), also occurs in the living state because of eye disease or trauma.

In the neural retina, two regions or portions that differ in function are recognized:

- The **nonphotosensitive region** (nonvisual part), located anterior to the ora serrata, lines the inner aspect of the ciliary body and the posterior surface of the iris (this portion of the retina is described in the sections on the iris and ciliary body).
- The **photosensitive region** (optic part) lines the inner surface of the eye posterior to the ora serrata, except where it is pierced by the optic nerve (see Fig. 24.1).

The site where the optic nerve joins the retina is called the **optic disc** or **optic papilla**. Because the optic disc is devoid of photoreceptor cells, it is a blind spot in the visual field. The **fovea centralis** is a shallow depression located about 2.5 mm lateral to the optic disc. It is the area of greatest visual acuity. The visual axis of the eye passes through the fovea. A yellow-pigmented zone called the **macula lutea** surrounds the fovea. In relative terms, the fovea is the region of the retina that contains the highest concentration and most precisely ordered arrangement of visual elements. The region of the retina surrounding the macula lutea may be affected in older individuals by **age-related macular degeneration** (see Folder 24.3).

Layers of the retina

Ten layers of cells and their processes constitute the retina.

Before discussing the **ten layers of the retina**, it is important to identify the types of cells found there. This identification will aid in understanding the functional relationships of the cells. Studies of the retina in primates have identified at least 15 types of neurons that form at least 38 different types of synapses. For convenience, neurons and supporting cells can be classified into four groups of cells (Fig. 24.9):

- **Photoreceptor cells**—the retinal rods and cones
- **Conducting neurons**—bipolar neurons and ganglion cells
- **Association neurons** and others—horizontal, centrifugal, interplexiform, and amacrine neurons
- **Supporting (neuroglial) cells**—Müller cells, microglial cells, and astrocytes

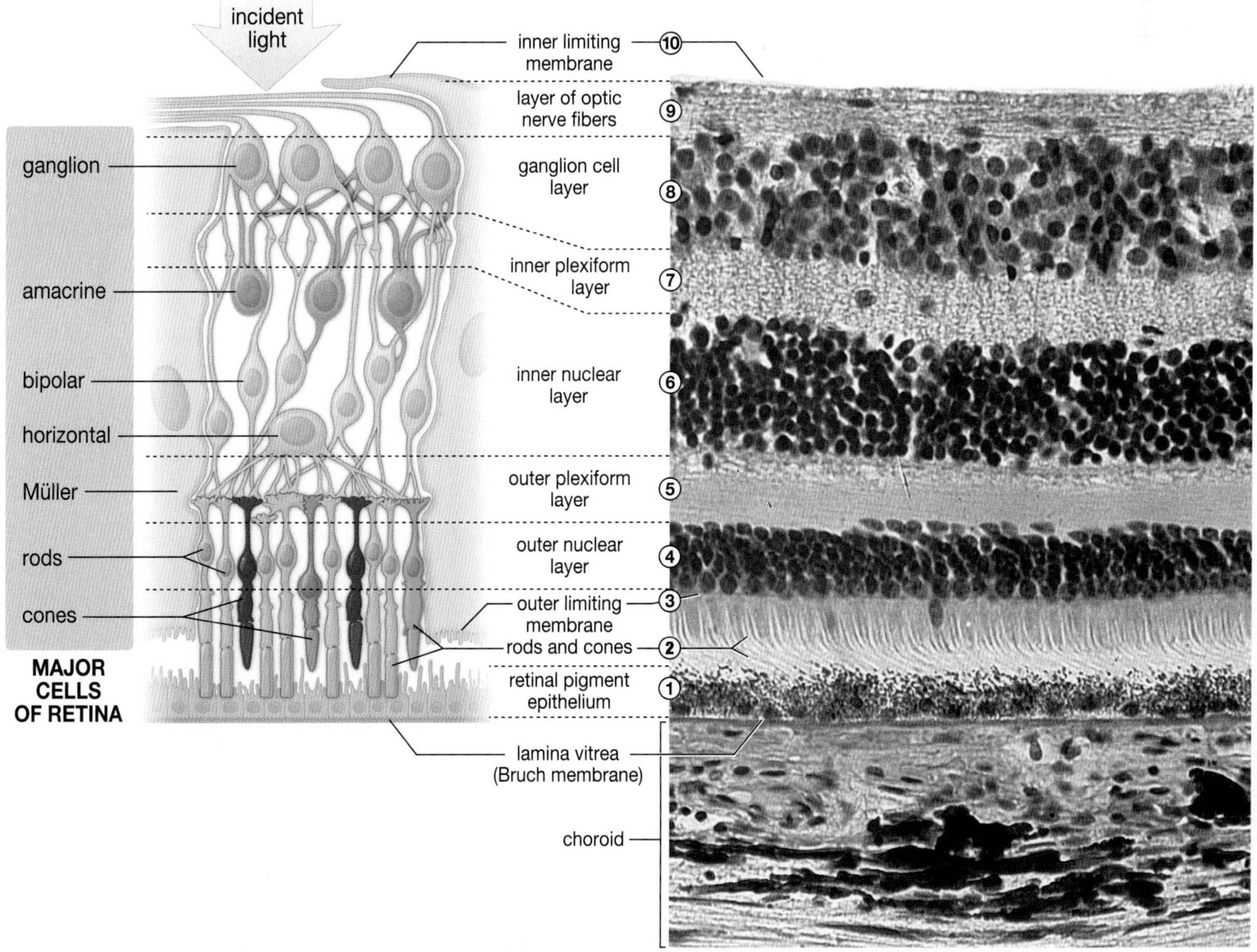

FIGURE 24.9. Schematic drawing and photomicrograph of the layers of the retina. On the basis of histologic features that are evident in the photomicrograph *on right*, the retina can be divided into 10 layers. The layers correspond to the diagram *on left*, which shows the distribution of major cells of the retina. Note that light enters the retina and passes through its inner layers before reaching the photoreceptors of the rods and cones that are closely associated with the retinal pigment epithelium. Also, the interrelationship between the bipolar neurons and ganglion cells that carry electrical impulses from the retina to the brain is clearly visible. Bruch membrane (lamina vitrea) separates the inner layer of the vascular coat (choroid) from the retinal pigment epithelium. ×440.

The specific arrangement and associations of the nuclei and processes of these cells form 10 retinal layers that can be seen with the light microscope. The layers of the retina can also be imaged and examined in living individuals using spectral-domain optical coherence tomography (see Folder 24.4). The 10 layers of the retina, from outside inward, are as follows (see Fig. 24.9):

1. **Retinal pigment epithelium (RPE)**—the outer layer of the retina, actually not part of the neural retina but intimately associated with it
2. **Layer of rods and cones**—contains the outer and inner segments of photoreceptor cells
3. **Outer limiting membrane**—the apical boundary of Müller cells
4. **Outer nuclear layer**—contains the cell bodies (nuclei) of retinal rods and cones
5. **Outer plexiform layer**—contains the processes of retinal rods and cones and processes of the horizontal, amacrine, and bipolar cells that connect to them
6. **Inner nuclear layer**—contains the cell bodies (nuclei) of horizontal, amacrine, bipolar, and Müller cells
7. **Inner plexiform layer**—contains the processes of horizontal, amacrine, bipolar, and ganglion cells that connect to each other
8. **Ganglion cell layer**—contains the cell bodies (nuclei) of ganglion cells
9. **Layer of optic nerve fibers**—contains processes of ganglion cells that lead from the retina to the brain
10. **Inner limiting membrane**—composed of the basal lamina of Müller cells

Each of the layers is more fully described in the following sections (see corresponding numbers).

The cells of the retinal pigment epithelium (layer 1) have extensions that surround the processes of the rods and cones.

The **RPE** is a single layer of cuboidal cells about 14 µm wide and 10–14 µm tall. The cells rest on Bruch membrane of the choroid layer. The pigment cells are tallest in the fovea and adjacent regions, which account for the darker color of this region.

Adjacent RPE cells are connected by a junctional complex consisting of gap junctions and elaborate zonulae occludentes and adherentes. This junctional complex is the site of the **blood–retina barrier**. This barrier makes the retinal vessels impermeable to molecules larger than 20–30 kDa.

The pigment cells have cylindrical sheaths on their apical surface that are associated with, but do not directly contact, the tip of the photoreceptor processes of the adjacent rod and cone cells. Complex cytoplasmic processes project for a short distance between the photoreceptor cells of the rods and cones. Numerous elongated melanin granules, unlike those found elsewhere in the eye, are present in many of these processes. They aggregate on the side of the cell nearest the rods and cones and are the most prominent feature of the cells. The nucleus with its many convoluted infoldings is located near the basal plasma membrane adjacent to Bruch membrane.

The cells also contain material phagocytosed from the processes of the photoreceptor cells in the form of lamellar debris (lipofuscin) contained in residual bodies or phagosomes. These lipofuscin granules reside in the basal cytoplasm of the RPE cell and are relatively difficult to detect in routine hematoxylin and eosin (H&E) preparation. Because the lipofuscin pigment is fluorescent, it can be clearly seen in the UV fluorescent microscope. A supranuclear Golgi apparatus and an extensive network of smooth-surfaced endoplasmic reticulum (sER) surround the melanin granules and residual bodies that are present in the cytoplasm.

The **RPE** serves several important functions, including the following:

- It **absorbs light** passing through the neural retina to **prevent reflection** and resultant glare.
- It isolates the retinal cells from blood-borne substances. It serves as a major component of the **blood–retina barrier** via tight junctions between RPE cells.
- It participates in **restoring photosensitivity** to visual pigments that were dissociated in response to light. The metabolic apparatus for visual pigment resynthesis is present in the RPE cells.
- It **phagocytoses and disposes of membranous discs** from the rods and cones of the retinal photoreceptor cells.

The rods and cones of the photoreceptor cell (layer 2) extend from the outer layer of the neural retina to the pigment epithelium.

The **rods** and **cones** are the outer segments of photoreceptor cells whose nuclei form the outer nuclear layer of the retina (Figs. 24.9 and 24.10). The light that reaches the

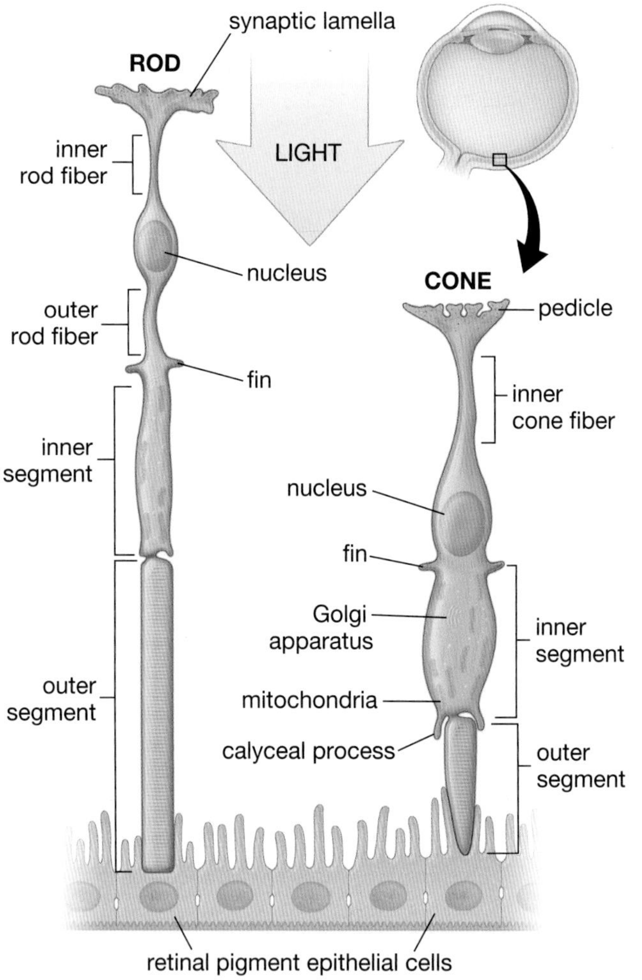

FIGURE 24.10. Schematic diagram of the ultrastructure of rod and cone cells. The outer segments of the rods and cones are closely associated with the adjacent pigment epithelium.

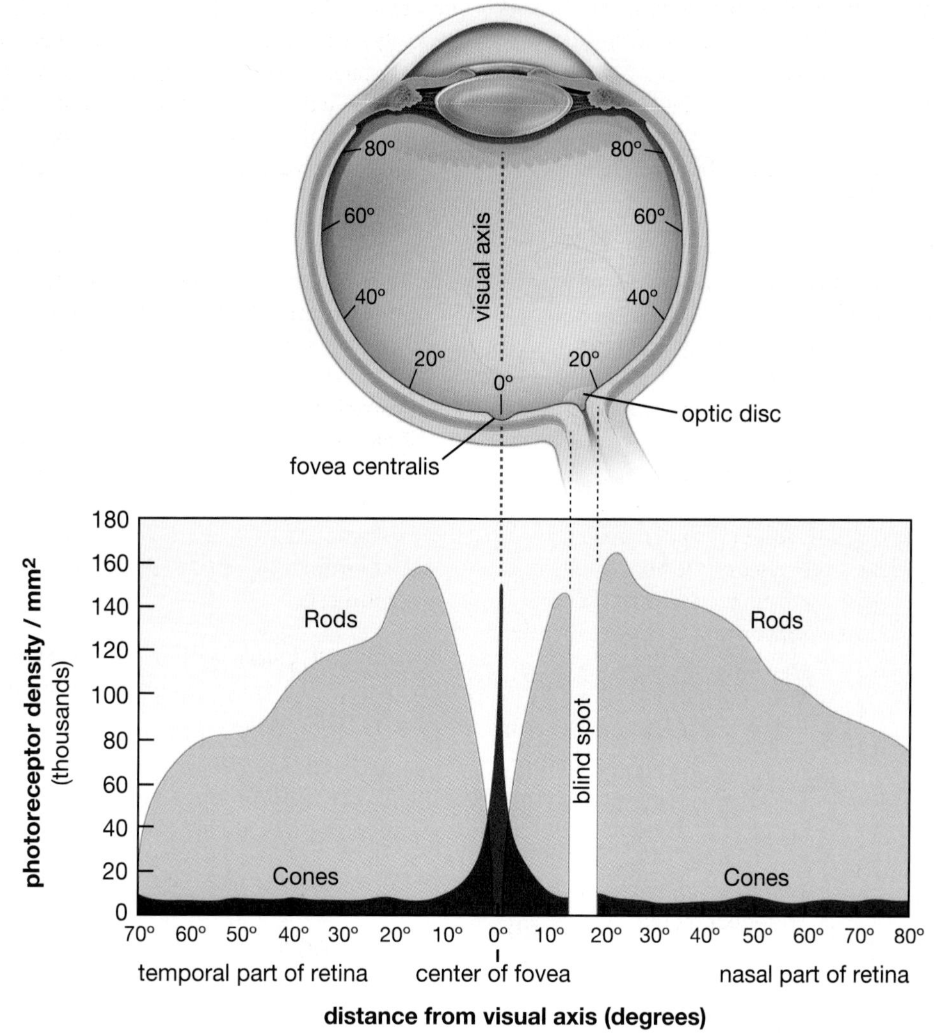

FIGURE 24.11. Distribution of rods and cones in the human eye. This graph shows the density of rods and cones per mm^2 across the retina. The peak number of cones occurs in the fovea centralis, where it reaches ~150,000 cones/mm^2. Rod density peaks about 20 degrees from the visual axis and is roughly the same as that of cones. Rods density decreases toward the periphery of the retina. Note that there are no photoreceptors at the optic disc.

photoreceptor cells must first pass through all of the internal layers of the neural retina. The rods and cones are arranged in a palisade manner; therefore, in the light microscope, they appear as vertical striations.

The retina contains approximately **120 million rods** and **7 million cones**. They are not distributed equally throughout the photosensitive part of the retina. The **highest density of cones** is detected in the **fovea centralis**, which corresponds to the highest visual acuity and best color vision (Fig. 24.11). The highest density of rods is outside the fovea centralis, and their density steadily decreases toward the periphery of the retina. Rods are not present in the fovea centralis nor at the optic disc, which is devoid of any photoreceptors (see Fig. 24.11). The rods are about 2 μm thick and 50 μm long (ranging from about 60 μm at the fovea to 40 μm peripherally). The cones vary in length from 85 μm at the fovea to 25 μm at the periphery of the retina.

Rods are sensitive in low light and produce black-and-white images; cones are less sensitive in low light and produce color images.

Functionally, the **rods** are more **sensitive to light** and are the receptors used during periods of low light intensity (e.g., at dusk or at night). The rod pigments have a maximum absorption at 496 nm of visual spectrum, and the image provided is one composed of gray tones (a "black-and-white picture"). In contrast, the **cones** exist in **three classes: L, M, and S** (long-, middle-, and short-wavelength sensitive, respectively) that cannot be distinguished morphologically. They are less sensitive to low light but more sensitive to red, green, and blue regions of the visual spectrum. Each class of cones contains a different visual pigment molecule that is activated by the absorption of light at the **blue** (420 nm), **green** (531 nm), and **red** (588 nm) ranges in the color spectrum. Cones provide a visual image composed of color by mixing the appropriate proportion of red, green, and blue light. For a description of different types of color blindness, see Folder 24.5.

Each rod and cone photoreceptor consists of three parts:

- The **outer segment** of the photoreceptor is roughly cylindrical or conical (hence, the descriptive name **rod** or **cone**). This portion of the photoreceptor is intimately related to microvilli projecting from the adjacent pigment epithelial cells.
- The **connecting stalk** contains a cilium composed of nine peripheral microtubule doublets extending from a basal body. The connecting stalk appears as the constricted

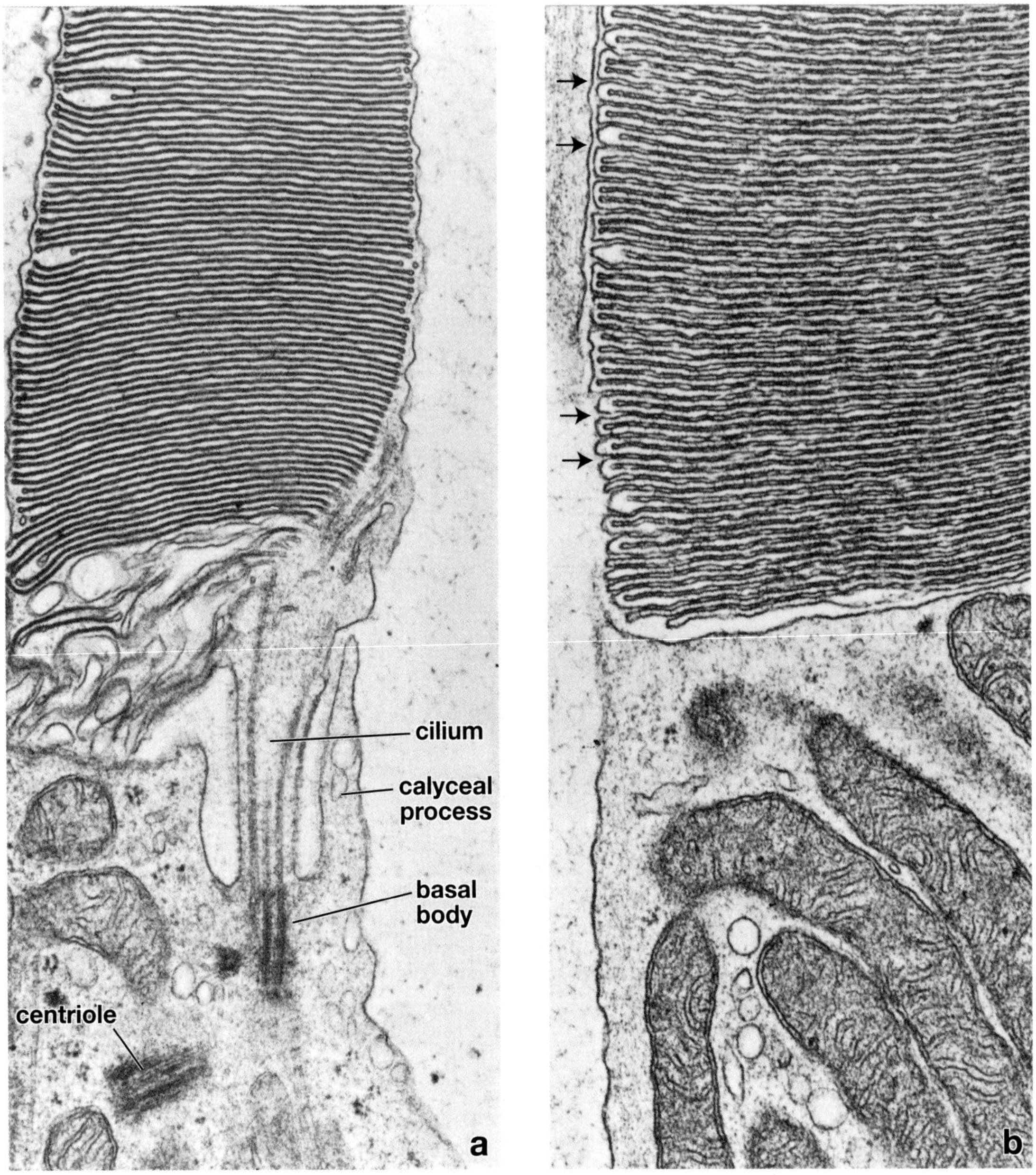

FIGURE 24.12. Electron micrographs of portions of the inner and outer segments of cones and rods. a. This electron micrograph shows the junction between the inner and outer segments of the rod cell. The outer segments contain the horizontally flattened discs. The plane of this section passes through the connecting stalk and cilium. A centriole, a cilium and its basal body, and a calyceal process are identified. ×32,000. **b.** Another electron micrograph shows a similar section of a cone cell. The interior of the discs in the outer segment of the cone is continuous with the extracellular space (*arrows*). ×32,000. (Courtesy of Dr. Toichiro Kuwabara.)

region of the cell that joins the inner to the outer segment. In this region, a thin, tapering process called the **calyceal process** extends from the distal end of the inner segment to surround the proximal portion of the outer segment (see Fig. 24.10).

- The **inner segment** is divided into an outer **ellipsoid** and an inner **myoid portion**. This segment contains a typical complement of organelles associated with a cell that actively synthesizes proteins. A prominent Golgi apparatus, rER, and free ribosomes are concentrated in the myoid region. Mitochondria are most numerous in the ellipsoid region. Microtubules are distributed throughout the inner segment. In the outer ellipsoid portion, cross-striated fibrous rootlets may extend from the basal body among the mitochondria.

The outer segment is the site of photosensitivity, and the inner segment contains the metabolic machinery that supports the activity of the photoreceptor cells. The outer segment is considered a highly modified cilium because it is joined to the inner segment by a short connecting stalk containing a basal body (Fig. 24.12a).

With the TEM, 600–1,000 regularly spaced horizontal **membranous discs** are seen in the outer segment (Fig. 24.12). In rods, these discs are membrane-bound structures measuring about 2 μm in diameter. They are enclosed within the plasma membrane of the outer segment (see Fig. 24.12a). The parallel membranes of the discs are about 6 nm thick and are continuous at their ends. The central enclosed space is about 8 nm across. In both rods and cones, the membranous discs are formed from repetitive

FOLDER 24.4 CLINICAL CORRELATION: CLINICAL IMAGING OF THE RETINA

The standard ophthalmoscopic examination of the eye has been recently supplemented by a new examination technique that utilizes **spectral-domain optical coherence tomography** (SD OCT). This noninvasive and noncontact examination is not only useful in visualizing the retinal surface, but it also provides a high-resolution cross-sectional image of the retina in vivo. All histologic layers of the retina can be easily differentiated with SD OCT (Fig. F24.4.1), and they can be objectively measured for tissue thickness and change. SD OCT technology is based on comparisons of spectral characteristics of the reflected light beam from the retina with those of the reference beam. For this purpose, an infrared laser beam (~840 nm wavelength with 50 nm bandwidth) is used that is able to produce images at 5-μm resolution. The laser beam passes through the structures of the eye and is partially absorbed and partially reflected depending on tissue characteristics. The reflected light is detected by a multichannel spectrometer, and the interference pattern is compared to the reference beam using complex computer algorithms. The spectral differences are used to construct the cross-sectional (line) scans as shown in Figure F24.4.1 or the three-dimensional images of the retina as shown in Figure F24.4.2. Introduced in the 1990s, the SD OCT has revolutionized the management and diagnosis of many eye diseases. SD OCT established itself as an imaging modality of choice in **glaucoma** (measurement of optic nerve and retinal nerve fiber layer) and retinal diseases. It is used for the early and accurate detection of **macular degeneration**, **retinal detachment**, **macular holes**, **epiretinal membranes**, and **optic disc pits** and for the detection of fluid accumulation within the retina that occurs in conditions such as **diabetic retinopathy**, **cystoid macular edema**, and **central serous choroidopathy**.

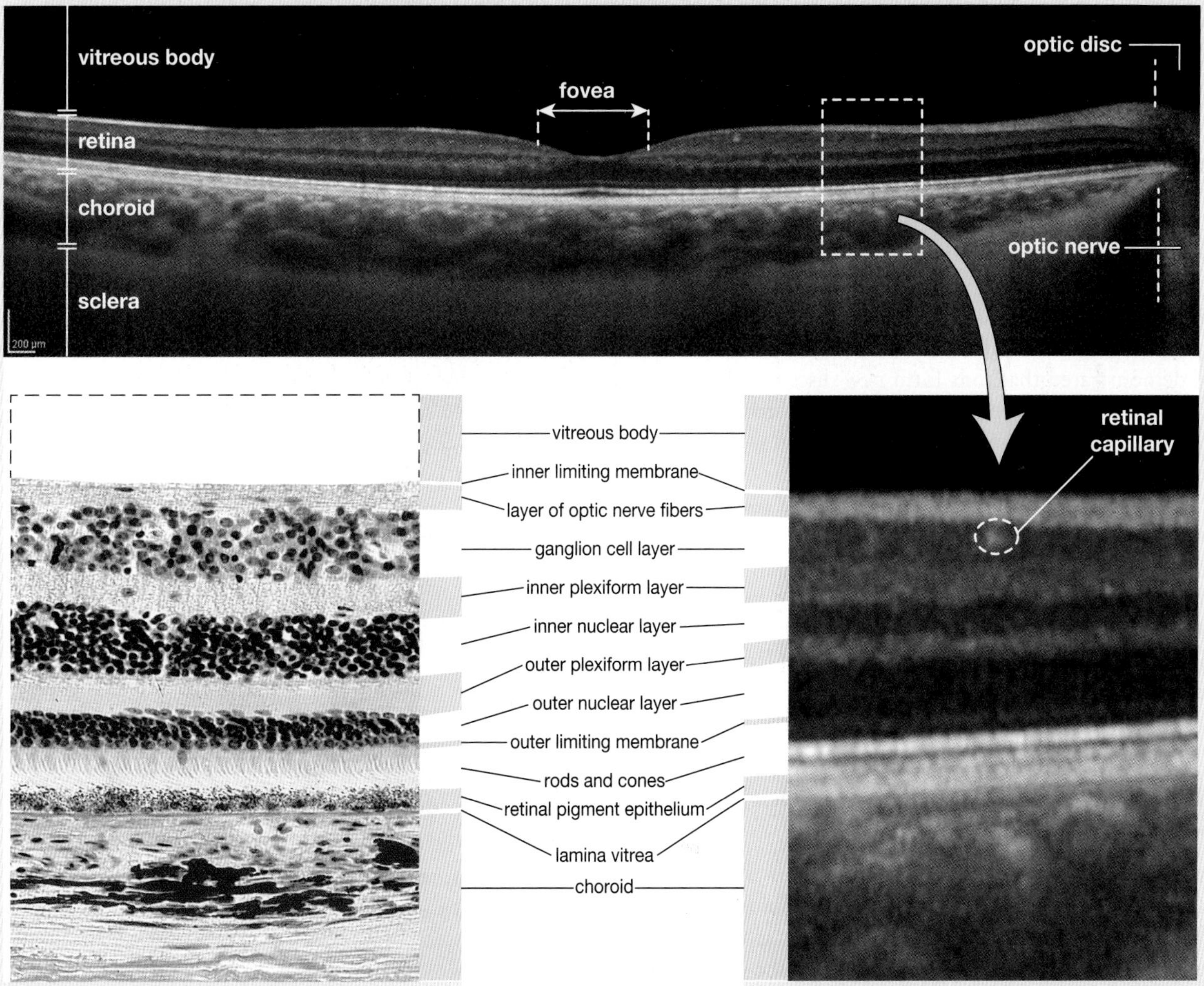

FIGURE F24.4.1. Spectral-domain optical coherence tomography (SD OCT) cross-sectional (line) image of the retina in a healthy eye. The *upper* image represents a normal cross-sectional image of the retina containing fovea and optic disc on the *right* side of the image. The optically transparent vitreous body is invisible and appears as the *black* region in the upper part of the image. Hyperreflective and hyporeflective bands of retinal tissue correspond to the histologic layers of the retina. Note the photoreceptor layer containing rods and cones as well the retinal pigment epithelium are well defined and are separated from the choroid layer containing blood vessels. (Courtesy of Drs. Andrew J. Barkmeier and Denise M. Lewison.)

(*continued*)

FOLDER 24.4

CLINICAL CORRELATION: CLINICAL IMAGING OF THE RETINA (*continued*)

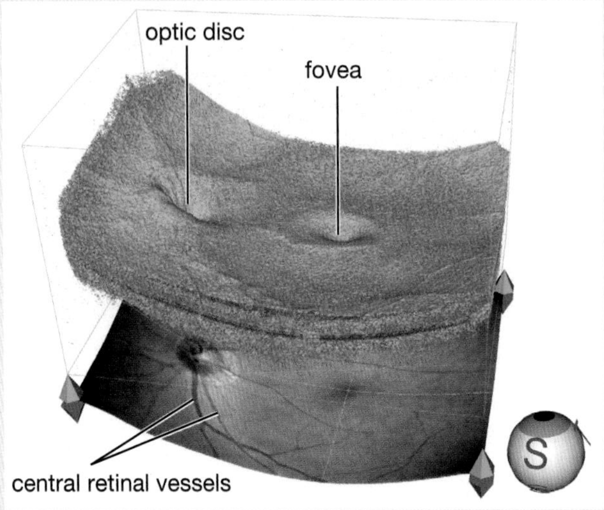

FIGURE F24.4.2. Spectral-domain optical coherence tomography (SD OCT) three-dimensional image of the retina of a healthy right eye. The scan area is ~12 mm × 9 mm in size and includes a portion of the optic disc (*on the left*) and fovea (*on the right*). A three-dimensional data set is acquired from four scans (two vertical and two horizontal), which is then processed with a motion-correction technology (MCT) algorithm. The MCT algorithm analyzes and compares the vascular pattern in each of the scans and reduces artifacts and image distortions associated with eye movement. This image has two parts. The upper false-color image (optical densities are coded in different colors) shows the surface and thickness of all layers of the retina and represents a motion-corrected, three-dimensional volume rendering of the entire data set. The lower grayscale vascular map image (optical densities are coded in grayscale) is a two-dimensional image created by summing all the pixels in each column. It is curved to match the curvature of the eye. The letters S (for superior) and T (for temporal) on the eye orientation icon in the *lower right corner* provide reference to the positioning of the scan in the patient's eye. (Image courtesy of Dr. Pravin Dugel, Phoenix, Arizona.)

transverse infolding of the plasma membrane in the region of the outer segment near the cilium. Autoradiographic studies have demonstrated that rods form new discs by infolding of the plasma membrane throughout their life span. Discs are formed in cones in a similar manner but are not replaced on a regular basis.

Rod discs lose their continuity with the plasma membrane from which they are derived soon after they are formed. They then pass like a stack of plates, proximally to distally, along the length of the cylindrical portion of the outer segment until they are eventually shed and phagocytosed by the pigment epithelial cells. Thus, each rod disc is a membrane-enclosed compartment within the cytoplasm. Discs within the cones retain their continuity with the plasma membrane (Fig. 24.12b).

Rod cells contain the visual pigment rhodopsin; cone cells contain the visual pigment iodopsin.

Rhodopsin (also called **visual purple**) is a 39-kDa protein in rod cells that initiates the visual stimulus when it is bleached by light. Rhodopsin is present in globular form on the outer surface of the lipid bilayer (on the cytoplasmic side) of the membranous discs. In the cone cells, the visual pigment protein on the membranous discs is the photopigment **iodopsin**. Each cone cell is specialized to respond maximally to one of three colors: red, green, or blue. Both rhodopsin and iodopsin contain a membrane-bound subunit called an **opsin** and a second small light-absorbing component called a **chromophore**. The opsin of rods is **scotopsin**; the opsins of cones are **photopsins**. The chromophore of rods is a vitamin A–derived carotenoid called **retinal**. Thus, an adequate intake of **vitamin A** is essential for normal vision. Prolonged dietary deficiency of vitamin A leads to the inability to see in dim light (**night blindness**).

The interior of the discs of cones is continuous with the extracellular space.

The basic difference in the structure of the rod and cone discs—that is, continuity with the plasma membrane—is correlated with the slightly different means by which the visual pigments are renewed in rods and cones. Newly synthesized rhodopsin is incorporated into the membrane of the rod disc as the disc is being formed at the base of the outer segment. It then takes several days for the disc to reach the tip of the outer segment. In contrast, although visual proteins are constantly produced in retinal cones, the proteins are incorporated into cone discs located anywhere in the outer segment.

Vision is a process by which light striking the retina is converted into electrical impulses that are transmitted to the brain.

The impulses produced by light reaching the photoreceptor cells are conveyed to the brain by an elaborate network of nerves. The conversion of the incident light into electrical nerve impulses is called **visual processing** and involves several steps:

- A photochemical reaction occurs in the outer segment of the rods and cones. In the dark, **rhodopsin** molecules contain a chromophore called retinal in its isometric form of **11-*cis*-retinal**. When rods are exposed to light, the 11-*cis*-retinal undergoes a conformational change from a bent to a more linear molecule called **all-*trans*-retinal**. The conversion of 11-*cis*-retinal to all-*trans*-retinal activates opsin, which results in the release of all-*trans*-retinal into the rod's cytoplasm (a reaction called **bleaching**).

- The activated **opsin** interacts with a G-protein called **transducin**, which subsequently activates phosphodiesterase that breaks down **cyclic guanosine monophosphate (cGMP)**. In the dark, high levels of cGMP molecules produced in the photoreceptor cells by guanylyl cyclase are bound to the cytoplasmic surface of **cGMP-gated Na^+ channels**, causing them to stay open. Steady influx of Na^+ into the cells results in **depolarization** of the plasma membrane and continuous **release of the neurotransmitter (glutamate)** at the synaptic junction with the bipolar neurons (Fig. 24.13).
- A decrease in the concentration of cGMP within the cytoplasm of the inner segment of the photoreceptor cells is due to the action of phosphodiesterase. Dissociation of cGMP from Na^+ channels effectively closes the channels and reduces the influx of Na^+ into the cell, resulting in **hyperpolarization** of the plasma membrane. The hyperpolarization causes a **decrease of glutamate secretion** at the synapses with bipolar cells, which is detected and conveyed as electrical impulses (see Fig. 24.13).

Released retinal from opsin is converted back to its original conformation in the RPE cells and Müller cells.

After release, all-*trans*-retinal is converted to all-*trans*-retinol in the cytoplasm of rods and cones and then transported to the cytoplasm of RPE cells (from rods) or both RPE cells and Müller cells (from cones). The energy for this process is provided by the mitochondria located in the inner segment of these photoreceptors. Both Müller cells and RPE cells participate in a multistep conversion of all-*trans*-retinol to 11-*cis*-retinal, which is transported back to the photoreceptor cells for the resynthesis of rhodopsin. The **retinal pigment epithelium–specific protein 65 kDa (RPE65)** is involved in this conversion; thus, the visual cycle can begin again.

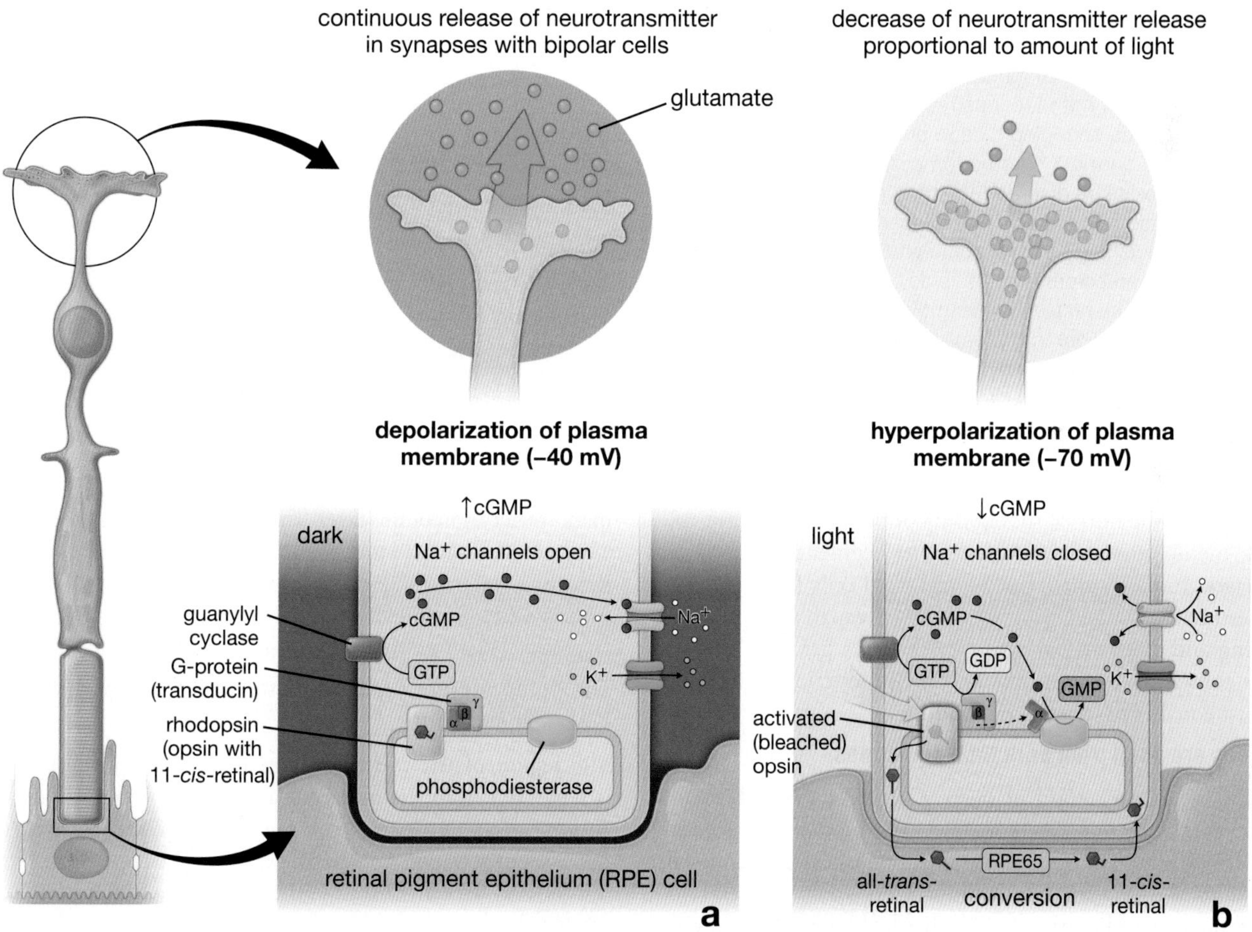

FIGURE 24.13. Schematic diagram of visual processing in the photoreceptor cell. a. In the dark, high levels of cGMP generated by guanylyl cyclase are present in the cytoplasm of the rod. Some of the cGMP molecules are bound to the cytoplasmic surface of cGMP-gated Na^+ channels, causing them to stay open and resulting in continuous influx of Na^+ and depolarization of the plasma membrane. This results in a steady release of glutamate, a neurotransmitter, in the synaptic junctions with bipolar neurons. Also in the dark, rhodopsin molecules that contain 11-*cis*-retinal are inactive. **b.** After exposure to light, 11-*cis*-retinal undergoes a conformational change to all-*trans*-retinal. This conversion activates opsin (a reaction called *bleaching*) and releases all-*trans*-retinal into the rod's cytoplasm. The activated opsin interacts with G-protein, which subsequently activates phosphodiesterase that breaks down cGMP, effectively lowering the concentration of cGMP in the cell. In this condition, cGMP molecules dissociate from Na^+ channels, resulting in their closing and hyperpolarization of the plasma membrane. This results in a decrease in glutamate secretion, which is detected by the bipolar neurons and conveyed as electrical impulses to the brain. The released retinal from opsin is converted to its original conformation in retinal pigment epithelial (*RPE*) cells by the RPE65 enzymatic complex and is recycled to the photoreceptor cell. *cGMP*, cyclic guanosine monophosphate; *GDP*, guanosine diphosphate; *GMP*, guanosine monophosphate; *GTP*, guanosine triphosphate.

FOLDER 24.5 CLINICAL CORRELATION: COLOR BLINDNESS

In individuals with normal color vision, the three primary colors (red, green, and blue) are combined to achieve the full spectrum of color vision. These individuals are called **trichromats** and possess three independent channels for conveying color information that are derived from three different classes of cones (L—red sensitive; M—green sensitive; and S—blue sensitive). Approximately 90% of trichromats can apperceive any given color from impulses generated in all three classes of cones. Some individuals have an impairment of normal color vision, which occurs when one of the cones is altered in its spectral sensitivity. For example, about 6% of trichromats matches colors with an unusual proportion of red and green. These individuals are called **anomalous trichromats**.

Color blindness is a condition in which individuals are missing or have a defect in a specific class of cones. True color-blind individuals are **dichromats** and have a defect either in the L, M, or S cones. In this condition, the affected cones are completely missing. Dichromats can only distinguish different colors by matching the impulses generated by the two remaining normal classes of cones.

Three major types of color blindness have been identified:

- **Protanopia** is characterized as a defect affecting the long-wavelength L cones responsible for red vision. The genes encoding L cone photoreceptor proteins are located on the X chromosome; therefore, protanopia is a sex-linked disorder affecting mainly males (1% of the male population). These individuals have difficulty distinguishing between blue and green as well as red and green colors; thus, this color vision deficiency is a serious risk factor in driving (Fig. F24.5.1).
- **Deuteranopia** is characterized as a defect affecting the middle-wavelength M cones responsible for green vision. Deuteranopia is the most common form of color blindness, affecting about 5% of the male population. It is also a sex-linked disorder because the genes encoding M cone photoreceptor proteins are located in the same region of the X chromosome as the genes for L cones. Similar to protanopia, red and green are the main problem colors (see Fig. F24.5.1).
- **Tritanopia** is characterized as a defect affecting the short-wavelength S cones responsible for blue vision (see Fig. F24.5.1). The defect is autosomal and involves mutation of a single gene encoding S cone photoreceptor proteins that reside on chromosome 7. This color blindness occurs very rarely (1 in 10,000) and affects women and men equally.

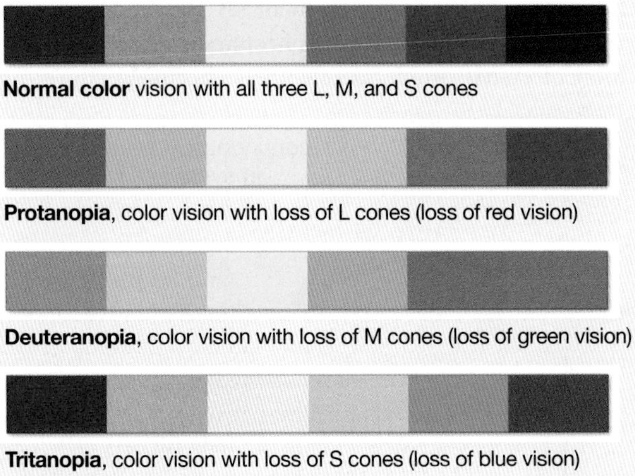
Normal color vision with all three L, M, and S cones
Protanopia, color vision with loss of L cones (loss of red vision)
Deuteranopia, color vision with loss of M cones (loss of green vision)
Tritanopia, color vision with loss of S cones (loss of blue vision)

FIGURE F24.5.1. Color blindness. This chart shows the six-color spectrum in normal color vision and in individuals with the three types of color blindness.

During the normal functioning of the photoreceptor cells, the membranous discs of the outer segment are shed and phagocytosed by the pigment epithelial cells (Fig. 24.14). It is estimated that each of these cells is capable of phagocytosing and disposing of about 7,500 discs per day. The discs are constantly turning over, and the production of new discs must equal the rate of disc shedding.

Discs are shed from both rods and cones.

In rods, after a period of sleep, a burst of **disc shedding** occurs as light first enters the eye. The time of disc shedding in cones is more variable. The shedding of discs in cones also enables the receptors to eliminate superfluous membrane. Although not fully understood, the shedding process in cones also alters the size of the discs so that the conical form is maintained as discs are released from the distal end of the cone.

The outer limiting membrane (layer 3) is formed by a row of zonulae adherentes between Müller cells.

The **outer limiting membrane** is not a true membrane. It is a row of zonulae adherentes that attaches the apical ends of Müller cells (i.e., the end that faces the pigment epithelium) to each other and to the rods and cones (see Fig. 24.9). Because Müller cells end at the base of the inner segments of the receptors, they mark the location of this layer. Thus, the supporting processes of Müller cells, on which the rods and cones rest, are pierced by the inner and outer segments of the photoreceptor cells. This layer is thought to be a metabolic barrier that restricts the passage of large molecules into the inner layers of the retina.

The outer nuclear layer (4) contains the nuclei of the retinal rods and cones.

The region of the rod cytoplasm that contains the nucleus is separated from the inner segment by a tapering process of the cytoplasm. In cones, the nuclei are located close to the outer segments, and no tapering is seen. The cone nuclei stain lightly and are larger and more oval than rod nuclei. Rod nuclei are surrounded by only a thin rim of cytoplasm. In contrast, a relatively thick investment of cytoplasm surrounds the cone nuclei (see Fig. 24.10).

The outer plexiform layer (5) is formed by the processes of the photoreceptor cells and neurons.

The **outer plexiform layer** is formed by the processes of retinal rods and cones and the processes of horizontal, interplexiform, amacrine, and bipolar cells. The processes allow the electrical coupling of photoreceptor cells to these specialized interneurons via synapses. A thin process extends

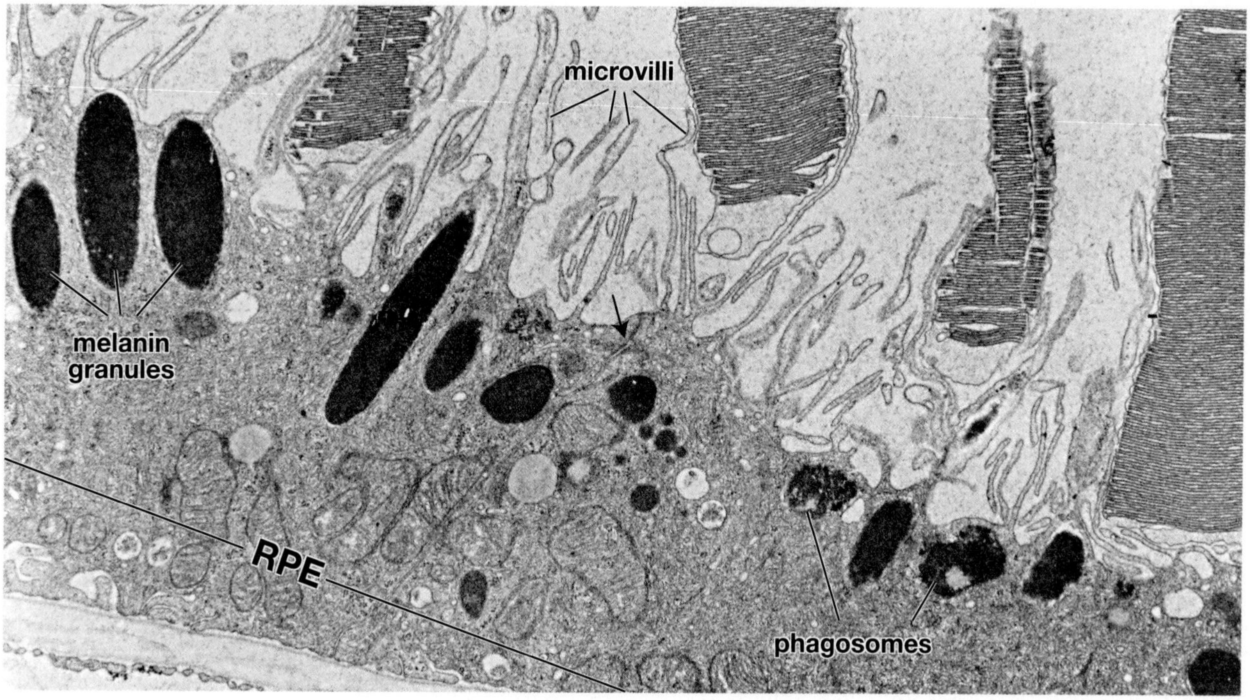

FIGURE 24.14. Electron micrograph of the retinal pigment epithelium in association with the outer segments of rods and cones. Retinal pigment epithelial (*RPE*) cells contain numerous elongated *melanin granules* that are aggregated in the apical portion of the cell, where the *microvilli* extend from the surface toward the outer segments of the rod and cone cells. The retinal pigment epithelial cells contain numerous mitochondria and *phagosomes*. The *arrow* indicates the location of the junctional complex between two adjacent cells. ×20,000. (Courtesy of Dr. Toichiro Kuwabara.)

from the region of the nucleus of each rod or cone to an inner expanded portion with several lateral processes. The expanded portion is called a **spherule** in a rod and a **pedicle** in a cone. Normally, many photoreceptor cells converge onto one bipolar cell and form interconnecting neural networks. Cones located in the fovea, however, synapse with a single bipolar cell. The fovea is also unique in that the compactness of the inner neural layers of the retina causes the photoreceptor cells to be oriented obliquely. Horizontal cell dendritic processes synapse with photoreceptor cells throughout the retina and further contribute to the elaborate neuronal connections in this layer.

The inner nuclear layer (6) consists of the nuclei of horizontal, amacrine, bipolar, interplexiform, and Müller cells.

Müller cells form the scaffolding for the entire retina. Their processes invest the other cells of the retina so completely that they fill most of the extracellular space. The basal and apical ends of Müller cells form the inner and outer limiting membranes, respectively. Microvilli extending from their apical border lie between the photoreceptor cells of the rods and cones. Capillaries from the retinal vessels extend only to this layer. The rods and cones carry out their metabolic exchanges with extracellular fluids transported across the blood–retina barrier of the RPE.

The four types of conducting cells—bipolar, horizontal, interplexiform, and amacrine—found in this layer have distinct orientations (see Fig. 24.9):

- **Bipolar cells** and their processes extend to both the inner and outer plexiform layers. In the peripheral regions of the retina, the axons of bipolar cells pass to the inner plexiform layer where they synapse with several ganglion cells. Through these connections, the bipolar cells establish communication with multiple cells in each layer, except in the fovea, where they may synapse only with a single ganglion cell to provide greater visual acuity in this region.
- **Horizontal cells** and their processes extend to the outer plexiform layer where they intermingle with processes of bipolar cells. The cells have synaptic connections with rod spherules, cone pedicles, and bipolar cells. This electrical coupling of cells is thought to affect the functional threshold between rods and cones and bipolar cells.
- **Amacrine cells'** processes pass inward, contributing to a complex interconnection of cells. Their processes branch extensively to provide sites of synaptic connections with axonal endings of bipolar cells and dendrites of ganglion cells. Besides bipolar and ganglion cells, the amacrine cells synapse in the inner plexiform layer with interplexiform and other amacrine cells (see Fig. 24.9).
- **Interplexiform cells** and their processes have synapses in both inner and outer plexiform layers. These cells convey impulses from the inner plexiform to the outer plexiform layer.

The inner plexiform layer (7) consists of a complex array of intermingled neuronal cell processes.

The **inner plexiform layer** consists of synaptic connections between axons of the bipolar neurons and dendrites of ganglion cells. It also contains synapses between intermingling processes of amacrine cells and bipolar neurons, ganglion cells, and interplexiform neurons. The course of these processes is parallel to the inner limiting membrane, thus giving the appearance of horizontal striations to this layer (see Fig. 24.9).

The ganglion cell layer (8) consists of the cell bodies of large multipolar neurons.

The cell bodies of large **multipolar nerve cells**, measuring as much as 30 μm in diameter, constitute the ganglion cell layer. These nerve cells have lightly staining round nuclei with prominent nucleoli and Nissl bodies in their cytoplasm. An axonal process emerges from the rounded cell body, passes into the **nerve fiber layer**, and then enters **the optic nerve**. The dendrites extend from the opposite end of the cell to ramify in the inner plexiform layer. In the peripheral regions of the retina, a single ganglion cell may synapse with 100 bipolar cells. In marked contrast, in the macular region surrounding the fovea, the bipolar cells are smaller (some authors refer to them as *midget bipolar cells*), and they tend to make one-to-one connections with ganglion cells. Over most of the retina, the ganglion cells are only a single layer of cells. At the macula, however, they are piled as many as eight deep, although they are absent over the fovea itself. Scattered among the ganglion cells are small neuroglial cells with densely staining nuclei (see Fig. 24.9).

The layer of optic nerve fibers (9) contains axons of the ganglion cells.

The axonal processes of the ganglion cells form a flattened layer running parallel to the retinal surface. This layer increases in depth as the axons converge at the **optic disc** (Fig. 24.15). The axons are thin, nonmyelinated processes measuring as much as 5 μm in diameter (see Fig. 24.9). The retinal vessels, including the superficial capillary network, are primarily located in this layer.

The inner limiting membrane (layer 10) consists of a basal lamina separating the retina from the vitreous body.

The **inner limiting membrane** forms the innermost boundary of the retina. It serves as the basal lamina of Müller cells (see Fig. 24.9). In younger individuals, reflections from the internal limiting membrane produce a **retinal sheen** that is seen during ophthalmoscopic examination of the eye. In older individuals, a semitranslucent sheet of cells and extracellular matrix can be formed on the inner surface of the retina in conjunction with the inner limiting membrane. This condition is called **epiretinal membrane (ERM)** or **macular pucker** and is responsible for variable clinical symptoms, including optical distortion and blurred vision. ERM is initially formed by cells from within the retina (RPE cells, Müller cells, and astrocytes) that begin proliferating and migrating onto the surface of the internal limiting membrane. Later, the membrane is infiltrated by macrophages, fibroblasts, and myofibroblasts. To prevent damage to the underlying retina, surgical removal of the ERM may be performed.

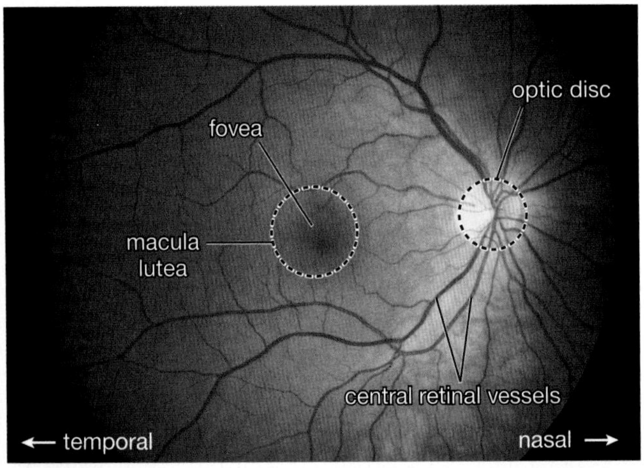

FIGURE 24.15. Normal view of the fundus in ophthalmoscopic examination of the right eye. The site where the axons converge to form the optic nerve is called the *optic disc*. Because the optic disc is devoid of photoreceptor cells, it is a blind spot in the visual field. From the center of the optic nerve (clinically called the *optic cup*), *central retinal vessels* emerge. The artery divides into upper and lower branches, each of which further divides into nasal and temporal branches (note the nasal and temporal directions on the image). Veins have a similar pattern of tributaries. Approximately 17 degree or 2.5 times optic disc diameters lateral to the disc, the slightly oval-shaped, blood vessel–free, and pigmented area represents the macula lutea. The *fovea centralis*, a shallow depression in the center of the *macula lutea*, is also visible. (Courtesy of Dr. Renzo A. Zaldivar.)

Specialized regions of the retina

The **fovea (fovea centralis)** appears as a small (1.5 mm in diameter), shallow depression located at the posterior pole of the visual axis of the eye. Its central region, known as the **foveola**, is about 200 μm in diameter (see Fig. 24.15). Except for the photoreceptor layer, most of the layers of the retina are markedly reduced or absent in this region (see Fig. 24.6). Here, the photoreceptor is composed entirely of cones (~4,000) that are longer and more slender and rod like than they are elsewhere. The fovea is the area of the retina specialized for the discrimination of details and color vision. The ratio between cones and ganglion cells is close to 1:1. Retinal vessels are absent in the fovea, allowing light to pass unobstructed into the cones' outer segments. The adjacent pigment epithelial cells and choriocapillaris are also thickened in this region.

The **macula lutea** is the area surrounding the fovea and is approximately 5.5 mm in diameter. It is yellowish because of the presence of yellow pigment (xanthophyll). The macula lutea contains approximately 17,000 cones and gains rods at its periphery. Retinal vessels are also absent in this region. Here, the retinal cells and their processes, especially the ganglion cells, are heaped up on the sides of the fovea so that light may pass unimpeded to this most sensitive area of the retina.

Vessels of the retina

The **central retinal artery** and **central retinal vein**, the vessels that can be seen and assessed with an ophthalmoscope, pass through the center of the optic nerve to enter the bulb of the eye at the optic disc (see Fig. 24.2 and pages 982-983, the section on the development of the eye). The central retinal artery provides nutrients to the inner retinal layers. The artery branches immediately into the upper and lower branches, each of which divides again into nasal and temporal branches (see Fig. 24.15). Veins undergo a similar pattern of branching. The vessels initially lie between the vitreous body and the inner limiting membrane. As the vessels pass laterally, they also move deeper within the inner retinal layers. Branches from these vessels form a capillary plexus that reaches the inner nuclear layer and, therefore, provides nutrients to the inner retinal layers (layers 6–10; see pages 993-994). Nutrients to the remaining layers (layers 1–5) are provided by diffusion from the vascular choriocapillary layer of the choroid. The branches of the **central retinal artery** do not anastomose and, therefore, are classified as **anatomic end arteries**. Evaluation of the retinal vessels and appearance of the optic disc during ophthalmoscopy not only gives important information on the state of the eye but also may reveal early clinical signs of a number of conditions, including increased **intracranial pressure**, **hypertension**, **glaucoma**, and **diabetes**.

Crystalline Lens

Like the lens in a camera, the basic function of the eye lens is to transmit and focus light onto the retina.

The **lens** is a transparent, biconvex structure that has no vessels or nerves and is almost totally devoid of connective tissue, except for an enveloping capsule of basal lamina. It is suspended between the edges of the ciliary body by the **zonular fibers**. The pull of the zonular fibers keeps the lens in a flattened condition. Release of tension causes the lens to widen or **accommodate** to bend light rays originating close to the eye so that they focus on the retina.

The lens has three principal components (Fig. 24.16):

- The **lens capsule** is a thick basal lamina that surrounds the outer surface of the lens. It originates as the basal lamina of the embryonic lens vesicle. The anterior part of the capsule is thick, measuring approximately 10–20 μm, and is produced by the anterior lens cells. The posterior part of the capsule is much thinner, measuring approximately 5–10 μm. The lens capsule, composed primarily of type IV collagen and proteoglycans (i.e., laminin, entactin, perlecan), is elastic. It is thickest at the equator where the zonular fibers attach to it.
- The **subcapsular epithelium** is derived from the epithelial cells of the anterior part of the embryonic lens vesicle. It represents a single cuboidal layer of **lens epithelial cells** present only on the anterior surface of the lens. The epithelial cells of the posterior part of the vesicle elongate anteriorly and form the **primary lens fibers** that fill the cavity of the optic vesicle.
- **Secondary lens fibers (lens fiber cells)** are formed at the periphery near the **lens equator**. Here, epithelial cells proliferate and migrate along the posterior lens capsule to differentiate into mature lens fiber cells. In the center of the lens, epithelial cells are quiescent. As lens fiber cells differentiate, they undergo massive elongation and lose all of their organelles, including nuclei, forming the **organelle-free zone**.

Gap junctions connect the cuboidal cells of the subcapsular epithelium. They have few cytoplasmic organelles and stain faintly. The apical region of the cell is directed toward the internal aspect of the lens and the **lens fibers**, with which they form **junctional complexes**. The lens increases in size during normal growth and then continues to produce new lens fibers at an ever-decreasing rate throughout life. The new lens fibers develop from the subcapsular epithelial cells located near the equator (see Fig. 24.16) are laid down peripherally as concentric lamellae in an onion-like arrangement. Cells in this region increase in height and then differentiate into lens fibers.

As the lens fibers develop, they become highly elongated and appear as thin, flattened structures. They lose their nuclei and other organelles as they become filled with proteins called **crystallins**. Mature lens fibers attain a length of 7–10 mm, a width of 8–10 μm, and a thickness of 2 μm. In the adult lens, only lens fibers in the outermost region maintain their nuclei and organelles. Near the center, in the **lens nucleus**,

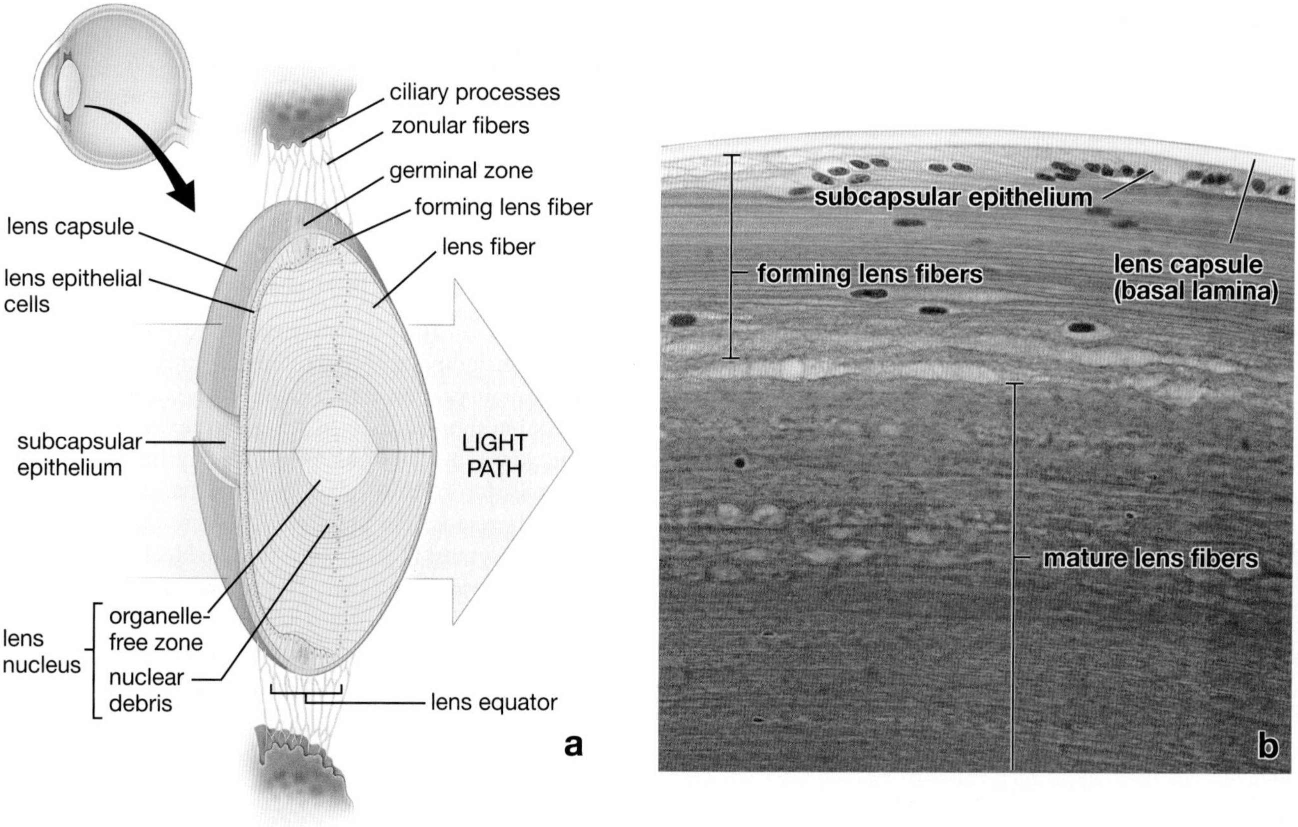

FIGURE 24.16. Structure of the lens. a. This schematic drawing of the lens suspended from ciliary processes by zonular fibers indicates its structural components. Note that the capsule of the lens is formed by the basal lamina of the lens fibers and the subcapsular epithelium located on the anterior surface of the lens. A strip of capsule was removed on this drawing to show underlying epithelium. Also note the location of the germinal zone (*yellow*) at the lens equator, where cells divide and differentiate into the lens fiber cells. The organelle-free center of the lens is occupied by the lens nucleus. **b.** This high-magnification photomicrograph of the germinal zone of the lens (near its equator) shows the active process of lens fiber formation from the *subcapsular epithelium*. Note the thick *lens capsule* and the underlying layer of nuclei of lens fibers during their differentiation. The *mature lens fibers* do not possess nuclei. ×570.

FOLDER 24.6
CLINICAL CORRELATION: CONJUNCTIVITIS

Conjunctivitis, otherwise known as *pinkeye*, is an inflammation of the conjunctiva. It may be localized in either the palpebral conjunctiva or the bulbar conjunctiva. Individuals may present with relatively nonspecific symptoms and signs that include redness, irritation, and watery discharge from the eye (Fig. F24.6.1). The symptoms can also mimic a foreign-body sensation. Extended use of contact lenses can cause allergic or bacterial conjunctivitis and may be the first sign of more serious ocular disease (i.e., corneal ulcer). In general, symptoms that last <4 weeks are classified as **acute conjunctivitis**, and those extending for a longer period are referred to as **chronic conjunctivitis**.

Acute conjunctivitis is most commonly caused by bacteria; a variety of viruses, including HIV, varicella-zoster virus (VZV), and herpes simplex virus (HSV); or allergic reactions. Bacterial conjunctivitis often causes an opaque purulent discharge containing white cells and desquamated epithelial cells. On eye examination, the purulent discharge and conjunctival papillae help differentiate between bacterial and viral etiology. Viral conjunctivitis is most common in adults. Clinically, it presents as a diffuse pinkness of the conjunctiva with particularly numerous lymphoid follicles on the palpebral conjunctiva, often accompanied by enlarged preauricular lymph nodes. Viral conjunctivitis is very contagious and usually associated with a recent upper respiratory infection. Patients need to be advised to avoid touching their eyes, to wash their hands frequently, and to avoid sharing towels and washcloths.

Bacterial conjunctivitis is usually treated with antibiotic eye drops or ointments. For viral conjunctivitis, no antimicrobial therapy is needed. However, conservative management with artificial tears to keep the eye lubricated may relieve symptoms. For severe cases, topical corticosteroid drops may be prescribed to reduce the discomfort of inflammation. However, prolonged use of corticosteroid drops increases the risk of side effects. Antibiotic drops may also be used for the treatment of secondary infections. Viral conjunctivitis usually resolves within 3 weeks. However, in the worst cases, it may take more than a month.

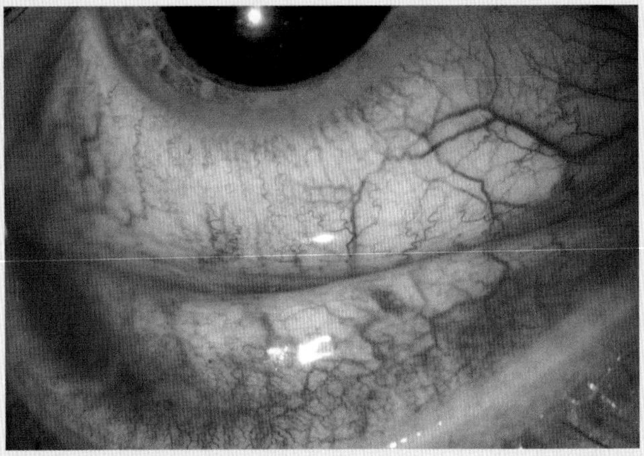

FIGURE F24.6.1. Conjunctivitis. This photograph of the lower part of the eyeball with reflected lower eyelid shows an infected conjunctiva. The enlarged blood vessels of the conjunctiva are responsible for moderate redness of the eye with conjunctival swelling. Moderately, clear (in allergic conjunctivitis) or purulent (in bacterial conjunctivitis) discharge is visible. (Courtesy of Dr. Renzo A. Zaldivar.)

the fibers are compressed and condensed to such a degree that individual fibers are impossible to recognize. The lens nucleus is an organelle-free zone and is composed of primary lens fiber cells laid down during embryonic and fetal development. The lens fibers are joined at their apical and basal ends by specialized junctions called **sutures**. Despite its density and protein content, the lens is normally transparent (see Fig. 24.16). The high density of lens fibers makes it difficult to obtain routine histologic sections of the lens that are free from artifacts.

Changes in the lens are associated with aging.

With increasing age, the lens gradually loses its elasticity and ability to accommodate. This condition, called **presbyopia**, usually occurs in the fourth decade of life. It is easily corrected by wearing reading glasses or using a magnifying lens.

Loss of transparency of the lens or its capsule is also a relatively common condition associated with aging. This condition, called **cataract**, may be caused by conformational changes or cross-linking of proteins. The development of a cataract may also be related to disease processes, metabolic or hereditary conditions, trauma, or exposure to a deleterious agent (such as ultraviolet radiation). Cataracts that significantly impair vision can usually be corrected surgically by removing the lens and replacing it with a plastic lens implanted in the posterior chamber.

Vitreous Body

The vitreous body is the transparent jelly-like substance that fills the vitreous chamber in the posterior segment of the eye.

The **vitreous body** is loosely attached to the surrounding structures, including the inner limiting membrane of the retina. The main portion of the vitreous body is a homogeneous gel containing approximately 99% water (the vitreous humor), collagen, glycosaminoglycans (principally hyaluronan), and a small population of cells called **hyalocytes**. These cells are believed to be responsible for the synthesis of collagen fibrils and glycosaminoglycans. Hyalocytes in routine H&E preparations are difficult to visualize. Often, they exhibit a well-developed rER and Golgi apparatus. Fibroblasts and tissue macrophages are sometimes seen in the periphery of the vitreous body. The **hyaloid canal** (or **Cloquet canal**), which is not always visible, runs through the center of the vitreous body from the optic disc to the posterior lens capsule. It is the remnant of the pathway of the hyaloid artery of the developing eye.

■ ACCESSORY STRUCTURES OF THE EYE

The primary functions of the eyelids are to cover, protect, and lubricate the eyes.

The **eyelids** represent folds of modified skin containing highly modified epidermal appendages to cover, protect, and lubricate

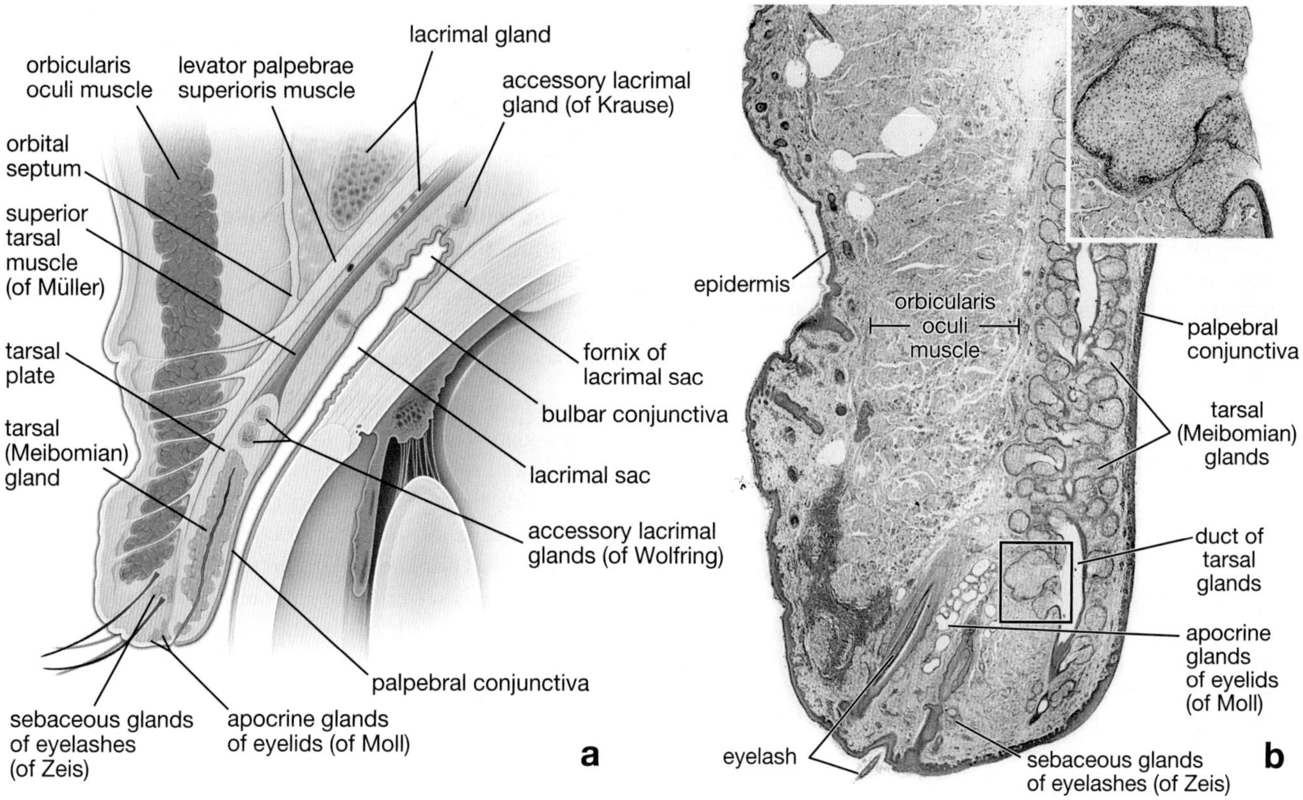

FIGURE 24.17. Structure of the eyelid. a. This schematic drawing of the eyelid shows the skin, associated skin appendages, muscles, tendons, connective tissue, and conjunctiva. Note the distribution of multiple small glands associated with the eyelid and observe the reflection of the palpebral conjunctiva in the fornix of the lacrimal sac to become the bulbar conjunctiva. **b.** Photomicrograph of a sagittal section of the eyelid stained with picric acid for better visualization of epithelial components of the skin and the numerous glands. In this preparation, muscle tissue (i.e., *orbicularis oculi muscle*) stains *yellow*, and the epithelial cells of the skin, conjunctiva, and glandular epithelium are *green*. Note the presence of numerous glands within the eyelid. The *tarsal (Meibomian) gland* is the largest gland, and it is located within the dense connective tissue of the tarsal plates. This sebaceous gland secretes into ducts opening onto the eyelids. ×20. **Inset.** Higher magnification of a tarsal gland from the *boxed area* showing the typical structure of a holocrine gland. ×60.

the anterior portions of the eyes. The anterior surface of the eyelid is covered by thin **skin**, and its posterior surface is lined by a specialized mucous membrane, the **conjunctiva**. The skin of the eyelids is loose and elastic to accommodate their movement. Within each eyelid is a flexible support, the **tarsal plate**, consisting of dense fibrous and elastic tissue. In the upper eyelid, the lower free edge of the tarsal plate extends to the lid margin, and its superior border serves for the attachment of smooth muscle fibers of the **superior tarsal muscle (of Müller)**. The undersurface of the tarsal plate is covered by the conjunctiva (Fig. 24.17). The striated **orbicularis oculi muscle**, a facial expression muscle, forms a thin oval sheet of circularly oriented skeletal muscle fibers overlying the tarsal plate. In addition, the connective tissue of the upper eyelid contains tendon fibers of the **levator palpebrae superioris muscle** that open the eyelid (see Fig. 24.17). A mucocutaneous junction between eyelid skin and conjunctiva occurs near the lid margin. The **eyelashes** emerge from the most anterior edge of the lid margin. They are short, stiff, curved hairs and may occur in double or triple rows. The lashes on the same eyelid margin may have different lengths and diameters.

The conjunctiva lines the space between the inner surface of the eyelids and the anterior surface of the eye without covering the cornea.

The **conjunctiva** is a thin, transparent mucous membrane that extends from the corneoscleral limbus located on the peripheral margin of the cornea across the sclera (**bulbar conjunctiva**) and covers the internal surface of the eyelids (**palpebral conjunctiva**). The palpebral conjunctiva merges with the bulbar conjunctiva at the fornices of the conjunctival sac; this part is called the **forniceal conjunctiva** (Fig. 24.18). Bulbar, palpebral, and forniceal

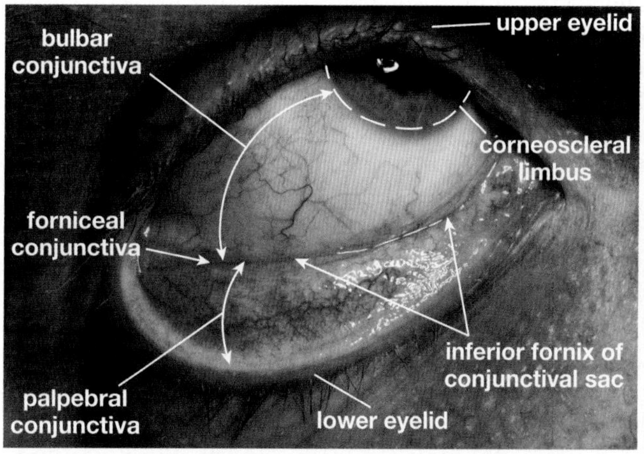

FIGURE 24.18. Conjunctiva and conjunctival sac. This photograph of the lower part of the eyeball with a reflected lower eyelid shows different regions of the conjunctiva that line the conjunctival sac. The area shown is located between the inner surface of the eyelid and the anterior surface of the eye. The bulbar conjunctiva extends from the corneoscleral limbus covering the sclera of the eye (it does not cover the cornea) to its reflections onto the internal surface of the eyelid, at which point it is called the *palpebral conjunctiva*. This photograph shows the inferior point of reflection onto the lower eyelid (called the *inferior fornix* of the conjunctival sac). The conjunctiva in these regions is recognized as the forniceal conjunctiva.

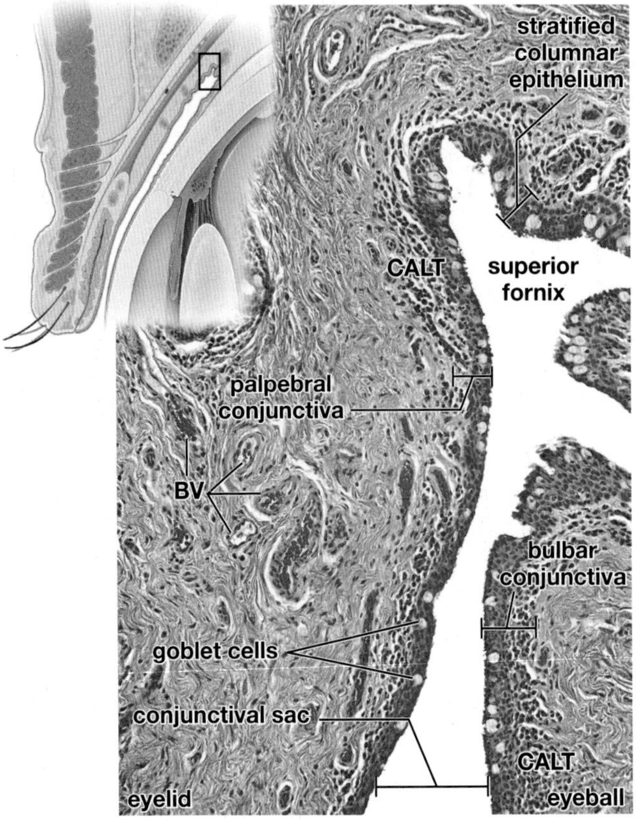

FIGURE 24.19. Superior fornix of the conjunctival sac. This low-magnification hematoxylin and eosin (H&E)-stained specimen was obtained from the superior fornix of the conjunctival sac as indicated by the *rectangle* in the inset. The palpebral conjunctiva lines the inner surface of the eyelid, and in the superior fornix of the conjunctival sac, it reflects onto the eyeball (bulbar conjunctiva). This reflection is identified as the forniceal conjunctiva and is composed of stratified columnar epithelium containing numerous goblet cells. Accumulations of lymphatic tissue called *conjunctiva-associated lymphatic tissue* (*CALT*) are clearly visible. There are numerous blood vessels (*BV*) underlying the palpebral conjunctiva. ×120. (Courtesy of Dr. Nick Mamalis, University of Utah, Moran Clinical Ophthalmology Resource for Education [CORE], Salt Lake City, Utah.)

conjunctiva form a conjunctival sac, a space between the eyelid and eyeball that opens anteriorly at the palpebral fissure. The conjunctival sac can hold fluid up to 30 μL. Because a standard eyedropper dispenses about 50 μL of suspended medicine per drop, one drop is more than enough to overfill the conjunctival sac.

The conjunctiva consists of a **stratified columnar epithelium** containing numerous **goblet cells** and rests on a lamina propria composed of loose connective tissue. The goblet cells secrete a component of the tears that bathe the eye. Melanocytes are present in the basal epithelial layer and, like melanocytes in the skin, transfer melanosomes into neighboring epithelial cells. Accumulation of diffuse lymphatic tissue is evident, especially deep to the forniceal conjunctiva (Fig. 24.19). These specialized collections of T and B lymphocytes underlying the conjunctiva are called **conjunctiva-associated lymphatic tissue (CALT)** (Fig. 24.20). It functions to recognize and process antigens and trigger an appropriate immune response against the microbial invasion of the ocular surface. The conjunctiva is supplied with blood by the branches of arteries of the eyelid (marginal tarsal arcades) and from the eyeball (anterior ciliary arteries). The conjunctiva receives sensory innervation from the branches of the trigeminal nerve. **Conjunctivitis**, an inflammation of the conjunctiva, commonly called **pinkeye**, is characterized by redness, irritation, and watering of the eyes. For more clinical information about this condition, see Folder 24.6.

Secretions from modified glands in the eyelid provide additional protection to the eye.

In addition to eccrine sweat glands, which discharge their secretions directly onto the skin, the eyelid contains four other major types of glands (see Fig. 24.17):

- The **tarsal glands (Meibomian glands)**, long sebaceous glands embedded in the tarsal plates, appear as vertical yellow streaks in the tissue deep into the conjunctiva. Their elongated ducts open at the lid margin behind rows of eyelashes. About 25 tarsal glands are present in the upper eyelid, and 20 are present in the lower eyelid. The sebaceous secretion of the tarsal glands produces an oily layer on the surface of the tear film that retards the evaporation of the normal tear layer. Blockage of the tarsal gland secretion leads to **chalazion** (tarsal gland lipogranuloma), an inflammation of the tarsal gland. It presents as a painless cyst usually on the upper eyelid that disappears after a few months without therapeutic intervention.
- **Sebaceous glands of eyelashes (glands of Zeis)** are small, modified sebaceous glands that are connected with and empty their secretion into the follicles of the eyelashes. Bacterial infection of these sebaceous glands causes a **stye** (also called a **hordeolum**), a painful tenderness and redness of the affected area of the eyelid.

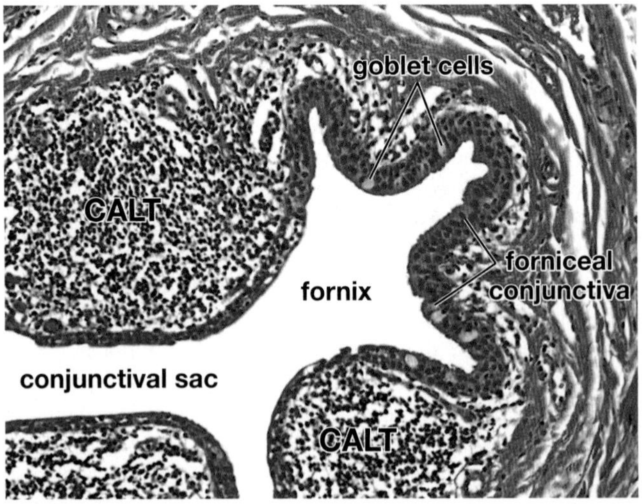

FIGURE 24.20. Forniceal conjunctiva. This high-magnification hematoxylin and eosin (H&E)-stained specimen shows the fornix of the conjunctival sac. The forniceal conjunctiva shows a typical pattern of the stratified columnar epithelium containing goblet cells that rests on a lamina propria composed of loose connective tissue. The stratified columnar epithelium farther away from the fornix may change into columnar stratified or squamous stratified nonkeratinized epithelium (*lower right corner of conjunctival sac*). Note the accumulations of diffuse lymphatic tissue deep into the conjunctiva known as *conjunctiva-associated lymphatic tissue* (*CALT*). ×220. (Courtesy of Dr. Nick Mamalis, University of Utah, Moran Clinical Ophthalmology Resource for Education [CORE], Salt Lake City, Utah.)

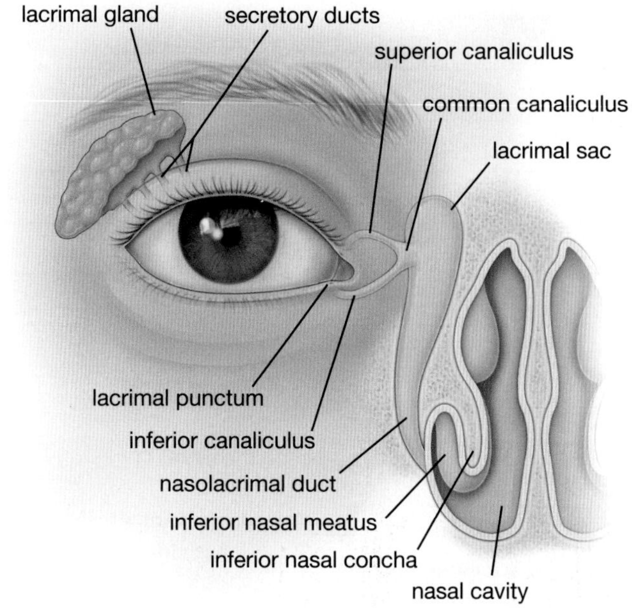

FIGURE 24.21. Schematic diagram of the eye and lacrimal apparatus. This drawing shows the location of the lacrimal gland and components of the lacrimal apparatus, which drains the lacrimal fluid into the nasal cavity.

- **Apocrine glands of eyelashes (glands of Moll)** are small sweat glands with unbranched sinuous tubules that begin as a simple spiral.
- **Accessory lacrimal glands** are compound serous tubuloalveolar glands that have distended lumina. They are located on the inner surface of the upper eyelids (**glands of Wolfring**) and in the fornix of the conjunctival sac (**glands of Krause**).

All glands of the human eyelid are innervated by neurons of the autonomic nervous system, and their secretion is synchronized with the lacrimal glands by a common neurotransmitter, vasoactive intestinal polypeptide (VIP).

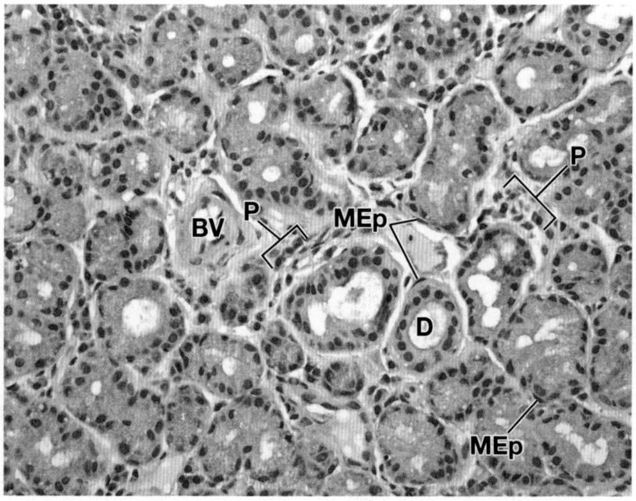

FIGURE 24.22. Photomicrograph of lacrimal gland. The lacrimal gland consists of tubuloacinar serous secretory units. The acini are lined with serous secretory columnar cells. Myoepithelial cells (*MEp*) are present below the epithelial cells within the basal lamina. Cytoplasm of the secretory cells contains small lipid droplets and mucin-containing granules. Intralobular ducts (*D*) lined by serous cells also contain myoepithelial cells. Occasional plasma cells (*P*) and lymphocytes are present between acini of the lacrimal gland. *BV*, blood vessels. ×450.

The lacrimal gland produces tears that moisten the cornea and flow to the nasolacrimal duct.

Tears are produced by the **lacrimal glands** and, to a lesser degree, by the accessory lacrimal glands. The lacrimal gland is located beneath the conjunctiva on the upper lateral side of the orbit (Fig. 24.21). The lacrimal gland consists of several separate lobules of tubuloacinar serous glands. The acini have large lumina lined with columnar cells. Myoepithelial cells, located below the epithelial cells within the basal lamina, aid in the release of tears (Fig. 24.22). Approximately 12 ducts drain from the lacrimal gland into the reflection of conjunctiva just beneath the upper eyelid, known as the **fornix of the conjunctival sac**.

Tears drain from the eye through **lacrimal puncta**, the small openings of the **lacrimal canaliculi**, located at the medial angle. The upper and lower canaliculi join to form the **common canaliculus**, which opens into the lacrimal sac. The sac is continuous with the **nasolacrimal duct**, which opens into the nasal cavity below the inferior nasal conchae. A pseudostratified ciliated epithelium lines the lacrimal sac and the nasolacrimal duct. **Dacryocystitis** is an inflammation of the lacrimal sac that is frequently caused by an obstruction of the nasolacrimal duct. It can be acute, chronic, or congenital. It usually affects older individuals and is most often secondary to stenosis (narrowing) of the lacrimal canaliculi.

Tears protect the corneal epithelium and contain antibacterial and UV-protective agents.

Tears keep the conjunctiva and corneal epithelium moist and wash foreign material from the eye as they flow across the corneal surface toward the medial angle of the eye (see Fig. 24.21). The thin film of tears covering the corneal surface is not homogeneous but a mixture of products secreted by the lacrimal glands, the accessory lacrimal glands, the goblet cells of the conjunctiva, and the tarsal glands of the eyelid. The tear film contains proteins (tear albumins and lactoferrin), enzymes (lysozyme), lipids, metabolites, electrolytes, and medications, the latter secreted during therapy.

The tear cationic protein lactoferrin increases the activity of various natural antimicrobial agents, such as lysozyme.

The eye is moved within the orbit by coordinated contraction of extraocular muscles.

Six muscles of the eyeball (also called **extraocular** or **extrinsic muscles**) attach to each eye. These are the medial, lateral, superior, and inferior rectus muscles and the superior and inferior oblique muscles. The superior oblique muscle is innervated by the trochlear nerve (cranial nerve IV). The lateral rectus muscle is innervated by the abducens nerve (cranial nerve VI). All of the remaining extraocular muscles are innervated by the oculomotor nerve (cranial nerve III). The combined, precisely controlled action of these muscles allows vertical, lateral, and rotational movement of the eye. Normally, the actions of the muscles of both eyes are coordinated so that the eyes move in parallel (called **conjugate gaze**).

101 HISTOLOGY NOTEBOOK

EYE

OVERVIEW OF THE EYE

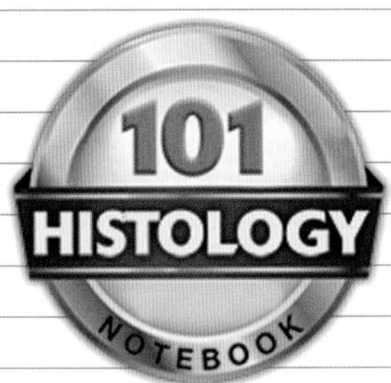

- The **eye** is a paired, specialized sensory organ that provides the sense of sight.
- The tissues of the eye are derived from **neuroectoderm** (retina), **surface ectoderm** (lens, corneal epithelium), and **mesoderm** (sclera, corneal stroma, vascular coat).
- The eyeball is composed of three structural layers: the outer **corneoscleral (fibrous) coat** consisting of the transparent cornea and the opaque white sclera; the middle **vascular coat** consisting of the choroid, ciliary body, and iris; and the inner layer, the **retina**.
- The layers of the eye and the lens serve as boundaries for three chambers: the **anterior chamber** and **posterior chamber**, which are filled with **aqueous humor**, and the **vitreous chamber**, which is occupied by a transparent gel, the **vitreous body**.
- **Aqueous humor** is secreted by the ciliary processes into the posterior chamber. From there it flows through the pupil into the anterior chamber, where it drains inside the **iridocorneal angle** to the **scleral venous sinus (canal of Schlemm)**.

COATS IN THE WALL OF THE EYE

- The **cornea** is transparent and consists of five layers (beginning from the anterior surface): **corneal epithelium** (nonkeratinized stratified squamous epithelium), **Bowman membrane** (anterior basement membrane for corneal epithelium), a thick avascular **corneal stroma**, **Descemet membrane** (posterior basement membrane for corneal endothelium), and **corneal endothelium.**
- The **sclera** is opaque and consists predominantly of dense connective tissue. It communicates with the cornea at the **corneoscleral limbus**, which contains **corneolimbal stem cells.**
- The **iris** arises from the ciliary body, and the diameter of its opening (**pupil**) is controlled by smooth muscle fibers of the **sphincter pupillae muscle** and the myoepithelial cell layer of the **dilator pupillae muscle.** Its posterior surface is covered by pigment epithelium and contains a stroma that is abundant with melanocytes.
- The **ciliary body** is located between the iris and the choroid. It contains **ciliary processes** that secrete aqueous humor, anchors **zonular fibers** that suspend the lens, and contains **ciliary muscle** that alters the shape of the lens during **lens accommodation.**
- The **lens** is a transparent, avascular, biconvex structure that is suspended between the edges of the ciliary body. It consists of a **lens capsule, subcapsular epithelium**, and **lens fiber cells.**
- The **choroid** is part of the vascular coat and has an inner **choriocapillary layer** containing blood vessels that provide nutrients to the retina and an outer **Bruch membrane** that serves as the basal lamina for both the endothelial and RPE cells.
- The **retina** is derived from the inner and outer layers of the optic cup. It consists of two basic layers: the **neural retina** is the inner layer containing photoreceptor cells, and the **retinal pigment epithelium (RPE)** is the outer layer that attaches to the choroid.

RETINA

- The **retina** contains 10 layers of cells and their processes. Major cells in the retina include **photoreceptors** (rods and cones), **conducting neurons** (bipolar neurons and ganglion cells), **association neurons**, and **supporting cells** (e.g., Müller cells).
- **Retinal pigment epithelium** (layer 1) is the outermost layer of the retina and **absorbs scattered light**, contributes to the **blood–retina barrier**, **restores photosensitivity** to visual pigments, and **phagocytoses membranous discs** from the rods and cones.
- **Rods** (layer 2) are most numerous (120 million) in the retina and detect light intensity with their cylindrical outer segments. **Cones** (layer 2) are less numerous (7 million) and, with their conical outer segment, detect three different wavelengths of light corresponding to the primary colors: blue, green, and red.
- Rods contain the visual pigment **rhodopsin** that consists of **opsin** and a small light-absorbing compound, **retinal**. Cone cells contain the visual pigment **iodopsin**.
- Conversion of light into nerve impulses in the photoreceptors is called **visual processing**. It involves a photochemical reaction based on the conversion of **11-cis-retinal** into **all-trans-retinal** in the rhodopsin. This results in the activation of opsin, which, in turn, activates G-protein and initiates hyperpolarization of the photoreceptor cell membrane that is detected by the bipolar neurons as a nerve impulse.
- The **outer limiting membrane** (layer 3) is formed by a row of zonulae adherentes between Müller cells.
- The **outer nuclear layer** (layer 4) contains the nuclei of rods and cones, and the **outer plexiform layer** (layer 5) contains their processes, which synapse with the horizontal, amacrine, and bipolar cells (the nuclei of which reside in the **inner nuclear layer** [layer 6]).
- Axons from cells in the outer plexiform layer synapse in the **inner plexiform layer** (layer 7) with ganglion cells, the cell bodies of which reside in the **ganglion cell layer** (layer 8). These cells send axons to the **layer of optic nerve fibers** (layer 9), which forms the optic nerve.
- The **inner limiting membrane** (layer 10) consists of a basal lamina separating the retina from the vitreous body.

ACCESSORY STRUCTURES OF THE EYE

- The **eyelids** consist of skin, tarsal plates, part of the **orbicularis oculi muscle**, tendon fibers of the **levator palpebrae superioris muscle** (in the upper eyelid), and the palpebral conjunctiva.
- The **conjunctiva** consists of **stratified columnar epithelium** with **goblet cells**. It lines the space between the inner surface of the eyelid and the anterior surface of the eye lateral to the cornea.
- A diffuse lymphatic tissue called **conjunctiva-associated lymphatic tissue (CALT)** is underlying conjunctiva at the superior and inferior fornices of the conjunctival sac.
- The **tarsal glands (Meibomian glands)** are long sebaceous glands embedded in the tarsal plates of the upper and lower eyelids.
- The **lacrimal gland** produces tears that moisten the cornea and flow to the nasolacrimal duct and into the nasal cavity.

PLATE 24.1 ■ EYE I

The human **eye** is a complex sensory organ that provides sight. The wall of the eye consists of **three concentric layers or coats**: the **retina**, the inner layer; the **uvea**, the middle or vascular layer; and the **corneosclera**, the outer fibrous layer. The eye is often compared to a simple camera with a lens to capture and focus light, a diaphragm to regulate the amount of light, and film to record the image. In the eye, the **cornea** and **lens** concentrate and focus light on the **retina**. The **iris**, located between the cornea and lens, regulates the size of the pupil through which light enters the eye. **Photoreceptor cells (rods and cones)** in the retina detect the intensity (rods) and color (cones) of the light that reaches them and encode the various parameters for transmission to the brain via the optic nerve (cranial nerve II).

The eye measures 25 mm in diameter. It is suspended in the bony orbit by six extrinsic striated muscles that control its movement. The extraocular muscles are coordinated so that both eyes move synchronously, with each moving symmetrically around its own central axis. A thick layer of adipose tissue partially surrounds and cushions the eye as it moves within the orbit.

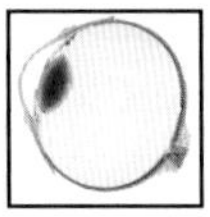

Modified drawing of human eye, meridional perspective by E. Sobotta.

The innermost layer is the **retina** (*R*), which consists of several layers of cells. Among these are receptor cells (rods and cones), neurons (e.g., bipolar and ganglion cells), supporting cells, and a pigment epithelium (see Plate 24.2, page 1012). The receptor components of the retina are situated in the posterior three-fifths of the eyeball. At the anterior boundary of the receptor layer, the **ora serrata** (*OS*), the retina becomes reduced in thickness, and nonreceptor components of the retina continue forward to cover the posterior or inner surface of the **ciliary body** (*CB*) and the **iris** (*I*). This anterior nonreceptor extension of the inner layer is highly pigmented, and the pigment (melanin) is evident as the black inner border of these structures.

The **uvea**, the middle layer of the eyeball, consists of the choroid, the ciliary body, and the iris. The choroid is a vascular layer; it is relatively thin and difficult to distinguish in the accompanying figure, except by location. On this basis, the **choroid** (*Ch*) is identified as being just external to the pigmented layer of the retina. It is also highly pigmented; the choroidal pigment is evident as a discrete layer in several parts of the section.

Anterior to the ora serrata, the uvea is thickened; here, it is called the ciliary body (*CB*). This contains the ciliary muscle (see Plate 24.3, page 1014), which brings about adjustments of the lens to focus light. The ciliary body also contains processes to which the zonular fibers are attached. These fibers function as suspensory ligaments of the lens (*L*). The iris (*I*) is the most anterior component of the uvea and contains a central opening, the pupil.

The outermost layer of the eyeball, the **fibrous layer**, consists of the **sclera** (*S*) and the **cornea** (*C*). Both of these contain collagenous fibers as their main structural element; however, the cornea is transparent, and the sclera is opaque. The extrinsic muscles of the eye insert into the sclera and affect the movements of the eyeball. These are not included in the preparation, except for two small pieces of a muscle insertion (*arrows*) in the *lower left* and *top center* of the illustration. Posteriorly, the sclera is pierced by the emerging **optic nerve** (*ON*). A deep depression in the neural retina lateral to the optic nerve (above the *ON* in this figure) is the fovea centralis (*FC*), the thinnest and most sensitive portion of the neural retina.

The lens is considered in Plate 24.4 (page 1016). Just posterior to the lens is the large cavity of the eye, the **vitreous cavity** (*V*), which is filled with a thick jelly-like material, the vitreous humor or body. Anterior to the lens are two additional, fluid-filled chambers of the eye, the **anterior chamber** (*AC*) and the **posterior chamber** (*PC*), separated by the iris.

AC, anterior chamber	**I,** iris	**R,** retina
C, cornea	**L,** lens	**S,** sclera
CB, ciliary body	**ON,** optic nerve	**V,** vitreous cavity
Ch, choroid	**OS,** ora serrate	**arrows,** muscle insertions
FC, fovea centralis	**PC,** posterior chamber	

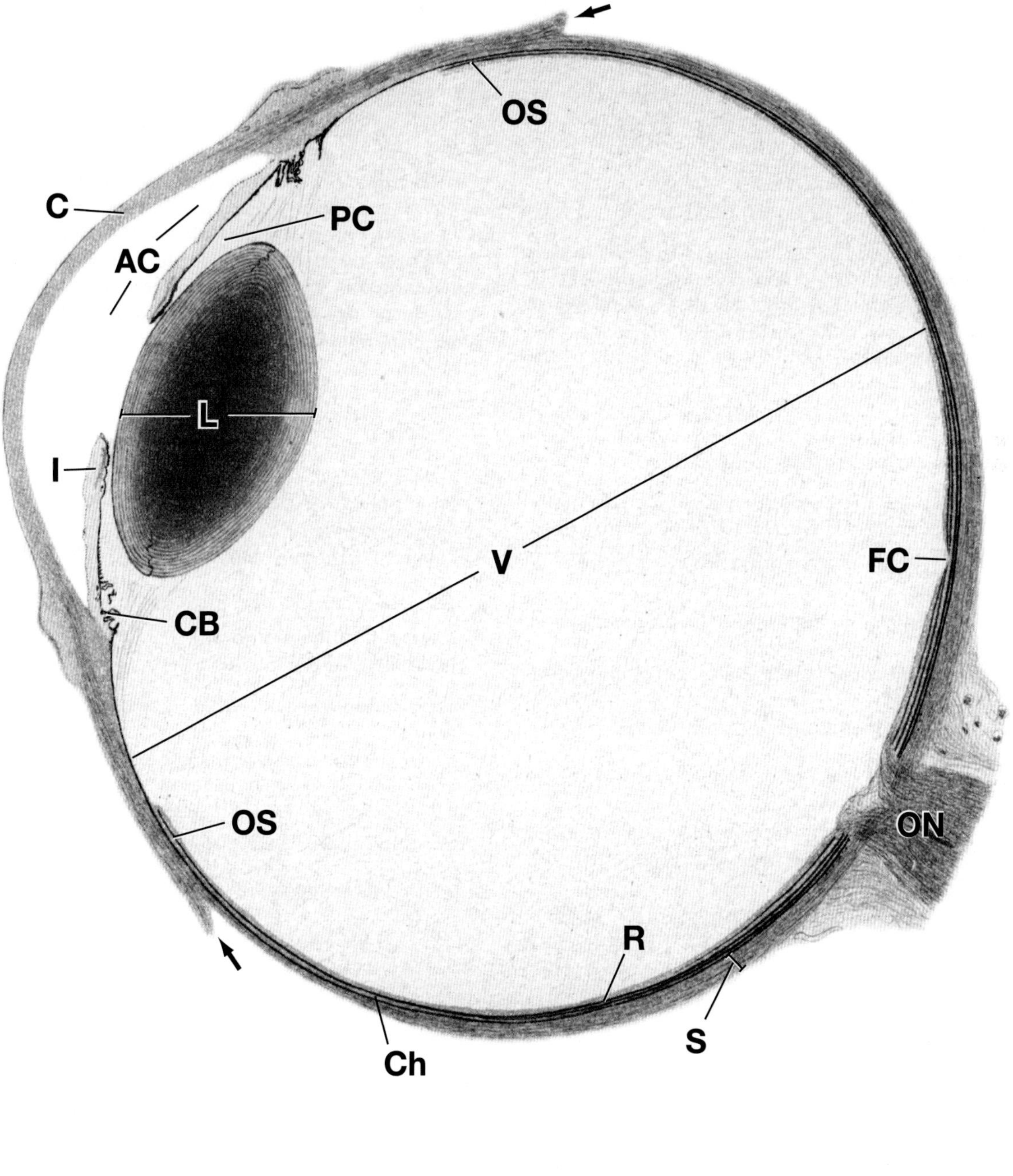
C
AC
PC
OS
L
I
V
FC
CB
OS
ON
R
S
Ch

PLATE 24.2 ■ EYE II: RETINA

The **retina** and **optic nerve** are projections of the forebrain. The fibrous cover of the optic nerve is an extension of the meninges of the brain. The neural retina is a multilayered structure consisting of photoreceptors (rods and cones); neurons, some of which are specialized as conducting and associating neurons; and supporting cells (**Müller cells**). External to the neural retina is a layer of simple columnar **retinal pigment epithelium (RPE)**. The Müller cells are comparable to neuroglia in the rest of the central nervous system. Processes of Müller cells ramify virtually through the entire thickness of the retina. The internal limiting membrane is the basal lamina of these cells; the external limiting membrane is actually a line formed by the junctional complexes between processes of these cells and the **photoreceptor cells**.

The neurons of the retina are arranged sequentially in three layers: (1) a deep layer of rods and cones; (2) an intermediate layer of **bipolar**, **horizontal**, and **amacrine** cells; and (3) a superficial layer of **ganglion** cells. Nerve impulses originating in the rods and cones are transmitted to the intermediate layer and then to the ganglion cells. Synaptic connections occur in the **outer plexiform layer** (between the rods and cones and the intermediate neuronal layer) and the **inner plexiform layer** (between the intermediate layer and the ganglion cells), resulting in summation and neuronal integration. Finally, the ganglion cells send their axons to the brain as components of the optic nerve.

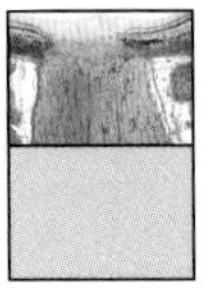

Optic disc and nerve, eye, human, hematoxylin and eosin (H&E) ×65.

The site where the optic nerve leaves the eyeball is called the **optic disc** (*OD*). It is characteristically marked by a depression, evident here. Receptor cells are not present at the optic disc, and because it is not sensitive to light stimulation, it is sometimes referred to as the *blind spot*.

The fibers that give rise to the optic nerve originate in the retina, more specifically, in the ganglion cell layer (see later). They traverse the sclera through a number of openings (*arrows*) to form the **optic nerve** (*ON*). The region of the sclera that contains these openings is called the **lamina cribrosa** (*LC*) or cribriform plate. The optic nerve contains a central artery and vein (not seen here) that also traverse the lamina cribrosa. Branches of these blood vessels (*BV*) supply the inner portion of the retina.

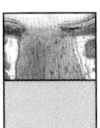

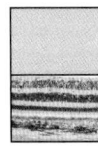

Retina, eye, human, H&E ×325.

On the basis of structural features that are evident in histologic sections, the retina is divided into 10 layers, from posterior to anterior, as listed herein and labeled in this figure:

1. **Retinal pigment epithelium** (*RPE*), the outermost layer of the retina
2. **Layer of rods and cones** (*R&C*), the photoreceptor layer of the retina
3. **External limiting membrane** (*ELM*), a line formed by the junctional complexes of the photoreceptor cells
4. **Outer nuclear layer** (*ONL*), containing nuclei of rod and cone cells
5. **Outer plexiform layer** (*OPL*), containing neural processes and synapses of rod and cone cells with bipolar, amacrine, interplexiform, and horizontal cells
6. **Inner nuclear layer** (*INL*), containing nuclei of bipolar, horizontal, interplexiform, amacrine, and Müller cells
7. **Inner plexiform layer** (*IPL*), containing processes and synapses of bipolar, horizontal, interplexiform, amacrine, and ganglion cells
8. **Layer of ganglion cells** (*GC*), containing cell bodies and nuclei of ganglion cells
9. **Nerve fiber layer** (*NFL*), containing axons of ganglion cells
10. **Internal limiting membrane** (*ILM*), consisting of the external (basal) lamina of Müller cells

This figure also shows the innermost layer of the choroid (*Ch*), a cell-free membrane, the lamina vitrea (*LV*), also called Bruch membrane. Electron micrographs reveal that it corresponds to the basement membrane of the pigment epithelium. Immediately external to the lamina vitrea is the capillary layer of the choroid (lamina choriocapillaris). These vessels supply the outer part of the retina.

BV, blood vessels
Ch, choroid
ELM, external limiting membrane
GC, layer of ganglion cells
ILM, internal limiting membrane
INL, inner nuclear layer (nuclei of bipolar, horizontal, amacrine, and Müller cells)
IPL, inner plexiform layer
LC, lamina cribrosa
LV, lamina vitrea
NFL, nerve fiber layer
OD, optic disc
ON, optic nerve
ONL, outer nuclear layer (nuclei of rod and cone cells)
OPL, outer plexiform layer
RPE, retinal pigment epithelium
R&C, layer of rods and cones
arrows, openings in sclera (lamina cribrosa)

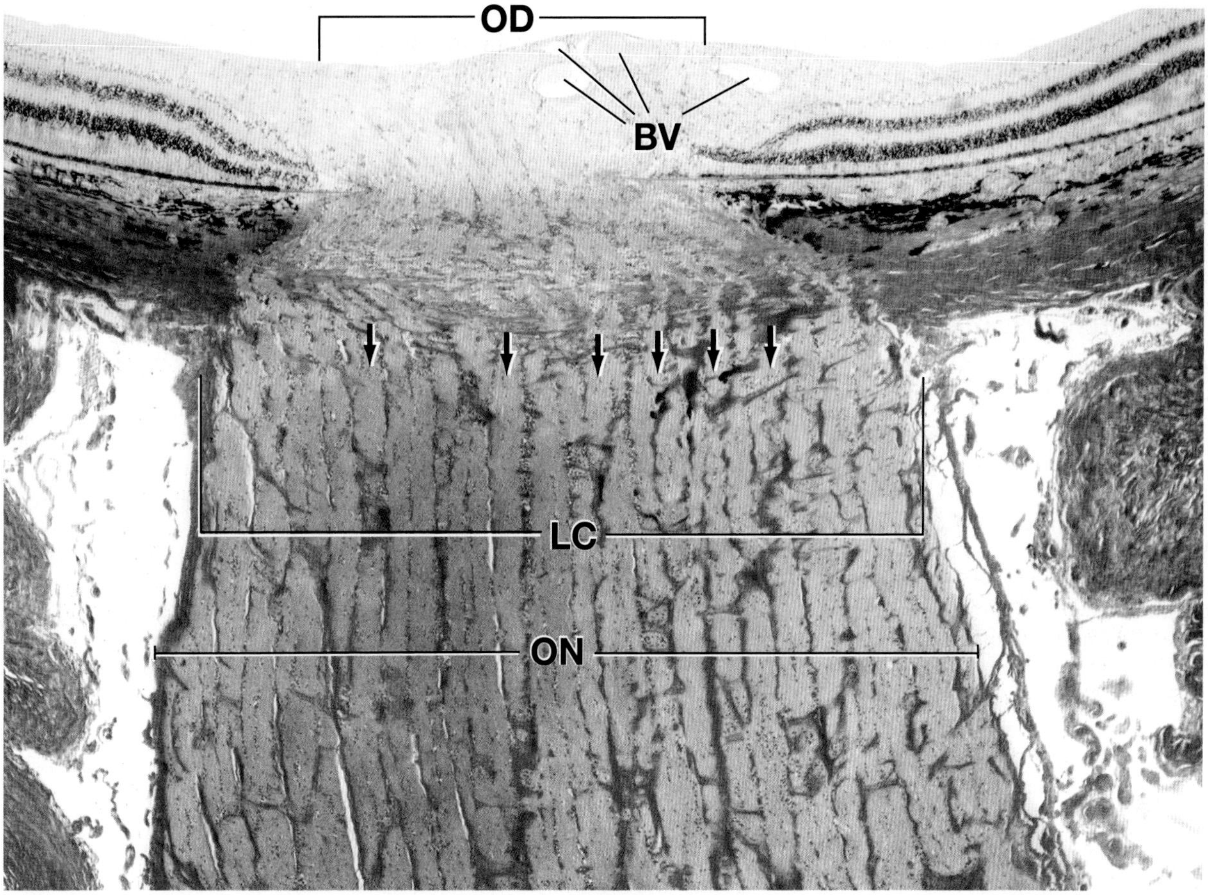
OD
BV
LC
ON

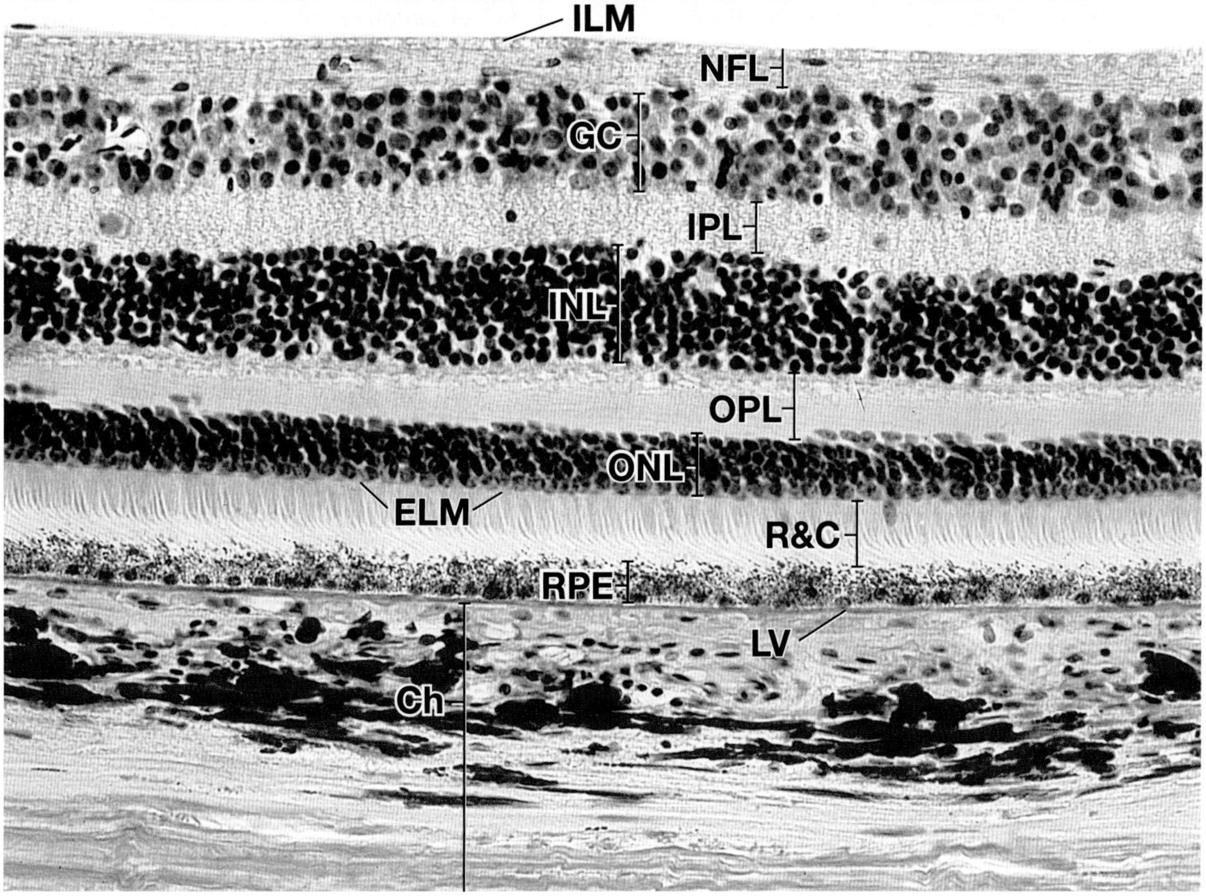
ILM
NFL
GC
IPL
INL
OPL
ONL
ELM
R&C
RPE
LV
Ch

PLATE 24.3 ■ EYE III: ANTERIOR SEGMENT

The **anterior segment** is that part of the eye anterior to the **ora serrata**, the most anterior extension of the neural retina, and includes the **anterior** and **posterior chambers** and the structures that define them. These include the cornea and sclera, the iris, the lens, the ciliary body, and the connections between the basal lamina of the ciliary processes and the lens capsule (thick basal lamina of the lens epithelium) that form the suspensory ligament of the lens, the **zonular fibers**. The posterior chamber is bounded posteriorly by the anterior surface of the lens and anteriorly by the posterior surface of the iris. The ciliary body forms the lateral boundary. Aqueous humor flows through the pupil into the anterior chamber, which occupies the space between the cornea and the iris, and drains into the **canal of Schlemm**.

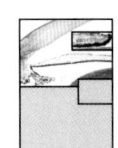

Anterior segment, eye, human, hematoxylin and eosin (H&E) ×45; inset ×75.

A portion of the **anterior segment** of the eye, shown in this figure, includes parts of the cornea (*C*), sclera (*S*), iris (*I*), ciliary body (*CB*), anterior chamber (*AC*), posterior chamber (*PC*), lens (*L*), and zonular fibers (*ZF*).

The relationship of the cornea to the sclera is illustrated to advantage here. The junction between the two (*arrows*) is marked by a change in staining, with the substance of the cornea appearing lighter than that of the sclera. The **corneal epithelium** (*CEp*) is continuous with the **conjunctival epithelium** (*CjEp*) that covers the sclera. Note that the epithelium thickens considerably at the corneoscleral junction and resembles that of the oral mucosa. The conjunctival epithelium is separated from the dense fibrous component of the sclera by a loose vascular connective tissue. Together, this connective tissue and the epithelium constitute the conjunctiva (*Cj*). The epithelial–connective tissue junction of the conjunctiva is irregular; in contrast, the undersurface of the corneal epithelium presents an even profile.

Just lateral to the junction of the cornea and sclera is the **canal of Schlemm** (*CS*; see also the next figure). This canal takes a circular route about the perimeter of the cornea. It communicates with the anterior chamber through a loose trabecular meshwork of tissue, the spaces of Fontana. The canal of Schlemm also communicates with episcleral veins. By means of its communications, the canal of Schlemm provides a route for the fluid in the anterior and posterior chambers to reach the bloodstream.

The *inset* shows the tip of the iris. Note the heavy pigmentation on the posterior surface of the iris, which is covered by the same double-layered epithelium as the ciliary body and ciliary processes. In the ciliary epithelium, the outer layer is pigmented and the inner layer is nonpigmented. In the iris, both layers of the iridial epithelium (*IEp*) are heavily pigmented. A portion of the iridial constrictor muscle (*M*) is seen beneath the epithelium.

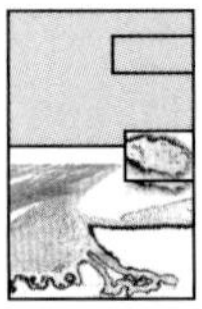

Anterior segment, eye, human, H&E ×90; inset ×350.

Immediately internal to the anterior margin of the sclera (*S*) is the **ciliary body** (*CB*). The **iris** (*I*) arises from the anterior border of the ciliary body. The inner surface of the ciliary body forms radially arranged, ridge-shaped elevations, the **ciliary processes** (*CP*), to which the zonular fibers (*ZF*) are anchored. From the outside, the components of the ciliary body are the ciliary muscle (*CM*), the connective tissue (vascular) layer (*VL*) containing small arteries (*A, inset*) and veins (*V, inset*) representing the choroid coat in the ciliary body, the lamina vitrea (*LV, inset*), and the ciliary epithelium (*CiEp, inset*). The ciliary epithelium consists of two layers (*inset*), the pigmented layer (*PE*) and the nonpigmented layer (*npE*). The lamina vitrea is a continuation of the same layer of the choroid; it is the basement membrane of the pigmented ciliary epithelial cells.

The **ciliary muscle** is arranged in three patterns. The outer layer is immediately deep into the sclera and contains the meridionally arranged fibers of Brücke. The outermost of these fibers continues more posteriorly into the choroid and is referred to as the *tensor muscle of the choroid.* The middle layer is the radial group. It radiates from the region of the sclerocorneal junction into the ciliary body. The innermost layer of muscle cells is circularly arranged. These are seen in cross section. The circular artery (*CA*; barely discernible) and vein (*CV*) for the iris, also cut in cross section, are just anterior to the circular group of muscle cells.

A, artery
AC, anterior chamber
C, cornea
CA, circular artery
CB, ciliary body
CEp, corneal epithelium
CiEp, ciliary epithelium
Cj, conjunctiva
CjEp, conjunctival epithelium
CM, ciliary muscle
CP, ciliary processes
CS, canal of Schlemm
CV, circular vein
I, iris
IEp, iridial epithelium
L, lens
LV, lamina vitrea
M, iridial constrictor muscle
npE, nonpigmented layer of ciliary epithelium
PC, posterior chamber
PE, pigmented layer of ciliary epithelium
S, sclera
V, vein
VL, vascular layer (of ciliary body)
ZF, zonular fibers
arrows, junction between cornea and sclera

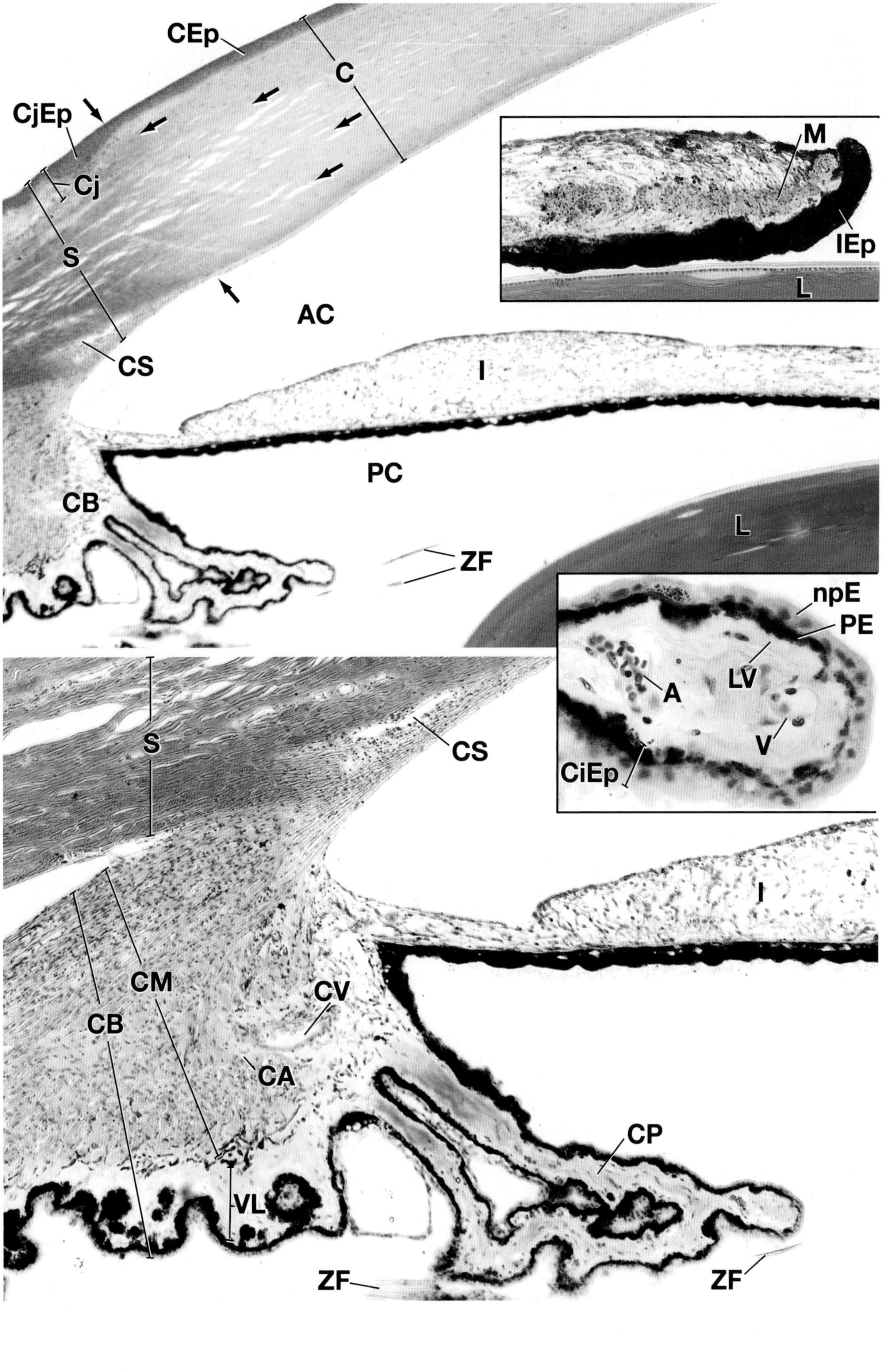
CEp
C
CjEp
Cj
S
AC
CS
I
PC
CB
ZF
L
M
IEp
L
npE
PE
LV
A
V
CiEp
S
CS
I
CM
CB
CV
CA
CP
VL
ZF
ZF

PLATE 24.4 ■ EYE IV: SCLERA, CORNEA, AND LENS

The transparent **cornea** is the primary dioptric (refractive element) of the eye and is covered with nonkeratinized stratified squamous epithelium. Its stroma consists of alternating lamellae of collagen fibrils and fibroblasts (**keratocytes**). The fibrils in each lamella are extremely uniform in diameter and uniformly spaced; fibrils in adjacent lamellae are arranged at approximately right angles to each other. This orthogonal array of highly regular fibrils is responsible for the transparency of the cornea. The posterior surface is covered with a single layer of low cuboidal cells, the **corneal endothelium**, which rests on a thickened basal lamina called **Descemet membrane**. Nearly all of the metabolic exchanges of the avascular cornea occur across the endothelium. Damage to this layer leads to corneal swelling and can produce temporary or permanent loss of transparency.

The **lens** is a transparent, avascular, biconvex epithelial structure suspended by the zonular fibers. Tension on these fibers keeps the lens flattened; reduced tension allows it to fatten or **accommodate** to bend light rays originating close to the eye to focus them on the retina.

Corneoscleral junction, eye, human, hematoxylin and eosin (H&E) ×130.

This low-magnification micrograph shows the full thickness of the sclera just lateral to the **corneoscleral junction** or limbus. To the *left* of the *arrow* is sclera; to the *right* is a small amount of corneal tissue. The **conjunctival epithelium** (*CjEp*) is irregular in thickness and rests on a loose vascular connective tissue. Together, this epithelium and underlying connective tissue represent the **conjunctiva** (*Cj*). The white opaque appearance of the sclera is due to the irregular dense arrangement of the collagen fibers that make up the stroma (*S*). The **canal of Schlemm** (*CS*) and small blood vessels (*BV*) are seen at the *left* close to the inner surface of the sclera near the border with anterior chamber (*AC*) of the eye.

Corneoscleral junction and canal of Schlemm, eye, human, H&E ×360.

Uppermost figure is a higher magnification micrograph showing the transition from the corneal epithelium (*CEp*) to the irregular and thicker conjunctival epithelium (*CjEp*) covering the sclera. Note that Bowman membrane (*B*), lying under the corneal epithelium, is just discernible but disappears beneath the conjunctival epithelium. The next figure shows a higher magnification of the canal of Schlemm (*CS*) than does the *top left* figure. That the space shown here is not an artifact is evidenced by the endothelial lining cells (*En*) that face the lumen.

Cornea, eye, human, H&E ×175.

This low-magnification micrograph shows the full thickness of the **cornea** (*C*) and can be compared with the sclera shown in the figure at the *left*. The **corneal epithelium** (*CEp*) presents a uniform thickness, and the underlying stroma (*S*) has a more homogeneous appearance than the stroma of the sclera (the white spaces seen here and in the figure at the *left* are artifacts). Nuclei (*N*) of the keratocytes of the stroma lie between lamellae. The corneal epithelium rests on a thickened anterior basement membrane called **Bowman membrane** (*B*). The posterior surface of the cornea facing the anterior chamber (*AC*) is lined by a simple squamous epithelium called the **corneal endothelium** (*CEn*); its thick posterior basement membrane is called **Descemet membrane** (*D*).

Corneal epithelium and endothelium, eye, human, H&E ×360.

Uppermost is a higher magnification micrograph showing the **corneal epithelium** (*CEp*) with its squamous surface cells, the very thick homogeneous-appearing **Bowman membrane** (*B*), and the underlying stroma (*S*). Note that the stromal tissue has a homogeneous appearance, a reflection of the dense packing of its collagen fibrils. The flattened nuclei belong to the keratocytes. Lowermost figure shows the posterior surface of the cornea. Note the thick homogeneous **Descemet membrane** (*D*) and the underlying **corneal endothelium** (*CEn*).

Lens, eye, human, H&E ×360.

This micrograph shows a portion of the lens near its equator. The lens consists entirely of epithelial cells surrounded by a homogeneous-appearing **lens capsule** (*LC*) to which the zonular fibers attach. The lens capsule is a very thick basal lamina of the epithelial cells. Simple cuboidal lens epithelial cells are present on the anterior surface of the lens, but at the lateral margin, they become extremely elongated and form layers that extend toward the center of the lens. These elongated columns of epithelial cytoplasm are referred to as **lens fibers** (*LF*). New cells are produced at the margin of the lens and displace the older cells inwardly. Eventually, the older cells lose their nuclei, as evidenced by the deeper portion of the cornea in this micrograph.

AC, anterior chamber
B, Bowman membrane
BV, blood vessels
C, cornea
CEn, corneal endothelium
CEp, corneal epithelium
Cj, conjunctiva
CjEp, conjunctival epithelium
CS, canal of Schlemm
D, Descemet membrane
En, endothelial lining cells
LC, lens capsule
LF, lens fibers
N, nuclei
S, stroma

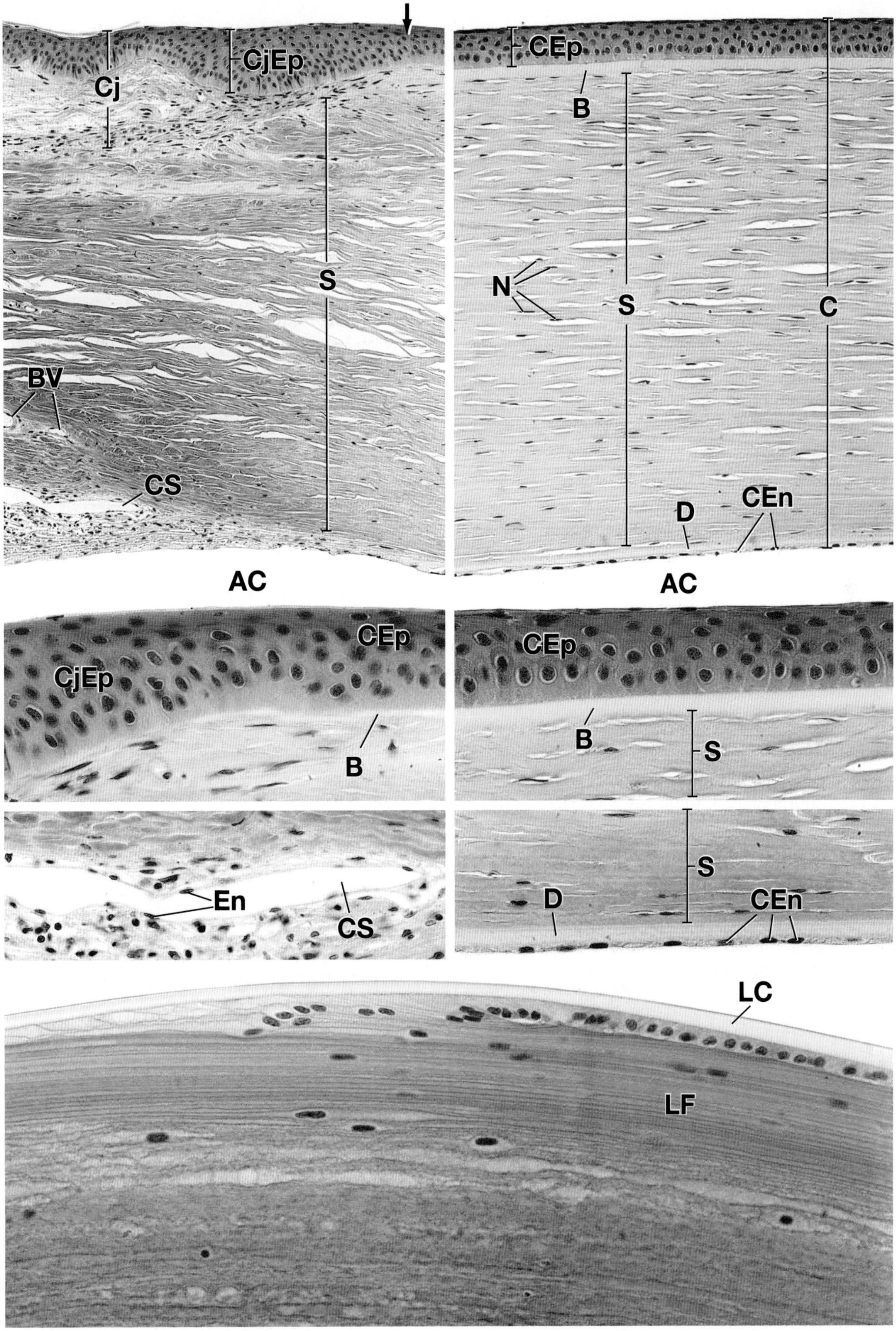
CjEp
Cj
S
BV
CS
AC
CEp
B
N
S
C
D
CEn
AC
CEp
CjEp
B
CEp
B
S
En
CS
S
D
CEn
LC
LF

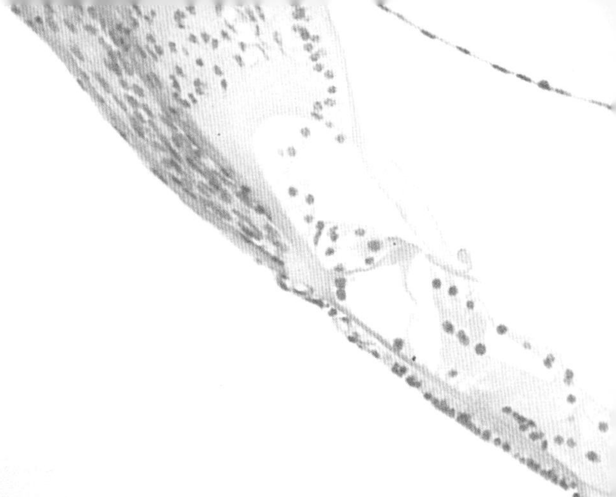

25 EAR

■ OVERVIEW OF THE EAR

The **ear** is a three-chambered sensory organ that functions as an **auditory system** for sound perception and as a **vestibular system** for balance. Each of the three divisions of the ear—the **external ear**, **middle ear**, and **internal ear**—is an essential part of both systems (Fig. 25.1). The external and middle ears collect and conduct acoustic energy to the internal ear, where auditory sensory receptors convert that energy into electrical impulses. The sensory receptors of the vestibular system respond to gravity and movement of the head. They are responsible for the sense of balance and equilibrium and help coordinate movements of the head and eyes.

The ear develops from surface ectoderm and components of the first and second pharyngeal arches.

The internal ear is the first of the three ear divisions to begin development. At the end of the third week, a thickening of **surface ectoderm** that appears on each side of the myelencephalon develops into the **otic placode**. Early in the fourth week, the otic placode invaginates and then pinches off to form the **otic vesicle (otocyst)**, which sinks deep to the surface ectoderm into the underlying mesenchyme (Fig. 25.2). The otic vesicle serves as a primordium for the development of the epithelia that line the membranous labyrinth of the internal ear. Later, development of the first and part of the second pharyngeal arch provides structures that augment hearing. The endodermal component of the **first pouch** gives rise to the **tubotympanic recess**, which ultimately develops into the **auditory tube (Eustachian tube)** and the **middle ear** and its epithelial lining. The corresponding ectodermal outgrowth of the **first pharyngeal groove** gives rise to the **external acoustic meatus** and its epithelial lining (see Fig. 25.2). The connective tissue part of the pharyngeal arches produces the ossicles ("ear bones"). The **malleus** and **incus** develop from the first pharyngeal arch and the **stapes** from the second pharyngeal arch. The sensory epithelia of the membranous labyrinth that originates from the otic vesicle link with cranial nerve VIII, which is an outgrowth of the central nervous system. The auricle of the external ear develops from six **auricular hillocks** located at the dorsal ends of the first and second pharyngeal arches surrounding the first pharyngeal cleft. The cartilaginous, bony, and muscular structures of the ear develop from the mesenchyme surrounding these early epithelia.

■ EXTERNAL EAR

The auricle is the external component of the ear that collects and amplifies sound.

The **auricle (pinna)** is the oval appendage that projects from the lateral surface of the head. The characteristic shape of the auricle is determined by an internal supporting structure of elastic cartilage. Thin skin with hair follicles, sweat glands, and sebaceous glands cover the auricle. The auricle is considered a nearly vestigial structure in humans, compared with its development and function in other animals. Nevertheless, it is essential in collecting the sound and directing it into the external acoustic meatus.

The external acoustic meatus conducts and amplifies sounds on the way to the tympanic membrane.

The **external acoustic meatus** is an air-filled tubular space that follows a slightly S-shaped course for about

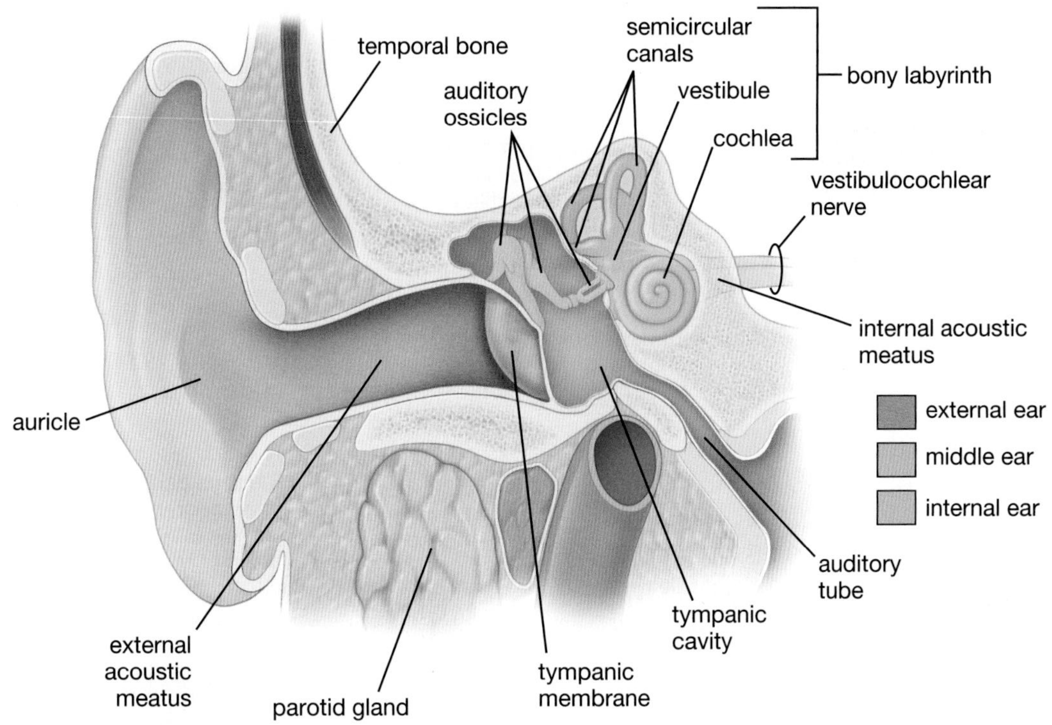

FIGURE 25.1. Three divisions of the ear. The three divisions of the ear are represented by different colors and consist of the external ear (auricle and external acoustic meatus; *pink*), the middle ear (tympanic cavity, auditory ossicles, tympanic membrane, and auditory tube; *green*), and the internal ear containing the bony labyrinth (semicircular canals, vestibule, and cochlea; *blue*) and the membranous labyrinth (not visible).

25 mm to the **tympanic membrane (eardrum)**. Because of its length, the external acoustic meatus can amplify sounds with frequencies of 2,000–5,000 Hz. By passively conducting sounds at this frequency and acting as a **resonator**, the external acoustic meatus increases the sound pressure at the tympanic membrane by approximately a **factor of 2**.

The wall of the meatus is continuous externally with the auricle. The wall of the lateral one-third of the meatus is cartilaginous and is continuous with the elastic cartilage of the auricle. The medial two-thirds of the meatus are contained within the temporal bone. Both parts of the meatus are lined by skin, which is also continuous with that of the auricle.

The skin in the lateral part of the meatus contains hair follicles, sebaceous glands, and **ceruminous glands**, but no eccrine sweat glands. The coiled tubular ceruminous glands closely resemble the apocrine glands found in the axillary region. Their secretion mixes with that of the sebaceous glands and desquamated cells to form **cerumen**, or **earwax**. Because the external acoustic meatus is the only blind pouch of the skin in the body, the earwax provides the means to evacuate desquamating cells from the stratum corneum, thus preventing their accumulation in the meatus. The **cerumen** lubricates the skin and coats the meatal hairs to impede the entry of foreign particles into the ear. It also provides some antimicrobial protection from bacteria, fungi, and insects. Excessive accumulation of cerumen (**impacted cerumen**) can plug the meatus, resulting in **conductive hearing loss**. The medial part of the meatus located within the temporal bone has thinner skin and fewer hairs and glands.

■ MIDDLE EAR

The middle ear is an air-filled space that contains three small bones, the ossicles.

The **middle ear** is located in an air-filled space, called the **tympanic cavity**, within the temporal bone (Fig. 25.3). It is spanned by three small bones, the **auditory ossicles**, which are connected by two movable joints. The middle ear also contains the **auditory tube (Eustachian tube)**, which opens to the nasopharynx as well as the muscles that attach to the ossicles.

The tympanic cavity has a roof, floor, and four walls: anterior, posterior, lateral, and medial. The tympanic cavity contains an opening of the auditory tube and is bound anteriorly by a thin layer of bone that separates it from the internal carotid artery. The posterior wall of the tympanic cavity is formed by the spongy bone of the **mastoid process**, which contains the **mastoid antrum** and other, smaller, air-filled spaces called **mastoid air cells**. The middle ear is bound laterally by the **tympanic membrane** and medially by the bony wall of the internal ear. The floor and roof of the tympanic cavity are both formed by a thin layer of bone, which separates them from the internal jugular vein and middle cranial fossa, respectively.

The middle ear is a mechanical energy transformer. Its primary function is to convert sound waves (air vibrations) arriving from the external acoustic meatus into mechanical vibrations that are transmitted to the internal ear. Two openings in the medial wall of the middle ear, the **oval (vestibular) window** and the **round (cochlear) window**, are essential components in this conversion process.

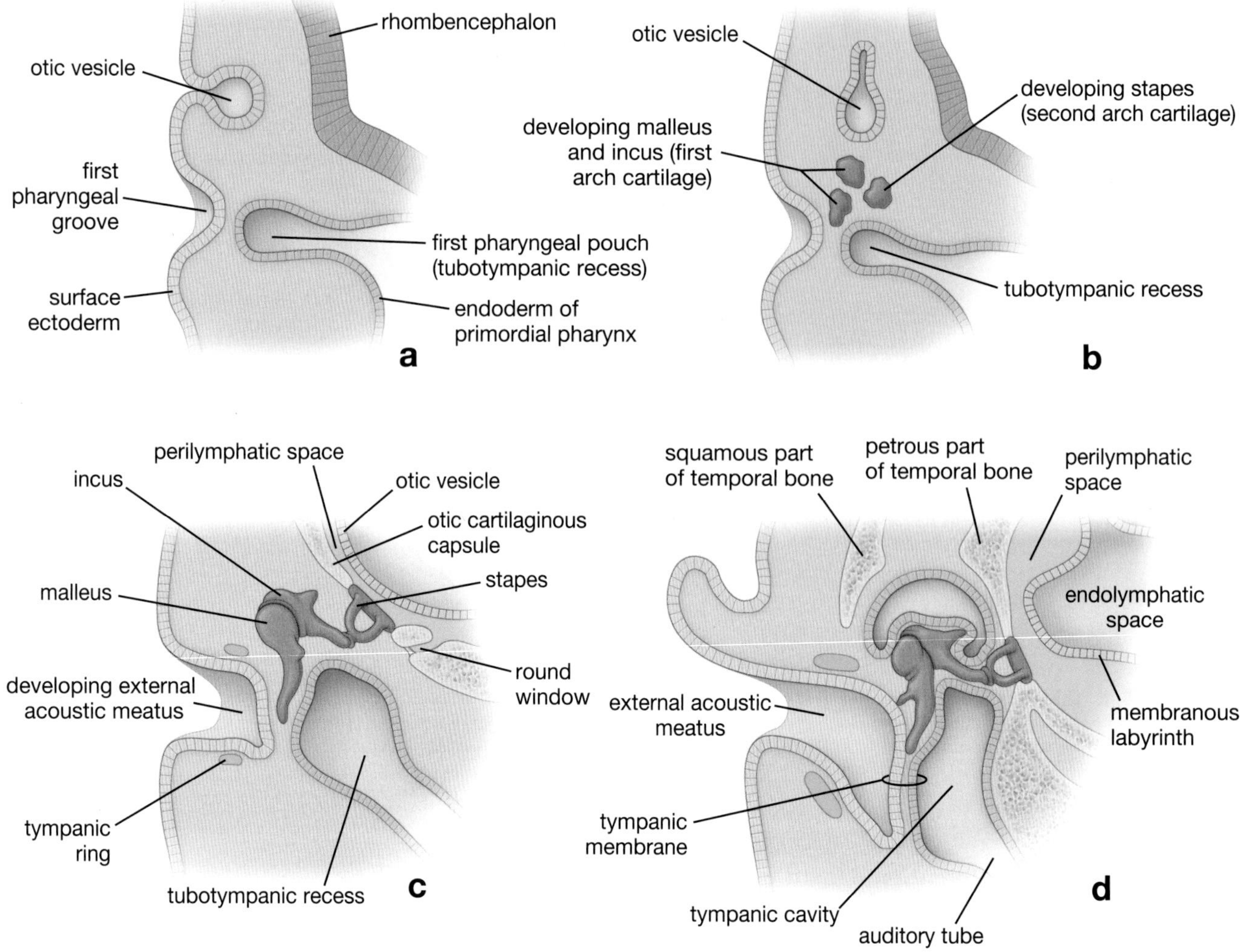

FIGURE 25.2. Schematic drawings showing development of the ear. a. This drawing shows the relationship of the surface ectoderm–derived otic vesicle to the first pharyngeal arch during the fourth week of development. **b.** The otic vesicle sinks deep into the mesenchymal tissue and develops into the membranous labyrinth. Note the development of the tubotympanic recess lined by endoderm into the future middle ear cavity and auditory tube. In addition, accumulation of mesenchyme from the first and second pharyngeal arches gives rise to the auditory ossicles. **c.** At this later stage of development, the first pharyngeal groove grows toward the developing tubotympanic recess. The auditory ossicles assume a location inside the tympanic cavity. **d.** This final stage of development shows how the tympanic membrane develops from all three germ layers: surface ectoderm, mesoderm, and endoderm. Note that the wall of the otic vesicle develops into the membranous labyrinth.

The tympanic membrane separates the external acoustic meatus from the middle ear.

The intact **tympanic membrane** is a semitransparent, thin (about 0.1 mm) membrane approximately 1 cm in diameter that has an average surface area in humans of about 65 mm^2. It is shaped like an irregular flat cone, the apex of which is located at the **umbo** that corresponds to the tip of the manubrium of the malleus. The tympanic membrane at the end of the external acoustic meatus is tilted anteriorly and inferiorly. Thus, orientation of the tympanic membrane has been compared to the position of a miniature satellite dish tuned to receive signals coming from the ground in front of the body and to the side of the head. During otoscopic examination of a normal ear, the tympanic membrane is a semitransparent light gray color and has a visible concavity toward the external acoustic meatus. Owing to its concavity, light from the otoscope reflects off the tympanic membrane as a triangular **cone of light** (light reflex) that radiates anteriorly and inferiorly from the umbo (Fig. 25.4). The malleus is one of three small auditory ossicles residing in the middle ear and is the only one that attaches to the tympanic membrane (see Fig. 25.1).

The **tympanic membrane** forms the medial boundary of the external acoustic meatus and the lateral wall of the middle ear (Fig. 25.5). From outside to inside, the three layers of the tympanic membrane are

- the skin of the external acoustic meatus (epidermis composed of stratified squamous keratinized epithelium)
- a core of connective tissue with an outer layer of radially and inner layer of circularly arranged collagen fibers, and
- the mucous membrane of the middle ear (composed of simple cuboidal epithelium).

The larger, lower part of the tympanic membrane (**tense part** or **pars tensa**) is tightly stretched and has a thick middle core that contains radial and circular collagen fibers and gives the membrane its shape and smooth appearance. The smaller, upper part of the tympanic membrane that lies superior to the lateral process of the malleolus is loose (**flaccid part** or **pars flaccida**) and lacks a prominent middle fibrous layer (see Fig. 25.4). Sound waves cause the tympanic membrane to vibrate, and these vibrations are transmitted through the ossicular chain of three small bones that link the external ear to the internal ear.

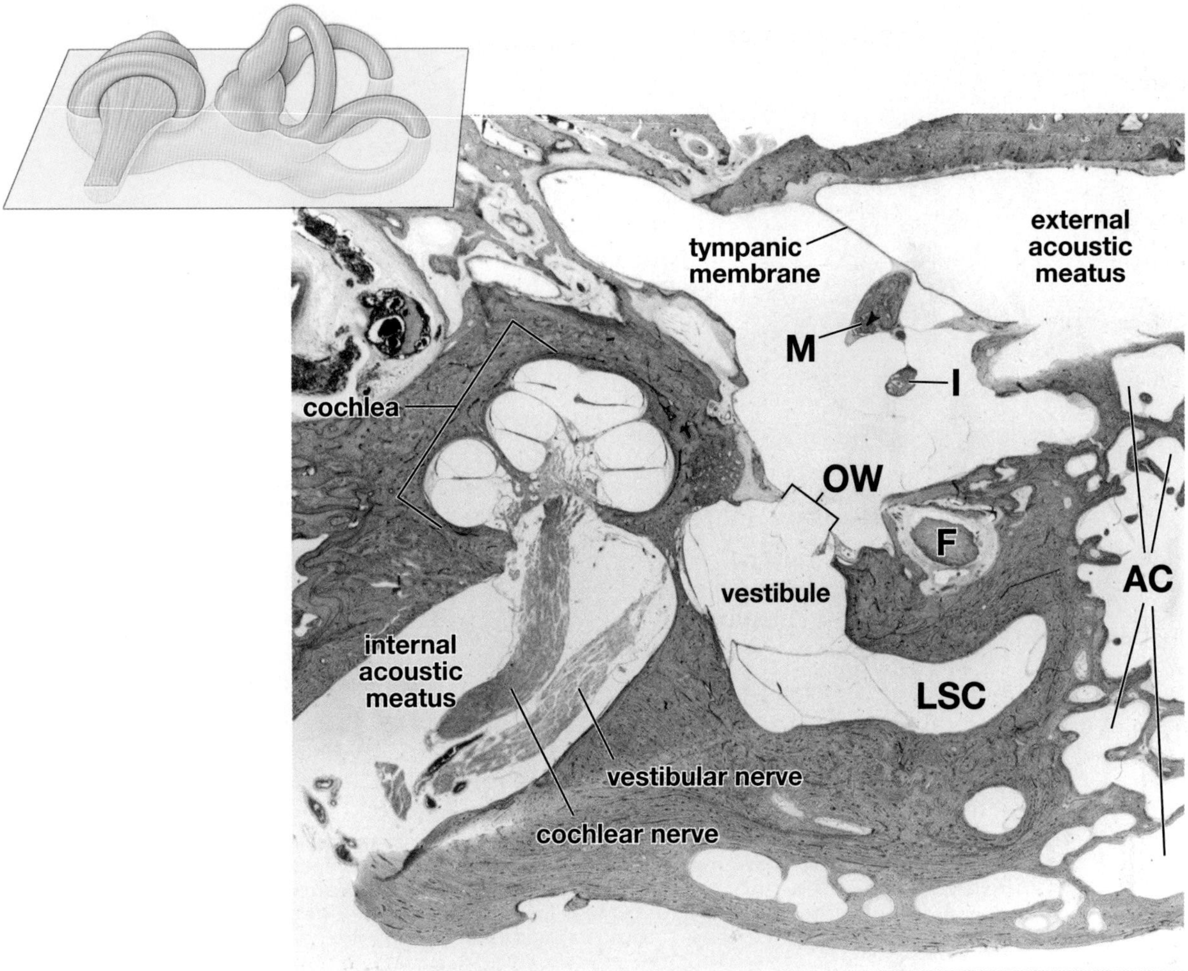

FIGURE 25.3. Horizontal section of a human temporal bone. The relationships of the three divisions of the ear within the petrous part of the temporal bone are shown. Note the orientation icon that shows the plane of section. The *tympanic membrane* separates the *external acoustic meatus* from the tympanic cavity. Within the tympanic cavity, sections of the malleus (*M*) and incus (*I*) can be seen. The posterior wall of the tympanic cavity is associated with the mastoid air cells (*AC*). The lateral wall of the cavity is formed principally by the tympanic membrane. The opening to the internal ear or oval window (*OW*) is seen in the medial wall of the cavity (the stapes has been removed). The facial nerve (*F*) can be observed near the oval window. The *cochlea*, vestibule, and a portion of the lateral semicircular canal (*LSC*) of the bony labyrinth are identified. The *cochlear* and *vestibular nerves* are divisions of cranial nerve VIII and can also be observed within the *internal acoustic meatus*. *Inset* in the upper left of the photomicrograph shows the plane of the section through the bony labyrinth. ×65.

Tympanic membrane perforations are caused by a rupture in the tympanic membrane that creates a connection between the external auditory meatus and the middle ear. This rapture can be attributed to infections, mechanical injury, or rapid changes in pressure, leading to sudden ear pain (otalgia), ear discharge (otorrhea), ringing in the ears (tinnitus), and a sensation of feeling off-balance (vertigo). Most perforations resolve spontaneously without complications; however, some may cause transient or permanent **hearing impairment**.

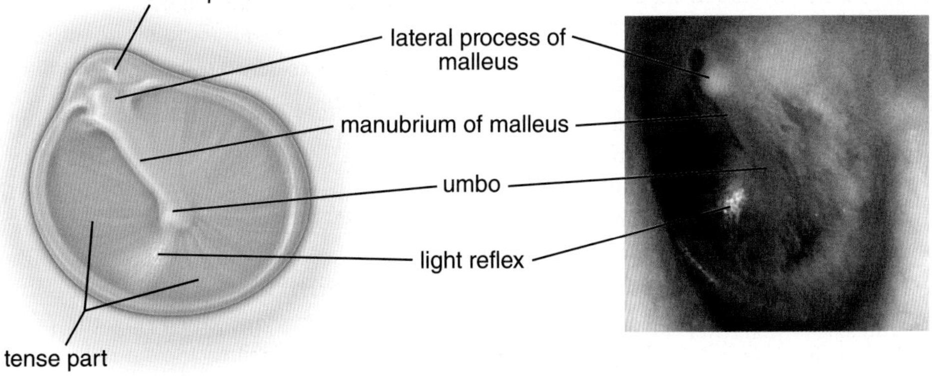

FIGURE 25.4. The tympanic membrane in otoscopic examination of the external ear. This diagram and photograph show the left tympanic membrane seen with an otoscope during examination of the external acoustic meatus. The landmarks of the tympanic membrane include the manubrium of the malleus with its visible attachment to the tense part of the membrane, umbo at the tip of the manubrium, and projecting lateral process of the malleus. A small, flaccid part of the tympanic membrane is located above the lateral process of the malleolus. Note the cone of light (light reflex) that is usually seen extending anteroinferiorly from the umbo of the tympanic membrane. (Courtesy of Dr. Eric J. Moore.)

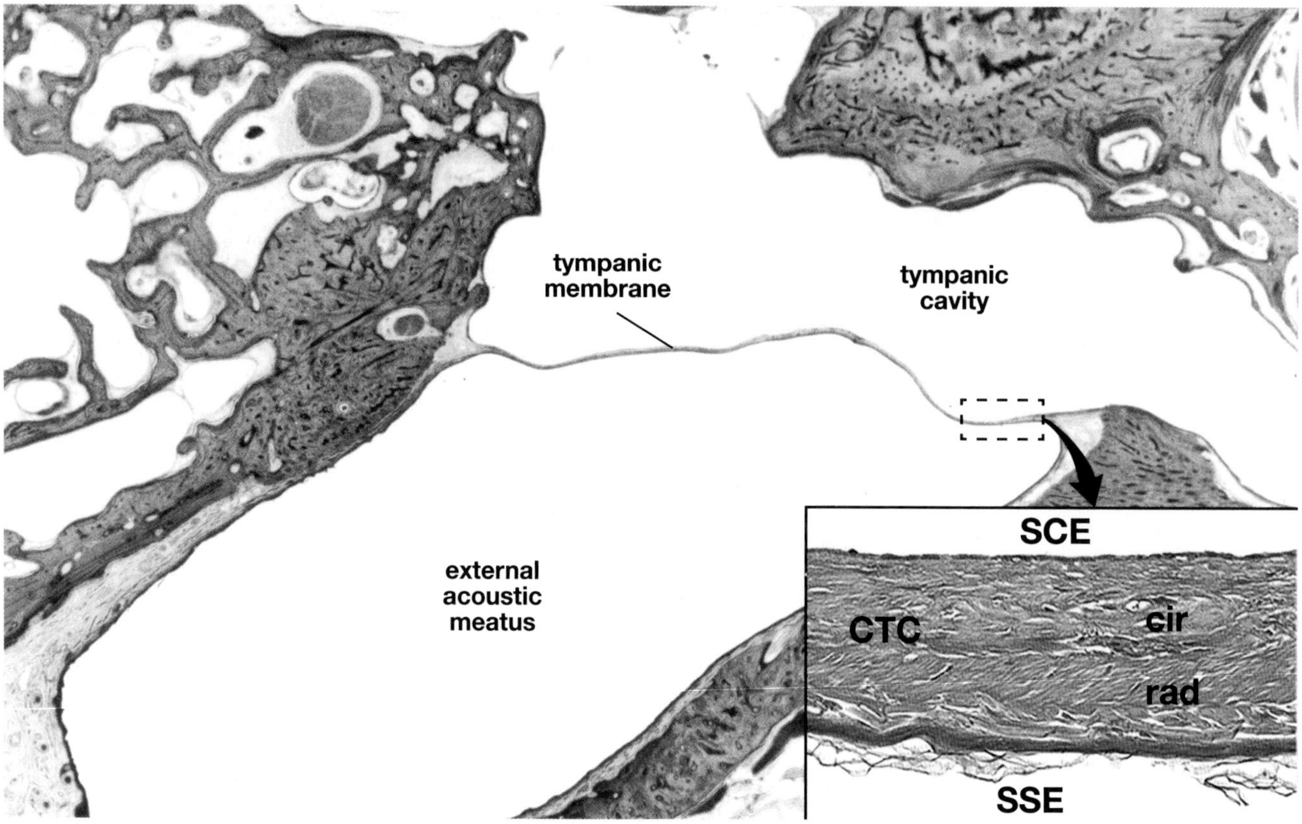

FIGURE 25.5. Cross section through a human tympanic membrane. This photomicrograph shows the *tympanic membrane, external acoustic meatus,* and *tympanic cavity.* ×9. **Inset.** Higher magnification of the tympanic membrane. The outer epithelial layer of the membrane consists of stratified squamous keratinized epithelium (*SSE*), and the inner epithelial layer of the mucous membrane consists of low simple cuboidal epithelium (*SCE*). A middle layer of connective tissue core (*CTC*) lies between the two epithelial layers. The dense irregular connective tissue core is formed by two layers: the outer layer in which fibers are radially arranged (*rad*) and the inner layer with circumferentially arranged fibers (*cir*). ×190.

The auditory ossicles connect the tympanic membrane to the oval window.

The **three auditory ossicles** or bones—the malleus, the incus, and the stapes—cross the space of the middle ear in series and connect the tympanic membrane to the oval window (Fig. 25.6). These bones work like a lever system that increases the force transmitted from the vibrating tympanic membrane to the stapes by decreasing the ratio of their oscillation amplitudes. The ossicles help convert sound waves to mechanical vibrations (hydraulic waves) in tissues and fluid-filled chambers. Movable synovial joints connect the bones, which are named according to their approximate shape:

- The **malleus (hammer)** attaches to the tympanic membrane and articulates with the incus.
- The **incus (anvil)** is the largest of the ossicles and links the malleus to the stapes.
- The **stapes (stirrup)**, the footplate of which fits into the oval window. The footplate in the human stapes measures approximately 3 mm × 1 mm and has an average surface area of 3 mm^2. It acts like a small piston on the cochlear fluid, creating hydraulic waves to represent the air-pressure fluctuations of the sound wave.

Diseases that affect the external acoustic meatus, tympanic membrane, or ossicles are responsible for **conductive hearing loss** (see Folders 25.1 and 25.2).

Two muscles attach to the ossicles and affect their movement.

The **tensor tympani muscle** lies in a bony canal above the auditory tube; its tendon inserts on the malleus. Contraction of this muscle increases tension on the tympanic membrane. The **stapedius muscle** lies in a bony eminence on the posterior wall of the middle ear; its tendon inserts on the stapes. Contraction of the stapedius tends to dampen the movement of the stapes at the oval window. The stapedius is only a few millimeters long and is the smallest skeletal muscle.

The two muscles of the middle ear are responsible for a protective reflex called the **attenuation reflex** or **acoustic reflex**. In response to intense sound, involuntary contraction of the muscles makes the chain of ossicles more rigid, thus reducing the transmission of vibrations to the internal ear. The muscles will contract on both sides, regardless of which ear is stimulated. This reflex protects the internal ear from the damaging effects of very loud sounds. In certain conditions, such as impulse noise (i.e., fireworks or gun fire), the attenuation reflex is ineffective.

The auditory tube connects the middle ear to the nasopharynx.

The **auditory (Eustachian) tube** is a narrow flattened channel approximately 3.5 cm long. This tube is lined with ciliated pseudostratified columnar epithelium, about one-fifth of which is composed of goblet cells. It vents the middle ear to nasopharynx, equalizing the pressure of the middle ear with atmospheric pressure. In addition, the auditory tube is responsible for draining the secretion produced by the mucous membrane of the middle ear towards the nasopharynx with the aid of the ciliated pseudostratified columnar epithelium. The auditory tube is normally closed; its walls are pressed together but they separate during yawning, chewing, swallowing, and when individual holds the nose

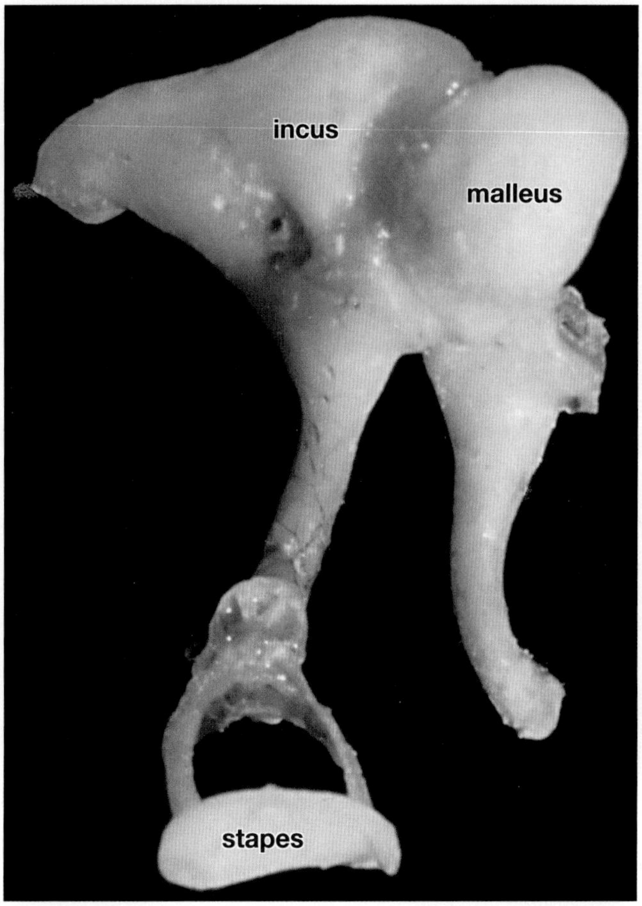

FIGURE 25.6. Photograph of the three articulated human auditory ossicles. The three ossicles are the malleus, the incus, and the stapes. ×30.

and blows. Children are more vulnerable to the middle ear infections, due to the immature development of their auditory tubes which are shorter, narrower, and more horizontal than in the adults. It is common for infections to spread from the pharynx to the middle ear via the auditory tube (causing **otitis media**). A small mass of lymphatic tissue, the **tubal tonsil**, is often found at the pharyngeal orifice of the auditory tube.

The mastoid air cells extend from the middle ear into the temporal bone.

A system of **air cells** projects into the mastoid portion of the temporal bone from the middle ear. The epithelial lining of these air cells is continuous with that of the tympanic cavity and rests on periosteum. This continuity allows infections in the middle ear to spread into **mastoid air cells**, causing **mastoiditis**. Before the development of antibiotics, repeated episodes of otitis media and mastoiditis usually led to deafness.

The middle ear contributes to the amplification of mechanical forces generated by the vibration of the tympanic membrane.

All three ossicles in the tympanic cavity are involved in the **amplification of the mechanical force** that vibrates the tympanic membrane in two ways:

- The main amplification comes from **differences in the surface area** between the tympanic membrane and the footplate of the stapes. The **tympanic membrane** has a surface area of approximately **65 mm²**, whereas the footplate of the **stapes** has a surface area of about **3 mm²**. Sound waves apply force to every square millimeter of the tympanic membrane, and this energy is transferred via the chain of ossicles to the much smaller area of the footplate. Therefore, the pressure applied to the cochlear fluid by the footplate is **about 22 times** the pressure applied to the tympanic membrane (Fig. 25.7).
- Additional amplification comes from the arrangement of **auditory ossicles** that act as **levers** that multiply the mechanical force applied to the stapes. Because the pivot point of the ossicle chain is located farther from the tympanic membrane than from the stapes, the amplification of the mechanical force at the oval window is increased by a factor of **approximately 1.3**. This lever system is adjustable by the action of muscles in the tympanic cavity and may attenuate loud sounds to protect the ear (see Fig. 25.7).

Under normal conditions, the acoustic energy entering the ear is amplified **approximately 60 times**, allowing humans to detect frequencies between 2,000 and 5,000 Hz. The degree of amplification is calculated by multiplying the amplification factors contributed by the external acoustic meatus (~2 times) as described earlier on pages 1018-1019, the surface area differences between the tympanic membrane and the footplate of stapes (~22 times), and the basic lever action of ossicles (~1.3 times). However, this calculation ($2 \times 22 \times 1.3 = 57.2$) must be used with caution owing to variability in the mechanical function of the middle ear and its components, such as ossicular joints, ligaments, muscles, and air volumes, as well as varying frequencies of sound.

■ INTERNAL EAR

The internal ear consists of two labyrinthine compartments, one contained within the other.

The **bony labyrinth** is a complex system of interconnected cavities and canals in the petrous part of the temporal bone. The **membranous labyrinth** lies within the bony labyrinth and consists of a complex system of small sacs and tubules that also form a continuous space enclosed within a wall of epithelium and connective tissue.

There are three fluid-filled spaces in the internal ear:

- **Endolymphatic spaces** are contained within the membranous labyrinth. The **endolymph** of the membranous labyrinth is similar in composition to **intracellular fluid** (it has a high K^+ concentration and a low Na^+ concentration). The endolymph is produced in the stria vascularis, a specialized area of the cochlear duct (see pages 1032-1034). It drains via the endolymphatic duct to the endolymphatic sac, which terminates in the epidural space of the posterior cranial fossa.
- The **perilymphatic space** lies between the wall of the bony labyrinth and the wall of the membranous labyrinth. The **perilymph** is similar in composition to **extracellular fluid** and **cerebrospinal fluid** (it has a low K^+ concentration and a high Na^+ concentration). Perilymph is produced as

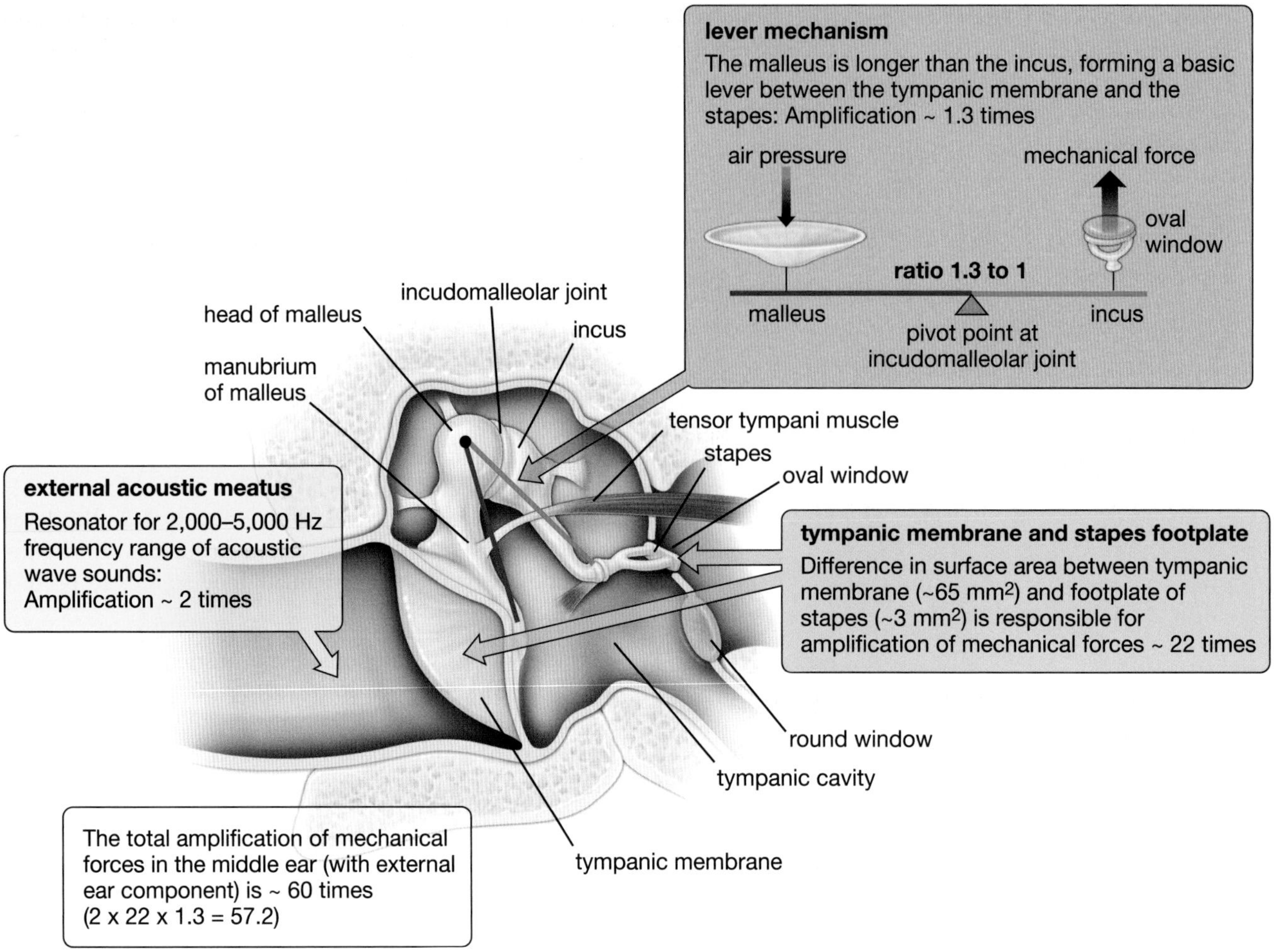

FIGURE 25.7. Summary of amplification of sound entering the ear. This drawing shows the external and middle ear structures and their contributions to the amplification of sound entering the ear. Note that the largest amplification comes from the difference in the surface area between the tympanic membrane (65 mm^2) and the footplate of the stapes (3 mm^2). This surface area difference results in ~22 times the amplification of the pressure applied by the footplate of the stapes. Another source of amplification comes from the external acoustic meatus and middle ear. The external acoustic meatus acts as a resonator that increases the sound pressure acting on the tympanic membrane by ~2 times. Finally, the arrangement of auditory ossicles resembles a basic lever that multiplies the applied mechanical force acting on the footplate of the stapes by ~1.3 times. By multiplying these three amplification factors, the acoustic energy entering the ear is amplified ~60 times.

FOLDER 25.1

CLINICAL CORRELATION: OTOSCLEROSIS

Otosclerosis is one of the most common causes of acquired hearing loss. It is reported that ~13% of the U.S. population has nonclinical otosclerosis (histologic otosclerosis); however, the incidence of clinical disease ranges from 0.5% to 1.0%. Individuals with clinical otosclerosis have progressive hearing loss. Symptoms usually become apparent between ages 20 and 45 years. Otosclerosis is characterized by the abnormal overgrowth of bone that uniquely affects the temporal bone and ossicles. Although the cause of bone overgrowth in otosclerosis is unknown, recent studies suggest an association with measles virus infection. In otosclerosis, mature bone in the area of the oval window on the medial wall of the tympanic cavity, which separates the middle ear from the internal ear, is removed by osteoclasts and replaced with much thicker immature (woven) bone. Because the footplate of the stapes normally resides and freely vibrates within the oval window to allow the transmission of sound into the internal ear, bone remodeling in this area results in fixation of the stapes into the surrounding bone. The "frozen" stapes cannot vibrate, which prevents sound waves from reaching the perilymphatic fluid space of the internal ear and causes conductive hearing loss. Treatment of otosclerosis includes several options: pharmacologic treatment to suppress bone remodeling with fluorides and bisphosphonates, amplification of sounds with hearing aids, and surgical removal of the stapes (**stapedectomy**) with subsequent implantation of a prosthesis between the incus and the oval window. Surgery is usually the most effective method of managing otosclerosis; >90% of patients experience a complete reversal of their hearing loss.

an ultrafiltrate from the periosteal microvasculature within the bony labyrinth. It drains via a narrow channel within the temporal bone, called the *cochlear aqueduct*, directly into the cerebrospinal fluid contained within the subarachnoid space of the cranial cavity.
- The **cortilymphatic space** lies within the tunnels of the organ of Corti of the cochlea. It is a true intercellular space. The cells surrounding the space loosely resemble an absorptive epithelium. The cortilymphatic space is filled with **cortilymph**, which has a composition similar to that of **extracellular fluid**.

Structures of the Bony Labyrinth

The bony labyrinth consists of three connected spaces within the temporal bone.

The three spaces of the bony labyrinth, as illustrated in Figure 25.8, are the

- **semicircular canals**,
- **vestibule**, and
- **cochlea**.

The vestibule is the central space that contains the utricle and saccule of the membranous labyrinth.

The **vestibule** is the small oval chamber located in the center of the bony labyrinth. The **utricle** and **saccule** of the membranous labyrinth lie in elliptical and spherical recesses, respectively. The **semicircular canals** extend from the vestibule posteriorly, and the **cochlea** extends from the vestibule anteriorly. The oval window into which the footplate of the stapes inserts lies in the lateral wall of the vestibule.

The semicircular canals are tubes within the temporal bone that lie at right angles to each other.

Three semicircular canals, each forming about three-quarters of a circle, extend from the wall of the vestibule and return to it. The semicircular canals are identified as anterior, posterior, and lateral and lie within the temporal bone at approximately right angles to each other. They occupy three planes in space—sagittal, frontal, and horizontal. The end of each semicircular canal closest to the vestibule is expanded to form the **ampulla** (Fig. 25.9a and b). The three canals open into the vestibule through five orifices; the anterior and posterior semicircular canals join at one end to form the **common bony limb** (see Fig. 25.9a).

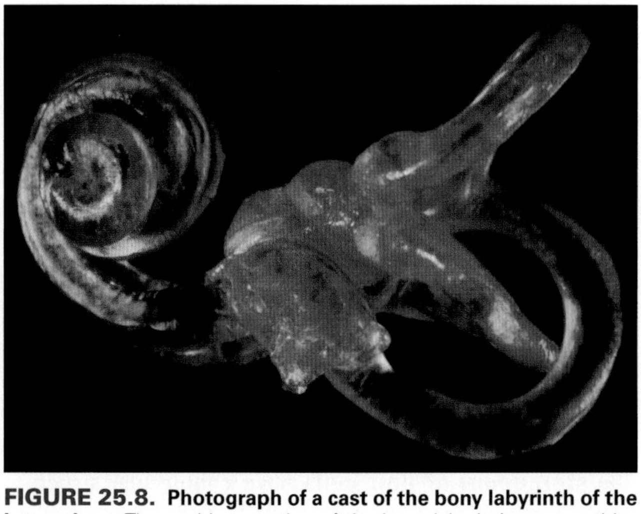

FIGURE 25.8. Photograph of a cast of the bony labyrinth of the internal ear. The cochlear portion of the bony labyrinth appears *blue green*; the vestibule and semicircular canals appear *orange red*. (Courtesy of Dr. Merle Lawrence.)

The cochlea is a cone-shaped helix connected to the vestibule.

The spiral lumen of the **cochlea**, called the **cochlear canal** (like the semicircular canals), is continuous with that of the vestibule. It connects to the vestibule via two openings, the **round window** and the **oval window**, both of which are located on the side opposite the openings of the semicircular canals. Between its base and the apex, the cochlear canal makes approximately 2.75 turns around a central core of spongy bone called the **modiolus** (Plate 25.1, page 1042). A sensory ganglion, the **spiral ganglion**, lies in the modiolus. A thin membrane (the secondary tympanic membrane) covers the round window, whereas the footplate of the stapes is positioned within the oval window. These two openings are located at the base of the cochlear canal.

Structures of the Membranous Labyrinth

The membranous labyrinth contains the endolymph and is suspended within the bony labyrinth.

The **membranous labyrinth** consists of a series of communicating sacs and ducts containing endolymph. It is suspended within the bony labyrinth (Fig. 25.9c), and the remaining space is filled with perilymph. The membranous labyrinth is composed of two divisions: the **cochlear labyrinth** and the **vestibular labyrinth** (Fig. 25.9d).

The vestibular labyrinth contains the following:

- Three **semicircular ducts** lie within the semicircular canals and are continuous with the utricle.
- The **utricle** and the **saccule**, which are contained in recesses in the vestibule, are connected by the membranous **utriculosaccular duct**.

The cochlear labyrinth contains the **cochlear duct**, which is contained within the cochlea and is continuous with the saccule (see Fig. 25.9c and d).

Sensory cells of the membranous labyrinth

Specialized sensory cells are located in six regions in the membranous labyrinth.

Six sensory regions of membranous labyrinth are composed of sensory **hair cells** and accessory **supporting cells**. These regions project from the wall of the membranous labyrinth into the endolymphatic space in each internal ear (see Fig. 25.9d):

- Three **cristae ampullares (ampullary crests)** are located in the membranous ampullae of the semicircular

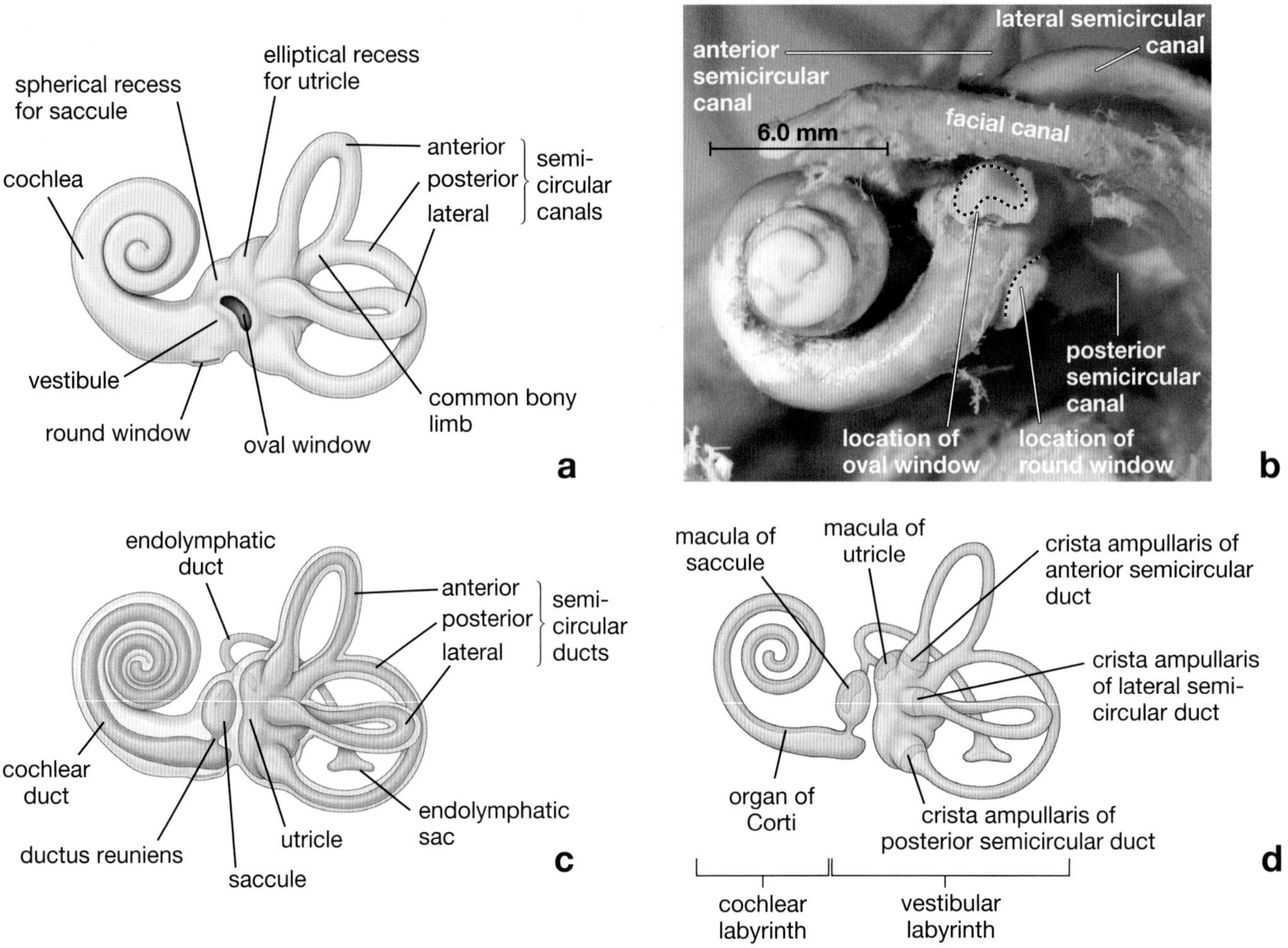

FIGURE 25.9. Diagrams and photograph of the human internal ear. a. This lateral view of the left bony labyrinth shows its divisions: the vestibule, cochlea, and three semicircular canals. The openings of the oval window and the round window can be observed. **b.** This photograph of a cast obtained by injection of polyester resin into the human internal ear shows an authentic shape of the bony labyrinth. Note that the cast material is pouring out of the cochlea through the oval and round windows. Also, in this image, the cast of the facial canal that contains the facial nerve is visible. ×5. (Courtesy of Dr. Elsa Erixon.) **c.** Diagram of a membranous labyrinth of the internal ear lying within the bony labyrinth. The cochlear duct can be seen spiraling within the bony cochlea. The saccule and utricle are positioned within the vestibule, and the three semicircular ducts are lying within their respective canals. This view of the left membranous labyrinth allows the endolymphatic duct and sac to be observed. **d.** This view of the left membranous labyrinth shows the sensory regions of the internal ear for equilibrium and hearing. These regions are the macula of the saccule and macula of the utricle, the cristae ampullares of the three semicircular ducts, and the spiral organ of Corti of the cochlear duct.

ducts. They are sensitive to the angular acceleration of the head (i.e., turning the head).

- Two maculae, one in the utricle (**macula of utricle**) and the other in the saccule (**macula of saccule**), sense the position of the head and its linear movement.
- The **spiral organ of Corti** projects into the endolymph of the cochlear duct. It functions as a sound receptor.

Hair cells are epithelial mechanoreceptors of the vestibular and cochlear labyrinth.

The **hair cells** of the vestibular and cochlear labyrinths function as **mechanoelectrical transducers**; they convert mechanical energy into electrical energy that is then transmitted via the vestibulocochlear nerve to the brain. The hair cells derive their name from the organized bundle of rigid projections at their apical surface. This surface holds a **hair bundle** that is formed by rows of stereocilia called *sensory hairs*. The rows increase in height in one particular direction across the bundle (Fig. 25.10). In the vestibular system, each hair cell possesses a single true cilium called a **kinocilium**, which is located behind the row of longest stereocilia (Fig. 25.11). In the auditory system, the hair cells lose their cilium during development but retain the **basal body**. The position of the kinocilium (or basal body) behind the longest row of stereocilia defines the polarity of this asymmetric hair bundle. Therefore, movement of the stereocilia toward the kinocilium is perceived differently than movement in the opposite direction (see later).

Stereocilia of hair cells are rigid structures that contain mechanoelectrical transducer channel proteins at their distal ends.

The **stereocilia of hair cells** have a molecular structure similar to those described on pages 127-128. Tightly packed **actin filaments** cross-linked by **fimbrin** and **espin** (actin-bundling proteins) form their internal core structure.

Espins provide the most rigid cross-linking for stereocilia; mutations that alter their structure cause cochlear and vestibular dysfunction. The high density of actin filaments and the extensive cross-linking pattern impart rigidity and stiffness to the shaft of the stereocilium. The shaft tapers at its proximal end near the apical surface of the cell, where the core filaments of each stereocilium are anchored within the terminal web (cuticular plate). When stereocilia are deflected, they pivot at their proximal ends like stiff rods (see Fig. 25.11).

Transmission electron microscope examination of the distal free end of the stereocilium reveals an electron-dense plaque at the cytoplasmic site of the plasma membrane. This plaque represents the **mechanoelectrical transducer (MET) channel complex**. A fibrillar cross-link called the **tip link** connects the tip of the stereocilium with the shaft of an adjacent longer stereocilium (see Fig. 25.11). These tip links are anchored to mechanically gated ion channels on both ends. The upper insertion of the tip link to the shaft of neighboring stereocilium contains a cluster of motor proteins (unconventional myosin VIIa) that maintains a resting tension on the tip link. The lower insertion to the distal free end of the stereocilium is connected to the MET channel complex. The tip link is composed of **cadherin-23** (CDH23) and **protocadherin-15** (PCDH15); however, the molecular composition of the MET channel complex remains elusive. Recently, two transmembrane channel-like (TMC) proteins, TMC1 and TMC2, have been identified in the MET channels that are expressed in developing hair cells. Mutations in the genes encoding TMC1 cause **deafness** in humans.

The tip link plays an important role in activating the MET channel complex at the tip of the stereocilia and opening additional transduction K^+ channels at the site of its attachment to the shaft of neighboring stereocilium (see Fig. 25.11). The molecular structure of the transduction K^+ channels is unknown.

A mutation that disrupts the gene that encodes the actin-bundling protein **espin** causes cochlear and vestibular symptoms in experimental mice. They lose their hearing early in life; these animals also spend most of their time walking or spinning in circles. The stereocilia of these animals do not maintain the rigidity necessary for the proper functioning of the **MET channels**. In humans,

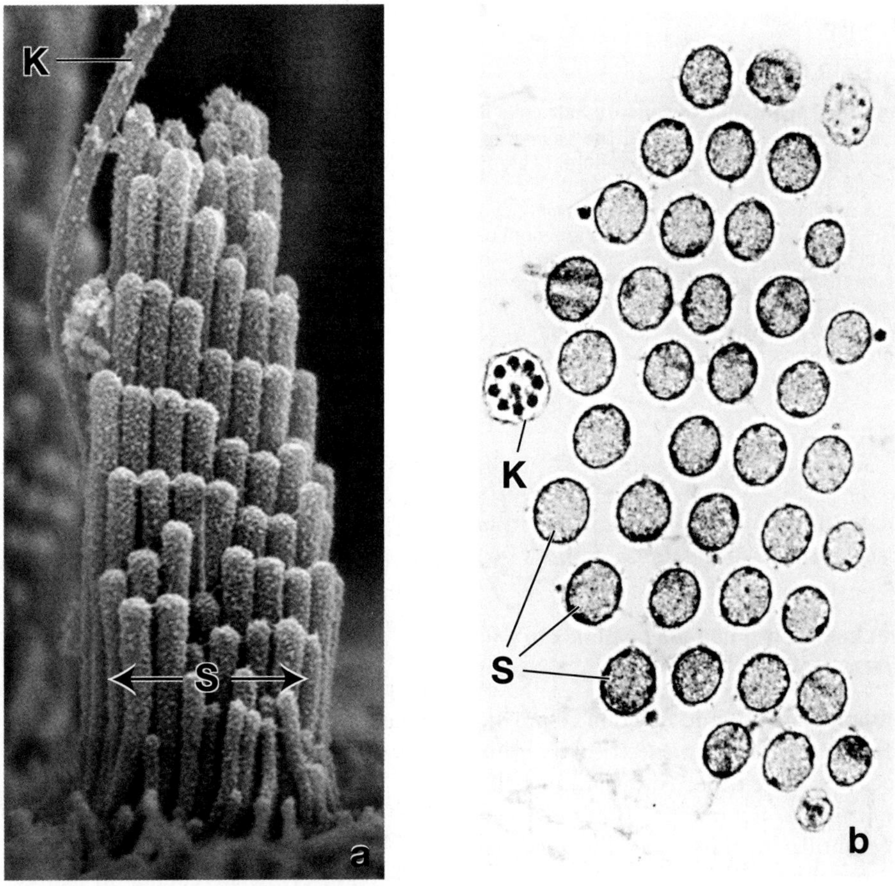

FIGURE 25.10. Electron micrographs of the kinocilium and stereocilia of a vestibular sensory hair cell. a. Scanning electron micrograph of the apical surface of a sensory hair cell from the macula of the utricle. Note the relationship of the kinocilium (*K*) to the stereocilia (*S*). ×47,500. **b.** Transmission electron micrograph of the kinocilium (*K*) and stereocilia (*S*) of a vestibular hair cell in cross section. The kinocilium has a larger diameter than the stereocilia. ×47,500. (**a.** Reprinted with permission from Rzadzinska AK, Schneider ME, Davies C, et al. An actin molecular treadmill and myosins maintain stereocilia functional architecture and self-renewal. *J Cell Biol.* 2004;164:887–897. **b.** Reprinted with permission from Hunter-Duvar IM, Hinojosa R. Vestibule: sensory epithelia. In: Friedmann I, Ballantyne J, eds. *Ultrastructural Atlas of the Inner Ear.* Butterworth; 1984.)

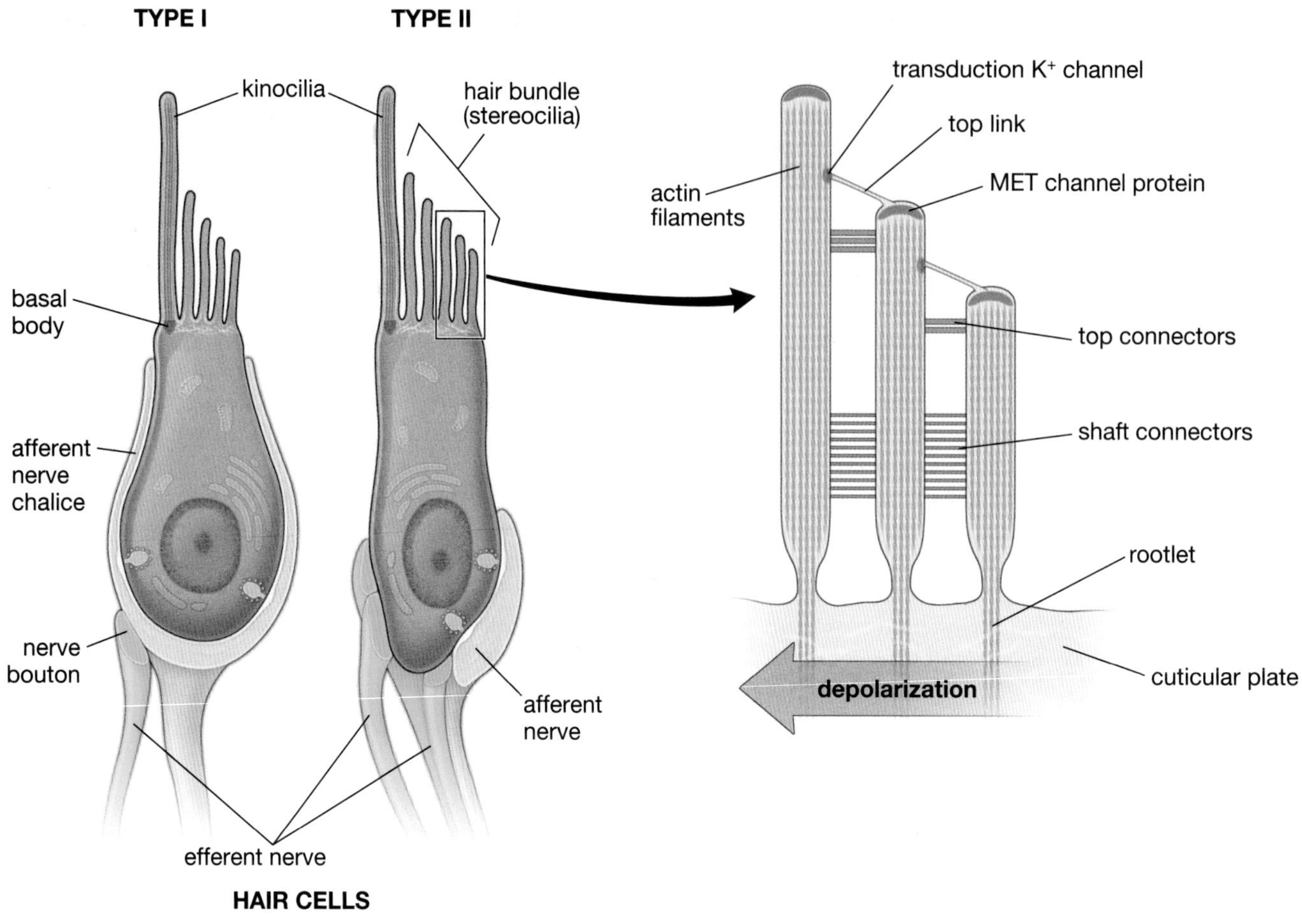

FIGURE 25.11. Diagram of two types of sensory hair cells in the sensory areas of the membranous labyrinth. The type I hair cell has a flask-shaped structure with a rounded base. The base is enclosed in a chalice-like afferent nerve ending containing several ribbon synapses in addition to several synaptic boutons for efferent nerve endings. Note the apical surface specializations of this cell, which include a kinocilium and hair bundle. The apical cytoplasm of hair cells contains basal bodies for the attachment of the kinocilium and a terminal web for the attachment of stereocilia. The type II hair cell is cylindrical and possesses several nerve terminals at its base for both afferent and efferent nerve fibers. The apical surface specializations are identical to those of the type I cell. The molecular organization of the stereocilia is depicted in the diagram on the *right*. The top link connects the lateral plasma membrane of the stereocilium shaft (where K^+ transduction channels are located) with the tip of the shorter stereocilium (where the mechanoelectrical transduction [*MET*] channel protein is located). Movement of the stereocilia toward the kinocilium opens the *MET* channels, causing depolarization of the hair cell, whereas movement in the opposite direction (away from the kinocilium) causes hyperpolarization. Note that the proximal end of each stereocilium is tapered and its narrow rootlets are anchored within the terminal web (cuticular plate) of the hair cell. Several other fibrillar connectors between neighboring stereocilia are also shown.

mutations in a gene located on chromosome 1 that encodes espin are associated with deafness without vestibular involvement.

All hair cells use mechanically gated ion channels to generate action potentials.

All hair cells of the internal ear appear to function by moving (pivoting) their rigid stereocilia. Mechanoelectrical transduction occurs in stereocilia that are deflected toward its tallest edge (toward the kinocilium, if present). This movement exerts tension on the fibrillar tip links, and the generated force is used to open **mechanically gated ion channels** near the tip of the stereocilium. This allows for an influx of K^+, causing depolarization of the receptor cell. This depolarization results in the opening of voltage-gated Ca^{2+} channels in the basolateral surface of the hair cells and the secretion of a neurotransmitter that generates an action potential in afferent nerve endings. Movement in the opposite direction (away from the kinocilium) closes the MET channels, causing hyperpolarization of the receptor cell. The means by which stereocilia are deflected varies from receptor to receptor; these are discussed in the sections describing each receptor area.

Hair cells communicate with afferent nerve fibers through ribbon synapses, a specialized type of chemical synapse.

Deflection of the stereocilia on hair cells generates a high rate of prolonged impulses that are quickly transmitted to the afferent nerve fibers. To ensure rapid release of the glutamate neurotransmitter from synaptic vesicles, hair cells possess specialized **ribbon synapses** that contain unique organelles called **ribbons**. In electron microscopy, ribbons appear as ovoid, 30-nm-thick, electron-dense plates that are anchored to the presynaptic membrane by electron-dense structures (Fig. 25.12). This arrangement allows the ribbons to float just above the presynaptic plate like balloons on a short leash. The ribbons tether a large number of synaptic vesicles on their surface that are primed for fusion with the presynaptic membrane, which contains a high density of voltage-gated Ca^{2+} channels (see Fig. 25.12). After activation of the Ca^{2+} channels, the ribbon serves as a fast-moving conveyor belt, delivering the vesicles to the presynaptic membrane for fusion. The tethered pool of synaptic vesicles is approximately fivefold greater than the pool of the remaining vesicles. The ribbons contain several proteins, including the active-zone protein RIM that interacts with rab3, a GTPase enzyme expressed on the surface of synaptic vesicles. Other proteins of the ribbon complex include presynaptic matrix proteins, such as RIBEYE, Bassoon, and Piccolo. A hair cell typically contains about 10–20 ribbons. These ribbon synapses are also found in the photoreceptors and bipolar cells of the retina.

Two types of hair cells are present in the vestibular labyrinth.

Both **hair cell** types are associated with **afferent** and **efferent nerve endings** (see Fig. 25.11). **Type I hair cells** are flask shaped, with a rounded base and thin neck, and are surrounded by an afferent nerve chalice and a few efferent nerve fibers. **Type II hair cells** are cylindrical and have afferent and efferent bouton nerve endings at the base of the cell (see Fig. 25.11).

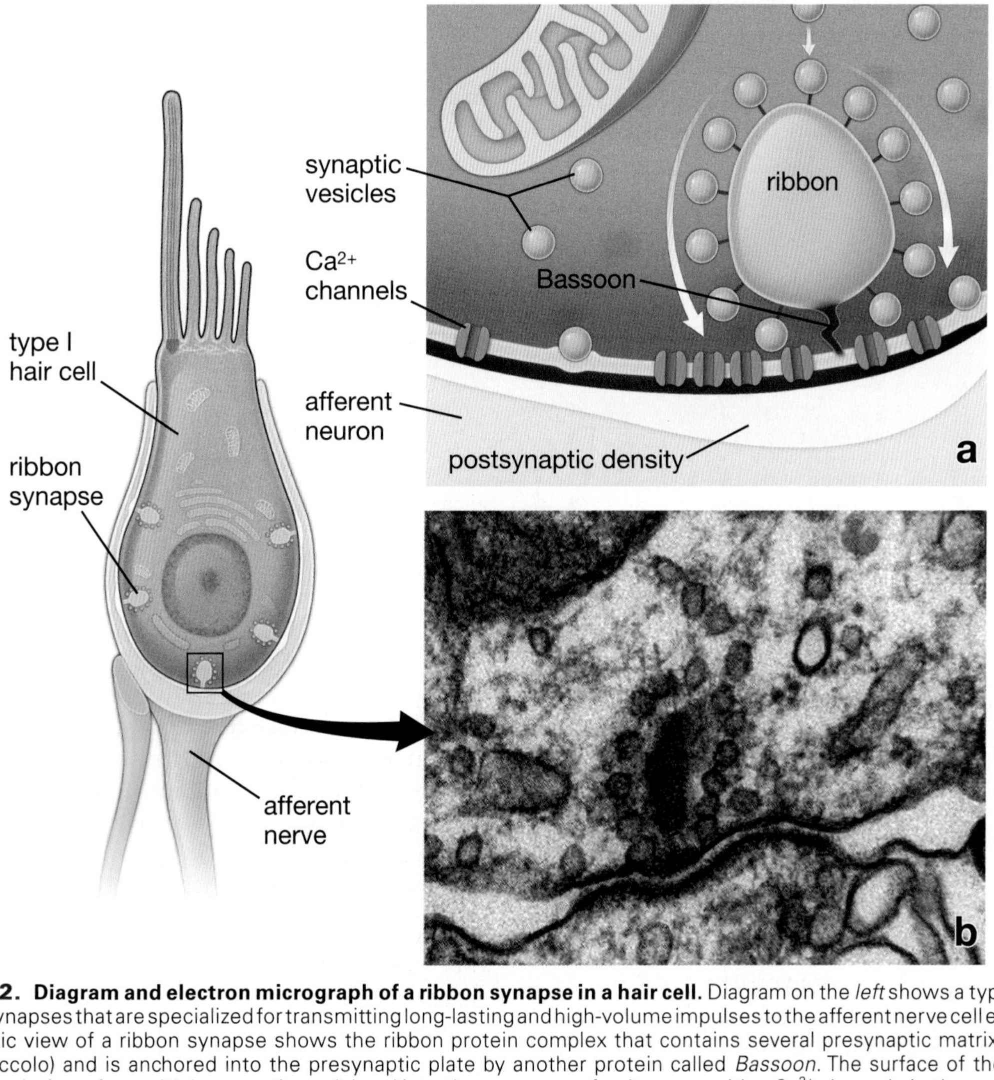

FIGURE 25.12. Diagram and electron micrograph of a ribbon synapse in a hair cell. Diagram on the *left* shows a type I hair cell with several ribbon synapses that are specialized for transmitting long-lasting and high-volume impulses to the afferent nerve cell endings (*yellow*). **a.** This schematic view of a ribbon synapse shows the ribbon protein complex that contains several presynaptic matrix proteins (RIM, RIBEYE, and Piccolo) and is anchored into the presynaptic plate by another protein called *Bassoon*. The surface of the ribbon serves as the tethering platform for multiple synaptic vesicles. Note the presence of voltage-sensitive Ca^{2+} channels in the presynaptic membrane next to the attachment of the ribbon. Upon influx of Ca^{2+}, the ribbon accelerates movement of the attached vesicles toward the presynaptic membrane for fusion (similar to the action of a fast-moving conveyor belt). **b.** This electron micrograph of a ribbon synapse from a mouse cochlear hair cell shows the ribbon protein complex with attached synaptic vesicles. ×27,400. (Reprinted with permission from Neef A, Khimich D, Pirih P, et al. Probing the mechanism of exocytosis at the hair cell ribbon synapse. *J Neurosci.* 2007;27:12933–12944.)

Sensory receptors of the membranous labyrinth

The crista ampullaris senses angular movements of the head.

Each ampulla of the semicircular duct contains a **crista ampullaris**, which is a sensory receptor for angular movements of the head (Figs. 25.13 and 25.14). The crista ampullaris is a thickened transverse epithelial ridge that is oriented perpendicularly to the long axis of the semicircular canal and consists of the epithelial hair cells and supporting cells (Plate 25.1, page 1042).

A gelatinous protein–polysaccharide mass, known as the **cupula**, is attached to the hair cells of each crista (see Fig. 25.13). The cupula projects into the lumen and is surrounded by endolymph. During rotational movement of the head, the walls of the semicircular canal and the membranous semicircular ducts move, but the endolymph contained within the ducts tends to lag behind because of inertia. The cupula, projecting into the endolymph, is swayed by the movement differential between the crista fixed to the wall of the duct and the endolymph. Deflection of the stereocilia in the narrow space between the hair cells and the cupula generates nerve impulses in the associated nerve endings.

The maculae of the saccule and utricle are sensors of gravity and linear acceleration.

The **maculae** of the saccule and utricle are innervated sensory thickenings of the epithelium that face the endolymph of the saccule and utricle (see Figs. 25.14 and 25.15). As in the cristae, each macula consists of **type I** and **type II hair cells**, supporting cells, and nerve endings associated with the hair cells. The maculae of the utricle and saccule are oriented at right angles to each another. When a person is standing, the macula of the utricle is in a horizontal plane and the macula of the saccule is in a vertical plane.

Hair cells are polarized with respect to the **striola**, an imaginary plane that curves through the center of each macula (see Fig. 25.15). On each side of the striola, the kinocilia of the hair cells are oriented in opposite directions, facing toward the striola in the utricle and turning away from the striola in the saccule. Owing to polarization of the hair cells, the maculae of the saccule and utricle are sensitive to multiple directions of linear accelerations.

The gelatinous polysaccharide material that overlies the maculae is called the **otolithic membrane** (see Fig. 25.15). Its outer surface contains 3- to 5-μm crystalline bodies of calcium carbonate and a protein (Fig. 25.16). **Otoliths**, also

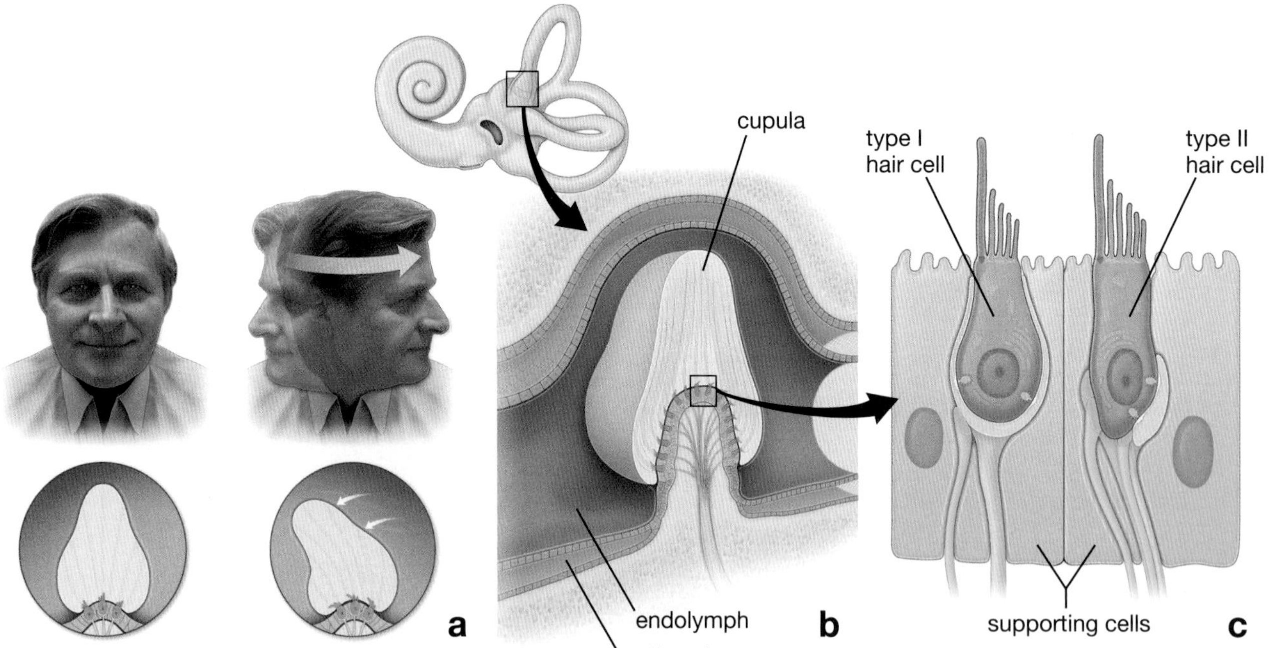

FIGURE 25.13. Diagram of function and structure of the crista ampullaris within a semicircular duct. a. As shown in this drawing, the crista ampullaris functions as the sensor for angular movement of the head. For example, when the head of the individual shown in this diagram rotates toward the left side, the bony labyrinth also rotates at the same speed together with the head. However, the endolymph lags behind due to its own fluid inertia. Because the crista ampullaris is attached to the wall of the bony labyrinth, it will be swayed by the lagging endolymph in the opposite direction to the movement of the head. **b.** The structure of the crista ampullaris includes sensory epithelium and large cupula made of a gelatinous protein–polysaccharide mass that projects toward the nonsensory wall of the ampulla. Note that the membranous ampulla is filled with endolymph and is surrounded by perilymph. **c.** The sensory epithelium of the crista ampullaris is composed of both type I and type II hair cells and supporting cells. The stereocilia and kinocilium of each hair cell are embedded in the cupula. Their mechanical deflection opens the K^+ channels, causing depolarization of the cell.

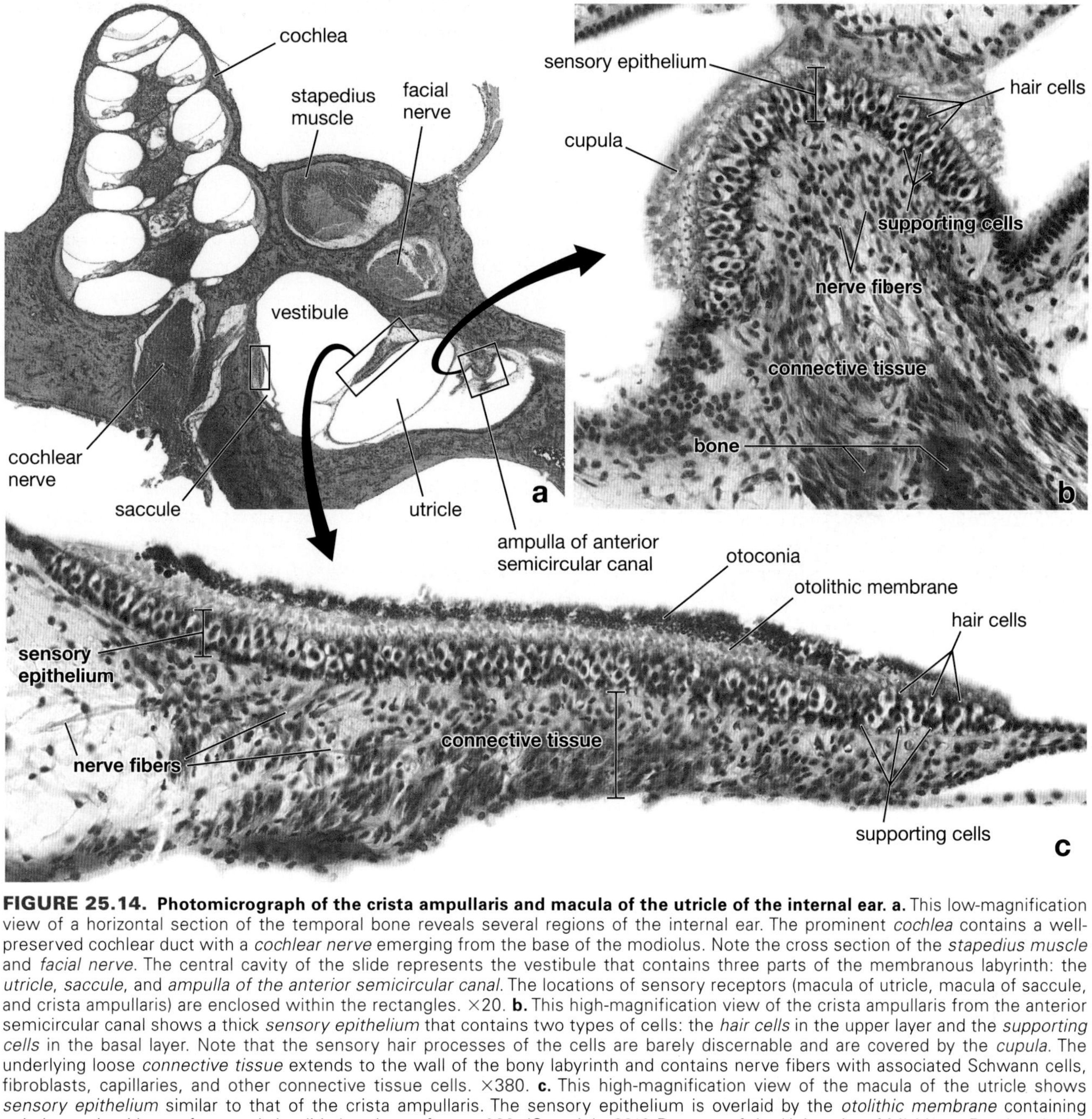

FIGURE 25.14. Photomicrograph of the crista ampullaris and macula of the utricle of the internal ear. a. This low-magnification view of a horizontal section of the temporal bone reveals several regions of the internal ear. The prominent *cochlea* contains a well-preserved cochlear duct with a *cochlear nerve* emerging from the base of the modiolus. Note the cross section of the *stapedius muscle* and *facial nerve*. The central cavity of the slide represents the vestibule that contains three parts of the membranous labyrinth: the *utricle*, *saccule*, and *ampulla of the anterior semicircular canal*. The locations of sensory receptors (macula of utricle, macula of saccule, and crista ampullaris) are enclosed within the rectangles. ×20. **b.** This high-magnification view of the crista ampullaris from the anterior semicircular canal shows a thick *sensory epithelium* that contains two types of cells: the *hair cells* in the upper layer and the *supporting cells* in the basal layer. Note that the sensory hair processes of the cells are barely discernable and are covered by the *cupula*. The underlying loose *connective tissue* extends to the wall of the bony labyrinth and contains nerve fibers with associated Schwann cells, fibroblasts, capillaries, and other connective tissue cells. ×380. **c.** This high-magnification view of the macula of the utricle shows *sensory epithelium* similar to that of the crista ampullaris. The sensory epithelium is overlaid by the *otolithic membrane* containing a darker stained layer of *otoconia* (otoliths) on its surface. ×380. (Copyright 2010 Regents of the University of Michigan. Reprinted with permission.)

called **otoconia**, are heavier than endolymph. The outer surface of the otolithic membrane lies opposite the surface in which the stereocilia of the hair cells are embedded. The otolithic membrane moves on the macula in a manner analogous to that by which the cupula moves on the crista. Stereocilia of the hair cells are deflected by gravity in the stationary individual when the otolithic membrane and its otoliths pull on the stereocilia. They are also displaced during linear movement when the individual is moving in a straight line and the otolithic membrane drags on the stereocilia because of inertia. In both cases, movement of the otolithic membrane causes the stereocilia to move toward the kinocilium, activating MET channels. This depolarizes hair cells and generates an action potential. Displacement of stereocilia in the opposite direction away from the kinocilium causes hyperpolarization of hair cells and inhibits the generation of the action potential.

The spiral organ of Corti is the sensor of sound vibrations.

The **cochlear duct** divides the cochlear canal into three parallel compartments or scalae:

- **Scala media**, the middle compartment in the cochlear canal
- **Scala vestibule**
- **Scala tympani**

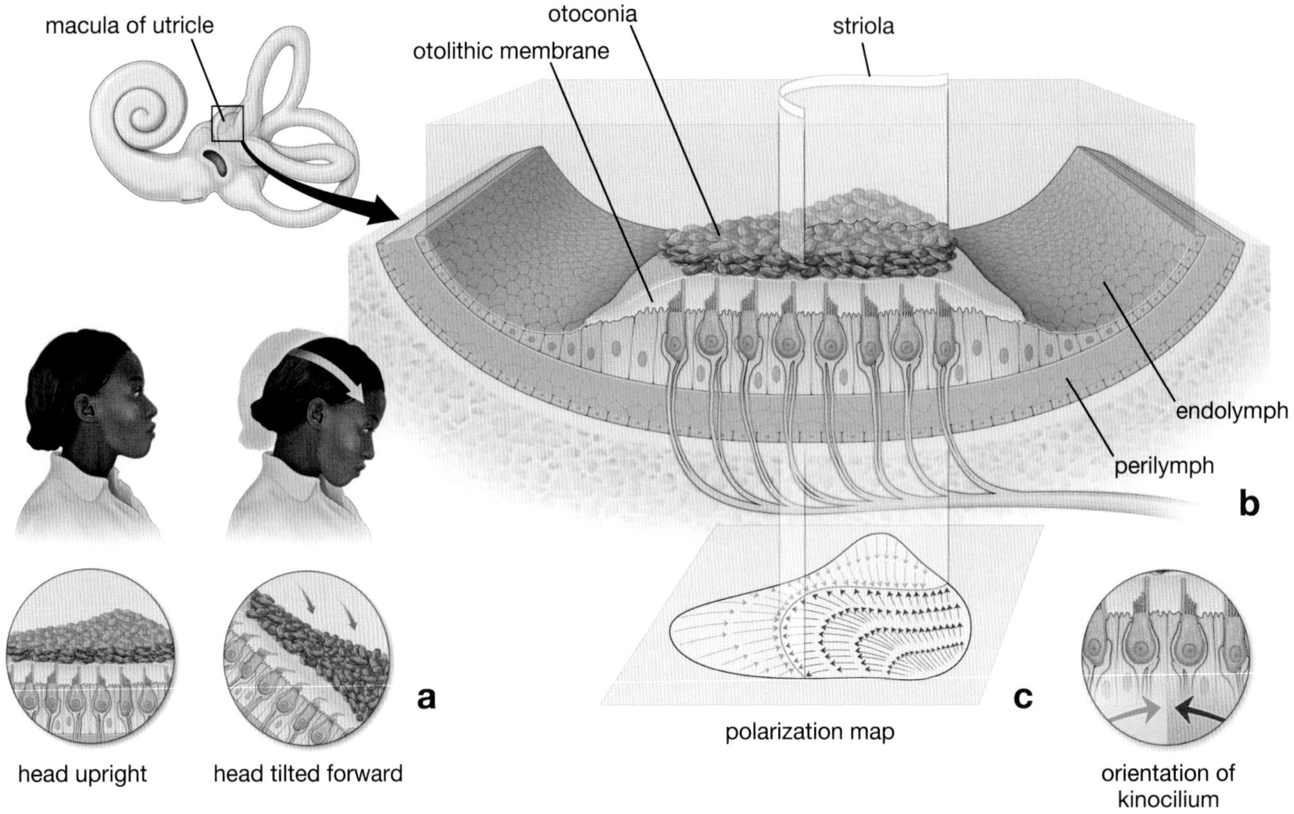

FIGURE 25.15. Diagram of function and structure of the macula within the utricle. a. As shown in this drawing, the macula of the utricle (as well as macula of the saccule) functions as a sensor for gravity and linear acceleration. For example, when the head of the individual shown in this diagram is tilted forward, tiny crystals of calcium carbonate called *otoconia* are shifted on the surface of the otolithic membrane. This movement is detected by the underlying hair cells. **b.** The macula is composed of a sensory epithelium containing both type I and type II hair cells. The hair cell processes are embedded in the gelatinous polysaccharide otolithic membrane. The luminal surface of the membrane is covered by otoconia that are heavier than endolymph. **c.** As visible on the map below the macula, the hair cells are polarized with respect to the striola, an imaginary plane that curves through the center of each macula. Note that on each side of the striola, the kinocilia of the hair cells are oriented in opposite directions facing toward the striola (see direction of the *blue* and *green arrows* on the polarization map of the utricle). This arrangement is only seen in the utricle because in the macula of the saccule, the kinocilia of the hair cells are turned away from the striola.

The **cochlear duct** itself is the **scala media** (Fig. 25.17). The scala vestibuli and scala tympani are the spaces above and below, respectively, the scala media. The scala media is an **endolymph-containing space** that is continuous with the lumen of the saccule and contains the spiral organ of Corti, which rests on its lower wall (see Fig. 25.17).

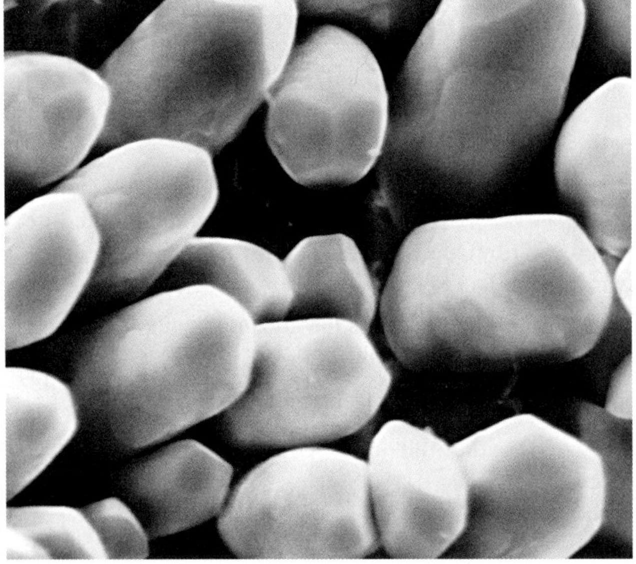

FIGURE 25.16. Scanning electron micrograph of human otoconia. Each otoconium has a long cylindrical body with a three-headed facet on each end. ×5,000.

The **scala vestibuli** and the **scala tympani** are **perilymph-containing spaces** that communicate with each other at the apex of the cochlea through a small channel called the **helicotrema** (see Fig. 25.17b). The scala vestibuli begins at the **oval window**, and the scala tympani ends at the **round window**.

The scala media is a triangular space with its acute angle attached to the modiolus.

In transverse section, the **scala media** appears as a triangular space with its most acute angle attached to a bony extension of the modiolus, the **osseous spiral lamina** (see Fig. 25.17). The upper wall of the scala media, which separates it from the scala vestibuli, is the **vestibular (Reissner) membrane** (Fig. 25.18). The lateral or outer wall of the scala media is bordered by a unique epithelium, the **stria vascularis.** It is responsible for the production and maintenance of endolymph. The stria vascularis encloses a complex capillary network and contains three types of cells (Fig. 25.19). The marginal cells, primarily involved in K^+ transport, line the endolymphatic space of the scala media. Intermediate pigment-containing cells are scattered among capillaries. The basal cells separate stria vascularis from the underlying spiral ligament. The lower wall or floor of the scala media is formed by a relatively flaccid **basilar membrane** that increases in width and decreases in stiffness as it coils from the base to apex of the cochlea. The spiral organ of Corti rests on the basilar membrane and is overlain by the **tectorial membrane**.

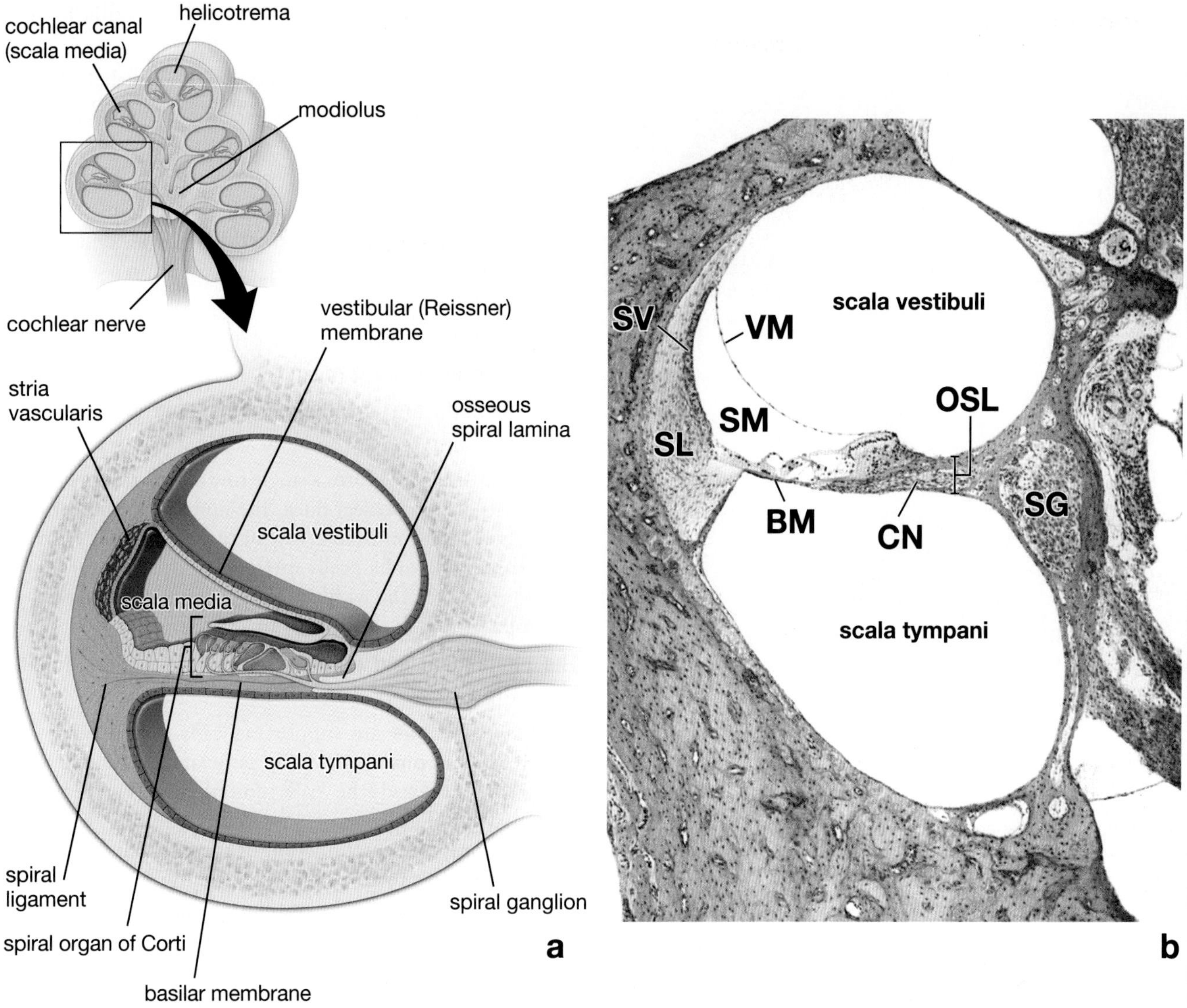

FIGURE 25.17. Schematic diagram and photomicrograph of the cochlear canal. a. Cross section of the basal turn of the cochlear duct is shown in the *box* on the smaller orientation view. This view of a midmodiolar section of the cochlea illustrates the position of the cochlear duct within the 2.75 turns of the bony cochlea. Observe that at the top of the cochlea, the scala vestibuli and scala tympani communicate with each other at the helicotrema. The scala media and the osseous spiral lamina divide the cochlea into the scala vestibuli and the scala tympani, which are filled with perilymph. The scala media (the space within the cochlear duct) is filled with endolymph and contains the organ of Corti. **b.** This photomicrograph shows a section of the basal turn of the cochlear canal. The osseous spiral lamina (*OSL*) and its membranous continuation, the basilar membrane (*BM*) as well as the vestibular membrane (*VM*) are visible. Note the location of the *scala vestibuli*, the scala media (*SM*) or cochlear duct, and the *scala tympani*. The three walls of the scala media are formed by the basilar membrane inferiorly, the stria vascularis (*SV*) and underlying spiral ligament (*SL*) laterally, and the vestibular membrane superiorly. The spiral organ of Corti resides on the inferior wall of the cochlear duct. Dendrites of the cochlear nerve (*CN*) that originate in the spiral ganglion (*SG*) enter the spiral organ of Corti. The axons of the spiral ganglion cells form the cochlear part of the vestibulocochlear nerve. ×65.

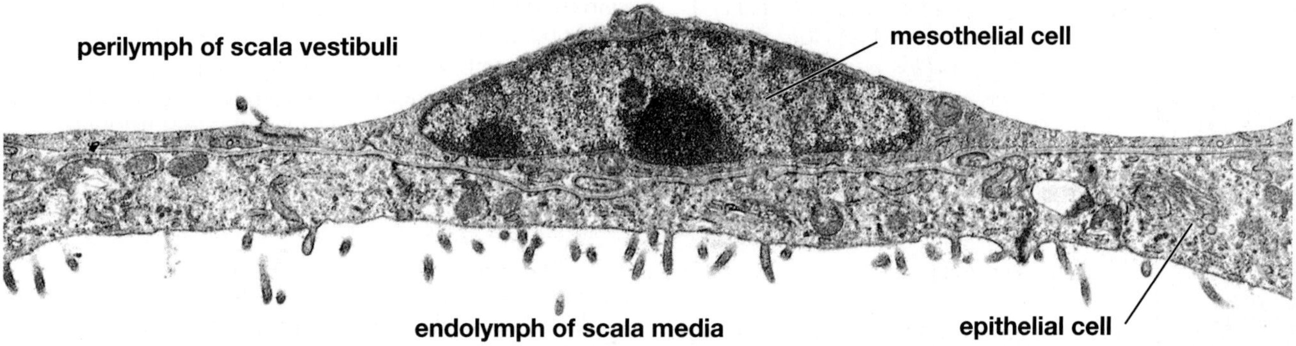

FIGURE 25.18. Transmission electron micrograph of the vestibular (Reissner) membrane. Two cell types can be observed: a mesothelial cell, which faces the scala vestibuli and is bathed by perilymph, and an epithelial cell, which faces the scala media and is bathed by endolymph. ×8,400.

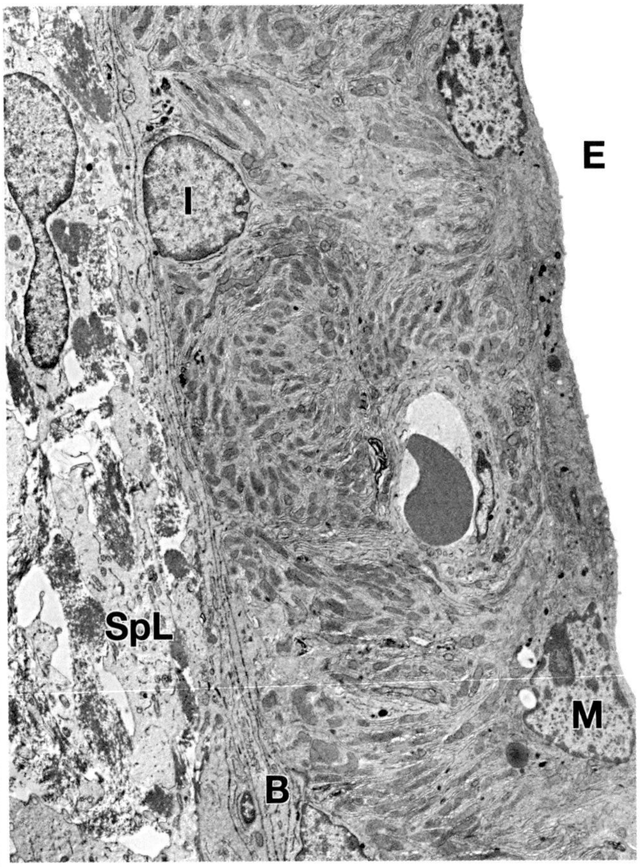

FIGURE 25.19. Transmission electron micrograph of the stria vascularis. The apical surfaces of the marginal cells (*M*) of the stria are bathed by endolymph (*E*) of the scala media. Intermediate cells (*I*) are positioned between the marginal cells and the basal cells (*B*). The basal cells separate the other cells of the stria vascularis from the spiral ligament (*SpL*). ×4,700.

The spiral organ of Corti is composed of hair cells, phalangeal cells, and pillar cells.

The **spiral organ of Corti** is a complex epithelial layer on the floor of the scala media (Fig. 25.20 and Plate 25.2, page 1044). It is formed by the following:

- **Inner hair cells** (close to the spiral lamina) and **outer hair cells** (farther from the spiral lamina)
- **Inner phalangeal (supporting) cells** and **outer phalangeal cells**
- **Pillar cells**

Several other named cell types of unknown function are also present in the spiral organ.

The hair cells are arranged in inner and outer rows of cells.

The **inner hair cells** form a single row of cells throughout all 2.75 turns of the cochlear duct. The number of cells forming the width of the continuous row of **outer hair cells** is variable. Three ranks of hair cells are found in the basal part of the coil (Fig. 25.21). The width of the row gradually increases to five ranks of cells at the apex of the cochlea.

The phalangeal and pillar cells provide support for the hair cells.

Phalangeal cells are supporting cells for both rows of hair cells. The phalangeal cells associated with the inner hair cells surround the cells completely (Fig. 25.22a). The phalangeal cells associated with the outer hair cells surround only the basal portion of the hair cell completely and send apical processes toward the endolymphatic space (Fig. 25.22b). These processes flatten near the apical ends

FOLDER 25.2

CLINICAL CORRELATION: HEARING LOSS—VESTIBULAR DYSFUNCTION

Several types of disorders can affect the auditory and vestibular system and result in deafness, dizziness (vertigo), or both. Auditory disorders are classified as either sensorineural or conductive. **Conductive hearing loss** results when sound waves are mechanically impeded from reaching the auditory sensory receptors within the internal ear. This type of hearing loss principally involves the external ear or structures of the middle ear. Conductive hearing loss is the second most common type of loss after sensorineural hearing loss, and it usually involves a reduction in sound level or the inability to hear faint sounds. Conductive hearing loss may be caused by otitis media (ear infection); in fact, this is the most common cause of temporary hearing loss in children. Fluid that collects in the tympanic cavity can also cause significant hearing problems in children. Other common causes of conductive hearing loss include excess wax or foreign bodies in the external acoustic meatus or diseases that affect the ossicles in the middle ear (otosclerosis; see also Folder 25.1). In many cases, conductive hearing loss can be treated either medically or surgically and may not be permanent.

Sensorineural hearing impairment may occur after injury to the auditory sensory hair cells within the internal ear, cochlear division of cranial nerve VIII, nerve pathways in the central nervous system (CNS), or auditory cortex. Sensorineural hearing loss accounts for about 90% of all hearing loss. It may be congenital or acquired. Causes of acquired sensorineural hearing loss include infections of the membranous labyrinth (e.g., meningitis, chronic otitis media), fractures of the temporal bone, acoustic trauma (i.e., prolonged exposure to excessive noise), and administration of certain classes of antibiotics and diuretics.

Another example of sensorineural hearing loss often results from aging. Sensorineural hearing loss not only involves a reduction in sound level but also affects the ability to hear clearly or to distinguish speech. A loss of the sensory hair cells or associated nerve fibers begins in the basal turn of the cochlea and progresses apically over time. The characteristic impairment is a high-frequency hearing loss termed **presbycusis** (see presbyopia, page 1004).

In selected patients, the use of a **cochlear implant** can partially restore some hearing function. The cochlear implant is an electronic device consisting of an external microphone, amplifier, and speech processor linked to a receiver implanted under the skin of the mastoid region. The receiver is connected to the multielectrode intracochlear implant inserted along the wall of the cochlear canal. After considerable training and tuning of the speech processor, the patient's hearing can be partially restored to various degrees ranging from recognition of critical sounds to the ability to converse.

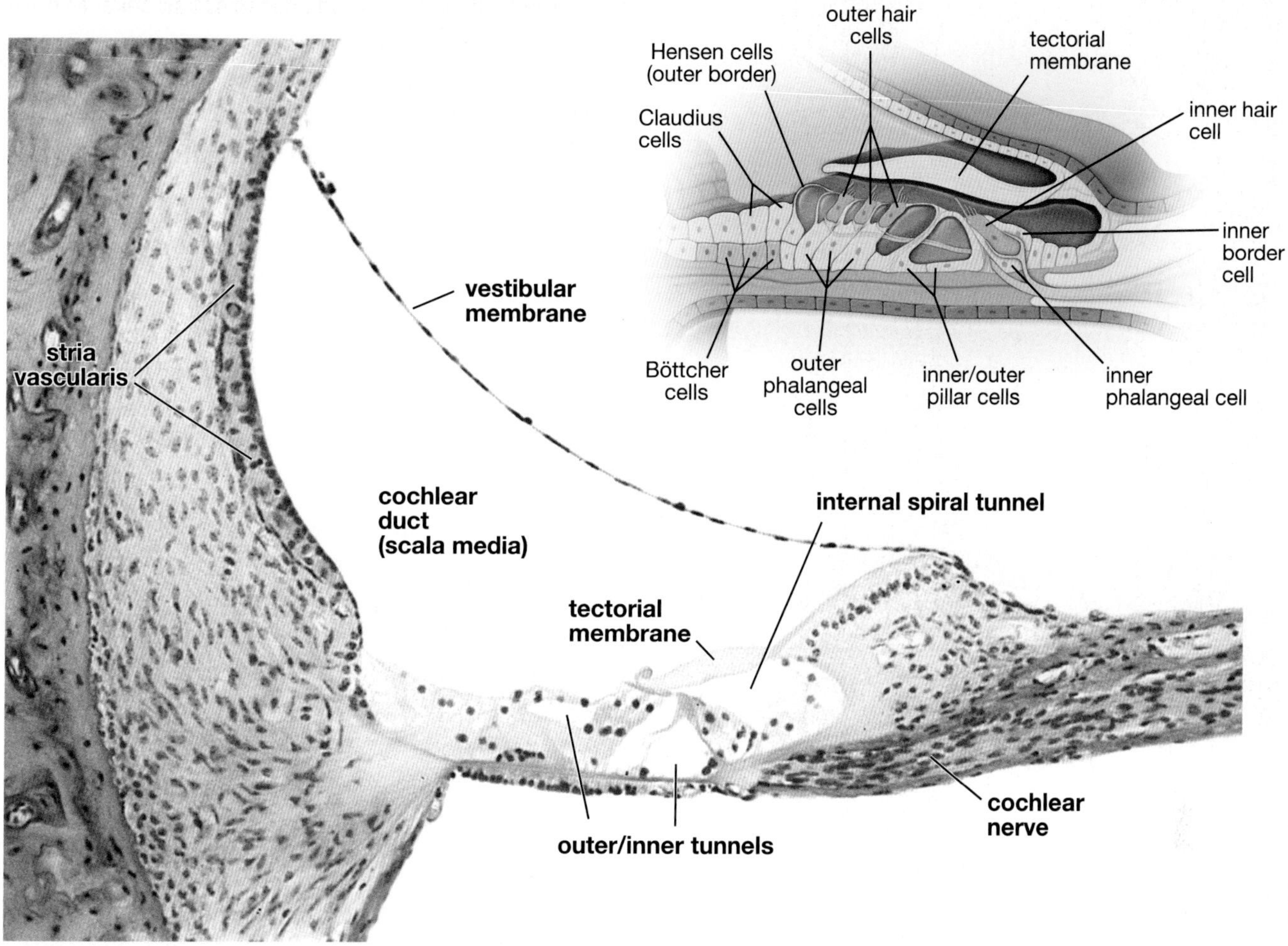

FIGURE 25.20. Photomicrograph of the vestibular duct and spiral organ of Corti. This higher magnification photomicrograph of the cochlear duct shows the structure of the spiral organ of Corti. Relate this structure to the *inset*, which labels the structural features of the spiral organ. ×180. **Inset.** Diagram of the sensory and supporting cells of the spiral organ of Corti. The sensory cells are divided into an inner row of sensory hair cells and three rows of outer sensory hair cells. The supporting cells are the inner and outer pillar cells, inner and outer (Deiters) phalangeal cells, outer border cells (Hensen cells), inner border cells, Claudius cells, and Böttcher cells.

of the hair cells and collectively form a complete plate surrounding each hair cell (Fig. 25.23).

The apical ends of the phalangeal cells are tightly bound to one another and to the hair cells by elaborate tight junctions. These junctions form the **reticular lamina** that separates the endolymphatic compartment from the true intercellular spaces of the organ of Corti (see Figs. 25.20 and 25.22b). The extracellular fluid in this intercellular space is **cortilymph**. Its composition is similar to that of other extracellular fluids and to perilymph.

Pillar cells have broad apical and basal surfaces that form plates and a narrowed cytoplasm. The inner pillar cells rest on the tympanic lip of the spiral lamina; the outer pillar cells rest on the basilar membrane. Between them, they form a triangular tunnel, the **inner spiral tunnel** (see Fig. 25.20).

The tectorial membrane extends from the spiral limbus over the cells of the spiral organ of Corti.

The **tectorial membrane** is attached medially to the modiolus. Its lateral free edge projects over and attaches to the organ of Corti by the stereocilia of the hair cells. It is formed from the radially oriented bundles of collagen types II, V, and IX embedded in a dense amorphous ground substance. Glycoproteins unique to the internal ear, called **otogelin** and **tectorin**, are associated with the collagen bundles. These proteins are also present in the otolithic membranes overlying the maculae of the utricle and saccule as well as in the cupulae of the cristae in the semicircular canals.

Sound Perception

As described on pages 1018-1019, sound waves striking the tympanic membrane are translated into simple mechanical vibrations. The ossicles of the middle ear convey these vibrations to the cochlea.

In the internal ear, the vibrations of the ossicles are transformed into waves in the perilymph.

Movement of the stapes in the oval window of the vestibule sets up vibrations or traveling waves in the perilymph of the scala vestibuli. The vibrations are transmitted through the vestibular membrane to the scala media (cochlear duct),

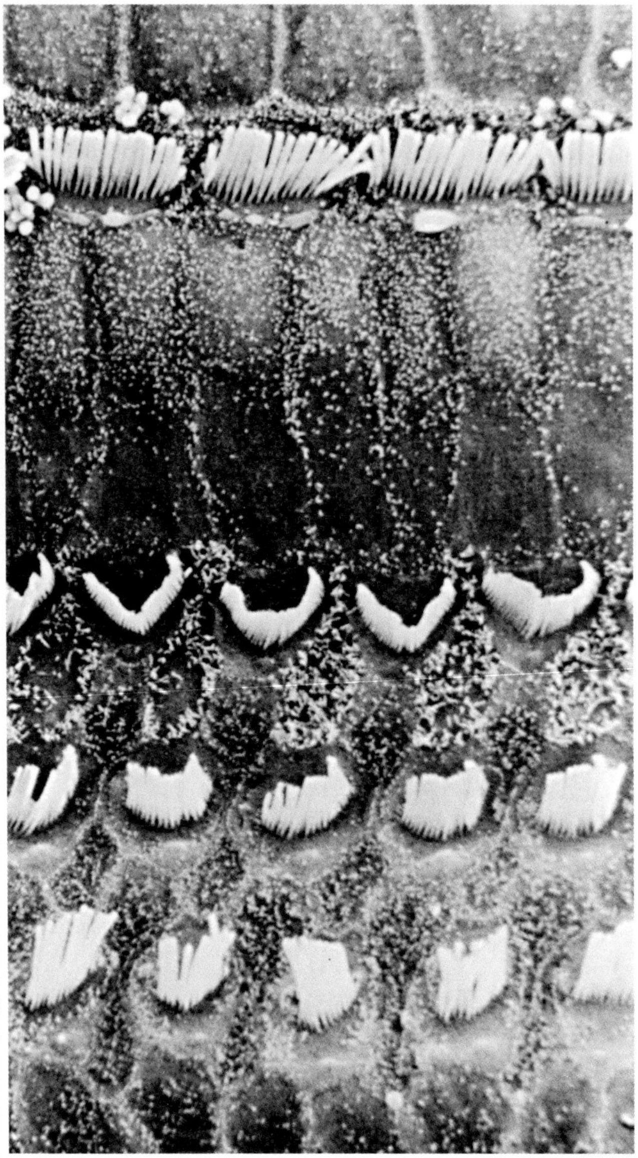

FIGURE 25.21. Scanning electron micrograph of the spiral organ of Corti. This electron micrograph illustrates the configuration of stereocilia on the apical surfaces of the inner row and three outer rows of the cochlear sensory hair cells. ×3,250.

which contains endolymph, and are also propagated to the perilymph of the scala tympani. Pressure changes in this closed perilymphatic–endolymphatic system are reflected in movements of the membrane that covers the round window in the base of the cochlea.

As a result of **sound vibrations** entering the internal ear, a traveling wave is set up in the basilar membrane (Fig. 25.24). A sound of a specified frequency causes displacement of a relatively long segment of the basilar membrane, but the region of maximal displacement is narrow. The point of maximal displacement of the basilar membrane is specified for a given frequency of sound and is the morphologic basis of frequency discrimination. High-frequency sounds cause maximal vibration of the basilar membrane near the base of the cochlea; low-frequency sounds cause maximal displacement nearer the apex. Amplitude discrimination (i.e., perception of sound intensity or loudness) depends on the degree of displacement of the basilar membrane at any given frequency range. Thus, coding acoustic information into nerve impulses depends on the vibratory pattern of the basilar membrane.

Movement of the stereocilia of the hair cells in the cochlea initiates neuronal transduction.

Hair cells are attached through the **phalangeal cells** to the basilar membrane, which vibrates during sound reception. The **stereocilia** of these hair cells are, in turn, attached to the tectorial membrane, which also vibrates. However, the **tectorial membrane** and the **basilar membrane** are hinged at different points. Thus, a shearing effect occurs between the basilar membrane (and the cells attached to it) and the tectorial membrane when sound vibrations impinge on the internal ear.

Because they are inserted into the tectorial membrane, the stereocilia of the hair cells are the only structures that connect the basilar membrane and its complex epithelial layer to the tectorial membrane. The shearing effect between the basilar membrane and the tectorial membrane deflects the stereocilia and thus the apical portion of the hair cells. This deflection activates **MET channels** located at the tips of stereocilia and generates action potentials that are conveyed to the brain via the **cochlear nerve** (cochlear division of the vestibulocochlear nerve, cranial nerve VIII).

Innervation of the Internal Ear

The vestibular nerve originates from the sensory receptors associated with the vestibular labyrinth.

The **vestibulocochlear nerve (cranial nerve VIII)** is a special sensory nerve and is composed of two divisions: a vestibular division called the *vestibular nerve* and a cochlear division called the *cochlear nerve*. The **vestibular nerve** is associated with equilibrium and carries impulses from the sensory receptors located within the vestibular labyrinth. The **cochlear nerve** is associated with hearing and conveys impulses from the sensory receptors within the cochlear labyrinth (Fig. 25.25).

The cell bodies of the bipolar neurons of the **vestibular nerve** are located in the **vestibular ganglion (of Scarpa)** in the internal acoustic meatus. Dendritic processes of the vestibular ganglion cells originate in the cristae ampullares of the three semicircular ducts, the macula of the utricle, and the macula of the saccule. They synapse at the base of the vestibular sensory hair cells, either as a chalice around a type I hair cell or as a bouton associated with a type II hair cell. The axons of the vestibular nerve originate from the vestibular ganglion, enter the brainstem, and terminate in four vestibular nuclei. Some secondary neuronal fibers travel to the cerebellum and to the nuclei of cranial nerves III, IV, and VI, which innervate the muscles of the eye.

The cochlear nerve originates from the sensory receptors of the spiral organ of Corti.

Neurons of the **cochlear nerve** are also bipolar, and their cell bodies are located in the **spiral ganglion of Corti** within the modiolus. Dendritic processes of spiral ganglion cells exit the modiolus through the small openings in the bony spiral lamina and enter the spiral organ. Approximately 90% of dendrites originating from the spiral ganglion cells synapse with the inner hair cells; the remaining 10% of dendrites synapse with

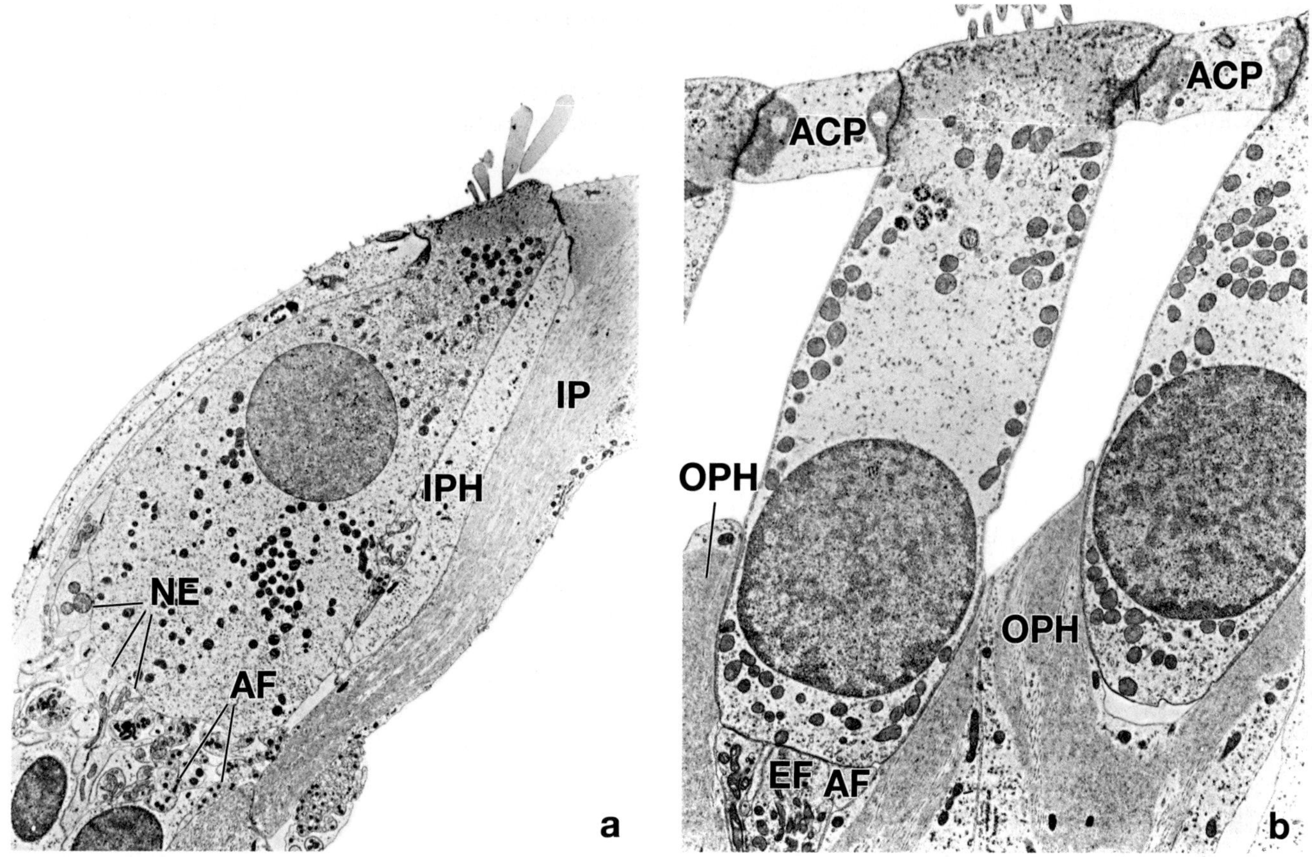

FIGURE 25.22. Electron micrograph of an inner and outer hair cell. a. Observe the rounded base and constricted neck of the inner hair cell. Nerve endings (*NE*) from afferent nerve fibers (*AF*) to the inner hair cells are seen basally. *IP*, inner pillar cell; *IPH*, inner phalangeal cell. ×6,300. **b.** Afferent (*AF*) and efferent (*EF*) nerve fiber endings on the base of an outer sensory hair cell are evident. Outer phalangeal cells (*OPH*) surround the outer hair cells basally. Their apical projections form the apical cuticular plate (*ACP*). Note that the lateral domains in the middle third of the outer hair cells are not surrounded by supporting cells. ×6,300. (Reprinted with permission from Kimura RS. Sensory and accessory epithelia of the cochlea. In: Friedmann I, Ballantyne J, eds. *Ultrastructural Atlas of the Inner Ear*. Butterworth; 1984.)

the outer hair cells of the spiral ganglion. The axons of the spiral ganglion cells form the cochlear nerve, which enters the bony cochlea through the modiolus to appear in the internal acoustic meatus (see Fig. 25.25). From the internal acoustic meatus, the cochlear nerve enters the brainstem and terminates in the cochlear nuclei of the medulla. Nerve fibers from these nuclei pass to the geniculate nucleus of the thalamus and then to the auditory cortex of the temporal lobe.

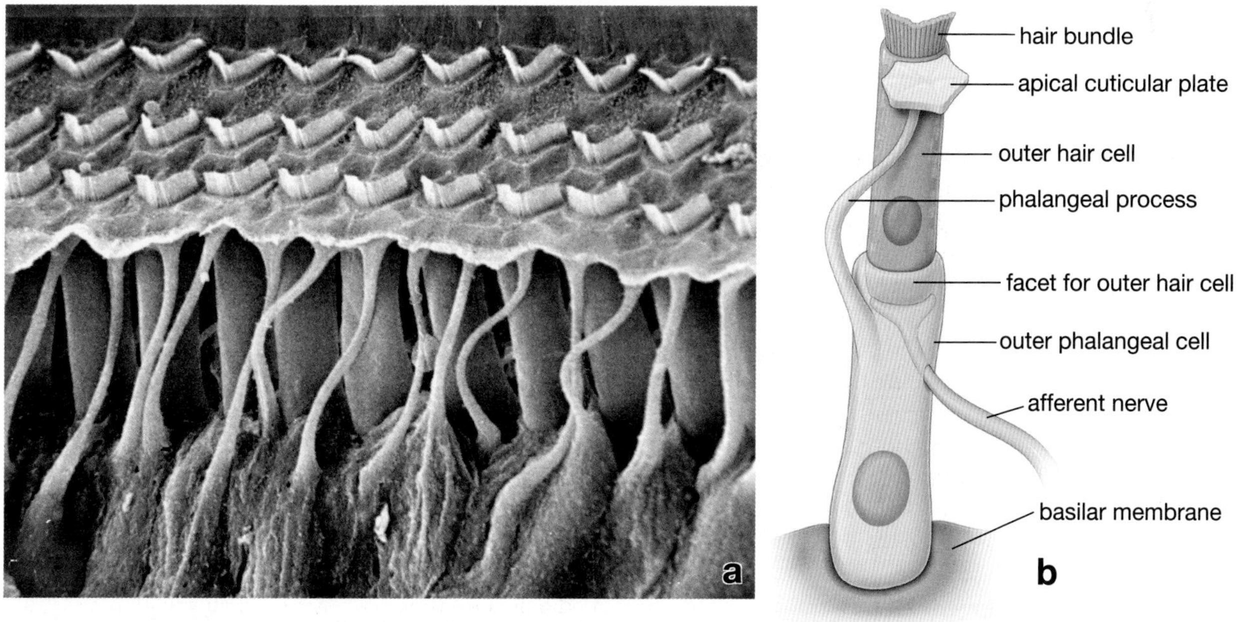

FIGURE 25.23. Structure of the outer phalangeal cell. a. This scanning electron micrograph illustrates the architecture of the outer phalangeal (Deiters) cells. Each phalangeal cell cups the basal surface of an outer hair cell and extends its phalangeal process apically to form an apical cuticular plate that supports the outer sensory hair cells. ×2,400. **b.** Schematic drawing showing the relationship of an outer phalangeal cell to an outer hair cell.

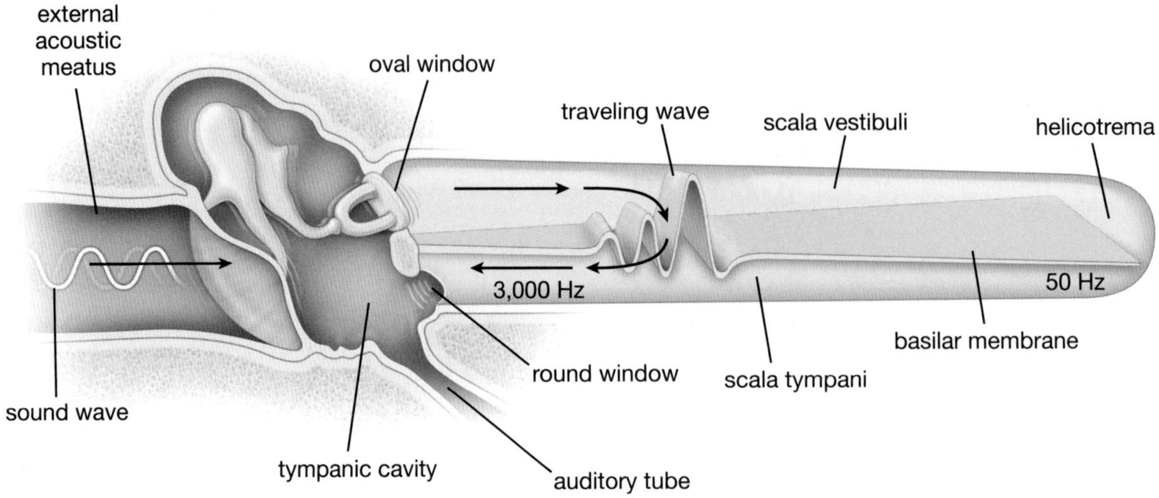

FIGURE 25.24. Schematic diagram illustrating the dynamics of the three divisions of the ear. The cochlear duct is shown here as if straightened. Sound waves are collected and transmitted from the external ear to the middle ear, where they are converted into mechanical vibrations. The mechanical vibrations are then converted at the oval window into fluid vibrations within the internal ear. Fluid vibrations cause displacement of the basilar membrane (traveling wave) on which rest the auditory sensory hair cells. Such displacement leads to stimulation of the hair cells and a discharge of neural impulses from them. Note that high-frequency sounds cause vibrations of the narrow, thick portion of the basilar membrane at the base of the cochlea, whereas low-frequency sounds displace basilar membrane toward the apex of the cochlea near its helicotrema.

The organ of Corti also receives a small number of efferent fibers conveying impulses from the brain that pass parallel to the afferent nerve fibers of the vestibulocochlear nerve (olivocochlear tract, cochlear efferents of Rasmussen). Efferent nerve fibers from the brainstem pass through the vestibular nerve. They synapse either on afferent endings of the inner hair cell or on the basal aspect of an outer hair cell. Efferent fibers are thought to affect the control of auditory and vestibular input to the central nervous system, presumably by enhancing some afferent signals while suppressing other signals. Damage to the organ of Corti, cochlear nerve, nerve pathways, or auditory cortex is responsible for **sensorineural hearing loss** (see Folder 25.2).

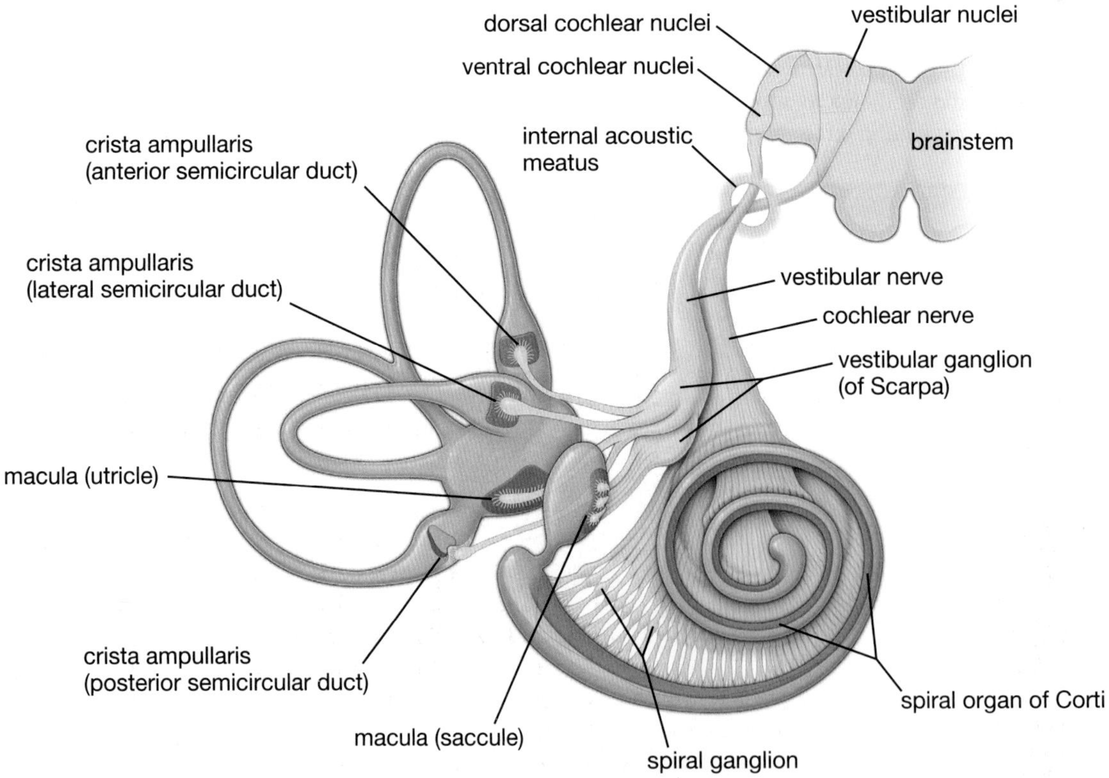

FIGURE 25.25. Diagram illustrating the innervation of the sensory regions of the membranous labyrinth. Note that cochlear and vestibular nerves form the vestibulocochlear nerve (cranial nerve VIII). The cochlear nerve carries the sound impulses from the spiral organ of Corti located within the cochlear duct; the vestibular nerve carries balance information from the three cristae ampullares of the semicircular canals, utricle, and saccule. The cell bodies of these sensory fibers are located in the spiral ganglion (for hearing) and vestibular ganglion (for equilibrium).

FOLDER 25.3

CLINICAL CORRELATION: VERTIGO

The sensation of rotation without equilibrium (**dizziness, vertigo**) signifies dysfunction of the vestibular system. Causes of vertigo include viral infections, certain drugs, and tumors such as **acoustic neuroma**. Acoustic neuromas develop in or near the internal acoustic meatus and exert pressure on the vestibular division of cranial nerve VIII or branches of the labyrinthine artery. Vertigo can also be produced normally in individuals by excessively stimulating the semicircular ducts. Similarly, excessive stimulation of the utricle can produce motion sickness (seasickness, carsickness, or airsickness) in some individuals.

The most common vestibular disorder is **benign paroxysmal positional vertigo (BPPV)**. In this condition, otoconia become detached from the macula of the utricle and lodge in one of the three cristae ampullares. The anatomic position of the posterior semicircular canal (it has an opening inferior to the macula) makes it the most common site for the detached otoconia to enter (81%–90%). The otoconia remain either free floating within the canal (**canalithiasis**) or are attached to the cupula (**cupulolithiasis**), causing inappropriate movement of the stereocilia at the apical surface of the receptor hair cells. Individuals with BPPV report episodes of an erroneous sensation of spinning evoked by certain movements of the head. Otoconia may detach following trauma or viral infections, but in many instances, it occurs idiopathically.

Some diseases of the internal ear affect both hearing and equilibrium. For example, people with **Ménière disease** initially complain of episodes of dizziness and tinnitus (ringing in the ears) and later develop low-frequency hearing loss. The causes of Ménière disease are related to blockage of the cochlear aqueduct, which drains excess endolymph from the membranous labyrinth. Blockage of this duct causes an increase in endolymphatic pressure and distension of the membranous labyrinth (endolymphatic hydrops).

Blood Vessels of the Membranous Labyrinth

Arterial blood is supplied to the membranous labyrinth by the labyrinthine artery; venous blood drainage is to the venous dural sinuses.

The blood supply to the external ear, middle ear, and bony labyrinth of the internal ear is from vessels associated with the external carotid arteries. The **arterial blood supply** to tissues of the membranous labyrinth of the internal ear is from the intracranial **labyrinthine artery**, a common branch of the anterior inferior cerebellar or basilar artery. The labyrinthine artery is a terminal artery: It has no anastomoses with other surrounding arteries. Branches of this artery are exactly parallel to the distribution of the superior and inferior parts of the vestibular nerve.

Venous drainage from the cochlear labyrinth is via the posterior and anterior spiral modiolar veins that form the **common modiolar vein**. The common modiolar vein and the vestibulocochlear vein form the vein of the cochlear aqueduct, which empties into the inferior petrosal sinus. Venous drainage from the vestibular labyrinth is via **vestibular veins** that join the vein of the cochlear aqueduct and by the vein of vestibular aqueduct, which drains into the sigmoid sinus.

HISTOLOGY 101 NOTEBOOK

EAR

OVERVIEW OF THE EAR

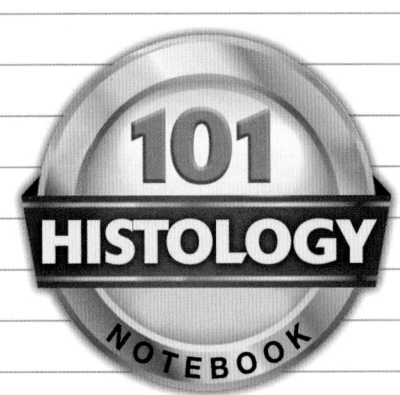

- The **ear** is a paired specialized sensory organ that is responsible for sound perception and balance.
- Tissues of the ear are derived from **surface ectoderm** (epithelia lining of the membranous labyrinth) and components of the **first pharyngeal pouch** (auditory tube and middle ear cavity), **first pharyngeal groove** (external acoustic meatus), **first pharyngeal arch** (malleus, incus, and anterior part of the auricle), and **second pharyngeal arch** (stapes and posterior part of the auricle).

EXTERNAL EAR

- The **auricle** is the external component of the ear that collects and amplifies sound.
- The **external acoustic meatus** extends from the auricle to the tympanic membrane. It is lined by skin that contains hair follicles as well as sebaceous and ceruminous glands (which produce **cerumen**, or **earwax**).

MIDDLE EAR

- The **middle ear** is an air-filled space lined by a mucous membrane that contains three **auditory ossicles** (malleus, incus, and stapes). It is separated from the external acoustic meatus by the tympanic membrane and is connected by the **auditory (Eustachian) tube** to the nasopharynx.
- The middle ear **amplifies mechanical forces** generated by the vibration of the tympanic membrane.
- The **tympanic membrane** is composed of skin of the external auditory meatus, a thin core of connective tissue, and mucous membrane of the middle ear.
- The auditory ossicles (**malleus, incus**, and **stapes**) cross the space of the middle ear in series and connect the tympanic membrane to the oval window. Movement of the ossicles is modulated by the **tensor tympani muscle** that inserts to the malleus and the **stapedius muscle** that inserts to the stapes.

COMPARTMENTS OF THE INTERNAL EAR

- The **internal ear** consists of two compartments within the temporal bone: the **bony labyrinth** and the **membranous labyrinth**, which is contained within the bony labyrinth.
- The internal ear has three fluid-filled spaces: the **endolymphatic space** within the membranous labyrinth (which has a high K^+ and a low Na^+ concentration), the **perilymphatic space** between the wall of the bony and membranous labyrinth (which has a low K^+ and a high Na^+ concentration), and the **cortilymphatic space** that lies within the tunnels of the organ of Corti of the cochlea.
- The **bony labyrinth** consists of three connected spaces: **semicircular canals**, **vestibule**, and **cochlea**, each containing different parts of the membranous labyrinth.
- The **membranous labyrinth** consists of a series of communicating sacs (**utricle**, **saccule**, and endolymphatic sac) and ducts (**three semicircular ducts**, **cochlear duct**, utriculosaccular duct, endolymphatic duct, and ductus reuniens) that contain **endolymph**.

SENSORY RECEPTORS OF THE MEMBRANOUS LABYRINTH

- Specialized sensory cells are located in six regions in the membranous labyrinth: three **cristae ampullares** in the ampullae of the semicircular ducts (receptors for angular acceleration of the head), two **maculae in** the utricle and saccule (receptors for position of the head and its linear movements), and the **spiral organ of Corti** (receptors for sound).
- Utricle and saccule maculae contain **hair cells** that are epithelial mechanoreceptors. These hair cells contain **hair bundles** on their apical surfaces (formed by rows of stereocilia with a single kinocilium) and are overlaid with a gelatin-like **otolithic membrane** that contains otoliths (otoconia).
- Movement of the **otoliths** is detected by the hair bundles, which activate **mechanically gated ion channels** to generate an action potential.
- Sensory receptors in the **crista ampullaris** are also covered by a gelatin-like mass without otoliths called the **cupula**. The cupula is deflected during the flow of endolymph through the semicircular canal. Movement of the cupula stimulates **mechanically gated ion channels** to generate an action potential.
- The **cochlear canal** is divided into three parallel compartments: **scala media** or **cochlear duct** (the middle compartment filled with endolymph that contains the spiral organ of Corti), **scala vestibuli**, and **scala tympani** (both containing perilymph).
- The **scala media** is a triangular space with its lower wall forming the **basilar membrane** on which the spiral organ of Corti resides. The upper wall (**vestibular membrane**) separates the scala media from scala vestibuli, and the lateral wall contains the **stria vascularis** that produces endolymph.
- The **spiral organ of Corti** is composed of **hair cells** (arranged in inner and outer rows), supportive **phalangeal cells**, and **pillar cells**. Movement of the stereocilia on hair cells during interaction with the overlying **tectorial membrane** generates electrical impulses that are transmitted to the cochlear nerve.
- **Sound waves** are transmitted from the vibrating tympanic membrane by the ossicles to the oval window, where they produce movement (waves) of the perilymph in the scala vestibule. This movement deflects the basilar membrane and spiral organ of Corti to generate electrical nerve impulses, which are perceived by the brain as sounds.
- Nerve impulses from the cristae ampullares and maculae travel with the **vestibular nerve**, and the impulses from the spiral organ of Corti travel with the **cochlear nerve**. These two nerves join together in the internal acoustic meatus to form the **vestibulocochlear nerve (cranial nerve VIII)**.

PLATE 25.1 ■ EAR

The **internal ear**, located in the temporal bone, consists of a system of chambers and canals that contain a network of membranous channels. These are referred to, respectively, as the **bony labyrinth** and **membranous labyrinth.** In some areas, the membranous labyrinth forms the lining of the bony labyrinth; in others, they are separated. Within the space lined by the membranous labyrinth is a watery fluid called **endolymph.** External to the membranous labyrinth, that is, between the membranous and bony labyrinths, is an additional fluid called **perilymph.**

The bony labyrinth is divided into three parts: **cochlea, semicircular canals,** and **vestibule.** The cochlea and semicircular canals contain membranous counterparts of the same shape; however, the membranous components of the vestibule are more complex in form, being composed of ducts and two chambers, the **utricle** and **saccule.** The cochlea contains the receptors for hearing (the **organ of Corti**); the semicircular canals contain the receptors for movement of the head; and the utricle and saccule contain receptors for position of the head.

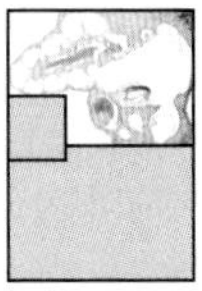

Internal ear, ear, guinea pig, hematoxylin and eosin (H&E) ×20.

In this section through the **internal ear**, bone surrounds the entire internal ear cavity. Because of its labyrinthine character, sections of the internal ear appear as a number of separate chambers and ducts. However, these structures are all interconnected (except for the perilymphatic and endolymphatic spaces, which remain separate). The largest chamber is the **vestibule** (*V*). The left side of this chamber (*black arrow*) leads into the **cochlea** (*C*). Just below the *black arrow* and to the right is the oval ligament (*OL*) surrounding the base of the stapes (*S*). Both structures have been cut obliquely and are not seen in their entirety. The facial nerve (*FN*) is in an osseous tunnel to the left of the oval ligament. The communication of the vestibule with one of the semicircular canals is marked by the *white arrow*. Note the crista ampullaris (*CA*) that is projecting into the lumen of the semicircular canal. At the *upper right* are cross sections of the membranous labyrinth passing through components of the semicircular duct system (*DS*).

The cochlea is a spiral, cone-shaped structure. The specimen illustrated here makes 3½ turns (in humans, there are 2¾ turns). The section goes through the central axis of the cochlea. This consists of a bony stem called the **modiolus** (*M*). It contains the beginning of the cochlear nerve (*CN*) and the spiral ganglion (*SG*). Because of the plane of section and the spiral arrangement of the cochlear tunnel, the tunnel is cut crosswise in seven places (note 3½ turns). A more detailed examination of the cochlea and the organ of Corti is provided in Plate 25.2 (page 1044).

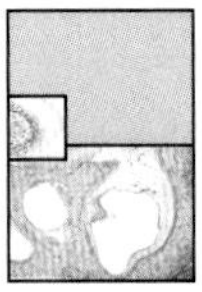

Semicircular canal, ear, guinea pig, H&E ×85; inset ×380.

A higher magnification of one of the semicircular canals and of the **crista ampullaris** (*CA*) within the canal seen in the *lower right* corner of the previous figure is provided here. The receptor for movement, the crista ampullaris (note its relationships in the previous figure), is present in each of the semicircular canals. The epithelial (*EP*) surface of the crista consists of two cell types, supporting cells and receptor hair cells. (Two types of hair cells are distinguished with the electron microscope.) It is difficult to identify the hair and supporting cells on the basis of specific characteristics; they can, however, be distinguished on the basis of location (see *inset*), as the **hair cells** (*HC*) are situated in a more superficial location than the supporting cells (*SC*). A gelatinous mass, the cupula (*Cu*), surmounts the epithelium of the crista ampullaris. Each receptor cell sends a hair-like projection deep into the substance of the cupula.

The epithelium rests on a loose, cellular connective tissue (*CT*) that also contains the nerve fibers associated with the receptor cells. The nerve fibers are difficult to identify because they are not organized into a discrete bundle.

C, cochlea
CA, crista ampullaris
CN, cochlear nerve
CT, connective tissue
Cu, cupula
DS, duct system (of membranous labyrinth)
EP, epithelium
FN, facial nerve
HC, hair cell
M, modiolus
OL, oval ligament
S, stapes
SC, supporting cell
SG, spiral ganglion
V, vestibule
black arrow, entry to cochlea
white arrow, entry to semicircular canal

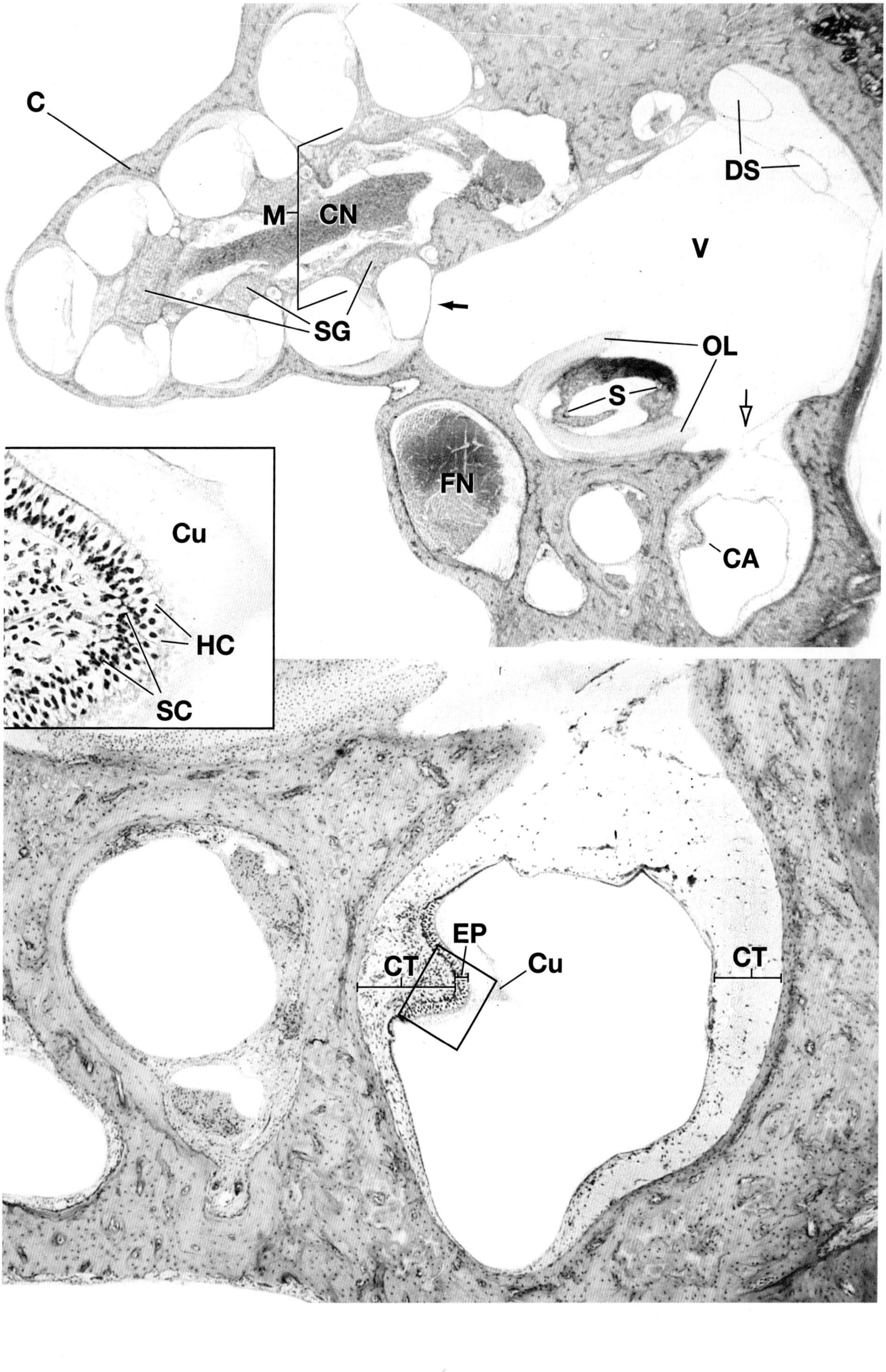
C
M
CN
SG
DS
V
OL
S
FN
CA
Cu
HC
SC
EP
CT
Cu
CT

PLATE 25.2 ■ COCHLEAR CANAL AND ORGAN OF CORTI

The **hair cell**, a nonneuronal mechanoreceptor, is the common receptor cell of the vestibulocochlear system. Hair cells are epithelial cells that possess numerous **stereocilia**, modified microvilli also called **sensory hairs**. They convert mechanical energy to electrical energy that is transmitted via the vestibulocochlear nerve (cranial nerve VIII) to the brain. Hair cells are associated with afferent, as well as efferent, nerve endings. All hair cells have a common basis of receptor cell function that involves bending or flexing of their stereocilia. The specific means by which the stereocilia are bent varies from receptor to receptor, but in each case, stretching of the plasma membrane caused by the bending of the stereocilia generates transmembrane potential changes that are transmitted to the afferent nerve endings associated with each cell. Efferent nerve endings on the hair cells serve to regulate their sensitivity.

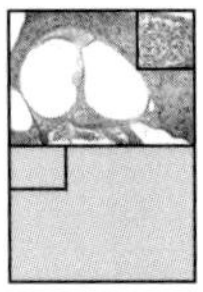

Cochlear canal, ear, guinea pig, hematoxylin and eosin (H&E) ×65; inset ×380.

A section through one of the turns of the cochlea is shown here. The most important functional component of the cochlea is the organ of Corti, enclosed by the *rectangle* and shown at higher magnification in the next figure. Other structures are included in this figure. The spiral ligament (*SL*) is a thickening of the periosteum on the outer part of the tunnel. Two membranes, the basilar membrane (*BM*) and the vestibular membrane (*VM*), join with the spiral ligament and divide the cochlear tunnel into three parallel canals, namely, the **scala vestibuli** (*SV*), the **scala tympani** (*ST*), and the **cochlear duct** (*CD*). Both the scala vestibuli and the scala tympani are perilymphatic spaces; these communicate at the apex of the cochlea. The cochlear duct is the space of the membranous labyrinth and is filled with endolymph. It is thought that the endolymph is formed by the portion of the spiral ligament that faces the cochlear duct, the stria vascularis (*StV*). This is highly vascularized and contains specialized "secretory" cells.

A shelf of bone, the osseous spiral lamina (*OSL*), extends from the modiolus to the basilar membrane. Branches of the cochlear nerve (*CN*) travel along the spiral lamina to the modiolus, where the main trunk of the nerve is formed. The components of the cochlear nerve are bipolar neurons whose cell bodies constitute the spiral ganglion (*SG*). These cell bodies are shown at higher magnification in the *inset* (*upper right*). The spiral lamina supports an elevation of cells, the limbus spiralis (*LS*). The surface of the limbus is composed of columnar cells.

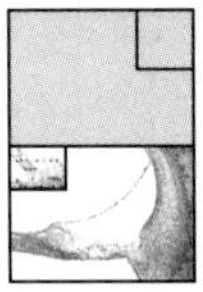

Organ of Corti, ear, guinea pig, H&E ×180; inset ×380.

The cross section of the **cochlear canal** (*CD*) visible in this image appears as a triangular space. The upper wall (roof) of this canal is formed by the vestibular membrane (*VM*) that separates it from the scala vestibuli (*SV*). The lateral (outer) wall of the cochlear canal is bordered the stria vascularis (*StV*) and underlying spiral ligament (*SL*). The lower wall (or floor) is formed by the basilar membrane, an extension of the osseous spiral lamina with visible branches of the cochlear nerve (*CN*). The basilar membrane supports the spiral **organ of Corti**. The components of the organ of Corti, beginning at the limbus spiralis (*LS*), are as follows: inner border cells (*IBC*), inner phalangeal and hair cells (*IP&HC*), and inner pillar cells (*IPC*). The sequence continues, repeating itself in reverse as follows: outer pillar cells (*OPC*), hair cells (*HC*) and outer phalangeal cells (*OP*), and outer border cells or cells of Hensen (*CH*). Hair cells are receptor cells; the other cells are collectively referred to as *supporting cells*. The hair and outer phalangeal cells can be distinguished in this figure by their location (see *inset*) and because their nuclei are well aligned. Because the hair cells rest on the phalangeal cells, it can be concluded that the upper three nuclei belong to outer hair cells, whereas the lower three nuclei belong to outer phalangeal cells.

The supporting cells extend from the basilar membrane (*BM*) to the surface of the organ of Corti (this is not evident here but can be seen in the *inset*), where they form a reticular membrane (*RM*). The free surface of the receptor cells fits into openings in the reticular membrane, and the "hairs" of these cells project toward, and make contact with, the tectorial membrane (*TM*). The latter is a cuticular extension from the columnar cells of the limbus spiralis. In ideal preparations, nerve fibers can be traced from the hair cells to the cochlear nerve (*CN*).

In their course from the basilar membrane to the reticular membrane, groups of supporting cells are separated from other groups by spaces that form spiral tunnels. These tunnels are named the inner tunnel (*IT*), the outer tunnel (*OT*), and the internal spiral tunnel (*IST*). Beyond the supporting cells are two additional groups of cells, the cells of Claudius (*CC*) and the cells of Böttcher (*CB*).

BM, basilar membrane
CB, cells of Böttcher
CC, cells of Claudius
CD, cochlear duct
CH, cells of Hensen
CN, cochlear nerve
HC, hair cells
IBC, inner border cells
IPC, inner pillar cells
IP&HC, inner phalangeal and hair cells
IST, internal spiral tunnel
IT, inner tunnel
LS, limbus spiralis
OP, outer phalangeal cells
OPC, outer pillar cells
OSL, osseous spiral lamina
OT, outer tunnel
RM, reticular membrane
SG, spiral ganglion
SL, spiral ligament
ST, scala tympani
StV, stria vascularis
SV, scala vestibule
TM, tectorial membrane
VM, vestibular membrane

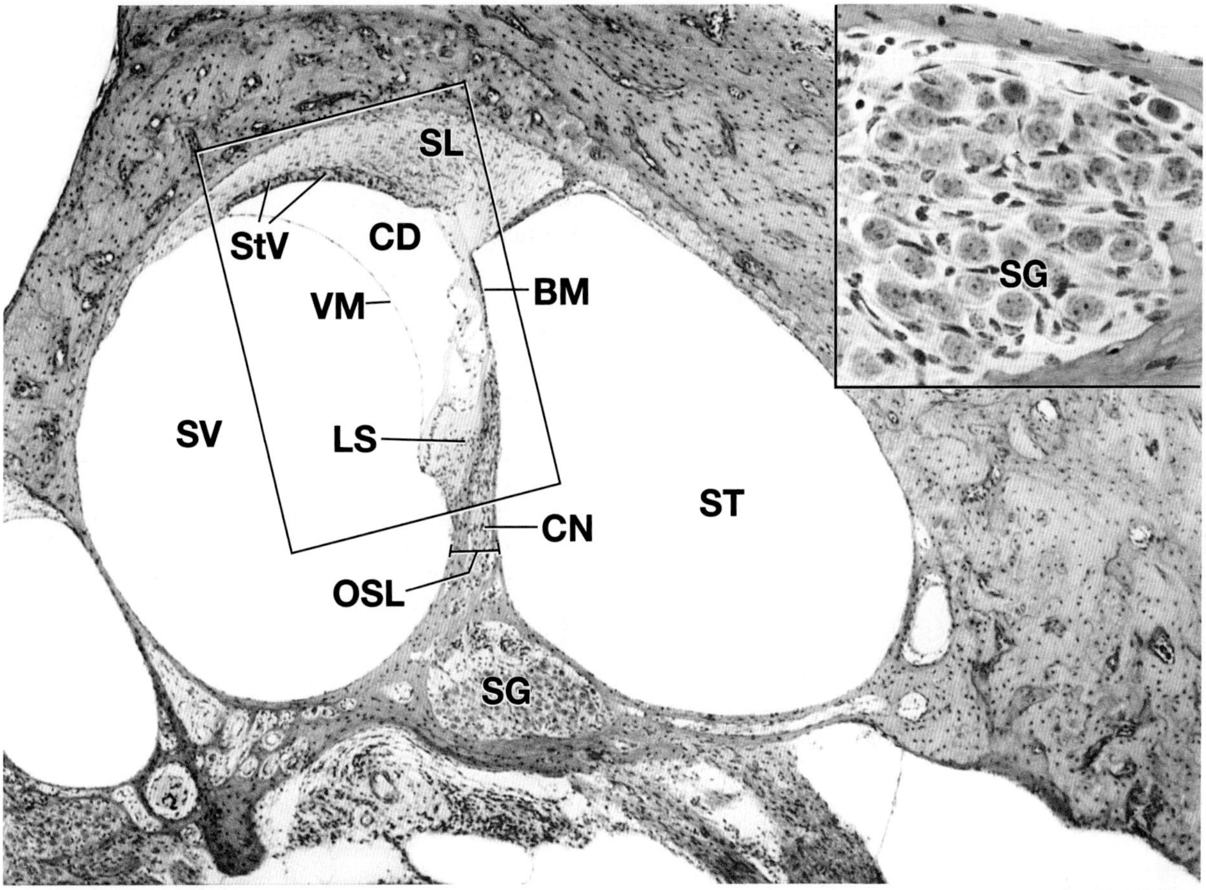
SL
StV
CD
VM
BM
SV
LS
ST
CN
OSL
SG
SG

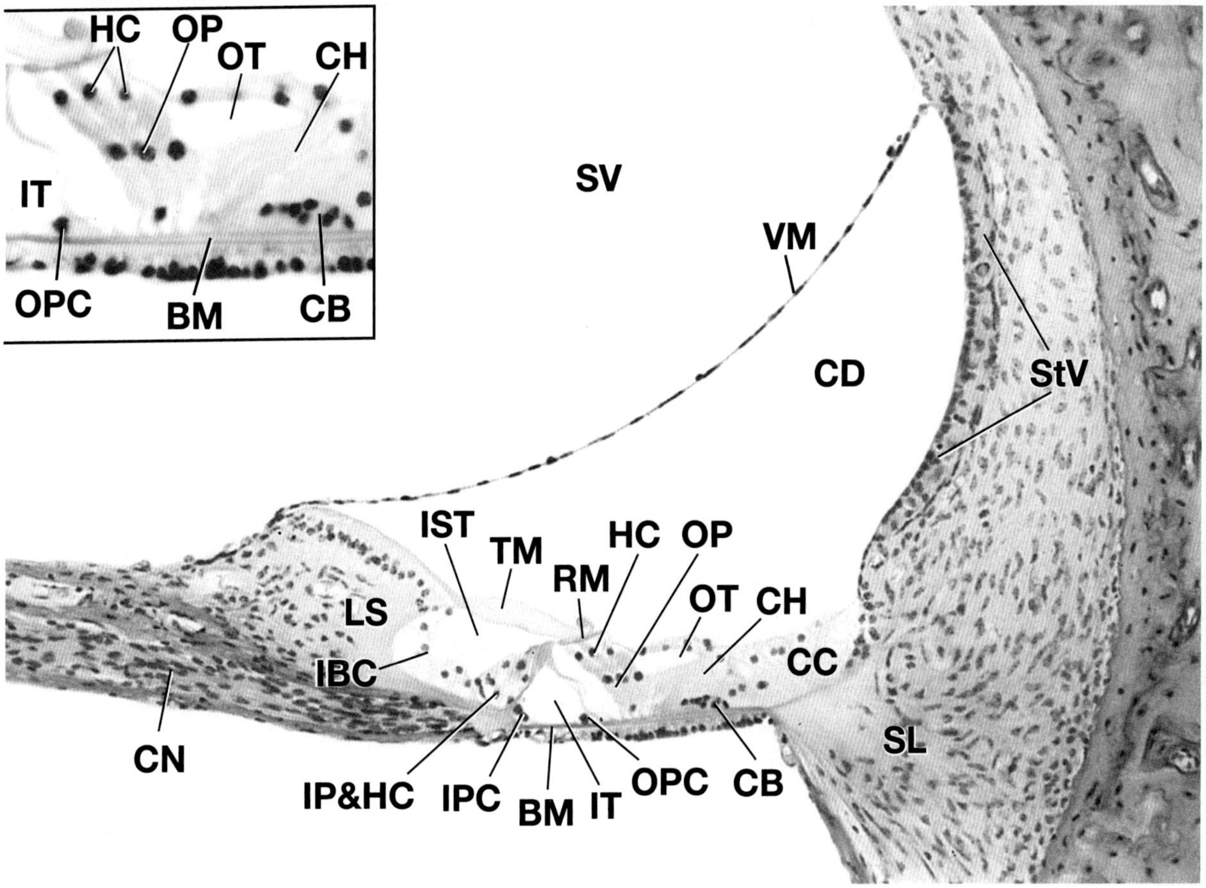
HC
OP
OT
CH
IT
OPC
BM
CB
SV
VM
CD
StV
IST
TM
HC
OP
RM
OT
CH
LS
IBC
CC
SL
CN
IP&HC
IPC
BM
IT
OPC
CB

INDEX

NOTE: Page numbers in *italics* designate figures; page numbers followed by *f* designate folders; page numbers followed by *p* designate plates; page numbers followed by *t* designate tables.

B

J

K

M

QUADM0823